FOURTH EDITION

PHARMACOTHERAPEUTICS FOR ADVANCED PRACTICE NURSE PRESCRIBERS

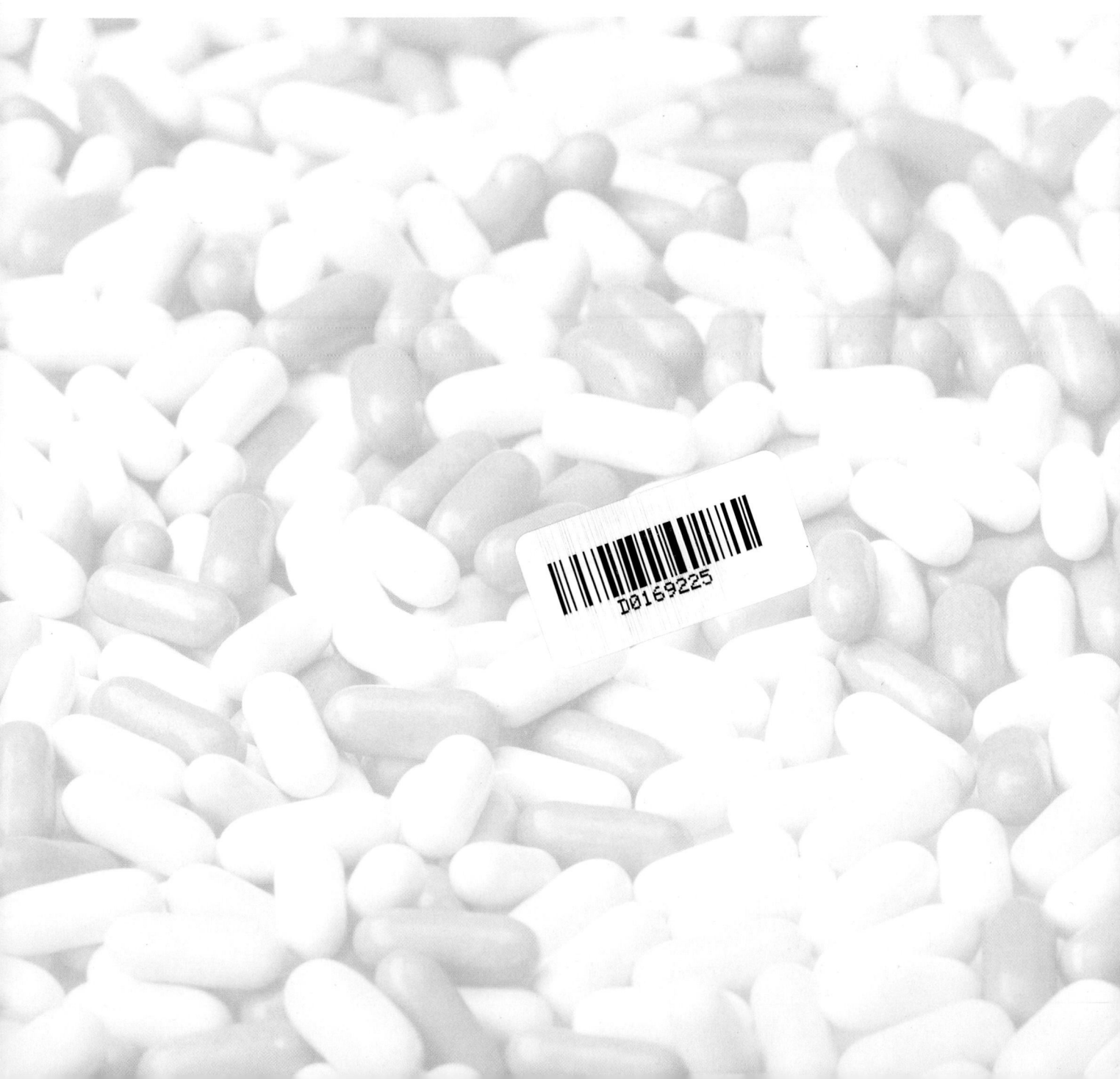

FOURTH EDITION

PHARMACOTHERAPEUTICS FOR ADVANCE PRACTICE NURSE PRESCRIBERS

Teri Moser Woo, RN, PhD, CPNP-PC, FAANP

Associate Professor of Nursing
Associate Dean for Graduate Nursing Programs
Pacific Lutheran University
School of Nursing
Tacoma, WA
and
Pediatric Nurse Practitioner
Kaiser Permanente Northwest Region

Marylou V. Robinson, PhD, FNP-C

Associate Professor
University of Colorado Anschutz Medical Campus
College of Nursing
Aurora, CO

F.A. Davis Company · Philadelphia

F. A. Davis Company
1915 Arch Street
Philadelphia, PA 19103
www.fadavis.com

Copyright © 2016 by F. A. Davis Company

Printed in the United States of America

Last digit indicates print number: 10 9 8 7 6 5 4 3

Senior Acquisitions Editor: Susan R. Rhyner
Developmental Editor: Jennifer Schmidt
Director of Content Development: Darlene D. Pedersen, MSN, FNP, BC
Content Project Manager: Echo K. Gerhart
Design & Illustration Manager: Carolyn O'Brien

As new scientific information becomes available through basic and clinical research, recommended treatments and drug therapies undergo changes. The author(s) and publisher have done everything possible to make this book accurate, up to date, and in accord with accepted standards at the time of publication. The author(s), editors, and publisher are not responsible for errors or omissions or for consequences from application of the book, and make no warranty, expressed or implied, in regard to the contents of the book. Any practice described in this book should be applied by the reader in accordance with professional standards of care used in regard to the unique circumstances that may apply in each situation. The reader is advised always to check product information (package inserts) for changes and new information regarding dose and contraindications before administering any drug. Caution is especially urged when using new or infrequently ordered drugs.

Library of Congress Cataloging-in-Publication Data

Woo, Teri Moser, 1962- , author.
  [Pharmacotherapeutics for nurse practitioner prescribers]
  Pharmacotherapeutics for advance practice nurse prescribers / Teri Moser Woo, Marylou V. Robinson. — Fourth edition.
      p. ; cm.
  Preceded by Pharmacotherapeutics for nurse practitioner prescribers / Teri Moser Woo, Anita Lee Wynne. 3rd ed. c2011.
  Includes bibliographical references and index.
  ISBN 978-0-8036-3827-3 (alk. paper) — ISBN 0-8036-3827-2 (alk. paper)
  I. Robinson, Marylou V., author. II. Title.
  [DNLM: 1. Pharmacological Phenomena—Nurses' Instruction. 2. Drug Prescriptions—Nurses' Instruction. 3. Drug Therapy—nursing. 4. Nurse Practitioners. QV 4]
  RM300
  615'.1–dc23
                                                                          2015020959

I would like to dedicate this book to my family.
My husband, John, and my three sons, Michael,
Patrick, and Nicholas, have been wonderfully
supportive as I have completed this project.
TMW

To my students who continually impress me with their
idealism and inspire me to always strive for excellence.
MVR

The increasing volume of pharmacology-related information presents a challenge to acquire and maintain current knowledge in the area of pharmacotherapeutics. The number of new drugs coming on the market each year, the changes in "the best" drugs to use for any given disease state based on the latest research, the influence on patient and practitioner alike of advertising and promotion, and restricted formularies create competing pressures on the prescriber. This book is designed to provide nurse practitioner students and the nurse practitioner in the primary care setting with a thorough, current, and usable pharmacology text and reference to address these challenges.

The design of this book assumes knowledge of basic pharmacology from one's undergraduate education in nursing. Although a brief review of basic pharmacology is presented in **Chapter 2**, the focus of the book is on advanced pharmacology and the role of the advanced practice nurse in pharmacotherapeutics. The authors of the text are practicing nurse practitioners, pharmacists, or selected specialists in a field. The book is by advanced practice registered nurses, for advanced practice registered nurses.

ORGANIZATION

This book is organized around four distinct content areas: The Foundation, Pharmacotherapeutics with Single Drugs, Pharmacotherapeutics with Multiple Drugs, and Special Drug Treatment Considerations.

The Foundation

The 13 chapters in Unit I provide the foundation of advanced pharmacology and the link between this knowledge and professional practice. Chapter 1 discusses the role of the advanced practice registered nurse (APRN) in both the United States and Canada as prescriber and the knowledge needed to actualize this role. Current issues about the evolving role and education of these providers are also presented in this edition, including discussion of the Doctorate of Nursing Practice.

Discussion of the roles of other advanced practice nurses in prescribing is included. Factors involved in clinical judgment related to prescribing are a central focus, and collaboration with other health-care providers is also presented.

The pharmacology knowledge required for rational drug selection requires more depth than that given in undergraduate pharmacology, where the focus is on safe administration of drugs prescribed by someone else. Advanced pharmacology information on receptor reserve and regulation, bioavailability and bioequivalence, metabolism of drugs, including a focus on the cytochrome P450 microsomal enzyme system, half-life, and steady state are provided in **Chapters 2** and **8**. Information central to the prescribing role includes an in-depth discussion of volume of distribution and therapeutic drug monitoring. Volume of distribution is important in prescribing drugs with very large or very small volumes of distribution and for selecting drugs for patients with cardiac or renal failure, during pregnancy, or when a patient is underweight or obese. Knowing what tests to order and when to order them to assess plasma drug levels by bioassay and to monitor for adverse drug reactions are necessary in making choices about when or if dosage alterations are required or drugs need to be stopped. These topics are also covered in **Unit I**.

Legal and professional aspects of the prescriber role are presented in **Chapter 4**. Issues surrounding the legal authority of the APRN to prescribe a drug, the conditions under which the prescription may be written, and how to write the prescription are presented. Risk management issues are also discussed, including informed consent, dealing with multiple providers, and substance abuse and drug-seeking behaviors.

Nurse practitioners have a history of high levels of patient satisfaction with the care provided. This is related, in part, to their holistic approach to each patient. Several chapters are devoted to information that reflects this approach. Cost, knowledge deficits, dealing with complex treatment regimens, and negotiating a shared responsibility for drug management are discussed in **Chapter 6**. Many patients choose to use complementary therapies such as herbal remedies. **Chapter 10** discusses herbal therapy and other complementary therapies.

A relatively new area in pharmacotherapeutics is ethnopharmacology. As more research is done in this area, treatment guidelines are beginning to include which drugs are best for different racial groups. Cultural and ethnic considerations in prescribing drugs are the subject of **Chapter 7**. Pharmacogenomics involves the influence of both race/ethnicity and individual genetic make-up on drug metabolism. **Chapter 8** provides a discussion of the role of pharmacogenomics in prescribing.

Consideration of drug and food interactions has long been a part of nursing knowledge, but the interrelationship between nutrition and drug therapy beyond these interactions has been largely overlooked. **Chapter 9** provides a discussion of this interrelationship, including nutritional supplementation and nutrition as therapy.

In an age of integrated use of technology, the APRN must be able to acquire information about drugs and to deliver care to patients using technology. The use of electronic health records (EHR) to aid in prescribing decision making is found in **Chapter 11**.

Cost issues cannot be ignored when making prescribing decisions. **Chapter 12** provides a discussion of pharmacoeconomics.

Over-the-counter drugs may be prescribed by the APRN or chosen by patients on their own. These drugs are often erroneously perceived to be less powerful and have fewer adverse reactions than prescription drugs. Understanding their role in pharmacotherapeutics is the focus of **Chapter 13**.

Pharmacotherapeutics With Single Drugs

The next two units are organized around specific drugs and the diseases they are used to treat. The chapters in Unit II are organized to provide easy access to information based on specific drug classes. Many practitioners have a personal formulary of drugs they use for disease processes that they commonly see. When presented with a patient requiring drug therapy, they know the class of drug from which they will make a rational drug choice. The information they seek is about drugs within that class that would be most appropriate for their patient.

Pharmacokinetics, pharmacodynamics, and pharmacotherapeutics for each drug class are discussed in the chapters in Unit II. The chapters include tables with easy-to-access information on the pharmacokinetic properties of each drug, drug interactions, clinical use and dosing, and available dosing forms. A major focus is on rational drug selection and on monitoring parameters. Patient education specific to each drug class is provided—designed around administration of the drug, adverse drug reactions to monitor for and what to do if they occur, and lifestyle modifications that complement the drug therapy.

To provide the most up-to-date, accurate, and relevant information possible, contributors to this unit are practicing clinicians and the newest published guidelines are consistently used. The "Clinical Pearls" features, drawn from the daily practice of these contributors, are incorporated throughout the text. Drugs currently in development that may influence drug choices in the near future are also included in the "On the Horizon" features.

Pharmacotherapeutics With Multiple Drugs

The chapters in Unit III provide drug information from the viewpoint of the disease processes they are commonly used to treat. Patients often have complex health and illness issues and treatment needs requiring multiple drugs in different drug classes. Unit III facilitates acquisition of complex prescribing knowledge by providing information from a disease process format. The diseases in this unit are those commonly seen in primary care and for which multidrug therapy from more than one drug class may be recommended.

Pharmacotherapeutics is discussed in Unit III in relation to the pathophysiology of the disease and the goals of treatment. Each chapter explores how patient variables, economic considerations, concurrent diseases, and drug characteristics influence rational drug selection. Evaluating outcomes along with guidelines for consultation and referral are included. Where relevant, the newest published professional guidelines are incorporated. Each patient is unique and no set of guidelines or treatment algorithm applies to each patient. However, these tools, drawn from the clinical knowledge and experience of experts in a given specialty, are helpful in rational drug selection, especially for the student and novice practitioner. Clinically based case studies, provided in an online supplement to this edition, provide a framework for application of pharmacotherapeutic knowledge.

Special Drug Treatment Considerations

Unit IV focuses on special populations. Age-related variables are explored in **Chapter 50**, "Pediatric Patients," and **Chapter 51**, "Geriatric Patients." Gender variables are considered in **Chapter 48**, "Women as Patients," and **Chapter 49**, "Men as Patients."

The final chapter in the book deals with one of the most common yet often perplexing issues with which prescribers deal: pain. **Chapter 52** focuses on management of both acute and chronic pain across the age continuum. The fourth edition includes the most current information on newer drugs used to treat chronic pain and new pain assessment tools for patients with dementia. The chapter includes a discussion of the legal aspects of prescribing related to drug-dependent patients and includes coverage of Material Risk Assessment and Pain Management Contract documents.

FEATURES

Throughout the text, care has been taken to provide the reader with a consistent and logical presentation of material. Visual appeal is provided through the generous use of tables, illustrations, and flowcharts. Other features are unique to the specific units:

Unit I chapters

In-depth pharmacology base for advanced pharmacotherapeutics
Herbal and complementary therapies
Ethnopharmacology and pharmacogenomics
Nutrition and nutraceuticals as therapy
Pharmacoeconomics
Information technology including EHR and how it is used in a busy practice

Unit II chapters

Tables for ease of access to information
  Pharmacokinetics tables
  Drug Interactions tables
  Dosage Schedule tables
  Available Drug Dosage Forms
Rational drug selection and monitoring parameters
Patient Education
Clinical Pearls
On the Horizon feature

Unit III chapters

Integration of pathophysiology and pharmacotherapeutics
Integration of professional treatment guidelines
Drugs Commonly Used tables
Patient Education displays

Unit IV chapters
Variables related to special populations
Pediatrics
Geriatrics
Women
Men
Pain management

SUMMARY

Every effort has been made to make this text as comprehensive, accurate, and user-friendly as possible. The generous use of tables for ease of access to information, the focus on rational drug selection, the inclusion of often hard-to-find monitoring parameters, and the integration of patient education throughout the text are examples of this user-friendly approach. The authors hope that you will find this a valuable resource both as a student and in your practice.

TMW
MVR

ACKNOWLEDGMENTS

I would like to acknowledge my mentors who have supported me throughout my nursing career. Included in this list are Dr. Sheila Kodadek, who has been my mentor and friend throughout my nursing career, and the late Dr. Terry Misener.

TMW

TERI MOSER WOO, RN, PHD, CPNP-PC, FAANP

Teri has been a pediatric health-care provider for 30 years. She received her BSN from Oregon Health Sciences University (OHSU) in 1984. Teri earned an MSN in Childrearing Family Nursing in 1989 and a post-Masters Pediatric Nurse Practitioner Certificate in 1993 from OHSU. In 2008, she earned a PhD in Nursing from the University of Colorado College of Nursing, Denver. Teri was president of the Oregon Pediatric Nurse Practitioner Association from 1998 to 2000 and from 2011 to 2013 and is a Fellow in the American Academy of Nurse Practitioners. She is an Associate Professor and Associate Dean for Graduate Nursing Programs at Pacific Lutheran University School of Nursing in Tacoma, Washington. Teri continues to practice as a Pediatric Nurse Practitioner for Kaiser Permanente in pediatric ambulatory care.

MARYLOU V. ROBINSON, PHD, FNP-C

Marylou V. Robinson received her BSN from the Walter Reed Army Institute of Nursing, University of Maryland; her Master's as a CNS from The Catholic University of America, her post-Master's as an FNP from Pacific Lutheran University, and her PhD from Oregon Health & Science University. After a 22-year U.S. Army career spanning from Vietnam to Desert Storm, she joined academia. Currently, she is an Associate Professor at the University of Colorado College of Nursing at the Anschutz Medical Campus. She has been a National Ski Patroller for over 26 years.

Erin Anderson, MSN, CPNP

Pediatric Urology
Oregon Health & Science University
Portland, OR

Cally Bartley, MSN, FNP-C

Instructor
School of Medicine, Department of Dermatology
University of Colorado Anschutz Medical Campus
Aurora, CO

Jane M. Carrington, PhD, RN

Assistant Professor
College of Nursing
University of Arizona
Tucson, AZ

Diana L. Dewell, ARNP, ANP

Family Medicine Clinic
Madigan Healthcare System
Fort Lewis, WA

Gina Dobbs, MSN, CRNP

Nurse Practitioner and Sub-Investigator
1917 HIV/AIDS Outpatient/Research Clinic
University of Alabama at Birmingham
Birmingham, AL

Krista Estes, DNP, FNP-C

Assistant Professor
College of Nursing
University of Colorado Anschutz Medical Campus
Aurora, CO

Teral Gerlt, MS, RN, WHCNP-E

Instructor
School of Nursing
Oregon Health & Science University
Portland, OR

Theresa Granger, PhD, ARNP, FNP

Visiting Professor
Chamberlain College of Nursing
Downers Grove, IL

Lorena C. Guerrero, PhD, MN, ARNP, FNP-BC

Assistant Professor
School of Nursing
Pacific Lutheran University
Tacoma, WA

Anne Hedger, DNP, ACNP-CS, ANP-CS, CPNP-AC, ENP-BC, CCRN

Associate Clinical Professor
Acute Care Curriculum Coordinator/AGACNP Program
School of Nursing
Boise State University
Boise, ID

Leila N. Jones, MSN, BA, RN

Madison House—Genesis Healthcare
Madison, CT

Jennifer Jordan, RPh, PharmD, BCPS

Associate Professor
School of Pharmacy
Pacific University
Hillsboro, OR

Tracy Klein, PhD, FNP, ARNP, FAANP, FRE, FAAN

Assistant Professor, College of Nursing
Washington State University, Vancouver
Vancouver, WA

Ashim Malhotra, BPharm, PhD

Assistant Professor
School of Pharmacy
Pacific University
Hillsboro, OR

Theresa Mallick-Searle, MS, RN-BC, ANP-BC

Division of Pain Medicine
Stanford Health Care
Redwood City, CA

Fujio McPherson, RN, DAOM, MSN, FNP, LAC

Internal Medicine Clinic
Madigan Army Medical Center
Fort Lewis, WA

Benjamin J. Miller, PhD, MN, ARNP, FNP, ACNP

Assistant Professor
College of Nursing
Seattle University
Seattle, WA

Anne E. Morgan, PharmD

Clinical Pharmacy Specialist, Department of Neurology
University of Colorado Hospital
Aurora, CO

Joan Nelson, DNP, RN

Associate Professor
College of Nursing
University of Colorado Anschutz Medical Campus
Aurora, CO

Priscilla Nodine PhD, CNM

Assistant Professor
College of Nursing
University of Colorado Anschutz Medical Campus
Aurora, CO

Kristen Lambert Osborn, MSN, CPNP–AC/PC

Pediatric Nurse Practitioner
UAB Division of Pediatric Hematology and Oncology
Children's of Alabama
Birmingham, AL

James L. Raper, DSN, CRNP, JD, FAANP, FAAN

HIV/AIDS Outpatient, Research and Dental Clinic
Associate Professor of Medicine & Nursing
University of Alabama at Birmingham
Birmingham, AL

Peter J. Rice, PharmD, PhD, BCPS

Professor
Skaggs School of Pharmacy and Pharmaceutical Sciences
University of Colorado Anschutz Medical Campus
Aurora, CO

Laura Rosenthal, DNP, ACNP

Assistant Professor
College of Nursing
University of Colorado Anschutz Medical Campus
Aurora, CO

Ruth Schaffler, PhD, FNP

Emeriti Associate Professor
School of Nursing
Pacific Lutheran University
Tacoma, WA

Tracy Scott, DNP, FNP

Assistant Professor
Department of Family Medicine
School of Medicine
University of Colorado Anschutz Medical Campus
Aurora, CO

Kathy Shaw, DNP, RN, CDE

Assistant Professor
College of Nursing
University of Colorado Anschutz Medical Campus
Aurora, CO

R. Brigg Turner, PharmD, BCPS

Assistant Professor
School of Pharmacy
Pacific University
Hillsboro, OR

Connie Valdez, PharmD, MSEd, BCPS

Associate Professor, Department of Clinical Pharmacy
Skaggs School of Pharmacy and Pharmaceutical Sciences
University of Colorado Anschutz Medical Campus
Aurora, CO

Mary Weber, PhD, PMHNP-BC, FAANP

Associate Professor
College of Nursing
University of Colorado Anschutz Medical Campus
Aurora, CO

Marianne Adam, PhD, RN, CRNP

Assistant Professor
Moravian College
Bethlehem, PA

Nancy Beckham, PhD, FNP-C

Associate Professor
Gonzaga University
Spokane, WA

Christopher W. Blackwell, PhD, ARNP, ANP-BC, AGACNP-BC, CNE

Associate Professor
College of Nursing
University of Central Florida
Orlando, FL

Sharon Chalmers, PhD, CNE, APRN-BC

Associate Professor
University of North Georgia
Dahlonega, GA

Patsy E. Crihfield, DNP, APRN, FNP-BC, PMHNP-BC, PMHS

Chair of Nurse Practitioner Tracks, Graduate Program
Union University
Germantown, TN

Linda Dayer-Berenson, PhD, MSN, CRNP, CNE, FAANP

Associate Clinical Professor
Drexel University–CNHP
Philadelphia, PA

Carolynn A. DeSandre, PhD, CNM, FNP-BC

Assistant Professor
University of North Georgia
Dahlonega, GA

Abimbola Farinde, PharmD, MS

Clinical Pharmacist Specialist
Webster, TX

Joan Parker Frizzell, PhD, CRNP, ANP-BC

Associate Professor
School of Nursing & Health Sciences
La Salle University
Philadelphia, PA

Tammy Gilliam, DNP, APRN-BC, FNP

Assistant Professor of Nursing/Adjunct Faculty
University of South Carolina/USC Upstate
Spartanburg, SC

Cathy R. Kessenich, DSN, ARNP, FAANP

Professor of Nursing, MSN Program Director
University of Tampa
Tampa, FL

Pamela King, PhD, APRN, FNP, PNP

MSN Program Director
Spalding University
Louisville, KY

Angela I. Kulesza, DNP, NP-C

Assistant Professor School of Nursing, Science and Health
    Professions
Regis College
Weston, MA

Christine Nelson-Tuttle, DNS, RN, PNP-BC

Associate Professor, Undergraduate Chair
St. John Fisher College
Rochester, NY

David G. O'Dell, DNP, ARPN, FNP-BC

Graduate Nursing Program Director
South University
Royal Palm Beach, FL

JoAnne Pearce, MS, PhDc, RN, APRN

Director of Nursing Programs
Idaho State University, College of Technology
Pocatello, ID

CONTENTS

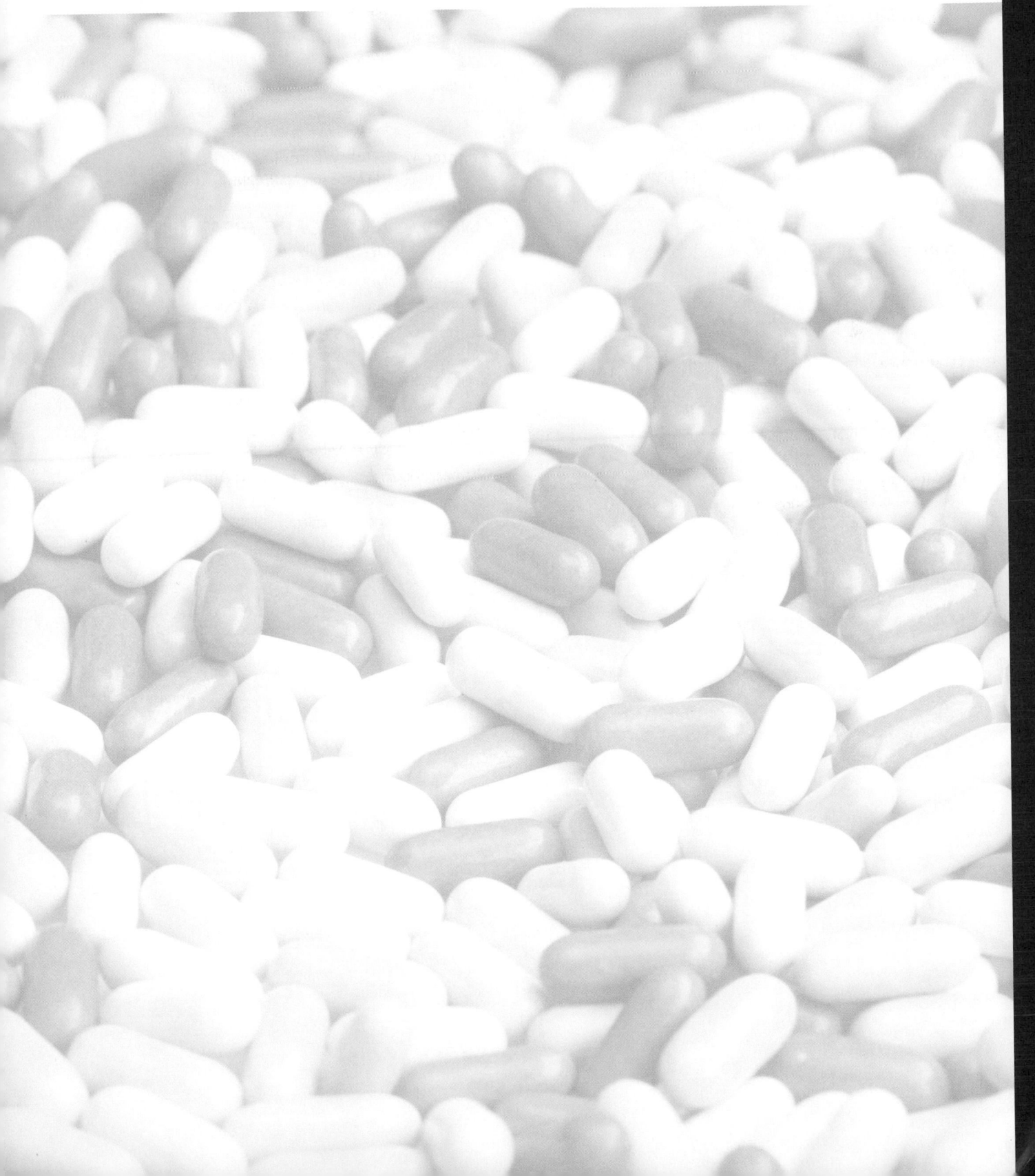

THE FOUNDATION

CHAPTER 1

THE ROLE OF THE ADVANCED PRACTICE NURSE AS PRESCRIBER

Teri Moser Woo • Marylou Robinson

Nurses have been administering medications prescribed by another provider for many years. The knowledge base to safely perform this activity has been an integral part of basic nursing education. With the advent of the advanced practice nurse, the role of the nurse in relation to medications has evolved to include prescribing the medications as well as administering them. The prescriber role requires additional knowledge beyond that taught in undergraduate nursing programs. More than that, it requires the willingness and ability to assume a different level of responsibility for this activity. Advanced practice nurses other than nurse practitioners (NPs) may gain prescriptive authority or prescribe under protocol; therefore, the term *advanced practice registered nurse* (APRN) will be used in this chapter to include NPs, certified nurse midwives (CNMs), certified registered nurse anesthetists (CRNAs), and clinical nurse specialists (CNSs) with prescribing authority, as determined by the individual state nurse practice act. The focus of the discussion will remain primary care prescribing.

ROLES OF REGISTERED NURSES IN MEDICATION MANAGEMENT

Registered Nurses

Experienced registered nurses (RNs) often find themselves in the position of discussing what might be the "best" drug a patient should receive with a physician or other prescribing provider. The RN is an advocate for the patient and his or her input should be sought and highly valued in the prescribing process. Collaboration between the nurse and prescriber improves patient safety and the quality of care the patient receives; however, the responsibility for the final decision regarding which medication to prescribe remains with the prescriber.

Advanced Practice Registered Nurses

APRNs have a higher level of responsibility related to pharmacotherapeutics than RNs. The nature of this responsibility depends on whether the APRN can prescribe medications. States vary in their laws related to prescriptive authority for APRNs. Twenty-one states have fully independent prescribing by nurse practitioners (AANP, 2013b; National Council of State Boards of Nursing, 2015). Some states have full or limited prescribing allowed by CNSs, including Alaska, Colorado, Connecticut, Hawaii, Iowa, Idaho, Minnesota, Montana, Nevada, New Mexico, North Dakota, Oregon, Utah, Vermont, Washington, DC, and Wyoming (National Council of State Boards of Nursing, 2015).

Because nonprescribing APRNs have in-depth knowledge of the drugs used in their specialty areas, their collaboration with the health-care providers who are prescribing is valuable. They may assist in determining the pharmacotherapeutic protocols for their patients and may be credentialed by their organization to select drugs within those protocols to be administered to their patients. These roles related to pharmacotherapeutics represent an intermediate level of responsibility between the staff RN, who administers drugs chosen by another provider, and the NP, who prescribes a drug without the need for a protocol. APRNs also collaborate with other providers in designing and implementing research protocols to test the efficacy of a new drug. They also have a central role in educating nurses and other providers in the appropriate use of these new drugs.

ROLES AND RESPONSIBILITIES OF APRN PRESCRIBERS

APRNs exist in a range of practices and include certified RN anesthetists, certified nurse midwives, and others whose title includes the words *nurse practitioner* or *advanced practice registered nurse*. The responsibility for the final decision on which drug to use and how to use it is in the hands of the APRN prescriber. The degree of autonomy in this role and the breadth of drugs that can be prescribed vary from state to state based on the nurse practice act of that state. Every year, the January issue of the *Nurse Practitioner* journal and an issue of the *American Journal for Nurse Practitioners* present a legislative update providing a summary of each state's practice acts as they relate to titling, roles, and prescriptive authority. As of January 2015 (Philips, 2015), the following were true of NP regulation of practice and prescribing authority:

- All states have title protection for NPs.
- Only Oregon has mandated third-party reimbursement parity for NP services.
- In all but five states, the control of practice and licensure is within the sole authority of the state's board of nursing. These five states have joint control in the board of nursing and the board of medicine.
- Scope of practice is determined by the individual NP's license under the nurse practice act of the licensing

jurisdiction. Some have a graduated scope based on experience level. New prescribers need to understand that their employment sites may restrict this legal scope of practice but cannot extend it.

- In 17 states and the District of Columbia, NPs have independent scope of practice and prescriptive authority without a requirement or attestation for physician collaboration, consultation, delegation, or supervision.
- Six states have full autonomous practice and prescriptive authority following a period of postlicensure/postcertification supervision or collaboration.

The 2010 Institute of Medicine's (IOM) publication *Future of Nursing: Leading Change, Advancing Health* called for removing scope of practice barriers and allowing NPs to practice to the full extent of their education and training (IOM, 2010). Many states are responding to this call, with the expectation that the above list will be significantly modified in years to come.

ADVANCED KNOWLEDGE

General knowledge about the pharmacokinetics and pharmacodynamics of drugs, how to administer them safely, and what to teach the patient is learned in undergraduate nursing courses and subsequently refined in practice. Additional knowledge, critical thinking, and assumption of a higher level of legal responsibility are required to assume the prescriber role. Knowledge of medicine, pharmacology, and nursing intertwine in the NP role. As a prescriber, it becomes the role and responsibility of the NP to determine the diagnosis for which the drug will be ordered, prescribe the appropriate drug, monitor the expected outcome of the drug, and incorporate a holistic assessment of the impact of disease and therapy on patient lives.

The APRN role requires advanced knowledge about pathophysiology, medical diagnoses, and pharmacology to choose an appropriate drug. Determining the medical diagnosis is not within the scope of this book, but rational drug selection requires knowledge of the disease processes (medical diagnoses) for which a drug may be prescribed and the mechanism of action of a specific drug and how it affects this disease process. Rational drug selection is discussed throughout the book.

The prescriber role requires advanced pharmacology knowledge beyond that taught in basic nursing education. Knowledge required for rational drug selection includes, for example, bioequivalence and cost when deciding whether to use a generic form of a given drug; the enzyme systems used to metabolize a drug for deciding about potential drug interactions; and the pharmacokinetics of a drug for determining the loading, maintenance, and tapering doses. The terms may sound familiar, but the underlying depth of information and the role of this information in determining the best drug to prescribe are beyond basic nursing pharmacology knowledge. Volume of distribution, for example, receives little discussion in undergraduate nursing pharmacology texts, but it is often critical in determining dosage for drugs with very large or small volumes of distribution and in selecting drugs for patients with cardiac or renal failure, pregnant patients, or patients who are underweight or obese. Assessment of plasma drug levels by bioassay may be a familiar concept, but the use of this knowledge to determine whether a drug should be prescribed or the prescription altered will be new. The RN may know a given drug's effect on renal functioning, but the prescribing APRN needs to know what tests to order and when to order them to appropriately monitor that functioning, as well as when or if to alter the dosage or stop the drug. Diagnostic tests and their role in drug monitoring may be briefly covered in a basic nursing pharmacology course, but appropriate modification of drug therapy based on results is added knowledge that an APRN needs to be a safe prescriber.

A nurse who is studying to be an APRN will need additional knowledge about prescriptive authority. Does the chosen drug fit within the legal authority of an APRN to prescribe in his or her state? What are the conditions under which the prescription may be written, and how does one correctly write it? What constraints may be in place because of the patient's health insurer or lack of health insurance?

Additionally, the APRN needs to be aware of new drugs that come on the market, medication alerts, and label changes due to postmarketing analysis. In 2014 there were a record 41 novel new drug entities approved by the U.S. Food and Drug Administration (FDA), with an average of 25 new drugs approved annually (U.S. Food and Drug Administration Center for Drug Evaluation and Research, 2015). The FDA sends out alerts to health-care providers via the Med-Watch Safety Alert system as new information becomes available from post-marketing surveillance and modifies drug labels as appropriate. Ever-changing drug information requires the APRN to remain up-to-date on drug information at all times.

BENEFITS OF AN APRN AS PRESCRIBER

Although the focus of this book is on pharmacotherapeutic intervention, alternative treatment options are also part of the armamentarium that can be used to treat a given disorder and may interact with the pharmacotherapeutic intervention. Discussion of common therapies that may be chosen as treatment options or that are integral to drug therapy is integrated throughout the drug-specific and disease-specific chapters.

Some therapies have traditionally been part of what all nurses teach, and they remain central to the role of the APRN, for example, lifestyle management issues for a cardiac patient, relaxation techniques for a patient experiencing stress, and appropriate exercise for a patient with low back pain or arthritis. Herbal therapies have been part of the health practices of people throughout history, but it is only recently that health-care providers have acknowledged them and considered them in planning treatment. If the APRN chooses to use herbal therapy or the patient is using this therapy as suggested by another provider, there must be reliable resources

about the therapy and its impact on prescribing. This book includes a separate chapter on herbal therapy and the uses of complementary therapies and also integrates the use of herbal interventions throughout.

Nutrition is also a common issue in nursing, but often the nurse's knowledge of nutrition related to pharmacology is limited to food–drug interactions or the low-sodium diet for a patient with hypertension. Knowledge regarding how foods and nutrition affect drug prescribing is integrated throughout the book; how foods are used as therapy is included in Chapter 9, "Nutraceuticals."

Choosing among pharmacological and other treatment options also involves advanced knowledge. The right choice depends on accurate information about the patient and his or her situation and the effects of any alternative treatment options on health outcomes. Choices also depend on the patient's culture, preferences for different health outcomes, attitudes toward taking risks, and willingness to endure often uncomfortable adverse drug effects during treatment for some possible future benefit.

Characteristic of APRNs and their practice are consideration of the whole patient, the joint setting of therapeutic goals with other members of the health-care team, and the inclusion of the patient in each decision about care. This holistic approach remains a central element in APRN practice and is often cited by patients and other providers as a hallmark and distinguishing feature of APRN practice when compared with other primary care providers. Adherence to a drug treatment regimen has traditionally been less than optimal. Statistics cited often place patient adherence (taking the drugs as prescribed) at less than 50 percent. Research shows that adherence is better for prescriptions given by NPs than by physician assistants (Manhattan Research, 2013). The reasons for the difference include consideration of the whole patient and inclusion of the patient in decision making. Another factor in improved adherence is patient education; APRNs spend more time than other providers in teaching their patients about the disease process and the relationship of the treatment regimen to it (Gielen, Dekker, Frecke, Mistiaen, & Krozen, 2013; Manhattan Research, 2013). Each of these important aspects of drug choice and utilization is covered in this book.

CLINICAL JUDGMENT IN PRESCRIBING

Prescribing a drug results from clinical judgment based on a thorough assessment of the patient and the patient's environment, the determination of medical and nursing diagnoses, a review of potential alternative therapies, and specific knowledge about the drug chosen and the disease process it is designed to treat. In general, the best therapy is the least invasive, least expensive, and least likely to cause adverse reactions. Frequently, the best choice is to have lifestyle, nonpharmacological, and pharmacological therapies working together. When the choice of treatment options is a drug, several questions arise.

Is There a Clear Indication for Drug Therapy?

In the age of health-care reform and increased awareness of the limitations of drugs, whether a medication is the best option for treatment has become an important question. For example, in treating acute otitis media, guidelines regarding the use of antibiotics has been evolving. A high percentage of otitis media infections resolve without intervention, so how does one know that the antibiotic was the cause of the cure? Of concern is organisms' resistance to antibiotics, with antibiotic overtreatment considered a contributing factor to resistance. Before drug therapy is chosen, the indication for and necessity of using a drug should be carefully considered.

What Drugs Are Effective in Treating This Disorder?

Several drugs may be effective in treating a condition, so which one is best for a particular patient? Even if only the most effective class of drug is considered, few classes of drugs include only one drug. How does one determine "best"; what are the criteria? Are there nationally recognized guidelines that can be used? The Agency for Health Care Quality (AHCQ), the National Institutes of Health (NIH), and many specialty organizations publish disease-specific treatment guidelines that include both pharmacological and nonpharmacological therapies.

What Is the Goal of Therapy With This Drug?

What is the best drug to achieve treatment goals? Various goals are possible in the choosing of therapy. The goal may be cure of the disease and short term in nature. If cure is the goal, troublesome adverse effects may be better tolerated and cost may be less of an issue. If the goal is long-term treatment for a chronic condition, adverse effects and costs take on a different level of importance, and how well the drug fits into the lifestyle of the patient can be a critical issue.

Under What Conditions Is It Determined That a Drug Is Not Meeting the Goal and a Different Therapy or Drug Should Be Tried?

At the onset of therapy, the provider and patient should have a clear understanding of what outcome or goal is expected of the medication prescribed. Follow-up and monitoring times are established to see how well treatment with the drug is meeting the goal. Often, monitoring parameters are published for a drug but may need to be adjusted based on the age or concurrent disease processes of the patient. Part of the decision-making process may include questions about when to consult with or refer the patient to a specialist.

Are There Unnecessary Duplications With Other Drugs That the Patient Is Already Taking?

The patient's medication history should be reviewed at each encounter to detect duplications or medications that may be discontinued. Sometimes drugs from different classes are given together to achieve a desired effect, and

this is a therapeutic choice. It may also be that the provider is not aware of the overlap, especially if the patient is seeing several different providers. For example, a patient who is on a diuretic to treat hypertension may be receiving potassium supplementation. Another provider may decide to use an angiotensin-converting enzyme (ACE) inhibitor to treat heart failure. An ACE inhibitor can also be used to treat hypertension. Rather than a treatment regimen with three drugs, it may be possible to use a combination of an ACE inhibitor with a diuretic in one tablet, and because ACE inhibitors cause potassium retention, no supplemental potassium would be needed. Use of an integrated electronic health record can assist the provider in discovering duplication of therapy and collaborating with other providers to develop a simplified regimen.

Would an Over-the-Counter Drug Be Just as Useful as a Prescription Drug?

Increasing numbers of drugs are being moved from prescription to over-the-counter (OTC) status. This may lead to a reduction in cost for the patient, or it may increase patient costs due to insurance no longer paying for the medication. Patients may not consider OTC medications as "drugs" because they are not prescribed; therefore, a careful history of all medications would specifically ask about OTC medications.

What About Cost?

Who will pay for this drug? Can the patient afford it? Will the cost of the medication affect adherence to the treatment regimen? Cost is an issue for several reasons. Many insurance policies do not cover the cost of drugs or only provide partial coverage, so the patient must pay "out of pocket." The newer the drug, the more likely the cost is to be high based on the drug manufacturer's need to reclaim research and development costs while the corporation still holds the patent on that drug. Newest is not always best, and consideration of cost is a major factor in choosing between newer drugs and ones that have been around long enough to be available in generic form. Many insurance plans have larger co-pays for name-brand drugs than for generic medications. Multiple national retail pharmacies have developed $4.00 prescription formularies. Awareness of what is on the local discount formulary may save the patient hundreds of dollars in prescription costs and may increase compliance. Factors likely to lead to poor adherence include a drug that is expensive in relation to a patient's finances, a drug that must be taken daily as part of a complex regimen, and a drug that is not covered by insurance.

Where Is the Information to Answer These Questions?

Nurses evaluate sources of drug information and learn which ones to trust. For an APRN, the sources of drug information expand to include the wide array of professional literature that ranges from the well-reputed journals to literature from specialty and professional organizations, the multitude of computerized drug databases (e.g., Micromedix, Lexicomp,

Epocrates), information from the U.S. Food and Drug Administration, and formula programs that can be accessed via a handheld device or computer.

The APRN prescriber needs to evaluate how reliable the drug information is. How can reliability be determined? Is the information source written by someone who may benefit from presenting biased information? Is the information source current? Today's "wonder drug" may be removed from the market tomorrow. Is the information relevant to the specific patient for whom the drug will be prescribed? If the information is a research report, what type of research design was used? Are there questions about the validity and reliability of the data? Are national or international guidelines used to inform prescribing or does the reference suggest prescribing outside established guidelines? To prescribe drugs appropriately, APRNs must be able to answer these questions; to answer them, they must master sources of information and use them on a regular basis.

COLLABORATION WITH OTHER PROVIDERS

No one member of the health-care team can provide high-quality care without collaborating with other team members. They most often collaborate with physicians, pharmacists, podiatrists, mental health specialists, therapists, and other providers, including APRNs who are not NPs, physician assistants (PAs), and other nurses.

Physicians

Collaboration with physicians has been something of a roller-coaster ride for NPs. Early in the development of the NP role, physicians were the teachers in the NP programs and accepted NPs as physician-extenders. As the role of the NP evolved to clearly indicate that it was advanced nursing practice, and as legislation made autonomy of practice possible, the relationship became more adversarial, with the American Medical Association (AMA) issuing statements regarding the NP and PA scope of practice (AMA, 2009), often for economic reasons. An AMA document, *AMA Scope of Practice Series: Nurse Practitioner,* stated, "It is the AMA's intention that these Scope of Practice Data Series modules provide the background information necessary to challenge the state and national advocacy campaigns of limited licensure health care providers who seek unwarranted scope-of-practice expansions that may endanger the health and safety of patients" (AMA, 2009, p 4). The AMA responded to the IOM *Future of Nursing* report by reiterating that NPs are not qualified to provide patient care because of lack of hours in clinical education (Patchin, 2010).

Although this struggle still continues at the national level (Patchin, 2010; American Academy of Nurse Practitioners [AANP], 2013; AMA, 2013), NPs and physicians do work together very effectively on an individual basis and in collegial care teams. In an era of health-care reform, our joint concerns about patient care decisions require us to be allies.

Physicians may offer insight or advice on pharmacological management from their experience. A physician's expertise related to pharmacology is based on understanding biochemistry and prescribing for a given pathophysiology. The emphasis is on the disease and the drug, with less emphasis on the impact on the patient. Patient education by physicians may be limited or left to a nurse or pharmacist.

APRNs traditionally approach prescribing drugs in a slightly different manner from that of physicians. As APRNs prescribe a drug for a given pathophysiology, their nursing background leads them to place equal emphasis on understanding the impact the drug will have on the patient. Patient education is a central focus of nursing and APRN practice. Knowledge and clinical experience shared from the mingling of medical and nursing perspectives are mutually beneficial to the providers and the patient. The APRN can benefit from the in-depth knowledge about the drugs in the physician's specialty area. The physician can benefit from APRNs' focus on the impact of the drug on the patient and from their patient education skills. In the age of health-care reform, increasing emphasis is being placed on these latter issues.

Pharmacists

Collaboration with pharmacists requires an understanding of the educational preparation for and evolution of the role of the pharmacist. The profession of pharmacy requires graduate-level preparation for all pharmacists with the granting of a practice doctorate, the Doctor of Pharmacy (PharmD). PharmDs have extensive knowledge about pathophysiology and take an active role in determining the best drug to prescribe. A PharmD can assist by offering expertise on the clinical management of patients, including available dosage forms, potential adverse reactions, and drug interactions. Both physicians and APRNs increasingly consult PharmDs for their knowledge of pharmacokinetics and pharmcotherapeutics when prescribing for complex patients. In some jurisdictions, PharmDs have some independent prescriptive authority.

Other APRNs

Collaboration with other NPs and APRNs who have prescriptive privileges has two major advantages. On a one-to-one basis dealing with individual patient issues, NPs and APRNs can share "clinical pearls" from their knowledge base and collaborate to improve the care of the patient. Collaboration on issues related to scope of practice and prescriptive privilege at the state and national level is critical to obtaining and maintaining the autonomy of practice needed to provide optimal patient care.

Physician Assistants

The focus of the PA's practice is similar to that of the physician, so both the APRN and the PA can benefit from interaction with each other in much the same way as from their interaction with physicians. Many PAs desire more autonomy in their practice, and the experience of APRNs in developing autonomy may be helpful. At this time, such autonomy does not exist, so it is important to know the laws that govern the practice of the PA as well as the APRN in the state to determine how collaboration can best occur.

Nurses Not in Advanced Practice Roles

APRNs regularly collaborate with other nurse colleagues who are not in advanced practice roles. Some have specialized knowledge, such as Certified Diabetes Educators (CDEs) and Wound and Ostomy Care Specialists (WOCS). These nurses and their assistants carry out the prescriptive orders of the APRN. For each of these care providers, it is important to remember their preparation and knowledge level and their legal responsibility in carrying out the APRN's orders.

RNs and licensed practical/vocational nurses function under their own licenses. Their preparation and responsibility are defined by the nurse practice act in each state. Whether they can legally take orders from an APRN is also delineated in these statutes. When prescribing drugs that others will administer, APRNs must know the nurse practice act in the state in which they practice. Medical assistants (MA) may have certification in the state that delineates their preparation, but they are generally not licensed. Their knowledge of drugs may be limited, if they have had any formal education in the area of pharmacology beyond administration. When prescribing drugs to be administered by MAs, APRNs must ensure that the MA clearly understands what they are to do; careful oversight is critical.

CANADIAN NURSE PRACTITIONER PRACTICE

There are over 3,000 APRNs in Canada (Canadian Nurses Association, 2015). As in the United States, where APRN scope of practice and regulation vary from state to state, NP scope of practice and regulation in Canada vary from province to province. NPs practice independently in most of the provinces with the exception of Prince Edward Island, where NPs must practice with a collaborating physician. The scope of practice for NPs also varies from province to province, as well as by practice setting. There are now pediatric, family practice, adult, and anesthesia NPs who can prescribe in Canada. Mental health NPs are working on prescriptive authority and currently must qualify as a prescribing NP in either adult, pediatric, or primary care.

In 2012, the Canadian federal government approved the New Classes of Practitioner Regulations (NCPR) under the Controlled Drugs and Substances Act that removed federal restrictions on NP authority to prescribe controlled substances. NCPR allows NPs to prescribe medications included in the Controlled Drugs and Substances Act when treating patients if they are authorized to do so under provincial/territorial legislation. Each individual province

and territory must individually implement the NP scope of practice to include prescribing controlled substances.

CURRENT ISSUES AND TRENDS IN HEALTH CARE AND THEIR EFFECT ON PRESCRIPTIVE AUTHORITY

Autonomy and Prescriptive Authority

The growth in autonomy and prescriptive authority for NPs and other APRNs is a source of pride. APRNs have now successfully overcome the "cannot prescribe," "cannot diagnose and treat," and "cannot admit" prohibitions to practice that have required so much time and energy to overturn in the past. More states are broadening and expanding the legal, reimbursement, and prescriptive authority to practice for all APRNs, including NPs. By January 2004, all states had recognized the NP title, scope of practice, and prescriptive authority in legislation. Momentum to full autonomy is gaining, with 26 states allowing independent practice for NPs and 21 states allowing independent full prescribing as of January 2015 (National Council of State Boards of Nursing [NCSBN], 2015). APRNs in other states have also gained recognition, although the scope of practice and prescriptive authority is often more restricted.

These gains are not written in stone, however, and can be reversed. Despite continuing research studies (Newland, 2009; Pearson, 2009; Gielen, 2013) that demonstrate the effectiveness of the role of the APRN in improving patient outcomes, barriers remain. Major concerns related to prescriptive authority must continue to be addressed. Not all states have legislation that permits APRNs to prescribe independently of any required physician involvement. Turf battles continue between APRNs and physicians at national and many state levels over physician supervision requirements and co-signatures on prescriptions. The advent of the doctorate of nursing practice (DNP) degree with its comparable level of education to that of other health-care providers and a focus on independent practice may address some of these issues about supervision. However, the American Medical Association continues to stress the need for physician supervision and final authority for the patient, even for APRNs who hold the DNP (Partin, 2008; AMA, 2010, 2013). This push for physician control occurs despite data from malpractice and malfeasance ratios that clearly show that the rationale for physician supervision is unfounded (Pearson, 2009).

Interdisciplinary Teams

In a study by Kaplan and Brown (2004), the top three barriers to effective prescriptive authority for NPs all related to interactions with physicians. Among the top twelve, two related to interactions with pharmacists. It is time to put this battle behind us and work together to create teams of health-care professionals who work together to foster excellent health care for every patient. Such teams would provide care of higher quality with better patient outcomes if the strengths of each team member were fully utilized. Research and systematic reviews comparing care given by such teams with that given by physicians alone supports this assertion (Gielen, 2013). The Institute of Medicine Committee on Health Professions Education (2003) states, "All health professionals should be educated to deliver patient-centered care as members of an interdisciplinary team, emphasizing evidence-based practice, quality improvement approaches and informatics" (p 45).

Level of Education of Team Members

One of the issues to be addressed in interdisciplinary teams is the level of education of the various providers. When the levels of education differ, issues of collegiality, collaboration, and, especially, supervision arise. Medicine has been at the practice doctorate level for more than 50 years. Pharmacists have moved the level of education to enter their profession to the practice doctorate (PharmD). APRNs are now addressing this issue. Recognizing that gaps exist between what is taught in master's-level education programs and the knowledge that is needed for practice, in 2004 the American Association of Colleges of Nurses (AACN) in collaboration with the National Organization of Nurse Practitioner Faculties (NONPF) formed a task force to develop the practice doctorate, and publish core content and competencies for such educational preparation. The title granted to the practice doctorate in nursing is the doctor of nursing practice. In 2006, the AACN organization published *The Essentials of Doctoral Education for Advanced Nursing Practice* (http://www.aacn.nche.edu). In April 2006, NONPF published the entry-level competencies for the graduate of a DNP program (http://www.nonpf.com). These competencies were replaced by NONPF in 2011/2012 with a common document that encompassed all competencies expected of NPs entering practice after graduation. Competencies related to scientific foundation, leadership, quality, practice inquiry, technology and information literacy, policy, understanding of health delivery systems, ethics, and practice are core to all NPs (NONPF, 2011/12).

A date of 2015 was set by the AACN for the educational preparation of all APRNs, including CRNAs, CNMs, CNSs, and NPs, to be at the doctoral level. A 2014 Rand study, "The DNP by 2015" (Auerbach et al., 2014), sponsored by AACN, found that of the 400 schools offering APRN education, 30 percent offered BSN to DNP programs and 58 percent had MSN to DNP programs. Barriers identified by schools that had not adopted the DNP include that the DNP is an option—not a requirement—for practice. Internal or institutional barriers included faculty resources and clinical sites.

In 2014, there were 241 DNP programs with 14,699 students enrolled (http://www.aacn.nche.edu/dnp). An additional 59 DNP programs were in the planning stages. In 2014, the AACN convened a group to evaluate the recognized variance that occurs within and across programs in order to establish more consistency in graduate outcomes and capstone projects, with the outcome not available as this text went to print. This move to the same level of education as other members of the health-care provider team will address some of the issues surrounding the interdisciplinary team. The content of this book is consistent with the recommendations of both the AACN and the NONPF related to the knowledge base in pharmacotherapeutics for DNP-prepared nurses.

Reimbursement

The passage of legislation and the adoption of regulations related to reimbursement is evolving, with the Affordable Care Act rollout creating an opportunity for APRNs to address reimbursement parity. However, the reimbursement by third-party payers continues to be a practice barrier for many nurses in advanced practice. In 2013, Oregon was the first state to pass payment parity for APRNs.

The transfer of additional accountability for Medicaid from the federal government to the states also has the potential to jeopardize the implementation of federal mandates for services and access to APRNs as providers, especially if APRNs are seen as primary care providers only to underserved populations that are financially undesirable to physicians. APRNs must be careful that they not be seen as physician-substitutes or physician-extenders but rather as APRNs who bring a different perspective and science to patient care; otherwise, the current autonomy we enjoy and the level of autonomy we hope to attain may disappear.

Private-sector and government restructuring of health care with a focus on cost control and for-profit groups has both positive and negative potential for the autonomy of the APRN. The negative aspect is that treatment options and decision making about their use are often transferred to the corporation or the government. This can limit the APRN's ability to determine treatment options, and the extra time the APRN takes to educate and counsel patients may be seen as a liability rather than as an asset. From a positive point of view, APRNs have demonstrated their ability to control costs and improve patient outcomes (Pearson, 2009). We must continue to conduct research on the ability of APRNs to provide competent, cost-effective, high-quality services to improve the health of our patients, whether in NP-only practices or in collaborative practices, and to share the findings of that research with the decision makers in the changing world of health care. Better yet, we must become decision makers.

APRNs and other providers must address these challenges and take control of their future in health care so that preferred outcomes are achieved rather than outcomes designed and implemented by others. This requires a commitment of time and energy from each APRN to work together with other providers and other nurses to deal with these issues at local, state, and national levels. Keeping current on new knowledge in pharmacology and on the latest drugs and their clinical applications is only part of the role of the health-care provider as prescriber. APRNs should join and support their professional organizations and engage in positive political activity to maintain the prescriptive authority already gained in each state and to extend autonomous prescriptive authority to all states.

REFERENCES

American Academy of Nurse Practitioners [AANP]. (2011). http://www.aanp.org/images/documents/practice/AANPIOMResponse92Date8_4_11.pdf

American Academy of Nurse Practitioners [AANP]. (2013a). Nurse practitioners challenge AMA recommendations on team-based care reimbursement. Retrieved from http://www.aanp.org/component/content/article/136-press-room/2013-press-releases/1394-nurse-practitioners-challenge-ama-recommendations-on-team-based-care-reimbursement

American Academy of Nurse Practitioners [AANP]. (2013b). State of practice environment. www.aanp.org/legislation-regulation/state-legistlation-regulation/

American Medical Association. (2009). AMA scope of practice series: Nurse practitioner. American Medical Association. AE13:08-0424rev: pdf:10/09

American Medical Association. (2010). AMA announces support for Healthcare Truth and Transparency Act. Retrieved from http://www.ama-assn.org/ama/pub/news/news/healthcare-truth-transparency.page

American Medical Association. (2013). AMA passes recommendations for payment models that support new approaches to team-based health care. *AMA Wire*. Retrieved from http://www.ama-assn.org/ama/pub/news/news/2013/2013-11-18-ama-passes-recommendation-for-payment-models.page

Auerbach, D.I., Martsolf, G., Pearson, M.L., Taylor, E.A., Zaydman, M., Muchow, A., Spetz, J. & Dower, C. (2014). The DNP by 2015: A study of the institutional, political, and professional issues that facilitate or impede establishing a post-baccalaureate Doctor of Nursing Practice program. Rand Health. Retrieved from http://www.aacn.nche.edu/dnp/DNP-Study.pdf

Canadian Nurses Association. (2015). Nurse practitioners. Retrieved from http://www.npnow.ca

Forchuck, C., & Kohr, R. (2009). Prescriptive authority for nurses: The Canadian perspective. *Perspectives in Psychiatric Care, 45*(1), 3–8.

Gielen, S., Dekka, J., Frecke, A., Mistiaen, P., & Krozen, M. (2013). The effects of nurse prescribing: A systematic review. *International Journal of Nursing Studies.* doi: 1016/ijnurstu.2013.12.003 online ahead of print.

Institute of Medicine. (2010). *The future of nursing: Leading change, advancing health.* Washington, DC: National Academies Press. Retrieved from http://www.iom.edu/Reports/2010/The-future-of-nursing-leading-change-advancing-health.aspx

Institute of Medicine Committee on Health Professions Education. (2003). *Health professions education: A bridge to quality.* Washington, DC: The National Academies Press.

Kaplan, L., & Brown, M. (2004). Prescriptive authority and barriers to NP practice. *Nurse Practitioner, 29*(3), 28–35.

Manhattan Research. (2013, 12 Sept.). Nurse practitioners are increasingly focused on promoting patient adherence. Taking the Pulse Nurses 2013 Study. Newswire. http://www.manhattanresearch.com/News-and-Events/Press-Releases/nps-patient-adherence

National Association of Nurse Practitioner Faculties. (2011/amended 2012). Nurse Practitioner Core Competencies. Retrieved from https://c.ymcdn.com/sites/nonpf.site-ym.com/resource/resmgr/competencies/npcorecompetenciesfinal2012.pdf

National Council of State Boards of Nursing. (2015). APRNs in the US. Retrieved from https://www.ncsbn.org/aprn.htm

Newland, J. (2009). NPs: The cornerstone of healthy patients. *Nurse Practitioner, 34*(5), 5.

Patchin, R. J. (2010). AMA responds to IOM report on future of nursing. American Medical Association. Retrieved from http://www.ama-assn.org/ama/pub/news/news/nursing-future-workforce.page

Partin, B. (2008). Advocacy in practice: Unite to fight AMA resolutions. *Nurse Practitioner, 33*(12), 11.

Pearson, L. (2009). The Pearson report: A national overview of nurse practitioner legislation and healthcare issues. *American Journal for Nurse Practitioners, 13*(2), 8–82.

Phillips, S. (2015) 27th annual legislative update: Advancements continue for APRN practice. *Nurse Practitioner, 40*(1), 16-42.

Scisney-Matlock, M., Makos, G., Saunders, T., Jackson, F., & Steigerwalt, S. (2004). Comparison of quality-of-hypertensive-care indicators for groups treated by physician versus groups treated by physician-nurse team. *Journal of the American Academy of Nurse Practitioners, 16*(1), 17–23.

U.S. Food and Drug Administration Center for Drug Evaluation and Research. (2015). Novel new drugs 2014 summary. U.S Food and Drug Administration. Retrieved from http://www.fda.gov/downloads/Drugs/DevelopmentApprovalProcess/DrugInnovation/UCM430299.pdf

CHAPTER 2

REVIEW OF BASIC PRINCIPLES OF PHARMACOLOGY

Peter J. Rice

PHARMACOLOGY—THE STUDY OF DRUGS

Pharmacology is the study of drugs and their actions. Pharmacologists, those who study drugs and their actions, consider a drug to be any chemical substance that produces a measurable biological response. So drugs include not only prescription medications but also nonprescription medications, botanicals, drugs of abuse, and poisons.

As we consider the variety of drugs and the measurable responses they produce, it will be helpful to think about what we would like to see in an ideal drug (Box 2-1). There are no perfect drugs—yet. But defining what would make an ideal drug will help us understand how medicines have developed over time, and what properties to consider as we compare one drug with another to choose the best medication.

HOW NEW DRUGS ARE DEVELOPED

Drugs are developed by pharmaceutical companies to help patients and to make money. The early part of the drug development process is called the preclinical stage. Identification of promising drugs and their testing in animals occur during this stage. Pharmaceutical companies will identify a drug target, starting sometimes with ingredients isolated from a plant (or organism in the case of antibiotics) with desirable medicinal properties, sometimes with a molecular target identified in the body to produce the desired response, and sometimes with a disease in need of treatment. It is common for companies to enlist medicinal chemists, who specialize in designing and synthesizing new drugs. Medicinal chemists can provide many new chemical compounds for the preclinical process. Each drug might have a small difference in its chemical structure that will change its drug properties. Many drugs are examined as pharmaceutical companies seek the elusive perfect

---

BOX 2–1 IDEAL DRUG PROPERTIES

- Convenient route of administration, probably taken by mouth
- Established dosage
- Immediate onset of action
- Produces a single desired biological action
- Produces no unwanted effects
- Convenient duration of action
- Dosage unaffected by loss of kidney or liver function or by disease state
- Improves quality of life
- Prolongs patient survival

---

drug with just the right combination of properties. Preclinical studies are performed on cells, isolated tissues and organs, and in laboratory animals to identify promising compounds.

Drugs approved by the Food and Drug Administration (FDA) must be both safe and effective and are screened by pharmacologists specializing in various aspects of drug activity. Toxicologists specialize in understanding the harmful effects of drugs and predicting as early as possible if a drug will be likely to harm patients. Ideally, drugs will produce their desired effects at dosages well below those needed to produce toxicity.

During the clinical stage of new drug development, pharmaceutical companies must establish the safety and effectiveness of new products in humans. Phase I clinical trials typically establish biological effects as well as safe dosages and pharmacokinetics in a small number of healthy patients. During phase II clinical trials, new drugs are used to treat disease in a small number of patients and to establish the potential of the drug to improve patient outcomes. If the drug still looks promising, phase III clinical trials will compare the new medication to standard therapy in a larger number of patients studied by at sites across the country. New drugs must be at least as good as, and it is hoped better than, other available therapies. Throughout the process, pharmaceutical companies work with the FDA.

After being approved by the FDA, drugs are continuously monitored through post-marketing surveillance, in which health professionals are encouraged to report adverse events, which are studied by both pharmaceutical companies and the FDA. During clinical trials, only several thousand patients receive a new drug. During the post-marketing period, a larger population of patients receives the drug, and sometimes much is learned about additional adverse effects that occur infrequently with use of the drug. Pharmacogenomics is the study of how individual variations in drug targets or metabolism affect drug therapy. Pharmacogenomic studies can identify factors that are responsible for beneficial or adverse effects in individual patients.

DRUG RESPONSES

Homeostasis is the tendency of a cell, tissue, or the body *not* to respond to drugs but instead to maintain the internal environment by adjusting physiological processes. Before a medication can produce a response, it often must overcome homeostatic mechanisms.

Drug effects depend on the amount of drug that is administered. If the dose is below that needed to produce a measurable biological effect, then no response is observed; any effects of the drug are not sufficient to overcome homeostatic capabilities. If an adequate dose is administered, there will be a measurable biological response. With an even higher dose, we may see a greater response. At some point, however, we will be unwilling to increase the dosage further, either because we have already achieved a desired or maximum response or because we are concerned about producing additional responses that might harm the patient.

Because pharmacology is the study of substances that produce biological responses, measurement of what happens when we administer medications is important. We will need ways to express and compare drug activity so that we can describe the action or effect of drugs, compare the effects of different drugs, and predict their pharmacological effects.

Dose–Response Curves

Drugs produce responses as a result of their chemical interactions with living systems. The relationship between the dose or concentration of a drug and its biological response follows the laws of chemistry. The law of mass action defines chemical interactions and forms the theoretical foundation for drug responses that occur through receptors that mediate drug responses. Simply stated, the higher the concentration of a drug at its site of action, the more the drug will bind to the receptor and the greater will be the response. With a greater number of drug molecules in the vicinity, more of them are likely to interact with the receptor.

It is simplest to think that drug responses are directly related to the fraction of receptors that are occupied, or bound, by a drug, so that 50% of the maximum response occurs at a blood level or concentration at which a drug occupies 50% of its receptors. But depending on the number of receptors in a tissue and the ability of drug binding to produce a change in the receptor conformation, far fewer receptors (less than 10%) may be needed to produce a maximum effect.

Types of Drug Responses

There are two basic types of drug responses: quantal and graded. These responses differ in how they are measured and dictate dosing decisions to achieve the desired effect.

Graded responses are biological effects that can be measured continually up to the maximum responding capacity of the biological system (Box 2-2). Most drug responses are graded. For example, changes in blood pressure are measured in millimeters of mercury (mm Hg), and patients may experience small or large changes in blood pressure following treatment with drugs. Graded responses are easier to manage clinically because we can see how each patient responds to a

BOX 2–2 EXAMPLES OF GRADED RESPONSES TO DRUGS

- Blood pressure
- Heart rate
- Diuresis
- Bronchodilation
- FEV1
- Pain (scale 1–10)
- Coma score

particular dose of medication and, if appropriate, alter the dosage to achieve a greater or lesser response. So if a patient's blood pressure is too low or too high when a particular blood pressure medication is administered, we can adjust the dosage based on the patient's individualized response to the medication.

Quantal effects are responses that may or may not occur (Box 2-3). For example, seizures either occur or they do not. The same is true for pregnancy, sleep, and death. If we designate a response as either occurring or absent, it is a quantal response. Prediction of drug dosages or blood levels that produce quantal effects is much more reliable for a population of patients than for an individual patient. Data from a population of patients must be used to establish appropriate doses or blood levels to predict quantal effects in a large number of patients. For example, oral contraceptive doses are high enough to prevent pregnancy (a quantal response!) in over 99% of women. Note that, even with anticonvulsants or oral contraceptives, we do not achieve a 100% response. Because of natural variation in drug metabolism and responses to drugs, there may always be individuals who fail to respond, even at higher dosages. In general, responses that are far outside the typical dose or concentration range occur in patients with unusual drug metabolism or receptor mutations.

The distinction between graded and quantal responses is not always fixed. Certainly, patients are either pregnant or not and either dead or alive. However, for some other quantal responses such as seizures, you can also count the number of occurrences. This can be helpful in adjusting medications to improve patient response with fewer or shorter seizures (a graded response), even though the goal is a seizure-free (quantal response) patient. We can also make graded responses quantal by considering such issues as "Did drug therapy lower

BOX 2–3 EXAMPLES OF QUANTAL RESPONSES TO DRUGS

- Convulsions
- Pregnancy
- Rash
- Sleep
- Death

blood pressure into the target range?" or "How many patients were headache-free?"

Expressing Drug Responses

Pharmacologists show the relationship between dose or concentration and drug effect using graphs that show the dose–response relationship, or dose–response curve. Graphs showing drug responses will show the response on the vertical axis and the concentration or dose on the horizontal axis. And for statistical reasons, because drug dosages extend over a large range, the horizontal axis is logarithmic, which means that it covers a larger dosage range and that numbers are distributed along the axis so that moving a certain distance right or left represents multiplying or dividing the dosage or blood level concentration by a fixed amount. Most dosage changes in patients are doubled or halved: a "logarithmic" adjustment.

Dose–response curves provide information on the relationship between dosage or concentration and responses for one or more drugs. To "read" a concentration–effect or dose–response curve, move from left to right along the horizontal axis; this represents an increasing dosage or concentration. At each dosage, the level of effect is shown by the vertical height of the curve. When concentration–response data are shown for two drugs or two responses on the same graph, we can compare the effects at each dose level.

Pharmacologists compare drugs and their actions in several ways, including potency, efficacy, intrinsic activity, and selectivity. Potency is the expression of *how much* drug is needed to produce a biological response (Fig. 2-1). Potency describes the difference in concentration or dosage of different drugs required to produce a similar effect. Drugs that are more potent require a lower dosage or concentration to produce the same response. For example, compare doses of nonprescription drugs that relieve headache: 200 mg ibuprofen, 325 mg aspirin, and 50 mg ketoprofen. Because ketoprofen requires the lowest dose, it has the highest potency. Drugs

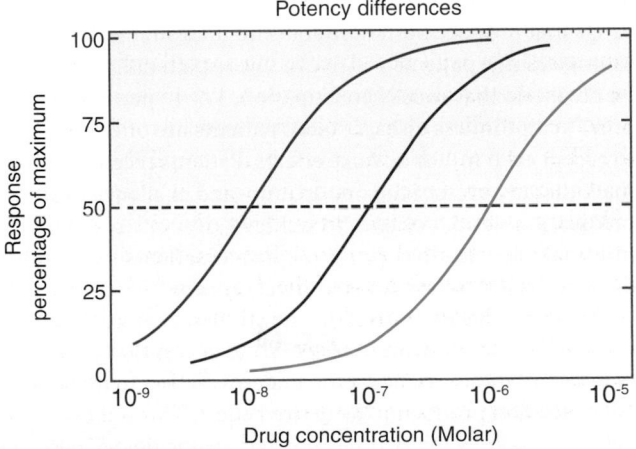

Figure 2–1. Concentration–effect curves for three drugs that differ in potency (i.e., the dose or concentration required to produce an effect). The drug concentration on the *x*-axis is expressed in molar units, representing the number of molecules in each liter of solution. The graded response is expressed as a percentage of maximum effect.

that differ in potency differ in their horizontal position on the dose–response curve.

Efficacy expresses the ability of a drug to produce a maximum effect at any dosage. Efficacy is the expression of the *maximum effect* a drug can produce. For example, consider the treatment of pain. There are many drugs that will relieve mild pain. No matter how high we increase the dosage, drugs that work well for mild to moderate pain are usually ineffective for treating more severe cancer-related pain, for example. Treatment of severe pain requires the use of stronger drugs, such as the opioid analgesics morphine or oxycodone. Morphine or oxycodone have higher efficacy for pain relief than ibuprofen. Drugs with high efficacy can produce greater effects than lower-efficacy drugs can.

Intrinsic activity is very similar to efficacy in that it represents the ability of a drug to produce a large response. Intrinsic activity, however, is used to describe the ability of a drug to produce a response once it has occupied specific receptors. Some drugs produce the maximum receptor stimulation once they occupy receptors; their response is limited by how many drug molecules occupy receptor sites. Other drugs with lower intrinsic activity can occupy the same number of receptors but will produce a lesser response. Drugs can also occupy receptors and produce no receptor stimulation; they merely block the action of neurotransmitters or other drugs.

Drug Selectivity

In clinical use, drugs produce responses that are desired and responses that are unwanted. Of course, we should be administering drugs with a goal in mind, and that goal should include a level of response, either graded or quantal. The level of unwanted response we are willing to accept typically depends on what we are treating and the type of undesired effect. Patients regularly accept all kinds of adverse effects from cancer chemotherapy when their life is on the line; cancer patients tolerate hair loss, nausea, vomiting, and generally feeling miserable because that is what goes along with killing cancer cells. Sometimes patients make surprising decisions regarding drugs that produce both desirable and undesirable effects; for example, some patients will live in severe pain rather than take an analgesic that causes constipation. For hypertension and other symptomless disease states, patients are often reluctant to accept even minor adverse effects. Patients receiving pharmacotherapy present the opportunity and challenge to adjust medications and dosages to achieve optimal results with minimal adverse effects and to educate patients to continue therapy even if minor adverse effects appear.

There are challenges to expressing drug selectivity. The most reasonable way to express *selectivity* is as a ratio of the dose or concentration producing the undesired effect to the dose or concentration producing the desired effect. This is the same as determining how many times the therapeutic dosage needs to be increased to produce the undesired effect. A medication that requires one tablet to produce the desired response and does not produce undesirable effects unless five tablets are used would have a selectivity ratio of 5. That is not a bad drug. But many drugs produce significant undesired effects at or slightly above the therapeutic dosage.

It would be nice if we could describe drug selectivity in a way to encourage optimal drug use. Would not a medication that has high selectivity and produces only the desired effects be the treatment of choice? There are problems, though, with consistently expressing selectivity based on desired and undesired effects. Medications often have more than one effect and might be used for any of their effects, so sometimes a particular effect is desired and sometimes it is undesired. Diphenhydramine is a very nice drug that is used as an antipruritic for itching, as an antihistamine for allergies, as an anticholinergic that dries secretions, and as a sleeping aid that produces drowsiness. Desired and undesired effects can differ for each patient, and if we compare dosages, there are several selectivity ratios.

The therapeutic index is a special ratio describing drug selectivity. The therapeutic index is the ratio of the lethal dose of a drug to the therapeutic dose of a drug. There are some limitations to the therapeutic index: it uses death, a really unacceptable adverse effect, and it uses data from animal studies. But the therapeutic index provides a fixed comparison for drug safety. The therapeutic index of drugs on the market is, of course, always greater than 1; a therapeutic index of less than 1 means that the drug kills before it cures. The therapeutic index ranges from 2 for some drugs (cancer chemotherapy, lithium carbonate) to 6,000 for others (penicillin in nonallergic patients).

Drug Responses in the Real World

Pharmacotherapy in real patients is different than what has already been described. The placebo effect is a pharmacological effect that is not due to the active ingredient. Placebos are tablets or capsules that contain no active ingredient; they are sometimes called "sugar pills" because they used to be filled with sugar. It is common for drug studies to have a placebo group to see if patients are responding to the active drug or just to the act of taking a medication (Fig. 2-2). The placebo group will also be monitored for adverse effects, which establishes the level in untreated patients. Placebo effects are relatively high in some disease states, such as depression, and very low in other disease states, such as cancer.

Dose–effect relationships in the real world do not start at zero response; they start at the response associated with the placebo effect. The level of response increases as the dose increases but rarely reaches 100%. Instead, the risk of toxicity will limit the maximum dosage, or another drug will be used if there is no satisfactory effect.

Brand Versus Generic Drugs

New drugs are patented to protect the innovator company for a period during which only it can manufacture the drug. New drugs are given a generic name that anyone can use to market the drug, but innovator companies will make up a brand name that only they can use to market their drug. During the years after a drug is released, it is marketed under the

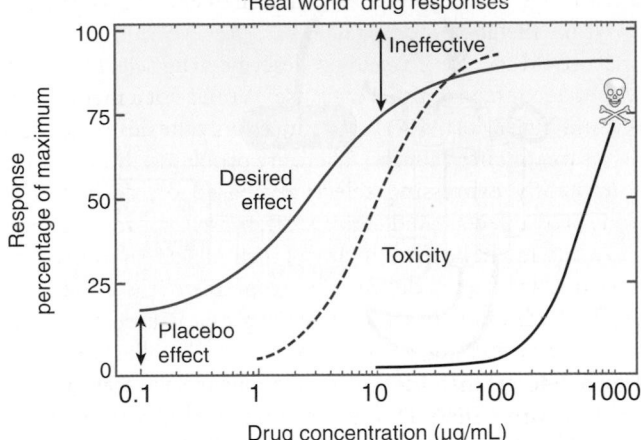

Figure 2–2. Theoretical representation of how drugs produce effects in clinical practice. Drug concentration (x-axis) increases from left to right. Some patients will respond at low dosages, either because of the placebo effect or sensitivity to the drug. As drug concentrations increase, greater numbers of patients will respond favorably but some will also respond adversely. At some dosage or concentration, the presence of toxic effects precludes the use of higher doses in patients.

brand name, and patients and practitioners often become familiar with the product under its brand name. Once the patent on the original drug expires, other companies can manufacture generic products that are designed to imitate the brand product. Once competition is allowed, generic manufacturers formulate similar dosage forms with the same active ingredient in the same amount.

Patients often wonder about the relationship between the effects of brand and generic preparations. Since brand and generic preparations contain the same active ingredient, the body treats the two exactly the same. Differences between brand and generic preparations can occur in the inactive ingredients of the tablet or capsule, such as coloring or filler materials.

Generic products are *supposed* to provide patients with the same dosage as brand-name products. Differences between brand and generic formulations result from differences in the time it takes for the different formulations to break apart in the stomach and dissolve prior to absorption. There are always differences in the speed, or rate, of absorption. The FDA rates generic formulations in its *Orange Book*, and products with an AB rating are considered to be similar enough to use as generic substitutes for brand-name products.

Because the differences between brand and generic products occur in the tablet/capsule disintegration and dissolution steps prior to absorption, brand and generic preparations in which the drug is already in solution, such as injectables, are similar in their rate and extent of absorption.

RECEPTORS

We can think of drug responses in a simple way. A favorite cartoon shows a mathematician solving a problem. The solution

begins with an equation that states the problem, and a gap follows in which the mathematician writes "and then a miracle happens," followed by the result. If we choose to think of drug responses as the predictable miracles that follow drug administration, then pharmacology would be no more than memorizing which responses go along with which drugs. A century ago, medical schools and pharmacy schools had departments of *materia medica*, a Latin way of describing the pairing of a drug with a response without necessarily knowing what happens in between. Today, we encounter the same knowledge level for many botanicals, and patients and health professionals alike will often consult manuals that list symptoms to be treated and the plant product that can produce that action.

If we choose to actually understand drug action and why drugs produce predictable sets of responses, we need to look at the biological molecules and the chemical principles that underlie responses to drugs. Almost all drugs act through receptors. Receptors are the large molecules, usually proteins, that interact with and mediate the action of drugs. Receptors are important because they determine the relationship between dose and effect, the selectivity of drugs, and the actions of pharmacological antagonists.

Pharmacologists tend to organize drug activity based on the receptors through which individual drugs act. There are several benefits to organizing the study of pharmacology around receptors. It simplifies the amount of material that needs to be memorized. Receptors provide a theoretical framework for understanding and predicting drug actions and the relationship between dose (or concentration) and effect. Also, receptors within the same "superfamily" often share properties.

Drug targets include enzymes, ion channels, cell surface receptors, nuclear hormone receptors, transporters, and DNA. In each case, chemical interactions take place between drug and receptor molecules. Receptors act through a number of mechanisms, including those described in the following sections. Chemical energy from the drug–receptor interaction is used to change the receptor in some way that alters physiological processes to produce cellular changes that result in a measurable response.

Because chemical interactions determine the activity of a drug at a particular receptor type, changes in chemical structure result in changes in pharmacological activity. The correlation of chemical structure with pharmacological activity is called the *structure-activity relationship* (SAR). SARs can be helpful in understanding receptors and for developing new drugs. There are separate, independent SARs for different drug properties (e.g., potency, selectivity, toxicity), so the fact that any one drug property changes for the better (or worse) does not necessarily mean that the change affects the other properties of the drug.

Ion Channel Receptors

Ion channel receptors transmit signals across the cell membrane by increasing the flow of ions and altering the electrical potential or separation of charged ions across the membrane. Ion channel receptors can produce responses with a rapid onset and short duration. For example, activation of ion channels by nicotinic receptors is responsible for muscle contraction. Muscle movement needs to start immediately and must stop at will to be effective. The nicotinic receptor consists of five subunits, which form a cylindrical structure with a hole in the center. When acetylcholine (ACh) binds to the two alpha subunits, a conformational change occurs, which momentarily opens the central channel, permitting sodium to enter and potassium to leave the cell (Fig. 2-3). Two binding sites for ACh result in a very steep concentration–effect curve, so a very small change in ACh concentration at the neuromuscular junction will produce dramatic openings in ion channels. Notice that the two ACh sites are a certain distance apart. This is important for the structure–activity relationship of drugs that blocks nicotinic receptor sites.

Ion channel receptors include receptors for ACh (nicotinic), gamma-aminobutyric acid (GABA), and excitatory amino acids (glycine, aspartate, glutamate, etc.).

Receptors Coupled to G Proteins

A number of different guanine nucleotide regulatory proteins (or G proteins) are present in cell membranes. G proteins share a similar structure in which seven regions of protein span the cell membrane to create a pocket (in which drugs can bind) and end with a receptor "tail" inside the cell (Fig. 2-4). Individual G protein receptors have the general G-protein structure but differ in their "binding site," the area that recognizes and binds to drugs, and in the intracellular portions of the G protein that control what happens after a drug is bound. Receptors are activated when specific drugs interact with the binding site, producing a conformational change, a sort of twist, in the G protein. Activation of receptors then produces intracellular changes in the binding of the G-protein receptor to other proteins that control response through other molecules called *second messengers.*

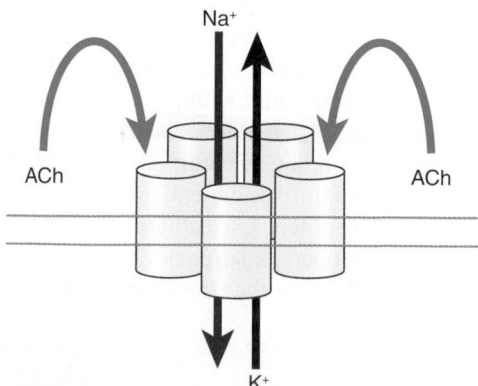

Figure 2–3. The nicotinic acetylcholine (ACh) receptor comprises five subunits that come together to form an ion channel receptor. When ACh binds to two sites on the receptor, the ion channel opens to let sodium (Na⁺) and potassium (K⁺) cross the cell membrane to initiate a response.

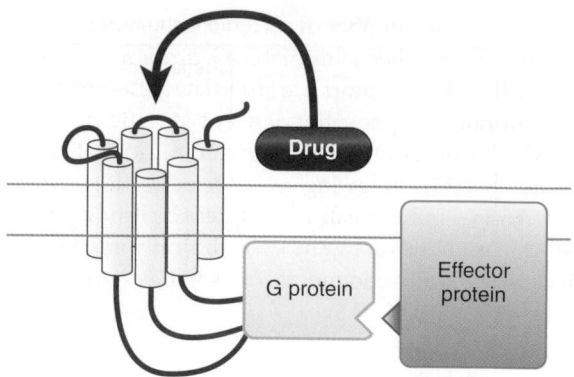

Figure 2–4. G-protein–coupled receptors are proteins that cross the cell membrane 7 times, creating a pocket in which drugs can interact. Bound drugs may stimulate the receptor to release a G protein that can interact with various effector proteins to produce physiological responses.

Second messengers include molecules such as cAMP (cyclic adenosine monophosphate), Ca^{++}, phosphoinositides, and diacylglycerols; each can be produced as a result of stimulating different G-protein–linked receptors. The conformational change in the G-protein receptor can also make intracellular parts of the receptor available for enzymes to phosphorylate. Phosphorylation, placing a phosphate group on a protein, is a way of marking it for activation or inactivation.

G proteins are made up of three major subunits (alpha [α], beta [β], gamma [γ]); minor variations (isotypes) of each subunit can result in a great deal of variation in G proteins just from different combinations of alpha, beta, and gamma subunits. Variation in G-protein subunits and receptors allows them to interact with a variety of drugs and produce different responses depending on which drug is recognized by the receptor, which subunits are involved, and which effector protein is altered. Individual cells and tissues can produce various types and amounts of G proteins. This is a homeostatic mechanism used by the body to adapt to disease states and drug treatment.

Receptors coupled to G proteins mediate the level of second messengers following the extracellular interaction of drug with the receptor. This receptor superfamily includes a large number of different receptors that recognize different drugs and activate or inhibit different second messengers. For example, beta-adrenoceptors mediate the effects of epinephrine (also called *adrenaline*) on the heart and make our hearts beat faster and stronger at scary movies.

In the prototype beta-adrenoreceptor system, interaction of epinephrine with the receptor displaces guanosine diphosphate (GDP) from the G protein, and its replacement by guanosine triphosphate (GTP) activates the G protein. The G protein uncouples from the receptor and stimulates the enzyme adenylyl cyclase to generate intracellular second messenger cAMP. Intracellular cAMP produces the pharmacological effect, such as making the heart beat stronger and faster, until the cAMP breaks down. Caffeine produces similar effects by inhibiting the breakdown of cAMP.

Changes in the number of receptors alter responsiveness to drugs. The number of available G-protein receptors decreases when the receptors are stimulated. Receptors in the cell membrane are phosphorylated at specific intracellular sites, which can lead to desensitization, or loss of receptors or responsiveness following receptor activation. These receptor changes influence drug treatment by limiting the time in which certain drugs can be used clinically and by placing patients at risk for rebound effects when certain drugs are discontinued.

Transmembrane Receptors

Transmembrane receptors consist of an extracellular hormone-binding domain and an intracellular enzyme domain that phosphorylates the amino acid tyrosine. When an active hormone binds to the extracellular binding site, the receptor conformation changes and two receptors bind to one another, activating the enzyme and sustaining the effect (Fig. 2-5). Different receptors catalyze the phosphorylation of tyrosine residues on various downstream signaling proteins.

The protein tyrosine kinase includes receptors for insulin, epidermal growth factor, and platelet-derived growth factor.

Intracellular Receptors Regulating Gene Expression

Lipid-soluble hormones can pass through the cell membrane and bind to intracellular receptors. The glucocorticoid receptor resides in the cytoplasm until it binds with a drug having glucocorticoid activity; binding of the drug displaces a stabilizing protein and permits the folding of the receptor into its active conformation. The receptor then moves to the nucleus, where it controls the transcription of genes by binding to specific DNA sequences (Fig. 2-6). Hormone receptors of this type include corticosteroids, mineralocorticoids, sex steroids, vitamin D, and thyroid hormones; these produce more sustained responses.

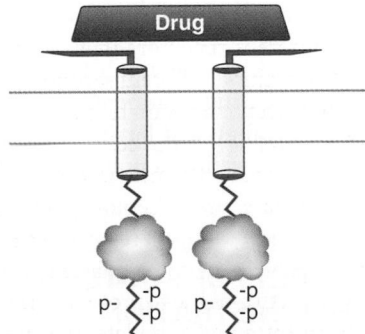

Figure 2–5. The insulin receptor is prototypical of tyrosine kinase receptors. These receptors are brought together by extracellular drug binding (insulin in the case of the insulin receptor), which activates the intracellular enzyme tyrosine kinase. Tyrosine kinase receptors activate one another by adding a phosphorus (P) to select sites on cellular proteins, which in turn activates a physiological response.

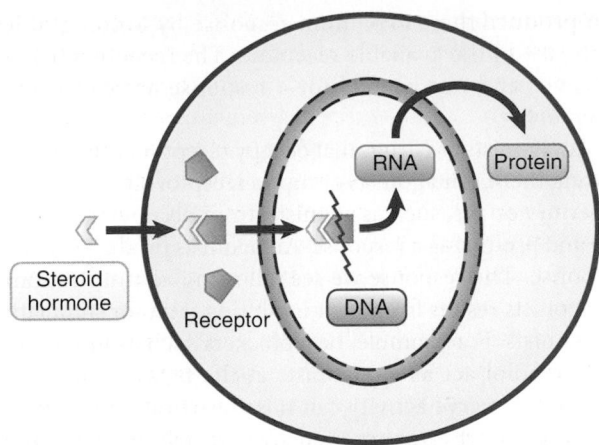

Figure 2–6. Steroid hormones diffuse through the cell membrane to interact with steroid receptors in the cytoplasm. The hormone–receptor pair relocates to the nucleus, where it can interact with DNA to effect RNA transcription and the synthesis of proteins.

Enzymes

Enyzmes are biological molecules that encourage specific chemical reactions in the body. For example, the enzyme acetylcholinesterase breaks a chemical bond in ACh to terminate its action and make acetic acid and choline (Fig. 2-7). A different enzyme can reassemble these molecules into ACh. Drugs can act to stimulate or inhibit specific enzymes. The anticoagulant heparin binds to an enzyme called antithrombin-III and increases its inactivation of clotting factors. The anticholesterol "statin" drugs are inhibitors of the enzyme HMG-Co-A (3-hydroxy-3-methyl-glutaryl coenzyme A) reductase, which controls cholesterol synthesis in the body. Antibiotics are frequently inhibitors of enzymes that are essential for bacteria to remain alive.

Drug Action at Receptors

Drugs can do three basic things once they bind to a receptor. Agonists, or full agonists, are drugs that produce receptor stimulation and a conformational change every time they bind. Full agonists do not need all of the available receptors to produce a maximum response. Some agonists

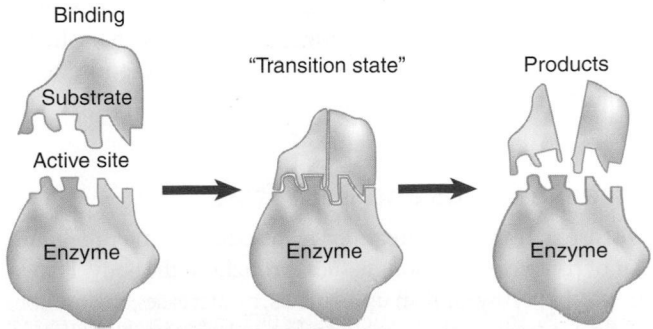

Figure 2–7. Enzymes bind to substrates and speed up biochemical reactions. Enzymes can serve as receptors to the substrate, which binds at the active site, or to drugs that control enzyme activity through binding at a different site.

can produce their maximum response by binding to less than 10% of the available receptors. The receptors that are left over and not needed for a response are called *spare receptors.*

Antagonists are drugs that occupy receptors without stimulating them. Antagonists occupy a receptor site and prevent other molecules, such as agonists, from occupying the same site and producing a response. Antagonists produce no direct response. The response we see following administration of antagonists results from their inhibiting receptor stimulation by agonists. For example, beta blockers such as propranolol and atenolol act as antagonists at the beta-adrenoceptor. Adrenergic nerve activity can raise heart rate, and patients with high heart rates experience a significant drop in heart rate following administration of beta blockers. The same administration may have little effect on patients who lack adrenergic nerve activity and already have a lower heart rate. The effect of antagonists is dependent on the background receptor activity that it can block.

Antagonists produce a shift in the concentration–effect relationship for agonists acting at that same specific receptor as the antagonist; they make agonists for the same receptor appear less potent. The effect of an antagonist is dependent on its blood levels and its affinity for the receptor. Most antagonists in clinical use are competitive reversible antagonists, and it is possible to overcome the antagonist effects with higher concentrations of the competing agonist. A very small number of antagonist drugs (e.g., echothiophate, phenoxybenzamine) act by irreversibly binding to the receptor; their antagonism remains until new receptors can be produced by the cell.

Partial agonists are drugs that have properties in between those of full agonists and antagonists. Partial agonists bind to receptors but when they occupy the receptor sites, they stimulate only some of the receptors. This is sometimes called *intrinsic activity.* So they can act as part agonist and part antagonist. Partial agonists would require all of the available receptors to produce their full response, and the maximum response for a partial agonist is less than that for a full agonist. The beta blockers acebutolol, penbutolol, and pindolol are partial agonists. Administration can block the effects of adrenergic nerves on heart rate, but partial agonist activity keeps heart rate from falling too low, as might occur following administration of a pure beta-adrenoceptor antagonist. So beta blockers with intrinsic sympathomimetic activity control heart rate within a range that is higher than the response to an antagonist and lower than the response to an agonist.

Disease States and Receptors

Disease states or drug treatment can selectively alter the number of receptors in various tissues throughout the body. For example, hyperthyroidism upregulates, or increases, the number of beta-adrenoceptors, making hyperthyroid patients more likely to have hypertension and a rapid heart rate. Treatment with some agonist drugs can cause the receptors to downregulate, or decrease, in response to receptor stimulation; this can

limit the duration over which the drug can be clinically useful. Treatment with some antagonist drugs can cause receptors to upregulate in response to the decrease in receptor stimulation; this can produce rebound effects if the antagonist is abruptly withdrawn.

Because the maximum response to partial agonists depends on the number of receptors, an increase in receptor number will increase the response of partial agonists.

Non-receptor Mechanisms

Not all drugs act through receptors. General anesthetics, sodium bicarbonate (which neutralizes stomach acid), and chelating agents (which bind to and remove metal ions in the blood) are some examples of drugs whose action is based on their physicochemical properties rather than interaction with receptors.

PHARMACOKINETICS

Pharmacokinetics is the branch of pharmacology dealing with the absorption, distribution through the body, metabolism, and excretion of drugs. Ideally, drugs will enter the body readily, go directly to their site of action, and have a favorable combination of metabolism and excretion that will make it easy to manage patients, even in the presence of kidney or liver disease.

Absorption

Medications produce little clinical effect when they remain inside the prescription bottle. To produce a biological effect, drugs must enter the body. Once inside the body, drugs can interact with various receptor molecules to produce physiological changes that result in clinical effectiveness.

The way in which medications are presented to the body affects the speed, the extent, and the duration of drug absorption. The route of administration also affects patient compliance, that is, their willingness to follow recommendations for taking a medication (Box 2-4). So choosing the route of administration can have important implications for drug therapy, and it is not surprising that a variety of routes of administration can be chosen based on the chemical properties of an individual drug, the condition of an individual patient, and the goal of drug treatment.

There is more to it than just having a medication enter the body. Patients can swallow a poorly formulated dosage

---

BOX 2-4 EFFECTS OF ROUTE OF ADMINISTRATION

- Compliance
- Bioavailability
- Onset of action
- Duration of action

form that travels through the intestines and arrives unchanged in the toilet. There is little biological effect from these "bedpan bullets" if the active medication never reaches its site of action.

Parenteral Administration

Medications may be administered parenterally, or by injection, when immediate effect is required, when the active ingredients are destroyed or not absorbed in the gastrointestinal tract or other routes, or when the patient is unable to take an oral medication. A major limitation of parenteral administration is that it requires needles, syringes, and sterile technique.

Drug absorption is greatest for intravenous (IV) injection. IV preparations use drugs that have been dissolved in aqueous solution and are sterile and ready to enter the bloodstream. Intramuscular or subcutaneous preparations may use drugs suspended in sterile media, which is usually aqueous but occasionally oil-based. When administered by IV injection, all the drug enters the bloodstream immediately. IV administration serves as the standard to which other routes of administration are compared when we consider bioavailability, the percentage of the administered drug that is absorbed. Although there are drawbacks to needles and the need for sterility, IV administration is used for its advantages of rapid or complete absorption and immediate drug action. A major disadvantage of IV administration is that, once administered, the dosage cannot be slowed or removed. IV administration is common for emergency drugs and in the hospital setting.

Oral Administration

Oral administration is the most convenient and common route of administration. In contrast to IV administration, orally administered drugs must go through a number of steps on their way to the bloodstream. Following oral administration, dosages, as tablets, capsules, or liquid, make their way to the stomach and continue to move into and through the small and large intestines on their way to the colon. Tablets or capsules must break apart, and their drug contents must dissolve in stomach acid or intestinal fluid before the drug can be absorbed. This takes time, so orally administered drugs may not act as fast as some other routes of administration. Orally administered drugs must pass through the lining of the intestines to enter the systemic circulation. Once absorbed, orally administered drugs travel to the liver, where they may be metabolized on their way to the bloodstream.

A number of related routes of administration overcome some of the problems encountered with oral dosing. Sublingual administration (under the tongue) and buccal administration (between the cheek and gum, as with chewing tobacco) allow drugs to have a more rapid onset of action and to avoid liver metabolism as they enter the bloodstream. Nitroglycerin sublingual tablets are used to treat chest pain; they can act within a minute or two and can help stop an anginal attack and avoid an emergency room visit. Buccal administration is not very common but is used with methyltestosterone and nicotine preparations.

Some medications are destroyed by stomach acid following oral administration or are absorbed too rapidly to be convenient medications. Enteric-coated formulations protect the medication in the stomach and only disintegrate and dissolve when they reach the gentler conditions of the intestinal tract. Sustained-release preparations allow a drug to dissolve slowly in the intestines so that medication is absorbed over a period of time. It is important not to crush these preparations before administration because that would destroy the formulation and speed absorption.

The use of oral medications may be limited when patients are nauseous, vomiting, or uncooperative. Administration of suppository preparations into the rectum allows drug absorption that is similar to oral administration. While rectal administration is appropriate for some medications and is used for some pediatric medications, it is not universally welcomed by patients.

Site of Administration

Administration of medication close to where it will act has some notable theoretical advantages. When medications are administered near their site of action, higher concentrations may be achieved while minimizing unwanted effects in other parts of the body. Topical administration allows medication to be concentrated in the skin when patients need an anti-inflammatory (e.g., hydrocortisone) or an antifungal (e.g., clotrimazole) medication for a skin condition. This is particularly advantageous in that drugs pass more easily through damaged skin, so more drug is available to the areas of the skin that need the medication. Multidose inhalers and nebulizers are commonly used to administer drugs (e.g., albuterol) directly into the lungs. Ophthalmic preparations are sterile preparations suitable for administration to the eye. Because the eye is particularly sensitive, ocular medications are typically buffered and isotonic so that they do not cause discomfort when administered. Aural preparations, intended for administration into the ear canal, do not meet the buffering and isotonicity requirements for ophthalmic administration.

Bioavailability

Because not all of the administered dosage may be dissolved or absorbed or survive liver passage, only a fraction of an administered dosage makes it to the bloodstream. This percentage of the administered dose that does enter the bloodstream is called the *bioavailability* of the dosage form. Bioavailability can range from less than 10% to more than 90% for oral dosing. When the bioavailability of an oral preparation is low, a higher dose will be given so that the amounts reaching the bloodstream are similar. For example, an oral dose of 500 mg of ciprofloxacin can be substituted for a 400 mg IV dose; ciprofloxacin has about 80% oral bioavailability.

Peak Blood Levels

The speed at which drugs enter the bloodstream affects the maximum blood level that is achieved following drug administration (Fig. 2-8). Rapid absorption leads to higher peak

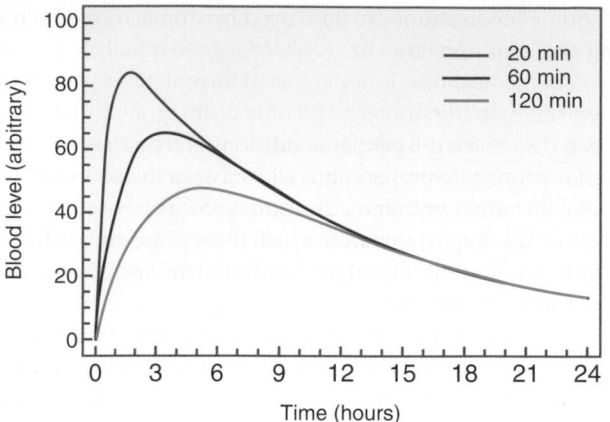

Figure 2–8. Blood levels for the same dose absorbed with peak-times of 20 minutes, 60 minutes, or 120 minutes. Rapid absorption results in faster effect, but blood levels are higher with a greater likelihood of toxicity.

blood levels, with a risk of greater toxicity and side effects. So rapid IV administration (e.g., "IV push") produces immediate drug effects but increases the risk of toxicity and adverse effects. For these reasons, some medications, such as aminoglycoside antibiotics, are administered by slow IV infusion over 30 to 60 minutes. This allows distribution to occur, keeps the blood level from getting too high, and minimizes toxicity.

Distribution

After a drug is absorbed, it still must reach its site of action to produce an effect. The process of drugs moving throughout the body is called *distribution*. Distribution of drugs can occur by transfer through the bloodstream and passive diffusion, or their distribution can be promoted or limited by the presence of transport systems that may selectively transport or exclude drugs based on size, charge, or chemical structure. Diffusion can influence the action of drugs; drugs can be effective only if they reach their site of action in adequate concentrations before they are metabolized.

Properties That Affect Distribution

Drugs can passively diffuse most readily when they are small and uncharged and also have the right balance between water and lipid solubility. Some of these properties will be related to the drug (e.g., molecular size and lipid:water solubility). Others will reflect drug properties as they present in an individual patient, such as pH, the acidity of the environment in which the drug finds itself. pH affects ionization of the drug. Of course, the drug may find itself in an acidic environment (pH ~2) in the stomach and more neutral environments in the intestine (pH 6–8) and blood (pH 7.4). The patient will also bring an environment that includes proteins inside the body to which the drug may bind.

Since passive diffusion represents transfer through partially permeable barriers, smaller molecules are better able to diffuse than larger molecules. Molecules with molecular weights of 500 or less are the best candidates for passive

diffusion. Molecules with molecular weights above 5,000 are expected to diffuse poorly.

Henderson–Hasselbalch Relationship

Acidity is an important property of biological environments. Acidity is measured as pH, defined as $-\log[H^-]$; lower pH is more acidic. Normal pH in the body is around 7.4; under conditions consistent with life, pH can range only about 0.3 units in either direction. Each 1 unit of pH change represents a 10-fold increase or decrease in the concentration of hydrogen ions, and each 0.3 pH unit change represents a 2-fold change in acidity.

Most drugs contain chemical functional groups, such as carboxylic acids and amines, that can exist in a neutral, uncharged form or as a charged form. The balance between the charged and uncharged forms depends on pH. At higher acidity, or lower pH, carboxylic acid groups are uncharged, but amine groups are charged. At low acidity, at higher pH under basic conditions, the amine groups are uncharged, but the carboxylic acid groups are charged. Each drug is unique, and the pH at which it exists half in the charged state and half in the uncharged state is defined as its pKa.

It is an important principle in pharmacology that passive diffusion through biological barriers occurs most readily when drugs are in the uncharged state. Since the pH of body fluids is limited to a relatively narrow range and the pKa is a fixed property for an individual drug, we can calculate the percentage of charged and uncharged molecules for a drug if we know its pKa. The pKa can be an important drug property that influences absorption, distribution, and excretion of the drug.

Passive diffusion is a process by which drugs cross some type of biological barrier, such as a cell membrane or through a layer of cells, based on the concentration difference on the two sides of the barrier. We expect that passive diffusion will proceed until the concentration of drug is equal on both sides, but that is not quite what happens. Instead, passive diffusion proceeds until the concentration of *unionized* drug is the same on both sides. As a result of this, pH differences can cause more drug to accumulate based on the fraction of unionized and ionized molecules. This is called *ion trapping*.

Protein Binding

Drugs passively diffuse and distribute when they are unbound and uncharged. Drugs can bind to a variety of proteins that are present in the bloodstream. These are often called *plasma proteins*. Many plasma proteins are produced in the liver, and their presence in the blood reflects liver function, nutritional status, and the effect of aging and disease. Albumin is a major protein in the blood and is measured as part of a typical blood analysis. Albumin has a molecular weight of 66,500 and is too large to be excreted by the kidneys in healthy patients, although in renal disease albumin is lost in the urine. Other plasma proteins include alpha-1-acid glycoprotein, cortisol-binding globulin, sex hormone–binding globulin, and lipoproteins.

Binding to plasma proteins serves several important functions. Drugs bound to plasma proteins can freely circulate in the bloodstream rather than be distributed by passive diffusion from their site of absorption, so plasma protein binding helps normalize concentrations throughout the body. Drugs that are bound to plasma protein can be protected from metabolism in the liver and from excretion by the kidneys, so plasma protein binding can extend the period of time that drugs remain in the body.

Plasma proteins can be altered by disease states. Patients with poor nutrition may not have the protein building blocks to produce adequate amounts of plasma proteins. Patients with cancer can be undernourished as the cancer cells feed off the body. Patients with liver disease may lack the cellular function to produce one or more of the plasma proteins. Plasma proteins can be affected by myocardial infarction, stress, and infection as well.

Plasma protein binding has advantages and disadvantages. As mentioned above, binding to plasma proteins can protect drugs from metabolism and excretion, extending the time the drugs remain in the body. But remember the general principle that drug action occurs through free, unbound drug. Protein binding, which may include binding to proteins that are not in the plasma, also prevents the interaction of drug molecules with their site of action. Plasma protein binding creates a reservoir of bound drug molecules that can unbind at any time to interact with drug receptors and produce responses.

Plasma protein binding occurs in the plasma and encourages retention of drug in the systemic circulation. So it may appear that blood levels of a drug are high, even if the drug is not at its active site. For example, when patients receiving digoxin, a cardiac glycoside used to slow and strengthen the heart, have clinical signs of toxicity and high blood levels, they can be given antibody fragments to digoxin (Digibind). The antibody fragments remain in the central circulation and bind to digoxin in the bloodstream, essentially pulling digoxin back into the bloodstream from its sites of action throughout the body. But since digoxin is binding to its antibody in the bloodstream, the blood concentration of digoxin rises even though there is much less free digoxin to produce pharmacological effects and toxicity. This illustrates how plasma protein binding holds drugs in the circulation and prevents their distribution to other sites in the body.

Binding to proteins is also the basis for a number of drug interactions. Drugs bound to plasma proteins cannot interact with their receptor. If a drug is very strongly bound to plasma proteins, then even a small change in the fraction that is bound can have significant pharmacological effects. Warfarin is an oral anticoagulant that is used to slow blood clotting in patients at risk for thrombosis. Warfarin is about 98% bound to plasma proteins; this means that only 2% of the drug is unbound and available to produce a pharmacological effect. What if the patient takes another drug that also binds to plasma proteins? If the binding of the second drug to plasma proteins displaces even a small fraction of warfarin, it can have a dramatic effect. If only an additional 2% of warfarin is displaced, for example, it would mean a doubling of circulating warfarin activity.

Transport Systems

Drug distribution is also influenced by transporters, membrane proteins that facilitate the movement of molecules across the cell membranes. Transport systems are often directional, and they can transport drugs into (influx) or out of (efflux) cells. In either case, the transport system can transfer molecules and can create and maintain a concentration difference between two sides of the cell membrane. For example, when some antibiotics diffuse into cancer cells, they are transported out by the multidrug resistance protein (MRP1), which maintains a concentration gradient with the drug outside the cell. The presence of MRP1 suggests that a variety of drugs that require intracellular access for activity will be ineffective because the transporter removes molecules from inside the cell as quickly as they can diffuse in.

Transport systems also form the basis for distribution into protected tissues. p-Glycoprotein, an efflux secretory transporter, is widely distributed and limits the entry of drugs into the brain, testes, intestines, and other sites. Depending on the site, inhibition of p-glycoprotein can result in increased intestinal absorption or distribution into the brain or testes.

Transport systems also affect distribution to sites of metabolism. Transport or diffusion of a drug into cells is required for intracellular metabolism, and transport systems can control how much of a drug is available to an intracellular enzyme for metabolism.

Volume of Distribution

The volume of distribution (V_D) is a hypothetical value that reflects the volume in which a drug would need to be dissolved to explain the relationship between dosage and blood levels. If we administer a dose of 100 mg and the plasma concentration is 2 mg/L, then it appears as though the drug is distributed in 50 liters. If we administer the same dose and the plasma concentration is 20 mg/L, then it appears as though the drug is distributed in a volume of 5 liters (Fig. 2-9).

Volume of distribution is important not only because it relates dosage to blood level but because it tells us something about where a drug might be distributed. Drugs that are confined to the bloodstream will have a volume of distribution equal to the blood volume. The plasma volume is really the smallest volume of distribution we will encounter, since it is not possible for drugs to confine themselves to part of the circulation volume. Plasma makes up about 4.5% of body weight, or about 3 L for an average person. Total body water is about 50% to 60% of body weight (35 to 40 L), depending on gender and body fat. Total body water is about two-thirds intracellular and one-third extracellular.

Volume of distribution is hypothetical, however, so it may also be higher than the amount of volume. For example, a volume of distribution can represent distribution into an amount of water greater than the total body volume; this suggests that much of the drug is bound somewhere outside the bloodstream.

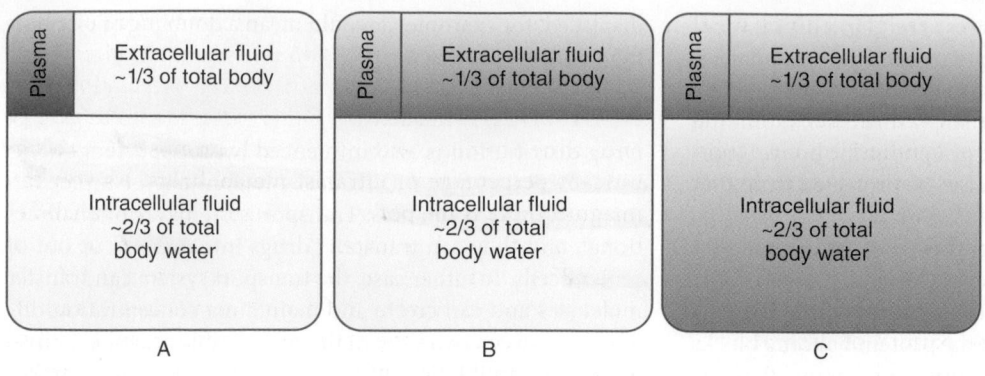

Figure 2–9. Drug concentration in the plasma following administration depends on the volume of distribution. If a drug is confined to plasma (A), then plasma concentration will be higher compared with distribution into extracellular fluid (B) or intracellular fluid (C). Dilution in increasing volumes is shown by shading of the areas containing a drug.

Concentration = amount/volume

Metabolism

Metabolism is an important factor in determining drug activity. When drugs are metabolized, they are chemically altered by enzymes into new molecules, called *metabolites*. Metabolism can increase or decrease the onset, duration of action, and toxicity of a medication. So it is important to know how metabolism affects drug activity and pharmacokinetics and how other drugs might interact to alter drug metabolism.

The body is a large container of enzymes that catalyze many different chemical reactions that are required to maintain life. If you think about it, one of the requirements for sustainable life is the ability to maintain a constant internal environment. All organisms are exposed to molecules that cannot be used for food or energy. If an organism cannot rid itself of a certain molecule, then that molecule can accumulate until it causes some sort of toxicity. Therefore, the human body has developed a series of enzymatic reactions directed at all sorts of molecules encountered during life. Drugs that are lipid soluble or weakly acidic or basic may not readily be excreted from the body. In general, the idea is to make these molecules more water soluble so they can be excreted by the kidneys.

Metabolism is the process of changing one chemical into another, and the process usually either creates or uses energy. Metabolism of drugs can occur in every biological tissue, but it occurs mostly in the smooth endoplasmic reticulum of cells in the liver. The liver is a major organ for drug metabolism because it contains high amounts of drug-metabolizing enzymes and because it is the first organ encountered by drugs once they are absorbed from the gastrointestinal tract. Metabolism by the liver following oral administration is called *first-pass metabolism* and is important in determining whether a drug can be orally administered.

There is a "family" of enzymes, cytochrome P450 (CYP; pronounced *sip*), that metabolizes drugs. Each of these CYP enzymes is responsible for a single type of metabolic reaction. A drug may undergo several of these biological transformations, or biotransformations, sometimes in different body tissues, before being excreted. Understanding drug metabolism through these CYPs can provide a framework for understanding metabolism in individual patients, as well as drug interactions with other medications and with food.

Phase I and Phase II Metabolism

Drug metabolism utilizes two types of reactions that prepare and tag molecules for excretion. Phase I reactions, or *nonsynthetic reactions,* involve oxidation, reduction, and hydrolysis reactions, which prepare the drug molecule for further metabolism. Phase I reactions introduce or unmask polar groups that, in general, improve water solubility and prepare drug molecules for further metabolic reactions. Phase I metabolism can result in metabolites with greater or lesser pharmacological activity. Many phase I metabolites

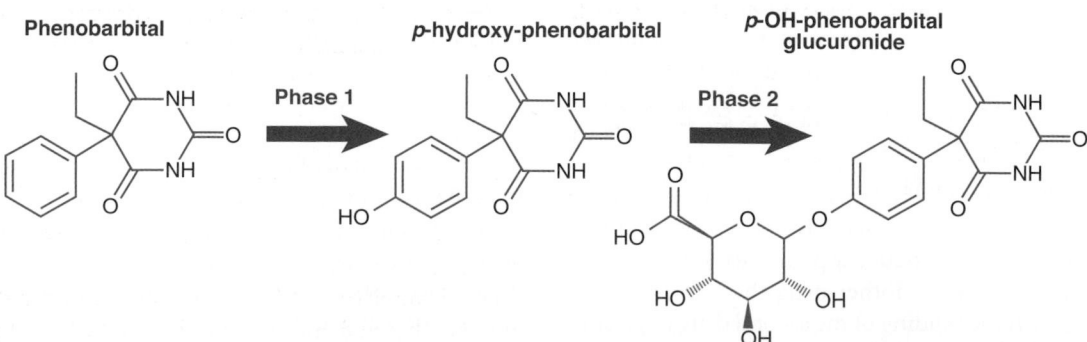

Figure 2–10. Metabolism of phenobarbital. Phase I metabolism adds an –OH to the molecule. A water-soluble glucuronide molecule is linked to this site during phase II metabolism.

are rapidly eliminated, whereas others go on to phase II reactions (Fig. 2-10).

Phase II reactions are called *synthetic* or *conjugation reactions* because drug molecules are metabolized and something is added to the drug to synthesize a new compound. Metabolites are linked, or conjugated, to highly polar molecules such as glucuronic acid, glycine, sulfate, or acetate by specific enzymes. Conjugation to these molecules makes metabolites more water soluble and more easily excreted by the kidneys. So the presence or activity of these enzymes can influence the pattern of drug activity and the duration of action for drugs.

Cytochrome P450

The most thoroughly studied drug metabolism reaction is the CYP P450 mixed-function oxidase reaction. This reaction catalyzes the metabolism of a large number of diverse drugs and chemicals that are highly lipid soluble. CYP transfers electrons from the oxidation of drugs to the electron transport system of the endoplasmic reticulum, a cell organelle. There are many forms of CYP that are products of separate and distinct genes and that catalyze different reactions. Over 50 human CYPs have been isolated so far. The CYPs are organized into numbered families based on their function. For example, the CYP1, CYP2, and CYP3 families metabolize a variety of drugs and steroids (Box 2-5). Subfamilies are designated by additional letters and individual enzymes by numbers. The CYP3As are the major subfamily expressed in the human liver and consist of three forms: CYP3A4, CYP3A5, and CYP3A7. The CYP3A7 enzyme is present in the fetus and appears to be discontinued after birth. CYP3A4 is a major drug-metabolizing enzyme, whereas CYP3A5 metabolizes the same drugs but is less active.

Single nucleotide polymorphisms (SNPs) are minor mutations in proteins that can result in metabolic activity changes. These alterations in DNA are sometimes associated with population groups and help explain why certain groups of patients are more or less sensitive to certain drugs. When SNP variations exist in the individual CYP enzyme, they are named by an asterisk and a number showing the order in which each SNP was identified. For example, there are several CYP2D6 isoforms: CYP2D6*1 (with no mutation), CYP2D6*3, CYP2D6*4, and up to CYP2D6*17. Metabolic activity for each isoform may be decreased, normal, or increased.

We inherit our drug-metabolizing enzymes from our parents, so it is possible to have two isoforms that differ in expression and activity. About 7% of the U.S. population lacks the CYP2D6 enzyme activity. Other patients exhibit a range of enzyme activities, with some ethnic groups having a significant percentage of ultrafast metabolizers. As you can imagine, there is the potential for a good deal of variability between individual patients.

CYP3A4 is a prominent enzyme that is responsible for metabolism of a number of drugs. It serves as an example of a CYP enzyme. Drugs that are metabolized by CYP3A4 include azole antifungals; the statin drugs that inhibit HMG-CoA (5-hydroxy-3-methylglutaryl-coenzyme A) reductase and lower cholesterol; the corticosteroids prednisone, prednisolone, and dexamethasone; the anticonvulsant carbamazepine; and many other drugs. Note the variety of drug classes and chemical structures that are metabolized by this enzyme.

Variations in CYPs and in their activity can result in marked differences in drug metabolism between individuals. Individual variation in drug metabolism contributes to drug–drug and some drug–food interactions. Enzyme induction occurs when drug treatment results in an increase in enzyme activity, usually limited to the enzymes responsible for metabolizing the drug. Enzyme induction results in an increase in metabolism that decreases the amount of drug and increases the amount of metabolite in the body.

Competition occurs when two different drugs are metabolized by the same enzyme. Often the enzyme can metabolize both drugs, but sometimes one drug will be preferentially metabolized, delaying the metabolism and extending the half-life of the competing drug.

Metabolism and Half-Life

The rate of drug metabolism depends on the blood levels of drug in relation to the affinity of the drug for its metabolism enzymes. Most drugs are present at concentrations below their K_m for metabolism (the concentration at which metabolism is half of maximum). Under these conditions, metabolism is related to drug concentration so that a fixed *fraction* of drug is metabolized per hour. This is called *first-order metabolism* and is characterized by a half-life, the time period over which the drug concentration will decrease by half. So, blood levels decrease 50% in one half-life, 75% in two half-lives, and 87.5% in three half-lives. As a general rule, drugs tend to be administered at dosing intervals that are close to their half-life.

Some drugs—ethanol is the prototype—are present at concentrations well above their K_m for metabolism. When this happens, enzymes act near to their maximal metabolic capacity and metabolize a constant *amount* of drug each hour. This is called *zero-order metabolism*.

Rarely but importantly, some drugs are present at blood concentrations that range from below to above the K_m for their metabolism. At lower doses or concentrations, they are metabolized like typical drugs, but at higher doses or concentrations their metabolism is limited. Phenytoin is a prototypical example of a drug with "mixed-order" or

---

BOX 2–5 DRUG-METABOLIZING ENZYMES (LISTED IN ORDER OF IMPORTANCE)

CYP3A
CYP2C
CYP1A
CYP2E
CYP2D

Michelis–Menten, pharmacokinetics. Above a certain level of phenytoin dosing (about 300 mg/day in adults), dosage must be adjusted by small amounts, which can produce disproportional increases in blood levels as metabolism changes from first order to zero order.

Patterns of Metabolism

It is important to remember that metabolism can change the pharmacological activity of drugs. We typically consider that drugs are pharmacologically active and that metabolism decreases the activity and promotes excretion (Fig. 2-11), so we expect to see inactive metabolites that have short half-lives and are rapidly excreted. This is not always the case, however.

Prodrugs are inactive compounds that rely on metabolism to become active. Prodrugs have advantages and disadvantages. The advantages may be in terms of their absorption or distribution. L-DOPA is a prodrug used to treat Parkinson's disease. The problem in Parkinson's disease is a lack of dopamine in the striatum of the brain. Dopamine, however, cannot pass through the blood–brain barrier, so it cannot be used to treat the neurotransmitter shortage in the brain. L-DOPA can pass into the brain and enter into cells, where it can be converted into dopamine.

Prodrugs can also have disadvantages. Terfenadine was one of the first nonsedating antihistamines and was quite popular at one time. First-pass metabolism by CYP3A4 biotransforms terfenadine, which is cardiotoxic, into fexofenadine, an effective antihistamine. When it was realized that inhibition of CYP3A4 could result in toxicity and death in some patients, terfenadine was withdrawn and replaced with fexofenadine, its active metabolite.

The prodrug terfenadine is cardiotoxic and relies on metabolism to produce more active antihistamine that is less cardiotoxic. Other prodrugs are pharmacologically inactive and rely on biotransformation to an active metabolite. Codeine is metabolized to the 12 times more potent opioid morphine by CYP2D6. Hydrocodone is metabolized to the more potent opioid hydromorphone by CYP2D6 as well. About 7% of the Caucasian population lack CYP2D6 activity. Administration of a prodrug requiring metabolism by CYP2D6 creates a situation in which the patient is receiving an inactive or poorly active drug. In the case of pain relievers, patients may be seeking stronger drugs, not because of abuse but because the drugs are not being biotransformed into their active metabolites. In contrast, patients with highly active CYP2D6 are at greater risk for toxicity following administration of codeine or hydrocodone.

Meperidine is an opioid analgesic that is used parenterally and orally to treat pain as well as post-operative shivering. It is metabolized by CYP2B6, 2C19, and 3A4. Meperidine remains present in the body a relatively short period of time; its half-life is 3 to 4 hours. Meperidine's metabolite, normeperidine, is more toxic and remains in the body for a much longer period of time; its half-life is 14 to 21 hours in patients with normal renal function and even longer in those with poor kidney function. This difference in half-lives creates a clinical situation in which meperidine is administered frequently and levels of normeperidine will rise until toxicity presents as irritability, tremors, delirium, and seizures in patients with poor renal function. The solution is to limit administration of meperidine so that normeperidine does not accumulate and to avoid meperidine use in at-risk patients.

Drug Interactions

Alterations in biotransformation are responsible for many drug–drug and drug–food interactions. There are a limited number of drug-metabolizing enzymes, and these enzymes can metabolize only one drug molecule at a time. Compounds compete for enzymes based on their chemical affinity; chemicals with higher affinity for a particular CYP or drug metabolism enzyme will be preferentially metabolized. So a drug that can be metabolized by multiple enzymes will be biotransformed by each enzyme in proportion to the affinity. When several drugs are metabolized by a single enzyme, each of the drugs will be metabolized in proportion to the affinity of each of the drug–enzyme interactions. If one drug monopolizes the enzyme, then it can block the biotransformation of other drugs, extending their time in the body and contributing to toxicity. So when we look for drug interactions, we often look for drugs that are metabolized by the same CYPs.

CYP3A4 is particularly problematic because it metabolizes so many different drugs. Consequently, there is a greater likelihood of interference with metabolism when a patient receives a number of drugs. In addition to other sites in the body, such as the liver, CYP3A4 activity is present in the cells lining the gastrointestinal tract and can be influenced by food as well as drugs. Grapefruit juice contains a substance that inhibits CYP3A4 and can sometimes markedly increase blood levels of drug in patients consuming grapefruit juice. Surprisingly, this interaction extends to patients consuming grapefruit juice within about a day prior to drug administration. This interaction can affect a number of drugs, such as

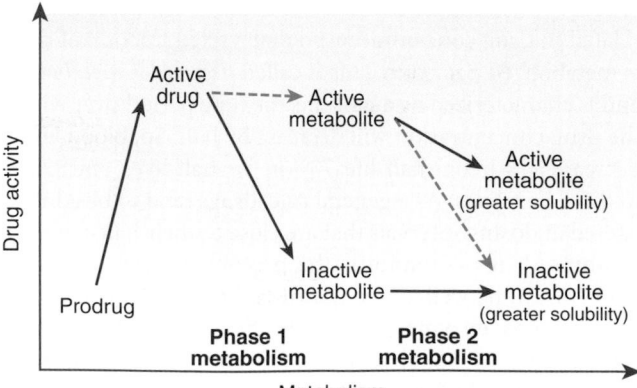

Figure 2–11. Typical effect of metabolism (solid arrows) on drug activity. Prodrugs are metabolized to active drugs that can undergo phase I and phase II metabolism, with metabolites varying in activity, compared with the parent drug, and in solubility, which increases the likelihood of renal elimination. Sometimes metabolism produces unusual effects (dashed arrows), such as drug metabolites that retain drug activity or accumulate in the body.

several older statin drugs that have increased blood levels in the presence of grapefruit juice. Higher blood levels are not always bad, but it is appropriate to counsel patients to avoid potential toxicity resulting from CYP3A4 interactions and inhibition.

Some drugs increase the expression of drug-metabolizing enzymes; this is called *enzyme induction*. Induction can be due to either increased enzyme synthesis or decreased enzyme degradation. Pharmacotherapy with phenobarbital, for example, effectively induces CYP1A2, CYP2A6, CYP2B6, CYP2C8, CYP2C9, and CYP3A4. Induction increases the biotransformation of drugs and can encourage variations in metabolism and generally increase the removal of drugs by metabolism.

In clinical practice, transport systems and metabolic enzymes work together in the biotransformation of drugs. Drugs are transported into cells where they can be metabolized. Patients can have genetic differences in their ability to transport drugs through cell membranes, leading to additional variation in metabolism and drug response.

We generally assume that metabolism of drugs results in a product that has less pharmacological activity and is more likely to leave the body. Metabolism, or biotransformation, can actually result in either an inactive or an active metabolite. Metabolites are generally excreted more rapidly, but sometimes metabolite excretion is delayed. Drugs may interact with more than one CYP enzyme to produce multiple metabolites with different levels of activity and excretion.

Excretion

Excretion is the process in which drugs are transferred from inside the body to outside the body. This makes excretion or elimination the opposite of absorption. Just as drugs pass a biological boundary between inside and outside for absorption, so they must pass in the opposite direction, though not necessarily in the same location, for elimination.

The locations at which drugs can pass from inside the body to outside include some sites that are familiar as sites of absorption, such as lung, skin, and intestines. There are also some unique sites where drugs are excreted but not absorbed. These include the kidney and the gallbladder. The principal organs for drug elimination are considered to be the kidneys, lung, biliary system, and intestines. Any individual drug may rely on one or more of these sites for elimination or on a different site, such as skin excretion or excretion into saliva or breast milk.

Renal Excretion

The kidney is the primary organ of excretion for most drugs. The general theme of metabolism is to produce drug metabolites that are more water soluble and more easily removed by the kidneys. The kidney can then remove these substances from the plasma and excrete them in the urine.

The kidney is a complex organ with several important functions, including excretion of waste products and maintenance of fluid and electrolyte balance in the body. The

strategy of the kidney is to allow removal of a large volume of plasma and then to take back the substances that the body needs. The result is urine. There are also transport mechanisms that can secrete substances into the urine. We will consider how drugs manage to end up in the urine.

Production of urine begins in the glomerulus of the kidney. The operational unit of the kidney is the nephron, and each of the approximately 1 million nephrons begins with a glomerulus (Fig. 2-12). The glomerulus is a specialized area of the nephron adapted for ultrafiltration, a process in which substances in the plasma pass through small holes, or pores, in the glomerular capillary membrane based on their size and charge. The structure of the glomerular capillary membrane permits filtration of smaller molecules while restricting the passage of compounds with larger molecular weights. As blood flows through the kidney and encounters the glomerulus, much of the fluid portion of the blood is filtered into the lumen, or center, of the nephron. The kidney is exceptionally efficient at what it does. Approximately 125 mL of blood flows through the glomeruli in the kidneys per minute, the glomerular filtration rate (GFR), and it is an important measure of renal function.

Glomerular filtration is the first step toward production of urine containing excreted drug. Filtration preserves plasma proteins while removing free drugs and other waste products from the plasma. The large volume of fluid filtered through the glomerulus is an ideal vehicle for drug removal. As the ultrafiltrate is formed, drugs that are free in the plasma and not bound to plasma proteins or blood cells are filtered. Filtration may be slower for drugs that are large because of the size of the pores through which filtration occurs; very large drugs may not be filtered at all. The pores of the glomerulus contain a fixed negative charge, so filtration may also be affected by drug charge.

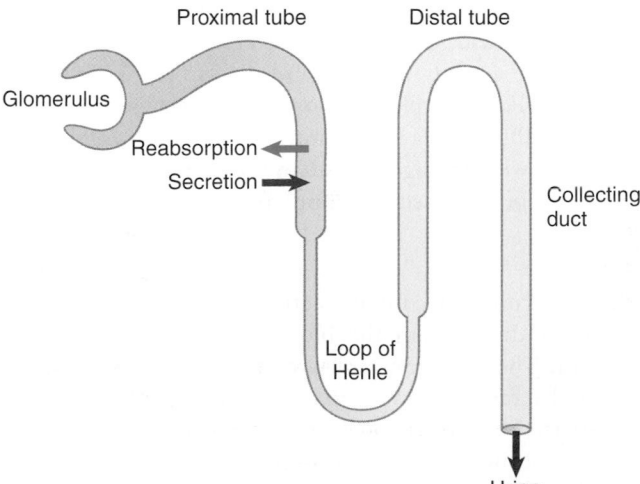

Figure 2–12. Diagram of the nephron, the functional unit of the kidney. Blood vessels flowing into the glomerulus provide blood, which is filtered into the lumen, the inner opening of the nephron. As fluid passes along the nephron, transporters can either reabsorb drugs (dark arrow) back into the blood or secrete (light arrow) drugs from blood into the lumen.

The glomerular filtrate in the nephron contains a variety of smaller molecules, including excreted drug and metabolites. As the filtrate moves through the lumen of the nephron, molecules are reabsorbed from the lumen into the blood. The extent to which a drug diffuses back across the nephron to reenter the circulation is one of the factors that determine urinary excretion of drug. The passive diffusion of substances back into the circulation is encouraged by the reabsorption of water that occurs along most of the nephron, creating a concentration gradient promoting reabsorption if the lipid solubility and ionization of the drug are appropriate.

The unionized or uncharged form of the drug will diffuse more readily, and the acidity of urine can influence the ionization and reabsorption of drugs. Acidification of the urine creates a situation that favors the excretion of basic drugs and metabolites, whereas basic urine encourages the excretion of acidic drugs and metabolites. Effects of urine acidity on drug elimination can have important clinical implications. Urine can be made acidic by administration of ammonium chloride and can be made basic by administration of sodium bicarbonate.

Tubular Reabsorption

In addition to reabsorption by passive diffusion, some substances filtered at the glomerulus are reabsorbed by active transport systems located primarily in the proximal tubule of the nephron. Active transport is important for endogenous substances that the body needs to recover from the glomerular filtrate, such as ions, amino acids, and glucose. The active transport systems are located on the luminal cell surface and transport substances into the cell, where they are passively transported into the plasma.

A small number of drugs may be actively reabsorbed. It is more common that drugs acting on tubular secretion do so by inhibiting active transport. Uricosuric agents such as probenecid and sulfinpyrazone inhibit the active reabsorption of uric acid. Substances that are actively reabsorbed can also be actively secreted and drugs may inhibit both processes. For example, low doses of salicylates, such as aspirin, inhibit tubular secretion and decrease total urate excretion, whereas higher doses inhibit tubular reabsorption and result in increased excretion of uric acid.

Tubular Secretion

The nephron also contains active secretory systems that transport drugs from the blood into the lumen of the nephron. There is a transport system that secretes organic anions and a transport system that secretes organic cations. The transporters are present on the plasma side of the tubular cells of the nephron, where they actively pump anions or cations into the cell. The substances then pass into the lumen by passive transport. The secretory capacity of these transporters can be saturated so that less drug is excreted at high drug concentrations. When two drugs are substrates for the same transporter, they compete with one another and decrease the rate at which each is excreted.

Active secretory systems for anions and cations are important because charged anions and cations are often strongly bound to plasma proteins and may not be readily excreted by glomerular filtration. Tubular secretion often contributes to the renal elimination of drugs that have short half-lives. Hydrochlorothiazide, furosemide, penicillin G, and salicylates are among the substrates for the organic anion transport system. The organic cation transport system actively secretes atropine, cimetidine, morphine, and quinine.

Renal Excretion of Drugs

The rate at which a drug is excreted by the kidneys depends on several factors. Renal blood flow influences the GFR, which is how much plasma is filtered per minute by the glomerulus. Filtration in the glomerulus depends on the molecular size, the charge, and the degree of protein binding, each of which influences how much drug passes through the glomerular basement membrane. Tubular acidity will influence the degree of reabsorption. Active reabsorption or active secretion into the urine may also influence excretion rate.

Renal excretion of drugs is typically well characterized. What is variable, however, is the level of renal function in an individual patient receiving a renally excreted medication. It is common to monitor renal function of patients in the clinical setting and to adjust dosages based on renal function and the renal contribution to drug excretion. Renal function is typically assessed from patient serum creatinine along with height, weight, age, and gender.

Biliary Excretion

In addition to metabolizing many drugs, the liver secretes about a liter of bile each day. Drugs can enter the bile and be excreted into the intestinal tract when bile is released to help digest food. Only small amounts of drug enter the bile by diffusion; instead, biliary excretion contributes to removal of some drugs. The biliary system includes three types of active transport. Organic cation and organic anion transporters are similar to those found in the renal tubules. The additional system is the bile acid transport system. Conjugated metabolites of drugs generally have enhanced biliary excretion. Cardiac glycosides, such as digoxin, are an example of drugs secreted into the bile.

Some drugs that are excreted in bile can be reabsorbed in the intestine. This creates a phenomenon called *enterohepatic cycling,* in which drug is excreted in the bile, absorbed from the intestines, and then excreted in the bile again. Enterohepatic cycling decreases the amount of drug that is actually excreted and extends the time that a drug remains in the body.

Other Sites of Excretion

Drug excretion is not limited to the kidneys and liver. Drugs can diffuse out of the body at various sites, and while these excretion sites are typically not major, they can be important for forensic or clinical reasons.

Pulmonary excretion can occur for any volatile material present in the body. Pulmonary excretion is important for anesthetic gases, such as nitrous oxide. Pulmonary excretion is also important following alcohol consumption. Ethanol distributes throughout the body and is readily excreted each time we breathe. Because the amount of ethanol exhaled in each breath is proportional to blood level, the Breathalyzer can be used to estimate blood levels of ethanol. Pulmonary excretion is also important for volatile ketones, which are produced in diabetic patients who are poorly controlled; the smell of ketones on a patient's breath can be an important clue that the patient may have diabetes and be at risk for diabetic ketoacidosis.

Substances can be excreted through the skin, although this is often a minor route of elimination. The skin has a large surface area through which excretion can occur; drugs may be incorporated into the hair and can be excreted through the sweat glands. Excretion of drugs into sweat and saliva is of minor importance for most drugs and depends on the diffusion of uncharged drug across the epithelial cells of sweat and salivary glands. Excretion into hair, sweat, and saliva is quantitatively unimportant but can be used to noninvasively detect drugs in the body. Interestingly, some drugs excreted into saliva can produce changes in taste. Excretion into saliva might help explain part of the pharmacological action of certain drugs, such as antibiotic erythromycin, in throat infections.

Drugs can also be excreted into the breast milk of nursing mothers. The concentration in the breast milk depends on drug properties such as lipid solubility and the degree of ionization and on patient properties such as the extent of active secretion into breast milk and the blood level of the drug in the mother. Low-molecular-weight drugs that are unionized can passively diffuse across the epithelial cells of the mammary gland and enter the breast milk. Because breast milk is more acidic than plasma, it tends to accumulate basic drugs.

Infants can be exposed to drugs through breast milk. The risk to the infant from drug exposure in breast milk depends on the amount and type of drug involved and the ability of the infant to metabolize the drug. Breastfeeding is discouraged when there is a potential for drug toxicity in the infant.

SUMMARY

The rational use of drugs is based on a foundation of chemical and physiological principles. Drugs interact with specific sites, called receptors, according to chemical laws; higher concentrations of drug produce more interactions and greater effects. How rapidly a drug is absorbed, distributed, metabolized, and excreted dictates local concentrations of drug that produce effects. The onset and duration of a drug effect reflect the pharmacokinetics of the drug and the properties of the receptor. Sound therapeutic decisions draw upon the unifying foundational principles of pharmacology.

REFERENCES

Burton, L., Lazo, J., & Parker, K. (2005). *Goodman & Gilman: The pharmacological basis of therapeutics* (11th ed.). New York: McGraw-Hill.

Kenakin, T. P. (2005, October). New bull's-eyes for drugs. *Scientific American, 293*(4), 50–57.

Rice, P. J. (2014). *Understanding drug action: An introduction to pharmacology.* Washington, DC: American Pharmacists Association.

CHAPTER 3

RATIONAL DRUG SELECTION

Teri Moser Woo

The process of prescribing medication requires a thoughtful, evidence-based approach to drug selection. The World Health Organization (WHO) definition of rational drug selection is that "patients receive medications appropriate to their clinical needs, in doses that meet their own individual requirements, for an adequate period of time, and at the lowest cost to them and their community" (WHO, 2013). WHO states that irrational use of medication is a "major problem" worldwide, with an estimated 50% of drugs prescribed, dispensed, or sold inappropriately (2013). Examples of irrational medication use outlined by the WHO include: polypharmacy, inappropriate prescribing of antimicrobials, overuse of injections versus oral preparations, and failure to follow guidelines when prescribing (2013). This chapter discusses the process of rational drug selection and the drug factors that influence drug selection as well as influences on rational prescribing.

THE PROCESS OF RATIONAL DRUG PRESCRIBING

Thoughtful prescribing requires a systematic process that is used every time a prescription is written. The WHO model for rational drug prescribing is one approach a provider can use (de Vries, Henning, Hogerzeil, & Fresle, 1994). The first step in the WHO process is an accurate diagnosis and a determination of the therapeutic objective, for example, treating an infection. The appropriate treatment is chosen with these factors in mind. It is critical that the provider collaborates with and educates the patient regarding the therapy. The chosen therapy then needs to be monitored to determine the effectiveness of the regimen (Box 3-1).

Define the Patient's Problem

The process of prescribing begins with the assessment of the patient and formulation of a working diagnosis and possible differential diagnosis. Early screening of high-risk patients maximizes the benefits of pharmacological treatment (WHO, 2012). Once the diagnosis is made the provider develops a plan of care. Is there a clear indication for drug therapy? What drugs are effective in treating this disorder? Differential diagnosis is not within the scope of this book, but the reader will find the diagnostic criteria and pathophysiology of common diseases treated with medications discussed in the chapters in Unit III.

Specify the Therapeutic Objective

Before deciding what medication to prescribe, it is important to clarify the therapeutic objective (de Vries et al, 1994). Is the goal to cure the disease? Relieve symptoms of disease? Replace deficiencies (i.e., insulin or iron)? Long-term prevention? Or is the goal treating the combination of two outcomes such as treating pain and inflammation. Sometimes the goal is to make the patient comfortable with palliative therapy. Maxwell suggests that the provider clarify whether the treatment goals are curative, symptom relieving, or preventive (2009). The WHO model recommends that the provider include the patient in this stage of the process so the patient is a partner in the treatment regimen (de Vries et al, 1994). Eliciting patient beliefs and preferences regarding the drug therapy is essential to successful drug therapy, especially in chronic diseases, such as diabetes, that require long-term drug treatment (Latter et al, 2010). When the goal is long-term therapy for a chronic disease, it is necessary to look at costs and how well the drug fits into the patient's lifestyle.

Choose the Treatment

Determining the drug treatment is actually a two-step process of first determining what would be the appropriate therapy based on evidence-based guidelines, then individualizing the drug choice for the specific patient (Richir, Tichelaar, Geijtemann, & de Vries, 2007). Individualizing the drug choice includes consideration of other drugs that the patient may be taking and potential interactions with the drug treatment choice being made. Richir and colleagues (2007) describe two types of reasoning used when choosing drug therapy: analytical and nonanalytical. Novice providers use an analytical approach, which is slow, time-consuming, systematic, and evidence-based. More experienced providers use their experience and pattern recognition to carry out a nonanalytical process in a faster, subconscious manner (Richir et al, 2007). When experienced

providers are confronted with a complex patient situation, they will use a more analytical, systematic approach to prescribing. Bissessur et al (2009) propose a model of therapeutic reasoning that incorporates these analytical or nonanalytical processes used to develop a course of treatment (Fig. 3.1).

Individualizing drug therapy requires examining the suitability of the drug for the patient. WHO recommends that the provider examine the drug and the dose, the dosage schedule, duration of treatment, effectiveness, and safety (de Vries et al, 1994). The criteria for examining a drug for appropriate prescribing are discussed later in this chapter. A mnemonic that new prescribers can use when learning to prescribe is proposed by Iglar, Kennie, and Bajcar (2007) and is summarized in Box 3-2. Table 3-1 provides an example of the use of the mnemonic.

Start the Treatment

Once the appropriate drug has been chosen, a prescription is written, and the patient must have the prescription dispensed at a pharmacy. The legal requirements for writing a prescription are discussed in Chapter 4.

Care should be taken when writing a prescription to make sure that the drug, dose, and schedule are accurate. At the time of writing the prescription, drug costs need to be

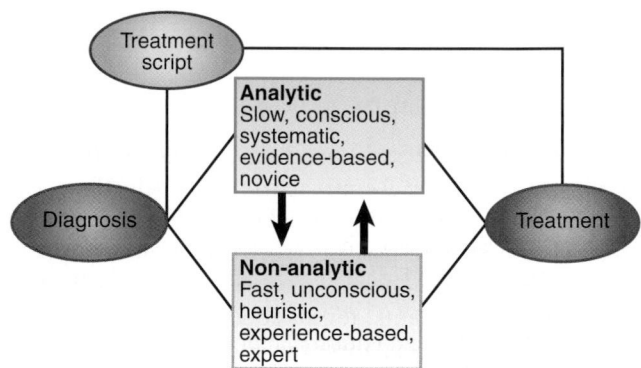

Figure 3–1. Hypothetical model of therapeutic reasoning. *Bissessur et al, 2009.*

Table 3–1   Example of the Use of the 'I Can PresCribE a Drug' Mnemonic

Case: A 23-yr-old female presents to the clinic with symptoms of a urinary tract infection (UTI). Urine analysis confirms initial diagnosis of UTI and a urine culture is pending.

Indication	Antibiotics are indicated in UTI treatment. Treatment guidelines for UTIs are found in Chapter 47. Sulfamethoxazole and trimethoprim (SMZ-TMP, Septra, Bactrim) is the recommended first-line drug in most patients.
Contraindications	SMZ-TMP is contraindicated in patients who are allergic or who have allergies to drugs with known cross-sensitivity to sulfa drugs (discussed in Chapter 24), porphyria, megaloblastic anemia due to folate deficiency.
Precautions	SMZ-TMP is Pregnancy Category C. Use cautiously in patients with G-6-PD deficiency, impaired renal function, or hepatic function. Potential drug–drug interactions should be evaluated.
Cost/Compliance	SMZ-TMP is on the $4 list of many retail pharmacies. It is dosed twice a day for 3 d for UTI. Fewer doses and shorter treatment length have higher compliance.
Efficacy	*E. coli* is the most common pathogen in UTI and is usually sensitive to SMZ-TMP. Culture results will need to be followed to determine sensitivity.
Adverse effects	Adverse effects of SMZ-TMP are discussed in Chapter 24.
Dose/**D**uration/**D**irection	Dose: 1 double-strength tablet twice a day. Duration: 3 d Direction: Drink plenty of fluids while taking SMZ-TMP.

addressed with the patient. If patients cannot afford to fill the prescription, they will not take the medication, regardless of how appropriate the drug is for the disease process. The pharmacoeconomic aspects of prescribing are discussed in depth in Chapter 12.

Educate the Patient

Up to 50% of patients do not take their medications as prescribed or they do not take them at all (Cohen, 2012). Poor medication adherence leads to worsening disease and death, as well as increased health-care costs; 33% to 69% of medication-related hospital admissions are related to poor adherence, at a cost of $100 billion per year (Osterberg & Blaschke, 2005). Patient education regarding the purpose of the medication, instructions for administration, and potential adverse drug effects will improve adherence to the medication regimen. Patient education should be tailored to the patient and presented in plain language (fifth- or sixth-grade reading level), with an understanding that nine out of 10 adults have difficulty reading health information (Centers for Disease Control and Prevention [CDC], 2013). Appropriate patient education is discussed for each drug category in the chapters in Unit II.

Monitor Effectiveness

Once the patient begins taking the prescribed medication, the chosen drug needs to be monitored for effectiveness. The WHO model describes two types of monitoring: passive and active (de Vries et al, 1994). Passive monitoring occurs when the patient is educated on the expected outcome of the drug therapy and is instructed to contact the provider if the treatment is not effective or if adverse

drug effects occur. This is common when short-term treatment, such as an antibiotic, is prescribed, and no test of cure is required. Active monitoring occurs when the provider schedules a follow-up examination to determine the effectiveness of the drug therapy (de Vries et al, 1994). Active monitoring may include evaluating therapeutic blood levels and making dosage adjustments, as is necessary in anticoagulant therapy or patients taking an antiseizure medication. Active monitoring may also include adding or subtracting medications from the treatment regimen based on the effectiveness of the treatment. Monitoring parameters are often published for a drug but may need to be adjusted based on age or concurrent disease processes.

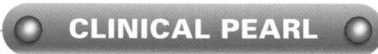
CLINICAL PEARL

Drugs don't work in patients who don't take them.
—C. Everett Koop, MD

At the follow-up visit, the provider will determine whether to continue the medication. If the treatment has been effective and the disease has been cured, the drug can be stopped. The treatment can also be effective but not curative, as in the case of chronic disease management. If the drug is working well for the patient, then it should be continued. If the medication is not effective or if the patient experiences significant adverse effects, the drug may need to be changed. Even an appropriately chosen medication will not work in every patient; therefore, evaluating the effectiveness of therapy and making adjustments as needed are essential.

DRUG FACTORS INFLUENCING DRUG SELECTION

Evidence-based guidelines are the gold standard for initial drug selection, but providers need to examine the drugs recommended in the guideline for their clinical utility with the individual patient. Selecting the appropriate drug treatment requires that the provider consider multiple factors regarding the drug and the patient who will be receiving the medication: pharmacokinetics, pharmacodynamics, therapeutic issues, safety, and cost (Spector & Vesell, 2002). Additionally, individual patient and provider factors may influence drug choice. The nurse practitioner should review and consider all seven of these criteria prior to prescribing (Spector & Vesell, 2002).

Pharmacodynamic Factors

The pharmacodynamics of a drug must be specific and selective to the target tissues affected by the disease to have the greatest therapeutic effect with the least adverse effects (Spector & Vesell, 2002). The ease of titration is influenced by the dose–response curve of the drug (Maxwell, 2009). The relationship between a drug's desired therapeutic effects and its adverse effects is called its *therapeutic index* (see Chap. 2). Drugs with a low or narrow therapeutic index may require close monitoring for toxicity or adverse effects, whereas drugs with a wide therapeutic index are fairly safe and require less monitoring. Antibiotics, for example, tend to have fairly wide therapeutic indices. Propranolol (Inderal) has such a wide therapeutic index that doses safely range from 20 mg to 320 mg.

Pharmacokinetic Factors

When deciding what drug in a class to prescribe, the pharmacokinetic properties of a drug may influence drug selection. For example, the bioavailability (BA) of different formulations may influence prescribing (Maxwell, 2009). The bioavailability of digoxin, for instance, varies between 60% and 100% depending on the formulation used. Because this drug has a very narrow therapeutic index, this difference in BA is critical in formulation choice. Another consideration is metabolism. Different drugs in a class may use different cytochrome P450 (CYP450) enzymes, which may influence metabolism or drug interactions. Drugs that are excreted almost exclusively by the kidney may not be appropriate for a patient with decreased renal function, such as the older adult. Therefore, a patient's renal function and the pharmacokinetics of the drug need to be evaluated during the drug selection process. Additionally, the dose–concentration curve and half-life will determine the dosing schedule, with fewer doses per day encouraging adherence to the drug regimen (Maxwell, 2009; Spector & Vesell, 2002). Pharmacokinetics are discussed in depth in Chapter 2.

Therapeutic Factors

The therapeutic impact of a drug is reviewed in the literature and observed in the individual patient. A nurse practitioner examines the evidence for the therapeutic impact of a selected drug, using evidence from clinical trials, clinical practice guidelines, and systematic reviews (including *Cochrane Reviews* or *Clinical Evidence Reviews*) to determine the impact of a drug. The effect of a drug on decreasing morbidity, mortality, and hospitalization is examined (Spector & Vesell, 2002) as well as the drug's ability to relieve symptoms and treat the disease process (Maxwell, 2009). Extrapolating results from randomized controlled trials (RCTs) should be done with caution because RCTs usually recruit patients who are relatively healthy with few comorbidities, whereas most patients are more complex (Maxwell, 2009).

Safety

The safety profile of a drug is taken into consideration and weighed against other factors when prescribing. Safety is initially determined in clinical trials and is outlined in the precautions and contraindications in the drug monograph. Safety may vary with the population. For example, a drug may be safe in a healthy elder but also be a teratogen; thus, it would be unsafe in pregnant women (Iglar et al, 2007). Safety may also vary with the disease process; for example, some drugs pose safety concerns in patients with liver or renal dysfunction. Contraindications to a drug in a specific patient population or allergy to the drug eliminate it from the potential drugs that can be prescribed for the patient.

The U.S. Food and Drug Administration (FDA) collects information on and monitors the safety of drugs via postmarketing surveillance by the MedWatch program (http://www.fda.gov/Safety/Medwatch). The FDA has a tiered system of safety announcements to promote drug safety. The agency gathers initial reports via MedWatch, then it issues an early communication about an "Ongoing Safety Review" while it collects and analyzes data (http://www.fda.gov). The FDA issues a "Public Health Advisory" when there is drug safety information that needs to be conveyed to patients or caregivers. When new drug information affects safe prescribing, the FDA may issue a "Letter to Health Care Professionals" or an "Information for Health Care Professionals" information sheet to provide specifics about the safety issue and factors to consider when making treatment decisions. When drugs are determined by the FDA to have serious safety issues, particularly ones that may lead to serious injury or death, the FDA may require a warning to be displayed prominently on the drug monograph, often referred to as a "Black Box" warning. Prescribers are responsible for keeping up-to-date on the latest drug safety information.

Cost

When prescribing, the nurse practitioner must consider the costs to the patient and the cost to the health-care system or to society at large. The cost to patients may be so high that they cannot afford prescriptions, and cost then becomes a barrier to adherence. Many insurance policies do not cover the cost of drugs, and patients must therefore pay out of pocket for their medications. Medicare patients with Part D coverage may reach the "donut hole," the coverage gap in drug costs where the proportion of out-of-pocket costs goes up to 50%. This coverage gap will slowly be decreased to 25% for generic drugs by 2020, but Medicare patients will still pay 50% of brand-name drug costs while in the coverage gap.

Increasingly, as soon as the patent on a brand-name drug expires, that drug may be made in a generic form. Prescribing generics when possible and knowing what drugs are on the $4 retail pharmacy prescription lists assists in keeping costs reasonable for the patient. For example, albuterol nebulizer solution (20 mL) is on the Walmart $4 list, whereas generic albuterol nebulizer solution (20 mL bottle) may cost $20. Knowing the approximate costs of medications and discussing with clients their out-of-pocket costs will improve adherence. Drug costs are shown in the Available Dosage Forms tables for each drug category in the chapters in Unit II.

Prescription drug spending has increased significantly over the past few years, from $239.9 billion in 2004 to $307.4 billion in 2010 (IMS Health, 2012). Although the out-of-pocket costs to patients may be acceptable to them, providers still need to consider the actual costs of the medications to the health system. Each prescriber plays a part in controlling prescription drug expenditures through thoughtful prescribing of the most cost-effective drug for the patient. The pharmacoeconomics of prescribing are discussed in depth in Chapter 12.

Patient Factors

Patient factors that may affect prescribing include drug adverse effects that influence adherence, health beliefs, values, and current drug therapy that may interfere with the new drug (Maxwell, 2009; Spector & Vesell, 2002). In addition to interference with the new drug, unnecessary duplications with other drugs being taken may occur. Any time a regimen can be simplified by reducing duplication, adherence is more likely. Other patient factors that affect prescribing are the patient's age (children and older adults), pregnancy, mental health diagnosis, or another disease. Beta blockers, for example, have adverse drug reactions (ADRs) that include anxiety, depression, and mental status changes. The drugs in this class that have higher central nervous system (CNS) penetration are more likely to have these ADRs. If a beta blocker is to be prescribed for a patient with a mental health diagnosis, it is best to use the ones that are less lipophilic because this subset of the drug class is less likely to exhibit these ADRs.

Previous Adverse Drug Reactions

ADRs can be a significant factor in nonadherence. Some patients, such as those with renal dysfunction, are at higher risk of experiencing ADRs. Exploration of previous experiences with medications will identify those at risk for ADRs (Maxwell, 2009). Listening to the patient and noting unusual responses is a proactive approach to prescribing. Remembering that each patient's response to a medication may differ and taking the time to carefully choose a medication that has the fewest ADRs will promote adherence. Chapter 5 provides an extensive discussion of ADRs.

Health Beliefs

Health beliefs and patient attitudes both affect the medication regimen. Patients who believe the medication is going to help them feel better or prevent long-term harm are more likely to adhere to the drug regimen and to have positive outcomes from taking the drug. Belief that one does not have asthma when symptoms are absent is more common among older asthmatics with poor health literacy, leading to nonadherence in use of asthma medications (Federman, Wisnivesky, Wolf, Leventhal, & Halm, 2010). Assessment of beliefs and attitudes is critical to medication adherence.

Current Drug Therapy

A patient's current drug therapy may affect the drug selected or the dosage prescribed because of the potential for drug interactions (Maxwell, 2009). Throughout this text potential drug interactions are listed for each drug category, with suggested alterations in therapy if needed. If a patient is on a complex medication regimen, consultation with a pharmacist or PharmD who has access to drug interaction software is warranted for patient safety.

Patient Age

Patients at the extremes of age, either the very young or the very old, have developmental pharmacokinetic differences that warrant careful prescribing. Infants have immature liver and renal functions that place them at risk for toxicity and ADRs and may require dosage adjustments based on age. Likewise, the elderly population has decreased liver and renal functions related to the physiological changes associated with aging, placing them at risk for increased ADRs. Prescribing for children is discussed in Chapter 50 and prescribing for geriatric patients is discussed in Chapter 51.

Pregnancy

Pregnant patients pose a challenge to the prescriber. Early in pregnancy, there is a risk for drugs being teratogenic to the fetus. The FDA has historically assigned a pregnancy category to prescription drugs, rating them as Pregnancy Category C, D, or X, known to cause fetal harm (U.S. Food and Drug Administration, 2009). The FDA has proposed a change in labeling to incorporate a pregnancy risk summary and clinical considerations to the drug label (U.S. Food and Drug Administration, 2011). Later in pregnancy, drugs may cause fetal adverse effects, such as tachycardia or stroke, or may cause the fetus to abort during premature labor. The National Library of Medicine TOXNET Developmental and Reproductive Toxicology Database (DART) is a Web-based databank of the latest information on the developmental and reproductive effects of drugs (http://toxnet.nlm.nih.gov). Drugs in pregnancy are discussed in the Precautions and Contraindications sections for each drug class and in Chapter 49.

Provider Factors

Ease of Prescribing or Monitoring

Providers often develop a personal formulary of drugs with which they are familiar and that they are comfortable prescribing (Maxwell, 2009). Unfamiliar medications require providers to research the drug and educate themselves in order to prescribe the drug safely. The amount of provider follow-up required, whether it is titrating doses or therapeutic monitoring, may influence prescribing decisions (Maxwell, 2009; Spector & Vesell, 2002).

Formularies

Many health insurance plans have restricted formularies; the provider must prescribe from the formulary or the patient may have significant additional out-of-pocket costs. The restricted formulary of many health plans requires that nurse practitioners move away from their personal formulary. Nurse practitioners need to be familiar with the formulary of medications they are allowed to prescribe from and to keep themselves updated as formularies change (Spector & Vesell, 2002).

INFLUENCES ON RATIONAL PRESCRIBING

Pharmaceutical Promotion

The pharmaceutical industry consistently ranks among the most profitable industries (Spitz & Wickham, 2012). Pharmaceutical companies fund many academic research studies, and there have been reports that some of these studies do not publish negative results of industry-sponsored clinical trials (Institute of Medicine, 2009). Pharmaceutical companies also offer free dinners, gifts, and free drug samples to providers to raise awareness of their products and to influence prescribing (Austed, Avorn, & Kesselheim, 2011). Gifts range from small items such as pens and coffee mugs to medical textbooks and equipment. The Institute of Medicine issued a report in 2009 regarding the conflicts of interest and noted the influence of meals and gifts on physician prescribing; the report stated, "Data suggest that these relationships may influence physicians to prescribe a company's medicines even when evidence indicates another drug would be more beneficial" (p 3).

There has been little research regarding the influence of pharmaceutical marketing on nurse practitioner (NP) prescribing practice. Blunt (2005) surveyed NPs (N = 393) regarding the influence of pharmaceutical company education and gifts, and 80% of respondents reported that they changed their prescribing practices after pharmaceutical company education or interaction with a drug representative. Ladd, Mahoney, and Emani (2010) surveyed NPs nationwide (N = 263) and found 90% believed it was acceptable to attend a lunch or dinner sponsored by the pharmaceutical industry, with 48% indicating they were more likely to prescribe a drug that was featured in the sponsored event. In focus groups exploring prescriptive decision making of geriatric nurse practitioners (GNPs), the GNPs reported skepticism regarding the information provided by pharmaceutical representatives. They noted that the studies presented to them often excluded geriatric patients from the sample, thus making the information provided of little use for their practice (Mahoney & Ladd, 2010). Mahoney and Ladd noted that the participants of their focus groups felt their nursing background influenced their prescribing and that GNPs have a more holistic approach to prescribing than do physicians. More research is needed regarding the influence of pharmaceutical marketing and education on NP prescribing.

In light of the influence that pharmaceutical marketing has on prescribing, professional organizations have issued statements regarding such marketing. The Institute of Medicine recommends that conflicts of interest and financial relationships be disclosed by those providing education and that providers limit the distribution of drug samples to patients who do not have financial access to medication (Institute of Medicine, 2009). The Pharmaceutical Research and Manufacturers of America (PhRMA) has developed its Code on Interactions with Healthcare Professionals, stating a commitment to high ethical standards in the marketing of pharmaceutical products (PhRMA, 2010). NP prescribers need to be aware of the influences of all aspects of pharmaceutical marketing on their prescribing.

When Prescribing Recommendations Change

The approach of expert providers may serve them well most of the time, but when guidelines change or new evidence becomes available, expert providers may need to be coached or reeducated regarding appropriate prescribing. Prior to the 1990s, antibiotics were widely prescribed for upper respiratory infections. The excessive and inappropriate use of anti-infectious agents became a major factor in drug resistance (Bishai, Morris, & Scanland, 2004; CDC, 2009; Linares, Ardanuy, Pallares, & Fenoll, 2010).

The emergence of antibiotic resistance due to antibiotic overprescribing led to a need to shift attitudes and prescribing patterns. The CDC developed the "Get Smart" campaign, and a similar STAR (Stemming the Tide of Antibiotic Resistance) campaign was conducted in the United Kingdom (Bekkers et al, 2010; CDC, 2009). The CDC employed an intervention involving collaboration with the medical professional organizations and intensive education regarding appropriate prescribing of antibiotics. The STAR program used Social Learning Theory, online learning, and context-bound learning to change attitudes about prescribing antibiotics (Bekkers et al, 2010; Simpson et al, 2009). Changing ingrained prescribing behavior is essential to reducing antibiotic resistance, and each prescriber is responsible for the thoughtful prescribing of antibiotics to prevent resistance.

The changing recommendations regarding prescribing antibiotics is just one example of how prescribing recommendations may change and of the necessity for prescribers to keep up-to-date on the current guidelines for prescribing.

REFERENCES

Austad, K., Avorn, J., & Kellelheim, A. (2011). Medical students' exposure to and attitudes about the pharmaceutical industry: A systematic review. *Plos Medicine, 8*(5), e1001037.

Bekkers, M. J., Simpson, S. A., Dunstan, F., Hood, K., Hare, M., Evans, J., et al, and the STAR Study Team. (2010). Enhancing the quality of antibiotic prescribing in primary care: Qualitative evaluation of a blended learning intervention. *BMC Family Practice, 11*(24). Retrieved from http://www.biomedcentral.com/1471-2296/11/34

Bishai, W., Morris, C., & Scanland, S. (2004). Treatment of community acquired pneumonia. *Clinician Reviews.* New York: Jobson Publishing. Retrieved November 29, 2010, from http://www.clinicianreviews.com/index.asp?page=/courses/3061/disclaimer.htm

Bissessur, S. W., Geijteman, E. C., Al-Dulaimy, M., Teunissen, P. W., Richir, M. C., Arnold, A. E., & de Vries, G. M. (2009). Therapeutic reasoning: From hiatus to hypothetical model. *Journal of Evaluation in Clinical Practice, 15*(6), 985–989.

Blunt, E. (2005). Do "pharma" perks sway patient care? *Holistic Nursing Practice, 19*(5), 242.

Centers for Disease Control and Prevention (CDC). (2009). Get smart: Know when antibiotics work. Treatment guidelines for upper respiratory tract infections. Retrieved from http://www.cdc.gov/getsmart/campaign-materials/treatment-guidelines.html

Centers for Disease Control and Prevention (CDC). (2013). Health literacy: Accurate, accessible and actionable health information for all. Retrieved from http://www.cdc.gov/healthliteracy/

Cohen, J., Christensen, K., & Feldman, L. (2012). Disease management and medication compliance. *Population Health Management, 15*(1), 20–28.

de Vries, T. P., Henning, R. H., Hogerzeil, H. V., & Fresle, D. A. (1994). *Guide to good prescribing.* WHO/DAP/94.11. Reprinted 2000. Geneva, Switzerland: World Health Organization.

Federman, A. D., Wisnivesky, J. P., Wolf, M. S., Leventhal, H., & Halm, E. A. (2010). Inadequate health literacy is associated with suboptimal health beliefs in older asthmatics. *Journal of Asthma: Official Journal of the Association for the Care of Asthma, 47*(6), 620–626.

Iglar, K., Kennie, N., & Bajcar, J. (2007). I can PresCribE a Drug: Mnemonic-based teaching of rational prescribing. *Family Medicine, 39*(4), 236–240.

IMS Health. (2012). Channel distribution by U.S. sales. IMS National Sales Perspectives. Retrieved from http://www.imshealth.com/deployedfiles/ims/Global/Content/Corporate/Press%20Room/Top-line%20Market%20Data/2010%20Top-line%20Market%20Data/2010_Distribution_Channel_by_Sales.pdf

Institute of Medicine. (2009). Conflict of interest in medical research, education, and practice. Report brief. Retrieved from http://www.iom.edu/~/imedia/Files/Report%20Files/2009/Conflict-of-Interest-in-Medical-Research-Education-and-Practice/COI%20report%20brief%20for%20web.pdf

Ladd, E., Mahoney, D., & Emani, S. (2010). "Under the radar": Nurse practitioner prescribers and pharmaceutical industry promotions. *The American Journal of Managed Care, 16*(12), e358–362.

Latter, S., Sibley, A., Skinner, T. C., Cradock, S., Zinken, K. M., Lussier, M. T., et al. (2010). The impact of an intervention for nurse prescribers on consultation to promote medicine-taking in diabetes: A mixed methods study. *International Journal of Nursing Studies, 47,* 1126–1138.

Linares, J., Ardanuy, C., Pallares, R., & Fenoll, A. (2010). Changes in antimicrobial resistance, serotypes and genotypes in *Streptococcus pneumoniae* over a 30-year period. *Clinical Microbiology and Infection, 16,* 402–410.

Mahoney, D. F., & Ladd, E. (2010). More than a prescriber: Gerontological nurse practitioners' perspectives on prescribing and pharmaceutical marketing. *Geriatric Nursing, 31,* 17–27.

Maxwell, S. (2009). Rational prescribing: The principles of drug selection. *Clinical Medicine, 9*(5), 481–485.

Osterberg, L., & Blaschke, T. (2005). Drug therapy: Adherence to medication. *New England Journal of Medicine, 353*(5), 487–497.

Pharmaceutical Research and Manufacturers of America (PhRMA). (2010). Code on interactions with healthcare professionals. Retrieved from http://www.phrma.org/code_on_interactions_with_healthcare_ professionals

Raebel, M. A., Carroll, N. M., Kelleher, J. A., Chester, E. A., Berca, S., & Macid, D. J. (2007). Randomized trial to improve prescribing safety during pregnancy. *Journal of the American Medical Informatics Association, 14,* 440–450.

Richir, M. C., Tichelaar, J., Geijtemann, E. C. T., & de Vries, T. P. G. M. (2007). Teaching clinical pharmacology and therapeutics with an emphasis on therapeutic reasoning of undergraduate medical students. *European Journal of Clinical Pharmacology, 64*(2), 217–224.

Scott, J. (2002). Using health belief models to understand the efficacy-effectiveness gap for mood stabilizer treatments. *Neuropsychobiology, 46*(Suppl. 1), 13–15.

Simpson, S. A., Butler, C. C., Hood, K., Cohen, D., Dunstan, F., Evans, M. R., and the STAR Study Team. (2009). Stemming the Tide of Antibiotic Resistance (STAR): A protocol for a trial of a complex intervention addressing the "why" and "how" of appropriate antibiotic prescribing in general practice. *BMC Family Practice, 10*(20). Retrieved from http://www.biomedcentral.com/1471-2296/10/20

Spector, R., & Vesell, E. S. (2002). A rational approach to the selection of useful drugs for clinical practice. *Pharmacology, 65,* 57–61.

Spitz, J., & Wickham, M. (2012). Pharmaceutical high profits: The value of R&D, or oligopolistic rents? *American Journal of Economics and Sociology, 71*(1), 1–36.

U.S. Food and Drug Administration. (2009). Pregnancy and lactation labeling. Retrieved from http://www.fda.gov/Drugs/DevelopmentApproval-Process/DevelopmentResources/Labeling/ucm093307.htm

U.S. Food and Drug Administration (2011). Summary of proposed rule on pregnancy and lactation labeling. Retrieved from http://www.fda.gov/Drugs/DevelopmentApprovalProcess/DevelopmentResources/Labeling/ucm093310.htm

Waller, D. G. (2005). Rational prescribing: The principles of drug selection and assessment of efficacy. *Clinical Medicine, 5,* 26–28.

World Health Organization (2012). The pursuit of responsible use of medicines: Sharing and learning from country experiences. Geneva, Switzerland: World Health Organization. Retrieved from http://apps.who.int/iris/bitstream/10665/75828/1/WHO_EMP_MAR_2012.3_eng.pdf

World Health Organization (WHO). (2013). Rational use of medicines. Retrieved from http://www.who.int/medicines/areas/rational_use/en/

CHAPTER 4

LEGAL AND PROFESSIONAL ISSUES IN PRESCRIBING

Tracy Klein

FEDERAL DRUG LAW

History

The Food, Drug, and Cosmetic Act of 1906 was the first federal law designed to protect the public by restricting the manufacture and distribution of drugs. The law designated that drugs must meet official standards for strength and purity and prohibited "the manufacture of adulterated or misbranded or poisonous or deleterious foods, drugs, medicines, and liquors" (U.S. Food and Drug Administration [FDA], 2010). Focusing primarily on how drugs were ultimately labeled or branded, it did not broadly prevent the manufacturing of unsafe or ineffective medications.

In 1937, a manufacturer marketed an elixir of sulfanilamide that used diethylene glycol as a solvent for the new antibiotic. Because its pharmacological effects were not tested, its toxicity went unnoticed until reports of more than 100 patient deaths were collected.

The public outcry for new laws resulted in the federal Food, Drug, and Cosmetic Act of 1938 (FDA, 2010). This act has three basic principles that restrict drug adulteration, misbranding, and the interstate commerce of an unapproved drug. It also created the FDA. As a regulatory agency, the FDA was initially charged with enforcing new laws requiring that drugs be checked before they went to market. From 1938 to 1962, the approval of new drugs was based on safety. In the early 1960s, the use of thalidomide by women in the early stages of pregnancy resulted in the birth of hundreds of deformed babies in Europe. A tragedy of this scale was avoided in the United States because the drug was not approved for marketing here. This situation spurred the passage of the Kefauver-Harris amendments in 1962 (FDA, 2010). These amendments required that both the safety and efficacy of a drug be proven before it is marketed. In addition, the act required that all drugs marketed from 1938 to 1962 be evaluated for efficacy. This study was performed by the National

Academy of Sciences/National Research Council and called the Drug Efficacy Study Implementation (DESI). Thousands of drugs were studied and ineffective drugs were withdrawn from the market.

Two additional acts have had considerable influence on improving drug availability and benefiting patients with rare diseases. The Orphan Drug Act of 1983 fosters orphan drug development for diseases so rare that the usual approval process would take decades to complete (FDA, 2010). The Drug Price Competition and Patent Term Restoration Act of 1984 expanded the number of generic drugs suitable for an abbreviated new drug application (ANDA). This makes it possible for generic drug companies to market generic versions of drugs by proving bioequivalence rather than duplicating the clinical trials needed for initial drug approval.

Another significant legislative act was the Pediatric Research Equity Act passed in 2003 (FDA, 2010). This act, referred to as the "Pediatric Rule," authorized the FDA to request pediatric studies of already marketed drugs or to require studies by others if the manufacturer refuses. Since the passage of the Pediatric Rule, several drugs in common use for children were removed from the market because their safety and efficacy had never been tested in pediatric subjects.

U.S. Food and Drug Administration Regulatory Jurisdiction

The FDA regulatory jurisdiction over drugs encompasses the standardization of nomenclature, the approval process for new drugs and new indications, official labeling, surveillance of adverse drug events, and methods of manufacture and distribution (FDA, 2012). The classification of a drug as a prescription or nonprescription medication is a matter of federal law. Products labeled with the legend "Caution: Federal law prohibits dispensing without a prescription" are regulated by the FDA and are referred to as *legend drugs*.

The FDA also regulates medical and electronic devices that meet criteria under the 1976 Medical Devices Amendment of the Food, Drug, and Cosmetic Act (FDA, 2012). Examples of medical and electronic devices include ultrasound imaging equipment, artificial joints, and HIV testing kits.

Prior to 1997, the FDA strictly limited direct-to-consumer advertisements (FDA, 2010). However, such advertising is now commonplace, and studies show it increasingly influences consumer and prescriber decision making regarding medications. The federal Food, Drug, and Cosmetic Act provides that the advertising of prescription drugs must conform to the labeling. Any advertisement that describes a drug's use must contain the generic name and amount of active ingredient, the name and address of the manufacturer, and a brief summary of the prescribing information. A prescription drug advertisement that implies incorrectly that a drug is the treatment of choice or is useful for an off-labeled indication is unlawful. Drug manufacturers are increasingly marketing prescription drugs to patients through print and electronic media, which has increased the demand on practitioners to prescribe advertised drug products.

The New Drug Approval Process

The U.S. system of new drug approvals is perhaps the most rigorous in the world. On average, it costs a company approximately $2.6 billion to get one new medicine from the laboratory to the pharmacist's shelf, according to a 2014 Tufts University analysis for its Center for the Study of Drug Development, which included costs for drugs that were never marketed as well as post-marketing research (DiMasi, Grabowski, & Hansen, 2014). As illustrated in Figure 4-1, it takes 8.5 years on average for an experimental drug to travel from laboratory preclinical trials to FDA approval (Duke Clinical Research Institute, 2010).

Preclinical Research

The process of synthesis and extraction identifies new molecules with the potential to produce a desired change in a biological system (e.g., to inhibit or stimulate an important enzyme, to alter a metabolic pathway, or to change cellular structure). The process may require research on the fundamental mechanisms of disease or biological processes, research on the action of known therapeutic agents, or random selection and broad biological screening. New molecules can be produced through artificial synthesis or extracted from natural sources (plant, mineral, or animal). The number of active pharmaceutical ingredients that can be produced based on the same general chemical structure runs into the hundreds of millions.

Biological screening and pharmacological testing use nonhuman studies to explore the pharmacological activity and therapeutic potential of compounds. These tests involve the use of animals, isolated cell cultures and tissues, enzymes, and cloned receptor sites, as well as computer models. If the results of the tests suggest potential beneficial activity, related compounds are tested to see which version of the molecule produces the highest level of pharmacological activity and demonstrates the most therapeutic promise, with the smallest number of potentially harmful biological properties.

Pharmaceutical dosage formulation and stability testing make up the process of turning an active compound into a form and strength suitable for human use. A pharmaceutical product can take any one of a number of dosage forms (e.g., liquid, tablets, capsules, ointments, sprays, patches) and dosage strengths.

Toxicology and safety testing determines the potential risk a compound poses to people and the environment. These studies use animals, tissue cultures, and other test systems to examine the relationship between factors such as dose level, frequency of administration, and duration of exposure to both the short- and the long-term survival of living organisms. Tests provide information on the dose–response pattern of the compound and its toxic effects. Most toxicology and safety testing is conducted on new molecular entities

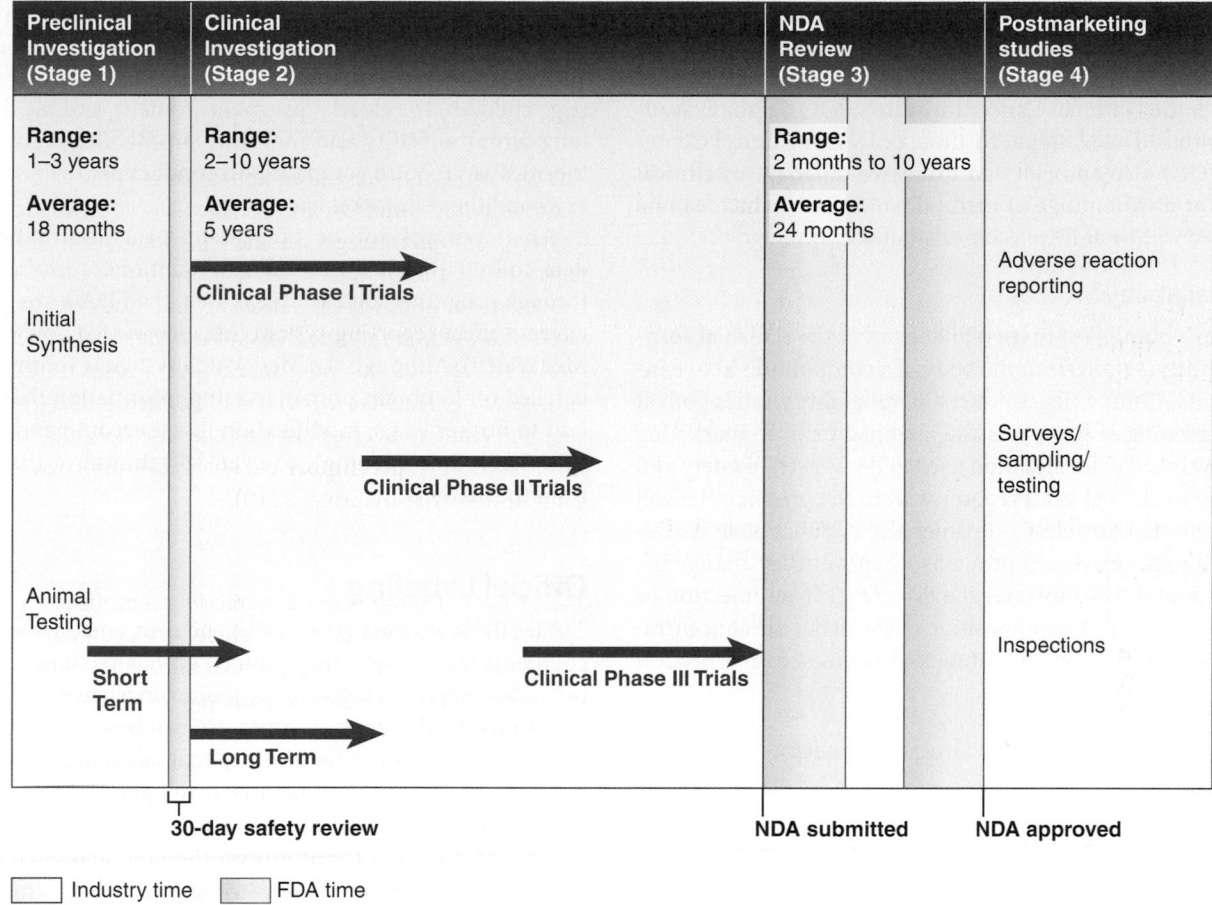

Preclinical Investigation (Stage 1)	Clinical Investigation (Stage 2)	NDA Review (Stage 3)	Postmarketing studies (Stage 4)
Range: 1–3 years	**Range:** 2–10 years	**Range:** 2 months to 10 years	
Average: 18 months	**Average:** 5 years	**Average:** 24 months	

Figure 4–1. New drug development timeline.

prior to their human introduction, but companies can choose to delay long-term toxicity testing until after the therapeutic potential of the product is established.

Clinical Studies

An investigational new drug (IND) application is filed with the FDA prior to human testing. The IND application is a compilation of all known information about the compound. It also includes a description of the clinical research plan for the product and the specific protocol for phase I study. Unless the FDA says no, clinical tests can begin 30 calendar days after submission. The FDA has formulated IND regulations for the clinical study of a new drug's safety and efficacy and has divided this evaluation into three phases:

1. Phase I clinical evaluation is the first testing of a new compound in subjects, for the purpose of establishing the tolerance of healthy human subjects at different doses; defining its pharmacological effects at anticipated therapeutic levels; and studying its absorption, distribution, metabolism, and excretion patterns in humans.
2. Phase II clinical evaluation is controlled studies performed on patients with the target disease or disorder to determine a compound's potential usefulness and short-term risks. A relatively small number of patients, usually no more than several hundred subjects, are enrolled in phase II studies.

3. Phase III trials are controlled and uncontrolled clinical trials of a drug's safety and efficacy in hospital and outpatient settings. Phase III studies gather precise information on the drug's efficacy for specific indications, determine whether the drug produces a broader range of adverse effects than those exhibited in the small study populations of phases I and II studies, and identify the best way of administering and using the drug for the purpose intended. If the drug is approved, this information forms the basis for deciding the content of the product label. Phase III trials verify that the acceptable risk/benefit ratio seen in phase II persists under conditions of anticipated usage and in groups of patients large enough to identify statistically and clinically significant responses.

Conferences between the sponsor and the FDA are held during all three phases of development. While an IND is in effect, the sponsor must report in writing to the FDA within 10 working days any serious and unexpected adverse reactions that may be drug related. The treatment IND program is part of the FDA's efforts to facilitate the development of significant new therapies. Under this program, treatment protocols using an investigational drug can be approved for life-threatening illnesses for which there is no comparable alternative therapy. Information on the availability of an investigational drug under a treatment IND is published in the

Journal of the American Medical Association and other public sources. Patients and families can learn about clinical trials and access to investigational drugs for cancer treatment through the National Cancer Institute's PDQ database available online. The National Institute of Health Clinical Center (NIH CC) also sponsors an extensive database of clinical trials for a wide range of medical conditions, which can be accessed online at http://clinicalstudies.info.nih.gov/.

Bioavailability Studies

Healthy volunteers are used to document the rate of absorption and excretion from the body of a compound's active ingredients. Companies conduct bioavailability studies both at the beginning of human testing and just prior to marketing to show that the formulation used to demonstrate safety and efficacy in clinical trials is equivalent to the product that will be distributed for sale. Companies also conduct bioavailability studies on marketed products whenever they change the method used to administer the drug (e.g., from injection or oral dose form), the composition of the drug, the concentration of the active ingredient, or the manufacturing process used to produce the drug.

Regulatory Review: New Drug Application

To market a new drug for human use, a manufacturer must have a new drug application (NDA) approved by the FDA. All information about the drug gathered during the drug discovery and development process is assembled in the NDA. During the review period, the FDA may ask the company for additional information about the product or seek clarification of the data contained in the application. The FDA has 60 days to determine whether the NDA will be filed for review. Once the FDA files the NDA, a team is assigned to review the drug sponsor's research on the safety and effectiveness of the drug. Usually, the FDA requests additional information, and the manufacturer needs from 1 to 5 years to complete any additional well-controlled trials necessary to support the claimed indications or prove the drug's safety.

Accelerated Approval of a New Drug Application

The timely availability of new drugs remains the subject of considerable debate. In December 1991, the FDA published new regulations to accelerate approval of certain new drugs that provide therapeutic benefit to patients with serious or life-threatening illnesses (FDA, 2010). The FDA can approve these drugs based on well-controlled clinical trials establishing that the product has an effect on a therapeutic endpoint that is likely to predict clinical benefit. The applicant is required to conduct post-marketing studies.

Postapproval Research

Clinical experience with a new drug may include no more than 1,000 to 2,000 patients. The detection of rare (less than 1 in 1,000) adverse drug reactions is not reliable until hundreds of thousands of patients have taken the drug. Clinical trials conducted after a drug is marketed (referred to as phase IV studies in the United States) are an important source of information on as-yet undetected adverse outcomes, especially in populations not included in the premarketing trials (e.g., children, the elderly, pregnant women), and the drug's long-term morbidity and mortality profile. Regulatory authorities can require companies to conduct phase IV studies as a condition of market approval.

An important source of postapproval information is data collected and submitted by practitioners in the field through programs such as MedWatch, the FDA's safety and adverse-effect reporting system (http://www.fda.gov/Safety/MedWatch). Although the MedWatch system is voluntary, it is relied on to obtain post-marketing information that may lead to further trials, modification in use recommendations (i.e., Black Box warning), or even withdrawal of the drug from the market.

Official Labeling

The legal distinction between a legend drug and an over-the-counter (OTC) drug is not founded on relative safety per se but rather involves a regulatory decision on whether adequate directions for the drug's proper use can be written for the layperson. If the FDA determines that adequate directions can be written, the manufacturer is not allowed to identify the drug with a prescription legend.

Conversely, for a prescription drug, the manufacturer's directions or FDA-approved labeling (the package insert) is intended for the prescriber, pharmacist, or nurse and provides a summary of information about the chemical and physical nature of the product, pharmacological indications and contraindications, means of administration, dosages, side effects and adverse reactions, how the drug is supplied, and any other information pertinent to safe and effective use. This summary, or official labeling, is developed through discussion between the FDA and the drug manufacturer. The material in the *Physician's Desk Reference* (PDR) is a verbatim presentation of the official labeling.

The FDA's jurisdiction over the uses of marketed drugs and doses extends only to what the manufacturer may recommend and must disclose in its labeling. The FDA is not charged with dictating how a prescriber should practice. The FDA is concerned with the marketing and availability of drugs that have demonstrated substantial evidence of an acceptable risk/benefit ratio for labeled indications. *The proper and efficacious therapeutic use of these drugs is the responsibility of the prescriber.*

Off-Label Use

The prescription of an FDA-approved drug for an off-label (unlabeled) indication may be initiated by patient need. Off-label use includes use of an FDA-approved drug in a dose or route for which it was not approved or for a clinical indication other than the FDA-approved use. Clinical support can be demonstrated for off-label use if the proposed use is based on rational scientific theory or controlled clinical studies. The FDA has made it clear that it neither has nor wants the authority to compel prescribers to adhere to FDA-approved use in all clinical situations. An example of off-label use is that of trazodone, which is an antidepressant, for sleep. In this example, a side effect of the medication (drowsiness) has been shown to have clinical efficacy for patients with difficulty sleeping whether or not they are clinically depressed. Although not FDA approved for insomnia, trazodone is commonly prescribed for this indication.

Nurse practitioners (NPs) are responsible for knowing the FDA indication and approval status of any drug they prescribe. However, a prescribing decision on how to use a drug must be based on what is best for the patient and then supported by available evidence. In professional liability suits, FDA-approved drug labeling may have evidentiary weight, but drug labeling is not intended to set the sole standard for what is good clinical practice. NPs must also be aware that Medicare and other insurers rarely cover off-label prescriptions and that consequently the patient may bear greater cost. Off-label prescribing can also result in increased or unknown risk to the patient (Gillick, 2009).

Controlled Substance Laws

The most comprehensive federal drug legislation is the Controlled Substances Act of 1970 (FDA, 2010). This law was designed to improve regulation of the manufacturing, distribution, and dispensing of drugs identified as "controlled" drugs by providing a closed system for legitimate providers of these substances. Every person who manufactures, distributes, prescribes, procures, or dispenses any controlled substance must register and obtain a registration number with the U.S. Drug Enforcement Administration (DEA). The *Practitioner's Manual: An Informational Outline of the Controlled Substances Act,* published in 2006, outlines regulations and requirements for controlled-drug prescribing. This pamphlet is available from the DEA or can be viewed online (http://www.deadiversion.usdoj.gov/pubs/manuals/pract/index.html). All those who regularly dispense and administer controlled substances during the course of their practice must maintain and keep on file for a minimum of 2 years accurate records of controlled drugs they purchase, distribute, administer, and dispense.

Many states have controlled substance acts patterned after federal law. Because differences are allowed in the scheduling of drugs among states (a state may be more restrictive but not less restrictive), NPs must become acquainted with the provisions of the regulations in the state in which they are licensed. NPs wanting authority to prescribe controlled substances must apply for state prescriptive authority prior to application for a federal DEA number. Applications for a DEA number may be obtained online through the DEA or though the state regional office. Before applying, it is important to verify with the state board of nursing or pharmacy if a state-issued prescribing number or certificate is also issued separately from the NP license.

For many years the DEA number was inappropriately used for other than controlled substances by pharmacies, primarily to bill insurance or track medications under a provider-unique identifier. Concern over this as well as the plethora of separate numbers used for Medicaid and Medicare billing led to the development and use of the National Provider Identifier number (NPI). The NP should obtain an NPI as soon as it is feasible. Application is free and available online. This number is unique to the provider and is used for all prescriptions that are billed through insurance, as well as for other billing services.

In an effort to control drug distribution, a classification system was developed to categorize drugs as "controlled" based on their potential for abuse, accepted medical use, and diversion potential. NPs must know the different classifications and schedules of controlled drugs as well as the associated prescribing rules and regulations. Controlled drugs are listed in five different schedules— I, II, III, IV, and V—to which different regulations apply. Controlled substance authority for NPs varies from state to state according to ability and autonomy of practice.

Table 4-1 presents the schedules, controls required, and examples of drugs.

Controlled Substance Prescribing Precautions

Prescribers should take precautions with controlled drug prescription pads and information included on the controlled substance prescription to minimize the chance for fraud and diversion of these drugs. The prescription pad (or prescription printer paper) should be stored in a locked area or locked drawer on the printer. Prescriptions should never be signed in advance or used as notepads. The prescriber's name, NPI number, address, and telephone number should be printed on the pads to allow verification by the dispensing pharmacist. Some states also require that the NP's license number appear on the prescription in addition to that of any supervising/collaborating practitioner. The DEA registration number must be designated on all controlled substance prescriptions, though individual states may permit a pharmacist to write in the DEA number if it is not initially provided. The prescription should be dated on the day it is written, indicating any authorized refills as allowed and clinically appropriate. It is helpful to spell out the quantity dispensed as well, using an Arabic numeral (e.g., "forty [40]") to discourage alterations in the intended quantity.

A prescription for a controlled substance may be directly faxed to the pharmacy as an additional precaution, with the exception of Schedule II controlled substances. A fax cannot be considered the original for Schedule II drugs unless the drug in question is (1) for a nursing home, (2) for a hospice, or (3) for parenteral medication for home IV administration.

As of 2009, tamper-proof prescription pads are required for prescriptions written for patients under Medicaid payment plans. State law incorporates the federal guidelines for what constitutes a tamper-proof prescription into any additional state-specific requirements for controlled substances, such as duplicate prescription pads. A practitioner may find

Table 4–1 Controlled Drug Schedules

Schedule	Controls Required	Drug Examples
I	No accepted medical use No legal use permitted For registered research facilities only	Heroin, LSD, mescaline, peyote, marijuana*
II	No refills permitted No telephone orders unless true emergency and followed up by written prescription within 7 days Electronic prescribing permitted as of 2011 with specific software and secure identification processes	Narcotics (morphine, codeine, meperidine, opium, hydromorphone, oxycodone, oxymorphone, methadone, fentanyl) Stimulants (cocaine, amphetamine, methylphenidate) Depressants (pentobarbital, secobarbital)
III	Prescription must be rewritten after 6 mo or 5 refills Telephone or fax prescription okay	Narcotics (codeine in combination with non-narcotic ingredients not to exceed 90 mg/tab; hydrocodone not to exceed 15 mg/tab) Stimulants (benzphetamine, chlorpheniramine, diethylpropion) Depressants (butabarbital) Anabolic steroids, testosterone
IV	Same as Schedule III Penalties for illegal possession are different	Pentazocine, phentermine, benzodiazepines, meprobamate
V	Same as all prescription drugs May be dispensed without a prescription unless regulated by the state	Loperamide, diphenoxylate Cough medications with less than 200 mg/100 mL Pregabalin

*Marijuana may be classified under individual state law as a Schedule II drug and used for medical purposes. It may not be "prescribed," however.

the use of tamper-proof prescription pads or paper to be advisable for all written prescriptions, because many drugs that have abuse potential are not currently federally controlled. Such drugs include tramadol, carisoprodol, and pseudoephedrine.

A few medications have such high abuse potential or potential for serious adverse effects that they should be prescribed very cautiously and with increased monitoring. The medications with high abuse potential that fall into this category include methadone, amphetamine, and scheduled appetite suppressants. Medications with especially problematic adverse-effect profiles include meperidine and butalbital. Medications with exceptionally narrow safety margins include secobarbital, pentobarbital, meprobamate, methadone, and ethchlorvynol. Medications with little established efficacy include carisoprodol, butalbital, and scheduled appetite suppressants.

Opioids such as morphine have legitimate clinical usefulness, and the practitioner should not hesitate to prescribe them when indicated for patients who require analgesia or symptomatic relief not provided by other analgesics. Methadone is also used for chronic pain management due to its cost and long half-life. However, methadone also has an extremely variable half-life (7 to 60 or more hours) that differs for individuals based on their metabolism. It therefore should not be a first-line therapy for pain management, especially for the less experienced practitioner. Buprenorphine is another long-acting opioid used for pain management. Both buprenorphine and methadone are legal to prescribe for pain management provided that an NP has his or her own Schedule II authority. However, it is not legal for an NP to prescribe methadone or buprenorphine for narcotic addiction, and such patients should be referred

to an MD or a state-registered clinic that specializes in addiction treatment.

A specific clinical challenge regarding controlled drug prescribing is the patient who has a history of drug or alcohol abuse or dependence and who needs management of pain, anxiety, and insomnia. Special attention should be given to patients with current dependence on opioids or other central nervous system depressants such as benzodiazepines. If a genuine symptomatic need is established by adequate diagnostic confirmation, evaluation, and periodic reevaluation and other analgesics or nondrug treatments are ineffective, then it is the practitioner's responsibility to prescribe appropriate pain control or refer to a specialized pain management clinic. When prescribing opioids, evaluation must be made of the patient using clinically available tools that have been validated, such as SOAPP (Screener and Opioid Assessment for Patients in Pain) or SOAPP-R (Screener and Opioid Assessment for Patients in Pain—Revised) (Butler, Fernandez, Benoit, Budman, & Jamison, 2008). In developing a pain treatment plan, it is important to consider that the effective dose will vary according to the degree of tolerance that the patient has developed.

For any patient, abrupt discontinuation can precipitate a withdrawal syndrome if the patient undergoes major surgical or medical trauma while dependent on the drug. Patients can be instructed in planned withdrawal or taper in conjunction with their surgical or hospital team. Withdrawal or taper of benzodiazapines requires particular clinical expertise and supervision. Unlike opioids, benzodiazapine withdrawal can result in seizures and significant mortality if managed improperly.

The practitioner must caution any patient for whom an antianxiety or hypnotic is prescribed about the potentiating effects of alcohol and other drugs. Practitioners should also be aware that benzodiazepines in particular have associated cautions due to their clinical effects and potential for abuse that contraindicate them for patients on methadone or with a current substance use disorder.

CONTROLLED SUBSTANCE MISUSE: PRESCRIBER EDUCATION

In standard clinical practice there are many opportunities for individuals to obtain excessive quantities of controlled drugs, either intentionally or as a result of duplicate prescribing, often by different prescribers. The problems and costs associated with misuse of controlled prescription drugs may have an impact on patients and their prescribers.

Principles for prescribers related to prescription drug misuse assessment include the following:

1. Acquisition and wide use of chemical dependence screening skills.

BOX 4–1 WEB RESOURCES FOR LEGAL AND ETHICAL ISSUES IN PRESCRIBING

National Cancer Institute Clinical Trials: http://www.cancer.gov/clinicaltrials

National Institute of Health Clinical Trials: http://clinicaltrials.gov/ct2/home

FDA MedWatch: http://www.fda.gov/Safety/MedWatch/default.htm

U.S. Drug Enforcement Administration: http://www.dea.gov

National Provider Identifier Number application: https://nppes.cms.hhs.gov/NPPES/Welcome.do

National Council of State Boards of Nursing: www.ncsbn.org

Institute for Safe Medication Practices: www.ismp.org

Opioid Assessment, Medication Agreement and Management Tools: http://www.painedu.org/tools.asp?Tool=11

---

2. Early and firm limit setting regarding indications for controlled drug prescribing.
3. Careful documentation of a confirmed diagnosis and the ruling out of chemical dependence before initiating a controlled prescription or drug subject to misuse.
4. Practice in "just saying no" and feeling comfortable in being firm without escalating the discussion into an argument with the patient.

Further discussion of pain medication abuse is found in Chapter 52.

Behavioral Red Flags

Almost every practice experiences the chemically dependent patient who uses dishonest mechanisms to obtain increasing supplies of controlled prescriptions. There are certain behaviors that are "red flags" for identifying patients who may be addicted or diverting their controlled medications. Passik and colleagues (1998) have listed behaviors that providers should be aware of that are predictive of addiction (Table 4-2).

Once a scam has worked in a given practice, that scam will continue to surface periodically in that office practice until the provider ceases to reinforce the scam. Drug enforcement investigators and patients who abuse prescription drugs commonly observe that the greater the ease of practicing scams and drug-seeking behavior in a provider's practice, the higher the prevalence of drug-abusing patients there will be in that practice. Dealing with scams consists of the following steps:

1. Learning to recognize the common scams.
2. Refusing to give in to scammers.
3. Practicing the skill of turning the tables on the scammer.

Scams are generally conducted to obtain more medications, more potent or higher-dosage formulations, higher street-value brands of drugs, a controlled drug without a chart or visit note, or to avoid noncontrolled alternatives. Most scams produce discomfort in providers, and patients using scams are often willing to push the practitioner if they encounter resistance to the scam. Patient-generated pressure to prescribe in the face of clinician hesitancy is one classic sign of a scam. Patients rarely argue pharmacology with providers unless the issue of prescribing

Table 4–2 Behaviors More and Less Predictive of Addiction

Probably More Predictive	Probably Less Predictive
Prescription forgery	Drug hoarding during periods of reduced symptoms
Selling prescription drugs	Aggressive complaining about need for higher doses
Stealing or borrowing another patient's drugs	Requesting specific drugs
Injecting oral formulation	Unapproved use of drug to treat another symptom
Obtaining prescription drugs from nonmedical sources	Obtaining similar drugs from other medical sources
Concurrent use of illicit drugs	Reporting psychic effects not intended by the provider
Unsanctioned dose escalations	Unsanctioned dose escalations one or two times
Recurrent prescription losses	Resistance to change in therapy associated with tolerable adverse effects, with expressions of anxiety related to return to severe symptoms
Evidence of deterioration in the ability to function at work, in the family, or socially, which appears to be related to drug use	
Repeated resistance to changes in therapy despite clear evidence of adverse physical or psychological effects from the drug	

Passik et al (2006).

controlled drugs is being contested. The clinical phenomenon of an initial no (refusal to prescribe by the practitioner) becoming a yes (eventual willingness to prescribe) if the patient brings the right pressure to bear on the practitioner is pathognomonic of prescription drug misuse.

Prescription altering and forging are a frequently encountered scam. Variations include stealing prescriptions, forging blank prescriptions, photocopying prescriptions, and rewriting prescriptions. Additional common prescription alteration strategies include changing the strength of a prescribed drug, the number of pills prescribed, the number of refills indicated, or the date of the prescription. Patients and staff members who have substance misuse issues may also call in prescriptions with the NP's DEA number, as current law permits phoned-in prescriptions for Schedules III–V.

Pressure to Prescribe

Another factor that increases the demand for controlled substances is the pressure to prescribe at every visit and the expectation that patients deserve a prescription for something at each visit or for each symptom offered. This process results in two well-known adverse situations: (1) overprescribing of antibiotics and resulting antibiotic resistance and (2) polypharmacy, especially of the elderly. It also may result in a tendency on the part of practitioners to prescribe higher-potency noncontrolled substances and then ultimately controlled drugs when patients persist with vague somatic complaints.

Enabling

Enabling refers to the powerful instinct in practitioners to do anything medically possible to enable patients with present or potential disability to live at a higher level of function. Unfortunately, the disease of chemical dependence has a bottomless appetite for enabling, also defined as behaviors on the part of a friend, family member, or health-care provider that shelter the chemically dependent individual from the adverse consequences of the disease. When the practitioners' enabling instincts interact with chemically dependent patients, the patients are often able to manipulate the practitioners to avoid the consequences of their disease process, thus permitting that disease to progress to further, more pathological levels. This is especially true when controlled drug prescribing is involved. A common statement from practitioners who have been manipulated into enabling and overprescribing to patients is "I was only trying to help." Chemical dependence is one disease process in which practitioners must strive against enabling tendencies, especially when prescribing controlled drugs.

When You Suspect a Patient Is Misusing Medications

Communication Barriers

Curricula in training programs over the past two decades have come to emphasize the clinical interview and practitioner–patient relationship-building skills. Skill building involves active learning strategies in the areas of verbal and nonverbal communication, empathy, and rapport building. Nursing socialization further emphasizes therapeutic patient advocacy, sometimes without the counterbalance of coaching nurses on how to say no and enforce boundary limitations. Therefore, many NPs feel acutely uncomfortable with conflict and interpersonal confrontation. It is obvious how the practitioners' fear and avoidance of confrontation play into the hands of chemically dependent patients, who have a stronger relationship with the prescription than they do with the practitioners.

Communication Skills

Practitioners must be able to identify common scams and defuse them efficiently and effectively. One strategy is to just say no and mean it. Chemically dependent patients have learned that the practitioners' enabling instincts and confrontation discomfort are so great that when NPs initially say no, it usually ultimately can be turned into a yes if enough pressure is applied. Thus, it is important to be able to mean no and to stick with it. A higher-level clinical skill is initially to say no and then to turn the tables on a patient who demands the prescription. This strategy is based on the clinical fact that patients who demand controlled drugs generally have a pathological relationship with that prescription because of underlying chemical dependence. By making the statement "I am feeling pressured by you to write a prescription today that is not clinically indicated. Because of this I am really concerned about you, and we need to talk about your use of alcohol or other substances," the NP can often effectively turn the tables and shift the discomfort to the patient while still refusing to prescribe.

Systemic Solutions to Problems of Controlled Substance Prescribing

Law enforcement and legislative efforts have produced few solutions to the problem of imbalance in controlled drug prescribing. Until recently, these approaches have targeted diversion of drugs and overprescribing. Results of duplicate and triplicate prescription policies, as well as stricter investigation and enforcement, led to decreased prescribing of controlled drugs across the board, even to patients in need of them for legitimate medical reasons. The development of more permissive policies and pain management guidelines by state legislatures and health regulatory boards increased prescribing for pain management; however, a concurrent 65% increase in hospitalizations in the United States for poisonings from prescription drugs (opioids, sedatives, and tranquilizers) ensued from 1999 to 2006 (Coben et al, 2010). Coben and colleagues report a 400% increase in admissions for methadone overdose. This increase is possibly due to inappropriate dosing and use of methadone for pain management, as well as by diversion of legitimately prescribed medications from the patient for whom it was originally prescribed.

Careful charting and documentation habits are essential for prescribing controlled drugs. Document clearly in a progress note (1) physical evaluation of the patient, (2) the diagnosis, (3) the clinical indications for treatment, (4) the written treatment plan, (5) the expected symptom outcomes, (6) informed consent and agreement for treatment from the patient, and (7) consultation and/or collaboration necessary to meet treatment goals and objectives. These strategies reduce, but do not eliminate, the risk of controlled drug diversion from one's practice.

PRESCRIBING TIPS

A few prescribing tips can help the practitioner reduce environmental facilitation of prescription misuse. First, collect and document a complete history and examination before prescribing controlled substances. Do not rely on patient-supplied history, x-rays, or medical records to confirm your assessment—obtain this information directly from the primary source. Passik and Weinreb (2000) advise use of the four "A's" to guide initial and ongoing assessment of medication efficacy: (1) analgesia measurement by use of pain scales or other assessment tools, (2) activities of daily living (ADLs) as measured by levels of physical and psychological functioning, (3) adverse effects, and (4) abuse issues.

Prescribe limited quantities without refills on a first visit, allowing additional time for patient assessment and confirmatory documentation. Educate medical and assistive staff in reinforcement of consistent clinic policies and procedures related to scheduling, forms, urine drug screening, records review and release, and refills. It is not uncommon for patients who do misuse substances to quickly identify the "weak link" among the treatment team and focus their energies on this person or process. Standardize expectations regarding after-hours calls, use of multiple providers, and weekend or early refills and post them where they are readily available.

Patients covered by insurance plans, including Medicaid and Medicare, can be limited to one pharmacy or one prescriber through their payment plan. Case managers can often be utilized to help review and manage medication use and advocate for access to additional options for pain management and control. Other tips include prescribing generic, longer-acting formulations of drugs that have less street value and writing out the quantity prescribed rather than using only numerals, which can be altered.

Medication Agreements

One tool for defining and implementing treatment objectives is the medication agreement. This written tool can be incorporated into treatment of chronic pain, particularly if long-term management with opioids is indicated. The agreement is not limited to opioid prescribing practice, however. A medication agreement can be used for treatment of pain or other conditions with medications that are not opioids but still have potential for patient misuse, such as benzodiazepines, tramadol, or other adjunctive medications. Formats can be found in the links at the end of this chapter and

in Chapter 52. These may be modified for individual clinic settings and client populations.

It is advisable to treat medication agreements under a "universal precaution" model of care, meaning that the NP develops and uses agreements that are expected of all patients requiring ongoing use of medications with potential for misuse. It is inequitable and a potential legal liability to pick and choose patients who will be asked to sign a medication agreement based on their age, income status, use of other controlled or illicit substances, or other personal characteristics. NPs are advised to familiarize themselves with urine drug and alcohol screens and their availability, cost, sensitivity, and specificity. In-office rapid screenings are now available that can be done quickly and without prior notice in order to confirm adherence to medication agreement criteria. An example of a pain medication use agreement is found in Chapter 52.

Prescription Drug Monitoring Programs

As of 2012, all but one state (Missouri) have an active or legislatively enabled Prescription Drug Monitoring Program (PDMP). A PDMP enables practitioners to query a confidential database of controlled substances statewide to evaluate whether a patient is currently receiving a prescription elsewhere. Some states also have regulations that permit cross-state sharing of this information, which has reduced the ability of patients who misuse controlled substances to obtain multiple prescriptions from multiple providers. For more information regarding these programs and how to access them, contact the local DEA office or state board of pharmacy or the Alliance of States with Prescription Drug Monitoring Programs (http://www.pmpalliance.org/).

STATE LAW

Jurisdiction

Federal law establishes whether a drug requires a prescription but does not dictate who may prescribe. The authority to prescribe is a function of state law. Unlike the uniform nature of federal law, prescriptive authority varies from state to state. The states have the authority to license health-care professionals. Although a state may sign a compact agreement permitting cross-state practice, as is the case with the Nurse Licensure Compact, there are no currently implemented cross-state agreements that cover NP practice.

Regulation of nursing education and practice is relatively recent. The NP role originated in the 1960s as an extension of the registered nurse (RN) role. States thereafter implemented a variety of methods for recognizing NP practice. Although the National Council of State Boards of Nursing recommends licensure as the appropriate level of regulation for the autonomy and authority of the NP role, some states still recognize NPs with certification, endorsement, or through delegated authority from a physician. States have authority under the states' "police power" to take regulatory action to protect public health, welfare, and safety, including emergency suspension or revocation of practice authority. The courts have consistently upheld professional licensing laws as legitimate use of this power. The purpose of these laws is to ensure that those who provide health-care services for a fee have demonstrated a minimum level of competency.

A license is always required for practice as an NP. The state Nurse Practice Act specifies the exact title that must be used for practice and on a prescription. NPs working in federal facilities such as the Veterans Administration or Indian Health Services need to have a state-based license that governs their scope of practice in that facility but may practice in a facility different from the state of origin under the same license. Persons practicing in a federal facility are also exempt from fees for DEA registration.

Each state has practice acts that set forth licensing requirements for health professionals, define the scope of practice, and prohibit unauthorized practice. These laws usually provide for a state board that governs each profession and establishes administrative rules of conduct for each profession. Prescriptive authority may be granted to a variety of types of health-care providers in a state, including optometrists, naturopaths, and clinical psychologists. Some states grant prescriptive authority to NPs solely through the board of nursing (plenary authority), whereas others require a joint process through a board of medicine or pharmacy. Some states require involvement of a board or authority other than the board of nursing only when controlled substances will be part of prescriptive authority.

Prescriptive authority exists as dependent and independent authority. Independent authority permits the prescriber to exert autonomous judgment. Dependent authority exists when the primary prescriber delegates the authority to another through a collaborative or supervisory agreement. These agreements usually involve written guidelines and/or a protocol for treatment. Some states limit authority by restricting prescribing to a written formulary. Other restrictions may apply, including limits on the geographic locations of the clinical site or limits on the number of doses or refills that may be authorized, or requiring written agreements with a practicing NP that spell out the scope of the prescribing authority. Dispensing, which means the release of a prescription from other than a pharmacy for a patient to take home, is an authority that some states grant with varying degrees of requirements to prescribing practitioners. All states permit NPs some degree of prescribing and all permit dispensing of samples with appropriate prescriptive authority.

Chapter 1 discusses the laws across states. Each year, the January issues of *Nurse Practitioner* and *The Journal for Nurse Practitioners* contains a review of the current state laws regarding prescriptive authority for advanced practice nurses. This review is useful in determining the current status of prescribing in each state.

Writing and Transmitting the Prescription

The Prescription Format

A number of directions need to be communicated in writing or verbally to the dispensing pharmacist to complete a prescription properly. Tools such as the Institute for Safe Medication Practice's (ISMP) *List of Error-Prone Abbreviations, Symbols and Dose Designations* (2012) can help prescribers decrease transmission errors. The following are suggestions to provide a complete, safe prescription:

1. Use preprinted prescription pads/electronic templates that contain the name, address, and telephone number and NPI number of the prescriber. This will allow the pharmacist to contact the prescriber if there are any questions about the prescription.
2. Designate the complete drug name, strength, dosage, and form.
3. Indicate the date of the prescription.
4. Use metric units of measure, such as milligrams and milliliters; avoid apothecary units of measure.
5. Avoid abbreviations.
6. Avoid the use of "as directed" or "as needed."
7. Include the general indication, such as "for infection."
8. Indicate "Dispense as Written" if generic substitution is not desired.
9. Include the patient weight, especially if pediatric or elderly.
10. Indicate if a safety cap is not required, as medications will be dispensed with them by default.

Examples of prescriptions are found in Figures 4-2 and 4-3.

As of April 1, 2008, all written prescriptions for covered outpatient drugs paid for by Medicaid must be designated on tamper-proof prescription paper. The required elements are adopted into state pharmacy law and include specific inks and papers. Contact the state board directly regarding state-specific prescription requirements.

The appropriate amount of drug and the refill authorization benefit the patient in terms of convenience and may reduce the cost of therapy. For acute therapies, the amount prescribed should be enough to cure the illness or maintain therapy until the next patient visit. Overprescribing is costly, permits inappropriate self-treatment with leftover doses, and contributes to the risk of accidental overdose. Patients cannot return unused drugs to the pharmacy for credit or disposal. Conversely, for the treatment of chronic illness, it is more economical to obtain a supply of medication for 90 days

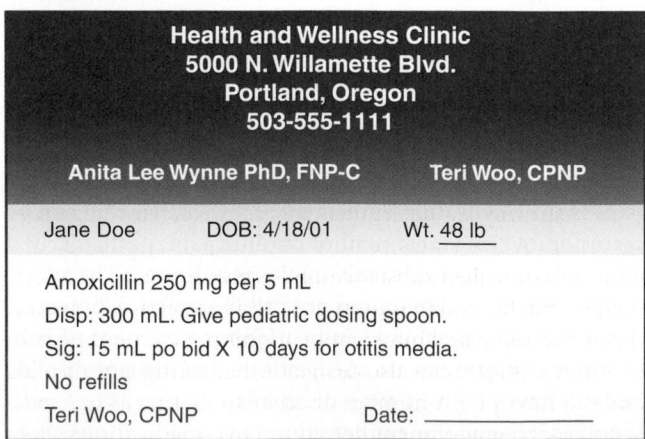

Figure 4–2. Sample prescription.

```
┌─────────────────────────────────────────┐
│         Health and Wellness Clinic       │
│           5000 N. Willamette Blvd.       │
│              Portland, Oregon            │
│                503-555-1111              │
│                                          │
│  Anita Lee Wynne PhD, FNP-C    Teri Woo, CPNP │
├─────────────────────────────────────────┤
│ John Doe       DOB: 6/5/51    Date: _____ │
├─────────────────────────────────────────┤
│ Oxycodone  5 mg                          │
│ Disp: 30 (thirty)                        │
│ Sig: 1 tablet q4–6h pm back pain.        │
│    Do not drive or use hazardous machinery until response │
│    is known. May produce drowsiness. Do not exceed │
│    6 tablets per day.                    │
│ No refills                               │
│ Anita Lee Wynne, FNP-C        DEA # on file in pharmacy │
└─────────────────────────────────────────┘
```

Figure 4–3. Sample prescription for controlled substance.

instead of repeated refills of smaller quantities. Mail-order pharmacies and insurance plans may require that a 90-day supply be dispensed with each prescription. It is judicious to prescribe small initial trial supplies until patient dosage and compliance can be determined, followed by larger refill quantities for chronic therapy.

Schedule II drugs may not be refilled and require a new prescription for each dispensed quantity. However, it is legal and acceptable to write 3 months' worth of prescriptions at one visit for established and stable patients. This is done by writing three separate prescriptions, each with the current visit date, and a statement "do not fill until__." The dates for the next 2- and 3-month refills can be filled in on each prescription, and these can be given to the patient in one visit, mailed, or left for pick up and signature.

What May Be Prescribed

Prescriptions are required for the majority of controlled drugs (state laws may permit the sale of Schedule V controlled substances without a prescription in limited quantities). They are also required for some medical devices, home-health and home-testing equipment, durable medical equipment, needles and syringes, and sometimes for Medicaid or Medicare coverage of OTC medications that are required for patient health. Prescriptions are required in order to compound medications for patient administration in strengths or formulas not otherwise available.

State-Specific Elements

State pharmacy law determines the required format for a prescription. A few states require duplicate or triplicate copy pads for controlled substances. NPs who prescribe in a state with mandated collaboration or supervision may need to indicate the name and information of this person on their prescriptions. A state can also designate that a drug is controlled and requires a DEA number or other special authority, even if the federal government does not. This is becoming true of pseudoephedrine, which is used for methamphetamine man-

ufacturing. A state may pass laws regarding medications that are more restrictive but may not pass laws more permissive than federal law. NPs must verify prescribing laws through their state board of nursing and pharmacy. Less commonly, a board of medicine may also be legally involved in an NP's prescribing practices and regulations.

Electronic Prescribing and Secure Prescribing

The days of "writing" a prescription may soon be over. Electronic prescribing is enjoying support and institutional funding as a method for decreasing medication error and increasing drug tracking and accountability. Electronic prescribing has been implicated, however, in medication errors as well. Prescribers may become exceedingly reliant on pre-populated protocols and dosages that may not apply to the individual patient's clinical circumstances. Most electronic health record systems have override features that are easy to implement, and this can be a benefit, but it can also be a danger in the wrong hands. It is critical that NPs who prescribe take responsibility for individually verifying appropriate doses and treatments. If in doubt, a pharmacist may be consulted directly, and many large universities run free consulting services for this purpose.

As of June 1, 2010, the DEA's revised "Electronic Prescriptions for Controlled Substances" regulation provides practitioners with the option of writing prescriptions for controlled substances electronically (DEA, 2010). The DEA outlines a certifying process required in order for prescribers and pharmacies to transmit electronic prescriptions for controlled substances. NPs will need to be aware of this issue, carefully follow state and federal legislation related to the area of electronic prescribing, and follow all DEA instructions regarding availability of prescribing software that is state-approved for electronic prescribing of controlled substances.

ETHICAL ASPECTS OF PRESCRIBING

Informed Consent

The notion of informed consent is shorthand for the doctrine of informed decision making, which proposes that patients have the right to make informed decisions about those things that will affect them. Although some question whether consent to medical procedures can ever be truly informed, the doctrine has been assimilated into American society's concept of what clinical practice should include. Informed consent should be obtained from a patient before all medical interventions, diagnostic as well as therapeutic. A patient may either agree to or refuse a proposed intervention; in both situations, the patient is making her or his own informed decision.

The provider who performs a specific service is responsible for obtaining consent to that specific service. The consent usually is given to the identified provider, as well as others working with him or her to perform the specific procedure or associated procedures. In general, a referring provider is not responsible for getting consent for a procedure performed by another provider. Some exceptions may apply, however, and practitioners who send patients for tests or consultations should inform them generally about the procedure and their clinical recommendations for requiring it.

Informed consent has four critical features: (1) a competent patient (2) who is provided adequate information with which to make a decision (3) and who voluntarily (4) consents to a proposed intervention. Although legal opinions tend to merge the concepts, it is helpful to consider competence as two related but distinct areas: legal competence and clinical competence. A patient must be both legally and clinically competent to give informed consent. In general, an adult is presumed to be legally competent unless declared incompetent in formal legal proceedings. To be clinically competent for medical decision making, a patient must be able to comprehend information that is provided, formulate a decision about a proposed intervention, and communicate that decision to the health-care team. Patients may be deemed legally competent to make certain types of decisions or give consent but not legally responsible for all decision making.

Clinical competence is also not an all-or-none phenomenon. A patient may be competent to make some choices but not others. Clinical competence may vary over time and is affected by the course of an individual's illness and therapies currently in use. Assistive devices and environmental modification may be important to maintaining and enhancing clinical competence. Hearing aids, interpreters, and communication boards may be key assistive devices to certain patients. Examples of environmental factors that affect clinical competence include sedative medications, presence of background noise for a patient with a hearing disability, and the side of approach to a patient with a visual field loss.

A medication agreement, as discussed in this chapter, may also outline informed consent for initial and ongoing treatment with medications that have the potential for side effects and habituation. Mental health medications have specific consent regulations due to the vulnerability of their target population. Other areas that may have specific consent procedures include prescribing medications for elderly or minor patients. Parental or partner involvement in prescribing determinations related to sexually transmitted infections, family planning, and birth control may be limited under specific state law, and a minor may give informed consent for some surgical or medical procedures even if a parent is not informed. These are sensitive areas of law that require specific study. Advice of an attorney may be required.

Prescribing for Self, Family, or Friends

State law varies regarding whether an NP can prescribe for family or friends. In order for a prescription to be clinically legitimate, a patient must be assessed and there must be a record of his or her assessment. It is clearly unethical to prescribe for oneself, and many states punish this with significant fines or board action. Although it may be technically legal to prescribe for family or friends, an NP needs to consider whether it is ethical. If the clinical circumstance requires a controlled substance, the judicious prescriber will refer a friend or family member to a colleague for confidential assessment and treatment. It is never considered ethical for a mental health provider to engage a family member or close friend in a clinically therapeutic relationship, whether or not prescribing is involved.

Sale of Pharmaceuticals and Supplements

It is illegal to sell pharmaceuticals that are designated as samples and provided to a clinic for free distribution to patients. Depending on the dispensing laws of the state, it may be permissible to stock and sell limited amounts of commonly prescribed medications within the practice setting. It may also be permissible to sell supplements such as prenatal vitamins or fish oil, especially if the prescriber is able to order them at a discount and pass the savings on to the patient. It may not be technically illegal but can be ethically questionable if the prescriber is selling medications with a broad profit margin to patients perceived as vulnerable.

NURSE PRACTITIONER ROLE OUTSIDE THE UNITED STATES

The NP role is expanding to health systems outside of the United States. As an example, in 2004–2006 the Canadian government funded the Nurse Practitioner Initiative to promote recognition, education, and utilization of NPs as primary care providers. Similar to U.S. states, Canadian provinces have individual practice acts that designate the parameters and autonomy of prescriptive authority. Prior to legislative recognition of the NP role, many provinces, such as Ontario, had provisions for a class of RN with expanded or extended practice permitting limited diagnosis and prescribing.

One significant difference in Canada, which is also true of the UK and its Nurse Practitioner movement, is that prescribing is supported by a national pharmacy system. Nationally adopted core competencies outlined in *The Canadian Nurse Practitioner Core Competency Framework* (Canadian Nurses Association, 2010) clearly articulate preparation of an NP who will be competent to select, prescribe, monitor, and dispense prescription medications. A national expert advisory committee (CEDAC) reviews and recommends drugs for provincial formularies based on efficacy and evidence-based review. Provinces develop formularies for prescribing, which may be further modified based on scope of practice for individual health professions. A provincial pharmacy network, known as PharmaNet, records all community prescriptions in a central database, which facilitates checking for duplication, contraindications, and interactions.

NPs have controlled substance prescribing ability in many Canadian provinces. They may also order laboratory tests, blood products, and other therapeutic interventions and diagnostics. Both NPs and pharmacists in the UK have prescribing ability, based on formularies or standards adopted based on national guidelines.

The NP role is expanding in other countries, such as Australia and New Zealand, to address primary care needs. In 2010, nurse practitioners in Australia gained approval to prescribe medicines designated by an "NP" on the Pharmaceutical Benefits Scheme (PBS) list of medications. In 2011, the Australian Controlled Substances Act was amended to allow prescribing of scheduled drugs. In 2013, the number of endorsed NPs in Australia passed 1,000. New Zealand has followed a similar pattern, with NPs gaining prescribing authority in 2013 and the ability to prescribe controlled substances in 2014.

REFERENCES

Barton, J. H., & Emanuel, E. J. (2005). The patents-based pharmaceutical development process: Rationale, problems, and potential reforms. *Journal of the American Medical Association, 294,* 2075–2082.

Butler, S. F., Fernandez, K., Benoit, C., Budman, S. H., & Jamison, R. N. (2008). Validation of the Revised Screener and Opioid Assessment for Patients with Pain (SOAPP-R). *Journal of Pain, 9*(4), 360–372.

Canadian Nurses Association. (2010). *The Canadian nurse practitioner core competency framework.* Retrieved from http://www2.cna-aiic.ca/CNA/documents/pdf/publications/Competency_Framework_2010_e.pdf

Coben, J. H., Davis, S. M., Furbee, P. M., Sikora, R. D., Tollitson, R. D., & Bossarte, R. M. (2010). Hospitalizations for poisoning by prescription opioids, sedatives, and tranquilizers. *American Journal of Preventive Medicine, 38*(5), 517–524.

DiMasi, J. A., Grabowski, H. G., & Hansen, R. W. (2014). Cost to develop and win marketing approval for a new drug is $2.6 billion. Tufts Center for the Study of New Drug Development. Retrieved from http://csdd.tufts.edu/news/complete_story/pr_tufts_csdd_2014_cost_study

Duke Clinical Research Institute. (2010). New drug development timeline. Clinical Trials Network Best Practices. Retrieved from https://www.ctnbestpractices.org/

Gillick, M. (2009). Controlling off-label medication use. *Annals of Internal Medicine, 150*(5), 344–347.

Hsu, J., Price, M., Huang, J., Brand, R., Fung, V., Hui, R., et al. (2006). Unintended consequences of caps on Medicare drug benefits. *New England Journal of Medicine, 354,* 2349–2359.

Institute for Safe Medication Practices. (2012). ISMP's List of Error-Prone Abbreviations, Symbols, and Dose Designations. Retrieved from http://www.ismp.org/tools/errorproneabbreviations.pdf

Oregon State Board of Nursing. (2012). *Prescriptive authority in Oregon for nurse practitioners and clinical nurse specialists.* Retrieved from http://www.oregon.gov/OSBN

Passik, S., & Portenoy, R. (1998). Substance abuse issues in palliative care. In A. Berger (Ed.), *Principles and practices of supportive oncology* (pp 513–530). New York: Lippincott-Raven.

Passik S., & Weinreb, H. (2000). Managing chronic nonmalignant pain: Overcoming obstacles to the use of opioids. *Advances in Therapy, 17*(2), 70–83.

Portenoy, R. K. (1996). Opioid therapy for chronic nonmalignant pain: Clinicians' perspective. *Journal of Law and Medical Ethics, 24*(4), 296–309.

U.S. Drug Enforcement Administration (DEA). (2006). *A practitioner's manual: An informational outline of the Controlled Substances Act.* Retrieved from http://www.deadiversion.usdoj.gov/pubs/manuals/pract/index.html

U.S. Food and Drug Administration (FDA). (2010). Milestones in food and drug law history. Retrieved from http://www.fda.gov/AboutFDA/WhatWeDo/History/Milestones/default.htm

U.S. Drug Enforcement Administration (DEA). (2010). State prescription drug monitoring programs. Retrieved from http://www.deadiversion.usdoj.gov/faq/rx_monitor.htm#4

U.S. Food and Drug Administration (FDA). (2012). What does FDA regulate? Retrieved from http://www.fda.gov/AboutFDA/Transparency/Basics/ucm194879.htm

CHAPTER 5

ADVERSE DRUG REACTIONS

Connie A. Valdez • Anne E. Morgan • Peter J. Rice

According to the U.S. Food and Drug Administration (FDA), over 2 million serious adverse drug reactions (ADRs) occur annually, resulting in emergency room visits, hospital admissions, and an estimated 100,000 deaths (FDA, 2009). It is estimated that 3% to 6% of all hospital admissions annually are for treatment of ADRs and that 10% to 15% of hospitalized patients experience an ADR (Gomes & Demoly, 2005). The total cost associated with ADRs has been estimated to range from $3.5 to $136 billion per year (Centers for Disease Control and Prevention [CDC], 2012; FDA, 2009;). In order to reduce morbidity and mortality associated with ADRs, it is important for practitioners to understand the causes and mechanisms of ADRs and develop practices to predict and prevent their occurrence.

An ADR is any undesirable or unintended effect following administration of a medical product, whether or not the effect is considered related to the medical product (FDA, 1995, 2009). Although ADRs are common, most are not severe and usually resolve when the drug is discontinued or the dose reduced, or they diminish as the body adjusts to the drug. For example, dry mouth from amitriptyline is a mild reaction that will resolve once the medication has been discontinued; dizziness from lisinopril is generally considered to be a common reaction that can be minimized by reducing the dose; an individual using diphenhydramine will notice that the sedative effects will diminish after about 2 to 3 weeks of consistent use. Unfortunately, some ADRs may be serious and/or persist for a significant duration of time even after the drug is discontinued. For example, isotretinoin can cause birth defects when used before or during pregnancy, and antipsychotics can cause tardive dyskinesia that endures after discontinuation of the medication. Since ADRs manifest in many forms, it is helpful to categorize the reactions based on type, onset, and severity.

MECHANISTIC CLASSIFICATION OF ADRS

There are two basic types of ADRs: pharmacological and idiosyncratic (Aronson & Ferner, 2003; Pirmohamed, Breckenridge, Kitteringham, & Park, 1998). A pharmacological reaction (Table 5-1) is often predictable based on the drug's mechanism of action and is typically dose-related (Aronson & Ferner, 2003; Edwards & Aronson, 2000; Pirmohamed et al, 1998). Idiosyncratic reactions are unpredictable and may be more likely to result in mortality (Aronson & Ferner; Edwards & Aronson; Pirmohamed et al, 1998).

Pharmacological ADRs are more common and comprise approximately 85% to 90% of reported ADRs (Pirmohamed et al, 1998). These reactions are often an exaggerated physiological response related to the pharmacology of the drug,

Table 5–1 Pharmacological Adverse Drug Reactions

85%–90%	Predictable and dose-dependent
10%–15%	Idiosyncratic: unpredictable and not dose-related

Table 5–2 Immune-Mediated Adverse Drug Reactions

Type I	IgE-mediated, immediate-type hypersensitivity Example: angioedema and anaphylaxis
Type II	Antibody-dependent cytotoxicity Example: heparin-induced thrombocytopenia
Type III	Immune complex hypersensitivity Example: Arthus reaction to tetanus vaccine
Type IV	Cell-mediated or delayed hypersensivity Example: Drug Rash, Eosinophilia and Systemic Syndrome

for example, hypotension from the beta blocker metoprolol, diarrhea from the fat-blocking drug orlistat, and insomnia from the stimulant methylphenidate. These adverse reactions are often managed by withdrawing the medication or reducing the dose. Pharmacological ADRs may also occur based on secondary pharmacology, such as weight gain from the atypical antipsychotic olanzapine, flatulence from the fiber supplement psyllium, or myopathy from the HMG Co-A reductase drug simvastatin. Because there is an interest in reducing adverse effects, preclinical trials are now focusing attention on secondary adverse effects to predict what may occur when the drug is administered to humans.

Idiosyncratic reactions are concerning because they are unpredictable, often serious, and may result in death (Pirmohamed et al, 1998). Idiosyncratic reactions are mediated by the immune system, receptor abnormalities, drug–drug interactions, abnormalities in drug metabolism, pharmaceutical variations, or unmasking of an abnormal biological system. Most commonly, idiosyncratic reactions are mediated by the immune system when a drug molecule is recognized as a foreign substance (Aronson & Ferner, 2003; Edwards & Aronson, 2000; Pirmohamed et al, 1998).

The hapten hypothesis describes how drugs may cause an immune-mediated hypersensitivity reaction. The hypothesis suggests that drugs are haptens, that is, low-molecular-weight chemicals that can become antigenic when they covalently bind to a carrier molecule, which is usually a protein (Chipinda, Hettick, & Siegel, 2011). Through this mechanism, individual patterns of metabolism may generate reactive metabolites that act as haptens to elicit an immune-mediated reaction. Penicillin is an example of a hapten with a low molecular weight that is able to bind to a protein and result in a Type I hypersensitivity (anaphylaxis) reaction.

Medications that are not haptens are also able to elicit an immune-mediated reaction through a different mechanism identified as the "pharmacologic interaction with immune receptors." For example, lidocaine, sulfamethoxazole, mepivacaine, celecoxib, carbamazepine, lamotrigine, and ciprofloxacin are chemically inert drugs, unable to covalently bind to proteins. However, these medications are able to "fit" into major histocompatibility complex (a set of surface molecules) and the T-cell receptor sandwich. This elicits a hypersensitivity reaction (Chipinda et al, 2011). Immune-mediated reactions can be further defined as Type I, II, III, or IV hypersensitivity reactions as described in Table 5-2 (Janeway, Travers, Walport, et al, 2001).

Type I immune-mediated reactions (IgE-mediated, immediate-type hypersensitivity) are provoked by reexposure to an antigen. A Type I reaction is an acute hypersensitivity reaction that may be local or systemic, involving the skin, bronchopulmonary system, nasopharynx tract, eyes, and/or gastrointestinal tract. It is caused by inducing the release of mediators (i.e., histamine, leukotrienes, and prostaglandins) from mast cells, basophils, and recruited inflammatory cells following antigen exposure, which then activates IgE. Although most cases are mild, symptoms may vary from mild to severe (allergic conjunctivitis, rhinitis, bronchospasm, urticaria, atopic dermatitis) and can be life-threatening (angioedema, anaphylactic shock). Symptoms may occur immediately, within minutes, or have a delayed onset where it may take several hours for symptoms to present following exposure to the provoking medication or antigen. For example, acute anaphylaxis may occur following the exposure to antibiotics (penicillin, cephalosporins, sulfonamides), neuromuscular blockers (suxamethonium, alcuronium, vecuronium, pancuronium, atracurium), and some chemotherapeutic agents (carboplatin, oxaliplatin) and monoclonal antibodies (cetuximab, rituximab). Management of Type I reactions usually involves administration of epinephrine, antihistamines, and corticosteroids.

Type II hypersensitivity reactions (antibody-dependent cytotoxicity) may affect a variety of organs and tissues. In the bloodstream and on the surface of cells, antibodies unite with antigens or haptens and induce destruction of cells and tissues through activation of the complement system or through removal by macrophages. Immune-mediated thrombocytopenia, also called *drug-induced immune thrombocytopenia* (DITP), is generally caused by medications but may also be caused by foods or herbal products. Most DITP reactions are associated with the formation of drug-dependent antibodies that bind to glycoprotein and cause an antibody–platelet reaction resulting in thrombocytopenia. Examples of medications with a risk of DITP include abciximab, argatroban, beta-lactam antibiotics, carbamazepine, eptifibatide, linezolid, phenytoin, quinine, quinidine, sulfonamide, rifampin, ranitidine, tirofiban, trimethoprim-sulfamethoxazole, valproic acid, and vancomycin (Aster, Curtis, McFarland, & Bougie, 2009; Burgess, Lopez, Gaudry, & Chong, 2000; Dihmess, et al,

2012; Gentilini, Curtis, & Aster, 1998; George et al, 1998; Kaufman et al, 1993; Nguyen, Reese, & George, 2011; Patel et al, 2010; Pedersen-Bjergaard, Andersen, & Hansen, 1996; Pedersen-Bjergaard, Andersen, & Hansen, 1997; Pedersen-Bjergaard, Andersen, & Hansen, 1998; Pereira et al, 2000; ten Berg et al, 2006; Von Drygalski et al, 2007).

DITP can also occur when heparin binds to platelet factor 4 (PF4) proteins resulting in the formation of an antigenic complex where IgG antibodies bind to the platelet. The antibody-coated platelets are viewed by the body as foreign and the body destroys the platelets via complement activation, causing thrombocytopenia. Hemolytic anemia and neutropenia occur by a similar mechanism. Hemolytic anemia occurs when a drug binds to antigens on the surface of red blood cells, resulting in complement activation and cell lysis. Examples of medications that cause hemolytic anemia include cephalosporins (e.g., cefotetan, ceftriaxone), penicillin and penicillin derivatives, NSAIDs, quinidine, quinine, and trimethoprim-sulfamethoxazole. Neutropenia or agranulocytosis can occur when antibodies unite with antigens on the surface of neutrophils. The reaction time generally occurs within minutes to hours following drug administration. Examples of common drugs that cause neutropenia or agranulocytosis include clozapine, antithyroid medications (e.g., methimazole, carbimazole), sulfasalazine, clomipramine, trimethoprim-sulfamethoxazole, ACE inhibitors, and H2 receptor antagonists (Alvir, Lieberman, Safferman, Schwimmer, & Schaaf, 1993; Casato et al, 1995; van der Klauw et al, 1999; Yunis, Lieberman, & Yunis, 1992). Treatment involves anti-inflammatory and immunosuppressive agents.

Type III hypersensitivity reactions (immune complex hypersensitivity) occur when aggregates of antigens and IgG and IgM antibodies create insoluble immune complexes in vessels or the blood that may be deposited in tissues (e.g., joints, kidneys). The reaction generally takes a week or more to occur and may present as serum sickness, drug fever, or vasculitis. The Arthus reaction is a local vasculitis reaction that causes severe pain, swelling, edema, induration, hemorrhage, and possibly necrosis, which can occur following tetanus/diphtheria toxoid (Td) vaccination. The risk of the Arthus reaction from the Td vaccine is elevated when a patient receives vaccination more frequently than every 10 years. The risk of developing more antibody–antigen immune complexes is higher if revaccination occurs when there is a high concentration of circulating tetanus antibodies. This is because the Arthus reaction results from deposition of immune complexes and complement activation. For this reason, it is recommended that individuals who have experienced an Arthus reaction following vaccination with tetanus toxoid do not receive Td more frequently than every 10 years, even if the vaccine is part of a protocol for wound management. The Arthus reaction can also occur with the 23 valent pneumococcal vaccine, and should this occur following the initial dose, revaccination is contraindicated (CDC MMRW, 1997). Other medications and treatments that can cause type III

hypersensivity reactions include streptokinase, monoclonal antibodies (e.g., rituximab, infliximab, alemtuzumab, omalizumab, natalizumab), rabies vaccine, antivenom, and other antitoxins. These reactions are treated with antihistamines and anti-inflammatory agents (NSAIDS and corticosteroids).

Type IV hypersensitivity reactions (cell-mediated or delayed-type hypersensitivity) are unlike other hypersensitivity reactions because they are not an antibody-mediated reaction but rather, a cell-mediated response that results in activation and proliferation of T cells. Type IV hypersensitivity reactions are the result of autoimmune and infectious diseases or contact dermatitis. These reactions generally occur within 2 to 3 days but may take days to weeks to occur. Following rechallenge, the reaction may occur within 24 hours.

The reaction may be in the form of contact dermatitis, morbilliform or maculopapular eruptions, Stevens–Johnson syndrome, toxic epidermal necrolysis, or drug-induced hypersensitivity syndrome. Drug-induced hypersensitivity syndrome (DiHS) is a severe reaction that not only causes rash but is frequently associated with fever (38° to 40°C), eosinophilia, and organ failure (i.e., lungs, kidney, liver, heart). DiHS is also known as DRESS (Drug Rash, Eosinophilia and Systemic Symptoms) (Ben m'rad et al, 2009; Cacoub et al, 2011; Peyrière et al, 2006). Examples of drugs that may cause DRESS include abacavir, allopurinol, carbamazepine, dapsone, minocycline, nevirapine, and phenobarbital. Corticosteroids and other immunosuppressive agents are used in treatment.

ADRs have also been categorized as Types A–F. Type A reactions are equivalent to pharmacological reactions, account for 85% to 90% of ADRs, are dose-dependent, and are predictable, whereas Type B reactions are idiosyncratic, account for 10% to 15% of ADRs, are not dose-dependent, and are not predictable (Rawlins, 1981). Adverse reactions have been further stratified by letters C through F. Type C reactions result from chronic medication use, Type D reactions are delayed, Type E reactions are from drug–drug interactions, and Type F reactions result from treatment failures.

TIME-RELATED CLASSIFICATION OF ADRS

One distinguishing feature of drug reactions is the correlation between administration and tissue exposure to onset of the reaction. The World Allergy Organization classifies immunological reactions as immediate or delayed. Symptom presentation that occurs within 1 hour following exposure is classified as an immediate reaction, whereas a delayed reaction occurs more than an hour following exposure (Johansson et al, 2004). Time-related reactions can be further categorized as rapid, first dose, early, intermediate, late, and delayed.

Rapid reactions occur during or immediately following the administration of a medication. These unintended adverse reactions generally occur when medications are administered improperly and are not necessarily related to being the first dose. For example, vancomycin can cause an adverse reaction known as red man syndrome when administered too rapidly (Aronson & Ferner, 2003). Phenytoin can cause can adverse reaction known as purple glove syndrome (blood vessel irritation and inflammation) when administered peripherally (Earnest, Marx, & Drury, 1983). Skin or tissue necrosis secondary to extravasation may occur with administration of chemotherapeutic agents. For example, hand-foot syndrome may occur when extravasation of chemotherapy occurs and damages the surrounding tissues in the hands and feet, causing redness, swelling, burning, blisters, ulcers, peeling skin, and difficulty when walking (Yokomichi et al, 2013). For these reasons, it is important for practitioners to be familiar with the proper administration technique of medications to avoid precipitation of these adverse reactions.

First-dose reactions occur following the first dose of a medication. For example, orthostatic hypotension is a common reaction that occurs following the first dose of doxazosin, which generally does not occur with repeated doses. Cytokine release syndrome can occur following the first dose of orthoclone OKT3. Patient education and monitoring are essential when administering medications that are known to have a first-dose reaction, especially to ensure continued adherence, as the reaction is unlikely to persist.

Early reactions occur early in treatment and generally resolve with continued treatment as the patient develops tolerance. These reactions typically do not require discontinuation of the drug but may simply require patients to adapt to the medications. It is often useful to initiate drugs likely to cause early reactions with low starting doses and sequentially titrate the dose upward to mitigate the severity and duration of side effects. Examples include gastrointestinal upset following the initiation of metformin or selective serotonin reuptake inhibitors. Immune hypersensitivities may occur following the first or subsequent dose. These reactions, however, often do require immediate discontinuation of the drug and possibly further medical attention, such as in the case of anaphylaxis resulting from administration of penicillin or its derivatives.

Intermediate reactions occur following repeated exposure to a medication. Examples include hyperuricemia from furosemide, hemolytic anemia from ceftriaxone, interstitial nephritis from penicillin G, and contact dermatitis from neomycin. Intermediate reactions are difficult to predict but should be monitored. Patients with predisposing factors or increased susceptibility for adverse reactions should be followed vigilantly while on therapy for occurrence of these reactions.

Late reactions occur after prolonged exposure to an offending agent. Examples include osteoporosis or thinning of the skin due to prolonged corticosteroid use or hypogonadism following prolonged use of opioids (Brennan, 2013). It may be possible to symptomatically treat late adverse drug reactions, but most are predictable and occur following repeated exposures. Thus, it is often recommended to remove the offending agent before the reaction is predicted to occur in order to manage this type of adverse effect. Late reactions also include reactions that occur when a dose of a chronic medication is reduced or withdrawn. For example, rapid discontinuation of oxycodone can cause the patient to experience symptoms of withdrawal (i.e., anxiety, insomnia, rhinorrhea, diaphoresis, tremor, vomiting, diarrhea, and/or tachycardia). A patient who takes clonidine or propranolol may experience rebound hypertension following withdrawal of the medication. These types of adverse drug reactions are relatively common and can often be avoided by thoughtful tapering of the drug, as they are a predictable extension of the drug's therapeutic effect.

Delayed reactions occur at variable time points following drug exposure and can even occur after the discontinuation of a drug. For example, drug-induced tardive dyskinesia may occur following prolonged exposure to antipsychotics or metoclopramide, with symptoms persisting for months to years following discontinuation of the precipitating drug (Tarsy & Baldessarini, 1984). Polyalkylimide implant injection (cosmetic filler) can cause swelling and tender nodules near the injection site as well as other symptoms (fever, arthritis, xerostomia) up to 12 months following the injection.

DOSE-RELATED ADRS

Adverse drug reactions may also be dose-related. This could be from administering an excessive dose or failing to adjust doses properly for age and organ function (i.e., renal insufficiency or liver failure). For example, a person with diabetes may become hypoglycemic after administering an excessive dose of insulin. An individual patient could experience lithium toxicity upon development of acute renal failure with no adjustment of the lithium dose.

SEVERITY OF ADRS

The severity of an adverse drug reaction varies based on the clinical effect and the outcome. The FDA defines serious ADRs as those that result in death, are life-threatening, result in hospitalization (new or prolonged), are disabling or incapacitating, produce congenital abnormality or birth defect, or require an intervention to prevent one of these outcomes. Any ADR that meets FDA criteria should be reported to the FDA MedWatch program (FDA, 2013).

In this chapter, the severity of ADRs will be further categorized as mild, moderate, and severe. Mild adverse events can typically be managed by dose reduction, discontinuation of the drug, or with no intervention if the reaction subsides following development of tolerance by the patient (Aronson & Ferner, 2003; FDA, 2013;). Moderate adverse events often require discontinuation of the drug and minimal medical intervention but typically do not cause permanent harm. An example of a moderate adverse reaction is drug-induced sunburn requiring an analgesic to treat the pain. Severe ADRs may be life-threatening and result in hospitalization, disability, birth defects, or even death and will require intensive medical intervention (FDA, 2013).

COMMON CAUSES OF ADRS

It is important for practitioners to realize that many ADRs are preventable. Approximately one-third result from medication errors and up to one-third from allergic reactions (Budnitz et al, 2006). Practitioners can reduce ADRs by being aware of specific drugs and drug classes that have a high incidence of ADRs. Budnitz and others evaluated ADRs that led to an emergency department visit. One single drug or drug class was the suspected cause in 94% of those cases. The top five drug classes responsible included insulins, opioid-containing analgesics, anticoagulants, amoxicillin-containing medications, and antihistamines or cold remedies. Additionally, the top five drug classes implicated in precipitating hospitalizations following admission to the emergency department included anticoagulants, insulins, opioid-containing analgesics, oral hypoglycemic medications, and antineoplastic agents. In the elderly population, one-third of all ADRs requiring treatment in the emergency department were due to only three medications: warfarin, insulin, and digoxin (Budnitz et al, 2006). In addition to the above medications, practitioners should be aware that antibiotics, sedatives, antipsychotics, and chemotherapeutic agents are also drug classes that have a high rate of ADRs (Bates et al, 1995; Evans, Lloyd, Stoddard, Nebeker, & Samore, 2005; Gurwitz et al, 2005; Woolcott et al, 2009).

One of the most common manifestations of ADRs is in the form of cutaneous skin reactions, ranging from mild skin rashes to life-threatening Stevens–Johnson syndrome. Out of the top 10 drugs linked to skin reactions, the majority are antibiotics. Specifically, the top 10 drugs linked to skin reactions are, in order, amoxicillin, trimethoprim-sulfamethoxazole, ampicillin, iopodate, blood products, cephalosporins, erythromycin, dihydralazine hydrochloride, penicillin G, and cyanocobalamin (vitamin B_{12}) (Roujeau & Stern, 1994).

RISK FACTORS

Multiple patient characteristics can increase an individual's risk of experiencing an adverse drug reaction (Aronson & Ferner, 2003). Risk factors for ADRs include genetic abnormalities, age, sex, polypharmacy (increasing the risk for drug–drug interactions), and concomitant medical conditions (increasing the chance for drug–disease interactions). Not all drug classes are susceptible to these risks, but an assessment should be made for all patients when starting or stopping medications to determine the relevance.

Genetics

Genetic features that affect the body's ability to metabolize medications can contribute to pharmacological and idiosyncratic reactions (FDA, 2009; Pirmohamed et al, 1998). Although rare, some people have DNA mutations that predispose them to develop adverse drug reactions. For example, if an individual has an alteration in liver enzyme activity secondary to a gene mutation, the rate at which affected medications are metabolized may be increased or decreased, thus altering the concentration of active, inactive, and potentially toxic drug products in the circulation. If drugs are not metabolized appropriately, patients can accumulate toxic or reactive metabolites, leading to adverse drug reactions, as is the case with acetaminophen. Malignant hyperthermia following administration of general anesthetics is an example of a receptor abnormality (mutations encoding for abnormal RYR1 or DHP receptors), which results in sustained muscle contraction from the unregulated movement of calcium from the sarcoplasmic reticulum into the intracellular space. Genetic factors can also increase the likelihood of a hapten-induced hypersensitivity reaction (Pichler, Naisbitt, & Park, 2011).

A common mediator for these immune responses is variation in the *HLA-B* alleles. For example, patients who express the *HLA-B*5701* allele are at a significantly increased risk of severe T-cell–mediated hypersensitivity reactions to the HIV medication abacavir. Additionally, the Han Chinese, who express *HLA-B*1502* or *HLA-B*5801* alleles, are at higher risk of hypersensitivity reactions to carbamazepine and allopurinol, respectively. For this reason, it is recommended that all patients receive genetic testing to confirm the presence or absence of the specific *HLA-B* allele prior to initiation of known high-risk medications (Panel on Antiretroviral Guidelines for Adults and Adolescents, 2013; Pichler et al, 2011).

Age

Children and the elderly are at higher risk of experiencing an ADR (Budnitz et al, 2006; Kongkaew, Novce, & Ashcroft, 2008). Children are at higher risk primarily because medication dosages must be tailored to their specific weight or body mass index. Inattention to weight-based dosing may cause harm. The very young may additionally have immature organ function, which further complicates dosing and increases the risk for an ADR (Kaushal et al, 2001).

Predictable underlying concerns in patients over 65 include taking more medications and taking them more often than younger patients. Also, elderly patients have decreased renal and hepatic function, resulting in decreased metabolism and clearance and causing an elevated drug concentration and risk of drug accumulation and toxicity. Patients over the age of 65 required hospitalization for treatment of ADRs 7 times more often than patients under the age of 65 (Budnitz et al, 2006). Hospitalizations in this age group due to ADRs were most commonly a result of unintentional overdoses (Budnitz et al, 2006). More than half of ADRs in hospitalized patients 70 years of age and older are considered to be preventable (Gray, Sager, Lestico, & Jalaluddin, 1998). Therefore, all prescribers working with these populations should take care to minimize polypharmacy, unless clinically necessary, to reduce the risk of drug–drug interactions, confusion between medications, and drug accumulation with insufficient renal and hepatic function. In addition, it has been shown that four out of five ADRs can be prevented by using prescriber computer order entry with clinical decision support and clinical pharmacist consultation in high-risk populations (Kaushal et al, 2001).

Gender

Women have more ADRs than men in part due to differences in body composition (impacting drug distribution, pharmacokinetic properties of medications, and hormonal fluctuation). Furthermore, ADRs may be related to pregnancy and lactation.

Drug Interactions

Similar to genetic differences in metabolism, drug–drug interactions can also affect the rate at which individuals metabolize medications. Some medications bind to certain enzymes in the liver and either speed up (induction) or slow down (inhibition) the rate of metabolism and clearance of drugs that flow through the same enzyme pathway. Both scenarios can cause problems, but most commonly drug inhibition leads to accumulation of drug and higher-than-desired concentrations in the circulation, often leading to ADRs. An additional interaction is the potential for two drugs to compete for metabolism, which increases the concentration of both medications and the risk of side effects.

Most drug interactions can be identified by reviewing patient medication profiles and using a drug interaction checker, such as Micromedex, Online Facts and Comparisons, or Lexicomp. These resources also provide recommendations based on the severity of the interaction. A review of therapy should be performed prior to the initiation of new medications. There is also the potential for foods to interact and affect metabolism. The best example of food–drug interactions is grapefruit reducing the clearance of simvastatin and increasing the risk of myopathy, or herbal products such as St. John's wort reducing clearance of cyclosporine (Aronson & Ferner, 2003; FDA, 2009).

Some drug–drug interactions can manifest rapidly (within 1 to 2 days). For example, when trimethoprim-sulfamethoxazole is added to warfarin, an anticoagulant, warfarin metabolism is reduced, resulting in an increase in the INR and prothrombin time. Ultimately, this increases the risk of bleeding and should be avoided, if possible, or adjustments should be made in monitoring warfarin frequency and dose. Many interactions, however, may take longer to present. For example, when the antiarrhythmic amiodarone is added to digoxin, amiodarone inhibits the

metabolism of digoxin. This interaction can take weeks to months before the full extent of the effect precipitates due to the long half-life of amiodarone. It requires diligence to appropriately adjust the digoxin dose and monitor serum concentrations. Although not all interactions are significant, clinicians should evaluate each interaction and determine clinical importance.

Medical Conditions

Many disease states alter the physiology of the body and affect drug metabolism, increasing the risk of ADRs (FDA, 2009). Liver and renal disease can decrease the metabolism and clearance of medications, resulting in increased serum concentrations. Medications that are extensively cleared from the body through the kidneys have specific dosage adjustments based on creatinine clearance. These recommendations should be followed to prevent drug accumulation. Heart failure decreases liver and kidney perfusion and can reduce metabolism and clearance. Similarly, thyroid dysfunction can alter drug metabolism; decreased thyroid function will reduce metabolic activity and increased function is likely to induce a faster metabolic rate. Additionally, other medical conditions, such as pregnancy, can create temporary changes in physiology that require dose adjustments or avoidance to prevent adverse reactions for the mother and/or child. Practitioners should be aware that medications can also affect various medical conditions. For example, indomethacin can precipitate an exacerbation of heart failure, aggravate gastroesophageal reflux, or worsen renal function in a patient with kidney disease. For these reasons, patients should always be assessed for past medical history and concomitant medical conditions upon initiation and/or changes of drug therapy.

DETECTION AND ASSESSMENT OF ADRS

Drugs or drug combinations suspected of producing adverse reactions will frequently be identified through drug interaction screening by pharmacists. It is important to remember that most (~90%) of identified drug interactions will not have clinical consequences for an individual patient but do represent a warning to monitor an individual patient for a potential problem. A smaller number (perhaps 2%) of identified drug interactions will have profound clinical consequences. The clinical challenge is that individual adverse reactions can present in patients without warning. It is appropriate for prescribers to work closely with pharmacists and other members of the health-care team to identify potential problems and monitor patients closely to optimize patient medications.

It can be difficult to determine causality between a drug and a potential adverse drug reaction. To aid in this distinction, several important elements should be considered. The presence of a temporal relationship between drug exposure and a reaction is often the first clue for causality

(Field, Furwitz, Harrold, Rothschild, Debellis, Seger et al, 2004). Some reactions, such as hypersensitivity reactions, occur almost immediately upon administration and can be easily linked to the drug being administered. This is more common with IV medications because they are directly administered into the bloodstream. Pharmacological and hypersensitivity reactions to oral medications are likely to present early but may subside after persistent exposure. Assuming no other changes in medications or health status, adverse reactions that present temporally with administration of a new drug can often be attributed to the drug in question.

Adverse reactions due to drug–drug or drug–disease interactions may be more difficult to discern because the interactions may not follow the timeline for initiation of the offending agent but may be more closely related to changes in disease status or alterations in interacting medications.

Responding to ADRs and Warnings

Many drugs suspected of causing an ADR are promptly discontinued and should be if the offending drug can be safely stopped, if the event is life-threatening or intolerable, if continuing the medication would worsen the patient's condition, and if there is a reasonable alternative medication. Drugs responsible for an adverse drug reaction may be continued in a patient if the drug is medically necessary and there is no acceptable alternative drug or if the problems are tolerable and reversible. Most adverse reactions that are related to dose and pharmacological effects will respond favorably to dosage adjustment.

If the ADR resolves following discontinuation of the medication, then the adverse event was likely caused by the discontinued medication. The only definitive indicator for causality is the recurrence of an adverse event following readministration of a potential drug offender. As long as no other medication changes are made and no change in the patient's health status occurs, the reappearance of an ADR following a rechallenge confirms causality.

Rechallenge is not a common practice and is generally not appropriate, especially for life-threatening ADRs. Also, patients are often reluctant to retry something that potentially caused an ADR. Therefore, although rechallenge is the gold standard for ADR detection, causality is often presumed based on temporal relationships, patient risk factors, and/or disappearance of the ADR following removal of the drug.

Assessing the causality of an adverse drug reaction involves consideration of several parameters relative to the reaction. Prior history of an ADR to the same or similar medications, literature reports, or a relationship in time between drug administration and the onset and resolution of the ADR support causality by an individual drug. The presence of alternative etiologies or absence of a relationship between dosing and the ADR support alternative explanations for the adverse reaction.

Naranjo ADR Probability Scale

Naranjo et al (1981) developed a framework for assessing the probability that an adverse reaction is related to administration of a particular drug. The Naranjo protocol, based on timing, prior history and reports, rechallenge, alternative causes, dose dependency, and objective evidence, defines the relationship between drug and adverse reaction as definite, probable, possible, or doubtful based on scoring. The Naranjo protocol is shown in Table 5-3.

ADR REPORTING

As drugs progress through preclinical and clinical trials, potential problems are identified based on the drug's pharmacology, toxicology, and pharmacokinetics. Exposure of patients to drugs during clinical trials identifies many adverse effects and their frequency. By the time a drug reaches the market,

Table 5–3 Naranjo Adverse Drug Reaction Scoring

Naranjo Adverse Drug Reaction Scoring	Yes	No	Not Known	Score
1. Are there previous *conclusive* reports on this reaction?	+1	0	0	
2. Did the adverse event appear after the suspected drug was administered?	+2	−1	0	
3. Did the adverse reaction improve when the drug was discontinued or a *specific* antagonist was administered?	+1	0	0	
4. Did the adverse reaction reappear when the drug was readministered?	+2	−1	0	
5. Are there alternative causes (other than the drug) that could on their own have caused the reaction?	−1	+2	0	
6. Did the reaction reappear when a placebo was given?	−1	+1	0	
7. Was the drug detected in the blood (or other fluids) in concentrations known to be toxic?	+1	0	0	
8. Was the reaction more severe when the dose was increased, or less severe when the dose was decreased?	+1	0	0	
9. Did the patient have a similar reaction to the same or similar drugs in any previous exposure?	+1	0	0	
10. Was the adverse event confirmed by any objective evidence?	+1	0	0	
			Naranjo Score (Total)	

Definite	>8
Probable	5–8
Possible	1–4
Doubtful	<1

however, it may have been studied in only several thousand patients. Because of this, it is likely that adverse events occurring in fewer than 1% of patients are not fully characterized.

Post-marketing surveillance becomes an important safety strategy. FDA post-marketing reporting programs seek to identify problems not identified prior to approval as well as any problems that may arise related to drug labeling or manufacturing. The FDA maintains a computerized database of adverse events for approved drugs and biologicals, the FDA Adverse Event Reporting System (FAERS). MedWatch is the FDA's safety information and adverse event reporting program that provides health-care professionals with medical product information on prescription and nonprescription drugs, biologics, medical devices, and nutritional products.

As health professionals, we have an obligation to provide data to allow the FDA to monitor medication and vaccine safety. MedWatch allows health-care professionals and consumers to report adverse events and serious problems caused by FDA-regulated products. The Vaccine Adverse Events Reporting System (VAERS) is a separate program used to report adverse events related to vaccinations and like MedWatch allows voluntary reporting on adverse events by both health-care professionals and consumers. The FDA monitors adverse events and can respond with safety announcements, alerts, and/or removal from the market. The FDA publishes alerts in MedWatch (Fig. 5-1) and consumer publications.

To ensure a favorable balance between benefits and risks for certain drugs or biologicals, the FDA requires manufacturers

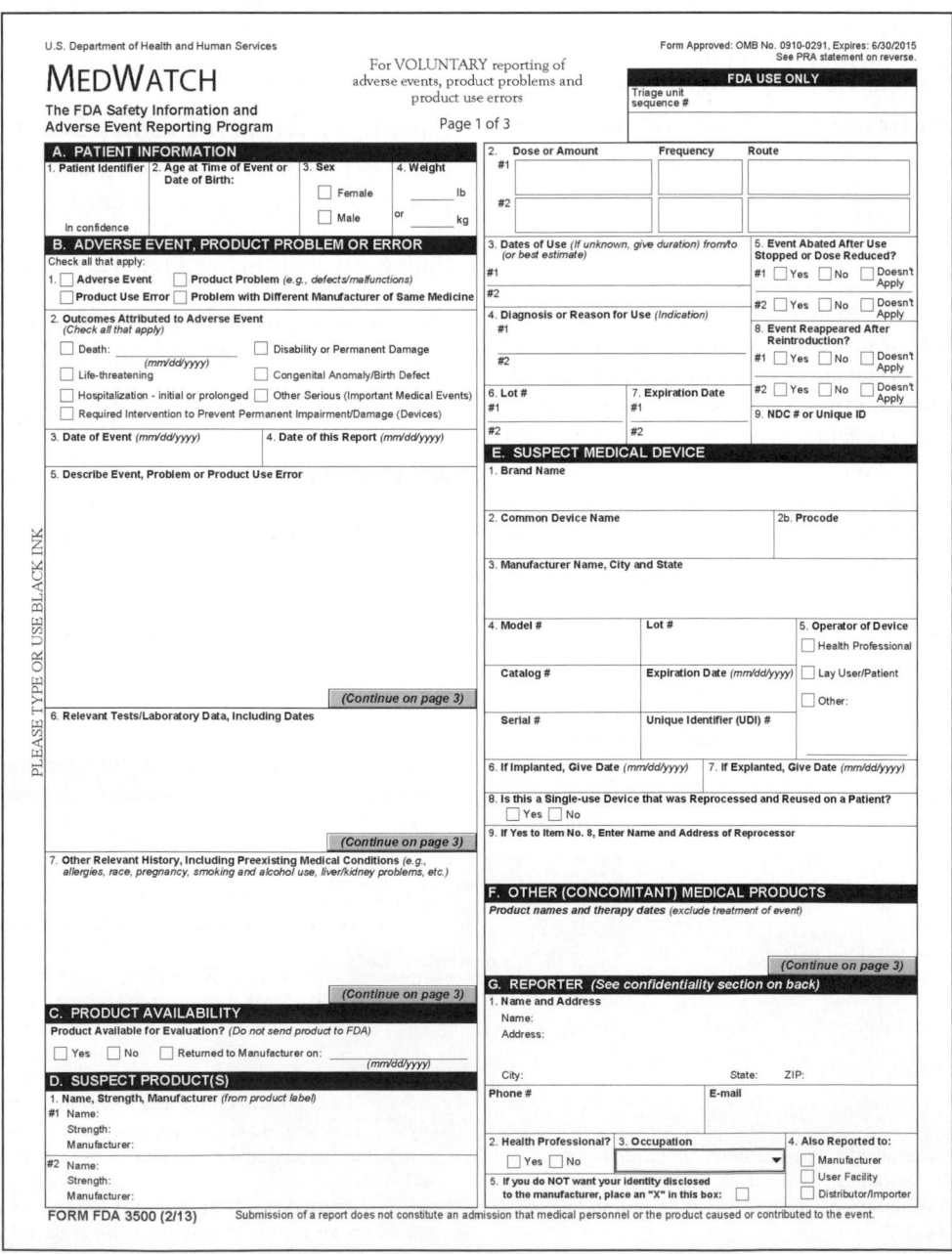

Figure 5–1. The FDA MedWatch form provides a mechanism for health professionals to report ADRs. *Source: U.S. Food and Drug Administration, www.fda.gov/Safety/MedWatch*

BOX 5–1 COMMON DRUGS WITH REMS

- Isotretinoin
- Extended-release and long-acting opioid analgesics
- Rosiglitazone
- Testosterone
- Verenicline
- Metoclopramide
- Mifepristone
- Buprenorphine and naloxone
- Naltrexone

to implement a Risk Evaluation and Mitigation Strategy (REMS). A REMS protocol is composed of various actions (called ETASU: elements to assure safe use), including letters to prescribers; additional patient information; and required patient, prescriber, and/or pharmacy registration and training. REMS are required for many drugs, including those listed in Box 5-1.

SUMMARY

Adverse drug reactions are an unavoidable reality with pharmacotherapy. Fortunately, many ADRs respond well to dosage adjustment or discontinuation of the offending agent. Strategies such as drug interaction screening and conscientious monitoring and reporting of adverse responses can identify at-risk patients and help minimize the incidence of ADRs.

REFERENCES

Alvir, J. M., Lieberman, J. A., Safferman, A. Z., Schwimmer, J. L., & Schaaf, J. A. (1993). Clozapine-induced agranulocytosis. Incidence and risk factors in the United States. *New England Journal of Medicine, 329*(3), 162–167.

Aronson, J., & Ferner, R. (2003). Joining the dots: New approach to classifying adverse drug reactions. *British Medical Journal, 327*(7425), 1222–1225.

Aster, R. H., Curtis, B. R., McFarland, J. G., & Bougie, D. W. (2009). Drug-induced immune thrombocytopenia: Pathogenesis, diagnosis, and management. *Journal of Thrombosis and Haemostasis, 7*(6), 911–918.

Bates, D. W., Cullen, D., Laird, N., Petersen, L. A., Small, S. D., Servi, D., et al. (1995). Incidence of adverse drug events and potential adverse drug events: Implications for prevention. *Journal of the American Medical Association, 274*, 29–34.

Ben m'rad, M., Leclerc-Mercier, S., Blanche, P., Franck, N., Rozenberg, F., Fulla, Y., et al. (2009). Drug-induced hypersensitivity syndrome: Clinical and biologic disease patterns in 24 patients. *Medicine, 88*(3), 131–140.

Brennan, M. (2013). The effect of opioid therapy on endocrine function. *American Journal of Medicine, 126*(3 Suppl 1), S12–S18.

Budnitz, D., Pollock, D., Weidenbach, K., Mendelsohn, A., Schroeder, T., & Annest, J. (2006). National surveillance of emergency department visits for outpatient adverse drug events. *Journal of the American Medical Association, 296*(15), 1858–1866.

Burgess, J. K., Lopez, J. A., Gaudry, L. E., & Chong, B. H. (2000). Rifampicin-dependent antibodies bind a similar or identical epitope to glycoprotein IX-specific quinine-dependent antibodies. *Blood, 95*(6), 1988–1992.

Cacoub, P., Musette, P., Descamps, V., Meyer, O., Speirs, C., Finzi, L., et al. (2011). The DRESS syndrome: A literature review. *American Journal of Medicine, 124*(7), 588–597.

Casato, M., Pucillo, L. P., Leoni, M., di Lullo, L., Gabrielli, A., Sansonno, D., et al. (1995). Granulocytopenia after combined therapy with interferon and angiotensin-converting enzyme inhibitors: Evidence for a synergistic hematologic toxicity. *American Journal of Medicine, 99*(4), 386–391.

Centers for Disease Control and Prevention. (2012, August 14). *Medication safety basics.* Retrieved from http://www.cdc.gov/MedicationSafety/basics.html

CDC MMRW Prevention of Pneumococcal Disease: Recommendations of the Advisory Committee on Immunization Practices (ACIP) April 04, 1997/46(RR-08);1–24.

Chipinda, I., Hettick, J., & Siegel, P. (2011). Haptenation: Chemical reactivity and protein binding. *Journal of Allergy (Cairo), 2011*, 839682.

Earnest, M. P., Marx, J. A., & Drury, L. R. (1983). Complications of intravenous phenytoin for acute treatment of seizures. Recommendations for usage. *Journal of the American Medical Association, 249*, 762–765.

Edwards, I., & Aronson, J. (2000). Adverse drug reactions: Definitions, diagnosis, and management. *The Lancet, 356*, 1255–1259.

Evans, R. S., Lloyd, J. F., Stoddard, G. J., Nebeker, J. R., & Samore, M. H. (2005). Risk factors for adverse drug events: A 10-year analysis. *Annals of Pharmacotherapy, 39*, 1161–1168.

Field, T., Furwitz, J., Harrold, L., Rothschild, J., Debellis, K., Seger, A., et al. (2004). Strategies for detecting adverse drug events among older persons in the ambulatory setting. *Journal of the American Medical Information Association, 11*(6), 492–498.

Gentilini, G., Curtis, B. R., & Aster, R. H. (1998). An antibody from a patient with ranitidine-induced thrombocytopenia recognizes a site on glycoprotein IX that is a favored target for drug-induced antibodies. *Blood, 92*(7), 2359–2365.

George, J. N., Raskob, G. E., Shah, S. R., Rizvi, M. A., Hamilton, S. A., Osborne, S., et al. (1998). Drug-induced thrombocytopenia: A systematic review of published case reports. *Annals of Internal Medicine, 129*(11), 886–890.

Gomes, E., & Demoly, P. (2005). Epidemiology of hypersensitivity drug reactions. *Current Opinion in Allergy and Clinical Immunology, 5*(4), 309–316.

Gray, S. L., Sager, M., Lestico, M. R., & Jalaluddin, M. (1998). Adverse drug events in hospitalized elderly. *The Journals of Gerontology. Series A, Biological Sciences and Medicine Sciences, 53*, M59–M63.

Gurwitz, J. H., Field, T. S., Judge, J., Rochon, P., Harrold, L. R., Cadoret, C., et al. (2005). The incidence of adverse drug events in two large academic long-term care facilities. *American Journal of Medicine, 118*, 251–258.

Janeway, C. A., Jr., Travers, P., Walport, M., et al. (2001). Allergy and hypersensitivity. In *Immunobiology: The immune system in health and disease* (5th ed.). Janeway, Jr., C. A., Travers, P., Walport, M., editors. New York: Garland Science. Available from: http://www.ncbi.nlm.nih.gov/books/NBK10756/

Johansson, S. G., Bieber, T., Dahl, R., Friedmann, P. S., Lanier, B. Q., Lockey, R. F., et al. (2004). Revised nomenclature for allergy for global use: Report of the Nomenclature Review Committee of the World Allergy Organization, October 2003. *Journal of Allergy and Clinical Immunology, 113*(5), 832–836.

Kaufman, D. W., Kelly, J. P., Johannes, C. B., Sandler, A., Harmon, D., Stolley, P. D., et al. (1993). Acute thrombocytopenic purpura in relation to the use of drugs. *Blood, 82*(9), 2714–2718.

Kaushal, R., Bates, D. W., Landrigan, C., McKenna, K. J., Clapp, M. D., Federico, F., et al. (2001). Medication errors and adverse drug events in pediatric inpatients. *Journal of the American Medical Association, 285*(16), 2114–2120.

Kongkaew, C., Novce, P. R., & Ashcroft, D. M. (2008). Hospital admissions associated with adverse drug reactions: A systematic review of prospective observational studies. *Annals of Pharmacotherapeutics, 42*(7), 1017–1025.

Naranjo, C. A., Busto, U., Sellers, E. M., Sandor, P., Ruiz, I., Roberts, E. A., et al. (1981). A method for estimating the probability of adverse drug reactions. *Clinical Pharmacology and Therapeutics, 30*(2), 239–245.

Nguyen, L., Reese, J. A., & George, J. N. (2011). Drug-induced thrombocytopenia. An updated systematic review, 2010. *Drug Safety, 34*(5), 437–438.

Panel on Antiretroviral Guidelines for Adults and Adolescents (2013). *Guidelines for the use of antiretroviral agents in HIV-1-infected adults and adolescents.* Retrieved from: http://aidsinfo.nih.gov/ContentFiles/AdultandAdolescentGL.pdf

Patel, N., VanDeWall, H., Tristani, L., Rivera, A., Woo, B., Dihmess, A. et al. (2012). A comparative evaluation of adverse platelet outcomes among Veterans' Affairs patients receiving linezolid or vancomycin. *Journal of Antimicrobial Chemotherapy, 67*(3), 727–735.

Pedersen-Bjergaard, U., Andersen, M., & Hansen, P. B. (1996). Thrombocytopenia induced by noncytotoxic drugs in Denmark 1968–91. *Journal of Internal Medicine, 239*(6), 509–515.

Pedersen-Bjergaard, U., Andersen, M., & Hansen, P. B. (1997). Drug-induced thrombocytopenia: Clinical data on 309 cases and the effect of corticosteroid therapy. *European Journal of Clinical Pharmacology, 52*(3), 183–189.

Pedersen-Bjergaard, U., Andersen, M., & Hansen, P. B. (1998). Drug-specific characteristics of thrombocytopenia caused by non-cytotoxic drugs. *European Journal of Clinical Pharmacology, 54*(9–10), 701–706.

Pereira, J., Hidalgo, P., Ocqueteau, M., Blacutt, M., Marchesse, M., Nien, Y. et al. (2000). Glycoprotein Ib/IX complex is the target in rifampicin-induced immune thrombocytopenia. *British Journal of Haematology, 110*(4), 907–910.

Peyrière, H., Dereure, O., Breton, H., Demoly, P., Cociglio, M., Blayac, J. P., et al. (2006). Variability in the clinical pattern of cutaneous side-effects of drugs with systemic symptoms: Does a DRESS syndrome really exist? *British Journal of Dermatology, 155*(2), 422–428.

Pichler, W. J., Naisbitt, D. J., & Park, B. K. (2011). Immune pathomechanism of drug hypersensitivity reactions. *J Allergy Clin Immunol, 127*(3), S74–S81.

Pirmohamed, M., Breckenridge, A., Kitteringham, N., & Park, B. (1998). Adverse drug reactions. *British Medical Journal, 316*(7140), 1295–1298.

Rawlins, M. D. (1981). Clinical pharmacology. Adverse reactions to drugs. *British Medical Journal (Clinical Research Edition), 282*(6268), 974–976.

Reese, J. A., Li, X., Hauben, M., Aster, R. H., Bougie, D. W., Curtis, B. R. et al. (2010). Identifying drugs that cause acute thrombocytopenia: An analysis using 3 distinct methods. *Blood, 116*(12), 2127–2133.

Roujeau, J. C., & Stern, R. S. (1994). Severe adverse cutaneous reactions to drugs. *New England Journal of Medicine, 331,* 1272–1285.

ten Berg, M. J., Huisman, A., Souverein, P. C., Schobben, A. F., Egberts, A. C., van Solinge, W. W., et al. (2006). Drug-induced thrombocytopenia: A population study. *Drug Safety, 29*(8), 713–721.

U.S. Food and Drug Administration, (1995). *Clinical safety data management: Definitions and standards for expedited reporting.* (ICH-E2A). Retrieved from http://www.fda.gov/downloads/Drugs/Guidances/ucm073087.pdf

U.S. Food and Drug Administration. (2009, April 30). *Preventable adverse drug reactions: A focus on drug interactions.* Retrieved from http://www.fda.gov/drugs/developmentapprovalprocess/developmentresources/druginteractionslabeling/ucm110632.htm

U.S. Food and Drug Administration. (2013, August 23). *Reporting serious problems to the FDA.* Retrieved from http://www.fda.gov/Safety/MedWatch/HowToReport/default.htm

van der Klauw, M. M., Goudsmit, R., Halie, M. R., van't Veer, M. B., Herings, R. M., Wilson, J. H., et al. (1999). A population-based case-cohort study of drug-associated agranulocytosis. *Archives of Internal Medicine, 159*(4), 369–374.

Von Drygalski, A., Curtis, B. R., Bougie, D. W., McFarland, J. G., Ahl, S., Limbu, I., et al. (2007). Vancomycin-induced immune thrombocytopenia. *New England Journal of Medicine, 356*(9), 904–910.

Woolcott, J. C., Richardson, K. J., Wiens, M. O., Patel, B., Marin, J., Khan, K. M., et al. (2009). Meta-analysis of the impact of 9 medication classes on falls in elderly persons. *Archives of Internal Medicine, 169,* 1952–1960.

Yokomichi, N., Nagasawa, T., Coler-Reilly, A., Suzuki, H., Kubota, Y., Yoshioka, R., et al. (2013). Pathogenesis of Hand-Foot Syndrome induced by PEG-modified liposomal doxorubicin. *Human Cell, 26*(1), 8–18.

Yunis, J. J., Lieberman, J., & Yunis, E. J. (1992). Major histocompatibility complex associations with clozapine-induced agranulocytosis. The USA experience. *Drug Safety, 7*(Suppl 1). 7–9.

CHAPTER 6

FACTORS THAT FOSTER POSITIVE OUTCOMES

Marylou V. Robinson • Teri Moser Woo

The goal of health-care providers is to help patients become healthier. When the patient does not or cannot follow recommendations or instructions that lead to this goal, the provider may become frustrated. Multiple clinical studies have revealed that even though providers expect adherence and positive outcomes, in reality these often do not happen. A change of perspective toward patient-centered care and patient participation in setting health-care goals may foster a positive change for adherence and positive outcomes.

Many questions arise when discussing adherence. Why do patients not adhere to instructions about taking their medications? What occurs outside the office setting to sabotage the best of intentions? What is the patient's responsibility, and what is the provider's? This chapter discusses the major issues in adherence and ways to foster positive outcomes.

OVERVIEW OF NONADHERENCE

The problem of poor adherence to drug therapy is widespread around the world (Brown & Bussell, 2011). In the United States, it is estimated that less than 50% of patients adhere to their drug regimen (New England Healthcare Institute [NEHI], 2009). Other studies report similar data (Brown & Bussell, 2011; Osterberg & Blaschke, 2005) with chronic disease patients more likely to have spotty adherence (NEHI, 2009). Those at highest risk include patients who have asymptomatic conditions, chronic conditions (Hayes, McCahon, Panahi, Hamre, & Pohlman, 2008; Mahat, Scoloveno, & Donnelly, 2007), cognitive impairment, psychiatric illness, or disorders requiring significant lifestyle changes (e.g., smoking cessation) (Myung, McDonnell, Kazinets, Seo, & Moskowitz, 2009) and those who are on complex regimens with multiple daily dosing and significant adverse reactions (Luthy, Peterson, & Wilkinson, 2008; Sarver & Murphy, 2009). When patients' interactions with the provider include poor communication (Zagaria, 2008), the risk of nonadherence is even higher. Wheeler, Roberts, and Neiheisel (2014) have synthetized much of the literature on adherence with much research left to be done on the multiple variables associated with whether medications are taken or not.

The health-care provider–patient relationship is not a parent–child relationship; it is one of setting and working toward realistic mutual goals. Providers cannot expect compliance unless patients have participated in realistic goal setting, including validating their belief they can follow the plan and identifying barriers that will impede those goals. Compliance implies an involuntary act of submission and provider-centric decision making. Adherence implies a voluntary act of negotiation and joint acceptance of a treatment regimen. Horne (2004) points out that "typically, over 30% of patients harbor strong concerns" about the need for their medication and the risk involved in taking it. What is more, the patient tends to overestimate the risk. If these issues are not addressed by open communication, surreptitious nonadherence is likely to result. This shift in attitude from compliance to adherence highlights the providers' essential focus upon their responsibility to educate patients about their diseases and drugs.

Nonadherence to pharmacological regimens can lead to failure to reach the desired treatment goal, which may be very costly. Patients who stop using their drugs have more complications from their disease, which results in total increased cost for themselves and the health-care system. The health-care system itself creates barriers to adherence by limiting access to health care; using restricted formularies; and having prohibitively high drug costs, co-payments, or both. Over $290 billion in unnecessary emergency room and health-care costs related to adherence issues are estimated to occur in the United States every year (NEHI, 2009). Mortality rates double for cardiovascular and diabetic patients who do not follow their treatment plans. Increasing insurance rates and co-pays contribute to this. The Affordable Care Act (ACA) is intended to remove some of these system barriers. Payment reform with an emphasis on quality outcomes is anticipated to also foster more prescriber attention to adherence factors.

Intentional Versus Nonintentional Nonadherence

Taking or not taking medications may be intentional or inadvertent. Unintentional nonadherence can be attributed to forgetfulness (especially if it is a side effect of a drug), dementia, mental health problems, simple procrastination, or an overextended lifestyle. Not perceiving the usefulness of a medication for symptom resolution is one source of intentional nonadherence. Whether people believe the medication is effective, are unaware of the subtlety of its actions, or become frustrated with a "lack of cure" can contribute to whether they take medications as prescribed. Drug cost may also be a factor in intentional nonadherence.

ADVERSE DRUG REACTIONS

Real or perceived adverse reactions directly affect the outcome of a prescribed drug regimen. If a patient reports a prescribed drug is causing a reaction, then the provider should explore alternative options to treating the problem. This response assures patients that the provider is willing to listen and work with them until the right drug or right dosage is prescribed. Patients might think that their skepticism about a drug will be interpreted as lack of confidence in the provider (Horne, 2004). It may be difficult for patients to tell providers that they have a different view of the drug. Encouraging open communication about these concerns and perceptions is important. Communication is discussed further below.

Certain adverse reactions are more likely to produce nonadherence than others. Oddly enough, serious adverse reactions such as severe hypotension or anaphylaxis are not among them. The ones most likely to produce nonadherence are the "irritating" ones that interfere with the patient's ability to carry out activities of daily living, including what he or she may do for a living. These reactions include headache, dizziness, anorexia, nausea and vomiting, constipation, sexual dysfunction, and diarrhea. Unfortunately, these are also the most common adverse reactions. What is a problematic adverse reaction for one person may not be for another. When looking for potential nonadherence, it is important to look for the adverse reactions that commonly cause nonadherence and talk to patients about them, but it is also important to ask which ones would be a problem for the individual patient and take these into consideration in making a drug choice.

ASYMPTOMATIC CONDITIONS

A variety of disease states are essentially asymptomatic until their later stages. Some of these can be treated with drugs in their early stages to prevent their progression. However, it may be difficult to convince a patient that he or she has a serious disease when there is no overt indication of the disorder except the provider's word. It is even more problematic when the drugs given to treat this "invisible" disorder produce "disease symptoms" themselves. One of the most common of these asymptomatic disorders is hypertension.

Uncontrolled hypertension contributes to increased risk for cardiovascular disease, including stroke, ischemic heart disease, and heart failure, yet adherence to antihypertensive medications is often poor (Rajpura & Nayak, 2013). Rajpura and Nayak report that 66% of elderly patients with hypertension did not take their medication as prescribed, with the reasons for not taking the medication including the patient's perception regarding the seriousness of the illness and beliefs or concerns about the medication. Beliefs about the benefits of the medication can outweigh cost as a reason for nonadherence.

Patients may realize through education that control of hypertension is very important to their health but may not adhere to the regimen secondary to the adverse reactions they experience to the drugs given to treat this disease. Antihypertensive drugs that have a rapid onset and short duration of action are not very desirable in long-term therapy secondary to possible large variations in blood pressure. If the patient misses one dose, the antihypertensive effect disappears, creating a possible rebound or adverse reaction. Since many of the drugs used to treat hypertension have these effects, nonadherence (including missed doses) is likely. Selecting a more "forgiving" drug that either does not depend on half-life or has a longer half-life will produce limited effect on the efficacy of the drug if doses are delayed or missed (Osterberg & Blaschke, 2005). Antihypertensives that require several dose titrations (e.g., alpha-adrenergic blockers) can be particularly troublesome (e.g., severe orthostatic hypotension) if the patient misses some doses and then restarts the drug, even if it is not at the full dose.

Erectile dysfunction (ED) is a highly publicized medical problem that may have as its root cause an adverse reaction to medications. Antihypertensives and psychotropic drugs have been implicated as the cause of ED. The provider must explore a change in medication if a patient is experiencing ED, anorgasmia, loss of libido, or other changes in sexual health.

Predicting probable adverse reactions of certain medications provides a basis for making an alternative treatment plan for individuals experiencing side effects. The provider looks at the tolerability profile of each drug and discusses it in selecting drugs for a particular patient. Tolerability is directly linked to patient adherence for both short- and long-term therapy and ultimately to the overall success of treatment.

CHRONIC CONDITIONS

One out of every two Americans has at least one chronic condition (Centers for Disease Control and Prevention [CDC], 2010). Chronic diseases account for three-fourths of the nation's 1.4 trillion dollars in medical care costs and one-third of the years of potential life lost before age 65 (CDC, 2010). Many variables, such as increased individual risk factors, a

lack of health-care resources for the poor and underserved, and environmental conditions that do not support the adoption and sustainability of healthy eating and physical activity impact chronic care onset and medication adherence. These factors may clinically express themselves differently from one person to another. As a result, the prescriber and members of a multidisciplinary health team must use a variety of approaches to positively intervene for persons living with chronic illness.

Ideally, the patient develops a pattern of taking drugs consistent with her or his activities of daily living; for example, taking the white pill before breakfast and the blue one at dinner. Weekends, vacations, visiting family, and unexpected events alter the pattern, leading to missed doses. Discuss methods for remembering how to take medication, such as calendars, phone or watch alarms, or day-of-the week pill organizers to assist patients in managing their medication regimen.

Building support mechanisms and setting up monitoring of drug taking for patients with chronic disease is critical to their adherence to their regimens. Kutzleb and Reiner (2006), for example, found significantly improved symptom control and disease self-management in patients with heart failure who received weekly telephone follow-up by nurse practitioners. Early phone contacts enable the provider to determine if the information shared in the clinic has been clearly understood and is being followed. Similar results were found with Web-based collaborative care for type 2 diabetes patients (Ralston et al, 2009). Such follow-up contacts not only help with adherence but also contribute to building a stronger patient–provider relationship. Factors influencing adherence in chronic illness are summarized in Table 6-1.

KNOWLEDGE DEFICIT AND PATIENT PERCEPTION

Understanding the disease state and the treatment regimen plays a role in adherence. Providing educational material alone, written or oral, cannot ensure that the patient will not

Table 6–1 Factors Contributing to Medication Adherence With Chronic Illness

Understanding treatment regimen	Beliefs in effectiveness
Fitting with current routine	Cultural relevancy (see Chap. 7)
Having the skills to carry out the regimen	The staging of disease and level of wellness
Fear of side effects	The ability to control side effects
Remembering to take the medications	Mental health
Family/caregiver support	Interaction with street drugs
Personal views of health	Trust in provider

Adapted from Frank, L., & Miramontes, H. (1998). *Health care provider adherence curriculum.* Pittsburgh, PA: AIDS Education and Training Centers Program.

have a knowledge deficit regarding the drug regimen or that she or he will be adherent. Today, providers feel pressured into having shorter visits with the patient, but more time spent with a patient is not the only component related to increased patient adherence. The quality of the communication and interaction that occur during that time is most important. Patients report greater adherence to a drug regimen if they feel that their concerns and specific points of knowledge deficit are addressed during the encounter. Post-encounter contacts by the office staff nurse, group visits, and tele-health may all be part of the solution to shorter encounters.

Keys to Patient Education

To be effective, patient education must:

- Be simple and focus on the critical points. What does the patient need to know to take this drug safely?
- Use language that is clear and understandable to the patient. This does not just mean "English versus Spanish," for example; it means reduced "medicaleze." It is important not to talk down to people who do understand the medical terms; however, never assume patients do or do not understand terms used. Likewise do not assume that a fellow health-care worker does not have knowledge deficits.
- Be in a form the patient can refer to as needed after the contact with the provider, such as an after-visit summary. Zagaria (2008) found many prepackaged materials are written at the 12th-grade reading level at least. Most patients read medical information at or below the 6th-grade reading level, and some do not read at all and are too embarrassed to tell the provider.
- Be in the order of use or preparation if steps therapy is used.
- Be inclusive of the family and caregivers. Health behaviors are learned and reinforced with the family, so a family-centered approach (Mahat et al, 2007; Tyler & Horner, 2008) that engages and supports parents and children has a better chance of improving adherence.

Patients may understand what you taught but not be able to follow through even when they want to do so.

Health and Cultural Beliefs

Other influences regarding a patient's knowledge deficit include culturally based health beliefs (see Chapter 7) and the relationship between the patient and the provider (Castro & Ruiz, 2009). Some patients do not want to share in the decision-making process. Their beliefs about health or their cultural beliefs may influence how they perceive their role in their care, and they may believe they need to do what the health-care provider tells them to do. To some others, the idea of having to share the control of taking care of themselves is foreign. Those patients who expect the provider to tell them what to do may perceive that the decision-sharing provider does not know what she or he is doing and may not return to that provider. Conversely, a mismatch can also occur between the patient who wants to be in control and a provider who presents information in an authoritarian manner.

Medical Terminology Literacy

Nearly 9 out of 10 adults have difficulty understanding health information (CDC, 2011). Certain populations are especially at risk for low health literacy. They include adults 65 years of age and older, minority populations, low-income individuals (who may read below the 5th-grade level), and immigrant populations whose English proficiency may be limited (U.S. Department of Health and Human Services, 2010; Zagaria, 2008). Using plain language makes it easier for patients to understand and use health information (CDC, 2012). Avoid using medical jargon and biomedical terminology when explaining disease processes and treatment plans. When in doubt as to whether the patient understood the information, ask the patient to repeat the information back to you in his or her own words. Remember that health literacy is not only about accessing and understanding the information but then being able to apply it to one's own personal health-care plan (Sakraida & Robinson, 2009).

Resources that may help the provider understand and address health literacy in their practice include the following:

- The Centers for Disease Control and Prevention health literacy Web site. http://www.cdc.gov/healthliteracy/.
- National Patient Safety Foundation. http://www.npsf.org/for-healthcare-professionals/programs/ask-me-3/.
- University of Arizona has a self-learning module for older adults with health literacy problems. http://www.healthlit.fcm.arizona.edu.

Written Handouts

The National Institutes of Health (NIH) has implemented the Clear Communication initiative to focus attention on health education materials that are accessible to specific audiences based on cultural competence and that incorporate plain language (NIH, 2013). Do not give patients written material without taking the time to explain it. Check all patient education materials to make sure they are written in plain language and meet the CDC and NIH recommendations for health education materials. Patient materials such as a drug insert may not be understood by the patient and may make patients anxious as they read how many adverse reactions may occur. The provider and pharmacist must work closely together to provide patients with plain-language information regarding their medication. Having open communication with patients and using plain language can enhance the positive outcomes from the drug regimen. Enhanced, clear communication forms a positive relationship between patient and provider. In an atmosphere of shared values, shared language (Castro & Ruiz, 2009), and mutual respect, adherence and positive patient outcomes occur.

COGNITIVE IMPAIRMENT AND PSYCHIATRIC ILLNESS

Communicating effectively with patients who have cognitive impairments (e.g., Alzheimer's disease) can be a challenge. Providers need to be able to count on the patient's ability to understand and remember education presented about the drug if adherence is to occur. Each person with cognitive impairment is unique, having a different constellation of abilities and needs for support in understanding and remembering. Assessing the abilities of each patient is important to maximizing adherence. This may involve working with a caregiver or guardian (see later).

Patients with psychiatric illnesses may have difficulty adhering to their drug regimen. Half of the patients with major depression for whom antidepressants are prescribed will not be taking the drugs 3 months after the initiation of therapy (Osterberg & Blaschke, 2005). Rates of adherence among patients with schizophrenia are between 50% and 60% (Lacro, Dunn, Dolder, Leckbane, & Jeste, 2002; Perkins, 2002), and among those with bipolar disorder, the rates are as low as 35% (Colom, et al, 2000). Three major factors are involved here. (1) Psychiatric illness has a social stigma. (2) The presence of symptoms may result in thoughts and behaviors that do not foster adherence—for example, paranoia, agitation, or depression. Finally, (3) the adverse effects with psychotropics—for example, dizziness, orthostatic hypotension, blurred vision, decreased central processing, and confusion—are effects commonly associated with nonadherence.

Longer-Acting Drugs

As with hypertension, selecting drugs with longer half-lives may reduce the likelihood of drug withdrawal symptoms and the return of illness. For example, fluoxetine (Prozac), a serotonin reuptake inhibitor used to treat depression, has a 2-week duration of action so that missing doses or stopping the drug altogether produces a long taper and gives the provider time to discover the problem and work to correct it. Fluphenazine (Prolixin) is a parenteral antipsychotic that also lasts 2 weeks and is very helpful in patients with schizophrenia. Other drugs are also being developed in depot formulations that are long acting and can be given intramuscularly. These agents combine better efficacy and tolerability with improved adherence.

Use of Reinforcements

Osterberg and Blaschke (2005) suggest the use of reinforcements such as monetary rewards or vouchers, frequent contact with the patient, and personalized reminders. Educational approaches appear to be most effective when combined with behavioral techniques and supportive services, including reinforcements. Regardless of the diagnosis, mental health patients require careful monitoring related to their adherence to drug therapy that may include help from family, friends, and other providers. Other patient groups also greatly benefit from the attention and support.

CAREGIVER'S ROLES

When the patient is a child, an adult with cognitive deficits or disabilities, or a person with mental illness, the patient's caregiver must be involved in the educational process. The caregiver can provide valuable information regarding the patient's responses to drugs or difficulties in adhering to the prescribed medication regimen, including adverse reactions. If the provider detects that the caregiver may be having difficulty in adhering to the drug regimen, it is possible that the caregiver may need to be provided one-on-one interventions to help foster positive outcomes for the patient.

The Pediatric Patient

Achieving full adherence in pediatric patients requires the cooperation not only of the child but also of a devoted, persistent, and adherent parent or caregiver (Mahat et al, 2007; Tyler & Horner, 2008). Adolescent patients create even more challenges, given the unique developmental, psychosocial, and lifestyle issues implicit in adolescence. Adherence rates in children and adolescents are similar to those seen in adults, with rates of adherence to drug regimens averaging about 50%. Special interventions for children are discussed in the chapter on pediatric patients (Chapter 51).

Caregiver's Quality of Life

The caregiver's quality of life may have a huge impact on the patient's quality of life. By exploring with the caregiver the psychological, physical, and social impact of giving care, the provider is acknowledging the difficulties the caregiver must face every day. Helping the caregiver find ways to "take a break" for herself or himself and showing concern for the caregiver as well as the patient will foster a positive relationship with the provider. Greater adherence and positive outcomes can be achieved by understanding the impact caregivers have on their patient and providing positive regard for their efforts.

Behavioral Therapy

Behavioral therapy can empower the caregiver to provide appropriate interventions. Discuss situations in which the patient does not cooperate with his or her care, including drug therapy. Help the caregiver to remember the times the patient did cooperate, and try to determine what the characteristics of the situation were that elicited that cooperation. Techniques to elicit cooperation can then become part of the routine care. An interdisciplinary approach is the best intervention for caregivers of patients having a multitude of consulting providers.

COMPLEXITY OF DRUG REGIMEN AND POLYPHARMACY

The number of drugs used to manage multiple complex disease processes increases the possibility of nonadherence, adverse reactions, and the chances of a decreased positive outcome for the patient. Thirty-two million Americans take three or more medications to treat a variety of ailments. Of Medicare-eligible patients, 51% take more than five medications, and more than half of these patients admit they take less medication than prescribed (PhRMA, 2011). Deciding what to do and when to do it can be complex and frustrating for all involved, patient and provider alike.

Collaborative management is an important method of encouraging adherence to a complex health-care regimen. Collaborative management is care that "strengthens and supports self-care in chronic illness while assuring that effective medical, preventive, and health maintenance interventions can take place" (von Korff, 1997, p 1097). The process of collaborative management is both dynamic and continuous. Collaborative management:

1. Begins with dialogue and mutual respect between the patient and the health-care team.
2. Is a starting point for care in chronic illness that includes choosing desirable and obtainable goals that provide direction for care management.
3. Is flexible in nature to enhance care and communication.
4. Does not end with regimen selection but progresses through stages in the direction of improving adherence, optimal health, and survival (Jani Stewart, Nolen, & Tavel, 2002, p 84).

Moreover, von Korff (1997, p 1098) further outlines the essential elements of health care central to such collaborative management. These essential elements are the following:

1. Collaborative definition of problems.
2. Targeting, goal setting, and planning.
3. Creating a continuum of self-management training and support services.
4. Active and sustained follow-up.

These four elements provide a unique manner for addressing not only medication adherence issues but also chronic illness care in general. For example, patients and providers may define problems differently. Patients may focus on functionality, subjective complaints, and lifestyle choices; providers may focus on disease prevention, medication therapy, nonadherence to recommendations, and risk factors related to prognosis. It is imperative that patients and providers have a mutual understanding of problems and understand one another's points of view (von Korff, 1997).

Personalized Drug Schedules

Education for the patient, written and oral, regarding the importance of following a daily schedule is the gold standard. Helping patients set up a personalized drug schedule devised only for them is one possible solution. Working with nursing staff at the clinic, a matrix of activities of daily living can be devised into which drug schedules can fit. Because the schedule is specific to that individual patient's life, it is easier for the patient and/or caregiver to follow and to remember.

Smartphones are used by 7 of 10 U.S. adults for symptom tracking or health-care monitoring (Pew Research Center, 2013). These high-tech "diaries" involve the patient in their own care and help provide an individualized method of refining medication plans.

Simplifying the Regimen

Multiple studies have been done relating adherence to the number of times a drug must be taken each day and the total number of drugs being taken daily. One study of diabetics (Morris, Brennan, MacDonald, & Donnan, 2000) found that for each increase in daily dosing frequency, there was a 22% decrease in adherence. Likewise, liver transplant patients were more adherent to once-daily dosing of the immunosuppressant tacrolimus than twice-daily dosing (Eberlin, 2013). A systematic review of 38 hypertension drug adherence trials involving 15,519 patients (Schroeder, Fahey, & Ebrahim, 2004) found that simplification of dosing regimens improved adherence between 8% and 19.6%. A literature review of 76 publications by Claxton, Cramer, and Pierce (2001) showed that adherence to once-daily dosing was 79%, twice a day was 69%, three times a day was 65%, and four times a day was 51%. The data on short-term use of antibiotics for respiratory infections are even more impressive, with nearly 100% adherence for once-daily dosing. When given an antibiotic dosing schedule of twice daily, at least one-third of patients missed one or more doses. As the number of doses increased, so did the nonadherence (Carlson, Stool, & Stutman, 2005). The ideal drug, it appears, would be taken once daily.

The combination of several medications into one tablet, a poly pill, helps adherence even in the population that is not mentally challenged (Thom, 2013). A meta-analysis of studies regarding the use of fixed-dose combination medications available for hypertension, tuberculosis, and HIV found a 24% to 26% decrease in noncompliance when combination medications are prescribed (Bangalore, Kamalakkannan, Parker, & Messerli, 2007). Consideration of whether the increased cost of fixed-dose combination medication is offset by better disease management due to increased adherence is part of the decision-making process when prescribing.

Sensory or Mobility Challenges

Patients need to be able to read the label and open pill bottles to easily self-administer medications. Large-print labels can increase safety for those with visual impairment. Easy-open lids and pillboxes increase ease of administration when a person has arthritis or impaired coordination or mobility. Prescribers need to anticipate sensory or mobility problems that affect self-administration of medications.

Cues as Reminders

There are multiple methods that can be employed to provide cues to remember to take medications. Some patients use a simple visual cue, such as putting their morning medication near the coffee pot to remind themselves to take their medication when they make the coffee. Pill containers can be purchased with compartments from once-daily to multiple times/day dosing and from weekly to monthly schedules. These containers not only serve as cues to take a drug but also help to monitor when a drug is or is not taken. Daily calendars with sections for each hour of the day can be marked with the name of the drug to be taken. Monthly calendars are sometimes needed for drugs not taken on a daily basis. Electronic technologies include reminders through mobile phones, personal digital assistants, and pillboxes with paging systems. Elders appear to profit the most from having multiple cues (Boron et al, 2013). A Cochrane review of the use of mobile phone messaging in the self-management of chronic disease demonstrated increased medication compliance (de Jongh, et al, 2012). For pediatric patients, stickers, which can be applied to a reminder board or chart, are also helpful. Keeping antihypertensive medications with the home blood pressure cuff may foster both medication adherence as well as self-monitoring of medication effect.

Scheduling Visits for Medication Follow-Up

Patients who miss appointments are often those who need the most help in improving their ability to adhere to a drug regimen. Such patients often benefit from clinical scheduling that matches their drug regimen. If a drug is prescribed for 2 weeks, the next appointment should be on the day after the drug should be completed. For chronic illness, clinic scheduling around the time for any laboratory work or doing physical assessments such as blood pressure can also include consideration for the time to fill the prescriptions. Matching the timing of refill intervals with appointment schedules is also patient-centered.

One-stop-shopping for medical care and prescription refills is a potential adherence strategy. Larger clinics with onsite pharmacies or even pharmacy-based convenience care clinics may provide the bonus of overcoming barriers to filling and refilling medications. Worksites with primary care clinics have nearly 10% better adherence rates (Sherman, et al, 2009).

FINANCIAL IMPACTS

Pharmacological interventions may be costly. Cost can have an impact on the ability and willingness of the patient to adhere to drug regimens. Even if the patient has access to financial assistance (e.g., Medicaid, insurance coverage for drugs), this does not ensure that the patient will view drugs as a primary financial need. Basic needs (e.g., food, housing) may take precedence over drugs in planning a monthly budget. This is especially true for older adults, who are frequently on fixed incomes and yet are the highest users of prescription and over-the-counter drugs. Over 50% of Medicare patients do not keep to their therapeutic regimens (Gould & Mitty, 2010).

Cost Versus Complications

Sipkoff (2005) reported a 3-year study that measured the medical effect of nonadherence on 8,000 people with chronic conditions, including hypertension, diabetes, and depression. Researchers found that study subjects who said they cut back on their prescriptions because of cost were 75% more likely to have suffered a significant decline in their overall health, and 50% were more likely to have had a heart attack, stroke, or chest pain episode than those who filled their prescriptions.

For newly diagnosed patients with chronic illnesses, high cost-sharing—that is, having a large co-payment for each prescription or having to pay up to a certain dollar amount before insurance pays the rest—has been shown to delay the initiation and continuation of drug therapy. A study of patients with hypertension found that 54.8% of the patients delayed initiating therapy when cost-sharing was doubled (Solomon, Goldman, Joyce, & Escarce, 2009).

Out-of-Pocket Versus Insurance

Having insurance that partially covers the cost of medications does not in itself guarantee appropriate utilization of this benefit. From a sample of 27,057 patients with type 2 diabetes, Dor and Encinosa (2004) estimated that the business cost saved by increasing a drug co-payment by as little as $6 would also increase the cost of diabetic complications related to increased nonadherence by $360 million per year, far exceeding the business savings of $31.2 million incurred by the co-payment increase (Lozada, 2005).

An increasing number of patients are either uninsured or underinsured. The hope is that the ACA will assist with this issue. Frustratingly, though, the Veteran's Administration has found that cheap or even free medication refills do not always produce adherence to treatment regimens. Mail-order pharmacy prescription refills are typically cheaper than monthly pickups at local pharmacy windows. Use of mail-order supplies had a higher adherence rate than those from retail agencies (Iyengar et al, 2013).

Family Versus Self

Patients who have several family members to support may view taking drugs for themselves as somehow being selfish. The child who has a chronic disease also affects the financial stability of the family, which may cause resentment from parents or siblings.

Generic Versus "New and Improved" Brand Name

Many patients see new drugs advertised on TV and the provider hears about them from the drug representative: "This new drug is so much better than the old one" or "This brand-name drug is so much better than a generic." There are times when a new drug has characteristics that make it better than anything else on the market, and generic drugs that are not bioequivalent may not be as effective as a brand-name drug. However, choosing a new or nongeneric formulation that is very expensive requires careful consideration. A brand-name drug may cost *hundreds* of times as much as the generic. Providers need to consider cost before prescribing a drug, even if the patient or the insurance provider appears to be able to cover the cost.

Public and Private Assistance

The issue of public assistance is certainly a complex and difficult one. Being aware of possible public programs available to assist financially is only a part of the whole picture. The provider also has to have knowledge of the patient and whether that patient will accept public assistance. Public assistance may not be an alternative if the patient or family views it as a social or cultural stigma that is unacceptable.

Prescribers should keep contact information on hand for large pharmaceutical companies that offer coupon reductions and home-delivery options. Many companies have need-based programs that result in no-cost medications for patients in temporary or even permanent financial crisis. During times of disaster, larger pharmacy chains provide rapid refills and low-cost substitutes for medications lost during floods, fires, and wind storms.

COMMUNICATION DIFFICULTIES

Finding common terminology is not the only communication difficulty. There are also speech, hearing, and language barriers. Communication barriers can create safety concerns, as well as frustration for the provider and patient.

Non–English Speakers and Interpreters

Language barriers may create difficulty in adhering to a drug regimen. Federal law requires that clinics provide an interpreter if the primary language is different from the provider's. Clinics are able to contact interpreters for a number of different languages via interpreter services or phone interpretation. The difficulty that arises is whether the interpreter is repeating exactly what the provider is saying and, in return, whether the interpreter is saying exactly what the patient is saying.

Professional certified medical interpreters are preferable. A patient may not want to share certain information with the family member who is the interpreter, and the family interpreter may not wish to give the provider certain information about the patient. Cultural norms play a major role here. When a professional interpreter is not accessible, every effort must be made to find a reliable interpreter. The provider can be held liable for poor outcomes if a lay interpreter is used and incorrect information is given to the patient.

Speech and Hearing Issues

Patients with hearing or speech difficulties should not be automatically classified as individuals who will have adherence problems. Patients with hearing difficulties may have learned to compensate by reading lips. If this is the case, the provider must stand directly in front of the patient and speak clearly, looking directly at the patient's face. Presbycusis (hearing loss due to age) is commonly associated with decreased ability to hear higher-pitched tones, often those within the range of the human voice. Speaking in low tones or finding a provider with a lower voice may improve the patient's ability to understand. Written instructions are necessary to ensure accurate information is conveyed to the patient.

Patients with speech difficulties include those who are deaf and those who have had strokes or laryngectomies that reduce their ability to produce speech. Sometimes, these patients have learned coping mechanisms or had speech therapy to enable them to communicate. The provider must discover what tools the patient uses/needs to communicate and use these to the patient's advantage. An interpreter should be provided for patients who use American Sign Language. Patients using speech-enhancing devices usually bring such items with them. In any case, special attention should be paid to ensure that these patients communicate effectively with the provider, and vice versa.

COMMUNICATION BETWEEN PROVIDERS

It can be challenging to coordinate health care for a patient who sees several different providers. Open lines of communication are a must between the patient and his or her provider(s) and among health-care providers. If a patient sees a specialist for whatever reason, ask the patient to request that the records of each visit be sent to the coordinating primary care provider. However, the patient or the specialist's staff does not always follow through on this request. A congenial call by the primary care provider will do much to secure these reports; coordinate care, regimens, and appointments; let patients know the provider thinks they are important; and let the specialists know who the primary care provider is, thus also enhancing the visibility and credibility of primary care practice.

Patients who see several health-care providers or who do not consistently have the same provider experience greater problems in adhering to treatment therapy. Encouraging repeat visits to the same provider increases communication and knowledge between the patient and the provider.

PATIENT'S RESPONSIBILITIES

Providers are responsible for determining the best plan of care for a patient and for working with the patient to actualize that plan of care. However, the plan of care should be mutually arrived at with the patient, and the patient carries some of the responsibility for its actualization. Not taking a drug, not taking it as prescribed, or premature discontinuance of a drug are common forms of nonadherence. Failure to fill or refill the prescription is another form of nonadherence. All of these are within the control and responsibility of the patient. Chronic illnesses create some of the greatest problems for the patient who has to adhere to ongoing therapy. Time, finances, and a desire to be perceived as healthy appear to have the greatest impact on compliance.

Self-monitoring has been shown to have positive effects on outcomes of drug regimens. For the patient with asthma, self-monitoring of peak expiratory flow rates can improve disease awareness and predict asthma flare-ups (see Chapter 31). Patients demonstrated better adherence after the first follow-up visits but gradually tapered off unless the importance of using the drugs was reiterated in follow-up visits. This technique can be utilized with other chronic diseases (e.g., diabetes, chronic obstructive pulmonary disease, cardiac disease, hypertension, depression) by reviewing whatever device is utilized for home management. Sarver and Murphy (2009) stress the importance of patient-centered versus disease-centered management strategies that include comprehensive patient and caregiver education and "solid partnerships between healthcare providers and patients."

Do not assume that the patient with a history of homelessness or substance abuse will not follow a treatment plan or that the well-educated, affluent patient will. The provider must find out if the patient actually wants to take the drug and is committed to adhering to a drug regimen. Patients have the responsibility to try to adhere to pharmacotherapeutics, but it is also the provider's responsibility to attempt to discover the barriers that are impeding a positive outcome.

MEASURING ADHERENCE

Adherence can rarely be measured by only one method. Methods that may be used include patient reports, clinical outcomes, pill counts, refill records, biological and chemical markers, and medication adherence tools.

Patient Reports

Patient reports are the easiest monitoring tool, but caution must be used when determining if the patient is actually pseudocompliant, telling the provider what the provider wants to hear rather than revealing the reality of nonadherence. Patients do not want to be scolded or chastised when nonadherence is discovered. Asking the "why" behind not taking meds helps to understand previously unknown or new barriers to adherence. Have the patient keep a drug diary to help him or her answer the following questions honestly:

- Did you fill your prescription?
- How often have you taken your drug in the past [number of days or weeks]?
- Have you missed any scheduled times to take the drug? If so, what was the reason? The answer to this question may give the provider insight into ways to improve adherence by removing barriers to it.
- Are there things we could do together to help you take your drugs?

Clinical Outcomes

In most cases, there is a clear clinical outcome being attempted by the use of drugs. Did the drug actually lower blood pressure or blood glucose? Did the patient have fewer asthma attacks or trips to the emergency room? Graphs or flow charts demonstrate the trajectory of outcomes and can be very convincing. If the clinical outcome was not met, adherence may be part of the problem, but remember, it is rarely the whole answer.

Pill Counts

Pill counts can be helpful in determining if the correct number of pills was taken between visits. Some new technologies dispense only one pill at a time, thereby reducing the risk that the patient may pour out pills to avoid being "caught." This type of dispensing can also be tied to reminders to take the pills. Bubble packs are cheap pill-counting methods that do not require fancy technology. If the patient has a caregiver, the caregiver can do the pill counts.

Refill Records

Records of refills can be monitored in the electronic health record or can be obtained from the pharmacy if the patient uses only one pharmacy to refill his or her prescriptions. Having clinic staff monitor whether refills are ordered as expected during the check in process can alert the provider to potential issues of adherence. Completing medication reconciliation as part of each patient encounter will uncover drugs not currently in use or duplication of prescriptions and may bring to light conflicting prescriptions from other providers.

Biological and Chemical Markers

Biological and chemical markers usually are laboratory tests or other diagnostic markers. Serum drug levels are mostly limited to measuring recent activity. Other biomarkers, such as Hb A1c, may be used to determine if a patient is taking the medication and whether the medication is effective.

Medication Adherence Scales

There are several medication adherence scales in the literature. None is considered the gold standard. The reader is directed to the literature for several scales currently in use. A review of four common scales is a good starting point

(Lavsa, Holzworth, & Ansani, 2011). The fastest to administer is the Medication Adherence Questionnaire (MAQ, also known as the Morisky 4), which is presented in Box 6-1. Because there are few questions and it is very easy to score, it is a popular tool to try to get to the source of adherence issues, including adverse drug effect and memory issues. The psychometrics include a reliability coefficient of $\alpha = 0.61$ (Lavsa, 2011). The addition of measuring self-efficacy is found in the Self-Efficacy for Appropriate Medication Use Scale (SEAMS), which has an alpha value of 0.89. Both the MAQ and the SEAMS have been validated in low-literacy populations.

PREDICTORS OF ADHERENCE

There is no end to the variety of factors that impact medication adherence. Wheeler, Roberts. and Neiheisel (2014) propose a model identifying predictors of medication adherence, which includes social, disease, financial, and health system factors that may influence medication adherence. There are additional elements that may influence adherence, including personal elements such as self-efficacy or health beliefs, and biomedical influences such as functional impact of the disease. While multiple elements influence adherence, each individual patient has unique elements that more greatly influence adherence at different points

of time (Fig. 6-1). The elements that influence adherence may be grouped into spheres of influence with elements of potential positive and/or negative contribution within those spheres. Determining which factors are impacting adherence at any point in time requires the advanced practice prescriber to conduct a complete nursing database concerning the elements that are playing into the current picture of adherence. These influences are not static; the elements are constantly in motion, with the importance of particular spheres of influence or several elements coming and going in duration and degree of impact on adherence to the therapeutic regimen. Every sphere plays a role in every patient's choices, abilities, and capabilities for self-care. A particular sphere or factor that may have played a key role previously can become more or less powerful in its influence. When previously reliable prescription adherence changes, the prescriber in tandem with the patient must return to the database to determine what new spheres and elements of influence might be at work.

Providers are encouraged to consider social factors and financial and health system factors when planning treatments in concert with patients. Planning must go beyond the disease factors that direct selection of therapeutic agents based on standard severity and degree of complexity of physiological effects. In concordance with the patient, the prescriber must weigh the pros and cons of different options, regimen complexity, and any concurrent medication or lifestyle challenges that may impact the patient's ability to adhere to the regimen. The relationship between prescriber and patient can make the difference in whether adherence is achieved or the issues previously discussed overshadow the plan and result in poor adherence. Predicting potential issues and exploring methods to overcome any objections are critical to promoting adherence.

SUMMARY

Patient education, enhanced communication between patient and provider and between providers, and consideration of multiple complicating social factors all contribute to fostering adherence and positive outcomes. Identifying patients at risk for nonadherence or those who actually are nonadherent, determining the cause of the nonadherence, facilitating the removal of the cause or barriers to adherence, and developing partnerships with patients to produce adherence and positive clinical outcomes are important roles for the prescribing provider. Table 6-2 provides a summary of adherence factors.

BOX 6–1 MORISKY SIMPLIFIED SELF-REPORT MEASURE OF ADHERENCE

Scoring: 0 = High Adherence; 1–2 Medium Adherence; 3–4 Low Adherence

1. Do you ever forget to take your medicine?
2. Are you careless at times about taking your medicine?
3. When you feel better do you sometimes stop taking your medicine?
4. Sometimes if you feel worse when you take your medication, do you stop taking it?

Adapted from Jani, A. A., Stewart, A., Nolen, R. D., & Tavel, L. (2002). Medication adherence and patient education. Florida AIDS Education & Training Center. In *HIV/AIDS primary care guide* (p 87). Gainesville, FL: University of Florida Press.

Five spheres of influence and multiple factors that impact adherence and self-management. M. Robinson, 2015.

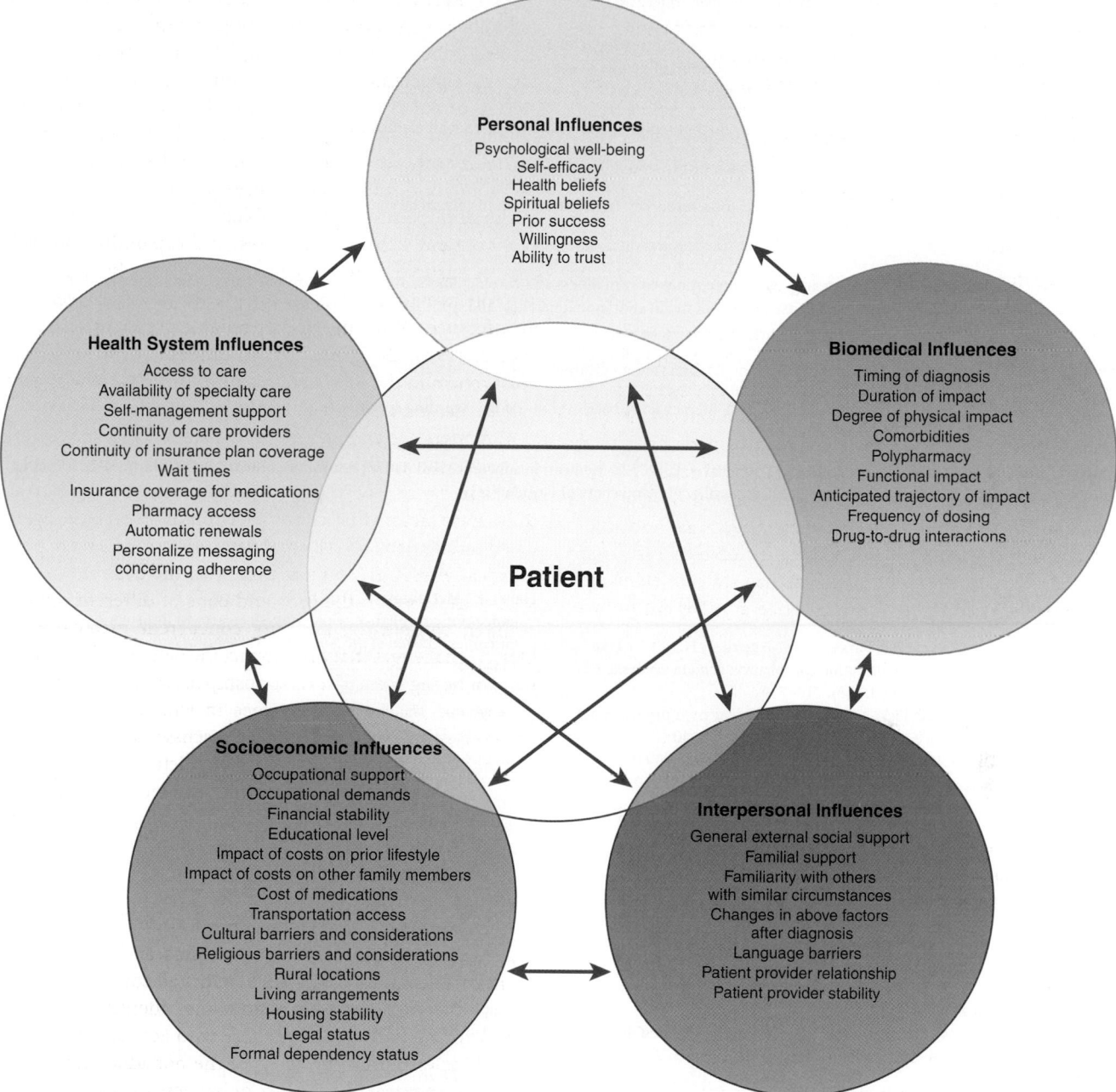

Figure 6–1. Five spheres of influence and multiple factors that impact adherence and self-management. *Robinson, M. (2015). Derived from Wheeler, K. J., Roberts, M. E., & Neiheisel, M. B. (2014). Medication adherence part two: Predictors of nonadherence and adherence.* Journal of the American Association of Nurse Practitioners, 26*(4), 225–232.*

Table 6–2   Factors Influencing Adherence

General Health Status	Medical History, Nutritional Assessment, and Comorbidities
Life goals	To understand deeper issues such as • what gives meaning to a patient's life • the context of illness and treatment on a patient's life • the patient's definition of quality of life • a patient's attitudes and motivations based on one's self-perception
Medication history	Past experience, current regimens, and side effects from all medications
Comorbidities	Psychiatric, substance use, and medical illnesses
Social stability	Housing status, food resources, transportation needs, financial status, and insurance status
Employment status	Type of job, constraints, and disclosure issues
Health beliefs & cultural background	Language and perceptions toward illness and chronic illness, diagnosis, prognosis, role of medications, understanding of consequences of medication nonadherence, and spiritual/religious orientation in reference to one's life and health goals
Family & social support	Identification of personalized medication facilitator and network of social support
Educational background	Educational level, literacy level, baseline knowledge regarding specific chronic illness, medications, and importance of adherence

Adapted from Jani, A. A., Stewart, A., Nolen, R. D., & Tavel, L. (2002). Medication adherence and patient education. Florida AIDS Education & Training Center. In *HIV/AIDS primary care guide* (p 86). Gainesville, FL: University of Florida Press.

REFERENCES

Bangalore, S.. Kamalakkannan, G., Parkar, S., & Messerli, F. H. (2007). Fixed-dose combinations improve medication compliance: A meta-analysis. *The American Journal of Medicine, 120*(8), 713–719.

Boron, J. B., Rogers, W. A., & Fisk, A. D. (2013). Everyday memory strategies for medication adherence. *Geriatric Nursing, 34*(5), 395–401

Brown, M., & Bussell, J. (2011, April). Medication adherence: WHO cares? *Mayo Clinic Proceedings, 86*(4), 304–314. doi: 10.4065/mcp.2010.0575

Carlson, L., Stool, S., & Stutman, F. (2005). Adherence and dosing. *Sound Advice, 1*(12), 1–12.

Castro, A., & Ruiz, E. (2009). The effects of nurse practitioner cultural competence on Latina patient satisfaction. *Journal of the American Academy of Nurse Practitioners, 21*(5), 278–286.

Centers for Disease Control and Prevention (CDC). (2011). Health literacy. Retrieved from http://www.cdc.gov/healthliteracy/index.html

Centers for Disease Control and Prevention (CDC). (2012). Health literacy: Plain language. http://www.cdc.gov/healthliteracy/developmaterials/PlainLanguage.html

Claxton, A., Cramer, J., & Pierce, C. (2001). A systematic review of the association between dose regimens and medication compliance. *Clinical Therapeutics, 23*, 1296–1310.

Colom, F., Vieta, E., Martinez-Aran, A., Reinares, M., Benabarre, A., & Gasto, C. (2000). Clinical factors associated with treatment noncompliance in euthymic bipolar patients. *Journal of Clinical Psychiatry, 61*, 549–555.

de Jongh, T., Gurol-Urganci, I., Vodopivec-Jamsek, V., Car, J., & Atun, R. (2012). Mobile phone messaging for facilitating self-management of long-term illness. *The Cochrane Database of Systemic Reviews, 12. Cochrane*, CD007459.

Dor, A., & Encinosa, W. (2004). How Does Cost-Sharing Affect Drug Purchases? Insurance Regimes in the Private Market for Prescription Drugs. The National Bureau of Economic Research (NBER), NBER Working Paper No. 1038. Retrieved from http://www.nber.org/papers/w10738

Eberlin, M. (2003). Increased medication compliance of liver transplant patients switched from a twice-daily to a once-daily tacrolimus-based immunosuppressive regimen. *Transplantation Proceedings, 45*(6), 2314–2320.

Gould, E., & Mitty, E. (2010). Medication adherence is a partnership, medication compliance is not. *Geriatric Nursing, 31*(4), 290–298.

Hayes, E., McCahon, C., Panahi, N., Hamre, T., & Pohlman K. (2008). Alliance not compliance: Coaching strategies to improve type 2 diabetes outcomes. *Journal of the American Academy of Nurse Practitioners, 20*(3), 155–162.

Horne, R. (2004). Non-adherence with drugs more likely if patients' beliefs are ignored. *The Pharmaceutical Journal, 273*(7320), 525.

Iyengar, R., Henderson, R., Vasaria, J., & Frazee, S. G. (2013). Dispensing channel and medication adherence: Evidence across 3 therapy classes. *American Journal Managed Care, 19*(10), 798–804.

Kutzleb, J., & Reiner, D. (2006). The impact of nurse-directed patient education on quality of life and functional capacity in people with heart failure. *Journal of the American Academy of Nurse Practitioners, 18*(3), 116–123.

Lacro, J., Dunn, L., Dolder, C., Leckbanc, S., & Jeste, D. (2002). Prevalence of and risk factors for medication nonadherence in patients with schizophrenia: A comprehensive review of recent literature. *Journal of Clinical Psychiatry, 63*, 892–909.

Lavsa, S. M., Holzworth, A., & Ansani, N. T. (2011). Selection of a validated scale for measuring medication adherence. *Journal of the American Pharmacists Association, 51*(1), 90–94.

Lozada, C. (2005). Effects of co-payment on prescription drug demand. *National Bureau of Economic Research.* Retrieved October 20, 2005 from http://www.nber.org/digest/apr05/w10738.html

Luthy, K., Peterson, N., & Wilkinson, J. (2008). Cost-efficient treatment options for uninsured or underinsured patients for five common conditions. *Journal for Nurse Practitioners, 4*(8), 577–584.

Mahat, G., Scoloveno, M., & Donnelly, C. (2007). Written educational materials for families of chronically ill children. *Journal of the American Academy of Nurse Practitioners, 19*(9), 471–476.

Morris, A., Brennan, G., MacDonald, T., & Donnan, P. (2000). Populations-based adherence to prescribed medication in type 2 diabetes: A cause for concern. *Diabetes Care, 23*, 1278–1283.

Myung, S., McDonnell, D., Kazinets, G., Seo, H., & Moskowitz, J. (2009). Effects of web- and computer-based smoking cessation programs: Meta-analysis of randomized controlled trials. *Archives of Internal Medicine, 169*(10), 929–937.

National Institute of Health (NIH). (2013). Clear Communication. Retrieved from http://www.nih.gov/clearcommunication/

New England Healthcare Institute. (2009). Thinking outside the pillbox: A system-wide approach to improving patient medication adherence for chronic disease. www.nehi.net/

Osterberg, L., & Blaschke, T. (2005). Adherence to medication. *New England Journal of Medicine, 353*(5), 487–497.

Perkins, D. (2002). Predictors of noncompliance in patients with schizophrenia. *Journal of Clinical Psychiatry, 63,* 1121–1128.

Pew Research Center (2013, January 28). Tracking for health. http://pewinternet.org/Press-Releases/2013/Tracking for Health

Pharmaceutical Research and Manufacturers of America (PhRMA) (2011). Key stats on medication adherence. www. PhRMA. org

Rajpura, J. R., & Nayak, R. (2013). Role of illness perceptions and medication beliefs on medication compliance of elderly hypertensive cohorts. *Journal of Pharmacy Practice.* Published online July 4, 2013. http://jpp.sagepub.com/content/early/2013/07/04/0897190013493806

Ralston, J., Hirsch, I., Hoath, J., Mullen, M., Cheadle, A., & Goldberg, H. (2009). Web-based collaborative care for type 2 diabetes: A pilot randomized trial. *Diabetes Care, 32*(2), 234–239.

Sakraida, T. J., & Robinson, M. V. (2009). Health literacy self-management by patients with T2DM and stage 3 CKD. *Western Journal of Nursing Research, 31* (5), 627–647. doi:10.1177/0193945909334096

Sarver, N., & Murphy, K. (2009). Management of asthma: New approaches to establishing control. *Journal of the American Academy of Nurse Practitioners, 21*(1), 54–65.

Schroeder, K., Fahey, T., & Ebrahim, S. (2004). How can we improve adherence to blood pressure lowering medication in ambulatory care? Systematic review of randomized controlled trials. *Annals of Internal Medicine, 164,* 722–732.

Sherman, B. W., Frazee, S. G., Fabius, R. J., Broome, R. A., Manfred, J. R., & Davis, J. C. (2009) Impact of workplace health services on adherence to chronic medications. *American Journal of Managed Care, 15*(7), e 53–e59.

Sipkoff, M. (2005). Generics linked to improved compliance due to lower cost. *Drug Topics: The Online Newsmagazine for Pharmacists.* Retrieved October 20, 2005 from http://www.drugtopics.com/drugtopics/article/articleDetail.jsp?id=152724

Solomon, M., Goldman, D., Joyce, G., & Escarce, J. (2009). Cost sharing and the initiation of drug therapy for the chronically ill. *Archives of Internal Medicine, 169*(8), 740–748.

Thom, S., et al. (2013). Effects of a fixed-dose combination strategy on adherence and risk factors in patients with or at high risk of CVD: The UMPIRE randomized clinical trial. *Journal of the American Medical Association, 310*(9), 918–929. doi: 10.1001/jama.2013.277064.

Tyler, D., & Horner, S. (2008). Family-centered collaborative negotiation: A model for facilitating behavioral change in primary care. *Journal of the American Academy of Nurse Practitioners, 20*(4), 194–203.

U.S. Department of Health and Human Services, Office of Disease Prevention and Health Promotion. (2010). *National action plan to improve health literacy.* Washington, DC: Author.

Wheeler, K., Roberts, M., & Neiheisel, M. (2014). Medication adherence part two: Predictors of nonadherence and adherence. *Journal of the American Association of Nurse Practitioners, 26*(4), 225–232. doi: 10.1002/2327-6924.12105

World Health Organization (WHO). (2003). Adherence to long term therapies: Evidence for action. www.worldhealthorganization.

Zagaria, M. (2008). Health literacy: Striving for effective communication. *The American Journal for Nurse Practitioners, 12*(9), 23–26.

CHAPTER 7

CULTURAL AND ETHNIC INFLUENCES IN PHARMACOTHERAPEUTICS

Lorena C. Guerrero • Leila M. Jones

The United States has been described as a melting pot of races and cultures. Its total population in 2010 was 308,745,538, and data indicate that the U.S. population is 72.4% white, 16.3% Hispanic, 12.6% black or African American, 4.8% Asian, 0.9% American Indian or Alaska Native, 0.2% Native Hawaiian or other Pacific Islander, 6.2% other race, and 2.9% of two or more races (U.S. Census Bureau, 2010a). With over 43.9% of our population being ethnic or racial minorities, the health-care provider must be versed in pharmacotherapeutic and other health topics that affect the health and well-being of diverse and growing segments of the population.

U.S. DEMOGRAPHICS

The U.S. Census Bureau (2012a) predicts that by 2060 the United States will become an equally diverse nation; that is, although the white non-Hispanic population will remain the largest group, other ethnic groups will also represent a large portion of the population. In fact, the U.S. census data show five states with "minority-majority" populations in 2012. These include Hawaii (77.2% minority), the District of Columbia (64.5%), California (60.6%), New Mexico (60.2%), and Texas (55.5%) (U.S. Census Bureau, 2013a). Projections for minority groups (one race/ethnic group only and not mixed in with other ethnic groups) show significant growth. By 2060, the Hispanic population will represent 31% of the population, African American 15%, Asian 8.2%, two or more races 6.4%, American Indian/Alaska Native 1.5%, and Native Hawaiian/Pacific Islander 0.3% (U.S. Census Bureau, 2012b). In addition, a growing percentage of the total American population, 13%, are those born in another country. Among the foreign-born population, people born in Latin America and the Caribbean represent the majority, with 53.1%, followed by Asians at 28.2% (U.S. Census Bureau, 2012c).

Consistent with the growth of the foreign-born population is the growth in the number of people who have limited English proficiency (LEP), defined by the U.S. Census Bureau as any person age 5 and over who reported speaking English "less than very well." As of 2010, 9% of the U.S. population (over 25.2 million people) are in this category. Of these individuals, 65.5% speak Spanish, followed by Chinese (6.1%). States with over 1 million or more LEP persons are California (27.3%), Texas (13.3%), New York (9.7%), Florida (8.4%), Illinois (4.6%), and New Jersey (4.1%) (Pandya, Batalova, & McHugh, 2011).

Being in the LEP category and having minority status have been shown to be risk factors for low health literacy. These factors make it difficult for patients to understand English and result in confusion over medical language, difficulty in completing forms, and/or possibly limited access to health-care providers. All of these factors create barriers in the health-care interaction, which can exacerbate communication errors between the patient and the provider (U.S. Department of Health and Human Services, 2013). Health literacy and English language proficiency have been shown to be strong factors in the delivery of high-quality health care. Prescribers have a duty to ensure that patients understand how to take medication. Masland, Kang, and Ma (2011) found that the odds of Chinese, Korean, Mexican, and Central American patients living in California experiencing difficulty in understanding prescription labels were 3 and 4 times those of their white American counterparts. Other patient factors that increased these odds were a history of disability, low education level, low income, and recent immigration (Masland et al, 2011).

This chapter presents relevant information about these fast-growing minority groups that practitioners in the United States need to consider when making prescribing decisions for people who may have cultural origins different from the prescriber's. The shifting of the U.S. population away from a Western European racial majority impacts every decision the provider makes when caring for a more heterogeneous group of patients. Health-care providers must be knowledgeable about specific racial and ethnic factors that may influence health disparities and adapt their practice to meet the health-care needs of a diverse populace.

U.S. Demographic Groupings

The American Anthropological Society (AAS) has raised several pertinent issues related to both racial and cultural heritage in the United States. Although the U.S. Census Bureau collects data based on seven distinct groupings, the AAS states that the United States is home to at least 26 different and distinct racial and cultural groupings; the U.S. Census Bureau lists 184 ethnic groups. It is not possible within this chapter to delineate all of these groupings, so we have used the 7 that are delineated by the census. Readers should understand, however, that these are artificial groupings and that people listed within a specific group may be very different from one another; for example, Japanese, Chinese, Vietnamese, Filipinos, and Asian Indians are all grouped under the umbrella category "Asian," yet within these ethnic groups there are differences in the manner in which they metabolize certain drugs (Purnell, 2013).

Health Disparities in the United States

The Centers for Disease Control and Prevention (CDC) defines health disparities as "differences in health outcomes and their determinants between segments of the population, as defined by social, demographic, environmental, and geographic attributes" (CDC, 2011, p 11). In addition to the diversity among racial groups are the existing health disparities that continue to affect racial and ethnic minorities. Long-standing inequalities in the medical treatment of ethnic and racial minority groups by the health-care system, as identified by the Institute of Medicine (IOM), are on the increase (IOM, 2012). Other current research documents significant gaps in health between segments of our society—among racial and ethnic minorities in particular.

The IOM identifies several factors that have an influence on these differences, such as socio-political-historical background; social policies that influence individual health-care interactions; financial and organizational structures in the health-care system that promote illness and poorly controlled chronic diseases instead of prevention; the settings in which health care is delivered, which focus mainly on acute care versus promoting the health of communities and populations; and the nature of the health-care workforce, which at this time does not reflect the current racial and ethnic minority makeup of the United States. Together, these factors contribute to the continuation of health disparities. Health-care practitioners must be aware of local, state, and national statistics that describe health disparities and work toward the reduction, and ultimately the elimination, of these disparities with the goal of improving the overall health of patients, the communities they live in, the nation, and the world.

Cultural Influences on Care

Equally important to understanding health disparities is having knowledge of cultural factors that may impact the well-being of patients. Knowing who makes the decisions in the family about health care and if this person supports the use of the prescribed drug and the plan of care, how the patient and family members view health and illness and their views on the management plan, and cultural factors that may create challenges in adhering to the treatment plan are all important to helping clients improve and/or maintain their health. Although each person with a specific cultural heritage is unique and may not subscribe to all or even most of the health beliefs and health practices of that cultural group, it is important to know what is common to members of the group and in particular what risk factors the group shares. Cultural heritage plays an important role in helping to explain values, attitudes, beliefs, customs, language preferences, and behaviors that influence health practices (Giger, 2013). Socioeconomic factors also influence prescription choices and they may supersede cultural and racial differences. For this reason, we discuss the cultural factors to be taken into account, including background socioeconomic data, such as current demographics, median income, education, and employment (since many patients obtain health insurance through their employment) as well as LEP status, percent foreign-born (if applicable), and health-care utilization.

This chapter focuses on both cultural and ethnopharmacological factors that influence the practitioner's choice of drugs. Pharmacogenetics, described in Chapter 8, also influences prescription choice. The data provided here are based on evidence derived from drug research and on the pharmacokinetics of those drugs most likely to exhibit differences. In using this information, it is important to keep in mind that most Americans are not of any "pure" cultural or racial background and that patients must be treated as unique individuals.

The United States is a constantly changing and evolving cultural mosaic made up of individuals who represent a variety of ethnic and racial backgrounds, each having its own culture and beliefs that influence health. How much of the material presented in this chapter on the cultural values, beliefs, and practices of different ethnic and racial minority groups continues to be valid in the 21st century is unknown. There is little empirical research to support the information on cultural beliefs and practices presented here, although every effort has been made to locate current evidence-based research. The reader should understand that the majority of our sources are found in cultural and anthropological texts that do not clearly state where the information originated or if it is still relevant to today's health-care consumer. Thus, we caution readers that our descriptions may be outdated and may not apply to all members of that particular group. Further research is needed to discover whether the long-reported cultural values, beliefs, and practices continue to represent the majority of the ethnic and minority populations discussed. The reader should acknowledge that culture is a living concept that is evolving and changing and that patients may represent a kaleidoscope of these ever-changing cultural beliefs and practices (Purnell, 2013).

TRANSCULTURAL NURSING CARE THEORIES

Cultural awareness allows the provider to be aware of and open to the differences between patients, regardless of their culture. Madeleine Leininger, in her Culture Care Sunrise model, focuses on assessing the patient in his or her environmental context, which includes seven major areas: technological, religious, social and kinship, cultural value, political/legal, and economic and educational factors (Leininger, 2004). Purnell (2013) expands this model to other factors, including health-care practices, attitudes toward health-care practitioners, high-risk health behaviors, and knowledge about current health disparities for diverse ethnic and cultural groups. The provider should consider all of these factors in planning and implementing treatment regimens that are unique to each patient—regardless of racial or ethnic minority group. For example, the provider would assess the patient's economic resources and education as well as culture before planning care. Several studies have shown that patients do not adhere to medications for several reasons, such as economic factors (high co-payments or lack of prescription coverage from health insurance), prescriptions delivered electronically, and new prescriptions (Shrank et al, 2010). This is especially true of ethnic minorities who lack prescription benefits; they have been reported to be more likely than whites to not take prescribed medications because of cost (Jacobs, Shepard, Suaya, & Stone, 2004).

In providing transcultural care, Leininger states that the provider must decide which preservation/maintenance, accommodation/negotiation, or repatterning/restructuring actions should be undertaken. For example, when a Hispanic patient is newly diagnosed with diabetes, the provider structures care to preserve relevant values that are important to the patient while negotiating changes in behavior, such as food choices and other lifestyle modifications. The client will need to change or greatly modify some behaviors in order to have optimal health outcomes. Practitioners should use frameworks such as those presented by Leininger or Purnell that allow them to provide evidence-based, individualized, and culturally appropriate care regardless of the ethnic or cultural group to which the patient belongs.

STANDARDS OF CULTURAL COMPETENCY

According to the Institute of Medicine (2012), the main factor affecting health disparities is the cultural competence of the health practitioner. The National Standards for Culturally and Linguistically Appropriate Services in Health and Health Care (referred to as the enhanced National CLAS Standards) were developed as a way to address and correct the inequities that exist in the delivery of health care to culturally and ethnically diverse populations. These standards offer a blueprint for health-care professionals and organizations to implement culturally and linguistically appropriate services (Office of Minority Health, 2013b).

National CLAS Standards were originally published in the Federal Registry in 2000 by the U.S. Office of Minority Health in response to a 1994 federal law mandating CLAS Standards for all organizations receiving federal funds, such as Medicaid and Medicare. Recently, the National CLAS Standards have undergone a revision, referred to as the Enhanced National CLAS Standards. These standards were further revised in response to research on health and health-care disparities and changing demographics, as well as legal and accreditation requirements. National CLAS Standards have gained recognition as an important way to help health-care professionals and organizations address the persistent health disparities that plague our nation's diverse communities by improving access and advancing health equity (Office of Minority Health, 2013b).

The new focus on national accreditation standards for professional licensure in the fields of medicine and nursing, as well as health-care policies recently passed by Congress, such as the Affordable Care Act, have also added to the importance of cultural and linguistic competency as part of high-quality health care and services in hopes of decreasing and eradicating health disparities (Putsch, SenGupta, Sampson, & Tervalon, 2003).

A notable change in the new 2013 version of the Enhanced National CLAS Standards is the definition of culture as "the integrated pattern of thoughts, communications, actions, customs, beliefs, values, and institutions associated, wholly or partially, with racial, ethnic, or linguistic groups, as well as with religious, spiritual, biological, geographical, or sociological characteristics" (Office of Minority Health, 2013b). Culture is further defined as a dynamic concept in which individuals may self-identify with more than one culture over the course of their lifetimes. For the first time, the Enhanced National CLAS Standards also include an explicit definition of health, as encompassing "many aspects, including physical, mental, social, and spiritual well-being and occurring along a continuum that can range from poor to excellent " (Office of Minority Health, 2013b). And finally, the Enhanced National CLAS Standards include not only a discussion on how the standards can lead to health equity for all individuals but are also specifically aimed at those of diverse racial, ethnic, and cultural backgrounds (Office of Minority Health, 2013b). The Enhanced National CLAS Standards add a broader definition of culture and health that is in line with nursing's view of health.

The Enhanced National CLAS Standards were developed to reach a broader audience, including patients, consumers, clients, recipients of care, families, caregivers, and even communities. The standards mandate language access services and organizational supports for cultural competence, which are included under culturally competent care. Three types of standards—mandates, guidelines, and recommendations—help providers meet the varied needs of culturally and linguistically diverse populations. These standards call for the provision of professional language assistance services for translation rather than ad hoc interpreters such as family and friends. The standards encourage the education and training of staff members and the provision of culturally appropriate and easily understood teaching materials, including those for adults with low literacy levels. They encourage collaboration with the communities served by the organization and stringent

assessment practices. Other organizations have approved strategies for CLAS implementation. In 2009, the Joint Commission, an organization that accredits health-care organizations such as hospitals and clinics, implemented requirements that help address communication, cultural competence, and patient- and family-centered care (Joint Commission, 2013).

Key to the understanding of the treatment plan is the patient's ability to understand what the health-care provider wishes to communicate through oral and written methods. Not only does the federal government and the Joint Commission require that cultural and linguistic standards be met and followed according to the CLAS Standards, but it is the duty of the prescriber to ensure that the correct information is elicited in order to make a proper diagnosis and that the patient is educated about the agreed-upon treatment plan. This is particularly important when providers care for people with LEP.

Although the majority of the U.S. population speaks English, many speak languages other than English. Immigrants have increased the number of people who are categorized as LEP. Prescribers must be aware of how well these groups are able to participate in the health-care visit, understand written and verbal instructions, and interact with the English-speaking majority. The Census Bureau determines LEP by asking three questions on its yearly American Community Survey and the decennial census: (1) whether there is someone in the household who speaks a language other than English, (2) what the foreign language is (write-in response), and (3) degree of English-speaking ability (self-rated as *very well, well, not well,* and *not at all*). Respondents who self-identify themselves as anything other than "very well" are required to have an interpreter.

As of 2010, 21% of the population (ages 5 and over) in the United States spoke a language other than English (but did not necessarily describe themselves as LEP); 62% reported speaking Spanish, 4.8% percent spoke Chinese, 2.6% spoke Tagalog, 2.3% spoke Vietnamese, and 2.1% spoke French (U.S. Census Bureau, 2010). As previously reported, over 25.2 million people are considered LEP; the primary language of the majority of these is Spanish (65.5%), followed by Chinese (6.1%). On further analysis, only 25.9% of the Spanish-speaking population reported speaking English *not well* and *not at all*, and 29.6% of the Chinese-speaking population, 7.2% of the Tagalog-speaking population, 33.1% of the Vietnamese-speaking population, and 6.5% of the French-speaking population describe their English skills as in the same manner. In fact, the percentages of other Asian groups who report speaking English *not well* and *not at all* are 28.4% for Korean speakers, 29.5% for Mon-Khmer/Cambodian speakers, and 27% for Laotian speakers. Providers must familiarize themselves with changing trends in their local service areas to be able to meet the needs of LEP patients and fully understand and communicate all pertinent information regarding the treatment plan (Pandya et al, 2011).

Providers must ensure that proper interpreter services are used to meet the CLAS Standards or risk losing Medicaid and Medicare funding. LEP patients who utilize interpreter services, rather than ad hoc interpreters such as family members, engage in more recommended preventive health services, make additional office visits, and fill more prescriptions (Jacobs et al, 2004). The importance of ensuring proper communication and understanding among LEP patients cannot be overemphasized and is an important factor that affects the health-care visit and patient adherence.

In order to meet the changing needs of diverse populations, prescribers must become culturally competent. According to Purnell (2013), cultural competence in health care is "having the knowledge, abilities, and skills to deliver care congruent with the patient's cultural beliefs and practices" (p 7). Becoming culturally competent involves having not only an understanding of the patient's culture but also knowledge of one's own culture and personal values and the ability to detach from preconceived ideas and beliefs that can influence attitudes and behaviors toward patients from diverse backgrounds (Purnell, 2013). Ethnocentrism can influence the relationship between the patient and the prescriber by creating barriers to providing culturally competent care. Although the Human Genome Project (2003) showed that only one-tenth of a percent of genetic variations are responsible for differences among humans, Purnell (2013) states that these differences may be significant when conducting health assessments and prescribing medications.

Accreditation bodies like the American Association of Colleges of Nursing (AACN) have also called for cultural competence in nursing education. The Essentials of Doctoral, Master's and Baccalaureate Education for Professional Nursing Practice (AACN, 2006, 2008, 2010) urges the integration of cultural competence standards in both undergraduate and graduate nursing education with the aim of supporting patient-centered care that addresses patient differences in values, preferences, and expressed needs, which may influence health outcomes. According to the AACN, nursing professionals should understand the interrelationship among the concepts of social justice, a commitment to the health of vulnerable populations, and the elimination of health disparities through an understanding of cultural, physiological, ecological, pharmacological, and genetic factors that affect people. In particular the AACN document (2006, 2008) calls for nursing professionals to be able to discuss the effect of drugs on specific ethnic and racial groups.

ELIMINATING HEALTH DISPARITIES

Since the inception of the Healthy People 10-year national objectives initiative in 1979, the focus of national health goals has moved toward improving the health of all Americans. The program has also identified the significant problem of health disparities that affect a disproportionate amount of our ethnic and minority populations. Although health indicators such as life expectancy and infant mortality (markers that are often used as proxy measures to compare the health and well-being of populations across and within countries) have improved for the majority of nonminority Americans, ethnic and racial minorities continue to experience a disproportionate burden of preventable diseases, death, and disability (CDC, 2013a).

Even though the United States spends $2.5 trillion annually on health care (CDC, 2012a), it consistently falls short of other industrialized Western countries in infant mortality rankings. As of 2011, the United States failed to meet the *Healthy People 2020* goal of fewer than 6.0 infant deaths per 1,000 live births (U.S. Department of Health and Human Services, 2013). Other countries that spend much less on health care per capita, such as Cuba and Singapore, have continued to report lower infant mortality rates than the United States (Central Intelligence Agency, 2012). Contributing to this poor standing is the rate of African American infant mortality, which is 2.3 times the rate for the white non-Hispanic population (Office of Minority Health, 2013a). Another example is the age-adjusted asthma mortality rate, which is significantly higher among non-Hispanic blacks (3.3 deaths per 100,000 persons) compared to non-Hispanic whites (1.1 deaths per 100,000 persons) (National Center for Health Statistics, 2010). Non-Hispanic blacks are more likely to have severe asthma, have more asthma control problems, and visit the emergency department more often, all of which influence asthma morbidity and mortality (Mosen et al, 2010).

The U.S. Department of Health and Human Services urges health practitioners to understand issues related to social justice and globalization that impact health care so that they can make a conscious effort to work toward eliminating health disparities. In order to positively influence the health of patients, and ultimately populations, health-care practitioners must be aware of socioeconomic, personal, and cultural factors that may affect adherence to treatments. The World Health Organization and the CDC recognize several factors, called *determinants of health*, that influence health disparities and contribute to a person's current health status: (1) biology and genetics, (2) individual behavior, (3) social environment, (4) physical environment, and (5) health services (CDC, 2013). The interrelationship of these factors requires practitioners to be aware of physical, psychological, spiritual, cultural, and environmental factors, as well as to be conscious of the social and political context in which health can be optimized and/or threatened.

ETHNOPHARMACOLOGY

A factor only recently being incorporated into pharmacotherapeutic decision making is that of ethnopharmacology—the study of racial differences in drug metabolism and response. Practitioners may be aware and guidelines may sometimes specify that certain drugs are less or more efficacious or may have different side effects with certain racial groups. As the cost of gene sequencing decreases, more research has been done that demonstrates the underlying genetic reasons for these differences in efficacy. Large studies are being conducted that include gene mapping of global populations and determining pharmacogenomically relevant markers of drug response, which provide evidence for predicting variations in drug response based on ethnic background (Ramos et al, 2014). Research implicates multiple cytochrome enzyme systems (CYP450, CYP 2D9, and others) in the differences in drug metabolism and response, but these enzymes are not the only sources of racial differences. The expectation is that more information will be gained in the area of ethnic differences in drug pharmacokinetics because of the National Institutes of Health's (NIH) mandate for inclusion of women and minorities in funded clinical research (NIH, 2013).

The pharmacokinetic factors that can be expected to potentially exhibit racial differences are (1) bioavailability for drugs that undergo gut or hepatic first-pass metabolism, (2) protein binding, (3) volume of distribution, (4) hepatic metabolism, and (5) renal tubular secretion. Absorption, filtration at the glomerulus, and passive tubular reabsorption would not be expected to exhibit such differences. Because there is little research evidence on racial differences for relatively few drugs, it is often necessary to conjecture whether these differences might exist. For example, a drug that is eliminated entirely by the kidney through filtration and reabsorption and is not highly protein bound is very unlikely to exhibit racial differences. Conversely, a drug that undergoes significant hepatic first-pass metabolism and is highly protein bound is more likely to exhibit pharmacokinetic differences between racial groups.

This chapter will identify and discuss cultural and ethnic influences on pharmacotherapeutics that play a role in influencing the health outcomes of the patients who trust their care and well-being to the health-care practitioner.

AFRICAN AMERICANS

Cultural Factors

Demographics

According to the U.S. Census Bureau, in 2011 those who designated themselves as African American alone and/or in combination with another race made up 13.6% of the population, and their numbers are increasing faster than the overall growth of the population (CDC, 2011a). The U.S. Census Bureau predicts that by 2060, African Americans will make up 18.4% of the population (CDC, 2011a). As a group, African Americans are young (33.9% under age 20) and more likely to be unmarried (68.8%) and female (53.1%). The majority of African Americans (55%) live in the South. The proportion below the poverty line in 2011 was 27.6%, and the mean household income was $32,329 (CDC, 2011a; U.S. Census Bureau, 2011a).

Education and Employment

In 2011, 82.5% of those who identify as African American have a high school diploma or equivalent, 13.3% have a bachelor's degree, and 6.8% hold an advanced degree (U.S. Census Bureau, 2011a). More African American women than African American men earn a bachelor's degree or higher (respectively, 21.6% compared to 18.2%). According to the U.S. Department of Labor (2012a), the unemployment rate is more than twice that of white Americans (15.8% versus 7.9%) and higher than that of any other ethnic group. In this group, men are more likely than women to be unemployed, at a rate

of 16.7% compared to 13.2%. Additionally, African Americans earn less than their white counterparts, with a median weekly salary of $653, approximately $200 less than the median weekly salary for white Americans. African Americans (along with other minority populations) are more likely to be employed in hazardous occupations (CDC, 2011a). A significantly higher number of households have non-Hispanic black women designated as female head of household (27.5%) than do non-Hispanic Asian (7.8%), non-Hispanic white (9.0%), and non-Hispanic Native Hawaiian/Other Pacific Islander (10.5%) households (U.S. Census Bureau, 2013b). These data support the potential for a difficult reality for many African American families as they continue to face socioeconomic challenges that other racial and ethnic minorities may not.

Family Relationships

Although over half of African Americans are raised in single-parent homes, a strong kinship bond among family members exists. The female is the dominant family force, and the grandmother is often the major decision maker. Sickness can bring families together, and extended and nuclear family members take care of one another (Purnell, 2013). Ever alert for signs of discrimination, they may see health-care providers as "outsiders" in health decisions.

Research has shown that family dynamics affect the course of psychiatric illnesses such as schizophrenia and are as well a factor in contributing to poor outcomes, which vary by race and ethnicity. For example, Lawson (2008) describes family behaviors (such as high emotionality, family intrusiveness, and critical comments) that are normally identified as "toxic" and causing poor outcomes among European American families are instead thought of as protective factors in African American families. African American patients experiencing schizophrenia will view their families as supportive, and therefore the practitioner may wish to continue family involvement in the therapeutic treatment plan to maximize compliance.

Health-Care Utilization

In 2011, 46.7% of African Americans, compared to 65.8% of whites, had employer-sponsored health insurance; and 18.8% of African Americans, compared to 11.1% of non-Hispanic whites, were uninsured (CDC, 2011d, 2012a). Beal, Doty, Hernandez, Shea, and Davis (2007) found that more African Americans (21%) than whites had no usual source of health care and that cost considerations for prescription drugs are especially important in this group. African Americans use hospital clinics and emergency rooms as their care providers more than any other ethnic group, perhaps in part because of their urban residence (Purnell, 2013).

Health-care utilization is also influenced by the types of jobs that people hold. African American males are twice as likely as non-Hispanic white males to work in service-related occupations, such as laborers, fabricators, and operators. These occupations result in higher injury rates (approximately by a third) among African American males and females when compared to white non-Hispanic workers (CDC, 2011c).

In addition to lacking health insurance, many African Americans have a long-standing distrust of the modern health-care system, in part due to the Tuskegee experiment with syphilis conducted by the U.S. Public Health Service from 1932 to 1972. This study withheld treatment from the African American patients it enrolled long after 1947, when treatment with penicillin became the drug of choice, only for the sole purpose of learning more about the long-term effects of syphilis on the body (CDC, 2013b). Despite public apologies from the U.S. government by President Bill Clinton and the Surgeon General in 1997, many African Americans still harbor a suspicion of government-provided health care. This also has implications for recruiting African Americans for research studies, because this population may choose to abstain from participation (CDC, 2013b; Soto, Dawson-Andoh, & BeLue, 2011). Prescribers should familiarize themselves with published clinical studies and evaluate whether they meet the NIH requirements that NIH-sponsored research adequately address its inclusion guidelines concerning recruitment of women, minorities, and children.

Additional factors that may influence health-care utilization is a shortage of African American providers, a belief that pain is inevitable and should be endured, the use of folk practitioners instead of traditional Western medicine, and the view that nurses are less important than physicians (Purnell, 2013).

Health Status and Other Biological Variables

The gap in life expectancy between African Americans and white Americans is narrowing but still exists. African Americans' life expectancy is shorter than the average American's by 4.7 years (National Center for Health Statistics, 2010).

This population continues to experience significant health disparities in the rate of preterm birth, low birth weight, and infant mortality. According to the U.S. Office of Minority Health, maternal mortality rates are over twice (2.3 times) those of other ethnic groups, such as non-Hispanic whites (2013c). In 2004, Sudden Infant Death Syndrome (SIDS) was the third leading cause of death for African American infants under the age of 12 months (111.5 versus 48.8 per 100,000), a rate that is 2.3 times greater than that of non-Hispanic whites. Researchers believe that factors influencing SIDS rates among this population include low rates of acceptance of current guidelines, which call for infants to be put "Back to Sleep"; continuation of myths passed down through generations, often by well-meaning mothers and grandmothers, that infants sleep better in a prone position; and the continued reluctance by this population to follow current research demonstrating that placing infants on their backs decreases the rate of SIDS by 50% (American Lung Association, 2007). Practitioners can help African American mothers make informed choices by offering clear instructions, addressing these myths, and offering research-based education whenever possible on the positive results of the "Back to Sleep" program.

African American women experience preterm birth (described as a birth before 37 weeks gestational age) at a rate of 17.4 per 1,000 births (compared to 10.9 per 1,000 for white non-Hispanics) and deliver an infant classified as low birth weight (a birth that is less than 2,500 grams) at almost twice the rate of the non-Hispanic white population (13.6% versus 7.2%). Some Southern states with high African American populations, such as Alabama, Louisiana, and Mississippi, have some of the highest premature rates of the nation: 14.9%, 15.6%, and 16.9%, respectively (March of Dimes, 2013). In addition, the African American population has the second-highest pregnancy rates in the nation for females ages 15 to 19 (47.3 versus 21.7 per 1,000 for white non-Hispanics) (Office of Adolescent Health, 2013).

The patterns of illness in the African American population include a higher prevalence of coronary heart disease, hypertension, stroke, obesity, type 2 diabetes mellitus, and HIV infection. When compared to their non-Hispanic white counterparts, the prevalence and age-adjusted mortality rate for diabetes and hypertension are 2 times higher, with an overall risk of being diagnosed with diabetes that is 77% higher than the risk for the general population, and a risk for stroke that is 1.7 times higher (Purnell, 2013). In 2011, the percentage of African Americans of all ages who reported their health as fair or poor was 14.2% (CDC, 2011a), versus 9.9% for the non-Hispanic white population (CDC, 2011b). These statistics demonstrate that the African American population may present with more chronic health problems that prescribers must address effectively.

Several risk factors for chronic health problems like coronary artery disease exist in the African American population: cigarette smoking, obesity, and poor dietary choices. The prevalence of cigarette smoking, a risk factor for heart disease, is similar in the African American and non-Hispanic white populations; 19.4% of blacks smoke as do 20.6% of non-Hispanic whites. However, while the non-Hispanic white population has seen a decrease in the number of smokers, this is not true for the African American population, where there has been no significant decline in the overall smoking rate from 2005 to 2011. In particular, black men make up 24.2% of smokers, versus 21.6% overall for male smokers in the general U.S. population (CDC, 2013c). In an 8-year study, Haiman et al (2006) found that African American and Native Hawaiian smokers (smoking 20 cigarettes or less per day) had a significantly higher risk of developing lung cancer when compared with white, Japanese American, and Latino smokers with similar smoking rates. The authors suggest that this may be related to smoking behavior (such as African Americans tending to inhale more nicotine than whites) and/or susceptibility to tobacco carcinogens.

Another cardiovascular risk factor, obesity, is more prevalent in the African American population, affecting 37.6% of men and 54.2% of women. Purnell (2013) believes that the reason for this is due to the African American diet, which contains more animal fat, less fiber, and fewer fruits and vegetables and includes traditional items like chitterlings, fried okra, ham hocks, corn, mustard, collard and kale greens, which are often cooked with pork fat. Foods are often prepared by frying or barbecuing and are often accompanied by gravies and sauces, which may add calories, fat, and salt. Practitioners need to understand that changing cooking and eating habits may be difficult, for the negative view of obesity that predominates in the American culture may not be shared by African Americans: a bigger body habitus is often viewed as a healthy body—particularly in women (Purnell, 2013).

Diets high in fat, cholesterol, and salt may also contribute to the increase in hypertension. For example, approximately 37% of African American men and 44% of women have hypertension (CDC, 2011a). When compared to other ethnic groups, hypertension in the African American population is normally more severe, is often resistant to treatment, occurs earlier in life, and leads to significantly worse target organ damage (Purnell, 2013).

African Americans also have the lowest immunization rates for infections like tetanus and the second-lowest rates after Hispanics for influenza and pneumococcus infections (CDC, 2008). These low vaccination rates may contribute to lower-respiratory infections and be the reason for such infections being the seventh leading cause of death for this population. On a positive note, the African American population has greater bone density than other ethnicities and therefore suffers less osteoporosis (National Center for Health Statistic, 2010).

Health data clearly demonstrate disparities in HIV in both new infections and death rates for the African American population. Although this population accounts for 12.6% of the U.S. population, it accounts for 44% of new HIV cases. In particular, young, gay, bisexual, and other African American men who have sex with men (MSM) are affected disproportionately. For 2010, African American MSM accounted for 70% percent of the black men newly diagnosed with HIV. This rate is 7 times higher than that for whites, 2 times higher than the rate for Hispanic men, and almost 3 times as high as the rate for black women (CDC, 2011a). More than two-thirds of black men who reported engaging in MSM sexual behavior in a low-income, high-HIV-prevalence community identified themselves as heterosexual (43%) or bisexual (24%), and over 71% of MSM reported having sex with women. Therefore, providers must have greater tolerance and acceptance of sexual diversity, provide health promotion education, and focus on HIV screening among the African American population.

Another disparity between African Americans and the general population involves susceptibility to pain. Interestingly, research indicates that African American and Hispanic patients experience pain differently than their non-Hispanic white counterparts. Rahim-Williams et al (2007) found that both racial groups had lower pain tolerance levels for contact heat and cold; however, there was no difference between minority and non-Hispanic white populations' tolerance of ischemic pain (pain experienced from an application of a tourniquet). Additionally, there was no difference in pain threshold (defined as the pressure level at which pressure pain was felt) between the racial groups. This may have implications for achieving adequate pain management goals.

Prescribers may need to keep these differences in mind when treating African American and Hispanic patients.

African Americans also have an increased risk (as high as 4 times that of European Americans and Latinos) of being diagnosed with schizophrenia (Blow et al, 2004). This increased risk may be due to a possible genetic predisposition as well as to environmental risk factors. Lawson (2008) proposes that polymorphisms of the synapsin III and NOTCH 4 genes found in African Americans with schizophrenia, but not as yet identified in European Americans, as well as environmental factors may increase the risk for schizophrenia. Another difference between these populations is that African Americans respond differently than whites to alcohol, psychotropic drugs, and caffeine: they reach higher blood levels, have a faster therapeutic response, and a higher rate of extrapyramidal effects than do non-Hispanic whites (Purnell, 2013).

Blacks have a higher number of asthma visits to the emergency department, 18.6 per 100,000 versus 5.6 for whites, and also experience a higher asthma-related death rate of 2.7 per 10,000 versus 1.4 for whites. But prescribers are falling short of the Healthy People 2020 target in providing black patients with key asthma education and management strategies, such as proper use of an inhaler (Alkinbami, Moorman, & Liu, 2011).

The U.S. Office of Minority Health attributes the poor health outcomes for African Americans to, among other things, "discrimination, cultural barriers, and lack of access to health care" (National Center for Health Statistics, 2010, p 2). In addition, a large body of literature, including Johnson (2006) and Soto and colleagues (2011), attributes psychopathology among the African American population to stress arising from racism, unequal treatment, and anxiety over experiences of racism, which may lead to poorer health status from the continued overactivation of the stress response and poorer overall health.

Health Beliefs and Practices

For a significant portion of the African American population, health is a gift from God, and illness and suffering are God's will or are caused by evil influences. Because God's will is the source of the illness, African Americans rely heavily on the healing powers of religious ritual and the advice of their religious leaders. They take their religion seriously and engage in prayer for many reasons. Folk healers and folk medicine—such as cod liver oil to prevent colds, sulfur and molasses in the spring to promote health, and copper or silver bracelets to protect from harm—are often used as are herbal remedies. Allopathic health care is not considered for prevention (Purnell, 2013).

Regional differences are often a factor in attitudes toward health issues for all ethnic groups, including African Americans. Those who were raised in the southeastern part of the United States are more likely to subscribe to health beliefs and practices common to that region than are African Americans raised elsewhere. Prescribers should become familiar with regional differences and assess each patient's unique attitudes in order to meet the health-care needs of that particular patient.

Racial Differences in Drug Pharmacokinetics and Response

African Americans appear to have been studied more than other ethnic groups in relation to ethnopharmacology, which has resulted in a larger body of knowledge about racial differences in pharmacokinetics for this group. This intense interest in ethnic pharmacology led to the first drug being approved by the U.S. Food and Drug Administration (FDA) in 2005 specifically for adjunctive treatment of heart failure in patients who self-identify as African American. BiDil is a fixed-dose combination of two generic drugs, hydralazine and isosorbide dinitrate, the first drug labeled exclusively for a specific race (Brody & Hunt, 2006). In an extensive review of ethnic variation and the significance of CYP 2C9 and CYP 2C19, Rosemary and Adithan (2007) discovered that the presence of CYP 2C9 *2 and *3 alleles required a 29% reduction in warfarin dose in African Americans.

Some black persons may be ultrarapid metabolizers of substrates of CYP 2D6. The prevalence of ultrarapid CYP 2D6 metabolizers among the African American population is 3.4%, similar to Caucasians, but the prevalence of ultrarapid CYP 2D6 metabolizers among Africans of Ethiopian descent is 29% (U.S. Food and Drug Administration [FDA], 2012). The impact of ethnic differences is seen in the case of codeine metabolism, where codeine is metabolized into morphine at a more rapid pace, leading to higher serum morphine levels and risk for morphine toxicity. Differences have also been demonstrated between African Americans and whites in plasma protein binding (Johnson & Livingston, 1997). This study found increased unbound fractions of drugs bound to albumin, a common binding site for many drugs. The researchers were careful to point out, however, that differences in protein concentrations might also explain the racial differences. At the time of this publication, no more recent research was found, indicating that further study is needed in this area. A large number of drugs could be affected by this racial difference if the findings can be replicated.

Hypertension has a high prevalence in African Americans. One reason behind this phenomenon appears to be salt sensitivity (Weinberger, 1993), which is often cited as the reason to use diuretics as first-line therapy for this ethnic group. In a study looking at the use of beta-adrenergic blockers to treat hypertension in African Americans, Prisant and Mensah (1996) found that not all African Americans are salt sensitive. When salt sensitivity was controlled for, there was no racial difference in efficacy when beta-adrenergic blockers were used with diuretics as combination therapy for hypertension. This study suggests that beta-adrenergic blockers should be given to some African Americans for certain indications, such as myocardial infarction prophylaxis.

To further confuse the issue of beta-adrenergic blockers, studies have been done related to racial differences in nucleotide-mediated smooth muscle relaxation (vasodilation) in response to nitric oxide. Studies by Cardillo, Kilcoyne, Cannon, and Panza (1998, 1999) support a difference between African Americans and whites in vasodilation response. The vasodilation effect of beta-adrenergic blockers stems from the combination of direct smooth muscle stimulation and endothelial nitric oxide release. Specifically, variations on a gene that codes for nitric oxide synthase, NOS3, has been found to correlate with left ventricular remodeling in African Americans with heart failure (McNamara et al, 2009). A variation on a similar gene, *eNOS4*, appears to influence the relationship between plasma nitric oxide levels and blood pressure (Li et al, 2004). Other drugs dependent on nitric oxide for their action include the nitrates. Both drug classes may not be efficacious or may require dosage alterations to achieve efficacy in African Americans.

The utilization of beta-adrenergic blockers in African Americans with heart failure is supported by Yancy, Laskar, and Eichhorn (2004) and Shekelle, et al (2003). Following a review of the literature, the authors recommended that, barring specific contraindications, beta-adrenergic blockers be used for any patient with left ventricular dysfunction in heart failure. Additionally, beta-adrenergic blockers used in conjunction with angiotensin converting enzyme (ACE) inhibitors in African Americans can be effective in treating heart failure (Yancy et al, 2004).

A study by Weir and colleagues (1998) also demonstrated that controlling for salt sensitivity affected response to two other classes of drugs (ACE inhibitors and calcium channel blockers). Calcium channel blockers are recommended second-line therapy for African Americans. African Americans who were salt sensitive had more lowering of blood pressure with isradipine (a calcium channel blocker) than with enalapril (also a calcium channel blocker). Therefore, differences appear to be not only between drug classes but also within them.

ACE inhibitors are also useful in treating hypertension, but African Americans appear to have less renin-dependent hypertension, and these drugs are less useful with that group. A study by Mitchell and colleagues (1997) confirmed racial differences in the renal hemodynamic response to chronic use of ACE inhibition that was independent of diuretic use and the magnitude of blood pressure lowering. More recent research into the use of ACE inhibitors in African Americans found that those homozygous for a variation at gene G12269A exhibited faster response to the ACE inhibitor Ramipril than those who were heterozygous (Bhatnagar et al, 2007). In this case, the authors are careful to stress that this area should be further researched before the information is utilized in clinical practice.

A serious adverse reaction to ACE inhibitors that contraindicates their use is angioedema. It is thought to be related to the reduced breakdown of bradykinin in patients taking this class of drugs. A study by Gainer, Nadeau, Ryder, and Brown (1996) concluded that African Americans show racial differences in the kallikrein-kinin system and are more sensitive to bradykinin, placing them at increased risk of ACE inhibitor–associated angioedema, independent of dose or concurrent drugs.

Diabetes mellitus has a higher prevalence in African Americans. The Bogalusa Heart Study Twentieth Anniversary Symposium (1995) suggested that elevated insulin levels observed in African American adolescents, especially girls, may be attributed to their decreased hepatic insulin clearance. This suggests consideration of drugs that affect hepatic insulin clearance (e.g., metformin [Glucophage]) for treating African Americans with type 2 diabetes. Stephens, Gillapsy, Clyne, Mejia, and Pollack (1990) also found racial differences in the incidence of end-stage renal disease associated with diabetes, which suggests that more aggressive management may be needed to prevent this complication.

Cryer and Feldman (1996) studied racial differences in gastric function between African Americans and whites. Gastric bicarbonate secretion was significantly higher in African Americans, making their gastric pH also higher. This might be a factor in the absorption of drugs that require highly acidic media for absorption. In the same study, mucosal biopsies demonstrated a much higher prevalence of *Helicobacter pylori* infection and chronic active superficial gastritis in African Americans. Even those who were negative for this infection had differences in gastric bicarbonate secretion.

As previously mentioned, African Americans are more likely to develop lung cancer when compared with European Americans (Haiman, et al., 2006). Berg, Mason, Boettcher, Hatsukami, and Murphy (2010) found that African Americans using a nicotine patch and abstaining from smoking metabolized nicotine differently from European Americans, as evidenced by lower urine excretion levels of nicotine and cotinine (a metabolic derivative of nicotine). This may have implications for African Americans who are quitting smoking using a nicotine patch.

Current biological evidence regarding psychotherapy agents points to decreasing the dosages of psychotropic medications and when possible prescribing atypical antypsychotics when formulating treatment plans for African American patients. In particular, Lawson (2008) describes that first-generation antipsychotics metabolized by the CYP450 2D6 isoenzyme show ethnic variation. African Americans (as well as European, Asian, and Hispanic Americans) demonstrate a reduced activity of this enzyme, which results in slower drug metabolism. Patients with this variation may experience increased extrapyramidal side effects when given a standard dose. Newer second-generation antipsychotic agents are not mainly metabolized through the CYP450 1A2 isoenzyme system, with CYP450 2D6 as a minor pathway. Thus, the adage of "start low, and go slow" applies to the treatment of African Americans when prescribing and choosing antipsychotics (Lawson, 2008).

Finally, a study by Carmel (1999) looked at racial differences in cobalamin and homocysteine levels between African Americans and whites. The study raised concern about potential underreporting and undertreatment of pernicious anemia because African Americans have significantly higher serum cobalamin levels than do whites. They also have significantly lower homocysteine levels, metabolize homocysteine more efficiently, and do not show the same benefit from vitamin therapy in treating this anemia. A further question raised related to the prescription of folate: "Given their lower rate of neural tube defects, possibly lower homocysteine levels, more efficient homocysteine metabolism, and lesser impact of vitamin therapy on it, does the untargeted promotion of high folate intake provide less benefit to blacks than to whites while exposing them to an equal risk for adverse effects because of unrecognized pernicious anemia?" (Carmel, 1999, p 90).

AMERICAN INDIAN/ALASKA NATIVE GROUPS

Cultural Factors

Demographics

American Indian and Alaska Native (AI/AN) peoples are a diverse group; more than 560 different tribes are recognized by the federal or state governments and, in addition, there are others that are not so recognized. Including individuals who identified as AI/AN in combination with another race, the U.S. Census in 2011 found that this group represents 1.6% of the population and that its numbers are increasing faster than the growth in the overall population (26.7% versus 9.7%, respectively) in part due to higher fertility rates than other racial/ethnic groups and living arrangements that include extended families (U.S. Census Bureau, 2012d). One problem in reporting the accurate size of the American Indian population is the tendency of this group to count members as part of an AI/AN tribal group by a blood quorum; that is, an individual must be at least a certain percentage American Indian or Alaska Native in order to be recorded and counted. Membership in the tribe would qualify the individual for health-care services provided by the Indian Health Service. Interracial marriages are also common, and the children are often documented as being of the race of the non-Indian parent. However, a shift toward recognition and taking pride in American Indian heritage has occurred (Purnell, 2013). The 2000 census permitted individuals to list more than one race, allowing children of mixed-race couples to avoid having to choose to be identified as one race or another.

As a group, the AI/AN are young (30.5% of the population is under the age of 18), undereducated (17.3% of those 25 years and older have a bachelor's degree or higher), and poorer than the rest of the U.S. population (median household income is $37,095, and 26.4% live below the federal poverty level (U.S. Census Bureau, 2012d). In addition, the AI/AN population is divided in residence, with 60% living in urban areas and fewer than a quarter living on the reservation and tribal lands (Office of Minority Health, 2012a).

Education and Employment

Over 81% of American Indian and Alaska Native adults (25 years of age or older) have at least a high school diploma or equivalency, 11.2% have a bachelor's degree, and 6.1% have achieved a graduate degree (U.S. Census Bureau, 2012d).

Overall, 17.3% of American Indians and Alaska Natives have a bachelor's degree or higher, compared with 34.5% of non-Hispanic white Americans (National Center for Education Statistics, 2012; U.S. Census Bureau, 2011b). In 2011, the unemployment rate among this population group was at 14.6%, the second-highest of any racial group in the United States (the highest being African Americans, unemployed at a rate of 15.8%, and significantly higher than the non-Hispanic white unemployment rate of 7.9%). The U.S. Department of Labor explains that higher levels of education tend to lead toward higher levels of employment for a racial group, which may help to explain the large unemployment rate among Native Americans and Alaska Natives (U.S. Department of Labor, 2012).

Family Relationships

The average American Indian family household has four to five members, making it the largest family size of any of the ethnic minority groups. Women head 25% of the households and the nuclear family is often comprised of extended relatives living under one roof, including relatives from both parental sides. Elder members usually assume leadership and decision-making roles. Some tribal groups are matriarchal while some are patriarchal, with the leadership and the health decision making coming from the sex that matches the leadership orientation, often with the help of spiritual leaders or medicine people (Purnell, 2013).

Many tribes have an established clan system whereby members of the tribe help to rear children, participate in general family life and customs of the tribe, and help make decisions for members of the clan. Marriage definitions in the AI/AN population may also not follow the traditions governing marriage and having children "out-of-wedlock" that exist in the predominant American culture. For example, 58.4% of births occur to women who have never been married versus 33.2% in the general population, yet these women may have a strong cultural identity and support from numerous clan members (National Healthy Marriage Resource Center, 2008). Prescribers should try to determine the unique histories, environments, and cultural beliefs of the specific tribal groups from which their patients originate in order to understand the family structure, decision making, and leadership style of AI/AN patients so as to ensure optimal treatment plans.

Health-Care Utilization

In 1824, the Bureau of Indian Affairs (BIA) was given the responsibility to "enhance the quality of life, to promote economic opportunity, and to carry out the responsibility to protect and improve the trust assets of American Indians, Indian tribes and Alaska Natives" (U.S. Department of the Interior, 2012, p 1). Numerous treaties, laws, Supreme Court decisions, and Executive Orders have assured the provision of health-care services for the 566 federally recognized tribes and their descendants.

Since 1954, the U.S. Department of Health, Education and Welfare, known today as the U.S. Department of Health and Human Services, has been responsible for providing no-cost comprehensive health-care services to American Indians and Alaska Natives under the direction of the Indian Health Service (IHS). Unfortunately, the IHS is severely underfunded when compared to other government health-care agencies. The IHS receives only $2,130 per person (pp) compared with $3,985/pp for the Bureau of Prisons, $5,010/pp for Medicaid, $5,234/pp for the Veterans Administration, and $7,631/pp for Medicare (Wilner, 2008). Approximately 70% of all members of the group who claim American Indian heritage receive IHS funded care.

Some tribes have chosen to take over the provision of health care from the IHS under the provisions of the 1975 Indian Self-Determination and Education Assistance Act, often because of the long-held deep suspicion of the federal government. In addition, only 22% of AI/AN live on the reservations or trust lands and an overwhelming 60% live in metropolitan areas away from IHS sites. Since 1972, the IHS has expanded its funding of health-related activities in off-reservation settings to help meet the needs of patients living away from reservations or trust lands. According to the IHS, 41% of AI/AN reported having private health insurance coverage, 36.7% relied on Medicaid coverage, and 29.2% had no health insurance coverage in 2010 (Office of Minority Health, 2012a); the percentage of non-Hispanic whites who had no health insurance in the same year was 16.3% (U.S. Census, 2013d).

Health Status and Other Biological Variables

Health disparities are prevalent in this minority group as demonstrated by the high rates of alcoholism (552% higher), diabetes (182% higher), unintentional injuries (138% higher), homicide (83% higher), and suicide (74% higher), when compared to the Caucasian population (IHS, 2013a, b). Among young males age 15–34, suicide is the second leading cause of death, which is 2.5 times higher than the national average for the same age group (CDC, 2012b). The infant mortality rate is 65% higher than that of whites, and the rate of sudden infant death syndrome is 2.4 times that of whites. Additionally, AI/AN infants have 2.3 times the rate of death from accidental injuries (MacDorman & Matthews, 2011).

These statistics ultimately influence the overall life expectancy of American Indians and Alaska Natives, which at 73.6 years is 4.1 years less than the overall U.S life expectancy for all races; life expectancy is 78.9 years for non-Hispanic whites (IHS, 2013a; Kaiser Family Foundation, 2013). Life expectancy within Arizona's American Indian population is 54.7 years (Wilner, 2008). The five top causes of mortality in 2009 were heart disease, cancer, injury, diabetes, and chronic liver disease/cirrhosis. Other causes, in descending order, are chronic lower respiratory diseases, cerebrovascular diseases, suicide, pneumonia and influenza, and kidney diseases (Kochanek, Xu, Murphy, Miniño, & Kung, 2011).

The higher a person's percentage of American Indian or Alaska Native genetic heritage, the more likely that individual is to manifest diabetes, almost exclusively type 2. The rate of type 2 diabetes is greatest in a subset of American Indians, the Pima Indians (Knowles, Saad, Pettitt, Nelson, & Bennett, 1993). Within this group, research has shown that genetic variants in the *PYY-Y2R* pathway were correlated with obesity among full-heritage Pima Indian men, which may relate to the increased rate of diabetes in this group. (Ma et al, 2005). Additional research on Pima Indians and Old Order Amish patients found that two variants of the *MBL2* gene, which encodes for mannose-binding lectin, are associated with a higher risk for type 2 diabetes (Muller et al, 2010). As more research is done regarding genetics, obesity, and type 2 diabetes in the Indian population, there will be an ever-increasing level of evidence to guide the care of this population. In order to address this health disparity, Congress has allocated over $150 million to the Special Diabetes Program for Indians (SDPI). This program has had a huge impact in the improvement of diabetes health outcomes in the AI/AN population. One of the most important improvements was a 10.8% decrease in the mean hemoglobin A1c level of AI/AN diagnosed with diabetes, which has resulted in a 40% reduction in diabetes complications (IHS, 2013b).

Navajo Neuropathy is a fatal autosomal recessive genetic disorder present in the Navajo population. Those with the illness display weakness, metabolic acidosis, neuropathy, and liver failure (Hodgins & Hodgins, 2013). Karadimas and colleagues (2006) examined incidences of Navajo Neuropathy and found that a mutation on the *MPV17* gene is associated with disease development. The authors suggest that this finding can be used in genetic testing.

Lactose intolerance is very common among American Indians, with between 79% and 100% of the population affected (Giger, 2013; Swagerty, Walling, & Klein, 2002). The NIH (2010) explains that actual percentages are difficult to determine, as much of the present data relies solely on self-report. Further research needs to be done in this field to determine more accurate statistics as well as investigate the cause of the variance between this group and Northern European whites, who have an estimated lactose intolerance prevalence of 2% to 15% (Swagerty et al, 2002).

Alcohol abuse is also prevalent among American Indians (Hodgins & Hodgins, 2013). A 2003 study conducted by Wall, Carr, and Ehlers (2003) found the rate of alcoholism among Mission Indians to be 60%, with men being more affected than women (72% versus 53%, respectively). Of this population, the percentage of Native American heritage was found to be important—those with more than 50% Native American heritage were more likely to be alcoholic when compared to those with less than 50% heritage. Additionally, they found that certain variations of *ADH2*, a gene for alcohol dehydrogenase, was a protective factor for alcoholism.

The AI/AN population has a higher prevalence of current smoking rates than any other minority or racial group. Only 20.6% of whites in the United States smoke cigarettes, but 31.5% of AI/AN use tobacco products, with men engaging in smoking behaviors more often than women (34.4% versus 29.1%, respectively). Unfortunately, there has been no significant documented change in the prevalence of smoking among the AI/AN compared to among the non-Hispanic white and black populations (CDC, 2013c). Therefore, prescribers should focus on discussing proven evidence-based interventions aimed at tobacco cessation with this population.

Health Beliefs and Practices

Practitioners must understand that the AI/AN population is characterized by a wide variance in cultural values, beliefs, and practices; the environments that they live in; and their socioeconomic circumstances. The AI/AN population's high-risk behaviors, such as alcoholism and higher smoking rates, may be due to alcohol metabolism issues and long-held sacred cultural traditions involving tobacco, which include the use of tobacco products for prayer, protection, respect, and healing (Cimino, Sayers, & Roods, 1999). For these populations, health is harmony with nature and oneself. Illness is disharmony and may be caused by a supernatural force or by violation of a restriction or prohibition. The illness is seen as an imbalance of mind, body, and spirit. Because the cause of the illness is external, illness-prevention practices that relate the cause of illness to the behavior of the patient are questioned. This is an interesting conflict, because self-control is considered to be a central attribute to maintaining harmony, and each person is accountable for his or her own health.

Many AI/AN maintain traditional beliefs regarding spiritual activities and their relationship to health (Giger, 2013). Traditional beliefs and Western medicine are often interwoven (Moghaddam & Momper, 2011). Western medicine is accepted but not seen as able to heal except when used in conjunction with native healing practices. Because the hospital is considered the place to die, the patient may resist hospitalization. Pain is supposed to be borne, so AI/AN may not request pain medication when needed. Practitioners should be mindful about educating the AI/AN community on the positive aspects of healing in regard to adequate pain control.

A belief in a Great Spirit pervades AI/AN views regarding life and their association in the natural world, where their focus is on the importance of balancing and achieving harmony with people, animals, plants, nature, weather, and supernatural forces (Giger, 2013). Giger (2013) describes an important philosophy among the Navajo called Blessing Way, a ceremonial song complex which attempts to restore harmony through stories, songs, rituals, prayers, symbols, and sand paintings. Medicine bags, which may contain medicine bundles—symbolic and sacral items such as corn pollen, feathers, stones, and arrowheads—and other instruments are used for healing and blessings. These bags may be worn or carried to protect a person from evil spirits or to promote wellness and harmony. The medicine person may also use negative powers, but only against the sick person's enemies. Native American/Alaska Native healing ceremonies that may include singing are often part of the healing ritual. Traditional care may be sought from a member of the family or a medicine man/woman who has the ability to use his or her powers of healing in conjunction with herbs and other rituals (Giger, 2013). Providers need to determine which herbal remedies a patient is using before prescribing modern medicines.

Racial Differences in Drug Pharmacokinetics and Response

Although a large portion of this ethnic group has health care provided by the U.S. Indian Health Service, little research has been done related to racial considerations in pharmacokinetics or other therapies. In the past, a few studies in the literature, which were found to be contradictory, were related to metabolism of alcohol (Bennion & Li, 1976; Chan, 1986). More recently, Gizer, Edenberg, Gilder, Wilhelmsen, and Ehlers (2011) investigated traits related to chromosome 4q near a cluster of alcohol dehydrogenase (ADH) genes. These genes encode enzymes of alcohol metabolism and may be responsible for variants in the *ADH1B* and *ADH4* genes, which may protect against the development of commonly seen symptoms associated with alcohol dependence in other ethnic/racial groups (Gizer et al, 2011). Another study, involving lipoproteins (Harris-Hooker & Sanford, 1994), reported that American Indians have a lower prevalence of coronary heart disease related to lower low-density lipoprotein (LDL) cholesterol and higher high-density lipoprotein (HDL) cholesterol levels. There may also be significant ethnic differences in the response to morphine in ventilated patients. Cepeda and colleagues (2001) found that despite higher levels of serum M6G levels in Caucasians, Native Indians were more susceptible to morphine depression of the ventilatory response than Caucasians. Providers should use caution when medicating this group to avoid an exaggerated response in the respiratory system.

Although research with the AI/AN groups has expanded since the last edition of this text, more research is needed to identify further racial/ethnic differences in drug pharmacokinetics in this ethnic group.

ASIAN AMERICANS

Cultural Factors

Demographics

The Asian cultural group is the most diverse of all the minority groups, encompassing over 50 distinct racial/ethnic subgroupings with over 30 different languages. Asians have many countries of origin (spanning East Asia, Southeast Asia, and South Asia), religious/spiritual affiliations, cultural backgrounds, health-care beliefs and practices, and immigration experiences. The top six Asian subgroups in the United States are Chinese, Filipino, Asian Indian, Vietnamese, Korean, and Japanese (U.S. Census Bureau, 2012c). In fact, in recognition of this diversity, the 2000 census divided this subgroup into two—one the "Asian American" group and the other the "Hawaiian and Other Pacific Islanders" group. Therefore, we discuss these two in separate sections in this edition of the text.

In the 2010 U.S. census, 5.6% of the population identified themselves as Asian, either alone or in combination with other races (U.S. Census Bureau, 2012a). This group includes people originating from the Far East, Southeast Asia, or the Indian subcontinent. The number of Asians, either alone or in combination with one or more other races, increased by 45.6% from 2000 to 2010 (U.S. Census, 2012b), and they have surpassed Hispanics as the fastest-growing ethnic minority immigrant group (PEW Research Center, 2013). This may be due to the changing national sociopolitical climate that has imposed more restrictions on southern border crossings and to changes in state laws (e.g., Arizona) that aim to verify the immigration status of Hispanics (PEW Research, 2010).

In the 2011 census study the median household income for those identifying as Asian American alone was $67,885, which is the highest of all minority groups in the United States, and the percentage of the population living in poverty was 12.8%, the lowest of all minority groups (U.S. Census Bureau, 2011b). However, as a reminder of the diversity of this group, the poverty levels ranged from low (among those of Indian, Japanese, and Filipino descent) to high (among those of Korean, Vietnamese, and Chinese descent). And although the averages give a positive picture, this group includes both extremes of health and socioeconomic indicators (PEW Research, 2012).

A high percentage (76.9%) of this population, age 5 and older, does not speak English at home, and large percentages are not fluent in English: 55% of Vietnamese, 46% of Chinese, 22% of Filipino, and 22% of Asian Indian (Pandya et al, 2011). Therefore, prescribers will need to have interpreter services available if their community has non-English–speaking Asian populations.

Education and Employment

Asian Americans as a group are better educated and better paid than the general U.S. population. The unemployment rate is lower than that of the general population and of each individual racial group, with 7% of Asians unemployed in the 2011 census, compared with an overall unemployment rate of 8.9% (U.S. Department of Labor, 2012a). About 49% were employed in managerial, professional, or other higher-paying jobs compared to 35% of white Americans (U.S. Department of Labor, 2012a).

In 2011, 85.1% of Asian American adults had at least a high school diploma, which is similar to the total population (85.9%), but 50% of Asian Americans compared to 28.5% of the total American population had at least a bachelor's degree. Additionally, 20.7% achieved a graduate degree or higher, compared with 10.6% of all Americans (U.S. Census Bureau, 2013a). These statistics demonstrate that as a whole, the Asian population is more affluent than other racial/ethnic minorities and in some instances may not be considered an at-risk group when they seek entry into higher education.

Family Relationships

Family relationships are strong, with extended (often multigenerational) families and an expectation of family loyalty from all members. Families are a source of strength. In Japanese families, the father is away from the home on business a great deal of the time, so the mother–eldest son relationship is very strong. Before the eldest son is of age, the mother is the dominant person in the home. Both nuclear and extended families are involved in decision making. In all Asian American groups, males are more "valued" than females, females are submissive to males, and respect for elders is taught at an early age. Individuals' wishes and needs are subordinated to the needs of the group. Spector (2004) says that adherence to Buddhism, Confucianism, and Taoism leads these Asian American families to avoid admitting physical or mental illness. Conflicts are handled within the family, and there is kinship solidarity in which the individual is expected to seek the input of elders in the family and from kin.

Health-Care Utilization

Researchers have found that there are substantial differences by country of birth in health-care access and utilization among Asian Americans. Recent Asian immigrants are less likely to have health-care coverage, which may result in less frequent visits to health-care providers. Asian groups overall, however, are well insured, with only 15.4% of U.S. Asians uninsured in 2011 (U.S. Census Bureau, 2013a). Asian Americans over age 65 make about half as many visits to health-care providers as their non-Hispanic white counterparts (Ye, Mack, Fry-Johnson, & Parker, 2012).

Health Status and Other Biological Variables

As a homogenous group, the health status of Asian Americans as a whole is excellent. They have a longer life expectancy and lower death rates from all causes than does the general population (Asian women have a life expectancy of 85.5 years—the largest of any other racial/ethnic minority group) (Office of Minority Health, 2012b). The illnesses that are experienced at higher levels than those in the general population include tuberculosis, stomach/colorectal cancer (among Japanese), and suicide (among elderly Chinese women). Southeast Asian refugees have a higher incidence of intestinal parasites, tuberculosis, and presence of hepatitis B antigen and more anemia than other Asian Americans or the general population. Overall, the leading causes of death are cancer, heart disease, stroke, accidents, and diabetes. Asian Americans have the highest rate of TB of any cultural group and twice the rate of the hepatitis B virus than white Americans (although this is decreasing). Sudden infant death syndrome is the fourth leading cause of infant mortality. Asian Americans also have a high rate of chronic obstructive pulmonary disease (Office of Minority Health, 2012b; Purnell, 2013).

Although Asian Americans have the lowest percentage of smoking rates among all of the racial/ethnic groups, 9.9% versus 20.6% for non-Hispanic whites, there exist marked differences among Asian subgroups. Asians of Korean and Vietnamese descent have the highest smoking rates among all of the Asian subgroups, 26.6% and 21.5%, respectively. The lowest smoking rates among the Asian population are found in the Chinese (8.8%), Asian Indian (11.9%), Japanese (12.1%), and Filipino (16.7%) populations. Gender differences for smoking rates also exist among the Asian subgroup populations. Women of Asian Indian descent have the lowest smoking rates (3.5%) and Korean

women have the highest rates (20.1%). Among men, those of Chinese ancestry have the lowest smoking rates (13.9%) while Korean men continue to have some of the highest smoking rates (37.4%) (CDC, 2013c).

Also important to note is that pneumonia/influenza is the fourth leading cause of death among Asians aged 65 and over and that case rates for tuberculosis (TB) (25.8 cases per 100,000) are the highest among any other ethnic/minority group, with Asians having the highest percentage of new TB cases among foreign-born persons living in the United States. However, recent research suggests that Asians may have a genetic component that somehow reduces their risk of chronic obstructive pulmonary disease (COPD) regardless of their smoking habits. In fact, rates of COPD are low in mainland China even though approximately one-third of that population smokes. In the United States, Asians are 60% less likely to be hospitalized for COPD than non-Hispanic whites (American Lung Association, 2007). These data clearly show that more research to further explore these differences among the different ethnic/minority groups is needed. In addition, practitioners should screen the Asian population for TB to help slow the spread of the disease.

Health Beliefs and Practices

Health beliefs and practices vary among different Asian American subgroups. Chinese and Vietnamese people have a fatalistic attitude and believe that health is a result of forces that rule the world: yin (cold) and yang (hot). Illness results when there is an imbalance in these forces. Illness is diagnosed by pulses (there are seven different ones), color and texture of the tongue, and other means not commonly used by allopathic medicine. Treatment is provided with the opposing force to achieve balance. For example, a "cold" illness (e.g., colic, diarrhea, or edema) is treated with "hot" herbs and foods. "Hot" illnesses (e.g., hypertension, blood diseases, or a cough) are treated with "cold" herbs and foods. Healers within the group are skilled at diagnosis and prescription of therapy. Such therapy may include acupuncture, acupressure, tai chi, moxibustion, or medicinal herbs.

Chapter 10 discusses herbal therapy, with the important caveat that one must understand and subscribe to a totally different view of health and illness to prescribe these herbs appropriately. "Chi" is innate energy, and lack of it results in fatigue and long illnesses. Asians may call on their ancestors for help, and the Vietnamese may use cupping with a heated cup or glass jar that is placed on the skin to create a vacuum. This practice leaves bruising and may be misinterpreted in children as child abuse. Asian populations may believe that mental illness and physical disabilities should be hidden. Women usually seek care from female providers. Older clients may appear willing to comply with prescribed therapies but then don't follow them; their respect for the provider prohibits them from discussing their unwillingness to follow the regimen.

Japanese beliefs are influenced by Shinto, a religious orientation. They believe that humans are inherently good and that evil is caused by outside spirits. Both Japanese and Vietnamese people believe that pleasing good spirits and avoiding evil ones help to maintain harmony and health. Evil is removed by purification rituals. Mental illness is taboo and often translates into acceptable somatic symptoms, and addictions are shameful (Purnell, 2013). Alcoholism and family violence are hidden but serious problems.

Filipinos also subscribe to the concept of yin and yang but believe that God's will and supernatural forces govern the universe and determine health and illness. Illness is punishment for violations of God's will. Amulets and religious medals may be worn as a shield from witchcraft or as a good-luck charm. Filipinos often engage in healing rituals and may perform sacrifices. The "evil eye" may be considered the reason for illness in infants and children. Filipinos are the most likely of the Asian American groups to be obese. They have high alcohol consumption and smoking rates.

All of these groups use combinations of allopathic and ethnically defined health and illness care. The allopathic approach, however, is often chosen last or to supplement ethnically defined care. In a study of college students who identified themselves as having an Asian or European background, Asian students had more negative views of medications than European students. Asian students were more likely to view medicines as "intrinsically harmful, addictive substances" and were less likely to believe in the benefits of modern medicine. All the students viewed taking prescribed medications more favorably if they had taken prescribed medications before (Horne et al, 2004, p 1307).

Racial Differences in Drug Pharmacokinetics and Response

Bertilsson (1995) first compared Asian Americans and whites on the basis of drug metabolism by the CYP450 2D6 and 2C19 isoenzyme systems. The CYP 2D6 isoenzyme system is responsible for metabolism of antiarrhythmics, antidepressants, and neuroleptics, among others. The mean activity of CYP 2D6 extensive metabolizers is lower in Asians and is the molecular genetic basis for slower metabolism of antidepressants and neuroleptics in Asians. This difference in metabolism requires lower doses of these drugs. The CYP 2C19 system is involved in the metabolism of acids (e.g., mephenytoin), bases (e.g., imipramine and omeprazole), and neutral drugs (e.g., diazepam). Diazepam (Valium) is partially demethylated by CYP 2C19, and the high frequency of mutated alleles in Asians is probably the reason that such populations have slower metabolism and are treated with lower doses of diazepam than are whites. Although other drugs in this same class have not been studied, it is likely that they have similar metabolic fates as diazepam. Omeprazole (Prilosec) is hydroxylated to a major extent by CYP 2C19, and there is an approximately 4-fold difference in oral clearance between Asians and whites. Hence, a lower dose for this drug is required for Asians (Vaz-da-Silva et al, 2005). Interestingly, when treating *H. pylori* in Chinese patients, success of a triple-drug therapy using a regimen of either esomeprazole or rabeprazole was not related to differences in the CYP2C19 gene (Lee et al, 2010).

Brooks, Enoch, Goldman, Li, and Yokoyama (2009) explained that those of East Asian descent (Japanese, Chinese, and Korean) have a propensity toward an aldehyde dehydrogenase-2 (ALDH2) deficiency, causing a "flush" to occur after drinking alcohol. This may occur despite the amount of alcohol ingested being minimal (O'Hara & Zhan, 2004). Chan (1986) also reported this "atypical" dehydrogenase, which he stated is present in 85% to 90% of Asian Americans. The deficiency in ALDH2 is caused by a genetic variance in the ALDH2 gene and can increase the patient's risk for developing esophogeal cancer (Brooks et al, 2009).

O'Hara and Zhan state that Asians have also been described as "fast acetylators." Recent studies have determined that Asian subgroups that originate in eastern Asia (Bangladesh, Thailand, Malaysia, China, Hong Kong, Korea, and Japan) have a higher percentage of fast acetylators than those from western Asia (Turkey, Russia, and Saudi Arabia). Researchers have determined an East–West geographic longitude, termed the Asian "fast acetylator longitude," that allows for prediction of acetylator status (Zaid et al, 2004). Hepatic acetylation is responsible for metabolism of many drugs, including cardiac and psychotropic drugs, and 78% to 93% of Asians are "fast acetylators" (Lin, Poland, Smith, Strickland, & Mendoza, 1991). This faster metabolism may require a more frequent or higher dose of drugs metabolized by acetylation to achieve efficacy.

Warfarin, a common anticoagulant, has a narrow window of therapeutic efficacy—too high a dose can cause excess bleeding, and too low a dose will not be effective as an anticoagulant. Moyer and colleagues (2009) conducted a literature review of articles exploring the genetic foundations of warfarin sensitivity. They found that among the two genes associated with sensitivity, Asians had a lower incidence of variance of the CYP 2C9 gene and increased variance of the *VKORC1* gene when compared to whites. The decrease in CYP 2C9 variance indicates a more "normal" warfarin metabolism, whereas the increase in *VKORC1* variance can mean an increased or a decreased sensitivity to warfarin (depending on the allele). A similar study found that a high occurrence of *VKORC1* variance led to prescribing lower doses of warfarin to achieve optimal results in Chinese patients when compared to New Zealand Europeans (Gladding et al, 2010).

For almost 50 years researchers have been aware of racial differences in response to antipsychotic drugs (Frackiewicz et al, 1997). An extensive review by Arranz and de Leon (2007) indicates Han Chinese may have enhanced response to atypical antipsychotics (risperdone) and no difference from Caucasians in their response to clozapine. Lee, Yang, and Hu (1998) found a lack of racial differences in lithium pharmacokinetics between Taiwanese Chinese bipolar patients and whites. In a study of antidepressant use, ethnic Chinese required significantly lower doses of sertraline (Zoloft) to achieve clinical efficacy than white patients (Hong Ng et al, 2006). "Despite controlling for weight, gender and dietary factors (alcohol, nicotine and caffeine) because of their possible influence on the metabolism of sertraline, the difference observed between ethnic groups remained statistically significant [$F(2,34) = 4.15$, $P < 0.05$]" (Hong Ng et al,

2006). These studies may indicate that atypical antipsychotics and selective serotonin reuptake inhibitors need to be dosed lower in Asian patients. Filipinos require lower doses of dopaminergics (levodopa) than do whites, and they develop dyskinesia more readily at comparable doses. This difference appears to be related to racial differences in erythrocyte catechol-o-methyltransferase (Rivera-Calimlim & Reilly, 1984).

Studies regarding the impact of pharmacogenetics on hypertension and response to antihypertensives were first published 20 years ago. In comparing Asian American children with African American, Hispanic, and white children, Liu and Levinson (1996) found a higher prevalence of elevated blood pressure in Asian Americans. Early studies supported the need for lower doses of beta-adrenergic blockers in Asians (Hui & Pasic, 1997; Matthews, 1995) and also ACE inhibitors and calcium channel blockers (Hui & Pasic, 1997), based in part on increased adverse drug reactions at doses used for whites. For example, Asian populations have an increased risk of a coughing side effect from angiotensin-converting enzyme inhibitors (Dikewicz, 2004). Interestingly, valsartan, an angiotensin II receptor blocker (ARB), has been shown to be equivalent to ACE inhibitor use in Indonesian and Taiwanese patients with hypertension (Black, Bailey, Zappe, & Samuel, 2009). Pharmacogenomic influences on the effectiveness of antihypertensive medications has become a focus of research in order to determine ethnic and individual response to medications (Johnson, 2010).

After organ transplant, patients are often given immunosuppressant medications to prevent organ rejection. One such medication is tacrolimus, a calcineurin inhibitor, which is metabolized by the protein products of the CYP 3A enzyme gene. Two single-neucleotide polymorphisms (SNPs) within CYP 3A, CYP 3A4*18B and CYP 3A5*3, are common in the Asian population. Among Chinese men, a combined genotype of CYP 3A4*1/*1- 9CYP3A5*3/*3 was associated with a change in the pharmacokinetics of tacrolimus (Shi et al, 2011). Patients with this genotype "may require lower [tacrolimus] doses to achieve target concentration levels" (Shi et al, 2011, p 621).

Of note is the fact there are ethnic differences among the Asian populations and ethnic minorities within the major Asian groups, with each having their own pharmacogenomic variant. For example, the Kyrgyz population in northwest China has three important pharmacogenetic variants from the Han Chinese, which are the majority ethnic group in China (Yunus et al., 2013). The drug-metabolizing enzyme activity of the Vietnamese differs from the Chinese (*CYP2A6*4* and *CYP2A6*5* differ), Koreans (*CYP2A6*5* and *CYP2A6*6*), Japanese (*CYP2A6*6*), and Malaysians (*CYP2A6*5*) (Viega et al, 2009).

NATIVE HAWAIIAN AND PACIFIC ISLANDERS

Cultural Factors

Demographics

According to the 2010 U.S. Census, the Native Hawaiian and Pacific Islander (NH/PI) population alone and in combination has seen incredible growth and has surpassed the rate of growth of the U.S. population by over 3 times, increasing by 35% from 399,000 to 540,000. This growth is especially evident for the NH/PI combination population rates because more than half (56%) of the NH/PI population declared a mixed combination with other racial groups, making up 0.4% of the total U.S. population. This is the second-fastest-growing racial group in the country after the Asian-alone or Asian-combination population. In addition, the NH/PI population is relatively young: 30% of NH/PI are under the age of 18 versus 23.5% of the U.S. population (U.S. Census Bureau, 2012e). The NH/PI population describes a wide array of people and customs whose origins may be Native Hawaiian, Guamanian or Chamorro, Samoan, or other Pacific Islander; Polynesian, such as Tahitian, Tongan, and Tokelauan; Micronesian, such as Marshallese, Palauan, and Chuukese; and Melanesian, such as Fijian, Guinean, and Solomon Islander.

The rulers of the Hawaiian islands were overthrown by a coup d'etat and the islands were subsequently annexed as a U.S. territory at the turn of the 20th century; Hawaii eventually became a state in 1959. It is important to note that although NH/PI originate from native lands, NH/PI have not been granted the same reparations, assistance, or group rights that have been afforded to other groups like American Indians and Alaska Natives and thus have significant health disparities.

Although traditionally the largest proportion of the NH/PI population has resided in the West (over 52% live in Hawaii and California), other parts of the United States have seen a tremendous growth in this population, particularly in the South and several Western states. In the southern states of Arkansas, Alabama, Delaware, North Carolina, Tennessee, Florida, Texas, Kentucky, Georgia, Oklahoma, Maryland, South Carolina, Virginia, and Louisiana, the NH/PI population grew by more than 50%. In the West, states such as Nevada, Alaska, Arizona, Idaho, Wyoming, Utah, Washington, Oregon, Montana, and New Mexico have also seen a 50% growth in the NH/PI population (U.S. Census Bureau, 2012e). Other localities that showed rapid growth include the District of Columbia, with a 68% growth rate, and counties in northern Alabama and northwest Arkansas, northern Utah, southern Nevada, Arizona, northern Georgia, Tennessee, North Carolina, and parts of Maryland, Virginia, and Texas, all of which experienced rapid growth of the NH/PI population (U.S. Census Bureau, 2012e).

There are significant economic disparities that must be addressed when formulating treatment plans for the NH/PI population. In 2011, the NH/PI poverty rate was 21.5% and the median income was $49,378, versus 13% and $55,305, respectively, for the non-Hispanic white population (U.S. Census Bureau, 2012e).

Education and Employment

The NH/PI attainment of a high school degree is similar to that of the non-Hispanic white population (85.1% versus 85.9%). However, only half continue on to college (14.5% versus 28.5%) or complete bachelor's degrees, and even fewer,

4.3%, of NH/PI, have completed a graduate/professional degree (versus 10.6% of non-Hispanic whites).

The average NH/PI family median income was $59,521 in 2010, versus $67,892 for non-Hispanic white families in the mainland United States, and 17% of NH/PI families, in comparison to 10.6% of non-Hispanic whites, were living at the poverty level during the 2010 census (Office of Minority Health, 2012c). The unemployment rate for this population in 2012 was 14%, considerably higher than the 7.9% rate for the non-Hispanic white population and 8.9% for the whole United States (U.S. Census Bureau, 2011a; U.S. Department of Labor, 2012a).

Family Relationships

The average family size for Hawaiian/Pacific Islanders is four and its organization is matriarchal with a belief in placing children in a position of prominence within the family (Liu & Almeda, 2011). Although there exists much diversity within the NH/PI populations in terms of family relationships, research describes four key pan-family values, beliefs, and practices that are commonly found in family practices across NH/PI subgroups.

The family interdependence is of utmost importance when forming a caring relationship with a patient from a NH/PI group. This interdependence is based on collectivism, relational orientation, familism, and family obligation. Collectivism is described as a predisposition to place group goals above those of the individual; relational orientation is defining the self as interdependent with others in the family unit; familism describes a family hierarchical system that includes extended family members as the basic social unit; and family obligation includes attitudes and behaviors expected of children. Children are expected to show respect and affection for older family members; seek their advice on important matters and accept their decisions; and maintain physical proximity, kinship, psychological and financial assistance, and emotional ties with parents, native Hawaiian elders (called *na kapuna*), and the extended family across the life span. These four cultural values, beliefs, and practices should influence the development of treatment plans that are culturally congruent with the NH/PI beliefs surrounding family relationships (Browne, Mokuau, & Braun, 2009; Yee, Debaryshe, Yuen, Kim, & McCubbin, 2013).

Health-Care Utilization

Data in the research literature on Native Hawaiian and Pacific Islanders is often limited due to a tendency to group this population with Asians and Pacific Islanders. Here we have attempted to distinguish among these groups because they often have different patterns of health risk and should not be viewed as homogeneous. For example, the Asian and Pacific Islander group's life expectancy is often reported as 80.3 years for the group as a whole (a level that is over 5 years higher than that of the total U.S. population), and this statistic includes the Japanese subgroup, which has one of the highest life expectancy rates—82.1 years (Kaiser Family Foundation,

2013). However, Native Hawaiians have one of the lowest life expectancy rates—68.3 years. For this reason, we have decided to treat this group separately from the Asian group in this edition.

Johnson, Oyama, LeMarchand, and Wilkens (2004) note that native Hawaiians die younger than Hawaiian residents of other ethnic groups. For example, in 2000, the age-adjusted death rates for Native Hawaiians due to heart disease, cancers, strokes, and diabetes were higher than for the general population in the state of Hawaii as a whole. In particular, diabetes age-adjusted death rates per 100,000 persons for the state of Hawaii were 16.3 versus 38.0 for Native Hawaiians and 155.8 versus 208.6 per 100,000 for cancer. McCubbin and Antonio (2012) state that the native Hawaiian population continues to have the highest rates of morbidity and mortality and chronic health conditions such as hypertension, diabetes, and asthma than other ethnic groups and have higher rates of smoking and drinking and more risk factors, such as overweight and obesity (Johnson et al, 2004).

Native Hawaiian children and adolescents also face significant health disparities: exposure to prenatal alcohol and tobacco use, late or no prenatal care, macrosomia as well as low birth rates, low rates of exclusive breastfeeding at 6 months, high rates of infant mortality, and high rates of obesity and physical, mental and sexual abuse (Liu & Almeda, 2011).

The leading causes of death in American Samoa, Guam, and the Federated States of Micronesia are similar to those in the United States, but patients must often travel long distances to Hawaii to obtain adequate treatment (Tseng, Omphroy, Cruz, Naval, & Haddock, 2004). The Pacific islands affiliated with the United States, such as Guam, have reported an increase in the number of chronic diseases. For example, diabetes was diagnosed in 9.1% of the population of Guam in 2009 (Ichiho, Gillan, & Aitaoto, 2013). Ichiho and colleagues describe risk factors for the leading causes of death in Guam (heart disease, cancer, and cerebrovascular accidents) to include poor diet, lack of physical activity, and lifestyle behaviors that are associated with overweight and obesity. These authors contend that significant advancements and the development of a territory-wide health plan and standards of care are needed to help address the prevention and control of such diseases.

Other areas in the Pacific, such as the Republic of Palau, reported cardiac arrest and respiratory arrest as the leading causes of death (Wong, Taoka, Kuartei, Demei, & Soaladaob, 2004), and in the Marshall Islands the leading cause of death was sepsis (Kroon, 2004).

Health Status and Other Biological Variations

There is limited data on the health status of Native Hawaiians and Pacific Islanders alone because many studies have small sample sizes and often include this group in a category labeled "Other Races," or results are often presented in conjunction with the Asian and the Native American group (American Lung Association, 2007). The NH/PI population has the second-highest tuberculosis rate after the Asian population

(15.9 per 100,000). In 2007, the TB rate was 21 times higher than that for white teenagers (American Lung Association, 2007; Office of Minority Health, 2012c). This population also has a high infant mortality rate.

Health Beliefs and Practices

In the Polynesian cultures, a Hawaiian philosophy called *Huna* is an important concept. One of the tenets of *Huna* is the seeking of harmony, love, and positive energy flow. The energy flow is believed to tap into the Universal Power that the Hawaiians call *mana*. The secret for attaining true health, happiness, prosperity, and success is the loving use of the power of *mana*. One of the ways that this can be achieved is through a Hawaiian massage, *lomi lomi*, that is delivered by a trained traditional healer. *Lomi lomi* is performed in a rhythmic and fluid motion that uses the practitioner's forearms as well as the hands to change the energy toward a positive flow. *Lomi lomi* is sometimes described as feeling like gentle waves moving over the body and is meant to relieve stress, stimulate blood and lymph flow, and assist in the elimination of wastes in the body (Lakainapali, 2013).

The cause of illness may be attributed to the stress of anger, guilt, recriminations, and lack of forgiveness. Families and individuals are encouraged to participate in *Ho'oponopono*, an ancient Hawaiian practice that leads to forgiveness and reconciliation. In other Polynesian cultures, illness may be attributed to a person's mistakes or errors, which may anger the gods. *Ho'oponopono* are family conferences in which interpersonal family relationships can be corrected through prayer, discussion, confession, repentance, and mutual restitution and forgiveness (Lakainapali, 2013).

The Native Hawaiian family, *'ohana*, is the core social unit within which the individual lives and interacts. It should be taken into account during the health-care transaction in order to aid NH/PI patients to meet their health-care goals (McGregor et al, 2003).

Racial Differences in Drug Pharmacokinetics and Response

Much current research on racial differences in pharmacokinetics has combined the Asian and NH/PI groups. However, Gladding and colleagues (2010) found in studying warfarin dosage in Chinese patients separately from Pacific Islanders that Chinese patients required lower doses of warfarin to achieve optimal results when compared to New Zealand Europeans and that Pacific Islanders had very few variants along the *CYP2C9* gene, requiring higher doses of warfarin (see Asian American section for further discussion of warfarin genetic variants).

HISPANIC AMERICANS

Cultural Factors

Demographics

The federal government considers race and ethnicity to be two separate constructs. Therefore, an individual can be of any race and self-identify as Hispanic. Individuals of Hispanic descent are not a homogeneous group. In fact, the group includes individuals who can trace their heritage to over 20 different Spanish-speaking countries of origin worldwide (Lopez, Gonzales-Barrera, & Cuddington, 2013). Hispanics are the largest minority group and make up 16.3% of the U.S. population (U.S. Census Bureau, 2010a), a figure that does not include the over 4 million residents of Puerto Rico. The Hispanic population is projected to more than double by 2060, from 53.3 million in 2012 to 128.8 million (U.S. Census Bureau, 2012a).

The majority of the Hispanic population is born in the United States (62.9%); only 37.1% is foreign-born, a 3% decrease since 2000 (PEW Research, 2012) that may be due to tougher border-crossing laws and enforcement of laws requiring official documents to cross the U.S. border. Although in 2008 the State Department implemented the use of passport cards, which are a less expensive and a more portable alternative to a passport for border crossings, the cards may still be a considerable expense for large Hispanic families, and some families may not qualify due to their undocumented status. Although the cards offer a lower-cost alternative to the traditional passport ($110), each card may cost from $40 to $55 for children and adults, respectively (U.S. Passport Cards, 2012).

In the United States, Hispanics include those of Mexican descent (63%), Puerto Ricans (9.2%), Cubans (3.5%), and people from Central and South America (CDC, 2012). The Hispanic population as a group is young, with 37.1% under age 20 compared to 22.4% for whites (U.S. Census Bureau, 2012a). Many Hispanic Americans live in the southwestern states, with over 50% living in California, Florida, and Texas (U.S. Census Bureau, 2010a). According to Lopez (2014), by March 2014, California will become the second state (behind New Mexico) where the Hispanic population is projected to become a plurality, meaning not that they are more than half of the population but make up the largest percentage of any other racial/ethnic group, surpassing the non-Hispanic white population.

Much heated debate has occurred recently regarding the unauthorized immigrant population in the United States. The majority (58%) of the 11.2 million unauthorized immigrants in 2010 were from Mexico. Of this population, approximately 5.5 million are children of unauthorized immigrants; 1 million of these children are foreign-born and 4.5 million are U.S.-born. It is important to note that the population of U.S.-born Hispanic children more than doubled from 2.1 million in 2000 (PEW, 2011).

Education and Employment

Hispanic subgroups differ in terms of socioeconomic data. For example, Hispanics of Mexican origin have a drastically lower college attainment rate (8%) than Hispanics from Cuba and South America (30% and 28%, respectively) (National Center for Education Statistics, 2010). As well, prescribers should be aware that there may be differences between U.S.-born Hispanics and Hispanic immigrants and Hispanic immigrants from different countries of origin. Hispanic patients may also display diverse levels of acculturation, even within the same family unit (Askim-Lovseth & Aldana, 2010). These factors add to the complexity of understanding and making treatment recommendations for this group.

Hispanics as a whole have lower socioeconomic status than that of the predominant white population. For example, as a group, the median household income in 2011 was $39,589 (compared to $55,305 for non-Hispanic whites), and the percentage of families below the poverty line was 25.8% compared to 11% for non-Hispanic whites. However, not all Hispanic subgroups have the same socioeconomic risk factors. For example, the national poverty rates ranged from a low of 16.2% for Cubans to a high of 26.3% for Dominicans. Among Hispanics, 74.3% of those age 5 and older spoke Spanish at home in 2011 (U.S. Census Bureau, 2011b).

In 2007, 61% of Hispanic adults compared to 89% of the total population had a high school education, 12.5% of Hispanic adults compared to 30.5% of the total population had at least a bachelor's degree, and 3.8% had advanced degrees (Office of Minority Health, 2013a). The unemployment rate for Hispanics in 2011 was 11.5%, the second-highest unemployment rate after African Americans. Within Hispanic subgroups, the unemployment rate for Hispanics from Puerto Rico was the highest (14.1%) and the rate for Cubans was slightly lower than the overall average (U.S. Department of Labor, 2012b). This statistic may not accurately reflect the migrant farm worker population nor the undocumented workers currently living in the United States, who do not qualify for unemployment benefits (U.S. Department of Labor, 2006).

Family Relationships

Familismo, the social structure in which the needs of the family as a group are viewed as more important than the needs of an individual family member, is the predominant social structure among Hispanic families. Strong kinship bonds often extend outside blood and marriage lines and include godparents, called *padrinos/compadres,* who are often established by ritual kinship. Thus, the family roles and titles of brother, sister, aunt, and uncle may not necessarily designate a true blood relative (Purnell, 2013). Hispanic families are often larger (average household size is 3.53 versus 2.55 for non-Hispanic whites) and made up of extended family members (U.S. Census Bureau, 2010b). Higher household size is due to higher fertility rates, continued migration, and the presence of other family members living in the home. This arrangement increases the resources that are available to benefit the family as a whole and serves as a major source of support in helping families mitigate socioeconomic stressors through the pooling of limited individual resources (Purnell, 2013).

Respect for parents and elders is taught early. Family is the major source of support for all its members and food is used to maintain family ties. There is respect for the elderly and infirm and for collective rather than individual achievement (Giger & Davidhizar, 2008). Religious leaders are also a source of support. Males and females have clearly differentiated roles. The father is the main decision maker in the family, but women, who are considered the primary healers in the group, decide health-related issues and provide health advice and remedies. Native healers (*curanderas/curanderos*) may be women or men (Giger, 2013; Purnell, 2013).

Health-Care Utilization

The combination of unemployment and undocumented workers means that this group has the highest percentage of people without health insurance (between 30% and 33% in 2008) and therefore lacks access to preventive care and health promotion (National Center for Health Statistics, 2010). Public health clinics and emergency departments are often used as the sites for primary health care.

Contrary to public belief, foreign-born Hispanics (specifically, the undocumented sector of the population) utilize fewer medical services and contribute less to health-care costs than the U.S.-born Hispanic population (Goldman, Smith, & Sood, 2006). Researchers attribute this to the Hispanic paradox, in which the foreign-born Hispanic population shares a better health status than the U.S.-born population despite having socioeconomic risk factors similar to those of other racial/ethnic groups and no health insurance (Goldman, Smith, & Sood). Recent debates in Washington, DC, have focused on undocumented, foreign-born Hispanic immigrants. However, empirical research does not support the case being made for the fiscal liabilities of providing care to this population. Researchers (Goldman, Smith & Sood; Hunt, Schneider, & Comer, 2004) have called for a dialogue on immigration that is based on empirical facts and looks at all sides of the immigration question, including both the positive and negative benefits of our mainly Hispanic immigrant population.

Health Status and Other Biological Variations

The National Center for Health Statistics (2008) data indicate that in 2008, 9.5% of Hispanics/Latinos were reported to be in fair or poor health. Obesity is a significant problem in the Hispanic population, with 69% of women and 70% of men over age 20 self-reporting as being overweight (National Center for Health Statistics, 2006b). Obtaining accurate health statistics on Hispanics is difficult because their data are often included with those of whites or go unreported owing to an undocumented status.

According to a National Health Interview Survey performed by the U.S. Department of Health and Human Services (2011), 11.8% of adults who identified as Hispanic reported having diabetes, which is greater than the 7.1% in adults who identified as non-Hispanic white. Specifically, Mexican adults reported having diabetes at a rate of 13.4%. Haffner and colleagues (1996), working with data from the Insulin Resistance Atherosclerosis Study (IRAS), studied racial differences in insulin resistance and insulin secretion and found that Hispanic patients had higher levels of insulin resistance and lower levels of insulin sensitivity when compared to non-Hispanic white patients. More recently, Hispanic Americans were found to demonstrate less insulin secretion yet be more insulin sensitive when compared with African Americans (Palmer et al, 2008).

Like African Americans, Hispanic patients experience pain differently than their non-Hispanic white counterparts. Rahim-Williams and colleagues (2007) found that both racial groups had lower levels of tolerance for contact heat and cold pain; however, there was no difference between minority and non-Hispanic white populations' tolerance of ischemic pain. Additionally, there was no difference in pain threshold for any of the three measures.

The leading causes of mortality for Hispanics are cardiovascular disease, cancer, accidents, stroke, and diabetes (CDC, 2008). Hispanics have higher rates of obesity; in 2006–2008, the age-adjusted estimated prevalence of obesity in Hispanic adults overall was 28.7% (versus 35.7% among non-Hispanic blacks and 23.7% for non-Hispanic whites). The obesity and overweight problem is also noted among Hispanic children. According to Singh and Kogan (2010), from 2006 to 2008, 43.3% of Hispanic children ages 6 to 17 were overweight (versus 39.6% of non-Hispanic blacks and 34% of non-Hispanic white children). Obesity rates are also highest among the Hispanic group, at 23.9%, versus 23.5% and 17.9% for non-Hispanic blacks and non-Hispanic whites, respectively. These data can have implications for metabolism and absorption of certain drugs.

The majority of Hispanics identify with the Roman Catholic Church. During an illness, Hispanic patients may use prayer, lighting of candles, and visiting shrines in order to influence a positive outcome (Giger, 2013). Even though there may be a strong religious tradition and connection with the Church, foreign-born Hispanics may choose to use contraception, but methods that are often less reliable, such as the rhythm method and condoms (Rocca & Harper, 2012), instead of more permanent methods, such as female sterilization, which Shih, Vittinghoff, Steinauer, and Dehlendorf (2011) found were used more often among U.S.-born Hispanics in California. However, Rocca and Harper (2012) state that this is due to lack of education regarding effectiveness rates among methods rather than religious beliefs. These data may have an influence on the higher birth and fertility rates seen among this population. In 2011, the birth rate for Central and South Americans was the highest of all Hispanic subgroups at 23 per 1,000 births, followed by Mexican (16.9), Puerto Rican (13.7), and Cuban (9.1) rates (per 1,000 births). In comparison, the non-Hispanic white birth rate was 10.7 and the black rate was 14.6 per 1,000 births (Martin, Hamilton, Osterman, Curtin, & Mathews, 2013).

Other health disparities include an increase in HIV/AIDS and the highest rate of diabetes among Puerto Ricans; a low rate of individuals who receive the flu vaccine; and more than twice the death rate from asthma than is seen in whites (CDC, 2008). Many pregnant Hispanic women do not seek prenatal care until late in their pregnancy; however, the rate of low birth weight is lower than that of whites except for a high rate among Puerto Ricans (OMH, 2010). Puerto Ricans also have low rates of prostate and breast cancer but a high rate of stomach and liver cancer.

Health disparities exist even within the Hispanic ethnic group. For example, 16.6% of Puerto Ricans suffer from asthma while only 4.9% of Hispanics of Mexican origin do (compared to 7.8% for non-Hispanic whites) (Akinbami et al, 2011). In the area of asthma prevention education, the data demonstrate that Hispanics of Mexican origin are least likely to have been given an asthma management plan, taught how to recognize early signs and symptoms of an asthma episode, advised on environmental controls, and taught how to properly respond to an asthma exacerbation (Akinbami et al, 2011). These data support the need for continued teaching by all health-care providers regarding known asthma education and management strategies that have been proven to decrease asthma morbidity and mortality.

Health Beliefs and Practices

The continued use of traditional medicine/folk medicine and traditional folk practitioners (*curanderos/curanderas*) is one of the most important variables leading to underutilization of Western medical care by many groups, including Hispanics (Ericksen, 2006). Patients may choose these traditional practices because they are often more accessible and affordable and have been used for many generations; patients also believe that traditional medicine and treatments are somehow gentler on the body (World Health Organization, 2002).

The prevalence of traditional medicine/complementary and alternative medicine (TM/CAM) has been documented to vary from 50% to 90% (Ortiz, Shields, Clauson, & Clay, 2010). Several studies have documented TM/CAM practices used by all subgroups of Hispanics, among which are medicinal herbs/teas (Factor-Litvak, Cushman, Kronenberg, Wade, & Kalmuss, 2001; Kronenberg, et al, 2006; Lagana, 2003); spiritual healing, religion, and prayer modalities and other traditional remedies (Palinkas & Kabongo, 2000; Upchurch & Chyu, 2005; Upchurch, et al, 2007); and visits to nutritionists and chiropractors (Factor-Litvak, Cushman, Kronenberg, Wade, & Kalmuss, 2001) . Several modalities of TM/CAM may be unfamiliar to prescribers. Ortiz, Shields, Clauson, and Clay (2010) report several studies described linden, sapodilla, and star anise as commonly used.

Hispanics are also more likely to engage in prayer as a form of TC/CAM, especially when feeling frustrated by lack of information regarding their disease processes and treatment options (Reyes-Ortiz, Rodriguez, & Markides, 2009). Prescribers should be prepared to ask Hispanic patients if they are engaging in TM/CAM practices and attempt to adequately assess for any potential drug interactions with other substances the patient may be taking or applying.

At the time that Spain was settling the New World, Spanish medicine was grounded in the humoral beliefs, that is, that the body was made up of four fluids: blood, phlegm, yellow bile, and black bile. These humors were further subdivided into the dualities of "wet and dry" and "hot and cold," which are classifications still used by many Hispanics to describe illness and wellness (Avila & Parker, 1999; Galanti, 2003). Diseases and illnesses, which can result from an imbalance of these forces, are either hot or cold and need to be treated with these concepts in mind. Illness may also be caused by several cultural ideas, such as *envidia* (jealousy), *mal ojo* (evil eye), *mal aire* (bad air), *nervios* (restlessness/anxiety), *caida de mollera* (fallen fontanel), and *susto* (magical freight), that can affect patients with physiological and/or psychological symptoms that vary in intensity and can be severe and life-threatening (Giger, 2013). For example, *caida de mollera* (fallen fontanel) may signal severe dehydration in an infant and requires medical treatment, and *mal ojo* (evil eye) is believed to be a condition that affects infants and children as a result of an individual thought to possess special powers who purposefully or involuntarily causes an illness by looking at or admiring but not touching a child. Practitioners can avoid being considered as inadvertently causing *mal ojo* by touching the child during the health-care visit (Giger, 2013). However, health-care providers can still be suspected of giving this look inadvertently. Although, several recently published texts (Giger, 2013; Romero, 2008) continue to state that these beliefs are common among the Hispanic population, providers should understand that few current empirical research studies give credence to their continuation among the Hispanic population living in the United States; also the beliefs may differ based on the acculturation level of the individual.

Health beliefs often have a strong religious association, with health being a gift from God as a reward for good behavior. Eating proper foods, working the proper amount of time, wearing religious medals, and sleeping with relics in the home are thought to prevent illness. Hispanics typically consult both traditional healers and allopathic providers and may or may not follow the modern medicine prescribed. For example, in one study only 53% percent of Hispanics with high blood pressure were taking antihypertensive medications. Hispanics also underuse preventive services and health promotion activities (Fordyce, 2003); in 2006, 43% of Hispanics had no medical home compared to 15% of whites (Beal, Doty, Hernandez, Shea, & Davis, 2007). When prescribing other drugs, understanding that *curanderas/curanderos* (traditional folk healers) treat illness with a variety of herbs and teas as well as recommend visits to shrines, medals, the use of candles, and promises to God to change behavior will reduce the risk for drug interactions. As with Asian medicinal therapies, it is important to understand that illness conditions are defined differently and that there are illnesses that have no correlate in allopathic medicine.

Racial Differences in Drug Pharmacokinetics and Response

A study that investigated the dose requirements using published warfarin dosing algorithms (derived from a mainly non-Hispanic white group) and genetic influences of warfarin in Hispanic versus non-Hispanic whites showed no pharmacokinetic differences in response. Specifically, researchers looked at the contribution of cytochrome *P450 2C9* (*CYP2C9*) and vitamin K epoxide reductase complex-1 (*VKORC1*) genotypes and their associated clinical factors to warfarin dose requirements. This study results suggests that factors influencing warfarin dose requirements in Hispanic

Caucasians are similar to those previously described in European Americans and that presently published dosing algorithms derived from non-Hispanic Caucasian cohorts are applicable to Hispanics living in the United States (Cavallari et al, 2011).

Asthma is the most common chronic illness among all children, with around 10% of all children afflicted. But Puerto Ricans have a much higher rate of asthma, with more than 20% afflicted compared with non-Hispanic whites. Conversely, only approximately 8% of Mexican American children are reported to have asthma. Similar statistics apply to Puerto Rican and Mexican adults in the United States (National Center for Health Statistics, 2002). This difference may be due to genetic differences between Puerto Ricans and Mexican Hispanics. Choudhry and colleagues (2005) studied the differences between Puerto Ricans and Mexicans with asthma in response to the drug albuterol and found there was a very strong association between the *Arg16* genotype and greater bronchodilator responsiveness for Puerto Ricans with baseline forced expiratory volume at 1 second (FEV_1) less than 80% of predicted, but not in those with FEV_1 greater than 80%. This association was not seen in the Mexican study participants, indicating that not all Hispanics respond to asthma medications in a similar fashion.

The *CYP2D6* gene is involved in metabolism of different medications, including dextromethorphan (a common cough suppressant). Research indicates that differing alleles on *CYP2D6* affect the rate of metabolism; however, research within the Mexican population is inconclusive. Mendoza and colleagues (2001) found that the *CYP2D6*4* variation occurs less often in Mexican Americans when compared to non-Hispanic whites and may be the cause of the lower rate of poor metabolism of drugs in Mexican Americans. Conversely, Alanis-Banuelos and colleagues (2006) found no difference in the rate of allele variation between the Mextizos of Durango, Mexico, and non-Hispanic whites. Further research needs to be completed in this area to provide conclusions.

Despite preliminary evidence of racial differences in insulin secretion and glucose metabolism and in factors associated with cardiovascular risk, evidence of differences within the Hispanic population in terms of drug pharmacokinetics and response to drugs is lacking. This may be related to the genetic variability among persons classified as Hispanic or to a lack of studies that focus on these differences.

NON-HISPANIC WHITES

Little discussion is needed of this segment of the population because most allopathic health care is currently directed at this group. Within this group, however, are some subgroups that require some discussion.

Whites of various ethnic backgrounds may hold beliefs in the "evil eye" and the curative powers of folk medicine. German, Polish, and Italian Americans also see stress and environmental changes as sources of illness. Along with Irish Americans, they have strong family ties, with the male as the dominant force and decision maker. Polish and Italian Americans may use folk

---

BOX 7–1 RESOURCES FOR CULTURALLY COMPETENT CARE

Center for Cross-Cultural Research

WESTERN WASHINGTON UNIVERSITY

Housed within an integral part of the Department of Psychology at Western Washington University, the Center for Cross-Cultural Research was started in response to the Euro-American bias in psychological theory, research, and practical applications. The mission of the Center for Cross-Cultural Research is to promote culture-related research, offer courses on culture, promote exchange between cultural scientists, and disseminate the results of culture research. http://www.wwu.edu/culture/

Cross Cultural Health Care Program

The mission of the Cross Cultural Health Care Program is to serve as a bridge between communities and health-care institutions to ensure full access to quality health care that is culturally and linguistically appropriate. http://www.xculture.org

Diversity Rx

Diversity Rx promotes language and cultural competence to improve the quality of health care for minority, immigrant, and ethnically diverse communities. http://www.diversityrx.org

National Center for Cultural Competence

The mission of the National Center for Cultural Competence (NCCC) is to increase the capacity of health and mental health programs to design, implement, and evaluate culturally and linguistically competent service delivery systems to address growing diversity, persistent disparities, and to promote health and mental health equity. http://nccc.georgetown.edu/

PharmGKB

The PharmGKB is managed by Stanford University and is a pharmacogenomics knowledge resource that encompasses clinical information including dosing guidelines and drug labels, potentially clinically actionable gene-drug associations and genotype-phenotype relationships. PharmGKB collects, curates and disseminates knowledge about the impact of human genetic variation on drug responses.

Transcultural Nursing Society

The mission of the Transcultural Nursing Society (TCNS) is to enhance the quality of culturally congruent, competent, and equitable care that results in improved health and well-being for people worldwide. The TCNS seeks to provide nurses and other health-care professionals with the knowledge base necessary to ensure cultural competence in practice, education, research, and administration. www.tcns.org

---

remedies and native healers. All four groups have strong religious ties, with Polish, Irish, and Italian Americans being mainly Roman Catholics. Religious medals and rituals are often used to promote health, prevent illness, and heal. Overall, an increasing percentage of the U.S. population is seeking alternative sources of health care or is self-medicating with herbal remedies; this is discussed in Chapter 10.

One interesting study by Gaskin, Spencer, Richard, Anderson, and Powe (2008) seems to defy the widely held belief that in the United States minorities receive poorer care than white Americans. Gaskin and colleagues found that "when whites and minorities were admitted to the hospital for the same reason or to receive the same hospital procedure, they receive the same quality of care."

SUMMARY

Consideration of demographic, socioeconomic, and cultural factors and recognition of the potential for drug interactions with herbs or foods that may be used in culture-specific healing practices are important in order to prescribe drugs for patients appropriately. Becoming culturally sensitive requires recognizing that cultural diversity exists, identifying and exploring one's own cultural beliefs, and being willing to modify health-care delivery to be more congruent with the patient's cultural background.

As can be seen from the research and other data discussed here, ethnopharmacology studies often present conflicting data. It is incumbent on prescribers to keep current in the literature and to take the time to review research studies for the validity and reliability of the methods and statistics used in the research and for its appropriateness to their patients. Box 7-1 describes sources of information for providers. Studies that report differences without stating a specific metabolic or biochemical relationship should be especially suspect. It is also important to focus on articles in journals with reputations for peer review and careful selection of research reports.

One quick way to review the literature in ethnopharmacology is to use a Web site (http://www.pharmgkb.org/aboutUs.jsp) sponsored by Stanford University Department of Genetics. It includes a full discussion of clinical information, including dosing guidelines and drug labels and potentially clinically actionable gene–drug associations and genotype–phenotype relationships, along with the research used to arrive at these conclusions.

REFERENCES

Akinbami, L. J., Moorman, J. E., & Liu, X. (2011). Asthma prevalence, health care use, and mortality: United States, 2005–2009. *National Health Statistics Reports, 32,* 1–15. Retrieved from http://www.cdc.gov/nchs/data/nhsr/nhsr032.pdf

Alanis-Banuelos, R. E., Bradley-Alvarez, F., Elizondo, G., Flores-Perez, C., Flores-Perez, J., & Lares-Asseff, I. (2006). CYP2D6 genotype and phenotype in Amerindians of Tepehuano Origin and Mestizos of Durango, Mexico. *Journal of Clinical Pharmacology, 46*(5), 527–536.

American Association of Colleges of Nursing. (2008). *Cultural competency in baccalaureate nursing education.* Washington, DC: Author.

American Association of Colleges of Nursing (2006). *Essentials of Doctoral Education for Advanced Nursing Practice.* Retrieved from www.aacn.nche.edu

American Association of Colleges of Nursing (2008). *Essentials of Baccalaureate Education in Nursing.* Retrieved from www.aacn.nche.edu

American Association of Colleges of Nursing (2010). *Essentials of Masters Education in Nursing.* Retrieved from www.aacn.nche.edu

American Cancer Society. (2005). Colorectal cancer facts and figures special edition 2005. Retrieved from http://www.cancer.org/research/cancerfactsfigures/colorectalcancerfactsfigures/colorectal-cancer-facts-figures-special-edition-2005

American Lung Association. (2007). State of lung diseases in diverse populations: 2007. Retrieved from http://www.lung.org/assets/documents/publications/lung-disease-data/SOLDDC_2007.pdf

Arranz, M. J., & de Leon, J. (2007). Pharmacogenetics and pharmacogenomics of schizophrenia: A review of the last decade of research. *Molecular Psychiatry, 12*(8), 707–747.

Askim-Lovseth, M. K., & Aldana, A. (2010). Looking beyond "affordable" health care: Cultural understanding and sensitivity—necessities in addressing the health care disparities of the U.S. Hispanic population. *Health Marketing Quarterly, 27,* 354–387.

Avila, E., & Parker, J. (1999). *Woman who glows in the dark: A curandera reveals traditional Aztec secrets of physical and spiritual health.* New York: Penguin Putman, Inc.

Beal, H. C., Doty, M. M., Hernandez, S. E., Shea, K. K., & Davis, K. (2007). Closing the divide: How medical homes promote equity in health care. The Commonwealth Fund.

Bennion, L., & Li, T. (1976). Alcohol metabolism in American Indians and whites: Lack of difference in metabolic rate and liver alcohol dehydrogenase. *New England Journal of Medicine, 294*(1), 9–13.

Berg, J. Z., Mason, J., Boettcher, A. J., Hatsukami, D. K., & Murphy, S. E. (2010). Nicotine metabolism in African Americans and European Americans: Variation in glucuronidation by ethnicity and UGT2B10 response. *Journal of Pharmacology and Experimental Therapeutics, 332*(1), 202–209.

Bertilsson, L. (1995). Geographic and interracial differences in polymorphic drug oxidation: Current state of knowledge of cytochromes P450 (CYP) 2D6 and 2C19. *Clinical Pharmacokinetics, 29*(3), 192–209.

Bhatnagar, V., O'Connor, D. T., Schork, N. J., Salem, R. M., Nievergelt, C. M., Rana, B. K., et al. (2007). Angiotensin-converting enzyme gene polymorphism predicts the time course of blood pressure response to to angiotensin-converting enzyme inhibition in the AASK trial. *Journal of Hypertension, 25*(10), 2082–2092.

Black, H. R., Bailey, J., Zappe, D., & Samuel, R. (2009). Valsartan: More than a decade of experience. *Drugs, 69*(17), 2393–2414. doi: 10.2165/11319460-000000000-00000

Blow, F. C., Zeber, J. E., McCarthy, J. F., Valenstein, M., Gillon, L., & Bingham, C. R. (2004). Ethnic and diagnostic patterns in veterans with psychoses. *Social Psychiatry and Psychiatric Epidemilogy, 39,* 841–851.

Bogalusa Heart Study Twentieth Anniversary Symposium. (1995). *American Journal of Medical Science, 310,* S1–S138.

Brody, H., & Hunt, L. M. (2006). Bidil: Assessing a race-based pharmaceutical. *Annals of Family Medicine, 4*(6), 556–560.

Brooks, P. J., Enoch, M. A., Goldman, D., Li, T. K., & Yokoyama, A. (2009). The alcohol flushing response: An unrecognized risk factor for esophageal cancer from alcohol consumption. *PLOS Medicine.* Retrieved from http://www.plosmedicine.org/article/info%3Adoi%2F10.1371%2Fjournal.pmed.1000050

Browne, C. V., Mokuau, L., & Braun, K. L. (2009). Adversity and resiliency in the lives of Native Hawaiian elders. *Social Work, 54*(3), 253–261.

Cardillo, C., Kilcoyne, C., Cannon R., III, & Panza, J. (1998). Racial differences in nitric oxide–mediated vasodilator response to mental stress in forearm circulation. *Hypertension, 31*(6), 1235–1239.

Cardillo, C., Kilcoyne, C., Cannon R., III, & Panza, J. (1999). Attenuation of cyclic nucleotide-mediated smooth muscle contraction in blacks as a cause of racial differences in vasodilator function. *Circulation, 99*(1), 90–95.

Carmel, R. (1999). Ethnic and racial factors in cobalamin metabolism and its disorders. *Seminars in Hematology, 36*(1), 88–100.

Cavallari, L. H., Momary, K. M., Patel, S. R., Shapiro, N. L., Nutescu, E., & Viana, M. A. (2011). Pharmacogenomics of warfarin dose requirements in Hispanics. *Blood, Cell, Molecules & Disease, 46*(2), 147–150. doi: 10.1016/j.bcmd.2010.11.005. Epub 2010 Dec 24.

Centers for Disease Control and Prevention. (2008). Vaccination coverage among U.S. adults: National immunization survey 2007. Retrieved from http://www.cdc.gov/vaccines/stats-surv/nis/downloads/nis-adult-summer-2007.pdf

Centers for Disease Control and Prevention. (2009). Differences in prevalence of obesity among Black, White, and Hispanic adults—United States, 2006–2008. *Morbidity and Mortality Weekly Report, 58*(27), 740–744. Retrieved from http://www.cdc.gov/mmwr/preview/mmwrhtml/mm5827a2.htm

Centers for Disease Control and Prevention. (2011a). Health of Black or African-American non-Hispanic population. http://www.cdc.gov/nchs/fastats/black_health.htm

Centers for Disease Control and Prevention. (2011b). Health of white non-Hispanic population. Retrieved from http://www.cdc.gov/nchs/fastats/white_health.htm

Centers for Disease Control and Prevention. (2011c). Occupational health disparities. Retrieved from http://www.cdc.gov/niosh/programs/ohd/

Centers for Disease Control and Prevention. (2011d). Black or African American populations. Retrieved from http://www.cdc.gov/minority-health/populations/REMP/black.html#Demographics

Centers for Disease Control and Prevention. (2012a). Health expenditures. Retrieved from http://www.cdc.gov/nchs/fastats/hexpense.htm

Centers for Disease Control and Prevention (2012b). Suicide: Facts at a glance. Retrieved from http://www.cdc.gov/ViolencePrevention/pdf/Suicide_DataSheet-a.pdf

Centers for Disease Control and Prevention. (2013a). Social determinants of health. Retrieved from http://www.cdc.gov/socialdeterminants/Definitions.html

Centers for Disease Control and Prevention. (2013b). U.S. Public Health Service syphilis study at Tuskegee. Retrieved from http://www.cdc.gov/tuskegee/timeline.htm

Centers for Disease Control and Prevention. (2013c). Cigarette smoking in the U.S.: Current cigarette smoking among U.S. adults aged 18 years and over. http://www.cdc.gov/tobacco/campaign/tips/resources/data/cigarette-smoking-in-united-states.html#populations

Central Intelligence Agency. (2012). *The world fact book: Infant mortality rates.* Retrieved from https://www.cia.gov/library/publications/the-world-factbook/rankorder/2091rank.html

Cepeda, S. M., Farrar, J. T., Roa, J. H., Boston, R., Meng, Q., Ruiz, F., et al. (2001). Ethnicity influences morphine pharamacokinetics and pharmacodynamics. *Clinical Pharmacology and Therapeutics, 70,* 351–361.

Chan, A. (1986). Racial differences in alcohol sensitivity. *Alcohol, 21*(1), 93–104.

Choudhry, S., Ung, N., Avila, P. C., Ziv, E., Nazario, S., Casal, J., et al. (2005). Pharmacogenetic differences in response to albuterol between Puerto Ricans and Mexicans with asthma. *American Journal of Respiratory and Critical Care Medicine, 171*(6), 563–570.

Cimino, E., Sayers, A. M., & Roods, R. (1999). The sacred use of tobacco. The University of Dayton Law School. http://academic.udayton.edu/health/syllabi/tobacco/native04.htm

Cryer, B., & Feldman, M. (1996). Racial differences in gastric function among African-Americans and Caucasian Americans: Secretion, serum gastrin and histology. *Professional Association of American Physicians, 108*(6), 481–489.

Dikewicz, M (2004). Cough and angioedema from angiotensin-converting enzyme inhibitors: New insights into mechanisms and management. *Current Opinion in Allergy and Clinical Immunology, 4*(4), 267–270.

Ericksen, A. (2006). Hispanic healthcare. *Healthcare Traveler*. Retrieved from http://healthcaretraveler.modernmedicine.com/healthcare-traveler/news/hispanic-healthcare-closer-look-travelers-perspective

Fordyce, M. (2003). Culture, ethnicity, and medications. *Aging Today, xxiv*(1), 9–12.

Frackiewicz, E., Srmek, J., Herrera, J., Kurtz, N., & Culter, N. (1997). Ethnicity and antipsychotic response. *Annals of Pharmacotherapeutics, 31*(11), 1360–1369.

Gainer, J., Nadeau, J., Ryder, D., & Brown, N. (1996). Increased sensitivity to bradykinin among African-Americans. *Journal of Allergy and Clinical Immunology, 98*(2), 283–287.

Galanti, G. A. (2003). *Caring for patients from different cultures* (3rd ed.). Philadelphia: University of Pennsylvania Press.

Gaskin, D. J., Spencer, C. S., Richard, P., Anderson, G. F., & Powe, N. R. (2008). Do hospitals provide lower-quality care to minorities than to whites? *Health Affairs, 27*(2), 518–527.

Giger, J. N. (2013). *Transcultural nursing: Assessment and intervention* (6th ed.). St. Louis, MO: Mosby.

Gizer, I. R., Edenberg, H. J., Gilder, D. A., Wilhelmsen, K. C., & Ehlers, C. L. (2011). Association of alcohol dehydrogenase genes with alcohol-related phenotypes in a Native American community sample. *Alcoholism Clinical and Experimental Research, 35*(11), 2008–2018.

Gladding, P., Mackay, J., Zeng, I., Stewart, R., Prabkahar, R., Webster, M., et al. (2010). A simulation of warfarin maintenance dose requirement using a pharmacogenetic algorithm in an ethnically diverse cohort. *Personalized Medicine, 7*(3), 319–325.

Haffner, S. M., D'Agostino, R., Saad, M. F., Rewers, M., Mykkänen, L., Selby, J., et al. (1996). Increased insulin resistance and insulin secretion in nondiabetic African Americans and Hispanics when compared with non-Hispanic Whites: The insulin resistance atherosclerosis study. *Diabetes, 45*, 742–748.

Haiman, C. A., Stram, D. O., Wilkens, L. R., Pike, M. C., Kolonel, L. N., Henderson, B. E., & LeMarchand, L. (2006). Ethnic and racial differences in the smoking-related risk of lung cancer. *New England Journal of Medicine, 354*(4), 333–342.

Harris-Hooker, S., & Sanford, G. (1994). Lipid, lipoproteins and coronary heart disease in minority populations. *Atherosclerosis, 108*(Suppl.), 83–104.

Hodgins, O., & Hodgins, D. (2013). American Indians and Alaska Natives. In L. D. Purnell (Ed.), *Transcultural health care: A culturally competent approach* (pp 449–451). Philadelphia, PA: F.A. Davis Company.

Hong Ng, C., Norman, T. R., Naing, K. O., Schweitzer, I., Kong Wai Ho, B., Fan, A., et al. (2006). A comparative study of sertraline dosages, plasma concentrations, efficacy and adverse reactions in Chinese versus Caucasian patients. *International Clinical Psychopharmacology, 21*(2), 87–92.

Horne, R., Graupner, L., Frost, S., Weinman, J., Wright, S. M., & Hankins, M. (2004). Medicine in a multicultural society: The effect of cultural background on beliefs about medications. *Social Science and Medicine, 59*(6), 1307–1313.

Hui, K., & Pasic, J. (1997). Outcome of hypertension management in Asian Americans. *Archives of Internal Medicine, 157*(12), 1345–1348.

Hunt, L. M., Schneider, S., & Comer, B. (2004). Should acculturation be a variable in health research? A critical review of research on U.S. Hispanics. *Social Science and Medicine, 59*, 973–986.

Ichiho, H. M., Gillan, J. W., & Aitaoto, N. (2013). An assessment of non-communicable diseases, diabetes, and related risk factors in the Territory of Guam: A systems perspective. *Hawaii Journal of Public Health, 72*(5), 68–76.

Indian Health Service. (2013a). Disparities. http://www.ihs.gov/newsroom/factsheets/disparities/

Indian Health Service. (2013b). Diabetes. http://www.ihs.gov/newsroom/factsheets/diabetes/

Institute of Medicine. (2012). How far have we come in reducing health disparities? Progress since 2000 workshop summary. Washington, DC National Academies Press. Retrieved from http://www.iom.edu/Reports/2012/How-Far-Have-We-Come-in-Reducing-Health-Disparities.aspx

Jacobs, E. A., Shepard, D. S., Suaya, J. A., & Stone, E. L. (2004). Overcoming language barriers in health care: Costs and benefits of interpreter services. *American Journal of Public Health, 94*(5), 866–869.

Johnson, A. B. (2006). Performance anxiety among African-American college students: Racial bias as a factor in social phobia. *Journal of College Student Psychotherapy, 20*, 31–38.

Johnson, J., & Burlew, D. (1996). Metoprolol metabolism via cytochrome P450 2D6 in ethnic populations. *Drug Metabolism Disposition, 24*(3), 350–355.

Johnson, J., & Livingston, T. (1997). Differences between blacks and whites in plasma binding of drugs. *European Journal of Clinical Pharmacology, 51*(96), 485–488.

Johnson, J. A. (2010). Pharmacogenomics of antihypertensive drugs: Past, present and future. *Pharmacogenomics, 11*(4), 487+.

Johnson, D. B., Oyama, N., LeMarchand, L., & Wilkens, L. (2004). Native Hawaiians' mortality, morbidity, and lifestyle: Comparing data from 1982, 1990, and 2000. *Pacific Health Dialogue, 11*(2), 120–130.

Joint Commission. (2013). Facts about advancing effective communication, cultural competence, and patient- and family-centered care. Retrieved from http://www.jointcommission.org/assets/1/18/Advancing_Effective_Comm.pdf

Kaiser Family Foundation, (2013). Life expectancy at birth (in years) by race/ethnicity. Retrievved from http://kff.org/other/state-indicator/life-expectancy-by-re/

Karadimas, C. L., Vu, T. H., Holve, S. A., Chronopoulou, P., Quinzii, C., Johnsen, S. D., et al. (2006). Navajo neuropathy is caused by a mutation in the MPV17 gene. *The American Journal of Human Genetics, 79*, 544–548.

Knowles, W. C., Saad, M. F., Pettitt, D. J., Nelson, R. G., & Bennett, P. H. (1993). Determinants of diabetes mellitus in the Pima Indians. *Diabetes Care, 16*(1), 216–227.

Kochanek, K. D., Xu, J., Murphy, S. L., Minino, A. M., & Kung, H. C. (2011). Deaths: Final data for 2009. *National Vital Statistics Reports, 60*(3), 1–116.

Lakainapali, L. (2013). Hawaiian Lomi Lomi massage. Retrieved from http://www.huna.org/html/lomilomi.html

Lawson, W. B. (2008). Schizophrenia in African Americans. In K. T. Mueser & D. V. Jeste (Eds.), *Clinical handbook of schizophrenia* (pp 616–623). New York: The Guildford Press.

Lee, C., Yang, Y., & Hu, O. (1998). Single-dose pharmacokinetic study of lithium in Taiwanese/Chinese bipolar patients. *Australia and New Zealand Journal of Psychiatry, 32*(1), 133–136.

Lee, V. W. Y., Chau, T. S., Chan, A. K. W., Lee, K. K. C., Waye, M. Y., Ling, T. K. W., et al. (2010). Pharmacogenetics of esomeprazole or rabeprazole-based triple therapy in Heliobacter pylori eradication in Hong Kong non-ulcer dyspepsia Chinese subjects. *Journal of Clinical Pharmacy and Therapeutics, 35*, 343–350.

Leininger, M. (2004). Leininger's Sunrise Enabler to Discover Culture Care. Retrieved April 24, 2006, from http://www.madeleine-leininger.com

Leininger, M. (2006). Madeline M Leininger's theory of culture care diversity and universality. In M. E. Parker (Ed.), *Nursing theories and nursing practice* (2nd ed.). Philadelphia: F.A. Davis.

Li, R., Lyn, D., Lapu-Bula, R., Oduwole, A., Igho-Pemu, P., Lankford, B., et al. (2004). Relation of endothelial nitric oxide synthase gene to plasma nitric oxide level, endothelial function, and blood pressure in African Americans. *American Journal of Hypertension, 17*(7), 560–567.

Lin, K., Poland, R., Smith, M., Strickland, T., & Mendoza, R. (1991). Pharmacokinetic and other related factors affecting psychotropic responses in Asians. *Psychopharmacology Bulletin, 27*(4), 427–437.

Liu, D. M., & Almeda, C. K. (2011). Social determinants of health for Native Hawaiian children and adolescents. *Hawaii Medicine Journal, 70*(11), 9–14.

Liu, K., & Levinson, S. (1996). Comparisons of blood pressure between Asian-American children and children from other racial groups in Chicago. *Public Health Reports, 111*(Suppl. 2), 65–67.

Lopez, M. H. (2014). In 2014, Latinos will surpass whites as largest racial/ethnic group in California. PEW RESEARCH Center. Retrieved from http://www.pewresearch.org/fact-tank/2014/01/24/in-2014-latinos-will-surpass-whites-as-largest-racialethnic-group-in-california/

Lopez, M. H., Gonzales-Barrera, A., & Cuddington, D. (2013). Diverse origins: The nation's 14 largest Hispanic-Origin groups. PEW Research

Center. Retrieved from http://www.pewhispanic.org/2013/06/19/diverse-origins-the-nations-14-largest-hispanic-origin-groups/

Ma, L., Tataranni, P. A., Hanson, R. L., Infante, A. M., Kobes, S., Bogardus, C., et al. (2005). Variations in peptide YY and Y2 receptor genes are associated with severe obesity in Pima Indian men. *Diabetes, 54,* 1598–1602.

MacDorman, M. F., & Matthews, T. J. (2011). Understanding racial and ethnic disparities in U.S. infant mortality rates. *National Center for Health Statistics Data Briefs, 74,* 1–8.

March of Dimes. (2013). Peristats. http://www.marchofdimes.com/peristats/Peristats.aspx

Martin, J. A., Hamilton, B. E., Osterman, M. J. K., Curtin, S. C., & Mathews, T. J. (2013). Births final data for 2012, Table 5. Births and birth rates, by Hispanic origin of mother and by race for mothers of non-Hispanic origin: United States, 1989–2012. *National Vital Statistics Reports, 62*(9), 1–87. Retrieved from http://www.cdc.gov/nchs/data/nvsr/nvsr62/nvsr62_09.pdf

Masland, M. C., Kang, S. H., & Ma, Y. (2011). Association between limited English proficiency and understanding prescription labels among five ethnic groups in California. *Ethnicity & Health, 16*(2), 125–144.

Matthews, H. (1995). Racial, ethnic and gender difference in response to medicines. *Drug Metabolism and Drug Interaction, 12*(2), 77–91.

McCubbin, L. D., & Antonio, M. (2012). Discrimination and obesity among Native Hawaiians. *Hawaii Journal of Public Health, 71*(12), 346–352.

McGregor, D. P., Morelli, P. T., Matsuoka, J. K., Rodenhurst, R., Kong, N., & Spencer, M. S. (2003). An ecological model of Native Hawaiian well-being. *Pacific Health Dialogue, 10*(2), 106–128.

McNamara, D. M., Tam, S. W., Sabolinski, M. L., Tobelmann, P., Janosko, K., Venkitachalam, L., et al. (2009). Endothelial nitric oxide synthase (NOS3) polymorphisms in African Americans with heart failure: Results from the A-HeFT trial. *Journal of Cardiac Failure, 15*(3), 191–198.

Mendoza, R., Wan, Y. J., Poland, R. E., Smith, M., Zheng, Y., Berman, N., et al. (2001). CYP2D6 polymorphism in the Mexican American population. *Clinical Pharmacology and Therapeutics, 70*(6), 552–560.

Mitchell, H., Smith, R., Cutler, R., Sica, D., Videen, J., Thompsen-Bell, S., et al. (1997). Racial differences in the renal response to blood pressure lowering during chronic angiotensin-converting enzyme inhibition: A prospective double-blind randomized comparison of fosinopril and lisinopril in older hypertensive patients with chronic renal insufficiency. *American Journal of Kidney Diseases, 29*(6), 897–906.

Moghaddam, J. F., & Momper, S. L. (2011). Integrating spiritual and western treatment modalities in a Native American substance user center: Provider perspectives. *Substance Use Misuse, 46*(11), 1431–1437.

Moyer, T. P., O'Kane, D. J., Baudhuin, L. M., Wiley, C. L., Fortini, A., Fisher, P. K., et al. (2009). Warfarin sensitivity genotyping: A review of the literature and summary of patient experience. *Mayo Clinic Proceedings, 84*(12), 1079–1094.

Muller, Y. L., Hanson, R. L., Bian, L., Mack, J., Shi., X., Pakyz, R., et al. (2010). Functional variants in MBL2 are associated with type 2 diabetes and pre-diabetes traits in Pima Indians and the Old Order Amish. *Diabetes, 59*(8):2080-5.

National Center for Education Statistics. (2010). Status and trends in the education of racial and ethnic groups. Retrieved from http://nces.ed.gov/pubsearch/pubsinfo.asp?pubid=2010015

National Center for Education Statistics. (2012). Percentage of persons age 25 and over with high school completion or higher and a bachelor's or higher degree, by race/ethnicity and sex: Selected years, 1910 through 2012. Retrieved from http://nces.ed.gov/programs/digest/d12/tables/dt12_008.asp

National Center for Health Statistics. (2002). A demographic and health snapshot of the U.S. Hispanic/Latino population: 2002 National Hispanic Health Leadership Summit. Retrieved April 26, 2006, from http://www.cdc.gov/NCHS/data/hpdata2010/chcsummit.pdf

National Center for Health Statistics. (2006a). Health of Hispanic/Latino population. Retrieved April 26, 2006, from http://www.cdc.gov/nchs/fastats/hispanic_health.htm

National Center for Health Statistics. (2006b). Health of Mexican American population. Retrieved April 26, 2006, from http://www.cdc.gov/nchs/fastats/mexican_health.htm

National Center for Health Statistics. (2010). Health, United States, 2008. Washington, DC. Retrieved August 20, 2010, from http://www.cdc.gov/nchs

National Center for Health Statistics. (2012). Summary of health statistics for U.S. adults: National health interview survey. (2011). Retrieved August 3, 2013, from http://www.cdc.gov/nchs/data/series/sr_10/sr10_256.pdf

National Healthy Marriage Resource Center. (2008). *Healthy marriage in culturally and ethnically diverse populations.* Retrieved from http://www.healthymarriageinfo.org/resource-detail/index.aspx?rid=3083

National Institutes of Health. (2010). National Institutes of Health: Consensus development conference statement.

National Institutes of Health. (2013). Inclusion of women and minorities as participants in research involving human subjects: Policy implementation page. Retrieved from http://grants.nih.gov/grants/funding/women_min/women_min.htm

Office of Adolescent Health. (2013). Trends in pregnancy and childbearing: Teen births. http://www.hhs.gov/ash/oah/adolescent-health-topics/reproductive-health/teen-pregnancy/trends.html

Office of Minority Health. (2012a). American Indian/Alaska Native profile. http://minorityhealth.hhs.gov/templates/browse.aspx?lvl=2&lvlID=52

Office of Minority Health. (2012b). Asian American/Pacific Islander profile. Retrieved from http://minorityhealth.hhs.gov/templates/browse.aspx?lvl=2&lvlID=53

Office of Minority Health. (2012c). Native Hawaiians and Pacific Islanders profile. Retrieved from http://minorityhealth.hhs.gov/templates/browse.aspx?lvl=2&lvlID=71

Office of Minority Health. (2013a). Infant mortality and African-Americans. Retrieved from http://minorityhealth.hhs.gov/templates/content.aspx?lvl=2&lvlID=51&ID=3021

Office of Minority Health. (2013b). National CLAS standards. Retrieved from http://minorityhealth.hhs.gov/templates/browse.aspx?lvl=2&lvlID=15

Office of Minority Health. (2013c). Hispanic/Latino profile. Retrieved from http://minorityhealth.hhs.gov/templates/browse.aspx?lvl=2&lvlID=54

O'Hara, E., & Zhan, L. (1994). Cultural and pharmacologic considerations when caring for Chinese elders: Knowledge of traditional Chinese medicine is necessary. *Journal of Gerontological Nursing, 30*(10), 11–16.

Ortiz, B. I., Shields, K. M., Clauson, K. A., & Clay, P. G. (2010). Complementary and alternative medicine use among Hispanics in the United States. *The Annals of Pharmacotherapy, 41*(6), 994–1004.

Palmer, N. D., Goodarzi, M. O., Langefeld, C. D., Ziegler, J., Norris, J. M., Haffner, S. M., et al. (2008). Qualitative trait analysis of type 2 diabetes susceptibility loci identified from whole genome association studies in the insulin resistance atherosclerosis family study. *Diabetes, 57,* 1093–1100.

Pandya, C., Batalova, J., & McHugh, M. (2011). Limited English proficient individuals in the United States: Number, share, growth, and linguistic diversity. Washington, DC: Migration Policy Institute. Retrieved from http://www.migrationinformation.org/integration/LEPdatabrief.pdf

PEW Research. (2010). Hispanics and Arizona's new immigration laws: Fact sheet. Retrieved from http://www.pewhispanic.org/2010/04/29/hispanics-and-arizona%E2%80%99s-new-immigration-law

PEW Research. (2011). Unauthorized immigrant population: National and state trends, 2010. Retrieved from http://www.pewhispanic.org/2011/02/01/unauthorized-immigrant-population-brnational-and-state-trends-2010/

Puri, A., Medhi, B., Panda, N. B., Puri, G. D., & Dhawan, S. (2012). Propofol pharmacokinetics in young healthy Indian subjects. *Indian Journal of Pharmacology, 44*(3), 402–406.

Putsch, B., SenGupta, I., Sampson, A., & Tervalon, M. (2003). Reflections on the CLAS standards: Best practices, innovations, and horizons. Office of Minority Health, The Cross Cultural Health Care Program. Retrieved from http://minorityhealth.hhs.gov/assets/pdf/checked/reflections.pdf

Prisant, L., & Mensah, G. (1996). Use of beta-adrenergic receptor blockers in blacks. *Journal of Clinical Pharmacology, 36*(10), 867–873.

Purnell, L. D. (2013). *Transcultural health care: A culturally competent approach,* (4th ed.). Philadelphia: F.A. Davis Company.

Rahim-Williams, F. B., Riley, J. L., Herrera, D., Campbell, C. M., Hastie, B. A., & Fillingim, R. B. (2007). Ethnic identity predicts experimental pain sensitivity in African American and Hispanics. *Pain, 129,* 177–184.

Ramos, E., Doumatey, A., Shriner, D., Haung, H., Chen, G., Zhou, J., et al. (2014). Pharmacogenomics, ancestry and clinical decision making for global populations. *The Pharmacogenomics Journal, 14*, 217–222.

Reyes-Ortiz, C. A., Rodriguez, M., & Markides, K. S. (2009). The role of spirituality healing with perceptions of the medical encounter among Latinos. *Journal of General Internal Medicine, 24*(3), 542–547.

Rivera-Calimlim, L., & Reilly, D. (1984). Difference in erythrocyte catechol-o-methyltransferase activity between Orientals and Caucasians: Difference in levodopa tolerance. *Clinical Pharmacology and Therapeutics, 35*(6), 804–809.

Rocca, C. H., & Harper, C. C. (2012). Do racial and ethnic differences in contraceptive attitudes and knowledge explain disparities in method use? *Perspectives in Sexual and Reproductive Health, 44*(3), 150–158.

Romero, M. G. (2008). Mental health counseling with Hispanics/Latinos: The role of culture in practice. In I. Marini & M. A. Stebnicki (Eds.), *The professional counselor's desk reference* (pp 1004). New York: Springer Company.

Rosemary, J., & Adithan, C. (2007). The pharmacogenetics of CYP2C9 and CYP2C19: Ethnic variation and clinical significance. *Current Clinical Pharmacology, 2*, 93–109.

Shekelle, P. G., Rich, M. W., Morton, S. C., Atkinson, S. W., Tu, W., Maglione, M., et al. (2003). Efficacy of angiotensin-converting enzyme inhibitors and beta-blockers in the management of left ventricular systolic dysfunction according to race, gender, and diabetic status. *Journal of the American College of Cardiology, 41*(9), 1529–1538.

Shi, X. J., Geng, F., Jiao, Z., Cui, X. Y., Qiu, X. Y., & Zhong, M. K. (2011). Association of the ABCB1, CYP3A4*18B and CYP3A5*3 genotypes with the pharmacokinetics of tacrolimus in healthy Chinese subjects: A population pharmacokinetic analysis. *Journal of Clinical Pharmacy and Therapeutics, 36*, 614–624.

Shih, G., Vittinghoff, E., Steinauer, J., & Dehlendorf, C. (2011). Racial and ethnic disparities in contraceptive method choice in California. *Perspectives on Sexual and Reproductive Health, 43*(3), 173–80. doi: 10.1363/4317311.

Shrank, W. H., Choudhry, N. K., Fischer, M. A., Avorn, J., Powell, M., Schneeweiss, S., et al. (2010). The epidemiology of prescriptions abandoned at the pharmacy. *Annals of Internal Medicine, 153*(10), 633–640.

Singh, G. K., & Kogan, M. D. (2010). Childhood obesity in the United States, 1976–2008: Trends and current racial/ethnic, socioeconomic, and geographic disparities. Health Resources and Services Administration, Maternal and Child Health Bureau. Rockville, MD: U.S. Department of Health and Human Services. Retrieved from http://www.hrsa.gov/healthit/images/mchb_obesity_pub.pdf

Soto, J. A., Dawson-Andoh, N. A., & BeLue, R. (2011). The relationship between perceived discrimination and generalized anxiety disorder among African-Americans, Afro-Caribbeans, and non-Hispanic whites. *Journal of Anxiety Disorders, 25*, 258–265.

Spector, R. E. (2004). *Cultural diversity in health and illness.* Upper Saddle River, NJ: Pearson Prentice Hall.

Stephens, G., Gillapsy, J., Clyne, D., Mejia, A., & Pollack, V. (1990). Racial differences in the incidence of end-stage renal disease in types I and II diabetes mellitus. *American Journal of Kidney Diseases, 15*(6), 562–567.

Swagerty, D. L., Walling, A. D., & Klein, R. M. (2002). Lactose intolerance. *American Family Physician, 65*(9), 1845–1850.

Tseng, C. W., Omphroy, G., Cruz, L., Naval, C. L., & Haddock, R. L. (2004). Cancer in the territory of Guam. *Pacific Health Dialogue, 11*(2), 57–63.

U.S. Census Bureau. (2010a). 2010 Census: Race and ethnicity. Retrieved from http://factfinder.census.gov/

U.S. Census Bureau. (2010b). Table AVG1. Average number of people per household, by race and ethnicity. Retrieved from https://www.census.gov/hhes/families/files/cps2011/tabAVG1

U.S. Census Bureau. (2011a).The black alone or in combination population in the United States: 2011. Retrieved from http://www.census.gov/population/race/data/ppl-bc11.html

U.S. Census Bureau. (2011b). American Fact Finder. Retrieved from http://factfinder2.census.gov/faces/nav/jsf/pages/index.xhtml.

U.S. Census Bureau. (2012a). U.S. Census Bureau projections show a slower growing, older, more diverse nation a half century from now. Retrieved from http://www.census.gov/newsroom/releases/archives/population/cb12-243.html

U.S. Census Bureau (2012b). The foreign-born population in the United States: 2010 American community survey reports. Retrieved from http://www.census.gov/prod/2012pubs/acs-19.pdf

U.S. Census Bureau. (2012c). 2010 Census shows Asians are fastest-growing race group. Retrieved from http://www.census.gov/newsroom/releases/archives/2010_census/cb12-cn22.html

U.S. Census Bureau. (2012d). Profile America Facts for Figures: American Indian and Alaska Native Heritage Month: November 2012. Retrieved from http://www.census.gov/newsroom/releases/archives/facts_for_features_special_editions/cb12-ff22.html

U.S. Census Bureau. (2012e). The Native Hawaiian and other Pacific Islander population: 2010. Retrieved from http://www.census.gov/prod/cen2010/briefs/c2010br-12.pdf

U.S. Census Bureau. (2013a). Asians fastest-growing race or ethnic group in 2012. Census Bureau reports. Retrieved from http://www.census.gov/newsroom/releases/archives/population/cb13-112.html

U.S. Census Bureau. (2013b). Highlights: 2011. http://www.census.gov/hhes/www/hlthins/data/incpovhlth/2011/highlights.html

U.S. Census Bureau. (2013c). American community survey: Families and living arrangements. Retrieved from http://www.census.gov/hhes/families/data/acs.html

U.S. Census Bureau. (2013d). Newsroom: American Indian and Alaska Native poverty rate about 50 percent in Rapid City, S.D., and about 30 percent in five other cities. Census Bureau reports. Retrieved from http://www.census.gov/newsroom/releases/archives/american_community_survey_acs/cb13-29.htm

U.S. Department of Health and Human Services. (2011). National diabetes statistics, 2011. Retrieved from http://diabetes.niddk.nih.gov/dm/pubs/statistics/

U.S. Department of Health and Human Services. Office of Disease Prevention and Health Promotion. *Healthy People 2020.* Washington, DC. Available at http://www.healthypeople.gov

U.S. Department of Health and Human Services. (2013). Health Resources and Service Administration. *About health literacy.* Retrieved from http://www.hrsa.gov/publichealth/healthliteracy/healthlitabout.html

U.S. Department of the Interior. (2012). Bureau of Indian Affairs. http://www.bia.gov/WhoWeAre/BIA/index.htm

U.S. Department of Labor Statistics. (2006). Employment status of foreign born and native born populations. Retrieved from http://www.bls.gov/news.release/forbrn.t01.htm

U.S. Department of Labor. (2012a). *Labor force characteristics by race and ethnicity, 2011.* Retrieved from http://www.bls.gov/cps/cpsrace2011.pdf

U.S. Department of Labor. (2012b). The Latino labor force at a glance. Retrieved from http://www.dol.gov/_sec/media/reports/HispanicLaborForce/HispanicLaborForce.pdf

U.S. Food and Drug Administration. (2012). FDA drug safety communication: Codeine use in certain children after tonsillectomy and/or adenoidectomy may lead to rare, but life-threatening adverse events or death. Retrieved from http://www.fda.gov/Drugs/DrugSafety/ucm313631.htm

U.S. Passport Card (2012). Retrieved from http://travel.state.gov/content/passports/english/passports/information/card.html

Vaz-da-Silva, M., Loureiro, A. I., Nunes, T., Maia, J., Tavares, S., Falcão, A., et al. (2005). Bioavailability and bioequivalence of two enteric-coated formulations of omeprazole in fasting and fed conditions. *Clinical Drug Investigations, 25*(6), 391–399.

Viega, M. I., Asimus, S., Ferreira, P. E., Martins, J. P., Cavaco, I., Riberr, V., Hai, T. N., et al. (2009). Pharmacogenomics of CYP2A6, CYP2B6, CYP2C19, CYP2D6, CYP3A4, CYP3A5 and MDR1 in Vietnam. *European Journal of Clinical Pharmacology, 65*(4), 355–363.

Wall, T. L., Carr, L. G., & Ehlers, C. L. (2003). Protective associations of genetic variations in alcohol dehydrogenase with alcohol dependence in Native American Mission Indians. *American Journal of Psychiatry, 160*(1), 41–46.

Weinberger, M. (1993). Racial differences in renal sodium excretion: Relationship to hypertension. *American Journal of Kidney Diseases, 21*(4), 41–45.

Weir, M., Chrysant, S., McCarron, D., Canossa-Terris, M., Cohen, J., Gunter, P., et al. (1998). Influence of race and dietary salt on the antihypertensive efficacy of an angiotensin-converting enzyme inhibitor or a calcium channel antagonist in salt-sensitive hypertensives. *Hypertension, 31*(5), 1088–1096.

Wilner, A. N. (2008). Pain management across cultures. *Medscape Neurology*. Retrieved from http://www.medscape.org/viewarticle/581930

Wong, V., Taoka, S., Kuartei, S., Demei, Y., & Soaladaob, F. (2004). Cancer in the Republic of Palau (Belau). *Pacific Health Dialogue, 11*(2), 64–69.

World Health Organization. (2002). WHO traditional medicine strategy 2002–2005. Retrieved from http://whqlibdoc.who.int/hq/2002/WHO_EDM_TRM_2002.1.pdf?ua=1

Yancy, C. W., Laskar, S., & Eichhorn, E. (2004). The use of beta-adrenergic receptor antagonists in the treatment of African Americans with heart failure. *Congestive Heart Failure, 10*(1), 34–37.

Ye, J., Mack, D., Fry-Johnson, Y., & Parker, K. (2012). Health care access and utilization among US-born and foreign-born Asian Americans. *Journal of Immigrant and Minority Health. 14*(5), 731–737.

Yee, B. W. K., Debaryshe, B. D., Yuen, S., Kim, S. Y., & McCubbin, H. I. (2013). Asian American and Pacific Islander families: Resiliency and lifespan socialization in a cultural context. http://uhfamily.hawaii.edu/publications/journals/aapifamiliesbookchapter.pdf

Yunis, Z., Liu, L., Wang, H., Zhang, L., Geng, T., Kang, L., et al. (2013). Genetic polymorphisms of pharmacogenomics VIP variants in the Kyrzyz population of northwest China. *Gene, 529*(1), 88–93.

Zaid, R. B., Nargis, M., Neelotpol, S., Hannan, J. M., Islam, S., Akhter, R., et al. (2004). Acetylation phenotype status in a Bangladeshi population and its comparison with that of other Asian population data. *Biopharmaceutics & Drug Disposition, 25*(6), 237–241.

CHAPTER 8

AN INTRODUCTION TO PHARMACOGENOMICS

Ashim Malhotra

Advances in health care have led to a significant improvement in patient survival in the past three decades. The introduction of more selective and potent therapeutic agents and optimal patient-care services have affected patient survival and quality of life significantly, with life expectancy rising from 70.9 years in 1970 (U.S. Department of Health, Education, and Welfare, 1974) to 77.7 years in 2006 (Arias, 2010). Drug therapy is often the most challenging aspect of care. Optimal drug treatment requires selection of the best possible agents with close monitoring of pharmacokinetics, pharmacodynamics, adverse drug reactions, and the cost of different agents. This chapter focuses on the pharmacogenomic influences on drug therapy. Adverse drug reactions (ADRs) are discussed in depth in Chapter 5, although this chapter will also discuss ADRs related to genetic polymorphisms.

Pharmacogenomics is the branch of science concerned with the identification of the genetic attributes of an individual that lead to variable responses to drugs. Interestingly, the science has evolved to also consider patterns of inherited alterations in defined populations, such as specific ethnicities, that account for variability in pharmacotherapeutic responses. For the purposes of this chapter, the term *pharmacogenomics* is used more generally to refer to genetic polymorphisms that occur in a patient population—for instance, in an ethnic group—as opposed to individual patients.

Until recently, the ultimate goal of pharmacogenomics had been the development of prediction models to forecast debilitating adverse events in specific individuals and, more recently, across populations based on similarities in age, gender, or more commonly, race or ethnicity, as contrasted with the rest of the population. However, in spite of this newer usage, pharmacogenomics may predict the extreme deviation of some patients from predictable pharmacokinetic and pharmacodynamic responses: the idiosyncratic response.

In recent practice, pharmacogenomic tools coupled with proteomics and other advanced molecular diagnostics are emerging as the cornerstone of individualized patient therapy, especially when differential genetic responses to xenobiotics are considered across specific ethnicities. For instance, a 2010 *New York Times* article described the cutting-edge genetic characterization of a patient's cells to identify the specific aberrant oncogenes responsible for cancer in this individual, who was subsequently administered chemotherapy specific to the identified altered molecular pathway (Kolata, 2012). This is the new and changing face of pharmacogenomics in the present century—enabling patient-centered and patient-specific pharmaceutical care.

Pharmacogenomics seeks to identify patterns of genetic variation that are subsequently employed to guide the design of optimal medication regimens for individual patients. Historically, the approach to drug therapy has been largely empiric and based on clinical studies that determined the maximally tolerated dose and reasonable toxicity in a narrowly defined population. This approach typically leads to the safe and effective administration of drugs for most individuals. However, with empiric therapy, interindividual (allotypic) variation in drug response occurs—with patient outcomes varying from a complete absence of therapeutic response to potentially life-threatening adverse drug reactions (ADRs).

Genetic differences may account in part for some of the well-documented variability in response to drug therapy. Obviously, many factors other than genetics—such as age, sex, other drugs administered, and underlying disease states—also contribute to variation in drug response. However, inherited differences in the metabolism and disposition of drugs and genetic polymorphisms in the targets of drug therapy (e.g., metabolizing enzymes or protein receptors) can have an even greater influence on the efficacy and toxicity of medications. Interestingly, age, gender, and endemic geographical differences may themselves emerge as phenotypic consequences of differential epigenetic control. This implies that heterogeneity in the control of gene expression based upon age, gender, and geographic location is itself a life-long changing process that is under the control of molecular "epigenetic" switches that either activate or inhibit groups of genes as a unit. Specific identification of these epigenetic controls in special populations, for instance differences in pediatric or geriatric protein expression in immune cells when compared to the general adult population, can provide valuable clues to how special populations based on age, gender, pregnancy, and even geographical location respond differentially to specific drugs. This information can then be incorporated in optimal therapeutic design.

With the publication in 2001 of Lander's and Venter's description of their groundbreaking effort to map the entire human genome, the Human Genome Project (HGP), about 95% of the sequence of all human DNA was established, resulting in the identification of Open Reading Frames (ORF) for many human proteins. A more recent development has been the discovery of single-nucleotide polymorphisms (SNPs), genetic differences that account for allotypic phenotype variations. About 1.4 million SNPs in humans have been identified through a mass effort by the SNP Consortium, which was funded by multiple pharmaceutical companies. The existence of the SNP Consortium is an excellent reminder of the significance of SNPs to drug companies, since SNPs may account for some of the differences in drug responses seen in pharmacotherapy in the population at large (Howe, 2009). With the identification of the individual SNPs, our understanding of pharmacogenetics and pharmacogenomics has exploded.

A study published in 2011 by Li, Zhang, Zhou, Stoneking, and Tang on the heterogeneity in drug-metabolizing genes in globally defined populations has provided profound insights and ever stronger evidence for the significance and relevance of SNP-induced variation in drug metabolism. This study compared differences in 283 drug-metabolizing enzymes and transporter genes across 62 globally distributed ethnic groups and demonstrated that patterns of emergence of SNPs in specific populations spread out across the world indicate positive selection at work and that these differences in SNPs importantly account for the differential drugs response in any given population (Li et al, 2011). Not only does this work support and explain the origin of genetic polymorphism in drug-metabolizing enzymes, it purports to provide an evolutionary rationale for such differences across ethnicities.

GENETICS REVISITED

An individual's genetic makeup (or genotype) is derived as a result of genetic recombination or "mixing" of genes from that individual's parents. All the DNA contained in any individual cell is known as the *genome* of the individual, a word formed by the combination of "gene" and "chromosome," and thus represents all the genes that individual can express. Interestingly, even though two unrelated people share about 99.9% of the same DNA sequences, the less than 0.1% difference between them translates into a difference of 3 million nucleotides. These variants, introduced above, are the SNPs (pronounced "snips") (Howe, 2009). The variability of the genome at these various SNPs accounts for nearly all of the phenotypic differences we see in each other.

The Human Genome Project has sought not only to identify and correlate SNPs with phenotypic differences but also to record and map haplotypes as well (Nebert, Zhang, & Vesell, 2008). Haplotypes are large portions of genetic material (around 25,000 base pairs) that tend to travel together. Understanding how SNPs and haplotypes make humans genetically unique is the current focus of much genetic research (Nebert et al, 2008). The completion of the Human Genome Project, as well as the mapping of SNPs and haplotypes, has allowed the field of pharmacogenomics to understand the variability of drug metabolism seen across individuals and populations. Box 8-1

BOX 8–1 **DEFINITIONS**

Genetic polymorphism: multiple differences of a DNA sequence found in at least 1% of the population

Genetics: the study of heredity and its variations

Genomics: the study of the complete set of genetic information present in a cell, an organism, or species

Pharmacogenetics: the study of the influence of hereditary factors on the response of individual organisms to drugs (Venes, 2005); the study of variations of DNA and RNA characteristics as related to drug response (U.S. Food and Drug Administration, 2010b)

Pharmacogenomics: the study of the effects of genetic differences among people and the impact that these differences have on the uptake, effectiveness, toxicity, and metabolism of drugs

SNP: single-nucleotide polymorphism

Source: Venes, D. (2005). *Taber's cyclopedic medical dictionary* (21st ed.). Philadelphia: FA Davis; U.S. Food and Drug Administration. (2010b). Table of valid genomic biomarkers in the context of approved drug labels. Retrieved from http://www.fda.gov/RegulatoryInformation/Guidances/ucm129286.htm

provides definitions of terms used in pharmacogenetics and pharmacogenomics.

Another interesting aspect of this discussion is the frequency with which the "mutant" gene copy is expressed. If the variant copy of a gene, such as is common for genes encoding Drug Metabolizing Enzymes (DME), is expressed in the equivalent of 1% or more of the population, the genetic variation is referred to as a polymorphic variation.

Standard adopted nomenclature is used in pharmacogenomics and pharmacogenetics. Of the various mutant variants of a specific gene, each variant is numerically and sequentially named starting with the "wild-type" or normal or nonmutated copy of the gene. Thus, for instance, *CYP2D6* written in italics refers to the normal copy of the gene, whereas *CYP2D6*1* (pronounced "star 1") refers to the first identified natural variant (mutant) copy of this gene.

HISTORY OF PHARMACOGENETICS

The Greek philosopher and mathematician Pythagoras recorded the first interindividual difference of drug administration in 510 BCE when he noted that some patients developed hemolytic anemia after ingesting the fava bean (Nebert et al, 2008). The term *pharmacogenetics* was first coined by Vogel in 1959, but not until1962 was pharmacogenetics defined as the study of heredity and the response to drugs by Kalow (Nebert et al, 2008). Since 1962, the term has been used to refer to the effects of genetic differences on a person's response to drugs.

Interest in pharmacogenetics emerged in the 1950s in response to the discovery of an abnormal butyrylcholinesterase enzyme in psychiatric patients who exhibited prolonged muscular paralysis after administration of succinylcholine before electroconvulsive therapy (Meyer, 2004). Also in the 1950s a connection was established between the development of hemolysis in African American males treated for malaria with primaquine and glucose-6-phosphate dehydrogenase deficiency (Beutler, 1959). Other seminal pharmacogenetic findings include the identification of the proportion of slow acetylators in certain ethnic groups, including 10% of the Japanese and Eskimos; 20% of the Chinese; and 60% Caucasians, blacks, and South Indians (Ellard, 1976), and attribution of peripheral neuropathy to slow acetylation of isoniazid in some patients treated for tuberculosis due to genetic diversity in the enzyme *N*-acetyltransferase (Fig. 8-1) (Yamamoto, Subue, Mukoyama, Matsuoka, & Mitsuma, 1999). The rate of acetylation of a drug such as isoniazid is clinically relevant because it determines the rate of elimination of the drug from the body. Thus, individuals known as slow acetylators will metabolize the drug slowly, allowing greater residence time in the body and enhanced toxicity. It is a pharmacogenomic variation, which is responsible for slow or fast acetylators as explained below.

PHARMACOGENOMICS

The ultimate promise of pharmacogenomics is the possibility that knowledge of the patient's DNA sequence might be used to enhance drug therapy to maximize efficacy, to target drugs only to those patients who are likely to respond, and to avoid ADRs. Increasing the number of patients who respond to a therapeutic regimen with a concomitant decrease in the incidence of ADRs is the promise of pharmacogenomic information. The long-term expected benefits of pharmacogenomics are selective and potent drugs, more accurate methods of determining appropriate drug dosages, advanced screening for disease, and a decrease in the overall cost to the health-care system in the United States caused by ineffective drug therapy.

GENETIC DIFFERENCES IN DRUG METABOLISM

Genetic differences in metabolism were first realized by the observation that sometimes very low or very high concentrations of drug were found in some patients despite their having been given the same amount of drug. Most genetic differences in drug metabolism have been found to be "monogenic" genetic polymorphisms, meaning that they arise from the variation in one gene (Nebert et al, 2008).

Genetic Polymorphism

A genetic polymorphism occurs when a difference in the allele(s) responsible for the variation is a common occurrence. An allele is an alternative form of a gene. A gene is called polymorphic when allelic variations occur throughout a given population at a stable rate of less than 1% (Howe, 2009). Under such circumstances, mutant genes will exist somewhat frequently alongside wild-type genes. The mutant genes will encode for the production of mutant proteins in these populations. The mutant proteins will, in turn, interact with drugs in different manners, sometimes slight, sometimes significant. Monogenic traits by themselves cannot explain the complexity of drug metabolism (Nebert et al, 2008). Genes interact on a complex level, yielding different responses depending on which genes are wild-type and which show mutant phenotypes. Sometimes these interactions can be very difficult to elucidate and may in fact be the source of seemingly unexplainable drug reactions. Figure 8-1 illustrates the relationship between genetic polymorphisms in drug metabolism and at drug receptors.

Four different phenotypes categorize the effects that genetic polymorphisms have on individuals: poor metabolizers (PMs) lack a working enzyme; intermediate metabolizers (IMs) are heterogeneous for one working, wild-type allele and one mutant allele (or two reduced-function alleles); extensive metabolizers (EMs) have two normally functioning alleles; and ultrarapid metabolizers (UMs) have more than one functioning copy of a certain enzyme (Belle & Singh, 2008). See Table 8-1 for the clinical implications of genetic polymorphisms.

Phase I and Phase II Metabolism

Drug metabolism generally involves the conversion of lipophilic substances and metabolites into more easily excretable water-soluble forms. Drug metabolism takes place

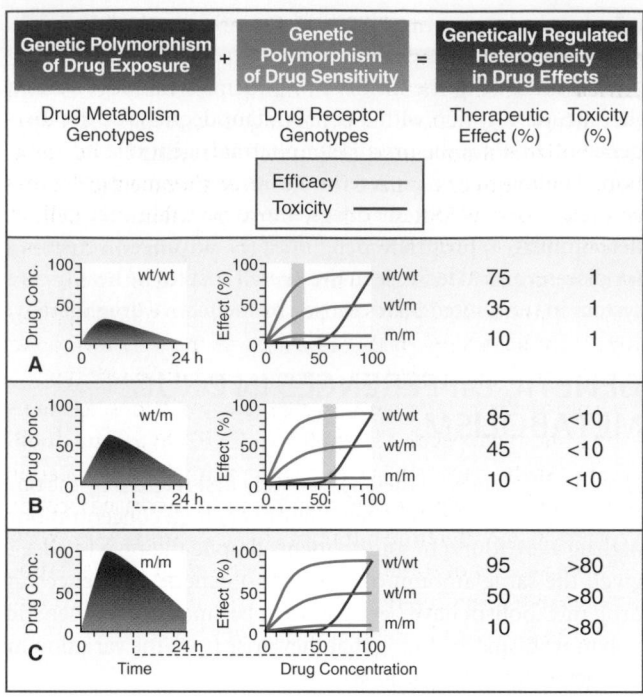

Figure 8–1. Genetic polymorphisms and drug metabolism/receptors.

Table 8–1   Clinical Implications of Genetic Polymorphisms

Metabolizer Phenotype	Effect on Drug Metabolism	Clinical Implications
Poor to intermediate metabolizers	Slow	Prodrug will be metabolized slowly into active drug metabolite. May have accumulation of prodrug. Active drug will be metabolized slowly into inactive metabolite. Potential for accumulation of active drug. Patient requires lower dosage of medication.
Ultrarapid metabolizers	Fast	Prodrug rapidly metabolized into active drug. No dosage adjustment needed. Active drug rapidly metabolized into inactive metabolites leading to potential therapeutic failure. Patient requires higher dosage of active drug.

mostly in the liver and is divided into two major categories, phase I (oxidation, reduction, and hydrolysis reactions) and phase II metabolism (conjugation reactions). A hallmark experiment in pharmacogenomics, diagrammed in Figure 8-2, illustrates how differences in the rates of the phase II metabolizing enzyme N-acetyltransferase (NAT-2) can affect the half-life and plasma concentration of drugs that are subject to NAT-2 metabolism (Meyer, 2004).

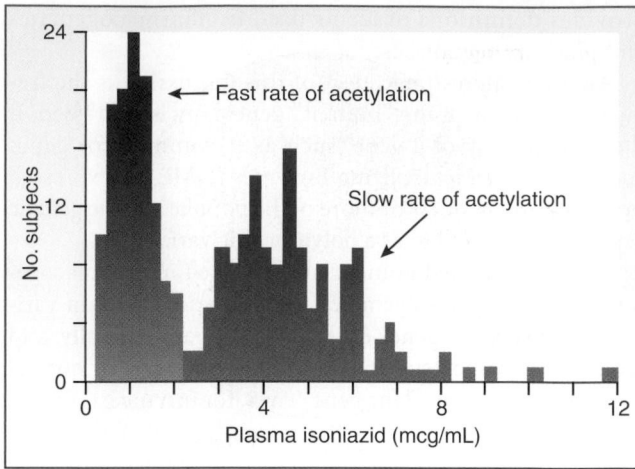

Figure 8–2. Pharmacogenomics of acetylation in isoniazid. Plasma isoniazid concentrations in 267 patients measured 6 hours post-dose. The bimodal distribution shows the effect of an *NAT-2* genetic polymorphism.

Phase I metabolism enzymes are responsible for approximately 59% of the adverse drug reactions cited in the literature (Phillips, Veenstra, Oren, Lee, & Sadee, 2001). In terms of evolution, the cytochrome P450 (CYP450) enzyme system was one of the first biocatalytic machineries to emerge on earth. These ubiquitous enzymes contain an iron-porphyrin ring center that is essential to the chemical reaction they catalyze. During this oxygenation reaction, the oxidative state of iron in the porphyrin ring changes, resulting in spectrophotometric absorption maxima observed at 450 nm, which contributed to their naming.

CYPs are generally located in the endoplasmic reticulum (ER) and the mitochondria in human cells, of which the ER isoforms are of particular importance to the field of drug metabolism. In terms of their organ distribution, they are found in greater amounts in the liver and the intestine and to a somewhat lesser extent in other organs, such as the skin, brain, lungs, and kidneys. Hepatic, renal, and intestinal ER CYPs are involved in the biotransformation of a plethora of drugs and endogenous substrates in humans mainly by oxygenation of the target substrate molecule and mediated by differential oxidation states of the central iron atom in the enzyme. Due to this oxygenation reaction, CYPs are classified as monooxygenases. The high genetic variability of the cytochrome *P450* enzymes constitutes the most important of the phase I metabolizing enzymes, with a total of 57 genes encoding for CYP450 enzymes. Of these, CYP2D6, CYP2C9, and CYP2C19 are highly polymorphic and account for upward of about 40% of hepatic phase I metabolism (Phillips et al, 2001) (Fig. 8-3 and Table 8-2).

Specific CYP450 Enzymes

CYP2D6

Up to 25% of drugs are metabolized via CYP2D6 (Belle & Singh, 2008). Phenotypic variations between some enzymes can have an astounding outcome on drug therapy. For example, a 1,000-fold difference has been observed in the rate of

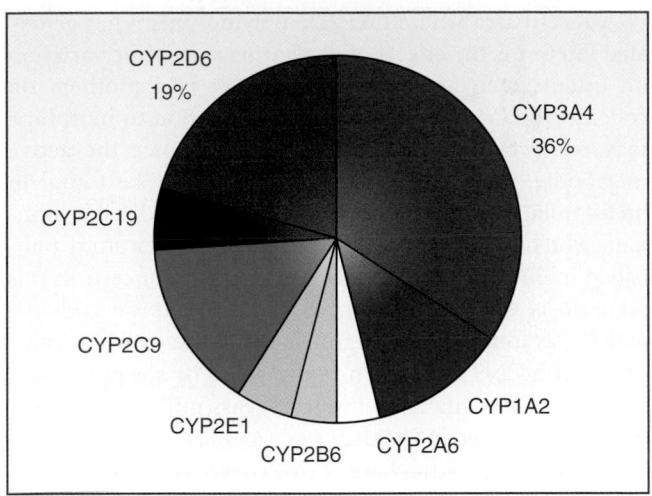

Figure 8–3. Proportion of drugs metabolized by CYP450 isoenzymes.

metabolism of some substrates due to differences in CYP2D6 isozymes. Figure 8-4 illustrates this difference within the European population for the CYP2D6 substrate nortriptyline.

Pharmacogenomic Variance of *CYP2D6*

CYP2D6 is a well-studied instance of a drug-metabolizing enzyme (DME) coding gene that exhibits polymorphism. The CYP2D6 gene product acts on many xenobiotics, including many common prescription drugs (Table 8-3) such as the selective serotonin reuptake inhibitors (SSRIs) fluoxetine, tricyclic antidepressants (TCAs), beta blockers (metoprolol), calcium channel blockers (diltiazem), theophylline (Phillips et al, 2001), and tamoxifen. Research has shown that while approximately 10% of Caucasians, up to 7% of

African Americans, and 4.8% of Asians have the "poor metabolizer" (PM) phenotype, 5% of Caucasians and 4.9% of African Americans have the "ultrarapid metabolizer" (UM) phenotype. For Asians, the percentage of CYP2D6 ultrarapid metabolizers shoots up to 21%, perhaps leading to the therapeutic failure of or the need for increased therapeutic dosages of drugs such as SSRIs in these target populations (Belle & Singh, 2008). Thirty-five percent of the population carries a nonfunctional 2D6 allele. This nonfunctional allele may increase the risk of ADRs, especially in patients with polypharmacy. Interestingly, of the 43 alleles of the CYP2D6 gene, about 5 alleles account for the poor metabolic phenotype.

Among the many reasons for genetic variations, an interesting one that specifically applies to CYP2D6 is gene duplication. As the name suggests, in some ethnicities duplication of the allele coding for 2D6 may result in increased protein expression and therefore ultrarapid metabolism and markedly reduced activity of some drugs. The percentage of population that shows gene duplication for CYP2D6 across different countries is shown in Figure 8-5.

CYP2D6 and Tamoxifen

Recently, the ameliorative effects that variable isoforms of CYP2D6 have on the metabolism and therapeutic efficacy of tamoxifen in some patients have received much attention. With reference to tamoxifen, the role of CYP2D6 is not so much the metabolism of this drug as it is to activate it by conversion to endoxifen inside the cell. Pharmacogenetic variation in CYP2D6 has been shown in clinical trials conducted in the United Kingdom and Germany to lead to variable therapeutic outcomes to tamoxifen treatment of estrogen-sensitive cancers (Schroth et al, 2009, 2010; Thompson et al, 2011).

Table 8–2 Medications and Their Receptors

Gene	Medications	Drug Effect Linked to Polymorphism
Drug-Metabolizing Enzymes		
CYP2C9	Tolbutamide, warfarin, phenytoin, NSAIDS	Anticoagulant effect of warfarin
CYP2D6	Beta blockers, antidepressants, antipsychotics, codeine, debrisoquine, dextromethorphan, encainide, flecainide, guanoxan, methoxyamphetamine, *N*-propylamaline, perhexiline, phenacetin, phenformin, propafenone, sparteine	Tardive dyskinesia from antipsychotics; narcotic side effects, efficacy, and dependence: imipramine dose requirement; beta blocker effect
Dihydropyrimidine dehydrogenase	Fluorouracil	Fluorouracil neurotoxicity
Thiopurine methyltransferase	Mercaptopurine, thioguanine, azathioprine	Thiopurine toxicity and efficacy; risk of second cancers
Drug Targets		
ACE	Enalapril, lisinopril, captopril	Renoprotective effects, cardiac indices, blood pressure, immunoglobulin A nephropathy
Potassium channels	Quinidine	Drug-induced long QT syndrome
HERG	Cisapride	Drug-induced torsade de pointes
KvLQT1	Terfenadine, disopyramide, mefloquine	Drug-induced long QT syndrome
hKCNE2	Clarithromycin	Drug-induced arrhythmia

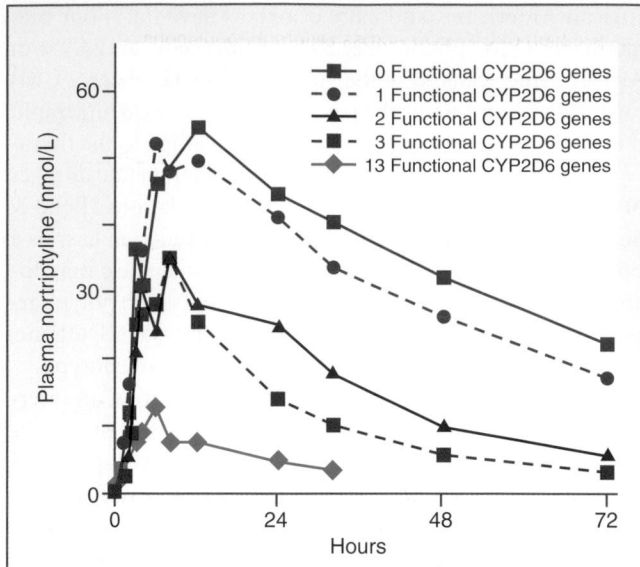

Figure 8–4. European population and the *CYP2D6* substrate nortriptyline.

Table 8–3 *CYP2D6*

Substrate	Inhibitors	Inducers
Codeine	Amiodarone	Carbamazepine
Dextromethorphan	Fluoxetine	Phenytoin
Metoprolol	Labetalol	Phenobarbital
Paroxetine	Paroxetine	Rifampin
Haloperidol	Propafenone	
Propranolol	Quinidine	
Risperidone	Sertraline	
Timolol	Cimetidine	
Amitriptyline		
Nortriptyline		
Clozapine		
Morphine		
Methadone		

CYP2D6 and Opioid Analgesics (Codeine)

Opioid analgesics such as codeine rely on CYP2D6 enzymes to convert them to their active form, morphine (Belle & Singh, 2008). Genetic polymorphisms of the CYP2D6 enzyme can greatly alter the effect that codeine has on patients who are PM or UM types. UM types may not experience the analgesic effects of the drug at normal therapeutic doses, and PMs may not be able to convert codeine to its active metabolite morphine, thus experiencing little or no clinical benefit. Other narcotics that are active when administered to patients may produce the effects of excess drug at even the lower end of therapeutic dosing. See Table 8-3.

A recent area where CYP2D6 polymorphism has generated interest is the effects of its pharmacogenomic variation on infants who are breastfed milk by UM mothers on codeine. In UMs, excessive codeine activation to morphine may cause fatal respiratory depression. Since the active metabolite, morphine, is lipophilic and may be found in breast milk, severe respiratory depression could result in infants who have not yet been weaned. However, a study published in 2012 demonstrated that the main concern in this scenario is CNS depression in UM mothers on codeine, which was found to be a significant risk factor when compared with CNS depression as measured by sleepiness and lethargy in the infants being fed breast milk by the same mothers (Sistonen et al, 2012).

In addition, fatalities have been observed in some pediatric patients following the administration of codeine for postoperative pain management after tonsillectomy and/or adenoidectomy procedures. In August 2012, the Food and Drug Administration (FDA) acknowledged that it was considering the lethal effects of codeine in some pediatric patients and estimated that "the number of "ultrarapid metabolizers" is generally 1 to 7 per 100 people, but may be as high as 28 per 100 people in some ethnic groups." Consequently, as recently as February 2013, the FDA issued a Black-Box Warning for the cautious use of codeine in children, particularly for pain management following surgery.

Genetic Testing for CYP2D6 Polymorphisms

There are commercially available tests that can provide immensely helpful information. One such test called the Tag-It system is described at the end of the chapter.

CYP2C9

CYP2C9 is the primary route of metabolism for about a hundred different drugs in humans. While some CYP2C9 substrates are the more common drugs, such as phenytoin, glipizide, and losartan, other drug substrates include those that evince a narrow therapeutic index, such as the coumarin-related anticoagulant agents warfarin and acenocoumarol.

CYP2C9 and Warfarin

Warfarin is one of the most effective, cheapest, and widely prescribed anticoagulant drugs that act by inhibiting the enzyme vitamin K epoxide reductase, which prevents the formation of functional vitamin K. This action in turn inhibits the activation of clotting factors in the liver, causing the anticoagulant effect. Warfarin is available as a racemic mixture, of which the *S*-enantiomer, which is the more bioactive form, is metabolized by CYP2C9. The presence of CYP2C9 mutations is associated with a reduction in the metabolism of *S*-warfarin. Clinically, warfarin maintenance dosing requirements are lower in patients with CYP2C9*2 polymorphisms and further reduced in patients with CYP2C9*3 variants (Gulseth, Grice, & Dager, 2009), making these two the most common "reduced function variants" for the CYP gene in terms of its effect on warfarin. The CYP2C9*2 variant evinces a 30% and the CYP2C9*3 variant a 90% reduction in warfarin clearance (Rettie,

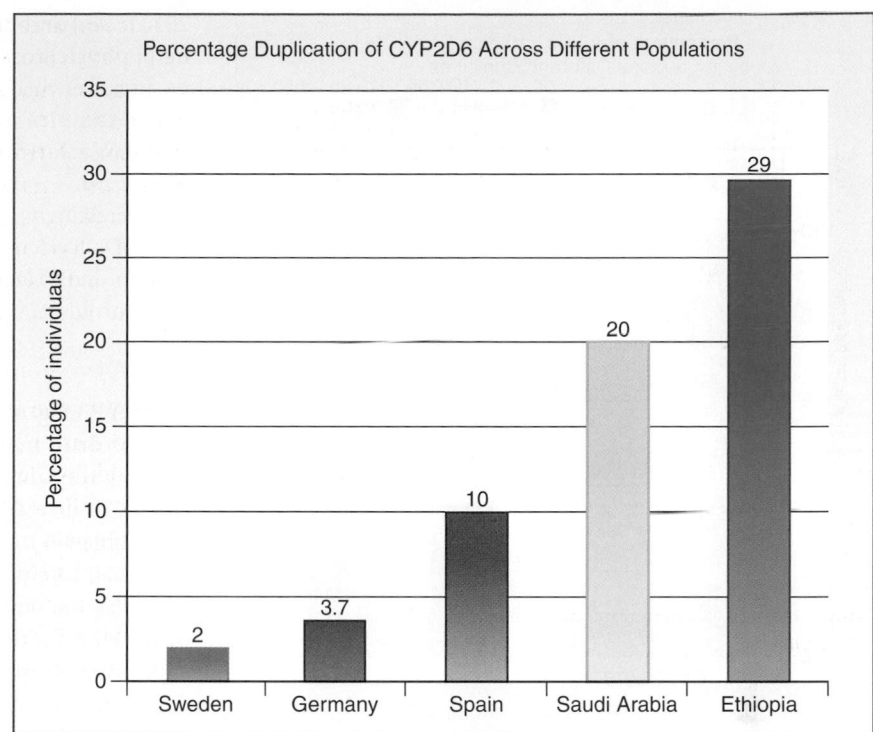

Figure 8–5. Percentage distribution of individuals across countries showing a duplication of an allele of CYP2D6. The figure explains the exaggerated metabolism of some drugs in the specified percentage of individuals belonging to certain ethnic backgrounds (generously assuming ethnic homogeneity in some countries) due to increased 2D6 activity.

Haining, Bajpai, & Levy, 1999), resulting in adjusted dose requirements in these patients compared with noncarriers.

In addition, patients with homozygous presentation of a CYP2C9 mutation appear to have a greater reduction in dosing requirement than do heterozygotes. Approximately one-third of the population carries at least one allele for the slow-metabolizing form of CYP2C9 (U.S. Food and Drug Administration, 2009). The clinical implications of altered warfarin metabolism can be significant; the clinical implications of pharmacogenomic variants are found later in this chapter. See Table 8-4.

In spite of the information outlined above, controversy exists in the field of pharmacogenetic testing over initiation or maintenance of anticoagulant therapy following an adverse cardiovascular event, in part due to some conflicting reports in the literature about the clinical effectiveness and relevance of pharmacogenomic variability in warfarin drug metabolism. However, recent studies on the pharmacogenomics of warfarin have included an analysis of the effects of polymorphism of CYP2C9 and vitamin K epoxide reductase (VKORC1) across populations in Europe, Asia, and elsewhere. Polymorphisms in these two genes account for nearly 40% of the differences in warfarin therapy across populations (Yip & Pirmohamed, 2013). Taken together, the data from these pharmacogenomic studies indicate a strong connection between the variant effects of CYP2C9 polymorphism and the metabolism and therapeutic efficacy of warfarin and acenocoumaral. CYP2C9 variation was reported to be important for the maintenance therapy of warfarin in a genome-wide association analysis in the Swedish and Japanese population (Cha et al, 2010).

Data from disparate research resources need to be organized to obtain clinically relevant information that assists in guiding the therapeutic rationale for the use of warfarin in special populations. One such approach would be to analyze studies on the frequency of allelic variation of the three drug-metabolizing genes for warfarin in selected populations. Thus, for the CYP2C9 gene, the frequency of allelic variation for CYP2C9*2 is about 10% in Caucasians, compared to less than 1% in Africans and Asians, while the frequency of allelic variation for CYP2C9*3 is about 6% in Caucasians, 4% in Asians, and less than 1% in Africans (Fig. 8-6). The frequency of allelic variation of the VKORC1 gene is substantially higher in all the three ethnicities compared with the mutational frequency of CYP2C9. For the specific VKORC1 (-1639) mutation, allelic frequency is 98% for Africans, 60% for Caucasians, and 2% for Asians; see Figure 8-7 (Voora & Ginsburg, 2012).

Table 8–4 *CYP2C (9 and 19)*

Substrate	Inhibitors	Inducers
S-warfarin	Amiodarone	Carbamazepine
Losartan	Cimetidine	Phenytoin
Diazepam	Chloramphenicol	Rifampin
Imipramine	Fluconazole	
Amitriptyline	Isoniazid	
Phenytoin	Ketoconazole	
Rosiglitazone	Zafirlukast	
	Fluoxetine	
	Fluvoxamine	
	Sertraline	
	Rosiglitazone	

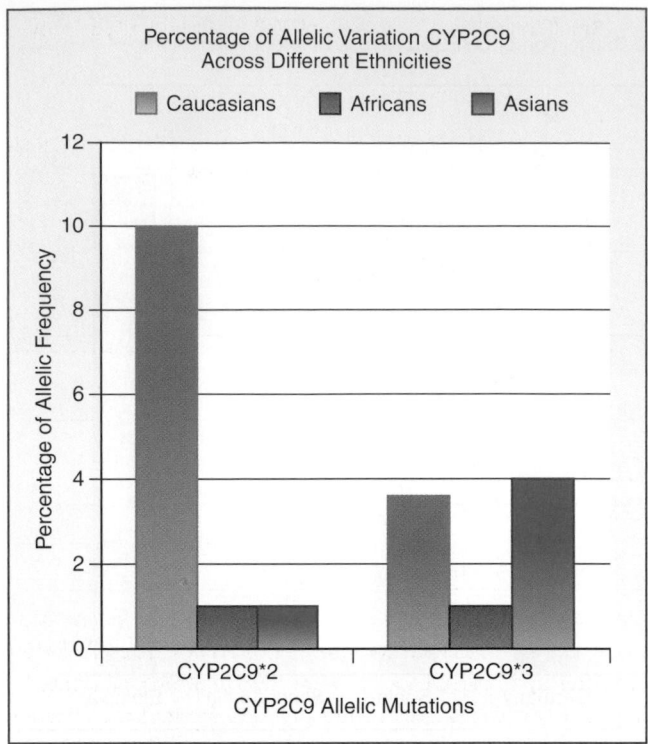

Figure 8–6. Percentage distribution of individuals across ethnicities exhibiting polymorphism in *CYP2C9*.

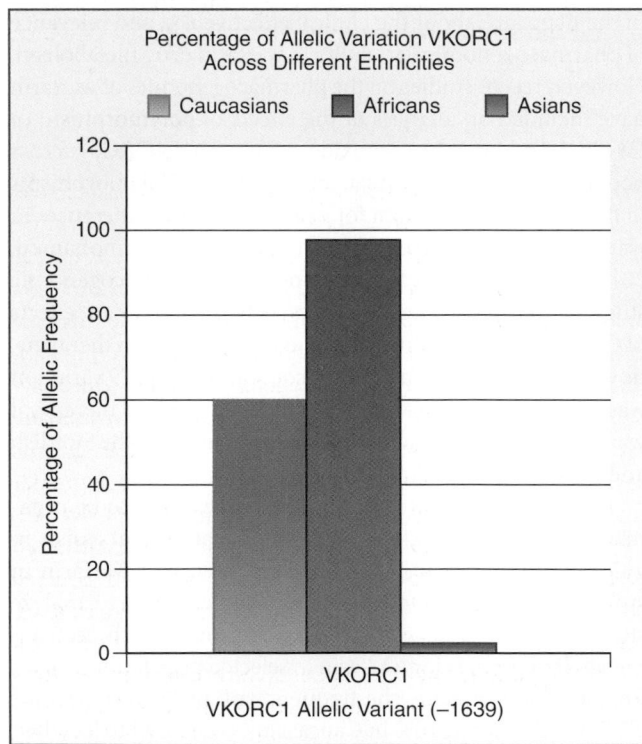

Figure 8–7. Percentage distribution of individuals across ethnicities showing variation in *VKORC1*.

The wealth of scientific data documenting evidence of *CYP2C9*2*, *CYP2C9*3*, and VKORC1 (-1639 G > A) polymorphisms affecting dose response to warfarin in different populations resulted in the FDA updating the label of the drug in 2007 and then again in 2010 (Finkelman et al,

2011). A number of algorithms have been published to help physicians in making a decision about warfarin dosing after pharmacogenetic testing, of which two prominent examples are the Gage algorithm and the International Warfarin Pharmacogenetics Consortium (IWPC) algorithm.

Interestingly, the nonsteroidal anti-inflammatory drugs (NSAIDs) celecoxib and flubiprofen have received "use with caution" in PM label warnings from the FDA owing to CYP2C9 polymorphism.

CYP3A4

The CYP3A group of isoenzymes is responsible for up to 50% of drug metabolism (Howe, 2009). CYP3A4 isoenzyme is responsible for metabolism of several important classes of drugs that are commonly used in primary care (see Table 8-1). Examples of these classes include azole antifungals, calcium channel blockers, antihistamines, anticonvulsants, antimicrobials, and corticosteroids. Both drug-related induction or inhibition of CYP450 3A4 isoenzyme may complicate drug therapy in patients (Howe, 2009). Predicting the onset and offset of these effects is very difficult. The time to onset and offset of drug–drug interactions is closely related to each drug's half-life and the half-life of enzyme production. Clinically significant drug interactions in this setting may increase the risk of toxicity. For example, amiodarone has a half-life of close to 60 days and requires months to reach steady state and inhibit the CYP450 enzyme system effectively (Table 8-5). Conversely,

Table 8–5 *CYP3A4*

Substrate	Inhibitors	Inducers
Cyclosporine, FK 506	Erythromycin	Carbamazepine
Corticosteroids	Clarithromycin	Phenobarbital
Erythromycin	Diltiazem	Rifampin
Felodipine, isradipine	Ketoconazole	Rifabutin
Nifedipine	Fluconazole	Phenytoin
Nisoldipine	Itraconazole	Corticosteroids
Nitrendipine	Quinidine	INH
Digoxin, quinidine	Grapefruit juice	St. John's wort
Verapamil	Cimetidine	
Warfarin	Indinavir	
Sildenafil	Fluoxetine	
Astemizole	Zileuton, zafirlukast	
Terfenadine	Verapamil	
Pioglitazone	Amiodarone	
R-warfarin	Corticosteroids	
	Fluvoxamine	

it takes less than 2 days for rifampin, which is a nonspecific CYP450 inducer with a shorter half-life, to decrease blood concentrations of many drugs to a subtherapeutic level and significantly increase the risk of therapeutic failure. Close monitoring is required when prescribing drugs that induce or inhibit CYP3A4 enzymes. See Table 8-5 for further information.

P-GLYCOPROTEIN

P-glycoprotein (Pgp) is a membrane-bound, ATP-dependent transport system responsible for the efflux of a variety of xenobiotics from cells to the extracellular fluid. This includes the ejection of drugs from cells, usually against their concentration gradients. Pgp, also known as multidrug resistance (MDR1) protein, is the product of the *ABCB1* and *ABCB4* genes and is a member of adenosine triphosphate (ATP)-binding family of proteins. Differential expression of Pgp may explain tissue-specific and temporal variations in efflux efficiency in different cells. In fact, chemoresistance in cancer therapeutics has been strongly linked with Pgp expression—the more Pgp protein expressed by the cell, the greater the efflux potential of xenobiotics such as anticancer drugs. In addition to differences in protein expression, polymorphic variation of the Pgp genes may also dynamically affect intracellular and plasma drug concentration. Over 50 SNPs within the *ABCB1* gene have been identified, which may lead to variability in drug responses (Reed & Parissenti, 2011).

Pharmaceutically relevant examples of this include the variation in drug response to agents such as antiepileptic drugs, select cardiovascular agents, and so on. Interestingly, P-glycoprotein at the site of the gastrointestinal (GI) tract effluxes hydrophilic drugs out of the cell and inhibits drug absorption through the GI tract (Howe, 2009). As drugs passively diffuse through the GI tract, Pgp pumps move drugs from cytoplasmic areas to extracellular fluid. Some examples of substrates of P-glycoprotein include carvedilol, diltiazem, and digoxin (Howe, 2009). Several antiepileptic drugs such as phenytoin, carbamezapine, lamotrizine, phenobarbital, valproic acid, and gabapentin are substrates or inhibitors of Pgp, but there is considerable controversy in the literature regarding these. In the case of digoxin, Pgp affects the level of digoxin available for absorption and elimination (Howe, 2009). P-glycoprotein inhibitors include verapamil, quinidine, cyclosporine, and ketoconazole (Howe, 2009). If an inhibitor of P-glycoprotein is administered, then blood levels of substrates will rise, as seen if quinidine is administered with digoxin.

Drugs can be categorized as reversible or suicidal inhibitors or P-glycoproteins. For example, calcium channel blockers and high-dose steroids are considered as reversible inhibitors of both P-glycoproteins and CYP450. However, grapefruit and ritonavir are suicidal agents for both P-glycoprotein and CYP450, meaning the effect of grapefruit juice will be prolonged, perhaps up to 24 hours. See Figure 8-8.

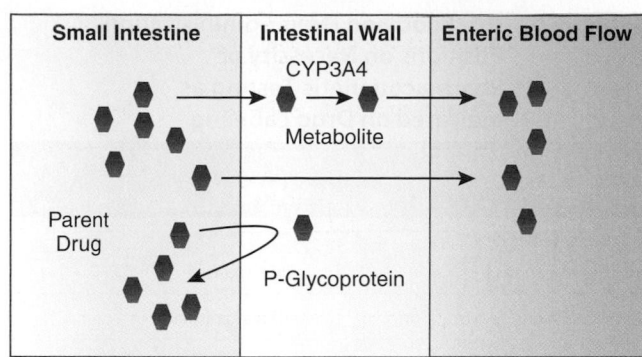

Figure 8–8. Drug–metabolism interactions.

CLINICAL IMPLICATIONS OF PHARMACOGENOMICS

Adverse Drug Reactions

One benefit of understanding pharmacogenomics is the possibility of a decrease in the number of ADRs. The CYPP450 enzymes in families 1 to 3 mediate 78% to 80% of all phase I–dependent metabolism of clinically used drugs (Spatzenegger & Jaeger, 1995). The polymorphic forms of CYPP450s are responsible for the development of idiosyncratic ADRs (Kalgutkar, Obach, & Maurer, 2007). According to Phillips and Van Bebber (2005), 56% of drugs cited in ADR studies are metabolized by polymorphic phase I enzymes, of which 86% are P450s.

Warfarin

In 2008, the package insert for warfarin was updated by the U.S. Food and Drug Administration to include application of pharmacogenomics to the dosing of warfarin. Previous work had identified variable metabolism by CYP2C9 as a major contributor to the variable response to the drug. In 2004, coding-region mutations in VCORC1, encoding a subunit of the vitamin K epoxide reductase complex (the pharmacological target for the drug), were found to cause a rare syndrome of warfarin resistance. Subsequently, the variants in VCORC1 have been found to account for a much greater fraction of variability in warfarin response (21%) than do variations in CYP2C9 (6%) (Gulseth et al, 2009). Although genetic testing prior to prescribing has not yet been required by the FDA, numerous warfarin dosing calculators exist on the Web where a clinician can insert clinical information about the patient, including genetic test results and indications, and a dosing regimen will be calculated or "individualized" for that patient (http://www.warfarindosing.com; http://www.globalrph .com/warfarin.htm).

Pharmacogenetic Testing Prior to Prescribing

The FDA now requires additional pharmacogenomic information on several drug package inserts (Table 8-6). Within the anticoagulant drug class, warfarin is a drug with

Table 8–6 U.S. Food and Drug Administration Positions on Necessity of Pharmacogenetic Testing as Indicated on Drug Labeling

Pharmacogenetic Biomarker	Drug
Test Required	
EGFR expression	Cetuximab
HER2/NEU overexpression	Trastuzumab
CCR-5-tropic HIV-1	Maraviroc
Presence of Philadelphia chromosome	Dasatinib
Test Recommended	
HLA-B*1502	Carbamazepine
HLA-B*5701	Abacavir
CYP2C9 variants	Warfarin
VKORC1 variants	Warfarin
Protein C deficiency	Warfarin
TPMT variants	Azathioprine, mercaptopurine, thioguanine
UGT1A1 variants	Irinotecan
G6PD deficiency	Rasburicase
Urea cycle disorders	Valproic acid
Information Only	
c-KIT expression	Imatinib
CYP2C19 variants	Voriconazole
CYP2C9 variants	Celecoxib
CYP2D6 variants	Atomoxetine, tamoxifen, fluoxetine
DPD deficiency	Capecitabine, fluorouracil
EGFR expression	Erlotinib
G6PD deficiency	Rasburicase, primaquine
NAT variants	Isoniazid, rifampin
Philadelphia chromosome	Busulfandeficiency
PML/RAR gene expression	Tretinoin

EGFR = epidermal growth factor receptor; HER2/NEU = v-erb-b2 erythroblastic leukemia viral oncogene homolog 2; CCR-5 = chemokine C-C motif receptor; HLA = human leukocyte antigen; CYP2C9 = cytochrome P-450 isoenzyme 2C9; VKORC1 = vitamin K epoxide reductase complex subunit 1; TPMT = thiopurine S-methyltransferase; UGT1A1 = uridine diphosphate-glucuronosyltransferase 1A1; c-KIT = v-kit Hardy-Zuckerman 4 feline sarcoma viral oncogene homolog; CYP2C19 = cytochrome P-450 2C19; CYP2D6 = cytochrome P-450 isoenzyme 2D6; DPD deficiency = dihydropyrimidine dehydrogenase; G6PD = glucose-6-phosphate dehydrogenase; NAT = N-acetyltransferase; PML/RAR = promyelocytic leukemia/retinoic acid receptor.cytochrome P-450 isoenzyme 2D6; DPD deficiency = dihydropyrimidine dehydrogenase; G6PD = glucose-6-phosphate dehydrogenase.
Source: Derived from U.S. Food and Drug Administration. (2010b). Table of valid genomic biomarkers in the context of approved drug labels. Retrieved from http://www.fda.gov/Drugs/ScienceResearch/ResearchAreas/Pharmacogenetics/ucm083378.htm

a narrow therapeutic index. In 2007, the FDA recommended an important label update suggesting genetic testing to prevent possibly fatal bleeding in patients with polymorphic variants of CYP2C9, the metabolizing enzyme, and VKORC1, the target enzyme of warfarin. Patients with CYP2C9 variations require more time to achieve the International Normalized Ratio, or INR, and are at an increased risk for bleeding (Sconce, 2005); they may also require lower doses of warfarin to achieve and maintain therapeutic INR (Limdi, 2007). Thus, if there are indications of inherited differences in these genes, the patient should be genotyped. However, monitoring INR is still as much of a requirement while dosing warfarin as before. While the FDA did not explicitly require genetic testing in patients prior to prescribing warfarin, the package labeling did show changes in dosage amounts. There is an FDA-approved genetic testing kit available, but others may also be used. Generally, cell samples are collected from the mouth or from blood. However, it should be emphasized that genetic testing is not the sole consideration, since patient-related factors such as age, sex, body weight, and some other parameters may need to be considered with the genetic results. A variety of online algorithms can aid physicians and hospital staff in making these dosage adjustments, as presented, for example, at www.warfarindosing.org.

The pharmacogenetic tests mentioned on drug labels can be classified as "test required," "test recommended," and "information only." Currently, four drugs are required to have pharmacogenetic testing performed before they are prescribed: cetuximab, trastuzumab, maraviroc, and dasatinib. Cetuximab treatment needs a confirmation of epidermal growth factor receptor (EGFR) expression. Trastuzumab therapy requires testing for HER2/NEU overexpression. Infection with CCR-5-tropic HIV-1 should be confirmed before initiation of therapy with maraviroc (an antiretroviral). Dasatinib is used for the treatment of patients with Philadelphia chromosome-positive acute lymphoblastic leukemia resistant to or intolerant of prior therapy (U.S. Food and Drug Administration, 2010b).

In December 2007, the FDA added a Black-Box Warning on the carbamazepine label, recommending testing for the HLA-B*1502 allele in patients with Asian ancestry before initiating carbamazepine therapy because these patients are at high risk of developing carbamazepine-induced Stevens–Johnson syndrome (SJS) or toxic epidermal necrolysis (TEN). Interestingly, although Asians or patients with Asian ancestry have been reported to have a strikingly high frequency (10 times higher than whites) of carbamazepine-induced SJS or TEN if they carry an HLA-B*1502 allele, other races carrying the allele do not seem to have the increased risk (U.S. Food and Drug Administration, 2007).

The anticancer agent irinotecan is a prodrug used for the treatment of colorectal cancer, small-cell lung cancer, and other solid tumors. The active metabolite of irinotecan is SN-38, a topoisomerase I inhibitor, and uridine diphosphate glucuronosyltransferase 1A1 (UGT1A1) plays a critical role in inactivating SN-38 (McLeod & Hoskins, 2007).

The low activity of the UGT1A1 enzyme may increase the risk for adverse events associated with irinotecan therapy (e.g., neutropenia) by increasing serum concentrations of the active metabolite. A polymorphism in the promoter region of the UGT1A1 gene determines patient exposure to SN-38 (McLeod & Hoskins, 2007). Patients homozygous for the polymorphism (UGT1A1*28) are at a 5-fold greater risk of irinotecan-related toxicity compared with patients with one or two normal alleles. Additionally, the FDA has approved a test for detection of the UGT1A1*28 genotype for irinotecan dosing. Additional genotype tests approved by the FDA and their implications are summarized in Table 8-7.

SUMMARY

We live in remarkable times, in which multiple therapeutic options are available for most common diseases. However, the selection of the optimal medication for an individual patient is still problematic. Practitioners still pick the "right" initial medication only half the time and ADRs are still unpredictable. In addition, the expense of new biological agents is such that even wealthy countries like the United States cannot afford to treat all patients.

The completion of the Human Genome Project has enabled the development of clinical tools for patient evaluation. Pharmacogenomics may allow identification of patients most likely to benefit from a given therapy and those patients for whom the cost and risk outweigh the benefits. Both the safety and efficacy of drug therapy may improve. In the future, genotyping may be used to personalize drug treatment for vast numbers of patients, decreasing the cost of drug treatment and increasing the efficacy of drugs and health in general.

Table 8–7 **FDA-Approved Diagnostic Test Commercially Available for Commonly Prescribed Pharmacologic Therapies**

Genetic Test	Drug	Benefit of Genetic Test
CYP2C9/ VCORC1	Warfarin	Reduce time to target INR; possibly decrease bleeding episodes
CYP2D6	Tamoxifen	Reduce therapeutic failure
	Codeine	Reduce GI toxicities/ improve pain control
	Oxycodone	Reduce GI toxicities/ improve pain control
	Tricyclic antidepressants	Reduce therapeutic failure
TMPT	Azathiaprine	Reduce myelosuppression
	6-mecappurine	Reduce myelosuppression
UGT1A1	Irinotecan	Reduce neutropenia

Source: Derived from McLeod, H. L., & Hoskins. J. M. (2007). Personalized drug therapy: The era of pharmacoeconomics. Retrieved from http://www .ipit.unc.edu/files/1233076125-one.pdf

REFERENCES

Arias, E. (2010). United States life tables, 2006. *National Vital Statistics Reports, 58*(21). Retrieved from http://www.cdc.gov/nchs/data/ nvsr/nvsr58/nvsr58_21.pdf

Belle, D. J., & Singh, H. (2008). Genetic factors in drug metabolism. *American Family Physician, 77*(11), 1553–1560.

Beutler, E. (1959). The hemolytic effect of primaquine and related compounds: A review. *Blood, 14*(2), 103–139.

Cha, P. C, Mushiroda, T., Takahashi, A., Kubo, M., Minami, S., Kamatani, N., et al. (2010). Genome-wide association study identifies genetic determinants of warfarin responsiveness for Japanese. *Human Molecular Genetics, 19*, 4735–4744.

Ellard, G. A. (1976). Variations between individuals and populations in the acetylation of isoniazid and its significance for the treatment of pulmonary tuberculosis. *Clinical Pharmacology and Therapeutics, 19*(5, Pt. 2), 610–625.

Evans, W. E., & Relling, M. V. (1999). Pharmacogenomics: Translating functional genomics into rational therapeutics. *Science, 286*, 487–491.

Finkelman, B. S., Gage, B. F., Johnson, J. A., et al. (2011). Genetic warfarin dosing: Tables versus algorithms. *Journal of the American College of Cardiology, 57*, 612–618.

Gulseth, M. P., Grice, G. R., & Dager, W. E. (2009). Pharmacogenomics of warfarin: Uncovering a piece of the warfarin mystery. *American Journal of Health Systems Pharmacists, 66*, 123–133.

Howe, L. A. (2009). Pharmacogenomics and management of cardiovascular disease. *The Nurse Practitioner, 34*(8), 28–35.

Kalgutkar, A. S., Obach, R. S., & Maurer, T. S. (2007). Mechanism-based inactivation of cytochrome P450 enzymes: Chemical mechanisms, structure-activity relationships and relationship to clinical drug-drug interactions and idiosyncratic adverse drugs reactions. *Current Drug Metabolism, 8*, 407–447.

Kolata G. In treatment of leukemia, glimpses of the future. *New York Times*. July 7, 2012.

Li, J., Zhang, L., Zhou, II., Stoneking, M., & Tang, K. (2011). Global patterns of genetic diversity and signals of natural selection for human ADME genes. *Human Molecular Genetics, 20*(3), 528–540.

McLeod, H. L., & Hoskins. J. M. (2007). Personalized drug therapy: The era of pharmacoeconomics. Retrieved from http://www.ipit.unc.edu/ files/1233076125-one.pdf

Meyer, U. A. (2004). Pharmacogenetics—five decades of therapeutic lessons from genetic diversity. *Nature Reviews, Genetics, 5*(9), 669–676.

Nebert, D. W., Zhang, G., & Vesell, E. S. (2008). From human genetics and genomics to pharmacogenetics and pharmacogenomics: Past lessons, future directions. *Drug Metabolism Reviews, 40*, 187–224.

Penny, M. A., & McHale, D. (2005). Pharmacogenomics and the drug discovery pipeline: When should it be implemented? *American Journal of Pharmacogenomics, 5*(1), 53–62. Review.

Peters, G. J., Smorenburg, C. H., & Van Groeningen, C. J. (2004). Prospective clinical trials using a pharmacogenetic/pharmacogenomic approach. *Journal of Chemotherapy, 16* (Suppl. 4), 2, 5–30.

Phillips, K. A., & Van Bebber, S. L. (2005). Measuring the value of pharmacogenomics. *Nature Reviews Drug Discovery, 4*(6), 500–509.

Phillips, K. A., Veenstra, D. L., Oren, E., Lee, J. K., & Sadee, W. (2001). Potential role of pharmacogenomics in reducing adverse drug reactions: A systematic review. *Journal of the American Medical Association, 286*(18), 2270–2279.

Rettie, A. E., Haining, R. L., Bajpai, M., & Levy, R. H. (1999). A common genetic basis for idiosyncratic toxicity of warfarin and phenytoin. *Epilepsy Research, 35*, 253.

Schroth, W., Goetz, M. P, Hamann, U., Fasching, P. A, Schmidt, M., Winter, S., et al. (2009). Association between *CYP2D6* polymorphisms and outcomes among women with early stage breast cancer treated with tamoxifen. *Journal of the American Medical Association, 302*, 1429–1436.

Schroth, W., Hamann, U., Fasching, P. A., Dauser, S., Winter, S., Eichelbaum, M., et al. (2010). *CYP2D6* polymorphisms as predictors of outcome in breast cancer patients treated with tamoxifen: Expanded polymorphism coverage improves risk stratification. *Clinical Cancer Research, 16*, 4468–4477.

Sistonen, J., Madadi, P., Ross, C. J., Yazdanpanah, M., Lee, J. W., Landsmeer, M. L., et al. (2012). Prediction of codeine toxicity in infants and their mothers using a novel combination of maternal genetic markers. *Clinical Pharmacology and Therapeutics, 91,* 692–699.

Spatzenegger, M., & Jaeger, W. (1995). Clinical importance of hepatic cytochrome P450 in drug metabolism. *Drug Metabolism Reviews, 27,* 397–417.

Suarez-Kurtz, G. (2005). Pharmacogenomics in admixed populations. *Trends in Pharmacology Science, 26*(4), 196–201.

Thompson, A. .M., Johnson, A., Quinlan, P., Hillman, G., Fontecha, M., Bray, S. E., et al. (2011). Comprehensive *CYP2D6* genotype and adherence affect outcome in breast cancer patients treated with tamoxifen monotherapy. *Breast Cancer Research and Treatment, 125,* 279–287.

U.S. Department of Health, Education, and Welfare. (1974). *Vital statistics of the United States, 1970* (Vol. 2, Sec. 5) (DHEW Publication No. HRA 74-1104). Retrieved from http://www.cdc.gov/nchs/data/lifetables/ life70.pdf

U.S. Food and Drug Administration. (2007). Information on carbamazepine (marketed as Carbatrol, Equetro, Tegretol and generics) with FDA alerts. Retrieved from http://www.fda.gov/Drugs/DrugSafety

U.S. Food and Drug Administration. (2009). Critical path initiative—warfarin dosing. Retrieved from http://www.fda.gov/ScienceResearch/Special-Topics/CriticalPathInitiative/FacesBehindCriticalPath/ ucm077473.htm

U.S. Food and Drug Administration. (2010a). E15 definitions for genomic biomarkers, pharmacogenomics, pharmacogenetics, genomic data and sample coding categories. Retrieved from http://www.fda.gov/Regulatory-Information/Guidances/ucm129286.htm

U.S. Food and Drug Administration. (2010b). Table of valid genomic biomarkers in the context of approved drug labels. Retrieved from www.fda.gov/Drugs/ScienceResearch/ResearchAreas/Pharmacogenetics/ucm083378.htm

Vermes, A., & Vermes, I. (2004). Genetic polymorphisms in cytochrome P450 enzymes. Effect on efficacy and tolerability of HMG0CoA Reductase inhibitors. *American Journal of Cardiovascular Drugs, 4*(4), 247–255.

Voora, D., & Ginsburg, G. S., (2012). Clinical applications of cardiovascular pharmacogenetics. *Journal of the American College of Cardiology, 60*(1), 9–20.

Walgren, R. A., Meucci, M. A., & McLeod, H. L. (2005). Pharmacogenomic discovery approaches: Will the real genes please stand up? *Journal of Clinical Oncology, 23*(29), 7342–7349.

Yamamoto, M., Subue, G., Mukoyama, M., Matsuoka, Y., & Mitsuma, T. (1999). Demonstration of slow acetylator genotype of *N*-acetyltransferase in isoniazid neuropathy using an archival hematoxylin and eosin section of a sural nerve biopsy specimen. *Journal of Neurological Sciences, 135*(1), 51–54.

Yip, V. L., & Pirmohamed, M. (2013). Expanding role of pharmacogenomics in the management of cardiovascular disorders. *American Journal of Cardiovascular Drugs, 13,* 151–162.

NUTRITION AND NUTRACEUTICALS

Teri Moser Woo

Eating is a part of daily life. The use of nutrition as therapy is beginning to take its rightful place in health promotion, disease prevention, and disease treatment because we now have significant knowledge about the importance of nutrition in these areas. We know that nutrition therapy can provide effective and efficient treatment when the medical condition affects nutritional needs or the diet affects the medical condition. When nutritional considerations are part of the plan of care, the health-care provider helps patients feel better; improves management of their health-care problems; and avoids complications that affect quality of life, productivity, and health-care costs. This chapter examines the role nutrition plays in pharmacotherapy, including the role of food intake on drug pharmacokinetics and the use of nutraceuticals (foods that claim to have a medicinal effect).

NUTRIENT–DRUG INTERACTIONS

Drugs do not create new bodily functions but rather interact with cellular function. Key to adequate cell function is the supply of needed nutrients. Because drugs are designed to improve altered cell function, it seems logical to conclude that nutritional factors can, in turn, affect pharmacological therapy. Clinically, health-care providers are concerned about the effect of drugs on the absorption, transport, metabolism, cellular uptake, and excretion of nutrients and the effect of nutrients on the pharmacokinetics of drugs. Additionally, some foods contain chemicals that may directly compete with medications; for example,

foods high in vitamin K compete with warfarin. Therefore, drug–nutrient interactions must be considered to utilize drugs effectively in the prevention and treatment of disease. Patient education must be provided about drug–food interactions, especially if there is a potential for adverse patient outcomes.

Influence of Diet on the Pharmacokinetics of Drugs

Drug Absorption

The most frequent type of drug–food interaction is the effect that food has on the gastrointestinal (GI) absorption of drugs. Drug absorption can be decreased, delayed, accelerated, or increased by food (Singh & Malhotra, 2004; Cvijic, Parojcic, & Langguth, 2014; Varum, Hatton, & Basit, 2013). Drug absorption takes place across the mucosa of the GI tract. The proximal part of the small intestine plays a significant role in drug and nutrient absorption, secondary to its large surface area. Drugs utilize the same transport mechanisms as nutrients: passive and facilitated diffusion, endocytosis, and active transport.

Several physiological factors affect drug absorption during the transport process: bioavailability—the percentage of drug available to produce a pharmacological effect—presystemic metabolism, gastric emptying time, concentration gradient, and absorptive surface area. Food in the GI tract at the time of drug administration affects absorption and bioavailability of the drug by changing the gastric emptying time through interaction within the GI lumen and by competitive inhibition.

The absorption of drugs can be increased or decreased, depending on the presence of food (Varum et al, 2013). Food decreases the amount of fluid in the GI tract, thus slowing down drug dissolution. Lack of food for an extended period—fasting for a day, for example—can decrease absorption secondary to vasoconstriction. Gastric emptying time also can influence drug absorption. However, the effect varies, depending on the type of drug preparation and the need for presystemic metabolism or dissolution. A drug that requires interaction in the stomach for disintegration and dissolution would have reduced absorption owing to the rapid gastric emptying time that might accompany a fasting state. Delayed gastric emptying that might occur with a meal high in fat would facilitate drug absorption because the drug is given more time for maximal disintegration and dissolution. Clearly, a change in gastric emptying can affect drug absorption, but the impact of the change is related to the dosage form and dissolution characteristics of the drug. A change in the drug form or time of administration can potentially affect bioavailability. Questioning the food intake of a patient who has had a change in the effectiveness of a pharmacological therapy can be an important part of the clinical decision-making process.

In addition, the effect of food on the pH of the stomach can change bioavailability. The degree of ionization that occurs when a drug is taken into the stomach is a function of GI pH. If a drug is a weak acid with best absorption in the nonprotonated (nonionized) state, then the low pH of the stomach is essential to drug absorption to allow the acid to remain nonionized and absorbable.

Chemical and physical changes in the drug can also occur as a result of interaction with food. These changes affect the absorption of the drug. Every nurse is aware of the need to advise patients to take tetracycline on an empty stomach or with foods that are not high in calcium, aluminum, iron, and magnesium because of decreased absorption, as the drug chelates with these minerals. The binding of phenytoin with enteral nutrition products that results in fluctuation of phenytoin levels has provided the impetus for the development of protocols that stop enteral nutrition before, during, and after delivery of this medication when the patient is tube fed. The bisphosphonate alendronate (Fosamax) demonstrates a 40% decrease in bioavailability when taken with food and a 60% decrease in bioavailability when administered with coffee or orange juice.

Additional physiological factors that may change a drug's absorption from the GI tract include food-induced changes in splanchnic blood flow, resulting in variation of drug absorption. As pointed out earlier, use of the same cellular transport proteins could result in competition for transport systems. Levodopa absorption is thought to be reduced with high-protein diets because of competition for the same transport system.

The potential for change in drug absorption by food or nutrients in the GI system is quite high. Drugs that have decreased absorption with food may need to be administered on an empty stomach, unless that is the desired effect, as when griseofulvin is given with a high-fat meal. When food

has no effect on drug bioavailability, then the drug may be administered without regard to food intake. Patient education regarding the coordination of medication administration and food intake should be integral to the prescribing process.

Drug Metabolism

The rate of drug metabolism in both the GI tract and the liver is affected by nutrient intake. A low-carbohydrate, high-protein diet may increase drug-metabolizing enzymes. Increasing intake of antioxidant cruciferous vegetables may increase the activity of these enzymes. Clinically, we see examples of the effect of foods on metabolism daily, as unexplained variability in drug response or therapeutic drug levels.

The cytochrome P450 (CYP450) system is the major enzyme group responsible for the metabolism of foreign chemicals that come into the body. Information is expanding about the clinically significant interactions between nutrients and drugs utilizing the CYP450 enzyme system. In addition, the CYP450 system has a significant amount of polymorphism associated with it; that is, there are between-individuals differences in the presence and/or function of a particular enzyme group. This difference reinforces the need to understand the nutrient effect on metabolizing enzymes. A more detailed discussion of the CYP450 system is provided in Chapter 8, including the genetic issues surrounding this system.

Grapefruit Juice and CYP3A4

Grapefruit juice influences the metabolism of many drugs because it contains components that inhibit CYP3A4, leading to alterations in the metabolism of drugs. Studies have determined that it is the furanocoumarins in the grapefruit juice that have been identified as CYP3A4 inhibitors, decreasing the first-pass metabolism of drugs (Gertz, Davis, Harrison, Houston, & Galetin, 2008; Mertens-Talcott, Zadezensky, De-Castro, Derendorf, & Butterweck, 2006; Paine et al, 2006). Ingestion of grapefruit juice leads to increased levels of calcium channel blockers, cyclosporine, tacrolimus, and the statins (Kuypers, 2009; Vaquero et al, 2010). The maximum inhibitory effect occurs if the grapefruit juice is ingested at the same time or within 4 hours of a drug (Gertz et al, 2008).

Foods and CYP1A2

Other foods or beverages that influence drug oxidation or conjugation reactions include indolic compounds in vegetables (cruciferous), methylxanthine-containing beverages (caffeine), and charcoal broiling. Cruciferous vegetables induce CYP1A2, an enzyme responsible for the metabolism of many drugs including theophylline. Patients who consume large amounts of cruciferous vegetables may have therapeutic failure if they are being treated with drugs that are metabolized by CYP1A2 (Peterson et al, 2009). Apiaceous vegetables (carrots, parsnips, celery or parsley family) inhibit CYP1A2 activity (Peterson, Lampe, Bammler, Gross-Steinmeyer, & Eaton, 2006). Tobacco smoking and charcoal-broiled meat induce CYP1A2 due to their high concentrations of olycyclic aromatic hydrocarbons (Larsen & Brosen, 2005). Patients will need to be educated regarding intake of foods that induce CYP1A2 if they are on a medication with a narrow therapeutic index, such as theophylline.

Drug Excretion

Certain foods can change urinary pH, which then increases or decreases the amount of the ionized form of a drug or metabolite. The half-life of some medications may be changed by altering urine pH (Ishmail, 2009). For example, gentamicin as a basic drug would be more likely to be reabsorbed in the renal tubule when there is an alkaline pH. Foods that alkalinize the urine include milk, vegetables, and citrus fruits. Foods that acidify the urine include meat, fish, cheese, and eggs (Ishmail, 2009).

Drug-Induced Nutrient Depletion

Another mechanism of interaction between drugs and nutrients is the effect drugs can have on nutrient absorption, synthesis, transport, storage, metabolism, and excretion. The side-effect profile of a drug taken over a period of time can be related to the effect of that drug on nutrient depletion. The number of potential drug-induced nutrient deficiencies is large and growing, and research in this area continues.

The mechanisms of action for drug-induced nutrient deficiencies are varied. As discussed previously, the GI changes due to dietary factors that affect drug absorption can also be induced by drugs and thus affect nutrient absorption. The alterations in gastric emptying time, changes in pH, mucosal irritation (enteropathy), and formation of complexes that can result from drug therapy often have an impact on nutrient absorption. For example, changes in the pH from antacid therapy or potassium therapy can reduce absorption of folic acid, iron, and vitamin B_{12}. Drugs can induce or inhibit metabolic processes and, as a result, affect nutrient metabolism and bioavailability. For example, phenytoin reduces the level of folic acid by inhibition of intestinal enzymes needed for folic acid absorption. Many metabolic pathways rely on specific nutrient availability; therefore, a deficiency results in cellular dysfunction. For example, the synthesis of vitamins, coagulation factors, and neurotransmitters can be affected by reduction in nutrient substrates.

Just as the nutrient can affect excretion of drugs, drugs can affect urinary secretion, reabsorption, and elimination of nutrients. For example, the commonly seen depletion of sodium, calcium, and potassium with loop diuretic use is the result of interference with renal reabsorption. Thus, drug-induced nutrient malabsorption, maldigestion, and vitamin antagonism are potential adverse reactions to commonly prescribed drugs.

Outcomes of Nutrient–Drug Interactions

The physiological and cellular basis for nutrient–drug interactions is strong. However, it is the outcome of the interaction that takes the spotlight. Does the interaction cause a change in the expected outcome of drug therapy or a nutrient deficiency that enhances the potential for adverse reactions or disease progression? Clinically, practitioners often overlook this area. If the expected outcome of drug therapy is not occurring or the adverse reaction profile is enhanced, the practitioner must know the key questions to ask to determine what is happening. It should be clear that a piece of the data needed is related to food and nutrient intake. Could the patient who became pregnant on the low-estrogen birth control pill have a reduction in drug bioavailability owing to food intake? Is the antidepressant not working secondary to high caffeine intake? Is the digoxin (Lanoxin) serum level low because of an aggressive bowel care program with high-fiber intake? And even more important, did the change in dietary fiber intake contribute to the digoxin toxicity the patient is experiencing?

An example of a food–drug interaction is one that occurs between warfarin and vitamin K–containing foods. Patients who are taking warfarin should not ingest foods high in vitamin K, as the combination may lead to therapeutic failure. Patients taking warfarin need to be educated regarding the vitamin K content of foods (Table 9-1). Warfarin and vitamin K interactions are further discussed in Chapter 18.

A high intake of food containing tyramine can result in enhanced norepinephrine synthesis—which can be problematic if the same patient is taking drugs that increase norepinephrine availability at the neurological synapse. For example, the adverse effect of acute hypertension associated with the use of monoamine oxidase inhibitors (MAOIs) is enhanced by intake of foods high in tyramine. The inhibition of aldehyde dehydrogenase by metronidazole results in a disulfiram-like reaction—flushing, headache, nausea, and abdominal or chest pain—when it is taken with alcohol or alcohol-containing products because of alteration in the alcohol metabolism.

Food contains many highly interactive ingredients that can have an impact on drug therapy. For example, the use of caffeine with known central nervous system (CNS) effects is problematic for patients utilizing psychotropic medications. The ability to manage the mental health problem becomes a challenge when high or variable levels of caffeine are consumed. Sorbitol, a common ingredient in sugar-free foods, has a significant effect on GI transit time and thus can influence the absorption of both drugs and nutrients.

Alcohol consumption is also associated with significant drug interaction problems. Alcohol can either induce or inhibit the CYP450 system enzymes, depending on the ingestion pattern. Chronic low levels cause enzymatic induction, whereas high binge intake or high chronic use, resulting in hepatic failure, inhibits the metabolizing enzymes. Therefore, the provider needs to know the patient's specific level of alcohol consumption to better understand the potential for interaction with drugs.

Clinical Decision Making

What can providers do to improve their skill in recognizing nutrient–drug interactions? The provider should consider the following:

1. Use up-to-date resources to evaluate the potential for drug–food interactions.

Table 9–1   Vitamin K Content in Common Foods

Food	Serving Size	Daily Value (%)
Foods High in Vitamin K (more than or equal to 200% DV)	**Eat No More Than 1 Serving per Day**	
Kale, fresh, boiled	1/2 cup	660
Spinach, fresh, boiled	1/2 cup	560
Turnip greens, frozen, boiled	1/2 cup	530
Collards, fresh, boiled	1/2 cup	520
Swiss chard, fresh, boiled	1/2 cup	360
Parsley, raw	1/2 cup	300
Mustard greens, fresh, boiled	1/2 cup	260
Foods Moderately High in Vitamin K (60% to 199% DV)	**Eat No More Than 2 Servings per Day**	
Brussels sprouts, frozen, boiled	1/2 cup	190
Spinach, raw	1 cup	180
Turnip greens, raw, chopped	1 cup	170
Green leaf lettuce, chopped	1 cup	125
Broccoli, raw, chopped	1 cup	110
Endive lettuce, raw	1 cup	70
Romaine lettuce, raw	1 cup	70

Source: Warren Grant Magnuson Clinical Center, National Institutes of Health Drug-Nutrient Interaction Task Force, 2003.

2. Seek out educational materials that can provide accurate and appropriate drug information to patients.
3. Consult with other practitioners, pharmacists, and registered dietitians to identify drug–nutrient interactions.
4. Get a complete patient profile in terms of drug, herb, and nutrient intake. Knowing all of the medications taken—prescribed, over-the-counter, herbal, vitamin, alcoholic, nutrient supplementation—is key to the identification of interaction potential.

The nurse practitioner must understand how the medication is taken in relation to food and fluids. How stable is food intake in terms of the substances known to affect drug absorption, such as fiber, protein, and fat? Clearly communicate to the patient the best routine for medication administration. The nurse practitioner needs to ensure that he or she and the patient read warning labels for instructions about mixing with food, using with nutritional supplements, and taking with fluid.

NUTRITIONAL MANAGEMENT

Consumers have shown increased interest and awareness of the importance of nutrition and nutrients in staying healthy. An outcome of this knowledge is increased use of nutrient supplementation. Nutritional supplementation is the use of vitamins, minerals, or other food factors to support health and prevent or treat disease. There are approximately 50 essential nutrients that must be acquired in the diet to maximize health. Although all nutritionists will explain that the interplay of these nutrients is significant to their role in the body, many still will recommend supplementation of specific nutrients or combinations of nutrients for individuals at risk. It is vital that providers include recommendations about how to utilize diet as part of the plan of care, but it is not uncommon that the ability to accomplish the recommendation by diet alone is difficult for given individuals. In addition, recommended diet alterations might not be best when considering other health problems. Therefore, the provider must become skilled in accurately advising patients about the benefits of nutraceuticals in maintaining health, preventing disease, and treating disease. Those individuals who might be on drug therapy that can induce nutrient deficiencies need specific recommendations about diet and nutrient supplementation to avoid additional drug adverse reactions.

A complete or focused nutritional assessment should be part of the information gathered during the patient interaction. Data from the diet history, anthropometric measurement, physical examination, and laboratory findings are useful for pharmacological decision making. Such team members as a clinical pharmacist and a registered dietitian are especially important in the care of patients with complex medical problems or pharmacological treatment plans. Disease-specific nutritional therapy is beyond the scope of this chapter; the American Dietetic Association (ADA) has developed medical nutrition therapy protocols for a variety of diagnoses (http://www.eatright.org) and the American Society of Parenteral and Enteral Nutrition (ASPEN) has developed clinical guidelines to reflect current, evidence-based approaches to the practice of nutrition support (http://www.nutritioncare.org).

Although much of the research surrounding use of supplements is not conclusive in terms of randomized clinical trials and is even sometimes contradictory, patients' use of nutritional supplementation is not waiting for conclusive outcomes. To partner with the patient who is interested in nutritional supplementation, nurse practitioners must have a clear understanding of the patient's philosophy surrounding nutritional supplementation and the recommendations of experts in the area. The ADA has developed a position statement about vitamin and mineral supplementation that provides a solid foundation for assisting patients with their nutrient supplementation decisions. The ADA supports obtaining nutrients through a wide variety of foods as the best way to promote health and reduce risk of disease (ADA, 2009).

However, the ADA also defines clearly in their position statement the circumstances in which supplementation is indicated. The following are populations that may warrant supplementation (ADA, 2009):

- Infants and children, including adolescents, need supplementation with 400 IU of vitamin D daily.
- Women of childbearing age who may become pregnant need 400 mcg/day of folic acid.
- Pregnant women need 600 mcg/day of folic acid, a multivitamin/mineral supplement, 27 mg/day of iron (60 mg/d if patient is anemic), and vitamin B_{12} if the patient is vegan or lacto-ovo-vegetarian.
- Older adults over age 50 need vitamin B_{12} 2.4 mcg/day and need to ensure adequate intake of vitamin D and calcium.
- Patients at risk for suboptimal vitamin D levels (older patients, patients with dark skin, patients who are not exposed to sufficient sunlight) should consume vitamin D–fortified foods and/or supplements.

The need to utilize nutritional supplementation is individualized and the nurse practitioner must guide patients to understand their need. Most important in this interaction between patient and practitioner is an open, honest discussion of the nutritional supplementation decision. Although vitamin supplementation is often inexpensive and unlikely to cause harm, the same cannot be said for many other nutrients for which there is no recommended daily allowance (RDA) and no established standard for supplementation. If you do recommend or prescribe a multiple vitamin and mineral supplement for an at-risk individual, it is important to frame the dosage needed around the RDA and recommended vitamin and mineral intake ranges.

NUTRACEUTICALS

As noted previously, nutraceuticals are foods that claim to have a medicinal effect on health. Nutraceuticals may also be referred to as functional foods, but the terms are not interchangeable; functional foods are foods that have health benefits, whereas neutraceuticals include dietary supplements (Crowe & Francis, 2013). There are five major categories of nutraceuticals used routinely in primary care: dietary fiber; vitamins and minerals; bioactive substances; fatty acids; and pre-, pro-, and symbiotics.

The list of nutraceuticals reviewed here is not exhaustive and is limited to those for which there are adequate safety and efficacy data to recommend their use. For a more expansive list of nutraceuticals with the current evidence, the reader is referred to the National Institutes of Health Office of Dietary Supplements (ODS) (http://ods.od.nih.gov). The ODS Web site contains extensive information for both providers and patients regarding nutraceuticals, including nutrient recommendations, a clinical trials database, and consumer safety information.

Fiber

Fiber is the term used to describe the substances in plants that the body cannot digest. According to the Institute of Medicine (2002), there are two types of fiber: dietary fiber and functional fiber. Dietary fiber is the nondigestible carbohydrates and lignin parts of the plant that are intrinsic and intact, whereas functional fiber is the nondigestible carbohydrates that have beneficial effects in human beings. Total fiber is the sum of the two types. The adequate intake for fiber recommendation is based on the fiber intake needed to decrease risk of coronary heart disease (ADA, 2008).

There are over 7.95 million visits per year to providers for constipation (Shah, Chitkara, Locke, Meek, & Talley, 2008). There have been controlled trials in chronically ill children (Daly, Johnson, & MacDonald, 2004), pregnant women (Jewell & Young, 2001), and women in the Nurses' Health Study (Dukas, Willett, & Giovanucci, 2003) that demonstrate a decrease in constipation with an increase in fiber in the diet. The American College of Gastroenterology recommends increased fiber intake to prevent constipation (Ward, 2010).

Dietary fiber intake may also lower cholesterol, improve cardiovascular health, and provide a feeling of fullness that may aid in weight loss. The National Health and Nutrition Examination Survey (NHANES) demonstrated a reduced lifetime risk of coronary heart disease and lower C-reactive protein level with increased fiber intake (Ning, Van Horn, Shay, & Lloyd-Jones, 2014). The American Heart Association (AHA) and the ADA both recommend increased fiber intake (at least 25 g/d) for cardiovascular health (ADA, 2008; AHA, 2014a).

Increased soluble fiber intake has been associated with a number of additional benefits, including better glucose control in diabetics and improved blood lipid levels (Aleixandre & Miguel, 2008; Vuksan, Rogovik, Jovanovski, & Jenkins, 2009), decreased risk of kidney stones in postmenopausal women (Sorensen et al, 2014), and improved bowel function and health-related quality of life in patients with Crohn's disease (Brotherton, Taylor, Bourguignon, & Anderson, 2014). Higher dietary fiber intake is associated with less periodontal disease and tooth loss in older male veterans (Schwartz, Kaye, Nunn, Spiro, & Garcia, 2012). Evidence that dietary fiber decreases cancer risk is inconsistent. Recommended fiber intake is found in Table 9-2.

Table 9–2 Recommended Fiber Intake

Gender/Age	Fiber (g/d)
1–3 yr	19
4–8 yr	25
Female 9–13 yr	26
Male 9–13 yr	31
Female 14–18 yr	29
Male 14–18 yr	38
Female 19–50 yr	25
Male 19–50 yr	38
Female 51 yr or older	21
Male 51 yr or older	30

Vitamins and Minerals

Vitamins and minerals are the most widely used supplements. When ingested as part of food sources, vitamins may be considered nutraceuticals. Evidence regarding recommended dosages and the preventive health properties of vitamins and minerals is constantly evolving. The most commonly recommended vitamins are discussed here and listed in Table 9-3. Iron is discussed in Chapters 18 and 27. More extensive information on vitamins and minerals may be found at the ODS Web site (http://ods .od.nih.gov).

Vitamin A

Vitamin A plays a critical role in vision, bone growth, reproduction, immune function, cell division and differentiation (ODS, 2013a). There are two types of vitamin A: preformed vitamin A, which is derived from animal sources, and provitamin A carotenoid, which is derived from plant sources. A

Table 9–3 Recommended Reference Intakes of Vitamins and Minerals

Nutrient	Age	RDA	Food Sources
Folate	Children: 1–3 yr 4–8 yr Adolescents aged 9–13 yr Adults Pregnancy	150 mcg/d 200 mcg/d 300 mcg/d 400 mcg/d 600 mcg/d	Enriched cereal grains, dark leafy vegetables, enriched and whole-grain breads and bread products, fortified ready-to-eat cereals
Riboflavin (Vitamin B$_{12}$)	Children: 1–3 yr 4–8 yr Adolescents aged 9–13 yr Adults Pregnancy	0.5 mg/d 0.6 mg/d 0.9 mg/d 1.3 mg/d 1.4 mg/d	Organ meats, milk, bread products, and fortified cereals
Thiamin (Vitamin B$_1$)	Children: 1–3 yr 4–8 yr Adolescents aged 9–13 yr Adult males Adult females Pregnancy	0.5 mg/d 0.6 mg/d 0.9 mg/d 1.2 mg/d 1.1 mg/d 1.4 mg/d	Enriched, fortified, or whole-grain products; bread and bread products, mixed foods whose main ingredient is grain, and ready-to-eat cereals
Vitamin A	Children: 1–3 yr 4–8 yr Adolescents aged 9–13 yr Adult males Adult females Pregnancy	300 mcg/d 400 mcg/d 600 mcg/d 900 mcg/d 700 mcg/d 770 mg/d	Liver, dairy products, fish, darkly colored fruits and leafy vegetables
Vitamin B$_6$	Children: 1–3 yr 4–8 yr Adolescents aged 9–13 yr 14–18 yr male 14–18 yr female Adult males 19–50 yr Adult males >50 yr Adult females 19–50 yr Adult females >50 yr Pregnancy	0.5 mg/d 0.6 mg/d 1.0 mg/d 1.3 mg/d 1.2 mg/d 1.3 mg/d 1.7 mg/d 1.3 mg/d 1.9 mg/d	Fortified cereals, beans, meat, poultry, fish, and some fruits and vegetables (bananas, spinach, avocados)

Table 9–3 Recommended Reference Intakes of Vitamins and Minerals—cont'd

Nutrient	Age	RDA	Food Sources
Vitamin C	Children:		Citrus fruits, tomatoes, tomato juice, potatoes, Brussels sprouts, cauliflower, broccoli, strawberries, cabbage, and spinach
	1–3 yr	15 mg/d	
	4–8 yr	25 mg/d	
	Adolescents aged 9–13 yr	45 mg/d	
	14–18 yr male	75 mg/d	
	14–18 yr female	65 mg/d	
	Adult males	90 mg/d	
	Adult females	75 mg/d	
	Pregnancy	85 mg/d	
Vitamin D	Children:		Fish liver oils, flesh of fatty fish, liver and fat from seals and polar bears, eggs from hens that have been fed vitamin D, fortified milk products, and fortified cereals
	< 1 yr	400 IU/d	
	1–3 yr	600 IU/d	
	4–8 yr	600 IU/d	
	Adolescents aged 9–18 yr	600 IU/d	
	Adults to age 70	600 IU/d	
	Adults > 70 years	800 IU/d	
	Pregnancy	600 IU/day	
Calcium	0–6 mo	210 mg	Milk, yogurt, cheese and other dairy products. Nondairy sources: Chinese cabbage, kale, broccoli, sardines
	7–12 m	270 mg	
	1–3 yr	500 mg	
	4–8 yr	800 mg	
	9–13 yr	1,300 mg	
	14–18 yr	1,300 mg	
	19–50 yr	1,000 mg	
	50+ yr	1,200 mg	
Iron	0–6 mo	0.27 mg/d	Chicken liver, oysters, beef, clams, turkey dark meat. Legumes, dark green vegetables. Fortified breads and cereals. Iron-fortified infant formula.
	7–12 mo	11 mg/d	
	1–3 yr	7 mg/d	
	4–8 yr	10 mg/d	
	9–13 yr	8 mg/d	
	14–18 yr male	11 mg/d	
	14–18 yr female	15 mg/d	
	19–50 yr male	8 mg/d	
	19–50 yr female	18 mg/d	
	19 to 50 yr pregnant	27 mg/d	
	50+ yr	8 mg/d	

healthy diet should contain a variety of carotenoid-rich fruits and vegetables.

Vitamin A deficiency is rare in the United States, but deficiencies may be found in developing countries. Vitamin A deficiency can lead to night blindness and decreased immune function. Vitamin A may reduce the severity and duration of diarrheal episodes in malnourished children in developing countries but not in well-nourished children (Imdad et al, 2011; ODS, 2013a). Vitamin A supplementation has also been found to decrease bronchopulmonary dysplasia in extremely low-birth-weight infants with no increase in mortality or neurodevelopmental disorder (Ambalavanan et al, 2005; Gadhia, Cutter, Abman, & Kinsella, 2014). Chronic alcoholism may lower vitamin A levels, and patients with chronic alcoholism may require supplementation. Patients with cystic fibrosis (CF) are predisposed to malabsorption and fat-soluble vitamin deficiency, with 10% to 40% of CF patients being vitamin deficient and requiring supplementation (Brei, Simon, Krawinkel, & Naehrlich, 2013).

Caution should be used to avoid excessive vitamin A supplementation, as toxicity may occur. Levels above recommended amounts may be teratogenic in pregnant women; vitamin A is labeled Pregnancy Category X if intake is greater than recommended amounts.

Vitamin B$_1$

Vitamin B$_1$ (thiamine) is a water-soluble vitamin critical for many body functions and is widely available in fortified breads and cereals. Deficiency of thiamine can lead to beriberi or Wernicke's encephalopathy. Alcoholic patients develop thiamine deficiency at 8 to 10 times the rate of the nonalcoholic population (Agabio, 2005). Wernicke's encephalopathy is a serious neurological illness in alcoholic patients and requires immediate high-dose levels of thiamine (500 mg IV TID for 2 days, then 500 mg/d IV or IM for 5 days). Patients should be given a daily 100 mg dose of oral thiamine until no longer considered at risk (Charness & So, 2009). Treatment for beriberi in children is IV thiamine 10 to 25 mg or 10 to 50 mg daily for 2 weeks, and in adults 50 mg IM/IV for several days or 5 to 30 mg/day for a month.

Vitamin B$_2$

Vitamin B$_2$, also known as riboflavin, is a water-soluble vitamin. Riboflavin deficiency is rare but may be seen in alcoholics, anorexic patients, and those with lactose intolerance who cannot drink milk or consume other dairy products. Riboflavin has been found to decrease headaches and migraines in some patients (Taylor, 2009). MigreLief, an over-the-counter product that contains feverfew, riboflavin, magnesium, and other vitamins, is a commonly used preventive headache medication. Doses of 25 to 400 mg of riboflavin daily are used for migraine prevention.

Vitamin B$_3$

Vitamin B$_3$, or niacin, is a water-soluble vitamin and antilipidemic. Niacin deficiency or pellagra results from inadequate intake. Pellagra is treated with 50 to 100 mg niacin three times daily. Use of niacin in the treatment of hyperlipidemia is discussed in Chapter 39.

Vitamin B$_6$

Vitamin B$_6$, also known as pyridoxine, is a water-soluble vitamin needed for protein and red blood cell metabolism, as well as glucose regulation. Vitamin B deficiency may lead to microcytic anemia, dermatitis with mouth sores and cracked lips, and glossitis (ODS, 2011a). Vitamin B$_6$ deficiency may be drug-induced by use of isoniazid (INH), cycloserine, or hydrazine, or caused by a diet that is deficient in vitamin B$_6$–containing foods (fortified cereals, potatoes, bananas, meat). Pyridoxine (vitamin B$_6$) 25 mg/day should be added to the regimen for pregnant patients to decrease the incidence of peripheral neuropathy associated with INH (American Thoracic Society, 2003). Pyridoxine (adults 100 to 200 mg/d in divided doses) may also be given prophylactically to patients on isoniazid, cycloserine, or hydrazine to prevent drug-induced neuritis. Vitamin B$_6$ supplements may reduce the symptoms of premenstrual syndrome, and nausea and vomiting associated with pregnancy (10 to 25 mg TID) (ODS, 2011a).

Vitamin B$_{12}$

Vitamin B$_{12}$ is a water-soluble vitamin that is essential for red blood cell formation and neurological function. Older adults and patients with reduced stomach acid levels, gastric bypass surgery, or intestinal disorders (celiac disease or Crohn's disease) may not absorb vitamin B$_{12}$ well and are at risk for deficiency (ODS, 2011b). Also, women who follow strict vegetarian diets without supplementation place their breastfed infant at risk for vitamin B$_{12}$ deficiency. Acid suppression medications (proton pump inhibitors or H2 receptor antagonists) and metformin reduce the absorption of vitamin B$_{12}$. vitamin B$_{12}$ deficiency will lead to megaloblastic anemia, fatigue, loss of appetite, and neurological changes (numbness and tingling in hands and feet). A complete discussion of vitamin B$_{12}$ replacement is found in Chapter 27 under the discussion of anemia.

Vitamin C

Vitamin C, also known as ascorbic acid, is a water-soluble vitamin that humans do not have the ability to synthesize so they must get adequate amounts of it in their diet. Patients with inadequate vitamin C intake may develop scurvy, with symptoms of fatigue, malaise, and gum inflammation or bleeding. Scurvy is rare in developed countries but may occur in cases of limited intake or limited food variety. Smokers and persons who are heavily exposed to secondary smoke have decreased vitamin C levels; therefore, it is recommended they take 35 mg more vitamin C per day than nonsmokers (ODS, 2013b). Other groups at risk of vitamin C deficiency are infants fed evaporated milk or boiled milk without additional supplementation of vitamin C, patients with malabsorption disorders, and patients with end-stage renal disease who are on hemodialysis (ODS, 2013b).

Vitamin C therapy has been studied for its effects on health because of its antioxidant and immune function action. It has been touted as prevention or treatment of the common cold since the 1970s, when Linus Pauling published his landmark study. A *Cochrane Review* in 2007 of 30 trials did not find that vitamin C decreases the incidence of colds in the general population (Douglas, Hemilä, Chalker, & Treacy, 2007).

The role of antioxidants in reducing the risk of cardiovascular disease has been studied extensively with mixed results. The Nurses' Health Study found an inverse relationship between coronary heart disease and vitamin C intake (Osganian et al, 2003). In the Physicians' Health Study, vitamin C supplementation for a 5.5-year period did not decrease the risk for cardiovascular disease mortality (Muntwyler, Heenekens, Manson, Buring, & Gaziano, 2002). However, a large ($N = 20,649$ men and women) study in Great Britain found those who had the highest vitamin C concentrations at baseline had a 42% lower risk of stroke, when controlling for age, sex, lifestyle, and other risk factors (Myint et al, 2008). A meta-analysis of 16 studies examining vitamin C intake, circulating vitamin C levels, and risk of stroke suggests lower stroke risk with higher vitamin C intake and levels (Chen, Lu, Pang, & Liu, 2013).

Studies of vitamin C as an antioxidant to prevent cancers show mixed results. In a long-term (10-year), large ($N = 77,721$) study of the effect of vitamin C supplementation on the development of lung cancer, there was no decreased risk of cancer in the group taking vitamin C (Slatore, Littman, Au, Satia, & White, 2007). A large, multiethnic study of Hispanic and non-Hispanic white women did not find any protective effects against breast cancer in women who took dietary antioxidants including vitamin C (Wang et al, 2009). Decreased cervical cancer was found in a smaller study ($N = 144$) of women who had higher intakes of the antioxidant vitamins A, C, and E; the isolated effects of vitamin C are not known (Kim et al, 2010). Because of the mixed results, there is no strong recommendation for vitamin C supplementation, beyond the recommended daily amounts, as prevention for cancer. Table 9-3 lists the recommended vitamin C intake levels for all ages.

Vitamin D

Vitamin D is a fat-soluble vitamin that is available in some foods, such as egg yolks and fatty fish (salmon and mackerel). The body synthesizes vitamin D when sunlight strikes the skin and triggers vitamin D synthesis. Vitamin D supplements, food sources, and the vitamin D synthesized from sunlight must be converted to an active form of drug in the liver and kidneys. The liver converts vitamin D into 25-hydroxyvitamin D, or calcidiol. The kidneys convert vitamin D into 1.25-dihydroxyvitamin D, or calcitriol. Vitamin D is critical to bone health as it is required for absorption of calcium from the intestinal tract and, when converted to calcitriol, regulates serum calcium and phosphate levels. It is a critical component in bone growth and remodeling. Vitamin D deficiency will lead to brittle bones that may become misshapen, a condition known as rickets in children and as osteomalacia in adults (ODS, 2011c).

Multiple studies link low vitamin D levels to increased asthma in adults and children. The use of oral corticosteroids places the patient at 20% to 40% higher risk of vitamin D deficiency (Korn et al., 2013). Vitamin D is an immunomodulator, which alters the development of immune cells, reduces airway remodeling and the inflammatory response, improves eosinophil function, and inhibits fibrotic mediators (Poon et al, 2013; Rance, 2013). Vitamin D supplementation may also improve asthma symptoms, particularly if the patient is deficient.

Serum levels of 25(OH)D can be drawn to determine whether the patient is vitamin D deficient. Table 9-4 lists ranges of 25(OH)D associated with deficiency and toxicity. Vitamin D is added to milk, most milk substitutes, infant formula, and dry cereal and is available in supplements as either vitamin D_2 or D_3. The use of vitamin D in the prevention and treatment of rickets, osteomalacia, and osteoporosis is discussed in depth in Chapter 38.

Vitamin K

Vitamin K, a critical component of blood clotting, is found in many foods and is synthesized by intestinal bacteria. Vitamin K deficiency is rare beyond the newborn period. Newborns are at risk for early vitamin K–deficiency bleeding, and the American Academy of Pediatrics recommends that all newborns receive vitamin K within the first 2 weeks of life (American Academy of Pediatrics [AAP] Committee on Fetus and Newborn, 2003), a recommendation it reaffirmed in 2009. The dose of vitamin K (phytonadione) recommended by the AAP is 0.5 mg to 1.0 mg IM, ideally given within the first hour of life (AAP Committee on Fetus and Newborn, 2003). Oral vitamin K is used by some countries and by some providers in the United States. The AAP notes that several countries have reported an increase in late-onset, vitamin K–deficiency bleeding in newborns who received oral vitamin K. The AAP recommends IM administration until further study of oral administration is conducted.

Warfarin interferes with the vitamin K–dependent clotting factors (II, VII, IX, and X), leading to decreased formation of clots. Vitamin K (phytonadione) is prescribed for patients who develop critically high INRs while on warfarin. Patients with an INR greater than 10 with no evidence of bleeding can be administered oral vitamin K (5–10 mg): if high INR with bleeding occurs, vitamin K (5–10 mg IV) is administered along with prothrombin complex (Guyatt et al, 2012).

Folate

Folate is a water-soluble vitamin that is critical to the production and maintenance of new cells. Folate is found in foods such as green leafy vegetables, citrus fruits, and dried legumes. Folic acid, the synthetic form of folate, is added to breads, flours, pastas, rice, and other grain products (ODS, 2012a). Folate deficiency occurs in times of increased demand, such as occurs in pregnancy and lactation, or when loss increases (malabsorption, alcohol abuse, dialysis, liver disease). Medications may interfere with folate utilization, leading to deficit (Box 9-1). Folic acid supplementation is recommended for all women of childbearing age (400 mcg/d),

Table 9–4   Serum 25-Hydroxyvitamin D [25(OH)D] Concentrations and Health*

ng/mL**	nmol/L**	Health Status
<10–11	<25–37.5	Associated with vitamin D deficiency, leading to rickets in infants and children and osteomalacia in adults
<10–15	<25–37.5	Generally considered inadequate for bone and overall health in healthy individuals
≥15	≥37.5	Generally considered adequate for bone and overall health in healthy individuals
Consistently >200	Consistently >500	Considered potentially toxic, leading to hypercalcemia and hyperphosphatemia, although human data are limited. In an animal model, concentrations ≤400 ng/mL (≤1,000 nmol/L) demonstrated no toxicity

* Serum concentrations of 25(OH)D are reported in both nanograms per milliliter (ng/mL) and nanomoles per liter (nmol/L).
** 1 ng/mL = 2.5 nmol/L
Source: Office of Dietary Supplements, 2010.

with extra given when a woman is pregnant (600 mcg/d) to prevent neural tube defects in the fetus (ODS, 2012a). Lactating women should take 500 mcg/day.

Folate is necessary for the normal maturation and functioning of red blood cells. Folate deficiency produces a macrocytic-normochromic anemia. Patients with folic acid–deficiency anemia commonly complain of glossitis, stomatitis, nausea and anorexia, and diarrhea, and a systolic ejection murmur may be heard. Oral folic acid is well absorbed, and doses of 1 to 2 mg/day result in correction of the deficiency in 4 to 5 weeks. Hemoglobin (Hgb) levels begin to rise within the first week, and anemia is completely corrected in 1 to 2 months.

Calcium

Calcium is a critical mineral in the function of the body, required for muscle contraction, blood vessel health, bone health, and normal nerve conduction. Maintaining calcium balance involves a complex relationship between adequate intake of calcium and vitamin D and endocrine system function. Populations at risk for calcium deficiency include postmenopausal women, amenorrheic women, women with female athlete triad, patients with lactose intolerance who cannot tolerate dairy products, and vegans. In the 2003–2006 NHANES study, the population groups with inadequate dietary calcium intake were females aged 9 to 13 years, 14 to 18 years, 51 to 70 years, and those over age 70 (Bailey et al, 2010). Calcium supplements were used by 43% of the NHANES 2003–2006 study population, leading to an adequate total calcium intake for all groups except for females in the 9- to 13-year-old and 14- to 18-year-old groups (Bailey et al, 2010). Recommended daily amounts of calcium are found in Table 9-3. The use of calcium for osteoporosis prevention is discussed in Chapter 38.

Iron

Iron is an essential mineral required for the regulation of cell growth and differentiation, as well as a component of oxygen transport. Patients with iron deficiency will develop microcytic-hypochromic anemia and have red blood cells that are small in size, pale, and low in hemoglobin. Iron-deficiency anemia (IDA) reduces the oxygen-carrying capacity of the blood, leading to fatigue and decreased immunity. Too much

iron can lead to iron toxicity; therefore, patients should be advised to take only the recommended amount for their age and condition (Table 9-3). The use of iron for the treatment of IDA is discussed in depth in Chapter 27.

Fatty Acids

The fatty acids are also called *essential* fatty acids. Fatty acids need to be consumed in food or via supplements, as the body cannot make them. The polyunsaturated fatty acid alpha-linolenic acid (ALA) is ingested in the diet and is an omega-3 fatty acid; linoleic acid (LA), also ingested from the diet, is an omega-6 fatty acid. Omega-3 is converted to the fatty acids eicosapentaenoic acid (EPA) and docosahexaenoic acid (DHA) in the body. Most Americans consume more omega-6 than omega-3 fatty acids, although it is recommended that more omega-3 than omega-6 should be consumed. Dietary sources of ALA are nuts, vegetable oils, and leafy green vegetables, whereas LA is found in vegetable oils and meat. Dietary sources of EPA and DHA are fish and organ meats (Vannice & Rasmussen, 2014).

The ODS conducted extensive evidence-based reviews to determine the best science regarding fatty acid supplementation. There is extensive evidence for the use of omega-3 fatty acids, either via the diet or supplementation, for its cardiovascular effects (Vannice & Rasmussen, 2014). Omega-3 fatty acid and its derivatives DHA and EPA have well-documented vascular protective effects, as well as anti-inflammatory effects.

Fish oil might have antiarrhythmic effects (ODS, 2004a) and consumption of omega-3 fatty acids, whether from fish or from supplements, reduces mortality and improves outcomes in patients with cardiovascular disease (Lee, O'Keefe, Lavie, Marchioli, & Harris, 2008; ODS, 2004b). In patients with diabetes, omega-3 fatty acids reduced triglyceride levels but have no significant effect on total cholesterol, high-density lipoprotein (HDL) cholesterol, low-density lipoprotein (LDL) cholesterol, fasting blood sugar, or glycosylated hemoglobin (ODS, 2004d).

Omega-3 fatty acids have received attention as a possible treatment for autism and attention deficit-hyperactivity disorder (ADHD). The theory is that either deficiency in omega-3 or an imbalance in the omega-3 to omega-6 fatty acid ratio is affecting neurocognitive development in children. It is clear that sufficient amounts of the essential fatty acids are crucial in central nervous development, with deficiency or imbalance found in multiple observational studies of children with neurocognitive issues (Schuchardt, Huss, Stauss-Grabo, & Hahn, 2009). This has led to the addition of DHA and ARA to commercial infant formulas (Enfamil LIPIL) to meet the need in the key developmental period of infancy.

In an extensive review of new and novel treatments for autism spectrum disorder, Rossignol (2009) rates omega-3 fatty acids with a C for supportive evidence (A to D scale; C indicates either one low-quality, randomized controlled trial or two case series reports). In another study by Meiri, Buchovsky, and Belmaker (2009), autistic children administered 1 g of omega-3 fatty acids daily demonstrated a 33% improvement on the Autism Treatment Evaluation Checklist.

Numerous studies of the use of omega-3 fatty acids in children with ADHD demonstrate improvement in ADHD scores (Schuchardt et al, 2009; Bloch & Qawasmi, 2011; Gillies, Sinn, Leach, & Ross, 2012). With these findings and the understanding of the need for essential fatty acids in neurological development, ensuring a diet that is rich in essential fatty acids throughout infancy and childhood is critical, with the trial of supplemental omega-3 fatty acids in children with autism or ADHD warranted.

Not all health claims for essential fatty acids are supported by evidence. For example, there is no supportive evidence for the use of omega-3 fatty acids in the care of asthma (ODS, 2004b), prevention of cancer or treatment after tumor removal (ODS, 2005a), or mental health disorders (including schizophrenia) (ODS, 2005b). Inconsistent findings in organ transplant patients warrant further study of omega-3 fatty acids in this population (ODS, 2005c). There was no reported improvement from the effects of omega-3 fatty acids in patients with rheumatoid arthritis in terms of patient report of pain, swollen joint count, erythrocyte sedimentation rate (ESR), and patient global assessment (ODS, 2004d). Research regarding the use of omega-3s in adult patients with cognitive decline is inconclusive (ODS, 2010e).

Recommended amounts of omega-3 fatty acids can be ingested in the diet by eating fatty fish or by taking fish oil capsules. The American Heart Association (2014b) recommends two servings a week of fatty fish such as salmon, mackerel, herring, lake trout, sardines, and albacore tuna for heart health. The recommended amount of omega-3 fatty acid from fish per day is 500 mg/day if there is no history of coronary heart disease (CHD), 1 g per day if there is a documented history of CHD, and 2 to 4 g/day to lower triglycerides (American Heart Association, 2014; Covington, 2004; Lee, O'Keefe, Lavie, Marchioli, & Harris, 2008). It may take 2 to 3 weeks for the effects of omega-3 to be seen. The National Heart Lung and Blood Institute (NHLBI) guidelines for reducing cardiovascular risk in children and adolescents recommend increasing dietary fish intake to increase omega-3 fatty acid intake (NHLBI, 2012). The studies of omega-3 for the treatment of ADHD and autism used 500 mg to 1 g/day.

Plant Sterols

Plant sterols are found in all plant-based foods as part of the structural components of the cell membrane (Ellegard, Andersson, Normen, & Andersson, 2007). Plant sterols are similar in structure to cholesterol but contain an extra methyl or ethyl group. When consumed in the diet, plant sterols compete with cholesterol in the intestine, reducing the amount of cholesterol that is absorbed (Devaraj & Jialal, 2006). Intake of 2 g/day of plant sterols has an associated 6% to 10% reduction in LDL cholesterol (Devaraj & Jialal, 2006; Ellegard et al, 2007). Combining plant sterols with cholesterol-lowering medications results in an additional 16% to 20% reduction in LDL (Berger, Jones, & Abumweis, 2004; Katan et al, 2003). The only adverse effect of plant sterols is reduced beta-carotene levels, which can be treated with an increased intake of carotene-containing fruits and vegetables (Berger et al, 2004; Devaraj & Jialal, 2006).

Plant sterols are present in edible oils (corn oil and canola oil have the highest amount), seeds, and nuts (Ellegard et al, 2007). There are many commercial food products available with added plant sterols, including margarine (Promise Active 1 g/serving, Benecol spread 0.85 g/serving, Smart Balance HeartRight 1.7 g/serving), orange juice (Minute Maid Heart Wise 1 g/serving), and milk (Smart Balance HeartRight 400 mg/serving). The recommended amount of plant sterols for LDL reduction is up to 2 g/day (Devaraj & Jialal, 2006). The NHLBI guidelines for children and adolescents is that plant sterols up to 2 g/d can be used as a replacement for the usual fat sources after age 2 years in children with familial hypercholesterolemia (NHLBI, 2012). Plant sterols may be combined with a low saturated fat and cholesterol diet, dietary fiber, and/or lipid-lowering drugs for an additive effect on reducing LDL cholesterol (Devaraj & Jialal, 2006).

Pre-, Pro-, and Symbiotics

Probiotics are nonpathogenic bacteria normally found in the intestinal microflora, the most common of which are *Lactobacillus acidophilus* and the *Bifidobacterium* species. Prebiotics are nondigestible food ingredients that stimulate growth of probiotic organisms, and symbiotics are a mixture of probiotics and prebiotics. Probiotics are used to restore the normal balance of gut flora that is disturbed with antibiotics, immunosuppressive medications, and other conditions (Weichert et al, 2012; Williams, 2010).

Probiotics have been used for many years and have been studied extensively for their health benefits and their effects on diarrhea. A *Cochrane Review* of the use of probiotics in rotavirus-associated acute diarrhea in children found probiotics reduced diarrhea severity and duration by 1 to 3 days (Allen, Okoko, Martinez, Gregorio, & Dans, 2004). Probiotics also reduce antibiotic-associated diarrhea in adults (D'Souza, Rajkumar, Cooke, & Bulpitt, 2002; Safdar, Barigala, Said, & McKinley, 2008; Tong, Ran, Shen, Zhang, & Xiao, 2006) and in children (Johnston, Supina, Ospina, & Vohra, 2007). It is reasonable to prescribe probiotics for patients with infectious or antibiotic-associated diarrhea.

Probiotics may also improve inflammatory bowel disorders and necrotizing enterocolitis (NEC). Premature infants have sterile guts when they are born and are at risk for bowel problems, including NEC. Multiple studies and reviews have found probiotics beneficial in preventing NEC and death in preterm infants (AlFaleh & Bassler, 2008; Bosante, Iacobelli, & Gouyon, 2013; Deshpande, Rao, Patole, & Bulsara, 2010; Fernández-Carrocera et al, 2013; Lin et al, 2008). Probiotics improved colic symptoms in a multicenter, double-blind, placebo-controlled trial of infants started on probiotics soon after birth (Indrio et al, 2014). Use of probiotics improved Symptom Severity Scores in patients with irritable bowel syndrome (Williams et al, 2008). Probiotics have also been found to improve eradication rates in patients being treated for *Helicobacter pylori* (Tong et al, 2006).

REFERENCES

Agabio, R. (2005). Thiamine administration in alcohol-dependent patients. *Alcohol and Alcoholism, 40*(2), 155–156.

Aleixandre, A., & Miguel, M. (2008). Dietary fiber in prevention and treatment of metabolic syndrome: A review. *Critical Reviews in Food Science and Nutrition, 48*, 905–912.

AlFaleh, K. M., & Bassler, D. (2008). Probiotics for prevention of necrotizing enterocolitis in preterm infants. *Cochrane Database of Systematic Reviews, 1*, CD005496.

Allen, S. J., Okoko, B., Martinez, E. G., Gregorio, G. V., & Dans, L. F. (2004). Probiotics for treating infectious diarrhea. *Cochrane Database of Systematic Reviews, 2*, CD003048.

Ambalavanan, N., Tyson, J. E., Kennedy, K. A., Hansen, N. I., Vohr, B. R., Wright, L. L., et al. (2005). Vitamin A supplementation for extremely low birth weight infants: Outcome at 18 to 22 months. *Pediatrics, 115*(3), e249–e254.

American Academy of Pediatrics Committee on Fetus and Newborn. (2003). Controversies concerning vitamin K and the newborn. Committee on Fetus and Newborn. *Pediatrics, 112*(1), 191–192.

American Dietetic Association. (2008). Position of the American Dietetic Association: Health implications of dietary fiber. *Journal of the American Dietetic Association, 108*(10), 1716–1731.

American Dietetic Association. (2009). Position of the American Dietetic Association: Nutrient supplementation. *Journal of the American Dietetic Association, 109*, 2073–2085.

American Heart Association. (2014a). Whole grains and fiber. *American Heart Association.* Retrieved from http://www.heart.org/HEARTORG/GettingHealthy/NutritionCenter/HealthyDietGoals/Whole-Grains-and-Fiber_UCM_303249_Article.jsp

American Heart Association. (2014b). Fish and omega-3 fatty acids. Retrieved from http://www.heart.org/HEARTORG/GettingHealthy/NutritionCenter/HealthyDietGoals/Fish-and-Omega-3-Fatty-Acids_UCM_303248_Article.jsp

American Thoracic Society. (2003). American Thoracic Society/Centers for Disease Control and Prevention/Infectious Diseases Society of America: Treatment of tuberculosis. *American Journal of Respiratory and Critical Care Medicine, 167*, 603–662.

Bailey, R. L., Dodd, K. W., Goldman, J. A., Gahche, J. J., Dwyer, J. T., Moshfegh, A. J., et al. (2010). Estimation of total calcium and vitamin D intakes in the United States. *Journal of Nutrition, 140*(4), 817–822.

Berger, A., Jones, P. J. H., & Abumweis, S. S. (2004). Plant sterols: Factors affecting their efficacy and safety as functional food ingredients. *Lipids in Health and Disease, 3*(5). Retrieved from http://www.lipidworld.com/content/3/1/5

Bloch, M. H., & Qawasmi, A. (2011). Omega-3 fatty acid supplementation for the treatment of children with attention-deficit/hyperactivity disorder symptomatology: Systematic review and meta-analysis. *Journal of the American Academy of Child and Adolescent Psychiatry, 50*(10), 991–1000.

Bonsante, F., Iacobelli, S., & Gouyon, J. (2013). Routine probiotic use in very preterm infants: Retrospective comparison of two cohorts. *American Journal of Perinatology, 30*(1), 41–46.

Brei, C., Simon, A., Krawinkel, M. B., & Naehrlich, L. (2013). Individualized vitamin A supplementation for patient with cystic fibrosis. *Clinical Nutrition, 32*(5), 805–810.

Brotherton, C. S., Taylor, A. G., Bourguignon, C., & Anderson, J. G. (2014). A high-fiber diet may improve bowel function and health-related quality of life in patients with Crohn's disease. *Gastroenterology Nursing: The Official Journal of the Society of Gastroenterology Nurses and Associates, 37*(3), 206–216.

Brulotte, J., Bukutu, C., & Vohra, S. (2009). Complementary, holistic, and integrative medicine: Fish oils and neurodevelopmental disorders. *Pediatrics in Review, 30*(4), e29–e33.

Charness, M. E., & So, Y. T. (2009, reviewed 2014). Wernicke's Encephalopathy. *UpToDate.* Wolters Kluwer Health. Retrieved from http://www.uptodate.com/contents/wernickes-encephalopathy

Chen, G. C., Lu, D. B., Pang, Z., & Liu, Q. F. (2013). Vitamin C intake, circulating vitamin C and risk of stroke: A meta-analysis of prospective studies. *Journal of the American Heart Association, 2*(6), e000329.

Crowe, K. M., & Francis, C. (2013). Position of the Academy of Nutrition and Dietetics: Functional foods. *Journal of the Academy of Nutrition and Dietetics, 113*(8), 1096–1103.

Cvijic, S., Parojcic, J., & Langguth, P. (2014). Viscosity-mediated negative food effect on oral absorption of poorly-permeable drugs with an absorption window in the proximal intestine: In vitro experimental simulation and computational verification. *European Journal of Pharmaceutical Sciences: Official Journal of the European Federation for Pharmaceutical Sciences.* Date of Electronic Publication April 18, 2014.

Daly, A., Johnson, T., & MacDonald, A. (2004). Is fibre supplementation in paediatric sip feeds beneficial? *Journal of Human Nutrition and Dietetics, 17*(4), 365–370.

Deshpande, G., Rao, S., Patole, S., & Bulsara, M. (2010). Updated meta-analysis of probiotics for preventing necrotizing enterocolitis in preterm neonates. *Pediatrics, 125*, 921–930.

Devaraj, S., & Jialal, I. (2006). The role of dietary supplementation with plant sterols and stanols in the prevention of cardiovascular disease. *Nutrition Reviews, 64*(7), 348–354.

Douglas, R. M., Hemilä, H., Chalker, E., & Treacy, B. (2007). Vitamin C for preventing and treating the common cold. *Cochrane Database of Systematic Reviews, 3*, CD000980.

D'Souza, A. L., Rajkumar, C., Cooke, J., & Bulpitt, C. J. (2002). Probiotics in prevention of antibiotics associated diarrhea: Meta-analysis. *BMJ: British Medical Association, 324*, 1361–1364.

Dukas, L., Willett, W. C., & Giovannucci, E. L. (2003). Association between physical activity, fiber intake, and other lifestyle variables and constipation in a study of women. *American Journal of Gastroenterology, 98*(8), 1790–1796.

Ellegard, L. H., Andersson, S. W., Normen, A. L., & Andersson, H. A. (2007). Dietary plant sterols and cholesterol metabolism. *Nutrition Reviews, 65*(1), 39–45.

Fernández-Carrocera, L., Solis-Herrera, A., Cabanillas-Ayón, M., Gallardo-Sarmiento, R., García-Pérez, C., Montaño-Rodríguez, R., et al. (2013). Double-blind, randomised clinical assay to evaluate the efficacy of probiotics in preterm newborns weighing less than 1500 g in the prevention of necrotising enterocolitis. *Archives of Disease in Childhood. Fetal and Neonatal Edition, 98*(1), F5–F9.

Gadhia, M. M., Cutter, G. R., Abman, S. H., & Kinsella, J. P. (2014). Effects of early inhaled nitric oxide therapy and vitamin A supplementation on the risk for bronchopulmonary dysplasia in premature newborns with respiratory failure. *The Journal of Pediatrics, 164*(4), 744–748.

Gertz, M., Davis, J. D., Harrison, A., Houston, J. B., & Galetin, A. (2008). Grapefruit juice–drug interaction studies as a method to assess the extent of intestinal availability: Utility and limitations. *Current Drug Metabolism, 9*, 785–795.

Gillies, D., Sinn, J. K. H., Leach, M. J., & Ross, M. J. (2012). Polyunsaturated fatty acids (PUFA) for attention deficit hyperactivity disorder (ADHD)

in children and adolescents. *Cochrane Database Systematic Review, 11*(7), CD007986.

Guyatt, G. H., Akl, E. A., Crowther, M., Gutterman, D. D., Schunemann, H. J., for the American College of Chest Physicians Antithrombotic Therapy and Prevention of Thrombosis Panel. (2012). Antithrombotic therapy and prevention of thrombosis, 9th ed: American College of Chest Physicians Evidence-based Clinical Practice Guidelines. *Chest, 141*(2), 7S–47S.

Imdad, A., Yakoob, M. Y., Sudfeld, C., Haider, B. A., Black, R. E., & Bhutta, Z. A. (2011). Impact of vitamin A supplementation on infant and childhood mortality. *BMC Public Health, 11*(Suppl 3), S20.

Indrio, F. et al (2014). Prophylactic use of a probiotic in the prevention of colic, regurgitation and functional constipation a randomized clinical trial. *JAMA Pediatrics, 168*(3), 228-233

Institute of Medicine, Food and Nutrition Board. (2002). *Dietary reference intakes: Energy, carbohydrates, fiber, fat, fatty acids, cholesterol, protein and amino acids.* Washington, DC: National Academies Press.

Ishmail, M. Y. M. (2009). Drug-food interactions and role of pharmacist. *Asian Journal of Pharmaceutical and Clinical Research, 2*(4), 1–10. Retrieved from http://ajpcr.com/Vol2Issue4/226.pdf

Jewell, D., & Young, G. (2001). Interventions for treating constipation in pregnancy. *Cochrane Database of Systematic Reviews, 2.* Edited Issue 1, 2009.

Johnston, B. C., Supina, A. L., Ospina, M., & Vohra, S. (2007). Probiotics for the prevention of pediatric antibiotic-associated diarrhea. *Cochrane Database of Systematic Reviews, 2,* CD004827.

Katan, M. B., Grundy, S. M., Jones, P., Law, M., Miettinen, T., & Paoletti, R. (2003). Efficacy and safety of plant sterols and sterols in the management of blood cholesterol levels. *Mayo Clinic Proceedings, 78*(8), 965–978.

Kim, J., Kim, M. K., Lee, J. K., Kim, J. H., Son, S. K., Song, E. S., et al. (2010). Intakes of vitamin A, C and E and beta-carotene are associated with risk of cervical cancer: A case-control study in Korea. *Nutrition and Cancer, 62*(2), 181–189.

Kuypers, D. R. J. (2009). Immunotherapy in elderly transplant recipients: A guide to clinical significant drug interactions. *Drugs and Aging, 26*(9), 715–737.

Larson, J. T., & Brosen, K. (2005). Consumption of charcoal-broiled meat as an experimental tool for discerning CYP1A2-mediated drug metabolism in vivo. *Basic & Clinical Pharmacology & Toxicology, 97*(3), 141–148.

Lee, J. H., O'Keefe, J. H., Lavie, C. J., Marchioli, R., & Harris, W. S. (2008). Omega-3 fatty acids for cardioprotection. *Mayo Clinic Proceedings, 83*(3), 324–332.

Lin, H. C., Hsu, H. C., Chen, H. L., Chung, M., Hsu, J. F., Lien, R., et al. (2008). Oral probiotics prevent necrotizing enterocolitis in very low birth weight preterm infants: A multicenter, randomized, controlled trial. *Pediatrics, 122,* 693–700.

Meiri, G., Bichovsky, Y., & Belmaker, R. H. (2009). Omega 3 fatty acid treatment in autism. *Journal of Child and Adolescent Psychopharmacology, 19*(4), 449–451.

Mertens-Talcott, S. U., Zadezensky, I., DeCastro, W. V., Derendorf, H., & Butterweck, V. (2006). Grapefruit-drug interactions: Can interactions with drugs be avoided? *Journal of Clinical Pharmacology, 46,* 1390–1416.

Muntwyler, J., Hennekens, C. H., Buring, J. E., Manson, J. E., & Gaziano, J. M. (2002). Vitamin supplement use in a low-risk population of U.S. male physicians and subsequent cardiovascular mortality. *Archives of Internal Medicine, 162,* 1472–1476.

Myint, P. K., Luben, R. N., Welch, A. A., Bingham, S. A., Wareham, N. J., & Khaw, K. T. (2008). Plasma vitamin C concentrations predict risk of incident stroke over 10 y in 20,649 participants of the European Prospective Investigation into Cancer Norfolk prospective population study. *American Journal of Clinical Nutrition, 8,* 64–69.

National Heart Lung and Blood Institute (2012). *Expert panel on integrated guidelines for cardiovascular health and risk reduction in children and adolescents.* NIH Publication No, 12-7486A. Retrieved from http://www.nhlbi.nih.gov/guidelines/cvd_ped/peds_guidelines_sum.pdf

Ning, H., Van Horn, L., Shay, C. M., & Lloyd-Jones, D. M. (2014). Associations of dietary fiber intake with long-term predicted cardiovascular disease risk and C-reactive protein levels (from National Health and Nutrition Examination survey data [2005–2010]). *The American Journal of Cardiology, 113*(2), 287–291.

Office of Dietary Supplements. (2004a). Health effects of omega-3 fatty acids on arrhythmogenic mechanisms in animal and isolated organ/cell culture studies. Retrieved from http://www.ahrq.gov/clinic/tp/o3arrtp.htm#Report

Office of Dietary Supplements. (2004b). Health effects of omega-3 fatty acids on asthma. Retrieved from http://www.ahrq.gov/clinic/tp/o3asthmtp.htm#Report

Office of Dietary Supplements. (2004c). Health effects of omega-3 fatty acids on cardiovascular disease. Retrieved from http://www.ahrq.gov/clinic/tp/o3cardtp.htm#Report

Office of Dietary Supplements. (2004d). Health effects of omega-3 fatty acids on lipids and glycemic control in type II diabetes and the metabolic syndrome and on inflammatory bowel disease, rheumatoid arthritis, renal disease, systemic lupus erythematosus and osteoporosis. Retrieved from http://www.ahrq.gov/clinic/tp/o3lipidtp.htm

Office of Dietary Supplements. (2005a). Effects of omega-3 fatty acids on cancer. Retrieved from http://www.ahrq.gov/clinic/tp/o3cantp.htm#Report

Office of Dietary Supplements. (2005b). Effects of omega-3 fatty acids on mental health. Retrieved from http://www.ahrq.gov/clinic/tp/o3menttp.htm#Report

Office of Dietary Supplements. (2005c). Effects of omega-3 fatty acids on organ transplantation. Retrieved from http://www.ahrq.gov/clinic/tp/o3organtp.htm#Report

Office of Dietary Supplements. (2011a). *Vitamin B$_6$: Dietary supplement fact sheet.* National Institutes of Health. Retrieved from http://ods.od.nih.gov/factsheets/VitaminB6-HealthProfessional/

Office of Dietary Supplements. (2011b). *Vitamin B$_{12}$: Dietary supplement fact sheet.* National Institutes of Health. Retrieved from http://ods.od.nih.gov/factsheets/VitaminB12-HealthProfessional/

Office of Dietary Supplements. (2011c). *Vitamin D: Dietary supplement fact sheet.* National Institutes of Health. Retrieved from http://ods.od.nih.gov/factsheets/VitaminD-HealthProfessional/

Office of Dietary Supplements. (2012a). *Folate: Dietary supplement fact sheet.* Retrieved from http://ods.od.nih.gov/factsheets/Folate-HealthProfessional/

Office of Dietary Supplements. (2013a). *Vitamin A: Health professional fact sheet.* National Institutes of Health. Retrieved from http://ods.od.nih.gov/factsheets/VitaminA-HealthProfessional/vitamin

Office of Dietary Supplements. (2013b). *Vitamin C: Health professional fact sheet.* National Institutes of Health. Retrieved from http://ods.od.nih.gov/factsheets/VitaminC-HealthProfessional/

Osganian, S. K., Stampfer, M. J., Rimm, E., Spiegelman, D., Hu, F. B., Manson, J. E., et al. (2003). Vitamin C and risk of coronary heart disease in women. *Journal of the American College of Cardiology, 42,* 246–252.

Paine, M. F., Widmer, W. W., Hart, H. L., Pusek, S. N., Beavers, K. L., Criss, A. B., et al. (2006). A furanocoumarin-free grapefruit juice establishes furanocoumarins as the mediators of the grapefruit juice–felodipine interaction. *American Journal of Clinical Nutrition, 83*(5), 1097–1105.

Peterson, S., Lampe, J. W., Bammler, T. K., Gross-Steinmeyer, K., & Eaton, D. L. (2006). Apiaceous vegetable constituents inhibit human cytochrome P-450 1A2 (hCYP1A2) activity and hCYP1A2-mediated mutagenicity of aflatoxin B1. *Food and Chemical Toxicology, 44*(9), 1474–1484.

Peterson, S., Schwarz, Y., Li, S. S., Li, L., King, I. B., Chen, C., et al. (2009). CYP1A2, GSTM1, GSTT1 polymorphisms and diet effects on CYP1A2 activity in a crossover feeding trial. *Cancer Epidemiology, Biomarkers & Prevention: A Publication of the American Association for Cancer Research, Cosponsored by The American Society of Preventive Oncology, 18*(11), 3118–3125.

Rance, K. (2013) The emerging role of vitamin D in asthma management. *Journal of the American Association of Nurse Practitioners, 26*(5), 263–267.

Rossignol, D. A. (2009). Novel and emerging treatments for autism spectrum disorders: A systematic review. *Annals of Clinical Psychiatry, 21*(3), 213–236.

Safdar, N., Barigala, R., Said, A., & McKinley, L (2008). Feasibility and tolerability of probiotics for prevention of antibiotic-associated diarrhea in hospitalized U.S. military veterans. *Journal of Clinical Pharmacy and Therapeutics, 33,* 663–668.

Schein, J. R. (1997). Cruciferous vegetables and drug metabolism. *European Journal of Drug Metabolism and Pharmacokinetics, 22*(1), 85–86.

Schuchardt, J. P., Huss, M., Stauss-Grabo, M., & Hahn, A. (2009). Significance of long-chain polyunsaturated fatty acids (PUFAs) for the development and behavior of children. *European Journal of Pediatrics, 169,* 149–164.

Schwartz, N., Kaye, E. K., Nunn, M. E., Spiro, A., & Garcia, R. (2012). High-fiber foods reduce periodontal disease progression in men aged 65 and older: The Veterans Affairs normative aging study/dental longitudinal study. *Journal of the American Geriatric Society, 60*(4), 676–683.

Shah, N. D., Chitkara, D. K., Locke, G. R., Meek, P. D., & Talley, N. J. (2008). Ambulatory care for constipation in the United States, 1993–2004. *American Journal of Gastroenterology, 103,* 1746–1753.

Singh, B. N. (1999). Effects of food on clinical pharmacokinetics. *Clinical Pharmacokinetics, 37*(3), 213–255.

Singh, B. N., & Malhotra, B. K. (2004). Effects of food on the clinical pharmacokinetics of anticancer agents: Underlying mechanisms and implications for oral chemotherapy. *Clinical Pharmacokinetics, 43*(15), 1127–1156.

Slatore, C. G., Littman, A. J., Au, D. H., Satia, J. A., & White, E. (2007). Long-term use of supplemental multivitamins, vitamin C, vitamin E, and folate does not reduce the risk of lung cancer. *American Journal of Respiratory and Critical Care Medicine, 177*(5), 524–530.

Sorensen, M. D., Hsi, R. S., Chi, T., Shara, N., Wactawski-Wende, J., Kahn, A. J., et al. (2014). Dietary intake of fiber, fruit, and vegetables decreases the risk of incident kidney stone in women: A Women's Health Initiative (WHI) report. *The Journal of Urology.* Published electronically May 21, 2014.

Taylor, F. R. (2009). Headache prevention with complementary and alternative medicine. *Headache, 49*(6), 966–968.

Tong, J. L., Ran, Z. H., Shen, J., Zhang, C. X., & Xiao, S. K. (2006). Meta-analysis: The effect of supplementation with probiotics on eradication rates and adverse events during *Helicobacter pylori* eradication therapy. *Alimentary Pharmacology & Therapeutics, 25,* 155–168.

Vaquero, M. P., Sanchez Muniz, F. J., Jimenez Redondo, S., Prats Olivan, P., Higueras, F. J., & Bastida, S. (2010). Major diet-drug interactions affecting the kinetic characteristics and hypolipidaemic properties of statins. *Nutrición Hospitalaria: Organo Oficial de la Sociedad Española de Nutrición Parenteral y Enteral, 25*(2), 193–206.

Varum, F. J., Hatton, G. B., & Basit, A. W. (2013). Food, physiology and drug delivery. *International Journal of Pharmaceutics, 457*(2), 446–460.

Vuksan, V., Rogovik, J., Jovanovski, E., & Jenkins, A. L. (2009). Fiber facts: Benefits and recommendations for individuals with type 2 diabetes. *Current Diabetes Reports, 9,* 405–411.

Wang, C., Baumgartner, R. N., Yang, D., Slattery, M. L., Murtaugh, M. A., Byers, T., et al. (2009). No evidence of association between breast cancer risk and dietary carotenoids, retinols, vitamin C and tocopherols in southwestern Hispanic and non-Hispanic white women. *Breast Cancer Research Treatment, 114,* 137–145.

Ward, A. (2010). Constipation and defecation problems. The American College of Gastroenterology. Retrieved from http://www.acg.gi.org/patients/gihealth/constipation.asp

Warren Grant Magnuson Clinical Center, National Institutes of Health Drug-Nutrient Interaction Task Force. (2003). Important information to know when you are taking: Coumadin and vitamin K. Retrieved from http://ods.od.nih.gov/Health_Information/Vitamin_and_Mineral_Supplement_Fact_Sheets.aspx

Williams, N. T. (2010). Probiotics. *American Journal of Health-System Pharmacy, 67,* 449–458.

Yetley, E. A. (2008). Assessing the vitamin D status of the U.S. population. *American Journal of Clinical Nutrition, 88,* 558S–564S.

CHAPTER 10

HERBAL THERAPY AND NUTRITIONAL SUPPLEMENTS

Fujio McPherson

Phytomedicine, defined as "the practice of using plants or plant parts to achieve a therapeutic cure" (Fetrow & Avila, 1999), is the oldest known form of medicine. Originally, plants were considered only for their nutritional value. However, from experience in plant production and awareness of plant behavior, noting the influence of climate and environmental changes on planting outcomes and the effects of specific plants in creating or removing various symptoms in the body, humans began to use plants as medicine.

In many cultures, herbal traditions are a part of a history that began well before the scientific dissection of plant cellular components. It is impossible to determine precisely when humans first discovered the medicinal use of any given plant, but through time and observation every culture developed a pharmacopoeia of herbal remedies. The Egyptians were widely respected for their use and recording of herbal remedies, many of which are still used today, including opium, cannabis, myrrh, frankincense, and fennel. The Greek and Roman use of herbs was based on the principles of the four humors that derived from the Indian and Chinese cultures. One of the oldest forms of herbal medicine was their use in altering states of consciousness in the shamanic traditions of South American and many of the Native American cultures. The Greeks also used hallucinogenic herbs, such as opiates, to heighten the healing powers within the body while the patient lay in an altered state of consciousness in Asclepian healing temples.

Today, the use of herbal medicine in the United States has grown significantly since the early 1990s. As determined by the 2007 National Health Interview Survey, 55.1 million adults in the United States had used herbs or supplements in the past 12 months, up from 50.6 million in the 2002 survey (Wu, Wang, & Kennedy, 2011). And up to 2.9 million children aged 4 to 17 years had used herbs or dietary supplements in the previous 12 months (Wu, Wang, & Kennedy, 2013). As mainstream medicine diverged from a predominantly plant-based pharmacopoeia to a synthesized, chemically based pharmacopoeia that is accompanied by a myriad of harmful side effects, a belief that herbal medicines are safer and have less harmful side effects has evolved to such a degree that many patients often abandon their use of synthetic medication for over-the-counter herbal substitutes. With limited regulation by the U.S. Food and Drug Administration (FDA), herbal formulas and products, which are classified as food sources, have become widely available.

Thus, allopathic providers are now faced with the challenge of drug and herbal interactions as well as by working with strong patient belief systems that can compromise management of the patient's condition. Providers need to consider the impact herbs may have on their medical and pharmaceutical management. In many cases, herbal therapy has proven to be very effective at either enhancing medical management of a disease and/or reducing the need for stronger pharmaceutical management, in some cases successfully replacing more harmful pharmaceutical drugs without the harmful side effects while achieving the same efficacy. For example, the root bark of *Hibiscus syriacus* has been used for many years in Asia as an antipyretic, antihelminthic, and antifungal agent. The results of a 2008 study indicated the herb had a significant and dose-dependent antiproliferative effect on lung cancer cells in vitro and in vivo (Cheng, Lee, Harn, Huang, & Chang, 2008).

Yet there are also many studies that identify potentially harmful effects of herbal therapy. Buettner, Mukamal, Gardiner, & Davis (2009) found lead levels to be 10% higher among women who used St. John's wort, Ayurvedic herbs, and some traditional Chinese herbs. Coenzyme Q10, a supplement commonly used to improve memory and cardiovascular function, was found to reduce the effectiveness of warfarin, and evidence is still inconclusive regarding its effect in reducing cardiovascular conditions like exercise-induced angina. When taken in doses higher than 3,000 mg per day for a prolonged period of time, CoQ10 can cause elevated liver enzymes.

Many studies support the argument that further research or regulation of herbal therapy is needed, but they also make clear that the safety and efficacious use of herbs in the treatment of specific disorders cannot be truly evaluated without considering the theories and principles of the traditional medicines of which they are a part. It is common knowledge that every pharmaceutical prescription has side effects that range from mild to life-threatening, so excluding the use of an herb solely due to its side effects is not only misguided but fails to consider the difference between herbal side effects and pharmaceutical side effects. For example, in Chinese medicine, an herb may be used for its cooling effect, and so the side effect that would indicate the herb is working properly would be the patient's display of symptoms of cold versus heat and a side effect of loose stools (which is an indication of cold) would actually be a positive sign rather than a negative side effect, as it would be considered by any Western research criteria. Most traditional herbal theories do not use scientific criteria in determining the use of an herb, and so allopathic medical practice does not recognize the theories and long traditions on which trained herbalists base their diagnoses and prescriptions of specific herbs and herbal formulas.

By definition, herbal therapy encompasses any plant source, which means that it also includes food. When the plant or a constituent of the plant is identified as a specific treatment for a disease or symptom, it is often referred to as an herb. And the designation of an herb as a medicine is based on how it is used. Herbs have long been considered one of the safest medicines to take and, like foods, can be classified by their effects on the body—mild, strong, or toxic. However, as mentioned, it is more important to understand the theory behind the herb before one can understand how it is used in the treatment of a disease. This includes understanding the various methods by which herbal preparations are prepared and manufactured. So it is imperative that nurse practitioners and other allopathic providers understand not only the name, ingredients, and source of a particular herb but also the various theories used in herbal medicine, or they should consult with clinicians who are trained in herbal medicine to better care for the patient who chooses to use herbal remedies.

This chapter serves as an introduction to phytomedicine. Because this is a relatively new area of study for Western health practitioners, the chapter includes definitions of terms and descriptions of the various principles involved in prescribing and using herbal medicines in North America. The purpose here is not to train readers to be herbalists but rather to introduce them to some of the major herbal theories used in the prescription of herbs, that is, the chapter is an introduction rather than a prescriptive resource.

OVERVIEW OF HERBAL MEDICINE

To understand the concept and theories of herbal medicine, it is important to examine the many herbal traditions practiced in the world today. For the purpose of this particular text, three traditions will be examined: Western herbal medicine, Ayurvedic herbal medicine, and traditional Chinese herbal medicine. Yet the reader is encouraged to explore other traditions of herbal medicine also, among them Unani medicine, homeopathic medicine, Native American traditional medicine, and shamanic herbal medicine.

DEFINITIONS

Medicinally an *herb* is any plant part or whole plant used for its therapeutic value. Yet many of the world's herbal traditions are not limited to plants only; mineral and animal substances are included as well. *Herbal medicine* is the art and science of using herbs for promoting health and preventing and treating illness. It has a written history that is more than 5,000 years old. Although the use of herbs in America has been overshadowed by dependence on modern medications in the last 100 years, 75% of the world's population relies primarily on traditional healing practices and the use of herbal medicine.

Pharmacognosy is the branch of pharmacology that uses the chemicals from plants, molds, fungi, insects, and marine animals for their medicinal value. Today, most pharmaceutical drugs are single chemical entities from plant sources that have been highly refined, purified, and synthesized into a single active component of the plant. Many of the drugs used in allopathic medicine were derived from plants in this way, including digitalis from foxglove, ephedrine from *Ephedra*, and ergotamine from *Claviceps purpurea*. In 1987, about 85% of modern drugs were originally derived from plants. However, only about 15% of all drugs are derived from plants today owing to advancements in synthetic reproduction and purification of plant constituents. In contrast, herbal medicines are prepared only from living or dried plants and contain hundreds to thousands of interrelated compounds, creating a type of synergy between its many constituents that science is now considering as the reason for the safety, effectiveness, and lower incidence of side effects of herbs (American Herbal Guild [AHG], 2006).

Western Herbal Medicine

The beginning of science-based herbal medicine can be traced back to the European Renaissance, when political independence from the Church and advances in science contributed greatly to the study of medicine. William Turner (1510–1568), regarded as "the father of British botany," was the first to scientifically study plants. John Gerrard (1545–1612), a surgeon and the author or *Gerard's Herbal*, studied over 1,000 plants and recorded his observations of their behavior and uses. But one of the most interesting scientists of this era was Nicolas Culpepper (1616–1654), who studied the relationship of herbs to astrology. Although he was ostracized by his peers at the time for his theories, his understanding of herbs from an energetic perspective influenced by factors other than the physical components of nutrients was very similar to the Eastern interpretation of plant-based medicine. Yet he fared much better than his female counterparts outside of the scientific community who used herbal medicine to heal. These female healers, branded as witches, were hunted down during the Inquisition, which effectively suppressed and eliminated this form of medicine and succeeded in denigrating the efforts of lay healers. Another pioneer in herbal medicine was Johann Wolfgang Von Goethe (1749–1832), a German herbalist who stated that the chemical mixture of the plant was the "open secret" to its effectiveness. Despite these setbacks, many of these early discoveries have survived and continue to be practiced today.

In Western herbology, herbs are primarily classified according to their therapeutic properties and the constituents of the plant. For example, the categories of diuretics, diaphoretics, and tonics allow Western herbalists to group herbs with similar qualities and then use them accordingly. This system is primarily based on the chemical constituents of the plant and remains the basis of Western pharmacology as well some of the herbal therapies used by many naturopathic physicians and other herbalists who base their practice on scientific examination of the plant.

What makes this form of herbal therapy different from Western pharmacology is that it is based on constituents taken from the plant instead of the synthetic modification commonly found in prescription drugs. One example is bromelain, a sulfhydryl proteolytic enzyme that is found in pineapple juice and in the pineapple stem. Bromelain activates the proteolytic activity at sites of inflammation and is commercially used as a natural anti-inflammatory agent (Pizzorno & Murray, 2006). Therefore, an herbal option to reduce inflammation can be bromelain or pineapple. Another example is the rhizome ginger commonly used in cooking. Ginger is considered a tonic, and one identified constituent of ginger root (*Zingiber officinale*) is the sesquiterpenes, which have significant antirhinoviral activity that is used to combat colds (Mills & Bone, 2000). Products made from ginger (e.g., teas, candy, lozenges) are used in the treatment of cold symptoms.

It is common to see the same plant being used in several different herbal theories, and although the principle actions are the same, the differences lie in how the plant is used and which parts. One example is cinnamon. Cinnamon (*C. zeylanicum*) is often referred to as "true cinnamon" or Ceylon cinnamon. However, a commercially related species known as cassia (*C. aromaticum*), or Saigon cinnamon (*C. loureiroi*), and *C. burmannii* are also labeled as cinnamon. True cinnamon (Ceylon cinnamon) comes from the thin inner bark; is finer, less dense, and more crumbly in texture; and is considered to be less strong than cassia. Cassia is derived from the entire bark layer, so it is thicker and has a much stronger, harsher flavor than cinnamon. This distinction is important because of a moderately toxic component called coumarin, which can cause liver and kidney damage in the high concentration that is found in higher doses of cassia compared to Ceylon cinnamon, in which the levels of coumarin are negligible.

Often used for its oil, cinnamon contains primarily cinnamic aldehyde but also has ethyl cinnamate, eugenol (found in the leaves), beta-carvophyllene, linalool, and methyl chavicol; it is used to cure colds and treat diarrhea and problems of the digestive system. It has been reported to be effective in the treatment of type 2 diabetes mellitus (Khan et al, 2003). In traditional Chinese medicine, cinnamon (Gui Zhi) is used to treat colds but is defined by its ability to release excess wind-cold conditions, warm and open channels and collaterals, and warm yang and is identified as being contraindicated in patients with yin deficiency or those having blood disorders because it stimulates blood circulation (Chen & Chen, 2001).

Traditional Chinese Medicine

The origins of traditional Chinese herbal medicine (TCM) are difficult to date; however, one of the oldest surviving texts that form the basis of TCM is the *Huangdi Neijing*, "The Inner Canon of Huangdi or Yellow Emperor's Inner Canon," first referenced in the *Book of Han*, in 111 CE. The *Huangdi Neijing* is composed of two texts, each with 81 chapters or treatises, and is primarily a written record of questions and answers between the mythical Huangdi (Yellow Emperor) and six of his ministers. The first text, the *Suwen*, covers the theoretical foundation of Chinese medicine and its diagnostic methods, and the second text, the *Spiritual Pivot*, discusses acupuncture therapy. The second important text in Chinese herbal medicine is the *Shang Hang Lun*, "Treatise on the Treatment of Acute Diseases Caused by Cold," written by Zhang Zhong-Jing (142–220 CE). The *Shang Hang Lun* describes the six stages of acute disease as an approach to the diagnosis and treatment of acute illness and is comprised of classical herbal formulas that can be used to treat them. Today, formulas contained in the *Shang Hang Lun,* such as Ge-Gen Tang, Shao Yao Gan Cao Tang, and Xiao Qing Long Tang, are still commonly used among TCM practitioners.

The *Huangdi Neijing* not only departed from the shamanic beliefs of the past but elaborated on the concepts of Daoist theory on which TCM is based. The Dao concept is that man is a microcosm of a larger macrocosm and to stay healthy or "in balance" there must be an intimate respect and understanding for the laws of nature and how those laws apply to man. Health or balance by definition results when there is a free flow of energy (qi). When qi is abundant and flowing freely, the body is able to heal itself and the patient will feel a balance of the mind, body, and spirit. Just as in nature, when there is enough water, nutrients, and sunlight, the plant will flourish and grow. Of course, knowing how to determine an imbalance (diagnosis before the presence of disease) or knowing the source of a disease resulting from an imbalance and how to prevent the progression of the imbalance, support self-healing, and treat the disease is the principle science of TCM.

There are a number of theories about how to interpret changes of balance in the human body, mind, and spirit. How TCM is practiced based on one or more of these theories often depends on the training of the practitioner and what the practitioner feels best suits the patient's condition. By understanding the basic principles of these TCM theories—yin and yang; the five elements; and the influence of environmental factors (wind, damp, hot and cold, dry, and wet)—along with the effects of diet, lifestyle, age, and emotions, a specific TCM diagnosis regarding the cause of imbalance can be determined and herbal therapy along with other treatment modalities like acupuncture, diet, counseling, movement, massage, and so on can be used to bring the body back into balance, promote self-healing, and treat diseases.

If there is one feature that distinguishes Western medicine from traditional Chinese medicine, it is the paradigm from which they view man and the role of plants. Instead of relying on science to identify the nature of disease and health, the Chinese look at nature from a Daoist perspective, paying attention to cycles of growth, the characteristics of the plant (according to taste and expression), the underlying condition of the individual consuming the herb, and most importantly the constitution of the individual.

In TCM, the herbs that represent energy (qi) are classified in a number of ways: by their amount of energy, quality, seasons in which they are at maximum strength, tastes, directions, and actions on the body (e.g., moving blood, reducing dampness or heat, breaking up stagnation, etc.). Traditionally, herbal formulas also include animal organs and minerals

for the same reasons. Using these principles, TCM practitioners use herbs to influence the imbalances unique to the patient. This symbiotic relationship is one of the most important aspects of TCM herbal medicine. Customizing the herbal formula and its properties to address the individual deficiencies or excesses assumes a more holistic approach to healing and the role of herbs in the treatment of diseases. For example, in TCM menopause is often considered a time of yin deficiency, so herbs that are yin in nature and that clear heat arising from deficient yin, such as mountain peony bark (*mu dan pi*) and phellodendron bark (*huang bai*), or formulas that contain each, are often recommended (Liu & Tseng, 2003). In doing so, TCM recognizes that if these herbs were applied inappropriately, for example, giving a yin herb to a yin excess patient, the herb could potentially make the condition worse even though the underlying condition is menopause. As mentioned, it is important to remember that TCM does not often restrict treatment to a single herbal therapy as does Western herbal medicine; it recognizes the principles of the Dao and concepts of change, so herbal therapy and formulas will often be changed within short intervals of time.

Although the focus of this chapter is herbal therapy, it is also important to remember that TCM places as much value on the power of food as it does on herbs in healing and never excludes food or herbs from the other aspects of TCM, which include the practice of acupuncture, energy movements (tai chi), massage (tui nai), and balance.

Ayurvedic Medicine

Ayurvedic medicine was developed in ancient India; it is defined as the study of life: *ayur* means "life" and *veda* means "to study." It is considered the oldest form of medicine in the world and is based on original texts derived from Vedic scriptures that date from 1500 BCE to 1200 BCE. Ayurvedic medicine eventually spread from India and influenced a number of cultures in the Far East, including TCM, Japanese acupuncture, Unani medicine, and the humoral medicine practiced by Hippocrates.

Although many of the teachings originate from knowledge that was handed down through generations of healers, many believe Ayurveda knowledge to be of divine origin received from the meditation of sages. Similar to TCM, Ayurvedic medicine encompasses a myriad of therapies based on the constitution of the individual and nature of the particular disease. But the use of herbal medicine is somewhat broader in that it is used in a number of different mediums and in delivery systems beyond the oral route. As well as being taken orally, herbs are used in body massage oils, in food preparation, and in aromatherapy, although the choice of therapy is still based on the individual and is linked to the patient's constitution and level of imbalance.

In Ayurvedic herbology, herbal therapy is interchangeable with food and spices, which are viewed as a sequence of herbal therapies that range from mild (food) to moderate (spices) to strong (herb). And their use depends on a person's constitution, classified according to a tridosha theory and the nature of the disease. In the tridosha system, all entities of matter, including people and plants, contain three *doshas*: *vata* (air/ether), which corresponds to the nervous system and movement; *pitta* (fire/water), representing transformation, circulation, warmth, and digestion; and *kapha* (water/earth), representing nourishment, solidity, and the formative aspects of tissue, fluid, and bone (Tiwari, 1995a).

Although all three doshas exist together, often plants and people are classified by the one that is most dominant in them, referred to as the person's "Prakruti," and specific to them as an individual. Treatment is then based on balancing the specific constitutional type for a particular patient, since each dosha is aggravated or pacified by certain therapies, herbs, and foods. So in Ayurvedic medicine (similar to TCM) herbal therapy actually begins with the use of food and spices that are consumed on a daily basis to maintain the balance of a given doshic constitution.

An example of this theory would be treating a person with a vata constitution and a vata disorder. Vata, meaning "wind," conceptually is made up of the elements of ether and air. Ether (space) affects the ability of air to gain momentum; if unrestricted, air can gain momentum and become forceful, so when balanced, a vata-type person will have free movement and flow (e.g., breathing will be strong, movement of the muscle and bones easy and light, movement of blood smooth, movement of thought and emotions easy, movement of the colon unimpeded). If unbalanced in either an excess or deficient condition, the person will experience either an excessive movement (e.g., manic behavior, diarrhea, nervousness) or deficient movement (e.g., constipation, depression, asthma). Therefore, the goal of therapy would be to counter the excess or deficiency first with food and spice and then support it with specific herbal therapy.

One Ayurvedic principle similar to the one used in homeopathic medicine is that "like increases like." Consequently, substances of similar doshas will increase those qualities in the body. A person experiencing an excess vata imbalance tends to be intolerant of dry or bitter substances (which are considered vata in nature); therefore, treatment would consist of avoiding foods that are dry and bitter and incorporating food like honey and rose hips and herbs like calamus or marshmallow root in the diet (Tiwari, 1995b). Similar to TCM, Ayurvedic treatment of imbalances within the tridoshic theory is not limited to herbal therapy alone. It also includes the five purification therapies (*panchakarma*), diet, aromatherapy, massage (*abyanga*), meditation, daily routine (*dinacarya*), and the practice of yoga.

It is important to remember that in most traditional cultures throughout the world herbal therapy is applied according to the energetic effects on the body and not on the individual constituents found in the plant. This in part recognizes the synergistic effects of the plant as being more important than the individual components. The conceptual model upon which clinical decisions and herbal recommendations are made is remarkably different from that of Western allopathic medicine. In the West, herbal medicines are often viewed strictly in terms of their actions, disregarding the energetic composition of the herb or the person consuming it. In the short term, this practice may result in a positive effect, but in the long and/or short term, it can often lead to poor or harmful effects. Therefore, it is important for Western clinicians who have an interest in herbal medicine or have patients who are taking herbal medicine to be aware of the different systems used to classify herbs and to recognize the importance of consulting with providers trained in a particular system. By doing so, practitioners can employ herbs efficiently and avoid the improper use of these therapies, which can either result in no effect or create an opposite and undesired effect.

HERBAL SAFETY

Today there are national standards and certification requirements for practitioners of TCM and naturopathic medicine (ND) for licensure to prescribe herbal therapy; however, state requirements may vary. In addition, herbal certification programs are now available, and guidelines for safe herbal practice have been established by the American Herbal Guild (AHG). The AHG is a nonprofit, educational organization founded in 1989 to represent the goals and voices of herbalists. It is the only peer-review organization in the United States for professional herbalists specializing in the medicinal use of plants. Herbalists from any tradition with sufficient education and clinical experience who demonstrate advanced knowledge in the medicinal use of plants and who pass the AHG credentialing process (a careful review by a multidisciplinary admissions board) receive professional status and the title Registered Herbalist, AHG. The AHG has also developed a code of ethics, continuing education programs, and specific standards for professional members as well as curriculum guidelines for herbal educational programs. The AHG Educational Guidelines recommend a curriculum with a minimum of 1,600 hours of total study, 400 of which should be in actual clinical work (AHG, 2006).

When considering herbal medicines it is important to understand that the development and preparation of medicines from plant and animal products can involve wide variations, based on the conditions of growth, harvesting, processing, storing, and shipping. Plants grown in the wild may be quite different from the same plants grown agriculturally. Methods of harvesting and weather variations in nature inevitably are different from those under controlled environments. In addition, variations in how plants are processed based on the drying and sterilizing techniques that are used have an effect on the potency of the herb. If products are not stored carefully, the inherent quality of the herb may be further compromised and it may be less effective.

In the United States, pharmaceuticals must meet a strict standard established by the FDA not only in the research and development stages but also in processing to maintain consistent standards of quality. Herbs, however, are regarded as food sources and do not come under the drug and pharmaceutical standards established by the FDA. However, many herbal manufacturers, particularly those in the United States, have adopted the FDA Good Manufacturing Practice (GMP) criteria for manufacturing, packing, and handling human food in the preparation of herbal medicines.

The GMP establishes federal guidelines for plant management, disease control, harvesting, storage, and distribution of foods, and herb manufacturers that meet these standards are authorized to display the GMP label on their products. Herbal products also provide supplement facts, active ingredients, and serving recommendations. The Dietary Supplement Health and Education Act (DSHEA) also requires dietary supplements (among which herbs are included) to carry this statement on the label: "This product has not been evaluated by the FDA. This product is not intended to diagnose, treat, cure, or prevent any disease." These measures have been taken to ensure the safety of herbal products and should be reviewed with each patient and practitioner who recommends or reviews a patient's use of herbs.

Evidence Grading

In an effort to evaluate herbal therapy, several systems have been developed to provide clinicians with methods for understanding the mechanism, use, and potential harmful effects of herbal therapy using an evidence-based system.

Natural Standard

Natural Standard (www.naturalstandard.com) is a complementary medicine grading system founded by clinicians and researchers from more than 100 academic institutions. It is designed to provide clinicians with the latest scientific data and expert opinion on complementary therapies, including herbal therapies, and is based on the Jadad scoring system of study quality (Jadad et al, 1996). A Jadad score of 0 to 5 is assigned, with 5 being the highest-quality study. In addition, a "magnitude of benefit" score is given to evaluate how strongly a study is able to show the benefit of a therapy. Natural Standard determines magnitude of benefit by subtracting the mean of the treatment group from the mean of the placebo group.

Taking into account the Jadad score, the magnitude of benefit, and other factors, Natural Standard grades the treatment. Grades reflect "the level of available scientific evidence in support of the efficacy of a given therapy for the specific indication." Treatments are also graded based on "evidence of harm." The Natural Standard's evidence rating scale is graded on a scale from A to F. A grade of "A" indicates that there is strong scientific evidence of the benefit of the therapy, whereas an "F" suggests that there is strong negative scientific evidence.

Healthnotes

Healthnotes' *The Natural Pharmacy* (2006) was designed as a reference for both practitioners and consumers. It evaluates the current state of the evidence in regard to herbs and nutritional supplements. This text is a culmination of the research contained in 25,000 articles in more than 600 peer-reviewed journals. In addition, chapters are contributed by a team of medical doctors, pharmacists, naturopaths, and chiropractors—all of whom have been in clinical practice. New editions of this manual are updated continually with the latest evidence-based information and recommendations. *The Natural Pharmacy* (2006) is notable for providing evidence that is based almost solely on human studies, as well as on information that specifically addresses contraindications to any herb or supplement. In addition, each recommendation is based on evidence derived from clinical, double-blind, meta-analyses or traditional empirical studies.

Rakel Evidence Versus Harm Scale

The Rakel Evidence Versus Harm Scale (Rakel, 2007) utilizes the Strength of Recommendation Taxonomy (SORT) (Ebell, Siwek, & Weiss, 2004) to rate the scientific evidence of a variety of integrated medicine treatments. The scale evaluates the strength of the evidence along with the evidence of potential harm. The evidence of benefit is graded from A to C, with "A" indicating that the evidence is "based on consistent, good quality, patient-oriented evidence." On the other hand, the potential harm of a therapy is graded from 1 (little or no risk of harm) to 3 (potential to result in death or permanent disability). An A rating represents that evidence is culled from systematic reviews or meta-analyses. It also incorporates Cochrane reviews of high-quality, randomized controlled trials that resulted in clear recommendations.

Cochrane Database of Systematic Reviews

Cochrane Database of Systematic Reviews (Cochrane Collaboration, n.d.) was created to help health-care providers keep up with and evaluate relevant scientific evidence. The Cochrane Collaboration produces reviews of evidence and creates a database of health-care interventions. The quality of the studies included in a review is evaluated using specific, predefined criteria. Most Cochrane reviews are based on randomized controlled trials and are statistically summarized into meta-analyses, showing a more thorough validation of clinical effect. Cochrane is considered one of the best sources of reliable evidence for and against specific treatments for specific conditions.

German Commission E Monographs

The German Federal Institute for Drugs and Medical Devices Commission E is a federal organization formed in 1978 to determine the efficacy and safety of herbs and supplements sold in Germany (National Institutes of Health, National Cancer Institute, n.d.). The commission is a multidisciplinary team of scientists, physicians, pharmacists, and herbal medicine experts who together review and analyze available data and form clinical recommendations based on the current evidence. To date, more than 300 herbs have been included in the recommendations and have been approved for clinical use in Germany.

Recommendations are published as monographs for each herb. Monographs include all pertinent botanical data, an explanation of mechanism (pharmacodynamic and pharmacokinetic action), and a complete therapeutic index (indications, contraindications, side effects, drug interactions, dosing, and duration). Additionally, the monographs include traditional uses, unapproved uses, and a summary of evidence. Commission E monographs are considered authoritative by experts in the field and have been reviewed for completeness and accuracy by the American Botanical Council (American Botanical Council [ABC], 2009).

The ABC is a nonprofit educational and research organization dedicated to the science of herbal medicine (American Botanical Council, 2009). It looks at evidence from both modern scientific and traditional perspectives. The ABC is comprised of an advisory council of experts and is affiliated with several natural medicine health science institutions and organizations. It maintains comprehensive databases; publishes a peer-reviewed journal (*Herbalgram*); and provides commentary, additions, and, in some cases, editor's notes for correction on all Commission E monographs. Although

specific herbal indications by Commission E are not based on a true evidence-graded system, the ABC considers them as having strong supportive evidence for inclusion within the context of *Herbalgram*.

The two evaluation systems that may be the most valuable to the primary care provider are Natural Standards and Rakel, since they provide a broad approach to recommended interventions for a given condition. Healthnotes, however, provides the most comprehensive data on individual supplements and serves as an expert source for clinical investigation of an herbal product. The Cochrane Database contains high-quality data reviews but is clinically the least useful for complementary and alternative medicine (CAM) evaluation because of its specificity in regard to what is reviewed.

Matrix for Evidence Grading

The following is a simple chart for comparing the various evidence-grading criteria for the treatment of several disorders.

Hypertension

CAM Therapy	Natural Standard	Healthnotes	Rakel	WHO	Commission-E
Acupuncture	Grade C			Category 1 (Essential & Primary HTN)	
Diet/Exercise	Grade B (Qi gong/yoga)		A1		
Mind-Body	Grade B		B1		
CoQ10	Grade B	3 Star	B2		
Fish oil (mixed EPA/DHA)	Grade A	3 Star	A2		Approved component
Calcium	Grade B	2 Star			
Magnesium		2 Star			
Garlic	Grade C	2 Star			Approved
Hawthorn (*Crataegus* spp.)	Grade D	1 Star	B1		Approved

Cochrane Summary:
- Review of calcium demonstrated positive effects but reviewers concluded data was insufficient due to poor study design and lack of heterogeneity between trials, leading to bias.
- Garlic review for peripheral arterial occlusion was inconclusive. No statistical significance in walking distances was seen.

*Tables not inclusive.

Clinical Implications for Practice: Hypertension

Herb/Supplement	Indications	Contraindications	Dose	Rakel Harm Scale
CoQ10	HTN	None	90–150 mg/qd	2
Fish oil (mixed EPA/DHA)	HTN	Coagulation (bleeding) disorders	3 g/qd	2
Calcium	HTN	Hypercalcemia, constipation, kidney stones, prostate cancer	800–1,500 mg/qd	
Magnesium	HTN	Caution in renal insufficiency	250–350 mg/qd	
Garlic	Hyperlipidemia	Allergy Caution with warfarin (WHO)	1–3 g/qd	
Hawthorn (*Crataegus* spp.)	Cardiac insufficiency/ heart failure	Allergy	Varies with form: tincture 35% ETOH 406 mL/TID Tea: 5–10 g/TID	1

*Dosing recommendation compiled from Healthnotes, Natural Standards, ABC Clinical recommendations, and Bastyr University clinical monographs.

Hypertension Commentary

Evidence supports the inclusion of mixed fish oil, CoQ enzyme 10, and probably calcium in the treatment of both essential and primary hypertension. Clinical consideration should also be given to incorporation of both acupuncture and mind–body techniques in addition to diet modification and exercise. Due to the broad systemic effects and safety profile of these interventions, supplemental therapy should be used to help control hypertension, prevent progression to advanced stages, and potentially decrease poly-pharmacy use.

Hyperlipidemia

CAM Therapy	Natural Standard	Healthnotes	Rakel	WHO	Commission- E
Acupuncture				Category 2	
Diet/Exercise	Grade B (Yoga)		A1		
Mind-Body	Grade C				
Plant sterols	Grade A	3 Star	A2		
Psyllium	Grade A	2 Star	A2		Approved as fiber for constipation and diarrhea
Fish oil (mixed EPA/DHA)	Grade A	3 Star	A2		Approved component
B vitamins	Grade A	3 Star (Niacin, B³)	A2		
Guggul (*Commifora mukul*)	Grade C	3 Star			Not approved
Fenugreek (*Trigonella foenum-graecum*)	Grade C	2 Star			Approved as appetite stimulator and digestive aid
Red yeast rice (*Monascus purpureus*)	Grade A	2 Star			
Garlic	Grade B	2 Star			Approved

Cochrane Summary:

- Omega-3 (fish oils) have strong evidence for lowering triglycerides and VLDL
- No conclusive data on dietary intervention for familial hyperlipidemia
- Plant sterol review currently pending
- Garlic protocol currently pending

*Tables not inclusive: Commission E approval is specific per condition unless otherwise noted.

Clinical Implications for Practice: Hyperlipidemia

Herb/Supplement	Indications	Contraindications	Dose	Rakel Harm Scale
Plant sterols	Hyperlipidemia	None (Caution in estrogen receptor + neoplasms)	2–3 g/qd	2
Psyllium	Hyperlipidemia	Caution in IBS	10–30 g/qd	
Fish oil (mixed EPA/DHA)	Hyperlipidemia HTN	Coagulation (bleeding) disorders	3 g/qd	2
Niacin (B³)	Hyperlipidemia Depression	Active liver disease, active ulcer or arterial bleeding	1 g/tid	2
Guggul (*Commifora mukul*)	Hyperlipidemia	Allergy, coagulation (bleeding) disorders and pregnancy/lactation	25 mg/bid (standardized extract guggulsterone)	
Fenugreek (*Trigonella foenum-graecum*)	Poor digestion Hyperlipidemia Diabetes I & II	Early pregnancy, hyperchlorhydia/GERD, and active peptic ulcer	Tincture: 30% ETOH, 3–5mL/tid	
Red yeast rice (*Monascus purpureus*)	Hyperlipidemia	Pregnancy and lactation	1200 mg/bid	
Garlic	Hyperlipidemia	Allergy Caution with warfarin (WHO)	1–3 g/qd	

*Dosing recommendation compiled from Healthnotes, Natural Standards, ABC Clinical recommendations, and Bastyr University clinical monographs.

Hyperlipidemia Commentary

There is strong evidence for diet and lifestyle modifications, combined with appropriate supplementation, for treating high cholesterol. Psyllium husk as fiber and mixed EPA/DHA fish oil should be considered as standard treatment due to the impact on both cholesterol and blood pressure. Niacin (B^3) is available in prescription form. Red yeast rice, garlic, and guggul can be considered as adjuncts, as these herbs also impact blood glucose levels and hematological clotting parameters. The cholesterol-lowering properties of red yeast rice are largely due to fungal metabolites known as monacolins, one of which, monacolin K, is identical to lovastatin and has been found to be effective at lowering cholesterol with minimal side effects (Becker, Gordon, Halbert, & French, 2009). However, guggul has been associated with elevated liver function tests and acute hepatitis (Grieco, Miele, Pompili, & Biolato, 2009). Therefore, the practitioner should still screen patients for liver abnormalities prior to starting these herbs and monitor them during therapy. Although the risks are lower, product uniformity, purity, labeling, and safety cannot be guaranteed, and it is the responsibility of the provider to solicit information from a particular company regarding their production process to ensure patient safety.

Challenges to Using an Evidenced-Based Model

Although evidenced-based medicine (EBM) is currently considered the "gold standard" of care for practice, using blind randomized controlled trials (RCTs) that are based on a statistical analysis to validate and determine efficacy of a particular medication or medical procedure may not be the most effective way to evaluate a holistic approach to care, particularly when it is deemed the only acceptable basis for health care. The value and role of the doctor is undermined, the psychological and social aspects of medicine are neglected, and sole reliance on EBM presents the danger of creating a utilitarian orthodoxy (Williams & Garner, 2002).

There are three factors that become problematic when evaluating CAM therapies, particularly herbal therapy. The first is that the Western scientific method applied to drug-based or pharmaceutical research is designed to measure single chemical components in relation to outcome. This model is used in the evaluation of Western herbs, but it does not reflect the philosophy and treatment parameters used in Ayurvedic or traditional Chinese medicine, which use the whole plant and consider only its nature and effect at reducing or enhancing the body's balance. Second, definitions used in CAM pose a unique problem for EBM researchers. The scientific method cannot be used to measure things that have yet to be physically defined by Western science. The concepts of qi or prana, representing universal energy or life force, are one example, but other concepts, such as yin and yang, vatta, kapha, and pita, also illustrate the complexity of analyzing concepts that do not have equivocal biomedical definitions. And the third challenge is that outcomes in traditional Chinese medicine and Ayurvedic medicine are determined largely by empirical, rather than experimental, diagnostic measures. Changes in a person's tongue coat and pulse or a change in symptoms often are enough to satisfy clinical management and evaluate the efficacy of an herbal formula.

Diabetes mellitus type 2 can serve as an example of the fundamental differences between these systems in disease diagnostic and treatment criteria. In biomedicine, diabetes is seen as a specific set of characteristics and laboratory markers. A fasting blood glucose of less than 126 mg/dL on more than one occasion would validate a diagnosis of this disease (Joslin Diabetes Center, 2007). In Oriental medicine, diabetes is comprised of seven possible patterns, none of which would be called "diabetes" and each of which would have a different parameter for the selection of an herbal treatment (Flaws & Lake, 2005).

In traditional CAM modalities, herbs are prescribed based on the phenotypical manifestation of the disease and the constitutional expression of the patient. This is in direct opposition to the drug model of herbal prescription currently being used in biomedicine. This model is based solely on the pharmacological understanding that relies, "perhaps erroneously, on a preference for empirical evidence gained from controlled clinical trials regardless of the underlying theory of disease and healing" (Tonelli & Callahan, 2001). The drug-based model of herbal medicine is a reductionist view, and it purposely ignores thousands of years of observational and empirical evidence that has been validated within many traditional medical models.

In a review of 19 randomized controlled trials that utilized ginseng, the authors found no mention or consideration of the traditional patterns used in TCM to determine appropriateness of herb selection (Yan, Engle, He, Jiao, & Gu, 2009). Ginseng, specifically *Panax ginseng*, or Ren Shen, is an herb traditionally used to support specific symptom manifestations of "qi deficiency," which is characterized by symptoms like fatigue, gas or bloating and loose stools, weakness, cold, sweating, bleeding, and prolapsed organs (Kaptchuk, 2000). In addition, several of the 19 trials utilized a different species of ginseng, which traditionally have different properties and applications. Analyzing the results as if looking through the lens of Oriental medicine theory, the reviewer found that positive results of ginseng were seen only in the conditions that corresponded to the traditional Chinese concept of qi deficiency. This demonstrated that biomedical evidence-based research, directed by traditional theory, may have a totally different outcome. Research that can employ these concepts can both improve study design and help validate traditional theory within a biomedical context.

Another challenge in herbal therapy is the use of polyherbal formulations common to traditional medical systems. Using the same type of analysis as just mentioned for a single herb, the criteria for evaluating a polyherbal formula would have to take into account numerous factors based on the traditional medicine model. Thus, patients who just want to take an herbal formula for a particular problem without the assistance of a trained herbalist are faced with the ongoing dilemma of deciding what herbal remedy(ies) are best suited for them.

COMMON HERBS

Today it is possible to find a health section with a variety of herbal remedies in most grocery or supplement stores in communities throughout the United States. These remedies are available without prescription or any particular guidance except what the consumer may gather from the label or other sources that may or may not be reliable. Therefore, it is very important that nurse practitioners, nurses, and other health professionals be aware of herbal therapy and be able to distinguish how they are to be used. For the purposes of this chapter, herbal therapy for a particular disease state will be discussed in three primary categories: Western, traditional Chinese medicine (TCM), and Ayurvedic medicine, along with the criteria for dispensing.

There are several other medicinal practices that use herbs to heal, for example, homeopathic herbal therapy, Bach Flower remedies, and Unani medicine. However, the purpose here is not to teach any particular style of herbal medicine but rather to use examples from TCM and Ayurvedic medicine to illustrate the differences in how herbal therapy is used and to encourage practitioners interested in using or recommending these herbs to understand the differences in order to refer to or consult with an herbalist, naturopath, TCM, or Ayurvedic practitioner whenever herbal therapy is considered. This section is not meant as a recommendation for prescribing to clients but rather as a guideline and reference.

Western Herbs

Mental Health Symptoms

The most common symptoms for which people use herbs are anxiety, difficulty in sleeping, depression or dysphoria, and forgetfulness and confusion. Like pharmaceutical drugs, some herbs may be beneficial for multiple symptoms.

Anxiety

Kava (ava, awa, kava-kava, kawa, kew, tonga) comes from the dried root of *Piper methysticum*, a member of the black pepper family. This shrub is native to the Pacific Islands and is commonly used by Hawaiians as a celebratory drink, just as alcohol is used in the West. But unlike alcohol, kava does not stimulate aggression and is not associated with hangovers. It is prepared as a drink from the pulverized root but also comes in tablet, capsule, and extract forms. This herb has been studied in human subjects and appears to have more than one active component that produces its effects. One component acts as a local anesthetic when chewed and produces intense muscle relaxation. It appears to act on the limbic system to suppress emotional excitability and produce mild euphoria without affecting memory or cognition. In therapeutic drug trials, kava seems to act on the gamma-amino butyric acid (GABA) receptor, like the benzodiazepines, and like the benzodiazepines, kava can reduce seizure activity and be used for sedation. Dose varies, depending on the form and the amount of active components retained in the preparation; studies indicate that 70 to 240 mg daily is the adult dose. Pharmacokinetics data are unavailable for kava, but users seem to prefer divided doses, usually 3 times a day. Unlike the benzodiazepines, it does not seem to produce dependence, but the studies are very limited.

When used short-term, kava seems to produce few adverse reactions, although these might include decreased motor reflexes, diminished judgment, and visual disturbances. Chronic use may decrease platelet count and cause dry, flaky skin; reddened eyes; shortness of breath; pulmonary hypertension; and weight loss. Because it seems to act like the benzodiazepines, it may potentiate alcohol, other sedatives, and GABA-nergic drugs such as phenobarbital and benzodiazepines. At higher doses, kava seems to block dopamine receptors and therefore to improve psychotic levels of anxiety as well as interact with antipsychotic drugs. It should not be used in pregnancy or when breastfeeding because its safety is uncertain during pregnancy (Volz, 1997). The FDA has issued a warning regarding the use of kava supplements leading to severe liver damage and the National Institute of Health National Center for Complementary and Alternative (NCCAM) suspended all NCCAM-funded studies of kava after the FDA warning (nccam.nih.gov/health/kava).

Mugwort (felon herb, wild wormwood, St. John's plant) comes from the root of the *Artemisia vulgaris* plant. It should not be confused with St. John's wort, which comes from a different plant. The name may have derived from the fact that it was commonly used to flavor beer before the use of hops. It is available as dried leaves and roots, fluid extract, tincture, or as a tea infusion, but only the root is used for its active constituents, which are believed to be from its volatile oil and acrid resin and tannins. It is a very versatile herb but its medicinal use lies more in its value as a nervine and emmenagogue (hastening menstrual flow when combined with pennyroyal and southernwood). When taken for anxiety and sedation, the usual dose is 5 mL of tincture 30 minutes before bedtime, although there are few studies that support this use. It does have an anticholinergic effect, observed in animal studies. In a recent study of mugwort, elements of alkaloids, coumarins, flavonoids, saponins, sterols, tannins, and terpenes were found with concentration-dependent (0.3 to 10 mg/mL) relaxation of spontaneous jejunum contractions, and a combination of anticholinergic and Ca(2+) antagonist mechanisms were found supporting its use in hyperactive gut and airway disorders, such as abdominal colic, diarrhea, and asthma (Khan & Gilani, 2009). This accounts for its use in the treatment of gastrointestinal problems and menstrual cramps.

One of the unique uses of mugwort comes from TCM, where it is applied topically and burned to treat pain and tonify deficient conditions. It is also used extensively in Japanese acupuncture as well as TCM, comes in several different forms, and is employed in a variety of ways (e.g., as a stick, directly on the skin, or by using a medium—holder, box, ginger—to hold it over acupuncture points or pain locations with or without needles). Adverse reactions to mugwort when taken internally include anaphylaxis and induction of premature birth or miscarriage or contact dermatitis if used topically. It should not be used during pregnancy or breastfeeding or by people who have clotting abnormalities or allergies to hazelnuts. Because there are no controlled studies on mugwort, no therapeutic claims can be made.

Passionflower (*Passiflora*, passion vines) has been used by many cultures as an herbal remedy for the treatment of anxiety. However, there are over 500 species of this flowering plant, which makes clinical trials inconsistent because they use different species. Two of the most common species used today are *P. incamata* (maypop), commonly used in Native American cultures, and *P. edulis* (passion fruit), used extensively in Central and South America. Despite the different species, passionflower is generally considered safe but it can cause drowsiness, dizziness, and confusion in some patients. As a dried herb, passionflower is generally well tolerated at 2 g, 3 to 4 times a day, and as an infusion of 2 g in 150 cc water 3 to 4 times a day. The tincture ratio is 1:5 (g/mL).

Insomnia

In addition to mugwort, melatonin, valerian, passionflower, and chamomile are used for sedation. Melatonin and valerian are discussed here. Melatonin is not an herb but a hormone produced by the pineal gland. Because it is a hormone, exogenous consumption over extended periods of time may act as negative feedback and suppress normally secreted melatonin. Melatonin is produced when serotonin is broken down in the pineal gland with the help of two enzymes: arylakylamine-N-acetyl transferase (AA-NAT) and hydroxyindole-O-methyl transerase (HIOMT). It is the AA-NAT that seems to be the rhythm enzyme, because when it is elevated, melatonin is elevated. Unfortunately, AA-NAT is rapidly destroyed and the production of melatonin is reduced by light.

Under physiological conditions, melatonin is released during the fourth stage of sleep along with prolactin and growth hormone. It is used to induce sleep via the same GABA-nergic mechanism as benzodiazepine sedatives and is widely used to prevent and treat jet lag. A single study identified the utility of melatonin in elderly people to help induce and maintain sleep, probably because the elderly usually have some degree of melatonin deficiency under normal circumstances. Used long-term, it can increase prolactin secretion, which can decrease luteinizing hormone, progesterone, and estradiol levels. Long-term use can also reset the sleep-wake cycle and contribute to disturbed sleep cycling.

Melatonin is available in tablets, capsules, extended-release capsules, and liquid forms. For difficulty in getting to sleep, 1 to 5 mg taken at bedtime is the usual dosage, but it should not be used more than three nights a week. In the elderly, the dosage is usually 1 to 2 mg taken 2 hours before bedtime. To prevent jet lag melatonin (2 mg to 5 mg) is taken at the target destination bedtime (10 PM to midnight) for 3 days prior to departure and for three days' post-travel (Morgenthaller et al., 2007). Adverse reactions include altered sleep patterns, confusion, headache, tachycardia, and hypothermia. Melatonin potentiates benzodiazepines. It also potentiates succinylcholine, thereby increasing the blocking action, which can be dangerous. Its content of active drug may vary widely in commercial melatonin, making it difficult to determine correct dosages (Brzezinski, 1997; Fetrow & Avila, 1999).

Valerian (all-heal, amantilla, setewale capon's tail, herba benedicta) is derived from the roots of *Valeriana officinalis*. It seems to inhibit uptake and increase presynaptic release of GABA; however, it is not readily absorbed, is highly unstable, and readily decomposes. Therefore, availability of the active drug is minimal when it is taken orally. German Commission E suggests valerian root for anxiety, restlessness, and difficulty in getting to sleep. Because of the instability, dosages are difficult to determine, especially among different brands. Usually 400 to 900 mg of extract at bedtime or 1 teaspoon of dried herb in tea several times a day is useful in inducing sleep. Commercial valerian tea at bedtime acts more as a relaxant and permits the person to fall asleep spontaneously. Valerian has no adverse reactions when used at the recommended level; however, overdosage at 2.5 g or more can cause cardiac disturbance, excitability, headache, insomnia, and nausea. It can potentiate alcohol and other CNS depressants if taken in large amounts. Because clinical trial studies are limited, it should not be used by pregnant or breastfeeding women, children, or patients with impaired liver function.

Depression

The popular media have touted the benefits of St. John's wort for depression, contributing to its great popularity. Kava, mugwort, and DHEA have also been used to treat mild depression. Because kava and mugwort have already been discussed, St. John's wort and DHEA are covered here.

St. John's wort is obtained from the tops and flowers of the *Hypericum perforatum* plant, which is common all over Europe, Asia, and the United States. The exact mechanism of action is still unknown but assumed to be related to inhibition of serotonin presynaptic uptake. Early studies showed inhibition of monamine oxidase (MAO) type A and minimally type B; however, this was later attributed to contaminants. In studies to determine effective dosages, St. John's wort was effective at blocking serotonin reuptake at much higher doses than could be achieved. St. John's wort also seems to act on the benzodiazepine receptor of GABA, inhibit norepinephrine reuptake, and block acetylcholine, as well as inhibit stress-induced corticotropin-releasing hormone, adrenocorticotropic hormone (ACTH), and cortisol and increase nighttime release of melatonin. Some reports have also indicated antiviral activity, including retroviruses (Chavez, 1997). With such a wide range of receptor activity, it is not surprising that it is used to treat depression, enuresis, gastritis, hypothyroidism, insomnia, kidney disorders, scabies, hemorrhoids, wounds, HIV infection, and Kaposi's sarcoma.

Most commonly, St. John's wort is used to relieve mild to moderate depression, less than would meet the criteria for a major depressive episode, or dysthymia. Therefore, it seems most effective for those who have sadness and lesser degrees of depression. When used for clinically diagnosed depression, St. John's wort is relatively ineffective and may dishearten or demoralize the person who is trying to avoid using more potent antidepressants. For standardized, commercially prepared St. John's wort, the usual dosage is 300 mg taken 3 times daily; because of the delayed neuroreceptor response, it may take 4 to 6 weeks to determine effectiveness. When St. John's wort is used as a tea, it requires 2 to 4 g of tea steeped in 1 to 2 cups of boiling water for 10 minutes and taken daily to be effective within 4 to 6 weeks.

There are a few adverse reactions, attributable to the anticholinergic blockade, including constipation, dry mouth, dizziness, gastrointestinal (GI) upset, restlessness, and insomnia. St. John's wort interacts with MAO inhibitors (MAOIs), tricyclic antidepressants, and serotonin reuptake inhibitors (SRIs) to cause serotonin syndrome. St. John's wort may decrease digoxin, phenytoin, and cyclosporine levels leading to therapeutic failure. Wafarin's effectiveness may be decreased. St. John's wort may lead to loss of virologic response and possible resistance to indinavir and other protease inhibitors. St. John's wort should be stopped 2 weeks prior to the beginning of treatment with the chemotherapy agent irinotecan and is contraindicated during therapy. St. John's wort reduces the effectiveness of oral contraceptives, increasing the risk of unintended pregnancy. Because there are inadequate studies available, St. John's wort should not be taken by children or pregnant or breastfeeding women. The primary care provider who determines that the patient meets the *Diagnostic and Statistical Manual of Mental Disorders, Fifth Edition* (2013) criteria for depression might advise the client to consider taking another kind of antidepressant if there are minimal results in 3 to 4 weeks.

Dehydroepiandrosterone (DHEA) is a steroid precursor found in plants from the yam family and is secreted by primate adrenal glands. Physiologically, DHEA is converted into androgens and estrogens (depending on the person's gender) and may raise the blood level of a precursor of the human growth hormone. There are many benefits attributed to DHEA, including immune enhancement and prevention of osteoporosis as well as antineoplastic, antiaging, and antidepressant benefits. Because few studies on humans are available, exact pharmacokinetics and pharmacodynamics are not known, but it does not seem to be readily absorbed through the GI tract. Similarly, it is difficult to determine dosage for the particular effect that is desired. At present, 50 mg daily is commonly used for depression, but serum levels should be checked, with an expected level of 3,600 ng/mL for men and 3,000 ng/mL for women. When used for depression, DHEA may have a 4-week lag time before an effect on depression is seen (Wolkowitz, 1997).

Because DHEA is a hormone-like drug, it may give negative feedback to the adrenal glands, thereby reducing production of endogenous hormones. Adverse reactions to be expected with an androsteroid include aggressiveness, hirsutism, insomnia, and irritability. Patients with hormone-sensitive cancers should be discouraged from using DHEA, as should pregnant and breastfeeding women. DHEA is likely to interact with other hormone therapy, such as estrogen replacement therapy. DHEA may be used by athletes to increase muscle mass, but it is a banned substance in college athletes by the National Collegiate Athletic Association (NCAA).

Confusion and Forgetfulness

Confusion and forgetfulness, along with other cognitive impairments, are often seen in dementia, depending on the root cause of the dementia. Additionally, people who are concerned about benign forgetfulness take herbs both to improve their cognitive abilities and to prevent memory problems. Common herbs used include ginkgo, ginseng, chaparral, and galanthamine. Ginseng and ginkgo, which are often taken together or combined in a single preparation, are used here as exemplars.

Ginseng (American ginseng, Asian ginseng, Chinese ginseng, five-fingers, Japanese ginseng, Jintsam, Korean ginseng, ninjin, seng and sang, schinsent) is from the *Panax quinquefolius* plant, especially the root. Asian ginseng should not be confused with Siberian ginseng, which seems to bind with estrogen receptors. Asian ginseng is usually dried or cured and is highly valued; American ginseng undergoes less processing and is not as widely sought.

Several compounds are biologically active, producing different effects. The mechanisms of action are not understood, but ginseng is said to have differing effects depending on the active component involved: anticonvulsant, analgesic, and antipsychotic effects; CNS-stimulating, anti-fatigue, hypertensive, and stress ulcer exacerbation; improvement of cardiac function; depression of cardiac function; antiarrhythmic activity; reduction of cholesterol and triglycerides; decrease in platelet adhesiveness; impaired coagulation; and increased fibrinolysis. The presumed focus of action is in the adrenal gland, although there are claims in popular literature that ginseng decreases thymus gland activity. Consequently, it is used as a sedative, aphrodisiac, antidepressant, hypnotic, and diuretic. It is also used to improve stress resistance, stamina, work efficiency, concentration, mental performance, and general feelings of well-being. Some studies found it decreased fasting blood sugar and hemoglobin to such a degree that some diabetics no longer needed insulin.

Ginseng comes in capsules, tea bags, and extract, and in some places ginseng root can be bought in bulk, such as in Asian markets. In processed form, however, it is difficult to standardize. Used for illness, it is usually taken at 0.5 to 2 g a day of dry root or 200 to 600 mg of extract daily in divided doses. For dementia in frail elderly people, it is usually taken at 0.4 to 0.8 g of dry root daily. There seems to be a lag time in achieving maximum effectiveness—up to 90 days to see full results. It seems to have minimal and mild adverse reactions, including dizziness, drowsiness, headache, and insomnia, although chest pain, diarrhea, hypertension, impotence, nervousness, agitation, palpitations, nausea, and vomiting have also been reported. It may potentiate insulin and oral hypoglycemics, and it interacts with MAOIs to cause headaches, tremors, and mania. There are more studies of ginseng than of other herbs to identify its effectiveness, yet the pharmacodynamics are elusive. The German Commission E considers ginseng to be an effective drug (Sorensen & Sonne, 1996; Wesnes et al, 1997).

Ginkgo (*Ginkgo biloba*) is an extract from the leaves of the ginkgo tree, with the toxic ginkgolic acid removed. It is available in many forms, including tablets, capsules, sublingual sprays, and even in juices and foods. It is believed to stimulate prostaglandin synthesis and thereby cause vasodilatation, increasing tissue perfusion and cerebral blood flow. Ginkgo has been used for centuries in Asian countries to improve mental alertness, and today is used in the treatment of cerebrovascular disease and peripheral vascular disease. Additionally, it is popularly taken to improve thinking ability, concentration, and memory.

Dosage for confusion and dementia symptoms is 120 to 240 mg daily in two or three divided doses. For vascular disease, 120 to 320 mg daily has been used, but there is a 4- to 6-week lag time before maximum effect is obtained. Adverse reactions include diarrhea, headache, nausea, vomiting, bruising, excessive bleeding, and seizures in overdose. Trying to use ginkgo leaves to make a home remedy is potentially dangerous because of the ginkgolic acid and the difficulty of determining the quantity of active ingredients. Because it reduces platelet-activating factor and erythrocyte aggregation, it should not be taken with anticoagulants or antiplatelet medications. The German Commission E approved ginkgo for the treatment of dementia and peripheral arterial occlusive disease (Fetrow & Avila, 1999).

Gastrointestinal Problems

Probably the most common use of home remedies is for GI upset, such as constipation, diarrhea, indigestion, and nausea. Because the underlying causes of these complaints are also common, the herbal medications used for them overlap. The herbs most often used for constipation are also incorporated into commercial OTC medications: cascara, castor bean, and senna.

Cascara sagrada is dried bark from the *Rhamnus purshiana* tree (found primarily in the Pacific Northwest and from Canada to California) that has been dried and aged for at least 1 year and up to 3 years. Cascara acts by increasing the smooth muscle tone of the large intestine and thus peristalsis. The FDA has approved cascara as a safe and effective laxative to be sold OTC. It is available in an extract or extract capsules. Although it is very safe, it may produce such adverse reactions as abdominal cramping, diarrhea, fluid and electrolyte imbalance, steatorrhea, vomiting, and vitamin and mineral deficiencies in long-term use. Cascara can be used in pregnancy but should not be used by breastfeeding women because it is excreted in milk and may cause serious diarrhea in the infant. Because a person can become dependent on cascara, it should be limited to short-term use.

Senna comes from the leaves and pods of the *Cassia* shrub. It is the active ingredient in OTC medications such as Senokot, Senokot-S, and Senolax and comes in capsules, tablets, and syrup. Dried senna leaves can also be made into a tea by adding 100 g of leaves to a liter of boiling water and steeping for 10 minutes. Sliced ginger or crushed coriander leaves make the tea more palatable. When senna enters the intestinal tract, bacteria convert it into a biologically active agent. Senna increases peristaltic action in the lower bowel. The usual adult dosage is about 340 mg taken at bedtime or 0.5 to 1 dram of syrup. Adverse reactions are similar to those of cascara: abdominal cramping, diarrhea, hypokalemia, and clubbing of the fingers with chronic use. Calcium channel blockers or indomethacin blocks the diarrheal effects. It is excreted in breast milk and should not be taken by breastfeeding woman. A patient with irritable bowel, hemorrhoids, GI inflammatory conditions, or prolapsed rectum should not use senna. Like cascara, it can be overused and create a laxative dependency.

Indigestion and heartburn plague Americans, as evidenced by the large amounts of medications sold to treat dyspepsia. In addition to antacids, common household herbs can be used effectively and safely. Caraway oil distilled from dried seeds of the *Carum carvi* herb or caraway water made from soaking 1 oz of crushed caraway seeds in a pint of cold water for 6 hours can be used for indigestion, flatulence, constipation, and menstrual cramps. Because of its mild action, it can be given to infants for colic. The usual dosage for adults is 1 to 4 drops of oil in a teaspoon of sweetened water; and for infants 1 to 3 tsp of caraway water. The only adverse reactions reported are diarrhea and mucous membrane irritation.

Licorice root has also been used for gastric irritation and dyspepsia. Licorice comes from the dried root of the *Glycyrrhiza glabra* shrub and is available in capsules, tablets, liquid extracts, chewing gum, tea, and candy. Studies indicate that glycyrrhetic acid is the active element that potentiates endogenous steroids and stimulates gastric mucus synthesis. It is a soothing and mild expectorant, mild laxative, and antispasmodic. Additionally, licorice has antiarrhythmic effects, lowers cholesterol and triglyceride levels, and may cause immunosuppression. The usual dose is 200 to 600 mg tablets taken daily for 4 to 6 weeks or licorice tea simmered for 5 minutes and taken 3 times a day after eating. Reported adverse reactions include mineralocorticoid effects of headache, lethargy, sodium and water retention, hypokalemia, and hypertension, as well as, in overdose, muscle weakness, heart failure, and cardiac arrest.

Licorice interacts with many medications: antihypertensives, diuretics, corticosteroids, digoxin, loratadine, procainamide, quinidine, and spironolactone. A patient who is taking licorice regularly should be warned against excessive and chronic use, especially when it is combined with diuretics. Licorice candy does not actually contain the herb but rather licorice flavoring, usually from anise oil.

Papaya enzymes, available in tablets and chewable tablets, are frequently used to prevent or treat common heartburn, although it is not effective with gastroesophageal reflux. Papaya is a proteolytic enzyme in the leaves, seeds, pulp, and latex of the *Carica papaya* tree. The clinical trials with humans have mostly focused on treating inflammation from trauma and surgery. It also has been used effectively as a debriding agent and for intradisk injections in patients with herniated disks. The dosage for inflammation is 10 mg 4 times a day for 1 week. Dosage for dyspepsia is variable and not standardized, but usually 4 to 5 tablets are taken immediately after eating. Adverse reactions are uncommon and limited to dermatitis, hypersensitivity, decreased heart rate and CNS activity, and perforation of the esophagus with excessive ingestion. No drug interactions have been reported. There have been no studies with pregnant and breastfeeding women, so it is safest to avoid use during pregnancy and breastfeeding.

Pain

Joint pain, soft tissue pain, and headache are frequent problems that people often treat with herbal and home remedies. There is little overlap in medications to treat each of these kinds of pain. Two products currently in health food stores are glucosamine and chondroitin, both of which are not herbal.

Glucosamine has been widely used for its anti-inflammatory and cartilage repair ability and is supported by in-vitro studies in the management of osteoarthritis. Glucosamine is thought to stimulate cartilage production and enhance rebuilding of damaged cartilage and has been demonstrated to provide relief of pain and rapid restoration of mobility and range of motion. There are two forms of glucosamine currently being sold as an herbal supplement: glucosamine sulfate (GS) and glucosamine HCL (GH). Both contain similar or equal concentrations of glucosamine, but GS has more salt content and GH has slightly higher concentrations of glucosamine. Although the effects are similar, glucosamine sulfate has been used in the majority of clinical trials; glucosamine HCL is often combined with other materials like chondroitin or MSM.

Glucosamine is a naturally occurring component found in shellfish; however, most of what is sold in the United States is synthetically made. It is sold under such names as Arth-X Plus, Glucosamine Mega, Joint Factors, and Nutri-Joint, in capsules or tablets in a range of dosages, so the upper limit advised is 1.5 g per day and the source an organic natural product. It has very few side effects and there is only rare occurrence of symptoms like constipation, diarrhea, drowsiness, headache, heartburn, nausea, and rash. There have been no drug interactions reported. Frequently, glucosamine is combined with chondroitin for greater efficacy.

Chondroitin is extracted from the cartilage of animals, often cows and pigs. It seems to stimulate chondrocyte metabolism and synthesis of collagen, improving the formation of cartilage. Other studies identified stimulation of hyaluronic acid in synovial cells in patients with rheumatic disease, resulting in increased viscosity and amount of synovial fluid. When it was used for up to 4 months, patients used much less pain medication and were doing weight-bearing exercises comfortably. Often combined with glucosamine, the dosage depends on the patient's weight: for patients under 120 lb, the recommended dosage is 1,000 mg of glucosamine and 800 mg of chondroitin; for patients 120 to 200 lb, the dosage is 1,500 mg of glucosamine and 1,200 mg of chondroitin. Used alone, the usual dose is 800 to 1,200 mg daily, taken in either divided doses or a single dose. Adverse reactions include dyspepsia, headache, motor restlessness, euphoria, nausea, and risk of internal bleeding. Chondroitin may potentiate anticoagulants. Because there have been no studies with pregnant or breastfeeding women, chondroitin should not be used by this population.

Tumeric (curcumin) is a rhizome from the ginger family, commonly used as a spice in Indian curry. It has been used for 2,000 years to treat conditions of inflammation, particularly in the gastrointestinal system. However, today turmeric is being used extensively for the treatment of chronic pain. Tumeric in food is considered safe but may come in many forms, most commonly as a standardized powder in which the recommended doses range from 400 to 600 mg, 3 times a day. Tumeric is often combined with bromelain or piper longum (black pepper) to increase its absorption from the GI tract. However, caution is advised when tumeric is combined with these agents due to their potential secondary risk of gastritis and increased absorption of other medications.

Wintergreen oil and liniments have been deemed effective in relieving pain from muscle strains, inflamed muscles, ligaments, and joints. Usually the oil is a combination of oil extracted from the leaves and bark of *Gaultheria procumbens* and methyl salicylate. Although there have been no studies of the efficacy of wintergreen, it is assumed to act through counterirritation, which masks pain, or through the analgesic and anti-inflammatory effects of the salicylate. The 10% wintergreen oil is applied to the skin no more often than 3 to 4 times a day. Overgenerous application can result in salicylate poisoning from absorption into the bloodstream. People who are allergic to aspirin or who are taking oral anticoagulants should not use it.

Feverfew is an interesting herb used most often to treat headache and migraines. It has also been used for toothache, joint pain, asthma, stomachache, menstrual problems, and threatening miscarriage. Feverfew (bachelors' button, featherfoil, Santa Maria, midsummer daisy) is extracted from the leaves of the feverfew plant, *Chrysanthemum parthenium*. The assumed mechanism of action is the inhibition of serotonin release from platelets. It is available in capsules, liquid, tablets, and dried leaves for tea. The feverfew research showed a decrease in the number, duration, and severity of migraines in a double-blind crossover study (Murphy, Hepinstall, & Mitchell, 1988). The average daily dose for the treatment of migraines was 543 mcg of parthenolide (the active component of feverfew); for migraine prevention, the dose was 25 mg daily of freeze-dried leaf extract. The most common adverse reactions were mouth ulcerations, hypersensitivity, and a withdrawal syndrome characterized by moderate to severe pain and joint and muscle stiffness.

Traditional Chinese Herbs

It is important to remember that traditional Chinese medicine does not isolate herbal medicine as the single remedy for any disorder but rather includes it as a part of four distinct methods of treatment that include herbal therapy, acupuncture, manipulative therapies (tui na), food, and exercise (qi-gong and tai chi). The application of herbs specifically is based on the nature and capabilities of the herb and the energies, flavors, movement, and meridian the herb affects.

The Four Energies

The four energies in herbal medicine are cold, hot, warm, and cool. The concept was derived from years of empirical research and observation of the direct effect of taking the herb over time. If the herb is effective in the treatment of a heat condition per se, it is classified as having a cooling energy. In the most basic sense herbs can be divided into yin (cooling) and yang (heating) energies. But since temperature can be a matter of interpretation, many TCM practitioners will refer to the herbal energy as extremely warm or slightly warm and extremely cold or slightly cold.

The Five Flavors

The five flavors refer to the effect the herb has on a person's sense of taste and are classified as pungent (or acrid), sweet, sour, bitter, and salty. Not only do the five flavors describe taste, they also exhibit properties that are medically useful. Pungent herbs can disperse and promote the flow of energy; sour herbs can constrict and obstruct; sweet herbs can slow down, tone up, and harmonize; bitter herbs can harden, dry up, and cause diarrhea; and salty herbs can soften up and promote downward movement. Often a question arises about things that are tasteless. Tasteless is still considered a flavor and tends to be classified with sweet; it can help disperse dampness and promote urination.

The Four Movements

The four movements of herbs are upward, downward, floating, and sinking. Pushing upward means that the herb has the capacity of lifting that which can no longer be supported, for example, prolapsed organs like the uterus or rectum. Pushing downward means the herb is capable of suppressing a rebellious symptom, for example, hiccups or a cough. Floating means the herb is capable of dispersing outward, as in inducing perspiration or a purging action. And sinking means the herb is capable of promoting diarrhea and directing excess energy down. Often the movement of an herb is a combination. Herbs that push upward and those that can float have the common function of moving upward and outward, by inducing perspiration and vomiting and elevating the yang energy. While the herbs that can push downward and those that can sink have the common function of moving downward and inward and relieving symptoms like vomiting or excess perspiration or diarrhea.

Meridian Routes

Meridian routes refer to the meridians the herb can enter and move through (or pathways of energy identified in TCM that correspond to the 12 organ systems). This is important to know because two herbs with the same energy and flavor can display two different actions because their meridian routes are different (e.g., two heating herbs may have different actions—one may be better for cold lung conditions while the other may work better for cold spleen conditions).

Actions

All Chinese herbs or herbal formulas have a number of common actions, but the actions are expressed differently than in Western medication. A Western medication will be classified as an antihistamine because it blocks the effects of histamine, but a Chinese herb will be classified by its action to clear heat, stop wind, or reduce fire. And a formula will have multiple actions that are designed specifically for the patient's condition; for example, one herb will clear lung heat, the other may

transform phlegm, and another cool blood. In this way, the formula can be changed as the patient's symptoms change. This is one argument against the prolific use of standardized formulas.

Herbal Formulas

In most cases, a syndrome will have more than one symptom and cannot be treated with a single herb. Thus, the primary method of herbal therapy used in TCM is the herbal formula. Although many practitioners will use their own formulas to treat patients, most will use established classic formulas with one or two modifications. The general format for herbal formulas is the use of three or more specific herbs. The primary herb that treats the major symptom is called the king herb; the second herb, called the subject herb, will reinforce the action of the king herb as well as treat the concurrent symptoms. Then there are herbs that are added to control undesirable effects of the first two, called the assistant herb; and the fourth herb, called the servant herb, may be one that can direct the formula to the affected region and harmonize the herbs in the formula.

How to Take Chinese Herbs

There are three common ways to taking TCM formulas. A decoction is considered the best method, although it is often not practical for many patients. Decoctions are made from raw herbs that are placed in a pot of water and cooked/boiled for an average of 20 minutes. The benefit of a decoction is that it is readily absorbed, takes effect more quickly, and can produce the best therapeutic effect. The second method of taking herbs is in the form of powders or granules, which can be dissolved in water. The quantity will depend on a patient's weight. The disadvantage of a powder is similar to that of most powdered drinks: they are difficult to dissolve completely and absorption is slower. The third and most common method of taking herbs is by tablet, normally prepared by a manufacturer. The advantage of tablets is the ease of taking the medication and convenience, but they have slow absorption rates, cannot be adjusted, and their quality depends on the manufacturing process.

Rules for Taking a Formula

In general, there are three rules for taking Chinese herbal formulas. The first is timing. To get the most effect from an herbal formula it is very important to know when and how to take the herb. Some herbs are better absorbed with food while others without. In addition, in accordance with TCM theory, there are certain times of the day when the energy of a certain organ system is higher. Depending on the action of the herb, and the organ condition, taking the herb during these times will improve the effect the herb has on the organ. The second rule is that temperature should be considered, depending on the condition being treated. If treating a cold condition, the temperature of the herbal formula should be hot; and if treating a heat condition, the herb may best be taken cold. The last rule is to refrain from taking herbal formulas with tea. Tea can obstruct the movement of the herb and reduce its effect. Tea is also cold in nature and can interfere with warming herbs. And third, tea contains caffeine and can excite the nervous system, cancelling the effect of calming herbs.

⬤ CLINICAL PEARL ⬤

TCM diagnosis

Although this text does not cover TCM diagnosis or an explanation of the disorder mentioned (e.g., spleen deficiency, heart fire, etc.), the general purpose of including the differential diagnosis is to demonstrate how diverse TCM diagnosis is and how it applies to the choice of herbal medicine prescribed. Please refer to TCM textbooks to further understand TCM diagnosis.

Insomnia

Depending on the source, according to TCM insomnia can be caused by several conditions; heart–spleen deficiency, heart–kidney disconnect, heart–gallbladder deficiency, phlegm fire, or just indigestion from eating too late in the evening. To illustrate the rationale behind the selection of an herbal formula and how each ingredient can be modified (added or removed) depending on the patient's clinical presentation, one of these differential diagnoses (heart–spleen deficiency) is presented here.

Heart–Spleen Deficiency

In TCM, insomnia is often associated with the heart because it is considered to be the place where the mind (shen) resides. And disturbances of the shen often result in the symptom of insomnia. Symptoms of a heart–spleen deficiency include sleeplessness and waking often, abdominal swelling, watery thin stools, low appetite, fatigue, impotence, night sweats, and palpitations. The treatment principle is to tone the heart and spleen and calm the mind.

Herbal Formula for Insomnia

Gui-Pi-Tang (restore the spleen decoction) is used for spleen qi deficiency with heart blood and yin deficiency, to tonify qi and blood, and to nourish the heart and strengthen the spleen. Therefore, the indications for its use are similar to those for heart–spleen deficiency: fatigue, palpitations, insomnia, poor sleep or dream-disturbed sleep, night sweats, but also anxiety, phobias, poor appetite, sallow complexion, poor memory, withdrawal, and early periods with loss of excess blood, continuous spotting, blood in the stool, and metrorrhagia.

Gui Pi Tang Ingredients

- Bai Zhu (*Rhizoma atractylodis macrocephalae*): 5 to 10 g; properties: aromatic, slightly acrid, nontoxic, sweet and warm; supplements the spleen and qi; dries dampness; enters the spleen and stomach channels; used in the treatment of indigestion and stomach disorders.
- Dang gui (*Angelica sinensis*): 12 g; properties: warm, bitter, sweet, slightly pungent; supports the liver and spleen; used as a tonic for female deficiencies and to enrich blood, promote circulation, stimulate appetite, improve muscle tone, stimulate the immune system, and moisturize dryness.
- Fu-shen (*Poria cocos*, a mushroom): 12 g; properties: sweet taste; used to calm the liver and heart and quiet the spirit; enters the heart, spleen, and lung channel; used for palpitations, fearfulness, and bad memory due to a frightful experience; considered a superb yin tonic.
- Gan cao (*Radix glycyrrhizae* or licorice root): 6 g; properties: sweet, neutral; tonifies the spleen and strengthens the qi, improving symptoms like fatigue, lack of appetite, loose stools, and shortness of breath; enters all 12 primary channels but particularly the lung, heart, spleen, and stomach; used to lessen the harsh and toxic nature of other herbs and protect the middle jiao (the primary source of digestion) and enhance the overall effects of a formula; often used with honey to treat drug poisoning or Xing Ren (*Semen armeniacaae amarum*) for lead poisoning.
- Huang qi (*Radix astragali membranacei* or *astragalus*): 20 g; properties: sweet, slightly warm; enters the lung and spleen channels; tonifies qi and blood; used to treat symptoms of spleen deficiency, can raise yang, tonify the wei qi (protective qi), treat spontaneous sweating, promote urination, and expel pus.
- Long yan rou (*Arillus euphoriae longanae* or flesh of the longan fruit, translated as "dragon eye flesh"): 15 g; properties: sweet and warm; enters the heart and spleen channel; actions are primarily to tonify the blood.
- Suan zao ren (*Ziziphus jujuba*, commonly called sour jujube seed): 10 to 18 g or 1.5 to 3 g in powder at bedtime; properties: the temperature and taste are neutral, sweet, and sour; supports several channels (gallbladder, heart, liver, spleen) and nourishes heart yin and blood, calms the spirit, and inhibits sweating; used to treat insomnia, irritability, dream-disturbed sleep due to yin and blood deficiency, as well as wind-damp bi syndrome, and wind-heat skin rashes/and itching and also given as a nourishing sedative.
- Yuan Zhi (*Radix polygalae tenuifoliae* or Chinese senega root): 6 g; properties: bitter, spicy, slightly warm; enters the heart, lung, and liver channels; used to nourish the heart and calm the shen.

The following are some of the single herbs that can be added to the formula:

- Bai zi ren (*Biota orientalis*, commonly called arbor vitae seed): 10 to 18 g every day; properties: the temperature and taste are neutral and sweet; supports several channels (heart, kidney, large intestine, and spleen) and is therefore used to nourish the heart, calm the spirit, as well as moisten the intestine and unblock the bowels; indications for its use include the treatment of insomnia/irritability/palpitations/anxiety/ and forgetfulness due to heart blood deficiency; also used to treat constipation due to yin and blood deficiency and night sweats due to yin deficiency.

- Yin Tonic Herbs
  - Bai he (commonly called lily bulb): 10 to 30 g daily; properties: the temperature and taste are cold, bitter, and sweet; supports heart and lung channel; used to moisten the lung, clear heat, calm spirit, heart, and stop cough; often used to treat menopause and also to treat dry cough and sore throat, insomnia, restlessness, and irritability and also used to treat qi and yin deficiency after a febrile disease.
  - Bai mu er (common name is fruiting body of tremella): 3 to 10 g of herb, soaked for 1 to 2 hours in soup until it is soft; properties: the temperature is neutral, sweet, and bland; supports the lung and stomach channel; used to tonify the lung and stomach, nourish yin, and generate fluids and also used to treat dry cough from lung heat and night sweats.

The herbal therapy above is just one example of the several differential diagnoses for the causes of insomnia according to the theories of TCM. It demonstrates the complexity of TCM herbal medicine and the diversity of choices and considerations available to the TCM herbal practitioner when choosing an herb or herbal formula specifically suited for the patient and the disease. The complexity of diagnosis is one of the reasons there is a long-standing debate among practitioners of TCM regarding the value of the standardized TCM formulas that are commonly found on the market today and the use of granules and raw herbs. Yet consumer behavior may ultimately determine the outcome of this debate because, as mentioned, raw herbs are difficult to prepare and to take because of the taste and consumers are more apt to take a pill than a preparation.

Ayurvedic Herbs

Ayurvedic herbology is based on the tridoshic theory that there exist six basic tastes (sweet, sour, salty, pungent, astringent, and bitter). When used correctly, these tastes (which are associated with all plants, herbs, and food) can be used to balance or counter an excess or deficient condition. Therefore, the first and basic principle in Ayurvedic medicine is the use of food, spices, and herbs not only to maintain good health but also to prevent and treat diseases. In general, sweet, sour, and salty tastes reduce vata, and bitter, pungent, and astringent tastes enhance it. Astringent, bitter, and sweet tastes reduce pitta; sour, salty, and pungent tastes enhance it. Bitter, pungent, and astringent foods reduce kapha; sweet, salty, and sour tastes enhance it. Based on these concepts, food, spices, and herbs with these specific effects are used to balance disharmonies in vata, pitta, and kapha conditions according to an excess or deficient condition.

For example, Ayurvedic medicine considers women to possess a greater amount of vata-type characteristics (tendency to be cold, dry, and light), which increase with age (old age is considered to be vata-dominant). Therefore, foods, spices, and herbs emphasizing sweet, sour, and salty tastes are often prescribed. However, taking into consideration the uniqueness in all of us, Ayurveda also recognizes that, as different as our body types are, so too are our nutritional requirements. For example, if you are a thin-framed, always-cold person with dry skin, you are considered to have a vata constitution and should eat a vata-balanced diet as a lifetime program. However, if you start to retain water, feel sluggish, and have excess mucus, you are demonstrating kapha imbalance and should avoid a sweet, sour, and salty diet to achieve balance.

Additional Approach to Choosing

Although tridoshic theory is the primary method used by Ayurvedic practitioners to individualize herbal therapy, they commonly use herbs and herbal formulas that target specific disorders when recommending commercial Ayurvedic herbs and herbal formulas.

Digestive Disorders

In Ayurvedic theory, most digestive disorders are a result of poor digestive "Agni" fire, which is responsible for absorbing nutrients in food, destroying pathogens, and converting food to be acceptable to our digestive systems. If Agni fire is weak, the body will not be able to perform these functions and food can become a negative pathogen for the body, creating toxins and undermining the immune system.

Herbs that enhance Agni fire are generally pungent, sour, or salty (e.g., black pepper, cayenne, or ginger). However, recommendations should be based on the condition of the Agni fire: if it is too high, herbs like aloe, barberry, and gentian are more appropriate; and if variable, spices like ginger, cumin, or rock salt are recommended. Generally, sustaining digestive fire is done with mild herbs (e.g., cardamom, turmeric, coriander, and fennel).

Ayurvedic formulas include the following:

Triphala is a blend of herbs or three fruits: amla (*Emblica officinalis*), bibitaki (*Terminalia belerica)*, and haritaki (*Terminalia chebula*). The fruits are dried, powdered, and mixed together and given as a general tonic and detoxifier. Triphala is taken every day to help balance all three doshas: each herb balances one of the three doshas—amla controls pitta, bibitaki controls kapha, and harataki controls vata. Triphala has traditionally been used to treat gastrointestinal disorder and restore bowel health. Most research has been done in animal trials; however, a 2007 study to evaluate the inhibitory activities of triphala against common bacterial isolates from HIV-infected patients supported an antibacterial activity by triphala against the bacterial isolates (Srikumar et al, 2007).

Trikatu mean "three herbs": ginger (*Zingiber officinale*), black pepper (*Piper nigrum*), and Indian long pepper (*Piper longum*). Used for its bitter taste, it is intended to rejuvenate the digestive fire as well as the respiratory tract.

Rejuvenative Disorders

In Ayurvedic theory, disorders that include symptoms of low energy, fatigue, lack of sexual motivation, anxiety, and impotence are often caused by vata (air) conditions. Therefore, tonification therapy will include an anti-vata diet, including foods like dairy products, ghee (clarified butter), nuts, okra, and meat. However, tonics like shatavari, chyavanprash, and aswagandha are commonly prescribed as well.

Shatavari root (*Asparagus racemosus,* "hundred husbands") is the main Ayurvedic tonic for women, with a role similar to that of the Chinese tonic dong quai. But it can also be used by men, having a similar role as ginseng, to treat impotence. Shatavari is a woody climber that has leaves that are like pine needles and white flowers with small spikes. It belongs to the *Liliaceae* family. By taste it is sweet, bitter, and cooling in nature; it is used as a nutritive and calming agent, to regulate menstrual flow, and to boost hormonal triggers, making it valuable in treating menopausal complaints such as vaginal atrophy and to increase female sexuality. Research on shatavari has found it to have multiple influences on the body, acting as an adaptogen, antitussive, antioxidant, antibacterial, immune-modulator, digestive, cyto-protective, galactogogue, anti-oxytocic (preventing the stimulation of involuntary muscles of the uterus), antispasmodic, antidiarrheal, and sexual tonic (Thomsen, 2002).

Amla fruit (*Emblica officinalis,* Indian gooseberry) is a small, very sour fruit that is the most widely used in Ayurveda as a general rejuvenative herb. This fruit is particularly high in vitamin C, with 20 to 30 times the amount found in oranges. The vitamin C in amla is also heat stable, surviving the cooling and drying process, making it an extremely powerful antioxidant. Amla is the principle ingredient in a jelly called *Chyavanprash* that has been used for over a thousand years to help rejuvenate the body and fortify the mind.

Aswagandha (*Withania somnifera* or "Indian ginseng") has been used for hundreds of years for its ability to restore vitality and strength. In Sanskrit the word means "the smell of a horse" and the herb has traditionally been used as a male tonic. Classified as an adaptogen, ashwagandha contains steroidal lactones, alkaloids, choline, fatty acids, amino acids, and a variety of sugars.

Herbs for Common Disorders

Table 10-1 presents additional information on herbal medicines for common health problems. Although many other herbs may be used for these disorders, the ones listed have all been studied in human trials. Others that are not listed in the

Table 10–1   Selective Herbal Agents Used for Common Conditions

Condition	Treatment
Candida	Garlic Berberine-containing herbs: Oregon grape, goldenseal, scutellaria, gentian, grapefruit seed extract Ginseng, astragalus, red clover, dandelion root, burdock root, asafetida, cumin
Constipation	Psyllium seeds, fennel, fenugreek, olive oil, cannabis seeds For constipation due to heat: turmeric, gentian, dandelion, Oregon grape, yellow dock Ayurvedic herb: triphala or rhubarb
Diarrhea	Blackberry root, raspberry leaf, agrimony, bayberry bark, oak bark, yarrow Spleen qi tonics: ginseng, *Codonopsis*, white atractylodes, and *Dioscorea* Cinnamon, ginger, or cardamom
Pain Headaches	Chinese herbs: Ligusticum (chuan xiong) or Chinese lovage Feverfew, chamomile, willow bark Western herbs: angelica Bupleurum, *Artemisia annua* (Sweet Annie) Menstrual headaches:, black cohosh, dandelion, chrysanthemum, and feverfew or the formula of dang gui, cooked rehmannia, white peony, and Ligusticum
Arthritis	Borage, capsicum, chondroitin, evening primrose oil, ginger glucosamine, turmeric
Insomnia	Chamomile, skullcap, valerian, or kava kava, passionflower, hops, ashwagandha to calm the nervous system, St. John's wort, lemon balm, schisandra, jujube dates
Benign prostatic hypertrophy	Nettle, pumpkin seed, saw palmetto
Menorrhagia	Shepherd's purse tincture, 3 to 6 drops every 2 h or a combination of cattail pollen, agrimony, mugwort, yarrow, shepherd's purse, raspberry, and blackberry leaves Building blood with iron floradix or blackstrap molasses, along with Chinese herbs dang qui, lycii, cooked rehmannia, and white peony
Dysmenorrhea	Combination of equal parts of vitex, wild yam, block cohosh, dang qui, sassafras, and licorice with ½ part ginger
Urinary tract infections	Cornsilk tea, parsley, dandelion, horsetail, cranberry, and for extreme burning, use goldenseal, gentian, gardenia

Source: Adapted from Tierra, L. (2003). *Healing with the herbs of life.* Berkeley, CA: Crossing Press; Fetrow, C. W., & Avila, J. R. (1999). *Professional's handbook of complementary and alternative medicines.* Springhouse, PA: Springhouse.

table are in use but have been reported on only in case or anecdotal reports.

HERBAL PREPARATIONS

Although understanding the use of herbs is important, proper preparation ensures their maximum effect. The following is a summary of several of the most common preparations and their proper use.

Bolus refers to a suppository inserted into the rectum. Common herbs used in this way are astringents such as white oak bark, bayberry bark; demulcents such as comfrey root or slippery elm; and antibiotics such as garlic, echinacea, chaparral, and golden seal.

Compress/fomentation are two terms that refer to the same treatment of applying herbs externally to the body. Especially effective for herbs that are too strong to take internally but that can be absorbed slowly in small amounts, compresses are used to treat many superficial ailments like swelling and pain and to stimulate circulation of blood or lymph in the area where the compress is applied.

Liniments are warming herbal extracts rubbed into the skin and are commonly used to relieve sore or strained muscles and treat conditions like arthritis or itchy skin.

Oils are concentrated extracts used for massaging the body. There are two types of oil preparations: *soothing emollients* that use herbs like calendula flower, lavender, lemon balm; and *warming and stimulating oils* that use herbs like ginger, peppermint, and eucalyptus. Oils are usually infused with a particular herb chosen with consideration of the moistening capacity of the oil: *nondrying oils* include jojoba, cocoa butter, and avocado; *semidrying oils* include safflower and sunflower; *drying oils* include soybean and linseed (flax).

Capsules or pills are one of the most popular preparations used in herbal therapy today because they are convenient and mimic Western medicine. They are entirely made up of herbs; however, capsules are generally twice more concentrated than pills.

Poultices and plasters are a topical application of herbs that have been powdered, crushed, or mashed and are usually applied moist, either hot or warm, and left on an area of the body for 12 to 20 hours. Caution must be taken to avoid skin reactions and burns.

Smoking mixtures are used for smoking herbs, like datura leaf for the treatment of asthma. Smoking of herbs should be done only occasionally, and patients should be warned about the risk of lung disease, as with any smoking habit.

Teas are the most well-known method of taking herbs. Although tea is generally considered a beverage, it can have the strongest medicinal effect of any preparation, making it suitable for the most serious illnesses. To be effective, the proportion of herbs to water must be greater than usual.

Tinctures are an alcoholic or vinegar extract of herbs. Their advantage is that they have a long shelf-life when stored in a cool, dry place, whereas dried herbs begin to lose potency after the first year. Tinctures tend to make herbs energetically "hotter," which affects the circulatory system. Consideration must be given to other chemical constituents found in alcohol, such as glycosides and sugars.

CONSIDERATIONS FOR THE APRN PRESCRIBER

There are many reasons people use herbal remedies instead of conventional medicines. Sometimes these reasons may not be consistent with those of Western medicine or supported by evidence-based studies; however, we have to respect the consumers' right to choose and acknowledge that consumers are using herbs at an ever-growing rate. Therefore, APNs and other health-care providers should be prepared to educate the patient about the many different concepts and herbal traditions and help guide them to the appropriate resource. In addition, providers need to educate themselves about the herbs that are commonly used by their patients and be aware of the growing amount of research being conducted to evaluate interactions with herbal therapy and allopathic medicines.

Because a product is natural does not mean it is risk-free. In the late 1980s, a particular brand of L-tryptophan tablets resulted in several cases of fatal eosinophilia myalgia, and from 1993 to 1997, several hundred cases of serious adverse effects were documented from ephedra in diet and weight-loss supplements. Yet some herbal preparations have been accepted and found to be relatively safe when used in combination with Western medication, such as astragalus and dong quai for the treatment of infections and menopause.

When consumers and nonherbalists speak either positively or negatively about any given herb, what they seriously fail to acknowledge is the many different herbal traditions and those practitioners who are either certified

---

BOX 10–1 WEB-BASED RESOURCES FOR HERBS AND ALTERNATIVE THERAPIES

- American Botanical Council, http://www.herbalgram.org
- American Herbalist Guild, http://www.americanherbalistsguild.com
- Biofeedback Certification Institute of America, http://www.bcia.org
- National Center for Complementary and Alternative Medicine, http://nccam.nih.gov
- Natural Standard: The Authority on Integrative Medicine, http://www.naturalstandard.com/
- Cochrane Database of Systematic Reviews, http://www.cochran.org

BOX 10–2 HERBAL RESOURCES

East West School of Herbology

P.O. Box 275
Ben Lomond, CA 95005
1-800-717-5010
herbcourse@planetherbs.com or www
.planetherbs.com
Sponsor of planetary herbal formulas that supplies
Western, Eastern, and Ayurvedic herbs.

Herb Pharm

Box 116
Williams, OR 97544
1-800-348-4372
Specializing in herbal tinctures.
www.herb-pharm.com

Spring Wind Herb Company

2325 4th Street #6
Berkeley, CA 94710
Good source for Chinese herbs.

Banyan Botanical

6705 Eagle Rock Ave, NE
Albuquerque, NM 87113
1-800-953-6424
www.banyanbotanicals.com
Good source for Ayurvedic herbs.

Mountain Rose Herbs

P.O. Box 50220
Eugene, OR 97405
1-800-879-3337
www.mountainroseherbs.com
Large selection of bulk organic herbs, spices, teas, essential oils, and bulk ingredients.

The Tao of Tea

3430 SE Belmont Street
Portland OR 97214
1-503-736-0198
www.taooftea.com
Good selection of herbal teas.

non-Western–based treatments that can meet their needs. However, professionals must also recognize their scope of practice and not venture into prescribing or recommending without adequate knowledge and training in other areas of therapy.

SUGGESTED READING

Western Herbs

Bach, P. A. *Prescription for herbal healing.* (2002). New York: Avery Books.
Kushi, M. (1977). *The book of macrobiotics: The universal way of health, happiness, and peace.* New York: Japan Publications Inc.
Pitchford, P. (2002). *Healing with whole foods: Asian traditions and modern nutrition* (3rd ed.). Berkeley, CA: North Atlantic Books.
Tierra, M. *Planetary herbology.* (1988). Santa Fe, NM: Lotus Press.
Weil, A.. (2004). *Health and healing: The philosophy of integrative medicine and optimum health.* New York: Houghton Mifflin Co.

Chinese Medicine

Beinfield, H., & Korngold, E. (1992). *Between heaven and earth: A guide to Chinese medicine.* New York: Ballantine Books.
Chen, J. K., & Chen, T. T. (2001). *Chinese medical herbology and pharmacology.* City of Industry, CA: Art of Medicine Press.
Chen, J. K., & Chen, T. T. (2008). *Chinese herbal formulas and applications.* City of Industry, CA: Art of Medicine Press.
Maciocia, G. (1989). *The foundations of Chinese medicine.* New York: Churchill Livingstone.

Ayurvedic Medicine

Lad, V. (1984). *A practical guide: The science of self healing.* Santa Fe, NM: Lotus Press.
Lad, V. (1999). *The complete book of Ayurvedic home remedies.* New York: Three Rivers Press.
Tiwari, M. (1995). *A life of balance: The complete guide to Ayurvedic nutrition and body types with recipes.* Rochester, VT: Healing Arts Press.
Tiwari, M. (1995). *Ayurveda secrets of healing.* Santa Fe, NM: Lotus Press.

General Recommendations

Blome, G. (1999). *Advanced Bach Fower therapy: A scientific approach to diagnosis and treatment.* Rochester, VT: Healing Arts Press.
Buhner, S. H. (2002). *The lost language of plants: The ecological importance of plant medicines to life on earth.* White River Junction, VT: Chelsea Green Publishing.
Cowan, E. (1995). *Plant spirit medicine.* Columbus, NC: Swan-Raven & Company.
Pollan, M. (2007). *The omnivore's dilemma: A natural history of four meals.* New York: Penguin Books.
Tierra, L. (2003). *Healing with the herbs of life.* Berkeley, CA: Crossing Press.

REFERENCES

Adams, K., Lindell, K., Kohlmeier, M., & Zeisel, S. H. (2006). Status of nutrition education in medical schools. *American Journal of Clinical Nutrition, 83* (Suppl.), 941S–944S.
American Botanical Council. (2009). Commission E monographs. February 24, 2009, from www.herbalgram.org
American Herbalist Guild. Retrieved February 1, 2009, from http://www.americanherbalistsguild.com
Barnes, P. M., Bloom, B., & Nahim, R. L. (2008, December). Complementary and alternative medicine use among adults and children: United States, 2007, *National Health Statistics Report, 10*(12), 1–23.

in herbal therapy or trained in a given medical discipline that has a history of using herbal therapy but that does not fall within the definitions of Western medicine. Often, it is a failure to evaluate a specific herbal theory or or to consult a practitioner of herbal medicine that leads to many of the adverse effects cited in clinical research and by consumers.

Health-care professionals need to keep an open mind to all the possible ways of treating health problems, and that ultimately may require the inclusion or consideration of medical systems that are not commonly practiced in Western culture. Primary care providers may need to explore the resources that are available to the public at large, critique the information, and assist the patient in finding practitioners of

Barnes, P. M., & Bloom, B. (2008, December). National Institute of Health. Retrieved April 17, 2009, from National Center for Complementary and Alternative Medicine, http://nccam.nih.gov/news/camstats/2007/camsurvey_fs1.htm

Bastyr University. (2008). Bastyr University Catalog 2008–2009 [Brochure]. Kent, WA: Author.

Becker, D. J., Gordon, R. Y., Halbert, S. C., & French, B. (2009). Red yeast rice for dyslipidemia in statin-intolerant patients: A randomized trial. *Annals of Internal Medicine, 150*(12), 830–839.

Biofeedback Certification Institute of America (n.d.). Entry level general biofeedback certification information. Retrieved April 28, 2009, from http://www.bcia.org

Biomedical Acupuncture Institute (2005). Biomedical acupuncture course descriptions. Retrieved May, 30, 2009, from www.biomedicalacupuncture.com

Brzezinski, A. (1997). Melatonin in humans. *New England Journal of Medicine, 336,* 186–195.

Buettner, C., Mukamal, K. J., Gardiner, P., & Davis, R. B. (2009). Herbal supplement use and blood levels of United States adults. *Journal of General Internal Medicine, 24*(11), 1175–1182.

Chavez, M. L. (1997). Saint John's wort. *Hospital Pharmacy, 32,* 1621–1632.

Chen, J. K., & Chen, T. T. (2001). *Chinese medical herbology and pharmacology.* City of Industry, CA.: Art of Medicine Press.

Cheng, Y. L., Lee, S. C., Harn, H. J., Huang, H. C., & Chang, W. L. (2008). The extract of Hibiscus syriacus inducing apoptosis by activating p53 and AIF in human lung cancer cells. *American Journal of Chinese Medicine, 36*(1), 171–184.

Cochrane Collaboration. (n.d.). The Cochran database of systematic reviews. Retrieved January 15, 2009, from http://www.cochran.org

Demory-Luce, D., & McPherson, R. S. (1999). Nutritional knowledge and attitudes of physician assistants. *Topics in Clinical Nutrition, 14*(2), 71–82.

Dietary Supplement Health and Education Act of 1994. Retrieved February 1, 2006, from http://www.cfsan.fda.gov/dms/dietsupp.html

Ebell, M. H. Siwek, J., & Weiss, B. D. (2004). Strength of recommendations taxonomy (SORT): A patient centered approach to grading evidence in the medical literature. *American Family Physician, 69,* 548–556.

Eisenberg, D. F., Davis, R. B., & Ettner, S. L (1998). Trends in alternative medicine use in the United States, 1990–1997. *Journal of the American Medical Association, 280*(18), 1569–1575.

Fetrow, C. W., & Avila, J. R. (1999). *Professional's handbook of complementary & alternative medicines.* Springhouse, PA: Springhouse.

Flaws, B., & Lake, J. (2005). *The treatment of modern Western diseases with Chinese medicine; A textbook and clinical manual* (2nd ed.). Boulder, CO: Blue Poppy Press.

Forgues, E. (2009). Methodological issues pertaining to the evaluation of the effectiveness of energy-based therapies, avenues for a methodological guide. *Journal of Complementary and Integrative Medicine, 6*(1), 1–19.

Fortin, M., Bravo, G., Hudon, C., Vanasse, A., & Lapointe, L. (2005). Prevalence of multimorbidity among adults seen in family practice. *Annals of Family Medicine, 3,* 223–228.

Gaby, A. R. (2006). *The natural pharmacy revised and updated 3rd edition: Complete A–Z reference to natural treatments for common health conditions.* New York: Three Rivers Press.

Grieco, A., Miele, L., Pompili, M., & Biolato, M. (2009). Acute hepatitis caused by a natural lipid-lowering product: When "alternative" medicine is no "alternative" at all. *Journal of Hepatology, 50*(6), 1273–1277. Epub 2009 Mar 31.

Hamilton, J. L., Roemheld-Hamm, B., Young, D. M., Jalba, M., & DiCicco-Bloom, B. (2008). Complementary and alternative medicine in US family medicine practices: A pilot qualitative study. *Alternative Therapies in Health & Medicine, 14*(3), 22–27.

Hayes, M., Buckley, D., & Judkins, D. Z. (2007). Are any alternative therapies effective in treating asthma? *Journal of Family Practice, 56*(5), 385–389.

Hirschkorn, K. A., & Bourgeault, I. L. (2008). Structural constraints and opportunities for CAM use and referral by physicians, nurses, and midwives. *Health: An Interdisciplinary Journal for the Social Study of Health, Illness & Medicine, 12*(2), 193–213.

Hoffer, J. L. (2003). Complementary or alternative medicine: The need for plausibility. *Journal of the Canadian Medical Association, 168*(2), 180–182.

Institute for Functional Medicine. (2006). *Textbook of functional medicine.* Gig Harbor, WA: Author.

Institute for Functional Medicine. (2009). Functional medicine certification program [Brochure]. Gig Harbor, WA: Author.

JABF. (2003) Mind-body medicine in primary care. *Journal of the American Board of Family Practice, 16*(2), 131–147.

Jadad, A. R., Moore, R. A., Carroll, D., Jenkinson, C., Reynolds, D. J., Gavaghan, D. J., et al. (1996). Assessing the quality of reports of randomized clinical trials: Is blinding necessary? *Controlled Clinical Trials, 17*(1), 1–12.

Joslin Diabetes Center and Joslin Clinic. (2007, January 12). *Joslin Diabetes Center clinical guideline for pharmacological management of type 2 diabetes.* Boston: Joslin Diabetes Center; Publication Department.

Jenkins, J. J., Jonkman, E., Leonard, J. H., Petrini, J. O., & van Lier, J. J.(1997). The cognitive, subjective, and physical effects of a ginkgo biloba/panax ginseng combination in health volunteers with neurasthenic complaints. *Psychopharmacology Bulletin, 33*(4), 677–683.

Kennedy, J. (2005, November). Herb and supplement use in the US adult population. *Clinical Therapy, 27*(11), 1847–1858.

Khan, A. U., & Gilani, A. H. (2009). Antispasmodic and bronchodilator activities of Artemisia vulgaris are dedicated through dual blockade of muscarinic receptors and calcium influx. *Journal of Ethnopharmcology, 126*(3), 480–486.

Khan, A., Safdar, M., Alie Khan, et al. (2003). Cinnamon improves glucose and lipids of people with type 2 diabetes. *Diabetes Care, 26*(12), 3215–3218

Kleronomos, C. A. (2009). *Complementary and alternative medicine course development: Evidence for primary care.* Unpublished scholarly project submitted in partial fulfillment of the requirements for MSN, Seattle University.

Lad, V. (2002). *Textbook of ayurveda: Fundamental principles.* Albuquerque, NM: Ayurvedic Press.

Lino, M., Dinkins, J., & Bente, L. (1999). Household expenditures on vitamins and minerals by income level. *Family Economics and Nutrition Review,* 1–6.

Liu, C., & Tseng, A. (2003). *Chinese herbal medicine: Modern applications of traditional formulas.* Boca Raton, FL: CRC Press.

Ma, Y. (2007). Biomedical acupuncture: An evidence-based acupuncture model. *Medical Acupuncture, 19*(4), 217–223.

Maciocia, G. (2005). *The foundations of Chinese medicine* (2nd ed.). Philadelphia: Churchstone Livingstone.

Mills, S., & Bone, K. (2000). *Principles and practice of phytotherapy: Modern herbal medicine.* Philadelphia: Churchill Livingstone.

Morgenthaller, TI, Lee-Chiong, T., Alessi, C., Friedman, L., Aurora, R. N., Boehlecke, B., et al. Standards of Practice Committee of the AASM. (2007). Practice parameters for the clinical evaluation and treatment of circadian rhythm sleep disorders. An American Academy of Sleep Medicine Report. *Sleep, 30*(11), 1445-1459.

Murphy, J. J., Heptinstall, S., & Mitchell, J. R. (1988). Randomized, double-blind, placebo-controlled trial of feverfew in migraine prevention. *The Lancet, 2,* 189–192.

National Center for Complementary and Alternative Medicine. (2008). The use of complemenatary and alternative medicine in the United States. Retrieved January 19, 2009, from http://nccam.nih.gov/

National Institutes of Health: National Cancer Institute (n.d.). Definition: German Commission E. Retrieved March 14, 2009 from www.cancer.gov

Natural Standard. (2009). *Natural standard integrative medicine database.* http://www.naturalstandard.com/

Pizzorno, J. E., & Murray, M. T. (2006). *Textbook of natural medicine* (3rd ed.). St. Louis, MO: Churchill Livingstone Elsevier.

Porter, S., & O'Halloran, P. (2009). The postmodernist war on evidence-based practice. *International Journal of Nursing Studies, 46*(5), 740–748.

Prout, L. (2000). *Live in the balance.* New York: Marlowe.

Rakel, D. (2007). *Integrative medicine* (2nd ed.). Philadelphia: Saunders Elsevier.

Rakel, D. P., Guerrera, M. P., Bayles, B. P., Desai, G. J., & Ferrara, E. (2008). CAM education: Promoting a salutogenic focus in health care. *Journal of Alternative Complementary Medicine, 14*(1),87–93

Rotblatt, M., & Ziment, I. (2002). *Evidence-based herbal medicine*. Philadelphia: Hanley & Belfus.

Schwartz, L. (2000). Evidence-based medicine and traditional Chinese medicine: Not mutually exclusive. *Medical Acupuncture, 12*(1), 38–41.

Srikumar, R., Parthasarathy, N. J., Shankar, E. M., et al. (2007). Evaluation of the growth inhibitory activities of Triphala against common bacterial isolates from HIV infected patients. *Phytotherapy Research, 21*(5), 476–480.

Sorensen, H., & Sonne, J. (1996). A double-masked study of the effects of ginseng on cognitive function. *Current Therapy Research, 57*, 959–968.

Thomsen, M. (2002). Shatavari-Asparagus racemosus. Weblink: www.Phytomedicine.com

Tierra, M. (1989). *Planetary herbology*. Twin Lakes, WI: Lotus Press.

Tiwari, M. (1995a). *Ayurveda: A life of balance*. Rochester, VT: Healing Arts Press.

Tiwari, M. (1995b). *Ayurveda: Secrets of healing*. Twin Lakes, WI: Lotus Press.

Tonelli, M., & Callahan, T. (2001). Why alternative medicine cannot be evidence-based. *Academic Medicine, 76*(12), 1213–1220.

U.S. Centers for Disease Control and Prevention: National Center for Health Statistics (2008). Americans make nearly four medical visits a year on average. Retrieved November 17, 2008, from http://www.cdc.gov/nchs/about.htm

U.S. Food and Drug Administration. (2009). Quality systems regulation. http://www.fda.gov/cdrh/comp/gmp.html

University of Arizona: Arizona Center for Integrative Medicine. (2009). Fellowship. Retrieved April 7, 2009, from http://www.integrativemedicine.arizona.edu

Viskoper , R., Shapira, I., Priluck, R., Mindlin, R., Chornia, L., Laszt, A., et al. (2003). Non-pharmacological treatment of resistant hypertensives by device-guided slow breathing exercises. *American Journal of Hypertension, 16*, 484–487.

Volz, H. P. (1997). Kava-kava extract WS-1490 versus placebo in anxiety disorders: A randomized placebo-controlled 25-week outpatient trial. *Pharmacopsychiatry, 30*, 1–5.

Wesnes, K. A., Faleni, R. A., Hefting, N. R., Hoogsteen, G., Houben, & Weisfeld, V. (2009). Summit on integrated medicine and health of the public: Issue background and overview. *Institute of Medicine Summit on Integrative Medicine and the Health of the Public*, 1–16.

Williams, D. D. R., & Garner, J. (2002). The case against "the evidence": A different perspective on evidence-based medicine. *British Journal of Psychiatry, 180*, 8–12.

Wolkowitz, O. M. (1997). Dehydroepiandrosterone treatment of depression. *Biological Psychiatry, 41*, 311–318.

World Health Organization. (2003). Acupuncture: Review and analysis of reports on controlled clinical trials. Retrieved December 28, 2008, from http://www.who.int/en/

Wu, C. H., Wang, C. C., & Kennedy, J. (2011). Changes in herb and dietary supplement use in the US adult population: A comparison of the 2002 and 2007 National Health Interview Surveys. *Clinical Therapeutics, 33*(11), 1749–1758.

Wu, C. H., Wang, C. C., & Kennedy, J. (2013). The prevalence of herb and dietary supplement use among children and adolescents in the United States: Results from the 2007 National Health Interview Survey. *Complementary Therapies in Medicine, 21*(4), 358–363.

Yan, J., Engle, V., He, Y., Jiao, Y., & Gu, W. (2009). Study designs of randomized controlled trials not based on Chinese medicine theory are improper. *Chinese Medicine, 4*(1). http://nccam.nih.gov/news/camstats/2007/camsurvey_fs1.htm#natural

CHAPTER 11

INFORMATION TECHNOLOGY AND PHARMACOTHERAPEUTICS

Jane M. Carrington

OVERVIEW

According to the essentials for Doctoral Education for Advanced Nursing Practice (DNP), established by the American Association of Colleges of Nursing (2006), graduates of these programs are trained to use information systems and patient-care technologies to improve and transform patient care. The federal government has also instituted the Healthcare Information Technology for Economic and Clinical Health (HITECH) provision of the American Recovery and Reinvestment Act (ARRA) of 2009, whereby providers, including advanced practice nurses (APN), are to be meaningful users of technology to increase patient safety and reduce health-care costs. Regardless of the practice setting, reimbursement is now connected to the provider's ability to use the electronic health record, computerized provider order entry, and clinical decision support. Furthermore, providers are also held to revised patient privacy standards, which will influence patient education and patient engagement.

This chapter will review the technologies that are involved in pharmacotherapeutics and that are essential to meaningful use. In addition, the chapter also discusses items that are essential to increased patient safety: medication reconciliation, sustaining all elements of patient privacy, supporting patients' use of the personal health record, patient education, and quality matters.

INTRODUCTION

The literature contains an abundance of evidence that the health-care system is inefficient and can ultimately be a threat to patient safety. The often cited report out of the Institute of Medicine (IOM), *To Err is Human: Building a Safer Health System*, brought to light the astonishing statistics that up to 98,000 lives are lost each year in our nation's hospitals due to medical errors (Kohn, Corrigan, & Donaldson, 1999). This report was the impetus for both legislative and regulatory initiatives that were designed to ultimately increase patient safety. One of these initiatives is ARRA. The goal of ARRA is to provide affordable health care by means of health information technology. The act states that reimbursement for care delivery will be attached to adoption and compliance with the electronic health record (EHR) beginning in 2015 and that health-care providers are to become meaningful users of EHR. Health-care providers are defined as meaningful users when they have effectively adopted EHR to improve patient safety and quality of care, engage patients in their care, improve care coordination, and protect patient health information (ARRA, 2009).

The EHR Incentive Program is a list of meaningful-use objectives to assist providers regardless of the type of practice (hospital, critical access hospital, primary care, and so forth) to become meaningful users. Of these 14 objectives, 9 directly involve the process of ordering or prescribing medications,

2 contribute to the process, and 2 are indirectly related. Table 11-1 is a list of the objectives and their relationship to pharmacotherapeutics. The objectives for professional meaningful use serve as organizers for this chapter (see Table 11-1), which will discuss the EHR, information storage and exchange, computerized provider order entry (CPOE), clinical decision support (CDS), patient privacy, and patient safety.

THE ELECTRONIC HEALTH RECORD

A number of definitions of EHR have been used in the literature, but for this chapter, the EHR is a computerized patient record in which all members of the health-care team enter patient information. This definition is all-encompassing, as it includes elements of an earlier definition of the electronic medical record (clinician based) and EHR that contained information generated by patients, family members, and other services (Garets & Davis, 2006). The broadest of definitions for EHR thus accounts for the diversity of practice settings and the inclusion of patients and family in their own care.

It can be argued that regardless the size of the practice, from a small private practice to larger organizations, the EHR can improve the quality of care patients receive, assist in measuring outcomes, and improve organizational efficiency (Chaudhry et al, 2006). Despite these advantages, the implementation of the EHR has been impeded by its cost. For example, hospitals have reportedly paid over $10 million in up-front costs to implement the EHR (Doyle, 2009). Doyle further suggests that health-care organizations should keep their EHR budget to within 1.5% of their annual operating expenses. Staying within this guideline may yield more offsetting costs, however. Budget estimates will soon include the money recouped through ARRA.

EHRs can be implemented within a practice or hospital or implemented across an entire health-care system that includes clinics, hospitals, and offices in one system. The larger implementation has the advantages of a single-vendor EHR, mechanisms for large data storage, and the exchange of patient information from provider to provider and across care settings. The smaller site implementations have internal communication advantages within the practice or hospital; however, they may lack the ability to exchange patient information with outside agencies due to incompatible interfaces between different vendors.

Information Storage and Exchange

Following adoption of the EHR, providers have access to vast amounts of patient data. Unlike data from the early electronic medical records, where the patient information is in the form of individual medical records akin to separate file documents, the EHR can provide data from a clinical warehouse and

Table 11–1 Core Elements for Meaningful Use for Providers

Core Element	Measures	Associated with Pharmacotherapeutics
Use of CPOE*	>30% medication orders created using CPOE	Yes
Drug-drug and drug-allergy interaction checks	Full functionality	Yes
Up-to-date problem list of diagnosis	>80% of patients	Contributing
Generate and transmit prescriptions electronically (eRx)	Exclusions for smaller practices and availability of a pharmacy	Yes
Active medication list	>80% patients	Yes
Active medication allergy list	>80% patients	Yes
Record demographics (language, gender, race, ethnicity, date of birth)	>50% patients	Contributing
Record changes in (height, weight, blood pressure, BMI, growth charts for pediatrics)	>50% patients	Yes
Smoking status for patient 13 years and older	>50% patients	Indirect
Report ambulatory clinical quality measures	Complete	Indirect
Implement one clinical decision support rule	One clinical decision support rule	Yes
Provide patients with electronic copy of health information	>50% of all patients who request, provided within 3 business days	Yes
Provide clinical summaries for patients	>50% patients within 3 business days	Yes
Protect electronic health information	Conduct a review to reflect success with this objective	Yes

CPOE = Computerized Provider Order Entry
Adapted from https://www.cms.gov/Regulations-and-Guidance/Legislation/EHRIncentivePrograms/downloads/EP-MU-TOC.pdf. Retrieved June 11, 2013.

recall the data in aggregate. The strength of this capability is evident in the scope for potential search questions. Using the EMR, a search question could be: "all admissions for diabetes for Jones, MR# (number)." Compare this to the EHR in a clinical warehouse: "all patients >65, diagnosis of congestive heart failure, with potassium levels of 2.9, with readmission <30 days." Both searches can provide the provider useful results; however, the relational clinical data warehouse has the potential for influencing broader care decisions, including establishing benchmark data and tracing the impact of quality improvement programs, which inform the root-cause analysis of suspected or known problems. Contents of the data warehouse can vary but may include: patient visits (in- and outpatient), surgeries, test results, and billing (Einbinder, Scully, Pates, Schubart, & Reynolds, Summer 2001).

These data in aggregate are useful at the local level, but what about regional or multiple health-care organizations? Can comparisons in care and outcomes be made available? Regional health information organizations (RHIOs) are designed to address these questions.

A RHIO unites patient-care stakeholders within a defined region for the purpose of improving care (HRSA, np). Critical issues must be resolved for the RHIO to survive. First, agreement on what patient data will be collected. For example, data could be collected on specific diagnoses and medications and then combined with data on ambulatory care, acute care facilities, and home-health care. Second, who should be members of the RHIO must also be agreed upon. For example, representatives from ambulatory, acute, home care, public health, and payers can be included. A strong RHIO would have stakeholder representation that would best appreciate the patient data so that its measures become more significant and potential changes in care could be developed. Third, the RHIO must be able to sustain itself through successful funding. In the United States, RHIOs use federal grant monies or fees from members (Adler-Milstein, McAfee, Bates, & Jha, 2007). Finally, standards for maintaining privacy when exchanging patient information must be established. RHIOs are not excluded from state and federal privacy standards (Solomon, 2007). Unfortunately, RHIOs face challenges to endure in our economy and our independent health-care systems. One possible solution is

building the RHIO according to business models designed to sustain themselves beyond the timeframe of government funding (Osterwalder, Pigneur, & Tucci, 2005).

The next level of organization is provided through the electronic Health Information Exchange (HIE), which is part of the HITECH Act of 2009. The HIE supports access by providers and patients to patient medical information in order to ultimately improve the quality and safety of patient care and reduce costs by connecting RHIOs (Adler-Milstein, Bates, & Jha, 2011; HealthIT, np; Overhage, Evans, & Marchibroda, 2005). The goal of this program is to increase the completeness of patient records, which would lead to reduced readmissions and medication errors, reduce duplicative tests, and lead to more timely diagnoses (HealthIT, np). HIE has the potential of connecting RHIOs across zip codes, city and county borders, and the states. It is a concerted effort to interconnect patient information in a highly mobile society (Vest & Gamm, 2010). It is not uncommon for patients to initiate care for a diagnosis in one state and then for a variety of reasons, continue care in another state. Consider the retirees who winter in one region of the United States and summer in another region. The HIE permits the exchange of health information in both locations.

Computerized Provider Order Entry

Computerized provider order entry (CPOE) is an application that supports orders entered in the EHR by providers. According to the The Leapfrog Group (2008), it is considered the piece of technology the most helpful for reducing medication errors. The reduction of errors has been attributed to increased legibility, decreased use of unapproved abbreviations, and fewer incidences of incomplete orders (Devine, et al, 2010). Unfortunately, a mere 10% of our nation's hospitals had implemented CPOE as of 2010 (HIMSS Analytics, 2010), which is especially concerning given that CPOE has been in existence in some form along with the EHRs for over 40 years (Goolsby, 2002). The current decade has seen an acceleration of adoption and use of EHRs and CPOE.

Table 11-2 contains a brief review of the literature demonstrating the established advantages and disadvantages of

Table 11–2   Advantages and Disadvantages of Computerized Provider Order Entry

Resource	Advantages	Resource	Advantages
Franklin, O'Grady, Donyai, Jacklin, & Barber (2007)	Positive impact on error reduction using electronic prescribing and administration systems	Campbell, Sittig, Ash, Guappone, & Dykstra (2006)	Additional work, difficult information gathering, difficult workflow
Shulman, Singer, Goldstone, & Bellingan (2005)	Reduction in medication errors compared to manual system	Koppel et al (2005)	Fosters errors
Raebel, Carrlo, Kelleher, Chester, Berga, & Magid (2007)	Reduced error for pregnant women; did not stop errors completely	Walsh et al (2006)	Found errors with system; duplicate medication orders, menu selection errors, incorrect abbreviations, order set errors
Vaidya, Sowan, Mills, Socken, Gaffoor, & Hilmas (2006)	Pediatric ICU, chemotherapy-error reduction		

CPOE. From this very brief review of the literature, research suggests that CPOE has the potential for reducing medication errors. Prior to implementation of CPOE, providers must take into account changes in workflow between a manual system and a computerized system. For example, the workflow or process of providing care in a health-care system using paper records is different from that of a system using electronic systems. Starting with obtaining patient information, the provider locates the chart, reads information, visits the patient, and writes updates, and then goes on to the next patient. Using an electronic system, signing on to a computer gives ready access to all the patient's information. Updates can be entered during the visit, reducing the risks of error due to forgetfulness.

Electronic health systems require extensive training and testing at each stage of design, construction, and implementation. Failure to do any of these well has the potential for catastrophic error and results in failure to adopt the system, ultimately resulting in failure to meet the requirements for meaningful use.

CLINICAL DECISION SUPPORT SYSTEMS

Clinical decision support systems (CDSS) are generally considered to be expert systems with defined decision aids that require two or more items of patient data to generate advice (Johnston, Langton, Haynes, & Mathieu, 1994). Clinical decision support systems can stand alone within the EHR, like CPOE, or can function with CPOE, and the two applications together increase patient safety by reducing adverse drug errors (ADE). Killbridge, Campbell, Cozart, & Mojarrad (2006) determined that these technologies, when combined, detected ADEs at a rate 3.6 times greater than a manual system. For example, CDSS function within the EHR to alert the health-care provider to patient allergies, drug-drug issues, and laboratory/medication inconsistencies. The extent to which the alerts are set is dependent upon the vendor system and agreement of the stakeholders (providers, pharmacists, laboratory personnel, etc.). Once an ADE has occurred, a root-cause analysis may shed light on the elements of the health-care system that led to the error and may result in a modification of an alert or the development of a new alert.

Depending on the number of patients seen by a provider and the medication list and tests entered into the system, alert fatigue may occur. Alert fatigue is the result of excessive alerts or clinical warnings resulting in providers potentially ignoring clinically useful alerts and thereby threatening patient safety (Avery et al, 2005). The challenge in resolving alert fatigue is finding the balance between the legal responsibilities of the vendor providing the alert mechanism and using principles of human–computer interaction to reduce alert fatigue.

Software developers who market their products in the United States are regarded by the Food and Drug Administration as providers of a medical device (Kesselheim, Cresswell, Phansalkar, Bates, & Sheikh, 2011). This presents legal risks to providers who ignore alerts that result in harm to the patient. To improve provider appreciation for alerts and reduce alert fatigue, researchers have suggested that alerts should be parsimonious (fewer words that still convey the message), while others have suggested a staged implementation, for example, first implementing alerts for drug allergy, then drug dosing, followed by drug-drug interaction, and finally formulary support followed by alerts for specific patient types, laboratory testing, and drug-disease alerts (Kesselheim et al, 2011; Kuperman et al, 2007).

The process for the provider of making therapeutic decisions connects each of these technologies and systems (EHR, CPOE, CDS, RHIOs, HIE). Regardless of the size of the practice (office, clinic, large health-care organization), the provider is responsible for the adoption of these technologies and for functioning as a meaningful user of them. From patient assessment to recording the information in the EHR, prescribing or ordering medications supported by CPOE, acknowledging alerts, and information storage for the RHIOs and HIE, what appears to be a linear task is a process and part of a larger information and health-care system.

PATIENT SAFETY

Patient safety is the ultimate goal of care for a provider. Complementary to this goal is the reduction of health-care costs. The health-care system in the United States is complex. Providers who are also patients have a frontline view of the complexities. From untangling payer documents to dissecting hospital bills, seeking care has become a quagmire for patients. By using technology and striving to meet standards for meaningful use, providers are poised to facilitate patient understanding. The following sections will present information on technology and patient safety for pharmacotherapeutics.

MEDICATION RECONCILIATION

According to the CMS and EHR Incentive Program (np) Meaningful Use Core Measure 14, medication reconciliation is the process of identifying and listing the most accurate list of medications that the patient is taking, including the name of the medication, current dose, frequency, and route. Furthermore, for this standard to be met, medication reconciliation must be done for each encounter after long gaps in care, changes in medications, or other reasons as determined by the provider. This standard also includes when patient care is transferred from one provider to another or when the care setting changes (in- or outpatient, home health, and so forth).

The patient may be taking several medications and only know them by color, size of the pill, number taken per day, and by some unofficial nickname "my water pill," for example. Storing medication records in the EHR reduces the challenge of medication reconciliation. As described previously, using an EHR that is connected across an entire health-care system supports this standard. In this case, the information entered at one location appears when another provider within the same care system signs on to the system. For stand-alone EHR systems (those that are not connected), the provider is dependent on the exchange of patient information (using portable storage devices or paper) and on the patient as a historian. Once medications are accurately entered into the system, manually updating per encounter or patient transfer is then required to meet this standard.

In the case of controlled substances, it is possible to track individual prescriptions by date, substance, and provider using a state database. These databases are now accessible in almost every state but are not searchable across state lines. Providers individually enroll in the system to gain access, which in most states requires a prescriptive license and Drug Enforcement Agency (DEA) number. The database returns information that can provide a picture of "doctor shopping"—multiple providers dispensing controlled medication to the same patient—and evidence of urgent care or emergency room dispenses. This evidence can be used to track adherence to pain/controlled substance contracts and those who are under care for addiction issues.

PATIENT PRIVACY

In 1996, the Health Insurance Portability and Accountability Act (HIPAA) established the standard for patient privacy. The act encompasses a number of statutes that apply to insurance and the patient and includes the privacy rule. The privacy rule includes the Protected Health Information (PHI) statute and a number of others that apply to providers (Terry, 2009). This standard was updated in 2013 to take into account the vast changes in health care that have taken place in the past 17 years. Along with the expansion of aspects of privacy for patient information now covered and an increase in penalties for violations, HIPAA also includes an expansion of patient rights. According to the U.S. Department of Health and Human Services (2013), patients can now ask for a copy of their electronic health record and can expect to receive the copy in an electronic format. As stated by the department, this provision of the revised HIPAA standard implies that providers must now have the capability to provide patients with copies of their health record, which may include, for example, digital recording, e-mail, or electronic storage devices.

Despite efforts to fully implement and adopt the EHR, the portion that involves the personal health record (PHR) has received less national attention. This is curious because of our national experience with disasters that have revealed the fragility of health-care records. Thankfully, these losses appear to be infrequent; however, the damage can last for years.

The EHR and data storage systems provide solutions for health-care organizations and office practices; however, patients have often been in the care of a variety of providers in their lifetimes, especially those with complex health histories and chronic illnesses. Because it is specific to pharmacotherapeutics, the PHR may assist in maintaining the medication health records of patients. The PHR captures health data entered by patients and consumers of health care and, in some cases, the care provider (Tang, Ash, Bates, Overhage, & Sands, 2006). PHRs can be as sophisticated as those "tethered" to the EHR, be stand-alone systems purchased by the patient, or be as simple as a paper document or spreadsheet.

The tethered EHR is supported by a number of vendors and made available by health-care organizations. This type of PHR allows data from the EHR to populate the PHR, for example, laboratory results, radiology results, surgical pathology, and medication changes. These PHRs also support patients contacting their providers via e-mail and scheduling or rescheduling appointments, to name a few functions. In some cases, the PHR tethered to the EHR may also be connected to the neighborhood pharmacy. This feature has the potential of supporting interprofessional communication with the patient regarding their medications. Patients have expressed satisfaction with tethered systems and were generally positive about having electronic access to their EHR and messaging their providers (Hassol et al, 2004).

Stand-alone PHRs, or those not connected to the EHR, require patients to enter their own health and medication information. While this is better than not having a PHR, it lacks the features mentioned above. This type of PHR places additional responsibility on the patient for entering accurate health information. The positive outcome can be the improved self-care accountability that comes with being a partner in one's own health. These systems can often be downloaded on a portable drive for provider access during appointments and in- and outpatient events. At the simplest level, a "recording" glucometer or peak flow meter can be considered a technological aid for gathering information. Providers should acknowledge the individual effort patients extend in gathering this data and reinforce that they are major partners in creating the therapeutic plan.

PATIENT EDUCATION

Providers are responsible for patient education. Educating by providing patients with a copy of their health information might be considered one way to satisfy the meaningful use objective. Specific to pharmacotherapeutics, patients should receive education regarding their medications and changes in medication therapy during the visit or inpatient stay. The challenge is making time in a busy practice to meet this objective. One solution is to use a "patient instructions" feature within the documented plan of care. This section can be printed out as an after-visit summary provided at discharge while the data is simultaneously recorded in the clinical note.

Having an EHR that features medication education handouts in the practice or at the health-care organization is also useful. This information can be tailored to the specific needs of the patient and printed or e-mailed (or both) for the patient's handy reference. These applications require updating to remain current, which is usually done by the vendor or internal support personnel.

Another option is the use of computing tablets or smartphones to download applications designed for patient education. As of 2012, there existed nearly 30,000 applications, or "apps," related to health care designed for both the Apple and Android platforms (Bresnick, 2012).

Bresnick estimates that over half of the adults in the United States use smartphones that are capable of uploading these apps. The provider can use a computing pad or smartphone with an app and teach the patient about the medication, as well as other issues that emerged during the visit. Examples of long-established products are *Epocrates* and *MicroMedix*. These and many others supply both provider-level information and simpler patient handouts. In lieu of these formal pharmacology aids, a simple search on the Internet or using a smart device will reveal the apps available for use with pharmacotherapeutics and patient education.

The Internet as a source of information for patients is both wonderful and challenging. It contains a vast amount of information—some accurate, some less so. For a provider, patient education includes assisting patients to understand what Web sites contain accurate and useful information associated with health and pharmacotherapeutics. Table 11-3 lists those sites that suggest how to screen for accuracy, and each provides a list for users to scan and apply to health-related Web sites.

All sites listed in Table 11-3 are consistent with each other in terms of search criteria, and the table includes pointers from the Setting Priorities for Retirement Years (SPRY) Foundation , and information about whether the site includes the options "Contact us" and "Copyright" when scanning for

accuracy of information. MedlinePlus has taken an additional step by including the provider in the screening. On its Web site, Medline Plus suggests that patients consult with their provider to validate the information on the site. Providers can also search the Internet to identify Web sites that meet the standard and provide patients with an appropriate list during a visit. This information can also be part of the assessment "what have you learned about your medications (or topic) on the Internet?" This creates an opportunity for discussion with the patient and for gathering added information to enhance care.

QUALITY IMPROVEMENT

As a nation, we are over a decade beyond the 1999 IOM report and yet a significant number of people continue to die each year due to medication errors (Landrigan et al, 2010). The original emphasis on quality improvement in EHR documentation was not initially linked with patient safety. The fortunate outcome is that both are inextricably interlocked. For this reason, the process of pharmacotherapeutics does not conclude when the patient walks out the door or is discharged from hospital care.

The first step in the process of pharmacotherapeutics may be assessing a patient, followed by entering the prescription or medication order in the EHR, educating the patient, and

Table 11–3 Suggestions for Screening Web Sites

Web Site/Source	Screening Suggestions
Medical Library Association (MLA) http://www.mlanet.org/resources/userguide.html (Included list of useful Web sites on their site; very helpful information)	1. Sponsor of site 2. Regularly updated 3. Factual, look for sources 4. Stated audience
National Network of Libraries of Medicine (NN/LM) http://nnlm.gov/outreach/consumer/evalsite.html	1. Accuracy—source verification 2. Authority—who published the page? 3. Bias/objectivity—presented with what point of view? 4. Currency/timeliness 5. Information complete?
MedlinePlus http://www.nlm.nih.gov/medlineplus/healthywebsurfing.html	1. Consider source 2. Quality of site 3. Critical viewer—question message 4. Evidence—sources of information 5. Currency—latest updates 6. Bias—what is the purpose of Web site/information? 7. Privacy protection—search for policy 8. Consult with provider
Setting Priorities for Retirement Years Foundation (SPRY) http://www.spry.org/sprys_work/education/EvaluatingHealthInfo.html	1. Accuracy 2. Who wrote the information? 3. Is the site copyrighted? (Legal ownership of content) 4. "Contact Us" or equivalent 5. Web site support 6. Disclaimers and caution statements by Web site sponsors 7. Up-to-date information 8. Intended audience 9. Completeness of information 10. Written with clarity

reassessing for effectiveness. This process continues to include quality improvement, which involves using data to monitor patient outcomes and using improvement methods to design and test changes to continuously strive to improve the quality of patient care (Cronenwett et al, 2007).

APNs are clinical leaders and are responsible for assessing their practice for quality and patient safety. Those who hold the DNP degree have the education required to facilitate such assessments at all levels of the practice. The health-care organization or fellow practice providers will turn to these clinical leaders to explore troubling outcomes or questions regarding the best evidence-based practice. An in-depth discussion of the process of quality improvement, program evaluation, and creation of a program with logic models, however, is outside the scope of this chapter, which is focused on the use of technology to explore and challenge current practice.

Box 11-1 lists sample questions specific to pharmacotherapeutics that may initiate discussion within a practice and begin the process of quality improvement. The question may arise from observation: "I have seen this same reaction with five other patients," or "In my practice, our patients are not doing as well on this medication; are we using it correctly?" The first place to then turn may be the EHR database. Based on these examples, the search could be: "patients >65 years of age, male, diagnosis congestive heart failure with type 2 diabetes, currently prescribed XXX medication." This search may then provide the information necessary for establishing a pattern of patient responses to medications. From there, technology can assist with a comprehensive literature review specific to the practice question. If the technology is not available within the practice, hospital libraries most often will have computers with access to the Internet for searches and access to specific articles. When teaching patients about a specific medication, the APN may discover that an important point is being missed or not well understood. The APN provider can then design a quality improvement plan that will include education for both staff and providers, institute changes in practice policies and workflow, and create an evaluation plan for key quality outcomes.

CONCLUSION

This chapter has presented information regarding the intersection between technology and pharmacotherapeutics, including elements involved in the meaningful use of guidelines that are directly related to medications, in the hope of reducing medication errors, a leading cause of patient deaths in the United States. To be a meaningful user, the APN has the professional responsibility to appropriately use the EHR, CPOE, and CDS to increase patient safety and reduce health-care costs.

The professional responsibility of the ANP provider expands beyond the obvious process of pharmacotherapeutics to include patient safety. Patient safety includes medication reconciliation, sustaining all elements of patient privacy, supporting patients' use of the PHR, patient education, and quality improvement. Again, technology supports each of these elements of patient safety.

REFERENCES

Adler-Milstein, J., Bates, D. W., & Jha, A. K. (2011). A survey of health information exchange organizations in the United States: Implications for meaningful use. *Annals of Internal Medicine, 154,* 666–671.

Adler-Milstein, J., McAfee, A. P., Bates D. W., & Jha, A. K. (2007) The state of regional health information organizations: Current activities and financing. *Health Affairs Web Exclusive,* w60–w69.

American Association of Colleges of Nursing (October, 2006). The essentials of doctoral education for advanced nursing practice. Retrieved from http://www.aacn.nche.edu/publications/position/DNPEssentials.pdf

Avery, A. J., Savelyich, B. S., Sheikh, A., Cantrill, J., Morris, C. J., Fernanco, B., et al. (2005). Identifying and establishing consensus on the most important safety feature of GP computer systems: E-Delphi study. *Informatics in Primary Care, 13*(1), 3–12.

Bresnick, J. (2012). Physicians use mobile health apps for research and patient education. EHR Intelligence. Retrieved from http://ehrintelligence.com/2012/11/16/physicians-use-mobile-health-apps-for-research-and-patient-education/

Campbell, E. M., Sittig, D. F., Ash, J. S., Guappone, K. P., & Dykstra, R. H. (2006). Types of unintended consequences related to computerized provider order entry. *Journal of the American Medical Informatics Association, 13,* 547–556.

Chaudhry, B., Wang, J., Wu, S., Maglione, M., Mojica, W., Roth, E., et al. (2006). Review: Impact of health information technology on quality, efficiency, and costs of medical care. *Annals of Internal Medicine, 144*(10), 742–752.

CMS and EHR Incentive Program (np). Retrieved from http://www.cms.gov/Regulations-and-Guidance/Legislation/EHRIncentivePrograms/downloads/Stage2_EPCore_14_MedicationReconciliation.pdf

Cronenwett, L., Sherwood, G., Barnsteiner, J., Disch, J., Johnson, J., Mitchell, P., et al. (2007). Quality and safety education for nurses. *Nursing Outlook, 55*(3), 122–131. Retrieved from http://www.unc.edu/courses/2009fall/nurs/379/960/%20M10%20Safety%20and%20Quality%2009/cronenwett%20Quality%20and%20Safety%20Educ%20for%20Nurses.pdf

Devine, E. B., Hansen, R. N., Wilson-Norton, J. L., Lawless, N. M., Fisk, A. W., Blough, D. K., et al. (2010). The impact of computerized provider order entry on medication errors in a multispecialty group practice. *Journal of the American Medical Informatics Association, 17*(1), 78–84.

Doyle, M. J. (2009). Open source will help drive EHR costs down. *Health Management Technology, 30*(9), 10–11.

EHR Incentive Program (np). Eligible professional meaningful use table of contents core and menu set objectives stage 1. Retrieved from https://www.cms.gov/Regulations-and-Guidance/Legislation/EHRIncentivePrograms/downloads/EP-MU-TOC.pdf

Einbinder, J. S., Scully, K. W., Pates, R. D., Schubart, J. R., & Reynolds, R. R. (Summer 2001). Case study: A data warehouse for an academic medical

---

BOX 11–1 SAMPLE QUESTIONS FOR QUALITY IMPROVEMENT

1. In this practice, are we consistent in ordering specific laboratory tests at specific time intervals for patients on medication XXX with a diagnosis of XXX?
2. Are patients who take medication XXX receiving education about nutrition, what to exclude from a diet?
3. For this diagnosis, are patients avoiding readmission with XXX medication?
4. In this practice, are we consistent in how we educate patients about medication XXX?

center. *Journal of Healthcare Information Management 15*(2), 165–175. Retrieved from http://www.di.ubi.pt/~ddg/aulas/licenciatura/dwdm/artigos/Case-Study-A-Data-Warehouse-for-an-Academic-Medical-Center.pdf

Franklin, B. D., O'Grady, K., Donyai, P., Jacklin, G., & Barber, N. (2007). The impact of a closed-loop electronic prescribing and administration system on prescribing errors, administration errors and staff time: A before and after study. *Quality and Safety Health Care, 16*, 279–284.

Garets D., & Davis, M. (2006). Electronic medical records vs. electronic health records: Yes, there is difference. Retrieved from www.himssanalytics.org/docs/WP_EMR_EHR.pdf

Goolsby, K. (2002). CPOE odyssey: The story of evolving the world's first computerized physician order entry system and implications for today's CPOE decision makers. Retrieved from www.outsourcing-information-technology.com/cpoe.html

Hassol, A., Walker, J. M., Kidder, D., Rokita, K., Young, D., Pierdon, S., et al. (2004). Patient experiences and attitudes about access to a patient electronic health care record and linked web messaging. *Journal of the American Medical Informatics Association, 11*(6), 505–513.

HealthIT (np). Retrieved from http://www.healthit.gov/providers-professionals/health-information-exchange/what-hie

HIMSS Analytics. (2010). EMR adoption model. Retrieved from www.himssanalytics.org

H.R. 1-111th Congress: American Recovery and Reinvestment Act of 2009 (2009). In GovTrack.us (database of federal legislation). Retrieved from http://www.govtrack.us/congress/bills/111/hr1

HRSA (np). What is a regional health information organization (RHIO)? Retrieved from http://www.hrsa.gov/healthit/toolbox/RuralHealthITtoolbox/Collaboration/whatisrhio.html

Johnston, M. E., Langton, K. B., Hynes, R. B., & Mathieu, A. (1994). Effects of computer-based clinical decision support systems on clinical performance and patient outcome: A clinical appraisal of research. *Annals of Internal Medicine, 120*, 135–142.

Kesselheim, A. S., Cresswell, K., Phansalkar, S., Bates, D. W., & Sheikh, A. (2011). Clinical decision support systems could be modified to reduce 'alert fatigue' while still minizing the risk of litigation. *Health Affairs, 30*(12), 2310–2317.

Kilbridge, P. M., Campbell, U. C., Cozart, H. B., & Mojarrad, M. G. (2006). Automated surveillance for adverse drug events at a community hospital and an academic medical center. *Journal of the American Medical Informatics Association, 13*(4), 372–377.

Kohn, L. T., Corrigan, J. M., Donaldson, M. S. (Eds.) (1999). *To err is human: Building a safer health system.* Washington, DC: National Academy Press.

Koppel, R., Metley, J. P., Cohen, A., Abaluck, B., Localia, A. R., Dimmel, S. E., et al. (2005). Role of computerized physician order entry systems in facilitating medication errors. *Journal of the American Medical Informatics Association, 13*, 547–556.

Kuperman, G. J., Bobb, A., Payne, T. H., Avery, A. J., Gandhi, T. K., Burns, G., et al. (2007). Medication related clinical decision support in computerized provider order entry systems: A review. *Journal of the American Medical Informatics Association, 14*(1), 29–40.

Landrigan, C. P., Parry, G. J., Bones, C. B., Hackbarth, A. D., Goldmann, D. A., & Sharek, P. J. (2010). Temporal trends in rates of patient harm resulting from medical care. *New England Journal of Medicine, 363*(22), 2124–2134.

The Leapfrog Group. (2008, April 9). Factsheet computerized physician order entry. Retrieved from http://www.leapfroggroup.org/media/file/Leapfrog-Computer_Physician_Order_Entry_Fact_Sheet.pdf

Osterwalder, A., Pigneur, Y., & Tucci, C. L. (2005). Clarifying business models: Origins, present, and future of the concept. *Communications of the Association for Information Systems, 16*, 1–40.

Overhage, J. M., Evans, L., & Marchibroda, J. (2005). Communities' readiness for health information exchange: The national landscape in 2004. *Journal of the American Medical Informatics Association, 12*(5), 107–112.

Raebel, M. A., Carrlo, N. M., Kelleher, J. A., Chester, E. A., Berga, S., & Magid, D. J. (2007). Randomized trial to improve prescribing safety during pregnancy. *Journal of the American Medical Informatics Association, 14*, 495–498.

Shulman, R., Singer, M., Goldstone, J., & Bellingan, G. (2005). Medication errors: A prospective cohort study of hand written and computerized physician order entry in the intensive care unit. *Critical Care, 9*, R516–R521.

Solomon, M. R. (2007). Regional health information organizations: A vehicle for transforming health care delivery. *Journal of Medical Systems, 31*, 35–47.

Tang, P. C., Ash, J. S., Bates, D. W., Overhage, J. M., & Sands, D. Z. (2006). Personal health records: Definitions, benefits, and strategies for overcoming barriers to adoption. *Journal of the American Medical Informatics Association, 13*(2), 121–126.

Terry, K. (2009) Patient privacy—The new threats. *Physicians Practice, 19*(3). Retrieved from http://www.physicianspractice.com/patient-privacy-%E2%80%94-new-threats

U.S. Department of Health and Human Services. (2013, January 17). New rule protects patient privacy, secures health information. Retrieved from http://www.hhs.gov/news/press/2013pres/01/20130117b.html

Vaidya, V., Sowan, A. K., Mills, M.E., Socken, K., Gaffoor, M., & Hilmas, E. (2006). Evaluating the safety and efficiency of a CPOE system for continuous medication infusions in a pediatric ICU. *American Medical Information Association Proceedings, USA*, 1128.

Vest, J. R., & Gamm, L. D. (2010). Health information exchange: Persistent challenges and new strategies. *Journal of the American Medical Informatics Association, 17*, 288–294.

Walsh, K. E., Adams, W. G., Bouchner, H., Vinci, R. J., Chessare, J. B., Cooper, M. R., et al. (2006). Medication errors related to computerized order entry for children. *Pediatrics, 118*, 1872–1879.

PHARMACOECONOMICS

Teri Moser Woo

Today more than ever, third-party payers, health-care providers, government regulators, and patients are demanding that new drug treatments be not only clinically more effective but also cost-effective. Angiography, stent placement, transplantation, and use of monoclonal antibodies for the treatment of oncological disorders have become relatively routine treatments. After transplantation, patients who were dialysis-dependent are restored to relatively normal lives and are able to contribute to society. These accomplishments do not come without cost to the patient or society.

Pharmacoeconomics provides a framework for evaluating drug treatments in terms of comparing one treatment against another and whether the treatment is providing "value for the money" spent (Hay, 2008). Pharmacoeconomic evaluations of medical and surgical procedures have very seldom taken into account factors other than the actual cost to the health-care system of pharmaceutical agents (Berger & Teutsch, 2005; Tunis, 2009). This approach underestimates the real cost of drug treatment, which depends on adherence, efficacy of therapeutic agents, hospitalizations and treatment for adverse drug reactions, and finally productive life years. Also, a disturbing trend in modern medicine is the achievement of excellent short-term benefits that have relatively little long-term impact on comorbid conditions, drug toxicities, or drug nonadherence. The introduction of "me-too drugs"

(similar drugs developed by multiple drug companies) and the number of highly promoted drugs also distort the facts about the actual cost of drug therapy.

Prescription drug spending has increased significantly over the past few years, from $239.9 billion in 2004 to $320 billion in 2011 (IMS Health, 2012). Health-care organizations and pharmacy benefits managers have tried to control drug costs by using generic drugs and strict formularies. Generic-drug sales accounted for 71.2% of drug sales in 2010, up from 49.4% in 2005 (Pal, 2013). Although generic drugs have a place in health care, the decision to use them should be based on more than just cost-cutting reasons. However, with today's cost-consciousness in health-care delivery, quality of care may be compromised in exchange for lower cost. Health care has become more like a business with a bottom line, but medicine cannot be just a business. Now, more than at any time in history, we are responsible for distinguishing between excellent care and inappropriate cost cutting. Factors that influence pharmacoeconomics are found in Table 12-1.

PHARMACOECONOMIC STUDIES

Pharmacoeconomic studies were originally designed to study the cost to the health-care system of drug therapy. Clinical studies evaluate the safety and efficacy of a drug therapy,

Table 12–1 Factors Influencing Pharmacoeconomic Outcomes

Research Type
Clinical outcomes
Efficacy
Safety
Adverse drug reaction
Drug-drug reaction
Hospital admission, clinic visits
Humanistic outcomes
Patient satisfaction with care
Quality of life measured by validated instrument
Economic outcomes
Cost associated with immunosuppressive therapy
Cost to treat adverse drug reactions
Cost to treat drug-drug interactions
Cost to treat long-term toxicity (nephrotoxicity, hypertension)
Cost of laboratory work-ups

whereas pharmacoeconomic studies investigate the dollar value of patient care. Pharmacoeconomic studies are an increasing trend in all fields of health care; these studies should focus primarily on clinical and humanistic outcomes and secondarily on economic factors. Unfortunately, most pharmacoeconomic drug studies have focused solely on economic outcomes, with little attention paid to clinical efficacy, safety, and humanistic outcomes. All health-care providers must understand the limitations of these pharmacoeconomic studies.

The criteria routinely used in the study of pharmacoeconomics include cost-minimization, cost-benefit, and cost-effectiveness. The information obtained from a well-designed, on-site (local) pharmacoeconomic study should help health-care providers make important decisions regarding which protocol, treatment, services, and drugs should be used. A well-designed study should include several components (Table 12-2).

Components of Well-Designed Studies

Pharmacoeconomics is the analysis of the costs and consequences of any given health-care–related treatment or service. Pharmacoeconomic analysis may involve several different studies, each performed to answer different and specific types of questions. For any given analysis, knowing the *point of view*—whether a third-party payer, hospital, or government is determining the cost to society—is critical. Along with point of view, one should have a good understanding of the various *types of costs* and which are included in each type of analysis.

Direct costs are those that can be directly attributed to the treatment or disease state in question. They can include factors such as the acquisition price of medications, health-care provider time, or the cost of diagnostic tests. Direct, nonmedical costs must also be considered. This latter category includes transportation to the medical facility or child-care expenses incurred while receiving treatments. Direct costs can further be divided into fixed and variable costs, but because fixed costs are usually associated with overhead and are not influenced by the treatment or disease state, they are often excluded in a pharmacoeconomic analysis.

Besides direct costs, *indirect costs* associated with the therapy must be considered in an analysis. These costs derive from morbidity and mortality and include things such as loss or reduction of wages owing to illness or the costs associated with premature death.

Indirect costs can be calculated by two different methods, each having its own inherent flaws. The human capital method assumes losses based on an individual's capacity to earn money and is therefore skewed against the elderly, homeless, and unemployed. The second method is the willingness-to-pay method. In this method, the patient is asked how much money he or she would be willing to spend to reduce the likelihood of a particular illness. This method tends to have a wide range of answers and is often not realistic.

Intangible costs are very difficult to measure. They are related to nonfinancial outcomes and are hard to express monetarily. Included here are things such as inconvenience, pain and suffering, and grief. These costs are included in the willingness-to-pay calculation, but not the human capital calculation.

Table 12–2 Commonly Used Pharmacoeconomic Research Methodologies

Method	Outcome	Examples
Cost-minimization	Outcome must be clinically identical in similar patient population All social costs should be considered	Adalat CC vs. Procardia XL Generic azathioprine vs. brand-name azathioprine
Cost-effectiveness	Different clinical outcome Justify the incremental cost increase for the therapeutic benefit from extra costs associated with treatment	Antilymphocyte induction vs. no induction
Cost-benefit	Expressing clinical outcome purely in monetary units Assigns a dollar value to specific disease state Unethical and should be avoided	10 mm Hg reduction in blood pressure worth $100

Cost-of-Illness Analysis

Cost of illness identifies the costs of a specific disease in a given population. It is a good baseline number when looking at different treatment or prevention strategies. The total for the cost-of-illness evaluation includes the cost for the medical resources used to treat the specified illness, the cost of nonmedical resources, and the loss of productivity by the patient. Intangible costs, such as pain and suffering, are difficult to quantify and thus are not included in this calculation. For many disease states, including diabetes and certain cancers, the cost-of-illness number has already been calculated. According to the American Diabetes Association (2013), the cost of diabetes in the United States was estimated at $245 billion in 2012, up from $174 billion in 2007, a 41% increase in 5 years. (*Note*: This is strictly an estimate of economic burden and does not distinguish among treatment options.)

Cost-Minimization Analysis

Cost-minimization analysis is very straightforward. It looks at two or more treatment alternatives that are considered equal in efficacy and compares the cost of each alternative in dollars. It assumes that evidence supporting the efficacy of each alternative already exists and strictly looks at which would be the least costly to administer. An example of this is a comparison between two or more generic medications in the same therapeutic class for treatment of the same condition. (*Note*: The costs are not just related to acquisition of the product, but include costs for any preparation, administration, or monitoring needed.) A comparison of heparin and its counterpart, the low-molecular-weight enoxaprin, is a good example. Heparin is inexpensive, but patients receiving it have associated laboratory costs, technician time, and pharmacist dosage adjustments that must be figured into the cost. Although enoxaprin is more expensive to acquire, the lack of need for laboratory monitoring may help to bring the overall cost of enoxaprin down to be about equal to that of heparin. Therefore, cost-minimization analysis applied to pharmaceuticals reveals that generics are not necessarily always the least costly alternative.

Cost-Effectiveness Analysis

Unlike cost-minimization analysis, cost-effectiveness analysis compares two or more treatments or programs that are not necessarily therapeutically equivalent. This type of analysis compares various treatment costs with a specific therapeutic outcome. The outcome is usually a nondollar unit, such as a mm Hg drop in blood pressure or number of cases cured. One of the following three conditions must be met for a treatment to be considered cost-effective: the alternative treatment may be less expensive and at least as effective as its comparator; it may be more expensive but provide an additional benefit worth the cost; or it may be less expensive and less effective in a situation in which the extra benefit is not worth the extra cost.

This method aims to find and promote the most efficient therapy for the given problem and find the best health care for each dollar spent. An example of this type of analysis is a comparison of two different regimens for treating hypertension. Regimen A might consist of three medications and decrease systolic blood pressure by an average of 35 points. Regimen B, consisting of two medications that cost significantly less per month than regimen A, lowers systolic blood pressure by 20 points. To determine which is more cost-effective, the analysis team must decide if the extra drop in blood pressure is worth the added cost of regimen A.

For example, one cost-effectiveness model for long-acting risperidone examined the cost of the longer-acting formula versus increased compliance with a simpler dosing schedule, factoring in the economic implications of poorly managed schizophrenia (Haycox, 2005). Another example is a comparison of the costs of colchicine and NSAIDS for the treatment of gout, where the monthly cost of colchicine is much higher than NSAIDS (Wertheimer, Davis, & Lauterio, 2011). When the total cost of treatment, including treating gastrointestinal complications in a patient taking NSAIDS, is calculated, colchicine is more cost-effective (Wertheimer et al, 2011).

Cost-Benefit Analysis

In cost-benefit analysis (CBA), the costs of a specific treatment or intervention are calculated and then compared with the dollar value of the benefit received. One way to think about this analysis is whether or not a given benefit will exceed the cost needed to implement it. Many CBAs will look at two separate interventions or programs and determine which produces a greater benefit for the money. The two benefits may or may not be similar. The results of a CBA can be described in two different formats. The first is a ratio and the second is the dollar difference between the two. If a specific treatment is valued at $5,000 and the benefit is determined to be $50,000, one could determine that the cost-benefit ratio was 10:1 (benefit divided by cost) or the benefit of this specific treatment is $45,000 (benefit minus cost). The net benefit (or cost) is more commonly used than a ratio, because a 10:1 ratio could imply numbers with vastly different benefits (i.e., $1,000,000 to $100,000 versus $40 to $4).

One of the challenges of this type of analysis is that the benefits are often perceived; thus, it is difficult to quantify them. A common use of CBA is for budgeting purposes. A pharmacy can determine whether an existing anticoagulation program is worth keeping or whether that money would be better spent on a new hypertension clinic or diabetes education program.

Cost-Utility Analysis

In cost-utility analysis, the costs of the treatment choice are in dollars and the outcomes are expressed in terms of patient preference or quality-adjusted life years (QALY). A full year at full health is considered 1 QALY, whereas various diseases and their treatments produce a lower number (0.01–0.99).

These QALY values are quite subjective, and agreement on a scale to measure utility is lacking. The best use for this analysis is when quality of life is the most important factor to be considered; the analysis is commonly used in situations in which the treatment option can be life-extending but have significant side effects. Cancer treatment options are often reviewed with CBA. A chemotherapy treatment regimen, for example, may bring about a 6-month extension of life expectancy, but if the patient is too nauseated to get out of bed or eat, it may not be worth the extra 6 months.

IMPACT OF GENERIC DRUGS ON DRUG THERAPY

Drug pricing in today's health-care system is complex. The goal is to reduce drug acquisition costs to the lowest possible amount without affecting quality of care. Most pharmacies can control acquisition costs by purchasing generic drugs. However, in some situations, brand-name drugs are less expensive than generic-drug products owing to internal bidding, group purchasing, and negotiations with vendors. The cost of generic drugs and single-source, brand-name drugs to pharmacies and patients differs and is driven by market-force competition for the limited pool of dollars.

Although most drugs are sold for 15% to 20% less than the average wholesale price (AWP) and prices vary widely, AWP is routinely used for comparing different agents. A common method for determining reimbursement and controlling health-care system costs used by the Federal Health Care Financing Administration (HCFA) and private payers is the maximum allowable cost (MAC). Although drug pricing is complex, most pharmacy benefits groups are still businesses that seek profits. According to the MAC list prices, most pharmacy benefits groups select a drug with the lowest acquisition cost regardless of generic or brand-name status to reduce the cost of drug therapy. In most cases, pharmacy benefits groups pass this cost savings on to the patients by means of substantially lower co-payments for generic drugs.

Many benefit plans have a two- or three-tiered benefit, in which the patient pays a greater co-payment for brand-name drugs than for generic equivalent prescriptions. Most pharmacy benefits groups have maximum annual benefits for brand-name drugs ranging from $1,500 to $2,000 per year. The generic-drug benefit is unlimited and the purchase of generic drugs will not count against the $2,000 annual ceiling. For many generic drugs, the AWP is at least 50% that of the brand-name drug. Therefore, in general, co-payments are usually 50% of the wholesale price for single-source brand-name drugs. Patients may also take advantage of the numerous prescription programs offered by many large retail pharmacies where they can get a month's supply of a generic drug for $4 and not have to be concerned about their prescription coverage.

Generic medications are available to treat the most common diseases seen in primary care, including diabetes, hypertension, asthma, and common infections; therefore, patients benefit from the prescription of generic equivalents

(IMS Health, 2012). Lipitor, the number-one-selling drug in 2011, with sales of $7,668,425,000, went off patent in November 2011, which has provided savings to consumers (Bartholow, 2012). The availability of less costly generic-drug products for expensive agents would ease financial burdens for most patients, enabling them to comply with their treatments. Increased compliance may decrease health-care utilization in these patients, allowing greater access to health care for other patients. In addition, most patients can easily be stabilized on a generic-drug product with a narrow therapeutic index as well as on an innovator brand.

Generic Substitution

As health-care system costs continue to escalate, accountability in health-care spending and patient outcomes as a measure of effectiveness of health-care delivery has become crucial. Decreasing the total cost of drug therapy while improving outcomes has become a challenging responsibility for health-care providers. Today, generic substitution for brand-name drugs is a common practice in most health-care organizations in order to decrease the total cost of pharmacotherapy. In 2011, 80% of all prescriptions in the United States were filled with generic drugs, yet generic drugs accounted for only 27% of dollars spent on prescriptions (IMS Institute for Healthcare Informatics, 2012).

The practice of generic-drug substitution has been an emotional issue for health-care providers, payers, and patients. Health-care providers are under pressure from both innovator companies and payers. Innovator companies that have supported the field of medicine over the past two decades through educational grants and clinical drug studies apply subtle pressure on health-care providers to continue to prescribe brand-name drugs only. The critical issue in using generic drugs involves justifying conversion from a brand-name drug to a generic agent in stable patients or using the drug de novo in terms of safety, efficacy, and economics. To help address this issue, the generic bioequivalence standards and different methods of studying pharmacoeconomics should be considered.

Generic Bioequivalence

The U.S. Food and Drug Administration (FDA) regulates the manufacturing of generic drugs by setting rigorous standards for bioequivalence and is responsible for protecting patients and assuring prescribers that generic-drug products truly are "equivalent" to those of the innovator pharmaceutical companies. To gain FDA approval (FDA, 2013), a generic drug must:

- Contain the same active ingredients as the innovator drug. Active ingredients make the drug effective against the disease or condition it is treating.
- Come in the same dosage form. If the brand name is a capsule, the generic should be a capsule too.
- Be administered in the same way. If the brand name is taken orally, the generic should be taken orally too.

- Be identical in strength.
- Have the same conditions of use.
- Be bioequivalent (an equal rate and extent of drug absorbed in the bloodstream).
- Meet the same standards for identity, strength, purity, and quality.
- Be manufactured under the same standards that the FDA requires for the manufacture of innovator products.

The FDA monitors complaints regarding generics. In the case of Budeprion XL 300 mg, a generic form of Wellbutrin XL, the FDA even conducted studies to determine Budeprion XL 300 was not bioequivalent to Wellbutrin XL 300 (FDA, 2013). These strict standards for generic medications ensure the availability of safe generic equivalents for the public.

Pharmaceutical Equivalents

Drug products are considered pharmaceutical equivalents when both agents contain identical amounts of active ingredients in the same salt or ester form, dosage form, and route of administration and possess identical disintegration times and dissolution rates.

Therapeutic Equivalents

Drug products are considered therapeutically equivalent when the generic drugs are pharmaceutical equivalents and show the same efficacy and safety profile as that product whose efficacy and safety has been established.

Bioequivalence

Bioequivalence is defined as pharmaceutical equivalents that display the same rate and extent of absorption. Biological equivalence means delivering the same amount of active drug moiety to the site of action when generic and innovator drugs are administered at the same molar dose under similar conditions. Only therapeutically equivalent drug products of those already FDA-approved are safe and should be considered for generic substitution in most patients.

APPLYING PHARMACOECONOMICS TO PRACTICE

Generic-drug versus brand-name drug prescribing is discussed in this section, using clinical examples of and rationales for generic substitution. An explanation of Medicare Part D will demonstrate why prescribers need to be familiar with their patients' prescription drug coverage, as it may affect compliance.

Prescribing Generic Versus Brand-Name Medications

Generic drugs that are considered therapeutic equivalents may be exchanged for brand-name drugs with confidence. Pharmacists may substitute a generic equivalent for a brand name unless the prescriber specifies "Dispense as Written"

on the prescription. Shrank and colleagues (2011) studied 5.6 million prescriptions written for 2 million patients and found there was a greater chance that the prescription was not filled if "Dispense as Written" was on the prescription or requested by the patient. It is critical to discuss pharmacy benefit coverage with the patient before prescribing a drug as "Dispense as Written."

Many retail stores offer prescription programs in which a select list of generic drugs are offered for $4 for a 30-day supply and $10 for a 90-day supply. This may be a substantial savings for patients, especially those without prescription drug coverage or with a high co-payment for their medications. For example, generic metformin 500 mg tablets are $4 for a 30-day supply, whereas the retail price for the brand-name Glucophage is $70 for the same 30-day supply. The caveat is that the patient must live near or have transportation to one of the retail pharmacies that have retail drug programs, such as Walmart, Target, Kroger, and Sam's Club stores.

Medicare Part D

In 2004, Congress added a prescription drug benefit to the Medicare program called Medicare Part D. Part D was enacted to assist seniors with the high cost of their medications, but the implementation has been confusing for many. When initially passed, Part D covered 75% of drug costs once the patient paid a deductible of $250 per year. Prescriptions that cost between $250 and $2,250 require the patient to pay 25% of the price of the medication. Once the patient's medication costs reach $2,250, the patient pays 100% of the costs of the medication until the total reaches $5,100. The coverage gap between $2,250 and $5,100 has been referred to as the "donut hole" point of coverage. After the patient reaches $5,100 in drug costs, Part D provides 95% coverage for drug costs for the remainder of the calendar year. The Affordable Care Act gradually narrows the gap and decreases the amount paid by Medicare recipients in the "donut hole." In 2013, the gap is $2,970 to $4,750, and Medicare enrollees get a 52.5% discount on brand-name drugs and 70% on generic-drug costs during the gap in the coverage period (Medicare.gov, 2013). Drug costs in the gap will be gradually reduced from 100% to 25% by 2020.

Part D has increased the use of essential drugs such as statins, warfarin, and clopidogrel among elders who did not have drug coverage before the prescription benefit plan was implemented (Schneeweiss et al, 2009). Schneeweiss and colleagues noted a 5% decline in the proportion of patients filling their clopidogrel prescription when patient drug costs reached the coverage gap. Similarly, a 4.8% decline in warfarin and a 6.3% decline in statin prescription refills were noted (Schneeweiss et al, 2009). Duru and colleagues (2010) examined cost-related noncompliance among diabetics covered by Part D and found noncompliance among beneficiaries using insulin increased when their benefits during the gap did not have generic-drug coverage. Providers must work with patients to determine if less expensive but equally effective prescriptions can be used to prevent patients with limited means from reaching the point of having to pay the full amount for their prescriptions, because paying the full amount may decrease compliance, increasing the overall cost of care due to poor outcomes.

CONCLUSION

Pharmacoeconomics is the study of the appropriate application of drug utilization for the treatment of a specific disease. Pharmacoeconomic studies characterize the improved outcomes while justifying additional drug expenditures. Because the value and economics of many approved drugs are unknown at the time, the true impact of new drug substitution on the cost and care of most patients with complicated conditions is also unknown. In theory, if a therapeutically equivalent and less expensive product is available, it should be substituted; this may substantially affect the cost of drug therapy and overall health-care costs. Applying pharmacoeconomics to prescribing practice involves understanding the impact of drug costs on patients and making an educated prescribing decision to ensure the best outcome.

REFERENCES

American Diabetes Association. (2013). The cost of diabetes. American Diabetes Association. Retrieved from http://www.diabetes.org/advocate/resources/cost-of-diabetes.html

Bartholow, M. (2012). Top 200 drugs of 2011. *Pharmacy Times.* Retrieved from http://www.pharmacytimes.com/publications/issue/2012/July2012/Top-200-Drugs-of-2011

Berger, M. L., & Teutsch, S. (2005). Cost-effectiveness analysis: From science to application. *Medical Care, 43*(Suppl. 7), II 49–II 53.

Duru, O. K., Mangione, C. M., Hsu, J., Steers, W. N., Quiter, E., Turk, N., et al. (2010). Generic-only drug coverage in the Medicare Part D gap and effect on medication cost-cutting behaviours for patients with diabetes mellitus: The translating research into action for diabetes study. *Journal of the American Geriatrics Society, 58*(5), 822–828.

Hay, J. W. (2008). Using pharmacoeconomics to value pharmacotherapy. *Clinical Pharmacology & Therapeutics, 84*(2), 197–200.

Haycox, A. (2005). Pharmacoeconomics of long-acting risperidone: Results and validity of cost-effectiveness models. *Pharmacoeconomics, 23*(Suppl. 1), 3–16.

IMS Health (2012). The US pharmaceutical market: Looking back and looking ahead! Retrieved from http://www.goldstandard.com/wp-content/uploads/The-US-Pharmaceutical-Market.pdf

IMS Institute for Healthcare Informatics (2012). The use of medicines in the United States: Review of 2011. Retrieved from http://www.imshealth.com/ims/Global/Content/Insights/IMS%20Institute%20for%20Healthcare%20Informatics/IHII_Medicines_in_U.S_Report_2011.pdf

Malone, D. (2005). The role of pharmacoeconomic modeling in evidence-based and value-based formulary guidelines. *Journal of Managed Care Pharmacy, 11*, S7–S10.

Medicare.gov. The Official U.S. Government Site for Medicare. (2013). Costs in the coverage gap. Centers for Medicare & Medicaid Services. Retrieved from http://www.medicare.gov/part-d/costs/coverage-gap/part-d-coverage-gap.html

Pal, S. (2013). Shifts in the generic-drug market: Trends and causes. *US Pharmacist, 38*(6 Suppl.), 6–10.

Schneeweiss, S., Patrick, A. R., Pedan, A., Varasteh, L., Levin, R., Liu, N., et al. (2009). *Health Affairs, 28*(2), w305–w316.

Shrank, W. H., Liberman, J. N., Fischer, M. A., Avron, J., Kilabuk, E., Chang, A., et al. (2011). The consequences of requesting "dispense as written." *The American Journal of Medicine, 124*(4), 309–317.

Tunis, S. L. (2009). A cost-effectiveness analysis to illustrate the impact of cost definitions on results, interpretations and comparability of pharmacoeconomic studies in the US. *Pharmacoeconomics, 27*(9), 735–744.

U.S. Food and Drug Administration. (2013). Generic drugs: Same medicine, lower cost. U.S. Department of Health and Human Services. Retrieved from http://www.fda.gov/forconsumers/consumerupdates/ucm340343.htm

Wertheimer, A. I., Davis, M. W., & Lauterio, T. J. (2011). A new perspective on the pharmacoeconimics of colchicine. *Current Medical Research & Opinion, 27*(5), 931–937.

OVER-THE-COUNTER MEDICATIONS

Teri Moser Woo

Patients are now taking a more active and informed role in their own health care. Thousands of self-help books, articles, Web sites, television commercials, and social media demonstrate the rapidly growing trend in self-care. Surveys consistently show that consumers are increasingly self-medicating with nonprescription drugs.

OVER-THE-COUNTER MEDICATIONS

An over-the-counter (OTC) drug has the following characteristics: (1) it must be safe (the benefit must outweigh the risks), (2) it has low potential for misuse or abuse, (3) it can be labeled, (4) the patient must be able to self-diagnose the condition for which the drug is being taken, and (5) it must be for a condition that the patient can manage without supervision by a licensed health professional (U.S. Food and Drug Administration Center for Drug Evaluation and Research [FDA CDER], 2012). The FDA CDER is responsible for ensuring that OTC drugs are properly labeled and that their benefits outweigh their risks. New OTC drug ingredients must undergo the New Drug Application process, just as prescription drugs do (FDA CDER, 2012). There are more than 80 therapeutic categories of OTC drugs and over 100,000 OTC drug products (FDA CDER, 2012).

In addition, there has been a dramatic increase in the number of prescription medications that have moved to OTC status, for a variety of reasons. Cohen, Paquette, and Cairns (2005) propose three motives for this: "pharmaceutical firms' desire to extend the viability of brand names, attempts by healthcare funders to contain costs, and the self-care movement" (p 39). A blockbuster drug such as the proton pump inhibitor Prilosec or the antihistamine Zyrtec can continue to reap large profits by moving to OTC status. Insurers often drop drugs from coverage when they become OTC and so have pushed for drugs to become OTC, as in the case of WellPoint's petitioning the FDA to designate three antihistamines (loratadine, cetirizine, and fexofenadine) as OTC (Cohen et al, 2005; Sullivan, Nair, & Patel, 2005). Clearly, when drugs are close to reaching the end of their patent, pharmaceutical firms and insurers are motivated to move the drug to OTC status.

Because patients are likely to treat many symptoms and conditions first with nonprescription drugs, the practitioner should assume that some therapy has been started when patients present for care and therefore should ask about OTC medication use. Patients are more likely to self-treat themselves or their children when they feel their illnesses are not serious enough to require medical care. Table 13-1 presents conditions for which OTC drugs are marketed.

Table 13–1 Conditions for Which OTC Drugs Are Marketed

Most frequently treated conditions	Acne, athlete's foot, cold sores, colds, cough, cuts, dandruff, headache, heartburn, indigestion, insomnia, premenstrual, sinusitis, sprains
Other conditions	Abrasions, aches and pains, allergic rhinitis, anemia, arthralgia, asthma, bacterial infection (superficial), boils, burns, candidal vaginitis, canker sores, chapped skin, congestion, conjunctivitis, constipation, contact lens care, contraception, corns, dental care, dermatitis (contact), diaper rash, diarrhea, dysmenorrhea, dyspepsia, feminine hygiene, fever, gastritis, gingivitis, hair loss, halitosis, head lice, impetigo, insect bites, jet lag, motion sickness, nausea, obesity, otitis (external), periodontal disease, pharyngitis, pinworms, prickly heat, psoriasis, ringworm, seborrhea, smoking cessation, sty, sunburn, swimmer's ear, teething, toothache, vomiting, warts, xerostomia

OTC = over-the-counter.

Nonprescription drug therapy should not be undervalued or underestimated in the current health-care environment. OTC medications are powerful drugs that should be considered just like prescription drugs with respect to their pharmacology, toxicology, contraindications, precautions, adverse effects, and drug interactions. Because many former prescription drugs have recently been converted to nonprescription (OTC) status, the same care and thought needed to monitor prescription drug use are necessary for nonprescription drugs.

This chapter discusses in general terms OTC drugs that patients commonly use and OTC drug adverse effects. For more specific information on these drugs, see the appropriate chapters in this book.

OTC MEDICATION SALES

Sales of OTC medications reported by the Consumer Healthcare Products Association were $33.1 billion in 2013 (Consumer Healthcare Products Association [CHPA], 2014a). CHPA data can be used to determine the common physical complaints patients self-treat with OTC medications. Over $4 billion was spent on cough and cold medications in 2008, representing the highest sales category (CHPA, 2014b.) Internal analgesics represented $3.99 billion in 2013 sales, indicating acute and chronic pain were common self-treated conditions. Self-treatment of heartburn led to $2.28 billion in sales of heartburn remedies in 2013, doubling in 5 years as multiple proton pump inhibitors became OTC. Other conditions commonly treated by OTC medications include constipation ($1.3 billion), acne ($617 million), and diarrhea ($225 million). Nicotine replacement products used for tobacco cessation represented $855 million in sales in 2013 (CHPA). The CHPA proposes that every dollar spent on OTC medications by consumers saves the U.S. health-care system $6 to $7, based on cost savings in clinical visits and drugs (CHPA, 2012).

SELF-PRESCRIBING OTC MEDICATIONS

Self-prescribing or self-medication is defined by the World Self Medication Industry as "the treatment of common health problems with medicines especially designed and labeled for use without medical supervision and approved as safe and effective for such use" (World Self-Medication Industry, n.d.). In order to safely self-medicate, the patient will need to accurately self-diagnose the condition and then take the appropriate medication, at the appropriate dose, for the correct duration, without creating interactions with other medication. Caregivers of children or those who are cognitively impaired need to accurately diagnose the ailment in the child or impaired person before choosing an OTC remedy. There is room for misdiagnosis and error in the process of self-medication.

Multiple studies have been conducted to investigate the process of self-medication with OTC medications. Pineles and Parente (2012) used the theory of planned behavior to explore belief about medications and the individual pain experience to predict intent to self-medicate with OTC analgesics. The authors discovered that patients tend to self-medicate when the patient values pain relief over harm and that 49% of the study participants reported taking more than the recommended dose of OTC analgesics (Pineles & Parente, 2012). In a telephone survey study of OTC topical corticosteroid use ($N = 2,000$), 83% of respondents were using the product consistent with labeling instructions (Ellis et al, 2005). Use of topical corticosteroids was usually short-term (less than 7 days) in both adults (92% used for ≤ 7 days) and in children (94%), and applied appropriately 4 times a day or less (adults 98%; children 97%) (Ellis et al, 2005). Pharmacists may be available for consultation, but even so, patients may not follow the direction of the expert pharmacist as to when to appropriately seek medical care rather than self-treat (Mehuys et al, 2009).

The FDA mandated a redesign of OTC drug labeling to ensure uniformity of labeling, consistent presentation of information, and use of lay language (FDA, 2014a). McDonald and others (2007) studied the use of the new FDA label by 137 adults and found that 61.2% were likely to read the medication label before taking an OTC analgesic. But despite being provided a pamphlet and the label regarding the use of the OTC analgesic, 25.4% were likely to give ibuprofen to a family member who takes an antihypertensive, 21.2% said they were likely to take another dose before the recommended time, and 27.7% were not likely to read the label before taking the medication (McDonald et al, 2007). Even if the consumer reads the label, its readability level is well above the average reading ability in the United States. Trivedi, Trivedi, and Hannan (2014) examined the labels of 40 OTC products (NSAIDS, antacids, laxatives, antihistamines, H2 blockers, proton pump inhibitors, sleep aids, and cough and cold medications) to determine the reading level. The authors found that the average Flesch–Kincaid reading ease score was 38 ($\pm$12), the average Flesch–Kincaid grade level score was 16 ($\pm$5), and the average Gunning–Fog grade level score was 17 ($\pm$5)—all were above the eighth-grade reading level of the average U.S. adult (Trivedi et al, 2014). There is clearly a need to revisit the OTC medication label to ensure the safe use of OTC medications.

HAZARDS OF OTC SELF-MEDICATION

Over-the-counter medications may be harmful if misused or may cause harmful interactions with prescription drugs. Acetaminophen has well-documented toxic effects on the liver if higher-than-recommended doses are taken. Patients may take higher doses due to the severity of symptoms or if they do not feel they are getting better with the recommended dose (Pineles & Parente, 2012). Patients may accidentally overdose on acetaminophen due to unknowingly taking two OTC medications that both contain acetaminophen or by taking OTC acetaminophen with prescription drugs that contain acetaminophen, such as Vicodin or Percocet. The FDA has been addressing acetaminophen toxicity by lowering the recommended daily dosage on OTC labels to 3 g per day and recommending providers only prescribe prescription acetaminophen combination drugs 325 mg per tablet or less (FDA, 2014b).

A concern with decongestant medications is their use in young children, specifically children under age 5. The safety and efficacy of these medications have been questioned after a number of reports of deaths of infants taking cold medications (U.S. Centers for Disease Control and Prevention, 2007). In October 2007, an FDA panel recommended that all pediatric cough and cold medications be relabeled as not indicated for use in children under age 4. In October 2007, manufacturers voluntarily removed all infant drop formulas of cough and cold medications from the market. In spite of the labeling change and withdrawal of infant formulations, one-third (33%) of parents surveyed by Hanoch, Gummermum, Miron-Shatz, & Himmelstein (2010) were not aware of the FDA recommendations, with 32.9% planning on continuing to administer OTC cough and cold medication to their young child. Use of decongestants in children is discussed in Chapters 17 and 50.

ADVERSE EFFECTS OF OTC SELF-MEDICATION

Self-medication with OTC products may lead to adverse effects, drug interactions, and potentially to abuse. Adverse effects and drug interactions are often listed on the label of the OTC medication, but as noted previously patients may not read or comprehend the label information.

Adverse Effects

All medications, whether prescription or OTC, have predictable and unpredictable adverse effects. When a prescriber is choosing a medication, this understanding of adverse effects is integral to the decision making and patient education regarding the medication. Likewise, when pharmacists fill a prescription, they will often discuss significant adverse effects with the patient. These safeguards are lost when a patient self-medicates with an OTC product.

Adverse effects of OTC medications may be mild, such as gastrointestinal upset, or severe, as in the case of gastrointestinal bleeding associated with NSAID or aspirin use. Exceeding treatment duration or taking the wrong dose increases the likelihood of adverse reactions (Schmeidl et al, 2014). The elderly are the most likely to be hospitalized due to adverse effects associated with OTC medication use (Villany, Fok, & Wong, 2011; Schmeidl et al, 2014).

Patients need to be educated regarding the adverse effects of OTC medications. Education includes reading the label carefully and asking questions of a pharmacist or the provider. Patients should be advised that some OTC medications may impair driving; most state laws do not differentiate between alcohol or prescription or OTC drugs in regard to impaired driving (American Automobile Association, 2011). Table 13-2 discusses OTC medications that may impair driving.

Table 13–2 Over-the-Counter Medications That May Impair Driving or Operating Machinery

Medication	OTC Products
Antihistamines: diphenhydramine, chlorpheniramine, brompheniramine, dexbrompheniramine, clemastine, cyproheptadine, doxylamine, pyrilamine (maleate)	Allergy medications Cold medications Sleep aids Menstrual cramp medications Motion sickness medications
Antimotility agents (loperamide)	Antidiarrheals
Antitussives (dextromethorphan)	Cough and cold medications
H2 antagonists (ranitidine, famotidine, nazatidine)	H2 antagonist/heartburn medications
NSAIDS (naproxen, ibuprofen)	NSAID analgesics
Alcohol	Cough and cold medications Expectorants Multivitamins with or without iron (liquid) Antihistamines (liquid forms) Motion sickness medications (liquid)

Drug Interactions

When patients receive a prescription from a provider or fill a prescription in the pharmacy, a review of current medications occurs and potential drug interactions are identified. When a patient self-medicates with an OTC medication, often no professional knowledgeable about drug interactions is involved. Patients may not be aware that OTC medications may interact with prescription or other OTC medications or alcohol.

Antacids

Antacids consist of a metallic cation and basic ion (calcium carbonate, magnesium hydroxide, etc.), which neutralize acidity in the stomach by raising the pH. The basic property of these drugs causes them to interact with most medications, by either binding with the drug molecule or altering pH and thus the absorption of drugs that need an acidic environment for optimal absorption. Most interactions can be avoided by separating the dosing of antacids by at least 2 hours from the dosing of the other oral medications. Intraluminal interactions occur in the stomach when an antacid chelates another drug or adsorbs another drug onto its surface.

The best-known antacid interaction is with tetracycline. Aluminum hydroxide and magnesium hydroxide have a strong affinity for tetracycline and form an insoluble and inactive chelate. This interaction can reduce the bioavailability of tetracycline by 90% and result in clinical failures. This chelation occurs with all other forms of tetracycline, including doxycycline and minocycline. Patients should not take any antacid until at least 2 hours after tetracycline administration. A similar interaction exists with the quinolone antibiotics, such as ciprofloxacin and ofloxacin. Antacids are discussed in Chapter 20.

Anticholinergics

The primary adverse effects of diphenhydramine and doxylamine are anticholinergic, such as dry mouth, constipation, blurred vision, and tinnitus. Older male patients may have difficulty in urinating. These effects may be additive with the anticholinergic effects of other drugs that are being taken. Older patients may develop delirium from modest doses of diphenhydramine.

Central Nervous System Depressants

Patients may be aware that their prescription medication may cause sedation, but they may not be aware of the additive central nervous system (CNS) sedating effects of OTC medication taken with their prescribed medication. Over-the-counter medications that contain alcohol, antihistamines, antitussives, or antidiarrheals may all cause additive sedation when taken with CNS-sedating medications.

NSAIDS and Aspirin

The cyclooxygenase inhibitors, including aspirin and the NSAIDS ibuprofen and naproxen, have a well-documented risk of gastrointestinal bleeding. When combined with antiplatelet or anticoagulant medications, the risk is significantly increased and may be life-threatening. Patients who are taking antiplatelet or anticoagulant medications should be educated to not take any OTC medication without consulting with a pharmacist or their provider.

ABUSE OF OTC MEDICATIONS

Over-the-counter medications have the potential for abuse. Many liquid products, such as cough and cold medications, expectorants, and liquid multivitamins or iron, contain alcohol. Common products like Geritol liquid vitamins contain 12% alcohol. Cough and cold medications may contain up to 25% alcohol. Dextromethorphan is abused for its ability to produce hallucinations and a dissociative state, with the peak age for abuse at 15 to 19 years (Drug Enforcement Administration, 2014; Wilson, Ferguson, Mazer, & Litovitz, 2011). Abuse of combination cough and cold medications that contain dextromethorphan may lead to toxic levels of multiple substances, including acetaminophen and anticholinergics.

Concern over the use of OTC decongestant medications to manufacture methamphetamine has led to changes in how the drugs are sold in the United States. The Combat Methamphetamine Epidemic Act, which is part of the 2006 U.S. Patriot Act, restricts the sales of all cough and cold products (including combination products) that contain the methamphetamine precursor chemicals ephedrine, pseudoephedrine, or phenylpropanolamine. The law specifically includes a daily and 30-day limit on retail store and Internet purchases of known methamphetamine precursors. All potential precursors are to be stored behind the counter in retail stores and retailers are required to ask for identification and keep a log of who is purchasing the drugs. Some states have additional restrictions; for example, Oregon and Mississippi have listed pseudoephedrine as a Schedule III drug under state law. Multiple states are enacting similar legislation to control the sales of pseudoephedrine (Office for State, Tribal, Local and Territorial Support Centers for Disease Control and Prevention, 2013). Internationally, countries including Mexico, Australia, New Zealand, and the United Kingdom are limiting unrestricted OTC sales of pseudoephedrine.

PATIENT EDUCATION REGARDING OTC MEDICATIONS

Given the concerns over OTC self-medication, providers are required to educate their patients about safe OTC use. Reading the label and following the label instructions are critical, but if patients do not understand the label, they should ask for assistance from a pharmacist or the provider. In a study of OTC medication consultation by pharmacy students in a community pharmacy, McConaha, Finole, Heasley, and Lunney (2012) found that only 37.6% of consumer participants initiated a consultation with the pharmacist, and that consultation resulted in significant cost savings by switching to a generic product and nonsignificant but clinically relevant prevention of OTC medication-related adverse outcomes. Educating patients that even though a medication is available over-the-counter, it still has the same concerns for adverse effect, drug interactions, and toxicity as prescription medication may increase safety when self-medicating (see Box 13-1).

SUMMARY

The provider must keep in mind that the prescription drug history, although very important, is usually not the only part of a patient's drug use. A careful history of both OTC medications and herbals is needed to avoid overlooking important aspects, such as adverse drug effects and drug interactions caused by these drugs and herbal products in tandem with any prescription drugs. Many people diagnose their own symptoms, select a nonprescription drug product, and monitor their own therapeutic response. This process is not often reliably reported when, during a routine health history, a patient is asked, "Do you take any medications?" Specific questions need to be asked.

Properly used, OTC medications are useful in self-care to relieve minor complaints and transient conditions. If used improperly or in combination with other medications, OTC medications can cause a multitude of problems, adverse drug events, and drug interactions.

BOX 13–1 PATIENT EDUCATION REGARDING OTC MEDICATIONS

- Read the label of the medication to determine dose, duration of treatment, adverse effects, and drug interactions.
- If you do not understand the label information, ask a pharmacist or your health care provider to clarify.
- Inform your provider and the pharmacist of any OTC medications you are taking, even medications you only take occasionally.
- Do not drive or operate machinery if you take sedating OTC medications. You may be charged with driving under the influence.
- Inform your provider if you have any adverse effects from the OTC medication.

BOX 13–2 OVER-THE-COUNTER MEDICATION RESOURCES

American College of Preventive Medicine
Over the Counter Medications Time Tool
http://www.acpm.org/?OTCMeds_ClinRef

Consumer Healthcare Products Association
www.chpa.org
http://otcsafety.org/

Scholastic OTC Literacy for Teachers
http://www.scholastic.com/otcliteracy/

U.S. Food and Drug Administration
Educational Resources: Understanding Over-the-Counter Medicine
http://www.fda.gov/Drugs/ResourcesForYou/Consumers/

REFERENCES

American Automobile Association (2011). State laws on medication use & driving. Retrieved from http://seniordriving.aaa.com/medical-conditions-medications/state-laws-medication-use-driving

Armstrong, S., & Cozza, K. (2003). Antihistamines. *Psychosomatics, 44*(5), 430–434.

Cohen, J. P., Paquette, C., & Cairns, C. P. (2005). Switching prescription drugs to over the counter. *BMJ: British Medical Association, 330*, 39–41.

Consumer Healthcare Products Association. (2012). *Value of OTC medicine to the United States.* Retrieved from http://www.chpa.org/ValueofOTCMeds2012.aspx

Consumer Healthcare Products Association. (2014a). OTC retail sales. Retrieved from http://www.chpa.org/OTCRetailSales.aspx

Consumer Healthcare Products Association. (2014b). OTC sales by category 2010–2013. Retrieved from http://www.chpa.org/OTCsCategory.aspx

Drug Enforcement Administration (2014). Dextromethorphan. Retrieved from http://www.deadiversion.usdoj.gov/drug_chem_info/dextro_m.pdf

Food and Drug Administration (2014a). The current over-the-counter medicine label: Take a look. Retrieved from http://www.fda.gov/drugs/resourcesforyou/ucm133411.htm

Food and Drug Administration (2014b). Limiting acetaminophen's strength in prescription medications. Retrieved from http://www.fda.gov/drugs/drugsafety/informationbydrugclass/ucm165107.htm

Food and Drug Administration Center for Drug Evaluation and Research (FDA CDER). (2012). Regulation of nonprescription products. Retrieved from http://www.fda.gov/aboutfda/centersoffices/officeofmedicalproductsandtobacco/cder/ucm093452.htm

Ellis, C. N., Pillitteri, J. L., Kyle, T. K, Ertischek, M. D., Burton, S. L., & Shiffman, S. (2005). Consumers appropriately self-treat based on labeling for over-the-counter hydrocortisone. *Journal of the American Academy of Dermatology, 53*(1), 41–51.

Hanoch, Y., Gummermum, M., Miron-Shatz, T., & Himmelstein, M. (2010). Parents' decision following the Food and Drug Administration recommendation: The case of over-the-counter cough and cold medication. *Child Care, Health and Development. 36*(6), 795–804.

McConaha, J.L., Finole, L.M., Heasley, J.E. & Lunney, P.D. (2012). Assessing student pharmacist impact on patient over-the-counter medication selection. *Journal of Pharmacy Practice. 26*(3), 280-287.

Mehuys, E., Van Bortel, L., De Bolle, L., Van Tongelen, I., Remon, J. P., & De Looze, D. (2009). Self-medication of upper gastrointestinal symptoms: A community pharmacy study. *Annals of Pharmacotherapy, 43*(5), 890–989.

Office for State, Tribal, Local and Territorial Support Centers for Disease Control and Prevention (2013). Pseudoephedrine: Legal efforts to make it a prescription-only drug. Retrieved from http://www.cdc.gov/phlp/docs/pseudo-brief112013.pdf

Pineles, L. L., & Parente, R. (2012). Using the theory of planned behavior to predict self-medication with over-the-counter analgesics. *Journal of Health Psychology, 18*(12), 1540–1549.

Qato, D. M., Alexander, G. C., Conti, R. M., Johnson, M., Schumm, P., & Lindau, S. T. (2008). Use of prescription and over-the-counter medications and dietary supplements among older adults in the United States. *Journal of the American Medical Association, 300*(24), 2867–2878.

Schmeidl, S., Rottenkolber, M., Hasford, J., Rottenkolber, D., Farker, K., Drewelow, B., et al. (2014). Self-medication with over-the-counter and prescribed drugs causing adverse-drug-reaction-related hospital admissions: Results of a prospective, long-term, multi-centre study. *Drug Safety, 37*(4), 225-35.

Sullivan, P., Nair, K., & Patel, B. (2005). The effect of the Rx-to-OTC switch of loratadine and changes in prescription drug benefits on utilization and cost of therapy. *American Journal of Managed Care, 6,* 374–382.

Trivedi, H., Trivedi, A., & Hannan, M. F. (2014). Readability and comprehensibility of over-the-counter medication labels. *Renal Failure, 36*(3), 473–477.

U.S. Centers for Disease Control and Prevention. (2007). Infant deaths associated with cough and cold medications—two states, 2005. *Morbidity and Mortality Weekly, 56*(1), 104.

Villanyi, D., Fok, M., & Wong, R.Y. (2011). Medication reconciliation: identifying medication discrepancies in acutely ill hospitalized older adults. *American Journal of Geriatric Pharmacotherapeutics, 9*(5), 339–344.

Wilson, M. D., Ferguson, R. W., Mazer, M., & Litovitz, T. L. (2011). Monitoring trends in dextromethorphan abuse using the National Poison Data System: 2000–2010. *Clinical Toxicology, 49*(5), 409–415.

Winkelman, J., & Pies, R. (2005). Current patterns and future directions in the treatment of insomnia. *Annals of Clinical Psychiatry, 1,* 31–40.

World Self-Medication Industry (n.d.). About self-medication. Retrieved from http://www.wsmi.org/aboutsm.htm

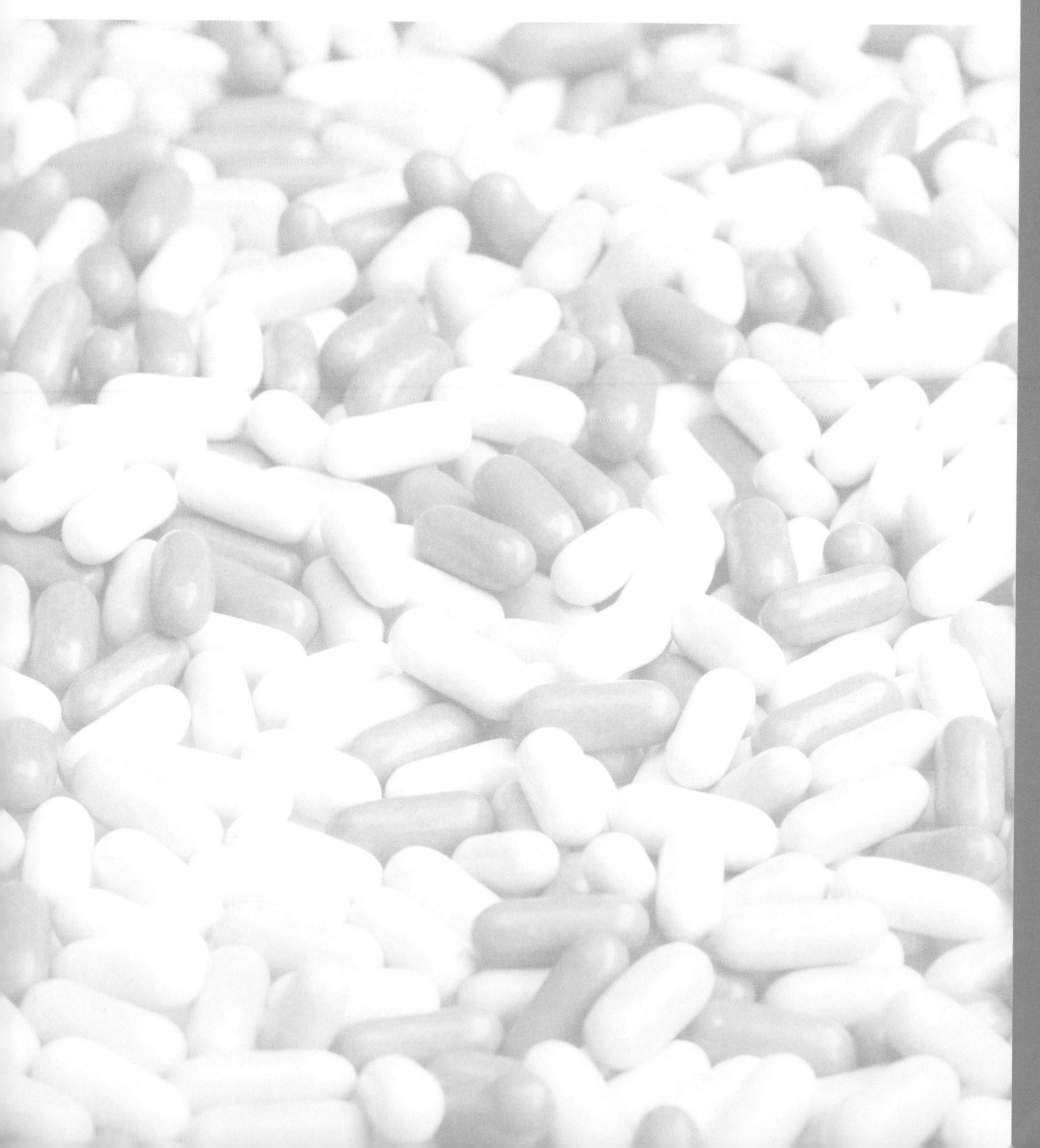

UNIT II

PHARMACOTHERAPEUTICS WITH SINGLE DRUGS

CHAPTER 14

DRUGS AFFECTING THE AUTONOMIC NERVOUS SYSTEM

Tracy Scott

The resting activity of most organs is maintained by opposing influences from the parasympathetic nervous system (PNS) and its neurotransmitter, acetylcholine (ACh), and the sympathetic nervous system (SNS) and its neurotransmitters, epinephrine, norepinephrine, and dopamine. Changes in resting activity can occur by increasing the activity of either the PNS or the SNS or by decreasing the activity of the opposing system (Fig. 14-1).

It is important to evaluate the risk for adverse drug effects when using these or any drugs. The drug may have a therapeutic effect on the target organ and an adverse effect on ancillary organs. An example of this may be damage to

the renal system or liver as medications are cleared from the body.

Drugs that affect the autonomic nervous system are used for a wide variety of diseases and in settings from intensive care to primary care. This chapter will focus on the drugs used in primary care to treat conditions typically managed by advanced practice nurses. Intravenous forms of the drugs are generally not used in primary care and are not discussed. Drugs such as peripherally acting alpha$_1$ agonists are used mainly as decongestants, and beta agonists are used mainly for their bronchodilating effects. These drugs are discussed in Chapter 17.

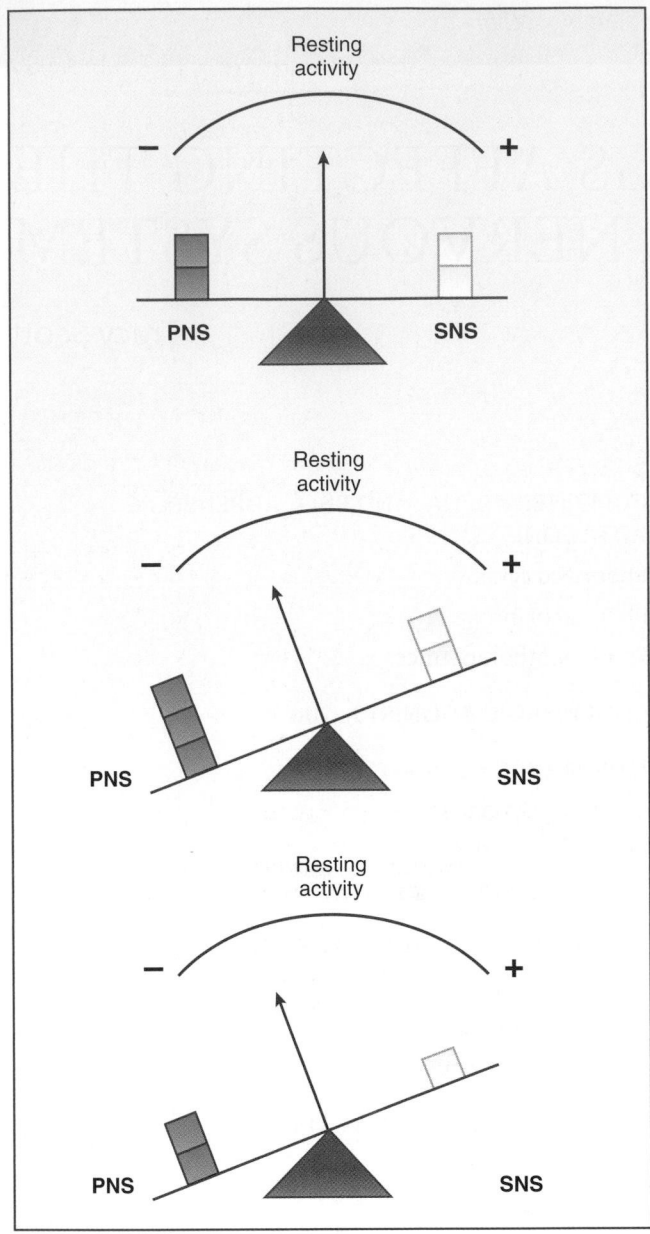

Figure 14–1. Resting activity and the autonomic nervous system.

ADRENERGIC AGONISTS

Through direct receptor binding to organs or tissues, promotion of norepinephrine release, or mimicking the action of norepinephrine or epinephrine, adrenergic agonists target the SNS by direct receptor binding to organs or tissues, promotion of norepinephrine release, or mimicking the action of norepinephrine or epinephrine. Four main receptor types are involved in this process: alpha$_1$, alpha$_2$, beta$_1$, and beta$_2$. Alpha$_1$ receptors are mostly associated with excitation or stimulation and are found mainly in the eye, salivary glands, arterioles, postcapillary venules, and gastrointestinal (GI) and genitourinary (GU) sphincters. Alpha$_2$ receptors are mostly associated with relaxation or with inhibition of norepinephrine release, and the majority are located in the presynaptic nerve terminals of smooth muscles, the islet

cells of the pancreas, salivary glands, skin, and mucosa. Beta$_1$ receptors, found mostly in the heart, brain, kidney, and lipocytes, are associated with stimulation of adenylyl cyclase via G$_S$-G-protein–coupled receptors to increase cAMP production. Beta$_2$ receptors are located in the smooth muscle of the eye, arterioles, venules, bronchioles, liver, pancreas, and GI and GU systems. They stimulate adenylyl cyclase, increase cAMP, and activate cardiac G$_1$ under certain conditions. Norepinephrine stimulates the alpha and beta$_1$ receptors, and epinephrine stimulates all four types of receptors (McCance & Huether, 2014). Centrally acting alpha$_2$ agonists are the relevant agonist drugs, and they are discussed here (Table 14-1).

ALPHA$_2$ AGONISTS: CENTRAL

Pharmacodynamics

Activation of central alpha$_2$ receptors results in inhibition of cardioacceleration and vasoconstriction centers in the brain. This action causes a decrease in peripheral outflow of norepinephrine, leading to decreases in peripheral resistance, renal vascular resistance, heart rate, and blood pressure. Because they lower blood pressure by reducing sympathetic function, they can produce compensatory effects on blood pressure, resulting in retention of sodium and expansion of blood volume through mechanisms that are not dependent on adrenergic nerves. For this reason, they may be given in combination with a diuretic. Centrally activating alpha$_2$ agonists are used largely as second-line or third-line drugs in the treatment of mild to moderate hypertension. Clonidine has several off-label uses, including treatment of withdrawal symptoms from opioid or alcohol based on its ability to lower the adrenergic stimulation that is associated with this withdrawal (WHO, 2009). It is also important to note that according to the BEERS criteria, drugs in this classification may be inappropriate for use in geriatric patients (AGS, 2012). The drugs in this class, commonly used to treat hypertension, are clonidine (Catapres), guanabenz (Wytensin), guanfacine (Tenex, Intuniv), and methyldopa.

Clonidine and other drugs in the class activate alpha$_2$ receptors in the medulla of the brain, reducing sympathetic tone and increasing parasympathetic tone, due to down regulation of alpha$_2$ receptors after chronic use. This results in a decrease in peripheral resistance, reduced heart rate, reduced blood pressure, and reduced renal vascular resistance. These medications should not be stopped abruptly because the relative "lack" of alpha$_2$ receptors impair the homeostatic balance that regulates SNS action. The prescriber should gradually taper the dose when discontinuing the medication over 4 days. Some of the common adverse reactions related to oral and transdermal doses of these medications include: bradycardia, AV block, palpitations, tachycardia, hallucinations, sleep disorders, contact dermatitis, dry mouth, orthostatic hypotension, constipation, nausea, urinary retention, decreased sexual activity, weight gain, leg cramps, and thrombocytopenia, with dry mouth being the most common adverse reaction (Food and Drug Administration [FDA], 2012).

Table 14–1 Actions of Autonomic Nervous System Based on Receptor

Organ or Tissue	Receptor	Adrenergic Effect	Receptor	Cholinergic Effect
Eye (radial muscle)	Alpha$_1$	Contraction (mydriasis)	M$_3$	None
Eye (ciliary muscle)	Beta$_2$	Relaxation for far vision	M$_3$	Contraction for near vision
Eye (sphincter muscle)	—	None	—	Contraction (miosis)
Lacrimal glands	—	None	—	Secretion
Nasopharyngeal glands	—	None	—	Secretion
Salivary glands	Alpha$_1$	Secretion of potassium and water	—	Secretion of potassium and water
Heart (SA node)	Beta$_1$	Increases heart rate	M$_2$	Decreases heart rate; vagus arrest
Heart (atria)	Beta$_1$	Increases contractility and conduction velocity	M$_2$	Decreases contractility; shortens action potential duration
Heart (AV junction)	Beta$_1$	Increases automaticity and propagation velocity	—	Decreases automaticity and propagation velocity
Heart (ventricles)	Beta$_1$	Increases contractility	—	None
Arterioles (coronary)	Alpha$_1$ Beta$_2$	Constriction Dilation	— —	Dilation
Arterioles (skin and mucosa)	Alpha$_1$ and alpha$_2$	Constriction	—	
Arterioles (skeletal muscle)	Alpha$_1$ Beta$_2$	Constriction Dilation	M$_3$ —	Dilation
Arterioles (cerebral)	Alpha$_1$	Constriction (slight)	—	None
Arterioles (pulmonary)	Alpha$_1$ Beta$_2$	Constriction Dilation	— —	None
Arterioles (renal)	Alpha$_1$ Beta$_1$ and beta$_2$	Constriction Dilation	— —	None
Veins (systemic)	Alpha$_1$ Beta$_2$	Constriction Dilation	—	None
Platelets	Alpha$_2$	Aggregation	—	None
Lungs (bronchial muscle)	Beta$_2$	Relaxation	M$_3$	Contraction
Lungs (bronchial glands)	Alpha$_1$ Beta$_2$	Decreases secretion Increases secretion	— —	Stimulation
GI (motility)	Alpha$_1$ and beta$_2$	Decrease	M$_1$	Increase
GI (sphincters)	Alpha$_1$	Contraction	M$_3$	Relaxation
GI (secretion)	—	M$_3$	Stimulation and increased secretion	
Liver	Alpha$_1$, alpha$_2$, and beta$_2$	Glycogenolysis and gluconeogenesis	—	Glycogen synthesis
Pancreas (islet cells)	Alpha$_2$ Beta$_2$	Decreases secretion Increases secretion	— —	None
Adrenal medulla	—		N and M$_3$	Secretion of epinephrine and norepinephrine (nicotinic effect)

Continued

Table 14–1 Actions of Autonomic Nervous System Based on Receptor—cont'd

Organ or Tissue	Receptor	Adrenergic Effect	Receptor	Cholinergic Effect
Kidney	Alpha$_1$ Beta$_1$	Decreases renin secretion Increases renin secretion	— —	None
Ureter (motility and tone)	Alpha$_1$	Increases	—	Decreases
Urinary bladder (detrusor)	Beta$_2$	Relaxation	—	Contraction
Urinary bladder (detrusor)	Beta3	Relaxation	-	
Urinary bladder (trigone and sphincter)	Alpha$_1$	Contraction	M$_3$	Relaxes
Uterus	Beta$_2$	Promotes smooth muscle relaxation	—	None
Male sex organs	Alpha$_1$	Ejaculation	M	Erection
Fat cells	Alpha$_2$ Beta$_1$	Inhibition of lipolysis Stimulation of lipolysis	— —	
Endothelium	—		M$_3$	Releases EDRF

Source: McCance & Huether, 2014; FDA, 2012.

   M = muscarinic receptors.

Guanabenz and guanfacine are also used to treat hypertension. Extended release guanfacine with a trade name of Intuniv is approved for use in the treatment of ADHD as both an adjunct therapy or monotherapy. Guanfacine also reduces sympathetic outflow by activating alpha$_2$ receptors in the brain but does not directly stimulate peripheral receptors, so blood pressure is reduced in both the supine and standing positions without alterations in normal postural mechanisms. The most common adverse reaction in monotherapy trials were somnolence, fatigue, nausea, lethargy, and hypotension. In the monotherapy trials, 12% of patients experienced adverse reactions, which resulted in their being discontinued from the trial. These adverse reactions were sedation, fatigue, hypotension, headache, and dizziness. In trials of adjunctive therapy, the most common reactions were somnolence, fatigue, insomnia, dizziness, and abdominal pain. In the trials of adjunctive therapy, only 3% of patients experienced adverse reactions leading to discontinuation from the trials (FDA, 2013a).

Methyldopa is an analogue of L-dopa. Because the pathways for its metabolism directly parallel the synthesis of norepinephrine (NE), its metabolite alpha-methyl-norepinephrine is stored in adrenergic nerve vesicles where it replaces NE. Stimulation of central alpha$_2$ receptors by this active metabolite produces a decrease in sympathetic outflow to the heart, kidneys, and blood vessels. In addition to the adverse effects associated with other drugs in the classification, rare cases of hemolytic anemia have been reported after taking methyldopa. A positive Coombs test has occurred in between 10% and 20% of patients taking methyldopa within 6 to 12 months of the initiation of therapy (FDA, 2004). The end result from the use of methyldopa is a decrease in blood pressure, peripheral resistance, and heart rate with a slight decrease in cardiac output. It also produces a reduction in renal vascular resistance.

Pharmacokinetics

Absorption and Distribution

Absorption following oral administration varies among the drugs in this classification. Clonidine is easily absorbed from the GI tract and the skin and is lipid-soluble, allowing it to rapidly enter the brain from the circulation. Guanabenz and guanfacine are also well absorbed. All of the drugs are widely distributed in body tissues. Both clonidine and methyldopa cross the placenta and are found in breast milk (FDA, 2004, 2012c). Methyldopa is not completely absorbed in the gut and is absorbed via an aromatic amino acid transport system (Skerjanec, Campbell, & Robertson, 1995).

Metabolism and Excretion

The liver, in varying degrees, metabolizes each of these drugs. Guanfacine has a significant first-pass effect. The drug is metabolized by CYP3A4 with about 50% of the oral dose metabolized to inactive sulfate metabolites and 50% eliminated unchanged in the urine. Methyldopa is also extensively metabolized by the liver to inactive metabolites, with only approximately 20% of the active drug appearing in the plasma. The kidney is the organ of excretion for each of these drugs. Patients with renal failure will experience increased adverse effects as methyldopa and its metabolites accumulate, resulting in prolonged hypotensive action. Approximately 50% of the clonidine dose is hepatically metabolized to inactive metabolites, and the remaining 50% is excreted unchanged in the urine (FDA, 2004, 2012,

2012c, 2013a). Table 14-2 shows the pharmacokinetics of these drugs.

Pharmacotherapeutics

Precautions and Contraindications

Cautious use is recommended in the presence of severe coronary insufficiency, recent myocardial infarction (MI), and renal function impairment. Because they cross the blood–brain barrier, methyldopa and clonidine are used cautiously in the presence of cerebrovascular disease. Clonidine should be used with caution with patients who are at risk for mental depression, and it should be discontinued if depression occurs. Clonidine should be avoided in patients at risk or with a history of bradycardia. Because they affect cognitive function, centrally acting alpha$_2$ agonists should be avoided or used with extreme caution in populations such as older adults for whom this adverse response creates a significant problem (FDA, 2004, 2012, 2012c).

Both guanabenz and clonidine are Pregnancy Category C. No adequate human studies have been done on guanabenz, and skeletal anomalies were found in the offspring of mice that were given the drug. Clonidine crosses the placenta and no well-controlled studies have been done in pregnant women. Both guanfacine and methyldopa are listed as Pregnancy Category B in oral form, but methyldopa is listed as Pregnancy Category C in an injectable form (FDA, 2004, 2012, 2012c).

Methyldopa appears in breast milk and should be used with caution in nursing women. Long-term follow-up of 195 participants and children born to women treated with methyldopa while pregnant did not find any significant effect on the children (FDA, 2004). All of the other drugs discussed in this category are not recommended for nursing mothers. Methyldopa and clonidine are available in pediatric doses. Methyldopa can be safely used in children, and sources vary regarding the safe use of clonidine in this age group (FDA, 2004, 2012).

Adverse Drug Reactions

The major adverse reactions related to this category of drugs is the effect they have on organs other than the targeted organ. These reactions include drowsiness, dry mouth, constipation, urinary retention, and impotence. Nightmares and insomnia have been associated with clonidine. Cardiac symptoms include hypotension, chest pain, and bradycardia. GI symptoms are more commonly associated with guanabenz and additionally include abdominal pain, vomiting, anorexia, and altered taste. Gynecomastia has also been associated with guanabenz and clonidine. All drugs in this class have also been associated with life-threatening rebound hypertension mediated by increased SNS activity after sudden withdrawal of these drugs. Clonidine and methyldopa have especially been noted to have this adverse reaction, which is exacerbated if the patient is also taking beta-adrenergic blockers (Table 14-3). All patients given these drugs should be warned about this possibility. If the drug must be withdrawn, it should be done gradually. All of the drugs in this class may result in pruritic rashes. The transdermal form of clonidine has also been associated with a rash that is an allergic reaction to the adhesive on the patch (FDA, 2004, 2012, 2012c).

Table 14–2 Pharmacokinetics: Selected Centrally Acting Alpha$_2$ Agonists

Drug	Onset	Peak	Duration	Protein Binding	Bioavailability	Half-Life	Elimination
Clonidine	Oral: 30–60 min	Oral: 3–5 h	Oral: 8 h	20%–40%		12–16 h: up to 41 h in impaired renal function	40%–60% unchanged in urine; 50% metabolized in liver
	Transdermal: 2–3 days	Transdermal: unknown	Transdermal: 7 days (8 h of effect after patch is removed)				
Guanabenz	60 min (onset of anti-HTN action)	2–5 h	12 h	90%		6 h: prolonged in renal impairment	<1% unchanged in urine
Guanfacine	1 h	1–4 h	24 h	70%	80%	*Adults:* 17 h; *Younger adults:* 13–14 h; *Older adults* 17–18 h	50% unchanged in urine; 70% in urine unchanged or as metabolites
Methyldopa	2–3 h	2–6 h	12–24 h	>20%	50%	1.8 h: blood pressure reduction is pronounced and prolonged in renal failure	Extensively metabolized in liver; 70% in urine as metabolites

Source: FDA, 2004, 2012, 2012c, 2013a.

Table 14–3 ▦ Drug Interactions: Centrally Acting Alpha₂ Agonists

Drug	Interacting Drug	Possible Effect	Implications
Clonidine	Alcohol, antihistamines, phenothiazines, barbiturates, benzodiazepines	Additive sedation	Avoid concurrent use
	Beta-adrenergic blockers	Attenuation or reversal of antihypertensive effect of clonidine; may result in life-threatening hypertension (HTN)	Avoid concurrent use; if patient is taking both drugs and withdrawal is required, withdraw beta-adrenergic blocker first to prevent excessive unopposed alpha stimulation that may lead to malignant HTN within 12 h
	Nitrates, other antihypertensives	Additive hypotensive effects	Avoid concurrent use
	Prazosin	Decreased antihypertensive effect of clonidine	Choose alternative drug
	TCAs	Block antihypertensive effects of clonidine and may result in life-threatening HTN	Choose alternative antidepressant
	Verapamil	Synergistic pharmacological and toxic effects; may result in atrioventricular block and severe hypotension	Choose alternative calcium channel blocker or antihypertensive
Guanabenz, guanfacine	Alcohol, antihistamines, phenothiazines, barbiturates, benzodiazepines	Additive sedative effects	Avoid concurrent use or choose alternative antihypertensive
	Alcohol, nitrates, other antihypertensives	Additive hypotension	Avoid concurrent use or monitor blood pressure closely
Methyldopa	Alcohol, antihistamines	Additive sedation	Avoid concurrent use
	Beta-adrenergic blockers	May result in life-threatening HTN	Less likely with beta₁ selective agents; see clonidine above for implications
	Haloperidol	Potentiate antipsychotic effects or may produce psychosis	Choose different antipsychotic
	Levodopa	Potentiate antihypertensive effects of methyldopa and central effects of levodopa in Parkinson's disease	Avoid concurrent use; choose alternative antihypertensive
	Lithium	Increased risk for lithium toxicity	Choose alternative antihypertensive
	Monoamine oxidase inhibitors (MAOIs)	Metabolites of methyldopa stimulate release of endogenous catecholamines that are usually metabolized by MAOIs; result is excessive SNS stimulation	Avoid concurrent use
	Nitrates, other antihypertensives	Additive hypotension	Avoid concurrent use
	Phenothiazines, sympathomimetics, barbiturates, amphetamines	May result in serious HTN	Avoid concurrent use
	Tolbutamide	Tolbutamide metabolism may be impaired, resulting in enhanced hypoglycemic effects	Choose alternative hypoglycemic
	TCAs	Attenuation or reversal of antihypertensive effect of methyldopa	Avoid concurrent use; choose alternative drugs for depression or HTN
	Herbals: licorice; yohimbe, ginseng	May affect electrolyte levels May decrease efficacy of methyldopa	Monitor blood pressure and inform patient

Source: FDA, 2004, 2012, 2012c.

Methyldopa has been associated with the development of a positive Coombs' test. Rarely, this is associated with hemolytic anemia (Wendell & Stanley, 2013). Perform a baseline Coombs' test, hemoglobin and hematocrit levels, and repeat them at 6 and 12 months after initiation of therapy (FDA, 2004).

Drug Interactions

All centrally acting alpha$_2$ agonists have additive sedative effects with central nervous system (CNS) depressants and additive hypotensive effects with other drugs that also reduce blood pressure (see Table 14-3). Tricyclic antidepressant (TCA) agents decrease the antihypertensive effects of all centrally acting alpha$_2$ agonists. Several other drugs used to treat psychoses interact with centrally acting alpha$_2$ agonists, resulting in toxicity, psychoses, or excessive SNS stimulation. Careful selection of the drugs to treat each condition is required.

Beta-adrenergic blockers interact with clonidine and methyldopa to produce potentially life-threatening hypertension if either clonidine or methyldopa is abruptly discontinued. They should not normally be used concurrently, but there are occasions, such as when beta-adrenergic blockers are used for MI prophylaxis, when use of both drugs is necessary. If withdrawal of one or both of these drugs is required because of adverse effects, the beta-adrenergic blocker is always withdrawn first to prevent excessive unopposed stimulation of alpha$_2$ receptors that can result in a hypertensive crisis in as little as 12 hours (FDA, 2004, 2012, 2012c).

Clinical Use and Dosing

Hypertension

Centrally acting alpha$_2$ agonists are used to treat mild to moderate hypertension and are second-line drugs usually chosen when other drugs are not effective in achieving blood pressure control. The exception is methyldopa, which is first-line therapy for pregnant patients. These drugs are not well suited for monotherapy because they produce troublesome adverse reactions in almost all patients who take them. Methyldopa and clonidine can be used effectively when combined with a diuretic to address the problems with sodium and water retention. Clonidine is now available in a combination tablet with chlorthalidone, a thiazide diuretic (Clorpres) (FDA, 2004, 2012, 2012c, 2013a).

Doses vary with each drug, but adverse reactions occur at higher doses and with older adults. Beginning with the lowest dose recommended for each drug, the dose is increased at weekly intervals until blood pressure control or the maximum dose is reached. To minimize the sedation, which is more common with clonidine and methyldopa, the dose may be divided, with a higher dose in the evening than in the morning. Smaller doses are required in renal impairment. Use of the low end of the dose range of guanfacine produces the least problems for patients with renal insufficiency (FDA, 2004, 2012, 2012c, 2013a).

Chapter 40 provides detailed discussion of the management of hypertension.

Unlabeled Uses of Clonidine

Clonidine has been evaluated for many off-label uses. It lowers the adrenergic stimulation associated with alcohol, heroin, and nicotine withdrawal and lessens the unpleasant symptoms of withdrawal. Attention deficit-hyperactivity disorder is associated with decreased stimulation of certain centers in the brain, and the stimulation of central alpha$_2$ receptors by clonidine has resulted in improved concentration and reduced behavioral symptoms in some children (Yoon, Cohn, Rocchini, Kershaw, & Clark, 2012).

Rational Drug Selection

Age

Only clonidine and methyldopa have pediatric doses and are approved for use with children. Clonidine works better in adults but should be used with caution in elderly patients. Dosage reductions may be required for methyldopa and clonidine when prescribed for older adults because of the risk for fluid retention and orthostatic hypotension (FDA, 2004, 2012).

Pregnancy

Traditionally, methyldopa was the drug of choice for pregnant women due to the longevity of experience by providers. Now other medications are also selected. Drugs used for the treatment of hypertension, including during pregnancy, are discussed in Chapter 40 and discussed in depth in the ACOG practice Bulletin No. 125 (ACOG, 2012).

Route of Administration

Patients who have difficulty taking pills, who have trouble remembering more frequent doses, or who for other reasons would have better adherence to the treatment regimen with a transdermal system can be given clonidine, the only antihypertensive currently available in a transdermal formulation (Table 14-4). Because the transdermal form of the medication results in lower serum levels (lack of a peak associated with oral administration), this dosage form may minimize many of the drug's bothersome adverse effects.

Monitoring

Clinical monitoring of blood pressure is appropriate for all drugs in this class as with any other antihypertensive drug. Baseline blood pressure should be taken before initiating therapy and with each change in dosage. Weight and other indicators of fluid status should also be monitored. (See Chapter 40 for further discussion of blood pressure monitoring.)

For patients who have or are at risk for renal impairment, dosage alterations are required. Assess serum creatinine prior to initiation of therapy and regularly thereafter for up to 1 year. Liver function studies should also be conducted prior to therapy and at 6 and 12 months. Methyldopa has been associated with hepatotoxicity (FDA, 2004, 2012, 2012c, 2013a).

Patient Education

Administration

The drug should be taken exactly as prescribed, at the same time each day, even if the patient is feeling well. Missed doses are taken as soon as they are remembered unless it is almost time for the next dose. Doses are not doubled These drugs must be withdrawn slowly over 2 to 3 days to prevent rebound hypertension, and missed doses increase the risk for

Table 14–4 ⊗ Schedule: Centrally Acting Alpha₂ Agonists

Drug	Indication	Form	Initial Dose	Maintenance Dose
Clonidine	Hypertension	**Tablets:** 0.1 mg (Catapres is scored) 0.2 mg (Catapres is scored) 0.3 mg (Catapres is scored) **Transdermal:** 0.1 mg patch 0.2 mg patch 0.3 mg patch **Transdermal:** Catapres-TTS 1: 0.1 mg/24 hr Catapres-TTS 2: 0.2 mg/24 hr Catapres-TTS 3: 0.3 mg/24 hr **Tablets:** (scored) Clonidine 0.1 mg Chlorthalidone 15 mg Clonidine 0.2 mg Chlorthalidone 15 mg Clonidine 0.3 mg Chlorthalidone 15 mg	*Adults:* 0.1 mg bid PO (older adults may need lower dose)	*Adults:* Increase in increments of 0.1 mg PO in weekly intervals; maintenance dose 0.1–0.3 mg bid; max dose: 1.2 mg bid
			Transdermal: Catapres-TTS 1 (0.1 mg)	After 1–2 wk, if desired blood pressure (BP) is not achieved, increase in increments of 0.1 mg/wk (Catapres-TTS comes in 2 [0.2 mg] and 3 [0.3 mg] patches)
			Children (12 yr and older): 0.1 mg bid	*Children:* Increase in 0.1 mg increments at weekly intervals; maintenance dose 0.1–0.3 mg bid; max dose: 2.4 mg/d
Clonidine HCl and Chlorthalidone (Clorpres) (B)	Hypertension		0.1 mg clonidine plus 15 mg chlorthalidone once or twice daily	Max dose 0.6 mg clonidine plus 30 mg chlorthalidone
Guanabenz	Hypertension	Tablets: 4 mg 8 mg (scored)	4 mg bid	Increase in increments of 4–8 mg/d every 1–2 wk until target BP achieved; max dose 32 mg bid
Guanfacine	Hypertension	**Guanfacine (G) (Tenex) (B)** **Tablets:** 1 mg 2 mg **(Intuiv)** **Tablets (extended-release):** 1 mg 2 mg 3 mg 4 mg	1 mg daily at bedtime	May increase to 2 mg qd after 3–4 wk if target BP not achieved; 2 mg dose may be given as 1 mg bid; max dose 3 mg qd
Methyldopa	Hypertension	Methyldopa **Tablets:** 250 mg 500 mg Methyldopa/ hydrochlorothiazide **Tablets:** 250 mg methyldopa/ 25 mg hydrochlorothiazide	*Adults:* 250 mg bid or tid for first 48 h	Increase in increments of 250 mg every 2 d until target BP is achieved: to minimize sedation, increase dose in evening; smaller doses should be used in renal impairment; maintenance dose 500–2,000 mg/d in 2–4 divided doses
			Children: 10 mg/kg/d in 2–4 divided doses	*Children:* max dose is 65 mg/kg or 3,000 mg, whichever is less

Source: FDA, 2004, 2012, 2012c, 2013a.

the occurrence of rebound hypertension. To prevent missing doses, patients should make certain they have enough medication available for weekends, holidays, and vacations (FDA, 2004, 2012, 2012c, 2013a).

Methyldopa has known interactions with several herbals; therefore, prescribers should ask patients about herbal use and be aware that drug interactions may occur. Drug–herbal interactions are listed in Table 14-3.

Instruct patients who are on the transdermal clonidine system in proper application of the patch. Apply the patch to a hairless area of intact skin on the upper arm or torso once every 7 days. Use a different site from the previous application. They should not cut or trim the patch. If the patch loosens, apply tape to secure it (FDA, 2011).

Adverse Reactions

Hypotension is the most common adverse reaction. Changing positions slowly, not exercising in hot weather, avoiding alcohol, and drinking an adequate amount of noncaffeinated fluid per day will decrease these reactions. For patients with heart failure, fluid intake should be discussed with the health-care provider.

Drowsiness and dry mouth are also common. Patients should avoid activities requiring mental alertness until their individual response to the drug is known. Dry mouth can be minimized by practicing good oral hygiene, chewing sugarless gum, or sucking on hard candy (FDA, 2004, 2012, 2012c, 2013a). Concurrent use of alcohol or other CNS depressants should also be avoided. Centrally acting alpha$_2$ agonists can produce additive sedation with these drugs.

Fluid retention is indicated by weight gain and swelling in the feet and ankles. Patients should report any weight gain of more than 2 lb (1 kg) in 1 day to the health-care provider. Fluid retention may be treated by the addition of a diuretic to the treatment regimen and consideration of salt intake (FDA, 2004, 2012, 2012c, 2013a).

Methyldopa has some unique adverse reactions. Jaundice may indicate hepatotoxicity and should be reported to the health-care provider. Decreased energy levels may indicate anemia. In the absence of another explanation for decreased energy, this symptom should also be reported to the health-care provider (FDA, 2004, 2012, 2012c, 2013a).

Lifestyle Management

Drugs control hypertension, but they do not cure it. Encourage patients to adhere to other interventions for management of hypertension, such as weight loss, aerobic exercise, a low-sodium diet, smoking cessation, and stress management (see Chapter 40).

ADRENERGIC ANTAGONISTS

Adrenergic antagonists act directly by blockading adrenergic receptors or indirectly by decreasing norepinephrine release within SNS terminals. Most of the clinically useful actions of these drugs result from the blockade of alpha$_1$ receptors in blood vessels, beta$_1$ receptors in the heart, and alpha$_1$ receptors in the bladder neck and prostate gland. Adrenergic antagonists are categorized on the basis of receptors that are blocked and include drugs that block only one receptor and those that block more than one receptor. The following section discusses antagonist drugs whose major effect is on alpha$_1$ and beta receptors outside the CNS (peripherally acting).

ALPHA$_1$ ANTAGONISTS

Alpha 1 antagonists include nonselective and selective types. Following are their differences and the drugs in each category.

Nonselective Alpha Antagonists

Nonselective alpha antagonists include phentolamine (Regitine) and phenoxybenzamine (Dibenzyline). These drugs have approximately equal affinities for both the postsynaptic alpha$_1$ receptors and the presynaptic alpha$_2$ receptors. Phenoxybenzamine blocks the receptors irreversibly, whereas the blockade by phentolamine is reversible. These drugs will result in lowered blood pressure as a result of the blockade of the postsynaptic alpha$_1$ receptors. In addition, blockade of the presynaptic alpha$_2$ receptors results in reflex cardiac stimulation because the negative feedback inhibition of neurotransmitter release is being blocked (FDA, 2009a). For this reason, these drugs are not used in the treatment of hypertension. They do have a role in the treatment of pheochromocytoma, in which they are used to prophylax against hypertensive crisis as a result of the release of norepinephrine from the tumor (Young, Kaplan, & Kebebew, 2013). Additionally, given by the intradermal route, they have a role in the treatment of extravasation of vasopressor drugs. Because these drugs are used almost exclusively by specialists, they are not discussed further here.

Selective Alpha$_1$ Antagonists

The alpha$_1$ antagonists reversibly block the effects of catecholamines at the postsynaptic alpha$_1$ receptors in vascular smooth muscle and in the smooth muscle of the bladder neck and prostate. These drugs are useful in lowering blood pressure as well as relieving outflow obstruction secondary to benign prostatic hypertrophy (BPH). Six drugs in this class are used clinically: doxazosin (Cardura), prazosin (Minipress), terazosin (Hytrin), tamsulosin (Flomax), alfuzosin (Uroxatral), and silodosin (Rapaflo). It should be noted that prazosin is not typically used to treat BPH due to the frequent dosing requirements and risk of cardiovascular side effects (McVary, Roehrborn, & Avins, 2011).Tamsulosin, alfuzosin, and silodosin have increased selectivity for the alpha$_1$ receptors in the prostate, and as a result these drugs have little effect on blood pressure while relieving symptoms associated with BPH (FDA, 2009c, 2010b, 2011a, 2012a).

Pharmacodynamics

Reversible alpha$_1$ antagonists block postsynaptic alpha$_1$ receptors in the vasculature, resulting in a decrease in both arterial and venous vasoconstriction. Because arteriole and venous tone are determined largely by the stimulation of alpha$_1$ receptors in vascular smooth muscle, the result is a decrease in peripheral vascular resistance and lowered blood pressure. Both supine and standing blood pressures are lowered, with the most pronounced effect on diastolic blood pressure. Orthostatic hypotension may result from their action on receptors in venous smooth muscle. Reflex tachycardia may result from compensatory mechanisms but is minimal. Since the remaining alpha$_1$ antagonists are more specific for the receptors found in the prostate, they do not cause reflex tachycardia. Prazosin and terazosin rarely produce reflex tachycardia. Chronic use of alpha$_1$ antagonists may result in compensatory increases in blood volume but at a fairly low rate of incidence. Studies of the newer selective blockers do not mention edema. Tamsulosin, silodosin, and alfuzosin have not been approved for treatment of hypertension (FDA, 2010b, 2011a, 2012a).

It should be noted that the ALLHAT (2002) trial compared doxazosin to chlorthalidone and found an increased risk of heart failure with doxazosin, so an alpha blocker is not recommended for initial monotherapy in hypertension.

The reduction in symptoms and improved urine flow rates in patients with BPH is related to relaxation of smooth muscle produced by the blockade of the alpha$_1$ receptors, which are densely located in the bladder neck and prostate gland. Blockade of these receptors decreases urethral resistance and may relieve the obstruction and improve urine flow and BPH symptoms. Because there are few alpha$_1$ receptors in the body of the bladder, these drugs are able to reduce bladder outflow obstruction without affecting bladder contractility.

Three subtypes of the alpha$_1$ receptors have been pharmacologically identified and cloned: alpha$_{1a}$, $_{1b}$, and $_{1d}$. Approximately 70% of the alpha$_1$ receptors in the prostate are subtype 1a and are also localized to the prostatic stroma (McCance & Huether, 2015). Presumably, if the efficacy of the selective alpha$_1$ blockers is mediated by the relaxation of the prostate smooth muscle, then the development of a selective alpha$_{1a}$ receptor antagonist would be advantageous. This would also result in fewer adverse drug reactions, which are theoretically mediated by the alpha$_{1b}$ and $_{1d}$ receptor subtypes. However, there is evidence that the selective alpha$_{1a}$ receptor antagonists relieve the lower urinary tract symptoms (LUTS) by a mechanism that is unrelated to prostate smooth-muscle relaxation. Therefore, an alpha$_1$ antagonist that does not demonstrate

selectivity for subtypes may still be useful in the treatment of BPH. This premise is borne out when looking at the available alpha$_1$ antagonists with indications for BPH. Large numbers of alpha$_1$ receptors are found in the base of the bladder and the prostate. The three subtypes of alpha$_1$ receptors identified as 1a, 1b, and 1d are selective for doxazosin, terazosin, and alfuzosin, and silodosin demonstrates a 583-fold selectivity for the alpha$_{1a}$ receptor subtype and 56-fold selectivity for the alpha$_{1d}$ receptor subtype (FDA, 2010b, 2011a, 2012a).

Pharmacokinetics

Absorption and Distribution

Five of the drugs in this class are well absorbed after oral administration (Table 14-5); silodosin is the exception. Tamsulosin is the most slowly absorbed. The absorption of alfuzosin was reduced by 50% when taken in a fasting state, so it should be administered with food. Taking tamsulosin in a fasting state increases bioavailability by 30% and increases C$_{max}$ by 40% to 70%. Since there is a risk for adverse effects when given in a fasting state, the dose should be administered 30 minutes following the same meal each day.

The bioavailability for silodosin is about 32% and the package insert recommends administering the drug with a meal. All drugs in this class are widely distributed in the body and all are highly protein bound. Doxazosin accumulates in breast milk with a concentration 20 times that in maternal plasma. Prazosin is found in small amounts in breast milk, and it is not known if terazosin is excreted in breast milk. No information about breast milk concentration is provided for tamsulosin, alfuzosin, or silodosin, which would not be given to female patients (FDA, 2009c, 2010b, 2011a, 2012a).

Metabolism and Excretion

Extensively metabolized by the liver, reversible alpha$_1$ antagonists are excreted in both feces and urine. Doxazosin has significant first-pass metabolism, and enterohepatic recycling of this drug causes plasma elimination to be biphasic. After morning dosing, the area under the curve (AUC) was 12% less than after evening dosing. The time to peak concentration after evening dosing occurred significantly later than after morning dosing. Doxazosin is primarily eliminated in the feces (FDA, 2009c).

Table 14–5 Selected Alpha$_1$-Adrenergic Antagonists

Drug	Onset	Peak	Duration	Protein Binding (%)	Bioavailability (%)	Half-Life	Elimination
Alfuzosin	Unknown	8 h	Unknown	82–90	49 (with food)	10 h	69% in feces; 24% in urine
Doxazosin	60–120 min	2–3 h	24 h	98	65	22 h	63% in bile/feces; 9% in urine
Prazosin	120–130 min	1–3 h	6–12 h	92–97	48–68	2–3 h	90% in bile/feces; 10% in urine
Silodosin	Unknown	2.6 h	Unknown	97	32	13.8 h	35.5% in urine; 55% in feces
Tamsulosin	Unknown	5 days	Unknown	94–99	>90	9–15 h	<10% unchanged in urine
Terazosin	15 min	1–2 h	12–24 h	90–94	90	9–12 h	60% in bile/feces; 40% in urine

Source: FDA, 2009c, 2010b, 2011a, 2012a.

Prazosin undergoes demethylation and conjugation in the liver, where a majority of the dose is eliminated via biliary excretion in the feces. Prazosin has four active metabolites that have approximately 10% to 15% of the activity of the parent drug and may contribute to the pharmacological effect of the drug. In the presence of renal failure, elimination half-life of this drug may be prolonged, protein binding decreased, and peak plasma levels increased (FDA, 2009b).

Terazosin has minimal hepatic first-pass metabolism to one active and three inactive metabolites. Nearly all of the circulating dose is in the form of the parent drug. Tamsulosin is extensively metabolized by CYP 450 enzymes; less than 10% of the dose is eliminated unchanged, but the specific isoenzymes have not been identified. The resulting metabolites undergo conjugation with glucuronide or sulfate and then are eliminated in the urine (FDA, 2011a).

Alfuzosin is extensively metabolized to inactive metabolites via CYP 3A4, and only about 11% of the administered drug is eliminated unchanged in the urine. The metabolites are eliminated primarily in the feces (FDA, 2010b).

Silodosin is metabolized by hepatic CYP 3A4, along with glucuronidation and alcohol and aldehyde dehydrogenase. Silodosin has an active metabolite that has a half-life of approximately 24 hours (FDA, 2012a).

Pharmacotherapeutics

Precautions and Contraindications

All the "azosin" drugs are contraindicated in the presence of volume depletion. Peripheral vasodilation caused by these drugs decreases venous return to the heart and may precipitate significant heart failure (HF). Several of the drugs are associated with fluid retention that may exacerbate HF (FDA, 2009b, 2010b, 2011a, 2012a).

The dosing for prazosin, doxazosin, terazosin, and tamsulosin does not need to be adjusted in renal or hepatic impairment. However, since each of these drugs is extensively metabolized by the liver and has significant potential for hypotensive events, it is prudent to start with the lowest dose and adjust based on clinical response. This approach is especially true for doxazosin because of the enterohepatic recycling discussed previously.

With creatinine clearance (CrCl) of less than 30 mL/min, limited safety data are available for alfuzosin; therefore, the drug should be used cautiously (FDA, 2009b, 2009c, 2010b, 2011a, 2012a). Alfuzosin should not be given to patients with mild to moderate hepatic impairment (Childs-Pugh classes B and C). Silodosin requires no adjustment of dose in patients with mild to moderate hepatic impairment but is not recommended in those patients with severe hepatic impairment (Childs-Pugh score equal to or greater than 10). For patients with CrCl greater than or equal to 50 mL/min, no dose adjustment is required for silodosin; for patients with CrCl 30 to 49 mL/min, the dose should be halved, and when the CrCl falls below 30 mL/min, the use of silodosin is not recommended (FDA, 2009b, 2010b, 2011a, 2012a).

Doxazosin, prazosin, and terazosin are Pregnancy Category C. Teratogenicity and reduced fertility have been demonstrated in animal studies. There are no adequate and well-controlled studies in pregnant women. Because of its high concentration in breast milk, doxazosin should not be given to nursing mothers. Prazosin has also been found in breast milk. Exercise caution when administering prazosin or terazosin to nursing mothers, and do so only when benefits clearly outweigh risks to the baby. Tamsulosin, alfuzosin, and silodosin are not prescribed to female patients. Safety and efficacy for use with children have not been established (FDA, 2009b, 2009c, 2010b, 2011a, 2012a).

Adverse Drug Reactions

Each of these drugs carries a risk for significant first-dose orthostatic hypotension that may result in syncope that tends to occur within 30 to 90 minutes of drug administration. This adverse reaction is decreased with continued doses but returns if therapy is interrupted for even a few doses, if the dosage is increased, or if another antihypertensive is added to the treatment regimen. The first dose should be given in the clinic or taken at bedtime. The "first-dose" reaction may be minimized by starting with a 1 mg dose and slowly increasing the dosage at 2-week intervals (Table 14-6). Terazosin exhibits this reaction most often, prazosin is average, and it occurs least with doxazosin (FDA, 2009b, 2009c, 2010b, 2011a, 2012a).

Fluid retention that results in peripheral edema occurs with several of these drugs. Close monitoring of weight changes may be needed, especially early in therapy. The addition of a diuretic to the therapy regimen may be required. Other adverse reactions are associated with alpha$_1$-adrenergic blockade (nasal congestion, blurred vision, dry mouth, constipation, impotence, and urinary frequency). Hypotensive symptoms of dizziness, headache, fatigue, tachycardia, and nausea are also potential adverse effects (FDA, 2009b, 2010b, 2011a, 2012a).

Drug Interactions

The major drug interactions result in decreased antihypertensive effects with the interacting drug or in additive hypotension, with increased risk for postural hypotension and falls. All six drugs have increased risk for postural hypotension when administered with acute alcohol ingestion, other antihypertensives, or nitrates. Doxazosin has the fewest published drug interactions and prazosin has the most. Cimetidine interacts with tamsulosin to decrease tamsulosin's effects. Alfuzosin is predominately metabolized by the CYP 3A4 isoenzyme systems, and other drugs also metabolized by this subsystem present a risk of interaction (FDA, 2009b, 2009c, 2010b, 2011a, 2012a). Table 14-7 depicts the common drug interactions.

Clinical Use and Dosing

Hypertension (HTN)

Alpha$_1$-adrenergic antagonists (except alfuzosin, tamsulosin, and silodosin, which are not approved to treat HTN) are the drugs of choice for treating HTN in older men with

Table 14–6 ✄ **Dosage Schedule: Selected Alpha₁-Adrenergic Antagonists**

Drug	Indication	Form	Initial Dose	Maintenance Dose
Doxazosin	Hypertension	Tablets: 1 mg, 2 mg, 4 mg, 8 mg	1 mg daily at bedtime	2–16 mg daily. Depending on standing blood pressure (BP), increase dose in 2 mg increments until target BP is achieved. Doses >4 mg increase risk of postural hypotension.
	BPH		1 mg daily at bedtime Extended-release form is 4 mg taken once daily at breakfast	1–8 mg daily. Depending on the urodynamics and BPH symptoms, the dose is increased to 2 mg and then to 4 mg and 8 mg/daily. The recommended maximum dose is 8 mg. The titration interval is 1–2 wk.
Prazosin	Hypertension	Generic capsules: 1 mg, 2 mg, 5 mg Minipress capsules: 1 mg, 2 mg, 5 mg	Adults: 1–2 mg bid or tid; take first dose at bedtime	Adults: 6–15 mg/daily in 2–3 divided doses. Depending on standing BP, increase dose in 1 mg increments, with the larger dose being given at bedtime until target BP is achieved. Doses >20 mg/d usually do not increase efficacy.
Silodosin	BPH	Capsules: 4 mg, 8 mg	8 mg once daily with a meal	No data are published about increasing dosage. Depending on standing BP, the starting dose may be 4 mg with increases to 8 mg as tolerated.
Tamsulosin	BPH	Capsules: 0.4 mg	0.1 mg daily 30 min prior to the same meal	May be increased after 2–4 wk to 0.8 mg daily
Terazosin	Hypertension	Generic tablets: 1 mg, 2 mg, 5 mg, 10 mg	1 mg daily at bedtime	1–5 mg daily. Depending on standing BP, increase dose in 1 mg increments until target BP is achieved. Doses >20 mg/daily do not increase efficacy.
	BPH		1 mg daily at bedtime	Increased in a stepwise fashion to 2, 5, and then 10 mg. Doses at 10 mg are usually required for clinical effect. Dose may be 10–20 mg daily. Four to 6 wk are required to assess for beneficial response, so this is the interval for dosage adjustment.
Alfuzosin	BPH	Tablet: 10 mg extended-release	10 mg daily after the same meal	10 mg daily after the same meal

Source: FDA, 2009c, 2010b, 2012a.

concomitant BPH. Their actions simultaneously improve both conditions. Doxazosin and terazosin also lower low-density lipoprotein levels. They also enhance insulin sensitivity, cause regression of left ventricular hypertrophy, and improve the activity of the fibrinolytic system, making them useful for patients with diabetes and heart failure. Because they do not aggravate bronchospastic disease, they are useful for patients with asthma. Alpha₁-adrenergic antagonists are usually not used for monotherapy because they cause troublesome adverse reactions in almost all patients who take them. They can be used effectively in combination with other drugs that address these adverse reactions (FDA, 2009b, 2009c, 2010b, 2011a, 2012a).

The Antihypertensive and Lipid-Lowering Treatment to Prevent Heart Attack (ALLHAT) trial was recently reevaluated in the face of information from new clinical trials, meta-analyses, and recent subgroup and explanatory analyses from ALLHAT. The reevaluation included special focus on studies related to the consequences of cardiovascular disease. Findings in the initial study and supported in the reevaluation show alpha₁-adrenergic antagonists are surpassed by thiazide-type diuretics as initial therapy for

reduction of cardiovascular and renal risk associated with hypertension (Wright et al, 2009). In the initial ALLHAT study, the drug used was doxazosin; this part of the study was discontinued early because so many subjects dropped out because of adverse effects and because the blood pressure lowering effect was the least. Given these data, it seems appropriate that this class of drugs be used mainly when a primary goal is treatment of BPH symptoms rather than hypertension.

To reduce "first-dose" postural hypotension, the dose is begun at 1 mg 1 to 2 times daily, depending on the drug (see Table 14-6). The dose is then gradually increased until target blood pressure is achieved or the maximum dose is reached. When the dose is increased, the first, larger dose is always given at bedtime to reduce orthostatic hypotension effects. Doxazosin has once-daily dosing. Postural hypotension effects are most commonly seen 2 to 6 hours after taking a dose. Measure the blood pressure at this time interval for the first dose and when increasing the dose to determine if the target blood pressure is being reached. Prazosin has a 2 to 3 times daily dosing schedule. Measure blood pressure 2 to 3 hours after dosing to see when maximum and minimum benefits

Table 14–7 ⚏ **Drug Interactions: Selected Alpha$_1$-Adrenergic Antagonists**

Drug	Interacting Drug	Possible Effect	Implications
Alfuzosin	Ketoanazole, itraconazole, ritoniver	Decrease metabolism and increase effects of alfuzosin	Avoid concurrent use
	Cimetidine, atenolol, dilitiazem	Increase level of alfuzosin and may increase effects of atenolol and dilitiazem	Monitor blood pressure and heart rate
	Antihypertensives, calcium channel blockers, nitrates, and alcohol	Increased hypotension risk	Monitor blood pressure or avoid concurrent use
Prazosin	Beta-adrenergic blockers	May enhance acute postural hypotension following first dose of alpha$_1$-adrenergic blocker	Select different alpha$_1$-adrenergic blocker. No adverse reaction seen with doxazosin or terazosin.
	Clonidine	May decrease antihypertensive effect of clonidine	Avoid concurrent use
	Indomethacin	Antihypertensive action of prazosin may be decreased	Select different alpha$_1$-adrenergic blocker or different NSAID. No adverse reaction with doxazosin or other NSAIDs.
Silodosin	Calcium channel blockers and thiazides	Increased incidence of dizziness and orthostatic hypotension	Exercise caution and monitor for adverse effects
	Azole antifungals, clarithromycin, and other strong CYP3A4 inhibitors	Ketoconazole increased C_{max} and AUC	Concomitant use with strong CYP3A4 inhibitors contraindicated
	Diltiazem, erythromycin, verapamil, and other moderate CYP3A4 inhibitors	May increase plasma levels	Exercise caution and monitor for adverse effects
	Phosphodiesterase type 5 inhibitors (e.g., sildenafil, tadalafil)	Increased incidence of orthostatic hypotension	Exercise caution and monitor for adverse effects
Tamsulosin	Cimetidine	May increase blood levels of tamsulosin, with increased risk for hypotension and toxicity	Select different histamine$_2$ blocker if one must be used
Terazosin	NSAIDs, sympathomimetics, estrogens	May decrease antihypertensive effects of terazosin	Avoid concurrent use or select doxazosin or another drug class for antihypertensive therapy
	Verapamil	Increases serum terazosin levels and may increase sensitivity to terazosin-induced postural hypotension	Avoid concurrent use
	Finasteride	Increase in peak plasma concentration and AUC of finasteride	Clinical significance unknown; monitor for adverse effects of finasteride
Doxazosin, prazosin, tamsulosin, terazosin, alfuzosin	Alcohol, antihypertensives, nitrates	Additive hypotension	Avoid concurrent use or administer first dose in the office and monitor blood pressure response closely

Source: FDA, 2009c, 2010b, 2011a, 2012a.

in blood pressure lowering result. If the response is substantially diminished at 24 hours on twice-daily dosing, consider increasing the dose or using a 3 times-a-day regimen. Measure blood pressure 2 to 3 hours after dosing for terazosin as well. Although terazosin usually has once-daily dosing, if the response is diminished, consider twice-daily dosing. When a diuretic is added to the treatment regimen of any of these drugs, the dose of the alpha$_1$-adrenergic antagonist is reduced for 2 to 3 days and then re-titrated to control the blood pressure (FDA, 2009b, 2009c, 2010b, 2011a, 2012a).

Benign Prostatic Hyperplasia

Tamulosin, alfuzosin, and silodosin have all been approved for treatment of symptoms of benign prostatic hyperplasia. The recommended dose of tamulosin is 0.4 mg once daily administered approximately 30 minutes following the same meal each day. If the patient fails to respond to this dose after 2 to 4 weeks, the dose is increased to 0.8 mg once daily. Alfuzosin is recommended at 10 mg of the extended-release tablet daily to be taken immediately after the same meal each day. The silodosin starting dose is 8 mg given once daily with a meal (FDA, 2009b, 2009c, 2010b, 2011a, 2012a).

Ureteral Stones

Doxazosin, tamsulosin, and terazosin have off-label use as adjunct treatment to promote ureteral stone expulsion. These drugs do so by reducing ureteral pressure, peristaltic frequency, and ureteral contractions. American Urological Association and European Association of Urology guidelines for the management of ureteral calculi indicate that the administration of these drugs can effectively accelerate the spontaneous passage of these stones (FDA, 2009b, 2009c, 2010b, 2011a, 2012a).

Rational Drug Selection

Doxazosin is less likely than the other two drugs to produce postural hypotension and fluid retention and may be used as monotherapy (FDA, 2009b, 2009c, 2010b, 2011a, 2012a). The overall cost of the treatment regimen is reduced if an additional drug is unnecessary.

Convenient Dosing and Tolerability

Terazosin and doxazosin are both longer-acting alpha$_1$-receptor antagonists, but both need to be titrated to the target dose because of hypotension issues. Tamsulosin is also a longer-acting alpha$_1$-receptor antagonist, but it produces a response without dose titration. Tamsulosin's disadvantage is an increased incidence of ejaculatory dysfunction. Alfuzosin is marketed as a slow-release formulation and thus has relatively low adverse drug reactions. It also does not require dose titration and has the advantage of not causing ejaculatory dysfunction. Silodosin does not require dose titration but has an increased incidence of ejaculatory dysfunction when compared with tamsulosin (FDA, 2009b, 2009c, 2010b, 2011a, 2012a).

Both doxazosin and terazosin offer once-daily dosing (see Table 14-6) and doxazosin is now available in an extended-release formulation for treating BPH. Prazosin requires dosing 2 to 3 times daily. Doxazosin is scored to allow the tablet to be broken in half, allowing dosages to be easily increased without a change in tablet size.

Tachycardia

Although all drugs in this class may exhibit reflex tachycardia due to their antihypertensive effects, prazosin is an exception to this. The antihypertensive effect is not usually accompanied by reflex tachycardia. Prazosin can also be mixed with concomitant administration of a diuretic or beta-adrenergic agent (FDA, 2009b, 2010b, 2011a, 2012a).

Indications

Doxazosin, prazosin, and terazosin are all approved to treat hypertension. Treatment of BPH symptoms is approved by the FDA only for doxazosin, tamsulosin, alfuzosin, silodosin, and terazosin, although dosage data for this indication are published for prazosin (FDA, 2009b, 2010b, 2011a, 2012a).

Monitoring

Clinical monitoring of symptoms according to guidelines for HTN (see Chapter 40) and for BPH is the main monitoring parameter. Fluid retention is monitored by weekly weighing and patient education about signs and symptoms of fluid overload to report (e.g., peripheral edema, weight gain of more than 1 kg in a 24-hour period). Reduced white blood cell (WBC) counts of 1% to 2.4% have been noted, although no patients became symptomatic with these lower counts. A baseline WBC is drawn prior to initiation of therapy and as part of regular physical examinations. This class of drugs is heavily metabolized by the liver, so baseline liver function tests are also recommended (FDA, 2009b, 2010b, 2011a, 2012a).

Cancer of the prostate gland and BPH often coexist and have the same symptoms. Patients who are to begin on alpha$_1$-adrenergic antagonist therapy for BPH should first have digital rectal examinations and the provider should consider obtaining prostate-specific antigen (PSA) levels, if indicated, to rule out prostate cancer. Research has indicated that doxazosin and terazosin do not affect PSA levels in patients treated for less than 3 years (FDA, 2009b, 2009c, 2010b, 2011a, 2012a).

Patient Education

Administration

The drug should be taken exactly as prescribed, at the same time each day, even if the patient is feeling well. The first dose at initiation of therapy and the first dose each time the dosage is increased should be taken at bedtime to minimize the first-dose effect (potential hypotension and syncope). Missed doses are taken as soon as they are remembered unless it is almost time for the next dose. Doses are not doubled. Drugs in this class that may be taken without regard to food intake are doxazosin, prazosin, and terazosin. Alfuzosin should be taken with food or after food intake and tamsulosin should be taken 30 minutes after food intake. Silodosin should be administered with a meal (FDA, 2009b, 2010b, 2011a, 2012a).

NSAIDs decrease the antihypertensive effects of most drugs in this class. Over-the-counter (OTC) medications that contain NSAIDs should be avoided. Advise the patient to consult the health-care provider before taking any OTC drug, especially cough, cold, and allergy remedies (FDA, 2009b, 2010b, 2011a, 2012a).

If the drug is given for BPH, teach the patient the signs and symptoms of BPH to monitor (urinary frequency, a feeling of incomplete bladder emptying, interruption of urinary stream, decreased size and force of stream, terminal urinary dribbling, and straining to start the flow of urine). Improvement in these symptoms may take 4 to 6 weeks (FDA, 2009b, 2010b, 2011a, 2012a).

Adverse Drug Reactions

Hypotensive reactions are the most common. In addition to taking the first dose at bedtime, teach patients to rise slowly from a supine position and to dangle their feet over the side of the bed before arising. Not exercising in hot weather and limiting alcohol intake can also decrease these reactions (FDA, 2009b, 2010b, 2011a, 2012a).

Nasal congestion and/or rhinitis may occur. It should not be treated with OTC antihistamines or other cold remedies without first consulting with the health-care provider. Drowsiness and dry mouth are also common. The patient should avoid activities requiring mental alertness until the patient's individual response to the drug is known. Drowsiness frequently subsides after 7 to 10 days of continuous therapy (FDA, 2009b, 2010b, 2011a, 2012a). Dry mouth can be minimized by practicing good oral hygiene, chewing sugarless gum, or sucking on hard candy.

The leading cause of nonadherence to a treatment regimen with alpha$_1$-adrenergic antagonists is inhibition of ejaculation and impotence. These reactions should be reported to the health-care provider, who may choose a different drug to treat the disorder or change the dosage.

Lifestyle Management

If the drug is being given for HTN, encourage the patient to adhere to additional interventions for reduction of blood pressure, such as weight loss, low-sodium diet, smoking cessation, regular exercise, and stress management. Further discussion of patient education related to HTN is found in Chapter 40. BPH is discussed in the "Men as Patients" chapter (Chapter 49).

BETA-ADRENERGIC ANTAGONISTS (BLOCKERS)

Beta-adrenergic antagonists (blockers) are used in the treatment of cardiac disorders such as heart failure and asymptomatic left ventricular dysfunction and after an acute myocardial infarction. They are also useful in a variety of other disorders, including essential tremor, migraine headache prophylaxis, and hyperthyroidism (Mann, 2013). They act by occupying beta-receptor sites and competitively preventing occupancy of these sites by catecholamines and other beta agonists. A major difference among these drugs is their selectivity for beta$_1$- and beta$_2$-receptor sites, and this difference has important clinical implications.

These drugs blockade beta-adrenergic receptors, and they are usually referred to in health-care literature as beta blockers. Because this term is easily recognized, *beta blocker* is used throughout this text to denote beta-adrenergic antagonists.

Pharmacodynamics

The highest concentration of B$_1$ adrenergic receptors are located in the heart, and when bound with norepinephrine and epinephrine they influence heart rate and myocardial contraction. The receptors are also found in the respiratory system and eyes (McCance & Huether, 2014). Blockade of beta-adrenergic receptors produces clinically significant action on the cardiovascular, renal, and respiratory systems and on the eye. This blockade also results in metabolic and endocrine effects.

Cardiovascular Effects

For the most part, the heart receptors are mainly beta$_1$ receptors. Blockade of these receptors acts at the sinoatrial (SA) node to decrease heart rate (negative chronotropism), in the atria and ventricles to decrease contractility (negative inotropism) and conduction velocity (negative dromotropism), and at the atrioventricular (AV) junction to slow conduction (McCance & Huether, 2014). Taken together, these effects decrease the incidence of angina, decrease cardiac rhythm disturbances associated with rapid rhythms, decrease both supine and standing blood pressure, and reduce reflex orthostatic tachycardia. In patients whose severely damaged hearts require sympathetic stimulation for adequate ventricular function, beta blockade may worsen the condition.

In the vascular system, beta blockade opposes beta$_2$-mediated vasodilation and may initially result in a rise in peripheral vascular resistance, but chronic drug administration leads to a fall in peripheral resistance through a possible central effect that causes reduced sympathetic outflow to the periphery. Up regulation of beta$_1$ receptors occurs with chronic use. These effects are key to the use of these drugs in the treatment of hypertension.

Renal Effects

Blockade of the beta$_1$ receptors in the juxtaglomerular apparatus of the kidney reduces the release of renin. This effect on the renin-angiotensin-aldosterone system (RAAS) leads to less angiotensin II–mediated vasoconstriction and aldosterone-mediated volume expansion, resulting in decreases in blood pressure (McCance & Huether, 2014).

Respiratory Effects

Beta$_2$ receptors are located throughout the body. In the lungs, blockade of these receptors interferes with endogenous adrenergic bronchodilator activity, which results in passive bronchial constriction. This increase in airway resistance is particularly problematic for patients with reactive airway diseases such as asthma (Hall, 2013).

Ocular Effects

Opthalmic beta blockers decrease intraocular pressure as a result of decreased aqueous humor manufacture or outflow. The exact mechanism by which these drugs reduce intraocular pressure is not established, but is thought to be achieved by reduction in the production of aqueous humor (FDA, 2009d). Topical use of beta blockers is discussed in Chapter 27.

Metabolic and Endocrine Effects

Beta$_2$-blockade effects on the liver lead to inhibition of lipolysis, resulting in increased triglycerides and cholesterol and decreased high-density lipoproteins. For patients with hyperlipidemia, beta$_2$ blockade may worsen the condition (Podrid, 2013).

Effects on the liver also lead to inhibition of gluconeogenesis. The action of epinephrine on the beta-adrenergic receptors impacts glucose metabolism by increasing glucose production through glycogenolysis and glyconeogenesis. The delivery of gluconeogenic substrates from peripheral stores restricts glucose uptake and inhibits insulin secretion (Podrid, 2013).

Effects on Other Systems

The effect of beta blockade on other body systems is the source of the adverse drug reactions that may cause nonadherence to the drug regimen. Data analysis indicates a small risk of sexual dysfunction in 5 out of every 1,000 patients. Fatigue was reported in 18 per 1,000 patients. Depression is frequently cited as an adverse effect of beta blockade but recent data does not support this reaction. Due to this recent data, fatigue, depression, and sexual dysfunction are not reasons to withhold beta blockers (Podrid, 2013).

Pharmacokinetics

Absorption and Distribution

All beta blockers are well absorbed when given orally and are widely distributed in body tissues (Table 14-8). All cross the placenta and enter breast milk. CNS penetration varies, based on lipid solubility, with minimal penetration for acebutolol, atenolol, nadolol, and pindolol and moderate penetration for timolol and metoprolol, with propranolol having the highest CNS penetration. Nebivolol is highly lipophilic and has CNS penetration, but the exact degree of penetration is not clear. Several factors may account for the antihypertensive response of nebivolol, including lower heart rate, a decrease in myocardial contractility, impact on sympathetic outflow to the periphery, suppression of renin activity, and decreased peripheral vascular resistance (FDA, 2007a, 2007b, 2007c, 2011b, 2011c, 2011, 2013).

Metabolism and Excretion

Most beta blockers are metabolized extensively by the liver and eliminated via the bile and feces. Dosages of most of these agents may need to be decreased in patients with hepatic impairment. Nebivolol, a new third-generation beta blocker, has several routes of metabolism and a metabolic fate that is heavily genetically based. Most of the population are extensive metabolizers (EM) of the drug and small percentages are poor metabolizers (PM). The half-life of the active isomer, d-nebivolol, is about 12 hours in the EM population and 19 hours in the PM population. Metabolism includes glucuronidation and hydroxylation by CYP2D6 and to a lesser extent dealkylation and oxidation via this same isoenzyme system. It has two active sterospecific isomers. The d-isomer is the most active and

Table 14–8 ❖ Pharmacokinetics: Selected Beta Blockers

Drug	Onset	Peak	Duration	Protein Binding (%)	Bioavailability (%)	Half-Life	Elimination
Acebutolol*	60 min	4–6 h	24–30 h	26	<50	3–4 h; (18–13 h for diacetolol, the active metabolite)	30%–40% in urine; 50%–60% in feces/bile
Atenolol	60 min	2–4 h	24 h	6–16	50–60	6–9 h	50% unchanged in urine; rest in feces
Metoprolol	15 min	90 min	13–19 h	12	50–77	3–7 h	<5% unchanged in urine
Nadolol	5 days†	3–4 h	17–24 h	30	30–50	20–40 h	Unchanged in urine
Nebivolol	15 min	1.5–4 h	UK	98	UK	12–19 h based on genetic differences	38%–67% in urine; 13%–44% in feces
Pindolol*	7 days†	1 h	24 h	40	100	3–4 h	60%–65% metabolites and 35%–40% unchanged drug in urine
Propranolol	30 min	60–90	6–12 h	90	30	3–5 h	<1% unchanged min in urine
Propranolol	UK	6 h	24 h	90	9–18	8–11 h	<1% unchanged ER in urine
Timolol	UK	1–3 h	12–24 h	10	75	4 h	Metabolites and unchanged drug in urine

Source: FDA, 2007a, 2007b, 2007c, 2011b, 2011c, 2011d, 2013.

UK = unknown.

*Intrinsic sympathomimetic activity. Pindolol more than acebutolol.

†Onset of cardiovascular effects.

PMs attain a 5-fold higher maximal drug concentration (C_{max}) and a 10-fold higher AUC of this isomer than EMs (FDA, 2011d).

Several beta blockers (acebutolol, atenolol, nadolol, and nebivolol) require dosage adjustment in patients with renal impairment. The dose of acebutolol should be decreased by 50% when CrCl is less than 50 mL/min and by 75% if CrCl is less than 25 mL/min. Because approximately 40% of atenolol is excreted unchanged in the urine, the dose of this drug will need to be adjusted if creatinine clearance falls below 35 mL/min. Because nadolol is excreted unchanged in the urine, dosing must be adjusted in renal impairment. The recommendation for dosing nadolol in this situation involves extending the dosing interval. Last, with CrCl less than 30 mL/min, nebivolol dosing should be started at 2.5 mg daily and titrated (FDA, 2007a, 2007b, 2007c, 2011, 2011b, 2011c, 2012b, 2013).

Pharmacotherapeutics

Precautions and Contraindications

Beta blockers are contraindicated for patients with respiratory conditions that include a bronchospastic component. Although there are beta$_1$-selective drugs that have less effect on the beta$_2$ receptors in the lungs, to date no beta blocker is sufficiently selective to beta$_1$ to completely reduce the risk of beta$_2$ blockade. Even beta$_1$-selective drugs show beta$_2$ effects at higher doses. Because of their relative beta$_1$ selectivity, low doses of acebutolol, atenolol, betaxolol, bisprolol, and metoprolol should be used cautiously for patients with bronchospastic disease who do not respond to any other hypertensive treatment. Nebivolol is also beta$_1$-selective, but no recommendation about its use in pulmonary disease has yet been made (FDA, 2007a, 2007b, 2007c, 2011, 2011b, 2011c, 2012b, 2013).

These drugs are also contraindicated for patients with AV block, because their actions to decrease heart rate and myocardial contractility result in increased reduction in cardiac output and worsened failure. Decreased cardiac output and the initial vasoconstrictive action of these drugs may also worsen peripheral vascular diseases. Recognition that beta-adrenergic stimulation is a factor in heart failure has resulted in the use of nonselective beta blockers in heart failure, where the class was formerly contraindicated, but should be used with caution (FDA, 2007a, 2007b, 2007c, 2011, 2011c, 2011d, 2012b, 2013). Chapter 36 discusses their use for this indication in more detail.

Older adults often have limited cardiac and renal reserves. Beta blockers are used to treat conditions common to older adults, but care must be taken with dosing. Closer monitoring of cardiac and renal status is required. Based on meta-analyses of previous studies, beta blockers are less efficacious than other first-line therapies for cardiovascular disorders in patients who are 60 years or older, especially for stroke prevention (Institute for Clinical Systems Improvement [ICSI], 2008). Use of these drugs as initial therapy for older adults should be restricted to situations in which there is another indication for their use.

Beta blockers may precipitate or exacerbate type 2 diabetes. Because of their effects on carbohydrate metabolism and their ability to mask the common symptoms of hypoglycemia, beta blockers must be used cautiously in patients with diabetes (Podrid, 2013). Beta blockers have been proven effective in the management of the ischemic and congestive cardiac disorders that are more common in patients with diabetes, so they do have a role. According to Colucci (2013), the use of beta blockers in patients with diabetes was found to improve survival in a meta-analysis that included 1,883 people with diabetes.

In cases of hyperthyroidism, there is an increase in beta-adrenergic activity. Beta blockers have been successful in relieving symptoms such as palpitations, tachycardia, tremors, anxiety, and heat intolerance in patients with hyperthyroidism. Beta blockers are recommended for most hyperthyroid patients who have no contraindications to beta blocker use (Ross, 2013).

The Pregnancy category of beta blockers varies. Atenolol is Pregnancy Category D; betaxolol, acebutolol, metoprolol, nadolol, nebivolol, timolol, and propranolol are Pregnancy Category C. All cross the placenta and can cause fetal or neonatal bradycardia, hypotension, hypoglycemia, or respiratory depression (FDA, 2007a, 2007b, 2007c, 2011b, 2011c, 2011d, 2012b, 2013). The use of beta blockers during pregnancy is controversial because there have been individual reports of early labor, bradycardia, and restricted fetal growth. It should be mentioned that myometrial relaxation during pregnancy is mediated by beta$_2$ receptor processes (August, 2013). Sotalol and pindolol are listed as Pregnancy Category B. Note, however, that neonates of mothers who received these latter drugs had reduced birthweight and decreased blood pressure and heart rate at birth (FDA, 2007b, 2011f).

Propranolol and metoprolol are excreted in breast milk and the manufacturer recommends using caution when administering to nursing mothers. All other beta blockers are excreted in larger amounts. Nursing mothers should be given these drugs only when benefits clearly outweigh risks (FDA, 2011c, 2013).

Beta blockers were an early drug of choice in the treatment of hypertension in children. Propranolol was the subject of original studies in this population, but more selective drugs such as atenolol and metoprolol are found to be better tolerated. Extended-release metoprolol was evaluated in a population of 140 children with hypertension and found to be effective (Mattoo, 2013).

Adverse Drug Reactions

Beta blockade affects target organs and nontarget organs and tissues alike. This wide range of effects results in many adverse reactions to these drugs, although most adverse reactions have been mild and transient and have rarely required withdrawal of therapy. The discussion here focuses on the adverse reactions on each organ system.

Cardiovascular Reactions

Bradycardia, CHF with concomitant pulmonary edema, and hypotension are the most common cardiovascular adverse reactions. They have been discussed here in the Precautions and Contraindications section.

Central Nervous System and Psychiatric Reactions

Fatigue, weakness, and dizziness are associated with reduced oxygen transport to the brain secondary to excessive hypotension. Anxiety, depression, drowsiness, insomnia, nightmares, and mental status changes are more common in those drugs that have higher CNS penetration and in older adults (FDA, 2007a, 2007b, 2007c, 2011b, 2011c, 2011d, 2012b, 2013).

Endocrine Reactions

Alterations in carbohydrate metabolism resulting in hyperglycemia, hypoglycemia, or unstable diabetes have been discussed in the Precautions and Contraindications section.

⊙ CLINICAL PEARL ⊙

For patients with diabetes who must take a **beta blocker**, the diaphoresis associated with hypoglycemia is not masked by these drugs. Patients should be taught to recognize this indication of possible hypoglycemia and test their blood glucose levels whenever unexplained diaphoresis occurs.

Gastrointestinal Reactions

Dry mouth is uncommon but may occur. It may be reduced by practicing good oral hygiene, chewing sugarless gum, or sucking on hard candy. Changes in GI motility may result in anorexia, nausea, vomiting, flatulence, and constipation or diarrhea (FDA, 2007a, 2007b, 2007c, 2011b, 2011c, 2011d, 2012b, 2013.

Genitourinary Reactions

One of the most likely reasons for nonadherence to a treatment regimen that includes beta blockers is the risk for impotence and decreased libido. This side effect may resolve with continued use of the medication (FDA, 2007a, 2007b, 2007c, 2011b, 2011c, 2011d, 2012b, 2013).

Respiratory Reactions

Bronchospasm and dyspnea have been discussed in the Precautions and Contraindications section. Nasal stuffiness may also occur.

Other Reactions

Less common adverse reactions include muscle and joint pain, pruritic rashes, and facial swelling (FDA, 2007a, 2007b, 2007c, 2011b, 2011c, 2011d, 2012b, 2013). These are not directly related to the actions of these drugs.

Drug, Food, and Laboratory Test Interactions

Drug Interactions

Many drug interactions occur with beta blockers. Before they are prescribed, Table 14-9 should be consulted. Common problems include additive hypotension with other antihypertensives, acute ingestion of alcohol or nitrates, bradycardia with digitalis, and altered effectiveness of hypoglycemic drugs. Concurrent use of several drugs found in OTC cold remedies (ephedrine, phenylephrine, pseudoephedrine) may result in unopposed alpha-adrenergic stimulation, causing excessive hypertension and tachycardia. Metoprolol, nebivolol, and propranolol have drug interactions in addition to those found with other beta blockers. The drug in this category with the fewest interactions is atenolol (FDA, 2007a, 2007b, 2007c, 2011b, 2011c, 2011d, 2012b, 2013).

Table 14–9 ▦ Drug Interactions: Selected Beta Blockers

Drug	Interacting Drug	Possible Effect	Implications
All beta blockers	Aluminum salts, barbiturates, calcium salts, cholestyramine, colestipol, NSAIDs, ampicillin, rifampin, salicylates	Decrease bioavailability and plasma levels of beta-adrenergic antagonists, possibly resulting in decreased pharmacological effect	Avoid concurrent use. Separate administration of cholestyramine or colestipol from administration of beta-adrenergic antagonist by 4 h.
	Calcium channel blockers	Potentiate effects of beta-adrenergic antagonists	Do not administer within 24 h of each other. If must give both, monitor for heart failure and decreased peripheral perfusion.
	Ciprofloxacin and other quinolones, cimetidine	Bioavailability of beta-adrenergic antagonists metabolized by CYP450 may be increased	Select different antibiotic or different beta-adrenergic antagonist
	Digoxin	Additive bradycardia	Avoid concurrent administration. If must give both, monitor closely for digitalis toxicity. May need to adjust doses of one or both.
	Antihypertensives, alcohol, nitrates	Additive hypotension	Avoid acute ingestion of alcohol. Monitor blood pressure (BP) closely.

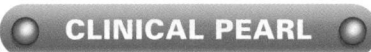

Table 14–9 ▓ Drug Interactions: Selected Beta Blockers—cont'd

Drug	Interacting Drug	Possible Effect	Implications
	Amphetamines, cocaine, ephedrine, epinephrine, norepinephrine, phenylephrine, pseudoephedrine	Concurrent use may result in unopposed alpha-adrenergic stimulation, resulting in excessive hypertension and bradycardia	Avoid concurrent use. Warn patients because many of these are included in OTC cold remedies
	Prazosin	Concurrent administration may potentiate postural hypotension	Avoid concurrent administration
	Sulfonylureas	Hypoglycemic effects of sulfonylureas may be attenuated	Select different hypoglycemic or antihypertensive. If they must be given together, monitor blood glucose closely.
	Clonidine	Life-threatening and fatal increases in BP have resulted after discontinuance of clonidine in patients also receiving beta-adrenergic antagonist or after simultaneous withdrawal	
Metoprolol, propranolol	Ranitidine	May increase bioavailability of metoprolol; other beta-adrenergic antagonists not affected	Select different histamine$_2$ blocker, but avoid cimetidine (see above)
	Hydralazine	Additive pharmacological effect	Avoid concurrent use or closely monitor effects
	MAOIs	Bradycardia may develop	Avoid concurrent use or use within 14 days of MAOI
	Propafenone	Plasma levels of metoprolol increased	Avoid concurrent use
	Benzodiazepines (BDZ)	Effects of BDZ increased by lipophilic beta-adrenergic antagonist	Change to atenolol. It does not interact.
	Seratonin reputake inhibitors (SRIs)	Certain SRIs may inhibit metabolism (CYP2D6) of these beta blockers leading to exessive beta blockades	Avoid concurrent use. Select different beta blocker.
	Thyroid hormone	Decrease actives of these beta blockers when patient is converted to euthyroid state	Monitor for decreased effects. Increase beta-blocker dose if needed.
Propranolol only	Acetaminophen	Decreased acetaminophen clearance	Avoid concurrent use or reduce dose
	Gabapentin	Increased gabapentin adverse responses	Avoid concurrent use
	Haloperidol	Hypotensive episodes	Select different antipsychotic
	Loop diuretics	Propranolol plasma levels and cardiovascular effects enhanced	Atenolol not affected. Use atenolol instead.
	Phenothiazines	Propranolol bioavailability and phenothiazine plasma levels increased, with potential toxicity	Selected different beta-adrenergic antagonist
	Warfarin	Increased anticoagulant effect	Select different beta-adrenergic antagonist
Nebivolol only	CYP2D6 inhibitors (e.g., fluoxetine, paroxetine, propafenone, quinidine)	Increased inhibition of CYP2D6 leading to increased plasma levels of nebivolol	Dose of nebivolol may need to be reduced
	Histamine 2 blockers (e.g., cimetidine)	Increased plasma levels of nebivolol metabolite by 23%	Avoid concurrent use
	Disopyramide	Clearance of disopyramide decreased leading to hypotension and sinus bradycardia	Avoid concurrent use or use caution and monitor closely if must coadminister
	Sildenafil	Decreased AUC and C_{max} of sildenafil by 21% and 23%, respectively	May require dosage adjustment

Source: FDA, 2007a, 2007b, 2007c, 2011b, 2011c, 2011d, 2013.

Life-threatening and fatal increases in blood pressure have been observed in patients taking clonidine and a beta blocker concurrently when the clonidine was withdrawn or when both the clonidine and the beta blocker were withdrawn. It is best to avoid using these drugs together, but if they are both given and withdrawal of one or both becomes necessary, taper the beta blocker first to avoid unopposed alpha stimulation and significant hypertension (FDA, 2007a, 2007b, 2007c, 2011b, 2011c, 2011d, 2012b, 2013).

Food Interactions

The beta blockers may be taken with or without food (FDA, 2007a, 2007b, 2007c, 2011b, 2011c, 2011d, 2012b, 2013).

Laboratory Test Interactions

Beta blockers may cause increased blood urea nitrogen (BUN), serum lipoprotein, potassium, triglyceride, and uric acid levels. They may also increase antinuclear antibody (ANA) titers and blood glucose levels (Podrid, 2013).

Clinical Use and Dosing

Regardless of the indication for which a beta blocker is given, there is no simple correlation between dose or plasma level and therapeutic effect. The dose-sensitivity range in clinical practice is wide because sympathetic tone and first-pass metabolism varies widely among individuals. Proper dosing requires titration (FDA, 2007a, 2007b, 2007c, 2011b, 2011c, 2011d, 2012b, 2013).

Angina

Atenolol, metoprolol, nadolol, and propranolol are indicated for long-term management of angina (Gibbons et al, 2003). Beta blockers lower blood pressure; reduce symptoms of angina; improve mortality; and reduce cardiac output, heart rate, and AV conduction. Both beta$_1$-selective and nonselective drugs affect the myocardial oxygen supply-demand equation on the demand side by decreasing the force of myocardial contractility, heart rate, and conduction velocity (National High Blood Pressure Education Program [NHBPEP], 2003). Nonselective agents, by a mechanism that is not clearly understood, decrease systemic vascular resistance and blood pressure, reducing afterload. Because they reduce myocardial oxygen demand, beta blockers are the drugs of choice for exertional angina. They are especially useful for patients with exertional angina whose lifestyle involves frequent vigorous activity, for patients with resting tachycardia, and for patients who have concomitant disease that might benefit from beta blockade (e.g., hypertension, post-MI migraine headaches). They do not improve myocardial oxygen supply, and propranolol has been reported to increase the risk for coronary artery vasospasm in some patients. Additional discussion of their use in patients with angina is found in Chapter 28.

To reduce the risk for adverse drug reactions, doses are started low and increased slowly, usually at no shorter than weekly intervals, based on resolution of symptoms. Dosage adjustment based on hepatic impairment and renal function is discussed in the metabolism and excretion section.

Hypertension

Initial drug therapy for hypertension is with a diuretic or a beta blocker in combination with a diuretic because they have been shown to reduce morbidity and mortality in numerous randomized controlled trials (RCT) (NHBPEP, 2003). Propranolol is now available in a combination form that includes hydrochlorothiazide. Beta blockers are also chosen because of reduced cost. They may be used in combination with other antihypertensives, largely to mitigate adverse effects. Atenolol, metoprolol, nadolol, and propranolol are the drugs most commonly chosen. Because of their relatively long half-lives, these drugs can be administered once daily, improving adherence. Pindolol and acebutolol have fewer myocardial depressant effects and do not increase cholesterol and triglyceride levels. Consideration of renal function is again important for dosing of some beta blockers (FDA, 2007a, 2007b, 2007c, 2011b, 2011c, 2011d, 2012b, 2013). Additional discussion of the use of beta blockers in hypertension management is found in Chapter 40.

Postmyocardial Infarction (MI) Prophylaxis

Use of beta blockers in post-MI prophylaxis has been shown to decrease mortality by 30% to 40%. They are most effective for patients who have had severe anterior MIs. The mechanism of action in MI prophylaxis appears to be related to limitation of infarct size, prevention of primary arrhythmic events, and protection from subsequent ischemia, and prevention of recurrent coronary occlusion. A clinical study of 1,395 patients in a double-blind, placebo-controlled trial found metoprolol to reduce 3-month mortality by 36% in patients with suspected or definite myocardial infarction. Atenolol, metoprolol, propranolol, and timolol have been shown to be effective for this indication. In a study of 1,456 patients, sotalol did not produce an increase in mortality rates at doses up to 320 mg/day in patients with a history of a recent MI and no ventricular arrhythmias. A second smaller study in a post-MI population did find suggestions of an increase in early sudden deaths (FDA, 2007a, 2007b, 2007c, 2011b, 2011c, 2011d, 2011f, 2012b, 2013).

Migraine Headache Prophylaxis

Propranolol in doses of 20 to 80 mg 3 or 4 times daily has proved effective in reducing the incidence of migraine headache in some patients. The mechanism of action is related to prevention of beta receptor–induced vasodilation and promotion of increased extracellular levels of serotonin. For propranolol, if a satisfactory response to the maximum dose is not obtained in 4 to 6 weeks, the drug should be gradually withdrawn because a longer trial is not associated with any better outcome (FDA, 2011c).

Glaucoma

Topical application of beta blockers in the treatment of glaucoma is discussed in Chapter 26.

Withdrawal of Beta Blockers

For all beta blockers, abrupt withdrawal can be life-threatening. It can result in severe angina, MI, ventricular arrhythmias, and death. The up-regulation of beta receptors with chronic use makes the system very sensitive to any SNS tone change. To withdraw any of these drugs, taper the dose by one-half every 4 days. Patients at high risk for serious consequences to rapid withdrawal include those with angina, coronary artery disease, and migraines (FDA, 2007a, 2007b, 2007c, 2011b, 2011c, 2011d, 2011f, 2012b, 2013).

Rational Drug Selection

Beta Selectivity

In selecting the most appropriate beta blocker, first consideration is usually given to beta$_1$ selectivity, sometimes referred to as "cardio selective." Atenolol, acebutolol, and metoprolol are beta$_1$-selective drugs. Nadolol, pindolol, propranolol, and timolol are nonselective drugs. Nebivolol, a third-generation beta blocker, is beta$_1$ selective in extensive metabolizers (EMs) and nonselective in poor metabolizers (PMs) (FDA, 2007a, 2007b, 2007c, 2011b, 2011c, 2011d, 2011f, 2012b, 2013).

The clinical significance of selectivity relates to the relative lack of action of beta$_1$-selective drugs on the beta$_2$ receptors. This relative lack of action makes beta$_1$-selective blockers more appropriate than nonselective agents for patients with chronic obstructive pulmonary diseases, asthma, peripheral vascular diseases such as Raynaud's syndrome, or diabetes mellitus. Among the beta$_1$-selective blockers, atenolol has greater selectivity than does metoprolol, which has greater selectivity than acebutolol (FDA, 2007a, 2007b, 2007c, 2011b, 2011c, 2011d, 2011f, 2012b, 2013).

Pharmacokinetics

The best choice of drug based on pharmacokinetics would be one with a long enough half-life to permit once-daily dosing, consistent bioavailability and limited interpatient variability in dosing, limited CNS penetration to reduce adverse reactions, and an excretion mechanism that does not require dosage adjustments so that extensive laboratory testing prior to initiation of therapy is not required. No one drug meets all these requirements, but several come close.

Atenolol, metoprolol, nadolol, and nebivolol have longer half-lives that permit once-daily dosing regimens, although metoprolol frequently has its best effects with twice-daily dosing. All other beta blockers have half-lives that require at least twice-daily dosing, with propranolol requiring 2 to 3 times daily dosing. Propranolol has a plasma half-life of 3 to 6 hours while the half-life of atenolol is 7 hours. It should be noted that this half-life is longer in elderly patients (FDA, 2007a, 2007b, 2007c, 2011b, 2011c, 2011d, 2011f, 2012b, 2013).

Atenolol and nadolol do not have significant hepatic first-pass effects. Acebutolol, metoprolol, and propranolol have significant first-pass effects and increased interpatient variability in the amount of drug that enters the patient's bloodstream. They also have short half-lives and require more frequent dosing. Timolol has some first-pass effects but the drug is about 75% bioavailable, so the first-pass effect is less significant. Pindolol does not have a significant first-pass effect (FDA, 2007a, 2007b, 2007c, 2011b, 2011c, 2011d, 2011f, 2012b, 2013).

Beta blockers that are excreted primarily by the kidney have increased half-lives in renal failure. Dosage adjustments are necessary. Atenolol, nebivolol, and nadolol fall into this category (Table 14-10). Although acebutolol has some excretion through the GI tract, its active metabolite is excreted through the kidneys, and the daily dose must be reduced in renal failure. Poor renal function has only minor effects on pindolol clearance, and the half-life of metoprolol is essentially unchanged (FDA, 2007a, 2007b, 2007c, 2011b, 2011c, 2011d, 2011f, 2012b, 2013).

Indications for Specific Drugs

Specific agents have been demonstrated to work with specific disorders. Other drugs in the class may not work as well. For example, propranolol is the only one proven useful in managing exertional or other stress-induced angina associated with idiopathic hypertrophic subaortic stenosis. A double-blind, placebo-controlled study of the effectiveness of propranolol in managing exercise-induced angina found it to be more effective than placebo (FDA, 2011c). The drug chosen should be backed by research that supports its use and an FDA approval for the intended use.

Monitoring

Monitoring parameters for beta blockers are essentially those used to monitor the disease process they are being used to treat (e.g., number of anginal attacks, lowering of blood pressure). For the drugs requiring dosage adjustments based on renal function, serum creatinine and/or creatinine clearance testing should be done prior to initiation of therapy. For drugs with significant first-pass effects, it may be appropriate to assess liver function before beginning therapy (FDA, 2007a, 2007b, 2007c, 2011b, 2011c, 2011d, 2011f, 2012b, 2013).

Patient Education

Administration

The patient should take the drug exactly as prescribed, even if feeling well. They should not skip or double doses. If a dose of atenolol, metoprolol, or nadolol is missed, it can be taken up to 8 hours before the next dose is due. Pindolol, propranolol, and timolol may be taken up to 4 hours before the next dose. Abrupt withdrawal may precipitate life-threatening arrhythmias, hypertension, and myocardial ischemia (FDA, 2007a, 2007b, 2007c, 2011b, 2011c, 2011d, 2011f, 2012b, 2013). The patient should make certain there is enough drug on hand to cover weekends or traveling and should carry identification describing the disease process and the medication regimen at all times.

Food may enhance the bioavailability of propranolol and metoprolol. They should be taken consistently either with food or on an empty stomach. Propranolol can be crushed and mixed with food, including oral solutions and semisolids, if it is consistently given with food. Food intake does not affect other beta blockers (FDA, 2007a, 2007b, 2007c, 2011b, 2011c, 2011d, 2011f, 2012b, 2013).

Patients should consult with the health-care provider before taking any OTC drugs, especially cold remedies. Several

Table 14–10 ⚔ Dosage Schedule: Selected Beta Blockers

Drug	Indication	Form	Initial Dose	Maintenance Dose
Acebutolol (Sectral)	Hypertension	Capsules: 200 mg Capsules: 400 mg	*Adults:* 400 mg/d in single or 2 divided doses *Older adults:* 200 mg/d in single or 2 divided doses	If target blood pressure (BP) not achieved in 1–2 wk, increase to 800 mg daily. Max dose is 1,200 mg. Reduce dosage by 50% if creatinine clearance (CCr) <50 mL/min; by 75% if CCr <25 mL/min.
	Ventricular arrhythmias		200 mg bid	Increase to 600–1,200 mg/d as needed to control arrhythmia
	Angina		300 mg tid	May increase to 400 mg tid if needed
Atenolol (Tenormin) (Canadian drug name: Apo-atenolol)	Hypertension	Tablets: 25 mg, 50 mg, 100 mg Atenolol/ Chlorthalidone (G)(Tenoretic) (B) Tablets: 50 mg atenolol/ 25 mg chlorthalidone, 100 mg atenolol/ 25 mg chlorthalidone	*Adults:* 25–50 mg daily *Children:* 0.8 mg/kg/d	If target BP not achieved in 1–2 wk, increase to 100 mg daily for adults and 1.5 mg/kg/d for children. Max dose for children is 2 mg/kg/d. Higher doses not likely to help in adults. Reduce dosage to 50 mg if creatinine clearance (CCr) 15–35 mL/min; 50 mg qod if CCr <15 mL/min.
	Angina		50 mg daily	If symptoms continue, increase to 100 mg daily. Some patients may need 200 mg. Reduce dosage to 50 mg if CCr 15–35 mL/min; 50 mg qod CCr <15 mL/min.
	MI (prophylaxis)		50 mg daily	50–100 mg daily (see note above re CCr)
Metoprolol (Lopressor) (Canadian drug names: Apo-Metoprolol, Betaloc)	Hypertension	Tablets: 25 mg, (G) 50 mg, 100 mg Tablets, extended-release: 25 mg, 50 mg, 100 mg, and 200 mg	*Adults:* 50–100 mg/d in single or divided doses (extended-release tablets: 50–100 mg daily) *Older adults:* 25 mg/d in single or divided doses	If target BP not achieved, increase at weekly intervals. Maintenance dose usually 100–450 mg/d. Does better in divided doses (extended-release tablets: 100–400 mg daily).
	Angina		100 mg/d in two divided doses (extended-release tablets: 100 mg daily)	If symptoms continue, increase in weekly intervals up to 400 mg/d in two divided doses (extended-release: up to 400 mg daily)
	MI (prophylaxis)		100 mg/d in two divided doses	100 mg/d in two divided doses
Nadolol (Corgard)	Hypertension	Tablets: 20 mg 40 mg (G) 80 mg (G) 120 mg 160 mg	40 mg daily	Increase in doses of 40–80 mg/d until target BP achieved. Maintenance dose usually 40–80 mg/d. Max dose 320 mg/d in divided doses. Increase dosage interval in renal impairment: CCr >50 = q 24 h; CCr 31–50 = q 24–36 h; CCr 10–30 = q 24–48 h; CCr <10 = q 40–60 h.
	Angina		40 mg daily	If symptoms continue, increase in 3–7 d intervals to 80–160 mg/d. Max dose is 240 mg/d. Increase dosage interval in renal impairment: CCr >50 = q 24 h: CCr 31–50 = q 24–36 h; CCr 10–30 = q 24–48 h; CCr <10 = q 40–60 h.

Table 14–10 ⊗ Dosage Schedule: Selected Beta Blockers—cont'd

Drug	Indication	Form	Initial Dose	Maintenance Dose
Nebivolol (Bystolic)	Hypertension	Tablets: 2.5, 5, 10, 20 mg	5 mg daily CCr <30 or moderate hepatic impairment = reduce dose to 2.5 mg daily	May increase dose at 2-wk intervals up to max dose of 40 mg/d. CCr <30 or moderate hepatic impairment = cautious upward titration.
Propranolol (Inderal) (Inderal LA) (InnoPran XL) (Canadian drug name: Apo-pranolol and Novopranolol)	Hypertension	Tablets (G): 10 mg, 20 mg, 40 mg, 80 mg Tablets (G): 60 mg, 90 mg Solution: 20 mg/ 5 mL <u>Propranolol CR Extended Release</u> Capsules: 60 mg, 80 mg, 120 mg, 160 mg <u>(InnoPran XL)(B)</u> Capsules: 80 mg, 120 mg <u>Propranolol/ Hydrochloro- thiazide (G) (Inderide) (B)</u> Tablets: 40 mg, 25 mg 80 mg/25 mg	*Adults:* 40 mg bid (SR = 80 mg daily) *Children:* 0.5 mg/kg/d in two divided doses	*Adults:* Usual maintenance dose is 120–240 mg bid or tid (SR = 120–160 mg daily); max dose = 640 mg/d *Children:* Max dose 16 mg/kg/d
	Angina		80–320 mg in two, three, or four divided doses (SR = 80 mg daily)	If symptoms continue; give 160 mg SR tablet; max dose, 320 mg SR
	MI (prophylaxis)		180–240 mg/d in 2–3 divided doses	
	Migraine prophylaxis		80 mg/d (SR)	160–240 mg/d in divided doses
Timolol (Blocadren)	MI (prophylaxis)	Tablets: 5 mg, 10 mg (G only), 20 mg		10 mg bid
	Migraine prophylaxis		10 mg bid	Maintenance dose 10–30 mg. May take up to 8 wk of maximum daily dose

Source: FDA, 2007a, 2007b, 2007c, 2011b, 2011c, 2011d, 2013.
SR = sustained release

drugs common in these preparations have drug interactions that result in hypertension and excessive bradycardia.

If these drugs are being taken for angina, beta blockers cannot relieve acute anginal attacks. If acute chest pain occurs, the patient should call 911 and go to the nearest hospital.

Adverse Reactions

Hypotensive reactions and bradycardia are the most common adverse reactions. Arising slowly from a supine position and dangling the feet over the side of the bed before standing will reduce postural hypotension. No exercise in hot weather and adequate hydration with noncaffeinated fluids will also reduce these problems (FDA, 2007a, 2007b, 2007c, 2011b, 2011c, 2011d, 2011f, 2012b, 2013). Assessment of blood pressure and pulse is necessary on a biweekly basis for those taking these drugs. Teach the patient home blood pressure and pulse monitoring and advise contacting the health-care provider if the pulse is less than 50 bpm or if the blood pressure changes suddenly.

Beta blockers may exacerbate diseases with a bronchospastic component. Teach patients to report wheezing or difficulty in breathing to the health-care provider immediately. Dizziness and drowsiness may occur with the drugs. Patients should avoid driving or other activities that require mental alertness until response to the drug is known. Insomnia can be reduced by not taking the last dose of the day late in the evening (FDA, 2007a, 2007b, 2007c, 2011b, 2011c, 2011d, 2011f, 2012b, 2013). Dry mouth responds to practicing good oral hygiene, chewing sugarless gum, or sucking on hard candy.

Depression and confusion have been associated with the beta blockers that have significant CNS penetration. The patient should report such problems, and a different beta blocker or a different class of drugs may be tried.

For diabetics, these drugs may mask the signs and symptoms of hypoglycemia and impair recovery from a hypoglycemic episode. Beta$_1$-selective drugs are less likely to cause this problem. The one indication of hypoglycemia that is not masked is diaphoresis. In the event of unexplained diaphoresis, the patient should check the blood glucose level immediately.

Beta blockers are contraindicated in the first trimester of pregnancy and must be withdrawn before delivery. Women of childbearing age should be given this warning. Other pregnancy considerations relate to the specific pregnancy category of the beta blocker being considered (FDA, 2007a, 2007b, 2007c, 2011b, 2011c, 2011d, 2011f, 2012b, 2013).

Nonadherence to a treatment regimen with a beta blocker is often caused by inhibition of ejaculation and impotence. If these occur, the patient should report them to the health-care provider, who may choose a different drug to treat the disorder or change the dosage.

Lifestyle Management

If the drug is being given for hypertension, encourage the patient to adhere to additional interventions for reduction of blood pressure, such as weight loss, a low-sodium diet, smoking cessation, regular exercise, and stress management. Further discussion of patient education is found in Chapter 40. Further discussion of patient education about angina is found in Chapter 28 and discussion of heart failure is found in Chapter 36.

COMBINED ALPHA- AND BETA-ADRENERGIC ANTAGONISTS

Drugs that exhibit blockade at both alpha and beta receptors have effects that would be expected from a combination of an alpha and a beta blocker. Because the alpha blockade predominates, however, they are less likely to produce significant reductions in heart rate or cardiac output. Alpha blockade also balances the tendency of beta blockers to produce reflex vasoconstriction.

Two drugs in this class are: carvedilol (Coreg) and labetalol (Normodyne). Both are used to treat hypertension, and carvedilol is also used to reduce progression of heart failure and to treat left ventricular dysfunction following an MI (FDA, 2010, 2011g). This section focuses on aspects of these drugs that are different from alpha-adrenergic antagonists and beta blockers. Aspects of these drugs that are similar to those of the other two classes are discussed only briefly.

Epinephrine also binds to both alpha and beta receptors and is used in the treatment of allergic reactions including anaphylaxis. The dose is delivered by subcutaneous injection. Auvi-Q is a brand which was approved in 2012 for this use and is available in auto-injectors for ease of use (FDA, 2012f).

Pharmacodynamics

These drugs combine selective alpha$_1$-adrenergic and nonselective beta blockade. The alpha and beta blockades decrease blood pressure; standing blood pressure is more affected than supine. They also decrease peripheral resistance by peripheral vasodilation (carvedilol more than labetalol). These combined effects decrease myocardial oxygen demand and lower cardiac workload. Single doses of labetalol have no significant effect on sinus rate, intraventricular conduction, or QRS duration. AV conduction time is only modestly prolonged. No significant change in cardiac output occurs. Labetalol has been associated with rare orthostatic hypotension. Carvedilol reduces orthostatic hypotension and exercise-induced reflex tachycardia. In hypertensive patients with normal renal function, it also decreases renal vascular resistance. Neither of these drugs demonstrates a significant effect on serum lipoproteins (FDA, 2010, 2011g).

Although beta blockade is useful in angina and hypertension, sympathetic stimulation is vital in some situations. For example, in patients with severely damaged hearts, adequate ventricular function may depend on sympathetic drive (FDA, 2010, 2011g).

Epinephrine (Auvi-Q) also decreases the vasodilation and vascular permeability, which are present during anaphylaxis. It causes bronchial smooth muscles to relax and relieves bronchospasm, wheezing, and dyspnea. Epinephrine decreases pruritis, angioedema, urticarial, and some of the genitourinary symptoms present with anaphylaxis.

Pharmacokinetics
Absorption and Distribution

Both carvedilol and labetalol are rapidly absorbed (Table 14-11). Carvedilol is more protein bound than labetalol. Both drugs are widely distributed in body tissues (FDA, 2010, 2011g). Epinephrine is given by injection and the onset is rapid and the duration short (FDA, 2012f).

Metabolism and Excretion

Carvedilol and labetalol undergo rapid hepatic first-pass metabolism resulting in bioavailabilities between 25% and 35%. Carvedilol is metabolized by CYP2D6 and 2C9 and labetolol undergoes glucoronidation and sulfation, which are not CYP meditated. Carvedilol undergoes more excretion in bile and feces than does labetalol (FDA, 2010, 2011g).

Pharmacotherapeutics
Precautions and Contraindications

Epinephrine is used in emergency situations in people who are at risk for anaphylaxis. There are no contraindications

Table 14–11 ⊞ **Pharmacokinetics: Combined Alpha-Beta Blockers**

Drug	Onset	Peak	Duration	Protein Binding	Bioavailability	Half-Life	Elimination
Carvedilol	1 h	1–2 h	12 h	>98%	25%–35%	7–10 h	Primarily in bile and feces: <2% unchanged in urine
Labetalol	20 min	1–4 h	8–12 h	50%	25% (increased by food and in older adults)	3–8 h	In bile and feces; 50%–60% as conjugates in urine

Source: FDA, 2010, 2011g.

listed by the FDA for use, but it should be used with caution in patients with cardiac arrhythmias, heart disease, hypertension, diabetes, or hyperthyroidism. Populations identified for cautious use are the elderly and pregnant women. People with Parkinson's disease may have a temporary worsening of symptoms following administration of epinephrine (FDA, 2012f).

For the oral drugs in the category, because they include nonselective beta blockade, alpha-beta blockers are contraindicated for patients with respiratory conditions that include a bronchospastic component. They are also contraindicated in overt, New York Heart Association (NYHA) class IV heart failure, greater than first-degree AV block, and severe bradycardia due to their negative inotropic effects. However, carvedilol has been shown to be effective in the management of NYHA class II and III heart failure because of its limited effects on heart rate and myocardial contractility while improving hemodynamics and cardiac performance (FDA, 2010, 2011g).

Cautions related to diabetes and thyroid disease and problems with withdrawal are similar to those of beta blockers. Although alpha-beta blockers produce less reflex vasoconstriction, caution is still required when these drugs are administered to patients with peripheral vascular disease (FDA, 2010, 2011g).

Like many beta blockers, these drugs are heavily metabolized by the liver, and use in patients with clinically manifested liver disease is not recommended. Hepatic injury has occurred rarely with both drugs, and onset of jaundice or hepatic dysfunction indicated by symptoms or elevations of liver function tests necessitates withdrawal of the drug (FDA, 2010, 2011g).

These drugs are Pregnancy Category C for the same reasons as beta blockers. Epinephrine should only be used in pregnancy if the benefit outweighs the risk. Small amounts of labetalol (0.004%) are excreted in breast milk, and the amount of carvedilol excreted in breast milk is unknown. Caution should be exercised in giving labetalol to nursing mothers, with careful consideration of benefits versus risk. Carvedilol should not be given to nursing mothers (FDA, 2010, 2011g, 2012f).

According to the American College of Obstetricians and Gynecologists (ACOG, 2012), labetalol may increase the risk of small for gestational age (SGA) infants if used to treat hypertension during pregnancy. A meta-analysis of studies evaluating the use of labetalol included atenolol and this may

have contributed to the finding of SGA. Consequently, ACOG finds the use of labetalol during pregnancy to treat chronic hypertension safe. It is reasonable to decrease the dosage or suspend treatment during pregnancy in those with mild hypertension defined as less than 150/100 mm Hg in the absence of comorbidities (ACOG, 2012).

Plasma levels of carvedilol average 50% higher in older adults than in young adults. Although there was no notable difference in adverse reactions in study subjects, it is advisable to monitor older patients more closely for adverse reactions such as dizziness, which places them at risk for falls (FDA, 2011g).

Safety and efficacy in children younger than 18 years of age have not been established for either drug. In a double-blind study discussed by the FDA on its pediatric exclusivity site, children ages 2 months to 17 years with chronic heart failure showed no significant effect of treatment with carvedilol on clinical outcomes after 8 months of follow-up (FDA, 2010, 2011g).

Adverse Drug Reactions

Adverse drug reactions are essentially the same as those seen with beta blockers, with the exception of fewer cardiac-related reactions (e.g., bradycardia, decreased contractility) and a lower incidence of CNS-related reactions. The risk for orthostatic hypotension is higher than with beta blockers and is related to the alpha$_1$-adrenergic blockade (FDA, 2010, 2011g). Adverse reactions to epinephrine include apprehensiveness, restlessness, tremor, anxiety, palpitations, dizziness, headache, and respiratory difficulties (FDA, 2012f).

Drug, Food, and Laboratory Test Interactions

Drug Interactions

Drug interactions are similar to those for beta blockers, with a few additions (Table 14-12). As with some of the other beta blockers, drugs that inhibit the CYP450 2D6 system increase plasma levels of carvedilol (FDA, 2010, 2011g).

Food Interactions

When carvedilol is taken with food, its rate of absorption is slowed, but the bioavailability is not affected. Taking it with food minimizes the risk for postural hypotension. Food slows the rate of absorption of labetalol but increases the absolute bioavailability. As a result, labetalol should be taken consistently with regard to food (FDA, 2010, 2011g).

Table 14–12 ▦ **Drug Interactions: Combined Alpha-Beta Blockers**

Drug	Interacting Drug*	Possible Effect	Implications
Carvedilol	Inhibitors of CYP450 2D6 (e.g., cimetidine, ciprofloxacin and other quinolones, quinidine, fluoxetine, paroxetine, propafenone)	Increased blood level of carvedilol	Avoid concurrent use
	Rifampin	Plasma concentration of carvedilol reduced by 70%	Avoid concurrent use
	Diphenhydramine	Inhibits metabolism of carvedilol leading to increased plasma concentrations and effects	Avoid concurrent use Warn patients related to OTC antihistamine
Labetalol	Beta agonists, theophylline	Labetalol can blunt the bronchodilator effect	A greater-than-normal dose of beta agonist may be required
	Cimetidine	Increases bioavailabity of labetalol	Avoid concurrent use
Epinephrine	Cardiac glycosides or diuretics		Observe for development of cardiac arrhythmias
	Tricyclic antidepressants, monoamine oxidase inhibitors, levothyroxine, antihistamines	Effects of epinephrine potentiated	Avoid concurrent use
	Beta-adrenergic blocking drugs		Avoid concurrent use
	Alpha-adrenergic blocking agents	Vasocontriction and hypertensive effects antagonized	Avoid concurrent use
	Ergot alkaloids	Reverses the pressor effects of epinephrine	Avoid concurrent use

Source: FDA, 2010, 2011g.

Laboratory Test Interactions

The presence of a labetalol metabolite in the urine may falsely increase urinary catecholamine levels measured by a nonspecific trihydroxyindole reaction. There have also been reversible increases in serum transaminases (4% of patients) and, rarely, reversible increases in BUN. Labetalol has also produced a false-positive test for amphetamine in a patient whose urine was screened for the presence of drugs (FDA, 2010, 2011g).

Clinical Use and Dosing

Hypertension

Both carvedilol and labetalol are used to treat essential hypertension either alone or in combination with other antihypertensive agents, especially thiazide-type diuretics. Both drugs are begun at a low dose, and dosage is increased until target blood pressure is achieved (Table 14-13). Carvedilol begins at 6.25 mg twice daily. Adjustments are made at 7- to 14-day intervals, based on standing systolic blood pressure. Labetalol is initiated at 100 mg twice daily and increased in 100 mg increments every 2 to 3 days until target blood pressure is achieved (FDA, 2010, 2011g).

Congestive Heart Failure

Carvedilol has an indication for treatment of heart failure in a narrow group of patients: mild to moderate (NYHA class II or III) heart failure of ischemic or cardiomyopathic origin, in conjunction with diuretics and (ACE) inhibitors, to reduce the progression of disease and increase survival (Packer et al, 2001). Treatment is begun at one-half the hypertension dosage (3.125 mg 2 times a day), with increases at 2-week intervals. The maximum dose is based on patient weight.

Withdrawal of the Alpha-Beta Blockers

As with beta blockers, abrupt withdrawal can be life-threatening. Angina has not been observed, but withdrawal can result in MI, ventricular arrhythmias, and death. To withdraw either of these drugs, taper the dose by one-half every 4 days over a period of 1 to 2 weeks. Patients at high risk for serious consequences due to rapid withdrawal include those with angina, coronary artery disease, and migraines (FDA, 2010, 2011g).

Age

Because of the risk for orthostatic hypotension, carvedilol and labetalol drugs should be used with caution in older adults (FDA, 2010, 2011g).

Concomitant Diseases

Carvedilol may be chosen when the patient has concomitant mild to moderate heart failure. Labetalol may be chosen when the patient cannot tolerate changes in heart rate but needs beta blockade (e.g., post-MI prophylaxis) (FDA, 2010, 2011g).

Table 14–13 ⊗ **Dosage Schedule: Combined Alpha-Beta Blockers**

Drug	Indication	Form	Initial Dose	Maintenance Dose
Carvedilol	Hypertension	Tablets: 3.125 mg, 6.25 mg, 12.5 mg, 25 mg Capsules: (extended-release) 10 mg, 20 mg, 40 mg, 80 mg	6.25 mg bid; if dose is tolerated using standing systolic blood pressure (BP) measured 1 h after the dose, maintain this dose for 7–14 d	After initial dose, increase to 12.5 mg bid if needed, based on trough BP using same standing systolic BP. Maintain this dose for 7–14 d before increasing to 25 mg if needed. When increasing dose, give first larger dose at bedtime or give with food to slow or to avoid orthostatic hypotension. Full antihypertensive effect seen in 7–14 d. Maximum dose is 50 mg.
	CHF		3.125 mg bid for 2 wk	Individualize dose and closely monitor during up-titration. If initial dose is tolerated, increase to 6.25 mg bid. Dose can then be doubled every 2 wk to the highest level tolerated by the patient. Maximum dose is 25 mg bid for <85 kg; 50 mg bid for > 85 mg. Transient worsening of CHF may be treated by increasing diuretic or reducing carvedilol dose.
	LV dysfunction following MI		6.25 mg bid	Increased after 3–10 d, based on tolerability, to 12.5 mg bid, then again to target dose of 25 mg bid
	Idiopathic cardiomyopathy (Children <62.5 kg)		6.25 mg daily	Increased as needed/tolerated. Max dose 75 mg/d. Continue for at least 6–8 mo.
	Idiopathic cardiomyopathy (Adults)		0.05 mg/kg bid	Increase dose twice at 2 wk intervals to 0.1 and 0.2 mg/kg bid. Max dose: 0.4 mg/kg.
	(Children > 62.5 kg)		3.125 mg bid	Increase twice at 2 wk intervals to 6.25 mg bid and 12.5 mg bid. Max dose 25 mg bid.
Labetalol	Hypertension	Tablets: 100 mg, 200 mg, 300 mg	*Adults:* 100 mg bid alone or added to a diuretic	If target BP is not achieved in 2–3 d, increase in increments of 100 mg bid every 2–3 d. Maintenance dose is usually 200–400 mg bid. Full antihypertensive effect seen within first 1–3 h of initial dose. Maximum dose 2,400 mg/d.
			Older adults: 100 mg bid	Maintenance dose is usually 100–200 mg bid.
Epinephrine (AUVI-Q)	Emergency treatment of allergic reactions (Type I) including anaphylaxis.	Injection: 0.3mg/ 0.3 mL prefilled auto-injector Injection: 0.15mg/0.15mL prefilled auto-injector	Patients greater than or equal to 30 kg (66 lb): Auvi-Q 0.3 mg Patients 15 to 30 kg (33– 66 lb): Auvi-Q 0.15 mg Inject Auvi-Q intramuscularly or subcutaneously into the anterolateral aspect of the thigh, through clothing if necessary. Each device is a single-use injection.	More than two sequential doses of epinephrine should only be administered under direct medical supervision.

Source: FDA, 2010, 2011g.

Monitoring

Liver function tests should be performed before initiating therapy, when adjusting dosage, and at the first indication of liver dysfunction (pruritus, dark urine, persistent anorexia, jaundice, upper-right quadrant tenderness, or unexplained flu-like syndrome). If the patient has laboratory evidence of liver injury, stop the drug and do not restart it (FDA, 2010, 2011g).

Renal function tests should be performed prior to initiating therapy and at regular intervals for any patients with a concomitant disease process that may impair renal function (FDA, 2010, 2011g).

Clinical monitoring of the disease process for which the drug was prescribed is also indicated. Discussion of such monitoring for hypertension is discussed in Chapter 40.

Patient Education

Administration

The patient should take the drug exactly as prescribed, at the same time each day, even if feeling well. Doses should not be skipped or doubled. If a dose of labetalol is missed, it should be taken up to 8 hours before the next dose is due. For carvedilol, the missed dose should be taken up to 4 hours before the next dose. Abrupt withdrawal may precipitate life-threatening arrhythmias, hypertension, and myocardial ischemia (FDA, 2010, 2011g). The patient should make certain there is enough drug on hand to cover vacations and holiday periods and should wear identification describing the disease process and the medication regimen at all times.

Carvedilol should be taken with food. This slows absorption and reduces the chance of orthostatic hypotension (FDA, 2010, 2011g). It is important to caution patients not to inject epinephrine into their hands, feet, or digits due to its strong vasoconstrictive properties. Epinephrine should not be injected into a vein and injection into the buttocks may not provide relief from an anaphylactic reaction (FDA, 2012f).

While taking an alpha-beta blocker, the patient should consult with the health-care provider before taking any OTC drugs, especially cold remedies. Several ingredients common in these preparations cause drug interactions that result in hypertension and excessive bradycardia.

Adverse Reactions

Hypotensive reactions and bradycardia are the most common adverse reactions. Alpha-beta blockers may exacerbate diseases with a bronchospastic component. Teach patients to report wheezing or difficulty in breathing to the health-care provider immediately.

Dizziness and drowsiness may occur with these drugs. Patients should avoid driving or other activities that require mental alertness until their response to the drug is known (FDA, 2010, 2011g).

For diabetics, these drugs may mask the signs and symptoms of hypoglycemia and impair recovery from a hypoglycemic episode. However, they are less likely to cause this problem because neither of these drugs is beta$_1$ selective.

Because alpha-beta blockers have beta-blocking activity, they are contraindicated in the first trimester of pregnancy and must be withdrawn before delivery (FDA, 2010, 2011g). Women of childbearing age should be counseled regarding these drugs. A leading cause of nonadherence to a treatment regimen with an alpha-beta blocker is inhibition of ejaculation and impotence. If these occur, they should be reported to the health-care provider, who may change the dosage or choose a different drug to treat the disorder.

Adverse reactions associated with epinephrine include apprehensiveness, tremor, anxiety, weakness, headache, difficulty breathing, and palpitations. Fatal arrhythmias may occur as well as rapid rises in blood pressure leading to cerebral hemorrhage, especially in elderly patients (FDA, 2012f).

Lifestyle Management

Lifestyle management is the same as for beta blockers. For patients with a history of severe allergic reactions it is important to avoid the allergen and keep an epinephrine injector with them at all time.

CHOLINERGIC AGONISTS

Cholinergic agonists, also known as parasympathomimetics or muscarinic agonists, promote or mimic the action of acetylcholine (ACh). These effects may be achieved either by direct agonist effect or indirectly by preventing the breakdown of ACh by acetylcholinesterase (AChE). As with adrenergic agonists, these drugs are not organ specific; when one organ is targeted for therapeutic reasons, the drug simultaneously produces effects in other organs. The targeted organ effects become the desired drug action, and the other organ effects become the adverse drug effects.

There are three categories of drugs in this class: muscarinic agonists, cholinesterase inhibitors, and ganglionic stimulants. Each category is discussed separately. The prototypic drug among ganglionic stimulants is nicotine, which is the only drug discussed in this category.

MUSCARINIC AGONISTS

Pharmacodynamics

Muscarinic receptors are located in the eye, heart, blood vessels, lung, GI tract, urinary bladder, and sweat glands. The results of stimulation of these receptors are depicted in Table 14-1. Their activation by muscarinic agonists modifies organ function by release of ACh from PNS nerves: (1) to activate muscarinic receptors on target organs to alter organ function and (2) to activate muscarinic receptors on nerve terminals to inhibit the release of their neurotransmitters (McCance & Huether, 2014).

There are five drugs in this group, each with a different susceptibility to breakdown by cholinesterase and different degrees of action at muscarinic and nicotinic receptors. ACh (Miochol) is highly susceptible to cholinesterase and very active at both types of receptors. Carbachol (Isopto Carbachol), pilocarpine (Isopto Carpine), and bethanechol (Urecholine) have negligible susceptibility to cholinesterase, and all three act at muscarinic receptors. Carbachol also acts at nicotinic receptors. Methacholine (Provocholine) has little susceptibility to cholinesterase and is very active at muscarinic receptors only (FDA, 2006, 2006b, 2008a, 2010a).

Muscarinic agonists are used clinically to treat glaucoma and to improve GI and urinary bladder tone. ACh lacks selectivity to target tissues and is so rapidly destroyed by cholinesterase that its half-life is too short for most clinical applications. Its use is restricted to dilation of the pupil for ophthalmic surgery. Methacholine is used only for diagnosis of bronchial airway hyper-reactivity by specialists familiar with its use for this purpose (FDA, 2008a). Neither of these drugs is discussed here.

Carbachol and pilocarpine are used to treat glaucoma and are discussed in Chapter 26. Pilocarpine comes in an oral form that can be used to increase salivary gland secretion for the management of xerostomia in patients who have undergone radiation therapy of the neck (FDA, 2006b, 2010a). This use is too restricted for discussion in this text. The only remaining drug in this category is bethanechol, and the remainder of this section discusses that drug.

Bethanechol increases the tone of the detrusor urinae muscle, and produces contractions strong enough to initiate micturation and empty the bladder. It stimulates gastric motility as well, increasing gastric tone and often restoring rhythmic peristalsis. Doses that stimulate micturation and increase peristalsis do not usually stimulate ganglia or voluntary muscles (NIH, 2012).

Pharmacokinetics

Absorption and Distribution

Bethanechol can be given orally or subcutaneously (SC). Effects appear in 30 to 90 minutes after oral administration and 5 to 15 minutes after SC administration. The effects peak in 60 minutes for the oral dose and 15 to 30 minutes for the SC dose. Duration of action is approximately 1 to 6 hours for the oral dose and 2 hours for the SC dose. The dose required to produce a therapeutic effect is significantly different by these two routes because bethanechol is a quaternary ammonium compound carrying a positive charge, which greatly impedes absorption from the GI tract. Because bethanechol is not destroyed by cholinesterase, its effects are more prolonged than those of ACh. Because of its selective nature, nicotinic symptoms of cholinergic stimulation are usually absent or minimal while the muscarinic effects are prominent (NIH, 2012).

Metabolism and Excretion

The metabolic rate and mode of excretion of bethanechol have not been elucidated. The drug does not cross the blood–brain barrier (NIH, 2012).

Pharmacotherapeutics

Precautions and Contraindications

Bethanechol is contraindicated in the presence of many diseases. It is contraindicated in peptic ulcer disease because at the usual therapeutic doses it can cause excessive secretion of gastric acid that could intensify gastric erosion and precipitate gastric bleeding and possible perforation. It is contraindicated in patients with intestinal obstruction because of its ability to increase GI peristalsis. Because of its ability to contract the bladder and increase pressure within the urinary tract, it is also contraindicated in the presence of urinary tract obstruction or weakness of the bladder wall. Stimulation of the muscarinic receptors in the lungs may result in bronchoconstriction, and therefore it is contraindicated in patients with latent or active bronchospastic disorders. Bethanechol can rarely cause hypotension and bradycardia especially when given subcutaneously. However, more typically, therapeutic doses have very little effect on heart rate, blood pressure, or peripheral circulation. It is contraindicated for patients with preexisting hypotension, bradycardia, or cardiovascular disease (NIH, 2012).

Bethanechol is also contraindicated in patients with hyperthyroidism. When initially given bethanechol, patients with hyperthyroidism react similarly to other patients by experiencing hypotension and bradycardia. However, the body reacts to the hypotension with the release of increased amounts of norepinephrine from sympathetic nerves, resulting in increased heart rate. Because the heart tissue of patients with hyperthyroidism is highly sensitive to norepinephrine levels, even small increases in the amount of norepinephrine can produce cardiac arrhythmias (NIH, 2012).

It is not known whether bethanechol can cause fetal harm when given to pregnant women or if it can affect reproductive capacity. It is Pregnancy Category C and should be used only when the benefits clearly outweigh the potential risk to the fetus. Whether bethanechol is excreted in breast milk is also unknown (NIH, 2012).

Adverse Drug Reactions

Adverse reactions are rare following oral administration, but more common after SC administration. GI, respiratory, and cardiac reactions were discussed in the Precautions and Contraindications section. Additional GI symptoms include abdominal pain, nausea, belching, and diarrhea. Other adverse reactions include increased tearing and miosis of the pupils and flushing that produces a feeling of warmth and a sensation of heat about the face (NIH, 2012).

Toxicity

Muscarinic poisoning can occur from overdosage and from ingestion of certain poisonous mushrooms. Early symptoms of poisoning are abdominal cramps, salivation, flushing, nausea, and vomiting. Atropine is the specific antidote. The preferred route of administration is SC to provide a rapid response. The recommended dose for adults is 0.6 mg repeated every 2 hours, based on clinical response. The recommended dose for children under the age of 12 is 0.01 mg/kg repeated every 2 hours, based on clinical response. The maximal single dose in children should not exceed 0.4 mg (NIH, 2012).

Drug Interactions

Additive drug interactions may occur with cholinesterase inhibitors. A critical fall in blood pressure may occur with ganglionic blockers. Quinidine, procainamide, and older phenothiazines such as chlorpromazine and thioridazine and histamine₁ blockers such as diphenhydramine and promethazine all have antimuscarinic activity. As a result, these drugs may antagonize the effects of bethanechol. Avoid concurrent administration of these drugs (NIH, 2012).

Clinical Use and Dosing

Urinary Retention

Bethanechol is used in primary care for neurogenic atony of the urinary bladder with retention. Oral dosing begins at 10 to 50 mg 3 or 4 times a day. The minimum effective dose is determined by giving 5 to 10 mg initially and repeating the dose every hour until a satisfactory response occurs or 50 mg is reached. SC dosing begins with 2.5 mg. The minimum effective dose is determined by injecting 2.5 mg initially and repeating every 15 to 30 minutes until satisfactory response is obtained or adverse reactions appear, but the maximum number of doses is four. The minimum effective dose is then given 3 or 4 times a day as needed (NIH, 2012).

Patient Education

Administration

To avoid nausea and vomiting, the patient should take the drug 1 hour before or 2 hours after a meal. The SC form is intended for subcutaneous use only and should never be given intramuscularly (IM) or IV because the resultant high drug levels can cause severe toxicity, evidenced by bloody diarrhea, bradycardia, profound hypotension, and cardiovascular collapse (NIH, 2012).

Adverse Reactions

This drug may cause abdominal discomfort, salivation, sweating, or flushing. Teach the patient to notify the health-care provider if these occur. The dose may be reduced or the drug discontinued (NIH, 2012).

Dizziness or lightheadedness may occur when the patient arises from a lying or sitting position. The probable cause is hypotension. Arising slowly from a supine position and dangling the feet over the side of the bed before standing will reduce postural hypotension. No exercise in hot weather and adequate intake of noncaffeinated liquids will also reduce these problems.

Bethanechol is contraindicated in patients with asthma and other diseases with a bronchospastic component. Teach the patient to report wheezing or breathing difficulties to the health-care provider immediately (NIH, 2012).

CHOLINESTERASE INHIBITORS

This class of drugs prevents the degradation of ACh by AChE, thereby enhancing the activity of ACh at cholinergic receptors. These inhibitors act as indirect cholinergic agonists, can intensify ACh activity at all cholinergic junctions (muscarinic, ganglionic, and nicotinic), and so have a wide range of responses and adverse reactions.

There are two basic categories of cholinergic inhibitors. (1) Reversible inhibitors produce effects of moderate duration. They include ambenonium (Myletase), demecarium (Humorsol), donepezil (Aricept), galantamine (Reminyl), pyridostigmine (Mestinon), physostigmine (Antilirium), rivastigmine (Exelon), and tacrine (Cognex). (Drugs in this group that are used for clinical diagnosis or for treatment of glaucoma are not discussed in this chapter.) (2) Irreversible inhibitors are highly toxic and, although they can be split from AChE, the split takes place extremely slowly and effects exist until new cholinesterase can be generated. They contain a phosphate atom and are referred to as organophosphate cholinesterase inhibitors. Because they are highly lipid-soluble, they can be absorbed even through the skin (FDA, 1982, 2001, 2008b, 2011e; NIH, 2008a, 2011).

Although it is not a cholinesterase inhibitor, memantine (Namenda) is used to treat Alzheimer's disease (AD). Because several of the reversible AChE inhibitors mentioned above are also used to treat Alzheimer's disease, memantine will also be discussed in this section (FDA, 2003b).

Pharmacodynamics

The reversible AChE inhibitors act as poor substrates for AChE. The process by which AChE breaks down ACh into choline and acetic acid takes place in two steps: (1) binding ACh to the active center of AChE and (2) splitting of the ACh, which regenerates free AChE. This reaction is rapid so that one molecule of AChE can break down a large amount of ACh in a relatively short time. The reversible AChE inhibitors follow this same process, except that it takes place slowly; the drug is bound to the active center of AChE for a relatively long time, preventing the regeneration of free AChE and preventing AChE from catalyzing the breakdown of more ACh. The slowing down of the inactivation of ACh results in an increased intrasynaptic concentration of ACh and intensified neural transmission at virtually all junctions where ACh is the neurotransmitter. In doses higher than the usual therapeutic doses, neostigmine and pyridostigmine can produce skeletal muscle stimulation and activation of muscarinic, ganglionic, and nicotinic receptors in the CNS. In therapeutic doses, they usually affect only muscarinic and nicotinic receptors at the myoneural junction without altering CNS function (FDA, 1982, 2001, 2008b, 2011e; NIH, 2008, 2011).

Tacrine, donepezil, rivastigmine, and galantamine, which are used to treat AD, are designed to alter CNS function. AD is associated with profound cholinergic depletion. All of these agents increase the availability of ACh in the brain by competitively inhibiting AChE but all are structurally dissimilar (FDA, 2006a, 2008b; NIH, 2008a, 2012b).

Tacrine is an acridine AChE inhibitor. Inhibition of AChE by tacrine is short-lived. In addition, the drug has more cholinergic activity in the periphery than do the other agents and, therefore, may have more peripheral cholinergic adverse drug reactions (ADR) associated with it. It may also act as a partial agonist at muscarinic receptors by blocking reuptake of dopamine, serotonin, and norepinephrine (NIH, 2008a).

Donepezil is a piperidine-type AchE inhibitor with increased affinity for the CNS and, thus, a decreased number of peripheral ADRs. It has a longer duration of inhibitory action than tacrine (NIH, 2012b). Rivastigmine is a potent, selective inhibitor of AChE in the cortex and hippocampus. The selectivity of this drug, like donepezil, for the brain accounts for the decreased number of peripheral cholinergic ADRs. Because of its carbamate structure, after binding to the esteratic site, the drug dissociates much more slowly from AChE than does ACh. Thus, it is considered to be a pseudo-irreversible inhibitor of the enzyme. This action also helps explain why that enzyme is inhibited for a much longer time frame than the plasma half-life would suggest (FDA, 2006a).

Galantamine is a natural tertiary alkaloid that reversibly inhibits AChE. Some evidence suggests that along with the AChE inhibition, the drug may enhance the effect of ACh on nicotinic receptors by binding at an allosteric site. Whether this effect results in increased clinical efficacy has not been demonstrated. Because these agents work to increase levels of ACh released from cholinergic neurons, as AD progresses and the patient has fewer functional cholinergic neurons, these drugs may have less effect (FDA, 2008b).

Persistent stimulation of the N-methyl-D-aspartate (NMDA) receptors by the excitatory amino acid glutamate may contribute to the symptomatology of AD. Memantine is a low to moderate, noncompetitive antagonist at NMDA receptors. It binds preferentially to the receptor-operated cation channels. The drug has low to negligible affinity for gamma-aminobutyric acid (GABA), benzodiazpine, dopamine, adrenergic, histamine, and glycine receptors. It does show antagonistic effects at the 5-HT3 (serotonin) receptor and blocks nicotinic ACh receptors, but with less potency. It does not effect the inhibition of AChE by donepezil, galantamine, or tacrine (FDA, 2003b).

Pharmacokinetics

Absorption and Distribution

Each of the AChE inhibitors differs in its pharmacokinetics (Table 14-14). Neostigmine and pyridostigmine carry a positive charge. This charge results in poor absorption from the GI tract. Oral doses must be much greater than SC doses to produce a therapeutic effect. Once absorbed, these drugs distribute to sites of action in the myoneural junction and at peripheral muscarinic receptors; they have limited ability to

Table 14–14 ▪ Pharmacokinetics: Selected Acetylcholinesterase Inhibitors

Drug	Onset	Peak	Duration	Protein Binding (%)	Bioavailability	Half-Life	Elimination
Donepezil	Within 6 wk*	4 h	24 h	94–96	100%	60–100 h	57% in urine; 15% in feces
Galantamine	Within 6 wk*	1 h; delayed 90 min by food	UK	18	90%	7 h	95% in urine; 5% in feces
Memantine	Within 6 wk*	3–7 h	UK	45	UK	60–80 h	82% unchanged in urine. Urine pH increase decreases elimination.
Memantine XR	Within 6 wk	9–12 h (even if capsule is opened to sprinkle on food)	UK	45	UK	60-80h	48% unchanged in urine; remainder in 3 plasma metabolites.
Neostigmine	45–75 min	UK	2–4 h	15–25	1%–2%	40–60 min	By enzymatic degradation
Pyrido-stigmine PO	30–35 min	UK	3–6 h	UK	11%–17%	3.7 h	By enzymatic degradation
Pyrido-stigmine SR	30–60 min	UK	6–12 h	UK	UK	3.7 h	By enzymatic degradation
Rivastigmine	Within 6 wk*	1 h; delayed 90 min by food	UK	40	36%	1.5 h	97% in urine as metabolites
Tacrine	Within 6 wk*	1–2 h	4–8 h	55	5%–30%; food reduces BA by 30%–40%	2–4 h	1% as unchanged drug in urine

Source: FDA, 1982, 2001, 2008b, 2011e; NIH, 2008a, 2011.

UK = unknown.

*Observable reduction in clinical symptoms.

cross the blood–brain barrier (FDA, 1982, 2001, 2008b, 2011e; NIH, 2008, 2011).

Tacrine is rapidly absorbed following oral administration but then undergoes extensive first-pass metabolism, resulting in an absolute bioavailibility of 5% to 30%. Absorption is significantly reduced when the drug is taken with food, and a 30% to 40% decrease in bioavailability results; therefore, it should be given on an empty stomach. Because it is lipid-soluble, it crosses the blood–brain barrier. Its drug concentration is highest in the brain. Women tend to have concentrations that are 50% higher than those of men, even when they take the same dose (NIH, 2008a).

Food has no effect on the absorption of donepezil; the disintegrating tablets and the solution are bioequivalent to its regular tablets. Total galantamine absorption is also not affected by food, but C_{max} is decreased by 25% and T_{max} is delayed 90 minutes when the drug is taken with food. Both donepezil and galantamine are well absorbed following oral administration, with a bioavailability of greater than or equal to 90%. Unlike tacrine, donepezil is concentrated in the CNS, with very little peripheral activity. Both drugs exhibit linear pharmacokinetics (FDA, 1982, 2001, 2008b, 2011e; NIH, 2008a, 2011).

Rivastigmine is completely absorbed following oral administration; however, its bioavailability is only 36%, indicating a significant first-pass effect. When taken with food, the absorption of rivastigmine is delayed and C_{max} is decreased by 30%. However, the AUC increases by about 30%. Thus this drug should be taken with food to maximize bioavailability. It also has nonlinear pharmacokinetics; doubling the dose from 3 to 6 mg twice daily results in a 3-fold increase in AUC (FDA, 2006a).

Memantine is highly absorbed following oral administration. Food has no effect on absorption. It has linear pharmacokinetics over the dosage range of the original formulation (FDA, 2003b).

Metabolism and Excretion

Neostigmine and pyridostigmine are degraded by AChE and metabolized by hepatic microsomal enzymes to inactive products, but only to a small extent. Both drugs are eliminated largely as unchanged drug in the urine: for neostigmine 50% to 70% of the dose is unchanged; pyridostigmine is mainly eliminated unchanged. Both drugs will potentially require dosing adjustment in renal impairment (NIH, 2011; FDA, 2001).

Tacrine is extensively metabolized by CYP 1A2 isoenzymes in the liver. The higher concentrations of drug in women may be related to decreased CYP 1A2 isoenzyme activity in women. Cigarette smoking also reduces this isoenzyme; smokers have higher drug concentrations than nonsmokers. The relatively high first-pass effect in the metabolism of tacrine is dependent on the dose administered. The CYP 1A1 system can be saturated at low doses. Once in the plasma, elimination is not dose-dependent. Although studies in patients with liver disease have not been done, it is reasonable to expect that hepatic dysfunction reduces

clearance of this drug. Dosing of this drug does not require adjustment in elderly patients or in patients with renal impairment (NIH, 2008a).

Donepezil is extensively metabolized by CYP 2D6 and 3A4 isoenzyme systems in the liver to two active and two less active metabolites. Approximately 57% of it is excreted in the urine and 15% in feces. Hepatic impairment has been shown to decrease clearance by 20%. Dosing of this drug does not require adjustment in elderly patients or in patients with renal impairment (NIH, 2012b).

Galantamine is extensively metabolized by CYP 2D6 and 3A4 isoenzymes. Approximately 20% of the dose is excreted as unchanged drug in the urine. Total renal elimination is 95%, with 5% eliminated in feces. Approximately 7% of the population has a genetic variation that leads to reduced levels of activity of CYP 2D6. However, there are no AUC changes seen in these individuals and no dosage adjustments are required. Galantamine clearance is decreased by about 25% in patients with moderate hepatic impairment, and these patients, as well as those with moderate renal impairment, probably should not have a dosage exceeding 16 mg/d (FDA, 2008b).

Rivastigmine is rapidly and extensively metabolized primarily by cholinesterase-mediated hydrolysis to one active metabolite. Evidence suggests that there is minimal involvement of the CYP450 system. Most of the drug is excreted as its metabolite in the urine. Moderate renal impairment reduces clearance by 64%, and moderate hepatic impairment reduces it by 60%. Dosage adjustment is not required in either scenario because the drug is usually titrated to tolerability. Nicotine use increases the clearance of this drug (FDA, 2006a).

Memantine undergoes little metabolism with the majority (57% to 82%) of an administered dose excreted unchanged in the urine. The remainder is converted primarily to three polar metabolites that possess minimal *N*-methyl-D-aspartate (NMDA) receptor antagonism. The CYP450 enzymes system does not play a significant role in its metabolism. Renal clearance involves active tubular secretion moderated by a pH-dependent tubular reabsorption. Although data on the effect of renal impairment are limited, based on its renal excretion, it is very likely that patients with moderate to severe renal impairment will have higher levels of the drug (FDA, 2003b).

Pharmacotherapeutics

Precautions and Contraindications

The only absolute contraindications for neostigmine and pyridostigmine are mechanical intestinal and urinary obstruction. The reasons are the same as those given for bethanechol. A relative contraindication is a history of reaction to bromides. Neostigmine and pyridostigmine are Pregnancy Category C because they may cause uterine irritability, and neonates may display muscular weakness. Use these drugs only when clearly needed and the benefits clearly outweigh the risks to the fetus. Neostigmine is ionized at physiological pH and is not expected to be excreted in breast milk. Pyridostigmine is excreted in breast milk and should not be used by breastfeeding women. Safety and efficacy have not been established for children (FDA, 2001; NIH, 2011).

Tacrine has been associated with hepatotoxicity. It is contraindicated for patients who have previously been treated with the drug and developed jaundice and for patients with abnormal transaminase levels or clinical jaundice with a serum bilirubin above 3 mg/dL. Patients who are unwilling or unable to avoid drinking alcohol should also not have this drug prescribed because concurrent use may have additive toxic effects on the liver. Unlike tacrine, donepezil, galantamine, and rivastigmine are not associated with hepatotoxicity. Memantine has been temporally associated with hepatic failure, but data are insufficient to document causality (FDA, 1982, 2001, 2008b, 2011e; NIH, 2008a, 2011).

Both tacrine and donepezil are Pregnancy Category C. There are no data to support findings that either of these drugs causes harm to the fetus. Safety has not been established in pregnancy. For rivastigmine, animal studies did not demonstrate teratogenicity with doses 2 to 4 times the maximal dose used in humans. Animal studies also showed that at doses 3 to 6 times the amount used for treatment, galantamine caused a slight delay in fetal development and some skeletal variations. Both rivastigmine and galantamine are Pregnancy Category B. Memantine is Pregnancy Category B because no adequate and well-controlled studies in pregnant women have been conducted (FDA, 1982, 2001, 2008b, 2011e; NIH, 2008a, 2011).

Drug clearance of rivastigmine and galantamine decreases in the presence of hepatic impairment and renal impairment. However, recommendations for both these drugs are to titrate to response and tolerability rather than specific dose recommendations. Administration of galantamine to patients with severe hepatic impairment or CrCl less than 9 mL/min is not recommended. In patients with renal impairment, no dosage adjustments are recommended for donepezil or tacrine. However, in patients with hepatic impairment donepezil should be titrated to response and tolerability, and tacrine should be discontinued when the transaminase levels are greater than 5 times the upper limit of normal (ULN) (FDA, 2006a, 2008b).

Because memantine undergoes little metabolism, no dosing adjustment is required in patients with hepatic impairment. No dosing adjustment is required in mild to moderate renal impairment, but with CrCl between 5 and 29 mL/min, the dosage should not exceed 14 mg. There are no specific recommendations for CrCl less than 5 mL/min (FDA, 2003b).

Cholinergic agonists are thought to have some potential to cause generalized seizures. Tacrine is also contraindicated for patients with a history of stroke, subdural hematoma, hydrocephalus, or CNS tumor because they are at increased risk for this adverse reaction (NIH, 2008a).

Cholinergic agonists and cholinesterase inhibitors tend to increase gastric acid secretion because of increased cholinergic activity. Monitor patients closely for indications of active or occult GI bleeding, especially patients at increased risk for developing ulcers (FDA, 1982, 2001, 2008b, 2011e; NIH, 2008, 2011).

All of these drugs should be used with caution for patients with a history of bronchospastic disorders, peptic ulcer disease, cardiovascular diseases that may worsen in the presence of hypotension or bradycardia, and hyperthyroidism. The reasons are the same as for muscarinic agonists and are based on the increased activity of ACh (FDA, 1982, 2001, 2008b, 2011e; NIH, 2008, 2011).

Adverse Drug Reactions

Each of these drugs differs in adverse reactions; however, all except memantine are associated with the adverse reactions common to all cholinergic agonists. (See precautions above.) In addition, muscle weakness, fasciculations, cramps, and spasms have been noted. Memantine has been associated with syncope, bradycardia, and hypotension; vertigo and ataxia; dyspnea and bronchospasm; and emotional lability and paranoid reactions in a small percentage of patients (FDA, 1982, 2001, 2003b, 2008b, 2011e; NIH, 2008, 2011).

Donepezil, galantamine, and rivastigmine are well tolerated, with few adverse reactions. The most common are headache, nausea, diarrhea, and insomnia. Patients with a history of frequent GI complaints may be prone to recurrence of these problems while taking these drugs. Because of their effects on the SA and AV nodes of the heart, bradycardia has been observed. As with tacrine, cholinergic-associated adverse reactions are usually dose-dependent and can be treated by temporarily reducing the dose or by taking the drug with meals, although the latter reduces bioavailability (FDA, 2006a, 2008b; NIH, 2012b).

Toxicity

The warning signs of overdose are very similar to common adverse reactions, and there is a narrow margin between the first appearance of adverse reactions and serious toxic effects. Adverse reactions such as excessive GI stimulation, excessive salivation, miosis, and fasciculations of voluntary muscles should be reported to the health-care provider immediately, and the drug will be temporarily discontinued. Atropine 0.5 to 1 mg IV may be required (FDA, 1982, 2001, 2008b, 2011e; NIH, 2008, 2011).

Hepatotoxicity

Tacrine has been associated with hepatotoxicity and it has been demonstrated that metabolites of tacrine are cytotoxic. A significant number of patients develop elevated serum transaminases (aspartate transaminase [AST] and alanine aminotransferase [ALT]). If the drug is promptly withdrawn, clinical evidence of liver injury is rare. To prevent liver injury in patients on this drug, monitor their liver function frequently. This topic is discussed in the Monitoring section (FDA, 1982, 2001, 2008b, 2011e; NIH, 2008a, 2011).

Drug Interactions

Synergistic effects occur between these drugs and other cholinergic agonists. Antagonistic effects occur with anticholinergic drugs. Neostigmine and pyridostigmine have increased risks for neuromuscular blockade with aminoglycoside antibiotics and succinylcholine. With the latter drug, respiratory support may be needed. These combinations should be avoided. Atropine and belladonna derivatives suppress many of the early warning symptoms of neostigmine and pyridostigmine overdose and toxicity. Given the narrow margin between therapeutic dose and overdose, this increased risk is unacceptable, and these drugs should not be given together. Corticosteroids and magnesium also interact with these drugs (FDA, 1982, 2001, 2008b, 2011e; NIH, 2008, 2011). Their interactions are presented in Table 14-15.

Many drug interactions for donepezil, galantamine, and tacrine occur because they undergo significant metabolism by the CYP enzyme systems of the liver. Any drug metabolized by the CYP 1A2 isoenzymes has interactions with tacrine, and those metabolized by 2D6 and 3A4 have interactions with donepezil and galantamine. The number of drugs metabolized by the 1A2 isoenzymes is relatively small, but the number metabolized by 2D6 and 3A4 is large. To date, these drug interactions have largely been in vitro and

Table 14–15 ▦ Drug Interactions: Selected Acetylcholinesterase Inhibitors

Drug	Interacting Drug	Possible Effect	Implications
Donepezil	Anticholinergics	Donepezil antagonizes activity of anticholinergics	Avoid concurrent administration
	Bethanechol, succinylcholine	Synergistic cholinergic activity	Reduce bethanechol dose if they must be given concurrently
	NSAIDs	Donepezil increases gastric acid secretion	Monitor for active or occult bleeding
	Furosemide, digoxin, warfarin	At concentrations of 0.3–10 mg/mL did not affect binding of these drugs	
	Ketoconazole, quinidine, other drugs metabolized by CYP450 2D6 and 3A4 isoenzymes	Potentially inhibit donepezil metabolism	Choose alternative "azole" or antiarrhythmic
	CYP2D6 and 3A4 inducers: carbamazepine, dexamethasone, phenobarbital, phenytoin, rifampin	Potentially increase rate of elimination	Avoid concurrent administration
Galantamine	Succinylcholine, bethanechol	Synergistic effect when combined	Memantine does not have this effect
	Cimetidine	Increased bioavailability of galantamine by 16%	Ranitidine does not have this effect
	Ketoconazole	Increased galantamine AUC by 30%	Select different antifungal
	Paroxetine	Increased bioavailability of galantamine by 40%	Avoid concurrent use
	Erythromycin	Increased galantamine AUC by 10%	Select different antibiotic
	Other inhibitors of CYP3A4: amitriptyline, fluoxetine, fluvoxamine, quinidine	Clearance of galantamine decreased by 25%–33%	Select different antidepressant or antiarrhythmic
	NSAIDs	Galantamine increases gastric acid secretion	Monitor for active or occult bleeding
Memantine	Amantidine, ketamine, dextromethorphan	Interaction not evaluated, but also NMDA antagonists	Use with caution
	Hydrochlorothiazide, cimetidine, ranitidine, quinidine, nicotine, triamterene	Potential altered plasma levels of both drugs since both use same renal cationic system for elimination	Avoid concurrent use or monitor for increased drug effects
	Drugs, diet, and clinical states that make urine alkaline	Clearance of memantine reduced by 80% under alkaline urine concentrations at pH 8. Can lead to accumulation of drug with increased adverse effects.	Use memantine with caution under these conditions
Neostigmine, pyridostigmine	Succinylcholine	Increase neuromuscular blocking; prolonged respiratory depression with extended periods of apnea	Provide respiratory support as needed or avoid concurrent use

Table 14–15 ▦ **Drug Interactions: Selected Acetylcholinesterase Inhibitors—cont'd**

Drug	Interacting Drug	Possible Effect	Implications
	Aminoglycoside antibiotics	Aminoglycosides have mild but definite nondepolarizing blocking action that may accentuate neuromuscular block	Choose different antibiotic or monitor closely for increased blockade
	Local and general anesthetics, antiarrhythmics	Decreased effects of neostigmine	Increase dose of neostigmine while patient is taking these drugs
	Atropine, belladonna derivatives	Suppress muscarinic symptoms of excessive GI stimulation, leaving only more serious symptoms of fasciculation and paralysis of voluntary muscles as signs of overdose	Avoid concurrent use. Margin of safety is already quite narrow, and this makes it narrower.
Corticosteroids	Decrease anti-AChE effects of neostigmine or pyridostigmine. Anti-AChE effects may increase after stopping steroids.	Avoid concurrent use or provide respiratory support as needed. Monitor respiratory status closely after stopping steroid.	
	Magnesium	Has direct depressant effect on skeletal muscle; may antagonize beneficial effects of neostigmine or pyridostigmine	Avoid concurrent use
	Methocarbamol	A single case report indicates this drug may impair effect of pyridostigmine	Only one case report. Monitor for possible effect.
Rivastigmine	No drug interactions based on no CYP450 activity		
	Anticholinergics	Rivastigmine may interfere with their activity	Avoid concurrent use. (See note below related to tacrine.)
	Cholinomimetics and other cholinesterase inhibitors	Synergistic effects	Avoid concurrent use
Tacrine	All drugs metabolized by CYP450 1A2 isoenzymes	May inhibit metabolism of tacrine	Avoid concurrent use, or monitor effects and adjust doses as needed
	Anticholinergics	Tacrine interferes with anticholinergic activity	Monitor for anticholinergic activity if they must be given together. *Note:* Many drugs have anticholinergic-like effects even if not anticholinergic drugs. These should also be watched.
	Cimetidine	Increases the peak plasma level of tacrine by 54% and the AUC by 64%	Choose different histamine$_2$ blocker
	Bethanechol, succinylcholine	Synergistic effects. Can cause bladder outlet obstruction	Avoid concurrent use
	Theophylline	Coadministration doubles theophylline elimination half-life and average plasma level	Monitor plasma theophylline levels and reduce theophylline dose if they must be given together
	NSAIDs	Increased risk for GI bleed	Monitor for occult bleeding with serial stool guaiac tests and hemoglobin determinations. May need to take antacids while on tacrine therapy.

Source: FDA, 1982, 2001, 2008b, 2011e; NIH, 2008, 2011.
  AUC = area under curve.

theoretical, but as these drugs are prescribed for larger numbers of patients, the interactions are likely to occur. Donepezil does not interact with furosemide, digoxin, and warfarin, drugs often prescribed for older adults who are also likely candidates for donepezil. The bioavailability of galantamine increases when given with erythromycin due to inhibition of CYP 3A4 by erythromycin. Because of its inhibition of both CYP 3A4 and 2D6, paroxetine increases the AUC of galantamine. Cimetidine increases the bioavailability of galantamine, but ranitidine does not (FDA, 2008b; NIH, 2008a, 2012b).

Memantine interacts with other NMDA receptor antagonists such as amantadine, ketamine, and dextromethorphan. Drugs that make urine alkaline reduce renal clearance of this drug and many drugs that use the same renal cation exchange system also interact with this drug to decrease its renal clearance (FDA, 2003b).

Clinical Use and Dosing

Myasthenia Gravis

Neostigmine and pyridostigmine are used to treat myasthenia gravis. In this disorder, an autoimmune process occurs in which the patient's immune system produces antibodies directed against nicotinic receptors on skeletal muscle, reducing the number of receptors by 70% to 90%, resulting in muscle weakness. Reversible cholinesterase inhibitors are the mainstay of treatment, preventing ACh inactivation and intensifying the effects of ACh on motor neurons. These drugs do not cure the disorder, but manage its symptoms; treatment is lifelong (FDA, 2001; NIH, 2011).

Establishing an optimal dose for treatment can be a challenge because these drugs produce widespread effects, not just at selected target organs. A small initial dose is administered, followed by other small doses until an optimal dose is reached. Signs of improvement that indicate optimal dosage include improved ability to swallow and to raise the eyelids (FDA, 2001; NIH, 2011).

The initial adult dose of neostigmine is usually 15 mg/day, and for children it is 2 mg/kg daily in divided doses given every 3 to 4 hours. The interval between dose increases is highly individualized. The average adult dose is 150 mg/day, but the maximum dose may approach 375 mg/day. Larger portions of the daily dose may be given 30 to 60 minutes prior to activities that produce greater fatigue, such as eating or shopping. For pyridostigmine, the initial adult dose is 60 mg/day, and for children it is 7 mg/kg divided into five or six doses daily (Armstrong & Schumann, 2003). Sustained-release tablets are available that require once- or twice-daily dosing. Regular tablets or syrup may be administered with extended-release tablets for optimal control of symptoms. Both of these drugs can be given parenterally if the patient has difficulty swallowing, but it is important to remember that, because of their first-pass effects, oral doses are 30 to 40 times greater than parenteral doses (FDA, 2001; NIH, 2011).

Reversal of Nonpolarizing Neuromuscular Blockade

By producing increased ACh at the myoneural junction, neostigmine and pyridostigmine can reverse the effects of nondepolarizing blocking agents. They cannot be used to counter the effects of succinylcholine because it is a depolarizing neuromuscular blocker. The most common application of this role is immediately post-operative and is determined by the anesthesiologist. Because it would probably not be used in primary care or by a nurse practitioner, this use is not discussed further.

Alzheimer's Disease (AD)

This disease is associated with a significant deficiency in brain levels of choline acetyltransferase, the enzyme responsible for the synthesis of ACh. In addition, cholinergic neurons in the brain's basal ganglia degenerate, resulting in a loss of cholinergic input to the muscarinic receptors in the frontal and temporal lobes of the cerebral cortex (Lai et al, 2001; Minger et al, 2000). Enhancing cholinergic activity with drugs is designed to counteract the decreased stimulation of the remaining cholinergic neurons. Donepezil, galantamine, rivastigmine, and tacrine are all used to treat AD by preventing the degradation of ACh by AChE. Another mechanism thought to contribute to AD symptoms is persistent stimulation of NMDA receptors by glutamate. Memantine relieves symptoms by blocking this stimulation (FDA, 2003b, 2006a, 2008b; NIH, 2008a, 2012b).

Tacrine is a centrally active, noncompetitive, reversible AChE inhibitor. Approximately 30% to 40% of AD patients who were able to complete their drug trials demonstrated modest improvement in cognitive and functional measures. Unfortunately, these improvements were not noted to last longer than 30 weeks, and many patients did not complete the trials because of the adverse reactions associated with this drug. The response was dose-related, and adverse reactions increase as the dose increases (NIH, 2008a).

Dosing of tacrine usually begins with 10 mg given 4 times daily between meals. Taking the drug with meals makes it more tolerable, but the bioavailability is decreased by 30% to 40%, requiring higher doses for the same effect. Doses are increased at 6-week intervals, based on liver function studies, to a maximum of 160 mg/day. The monitoring requirements are discussed later. An adequate response is defined as the lack of apparent disease progression for 6 months. It requires at least 8 weeks at doses greater than 120 mg/day. The highest-tolerated dose is the most efficacious (NIH, 2008a).

Tacrine was the first drug to show some success in treating AD. Because it has many adverse reactions and requires extensive monitoring because of its hepatotoxicity, tacrine is currently the least used of the drugs to treat AD (NIH, 2008a).

Donepezil is a piperidine-based derivative dissimilar from other AChE inhibitors in its pharmacokinetics and tolerability. It is also a centrally active, noncompetitive, reversible AChE inhibitor, but its duration of inhibitory action is longer than tacrine's. This longer duration of action permits once-daily dosing, which is a major advantage for this drug. Another advantage is its better adverse reactions profile. The most problematic adverse reaction is digestive complaints. This may require dosage reduction (NIH, 2012b).

Clinical trials (Pratt, 2002; Salloway, Pratt, & Perdomo, 2003; Winblad et al, 2001) showed improvement in cognitive function for as long as 2 years, but after this period there were indications that the drug did not prevent further long-term disease progression. The improvement was dose-related, and adverse reactions also increased with the increased dose. Many patients do not have real improvement. Of concern, many others have serious side effects (Howard et al, 2012).

The mean age of patients in clinical trials was 73 years; 80% of the patients were between 65 and 84 years of age and 49% were 75 years or older. Although there was no clinically significant difference in response compared to other age groups, the most adverse reactions were reported by patients 65 to 75 years of age and younger than 65 years of age (NIH, 2012b).

The recommended starting dose of donepezil is 5 mg daily at bedtime. Doses are increased at 4- to 6-week intervals to reduce adverse reactions. The maximum dose is 10 mg daily. The higher dose should be used if tolerated because it is more efficacious, especially for severe disease. Unlike tacrine, donepezil is not likely to cause hepatotoxicity and does not require assessment of liver function in order to increase the dose or frequent monitoring of liver function throughout therapy. Patients are monitored for indications of active or occult bleeding because of the potential for anticholinesterase inhibitors to increase gastric acid secretion (NIH, 2012b).

Galantamine is administered twice daily, preferably with morning and evening meals. The initial dose is 4 mg 2 times a day. After a minimum of 4 weeks of treatment, if the drug is well tolerated, the dose may be increased to 8 mg 2 times a day. A further increase to 12 mg 2 times a day should be attempted only after a minimum of 4 weeks at the previous dose. If therapy is interrupted for several days or longer, the dose must be reinitiated at 4 mg 2 times a day and increased based on the same titration as above. The usual maintenance dose is 8 to 12 mg 2 times a day. Based on the reduced clearance seen in patients with moderate hepatic or renal impairment, the dose for these patients generally should not exceed 16 mg/d (FDA, 2008b).

Razadyne, the brand-name form of galantamine, is also available in an extended-release formulation allowing for once-daily dosing. The initial dose for this formulation is 8 mg. The dosage is increased at 4-week intervals, as with the regular formulation. The usual maintenance dose is 16 to 24 mg daily. This formulation also carries a dosage restriction for hepatic and renal impairment (FDA, 2008b).

Rivastigmine is also administered twice daily, in the morning and evening with food. The starting dose is 1.5 mg 2 times a day. If the dose is well tolerated, it may be increased to 3 mg 2 times a day after 2 weeks of treatment. Subsequent increases to 4.5 and 6 mg 2 times a day also require a 2-week interval. Treatment interrupted for several doses is reinstituted at the 1.5 mg 2 times a day dose and titrated as above. The most effective dose in clinical trials was 3 to 6 mg 2 times a day (FDA, 2006a).

For patients who have difficulty swallowing, Exelon, the brand-name formulation of rivastigmine, is available in an oral solution and in a transdermal patch (FDA, 2006a). Dosing regimens for these two forms are shown in Table 14-16.

Memantine is started at 5 mg once daily with a target dose of 20 mg daily in the original formulation. Forest Laboratory has ceased production and only has a newer XR form available at press. The starting XR dose of 7 mg is increased in 7 mg increments weekly if the prior dose is tolerated, up to a max of 28 mg/d. Dosages may need to be reduced in patients with moderate renal impairment. The drug is not recommended for patients with severe renal impairment (FDA, 2003b). When a generic form becomes available the old method of increasing 5 mg per week in divided doses up to a max of 20 mg/d would be used.

Table 14-17 shows the clinical use and dosing schedules for all of these drugs. Only uses associated with primary care are presented. Only currently available memantine XR is listed.

Rational Drug Selection

Formulation

For neostigmine and pyridostigmine, formulation is a consideration (see Table 14-16). Difficulty in swallowing is a common problem for patients with myasthenia gravis. Pyridostigmine is available in a syrup form that can be used by many patients with this problem without having to resort to an injectable form. In addition, the syrup can be used for children to administer their individualized doses based on body weight (FDA, 2001; NIH, 2011).

For patients with Alzheimer's disease, rivastigmine has an oral-solution dosing formulation that permits it to be taken directly from the syringe or mixed with juice or water for those who have difficulty in swallowing tablets. Once mixed, the drug is stable for 4 or fewer hours. Rivastigmine is also available in a transdermal patch. Donepezil is available in an oral solution and in orally disintegrating tablets. Galantamine and memantine are also available in an oral solution (FDA, 2003b, 2006a, 2008b; NIH, 2008, 2012b).

Dosing Schedule

The dosing schedules of neostigmine and pyridostigmine are similar. Those of the drugs used to treat Alzheimer's disease are quite different. Donepezil has a once-daily dosing regimen. Galantamine, rivastigmine, and memantine are all 2 times a day doses, but galantamine is available in extended-release capsules that are dosed once daily. Rivastigmine can also be dosed once daily in the transdermal patch form. Tacrine requires four daily doses and is most effective on an empty stomach, which results in the doses being adjusted for meals. For patients who are older adults and who have a disease process that includes memory problems, or for patients whose caregivers are also older adults, this complex regimen may present adherence problems (FDA, 2003b, 2006a, 2008b; NIH, 2008a, 2012b). If there is no evidence of positive effect in six months, or when the patient

Table 14–16 ⚬ **Dosage Schedule: Acetylcholinesterase Inhibitors**

Drug	Indication	Form	Initial Dose	Maintenance Dose
Donepezil	AD	Tablets: 5 mg, 10 mg Orally disintegrating tablets: 5 mg, 10 mg Oral solution: 1 mg/mL	5 mg daily at bedtime for 4–6 wk	May increase to 10 mg daily after 4–6 wk. The higher dose should be used if tolerated because it is more efficacious, especially for severe AD.
Galantamine (G) (Razadyne) (B)	AD	Tablets: 4 mg, 8 mg, 12 mg Capsules (extended-release): 8 mg, 16 mg, 24 mg	4 mg twice daily with morning and evening meals	Increase dose to 8 mg twice daily after 4 wk of therapy if drug well tolerated. Titration to 12 mg twice daily only after another 4-wk interval. Maintenance dose 8–12 mg bid. If therapy interrupted for several days or longer, reinitiate at 4 mg and follow same titration. Dose should not exceed 16 mg/d for patients with moderate renal or hepatic impairment.
(Razadyne) ER (B)		Oral solution: 4 mg/mL	8 mg once daily in the morning	Increase to 16 mg daily after minimum of 4 wk. May increase to 24 mg daily after another 4-wk interval. Maintenance dose 16–24 mg daily. See above for renal and hepatic impairment.
Memantine	AD	Tablets: 5 and 10 mg	5 mg once daily	Target dose is 20 mg daily. Titrate up in 5 mg increments/d if prior dose tolerated. Use one week dose increases rate in divided doses
Memantine (NamendaXR only available at press)	AD	Tablets: 7, 14, 21 and 28mg, Oral solution: 2 mg/mL	7 mg once daily	Target dose is 28 mg daily. Titrate up in 7 mg increments/d if prior dose tolerated. Minimal interval for titration is 1 wk. Dosages may need to be reduced if moderate renal impairment. Not recommended for severe renal impairment.
Non-FDA	Postherpetic neuralgia (adults 20–78 yr)		21 mg daily in divided doses	Max dose 55 mg/d in divided doses for up to 9 wk
Non-FDA	Prevention of migraine headaches (adults 15–78 yr)		7 mg daily	May increase to 28 mg daily. Use for at least 2 mo.
Neostigmine	Myasthenia gravis	Tablets: 15 mg	*Adults:* Oral: 15 mg/d divided and given every 3–4 h. Increase dose in 15 mg increments at daily intervals until optimal response is achieved.	Usual dose is 150 mg/d divided and given every 3–4 h. Maximum dose is 375 mg/d
			SC/IM: 0.5 mg every 2–3 h	Usually needed short-term, and dose is 5 mg every 2–3 h
			Children: Oral: 2 mg/kg/d in 6–8 divided doses	Same maintenance dose
			SC/IM: 0.01–0.04 mg/kg every 2–3 h	Usually needed short-term. Same dose.

Table 14–16 ⚙ **Dosage Schedule: Acetylcholinesterase Inhibitors—cont'd**

Drug	Indication	Form	Initial Dose	Maintenance Dose
Pyridostigmine (G) (Mestinon) (B)	Myasthenia gravis	Tablets: 60 mg Syrup: 60 mg/5 mL	*Adults:* Oral: 60 mg/d divided and given every 3–4 h. Increase dose in 60 mg increments at daily intervals until optimal dose is achieved.	Usual dose is 600 mg/d divided and given every 3–4 h. Maximum dose is 1,500 mg/d.
			IM: one-third the oral dose	
			Children: Oral: 7 mg/kg/d divided into 5–6 doses	Same maintenance dose
			IM: 0.05–0.15 mg/kg/dose every 2–3 h	Usually needed short-term. Same dose.
Mestinon ER (B)		SR tablets: 180 mg	180 mg daily	Usual dose 180–540 mg daily or bid with dosing interval of at least 6 hr
Rivastigmine (G) (Exelon) (B) Exelon oral solution (B)	AD and dementia associated with Parkinson's disease	Capsules: 1.5 mg, 3 mg, 4.5 mg, 6 mg Oral solution: 2 mg/mL Transdermal patch: 4.6 mg/24 h 9.5 mg/24 h	1.5 mg twice daily in the morning and evening with food	Increase dose to 3 mg twice daily after 2 wk, if well tolerated. Titration to 4.5 mg and 6 mg twice daily also requires 2-wk interval. If several doses missed, reinitiate at 1.5 mg and follow same titration. Most effective dose for AD is 3–6 mg twice daily; for PD is 1.5–6 mg bid.
Exelon transdermal patch		Transdermal patch: 4.6 mg/24 h 9.5 mg/24 h	Initiate with the 4.6 mg/24 h patch applied once daily	After a minimum of 4 wk, and, if well tolerated, increase to 9.5 mg/24 h patch applied once daily. If adverse reactions cause intolerance, therapy should be discontinued for several days and restarted at the next lower dose. If treatment is interrupted for longer than several days, reinitiate with the lowest daily dose.
Tacrine (Cognex)	AD	Tablets: 10 mg, 20 mg, 30 mg, 40 mg	10 mg qid between meals for 4 wk; may be given with food, but bioavailability is decreased 30%–40%	If ALT remains unchanged, increase by 40 mg/d every 4 wk up to a maximum of 40 mg qid. Usual maintenance dose is 120 mg/d. Elevated ALT requires detailed dosing adjustments.

Source: FDA, 1982, 2001, 2008b, 2011e; NIH, 2008, 2011.
   ALT = alanine amino-transferase.

becomes noncommunicative, the drug should be tapered off over 4 weeks (Howard et al, 2012).

Adverse Reactions Profile

Neostigmine and pyridostigmine have similar adverse reaction profiles. Among the drugs used to treat Alzheimer's disease, tacrine and rivastigmine have the worst adverse reaction profiles and donepezil has the best (FDA, 2001, 2006a; NIH, 2008a, 2011).

Time to Recurrence of Disease Progression

Tacrine has been associated with loss of beneficial effects after about 30 weeks. Donepezil, galantamine, memantine, and rivastigmine have shown positive effects for at least 2 years

(FDA, 2001, 2006a; NIH, 2008a, 2011). There is no data to support using more than one medication together to increase effect (Howard et al., 2012).

Monitoring

Monitoring parameters for tacrine are complex and, at a minimum, continue for 9 months. Baseline liver function tests (total bilirubin, AST, and ALT) should be done prior to initiation of therapy. ALT levels, the ones most likely to indicate hepatotoxicity, should be monitored every other week for the first 16 weeks of therapy, then monthly for 2 months, and then every 3 months. If the ALT level remains less than double the upper limit of normal, then the dose may be left

Table 14–17 ❖ Pharmacokinetics: Selected Cholinergic Blockers

Drug	Onset	Peak	Duration	Half-Life	Elimination
Atropine PO	30 min	30–60 min	4–6 h	3 h	77%–94% in urine
Benztropine PO	1–2 h	Several days	6–10 h	Unknown	Unknown
Dicyclomine PO	1–2 h	60–90 min		9–10 h	80% in urine; 10% in feces
Darifenacin PO (extended-release tablets)	Unknown	7 h	Unknown	12–13 h for EM; 19 h for PM	60% in urine and 40% in feces
Fesoterodine PO (extended-release tablets)	Unknown	5 h	Unknown	7 h	70% in urine as active metabolite and 7% in feces
Propantheline	30–60 min	2–6 h	6 h	3–4 h	Inactivated in upper small intestine
Oxybutynin (tablets and syrup)	30–60 min	3–6 h	6–10 h	2–3 h	Unknown
Oxybutyin transdermal and gel	Within 24 h	36 h	3–4 d	7–8 h	<0.1% unchanged drug in urine
Oxybutynin XL	30–60 min	2–6 h	24 h	Unknown	<0.1% unchanged drug in urine
Scopolamine PO	30 min	1 h	4–6 h	8 h	Mostly metabolized by liver
Scopolamine transdermal	4 h	Unknown	72 h	9.5 h	Mostly metabolized by liver
Solifenacin PO	Unknown	3–8 h	Unknown	45–68 h	69% in urine; 23% in feces
Tolterodine	Unknown	1–2 h	12 h	1.9–3.7 h	77% in urine; 17% in feces
Tolterodine (LA)	Unknown	2–6 h	24 h	2.9–3.1 h	77% in urine; 17% in feces
Trihexyphenidyl	1 h	2–3 h	6–12 h	5.6–10.2 h	In urine
Trospium PO	Unknown	5–6 h	Unknown	20 h	85% in feces; 5.8% in urine. Active tubular secretion is a major factor in renal excretion.

Source: FDA, 2001a; NIH, 2006, 2008b, 2009, 2010a, 2011a, 2012d, 2012e, 2012f, 2012g.
EM = extensive metabolizers and PM = poor metabolizers.

unchanged or titrated upward as needed. If the ALT level is more than double the upper limit of normal, weekly monitoring of liver function is required. If the ALT level is 3 to 5 times the upper limit of normal, then weekly monitoring of liver function is required and the dose must be decreased by 40 mg/day. If the ALT level returns to the normal range with the reduced dose, then monitoring of ALT levels every other week is sufficient. Treatment is discontinued if the ALT concentration is more than 5 times the upper limit of normal (FDA, 2001, 2006a; NIH, 2008a, 2011).

Donepezil requires routine monitoring of blood chemistries and hematology. Baseline liver function studies seem advisable for galantamine and rivastigmine, but they are not required. Assessment of renal function is advisable for galantamine and memantine; dosage adjustments are based on renal function. Neostigmine and pyridostigmine do not have monitoring parameters beyond those of the disease process they are used to treat (FDA, 2001, 2006a; NIH, 2008, 2011).

Patient Education

Administration

Administration education differs for the two groups of drugs. All of the drugs should be taken exactly as prescribed. Doses should not be skipped or doubled up.

For neostigmine and pyridostigmine, patients may need to set a backup alarm to remind them to take a dose when the doses are every 3 to 4 hours. Taking the dose late may cause myasthenic crisis, and taking it early may result in cholinergic crisis. Because drug therapy is lifelong, it is important to establish a regimen that the patient can follow over time (FDA, 2011; NIH, 2011).

For donepezil, missed doses should be skipped and the schedule resumed the next day. Missed doses of galantamine, rivastigmine, and memantine should be skipped and the next dose taken as scheduled. Patients taking tacrine should deal with missed doses by taking them as soon as possible unless it is within 2 hours of the next dose. For all of these drugs, increasing the dose may not improve the symptoms, but it does increase the risk for adverse reactions. Abruptly discontinuing the drug may cause a decline in cognitive function (FDA, 2001, 2006a; NIH, 2008a, 2011).

Donepezil is available as a liquid preparation and as orally disintegrating tablets. Donepezil orally disintegrating tablets should be allowed to dissolve on the tongue and then followed with water (NIH, 2012b).

Rivastigmine oral solution comes with a dosing syringe kept in a protective case. Push down and twist the child-resistant closure to open the drug bottle. Insert the tip of the syringe into the opening in the white stopper. Invert the bottle and, while holding the syringe, pull the plunger out to the appropriate markings on the side of the syringe that indicates the dose. Teach the patient how to remove any large bubble from the syringe to avoid an inaccurate dose. The drug may be taken directly from the syringe or mixed in a small glass of water, cold fruit juice, or soda. Do not mix it with other liquids. The syringe should be stored in its protective case (FDA, 2006a).

Memantine and galantamine are also available in oral solutions. Both of these also have oral dosing devices (FDA, 2003b, 2008b).

The rivastigmine transdermal patch is applied once daily (24 hours apart) to a clean, dry area of skin that does not have hair. Although no recommendation is made by the drug manufacturer, it is probably advisable to rotate the site used (FDA, 2006a).

Adverse Reactions

All of these drugs have in common the adverse reactions associated with an increased amount of ACh: dizziness, miosis, lacrimation, excessive secretions in the respiratory and GI tracts, bronchospasm, bradycardia, abdominal cramps, nausea, vomiting, diarrhea, and excessive salivation. Because they have fewer peripheral effects, drugs used to treat Alzheimer's disease have fewer of the peripheral adverse reactions and more of those associated with the CNS. Patients and their caregivers should observe safety precautions related to the dizziness (FDA, 2001, 2006a; NIH, 2008, 2011).

Administration of neostigmine or pyridostigmine with food or milk helps to minimize adverse GI reactions. Patients with myasthenia gravis often have difficulty with swallowing. Sustained-release tablets must be swallowed whole. Immediate-release tablets may be crushed, and syrup forms of pyridostigmine are available to facilitate administration in this situation. The mottled appearance of the sustained-release form of pyridostigmine does not affect its potency (FDA, 2001; NIH, 2011).

Administration with food may reduce GI complaints for donepezil and does not affect its bioavailability. Although tacrine can also be administered with food, this decreases its bioavailability by 30% to 40% and may necessitate increased dosage. However, higher doses are associated with increased risk for adverse reactions. For patients with difficulty in swallowing, tacrine capsules can be dissolved in any aqueous solution. Orange juice masks the bitter taste best. Memantine and

galantamine can be administered without regard to food. Rivastigmine should be given with food (FDA, 2001; NIH, 2011).

Tacrine has adverse reactions associated with hepatotoxicity. Patients who experience jaundice, rash, or fever should contact the health-care provider immediately. The drug will be discontinued (NIH, 2008a).

Lifestyle Management

No specific lifestyle modifications are directly related to these drugs. Patients with myasthenia gravis should at all times wear identification describing the disease and the medication regimen.

CHOLINERGIC BLOCKERS

Cholinergic blockers are also referred to as parasympatholytics, muscarinic antagonists, and anticholinergics. The term *anticholinergic* can be deceiving because it implies blockade of all cholinergic receptors. In reality, cholinergic blockers produce selective muscarinic blockade against the actions of ACh. Because muscarinic receptors are found in many organs of the body (the eye, heart, blood vessels, lung, GI tract, urinary bladder, and sweat glands), and these drugs cannot be targeted at a single organ, they have many adverse reactions. Throughout this section, *cholinergic blocker* will be synonymous with *muscarinic blockade* unless otherwise stated.

There are several subtypes of cholinergic blockers based on the organs they are likely to target. Atropine is the prototype drug in this class and affects most muscarinic receptors. Its main use orally is as an adjunct to treatment of GI disorders. Other uses are more related to hospital-based care. Its oral use is discussed in this section. Scopolamine has actions similar to atropine except for increased CNS depression and ability to suppress motion sickness and emesis. The antispasmodic group of drugs is indicated for reduction of GI motility and urinary tract smooth muscle spasm. Ipratropium bromide (Atrovent) is used to treat acute exacerbations of asthma and other respiratory diseases such as chronic obstructive pulmonary disease (COPD). It is discussed in Chapter 17 with respiratory drugs and in Chapter 30 where the management of asthma and COPD are discussed. Mydriatic cycloplegics are used for ophthalmic procedures. This use is covered in Chapter 26. Centrally acting cholinergic blockers are used to treat Parkinson's disease and to counteract the extrapyramidal adverse reactions associated with some psychotropic drugs. They are briefly discussed here, but their uses for this indication are covered in Chapter 15.

Pharmacodynamics

Cholinergic blockers competitively block the actions of ACh at muscarinic receptors. They have no direct effect on the receptor. Their actions are based on preventing interaction of endogenous neurotransmitters from activating the receptor and thereby blocking the action associated with stimulation of these receptors. The results of the stimulation of these receptors are depicted in Table 14-1. Blockade produces clinically significant action on the cardiovascular, respiratory, urinary, GI, and central nervous systems; on exocrine glands; and on the eye. Different drugs in the class affect these systems to differing degrees.

Cardiovascular Effects

The sinoatrial (SA) node is very sensitive to muscarinic stimulation. Because stimulation of muscarinic receptors decreases heart rate, blockade increases heart rate. In the presence of high vagal tone, muscarinic blockade can significantly reduce the PR interval of the electrocardiogram (ECG) by blocking receptors in the atrioventricular (AV) node, increasing AV node conduction and decreasing the refractory period of the AV node. The effect on contractility and automaticity is minimal because control of these is primarily via the sympathetic nervous system. Blood vessels have no direct innervation from the parasympathetic nervous system (PNS); however, PNS stimulation does dilate coronary arteries.

Respiratory Effects

Both smooth muscle and secretory glands of the respiratory tract have vagal innervation and contain muscarinic receptors. Blockade of muscarinic receptors relaxes bronchial muscle resulting in bronchodilation, whereas blockade of receptors in the bronchial glands decreases bronchial secretions (Kaufman, 2013).

Exocrine Gland Effects

Muscarinic blockade is very effective in the salivary glands, resulting in dry mouth. It is used for this purpose preoperatively, but it is an unwanted effect in patients taking these drugs for such conditions as Parkinson's disease or urinary incontinence. Gastric acid secretions are less effectively blocked. The volume and amount of acid, pepsin, and mucin are reduced. Basal secretion is more affected than stimulated secretion. Sympathetic cholinergic fibers innervate eccrine sweat glands and many of these have muscarinic receptors. Cholinergic (muscarinic) blockers suppress thermoregulatory sweating (NIH, 2012c).

Urinary and Gastrointestinal Effects

Blockade of muscarinic receptors has extensive effects on smooth muscle in the gut and the urinary system. Gastrointestinal smooth muscle is affected from the stomach to the colon. In muscarinic blockade, the visceral walls are relaxed and both tone and peristalsis are diminished. This prolongs gastric emptying time and intestinal transit time. Smooth muscle of the ureters and bladder wall is relaxed with muscarinic blockade. This action is useful in treatment of urinary tract spasms, but it can precipitate urinary retention, especially in older adult males with benign prostatic hyperplasia (NIH, 2012c).

Central Nervous System Effects

At therapeutic doses, muscarinic blockade produces mild CNS excitation. At higher doses, scopolamine, and to a lesser extent atropine, can produce agitation, hallucinations, and delirium. The relative excess of cholinergic activity in parkinsonian tremor and extrapyramidal symptoms associated with antipsychotic drugs can be partially corrected by muscarinic blockade, especially if combined with a dopamine precursor (NIH, 2012c).

Optic Effects

The papillary constrictor depends on muscarinic receptor stimulation. Blockade of muscarinic receptors results in unopposed sympathetic dilator activity, producing mydriasis. Blockade of receptors on the ciliary muscle produces cycloplegia, which results in loss of the ability to accommodate for near vision (FDA, 2012c). Both effects allow complete retinal assessments during a fundoscopic exam.

Pharmacokinetics

Absorption and Distribution

Cholinergic blockers in the belladonna alkaloid group (atropine, scopolamine) are well absorbed from the gut and cross the conjunctival membrane (Table 14-17). When applied in a suitable vehicle, scopolamine is absorbed from the skin. In contrast, only about 10% to 30% of a dose of the drugs in the quaternary group (propantheline [Probanthine]) is absorbed after oral administration because these drugs have a positive charge, which decreases their ability to move across membranes. Benztropine (Cogentin), darifenacin (Enablex), fesoterodine (Toviaz), oxybutynin (Ditropan), solifenacin (Vesicare), tolterodine (Detrol), and trihexyphenidyl (Trihexy) are all well absorbed following oral administration and oxybutynin is also well absorbed from the skin. Less than 10% of trospium (Sanctura) is absorbed following oral administration (FDA, 2001a; NIH, 2006, 2008b, 2009, 2010a, 2011a, 2012d, 2012e, 2012f, 2012g).

The belladonna alkaloid group is widely distributed, with significant levels reaching the CNS within 30 to 60 minutes after administration. The quaternary group is widely distributed except to the CNS, where it is poorly taken up. The distribution of benztropine and trihexyphenidyl is not clearly known. Darifenacin (Enablex), fesoterodine (Toviaz), oxybutynin, solifenacin (VESIcare), and tolterodine are highly bound to plasma proteins and have large volumes of distribution. Trospium (Sanctura, Sanctura XR) has lower protein binding (50% to 85%) (FDA, 2001a; NIH, 2006, 2008b, 2009, 2010a, 2011a, 2012d, 2012e, 2012f, 2012g).

Metabolism and Excretion

Both the belladonna alkaloids and the quaternary groups are metabolized mostly by the liver and excreted in urine. Oxybutynin and solifenacin are metabolized by the CYP 3A4 isoenzyme system and tolterodine is metabolized by the CYP 2D6 isoenzyme system. Darifenacin and fesoterodine are metabolized by both the 3A4 and 2D6 systems. The metabolism of trospium is not clearly known but early studies suggest that the CYP isoenzyme systems are not inhibited in clinically relevant concentrations (FDA, 2001a; NIH, 2006, 2008b, 2009, 2010a, 2011a, 2012d, 2012e, 2012f, 2012g).

Pharmacotherapeutics

Precautions and Contraindications

Absolute contraindications to these drugs are few and based on their effects on various body systems. Cholinergic blockers are contraindicated in glaucoma, particularly angle-closure glaucoma, because of their ability to produce mydriasis and cycloplegia, thereby impeding the flow of aqueous humor. Cautious use is necessary in obstructive disorders of the GI and urinary tracts, including bladder outlet obstruction and BPH, based on the ability of these drugs to decrease tone and motility in these systems. Patients with hypertension and tachycardia or other cardiac arrhythmias require cautious use, based on the potential for these drugs to increase heart rate (FDA, 2001a; NIH, 2006, 2008a, 2009, 2010a, 2011a, 2012d, 2012e, 2012f, 2012g).

Older adults are particularly susceptible to the CNS effects of cholinergic blockers, with an increased risk for cognitive impairment and falls. Other drugs should be chosen when possible, or cholinergic blockers should be used with caution (FDA, 2001a; NIH, 2006, 2008a, 2009, 2010a, 2011a, 2012d, 2012e, 2012f, 2012g).

All drugs in this class except dicyclomine and oxybutynin are Pregnancy Category C. There are no well-controlled studies in pregnant women, and these drugs should be used only when potential benefits clearly outweigh the risk to the fetus. Dicyclomine and oxybutynin are Pregnancy Category B. No risk to the fetus has been shown in animal or human studies (FDA, 2001a; NIH, 2006, 2008a, 2009, 2010a, 2011a, 2012d, 2012e, 2012f, 2012g).

The quaternary group of drugs is not widely distributed in the body and is the least problematic for lactating women. All other cholinergic blockers either have wide distribution including breast milk or their distribution is not known. They should be avoided in nursing mothers unless clearly needed (FDA, 2001a; NIH, 2006, 2008a, 2009, 2010a, 2011a, 2012d, 2012e, 2012f, 2012g).

Safety and efficacy of many of these drugs have not been established in children. Atropine has safe dosing schedules down to infants weighing 7 pounds. Oxybutynin has safe dosing schedules for children older than 6 years of age with detrusor overactivity associated with a neurological condition. Tolterodine has been shown in studies to increase aggressive, abnormal, and hyperactive behavior and attention disorders in children and should not be used in children (FDA, 2001a; NIH, 2006, 2008b, 2009, 2010a, 2011a, 2012d, 2012e, 2012f, 2012g).

Adverse Drug Reactions

Adverse reactions to cholinergic blockers are based on their actions on tissues other than the target tissue or organ. The discussion here focuses on the adverse reactions on each organ system.

Cardiovascular

Cholinergic blockade eliminates the parasympathetic influence on the heart, resulting in tachycardia. This action can be used therapeutically to treat patients with bradycardia below 50 bpm. The belladonna alkaloids have the highest incidence of this adverse reaction (FDA, 2001a; NIH, 2006, 2008a, 2009, 2010a, 2011a, 2012d, 2012e, 2012f, 2012g).

Respiratory

Cholinergic blockers are sometimes used to produce relaxation of bronchial smooth muscle for patients with an acute exacerbation of asthma and with COPD, but their tendency to thicken and dry bronchial secretions can result in ineffective airway clearance and make patients more at risk for respiratory infection (FDA, 2001a; NIH, 2006, 2008a, 2009, 2010a, 2011a, 2012d, 2012e, 2012f, 2012g).

Exocrine Glands

Blockade of muscarinic receptors on sweat glands can produce anhidrosis. Because sweating is necessary for cooling the body, patients are at risk for hyperthermia. The effect on salivary glands produces xerostomia (dry mouth). This can be irritating and can impair swallowing. Practicing good oral hygiene, chewing sugarless gum, and using other methods to reduce this problem should be taught to patients (FDA, 2001a; NIH, 2006, 2008a, 2009, 2010a, 2011a, 2012d, 2012e, 2012f, 2012g).

Gastrointestinal and Urinary

Decreased tone and motility in the GI tract can lead to constipation, especially when the secretory function of the intestine is also reduced. Patients are taught to increase their intake of fluids and dietary fiber. Blockade of muscarinic receptors in the urinary tract reduces contractile force and pressure in the urinary bladder and increases tone in the urinary sphincter. These combined effects produce urinary hesitancy and urinary retention and increase the risk for urinary tract infection. Impotence has also been reported (FDA, 2001a; NIH, 2006, 2008a, 2009, 2010a, 2011a, 2012d, 2012e, 2012f, 2012g).

Eye

Mydriatic and cycloplegic action of cholinergic blockers results in increased intraocular pressure, blurred vision, and photophobia (FDA, 2001a; NIH, 2006, 2008a, 2009, 2010a, 2011a, 2012d, 2012e, 2012f, 2012g).

Central Nervous System

Cholinergic blockers that cross the blood–brain barrier produce varied adverse reactions, from mild excitation to dizziness and confusion and, in the case of scopolamine, CNS depression. These adverse reactions are more common in older adults (FDA, 2001a; NIH, 2006, 2008a, 2009, 2010a, 2011a, 2012d, 2012e, 2012f, 2012g).

Drug Interactions

Many drugs that are not cholinergic blockers can produce significant muscarinic blockade. These drugs include antihistamines, disopyramide, quinidine, phenothiazine antipsychotics, and TCAs. Additive or synergistic antimuscarinic effects occur when these drugs are given with cholinergic blockers. Additive CNS depression can occur with alcohol, antidepressants, opioids, and sedative-hypnotics (FDA, 2001a; NIH, 2006, 2008a, 2009, 2010a, 2011a, 2012d, 2012e, 2012f, 2012g).

Because cholinergic blockers alter transit time through the GI tract, they may alter the absorption of any orally administered drug. For drugs with a narrow therapeutic range or drugs that can reach toxic levels if retained too long in the GI tract, concurrent administration is not recommended.

Antacids and adsorbent antidiarrheals decrease the absorption of cholinergic blockers (FDA, 2001a; NIH, 2006, 2008a, 2009, 2010a, 2011a, 2012d, 2012e, 2012f, 2012g).

Drug interactions specific to each drug are presented in Table 14-18.

Table 14–18 ⠿ Drug Interactions: Selected Cholinergic Blockers

Drug	Interacting Drug	Possible Effect	Implications
Atropine, dicyclomine, propantheline, scopolamine	Other drugs with cholinergic blocking effects: antihistamines, disopyramide, quinidine, phenothiazines, TCAs, MAOIs	Additive cholinergic blocking adverse effects; antipsychotic effects of phenothiazines decreased	Avoid concurrent use or select drug in each category with the fewest cholinergic blocking properties. Adjust phenothiazine dose.
	Orally administered drugs	Atropine may alter absorption by slowing GI motility	Separate administration or select drugs that do not have narrow therapeutic ranges for which altered absorption would create a problem.
	Antacids	Decrease the absorption of the cholinergic blocker	Separate administration. Give cholinergic blocker first and then antacid at least 30 min later.
	Amantadine	Coadministration may result in increased cholinergic blocking adverse effects	Consider decreasing the dose of the cholinergic blocker
	Atenolol	Pharmacological effects of atenolol may be increased	Metoprolol and propranolol not affected. Substitute one of these if possible.
	Oral potassium	May increase GI mucosal lesions	Take with food and at least 8 oz water.
Benztropine, trihexyphenidyl	Other drugs with cholinergic blocking effects: antihistamines, disopyramide, quinidine, phenothiazines, TCAs	Additive cholinergic blocking adverse effects; antipsychotic effects of phenothiazines decreased	Additive cholinergic blocking adverse effects. Antipsychotic effects of phenothiazines decreased. Adjust phenothiazine dose.
	Bethanechol	Counteracts the cholinergic effects of bethanechol	Avoid concurrent use
	Antacids and antidiarrheals	May decrease absorption	Separate administration. Give cholinergic blocker first and then antacid or antidiarrheal at least 30 min later.
	Haloperidol	Worsens schizophrenic symptoms, increases risk for tardive dyskinesia, decreases blood levels of haloperidol	Avoid concurrent use for schizophrenic patients. Increase dose of haloperidol for others.*
	Levodopa	Decreased GI motility, increased deactivation of levodopa, and reduced intestinal absorption	Effectiveness of levodopa is reduced. May need to alter dose of levodopa if both must be given.
Darifenacin	Strong inhibitors of CYP3A4 (e.g., clarithromycin, azole antifungals, nefazone, and protease inhibitors) Moderate CYP3A4 inhibitors (e.g., diltiazem, erythromycin, fluconazole, verapamil) CYP2D6 substrates (e.g., felcainide, thioridazine, despiramine, imipramine) Digoxin	Darifenacin levels may be increased Mean C_{max} and AUC of interacting drug may increase Increased in digoxin levels (16%)	Dose of darifenacin should not exceed 7.5 mg when coadministered with these drugs No dosage adjustments recommended Use caution when darifenacin is given with drugs metabolized by CYP2D6 and that have a narrow therapeutic window If must coadminister, monitor digoxin levels closely

Table 14–18 ⠿ Drug Interactions: Selected Cholinergic Blockers—cont'd

Drug	Interacting Drug	Possible Effect	Implications
Fesoterodine, solifenacin	CYP3A4 inhibitors (e.g., clarithromycin, erythromycin, itraconazole, ketoconazole) CYP3A4 inducers (e.g., rifampin)	Increases the active metabolite of fesoterodine Coadministration decreases C_{max} and AUC of fesoterodine by 70% and 75%, respectively	For fesoterodine doses >4 mg/d and for solifenacin doses >5 mg/d are not recommended in patients taking these inhibitors No dosing adjustments recommended at this time
Oxybutynin	CNS depressants: alcohol, antihistamines, antidepressants, opioids, sedative-hypnotics	Additive CNS depression	Avoid concurrent administration or monitor closely for CNS effects. May need to alter dosage.
	Other drugs with cholinergic blocking effects: antihistamines, disopyramide, quinidine, phenothiazines, TCAs, MAOIs	Additive cholinergic blocking adverse effects; antipsychotic effects of phenothiazines decreased	Additive cholinergic blocking adverse effects. Antipsychotic effects of phenothiazines decreased. Adjust phenothiazine dose.
	Haloperidol	Worsens schizophrenic symptoms, increases risk for tardive dyskinesia, decreases blood levels of haloperidol	Avoid concurrent use for schizophrenic patients. Increase dose of haloperidol for others.*
	Atenolol	Bioavailability of atenolol increased; increased effects	Metoprolol and propranolol not affected. Substitute one of these if possible.
	Nitrofurantoin	Increased blood levels and bioavailability of nitrofurantoin	Choose different antibiotic to treat urinary tract infection if patient already on oxybutynin
Scopolamine	Alcohol, meperidine	Additive CNS depression	Unless desired therapeutic effect, may need to alter dose of one or both
Tolterodine	Erythromycin, ketoconazole, itraconazole, miconazole	May inhibit metabolism and increase effects of tolterodine	Avoid concurrent use
Trospium	Drugs that are eliminated by active renal tubular secretion (e.g., digoxin, procainamide, morphine, vancomycin, metformin, tenofovir)	May increase the serum concentration of trospium and/or the competing drug	If must coadminister, carefully monitor for adverse effects. For digoxin, monitor drug levels carefully.

Source: FDA, 2001a; NIH, 2006, 2008b, 2009, 2010a, 2011a, 2012d, 2012e, 2012f, 2012g.

*Administration of these drugs may be a therapeutic choice with phenothiazines to reduce extrapyramidal adverse reactions associated with phenothiazines.

Clinical Use and Dosing

Parkinson's Disease

First-line management of Parkinson's disease is accomplished with dopaminergics and dopamine agonists. Cholinergic blockers are useful adjuncts early in the course of the disease to control tremor by relaxing smooth muscle and oral secretion control. They are also useful for middle-aged patients who have tremor but little rigidity or bradykinesia and for control of salivation and drooling (FDA, 2001a; NIH, 2006, 2008a, 2009, 2010a, 2011a, 2012d, 2012e, 2012f, 2012g).

Trihexyphenidyl is one cholinergic blocker currently used as an adjunct to therapy with carbidopa/levodopa. The initial dose is 1 to 2 mg the first day, increased by 2 mg increments at 3- to 5-day intervals until a total of 6 to 10 mg are given daily (Table 14-19). Many patients receive maximum benefits at this dose, but postencephalitic patients often require doses

of 12 to 15 mg/day. The drug is best tolerated when the daily dose is divided into three doses and taken at mealtimes. High doses may be divided into four doses and taken at mealtimes and bedtime. Because of the relatively high dosage of sustained-release capsules, they are not used for initial therapy. Once patients have been stabilized on regular formulations, they may be switched to sustained release. Sustained-release capsules are administered in a once-daily dose after breakfast or in doses 12 hours apart (NIH, 2006).

When given concurrently with levodopa, the usual dose may need to be reduced. Conversely, trihexyphenidyl decreases the total bioavailability of levodopa. Careful adjustment of the doses of the two drugs is required, depending on adverse reactions and degree of symptom control (NIH, 2006).

Benztropine is also used for this indication. The dose is 1 to 2 mg/day with a range of 0.5 to 6 mg/day. Therapy is

Table 14–19 ⊗ **Dosage Schedule: Selected Cholinergic Blockers**

Drug	Indication	Form	Initial Dose	Maintenance and Maximum Dose
Atropine	Irritable bowel syndrome, peptic ulcer disease	Tablets: 400 mcg	*Adults:* 400 mg q 4–6 h	May increase to 600 mcg if needed
	(In children also used for frequent urination and bed-wetting)		*Children:* 7–16 lb = 0.1 mg; 17–24 lb = 0.15 mg 24–40 lb = 0.2 mg 40–65 lb = 0.3 mg 65–90 lb = 0.4 mg >90 lb = 0.4 mg q 4–6 h	Not to exceed 400 mcg. Use lowest effective dose.
Benztropine	Parkinson's disease	Tablets: 0.5 mg, 1 mg, 2 mg (Cogentin in 0.5 mg tablets only) Injection: 1 mg/mL	1–2 mg/d For postencephalitic patients: 2 mg/d	Increase in increments of 0.5 mg/d gradually at 5- or 6-d intervals until symptom relief. Use smallest dose that achieves effect. Maximum dose is 6 mg/d. Older adults and thin patients may not tolerate higher doses. Giving dose at bedtime is preferred.
	Drug-induced EPS		1–2 mg daily or bid PO or IM	1–2 mg PO provides relief in 1–2 d and prevents recurrence. If inadequate relief in that time, may increase to 2 mg tid. 1–2 mg IM provides rapid relief. Maximum dose by either route is 6 mg/d.
Darifenacin	For overactive bladder with symptoms of incontinence, urgency, and frequency	Tablets, extended-release:7.5 mg 15 mg	7.5 mg once daily	May increase to 15 mg once daily as early as 2 wk after starting therapy. In moderate hepatic impairment or when coadministered with strong CYP3A4 inhibitor, daily dose should not exceed 7.5 mg. Maximum dose: 15 mg/d.
Fesoterodine	For overactive bladder with symptoms of incontinence, urgency, and frequency	Tablets, extended-release: 4 mg 8 mg	4 mg once daily	May increase to 8 mg once daily based on individual response and tolerability. In severe renal insufficiency or when coadministered with strong CYP3A4 inhibitor, dose should not exceed 4 mg/d. This drug should not be given to patients with severe hepatic impairment.
Dicyclomine	Irritable bowel syndrome	Tablets: 10 mg Tablets: 20 mg Capsules: 10 mg and 20 mg Syrup: 10 mg/5 mL	80 mg/d in 4 equally divided doses	Increase to 160 mg/d in 4 divided doses
Oxybutynin	Antispasmodic for bladder instability and overactive bladder	Tablets: 5 mg (G) Syrup: 5 mg/5 mL XL tablets: 5 mg, 10 mg, 15 mg	*Adults:* 5 mg bid or tid immediate-release The XL formulation is recommended for overactive bladder and is given once daily. Transdermal formulation is used only in adults. Dose is 3.9 mg system applied twice weekly (every 3–4 d). *Frail elderly:* 2.5 mg bid or tid *Children >5 years of age:* 5 mg bid	*Adults:* 5 mg qid or 10 mg bid of the XL formulation *Children >5 years of age:* Maximum doses of 5 mg tid of immediate release and 20 mg/d of extended release

Table 14–19 ⊗ **Dosage Schedule: Selected Cholinergic Blockers—cont'd**

Drug	Indication	Form	Initial Dose	Maintenance and Maximum Dose
	Detrusor overactivity associated with a neurological condition		*Children 6 years of age and older:* 5 mg once daily of extended-release tablets *Children >5 years of age:* 5 mg bid of immediate-release tablets or syrup	*Children 6 years of age or older:* Dosage adjustments in 5 mg increments to achieve a balance of efficacy and tolerability up to a maximum of 20 mg/d *Children >5 years of age:* Dosage adjustments in 5 mg increments to achieve a balance of efficacy and tolerability up to a maximum of 5 mg tid
Propantheline	Peptic ulcer	Tablets: 7.5 mg (B)	15 mg 30 min before meals and 30 mg at bedtime	Same as initial dose
Scopolamine	Prevention of nausea and vomiting associated with motion sickness	Transderm-Scop: 1.5 mg disk	One transdermal disk applied to postauricular skin 4 h before antiemetic effect is desired	One disk delivers 0.5 mg/d for 3 days. If effect needed for >3 d, remove and replace with new disk.
Solifenacin	For overactive bladder with symptoms of incontinence, urgency, and frequency	Tablets: 5 mg 10 mg	5 mg once daily	May increase to 10 mg once daily based on patient response and tolerability. In severe renal impairment, moderate hepatic impairment or when coadministered with strong CYP3A4 inhibitor, daily dose should not exceed 5 mg. This drug should not be given to patients with severe hepatic impairment.
Mirabegron	For overactive bladder	25 mg or 50 mg oval coated tablet	25 mg once daily	May increase to 50 mg once daily in patients with no renal or hepatic impairment
Tolterodine (Detrol)	Antispasmodic for bladder instability	Tablets: 1 mg, 2 mg	1 mg bid	Usual dose 2 mg daily. Adult with impaired hepatic or renal function or on concurrent enzyme inhibitors may require dose reduction to 1 mg bid.
Detrol LA		Capsules (extended-release): 2 mg, 4 mg	2–4 mg daily	Usual dose 4 mg daily. Adult with impaired hepatic or renal function or on concurrent enzyme inhibitors may require dose reduction to 2 mg bid.
Trihexyphenidyl	Parkinson's disease Drug-induced EPS	Tablets: 2 mg, 5 mg Sequels (sustained-release) (Artane brand only): 5 mg Elixir: 2 mg/5 mL	1–2 mg/d tablets or elixir. Initial therapy usually not begun with sustained release.	Increase in increments of 2 mg at 3- to 5-d intervals until 6–10 mg/d. Postencephalitic patients may require 12–15 mg/d. All doses tolerated better when given in 3 divided doses with meals. Higher doses given in 4 divided doses with meals and at bedtime. After dosage is stabilized, sustained-release forms may be used. Total daily dose is same as other forms but can be given daily at breakfast or in 2 divided doses 12 h apart.
Trospium (Sanctura)	For overactive bladder with symptoms of incontinence, urgency, and frequency	Tablets: 20 mg	20 mg bid Take at least 1 h before meals or on an empty stomach.	May increase to a total daily dose of 60 mg. In severe renal impairment (CrCl <30 mL/min) dose is 20 mg once daily at bedtime.
Sanctura XR		Capsules, extended-release: 60 mg	60 mg daily in the morning. Take at least 1 h before morning meal or on an empty stomach.	Not recommended for patient with severe renal impairment (CrCl <30 mL/min)

Source: FDA, 2001a; NIH, 2006, 2008b, 2009, 2010a, 2011a, 2012d, 2012e, 2012f, 2012g.
EPS = extrapyramidal symptoms.

initiated with a 0.5 to 1 mg dose and increased in 0.5 mg increments until optimal benefits are achieved. Postencephalitic patients begin with 2 mg/day in one or more doses, which are increased by 0.5 mg/day until optimal benefits are reached (NIH, 2012d).

The long duration of action of benztropine makes it especially suitable for a bedtime medication, and some patients experience greatest relief by taking the entire dose at bedtime. Others do better with divided doses, from 2 to 4 times a day (NIH, 2012d).

Management of Extrapyramidal Symptoms (EPS) Secondary to Drug Therapy

Cholinergic blockers are the drugs of choice for treating akathisia arising from antipsychotic drugs. Both benztropine and trihexyphenidyl are used for this indication. Size and frequency of dosing are determined empirically within usual dosing recommendations (NIH, 2006, 2012d).

The initial dose of trihexyphenidyl for EPS is 1 mg in a single dose. If symptoms are not controlled within a few hours, the dose is gradually increased until control is achieved. Daily dosages range from 5 to 15 mg, although symptoms have been controlled on as little as 1 mg/day. An elixir form is available for patients who have difficulty with swallowing tablets. Control can be more rapidly achieved by temporarily reducing the dose of the antipsychotic drug when trihexyphenidyl therapy is initiated and then adjusting both drugs until the desired effects are achieved without EPS reactions (NIH, 2006).

Benztropine therapy is initiated with 1 to 2 mg daily or 2 times a day. Dosage titration is in 0.5 mg increments at 5- or 6-day intervals so that the smallest amount required for symptom relief is used. A dose of 1 to 2 mg 2 or 3 times a day usually provides symptom relief within 1 to 2 days. The maximum dose is 6 mg/day. Older adults and thin patients often cannot tolerate the higher doses. Benztropine also comes in an injectable form that can be used for patients with severe dystonic reactions or for those who cannot swallow a pill. The intramuscular dose is 1 to 2 mg, and relief of symptoms is rapid (NIH, 2012d).

For both of these drugs, after several weeks of therapy, the drug may be withdrawn to see if symptoms return and to determine the need for continued therapy. Some patients' symptoms will not return, and some drug-induced EPS reactions do not respond to these two drugs (NIH, 2006, 2012d).

Antispasmodic for Bladder Instability and Overactivity

Overactive bladder and urinary incontinence prevalence ranges from 10% to 50% in the general population (Parazzini, Lavezzari, & Artibani, 2002). Darifenacin, fesoterodine, oxybutynin, solifenacin, tolterodine, and trospium treat these disorders by exerting direct antispasmodic effects and inhibiting the muscarinic action of ACh on smooth muscle. Oxybutynin exhibits only one-fifth the cholinergic blocking activity of atropine, but has 4 to 10 times the antispasmodic activity.

No cholinergic blocking effects occur at the myoneural junction for any of these drugs. This combination of effects makes them especially useful to treat bladder spasms. Patients with conditions characterized by involuntary bladder contractions experience increased bladder capacity, diminished frequency of urination, and reduced urgency related to voiding. These effects are strongest for patients with uninhibited neurogenic bladder, including children with detrusor overactivity associated with a neurological condition. They are also extremely effective for patients who experience incontinence and are well tolerated in long-term administration (more than 2 years). Because oxybutynin increases blood levels and bioavailability of nitrofurantoin, a different antibiotic should be chosen to treat any concurrent urinary tract infection that may be associated with urinary retention. Assessment for bladder outlet obstruction should be done prior to prescribing because obstruction contraindicates the use of this drug (FDA, 2001a; NIH, 2006, 2008a, 2009, 2010a, 2011a, 2012d, 2012e, 2012f, 2012g).

For adults, the initial dose of oxybutynin is 5 mg 2 or 3 times a day of the regular formulation or the syrup and 5 to 10 mg daily for the extended-release (XL) formulation (Table 14-19). For frail elderly, the initial dose is 2.5 mg given 2 or 3 times a day because of a prolongation of the elimination half-life from 2 or 3 hours to 5 hours. Symptom response usually occurs with the first dose but may require up to a week for the full effect. If the desired effects have not occurred in 1 week, the dose is increased. Both the regular and extended-release formulations are similarly effective and tolerable (Diokno et al, 2003). The maximum dose is 20 mg/day for immediate release and 30 mg/day for extended release. For children, the initial dose is 5 mg 2 times a day for immediate-release tablets or syrup (for children more than 5 years of age) and 5 mg once daily for extended-release tablets (for children more than 6 years of age), with a maximum dose of 15 mg/day of immediate release and 20 mg/day of extended release. Adverse reactions are more likely with higher doses, and lifestyle modifications should be made concurrently to keep the dose as low as possible. For children and adults who have difficulty swallowing pills, the drug is available in syrup form. There is also a transdermal formulation that is used only in adults. This 3.9 mg system is applied twice weekly (NIH, 2012f).

The remaining drugs are used only in adults and have no dosages for children. Darifenacin, festerodine, and solifenacin are extended-release formulations and are taken once daily. The initial dose of darifenacin is 7.5 mg. If the desired effects do not occur in 2 weeks, the dose can be increased to 15 mg once daily. Fesoterodine is started at 4 mg once daily. It may be increased to 8 mg once daily based on patient response and tolerability. Solifenacin is initiated at 5 mg once daily with an increase to 10 mg once daily if symptoms require. The initial dose of trospium depends on its formulation. The immediate-release formulation dose is 20 mg 2 times a day. The extended-release formulation is initiated at 60 mg daily in the morning. Administration with a high-fat meal resulted in reduced absorption, with AUC and C_{max} values 70% and 80% lower than those obtained while fasting. All doses should be taken at least 1 hour before meals or on an empty stomach (FDA, 2001a; NIH, 2006, 2008a, 2009, 2010a, 2011a, 2012d, 2012e, 2012f, 2012g).

The newest drug approved for the treatment of overactive bladder in the adult population is mirabegron. Approved by the FDA in 2012, this drug works as an agonist of beta-3 adrenergic receptors and relaxes the detrusor smooth muscles of the urinary bladder to increase bladder capacity. The recommended dosage is 25 mg once daily and may be increased to 50 mg daily in patients who do not have renal or hepatic impairment. The medication may take up to 8 weeks to reach full effectiveness. This medication may cause increases in blood pressure and so should be used with caution in patients with poorly controlled hypertension. Mirabegron was evaluated for safety in a study of 2,736 individuals and another trial of 1,632 patients. The most common adverse effects were nausea, hypertension, constipation, dizziness, tachycardia, and headache. A small number of participants experienced atrial fibrillation (0.2%) and prostate cancer (0.1%) at a rate greater than placebo (FDA, 2012e).

Renal function is a factor in dosing most of these drugs. The dose should not exceed the initial dose in the case of severe renal impairment (CrCl less than 30 mL/min) for fesoterodine and solifenacine. No dosage adjustments are recommended in moderate renal impairment. Only the immediate-release formulation of trospium can be used in patients with severe renal impairment, but the dose must not exceed the initial dose (20 mg) (FDA, 2001a; NIH, 2006, 2008a, 2009, 2010a, 2011a, 2012d, 2012e, 2012f, 2012g).

Hepatic function is a dosing factor in all of these drugs. Doses should not exceed the initial dose for darifenacin and solifenacin in patients with moderate hepatic impairment. Cautious use in moderate hepatic impairment is recommended for fesoterodine. The metabolic pathway for trospium has not been fully defined and there is no information regarding the effect of severe hepatic impairment on exposure to this drug. Although caution should be used when administering trospium in circumstances of moderate or severe hepatic impairment, the drug is not contraindicated in this situation. All of these drugs except trospium are contraindicated in the presence of severe hepatic impairment. The initial dose of tolterodine is 1 mg 2 times a day with a usual dose of 2 mg daily for maintenance. Doses of 2 to 4 mg once daily of the extended-release capsules are used with a usual maintenance dose of 4 mg daily. Adults with impaired hepatic or renal function often require the lower dose both initially and for maintenance. Symptom relief is similar to oxybutynin (FDA, 2001a; NIH, 2006, 2008b, 2009, 2010a, 2011a, 2012d, 2012e, 2012f, 2012g).

Prevention of Nausea and Vomiting Associated With Motion Sickness

Scopolamine in a transdermal form is used for this indication. One disk is applied to the clean, dry, postauricular skin at least 4 hours before the antiemetic effect is desired. Over a space of 3 days, 0.5 mg is delivered. If therapy is required for more than 3 days, the original disk is removed and replaced with a new one. Only one disk is worn at a time. After application of the disk, the hands are washed with soap and water to prevent any traces of the drug from coming into direct contact with the eyes (FDA, 2001a).

Adjunct Therapy in Management of Irritable Bowel Syndrome and Peptic Ulcer Disease

Atropine is used for both indications. Dicyclomine is used for the management of irritable bowel syndrome in patients who do not respond to the usual interventions with sedation and diet (NIH, 2007). Propantheline is indicated for its antisecretory activity in the management of peptic ulcer disease (NIH, 2009).

The initial adult dose of atropine for both indications is 400 mcg every 4 to 6 hours. Doses may be increased, if necessary, to 600 mcg. For children, the dose is 10 mcg/kg every 4 to 6 hours. The dose is not to exceed 400 mcg. Children are especially sensitive to the adverse reactions associated with atropine, and every effort should be made to keep the dose as low as possible (NIH, 2012c).

Symptoms of poisoning in infants and children differ from adult symptoms. They include burning sensations in the mouth; difficulty in swallowing; rash; blurred vision; tachycardia; tachypnea; fever up to 109.8°F; muscle incoordination; and eventually seizure, respiratory paralysis, and death. The antidote for atropine poisoning is physostigmine (NIH, 2012c).

The only oral dose of dicyclomine shown to be effective is 160 mg/day in four equally divided doses. However, because of adverse effects, the initial dose is 80 mg/day in four equally divided doses. The dose is then increased if tolerated. For patients who have difficulty with swallowing, a syrup form is available with the same dosage range. A formulation for IM administration is also available. The dose is 80 mg/day in four equally divided doses (NIH, 2007).

The oral dose of propantheline for adults is 15 mg 30 minutes before meals and 30 mg at bedtime. For patients with mild manifestations, older adults, and patients of small stature, the dose is 7.5 mg 3 times a day. The safety and efficacy of this drug for treating peptic ulcer in children have not been established. There is a dosage schedule published for antisecretory and antispasmodic use in children, but it is an unlabeled use. The dose for children is 1.5 mg/kg a day in three or four divided doses for antisecretory indications and 2 to 3 mg/kg a day in four to six divided doses given every 4 to 6 hours for antispasmodic indications (NIH, 2009).

Rational Drug Selection

Aside from clinical indications, there are few parameters that assist in deciding which is the best drug to choose. Some are associated with slightly fewer adverse reactions, but all have several reactions that cause patients not to adhere to treatment regimens.

Formulation

In addition to the cost data, formulation can be an issue when speed is a major concern (e.g., severe dystonic symptoms in a patient who is taking an antipsychotic) or when the patient has difficulty in swallowing for any of a variety of reasons, including the progression of a disease process itself. Several drugs come in injectable or syrup forms. Oxybutynin has a transdermal formulation that may also address this issue.

Extended-release formulations may improve adherence by simplifying the treatment regimen (NIH, 2012f).

Monitoring

No specific monitoring parameters are required for cholinergic blockers beyond monitoring for adverse reactions and the monitoring parameters that are appropriate for the disease being treated.

Patient Education

Administration

Instruct the patient to take the drugs exactly as prescribed. If a dose is missed, take it as soon as remembered unless it is almost time for the next dose. Doses should not be doubled. Benztropine is administered with food or immediately after meals to minimize gastric irritation. The tablet may be crushed and administered with food if the patient has difficulty in swallowing. Atropine, dicyclomine, and propantheline are administered 30 to 60 minutes before a meal; oxybutynin is administered on an empty stomach (may be given with food to minimize GI irritation); and trihexyphenidyl is administered after a meal (may be given before a meal for patients with dry mouth or with the meal if GI distress occurs). Extended-release formulations must be swallowed whole and not crushed or chewed. Calibrated measuring instruments such as medicine cups or syringes should be used with liquid formulations to make certain the dose is accurate (FDA, 2001a; NIH, 2006, 2008a, 2009, 2010a, 2011a, 2012d, 2012e, 2012f, 2012g).

The scopolamine disk has specific instructions for its application. The disk is applied to clean, dry skin behind the ear at least 4 hours before the antiemetic effect is desired. It is left in place for up to 3 days. Only one disk at a time is worn. If longer effects are required, the disk is removed and replaced. Hands are washed with soap and water after application to make sure no trace of the drug comes in contact with the eyes. The same procedure is followed when removing the disk (FDA, 2001a).

Adverse Reactions

The following information is drawn from FDA and NIH sources (FDA, 2001a; NIH, 2006, 2008a, 2009, 2010a, 2011a, 2012d, 2012e, 2012f, 2012g):

- Cholinergic blockers have many adverse reactions because their actions are not organ-specific. Cardiovascular reactions include tachycardia. Teach patients to take their own pulses and report heart rates above 100 bpm. Dosage adjustments may be required. This adverse effect is especially problematic for patients who concurrently have coronary artery disease and for older adults.
- Cholinergic blockers tend to thicken and dry respiratory secretion. Advise the patients to drink at least 2 quarts of noncaffeinated fluid daily to maintain adequate hydration.
- Fluid and fiber intake are also important because these drugs may cause constipation and difficulty in voiding. Dry mouth can be relieved by practicing good oral hygiene, consuming cold drinks, sucking on hard candy, or chewing sugarless gum.
- The therapeutic goal for many of these drugs is to reduce gastric secretion. Substances that increase gastric acid secretion, such as alcohol, tobacco, caffeine, and aspirin, should be avoided.
- Activities that require visual acuity, mental alertness, and vigorous activity in warm weather can create problems. Cholinergic blockers may result in blurred vision, photophobia, and dizziness, and they reduce the sweating necessary to cool the body during exercise.

Lifestyle Management

Several of the disease processes for which these drugs are prescribed require lifestyle modifications. Incontinence can also be treated with a variety of therapies besides drugs. Bladder retraining, Kegel exercises, biofeedback, and other nonpharmacological therapies should also be used in treating many of these disorders.

REFERENCES

American College of Obstetricians and Gynecologists (ACOG). (2012). Practice Bulletin No. 125 : Chronic hypertension in pregnancy. *Clinical Management Guidelines for Obstetrician-Gynecologists, 119*(2pt 1), 396–407.

August, P. (2013). *Management of hypertension in pregnant and postpartum women.* In D. S. Basow (Ed.), *UpToDate,* Waltham, MA: UpToDate.

Basow, D. S. (Ed). (2013). *UpToDate.* Waltham, MA: UpToDate.

Colucci, W. (2013). *Use of beta blockers in heart failure due to systolic dysfunction.* In D. S. Basow (Ed.), *UpToDate.* Waltham, MA: UpToDate.

Dickstein, K., Cohen-Solai, A., Filippatos, G., McMurray, J., Ponikowski, P., Poole-Wilson, P., et al, and ESC Committee for Practice Guidelines. (2008). ESC guidelines for the diagnosis and treatment of acute and chronic heart failure 2008: The task force. *European Heart Journal, 29*(19), 2388–2442.

Howard, R., McShane, R., Lindesay, J., Ritchie, C., Baldwin, A., Barber, R, et al. (2012) Donepezil and Memantine for Moderate-to-Severe Alzheimer's Disease. New England Journal of Medicine. 2012 (3); 366:893-903.

Hunt, S., Abraham, W., Chin, M., Feldman, A., Francis, G., Ganiats, T., et al. (2005). ACC/AHA 2005 guideline update for the diagnosis and management of chronic heart failure in the adults: A report of the American College of Cardiology/American Heart Association Task Force on Practice Guidelines. Bethesda, MD.: American College of Cardiology Foundation, 82 p.

Kaufman, G. (2013). The pharmacology of bronchodilators. *Nurse Prescribing, 11*(3), 122–129.

Mann, J. (2013). *Choice of therapy in essential hypertension: Recommendations.* In D. S. Basow (Ed.), *UpToDate.* Waltham, MA: UpToDate.

Mattoo, T. (2013). *Treatment of hypertension in children and adolescents.* In *UpToDate,* D. S. Basow (Ed.).Waltham, MA: UpToDate.

McCance, K. L., & Huether, S. E. (2014). *Pathophysiology: The biologic basis for disease in adults and children,* 7th edition. St. Louis: Mosby.

National Institutes of Health (NIH). (2006). *Trihexyphenidyl.* U.S. National Library of Medicine: Daily Med. Retrieved from http://dailymed.nlm.nih.gov/dailymed/archives/fdaDrugInfo.cfm?archiveid=2670

National Institutes of Health (NIH). (2007). *Dicyclomine.* U.S. National Library of Medicine: Daily Med. Retrieved from http://dailymed.nlm.nih.gov/dailymed/archives/fdaDrugInfo.cfm?archiveid=3317

National Institutes of Health (NIH). (2008a). *Tacrine.* U.S. National Library of Medicine: Daily Med. Retrieved from http://dailymed.nlm.nih.gov/dailymed/archives/fdaDrugInfo.cfm?archiveid=9851

National Institutes of Health (NIH). (2008b). *Tolterodine.* U.S. National Library of Medicine: Daily Med. Retrieved from http://dailymed.nlm.nih.gov/dailymed/archives/fdaDrugInfo.cfm?archiveid=7788

National Institutes of Health (NIH). (2009). *Propantheline*. U.S. National Library of Medicine: Daily Med. Retrieved from http://dailymed.nlm.nih .gov/dailymed/archives/fdaDrugInfo.cfm?archiveid=13088

National Institutes of Health (NIH). (2010). *Nicotine (Comit)*. U.S. National Library of Medicine: Daily Med. Retrieved from http://dailymed.nlm.nih .gov/dailymed/archives/fdaDrugInfo.cfm?archiveid=15397

National Institutes of Health (NIH). (2010a). *Darifenacin*. U.S. National Library of Medicine: Daily Med. Retrieved from http://dailymed.nlm.nih .gov/dailymed/archives/fdaDrugInfo.cfm?archiveid=16949

National Institutes of Health (NIH). (2011). *Neostigmine*. U.S. National Library of Medicine: Daily Med. Retrieved from http://dailymed.nlm.nih .gov/dailymed/lookup.cfm?setid=6c3a7e99-cbde-43a8-acb9-6b414820cd46

National Institutes of Health (NIH). (2011a). *Trospium*. U.S. National Library of Medicine: Daily Med. Retrieved from http://dailymed.nlm.nih .gov/dailymed/archives/fdaDrugInfo.cfm?archiveid=64118

National Institutes of Health (NIH). (2012a). *Bethanechol*. U.S. National Library of Medicine: Daily Med. Retrieved from http://dailymed.nlm.nih .gov/dailymed/drugInfo.cfm?id=74639

National Institutes of Health (NIH). (2012b). *Donepezil*. U.S. National Library of Medicine: Daily Med. Retrieved from http://dailymed.nlm.nih .gov/dailymed/lookup.cfm?setid=98e451e1-e4d7-4439-a675-c5457ba20975

National Institutes of Health (NIH). (2012c). *Atropine sulfate*. U.S. National Library of Medicine: Daily Med. Retrieved from http://dailymed.nlm.nih .gov/dailymed/archives/fdaDrugInfo.cfm?archiveid=91425

National Institutes of Health (NIH). (2012c). *Donnatal*. U.S. National Library of Medicine: Daily Med. Retrieved from http://dailymed.nlm .nih.gov/dailymed/archives/fdaDrugInfo.cfm?archiveid=73719

National Institutes of Health (NIH). (2012d). *Benztropine*. U.S. National Library of Medicine: Daily Med. Retrieved from http://dailymed.nlm .nih.gov/dailymed/archives/fdaDrugInfo.cfm?archiveid=79054

National Institutes of Health (NIH). (2012e). *Fesoterodine*. U.S. National Library of Medicine: Daily Med. Retrieved from http://dailymed.nlm .nih.gov/dailymed/archives/fdaDrugInfo.cfm?archiveid=79806#S8.7

National Institutes of Health (NIH). (2012f). *Oxybutynine*. U.S. National Library of Medicine: Daily Med. Retrieved from http://dailymed.nlm.nih .gov/dailymed/archives/fdaDrugInfo.cfm?archiveid=71471

National Institutes of Health (NIH). (2012g). *Solifenicine*. U.S. National Library of Medicine: Daily Med. Retrieved from http://dailymed.nlm.nih .gov/dailymed/archives/fdaDrugInfo.cfm?archiveid=81852

Podrid, P. I. (2013). *Major side effects of beta blockers*. In D. S. Basow (Ed.), *UpToDate*. Waltham, MA: UpToDate.

Ross, D. (2013). *Beta blockers in treatment of hyperthyroidism*. In D. S. Basow (Ed.), *UpToDate*. Waltham, MA: UpToDate.

U.S. Food and Drug Administration (FDA). (1982). *FDA approved drug products: Demecarium*. Retrieved from http://www.fda.gov/ohrms/ dockets/dockets/98n0182/nom004b.pdf

U.S. Food and Drug Administration (FDA). (2001). *FDA approved drug products: Pyridostigmine*. Retrieved from http://www.accessdata.fda.gov/ drugsatfda_docs/label/2001/15193s18lbl.pdf

U.S. Food and Drug Administration (FDA). (2001a). *FDA approved drug products: Scopolamine*. Retrieved from http://www.accessdata.fda.gov/ drugsatfda_docs/label/2001/017874s18s27lbl.pdf

U.S. Food and Drug Administration (FDA). (2003b). *FDA approved drug products: Memantine*. Retrieved from http://www.accessdata.fda.gov/ drugsatfda_docs/label/2003/021487lbl.pdf

U.S. Food and Drug Administration (FDA). (2004). *FDA approved drug products: Methyldopa*. Retrieved from http://www.accessdata.fda.gov/ drugsatfda_docs/label/2004/13400s086lbl.pdf

U.S. Food and Drug Administration (FDA). (2006). *FDA approved drug products: Miochol*. Retrieved from http://www.accessdata.fda.gov/ drugsatfda_docs/label/2006/020213s010lbl.pdf

U.S. Food and Drug Administration (FDA). (2006a). *FDA approved drug products: Rivastigmine*. Retrieved from http://www.accessdata.fda.gov/ drugsatfda_docs/label/2006/020823s016,021025s008lbl.pdf

U.S. Food and Drug Administration (FDA). (2006b). *FDA approved drug products: Carbachol*. Retrieved from http://www.accessdata.fda.gov/ drugsatfda_docs/label/2004/16968s022lbl.pdf

U.S. Food and Drug Administration (FDA). (2007a). *FDA approved drug products: Acetabulol*. Retrieved from http://www.accessdata.fda.gov/ drugsatfda_docs/label/2007/018917s024lbl.pdf

U.S. Food and Drug Administration (FDA). (2007b). *FDA approved drug products: Pindolol*. Retrieved from http://www.accessdata.fda.gov/ drugsatfda_docs/label/2007/018285s034lbl.pdf

U.S. Food and Drug Administration (FDA). (2007c). *FDA approved drug products: Timolol*. Retrieved from http://www.accessdata.fda.gov/ drugsatfda_docs/label/2007/020963s010lbl.pdf

U.S. Food and Drug Administration (FDA). (2008a). *FDA approved drug products: Provocholine*. Retrieved from http://www.accessdata.fda.gov/ drugsatfda_docs/label/2010/200890s001lbl.pdf

U.S. Food and Drug Administration (FDA). (2008b). *FDA approved drug products: Galantamine*. Retrieved from http://www.accessdata.fda.gov/ drugsatfda_docs/label/2008/077605s000lbl.pdf

U.S. Food and Drug Administration (FDA). (2009a). *FDA approved drug products: Phentolamine*. Retrieved from http://www.fda.gov/downloads/ Drugs/GuidanceComplianceRegulatoryInformation/Enforcement ActivitiesbyFDA/WarningLettersandNoticeofViolationLettersto PharmaceuticalCompanies/UCM199745.pdf

U.S. Food and Drug Administration (FDA). (2009b). *FDA approved drug products: Prazosin*. Retrieved from http://www.accessdata.fda.gov/ drugsatfda_docs/label/2009/017442s033lbl.pdf

U.S. Food and Drug Administration (FDA). (2009c). *FDA approved drug products: Doxazosin*. Retrieved from http://www.accessdata.fda.gov/ drugsatfda_docs/label/2009/019668s021lbl.pdf

U.S. Food and Drug Administration (FDA). (2009d). *FDA approved drug products: Betaxolol*. Retrieved from http://www.accessdata.fda.gov/ drugsatfda_docs/label/2010/021114s003lbl.pdf

U.S. Food and Drug Administration (FDA). (2010). *FDA approved drug products: Labetalol*. Retrieved from http://www.accessdata.fda.gov/ drugsatfda_docs/label/2010/018716s026lbl.pdf

U.S. Food and Drug Administration (FDA). (2010a). *FDA approved drug products: Pilocarpine*. Retrieved from http://www.accessdata.fda.gov/ drugsatfda_docs/label/2010/200890s001lbl.pdf

U.S. Food and Drug Administration (FDA). (2010b). *FDA approved drug products: Alfuzosin*. Retrieved from http://www.accessdata.fda.gov/ drugsatfda_docs/label/2010/021287s016lbl.pdf

U.S. Food and Drug Administration (FDA). (2011). *FDA approved drug products: Catapres-TTS*. Retrieved from http://www.accessdata.fda.gov/ drugsatfda_docs/label/2012/018891s028lbl.pdf

U.S. Food and Drug Administration (FDA). (2011a). *FDA approved drug products: Tamsulosin*. Retrieved from http://www.accessdata.fda.gov/ drugsatfda_docs/label/2011/020579s027lbl.pdf

U.S. Food and Drug Administration (FDA). (2011b). *FDA approved drug products: Nadolol*. Retrieved from http://www.accessdata.fda.gov/ drugsatfda_docs/label/2011/018063s062lbl.pdf

U.S. Food and Drug Administration (FDA). (2011c). *FDA approved drug products: Propranolol*. Retrieved from http://www.accessdata.fda.gov/ drugsatfda_docs/label/2011/016418s080,016762s017,017683s008lbl.pdf

U.S. Food and Drug Administration (FDA). (2011d). *FDA approved drug products: Nebivolol*. Retrieved from http://www.accessdata.fda.gov/ drugsatfda_docs/label/2011/021742s013lbl.pdf

U.S. Food and Drug Administration (FDA). (2011e). *FDA approved drug products: Ambenonium*. Retrieved from http://www.accessdata.fda.gov/ drugsatfda_docs/label/2011/010155s023lbl.pdf

U.S. Food and Drug Administration (FDA). (2011f). *FDA approved drug products: Sotalol*. Retrieved from http://www.accessdata.fda.gov/ drugsatfda_docs/label/2011/019865s020lbl.pdf

U.S. Food and Drug Administration (FDA). (2011g). *FDA approved drug products: Carvedilol*. Retrieved from http://www.accessdata.fda.gov/ drugsatfda_docs/label/2011/020297s036lbl.pdf

U.S. Food and Drug Administration (FDA). (2012). *FDA approved drug products: Clonidine*. Retrieved from http://www.accessdata.fda.gov/ scripts/cder/drugsatfda/index.cfm?fuseaction=Search.Label_Approval History#labelinfo

U.S. Food and Drug Administration (FDA). (2012a). *FDA approved drug products: Silodosin*. Retrieved from http://www.accessdata.fda.gov/ drugsatfda_docs/label/2012/022206s008lbl.pdf

U.S. Food and Drug Administration (FDA). (2012b). *FDA approved drug products: Atenolol.* Retrieved from http://www.accessdata.fda.gov/drugsatfda_docs/label/2012/018240s032lbl.pdf

U.S. Food and Drug Administration (FDA). (2012c). *FDA approved drug products: Guanabenz.* Retrieved from http://www.accessdata.fda.gov/drugsatfda_docs/anda/98/74517_Guanabenz%20Acetate_Prntlbl.pdf

U.S. Food and Drug Administration (FDA). (2012d). *FDA approved drug products: Guanabenz.* Retrieved from http://www.accessdata.fda.gov/drugsatfda_docs/label/2012/202611s000lbl.pdf

U.S. Food and Drug Administration (FDA). (2012e). *FDA approved drug products: Mirabegron.* Retrieved from http://www.accessdata.fda.gov/drugsatfda_docs/label/2013/017963s068lbl.pdf

U.S. Food and Drug Administration (FDA). (2012f). *FDA approved drug products: Auvi-Q.* Retrieved from http://www.accessdata.fda.gov/drugsatfda_docs/label/2012/201739s000lbl.pdf

U.S. Food and Drug Administration (FDA). (2013a). *FDA approved drug products: Guanfacine.* Retrieved from http://www.accessdata.fda.gov/drugsatfda_docs/label/2013/022037s008lbl.pdf

Wendell, R., & Stanley, S. (2013). *Pathogenesis of autoimmune hemolytic anemia: Warm agglutinins and drugs.* In D. S. Basow (Ed.), *UpToDate.* Waltham, Ma: UpToDate.

World Health Organization (WHO). (2009). *Clinical guidelines for withdrawal management and treatment of drug dependence in closed settings.* Retrieved from http://www.wpro.who.int/publications/docs/Clinical Guidelines_forweb.pdf

Yoon, E. Y., Cohn, L., Rocchini, A., Kershaw, D., & Clark, S. J. (2012). Clonidine utilization trends for Medicaid children. *Clinical Pediatrics, 51*(10), 950–955. doi:http://dx.doi.org.ezp.waldenulibrary.org/10.1177/0009922812441661

Young, W., Kaplan, N., & Kebebew, E. (2013) *Treatment of pheochromocytoma in adults.* In D. S. Basow (Ed.), *UpToDate.* Waltham, MA: UpToDate.

CHAPTER 15

DRUGS AFFECTING THE CENTRAL NERVOUS SYSTEM

Teri Moser Woo

This chapter addresses drugs that affect the central nervous system (CNS) in two broad ways: to treat psychiatric conditions and to treat other neurological conditions. Traditionally, drugs to treat psychiatric conditions were developed serendipitously and were identified with the psychiatric diagnosis associated with the responsiveness.

As the neurophysiology of psychiatric symptoms has been researched more deliberately, it has become clear that drugs affect specific neuroreceptors and neurotransmitters in different parts of the brain to bring about a response. The response is not limited to a psychiatric diagnosis because the diagnoses are based not on neurophysiology but on behavioral presentations. Therefore, this chapter will try to make links between the traditional reference to drugs based on diagnoses (e.g., antidepressants) and their pharmacological mechanism of action (e.g., serotonin reuptake inhibitors).

Similarly, because some drugs that originally were used to treat a nonpsychiatric neurological condition have since been found to be useful in treating psychiatric conditions with similar neuropathological mechanisms (e.g., anticonvulsants used to treat mood lability), these drugs may be discussed in more than one section. This is because the brain functions in a very complex fashion but also has neurological redundancy, permitting efficiency in responsiveness.

This chapter focuses on drugs that affect the CNS. In addition, Chapter 29 focuses on drugs to treat anxiety and depressive disorders and Chapter 52 discusses pain management in greater depth. Some redundancy is necessary.

ANOREXIANTS

Anorexiants are short-term adjuncts to calorie-limiting, cognitive-behavioral, weight-loss programs for severely obese individuals. The anorexiants commonly in use today are non-amphetamine appetite suppressants that are chemically and pharmacologically related to amphetamines. In 2011, approximately 2.7 million patients received a prescription for an anti-obesity medication (Borders-Hemphill, U.S. Food and Drug Administration Division of Epidemiology, 2012). These drugs include phentermine (Adipex-P, Ionamin, Suprenza, Obenix, Oby-Cap, Phentercot, and Phentride), benzphetamine (Didrex), diethylpropion HCL (Tenuate), phendimetrazine tartrate (Bontril, Prelu-2, Plegine,), and lorcaserin (Belviq). A unique combination of phentermine and topiramate (Qsymia) is available for chronic weight management. Two formerly used drugs, fenfluramine (Pondimin) and dexfenfluramine (Redux), were removed from the market by the U.S. Food and Drug Administration (FDA) in 1997 because of potentially fatal cardiac and pulmonary adverse reactions. In October 2010, the FDA asked that the manufacturer voluntarily withdraw sibutramine (Meridia) from the U.S. market due to cardiovascular side effects.

Pharmacodynamics

Anorexiants are sympathomimetic amines and are thought to exert their action by stimulation of satiety centers in the hypothalamus and limbic region. They act through noradrenergic, dopaminergic, or serotonergic pathways. Lorcaserin promotes satiety by selectively activating 5-HT_{2C} receptors in the hypothalamus. The exact mechanism of action of topiramate in the combination of phentermine and topiramate is not known, although topiramate is known to cause appetite suppression and satiety.

Pharmacokinetics

Absorption and Distribution

After oral administration, anorexiants are absorbed in the stomach and small intestine, depending on whether they are in regular or extended-release form. They are lipid-soluble, widely distributed, and cross the blood–brain barrier. Diethylpropion and its metabolites cross the placental barrier and are Pregnancy Category C.

Metabolism and Excretion

Anorexiants are metabolized in the liver and excreted through the kidneys. Duration of action is 4 to 6 hours in the regular form and longer in extended-release forms. Half-lives vary from 8 to 20 hours.

Table 15-1 presents the pharmacokinetics of anorexiants.

Pharmacotherapeutics

Precautions and Contraindications

Anorexiants carry a high risk of tolerance and dependence, both physical and psychological, and they should be used cautiously with patients who have known histories of alcohol or drug dependence because of the high risk of cross-tolerance. Actively drinking alcoholics taking anorexiants have experienced depression, paranoia, and psychosis. Use of anorexiants should be limited to a maximum period of 6 months and discontinued at any sign of tolerance. Anorexiant use is contraindicated in patients who abuse substances such as cocaine, phencyclidine, and methamphetamine because of the potential for excessive adrenergic stimulation. Patients with diabetes may experience altered insulin or oral hypoglycemic dosage requirements.

Lorcaserin is a serotonergic drug, and patients may develop serotonin syndrome or Neuroleptic Malignant Syndrome-like reactions if coadministered with serotonergic

Table 15–1 ⠿ Pharmacokinetics: Anorexiants

Drug	Onset	Peak	Duration	Half-Life	Excretion
Phendimetrazine tartrate	—	—	4–6 h	1.9–9.8 h	Urine
Benzphetamine	—	—	4–6 h	—	Urine
Diethylpropion HCI	—	—	4–6 h	—	Urine
Phentermine	—	—	4–6 h	—	Urine
Lorcaserin		1.5–2 h		11h	Urine

drugs. Lorcaserin is Pregnancy Category X and is not approved in children under 18 years of age.

Adverse Drug Reactions

Adverse reactions to anorexiants include CNS overstimulation and agitation, confusion, insomnia, dizziness, hypertension, headache, palpitations, arrhythmias, dry mouth, mydriasis, dysuria, constipation, vomiting, diarrhea, and impotence. Patients taking high doses of anorexiants over a long period may experience dizziness, fatigue, and depression if the drug is suddenly withdrawn.

The most common adverse reactions to lorcaserin are headache, dizziness, fatigue, nausea, dry mouth, and constipation. Development of valvular heart disease has been reported with a slightly greater incidence (2.4% versus 2.0%) of valvular regurgitation noted over patients taking a placebo (Arena Pharmaceuticals GmbH, 2012). Cognitive impairment has been reported in 1.95% of patients in clinical trials (versus 0.5% for placebo). Potential adverse effects of lorcaserin include psychiatric disorders (euphoria, hallucination, and dissociation), potential risk of hypoglycemia in patients with type 2 diabetes mellitus on antidiabetic therapy, priapism, prolactin elevation, and hematological changes (leukopenia, lymphopenia, neutropenia, and decreased white blood cell count).

Drug Interactions

The potential exists for hypertensive crisis with coadministration of anorexiants and MAO inhibitors. Anorexiants may elevate serotonin levels and should not be prescribed to patients on other serotonergic agents because of the increased risk of serotonin syndrome (hyperthermia, agitation, restlessness, confusion, ataxia, myoclonus, tremor, rigidity, tachycardia, hypotension or hypertension, diaphoresis). The actions of adrenergic blockers, insulin, sulfonylureas, and phenothiazines may be antagonized during concomitant administration of anorexiants. Table 15-2 presents drug interactions.

Based on its pharmacologic mechanism of action on the serotonin 2C receptor, locaserin should be used with extreme caution with other drugs that work on serotonin, including triptans, MAOIs, including linezolid, an antibiotic which is a reversible nonselective MAOI; SSRIs; SNRIs; dextromethorphan; tricyclic antidepressants (TCAs), bupropion, lithium, tramadol, tryptophan, and St. John's wort (Arena Pharmaceuticals GmbH, 2012). Locaserin should also be used cautiously with drugs that are CYP 2D6 substrates because locaserin may increase exposure to the interacting drug.

Clinical Use and Dosing

Anorexiants are indicated for the treatment of morbid exogenous obesity in conjunction with a calorie-restrictive diet. The course of treatment should last no longer than 6 months. An alternative method of dosing is to use the drug for a few weeks followed by no drug for a period, suggested to be half the length of time with the drug, followed by reinstitution of the drug for a few more weeks. Evening dosing should be avoided because of the likelihood of insomnia. Lorcaserin may be administered in the evening as it is not a stimulant and should not affect sleep. Table 15-3 presents the dosage schedule and available dosage forms for anorexiants.

Rational Drug Selection

Significant increases in blood pressure, palpitations, and arrhythmias can occur with phentermine; thus, use is not advisable in hypertensive clients or those with cardiovascular disease. Diethylpropion causes less insomnia than does phentermine. Diethylpropion is considered one of the safest noradrenergic appetite suppressants and may be used in patients with mild to moderate hypertension or angina pectoris.

ANTICONVULSANTS

Seizures are the result of the abnormal discharge of neurons. Anything that disrupts the stability of the neuron may

Table 15–2 ⠿ Drug Interactions: Anorexiants

Drug	Interacting Drug	Possible Effect	Implications
All anorexiants	MAOIs	Hypertensive crisis	Do not prescribe during or within 14 d of use of MAOI
	Alcohol	CNS depression	Abstain from alcohol use
	Phenothiazines	Psychosis	Monitor for increased psychotic symptoms
	Insulin, sulfonylureas	Altered requirements	Monitor blood glucose
	Guanethidine	Antagonization of effect	Monitor for increased blood pressure
	Furazolidone	Serotonin syndrome	Monitor for symptoms of syndrome
Lorcaserin	Drugs that affect serotonin (triptans, MAOIs, linezolid, SSRIs, SNRIs, dextromethorphan, TCAs, bupropion, lithium, tramadol, tryptophan, and St. John's wort	Increased potential for serotonin syndrome	Use with extreme caution

Table 15–3 ⊗ Dosage Schedule: Anorexiants

Drug	Indications	Dosage	Available Dosage Forms
Benzphetamine (Didrex)	Short-term adjunctive treatment of exogenous obesity	25–50 mg daily; max 50 mg tid Not approved for children	Tablets: 50 mg, scored tablets
Diethylpropion (Tenuate, Tenuate Dospan)	Short-term adjunctive treatment of exogenous obesity	25 mg tid ac* or prn if needed; sustained-release: 75 mg q a.m.	Tablets: 25 mg Sustained-release: 75 mg
Phendimetrazine tartrate (Bontril PDM, Prelu-2)	Short-term adjunctive treatment of exogenous obesity	35 mg bid or tid 1 h ac; sustained-release: 105 mg daily 30–60 min before breakfast *Not for children*	Tablets: 35 mg Capsules: 35 mg Sustained-release: 105 mg
Phentermine (Zantryl, Adipex-P, Ionamin)	Short-term adjunctive treatment of exogenous obesity	*Adults*: 8 mg tid, 30 minutes ac or 15–37.5 mg daily before breakfast or 10–14 h before bedtime	Tablets: 8 mg, 30 mg, 37.5 mg Capsules: 15 mg, 30 mg, 37.5 mg
Lorcaserin (Belviq)	Adjunct to a reduced-calorie diet and increased physical activity for chronic weight management in adult patients	10 mg bid	10 mg tablets

*ac = *ante cibum* (before meals).

trigger abnormal activity and seizures. Many factors can precipitate seizures, including hyperventilation, sleep deprivation, sensory stimuli, emotional stress, and hormonal changes. Some drugs with anticonvulsant properties are increasingly being used in the treatment of mood disorders and will be discussed in that section of this chapter (e.g., valproates, gabapentin, lamotrigine). Phenobarbital, used to treat seizure disorders, will be discussed with sedative-hypnotics later in this chapter. Benzodiazepines, also used to treat seizures, will be discussed with anxiolytic drugs. Three major classes of antiepileptic drugs (AEDs), the hydantoins, iminostilbenes, and succinimides, are discussed here.

HYDANTOINS

The hydantoins—phenytoin (Dilantin), ethotoin (Peganone), and fosphenytoin (Cerebyx)—are the first-line treatment of choice for tonic-clonic and partial complex seizures and the least sedating drugs used to treat seizure disorders of any type. Phenytoin is the most commonly used.

Pharmacodynamics

Hydantoins inhibit and stabilize electrical discharges in the motor cortex of the brain by affecting the influx of sodium ions into the neuron during depolarization and repolarization, slowing the propagation and spread of abnormal discharges. They also affect the brainstem's contribution to grand mal seizures and have antiarrhymic properties.

Pharmacokinetics

Absorption and Distribution

The usual route of administration is oral. Absorption occurs in the small intestine and is slow, although the rate varies with the form of the drug. Hydantoins enter the brain quickly, and are then redistributed to other body tissues, saliva, and breast milk. The rate and degree of absorption from intramuscular (IM) administration is erratic, generally resulting in lower plasma levels than the oral route. Hydantoins are 87% to 93% protein bound. The therapeutic plasma level range is 10 to 20 mcg/mL and correlates well with treatment effect.

Metabolism and Excretion

Metabolism of hydantoins takes place in the liver; excretion, via the kidneys. Plasma half-lives range from 6 to 24 hours.

Table 15-4 presents the pharmacokinetics of hydantoins.

Pharmacotherapeutics

Precautions and Contraindications

Hydantoins are contraindicated under conditions of hypersensitivity. Phenytoin-induced hepatitis is a common hypersensitivity reaction. Other hypersensitivity reactions include fever, rash, arthralgias, and lymphadenopathy. Phenytoin may cause severe cardiovascular events and death has resulted from too-rapid IV administration. Phenytoin has a Black-Box Warning that IV administration should not exceed 50 mg/minute in adults and 1 to 3 mg/kg/minute in pediatric patients owing to risk of cardiovascular reactions associated with a too rapid rate of administration. Phenytoin is contraindicated in sinus bradycardia, sinoatrial block, second- and

Table 15–4 ❖ **Pharmacokinetics: Antiepileptic Drugs**

Drug	Onset	Peak	Duration	Half-Life	Excretion
Hydantoins					
Ethotoin (Peganone)	Rapidly absorbed	—	4–6 h	3–9 h	Urine
Fosphenytoin (Cerebyx)	—	—	—	12–29 h	Urine
Phenytoin (Dilantin)	Slow	4–12 h (extended) 1.5–3 h (rapid)	5 h	22 h	Urine
Iminostilbenes					
Carbamazepine		4–8 h Chronic use: 1.5 h		25–65 h Multiple dosing *Children:* 8–14 h *Adults:* 12–17h	Urine
Oxcarbazepine		4.5 h		2 h Metabolite 9 h	Urine
Succinimides					
Ethosuximide		2–4 h		Children 30 h *Adults:* 50–60h	Urine Small amounts in feces
Methsuximide	Rapid	1–4h		2.6–4h	Urine
Drugs That Affect GABA					
Gabapentin	—	2–2.5 h		*Adults:* 2.5–3.5 h Children 9 mo–12 y: 2.4 h Neonates: 2.4 h	80% to 90% excreted unchanged in urine
Tiagabine	Rapid Food slows absorption	45 min		7–9 h Patients on enzyme-inducing AEDs: 2–5 h	Urine 25% Feces 63%
Topiramate	Rapid	2 h			Urine
Lamotrigine		1.7–2.2		25.4–35.8h	Renal

third-degree atrioventricular block, and Stokes–Adams syndrome. It should be used cautiously in patients with hepatic or renal disease. Ethotoin is contraindicated in the presence of hepatic or hematological disorders.

Although fetal defects have been associated with use of hydantoins during pregnancy and it is classified as Pregnancy Category D, the overall risk of malformations in children exposed to phenytoin during pregnancy is 10%. Pregnant women who take phenytoin can decrease the risks to the fetus by taking 400 international units (IU) of folic acid per day. Some women with epilepsy have fewer seizures during pregnancy; in others, the risks to the woman who goes without the drug may outweigh any risks to the fetus. Hydantoins are present in breast milk; their safety during lactation has not been established.

Newborns who have been exposed to phenytoin in utero may experience decreased levels of vitamin K-dependent clotting factors, and it is critical that the mother receive vitamin K before delivery and that the newborn receives vitamin K at birth.

Rebound status epilepticus may result from abrupt discontinuation of these drugs. Phenytoin has a narrow therapeutic range and older adults or those with impaired liver function may manifest signs of toxicity at lower-than-usual doses. Use cautiously in patients with myocardial insufficiency and hypotension.

Adverse Drug Reactions

Possible adverse effects are multiple and may include CNS effects such as agitation, ataxia, confusion, dizziness, drowsiness, headache, and nystagmus; cardiovascular effects such as hypotension, tachycardia, atrial and ventricular conduction depression, and ventricular fibrillation; gastrointestinal (GI) effects such as nausea, vomiting, anorexia, altered taste, constipation, dry mouth, and gingival hyperplasia; and genitourinary effects such as urinary retention and reddish brown discoloration of the urine. Serious dermatologic reactions, including Stevens–Johnson syndrome and toxic epidermal necrolysis may occur. Other possible adverse effects include skin rashes (scarlatiniform or morbilliform), hyperglycemia, tinnitus, gynecomastia, coarsening of facial features and enlargement of the lips, hematopoietic changes, photophobia, and polyarthropathy.

Drug Interactions

Drug interactions consist of those that either increase or decrease the effect of the hydantoin and those that decrease the effect of the other drug. Interactions that increase hydantoin's effect because of increased metabolism, competition for binding sites, or for unknown reasons occur with benzodiazepines, cimetidine, disulfiram, tricyclic antidepressants, salicylates, and valproic acid. Conversely, interactions that decrease hydantoin's effect include barbiturates, rifampin, theophylline, influenza vaccine, pyridoxine, and antacids. Acute acohol intake may increase phenytoin serum levels, whereas chronic alcohol use may decrease levels. IV phenytoin should only be mixed with normal saline and should not be mixed with dextrose-containing IV solutions because a precipitate may form.

Concurrent administration causes the decreased effect of carbamazepine, estrogens, corticosteroids, haloperidol, methadone, levodopa, sulfonylureas, oral contraceptives, and cardiac glycosides.

Table 15-5 presents drug interactions.

Table 15–5 ▦ Drug Interactions: Hydantoins (Anticonvulsants

Drug	Interacting Drug	Possible Effect	Implications
All hydantoins	Allopurinol, cimetidine, diazepam, disulfiram, alcohol (acute intake), phenacemide, succinimides, valproic acid	Increased plasma level of hydantoins	May need to decrease hydantoin dose; monitor plasma level
	Barbiturates, carbamazepine, alcohol (chronic use), theophylline, antacids, calcium	Decreased plasma level of hydantoins	May need to increase hydantoin dose; monitor plasma level
	Corticosteroids, dicumarol, digitoxin, doxycycline, haloperidol, methadone, oral contraceptives, dopamine, furosemide, levodopa	Decreased effect of interacting drug	Monitor plasma levels where possible; monitor signs and symptoms
Iminostilbenes			
Carbamazepine	CYP 3A4 inhibitors: cimetidine, danazol, diltiazem, macrolides, erythromycin, troleandomycin, clarithromycin, fluoxetine, fluvoxamine, nefazodone, trazodone, loxapine, olanzapine, quetiapine, loratadine, terfenadine, omeprazole, oxybutynin, dantrolene, isoniazid, niacinamide, nicotinamide, ibuprofen, azoles (e.g., ketaconazole, itraconazole, fluconazole, voriconazole), acetazolamide, verapamil, ticlopidine, grapefruit juice, protease inhibitors, valproate	CYP 3A4 inhibitors inhibit carbamazepine metabolism and can thus increase plasma carbamazepine levels	
	CYP 3A4 inducers: cisplatin, doxorubicin HCl, felbamate, fosphenytoin, rifampin, phenobarbital, phenytoin, primidone, methsuximide, theophylline, aminophylline	CYP 3A4 inducers can increase the rate of carbamazepine metabolism leading to decreased plasma carbamazepine levels	
Oxcarbazepine	Carbamazepine, phenobarbital, phenytoin, valproic acid	Decreased oxcarbazepine levels	
Succinimides			
Ethosuximide	Phenytoin Valproic acid	Elevated phenytoin levels Increased or decreased ethosuximide levels	
Methsuximide	Carbamazepine, hydantoins (e.g., phenytoin) Lamotrigine	Methsuximide plasma concentrations may be reduced	

Table 15–5 ▦ Drug Interactions: Hydantoins (Anticonvulsants)—cont'd

Drug	Interacting Drug	Possible Effect	Implications
	Phenobarbital, primidone	Plasma concentrations of the active metabolite of primidone, phenobarbital, may be elevated by methsuximide	
Drugs That Affect GABA			
Gabapentin	No significant drug interaction		
Tagabine	Bupropion, gemfibrozil	Tiagabine plasma concentrations may be increased	
	Enzyme-inducing antiepileptic drugs (e.g., carbamazepine, phenobarbital, phenytoin, primidone)	Tiagabine clearance may be increased	
Topiramate	Phenytoin Ethinyl estradiol	Decreased plasma concentrations of Topiramate	
	Carbamazepine	Decreased ethinyl estradiol levels	
	Carbonic anhydrase inhibitors (e.g., zonisamide, acetazolamide, or dichlorphenamide)	May increase the severity of metabolic acidosis and may also increase the risk of kidney stone formation	If topiramate is given concomitantly with another carbonic anhydrase inhibitor, the patient should be monitored for the appearance or worsening of metabolic acidosis
Levetiracetam	No significant drug interactions		
Lamotrigine	Estrogen-containing oral contraceptive preparations containing 30 mcg ethinylestradiol and 150 mcg levonorgestrel Carbamazepine, Phenobarbital/Primidone, Phenytoin, Rifampin	Decreased lamotragine levels Decreased levonorgestcrel levels Decreased lamotrigine levels	Decreased lamotrigine levels approximately 50% Decrease in levonorgestrel component by 19%
	Valproate	Increased lamotragine levels	Decreased lamotrigine concentration approximately 40% Increased lamotrigine concentrations slightly more than 2-fold

Clinical Use and Dosing

Table 15-6 presents the indications and dosage schedules of hydantoins.

Rational Drug Selection

Hydantoins are used for the treatment of grand mal and psychomotor seizures. Phenytoin, however, may worsen absence seizures. Hydantoins are not the first-line treatment of status epilepticus, but IV phenytoin can be used for the control of grand mal types of seizures. Fosphenytoin is used for short-term (less than 5 days) management of seizures when oral use is not feasible. Ethotoin is dosed in 4 to 6 doses a day with food, spaced as evenly as possible, which may be a complex regimen for some patients.

Monitoring

Patients should be assessed for phenytoin hypersensitivity syndrome (fever, skin rash, lymphadenopathy), which usually occurs at 3 to 8 weeks. Baseline complete blood count, urinalysis, and liver function tests should be assessed prior to onset of treatment, with frequent reassessment during the first few months of treatment.

Plasma levels should be monitored, especially when drugs that increase plasma hydantoin, such as ibuprofen, are used. As well, other drugs that are negatively affected by concurrent administration with hydantoins may also require monitoring of the plasma level. Phenytoin may alter thyroid hormone demand, which may require monitoring.

Patients started on hydantoins or any AED should be monitored for suicidality (suicidal thoughts, depression, behavior changes).

Patient Education

The patient should be instructed to take the medication exactly as directed and to avoid missing doses. Abrupt withdrawal may lead to status epilepticus. Advise the patient to

Table 15–6 ⊗ Dosage Schedule: Selected Anticonvulsants

Drug	Indications	Dosage	Available Dosage Forms
Ethotoin (Peganone)	Generalized tonic-clonic or psychomotor seizures	*Adults:* Initially 1 g/d or less in 4–6 divided doses, spaced as evenly as possible, taken after food; increase gradually to usual maintenance dose of 2–3 g/d *Children:* Initial maximum dose of 750 mg/d in divided doses as with adult; usual maintenance dose of 500–1,000 mg/d	*Tablets:* 250 mg
Fosphenytoin (Cerebyx)	Status epilepticus	IV loading dose: 15–20 mg PE/kg diluted in 5% dextrose or 0.9% saline solution at rate of 100–150 mg PE/min (PE: phenytoin sodium equivalent units) Other measures such as IV diazepam will be needed Nonemergent loading dose and maintenance: loading dose 10–20 mg PE/kg IV or IM; maintenance 4–6 mg PE/kg/d at rate of 150 mg PE/min or less *Children:* usual range 100–400 mg/d	Solution for injection: 100 mg/2 mL, 500 mg/10 mL
Phenytoin (Dilantin)	Generalized tonic-clonic, psychomotor, and simple partial seizures; status epilepticus	*Adults:* Initial PO dose 1 g in 3 divided doses, then after 24 h, 300 mg/d in 1 dose (extended-release); IV loading dose of 10–15 mg/kg at rate of 50 mg/min; maintenance dose of 100 mg PO or IV every 6–8 h *Children:* 4–8 mg/kg/d PO in divided doses; 15–20 mg/kg IV at rate of 50 mg/min	*Chewable tablets:* 50 mg *Suspension:* *Extended-Release Capsules:* 30 mg, 100 mg, 200 mg, 300 mg *Injection:* 50 mg/mL

Drugs That Affect GABA

Drug	Indications	Dosage	Available Dosage Forms
Gabapentin (Neurontin) (Gralise) Gabapentin enaccarbil (Horizant)	Epilepsy	*Adults and children >12 yr:* The starting dose is 300 mg tid. The dose may be increased using 300 or 400 mg capsules, or 600 or 800 mg tablets tid up to 1,800 mg/day. Dosages up to 2,400 mg/ day have been well tolerated in long-term clinical studies. The maximum time between doses in the tid schedule should not exceed 12 h. *Children 3–12 yr:* The starting dose should range from 10–15 mg/kg/d in 3 divided doses, and the effective dose reached by upward titration over a period of approximately 3 d. The effective dose of gabapentin in patients 5 yr of age and older is 25–35 mg/kg/d and given in divided doses (tid). The effective dose in pediatric patients ages 3 and 4 yr is 40 mg/kg/d and given in divided doses (tid). Dosages up to 50 mg/kg/d have been well tolerated in a long-term clinical study. The maximum time interval between doses should not exceed 12 hr.	*Capsules:* 100 mg, 300 mg, 400 mg *Oral solution:* 50 mg/mL *Tablets:* 300 mg, 600 mg *Extended-release tablet:* 300 mg, 600 mg
	Postherpetic neuralgia	*Adults:* Therapy is initiated as a single 300 mg dose on day 1, 600 mg/d on day 2 (divided bid), and 900 mg/d on day 3 (divided tid). The dose can subsequently be titrated up as needed for pain relief to a daily dose of 1,800 mg (divided tid).	
Tiagabine (Gabitril)	Adjunctive therapy in adults and children 12 yr and older in the treatment of partial seizures	*Enzyme-induced adults and adolescents >12 yr:* Week 1: 4 mg q day Week 2: Increase dose by 4 mg/d, to 8 mg/d divided bid Week 3: Increase dose by 4 mg/d, to 12 mg/d divided tid Week 4: Increase dose by 4–16 mg/day divided bid or qid Week 5: Increase dose by 4–8 mg/day, to 20–24 mg/day divided bid or qid Week 6: Increase dose 4 mg/d, to 24–32 mg/d divided bid or qid Usual adult maintenance dose in induced patients: 32–56 mg/day divided bid or qid	*Tablets:* 2 mg, 4 mg, 12 mg, 16 mg
Topiramate (Topamax)	Monotherapy for epilepsy	*Adults and children ≥10 yr:* Week 1: 25 mg bid Week 2: 50 mg bid	*Tablets:* 25 mg, 50 mg, 100 mg, 200 mg *Sprinkle capsules:* 15 mg, 25 mg

Table 15–6 ⊗ **Dosage Schedule: Selected Anticonvulsants—cont'd**

Drug	Indications	Dosage	Available Dosage Forms
		Week 3: 75 mg bid Week 4: 100 mg bid Week 5: 150 mg bid Week 6: 200 mg bid	
	Adjunctive therapy for epilepsy, partial seizures, Lennox–Gastaut syndrome	*Adults age ≥17 yr:* Initial dose: 25–50 mg/d, titrate dose in 25–50 mg/d increments in weekly intervals to a dose of 200–400 mg/d *Pediatric patients (age 1 to 16 yr):* Initial dose of 1–3 mg/kg/d (max 25 mg) for a week. Dosage is increased by 1–3 mg/kg/d in 1–2 wk intervals. The dose is divided in bid dosing. The total recommended daily dose is 5–9 mg/kg/d. Dose titration is guided by clinical response.	
	Migraine prophylaxis	Week 1: 25 mg in p.m. Week 2 25 mg bid Week 3: 25 mg in a.m., 50 mg in p.m. Week 4: 50 mg bid The recommended dosage for migraine prophylaxis is 100 mg/d.	
Levetiracetam (Keppra) (Keppra XR)	Partial onset seizures	*Adults and adolescents ≥16 yr:* Initial dose 500 mg bid. Increase dose in increments of 1,000 mg/d every 2 wk until a maximum of 3,000 mg/d divided bid. *Children 4 yr to < 16 yr:* Initial dose 20 mg/kg in 2 divided doses (10 mg/kg bid). Increase dose every 2 wk by 20 mg/kg to the recommended daily dose of 60 mg/kg/d.	*Tablets:* 250 mg, 500 mg, 750 mg, 1,000 mg *Liquid:* 100 mg/mL *Extended-release tablet:* 500 mg, 750 mg
	Myoclonic seizures in patients ≥12 yr with juvenile myoclonic epilepsy	Initial dose of 1,000 mg/d (500 mg bid). Increase dose by 1,000 mg/d every 2 wk to the recommended dose of 3,000 mg/d.	
	Primary generalized tonic-clonic seizures	*Adults >16 yr:* Initial dose 1,000 mg/d divided bid (500 mg bid). Increase dose 1,000 mg/d every 2 wk to the recommended dose of 3,000 mg/d. *Pediatric patients age 6 yr to < 16 yr:* Initial dose 20 mg/kg/d divided bid (10 mg/kg bid). Increase dose 20 mg/kg/d every 2 wk to the recommended daily dose of 60 mg/kg/d divided bid.	
Lamotrigine (Lamictal) (Lamictal XR)	Epilepsy therapy in patients not taking enzyme-inducing AEDs	*Adults and children ≥12 yr:* Weeks 1 and 2: 25 mg/d Weeks 3 and 4: 50 mg/d Week 5: 100 mg/d Increase dose by 50 mg per day every 1–2 wk until the usual maintenance dose of 225–375 mg per day in 2 divided doses. *Children 2 yr to 12 yr:* Weeks 1 and 2: 0.3 mg/kg/d in 1 or 2 divided doses. The dosage should be rounded down to the nearest whole tablet and tablets should not be cut. Weeks 3 and 4: 0.6 mg/kg/d in 2 divided doses rounded down to the nearest whole tablet. Starting in week 5 the dose is increased every 1–2 wk by calculating 0.6 mg/kg/d; round this amount down to the nearest whole tablet and add this amount to the previously administered daily dose. The dose is titrated to effect, with an average daily dose of 4.5–7.5 mg/kg/d. Maintenance dose may need to be increased by as much as 50% in children who weigh less than 30 kg.	*Tablets:* 25 mg, 100 mg, 150 mg, 200 mg *Chewable tablets:* 2 mg, 5 mg, 25 mg *Orally disintegrating tablets (ODT):* 25 mg, 50 mg, 100 mg, 200 mg *Extended-release tablets:* 25 mg, 50 mg, 200 mg, 300 mg
	Patients taking enzyme-inducing AEDs (not valproate)	*Adults and children ≥12 yr:* Weeks 1 and 2: 50 mg/d Weeks 3 and 4: 100 mg/d in 2 divided doses	

Continued

Table 15–6 ⊗ Dosage Schedule: Selected Anticonvulsants—cont'd

Drug	Indications	Dosage	Available Dosage Forms
		Beginning in week 5 the dose is increased by 100 mg/d every 1–2 wk to the usual maintenance dose of 300–500 mg/d in 2 divided doses. *Pediatric patients 2 yr to 12 yr:* Weeks 1 and 2: 0.6 mg/kg/d in 2 divided doses, rounded down to the nearest whole tablet Weeks 3 and 4: 1.2 mg/kg/d in 2 divided doses, rounded down to the nearest whole tablet Beginning in week 5 the dose is increased by 1.2 mg/kg/d, rounded down to the nearest whole tablet and added to the previously administered daily dose. The usual daily maintenance dose is 5–15 mg/kg/d, with a maximum of 400 mg per day in 2 divided doses. The maintenance dose of lamotrigine may need to be increased by as much as 50% in children who weigh less than 30 kg.	
	Patients taking valproate	*Adults and children >12 yr:* Weeks 1 to 4: 25 mg per day Beginning in week 5 the dosage is increased 25–50 mg/d every 1–2 wk. The usual maintenance dose of lamotrigine in patients taking valproate alone is 100–200 mg/d. If patients are taking valproate and other drugs that induce glucuronidation, the usual maintenance dose is 100–400 mg/d. *Children age 2 yr to 12 yr:* Weeks 1 and 2: 0.15 mg/kg/d in 1 or 2 divided doses, rounded down to the nearest whole tablet. Children that weigh more than 6.7 kg and less than 14 kg 2 mg: every other day. Weeks 3 and 4: 0.3 mg/kg/d in 1 or 2 divided doses, rounded down to the nearest whole tablet. Week 5: Calculate 0.3 mg/kg/d and round this amount down to the nearest whole tablet and add this amount to the previously administered daily dose. The usual maintenance dose in children taking valproate is 1–5 mg/d with a maximum of 200 mg/d. The maintanence dose of lamotrigine may need to be increased by as much as 50% in children who weigh less than 30 kg.	
	Bipolar disease	*Adult patients with bipolar disorder not taking enzyme-inducing AEDs or valproate:* Weeks 1 and 2: 25 mg/d Weeks 3 and 4: 50 mg/d Week 5: 100 mg/d Week 6: 200 mg/d, which is the maintenance dose of lamotrigine *Adults taking enzyme-inducing AEDs (carbamazepine, phenytoin, phenobarbital or primidone) and not taking valproate:* Weeks 1 and 2: 50 mg/d Weeks 3 and 4: 100 mg/d in divided doses Week 5: 200 mg/d Week 6: 300 mg/d divided bid Week 7: 400 mg/d in divided doses *Adults with bipolar disease valproate:* Week 1 and 2: 25 mg every other day Weeks 3 and 4: 25 mg/d Week 5: 50 mg/d Week 6: Increase to the maintenance dose of 100 mg/d	
	Women taking oral contraceptives	Oral estrogen-containing contraceptives decrease lamotrigine levels by approximately 50%. If the patient is already taking lamotrigine and an oral contraceptive is started, the lamotrigine dose is increased 50 mg/d weekly. The lamotrigine dose may need to be twice the normal dose.	

wear a medical identification bracelet, to avoid hazardous situations if drowsiness occurs, and to report adverse effects to the clinician. Patients should avoid alcohol use while taking a hydantoin. Advise the patient to maintain good oral hygiene to prevent tenderness, bleeding, and gingival hyperplasia. Inform the patient that phenytoin may color the urine pink, red, or reddish brown but that this color change is not a cause for alarm. Advise diabetic patients to monitor blood glucose levels and report significant changes to the clinician.

IMINOSTILBENES

Carbamazepine (Tegretol) and oxcarbazepine (Trileptal, Oxtellar XR) are iminostilbene derivatives structurally related to TCAs. They are used to treat epilepsy, bipolar affective disorder, aggressive and assaultive behavior, and some neuralgias.

Pharmacodynamics

The exact mechanism of action of carbamazepine and oxcarbazepine is not known, but they are thought to affect the sodium channels, slowing influx of sodium in the cortical neurons and slowing the spread of abnormal activity. Carbamazepine exerts its effect by depressing transmission in the nucleus ventralis anterior of the thalamus. This area is associated with the spread of seizure discharge. Other actions not explained by effects on sodium channels include anticholinergic, antidiuretic, antidysrhythmic, and antidepressant activity.

Absorption and Distribution

Carbamazepine is absorbed through the stomach, the suspension being absorbed more quickly than the tablet form. Absorption from immediate-release tablets is slow and erratic because of its low water solubility. The drug is highly lipophilic, resulting in high body tissue binding. Oxcarbazepine is well absorbed after oral administration and is 67% protein bound, with its active metabolite 40% bound.

Metabolism and Excretion

Carbamazepine is metabolized in the liver and has the unique ability to induce its own metabolism (autoinduction). Due to autoinduction, initial concentrations within a therapeutic range may later fall despite good compliance. It also induces the metabolism of many CYP450 enzymes and other substrates. Excretion is through urine and feces.

Oxcarbazepine is metabolized into an active metabolite 10-monohydroxy metabolite, which is responsible for the pharmacologic effect of the drug. The metabolites of oxcarbazepine are excreted 95% in the urine, 4% in the feces, and 1% as unmetabolized oxcarbazepine. Oxcarbazepine does not autoinduce metabolism.

Onset, Peak, and Duration

Average peak blood levels of carbamazepine occur approximately 6 hours after administration. Half-life can be as long as 65 hours with initial dosing, but is typically 12 to 17 hours as administration continues. It is noteworthy that the half-life after a single dose is much longer than the half-life after long-term use. Steady state is attained in 2 to 4 days.

Oxcarbazepine peaks 3 to 13 hours (median 4.5 hours) after ingesting tablets and 6 hours after administration in suspension. Food has no effect on rate of absorption or time to peak. The half-life of oxcarbazepine is 2 hours, but its active metabolite has a half-life of 9 hours. Half-life is prolonged to 19 hours in patients with renal impairment.

Pharmacotherapeutics

Precautions and Contraindications

Contraindications include hypersensitivity to carbamazepine or TCAs, history of bone marrow suppression, and concurrent administration with MAOIs. Carbamazepine is Pregnancy Category D; teratogenic defects have occurred, including spina bifida. It is excreted in human milk but is not contraindicated during lactation.

Oxcarbazepine is Pregnancy Category C; it crosses the placenta and adverse effects have been noted in animal studies, but no well-designed human studies have been done. It is recommended that pregnant patients taking oxcarbazepine (Trileptal) be enrolled in the NAAED Pregnancy Registry (1-888-233-2334 or http://www.aedpregnancyregistry.org).

Carbamazepine has a Black-Box Warning regarding serious dermatological reactions, particularly among patients of Asian ethnicity. (Stevens–Johnson syndrome and toxic epidermal necrolysis) and the risk of developing aplastic anemia and agranulocytosis. Patients of Asian ethnicity should be screened for the presence of the HLA-B*1502 genetic variant prior to starting carbamazepine. Use with caution in patients with increased intraocular pressure because of its mild anticholinergic effects. Caution is also advised in patients with a history of previous adverse hematological reactions to any drugs and in those with cardiac, renal, or hepatic impairment.

The only contraindication to oxcarbazepine is hypersensitivity to oxcarbazepine.

Adverse Drug Reactions

Carbamazepine has a Black Box warning regarding the development of Stevens-Johnson Syndrome (SJS) and toxic epidermal necrolysis (TEN) in patients of Chinese ethnicity (1 to 6 per 1000) versus patients of caucasian ethnicity (1 to 6 per 10,000). There is a strong association with the HLA-B*1502 allele variant and the development of SJS/TEN. Patients from Asian countries are more likely to have the HLA-B*1502 variant and should be screened for the presence of HLA-B*1502 prior to beginning carbamazepine.

Carbamazepine has a Black-Box Warning due to its potential to cause blood dyscrasias, some potentially lethal. Although a transient decrease of the white blood cell count can occur and is manageable, carbamazepine can depress the bone marrow and lead to leukopenia, thrombocytopenia, agranulocytosis, and aplastic anemia. For that reason, a baseline blood screen that includes a complete blood count (CBC), chemistry, liver function tests, and thyroid-stimulating hormone (TSH) test should be obtained, followed by periodic monitoring. Follow-up studies should be more frequent initially, decreasing to every 3 to 4 months if the results remain normal or the CBC and differential are only minimally lowered.

Other adverse reactions to carbamazepine include hepatic damage and impaired thyroid function. Less serious early adverse events may include drowsiness, dizziness, blurred vision, ataxia, nausea, vomiting, dry mouth, diplopia, and headache.

The most common adverse effects (5% or greater incidence) observed in patients taking oxcarbazepine were dizziness, diplopia, somnolence, fatigue, nausea, vomiting, ataxia, abdominal pain, tremor, and dyspepsia. Hyponatremia (serum sodium less than 125 mEq/L) may occur, particularly in the first 3 months of therapy. Pediatric patients experienced effects similar to those of adults.

Drug Interactions

The interactions of most significance are those that increase the plasma level of carbamazepine to potentially toxic levels, such as the concurrent administration of propoxyphene, hydantoins, cimetidine, some antibiotics (erythromycin, clarithromycin), isoniazid, and verapamil. Interactions that can result in hepatic damage occur with coadministration of some anesthetics and with isoniazid. Interactions that decrease plasma levels of the other drug occur with beta blockers, succinimides, valproic acid, warfarin, haloperidol, doxycycline, and nondepolarizing muscle relaxants. Grapefruit juice increases serum levels and effects of carbamazepine.

Oxcarbazepine can inhibit CYP2C19 and induce CYP3A4/5, leading to increased levels of drugs metabolized by CYP2C19. Oxcarbazeine may decrease the effectiveness of hormonal contraceptives containing ethinylestradiol and levonorgestrel.

Table 15-7 presents drug interactions.

Clinical Use and Dosing

Table 15-8 presents the indications, dosage schedules, and available dosage forms of carbamazepine.

Rational Drug Selection

Carbamazepine is indicated in the treatment of partial complex seizures. It is also useful for generalized tonic-clonic seizures. Its relative lack of side effects compared to phenytoin and phenobarbital has resulted in increased use for a variety of seizure disorders. The drug is also used as a third-line mood stabilizer for bipolar patients who have not responded to lithium or divalproex (Depakote) and for patients unable to tolerate either of the others. Carbamazepine, in a dosage range of 100 to 300 mg at bedtime, can be used to treat restless legs syndrome. Carbamazepine is sometimes used to relieve the pain of trigeminal neuralgia.

Oxcarbazepine may be used as monotherapy or adjunctive therapy in the treatment if partial seizures in adults. Oxcarbazepine is approved as monotherapy for partial seizures in children age 4 and older, and adjunctive therapy for children age 2 and older with partial seizures.

Monitoring

Patients taking carbamazepine and oxcarbazepine should be monitored for seizure activity, severity, and duration. Adverse effects should be monitored, including CNS depression and suicidality or behavioral changes.

Table 15–7 ▦ Drug Interactions: Carbamazepine and Oxcarbazepine (Anticonvulsants)

Drug	Interacting Drug	Possible Effect	Implications
Carbamazepine	Anesthetics	Hepatic or renal damage	Ensure anesthetist is aware of carbamazepine use
	Cimetidine, propoxyphene, isoniazid, calcium channel blockers, fluoxetine, valproic acid, erythromycin, paroxetine, fluvoxamine, danazol, grapefruit juice, influenza vaccine, olanzapine, loxapine, ritonavir, nicotinamide	Increased plasma level of carbamazepine	Monitor plasma level
	Hydantoins, barbiturates, primidone, felbamate, rifampin, cisplatin, theophylline	Decreased plasma level of carbamazepine	Monitor level for possible dosage increase; monitor for seizure activity
	MAOIs	Hyperpyretic crisis	Do not give during or within 14 d of MAOI use
	Doxycycline, anticoagulants, warfarin, theophylline, haloperidol, acetaminophen, alprazolam, clozapine, anticonvulsants, clomipramine, phenytoin, primidone	Decreased effect of interacting drug	Monitor plasma levels when able; monitor for signs and symptoms of condition for which interacting drug was prescribed
	Lithium	Increased risk of neurotoxicity	Monitor plasma levels of both drugs; monitor for CNS-related adverse events
	Oral contraceptives	May decrease ethinyl, estradiol, and levonorgestrel availability	Use other birth control measures

Table 15–8 ⊗ Dosage Schedule: Carbamazepine and Oxcarbazepine (Anticonvulsants)

Drug	Indications	Dosage	Available Dosage Forms
Carbamazepine (Tegretol, Carbatrol)	Partial complex seizure disorder	*Adults and children >12 yr:* Initially 200 mg bid; increase by 200 mg/d at weekly intervals to maximum of 1,000 mg/d for children 12–15 yr; maintenance range: 800–1,200 mg/d 3–4 times/d *Children <12 yr:* Initially 100 mg bid; increase by 100 mg/d tid qid at weekly intervals to maximum of 1,000 mg/d: may also give at 20–30 mg/kg/d tid qid; maintenance range 400–800 mg/d	Tablets: 100, 200, 300, 400 mg Chewable tablets: 100, 200 mg Suspension: 100 mg/5 mL
	Trigeminal neuralgia	*Adults:* 100 mg bid on first day; increase by 200 mg/d at 100 mg every 12 h to maximum of 1,200 mg/d; maintenance range 200–1,200 mg/d, usually 400–800 mg/d: decrease dosage or discontinue every 3 mo	
	Bipolar disorder, aggressive/assaultive behavior	Same dosage guidelines as above until severe mood swings are stabilized and plasma level is within therapeutic range	
Oxcarbazepine (Trileptal)	Monotherapy or adjunctive therapy of partial seizures	*Adults PO:* 300 mg bid increased by 600 mg/d weekly up to 1,200 mg bid PO *Children (4–16 yr):* 4–5 mg/kg bid, increased over 2 wk	Tablets 150, 300, 600 mg Oral suspension 300 mg/5mL

Plasma carbamazepine levels should be monitored on a regular basis. The therapeutic range is 4 to 12 mcg/mL. Higher levels can lead to toxic symptoms consisting of the initial adverse effects and also hypertension, tachycardia, electrocardiogram (ECG) changes, stupor, agitation, nystagmus, urinary retention, respiratory depression, seizures, and coma. Children and elderly patients may develop toxicity at levels below 12.

Oxcarbazepine does not require serum level monitoring. Serum sodium levels should be monitored for the first 3 months of therapy, especially if the patient is taking other drugs that may cause hyponatremia.

Patient Education

Patients taking carbamazepine should be instructed to report to the clinician any symptoms such as skin lesions, bruising, fever, or sore throat. Carbamazepine should then be discontinued and another drug substituted. Tell the patient that administration with food may increase absorption, and because carbamazepine can be sedating, care should be exercised in situations in which mental and physical alertness is required for safety.

Oxcarbazepine may cause hyponatremia; therefore, patients should be educated regarding symptoms of hyponatremia, which include nausea, fatigue, headache, confusion, and increased seizures. Patients should report swelling of face, eyes, lips, or tongue, which may be symptoms of angioedema. Rash or mouth sores may be early symptoms of Stevens–Johnson syndrome.

Advise the patient that it is important to take the medication exactly as directed. If a dose is missed, the patient should take it as soon as possible but not right before the next scheduled dose and should not take double doses. Advise the patient to carry medical identification for the seizure disorder. Patients should report any mood changes or suidical thoughts.

SUCCINIMIDES

The succinimides are used for the treatment of absence seizures in children and adults. The succinimides include ethosuximide (Zarontin) and methsuximide (Celontin).

Pharmacodynamics

The succinimides exert their anticonvulsant effects by decreasing nerve impulses and transmission in the motor cortex. This produces a variety of effects, including an increase in the seizure threshold and reducing the electroencephalogram (EEG) spike-and-wave pattern of absence seizures.

Pharmacokinetics

Absorption and Distribution

Succinimides are administered orally and are thoroughly absorbed from the GI tract.

Metabolism and Excretion.

Succinimides are metabolized in the liver and excreted through the urinary tract, although a small amount of phensuximide is excreted in bile.

Onset, Peak, and Duration

There is a wide difference in half-lives, ranging from 30 hours in children and 60 hours in adults for ethosuximide, and 2.6 to 4 hours for methsuximide. Peak plasma levels are reached in 1 to 4 hours for methsuximide and in 3 to 7 hours for ethosuximide. Methsuximide has an onset of action of 15 to 30 minutes and a duration of 3 to 4 hours.

Pharmacotherapeutics

Precautions and Contraindications

Anticonvulsants in general are associated with fetal defects, but the succinimides, with careful monitoring of plasma levels, appear to be safe for use during pregnancy and are Pregnancy Category C. They are contraindicated, as are other anticonvulsants, during lactation.

Although uncommon, succinimides have caused blood dyscrasias and use should be preceded by a CBC with differential repeated at frequent intervals initially and less often as the patient continues on the medication without adverse effects. Liver function tests should also be obtained prior to instituting treatment.

Adverse Drug Reactions

The most common adverse reactions to the succinimides are GI distress, which can be relieved by taking the medication with food or milk, and CNS depression, characterized by sedation, ataxia, and lethargy. Other adverse reactions may include headache, rash, pruritus, and mood changes. Symptoms of toxicity are a worsening of these adverse reactions. Cases of systemic lupus erythematosus have been reported with the use of succinimides. All AEDs increase risk of suicidal ideation.

Drug Interactions

The most significant drug interactions are those that increase CNS depression, such as alcohol, opioid agonists, benzodiazepines, and CNS depressants. Succinimides may be given concurrently with other anticonvulsants but may antagonize them and contribute to tonic-myoclonic breakthrough seizures, therefore requiring the need for a higher dose of the other anticonvulsant.

Avoid concurrent use with TCAs and phenothiazines because an antagonistic effect on succinimides may lower the patient's seizure threshold. Haloperidol may change the pattern or frequency of seizures, necessitating an adjustment in dosage of the anticonvulsant. Succinimides may decrease the effectiveness of oral contraceptives; thus, the patient should be advised to use a backup birth control method.

Clinical Use and Dosing

Table 15-9 presents the indications, dosage schedules, and available dosage forms of succinimides.

Rational Drug Selection

Succinimides are the treatment of choice for childhood absence seizure disorders. They are sometimes used for the treatment of absence seizures in adults, but valproic acid becomes the primary treatment in adults. Methsuximide is equally effective as ethosuximide but may have more adverse reactions.

Monitoring

Plasma levels should be monitored. The normal therapeutic range of ethosuximide is 40 to 100 mcg/mL; levels over 150 mcg/mL are considered toxic. The therapeutic range for methsuximide is 10 to 40 mcg/mL, with levels greater than 40 mcg/mL considered toxic. In addition to monitoring seizure activity, evaluate liver, renal, and hematological studies periodically for adverse effects.

Patient Education

Advise the patient to avoid alcohol and, if sedation occurs, to avoid hazardous activities. To decrease stomach distress, succinimides should be taken with milk or food. Because adverse mood changes can occur while taking these medications, advise the client to report any behavioral changes to the clinician. Caution the client that withdrawal of the medication may precipitate absence seizures. Inform the client taking phensuximide that harmless changes in urine color may occur.

DRUGS THAT AFFECT GABA

The AEDs that affect gamma aminobutyric acid (GABA) include the benzodiazepines, gabapentin (Neurontin), topiramate (Topamax), and tiagabine (Gabitril). The AEDs that affect the inhibitory neurotransmitter GABA are also used for pain, including neuropathic pain (gabapentin) and migraine (topiramate).

Pharmacodynamics

The mechanism of action of the drugs that affect GABA is not well understood. Gabapentin is thought to be a GABA analogue that binds to unknown receptors in the brain; it does not bind to GABA receptors, nor does it mimic GABA. Topiramate may block sodium channels or potentiate GABA. Tiagabine may potentiate the action of GABA by blocking GABA reuptake into presynaptic neurons, allowing for more

Table 15–9 ⊗ **Dosage Schedule: Succinimides (Anticonvulsants)**

Drug	Indications	Dosage	Available Dosage Forms
Ethosuximide (Zarontin)	Absence seizures (petit mal)	*Adults and children >6 yr:* 500 mg daily or 250 mg bid; may increase by 250 mg every 4–7 d to maximum of 1.5 g/d	Capsules: 250 mg
		Children <6 yr: 250 mg daily or 125 mg bid; optimal dose 20 mg/kg/d; maximum dose 1.5 g/d	Syrup: 250 mg/5 mL
Methsuximide (Celontin)	Absence seizures (petit mal); second choice	*Adults and children:* Initially 300 mg/d; may increase by 300 mg/d increments at weekly intervals to maximum of 1.2 g/d in divided doses	Capsules: 150, 300 mg

GABA to be available to bind to postsynaptic neuronal receptors.

Pharmacokinetics

Absorption and Distribution

All the AEDs that affect GABA are rapidly absorbed after oral administration, and gabapentin plasma concentration peaks in 2 to 3 hours. Food increases absorption of gabapentin by 14% percent. Topiramate peaks 2 hours after oral administration and is not affected by food intake. Tiagabine peaks 45 minutes after ingestion if taken on an empty stomach. The drugs that affect GABA are widely distributed, including in the CNS and in breast milk. The pharmacokinetics of drugs that affect GABA are found in Table 15-10.

Metabolism and Excretion

Gabapentin is not metabolized; it is excreted unchanged in the urine (75% to 80%) and the feces (10% to 20%). Topiramate is not extensively metabolized, with minor amounts metabolized in the liver via hydroxylation, hydrolysis, and glucuronidation. The percentage of topiramate metabolized in the liver increases when coadministered with drugs that are enzyme inducers. Topiramate is eliminated 70% unchanged in the urine. Tiagabine is extensively metabolized in the liver, primarily by CYP 3A4, and undergoes enterohepatic recirculation. Tiagabine is eliminated as metabolites, 25% in the urine and 63% in the feces.

The half life of gabapentin is 4.7 hours in infants and children and 5.3 hours in adults. In adults with renal insufficiency (CrCl less than 30 mL/min), it may have a half-life of 52 hours. The half-life of topiramate in adults is 21 hours and in adults with renal impairment the half-life is 59 hours. The half-life of tiagabine in adults is 7 to 9 hours. In children age 3 to 10 years, the mean half-life is 5.7 hours. In children who are on enzyme-inducing AEDs, the half-life of tiagabine is 3.2 hours and in adults on enzyme-inducing AEDs the half-life is 2 to 5 hours.

Pharmacotherapeutics

Precautions and Contraindications

Gabapentin

Gabapentin is contraindicated in patients who are hypersensitive to it. Gabapentin should not be abruptly discontinued because it may precipitate status epilepticus; the dose should be decreased over at least a week.

Neuropsychiatric events such as behavior problems, hostility, aggressive behavior, thought disorder, including changes in school performance and hyperkinesias, have been reported in pediatric patients ages 3 to 12 years taking gabapentin. The safety and effectiveness of gabapentin has not been established in children younger than age 3 years.

AEDs including gabapentin increase the risk of suicidal behavior and ideation; patients should be monitored for emergence or worsening of depression, suicidal thoughts, or changes in behavior.

Gabapentin is Pregnancy Category C. Gabapentin is excreted in breast milk, and nursing infants may be exposed to up to 1/mg/kg/day. Gabapentin should be used in nursing women only if the benefits outweigh the risks. Monitor the infant for lethargy or other neurological effects.

Topiramate

Patients taking topiramate may have decreased concentrations of serum bicarbonate due to inhibition of carbonic anhydrase and increased renal bicarbonate loss, leading to hyperchloremic metabolic acidosis. In adults, doses as low as 50 mg per day of topiramate may result in low serum bicarbonate, with the incidence of decreased serum bicarbonate 30% in clinical trials when topiramate dosage was 400 mg per day. Low serum bicarbonate levels in children 2 to 16 years of age were reported in up to 67% of children receiving 6 mg/kg/day. Severe metabolic acidosis has been reported in infants receiving a topiramate dose of 5 mg/kg/day. Serum bicarbonate should be monitored at baseline and periodically throughout therapy.

Table 15–10 ✂ Pharmacokinetics: Tricyclic Antidepressants

Drug	Onset	Peak	Duration	Half-Life	Excretion
Amitriptyline HCl	45 min	2–12 h	Long-acting	31–46 h	Urine, feces
Amoxapine	90 min	2–4 wk	Long-acting	8–30 h	Urine
Clomipramine	4-7 h	2–4 wk	Long-acting	19–37 h	Urine
Desipramine HCl	2–5 d	2–3 wk	Long-acting	12–24 h	Urine
Doxepin HCl	2–8 d	2–4 wk	Long-acting	8–24 h	Urine
Imipramine HCl	2–4 h	2–4 wk	Long-acting	11–25 h	Urine, feces
Nortriptyline HCl	—	2–4 wk	Long-acting	18–44 h	Urine
Protriptyline HCl	8–12 h	24–30 h	Long-acting	67–89 h	Urine
Trimipramine maleate	—	—	Long-acting	9–11 h	Urine

An ocular syndrome consisting of acute myopia and angle closure glaucoma has been reported in adults and children taking topiramate. Symptoms usually occur within 1 month of starting topiramate. Patients who have eye pain or blurred vision should contact their provider immediately. The treatment is to discontinue topiramate as soon as possible.

A rare adverse effect of topiramate is oligohidrosis (decreased sweating) and hyperthermia. Most cases were reported in children and were associated with vigorous exercise and/or high environmental temperatures. Patients, especially children should be monitored for decreased sweating and hyperthermia, especially in warm weather. Use caution when prescribing drugs that predispose patients to heat-related disorders (anticholinergic drugs and carbonic anhydrase inhibitors).

AEDs including topiramate increase the risk of suicidal behavior and ideation; patients should be monitored for emergence or worsening of depression, suicidal thoughts, or changes in behavior.

Topiramate should not be abruptly discontinued because that may precipitate status epilepticus; it should be withdrawn gradually.

Topiramate is Pregnancy Category D and has been found to be teratogenic in animal studies. There is an increased risk of cleft lip and/or cleft palate in infants born to women who take topiramate during pregnancy. Topiramate is excreted in breast milk, with infant plasma concentrations of 10% to 20% of maternal concentrations. Infants ingesting topiramate via breast milk should be monitored for drowsiness, weight gain, and developmental milestones (Toxnet, 2011).

Tiagabine

Tiagabine is contraindicated in patients who are hypersensitive to it or any of its components. Post-marketing reports have shown that patients without epilepsy who are prescribed tiagabine may have seizure or status epilepticus. Seizures have been reported in doses as low as 4 mg per day. Most of these patients were taking other medications concomitantly, such as antidepressants, antipsychotics, stimulants, or narcotics. It is thought the concomitant drug lowered the seizure threshold. Seizures occurred soon after a dosage increase. Dosing recommendations for tiagabine are based on a study sample that was also taking enzyme-inducing AEDs, such as carbamazepine, phenytoin, primidone, and phenobarbital, leading to lower plasma tiagabine levels. Tiagabine should not be abruptly discontinued because that may precipitate increased seizure activity; it should be withdrawn gradually.

AEDs including tiagabine increase the risk of suicidal behavior and ideation; patients should be monitored for emergence or worsening of depression, suicidal thoughts, or changes in behavior.

Tiagabine is Pregnancy Category C. It has been found to be teratogenic in fetal rats. There are no adequately well-controlled studies in pregnant women. Tiagabine is excreted in breast milk and is not recommended in lactating women unless there are no other options for maternal treatment. Infants should be monitored for adequate weight gain and developmental milestones.

Tiagabine has been minimally studied in children and is not labeled for use in children younger than age 12.

Adverse Drug Reactions

The most common CNS adverse effects of gabapentin include somnolence (28% in clinical trials) and dizziness (21%). Less common CNS effects include ataxia (3.3%) and abnormal thinking (2.7%). In children 3 to 12 years of age, neuropsychiatric adverse effects of gabapentin include emotional lability (6%), hostility (5.2%), hyperkinesias (4.7%), and thought disorder, including problems with concentration and school performance (1.7%).

Peripheral edema occurred in 8.3% of patients taking gabapentin in clinical trials versus 2.2% in the control group.

The CNS adverse effects of topiramate include ataxia, parathesia, dizziness, somnolence, and difficulty concentrating. Patients in the treatment group also reported anorexia, difficulty with memory, confusion, depression, mood problems, and psychomotor slowing. In children, the most common CNS adverse effects are somnolence and fatigue. Weight loss was reported in 6% of patients taking 50 mg/day of topiramate and 16% of patients taking 400 mg/day.

There is an increase in incidence of kidney stones (2% to 4% greater than expected in clinical trials) in patients taking topiramate. Kidney stones were more prevalent in men and also occurred in children during clinical trials.

Hyperammonemia with and without encephalopathy has been observed in in clinical trials and in post-marketing reports in patients who were taking topiramate both with and without concomitant valproic acid use. Topiramate inhibits carbonic anhydrase, leading to renal bicarbonate loss, and may cause metabolic acidosis.

The adverse drug reactions most commonly reported for tiagabine were related to the CNS, including difficulty with concentration or attention, dizziness, light-headedness, somnolence, confusion, asthenia or lack of energy, and nervousness or irritability. Suicidal thinking has been reported, as previously mentioned.

Drug Interactions

Gabapentin does not interfere with the metabolism of commonly coadministered AEDs. Coadministration of naproxen increases absorption of gabapentin 12% to 15%. Gabapentin may increase the effects of alcohol and other CNS depressant drugs. Gabapentin may cause a false-positive urinary protein level with the N-Multistik SG test.

Clinical Use and Dosing

Dosing of gabapentin for seizures in children older than age 12 and in adults is 300 mg 3 times a day, which is titrated upward to the usual dose of 900 to 1,800 mg 3 times a day. Dosages up to 2,400 mg per day have been tolerated in long-term studies. Initial gabapentin dosing for children 3 to 12 years is 10 to 15 mg/kg/day divided into three doses per day; the dose is titrated up to a usual dose of 40 mg/kg/day in children 3 to 4 years, and 25 to 35 mg/kg/day in children 5 to 12 years. Neuropathic pain is treated in adults with a starting dose of 100 mg 3 times a day, with the dose titrated upward

300 mg per day at weekly intervals to a dose of at least 900 mg per day. The usual gabapentin dosage range for neuropathic pain is 1,800 to 2,400 mg per day, divided into three doses. The dose of gabapentin to treat post-herpetic neuralgia in adults is an initial dose of 300 mg per day; on day 2 the dose is 300 mg twice a day and on day 3 the dose is 300 mg 3 times a day. The dose is titrated up to 600 mg 3 times a day as needed to relieve pain. Dosage adjustment of gabapentin is required in patients with renal failure.

When topiramate is used as monotherapy for epilepsy in children age 10 years or older and in adults, the recommended dose is 400 mg per day in two divided doses. Patients should be titrated up to the recommended dosage. The topiramate starting dose is 25 mg twice a day for a week, then the dose is increased to 50 mg twice a day for a week. In week 3 the dose is 75 mg twice a day, and in week 4 the dose is 100 mg twice a day. In week 5 the topiramate dose is increased to 150 mg twice a day, and in week 6 the goal dosage of 200 mg twice a day is achieved. The recommended total daily dose in patients with partial onset seizures or Lennox–Gastaut Syndrome is 200 to 400 mg daily. In pediatric patients age 2 to 16 years with partial onset seizures, primary generalized tonic-clonic seizures, or seizures associated with Lennox–Gastaut syndrome, the topiramate dose is approximately 5 to 9 mg/kg/day in two divided doses. Pediatric dosing is started at 1 to 3 mg/kg/day (maximum 25 mg/day) in two divided doses and titrated up by 1 to 3 mg/kg/day at 1 to 2 week intervals to achieve clinical response. The usual maintenance dose of topiramate in children is 5 to 9 mg/kg/day, divided into twice-a-day dosing. In patients with renal impairment, half the usual dosage is recommended.

Tiagabine dosing depends on whether a patient is concurrently taking an enzyme-inducing AED. Use of tiagabine in patients not taking enzyme-inducing AEDs may result in serum concentration up to twice that of patients on enzyme-inducing AEDs. Tiagabine dosage adjustment is needed if an enzyme-inducing drug is added, discontinued, or has a dosage change. Avoid loading doses or rapid escalation of dose. The initial dose of tiagabine in adolescents age 12 to 18 years is 4 mg once daily for a week, then in week 2 the dose is 4 mg twice a day (8 mg/day total). Dosage is increased by 4 to 8 mg daily at weekly intervals until clinical response is achieved. The maximum dose of tiagabine in adolescents is 32 mg per day. The dosage for adults on enzyme-inducing AEDs is 4 mg once daily in week 1, then it is increased by 4 to 8 mg per day increments until the maximum daily dose of 32 to 56 mg per day divided in two to four doses is achieved. If a dose is missed, the patient should skip that dose and administer the next dose at the regularly scheduled time. Patients should not double the dose to catch up. If multiple doses of tiagabine have been missed, possible retitration may be required.

Rational Drug Selection

Drug selection of drugs that affect GABA is based on the type of seizure and possible drug interactions that may affect therapy.

Monitoring

Seizure frequency, duration, and severity are monitored with all AEDs, as should mood changes, signs of depression, anxiety, and suicidal thoughts. Patients taking gabapentin, topiramate and tiagabine do not require routine monitoring of serum drug levels.

Patients taking topiramate should have serum electrolyte, including sodium bicarbonate, monitored at baseline and periodically. Weight is monitored in all patients on topiramate as are body temperature and the ability to sweat, especially in warm weather. Serum ammonia levels should be drawn in any patient taking topiramate who exhibits any change in level of consciousness, unexplained lethargy, or vomiting.

Patient Education

Administration

Patients taking AEDs that affect GABA should take the medication exactly as prescribed to maintain consistent therapeutic levels. Missing doses may cause an increase in seizures. Withdrawal seizures may occur if any of these medications is abruptly discontinued; therefore, patients need to be warned to take their medication as scheduled and to not stop without discussing cessation with their provider.

Adverse Reactions

Patients and family members of patients taking AEDs should be warned about the potential neuropsychiatric adverse drug reactions (ADRs), including suicidal thoughts and action, and behavioral changes. Any changes should be reported to the prescriber immediately. Patients should also be warned about the possibility of somnolence, dizziness, or balance issues when starting on AEDs that affect GABA.

Patients taking topiramate will need to monitor their ability to sweat and monitor their temperature in warm weather. Any signs of confusion, unexplained vomiting, or mental status change in patients taking topiramate require investigation for elevated ammonia levels or metabolic acidosis.

Lifestyle Management

Patients who have seizures should get adequate sleep and exercise and avoid stressful situations that may trigger seizures.

LEVETIRACETAM

Levetiracetam (Keppra) is an antiepileptic indicated as an adjunct drug in the treatment of partial onset seizures in children and adults. It is its own unique drug class because it is chemically unrelated to other AEDs.

Pharmacodynamics

The exact mechanism of action of levetiracetam is not known. It does not appear to inhibit or affect GABA, nor does it affect calcium or sodium currents or channels. In vitro and in vivo recordings of epileptiform activity during clinical trials have shown that levetiracetam inhibits burst firing without affecting normal neuronal excitability, suggesting that levetiracetam may prevent epileptiform burst firing and spread of seizure activity.

Pharmacokinetics

Absorption and Distribution

Levetiracetam is almost completely absorbed after oral administration. Time to peak concentration is 1 hour in immediate-release tablets and 3 hours in extended-release tablets. Intake of a high-calorie, high-fat meal before administration delays time to peak in the extended-release levetiracetam by up to 2 hours. It is less than 10% protein bound.

Metabolism and Excretion

Levetiracetam is not extensively metabolized and does not use the cytochrome P450 enzymes. It is metabolized by hydrolysis of the acetamide group, which produces an inactive carboxylic acid metabolite. The half-life of levetiracetam is 7 hours. Levetiracetam is 68% eliminated renally; renal clearance is impaired in patients with renal dysfunction.

Pharmacotherapeutics

Precautions and Contraindications

The only absolute contraindication to the use of levetiracetam is sensitivity to the drug. Patients taking AEDs, including levetiracetam, are at increased risk for suicidal thoughts, depression, and unusual changes in mood and behavior. The mood changes can occur as early as 1 week from the onset of therapy and persist throughout the duration of therapy. Patients and caregivers should be informed of the risk for neuropsychiatric changes while taking levetiracetam and to report any changes in mood, suicidal thoughts, or behavioral changes. Levetiracetam may cause somnolence, fatigue, dizziness, and muscle coordination difficulties. Patients should be warned not to drive or operate heavy machinery until they know the effects of levetiracetam. There is a potential for withdrawal seizures if levetiracetam is abruptly stopped. Levetiracetam should be withdrawn slowly to prevent these.

Levetiracetam may cause a transient decrease in white blood count (WBC), with 3.2% of patients in the clinical trials experiencing a decreased WBC and 2.4% experiencing a decreased neutrophil count. Neutrophil counts returned to normal after continued use.

Levetiracetam is Pregnancy Category C, although there are no well-controlled trials in pregnant women. Administration of levetiracetam to rats led to minor fetal skeletal abnormalities. Altered pharmacokinetics during pregnancy may affect levetiracetam serum concentrations; with decreased serum concentration reported during pregnancy. Discontinuing AEDs during pregnancy may be harmful to the mother, so consultation with a perinatologist is warranted. Pregnant women who take levetiracetam during pregnancy should be reported and enrolled in North American Antiepileptic Drug Pregnancy Registry (888-233-2334).

Levetiracetam is FDA-approved for use in children age 1 month or older as adjunct therapy in partial seizures and as adjunctive therapy in children age 6 years and older with primary generalized tonic-clonic seizures.

Adverse Drug Reactions

The most common ADR reported in clinical trials of levetiracetam was somnolence, reported in 15% of patients. Dizziness is another common ADR (9% of patients). Behavioral changes are uncommon but significant in patients taking levetiracetam, including nervousness (4% of patients), anxiety (2%), hostility (2%), and emotional lability. Alopecia has been reported in post-marketing surveillance of levetiracetam, with recovery reported once the drug was discontinued.

As previously mentioned, suicidal thinking or behavior may occur in patients taking AEDs. In clinical trials of 11 different AEDs, patients randomized to one of the AEDs had approximately twice the risk of suicidal thoughts or behavior of the controls.

Drug Interactions

Levetiracetam is mostly unbound and does not use CYP 450 enzymes for metabolism, thereby decreasing the likelihood of drug interactions. Levetiracetam does not interact with phenytoin, valproate, carbamazepine, gabapentin, lamotrigene, or phenobarbital. It also does not interact with oral contraceptives or warfarin.

Clinical Use and Dosing

Levetiracetam is prescribed as adjunct therapy in adults and children age 1 month or older with partial onset seizures. It is indicated as adjunctive therapy in the treatment of primary generalized tonic-clonic seizures in adults and children age 6 years or older, and as adjunctive therapy for myoclonic seizures in adult patients and adolescents age 12 or older with juvenile myoclonic epilepsy Levetiracetam is added to a stable dosing regimen of an AED.

Rational Drug Selection

There are two forms of levetiracetam available, immediate-release and extended-release (Keppra XR) tablets. The immediate-release form is available in suspension or as tablets. The extended-release formula is FDA-approved for age 16 years and older. There is a significant cost difference between generic levetiracetam and the brand-name Keppra, with 60 tablets of 1,000 mg generic levetiracetam priced at $42 and 60 tablets of 1,000 mg Keppra priced at $848 (CostCo, www.costco.com).

Monitoring

Routine laboratory monitoring of patients on levetiracetam is not necessary. Efficacy is determined by a decrease in the mean weekly frequency of partial onset seizures.

Patient Education

Administration

Patients should take levetiracetam exactly as prescribed. Missing doses may cause an increase in seizures. Withdrawal seizures may occur if levetiracetam is abruptly discontinued; therefore, patients need to be warned to take their medication as scheduled and to not stop without discussing cessation with their provider.

Adverse Reactions

Patients and family members of patients taking levetiracetam should be warned about the potential neuropsychiatric ADRs, including suicidal thoughts and action, and behavioral changes. Any changes should be reported to the prescriber immediately. Patients should also be warned about the possibility of somnolence, dizziness, or balance issues when starting on levetiracetam.

Lifestyle Management

Patients who have seizures should get adequate sleep and exercise and avoid stressful situations that may trigger seizures.

LAMOTRIGINE

Lamotrigine (Lamictal) is used as adjunctive therapy in adults and children age 2 or older in the treatment of partial seizures, primary generalized tonic-clonic seizures, and generalized seizures associated with Lennox–Gastaut syndrome. Lamotrigine is approved for maintenance treatment of bipolar 1 disorder to delay occurrence of mood episodes in adults age 18 or older.

Pharmacodynamics

The exact mechanism of action of lamotrigine is not known. It is thought that lamotrigine affects voltage-sensitive sodium channels and inhibits presynaptic release of glutamate and aspartate in the neuron. The mechanism of action of lamotrigine in the treatment of bipolar disorder is not known.

Pharmacokinetics

Absorption and Distribution

Lamotrigine is well absorbed after oral administration. Lamotrigine chewable tablets have the same rate of absorption whether chewed or dissolved in water. Orally disintegrating tablets and regular tablets taken with water have the same rate and extent of absorption. Immediate-release lamotrigine peaks in 2 hours. Some patients may have a second peak at 4 to 6 hours due to enterohepatic recirculation. Extended-release lamotrigine peaks in 4 to 11 hours. The mean volume of distribution of lamotrigine is 0.9 to 1.3 L/kg after oral administration. Lamotrigine is 55% protein bound. It crosses the placenta and is excreted in breast milk.

Metabolism and Excretion

Lamotrigine is metabolized extensively in the liver via glucuronic acid conjugation. When lamotrigine is given alone, after multiple doses it induces its own metabolism resulting in a 25% decrease in half-life. Ninety-four percent of lamotrigine is excreted as metabolites in the urine and 2% is excreted in the feces.

Pharmacotherapeutics

Precautions and Contraindications

Lamotrigine is contraindicated in patients hypersensitive to the drug or its ingredients. Life-threatening hypersensitivity

reactions have occurred; these include multiorgan failure or dysfunction, hepatic abnormalities, and disseminated intravascular coagulation. Early symptoms of hypersensitivity, such as fever or lymphadenopathy, require evaluation and discontinuation if the reason for symptoms cannot be established. Blood dyscrasias, including neutropenia, leukopenia, anemia, thrombocytopenia, pancytopenia, and aplastic anemia have been reported in patients taking lamotrigine.

Lamotrigine has a Black-Box Warning regarding life-threatening rashes, including Stevens–Johnson syndrome, toxic epidermal necrolysis, and rash-related death. Pediatric patients are more likely to have serious rash than adults. Coadministration with valproate may increase the risk of rash. Exceeding recommended initial doses or exceeding recommended dosage escalation of lamotrigine increases risk of rash. Lamotrigine should be discontinued at the first sign of rash, unless clearly not drug related.

Patients taking AEDs, including lamotrigine, are at increased risk for suicidal thoughts, depression, and unusual changes in mood and behavior. The mood changes can occur as early as 1 week from the onset of therapy and persist throughout the duration of therapy. Patients taking lamotrigine for bipolar disorder may experience worsening of depression and emergence of suicidal ideation. Patients and caregivers should be informed of the risk for neuropsychiatric changes while taking lamotrigine and to report any changes in mood, suicidal thoughts, or behavior changes.

There is a potential for withdrawal seizures if lamotrigine is abruptly stopped. Lamotrigine should be withdrawn slowly (over at least 2 weeks) to prevent seizures.

Lamotrigine is Pregnancy Category C. Although not specifically found to be teratogenic, it decreases folate levels in animal studies. Lamotrigine should only be prescribed to pregnant women if the benefit outweighs the risk. Pregnant women who take lamotrigine during pregnancy should be referred to enroll in the North American Antiepileptic Drug Pregnancy Registry (888-233-2334). Providers may enroll patients in the Lamotrigine Pregnancy Registry by calling 1-800-336-2176.

Lamotrigine is excreted in breast milk. Breastfed infants of women taking lamotrigine have measurable serum levels of lamotrigine, which may be 30% to 50% of maternal levels. Neonates have limited ability to metabolize lamotrigine, placing them at higher risk of exposure. Lamotrigine has low protein binding, and maternal plasma levels may rise in the postpartum period, leading to elevated milk levels (LactMed, 2014). If there are no other therapeutic options to maternal lamotrigine use, then the infant should be monitored closely for drowsiness, poor suck, apnea, and rash. Consider measuring serum lamotrigine levels and platelet count in the infant. Infants may exhibit withdrawal symptoms if breastfeeding is abruptly discontinued (LactMed, 2014).

Lamotrigine is FDA-approved for use in children age 2 or older for the treatment of generalized tonic-clinic seizures, partial seizures, and Lennox–Gastaut syndrome. The safety and effectiveness in the treatment of bipolar disorder in patients younger than 18 has not been established.

Adverse Drug Reactions

As discussed in the Precautions and Contraindications section, lamotrigine has a Black-Box Warning regarding serious, possibly life-threatening rashes, including Stevens–Johnson. The incidence in pediatric patients age 2 to 16 years is 0.8% (8 in 1,000) and it is 0.3% in adults taking lamotrigine as adjunctive therapy. Any unexplained rash requires discontinuation of lamotrigine and investigation.

Multiorgan failure has been reported in patients taking lamotrigine, including hepatic failure. Blood dyscrasias may occur in patients taking lamotrigine. Reported abnormalities include neutropenia, anemia, thrombocytopenia, and pancytopenia. Rare reactions include aplastic anemia and red cell aplasia.

Patients taking lamotrigine for any reason may have increased suicidal thoughts or behavior. Monitor patients for mood changes or suicidal thoughts, especially those taking lamotrigine for bipolar disorder.

Abruptly discontinuing lamotrigine may cause withdrawal seizures. Patients may exhibit withdrawal seizures if they are taking lamotrigine for bipolar disorder also. To avoid withdrawal seizures, lamotrigine should be tapered off over 2 weeks.

Lamotrigine may cause increased seizures, including status epilepticus.

Drug Interactions

There are many drug interactions with lamotrigine due to enzyme induction that affect drug levels of both lamotrigine and the concurrently administered drugs. For example, the enzyme inducers carbamazepine, phenytoin, phenobarbital, and primidone decrease lamotrigine concentrations by approximately 40%.

Oral estrogen-containing contraceptives decrease lamotrigine levels by approximately 50%. If the patient is already taking lamotrigine and an oral contraceptive is started, the lamotrigine dose may need to be twice the normal dose. Lamotrigine decreases levonorgestrel levels by 19% when taken with combined oral contraceptives.

Rifampin decreases lamotrigine concentrations by 40% when taken concurrently.

The most concerning interaction with lamotrigine is with valproate. When valproate is administered concurrently with lamotrigine, there is an increased risk of life-threatening rash, such as Stevens–Johnson, developing. Valproate also increases lamotrigine levels by more than 2-fold.

Clinical Use and Dosing

Dosing of lamotrigine is dependant on the concurrent medications the patient may be taking. It is critical to follow recommendations for initial dosing and the escalation schedule to avoid the development of life-threatening rashes. There are Lamictal starter kits and Lamictal ODT Patient Titration kits available for the first 5 weeks of treatment if adherence to the escalation schedule is a concern.

Tablets should not be crushed or chewed. There is a chewable tablet that may be dissolved in water or juice if needed or oral disintegrating tablets (ODT). Do not prescribe partial portions of either regular or chewable tablets.

Dosing in Treating Seizures

Patients Not Taking Enzyme-Inducing AEDs

Patients age 12 or older and adults who are not taking enzyme-inducing AEDs (carbamazepine, phenytoin, primidone, or valproate) are started on 25 mg every day for 2 weeks. In weeks 3 and 4, the dosage is increased to 50 mg per day. In week 5, the lamotrigine dosage is increased 50 mg per day, and dosage increases by 50 mg per day every 1 to 2 weeks until the usual maintenance dose of 225 mg to 375 mg per day in two divided doses.

The dosage for children age 2 to 12 years with epilepsy who are not taking an enzyme-inducing AED begins with 0.3 mg/kg per day in one or two divided doses in weeks 1 and 2. The dosage should be rounded down to the nearest whole tablet and tablets should not be cut. In weeks 3 and 4, the dosage is 0.6 mg/kg per day in two divided doses rounded down to the nearest whole tablet. Starting in week 5, the dose is increased every 1 to 2 weeks by calculating 0.6 mg/kg/day, rounded down to the nearest whole tablet and added to the previously administered daily dose. The dose is titrated to effect, with an average daily dose of 4.5 to 7.5 mg/kg per day. A maintenance dose may need to be increased by as much as 50% in children who weigh less than 30 kg.

Patients Taking Enzyme-Inducing AEDs

For patients age 12 years and older taking carbamazepine, phenytoin, phenobarbital, or primidone and not taking valproate, the dose for the initial 2 weeks is 50 mg per day. In weeks 3 and 4, the dose is 100 mg per day in two divided doses. Beginning in week 5, the dose of lamotrigine is increased by 100 mg/day every 1 to 2 weeks to the usual maintenance dose of 300 to 500 mg per day in two divided doses.

The dosage in pediatric patients age 2 to 12 years taking carbamazepine, phenytoin, phenobarbital, or primidone and not taking valproate is 0.6 mg/kg/day in two divided doses, rounded down to the nearest whole tablet for the first 2 weeks. In weeks 3 and 4, the dose is 1.2 mg/kg/day in two divided doses, rounded down to the nearest whole tablet. Beginning in week 5, the dose of lamotrigine is increased by 1.2 mg/kg/day, rounded down to the nearest whole tablet and added to the previously administered daily dose. The usual daily maintenance dose is 5 to 15 mg/kg per day, with a maximum of 400 mg per day in two divided doses. The maintenance dose of lamotrigine may need to be increased by as much as 50% in children who weigh less than 30 kg.

Patients Taking Valproate

Valproate inhibits glucuronidation and decreases clearance of lamotrigine; therefore, the escalation schedule is slower. The initial dose of lamotrigine in patients older than age 12 is 25 mg per day for the first 4 weeks. Beginning in week 5, the dosage is increased 25 to 50 mg per day every 1 to 2 weeks. The usual maintenance dose of lamotrigine in patients taking valproate alone is 100 to 200 mg per day. If patients are taking valproate and other drugs that induce glucuronidation, the usual maintenance dose is 100 to 400 mg per day.

Children age 2 to 12 years taking valproate are started on 0.15 mg/kg per day of lamotrigine in one or two divided doses, rounded down to the nearest whole tablet for the first 2 weeks. Children who weigh more than 6.7 kg and less than 14 kg are given 2 mg of lamotrigine every other day for weeks 1 and 2. The dose for weeks 3 and 4 is 0.3 mg/kg/day in one or two divided doses, rounded down to the nearest whole tablet. Beginning in week 5, calculate 0.3 mg/kg/day of lamotrigine, rounded down to the nearest whole tablet and added to the previously administered daily dose. The usual maintenance dose of lamotrigine in children taking valproate is 1 to 5 mg/kg per day, with a maximum of 200 mg per day. The maintanence dose of lamotrigine may need to be increased by as much as 50% in children who weigh less than 30 kg.

Dosing in Bipolor Disease

The initial dosage of lamotrigine in adult patients with bipolar disorder who are not taking enzyme-inducing AEDs or valproate is 25 mg daily for the first 2 weeks. During weeks 3 and 4, the dose is increased to 50 mg per day. In week 5, the dose of lamotrigine is increased to 100 mg per day. In week 6, the dose is increased to 200 mg per day, which is the maintenance dose of lamotrigine.

For patients taking carbamazepine, phenytoin, phenobarbital, or primidone and not taking valproate, the dose to treat bipolar disease for the initial 2 weeks is 50 mg per day. In weeks 3 and 4, the dose is 100 mg daily in divided doses. In week 5, the dose increases to 200 mg per day. The dose is increased to 300 mg per day in week 6, with the dose divided into two doses per day. In week 7, the lamotrigine dose is increased to up to 400 mg per day in divided doses.

In bipolar patients taking valproate, the initial dose of lamotrigine is 25 mg every other day for the first 2 weeks. In weeks 3 and 4, the dose is increased to 25 mg daily. The lamotrigine dose is increased to 50 mg per day in week 5. In week 6, the lamotrigine is increased to the maintenance dose of 100 mg daily.

Patients Taking Oral Contraceptives

Oral estrogen-containing contraceptives decrease lamotrigine levels by approximately 50%. If the patient is already taking lamotrigine and an oral contraceptive is started, the lamotrigine dose is increased 50 mg per day weekly. The lamotrigine dose may need to be twice the normal dose.

Rational Drug Selection

Lamotrigine is the only drug in its class. Its use is determined by the type of seizures, concurrent medications, and patient profile. Consultation with a neurologist is warranted when prescribing lamotrigine.

Monitoring

Patients should be monitored closely for any newly occurring rash and for hypersensitivity reactions. Complete blood count and differential should be monitored, as well as renal and hepatic function. Patients need to be instructed to monitor seizure activity. Concurrent AED levels should be monitored as should signs of suicidality or mood changes. Bipolar patients should be monitored for worsening depressive symptoms.

Patient Education

Administration

Patients need to be instructed to take lamotrigine exactly as prescribed and should follow the escalation schedule exactly. Tablets should not be crushed or chewed. Chewable tablets are chewed and washed down with a small amount of juice or water or may be dissolved in a small amount of water or juice.

Adverse Drug Reaction

Any rash needs to be reported to the provider immediately and the patient examined. Patients and family members of patients taking levetiracetam should be warned about the potential neuropsychiatric ADRs, including suicidal thoughts and action and behavioral changes. Any changes should be reported to the prescriber immediately.

Lifestyle Management

Patients who have seizures should get adequate sleep and exercise and avoid stressful situations that may trigger seizures.

ANTIDEPRESSANTS

The antidepressants are usually identified in five classes: tricyclics (TCAs), selective serotonin reuptake inhibitors (SSRIs), monoamine oxidase inhibitors (MAOIs), serotonin-norepinephrine reuptake inhibitors (SNRIs), norepinephrine reuptake inhibitors (NRIs), and miscellaneous drugs that do not easily fit one of the other categories.

As of 2007, all categories of antidepressants carry an FDA Black-Box Warning regarding increased risk of suicidal thought and behavior. This is most likely to occur in children, adolescents, and young adults to age 24 and is most likely to occur in the first 2 months of treatment. It is emphasized that depression and other serious psychiatric illnesses are themselves important causes of suicide. Providers and patients and their families must weigh benefits versus risks and if antidepressants are prescribed, monitor closely for suicidal ideation and behavior.

TRICYCLIC ANTIDEPRESSANTS (TCAs)

The development of TCAs grew out of work with phenothiazines, to which they are structurally related. Prior to TCAs' availability in the 1960s, depression had been treated with stimulants and tranquilizers, both of which had some utility but left the basic mood disorder essentially unchanged. They were not overshadowed until the late 1980s, when the new SSRIs began to be widely marketed.

Although now used less frequently than in the past, amitriptyline (Elavil), nortriptyline (Pamelor, Aventyl), imipramine (Tofranil), doxepin (Sinequan), trimipramine maleate (Surmontil), amoxapine (Asendin), desipramine (Norpramin, Pertofrane), protriptyline HCL (Vivactil), and clomipramine (Anafranil) still have their individual usefulness. Essentially, the TCAs are equally efficacious as the newer drugs in treating depression, cost less, but have much more troublesome side effects. Also the TCAs are less safe in treating depression in those who are at high risk for suicide, because overdose can be fatal, whereas the newer antidepressants are much less likely to be fatal.

Pharmacodynamics

The TCAs act on the neurotransmitters serotonin and norepinephrine by inhibiting their reuptake at the presynaptic neuron. However, they also act on histamine (contributing to drowsiness and weight gain) and acetylcholine. Loxapine, an active metabolite of amoxapine, acts as an antipsychotic by blocking the dopamine receptor.

Pharmacokinetics

Absorption and Distribution

All the TCAs are administered orally, thoroughly absorbed, and highly lipophilic and protein bound. They have a fairly long half-life of elimination; therefore, steady state is achieved in approximately 5 days. There is a lag time of 2 to 4 weeks before remission of depressive symptoms becomes apparent. Half-life ranges from 8 to 90 hours but averages 24 to 36 hours. Table 15-10 includes the pharmacokinetics of TCAs.

Metabolism and Excretion

The TCAs undergo first-pass metabolism by the liver and are excreted by the kidneys. At least two (amitriptyline and imipramine) of the TCAs are metabolized into active metabolites that further extend the half-life and contribute to the difficulty in overdosage.

Pharmacotherapeutics

Precautions and Contraindications

Due to their direct alpha-adrenergic blocking effect and quinidine-like effect on the myocardium, TCAs are contraindicated with cardiovascular disorders. Similarly, due to their acetylcholine blocking effect they should be used with caution in those who have glaucoma, prostatic hypertrophy, or urinary incontinence. They should not be prescribed in combination with MAOIs or to individuals who have demonstrated hypersensitivity in this class.

Safety of use in pregnancy is unclear. TCAs are Pregnancy Category C and are excreted in low doses in breast milk.

Although rare, tardive dyskinesia and neuroleptic malignant syndrome have been reported, and are more likely with amoxapine use due to its dopaminergic effect.

As with any drug that affects the CNS, the TCAs should be titrated gradually in either direction. Nausea, headache,

vertigo, malaise, and nightmares have been noted following abrupt discontinuance of the drug or after large dose decreases.

The most significant risks related to TCA use are cardiac conduction disorder. At highest risk are children and the elderly; therefore, baseline ECG and periodic monitoring should be performed. The most common cardiovascular effect is sinus tachycardia due to the inhibition of norepinephrine reuptake and anticholinergic action. In addition, TCAs contribute to slowing of depolarization of the cardiac muscle, contributing to prolongation of the QRS complex and the PR/QT intervals.

TCAs can lower the seizure threshold of those with a seizure disorder or those taking medications that also decrease the seizure threshold. Because the index between therapeutic and toxic levels is narrow, great care needs to be taken when prescribing for a person who is depressed and has suicidal ideas. When treating such a person, the nurse practitioner needs to be alert for an energizing effect that precedes depressive symptom remission because this may contribute to sufficient activation to follow through with a suicidal plan. Such patients need to be monitored on a weekly basis, especially regarding suicidal thoughts and behaviors, and medication should be dispensed in only small amounts until suicidal risk decreases.

Finally, TCAs should be used with extreme caution if at all with the elderly. Due to their anticholinergic and norepinephrine effects, they can contribute to confusion, orthostatic hypotension, and falls.

Adverse Drug Reactions

Anticholinergic adverse effects are common and can include dry mouth, constipation, urinary hesitancy or retention, blurred vision, sedation, orthostatic hypotension, weight gain, nausea and vomiting, gynecomastia, and changes in libido. Patients newly prescribed a TCA should be cautioned about safety in a situation in which mental alertness is required until the full effect of the drug has been determined.

Drug Interactions

The most significant drug interactions are those that increase the plasma level of the TCA and thereby increase the risk of cardiotoxicity, such as can occur with the concurrent use of SRIs, cannabis, and sympathomimetics. Hyperpyrexia can occur with MAOIs and TCAs. Table 15-11 presents drug interactions.

Clinical Use and Dosing

The TCAs have shown efficacy in a variety of clinical conditions, including depression, panic disorder, enuresis, and chronic neuropathic pain. Due to their serotonergic and noradrenergic effects, they are especially helpful with anxiety disorders such as obsessive-compulsive disorder (clomipramine) and panic disorder (imipramine). Some TCAs, especially secondary and tertiary amines, contribute to significant drowsiness as a side effect; therefore, they are more commonly used for insomnia than they are for depression. Most notable of the TCAs used for insomnia include doxepin (Sinequan), amitriptyline (Elavil), and trazodone (Desyrel). Amitriptyline and imipramine are useful for neuropathic pain. Dosages are shown in Table 15-12.

Table 15–11 ⚏ Drug Interactions: Tricyclic Antidepressants

Drug	Interacting Drug	Possible Effect	Implications
All TCAs	SSRIs, anorexiants, cimetidine, oral contraceptives, charcoal, calcium channel blockers, protease inhibitors, propoxyphene, methylphenidate	Increased plasma level of TCA and increased risk of cardiotoxicity	Use with caution; monitor plasma levels of TCA
	Narcotics, barbiturates, antihistamines, alcohol, benzodiazepines, antipsychotics	Increased CNS depression; increased TCA plasma level; increased risk of cardiotoxicity	Use with caution; monitor plasma level of TCA
	Anticholinergics	Increased anticholinergic adverse reactions	Avoid concurrent use if possible
	Dicumarol	Increased prothrombin time	Monitor
	Carbamazepine, phenytoin	Increased plasma level of anticonvulsant	Monitor blood levels of anticonvulsants
	MAOIs	Hyperpyretic crisis, convulsions	Avoid concurrent use
	Guanethidine	Hypotension	Monitor blood pressure
	Clonidine	Hypertension	Monitor BP
	Levodopa	Hypertension, dyskinesia	Use different type of antidepressant
	Tamoxifen, nicotine, rifampin	Decreased TCA effect	May require higher dose
	Sympathomimetics	Hypertension, risk of arrhythmias	Avoid if possible
	Cannabis	Increased risk of cardiotoxicity, tachycardia, light-headedness, confusion, mood lability, delirium	Avoid

Table 15–12 ⚗ Dosage Schedule: Tricyclic Antidepressants

Drug	Indications	Dosage	Available Dosage Forms
Amitriptyline (Elavil)	Depression, insomnia	*Adult:* 75 mg/d in divided doses to maximum of 150 mg/d; may give entire dose at bedtime; hospitalized patients may require 200–300 mg/d.	Tablets: 10, 25, 50, 75, 100, 150 mg
		Adolescents and older adults: 10 tid or 25 mg at bedtime; maximum 100 mg/d.	Syrup: 10 mg/5 mL
Amoxapine (Asendin)	Depression, psychotic depression	*Adults and children >16:* 50 mg bid tid, gradually increasing to 200–300 mg/d/ if needed; maximum 400 mg/d. If total dose equals 300 mg or more, give in divided doses. *Older adults:* 25 mg bid tid; may gradually increase to maximum of 300 mg/d	Tablets: 25, 50, 100, 150 mg
Clomipramine (Anafranil)	OCD	*Adults:* 25 mg/d initially; increase over 2 wk to maximum or 250 mg/d. Give with food to minimize GI distress. May divide dose initially; give at bedtime for maintenance.	Capsules: 25, 50, 75 mg
		Children and adolescents: 25 mg/d initially; may gradually increase over 2 wk to maximum of 3 mg/kg/d or 100 mg, whichever is smaller, or for adolescents, to maximum of 3 mg/kg/d or 200 mg, whichever is smaller.	
Desipramine HCl (Norpramin)	Depression	*Adults:* 100–200 mg/d in single or divided dose; maximum 300 mg/d *Adolescents and older adults:* 25–100 mg/d maximum 150 mg/d	Tablets: 10, 25, 50, 75, 100, 150 mg
Doxepin HCl (Sinequan)	Depression, insomnia	*Adults:* 75–150 mg/d, preferably at hs; maximum 300 mg/d. Dilute concentrate with 120 mL of milk, water, or juice.	Capsules: 10, 25, 50, 75, 100, 150 mg Concentrate; 10 mg/mL
Imipramine HCl (Tofranil, Tofranil PM)	Depression, enuresis in children >6 yr	*Adults:* 50–150 mg/d at hs; maximum 200 mg/d. Hospitalized patients may require 250–300 mg/d.	Tablets: 10, 25, 50, 75
		Adolescents and older adults: 30–40 mg/d to maximum of 100 mg/d	Capsules: 75, 100, 125, 150

Continued

Table 15–12 ⊗ **Dosage Schedule: Tricyclic Antidepressants—cont'd**

Drug	Indications	Dosage	Available Dosage Forms
		Children: 1.5 mg/kg/d tid to maximum of 5 mg/kg/d. Increase by increments of 1–15 mg/kg/d at 3 to 5 d intervals.	
Nortriptyline HCl (Pamelor, Aventyl)	Depression	*Adults:* 25 mg tid qid to maximum of 100 mg/d	Capsules: 10, 25, 50, 75 mg
		Adolescents and older adults: 30–50 mg/d in divided doses	Solution: 10 mg/5 mL
Protriptyline HCl (Vivactil)	Depression	*Adults:* 100–200 mg/d in single or divided dose; maximum 60 mg/d. Make increase in a.m.	Tablets: 5, 10 mg
		Adolescents and older adults: 25–100 mg/d: maximum 150 mg/d	
Trimipramine maleate (Surmontil)	Depression	*Adults:* 75–150 mg/d in divided doses; maximum 200 mg/d. Hospitalized patients may require 250–300 mg/d. *Adolescents and older adults:* 50–100 mg/d	Capsules: 25, 50, 100 mg

Rational Drug Selection

Indications for the use of TCAs are depression, anxiety with sleep disturbance, enuresis in children 6 years or older, obsessive-compulsive disorder (OCD), and eating disorders. Prior to prescribing, the nurse practitioner needs to obtain a patient and family history of suicide and cardiovascular disease, as these are risk factors for adverse events. These drugs should be avoided with the elderly and used with caution with children.

Monitoring

A preliminary ECG should be done with QT correction and repeated after 3 weeks. Plasma levels can be assessed to assure delivery of an adequate dosage and to support patient adherence. Drugs with secondary active metabolites will show the plasma level in terms of each metabolite as well as a total level. Again, suicidal ideation must be monitored carefully during the first month after initiation, then periodically if residual depressive symptoms remain.

Patient Education

Advise the patient to avoid engaging in hazardous activities or using heavy machinery if drowsy or sedated. If the patient develops dry mouth, advise him or her to use sugarless candy or gum. If constipation develops, advise the patient to increase fluid and fiber intake and to use a bulking agent or stool softener.

MONOAMINE OXIDASE INHIBITORS (MAOIs)

MAOIs are infrequently used today in mental health nursing and psychiatry because safer drugs that are equally efficacious are available. If the nurse practitioner decides to prescribe these drugs, it is advisable to do so with expert consultation. These drugs are primarily reserved for the treatment of refractory unipolar depression. There are four MAOIs available: phenelzine (Nardil), isocarboxazid (Marplan), tranylcypromine (Parnate), and selegiline (Emsam), a transdermal preparation.

Pharmacodynamics

The MAOIs exert their effect by irreversibly inactivating the enzymes that metabolize norepinephrine, serotonin, and dopamine, thereby increasing the bioavailability of these neurotransmitters. In addition, they prevent the breakdown of tyramine, found in many foods that are aged or fermented. Because tyramine is toxic to humans, contributing to rapid extreme hypertension, these drugs require careful dietary restrictions. Selegiline transdermal (Emsam) requires dietary restriction only for doses above 9 mg in 24 hours.

Pharmacokinetics

Absorption and Distribution

The MAOIs are administered orally and are rapidly and thoroughly absorbed from the GI tract.

Metabolism and Excretion

There is a major first-pass effect of liver metabolism, and most of these drugs have P450 2D6 as a substrate. They are metabolized by the liver. Half-life is variable within 1 to 3 hours. TCA metabolites are excreted by the kidneys.

Onset, Peak, and Duration

Whereas SRIs and TCAs have long half-lives, requiring 3 to 4 weeks before full therapeutic benefits are evident, patients taking MAOIs may begin to experience relief of their depressive symptoms immediately or within approximately 14 days. Onset is 1 to 2 weeks; the peak for isocarboxazid and tranylcypromine is 0.7 to 3 hours and 1 to 2 hours for phenelzine.

Pharmacotherapeutics

Precautions and Contraindications

Contraindications include liver or kidney disease, hypersensitivity, congestive heart failure or arteriosclerotic disease, and age over 60 years. They should not be used with patients who are impulsive, cognitively impaired, or cannot follow the necessary dietary restrictions.

These drugs are rated Pregnancy Category C. They are excreted in breast milk, and safety has not been established. They have not been approved for use with children.

Postural hypotension and suppression of myocardial pain may occur.

Adverse Drug Reactions

Initial adverse effects may include insomnia, anxiety, and agitation as a result of the delayed metabolism of dopamine. In addition, dry mouth, blurred vision, urinary retention, and constipation occur because of anticholinergic activity. Most common side effects include dizziness, headache, insomnia, restlessness, and hypotension.

Clinical Use and Dosing

Because safer and more convenient drugs are available, the MAOIs are reserved for drug-resistant, refractory depressions.

Drug and Food Interactions

Because MAOIs inhibit the metabolism of norepinephrine, hypertensive crisis can occur if they are administered concurrently with other drugs or foods that raise blood pressure, including anticholinergics, sympathomimetics, stimulants, and foods containing tyramine. Tyramine is a precursor to dopamine, norepinephrine, and epinephrine. Foods that have been aged or fermented are rich in tyramine; therefore, dietary restrictions apply during use or within 14 days following discontinuance of the MAOI.

Symptoms of hypertensive crisis include headache, heart palpitations, stiff or sore neck, chest tightness, tachycardia, sweating, and dilated pupils. The crisis needs to be managed immediately, and the patient should remain standing until it is. Usual treatment is phentolamine (Regitine) 5 mg IV and then 0.25 to 0.5 mg IM every 4 to 6 hours. The prolonged metabolism of norepinephrine and the pressor effect of other drugs can lead to interactions resulting in hypotension and heart failure.

The 14-day restriction discussed previously also applies to initiating SRI or SNRI drug treatment. The increased amount of serotonin available due to inhibition of its metabolism by the MAOI leads to a risk of the potentially fatal serotonin syndrome. As a result of other drug interactions, particularly with meperidine, CNS depression can also occur. Table 15-13 presents drug interactions.

Rational Drug Selection

Use of MAOIs should be limited to conditions that are resistant to other forms of pharmacotherapy. Most notably, MAOIs have been used with treatment-resistant unipolar depression, panic disorder, and atypical depression associated with borderline personality disorder.

Monitoring

Periodic liver function tests should be performed and the drug discontinued if any abnormalities are found.

Patient Education

Advise the patient that strict dietary restrictions need to be followed. Provide a written list of foods to be avoided, including cheese, yogurt, sour cream, aged meat and meat products, dried fish and herring, alcoholic beverages, fermented vegetables such as sauerkraut, soy sauce, miso soup, bean curd, fava beans, avocados, bananas, raisins, caffeine, chocolate, and ginseng.

SELECTIVE SEROTONIN REUPTAKE INHIBITORS (SSRIs)

The SSRIs were first approved by the FDA in 1985 with the introduction of fluoxetine (Prozac) and quickly followed by paroxetine (Paxil), sertraline (Zoloft), fluvoxamine (Luvox), citalopram (Celexa), and most recently escitalopram (Lexapro).

Table 15–13 ⠿ Drug Interactions: Monoamine Oxidase Inhibitors

Drug	Interacting Drug	Possible Effect	Implications
All MAOIs	Anorexiants, venlafaxine, SSRIs, bupropion, bromocriptine, L-dopa, L-tryptophan, MAO-B inhibitor, sumatriptan	Increased serotonergic effect, possible serotonin syndrome	Avoid
	CNS depressants, meperidine, antipsychotics	Increased CNS depression	Use cautiously in hazardous situations
Amphetamines	Buspirone, L-dopa, reserpine, tetrabenazine, guanethidine, meperidine	Increased blood pressure and possible hypertensive crisis	Monitor blood pressure; avoid if possible
	Antihypertensives, propoxyphene, meperidine, diuretics, nitroglycerin, dextromethorphan	Hypotension agitation diaphoresis, vascular collapse	Monitor blood pressure; avoid concurrent administration if possible
	Insulin, sulfonylureas	Hypoglycemia	Monitor blood glucose and for signs and symptoms of hypoglycemia
	Carbamazepine	Increased carbamazepine level	Monitor level; use alternative anticonvulsant if possible
	TCAs and SSRIs	Seizures and delirium	Avoid

Vortioxetine (Brintellix), the newest SSRI, was approved by the FDA in 2013. Because of their safety and equitable efficacy, their use has exceeded the use of TCAs and MAOIs.

Pharmacodynamics

All the SSRIs affect the serotonin neurotransmitter in the synaptic cleft by blocking the serotonin transporter from returning remaining serotonin to the presynaptic cell. Although traditionally these drugs are referred to as *selective* serotonin reuptake inhibitors, each one has different effects on other neurotransmitters. For example, fluoxetine significantly affects dopamine that contributes to the development of side effects. Citalopram and escitalopram are probably the closest to a true serotonin selective reuptake inhibitor. Through this mechanism, more serotonin is available to bind with the postsynaptic receptors.

Pharmacokinetics

Absorption and Distribution

All of the SSRIs are given orally and thoroughly absorbed through the GI tract. They are all highly protein bound with variable biodistribution, ranging from 12 to 40 L/kg. Peak plasma levels range from 1 to 8 hours and have a positive correlation with parent half-life.

Metabolism and Excretion

The SSRIs have a significant first-pass effect in the liver and are metabolized predominantly by the CYP450 system. Consideration of the half-life requires consideration of active metabolites as well as the possibility of inhibiting the SSRI's own metabolism. For example, fluoxetine as the parent drug has a half-life of 1 to 3 days and its first metabolite, norfluoxetine, has an additional half-life of 4 to 16 days, resulting in an overall half-life of 4 to 16 days. Similarly, sertraline has a half-life of 24 to 26 hours but inhibits the P450 2D6 enzyme that is also the substrate for metabolism. Vortioxetine is metabolized primarily via CYP450 isozymes CYP2D6, CYP3A4/5, CYP2C19, CYP2C9, CYP2A6, CYP2C8 and CYP2B6. CYP2D6 poor metabolizers have approximately twice the vortioxetine plasma concentration of extensive 2D6 metabolizers. Table 15-14 presents the pharmacokinetics of SSRIs. Excretion of the SSRIs is primarily by the kidneys.

Pharmacotherapeutics

Precautions and Contraindications

Contraindications to use are limited to hypersensitivity to any of the drugs and concurrent or within 14 days of the administration of an MAOI. They should be used cautiously in patients with severe hepatic or renal impairment and should be avoided in the first and last trimesters of pregnancy. Although safety of use during pregnancy has not been definitively established, sertraline in particular has been used without adverse consequences. Risk versus benefit needs to be carefully considered, as it does during lactation as well. Caution is recommended. Fluvoxamine and vortioxetine are Pregnancy Category C, paroxetine is Pregnancy Category D, and the others are Category B. High doses of SSRIs have caused malformations and fetal death in animal studies. Neonates exposed to SSRIs in the late third trimester have demonstrated complications soon after birth, requiring hospitalization, respiratory support, and tube feedings.

Table 15–14 ⚏ **Pharmacokinetics: SNRIs, SSRIs, and Other Antidepressants**

Drug	Peak	Half-Life	Excretion
Trazodone	1–2 h	3–9 h	Urine, feces
Fluoxetine HCl	6–8 h	1–384 h	Urine
Fluvoxamine maleate	3–8 h	16 h	Urine
Levomilnacipran	6–8 h	12 h	Urine
Milnacipran	2–4 h	6-8 h	Urine
Nefazodone HCl	1 h	2–18 h	Urine, feces
Mirtazapine	12 h	20–40 h	Urine, feces
Bupropion HCl	2 h	21–37 h	Urine
Paroxetine HCl	5.2 h	21–33 h	Urine
Sertraline HCl	4.5–8 h	26 h	Urine
Venlafaxine	1–3 h	5–11 h	Urine
Vortioxetine	7–11 h	66 h	Urine
Citalopram	4 h	35 h	Urine
Escitalopram	5 h	27–32 h	Urine

All of the SSRIs have been studied in children and FDA-labeled according to safety and effectiveness. Fluoxetine is labeled effective for major depression in children age 8 to 17 years and effective in treating OCD in children age 7 to 17 years. The safety and effectiveness of escitalopram have been established for treating major depression in adolescents age 12 to 17 years. Fluvoxamine is approved for treating OCD in children and adolesents age 8 to 17 years; it is not approved for treating depression in children or adolescents. Paroxetine is not approved for use in children after studies indicated it is not effective for them. Sertraline is approved for the treatment of OCD in children age 6 to 17 years, but not for treatment of depression or panic disorder in children. Vortioxetine has not been studied for safety or effectiveness in children or adolescents.

Although clinical drug trials do not substantiate a link between SSRIs and suicidal thinking, there is clearly a greater risk of suicide within the first 3 weeks of taking SSRIs and other antidepressants. This is related to the lag time in receiving the full therapeutic effect while there is an increase in neurocognitive activation early in initiation of the drug. Therefore, patients have greater energy to act on suicidal thoughts.

Adverse Drug Reactions

Adverse reactions to this group of drugs depend on which receptors are affected but are usually relatively minor and transient. Most common are nausea and sometimes vomiting, headache, light-headedness, dizziness, dry mouth, increased sweating, weight gain or loss, exacerbation of anxiety, and agitation. Sexual side effects may occur in up to 35% of patients and manifest as diminished, delayed, or absent orgasm; premature ejaculation; and decreased libido. A patient may not experience the same sexual side effects with other SRIs, and it is reasonable to decrease the dosage or change to another medication if they develop.

A significant adverse effect is serotonin syndrome, which occurs in the presence of excessive serotonergic activity. Therefore, maximum recommended doses must be adhered to, adjunctive combinations of serotonergic agents must be avoided, and adequate time for titration when changing from one serotonergic to another must be provided. A safe guideline when making such a change is to allow five half-lives per dose decrease, so that titrating off a 20 mg dose of paroxetine would need 5 days at 10 mg before starting another serotonergic drug. Symptoms of serotonin syndrome are nausea, diarrhea, chills, sweating, hyperthermia, hypertension, myoclonic jerking, tremor, agitation, ataxia, disorientation, confusion, and delirium. It can progress to coma and death.

Several years after the SSRIs had been on the market, it became apparent that some have a significant withdrawal syndrome that can be very disturbing to patients. In fact, the shorter half-life drugs such as paroxetine, sertraline, citalopram, and escitalopram can show withdrawal symptoms with just one missed dose. These symptoms are nausea, dizziness, and paresthesias such as electric shock sensations or visual tracers with eye movements. Fluoxetine is the only SSRI that does not require gradual and slow tapering because of its long half-life and active metabolites. In fact, a single dose of fluoxetine as the last step in tapering off other SSRIs is helpful in avoiding withdrawal symptoms.

Drug Interactions

Significant drug interactions may occur. As previously mentioned, the most significant are with MAOIs and other serotonergic drugs. With MAOIs there needs to be at least a 14-day washout period before initiating an SSRI and at least a 21 day washout of fluoxetine before initiating an MAOI. Drugs that inhibit the P450 2D6 will increase the effects of the SRI, and many SRIs inhibit the 2D6 and 3A3/4 and will interact with drugs that use these enzymes as substrates. CNS depression can occur with alcohol, antihistamines, and opioid analgesics. Concomitant use of St. John's wort and/or SAMe (S-adenosylmethionine) may contribute to serotonin syndrome. SSRIs should not be prescribed with TCAs and require washout between drugs. The SSRI may increase the plasma level of the TCA, which increases the risk of cardiac conduction complications. Table 15-15 includes the drug interactions with the SRIs.

Clinical Use and Dosages

Table 15-16 includes the indications, dosages, and available dosage forms for the SRIs and non-TCA antidepressants.

Rational Drug Selection

The SRIs, with the exception of fluvoxamine, are indicated for the treatment of depressive, anxiety, and panic disorders; OCD; and bulimia. Fluvoxamine is FDA-approved for the treatment of OCD, although it is likely to be as effective as the others for the listed disorders. More recently, the FDA has approved the indication for premenstrual dysphoric disorder, post-traumatic disorder (PTSD), generalized anxiety disorder, and social phobia. Off-label uses include the treatment of anorexia, the depressive phase of bipolar disorder, chronic headaches and other types of pain, impulse control disorders, and trichotillomania.

The patient needs to be monitored closely during the first 2 to 3 weeks of initiation of SRIs, including regular assessment of suicidal thinking. There should be at least telephone contact on a weekly basis with an agreement to notify the prescriber immediately if suicidal thoughts occur or persist.

Monitoring

No specific monitoring is required, other than ongoing assessment of mood.

Patient Education

Advise the patient that these drugs may take as long as 3 to 4 weeks until their full therapeutic benefits become evident and that the initial adverse reactions, commonly including nausea, intermittent light-headedness, sedation, muscle restlessness, and sleep disruptions, should be minor and transient. Also, tell the patient to assess the level of sedation the drug can initially cause before engaging in hazardous activities. Patients also need to be reminded not to miss a dose or let their prescription run out before seeking a refill because of the withdrawal syndrome.

Table 15–15 ▦ Drug Interactions: Selective Serotonin Reuptake Inhibitors (SSRIs)

Drug	Interacting Drug	Possible Effect	Implications
All (SSRIs)	Anorexiants, ergotamine, tryptophan	Serotonin syndrome	Avoid; or use with caution
	MAOIs	Hypertensive crisis	Contraindicated
	Valproate carbamazepine	Increased level of anticonvulsant	Monitor plasma levels
	TCAs	Increased level of TCA, increased risk of cardiotoxicity	Monitor blood levels of TCA; use with caution
	Benzodiazepines	Increased plasma level of benzodiazepines with sedation and psychomotor/cognitive impairment	Avoid long-term use of benzodiazepines
	Beta blockers	Bradycardia, syncope, increased serum levels of SSRI	Warn patient
	Insulin	Increased insulin sensitivity	Monitor blood glucose
	Neuroleptics	Increased plasma level of neuroleptic	Monitor for adverse reactions
	Zolpidem	Hallucinations and delirium	Avoid
	Aspirin, NSAIDs	Risk of bleeding increased	Caution
	Alcohol	May potentiate alcohol effects	Avoid

Table 15–16 ✂ Dosage Schedule: Non-TCA Antidepressants

Drug	Indications	Neurotransmitters Affected	Dosage	Available Dosage Forms
Bupropion (Wellbutrin, Wellbutrin SR, Wellbutrin XL)	Depression, Seasonal Affective Disorder	Dopamine, norepinephrine	*Adolescents and adults:* 75–450 mg/d; give 2–3 times/d with 6 h intervals in between; no single dose to exceed 150 mg; increase at 3 to 4 d intervals Wellbutrin XL 150–300 mg qAM	Tablets: 75, 100 mg Sustained-release tablets: 75, 100 mg Extended-release: 150, 300 mg
Citalopram (Celexa)	Depression, anxiety (off-labeled)	Primary: serotonin Secondary: norepinephrine and dopamine	*Adults:* 20 mg qd; may increase in 20 mg increments at weekly intervals; maximum 60 mg/d *Older adults:* 20 mg/d	Tablets: 10, 20, 40 mg
Desvenlafaxine (Pristiq)	Depression	Serotonin Norepinephrine	*Adults:* 50 mg qam, max 100 mg/d	Tablets, extended-release: 50, 100 mg
Duloxetine (Cymbalta)	Depression, diabetic neuropathy, fibromyalgia, anxiety	Serotonin and norepinephrine	*Adults:* 40–60 mg/d max 60 mg 60 mg for neuropathy and fibromyalgia	Tablets: 20, 30, 60 mg
Escitalopram (Lexapro)	Depression, anxiety	Serotonin	*Adults:* 10 mg qam, max 20 mg qd *Children 12 and up:* 10 mg, may increase to 20 mg after 3 wk	5, 10, 20 mg tabs Oral solution 1 mg/mL
Fluoxetine (Prozac)	Depression, OCD, bulimia, panic disorder	Primary: serotonin Secondary: norepinephrine	*Adolescents and adults:* 20–80 mg/d; may increase slowly at 5 d intervals after 3 to 4 wk trial at lower dose; OCD may require a higher dose *Children 8–17:* 10 mg qd, increase by 10 mg in 1 wk. Slower titration with lower-weight children *Older adults:* Half dose	Capsules: 10,0 mg, 40 Liquid: 20 mg/5 mL Delayed-release capsules: 90 mg

Table 15–16 ⊗ **Dosage Schedule: Non-TCA Antidepressants—cont'd**

Drug	Indications	Neurotransmitters Affected	Dosage	Available Dosage Forms
Fluvoxamine (Luvox)	OCD, social anxiety disorder Depression (off-labeled)	Primary: serotonin Secondary: norepinephrine	*Adults:* 50–300 mg/d; dose >100 mg should be divided; increase in 50 mg increments every 4–7 d *Older adults:* half dose	Tablets: 50, 100 mg
Levomilnacipran (Fetzima)	Major depression	Serotonin and norepinephrine	*Adults:* 40 to 120 mg daily. Titration schedule: 20 mg qd x 2 days; then 40 mg qd. Adjust dose in increments of 40 mg q 2d. Maximum 120 mg daily.	Capsules: 20, 40, 80, or 120 mg
Milnacipran (Savella)	Fibromyalgia	Serotonin and norepinephrine	*Adults:* 100 mg (50 mg bid). Titration schedule: day 1: 12.5 mg once; days 2–3: 25 mg/d (12.5 mg bid); days 4–7: 50 mg/d (25 mg bid); after day 7: 100 mg/d (50 mg bid)	Tablets: 12.5 mg, 25 mg, 50 mg, 100 mg
Mirtazapine (Remeron, Remeron Soltabs)	Depression	Primary: histamine Secondary: serotonin and norepinephrine	*Adults:* 15–45 mg/d, preferably at bedtime Disintegrating Soltab: 15, 30, 45 mg Lower doses may increase sedation	Tablets: 15, 30, 45 mg
Nefazodone	Depression	Primary: serotonin Secondary: adrenergic	*Adults:* 200–600 mg/d in 2 divided doses; increase in 100–200 mg/d increments at weekly intervals	Tablets: 50, 100, 150, 200, 250 mg
Paroxetine (Paxil, Paxil CR)	Depression, OCD, panic disorder, social phobia, PTSD, anxiety, PMDD (CR)	Primary: serotonin; Secondary: norepinephrine	*Adolescents and adults:* 20–60 mg/d; panic disorder and OCD may require higher doses; taper off slowly *Older adults:* half dose	Tablets: 10, 20, 30, 40 mg Controlled-release: 12.5, 25 mg Oral suspension: 10 mg/5 mL
Sertraline (Zoloft)	Depression, OCD, GAD, PMDD, PTSD, social anxiety disorder	Primary: serotonin Secondary: norepinephrine	*Adolescents and adults:* 50–200 mg/d; increase at weekly intervals *Older adults:* half dose	Tablets: 25, 50, 100 mg Concentrate: 20 mg/mL
Trazodone (Desyrel)	Depression, off label for sleep	Primary: serotonin Secondary: adrenergic	*Adults:* 50–400 mg/d; increase in 50 mg increments every 3–4 d; take with food	Tablets: 50, 100, 150, 300 mg
Venlafaxine (Effexor)	Depression, PTSD, GAD, social anxiety disorder, panic disorder	Primary: serotonin Secondary: norepinephrine	*Adults:* 75–375 mg/d in divided doses. When discontinuing, taper off over a 2 wk period; increase in 75 mg increments at 4 d intervals; take with food Extended-release: 37.5, 75, 150 mg	Tablets: 25, 37.5, 50, 75, 100 mg
Vortioxetine (Brintellix)	Major depression	Serotonin	*Adults:* 10 mg/d, may increase to 20 mg/d	Tablet: 5, 10, 15, or 20 mg

SEROTONIN-NOREPINEPHRINE REUPTAKE INHIBITORS (SNRIs)

In the United States there are six SNRIs that have been approved by the FDA: venlafaxine (Effexor and Effexor XR), desvenlafaxine (Pristiq), duloxetine (Cymbalta), Milnacipran (Savella), and levomilnacipran (Fetzima). Milnacipran (Savella) was approved by the FDA in 2009 to treat fibromyalgia. Levomilnacipran (Fetzima) is the newest SNRI, approved for major depression in 2013. Nefazodone is a serotonin antagonist and reuptake inhibitor that also inhibits the reuptake of norepinephrine. It is available only in generic form. In 2004, the FDA added a Black-Box Warning related to liver toxicity in 1 out of 250,000 cases of those taking nefazodone and 21 deaths related to liver failure. It will not be discussed in detail in this chapter.

Pharmacodynamics

Venlafaxine and duloxetine both block the serotonin and norepinephrine transporters, thereby inhibiting the reuptake of the neurotransmitter and increasing the availability to bind with the postsynaptic receptors. At lower doses (75 mg), venlafaxine predominantly affects serotonin reuptake, contributing to greater reduction of anxiety more so than reduction of depressive symptoms. Duloxetine, however, appears to be a more potent and equal serotonin and norepinephrine reuptake inhibitor than venlafaxine is. The exact mechanism of action of milnacipran and levomilnacipran are unknown, but it is thought that they inhibit reuptake of serotonin and noepinephrine.

Pharmacokinetics

Absorption and Distribution

These drugs are rapidly absorbed after oral intake and metabolized extensively in the liver. The time needed to reach maximum plasma concentration is 2 hours for both venlafaxine and duloxetine. Venlafaxine has only 30% protein binding, whereas duloxetine has greater than 90%.

Metabolism and Excretion

Venlafaxine is metabolized by CYP450 2D6 with one active metabolite (O-desmethylvenlafaxine) and two less-active metabolites. Duloxetine is metabolized by CYP450 2D6 and 1A2. Venlafaxine has a half-life of 5 hours, and the active metabolite has a half-life of 11 hours. Steady state is achieved in 3 to 4 days. Duloxetine has a half-life of 12 hours, reaching steady state in 3 days. Both drugs are excreted mostly in the urine. Levomilnacipran is catalyzed primarily by CYP3A4 and is excreted renally. Fifty-five percent of milnacipran is excreted unchanged in the urine. Milnacipran is also metabolized into inactive metabolites that are excreted in the urine.

Pharmacotherapeutics

Precautions and Contraindications

As with other drugs used to treat depression, a major precaution is increased suicidal thinking during the first few weeks of initiation and change in dosage of the medication. The patient must be monitored at least weekly and assessed for suicide risk each time. Patients need to be monitored for mood lability and switching into a manic or hypomanic state. In addition, hypersensitivity contraindicates use.

The SNRIs venlafaxine, duloxetine, levomilnacipran, and milnacipran are rated as Pregnancy Category C. There are no well-controlled studies in pregnant women taking SNRIs. There have been reports of fetal mortality and skeletal malformations in rats and rabbits. Neonates of women who took SNRIs in the third trimester have developed complications soon after birth, requiring prolonged hospitalization, respiratory support, and tube feeding.

Both venlafaxine and duloxetine have been found in breast milk. There are no proven adverse effects in infants exposed to venlafaxine via breast milk, but it is recommended infants be monitored for weight gain and excessive sedation (LactMed, 2014). There is little information on the effects of duloxetine in breastfed infants. It is recommended that exclusively breastfed infants of mothers who take duloxetine be monitored for adequate weight gain, drowsiness, and developmental milestones (LactMed, 2014). Levomilnacipran is excreted in breast milk in rats, but has not been studied in lactating women, and the manufacturer recommends nursing women not take the medication while breastfeeding (LactMed, 2014). Milnacipran is excreted in breast milk and in a single study where lactating women were administered a single 50 mg dose of milnacipran, the maximum estimated infant dose via breast milk was 5% of maternal dose (Forest Laboratories, 2013).

Duloxetine may exacerbate narrow-angle glaucoma and should be used cautiously with these patients. Duloxetine has also shown increased serum transaminase levels and should not be used with patients with liver disorders.

Adverse Drug Reactions

The most common side effects with both venlafaxine and duloxetine include headache, somnolence, dizziness, insomnia, nervousness, nausea, dry mouth, constipation, and abnormal ejaculations. Appetite and weight decreases may occur. At higher doses, both drugs may contribute to elevated blood pressure. There was no effect shown to the QTc interval with either of these drugs.

The most common adverse effect of milnacipran in clinical trials was nausea in 37% of patients. Other common adverse effects include headache (18%), constipation (16%), hot flush (12%), dizziness (10%), hyperhidrosis (9%), and palpitations (7%). Male patients reported erectile dysfunction, decreased libido, and ejaculation failure.

Levomilnacipran most commonly may cause nausea (17%), constipation (9%), hyperhidrosis (9%), tachycardia (6%), erectile dysfunction (6%), and urinary hesitation (4%). Erectile dysfunction and urinary hesitation increase as the dose increases.

Drug Interactions

Drugs that inhibit CYP450 2D6 will interact with both venlafaxine and duloxetine, including fluoxetine and quinidine. With duloxetine, drugs that inhibit 1A2 will also interact, especially fluvoxamine and some quinolone antibiotics. There seems to be no interaction between alcohol and either venlafaxine or duloxetine; however, frequent use of alcohol may affect the liver function, and therefore duloxetine should not be used with patients who abuse or are dependent on alcohol.

Drugs that inhibit CYP3A4 (i.e., ketoconazole) may require adjustment of levomilnacipran dosage. Alcohol may cause an accelerated release of levomilnacipran extended-release, and it is recommended that levomilnacipran not be taken with alcohol.

Serotonin syndrome may occur if milnacipran is used concurrently with a triptan. If a triptan is clinically indicated, patients should be monitored closely. The catecholamines epinephrine and noepinephrine may cause paroxysmal hypertension and dysrhythmias if coministered with milnacipran, because milnacipran inhibits the reuptake of norepinephrine. Patients taking milnacipran and digoxin have reported postural hypotension and tachycardia. Clonidine's antihypertensive effect may be inhibited by milnacipran owing to inhabitation of norepinephrine reuptake.

Clinical Use and Dosing

These drugs are indicated in treating major depressive disorders and bipolar mood disorders. Venlafaxine is also approved for treating anxiety disorders such as generalized anxiety disorder, social phobia, and PTSD. Duloxetine is also approved to treat neuropathic pain and overactive bladder. It is likely that duloxetine, owing to its neurophysiological action, will eventually be approved for treating anxiety disorders as well.

Venlafaxine is available in extended-release (XR) form as well as in immediate-release form. The immediate-release form must be taken at least twice a day and has uncomfortable discontinuation symptoms if doses are missed, including paresthesias, dizziness, nausea, and vomiting. The initial dose for venlafaxine XR is 75 mg/day, which is increased to 150 to 300 mg/day in increments of 75 mg every 4 days. Severely depressed patients may require a higher dosage of 375 to 450 mg/day in divided doses to prevent side effects.

The initial dose of duloxetine is 20 mg/day, which is increased to 60 mg/day in increments of 20 mg every 4 days. There is no evidence that doses higher than 60 mg/day produce better results than 60 mg/day. Desvenlafaxine (Pristiq), an active metabolite of venlafaxine, is available only in extended-release capsules.

Levomilnacipran is indicated for major depressive disorder, with the recommended dose range of 40 mg to 120 mg daily. Patients should be started on 20 mg once daily for 2 days, then increased to 40 mg daily. The dose may be adjusted in increments of 40 mg every 2 days until efficacy is determined. The maximum dose is 120 mg daily. Withdrawal symptoms may be seen if levomilnacipran is discontinued abruptly; therefore it should be tapered if discontinued.

Milnacipran is indicated for treatment of fibromyalgia, with a recommended dose of 100 mg/day (50 mg twice daily). Patients may tolerate milnacipran better if the dose is titrated based on the following schedule: day 1: 12.5 mg once; days 2–3: 25 mg/day (12.5 mg BID); days 4–7: 50 mg/day (25 mg BID); after day 7: 100 mg/day (50 mg BID). Withdrawal symptoms are seen if milnacipran is abruptly discontinued; therefore it should be tapered when discontinuing.

Rational Drug Selection

Initially, it was thought that duloxetine would be especially effective for patients with melancholic depressions or the type of depressions with low energy, hypersomnia, low motivation, and social withdrawal. However, the results have been inconclusive about this selective and difficult-to-treat population. Both venlafaxine and duloxetine are more activating than the SSRIs and therefore are first-line drugs to use with patients who have the more sluggish types of depression. Venlafaxine also seems effective with adults who have both depression and attention deficit-hyperactivity disorder. Milnacipran is only used for fibromyalgia.

Monitoring

No specific serum level monitoring is available for the SNRIs. With duloxetine, liver function should be monitored once weekly, once monthly, biannually, and finally annually. All patients taking antidepressants need to be carefully monitored for suicidal risk as well as activation of hypomanic or manic symptoms.

Patient Education

Patients should be given written descriptions of side effects and ways to relieve them. Women of childbearing age need to be told to report if pregnant and should be tapered off medication, especially in the third trimester. As with the SSRIs, sudden discontinuation frequently results in uncomfortable withdrawal symptoms; and patients need to request refill prescriptions in an adequate amount of time to avoid running out.

ANTIPSYCHOTICS (APS)

Since 1952, when chlorpromazine (Thorazine) was first used to treat psychosis, there has been a substantial increase in the types of antipsychotic agents available. Antipsychotic drugs (APs) are generally divided into two major categories, although numerous specific classes exist. The older APs are variably termed *conventional*, *traditional*, or *typical* antipsychotics. They are also referred to as *neuroleptics* or *major tranquilizers*. The newer APs are generally termed *atypical antipsychotics*. In this chapter, the older APs will be termed typical APs and the newer agents will be termed atypical APs. The specific classes of APs and examples of these include the benzisoxazoles (paliperidone, risperidone, ziprasidone), piperidinyl-benzisoxazole (iloperidone), benzisothiazol (lurasidone), butyrophenones (haloperidol), dibenzoxazepines (loxapine), dibenzo-oxepino pyrroles (asenapine), dibenzodiazepines (clozapine), dibenzothiazepines (quetiapine), dihydroindolones (molindone), diphenylbutylpiperidines (pimozide), phenothiazines (chlorpromazine), quinolinones (aripiprazole), thienobenzodiazepines (olanzapine), and thioxanthenes (thiothixene).

Traditionally, it was believed that overstimulation of dopamine (D) receptors was at the heart of schizophrenia. This theory, called the dopamine hypothesis, formed the basis for understanding the effect of typical APs in reducing the positive symptoms of schizophrenia, such as hallucinations and delusions. A more current hypothesis is that schizophrenia involves overactivity of D_2 receptors in the basal ganglia, hypothalamus, limbic system, brainstem, and medulla, and underactivity of D_1 receptors in the prefrontal cortex. The overactivity of these D_2 receptors is thought to contribute to the positive symptoms of schizophrenia, whereas the underactivity of D_1 receptors explains the negative symptoms of schizophrenia, such as lack of motivation and social isolation. As new knowledge of the brain evolves, it is apparent that it is not a simple question of too much or too little of a neurotransmitter (NT), but where is there too much, too little, or an imbalance of neurotransmitters.

TYPICAL ANTIPSYCHOTICS

The phenothiazine group of typical APs includes chlorpromazine (Thorazine), thioridazine (Mellaril), fluphenazine (Prolixin), and fluphenazine decanoate, perphenazine (Trilafon), and trifluoperazine (Stelazine). Nonphenothiazine typical APs include haloperidol (Haldol) and haloperidol decanoate, thiothixene (Navane), loxapine (Loxitane), and molindone (Moban).

Pharmacodynamics

The typical APs block D_2 receptors in the basal ganglia, hypothalamus, limbic system, brainstem, and medulla and reduce the positive symptoms of schizophrenia. Typical APs, however, are less effective in treating the negative symptoms of schizophrenia, such as flat affect, decreased motivation, withdrawal from interpersonal relationships, and poor grooming and hygiene. Clinical effectiveness occurs when 60% to 70% of D_2 receptors are blocked. Too much dopamine blockade, however, leads to symptoms resembling those of parkinsonism. Prolactin elevation appears beyond 72% D_2 occupancy. As D_2 occupancy nears 78%, extrapyramidal symptoms (EPSs) are more prominent.

Pharmacokinetics

Absorption and Distribution

Typical APs are usually administered orally, although parenteral versions and long-acting decanoate forms of haloperidol and fluphenazine are available. The drugs are absorbed rapidly and distributed widely to adipose tissue. Onset of action varies among agents. Onset of oral agents is generally within 1 to 2 hours, IM injections within 10 to 30 minutes, and decanoate forms within 1 to 9 days.

Metabolism and Excretion

Typical APs are metabolized in the liver and excreted in the urine. Half-life varies widely among agents and types of agents. Because of their lipid solubility, several weeks may be required before their antipsychotic benefits become evident. Table 15-17 presents the pharmacokinetics.

Pharmacotherapeutics

Precautions and Contraindications

Typical APs may be grouped according to whether they are high or low potency. High-potency drugs such as haloperidol and fluphenazine carry an increased risk of causing EPSs, whereas low-potency drugs such as chlorpromazine and thioridazine carry less risk of EPSs but more risk of anticholinergic adverse reactions (dry mouth, constipation, urinary retention, blurred vision) and antiadrenergic effects (orthostatic hypotension).

Contraindications for use may include narrow-angle glaucoma, bone marrow depression, and severe liver or cardiovascular disease. These agents should be used cautiously in the presence of CNS tumors, epilepsy, diabetes mellitus, respiratory disease, and prostatic hypertrophy. Safety is not established in pregnancy and lactation.

All antipsychotic medications now have an FDA Black-Box Warning regarding increased mortality in elderly patients with dementia-related psychosis and are not approved for the treatment of such patients.

Adverse Drug Reactions

Typical APs have many adverse effects that make compliance a common issue. A life-threatening adverse reaction is

Table 15–17 ⁘ Pharmacokinetics: Typical Antipsychotics

Drug	Onset	Peak	Duration	Half-Life	Excretion
Chlorpromazine HCl	Erratic	2–4 h	Up to 6 mo	10–30 h	Urine
Fluphenazine	1 h	—	6–8 h	4.7–15.3 h	Urine
Fluphenazine decanoate	1 h; 1–3 d	2–4 h; 2–3 d	6–8 h; up to 4 wk	6.8–14.3 d	Urine
Perphenazine	Erratic	2–4 h	6 h	12–24 h	Urine
Trifluoperazine	Erratic	2–4 h	4–6 h	13 h	Urine and feces equally
Thioridazine HCl	Erratic	2–4 h	4–6 h	24–36 h	Urine
Thiothixene	Slow	2–8 h	Up to 12 h	34 h	Urine
Loxapine	20–30 min	2–4 h	12 h	5–19 h	Urine
Pimozide	—	6–8 h	—	55 h	Urine
Haloperidol	2 h	2–6 h	8–12 h	21–24 h	Urine
Haloperidol decanoate	3–9 d	—	Up to 4 wk	12–36 h; 3 wk	Urine, bile
Molindone HCl	Erratic	1.5 h	24–36 h	10–20 h	Urine and feces equally

neuroleptic malignant syndrome (NMS), characterized by fever up to 107°F, elevated pulse, diaphoresis, rigidity, stupor or coma, and acute renal failure. EPSs are among the most troublesome side effects and include pseudoparkinsonism (shuffling, pill-rolling, cog-wheeling, tremors, drooling, rigidity), akathisia (restlessness), dystonia (involuntary, painful movements), and tardive dyskinesia (TD) (involuntary buccolingual movements, difficulty speaking and swallowing, which may be irreversible). Antiparkinson, antihistamine, and anticholinergic drugs are given to counter EPSs. Other side effects of typical APs include sedation, weight gain, anticholinergic effects, photosensitivity, reduction of seizure threshold, orthostatic hypotension, sexual dysfunction, galactorrhea, and amenorrhea.

Drug Interactions

Drug interactions are many and varied, the most serious of which is CNS depression with concomitant use of CNS depressants. There may be additive hypotension with antihypertensives. Lithium in combination with a phenothiazine increases the risk of EPSs and masks the early signs of lithium toxicity. There is an increased risk of anticholinergic effects with other agents having anticholinergic properties. Table 15-18 presents drug interactions.

Clinical Use and Dosing

Typical APs are more effective in reducing the positive than they are the negative symptoms of schizophrenia. Typical APs may be more effective than atypical APs in treating very severe psychosis. Patients who need rapid control of agitation and dangerous psychosis can be treated with IV haloperidol. IM chlorpromazine also provides rapid sedation. Table 15-19 presents the indications and dosage schedules of typical APs.

Rational Drug Selection

The choice of a specific agent can be guided by past response to the medication, initial response, family history, and side-effect profile of the medication. Usually, EPSs can be decreased or eliminated by the addition of drugs such as benztropine (Cogentin), diphenhydramine (Benadryl), trihexyphenidyl (Artane), atenolol (Tenormin), or amantadine (Symmetrel). A decrease in the dose or a change to a different type of antipsychotic may also counter these effects. Some anticholinergic effects, such as constipation, can be addressed by nonpharmacological measures, such as increased fluid intake and dietary bulk.

The depot or decanoate form of medication may be used if compliance is an issue. It is usually administered every 2 to 4 weeks.

Monitoring

The motor function of individuals taking typical antipsychotics should be routinely assessed with the Abnormal Involuntary Movement Scale (AIMS), which rates various movements such as joint rigidity and balance numerically, thereby enabling the clinician, over time, to detect changes

Table 15–18 ⚏ Drug Interactions: Typical Antipsychotics

Drug	Interacting Drug	Possible Effect	Implications
All typical antipsychotics	Alcohol, antihistamines, barbiturates, hypnotics, narcotics, benzodiazepines	CNS depression	Avoid; monitor for adverse reactions
	Lithium	Increased risk of neurotoxicity and EPS	Monitor lithium levels and signs and symptoms of toxicity
	Lithium, antacids, cimetidine	Decreased antipsychotic effect	May require increased antipsychotic dose
	Anticholinergics	Increased anticholinergic effect; increased risk of hyperthermia	Monitor temperature
	Beta blockers	Increased effect of both drugs	Monitor for adverse reactions
	Dopaminergics	Antagonize antipsychotic effect	Avoid concurrent use
	Hypoglycemics	Decreased diabetic control	Monitor blood glucose closely
	Phenytoin	Increased toxicity of phenytoin	Monitor blood level of phenytoin; lower dose of antipsychotic may be needed
	Trazodone	Increased hypotension	Monitor postural hypotension; warn patient to change position slowly
	Diazoxide	Hyperglycemia	Monitor blood glucose
	TCAs	Increased sedation, risk of seizures, anticholinergic effect, serum levels of TCA, risk of arrhythmias	Use SSRI
	SSRIs	Increased antipsychotic levels	Monitor dose of antipsychotic
	Nicotine	Decreased antipsychotic levels	Monitor dose of antipsychotic

Table 15–19 ⊗ Dosage Schedule: Typical Antipsychotics

Drug	Indications*	Dosage	Available Dosage Forms
Chlorpromazine HCl (Thorazine)	Psychosis; acute severe agitation	*Adults:* PO: 25 mg tid, increase gradually to maximum of 400 mg/d IM: 25 mg initially; may repeat with 25–50 mg in 1 h: maximum 400 mg IM every 4–6 h; substitute with oral as soon as possible; give concentrate with 60 mL or more of diluent *Children:* PO: 0.5 mg/kg every 4–6 h as needed Rectal: 1 mg/kg every 6–8 h as needed IM: 0.5 mg/kg every 6–8 h as needed	Tablets: 10, 15, 25, 50, 100, 150, 200 mg Solution: 30, 100 mg/mL
Fluphenazine (Prolixin)	Psychosis; acute severe agitation	*Adults:* PO: 0.5–10 mg/d in divided doses at 6 to 8 h intervals *Older adults:* PO 1–2.5 mg/d: IM one-third to one-half oral dose starting with 1.25 mg Decanoate: 12.5–25 mg deep IM every 1–3 wk	Tablets: 1, 2.5, 5, 10 mg Elixer: 2.5 mg/5 mL
Perphenazine (Trilafon)	Psychosis; acute severe agitation	*Adults:* 4–16 mg 2–4 times daily to maximum of 64 mg/d. Prolonged dosage of greater than 24 mg/day should be reserved for hospitalized patients who can be monitored for EPS. *Older adults:* One-third to one-half adult dose *Children >12 yr:* Lowest adult dose possible	Tablets: 2, 4, 8, 16 mg Concentrate: 16 mg/5 mL Injection: 5 mg/mL
Trifluoperazine (Stelazine)	Psychosis; acute severe agitation	*Adults:* 2–5 mg bid to maximum of 40 mg/d. Most are managed on 15–20 mg/day. IM: 1–2 mg every 4–6 h has needed *Older adults:* Low end of adult dose *Children >6 yr:* 1 mg 1–2 times daily; adjust according to weight	Tablets: 1, 2, 5, 10 mg Concentrate: 10 mg/mL Injection: 2 mg/mL
Thioridazine (Mellaril)	Psychosis; acute severe agitation	*Adults:* 50–100 mg tid to maximum of 800 mg/d *Children >2 yr:* 0.5 to maximum of 3 mg/kg/d	Tablets: 10, 15, 25, 50, 100, 150, 200 mg 25, 100 mg/5 mL 30, 100 mg/mL
Thiothixene (Navane)	Psychosis; acute severe agitation	*Adults:* Initial dose of 2 mg tid (5 mg tid in severe conditions). The usual optimum dose is 15 mg/day in milder conditions and 20–30 mg/d in more severe cases; maximum 60 mg/d	Capsules: 1, 2, 5, 10, 20 mg Concentrate: 5 mg/mL
		IM: 16–20 mg 2–4 times/d to maximum of 30 mg/d	Injection: 2 mg/mL
Loxapine (Loxitane)	Psychosis; acute severe agitation	*Adults and children >15 yr:* 10 mg bid initially; may increase rapidly over 7–10 d to 60–100 mg/d to control symptoms. Lower dose to lowest to control symptoms, maintenance dose 20–60 mg/d.	Tablets: 5, 10, 25, 50 mg Concentrate: 25 mg/mL Injection: 50 mg/mL
		IM: 12.5–50 mg every 4–6 h until desired response; then start oral	
Pimozide (Orap)	Motor and phonic tics in patients with Tourette's disorder	*Adults and children >12 yr:* 1–2 mg/d in divided doses. Increase every other day to max of 10 mg/d. Doses above 4 mg/d (0.05 mg/kg/d in children) require CYP 2D6 genotyping; do not exceed 4 mg/d in poor CYP 2D6 metabolizers. ECG at baseline and periodically thereafter.	Tablets: 1, 2 mg
Haloperidol (Haldol)	Psychosis; acute severe agitation	*Adults:* 0.5–5 mg 2–3 times daily to usual maximum dose of 30 mg/d; some adults require 100 mg/d IM: 2–5 mg; may repeat after 60 min; substitute with oral as soon as feasible. First oral dose should be administered 12–24 h following last IM dose. Decanoate: Deep IM every 4 wk; initial dose 10–15 times oral dose; not to exceed 100 mg *Older adults:* Lower doses and slower titration *Children:* 0.05–15 mg/kg/d; may give in divided doses	Tablet: 0.5, 1, 2, 5, 10, 20 mg Concentrate: 2 mg/mL Injection solution: 5 mg/mL IM injection solution decanoate: 50, 100 mg/mL
Molindone HCl (Moban)	Psychosis; acute severe agitation	*Adults and children >12 yr:* 50–75 mg/d. Increase in 3 to 4 days to maximum of 225 mg/d. Maintenance: Mild: 5–15 mg 3–4 times daily; moderate 10–25 mg 3–4 times a day; severe 225 mg/d may be required	Tablet: 5, 10, 25, 50 mg Concentrate: 20 mg/mL

*Not for dementia-related psychosis in the elderly.

that represent early EPSs. Table 15-20 presents an AIMS checklist that the nurse practitioner may use to evaluate patients.

Typical APs may elevate prolactin levels because dopamine, which inhibits prolactin, is blocked. Patients should be monitored for the consequences of chronic prolactin elevation, such as galactorrhea, gynecomastia, amenorrhea, and sexual dysfunction.

Patient Education

Anticipate the need for refills before the patient runs out of medication. Teach the patient to avoid sudden withdrawal of the medication because EPSs can occur. Emphasize that it is important to take the medication as prescribed, because noncompliance is the leading cause of increased symptoms and hospitalization. Advise the patient to report any side effects of EPSs, TD, or NMS. Advise the patient to rise slowly to minimize orthostatic hypotension. Caution the patient to avoid taking alcohol or other CNS depressants concurrently with these drugs and to avoid driving or other activities requiring alertness, because medication may cause drowsiness. Advise the patient to wear sunscreen and protective clothing because photosensitivity and changes in skin pigmentation may occur.

ATYPICAL ANTIPSYCHOTICS

A number of atypical APs have been marketed since 1990. These drugs include aripiprazole (Abilify), asenapine (Saphris), clozapine (Clozaril), iloperidone (Fanapt), lurasidone (Latuda), olanzapine (Zyprexa, Zyprexa Zydis, IM), paliperidone (Invega, Invega Sustenna), quetiapine (Seroquel), risperidone (Risperdal, Risperdal M-Tabs, Risperdal Consta), and ziprasidone (Geodon). Atypical APs address both the positive and negative symptoms of schizophrenia. Some of the superiority in treating negative symptoms, as compared to typical APs, may be related to less interference with cognitive functioning. Because there is better patient tolerability than with the typical APs, patients are more likely to continue taking the atypical APs. These newer agents are characterized by less risk for EPSs, TD, and elevation of

prolactin levels. The atypical APs, however, are associated with unhealthy weight gain, which leads to a metabolic syndrome (abdominal obesity, high blood pressure, high cholesterol levels, and insulin resistance). Schizophrenia itself, as well as the atypical APs, increases the risk of diabetes. Before starting any atypical antipsychotic, patients should be assessed for waist circumference, body mass index (BMI), blood pressure (BP), fasting plasma glucose, and lipid profile. The practitioners should recheck BMI monthly and order laboratory work-ups at 3 months. After 3 months, the BMI should be checked quarterly and BP, laboratory work-ups, and waist circumference annually.

Pharmacodynamics

Although the mechanism of action for these APs is not precisely understood, the atypical APs are thought to block serotonin receptors in the cortex, which blocks the usual ability of serotonin to inhibit the release of dopamine. Thus, more dopamine is released to the prefrontal cortex, which reduces the negative symptoms of schizophrenia. All drugs with antipsychotic properties block dopamine D_2 receptors, but atypical APs generally have less D_2 blockade than the typical APs. Drugs with the least D_2 blockade (clozapine, olanzapine) have the lowest incidence of EPSs. Most of the atypical APs also variously affect adrenergic, histaminic, and cholinergic receptors. Drugs that are potent histamine H_1 receptor antagonists (olanzapine, clozapine) produce more weight gain and sedation. Drugs that block noradrenergic receptors (clozapine) produce more hypotension.

Pharmacokinetics
Absorption and Distribution

These drugs are commonly administered orally and are rapidly and completely absorbed. Parenteral or long-acting decanoate forms of olanzapine, risperidone, and ziprasidone also exist. Orally disintegrating tablets of olanzapine and risperidone are available and helpful when "cheeking" of medication is suspected.

Table 15–20 Abnormal Involuntary Movement Scale (AIMS) Checklist

Instructions: Rate on a scale from 1 to 5, with 1 being none and 5 being severe. Rate at each appointment initially, then decrease frequency unless patient is a male under age 25 or a female over age 70.

Abnormal Involuntary Movement	Scale	Notes
Holding arms outstretched to sides		
Arms outstretched to front with hands flat and parallel		
Walking in a straight line		
Fluidity of shoulder and elbow joints		
Touching each finger with thumb of both hands		
Sticking tongue out straight		
Rolling head laterally, front and back		

Metabolism and Excretion

All are metabolized in the liver and primarily excreted through the renal system.

Onset, Peak, and Duration

Onset of action is within a few days to a few weeks. These drugs reach their peak activity in approximately 1 to 6 hours and steady state within a few days. Half-lives vary widely. For example, clozapine peaks in 2.5 hours and has a half-life of 8 to 12 hours, whereas olanzapine peaks in 6 hours and has a half-life of 21 to 54 hours.

Pharmacotherapeutics

Precautions and Contraindications

Most atypical APs are not recommended in pregnancy (Pregnancy Category C), lactating women, or young children. Lurisidone is Pregnancy Category B. APs should be prescribed cautiously in the presence of hepatic or renal disease. Analysis of risk versus benefit is indicated in individuals who have hepatic or renal disease but who also have poor quality of life without treatment with an antipsychotic. Because of liver function decline, the geriatric population generally requires smaller doses. An additional contraindication is hypersensitivity.

Adverse Drug Reactions

Although the risk of developing EPSs, tardive dyskinesia, and neuroleptic malignant syndrome exists with any antipsychotic, it is significantly less with the atypical APs than it is with the typical APs. Atypical APs do have significant negative adverse effects, including seizures, weight gain, diabetes, hyperprolactinemia, dizziness, orthostatic hypotension, tachycardia, sleep disturbance, constipation, and rhinitis.

Specific adverse reactions may occur with individual agents. Because of the risk of potentially fatal agranulocytosis, clozapine is reserved for the treatment of severe schizophrenia refractory to complete trials of at least two different types of antipsychotics. Clozapine is available only through a patient management system in which a clinician and patient are both registered. A baseline CBC with differential is obtained prior to treatment, then monitored weekly or biweekly, depending on the length of time the patient has been taking clozapine, before the next week's medication is dispensed by the pharmacy. Monitoring should be continued for 4 weeks after clozapine is discontinued. The clinician must be aware of the indications of a falling white blood count (WBC) (fever, lethargy, bruising, sore throat, flu-like symptoms). A precipitous onset of agranulocytosis is potentially lethal within 24 to 72 hours and requires immediate attention.

Aripiprazole is relatively weight neutral and lacks any significant effect on QT intervals. It has good antidepressant properties but may be unpleasantly activating to some patients. Side effects include agitation, akathisia, nausea, tremor, insomnia, and headache.

Asenapine may cause somnolence and dose-related akathisia. Patients taking 10 mg daily of asenapine for bipolar disorder may report oral hypoesthesia (5% of patients versus 0% of placebo).

The most common adverse effects reported in clinical trials of iloperidone included tachycardia (12% in patients taking 20 to 24 mg/day), nausea and dry mouth (10%), dizziness (20% in patients taking 20 to 24 mg/day), somnolence (15% in patients taking 20 to 24 mg/day), and orthostatic hypotension (5%). There is a slight increase in EPS symptoms in patients taking iloperidone over placebo (13.5% to 15.1% versus 11.6% in placebo).

The dosage of risperidone should be titrated up slowly over a few days or longer to minimize adverse effects. Adverse effects may include orthostatic hypotension, bradykinesia, akathisia, agitation, and elevation of prolactin levels. Weight gain with risperidone is generally less than it is with clozapine or olanzapine.

The most problematic adverse effects of long-term use of olanzapine are sedation and weight gain. This weight gain appears to be associated with increased appetite, with much of the weight gain occurring in the first 6 months of drug therapy. Olanzapine is very sedating and should be taken at bedtime if possible. Olanzapine has a low incidence of EPSs.

The most common adverse effects of paliperidone reported in clinical trials included tachycardia (14% versus 7% in placebo), somnolence (11%), akathisia (10% versus 4% in placebo), and EPS symptoms (18% to 20%).

The most common side effects of quetiapine are dizziness and somnolence. Other side effects may be weight gain and orthostatic hypotension.

Ziprasidone appears to be well tolerated in general. It is unique among the atypical APs in that it does not cause significant weight gain, and may even result in weight loss and reduced triglyceride levels. Ziprasidone has a low incidence of EPSs. The most common side effects are drowsiness, dyspepsia, dizziness, constipation, and nausea. One concern with ziprasidone is that it is associated with mild to moderate QT interval prolongation in about 5% of patients taking this drug. Patients with a known history of arrhythmia should have a baseline and repeat ECG.

Drug Interactions

Concurrent use with fluvoxamine (1A2 inhibitor) may increase atypical AP levels. Use with alcohol and other CNS depressants results in increased sedation and orthostasis. Use with antihypertensives may increase orthostasis. Carbamazepine decreases serum levels of olanzapine and is contraindicated with clozapine. Ciprofloxacin (Cipro) is a potent 1A2 inhibitor and increases atypical antipsychotic levels. Smoking increases the rate of metabolism of APs, thereby potentially decreasing their effect. Combinations of APs may increase the risk of TD and NMS. Table 15-21 presents drug interactions.

Clinical Use and Dosing

Table 15-22 presents the indications, dosages, and available dosage forms of atypical APs.

Rational Drug Selection

Indications for use of the atypical APs include schizophrenia, schizoaffective disorder, depression or mania with psychotic

Table 15–21 ⊞ **Drug Interactions: Atypical Antipsychotics**

Drug	Interacting Drug	Possible Effect	Implications
All atypical antipsychotics	Antihypertensives CNS depressants Ciprofloxacin (Cipro)	Hypotension Increased CNS depression Potent 1A2 inhibitor	Monitor blood pressure, orthostasis Warn patient about drowsiness Increase atypical antipsychotic levels
Clozapine	Anticholinergics	Increased anticholinergic effect	Increase fluid intake; use hard candies for dry mouth; stool softener if needed; monitor for urinary retention
	Caffeine	Increased effect of clozapine	Monitor CNS depression, WBC
	Lithium	Increased risk of neurotoxicity and agranulocytosis	Monitor lithium level, WBC, and for signs and symptoms of neurotoxicity
	Carbamazepine	Decreased serum levels of olanzapine	Contraindicated with clozapine
Quetiapine	Glucocorticoids	Decreased effect of quetiapine	Avoid concurrent use
Clozapine, quetiapine	Phenytoin	Increased toxicity of phenytoin; decreased antipsychotic effect	Monitor phenytoin blood levels and for increased psychotic symptomatology
	Erythromycin, ketoconazole, itraconazole, fluconazole	Increased effect of antipsychotics	Monitor for increasing CNS depression
Olanzapine, quetiapine	Rifampin, SSRIs	Decreased effect of antipsychotics	Monitor for increased psychotic symptomatology
Olanzapine, quetiapine, risperidone	Carbamazepine	Increased toxicity of carbamazepine	Monitor plasma levels of carbamazepine
Paliperidone	Carbamazepine	Coadministration may decrease paliperidone levels	Monitor effectiveness of paliperidone and increase dose if necessary
	Dopaminergic	Antagonistic to effect of antipsychotics	Do not use if possible; increased dose may be required
Olanzapine, quetiapine, clozapine	Cimetidine	Increased effect of antipsychotics	Monitor for increasing CNS depression
Aripiprazole, iloperidone	Ketoconazole or other CYP3A4 inhibitors	Decreases metabolism and increases effects of antipsychotic	Reduce aripiprazole or iloperidone dose by 50%
Ziprasidone	Drugs that prolong QT interval	Potentially life-threatening cardiac changes	ECG monitoring
Lurasidone	Strong CYP 3A4 inducers (rifampin, avasimibe, St. John's wort, phenytoin, carbamazepine) Moderate CYP 3A4 inducers		Do not use concurrently May need to increase lurasidone dose
Lurasidone	Strong CYP3A4 inhibitors (ketoconazole, clarithromycin, ritonavir, voriconazole, mibefradiol, grapefruit and grapefruit juice) Moderate CYP3A4 inhibitors (diltiazem, atazanavir, erythromycin, fluconazole, verapamil)		Avoid concomitant use Reduce lurasidone dose by one-half
Iloperidone	Inhibitors of CYP 2D6: fluoxetine, paroxetine	Increased iloperidone levels	Reduce iloperidone level by one-half when coadministering
Asenapine	CYP 2D6 inhibitors or substrates	May enhance inhibitory effects	Coadminister with caution
Asenapine	Fluvoxamine	Increased asenapine levels	Coadminister with caution
Aripiprazole	Carbamazepine and other CYP3A4 inducers	Reduced aripiprazole levels	Double dose of aripiprazole if carbamazepine added
Aripiprazole	Quinidine or other 2D6 inhibitors (fluoxetine or paroxetine)	Increase levels of aripiprazole	Reduce aripiprazole by one-half original dose

Table 15–22 ⊗ Dosage Schedule: Atypical Antipsychotics

Drug	Indications	Dosage	Available Dosage Forms
Aripiprazole (Abilify)	Schizophrenia, psychotic disorders, acute agitation, acute mania, bipolar maintenance, adjunct to antidepressant treatment for major depression	*Adult dose:* 10–15 mg/d single dose, may increase dose at 2 wk intervals up to 30 mg/d Bipolar: 15 mg q d initially Depression adjunct: 2–5 mg/d, may increase by 5 mg q wk to max 15 mg *Children:* Schizophrenia age 12–17 yr 2 mg/d, increase to 5 mg after 2 d, then to target dose of 10 mg after 2 d, then 5 mg q d if needed to max 30 mg Bipolar age 10–17: 2 mg/d, increase to 5 mg after 2 d, then in 2 d, if needed to max of 10 mg. Abilify injection: 9.75 mg IM, may repeat in 2 h, max 30 mg/d	Tablets: 2 mg 5 mg 10 mg 15 mg 20 mg 30 mg Oral solution: 1 mg/mL Discmelt: 10, 15 mg Injection: 7. 5 mg/mL (IM)
Asenapine (Saphris)	Schizophrenia, acute bipolar mania	*Adults:* 5 mg bid, max 10 mg bid For acute mania: Initial 10 mg bid	Oral disintegrating tablets: 5, 10 mg
Clozapine (Clozaril)	Refractory severe schizophrenia	*Adults:* Initial dose: 25–50 mg/d increasing by 25 mg increments/d until target range of 300–450 mg/d; maximum dose 900 mg/d; can give once daily or in divided doses; do not increase dose until adequate time for response has been provided, usually a few weeks. See pharmacy titration schedule.	Tablets: 25, 100 mg
		Maintenance: Lowest dose possible to resolve psychotic symptoms Discontinuation: Taper slowly over 1–2 wk	25 mg (G) 100 mg (G)
Lurasidone (Latuda)	Schizophrenia	40 mg daily (maximum 80 mg/daily)	Tablet: 20 mg, 40 mg, 60 mg, 80 mg, 120 mg
	Depressive episodes associated with bipolar I disorder	20 mg daily as monotherapy or as adjunctive therapy with litihium or valproate. Maximum dose 120 mg daily.	
Iloperidone (Fanapt)	Schizophrenia	*Adults:* Start with 1 mg bid, increase to 2 mg bid on second day, then by 2 mg bid q day to target dose of 12–24 mg bid on day 7	1-, 2-, 4-, 6-, 8-, 10-, 12 mg tablets
Olanzapine (Zyprexa, Zyprexa Zydis (oral-disintegrating form) Zyprexa (IM)	Psychotic disorders, severe agitation, acute mania, bipolar maintenance	Schizophrenia: 5–10 mg daily in single dose; dosage adjustment should occur no less often than once weekly; 5 mg/d in debilitated patients or those with predisposition to hypotension Bipolar: Initially 10–15 mg qd, may increase by 5 mg/d to target dose 20 mg/d Bipolar maintenance: 5–20 mg/d Acute agitation: IM 2.5–10 mg/dose deep IM, 3 doses 2–4 h apart up to 3 in 24 h	Tablets: 2.5 mg 5 mg 7.5 mg 10 mg 15 mg 20 mg Zydis: 5 mg 10 mg 15 mg 20 mg IM: 10 mg vial (before reconstitution)
Paliperidone (Invega, Invega Sustenna)	Schizophrenia Schizoaffective disorder	*Adults:* 6 mg qam, increase by 3 mg q 4–5 days to max of 12 mg (lower doses for renal impairment) Invega Sustenna (IM): First establish tolerability with oral treatment, deep deltoid 234 mg day 1, in 1 wk, 156 mg. Maintenance injection: deltoid or gluteal 117 mg monthly (range 39–234 mg (lower doses for renal impairment).	Tabs (extended-release): 3, 6, 9 mg Invega Sustenna extended-release injection: 39, 78, 117, 156, 234 mg
Risperidone (Risperdal) (Risperidal M-TAB) (oral-disintegrating form) Risperdal Consta (IM)	Psychotic disorders, severe agitation, acute mania, autism-related irritability in children	Schizophrenia: *Adults:* Initial dose: 1 mg bid; increase (q 24 h) by 1 mg per dose to target dose of 4–8 mg/d; most efficacious in range of 4–6 mg/d *Children 13–17 yr:* 0.5 mg qd, increase by 0.5 mg q 24 h to target of 3 mg/d. Divide dose if somnolence occurs.	Tablets: 0.25 mg 0.5 mg 1 mg 2 mg 3 mg 4 mg

Table 15–22 ⊗ Dosage Schedule: Atypical Antipsychotics—cont'd

Drug	Indications	Dosage	Available Dosage Forms
		(Debilitated patients should begin with 0.5 mg bid and have the dose increased in 0.5 mg increments.) For bipolar I maintenance or adjunct to lithium or valproate: *Adult:* Range 1–6 mg/d *Children 10–17 yr:* 0.5 mg/day; increase dose after 4 days to 1.0 mg/day; target 2.5 mg/d, max 6 *For irritable autism symptoms age 5–16 yr:* 15 to 20 kg, 0.25 mg/d; increase in 4 d to 0.5 mg. Remain for 14 d, then may increase 0.25 mg q 2 wk. >20 kg: 0.5 mg; may increase in 4 d to 1 mg. Remain for 14 d then may increase 0.5 mg q 2 wk. Risperdal Consta for adults: After trial with oral only, give IM deep gluteal or deltoid. Give injection with oral dose for 3 wk, then stop oral. Every 2 wk, 25 mg IM; adjust q 4 wk if needed to max 50 mg q 2 wk injection.	Solution: 1 mg/1 mL M-TAB: 0.5 mg 1 mg 2 mg Consta: Long-acting injectable: 25 mg 37.5 mg 50 mg
Quetiapine (Seroquel, Seroquel XR)	Psychotic disorders, severe agitation, schizophrenia, acute mania, bipolar maintenance, bipolar depression, adjunct to major depressive disorder antidepressant treatment	*Adults:* Schizophrenia Seroquel: Initially 25 mg bid, day 1 and increase q d by 25–50 mg in divided doses to target of 300–400 mg/d (divided) by day 4. Then increase by 25–50 mg in 2-d intervals to max 800 mg; lower in the elderly or with hepatic impairment. XR formulation: Initially 300 mg in p.m. (3–4 h before hs), increase by 300 mg/d to range 400–800/d. Mania: 100 mg/d divided, increase by 100 mg/d (divided) to 400 mg by day 4, then 200 mg increments to 800 mg (divided) by day 6. Depression: 50 mg day 1 at hs, then increase by 100 mg qhs until 300 mg on day 4. May increase to 400 mg day 5 and 600 mg day 8 if needed. XR formulation: Mania— 300 mg in p.m. day 1, then 600 mg in p.m. day 2. Day 3 titrate to effective dose (range 400–800) Depression—50 mg day 1, 100 mg day 2, 200 mg day 3, and 300 mg day 4 Give evening dose 3–4 h before hs.	Tablets: 25 100, 200, 300, 400 mg XR tablets: 50, 150, 200, 300, 400 mg
Ziprasidone (Geodon)	Schizophrenia, severe agitation, mania	*Adults:* Must be taken with full meal for proper absorption. *Schizophrenia:* Initial dose: 20 mg bid may increase at 2-d intervals up to 80 mg bid *Mania:* Initial dose 40 mg bid, day 2 60–80 mg bid Injection: Severe agitation 10–20 mg IM to max 40 mg per day (10 mg q 2 h or 40 mg q 4 h), not to exceed 3 days	Capsules: 20 mg 40 mg 60 mg 80 mg IM: 20 mg vial (before reconstitution)

features, and severe agitation and delusions with dementia. Selecting one atypical antipsychotic over another may be based on specific patient risk factors, history of response to specific medications, or adverse effects experienced by the patient. Change from one AP to another should be accomplished by slowly titrating off the first medication and onto the second, with a washout period in between if possible. If the presence of psychotic symptoms makes a washout period unfeasible, overlap of medications should be at the lowest doses and for the shortest period of time possible.

Monitoring

No specific blood tests are available to determine the plasma level of these medications. Dosages are adjusted based on subjective information provided by the patient and the clinician's objective observations of the client.

Patient Education

Patients need to be informed of the possible adverse reactions that may be associated with individual agents. Patients taking clozapine, for example, need to know the signs and symptoms of agranulocytosis so that these symptoms can be promptly reported to the clinician. Advise the patient to change position slowly to prevent orthostatic hypotension. Provide safety instructions for driving and other activities that require alertness. Sugarless gums, candies, or ice chips may be used to alleviate symptoms of dry mouth. Alert the patient to avoid the use of alcohol or other CNS depressants. Advise of the potential for significant weight gain and increase in triglycerides, and assist the client in modifying diet and exercise regimes to counter these undesirable effects.

DOPAMINERGICS

The dopaminergics, also known as dopamine agonists, are the pharmacological treatment of choice for Parkinson's disease. These agents include amantadine (Symmetrel), bromocriptine (Parlodel), carbidopa-levodopa (Sinemet), carbidopa-levodopa-entacarpone (Stalevo), selegiline hydrochloride (Eldepryl), pramipexole (Mirapex), rasagiline (Azilect), ropinirole (Requip), and tolcapone (Tasmar). Amantadine is occasionally used to treat the parkinsonism-like EPS of the antipsychotic drugs, but to give a dopamine-enhancing drug to a patient with schizophrenia might cause psychotic symptoms to increase.

Pharmacodynamics

Dopamine and acetylcholine are the neurotransmitters primarily responsible for balance and coordinated musculoskeletal functioning, and each needs to balance the other for smooth functioning to take place. When dopamine depletion occurs, either idiopathically as in Parkinson's disease or because of inadequate synthesis or impaired storage, transmission, or reuptake, the classic signs of muscular rigidity, tremors, and psychomotor retardation appear. Excessive amounts of dopamine are thought to produce the positive symptoms of schizophrenia, such as hallucinations and delusions.

Amantadine is effective because it releases dopamine from storage, whereas the dopamine precursors levodopa and carbidopa-levodopa increase dopamine synthesis. When entacapone is given with levodopa and carbidopa, the plasma levels of levodopa increase and are higher and more sustained when given with just carbidopa. Bromocriptine and pergolide act as dopamine agonists at the postsynaptic receptor sites. Selegiline inactivates monoamine oxidase (MAO), which then leads to increased amounts of dopamine available in the CNS. Similarly, rasagiline acts as a selective, irreversible MAO inhibitor. Pramipexole and ropinirole act by stimulating dopamine receptors in the brain. The exact mechanism of action of tolcapone is unknown, but it is thought to enhance the pharmacokinetics of levodopa.

Pharmacokinetics

Absorption and Distribution

Dopaminergics are administered orally and are relatively rapidly and completely absorbed. These agents are widely distributed and enter breast milk.

Metabolism and Excretion

Variations occur in metabolism; for example, bromocriptine, levodopa, rasagiline, and tolcapone are metabolized in the liver, but amantadine is excreted unchanged in the urine. Selegiline has three active metabolites, including amphetamine and methamphetamine, and deaths have occurred when selegiline has been taken concurrently with meperidine. Dopaminergics are excreted through urine and feces. Table 15-23 presents the pharmacokinetics of dopaminergics.

Pharmacotherapeutics

Precautions and Contraindications

These agents are contraindicated in hypersensitivity and should be used cautiously in patients with a history of cardiac, psychiatric, or ulcer disease. Dopaminergics are Pregnancy Categories B and C; their safety of use during lactation and in children has not been determined. Selegiline is contraindicated with concurrent administration of meperidine. Renal impairment should be carefully assessed before using amantadine because it is excreted unchanged through the kidneys. Patients with underlying cardiac arrhythmias who have taken pergolide have experienced bradycardia and sinus tachycardia. Ropinirole and pramipexole should be used cautiously

Table 15–23 ❖ Pharmacokinetics: Dopaminergics

Drug	Onset	Peak	Duration	Half-Life	Excretion
Amantadine (Symmetrel)	48 h	4 h	—	18–24 h	Urine
Bromocriptine mesylate (Parlodel)	—	1–3 h	4–8 h	3–8 h	Feces (85%–98%), Urine
Carbidopa-levodopa (Sinemet)	—	1–3 h	4–6 h	—	Urine
Selegiline HCI (Eldepryl)	—	0.5–2 h	—	18–20 h	Urine
Pergolide (Permax)	—	—	—	—	Urine
Pramipexole (Mirapex)	—	2 h	8 h	8 h	Urine
Ropinirole (Requip)	—	—	8 h	6 h	Urine

in geriatric patients because of the increased risk of hallucinations. Carbidopa-levodopa is contraindicated in narrow-angle glaucoma and malignant melanoma. Tolcarpone is contraindicated in patients with liver disease.

Adverse Drug Reactions

Adverse effects may include nausea and vomiting, dizziness, postural hypotension, abdominal pain, dyspepsia, constipation, dry mouth, depression, insomnia, confusion, and hallucinations. Pramipexole and ropinirole may cause sleep attacks in which the patient has unexpected episodes of falling asleep. Tolcapone may cause severe hepatocellular injury, including liver failure.

Drug Interactions

Drug interactions among the dopaminergic agents are many and varied. For example, administration with MAO inhibitors may cause hypertensive crisis. Concurrent use with antihypertensives may increase hypotension. Concurrent use with antihistamines, phenothiazines, quinidine, and tricyclic antidepressants may increase anticholinergic effects. Phenothiazines, haloperidol, and phenytoin may decrease the effect of levodopa. Concurrent use of levodopa with pramipexole increases the risk of hallucinations and dyskinesia. Ropinirole is extensively metabolized by the liver's CYP450 CYP1A2 enzyme systems; thus, drugs that alter the activity of these enzyme systems may affect the activity of ropinirole. Concurrent administration of rasagiline and meperidine may lead to serotonin syndrome. Concurrent administration of rasagiline and dextromethorphan may lead to psychosis or bizarre behavior. Table 15-24 presents drug and food interactions.

Clinical Use and Dosing

Table 15-25 presents the indications and dosage schedule of dopaminergics.

Rational Drug Selection

Treatment with a dopamine agonist such as bromocriptine, pergolide, pramipexole, or ropinirole is recommended as the first-line therapy for patients with mild to moderate parkinsonism symptoms. As symptoms worsen over time, levodopa may be introduced. Combinations such as levodopa with amantadine or carbidopa-levodopa with selegiline may provide improved response over a single drug or in cases of deterioration in status. In late-stage therapy, a controlled-release preparation (Sinemet CR) may relieve "wearing off," the recurrence of severe symptoms hours after the dose of medication. Patients who take levodopa for several years may experience a decrease in the effectiveness of the drug and require a drug holiday to restore effectiveness. Some newer dopamine agonists, such as pramipexole, have been used in the treatment of resistant depression.

Monitoring

Monitor the effectiveness of the drug in managing parkinsonism symptoms. Assess for the "on-off" phenomenon in which symptoms suddenly worsen or improve. Monitor

Table 15–24 ▦ Food and Drug Interactions: Dopaminergics

Drug	Interacting Drug or Food	Possible Effect	Implications
All dopaminergics	Antihypertensives	Increased antihypertensive effect	Monitor for postural hypotension, blood pressure
	Oral contraceptives	Decreased effectiveness of oral contraceptives	Use backup contraception
	MAOIs, TCAs, opioids	Hypertensive crisis	Avoid concurrent use
Carbidopa-levodopa	Food	Increased plasma level of carbidopa-levodopa with sustained-release form	Avoid taking with food
	Anticholinergics	Increased adrenocorticotropic hormone (ACH) adverse effects and decreased effect of levodopa	Monitor eye pain/vision; effect of dopaminergic
	Haldol, hydantoins	Decreased effect of levodopa	Monitor eye pain/vision; effect of dopaminergic
Pramipexole, ropinirole	Levodopa	May increase effect of levodopa	Monitor for hallucinations, dyskinesia (may allow dosage reduction of levodopa)
Tolcapone	Drugs metabolized by COMT (methyldopa, apomorphine, dobutamine, isoproterenol)	May increase the effects of methyldopa, apomorphine, dobutamine, isoproterenol	Consider dosage reduction of concurrent drug
Rasagiline	Dextromethorphan	Psychosis/bizzare behavior	Avoid concurrent use
Rasagiline	Meperidine	Serious, sometimes fatal reactions	Wait 14 days between giving

Table 15–25 ⊗ **Dosage Schedule: Dopaminergics**

Drug	Indications	Dosage	Available Dosage Forms
Amantadine (Symmetrel)	Parkinson's disease; drug-induced EPS; parkinsonism syndrome following carbon monoxide poisoning	*Adults:* 100–200 mg bid; may increase to maximum of 400 mg/d in divided doses after several weeks without response after lower dose. In conjunction with levodopa: 100 mg qd bid	Capsules: 100 mg Syrup: 50 mg/5 mL
Bromocriptine mesylate (Parlodel)	Parkinson's disease	*Adult:* Initial dose 1.25 mg bid with meals; if dosage increase needed after 2 wk, increase by 2.5 mg/d in divided doses with meals; maintain at lowest dose producing optimal response; usual range 10–40 mg/d	Tablets: 2.5 mg Capsules: 5 mg
Carbidopa-levodopa (Sinemet)	Parkinson's disease; parkinsonism syndrome following carbon monoxide or manganese poisoning	*Adult:* 1 tab (25 mg carbidopa and 100 mg levodopa) tid or 1 tab (10 mg carbidopa and 100 mg levodopa) tid qid; may increase by 1 tab daily or every other day until maximum of 8 tabs/d. Tablets of various ratios may be used but maintain 70–100 mg carbidopa/d. CR form: 1 tab bid with minimum of 6 h between doses; increase as above; do not crush or chew tabs	Tablets: 10 mg carbidopa/100 mg levodopa 25 mg carbidopa/100 mg levodopa 25 mg carbidopa/250 mg levodopa Sustained-release tablets: 25 mg carbidopa/100 mg levodopa 50 mg carbidopa/200 mg levodopa
Selegiline HCl	Adjunctive treatment of Parkinson's disease with carbidopa-levodopa	*Adult:* 5 mg bid with breakfast and lunch; after 2–3 d, decrease dose of carbidopa-levodopa	Tablet: 5 mg
Pramipexole	Parkinson's disease	*Adult:* 0.125 mg tid initially, may increase 5–7 d up to 1.5–4.5 mg/d in 3 divided doses	Tablet: 0.125, 0.25, 0.5, 1, 1.5 mg
Ropinirole	Parkinson's disease	*Adult:* 0.25 mg tid for 1 wk, then 0.5 mg tid for 1 wk, then 0.75 mg tid for 1 wk, then 1 mg tid for 1 wk; then may increase by 1.5 mg/d each wk up to 9 mg/d; then may increase by up to 3 mg/d each wk up to 24 mg/d	Tablet: 0.25, 0.5, 1, 2, 4, 5 mg
Levodopa, carbidopa, entacapone (Stalevo)	Idiopathic Parkinson's disease	May substitute Stalevo for equal dose of carbidopa-levodopa. Individualize dose.	Tablet: Stalevo 50: 12.5 mg of carbidopa, 50 mg of levodopa and 200 mg of entacapone Stalevo 75: 18.75 mg of carbidopa, 75 mg of levodopa, and 200 mg of entacapone Stalevo 100: 25 mg of carbidopa, 100 mg of levodopa, and 200 mg of entacapone Stalevo 125: 31.25 mg of carbidopa, 125 mg of levodopa, and 200 mg of entacapone Stalevo 150: 37.5 mg of carbidopa, 150 mg of levodopa, and 200 mg of entacapone Stalevo 200: 50 mg of carbidopa, 200 mg of levodopa, and 200 mg of entacapone
Rasagiline (Azilect)	Idiopathic Parkinson's disease	*Adults:* 0.5 to 1.0 mg/d	Tablet: 0.5 mg, 1.0 mg
Tolcapone (Tasmar)	Used as adjunct to levodopa and carbidopa for idiopathic Parkinson's disease	*Adults:* 100 mg tid. Maximum 600 mg/d. Monitor liver function.	Tablet: 100 mg

CR = controlled release.

hepatic and renal function in patients on long-term therapy. Monitor patients on pramipexole and ropinirole for the occurrence of drowsiness and sleep attacks.

Patient Education

Advise the patient to exercise care when changing position to prevent postural hypotension and to avoid hazardous activities if drowsy or dizzy. Explain that gastric irritation may be decreased by taking medication with food but that high-protein meals may impair levodopa's effects. Caution patient to monitor skin lesions for any changes, because carbidopa-levodopa may activate malignant melanoma. Advise the patient that large amounts of vitamin B (pyridoxine) may interfere with the action of levodopa.

ANXIOLYTICS (ANTIANXIETY) AND HYPNOTICS

Drugs used to treat anxiety can be divided into three groups based on their pharmacological action: serotonergics, gaba-ergics, and dopaminergics. Traditionally, however, the benzodiazepines, such as diazepam or alprazolam, were regarded as the anxiolytics. The benzodiazepines affect the gamma amino butyric acid (GABA) receptors at a particular site within the receptor, whereas other gaba-ergics affect the receptor more globally. The net effect of inhibiting GABA is to slow down neurotransmission and thereby produce reduction in anxiety. Serotonin as a neurotransmitter has a calming effect as well, owing to the areas of the brain where there are high concentrations of these pathways. Finally, dopaminergics have an anxiolytic effect in a fashion similar to that of serotonin but in more specific areas of the brain. Therefore, the prescriber needs to select a drug based not only on the general class of drugs but also on the specific symptomatology produced by the neurophysiology.

Because the SSRIs and serotonin-dopamine antagonists are discussed elsewhere in this chapter, this section focuses on the gaba-ergics, including the benzodiazepines. There is one exception and that is buspirone (BuSpar), which is a partial serotonin receptor agonist. For greater depth of discussion regarding the treatment of anxiety, see Chapter 29.

BENZODIAZEPINES

Benzodiazepines have been frequently prescribed to treat anxiety and insomnia. However, because of the increased potential for tolerance and dependence on the newer variations, the CNS depressant-related adverse effects, and the development of buspirone, many clinicians are more cautious in assessing risks versus benefits for their patients than they might have been previously. The drugs in this class include the following:

- Alprazolam (Xanax, Xanax XR)
- Chlordiazepoxide (Librium)
- Clonazepam (Klonopin)
- Clorazepate (Tranxene)
- Diazepam (Valium)
- Halazepam (Paxipam)
- Lorazepam (Ativan)
- Oxazepam (Serax)

Benzodiazepines have also been extensively used as a muscle relaxant and for preanesthesia sedation, prevention and treatment of panic attacks, acute agitation and dystonia, emergency treatment of uncontrollable seizures, and treatment of restless leg syndrome.

Pharmacodynamics

Benzodiazepines are thought to exert their anxiolytic and sedative effects by increasing the action of GABA, an inhibitory neurotransmitter, thereby decreasing the effect of neuronal excitation. Within the GABA receptor is an area that the benzodiazepines bind to, referred to as the benzodiazepine receptor.

Pharmacokinetics

Absorption and Distribution

Benzodiazepines are rapidly and widely distributed following oral administration and reach their peak levels within 30 minutes to 6 to 8 hours. Chlordiazepoxide (Librium) and diazepam (Valium) are slowly and inconsistently absorbed after intramuscular administration, but lorazepam (Ativan) and midazolam are rapidly absorbed and widely distributed after IM injection. These drugs are lipid-soluble and highly protein bound, which means that they may have prolonged activity in obese people and compete with other protein-bound drugs for receptor sites.

Metabolism and Excretion

Benzodiazepines are metabolized in the liver and biotransformed by oxidation. Some (lorazepam and temazepam) are biotransformed by conjugation. These two mechanisms may influence the patient's reaction to the drug. Benzodiazepines that are metabolized by conjugation are better tolerated by patients with impaired liver function or who are elderly or are smokers, whereas those drugs metabolized by oxidation may have a prolonged effect in the elderly. Duration of effect is influenced by the lipid solubility and the half-life of the active metabolites more than the parent drug. Half-lives and active metabolites are included in Table 15-26.

Pharmacotherapeutics

Precautions and Contraindications

The development of dependence, which can be psychological as well as physical, is of concern with the benzodiazepines. Although dependence is usually related to dose (high) and duration of use (more than a few weeks), it can occur in the absence of these parameters. It is thought that alprazolam (Xanax) and lorazepam (Ativan) are more likely to cause dependence because of their high potency and rapid, short-term action but clonazepam (Klonopin) is less likely because of its long action.

Symptoms of withdrawal, which usually occur 1 to 2 days after the last dose of short-acting benzodiazepines and 5 to

Table 15–26 ⊞ **Pharmacokinetics: Benzodiazepines**

Drug	Onset	Peak	Duration	Half-Life	Excretion
Alprazolam	Intermediate	1–2 h	Intermediate	8–37	Urine
Chlordiazepoxide	Intermediate	0.5–4 h	Long	5–30 h	Urine
Clonazepam	Intermediate	1–4 h	Long	30–40	Urine
Clorazepate	Fast	1–2 h	Long	40–50 h	Urine
Diazepam	Very fast	0.5–2 h	Long	20–80 h	Urine
Lorazepam	Intermediate	2–4 h	Intermediate	10–20 h	Urine
Oxazepam	Slow	2–4 h	Intermediate	5–20 h	Urine

10 days after the last dose of the long-acting compounds, resemble withdrawal symptoms of other CNS depressants. Use of the drug should be gradually tapered rather than abruptly discontinued because of the risk of severe withdrawal symptoms. One strategy for tapering is to decrease the dose by 0.5 mg per week, and then by 0.25 mg per week for the last few weeks. Another is to substitute a long-acting benzodiazepine such as clonazepam in an equivalent dose for a short-acting one and then titrate down.

Benzodiazepines are contraindicated in pregnancy and lactation and in the presence of hepatic and renal disease, and they are not recommended for children younger than 6 years. Other contraindications include hypersensitivity to benzodiazepines and acute narrow-angle glaucoma.

Geriatric patients generally should not be prescribed benzodiazepines; if they are prescribed, they should be in very low doses due to their decreased rate of metabolism and consequent potential for accumulation.

These drugs are not the treatment of choice for depression or psychosis or in the absence of anxiety signs and symptoms.

Adverse Drug Reactions

Major adverse effects are due to the drugs' action as CNS depressants. The same concerns apply to their use as with other CNS depressants: excessive sedation, particularly initially, in a situation requiring mental and physical alertness, and the potential for cardiac and respiratory depression, especially in combination with other CNS depressants. Paradoxical anxiety, agitation, and acute rage may occur with benzodiazepines. Clonazepam may increase salivation. Other common side effects include dizziness, confusion, blurred vision, and hypotension.

Drug Interactions

Drug interactions of greatest concern are those involving other CNS depressants, such as barbiturates, alcohol, antihistamines, and neuroleptics, because of their additive effects. Benzodiazepines also increase the blood levels of TCAs and digitalis preparation. Table 15-27 includes drug interactions and possible effects.

Clinical Use and Dosing

Benzodiazepines are indicated for the short-term treatment of anxiety and anxiety-related disorders. Additional uses include muscle relaxants, emergency treatment of status epilepticus, irritable bowel syndrome, chemotherapy-induced nausea and vomiting, and restless leg syndrome. Because they have cross-sensitivity with alcohol and act as an anticonvulsant, the benzodiazepines are especially useful in alcohol withdrawal and delirium tremens. Table 15-28 includes dosages and available dosage forms for the benzodiazepines.

Rational Drug Selection

Diazepam is the treatment of choice for status epilepticus, administered by a parenteral route, preferably IV, because of the rapidity of absorption and effect. In acute alcohol withdrawal, care must be exercised so that cross-tolerance does not develop. Because dependence has occurred after as little as 4 to 6 weeks of use, these drugs should be not be used beyond the acute stage of alcohol withdrawal and should be slowly tapered to avoid withdrawal symptoms.

All of the benzodiazepines are equally efficacious and drug selection depends on the patient's and prescriber's preference and the patient's side-effect profile. For long-term treatment of anxiety, other classes of drugs should be considered first (e.g., buspirone or SSRIs); and if the benzodiazepine is necessary, then clonazepam is preferred due to its long half-life and daily dosing ability.

Monitoring

Increased blood levels of TCAs and digitalis may occur with concurrent use of benzodiazepines and should be monitored. In long-term use, periodic assessment of liver function and complete blood cell counts should be performed.

Patient Education

Advise the patient to avoid alcohol. Because drowsiness and impaired cognition may be an adverse effect, tell the patient to avoid taking a benzodiazepine before or during situations in which mental or physical alertness is required to maintain safety. Patients should also be advised to report ocular pain or changes in vision immediately.

Table 15–27 ⚏ Drug Interactions: Benzodiazepines

Drug	Interacting Drug	Possible Effect	Implications
All benzodiazepines	Digoxin	Increased level of digoxin	Monitor level; take pulse before giving digoxin
	TCAs	Increased plasma level of TCAs	Monitor level of TCA
	Barbiturates, nefazodone, fluoxetine, fluvoxamine, MAOIs, sertraline, antihistamines	Increased CNS depression	Avoid concurrent administration
	Clozapine	Increased sedation, salivation, hypotension, delirium, respiratory arrest	Avoid concurrent administration
Alprazolam	Cimetidine oc, disulfiram, omeprazole, macrolide antibiotics		Warn of increased effects
	Grapefruit juice	Decreased metabolism and increased effect of alprazolam	Use alternative juice
	Ketoconazole		Concurrent use contraindicated
Alprazolam, clonazepam	Carbamazepine	Decreased plasma level of benzodiazepines	Use alternative anticonvulsant
Clonazepam	Lithium	Increased sexual dysfunction	Warn of possible adverse effects
Clonazepam, diazepam, chlordiazepoxide	Phenytoin	Decreased plasma level and toxicity of phenytoin	Use alternative anticonvulsant
		Decreased clinical effect of benzodiazepines	Monitor phenytoin blood level; may need lower dose
Clonazepam, lorazepam	Valproate	Decreased metabolism and increased effect of benzodiazepines	May require lower dose of benzodiazepine
Diazepam	Phenobarbital	Additive CNS depression; increased metabolism of diazepam	May affect treatment of status epilepticus

SEROTONERGIC ANXIOLYTICS

Neurophysiologically, it makes sense that enhancing serotonin would contribute to relief of anxiety because of the areas of the brain that are heavily innervated by serotonin. However, there are 15 subtypes of serotonin receptors, some of which may actually contribute to anxiety. Buspirone is a serotonergic that is a member of the azapirones, a relatively new group of anxiolytics. Other drugs in this group are ipsapirone and gepirone, neither of which is approved for use in the United States for treatment of anxiety. These drugs exert their effects without the CNS depression and sedation of barbiturates and benzodiazepines but also without the anticonvulsant or muscle-relaxant qualities. Buspirone has little risk of dependence and few drug interactions, and it is considered relatively safe, even in high doses.

Pharmacodynamics

Buspirone has a similar chemical structure to butyrophenone antipsychotics such as haloperidol (Haldol) and was thought to be an atypical antipsychotic similar to clozapine (Clozaril) without the EPSs. However, further human studies showed that it had greater efficacy as an anxiolytic, through its action on the serotonin-1A (5-HT 1a) presynaptic and postsynaptic receptors. At the presynaptic 5-HT 1a receptor, buspirone is a full agonist, that is, it contributes to the channel's opening and permitting serotonin binding, thereby inhibiting neuron firing. Buspirone also is a partial agonist at the postsynaptic 5-HT 1a receptors. When there is an excess of serotonin, buspirone acts as an antagonist, but in a deficit state such as is presumed in anxiety and depression, it acts as an agonist.

Remembering that buspirone was originally thought to be an atypical antipsychotic, it is not surprising that buspirone inhibits the increase in dopamine D_2 receptors. However, the dopaminergic action is minor compared to the serotonergic effects. Buspirone has no effect on the GABA receptor and cannot be used as a substitute for benzodiazepines in withdrawal treatment.

Pharmacokinetics

Absorption and Distribution

Buspirone is rapidly absorbed and undergoes extensive first-pass metabolism. When taken with food, buspirone has a reduced first-pass effect, allowing for more active drug going directly into

Table 15–28 ⊗ Dosage Schedule: Benzodiazepines

Drugs	Indications	Dosage	Available Dosage Forms
Alprazolam (Xanax)	Anxiety disorder, panic disorder	Anxiety: 0.25–0.5 mg tid, maximum 4 mg/d Panic disorder: 0.5 mg tid, titrate q 3–4 d to 1–10 mg/d (mean 5–6 mg/d) Wean off slowly when discontinuing	Tablets: 0.25 mg, 0.5 mg, 1 mg, 2 mg Orally disintegrating tablets: 0.25 mg
			Intensol solution: 1 mg/mL concentrated solution to be mixed with liquid or semisolid food, using only the provided calibrated dropper Extended-release tablets (Xanax XR): 0.5 mg, 1 mg, 2 mg, 3 mg
Chlordiazepoxide (Librium)	Anxiety, alcohol withdrawal	Mild to moderate anxiety: 5–10 mg tid Severe anxiety: 20–25 mg tid Older adults: 5 mg 2–4 times daily	Capsules: 5, 10, 25 mg Powder for injection: 5, 10, 25, 100 mg
Clonazepam (Klonopin)	Seizure disorders, panic disorder,	Seizure disorder: 1.5 mg/d, increase 0.5 mg to 1.0 mg q3d to maxiumum of 20 mg/d Panic disorder: 0.25 mg bid, may increase q 3 d to a maximum of 1 mg/d	Tablets: 0.5 mg, 1 mg, 2 mg
Diazepam (Valium, Diastat)	Anxiety, alcohol withdrawal, skeletal muscle spasm, status seizures	Anxiety: 2–10 mg 2–4 times a day Acute alcohol withdrawal: 10 mg tid or qid during first 24 h, then 5 mg tid or qid Muscle spasms: 2–10 mg tid or qid Seizures: Age 2–5 yr: 0.5 mg/kg; age 6–11 yr: 0.3 mg/kg; ≥ 12 yr: 0.2 mg/kg	Tablets: 2, 5, 10 mg Oral solution: 5 mg/5 mL Intensol solution: 5 mg/5 mL Injection: 5 mg/5 mL Rectal gel: 10 mg, 20 mg rectal delivery system
Lorazepam (Ativan)	Anxiety	Anxiety: Initial dose: 2–3 mg/d divided bid or tid, increase to usual range of 2–6 mg/d Elderly: 1–2 mg/d in divided doses Short-term insomnia due to anxiety: 2–4 mg at bedtime	Tablets: 0.5, 1, 2 mg Intensol solution: 2 mg/mL Injection: 2 or 4 mg/mL
Oxazepam (Serax)	Anxiety, alcohol withdrawal	Mild to moderate anxiety: 10–15 mg tid or qid Severe anxiety: 15–30 mg tid or qid Older patients: 10 mg tid Alcohol withdrawal: 15–30 mg tid or qid	Capsules: 10 15, 30 mg

circulation. It has many metabolites that have no effect on anxiety symptoms, but at least one metabolite has noradrenergic effects, which may explain why buspirone is contraindicated in panic attacks (Schatzberg & Nemeroff, 2009). It has a short half-life, ranging from 1 to 10 hours, but a slow onset of action (up to 6 weeks); therefore, it requires multiple dosing during the day. It is highly protein bound and lipid-soluble, therefore having broad distribution in brain and adipose tissue.

Metabolism and Excretion

Buspirone is metabolized by oxidation in the liver and is a substrate for the CYP450 3A4 enzyme. It does not inhibit any of the CYP450 enzymes; therefore, it has few drug interactions. It is excreted in the urine and feces.

Onset, Peak, and Duration

For unknown reasons it takes 1 to 2 weeks for the onset of anxiolytic effects of buspirone and up to 6 weeks for maximum effects. It peaks in circulation in 0.7 to 1.5 hours and has an intermediate duration.

Pharmacotherapeutics

Precautions and Contraindications

Buspirone is contraindicated in patients with known hypersensitivity or in those with severe hepatic or renal disease. As mentioned previously, it is contraindicated in the treatment of panic disorder both because of its prolonged onset and possibility of exacerbating panic.

Buspirone is considered Pregnancy Category B. The extent of excretion in breast milk is not clear and use during lactation should be avoided. Although buspirone is not commonly thought to be sedating, as with other anxiolytics, drowsiness should be assessed prior to use in situations requiring cognitive or motor alertness in order to maintain safety.

Adverse Drug Reaction

Adverse effects are few and usually resolve with continued use. Most common are light-headedness, headache, insomnia, nausea, nervousness, and dry mouth. Akathisia and involuntary movements are possible although rare.

Drug Interactions

Interactions between buspirone and other serotonergic drugs such as MAOIs and SSRIs have the potential to cause serotonin syndrome with symptoms of nausea, diarrhea, chills, sweating, elevated temperature and blood pressure, agitation, ataxia, coma, and death.

Interactions with antipsychotic drugs, especially haloperidol, contribute to increased serum levels of haloperidol due to competition for metabolism. When combined with trazodone, there may be an increased ALT (alanine transaminase).

Drugs that inhibit CYP3A4 (erythromycin, ketoconazole, nefazodone, intraconazole, ritonavir) and grapefruit juice may increase serum levels of buspirone. Drugs that induce CYP3A4 (rifampin, dexamethasone, phenytoin, phenobarbital, carbamazepine) decrease buspirone levels.

Clinical Use and Dosing

Used primarily for anxiety, buspirone's usual dose is 15 mg per day (7.5 mg BID). Initially, the patient takes 5 mg 2 or 3 times a day for 4 days; then the dose is increased by 5 mg each dose to a maximum dose of 60 mg per day. It is available in 5, 10, and 15 mg tablets, bisected or trisected for easy titration. The tablets are small and may be difficult to handle for those with hand mobility problems.

Rational Drug Selection

Although buspirone can be used as the sole pharmacotherapeutic modality for anxiety, it is frequently used adjunctively with SSRIs in treatment-resistant depression because of the combined serotonergic mechanisms, that is, postsynaptic reuptake inhibition and receptor agonism. Buspirone is indicated in treating generalized anxiety disorder, depression with an overlay of anxiety, and situational anxieties that are long-lasting. It is essential, however, that the drug be taken daily; it cannot be used on an as-needed basis.

A positive response may begin within 7 to 10 days of starting the drug, but maximum benefits may not become evident for 3 to 6 weeks. It may be necessary to add a benzodiazepine in very low doses initially to relieve the patient's anxiety and fear about the anxiety.

Monitoring

No monitoring other than periodic reassessment of the drug's continued effectiveness is required.

Patient Education

To maintain safety, advise the patient to try the medication and observe the effects, especially drowsiness, before engaging in activities requiring mental or physical alertness. The patient also needs to be told of the prolonged onset and be offered nonpharmacological strategies for anxiety management during this time.

BARBITURATES

Before the benzodiazepines became standard treatment, anxiety was treated with a variety of drugs with different mechanisms of action. Barbiturates have been used historically as anxiolytics, sedative-hypnotics, and anticonvulsants. Because of tolerance and dependence problems associated with their use, the indications for short-acting barbiturates are limited to preanesthesia sedation, short-term treatment of insomnia, and uncomfortable seizure activity, such as status epilepticus. Long-acting phenobarbital (Solfoton, Mebaral) is the drug of choice for some types of epilepsy, the only indication for its long-term use.

Pharmacodynamics

Barbiturates are CNS depressants and can be short- (30 minutes to 4 hours), intermediate- (6 to 8 hours), or long-acting (10 to 12 hours). They produce sedation and sleep by decreasing sensitivity to stimuli in the reticular formation, a primitive area deep in the brainstem through which all the sensorimotor nerve tracts pass. They bind to $GABA_A$ receptors at a site other than the benzodiazepines and contribute to prolonged opening of the chloride ion channel. With a prolonged activation of the GABA in the reticular activating system, decreased motor stimulation and increased sleep would be expected.

Pharmacokinetics
Absorption and Distribution

Barbiturates are administered by oral, parenteral, and rectal routes. Their rate of absorption depends on the route of administration, but generally, salts are absorbed more rapidly than are acid forms. They are widely distributed, particularly to brain, kidney, and liver tissue and fluid.

Metabolism and Excretion

Barbiturates are metabolized in the liver by CYP450 2C19 enzymes. They induce their own metabolism, thereby increasing the rate of their metabolism and increasing the potential for tolerance. They are excreted in the urine, although up to 50% is eliminated unchanged. Table 15-29 includes the pharmacokinetics of the barbiturates.

These drugs are FDA Pregnancy Category D and should be avoided during pregnancy. Infant sedation has occurred when the lactating mother has used barbiturates. For women of childbearing age, care is needed to maintain birth control to prevent unwitting teratogenicity in the first trimester.

Pharmacotherapeutics
Precautions and Contraindications

Barbiturates combined with alcohol have contributed to many deaths, whether suicide or accident, because of the additive depressive effect each has on the other. Caution should be exercised in prescribing them for patients with a history of depression, suicide attempts, or alcoholism. If the clinician has any doubts about the patient's safety and there is no other medication option, no more than a week's worth of the drug should be supplied at a time and for as short a period as possible.

Because of the anxiolytic effect of the short-acting barbiturates, known as "downers" on the street, they may be abused. In addition to the hazard associated with the narrow

Table 15–29 ⚙ Pharmacokinetics: Barbiturates

Drug	Onset	Peak	Duration	Half-Life	Excretion
Pentobarbital	10–15 min	—	3–4 h	15–50 h	Urine, feces
	IV immediate				
Secobarbital	10–15 min	—	3–4 h	15–40 h	Urine, feces
	IV immediate				
Amobarbital	45–60 min	—	6–8 h	16–40 h	Urine, feces
Butabarbital	45–60 min	—	6–8 h	66–140 h	Urine, feces
Phenobarbital	30 min or more		10–16 h	53–118 h	Urine, feces
	IV: less than 5 min	IV: 15 min or more			

therapeutic index and the risk for combining them with other CNS depressants, particularly alcohol, the short-acting barbiturates secobarbital (Seconal) and pentobarbital (Nembutal) can cause physiological dependence quickly. Tolerance leads the individual to increase the dose. One gram can cause toxic adverse effects, and 2 to 10 grams can be fatal.

Withdrawal and detoxification are potentially fatal and should be accomplished extremely slowly. Withdrawal symptoms usually begin 8 to 12 hours after the last dose and can range from nausea and vomiting, confusion, and tremors to delirium and seizures, with the latter beginning approximately 16 hours after the last dose. If untreated, symptoms can last for several days.

Barbiturates are not recommended for children younger than 6 years. Other contraindications include barbiturate sensitivity, severely impaired liver function, nephritis, impaired pulmonary function with dyspnea or obstruction, and history of dependence on barbiturates, hypnotics, or alcohol. They should not be administered subcutaneously or intra-arterially.

Adverse Drug Reactions

Adverse reactions are due to the CNS depressant effects of the drug and can consist of persistent sedation and drowsiness, leading to safety concerns for patients in situations requiring alertness. Although respiratory depression and cardiac depression are dose-related, they are always a concern, especially in combination with other CNS depressants. Other adverse reactions may include agitation, particularly in young children and older adults, confusion, headache, insomnia, ataxia, skin rash, nausea and vomiting, bradycardia, dyspnea, and somnolence.

Rebound status epilepticus may follow abrupt withdrawal of barbiturates during daily administration for treatment of seizure disorders.

Drug Interactions

As discussed earlier, CNS depression may occur with concurrent use of drugs such as antihistamines, alcohol, benzodiazepines, valproic acid, and MAOIs. Table 15-30 includes the drug interactions with barbiturates.

Barbiturates may also decrease the efficacy of beta blockers, steroids, hormones, doxycycline, theophylline, protease inhibitors, dicumarol, exogenous corticosteroids, and vitamins K and D, due to the P450 enzyme induction of 2C19.

Clinical Use and Dosing

Phenobarbital and mephobarbital are effective in the treatment of some types of epilepsy—primarily tonic-clonic,

Table 15–30 ⚙ Drug Interactions: Barbiturates

Drug	Interacting Drug	Possible Effect	Implications
Barbiturates	Anticoagulants	Induces metabolism of anticoagulants and rebound bleeding when barbiturate stopped	Monitor bleeding times
	Antihistamines, alcohol, benzodiazepines	Increases CNS depression	Avoid concurrent administration
	Neuroleptics	Decreases effect of neuroleptic	Monitor for increase in psychotic symptoms
	Beta blockers, steroids, estrogen, doxycycline, protease inhibitors, valproate, theophylline, griseofulvin, quinidine, phenylbutazone	Induces metabolism and decreases effectiveness of drugs	Monitor blood levels where appropriate and assess effectiveness if concurrent administration unavoidable
	Caffeine	Antagonizes sedation and increases insomnia	Avoid coffee, tea, cola, and chocolate

simple partial, and complex partial seizures—because the reduction of response to stimuli raises the threshold of seizure activity. In addition to epilepsy, other indications for use include preanesthetic sedation and short-term treatment of insomnia. The latter indication, however, is a last resort because of the risk of dependence and the comorbidity of sleep disturbance and depression, raising the risk for suicide.

Other than parenteral administration of phenobarbital in medical emergencies such as eclampsia and status epilepticus, barbiturates are generally given orally. The short-, intermediate-, and long-acting forms have an onset of action ranging from 10 to 60 minutes, a duration of action from 3 to 16 hours, and half-lives from 24 to 100 hours. Table 15-31 includes the indications, dosage schedules, and available dosage forms for the barbiturates.

Rational Drug Selection

Although efficacious in the treatment of partial, tonic-clonic, and cortical focal seizures, phenobarbital and mephobarbital are not considered the first-line treatment of the medical

Table 15–31 ⚛ Dosage Schedule: Barbiturates

Drug	Indications	Dosage	Available Dosage Forms
Amobarbital sodium (Amytal)	Sedation, hypnotic, preanesthetic, acute convulsive episodes	Sedative: 30–50 mg bid to tid Hypnotic: 65–200 mg IM: 65–500 mg IV: do not exceed 50 mg/min *Children 6–12 yr:* 65–500 mg Single dose not to exceed 1 g	Injection: 0.5 g vials
Butabarbital sodium (Butisol)	Sedation, hypnotic, preanesthetic, acute convulsive episodes	Sedation: 15–30 mg tid to qid Hypnotic: 50–100 mg hs* Pre-operative sedation: 50–100 mg 60–90 min before surgery *Children:* 2–6 mg/kg/d; not to exceed 100 mg	Tablets: 30, 50 mg Solution: 30 mg/5 mL
Pentobarbital sodium (Nembutal)	Sedation, hypnotic, preanesthetic	IV: Initial dose of 100 mg in adult with proportional decrease of dose for children or debilitated adults. Wait for a full minute to assess effect before adding more. Not to exceed 200–500 mg for healthy adult. IM: Usual adult dose is 150–200 mg *Children:* 2–6 mg/kg as single injection; not to exceed 100 mg	Injection: 1 g/20 mL vial
Phenobarbital	Sedation, hypnotic, preanesthetic, treatment of partial and generalized tonic-clonic and cortical focal seizures status epilepticus	Epilepsy *Adults:* 60–100 mg/d *Children:* 3–6 mg/kg/d Acute convulsions *Children:* 200–320 mg IM/IV, repeat q6h prn *Children:* 4–6 mg/kg/d IM/IV for 7–10 d to blood level of 10–15 mcg/mL	Oral tablets: 15, 30, 100 mg Elixer: 20 g/5 mL
		Sedation *Adults:* 30–120 mg/d in divided doses; not to exceed 400 mg/24 h *Children:* 8–32 mg Hypnotic *Adult:* 100–200 mg *Children:* Dose based on age and weight Pre-operative sedation *Adults:* 100–200 mg IV 60–90 min before surgery *Children:* 1–3 mg/kg IM or IV Status epilepticus 15–20 mg/kg IV over 10–15 min; may require 15 min or more to achieve peak	
Secobarbital sodium (Seconal)	Sedation, hypnotic, pre-operative sedation, status epilepticus	Pre-operative sedation *Adult:* 200–300 mg 1–2 h before surgery or 1 mg/kg IM 10–15 min before surgery *Children:* 2–6 mg/kg not to exceed 100 mg or 4–5 mg/kg IM Hypnotic *Adult:* 100 mg at bedtime Status epilepticus *Children:* 15–20 mg/kg IV over 15 min	Capsules: 100 mg

*hs = *hora somni* (at bedtime).

emergencies mentioned previously, which also include seizures associated with meningitis and tetanus. The first choice in such situations is intravenous diazepam (Valium).

Phenobarbital for the treatment of epilepsy is usually prescribed in low doses so that dependence and tolerance are not significant concerns. Adults are treated with 50 to 100 mg 2 to 3 times per day, and children are prescribed 3 to 5 mg/kg per day. For uses other than treatment of tonic-clonic seizures and focal epilepsy, safer drugs are available.

Short-acting barbiturates are Schedule II controlled drugs and therefore may not be available to some nurse practitioners. Phenobarbital is Schedule IV and may be included on a state nurse practitioner formulary, depending on the individual state's rules and regulations.

Monitoring

The difference between therapeutic and toxic plasma levels is not wide, and levels should be monitored frequently. The therapeutic range is 15 to 40 mcg/mL. It is necessary to closely monitor blood levels when prescribing barbiturates with other drugs metabolized by CYP450 2D19.

Sedative-Hypnotics

Insomnia can be either a symptom within a syndrome or a specific type of sleep disorder. However, it should not be treated as an illness by itself. When patients complain about difficulty sleeping, it is necessary to further assess the kind of difficulty, that is, is the difficulty falling asleep (initial or onset insomnia), difficulty staying asleep (sleep maintenance insomnia), waking up too early and not being able to return to sleep (late or terminal insomnia), or waking up tired and not rested. Each of these components indicates different problems and is treated differently.

Onset insomnia frequently is a symptom of anxiety or agitated depression and better treated by sleep hygiene measures. Terminal insomnia again is common in depression and improves when the depression remits. Waking up tired and waking up several times during the night may be depression, pain, or other physical problem such as overactive bladder. Finally, other medical conditions (e.g., fibromyalgia, chronic obstructive pulmonary disease [COPD], cardiac arrhythmias) or medications (e.g., beta blockers, corticosteroids, bronchodilators) may contribute to sleep disturbances.

Insomnia may occur transiently, lasting only a few days; short-term, lasting 2 to 3 weeks; or chronic, lasting longer than 3 weeks and even years. Transient and short-term insomnia can often be treated with sleep hygiene only. Chronic insomnia should be treated with medication for a few months; then the patient should be tapered off the medication. If the problem persists, however, the practitioner should refer the patient for a sleep laboratory study before continuing with treatment.

Whatever the cause of the insomnia, sleep disturbance can contribute to other health problems and requires attentive decision making. Prior to considering medication, sleep hygiene measures should be the first resort. This includes limiting the bedroom and bed to purposes of sleep and sex only. Working in bed, watching television, eating in bed are all activities that disturb sleep and contribute to the perception that the bed is a battleground on which to fight sleep. In addition, the patient may be advised to establish a bedtime routine that includes comforting and relaxing measures an hour before going to bed. These may include a hot bath, a warm noncaffeine drink or high tryptophan snack, light reading, and relaxation or mild stretch exercises. More vigorous exercise should be avoided within 4 hours of going to bed, as should eating. If not asleep within 30 minutes, the patient should get up and read or do some simple tasks and return to bed when sleepy.

BENZODIAZEPINE HYPNOTICS

If sleep is still a problem after treating the underlying problem, the most common sedatives or hypnotics include benzodiazepines and nonbenzodiazepine gaba-ergics. The benzodiazepines most commonly used for sleep include the rapid-onset, slow-acting triazolam (Halcion); delayed-onset, intermediate-acting temazepam (Restoril) and estazolam (Prosom); and rapid-onset, long-acting flurazepam (Dalmane) and quazepam (Doral). They all have the potential for dependence and tolerance and should not be used more than 3 weeks at a time of daily dosing and no more than 3 times a week for no more than 3 months. The pharmacodynamics and pharmacokinetics are the same as for the benzodiazepine anxiolytics shown in Table 15-26.

NONBENZODIAZEPINE HYPNOTICS

Pharmacodynamics

There are three categories of nonbenzodiazepine hypnotics used to induce sleep. Nonbenzodiazepine hypnotics also act at the GABA receptor but not at the benzodiazepine site. There are four drugs in this class, including zolpidem (Ambien, Edluar, Intermezzo), zaleplon (Sonata), and eszopiclone (Lunesta) (zopiclone is not available in the United States). Ramelteon (Rozerem) is a melatonin receptor agonist with high affinity for melatonin MT1 and MT2 receptors, similar to exogenous melatonin.

The first orexin receptor antagonist suvorexant (Belsorma) was approved in 2014. Orexin, a neurotransmitter that regulates wakefulness, arousal, and appetite, is produced in the hypothalamus. The neurotransmitter, also called hypocretin, was discovered in 1998. An orexin receptor mutation is thought to cause narcolepsy. Suvorexant blocks the binding of orexin to the orexin A and orexin B recptors, promoting sleep.

Pharmacokinetics

Absorption and Distribution

The nonbenzodiazepine hypnotics are rapidly absorbed through oral administration and are protein bound differentially; that is, zaleplon is minimally protein bound but zolpidem is 92% protein bound. They have short half-lives, ranging from 1 hour (zaleplon) to 5.8 hours (eszopiclone) and short duration. Peak onset occurs in 0.5 to 1 hour. Ramelteon is rapidly absorbed after oral administration with a peak in 0.75 hours (range 0.5 to 1.0 hours); it is 82% protein bound. After oral administration on an empty stomach, suvorexant peaks in 2 hours (range 30 minutes to 6 hours). Peak onset of suvorexant is delayed by 1.5 hours if it is taken on an empty stomach.

Metabolism and Excretion

Zolpidem, zaleplon, and eszopiclone are extensively metabolized by aldehyde oxidase and the CYP450 3A4 isoenzymes. They are excreted by the kidneys. Ramelteon is metabolized by CYP1A2 and excreted in the urine (84%) and feces (4%). Suvorexant is metabolized primarily by CYP3A4, with CYP2C19 contributing to a minor portion of metabolism, and is excreted in the feces (66%) and urine (23%).

Pharmacotherapeutics

Precautions and Contraindications

All of the nonbenzodiazepine drugs are within Pregnancy Category C and should not be used during pregnancy or lactation. Use of sedative-hypnotics may lead to worsening of depression. Zolpidem, eszopiclone, and zaleplon are associated with withdrawal signs and symptoms when discontinued. All the drugs in this class may lead to abnormal thinking and behavioral changes, including bizarre behavior and complex behaviors such as "sleep driving" or other behaviors (eating food, having sex, making phone calls). Rare cases of angioedema have been reported with ramelteon. Suvorexant is contraindicated in patients with narcolepsy and should be used cautiously in patients with respiratory compromise. No sleeping medication should be used acutely beyond 3 weeks or chronically beyond 3 months without careful evaluation of the treatment plan. None of these medications is approved for use in children.

Adverse Drug Reactions

The most common side effects of nonbenzodiazepine hypnotics include headache, mild transient anterograde amnesia, dizziness, somnolence, and nausea. There may be daytime drowsiness, especially if taken 6 hours or less before it is necessary to awaken. Abnormal behaviors such as "sleep driving" or worsening of depression may occur. Older adults may be more sensitive to the adverse effects of these medications. Women are more sensitive to the effects of zolpidem and should be prescribed lower doses than men.

A dose-related worsening of suicidal ideation was reported in clinical trials of suvorexant. Mild cataplexy, including periods of leg weakness lasting seconds to minutes, may occur day or night. Sleep paralysis, the inability to move or speak, may occur for up to several minutes during the sleep-wake transition. Hypnagogic or hypnopompic hallucinations may occur with suvorexant.

Zolpidem, eszopiclone, and zaleplon are Schedule IV drugs and all exhibit withdrawal symptoms when used chronically and abruptly discontinued. Ramelteon is not a controlled substance and does not appear to cause physical dependence. Suvorexant is Schedule IV due to potential for abuse, but does not cause physical dependence.

Drug Interactions

The nonbenzodiazepine drugs have an additive effect with CNS depressants including benzodiazepines and alcohol. Drugs that induce CYP450 3A4 will decrease the blood levels of these hypnotics, including cimetidine, phenytoin, rifampin, and carbamazepine. Drugs that inhibit CYP450 3A4 will increase the blood levels of these hypnotics, including ketoconazole, clarithromycin, erythromycin, and protease inhibitors. Fluvoxamine, a strong CYP 1A2 inducer, increases the serum levels of ramelteon significantly and they should not be administered concurrently. Ketoconazole, a strong CYP3A4 inhibitor, increases ramelteon levels when coadministered. Concominent use of suvorexant and strong CYP3A4 inhibitors (e.g., ketoconazole, itraconazole, posaconazole, clarithromycin, nefazodone, ritonavir, saquinavir, nelfinavir, indinavir, boceprevir, telaprevir, telithromycin and conivaptan) should be avoided. The dose of suvorexant is decreased if a patient is on a moderate CYP3A4 inhibitor (e.g., amprenavir, aprepitant, atazanavir, ciprofloxacin, diltiazem, erythromycin, fluconazole, fosamprenavir, grapefruit juice, imatinib, verapamil). Likewise, fluconazole (CYP2C9 inhibitor) increases ramelteon levels. Suvorexant levels will be decreased when administered with CYP3A4 induducers.

Clinical Use and Dosing

The primary use of the nonbenzodiazepine gaba-ergics in this class is for sedation during episodes of insomnia. All have rapid onset and the patient should be warned to take the medication within 30 minutes of bedtime. Lower doses of all these drugs should be used with the elderly. The dose of zaleplon is 10 mg, and 5 mg in the elderly or small adults. Zolpidem is dosed at 5 mg for the elderly or women and 10 mg for men. The dose of Ambien CR (zolpidem extended-release) is 12.5 mg before bed, with elderly patients prescribed 6.5 mg daily. Zolpidem is available as a sublingual tablet for middle-of-the-night awakening with the maximum dose of 1.75 mg for women and elderly patients and 3.5 mg for men. The daily dose of eszopiclone is 2 to 3 mg before bed, with elderly patients prescribed 1 to 2 mg. The dose of the melatonin receptor agonist ramelteon is 8 mg taken 30 minutes before bed.

The recommended initial dose of suvorexant is 10 mg, taken within 30 minutes of bedtime and with at least 7 hours before wakening time. Only 1 dose of suvorexant should be taken each night. If 10 mg is tolerated but not effective, the dose can be increased to 20 mg once daily before bed. If the patient is on a moderate CYP3A4 inhibitor, the initial dose is 5 mg and should not exceed 10 mg once day.

Rational Drug Selection

There is little to distinguish between the nonbenzodiazepine drugs other than individual response. Ramelteon (Rozerem) is not a controlled substance and does not cause dependence; therefore it may be preferred for some patients. Care must be taken with patients who have a drug or alcohol abuse history that may contribute to psychological dependence.

Monitoring

No drug monitoring is needed or available. Ongoing monitoring of use is necessary to determine overuse.

Patient Education

Patients should be advised to take these drugs immediately before bedtime and to get at least 6 hours of sleep (7 hours with suvorexant). They should be advised to use caution if driving a vehicle or operating hazardous machinery until they know what effect the drug has for them. Patients should not combine these drugs with over-the-counter sleeping aids or alcohol.

MOOD STABILIZERS

Mood stabilizers are used with patients who have bipolar disorders with evidence of depressive and manic or hypomanic episodes. Bipolar disorders are distinctive from unipolar depression by virtue of mood swings and require medication not just for depression but to restore balance in the moods. Neurophysiologically, this is achieved by maintaining a regularity in nerve firing as opposed to the erratic firing that produces changes in behavior and mood. An oversimplified analogy is that bipolar disorder is like epilepsy, but the erratic firing occurs between the limbic system and the frontal cortex as opposed to the motor strip in clonic seizures. The most direct way to achieve regularity is by affecting the calcium channel on the nerve axon that permits influx of ions and stimulates the release of GABA.

Traditionally, bipolar disorder has been treated with lithium salts, first introduced in the mid-19th century and reintroduced in 1960. Although at the time it was not understood how it worked, more recently theories focus on lithium exchanging with sodium ions to propel the nerve impulse along the cell membrane. Currently, the theory underlying neuromodulation is that the catecholaminergic, indolaminergic, cholinergic, and gamma aminobutric acid systems interact to alter the pre- and postsynaptic receptors and postsynaptic activity. The most direct manner of affecting these systems is with the anticonvulsant drug classes; therefore, this section will focus on the anticonvulsants used in mood stabilization. Chapter 29 addresses additional approaches to the prominent depressive episodes.

Although traditionally medications to stabilize mood in bipolar disorders included lithium and anticonvulsants, more recently the atypical APs demonstrate mood stabilization through the combination neurotransmitter effects on dopamine and serotonin. A product released in 2003 departs from the standard because it combines fluoxetine and olanzapine in the brand-name form of Symbyax to provide mood stabilization. Because this drug is predominantly used in patients with mixed bipolar disorder, it will be discussed in greater detail in Chapter 29 along with anxiety and depression.

LITHIUM

Lithium's stabilizing effect on manic individuals was discovered in the mid-1940s, making it the earliest psychotropic drug available for use. Until recently it was considered the treatment of choice for classic bipolar mood disorder and is used as an adjunct for treatment-resistant unipolar depression.

Pharmacodynamics

Lithium carbonate (Lithobid, Eskalith) is a naturally occurring substance, similar to sodium in its lack of metabolism, its excretion through the renal system, and its affinity for the same binding sites. Both are widely distributed and interchangeable.

The relationship between sodium, lithium, and body fluid is inverse in that when sodium and fluids are depleted, as can occur during severe vomiting, prolonged heavy sweating, and diuretic use, the level of lithium is increased. The opposite also occurs, for example, as a result of water intoxication, which has the effect of decreasing the lithium level. Such variations in lithium concentration can also be the product of abrupt dietary changes or seasonal weather changes.

Lithium's mechanism of action is not completely understood but, because of the two substances' ability to substitute for each other, it is believed that lithium replaces sodium during depolarization in neuronal pathways, effectively stopping the transmission of electrical impulses. Additionally, it is suspected that lithium acts on the second messenger system postsynaptically to inhibit either the inositol monophosphatase enzyme to modulate the G proteins or the messenger RNA to alter the protein kinase C (Stahl, 2009).

Pharmacokinetics

Absorption and Distribution

Lithium is quickly absorbed through the GI tract after oral administration and shows no protein binding. Ingestion of food does not affect absorption. It is widely distributed throughout the body according to water volume. Distribution across the blood–brain barrier is slow.

Metabolism and Excretion

Lithium is one of the few psychopharmacological agents that is not metabolized by the liver and is essentially excreted into the urine unchanged. Because it is excreted by the kidneys, kidney function is critical in the use of lithium in treatment. The excretion half-life is between 10 and 50 hours.

Onset, Peak, and Duration

Lithium reaches maximum blood level within 0.5 to 3 hours and has a half-life of 17 to 36 hours. Steady state is achieved in 5 to 7 days.

Pharmacotherapeutics

Precautions and Contraindications

Because lithium is almost completely excreted through the renal system, it is essential that the presence of kidney disease be assessed before starting lithium. Baseline blood chemistry, including creatinine, blood urea nitrogen (BUN), and TSH levels, should be obtained. In the event of positive findings, a different drug should be used.

Lithium is contraindicated in children younger than 12 years because of insufficient clinical trials with young children. Lithium is rated Pregnancy Category C and should not be used with pregnant or lactating women without serious balancing of risks and benefits. When taken in the first trimester, there is a 10% chance of fetal abnormalities, including

Epstein's cardiac anomaly and tricuspid valve prolapse. When taken in the third trimester, there is a significant risk for neonatal lithium toxicity, hypertonicity, congenital hypothyroidism, and congenital goiter (Williams & Oke, 2000).

Extreme caution should be used when prescribing lithium to patients with sodium depletion or to those taking diuretics. Hypothyroidism and kidney failure may occur with long-term administration.

Adverse Drug Reactions

Early, transient adverse reactions may occur, including most commonly fine tremors of the fingers, nausea, dry mouth, headache, and drowsiness. Lithium may be taken with food to minimize GI distress, and the form of the drug may be changed to sustained release to minimize adverse effects associated with dosage peaks. Even at therapeutic blood levels, some patients may have ECG changes that are not necessarily indicative of underlying cardiac disease but should be monitored.

The index between therapeutic and toxic levels is narrow at the upper end, requiring frequent monitoring initially and in the event of significant changes in fluid balance, as often as daily if necessary. The therapeutic range is 0.6 to 1.5 mEq/L.

Indicators of toxicity, which can also occur at therapeutic levels, are coarse tremors of the hands that impair function, nausea and vomiting, diarrhea, confusion, stupor, polydipsia and polyuria, muscle weakness, and ataxia. If the lithium level is elevated enough, coma and death can result. Treatment for overdose is supportive, including ensuring adequate hydration and even dialysis. Because lithium overdose may contribute to arrhythmias, ECG monitoring is necessary.

Drug Interactions

Because the liver does not metabolize lithium, drug interactions due to the CYP450 system are not an issue. However, drug interactions associated with altering fluid balance and lithium concentrations may increase the risk for lithium toxicity. Diuretics may increase sodium excretion and increase lithium concentrations. NSAIDs and COX 2 inhibitors reduce renal elimination and elevate serum lithium levels. Lithium prolongs the effects of neuromuscular-blocking agents used before surgery and during electroconvulsive treatments (ECT). Concurrent use of etronidazole increases risk of lithium toxicity due to decreased renal excretion.

Decreased lithium levels may result with theophylline, concurrent use of sodium salts, and bulking agents such as Metamucil. Concurrent administration with anticonvulsants may increase toxicity of both drugs. Table 15-32 includes the drug interactions with lithium.

Clinical Use and Dosing

Table 15-33 includes the indications, dosage schedule, and available dosage forms for lithium.

Rational Drug Selection

Because of its long half-life, lithium takes 10 to 14 days to reach maximum efficacy; therefore, it is not indicated in the treatment of acute mania. Rather, it is indicated for maintenance of mood stability and prevention of mania or hypomania. A strategy for responding to acute mania would be to start a patient on lithium supplemented initially with a dopaminergic or serotonergic-dopaminergic drug such as haloperidol or risperidone and to discontinue the neuroleptic, if possible, when the required length of time for lithium to be become efficacious has elapsed and the mania has abated. Some clinicians raise the dosage initially to achieve a serum level of 1.2 mEq/L during an acute stage and back down to 0.8 mEq/L for maintenance. As a patient achieves and maintains stability, levels need not be obtained as frequently.

Table 15–32 ⣿ Drug Interactions: Lithium

Drug	Interacting Drug	Possible Effect	Implications
Lithium	Angiotensin-converting enzyme (ACE) inhibitors, antibiotics (ampicillin, doxycycline, tetracycline, spectinomycin), antihypertensives, metronidazole, NSAIDs, antimicrobials, diuretics, fluoxetine	Increased lithium level	Monitor lithium blood levels and for signs and symptoms of toxicity Avoid NSAIDs
	Caffeine, psyllium, urinary alkalizers, theophylline	Decreased lithium level	Monitor lithium blood level and recurrence of manic signs and symptoms for need to increase dose
	Anticonvulsants, calcium channel blockers, phenothiazines, haloperidol, methyldopa	Increased neurotoxicity	Avoid coadministration
	Benzodiazepines	Sexual dysfunction	Avoid
	SSRIs	Serotonin syndrome	Keep SSRI dose low
			Monitor for signs and symptoms of serotonin excess
	Acetazolamide, osmotic diuretics, theophyllines, urinary alkalizers	Increased renal excretion	Monitor PT response and lithium blood levels, adjust lithium dose
	Neuromuscular blocking agents, TCAs	Increased pharmacological effects of additive drugs	Adjust dosage accordingly

Table 15–33 🕸 **Dosage Schedule: Lithium**

Drug	Indications	Dosage	Available Dosage Forms
Lithium (Lithobid, Eskalith, lithium carbonate, Lithotabs)	Treatment of manic phase of bipolar disorders and prevention of manic episodes	Acute mania; 600 mg tid or 900 mg bid Extended-release Maintenance: 300 mg tid qid or 450 mg bid Controlled-release	Capsules (G): 150 mg 300 mg 600 mg Tablets: 300 mg Controlled-release tablets: 300 and 450 mg Syrup: 300 mg/15 mL Slow-release capsules 150 and 300 mg

Refractory unipolar depression = 300–600 mg daily.
G = generic.

Lithium is also prescribed for patients who have been resistant to adequate trials of the usual antidepressants based on the theory that the resistance is due to an underlying bipolar pathology. Adjunctive doses of lithium are frequently lower than they would be for bipolar disorder, with concomitantly lower risks.

Monitoring

Because signs and symptoms of toxicity may occur even at subtoxic blood levels, patients should always be assessed for tremors, nausea, and drowsiness. Lowering the dose will usually be sufficient to resolve the problems.

Blood levels should be obtained 14 days after beginning treatment and 14 days after every dosage change. Generally, routine blood levels are obtained every 3 to 6 months after stability is achieved. In the event of patient illness involving severe vomiting, diarrhea, prolonged high fever, or heatstroke, more frequent monitoring is needed as would also be the case in a planned dietary change or weight-loss plan. The procedure for obtaining an accurate lithium level is to have the sample drawn 12 hours after the last dose, usually the bedtime dose, before any morning dose has been taken. The patient need not be fasting, but the timing needs to be accurate within an hour to ensure standardization of interpretation of the results.

Routine blood counts with differential, chemistry screens, and thyroid panels should be obtained yearly. In addition, there should be a baseline ECG and annual ECG to ascertain arrhythmias.

Patient Education

Patients should be informed of the procedure for obtaining an accurate lithium level as described above. Advise the patient to report any illness involving severe vomiting, diarrhea, or prolonged fever. Also tell patients engaging in activities that produce copious sweating to increase their water intake and maintain an adequate salt intake. Women of childbearing age need to be advised of contraceptive strategies and that unplanned pregnancies may result in congenital malformations.

VALPROATES

Although valproate (Depakote) was approved for treatment of seizures in the 1960s, the FDA did not approve its use in mania until 1995. It is currently seen as the first- or second-choice drug in the treatment of bipolar disorder, especially in acute mania and maintenance for bipolar, manic disorder.

Pharmacodynamics

Although the exact mechanism is unknown, valproate blocks GABA uptake into presynaptic neurons without affecting the benzodiazepine binding site. It appears to enhance GABA function, thereby slowing down repolarization and reducing glutamate functioning at the sodium and calcium channels.

Pharmacokinetics

Absorption and Distribution

Valproate is administered orally and is rapidly absorbed by the GI tract. It has also been approved for IV administration for immediate treatment of seizures, but this route has not been used in rapid treatment of mania. It is 100% bioavailable with high protein binding. It reaches peak levels in 1 to 4 hours and has a half-life of 6 to16 hours. Valproate may be displaced by carbamazepine and warfarin, contributing to toxic side effects.

Metabolism and Excretion

Valproate is metabolized by the liver with several active metabolites. It is metabolized by P450 2C9, 2C19, and 2A6; possibly induces 2C9 and 2C19; and inhibits 2C9, 2D6, and 3A4. Such a complicated metabolism contributes to many drug interactions, as described below. It is excreted by the kidneys.

Onset, Peak, and Duration

Peak plasma levels occur within 1 to 4 hours, although when administered by syrup, the drug peaks sooner. Conversely, the enteric-coated version delays absorption and peaking.

Pharmacotherapeutics

Precautions and Contraindications

Contraindications include hypersensitivity and hepatic disease.

Use of these drugs during the first trimester of pregnancy is associated with neural tube defects including spina bifida. They are Pregnancy Category D. Their use should be restricted to cases in which the woman's life would be endangered without them and then only beyond the first trimester. They should be used with caution during lactation.

The plasma level range is 50 to 100 mcg/mL. Levels above 100 mcg/mL are thought to be toxic, although symptoms of toxicity can occur at blood levels within the normal range, and patients have been maintained on levels above 100 mcg/mL without apparent toxicity. Therefore, valproate has a wider safety margin than lithium. Symptoms of toxicity include dizziness, hypotension, tachycardia or bradycardia, drowsiness, visual hallucinations, and respiratory depression. Coma and death may result.

Although relatively uncommon, valproate may impair platelet aggregation so that bleeding time may be prolonged, and it may suppress bone marrow production. For this reason, a CBC with differential and platelets should precede use and be repeated with regularity initially and less frequently beyond the first 3 months as the patient continues to take the medication without adverse events.

Rare cases of hepatotoxicity and liver failure have occurred, primarily in children younger than 2 years who have been on combination antiepileptic drug therapy. Because bipolar disorder has not yet been diagnosed in children younger than 2 years, valproate has not been used for mood stabilization in this population.

Patients with diabetes taking valproate may show falsely positive ketone urine tests because the drug is partially excreted in the urine as a ketone metabolite. Any patient may have initially elevated liver enzymes, but this is usually transitory.

Adverse Drug Reactions

Valproate is well tolerated, and most adverse effects, such as GI distress, heartburn, and CNS depression, are mild and transient. Safety in situations requiring mental alertness is of concern initially, and the patient should be instructed to avoid potentially dangerous situations until the effect of the drug can be assessed. Alopecia has also been reported but the hair usually grows back, although with a different texture.

Drug Interactions

Many common drug interactions have to do with the competition with protein-binding sites and the P450 enzyme involvement. Valproates in combination with other CNS depressants can lead to an additive depressant effect. Bleeding time can be increased in combination with anticoagulants. Combinations of TCAs and valproates can lead to increased risk of cardiotoxicity. Combinations of valproates with carbamazepine or hydantoins may result in increased levels of these drugs and reduced efficacy of valproate. Chlorpromazine, cimetidine, erythromycin, rifampin, and salicylates may increase valproate serum levels. Table 15-34 includes the drug interactions with the valproates.

Clinical Uses and Dosages

Table 15-35 includes the indications, dosage schedule, and available dosage forms for the valproates.

Rational Drug Selection

Valproate psychiatric indications include the treatment of bipolar disorder, particularly the rapid cycling or mixed types, both for acute mania and prevention. It can be given in large doses in an acute state with minimal concern for toxicity.

Other uses include treatment of mood stability associated with borderline personality disorder or PTSD, anger and aggression, and adjunctive treatment for drug-resistant unipolar depression.

The usual adult dose is 750 to 3,000 mg/day taken initially in divided dose then once daily at bedtime if side effects are

Table 15–34 ⠿ Drug Interactions: Valproates

Drug	Interacting Drug	Possible Effect	Implications
Valproic acid and derivatives	CNS depressants	Increased sedation and disorientation	Warn patient about safety issues; avoid if possible
	Anticoagulants	Increased bleeding time	Monitor bleeding time
	Anticonvulsants	May increase plasma level of anticonvulsant, decrease valproate efficacy	Monitor plasma levels
	TCAs, barbiturates, diazepam, ethosuximide	Increased blood level and increased risk of cardiotoxicity	Monitor blood level
	Clonazepam	Increased risk of absence seizure	
	Lithium	Increased tremors	Decrease lithium dose
	Typical antipsychotics	Increased risk of neurotoxicity, sedation, EPS	Monitor for signs and symptoms of toxicity
	Antiviral	Decreased valproate level	Monitor plasma level of valproate
	Cimetidine, salicylates, rifampin, erythromycin	Increased plasma level and half-life of valproate	Monitor plasma level of valproate
	Lamotrigine	Decreased valproic levels, increased lamotrigine levels	Monitor plasma levels

Table 15–35 ⊗ **Dosage Schedule: Valproates**

Drug	Indications	Dosage	Available Dosage Forms
Valproic acid (Depakote, Depakene; Depacon)	Complex partial, simple (petit mal), absence seizure epilepsy; mania; migraine headache	*Adults:* 750 mg daily in divided doses; may increase rapidly to control acute mania to maximum of 60 mg/kg/d For migraine headache: 250 mg bid *Children and older adults:* Reduce dose Sprinkle capsule should not be chewed and not stored for future use once opened; take with food to prevent GI distress For acute mania: 60 mg IV infusion (20 mg/min or less) at same frequency as oral dose	Depakene: 250 mg capsule 250 mg/5 mL syrup Generic: 250 mg capsules 250 mg/5 mL syrup Depakote enteric-coated tablet: 125 mg 250 mg 500 mg 125 mg sprinkle capsule Extended-release Depakote 250 and 500 mg Depacon: 5 mg injection

tolerable. Maximum daily dosage is 60 mg/kg/day. Because it inhibits its own metabolism after reaching steady state, the drug begins to maintain a consistent blood level sufficient for single daily dosing.

Monitoring

Plasma levels should be assessed to help guide dosage adjustments, with a trough concentration of 50 to 125 mcg/mL. CBCs and chemistries should be obtained prior to onset of treatment and then every 3 months for 1 year. After 1 year, monitoring can be done annually.

Patient Education

Patients should be advised about the side effects, especially the possibility of bruising and delayed clotting initially. Patients who are prone to falls should especially be advised to tell their primary care provider and family members. Patients should be advised to avoid hazardous activities until their level of sedation is determined. Also, advise patients not to discontinue the drug abruptly.

NONCLASSIFIED MOOD STABILIZERS

The nonbenzodiazepine gaba-ergics used in the treatment of epilepsy have shown effectiveness in treating bipolar states, as might be expected based on the data about valproates. These include lamotrigine (Lamictal), gabapentin (Neurontin), and topiramate (Topamax). Only lamotrigine has been approved by the FDA for this use.

Pharmacodynamics

All of these drugs act in some way on GABA as well as other mechanisms. Lamotrigine also acts as a 5-HT_3 blocker and glutamate modulator as well as inhibits the sodium channels to slow down depolarization. Gabapentin does not act directly on GABA but instead seems to act as a GABA transporter inhibitor, thereby increasing the availability of GABA. As with lamotrigine, gabapentin decreases the excitatory amino acid neurotransmitter, glutamate. Finally, topiramate acts in a manner similar to gabapentin to enhance GABA functioning and interfere with glutamate by means of the sodium and calcium channels.

Pharmacokinetics

Absorption and Distribution

All three of the gaba-ergic drugs are readily absorbed through the GI tract and have between 80% to 90% bioavailability. Gabapentin's bioavailability decreases as the dose increases, however. Lamotrigine has the longest half-life at 25 hours, topiramate has 21 hours, and gabapentin is at 5 to 8 hours. Food does not alter absorption for any of these drugs.

Metabolism and Excretion

Lamotrigine is metabolized by glucuronidation; however, all three drugs are essentially excreted by the kidneys relatively unchanged. Neither gabapentin nor topiramate undergoes metabolism at all.

Pharmacotherapeutics

Precautions and Contraindications

All three of these drugs are rated Pregnancy Category C. Based on the pregnancy registry, there is no evidence of harm to the fetus; however, the database is insufficient to determine the risk. The prescriber would need to balance the risks and the benefits of treating a pregnant woman with these drugs. If it is necessary to use them, it serves the fetus best to wait until the second trimester. Although no detrimental effects have been reported to the breastfeeding newborn, each of these drugs is excreted in breast milk and exposes the healthy neonate unnecessarily to the drug.

These drugs have not been tested in children and should not be used to treat children younger than 2 years. There are no age-related differences in safety; however, dosages may need to be changed in the elderly to accommodate changes in renal clearance.

Topiramate has shown the effect of hyperchloremic non-anion gap metabolic acidosis and should be used cautiously with patients with eating disorders.

Adverse Drug Reactions

The gaba-ergic drugs have relatively few side effects. Those most commonly seen are somnolence, dizziness, ataxia, and fatigue. Gabapentin is associated with weight gain, whereas topiramate and to a lesser extent lamotrigine are associated with weight loss. In addition, diplopia, blurred vision, nausea, and rhinitis are not uncommon. Lamotrigine and topiramate have a rare incidence (0.8% in children; 0.3% in adults) of Stevens–Johnson syndrome occurring within the first 2 to 8 weeks of therapy that can be fatal. Topiramate has a 1% occurrence of renal calculi.

Drug Interactions

The gaba-ergics are minimally metabolized by the liver; there are few drug interactions. When given in conjunction with other antiepileptic drugs, such as carbamazepine or phenytoin, the half-life of lamotrigine is decreased, but with valproate the half-life is increased. Gabapentin reduces the bioavailability of antacids, but cimetidine increases the bioavailability of gabapentin. Gabapentin also increases the serum levels of contraceptives. Topiramate decreases the effectiveness of oral contraceptives, and carbonic anhydrase inhibitors may increase the risk of kidney stones.

Clinical Use and Dosing

The primary use of these non-benzodiazepine gaba-ergics is for epilepsy; however, lamotrigine has been approved for use in acute mania, maintenance and prophylaxis of mood lability, and may even reduce the incidence of depression in bipolar disorders. Gabapentin and topiramate have not been approved to treat bipolar disorders; however, indication for this is likely to be approved in the near future.

Rationale Drug Selection

Currently these three drugs are seen as a third line for the treatment of bipolar disorder and are often used in conjunction with other therapies for treatment-resistant bipolar conditions. They are safe and easy for patients to maintain treatment.

Monitoring

No routine serum levels are necessary. Patients should monitor skin appearances and report any rashes within the first 2 months of therapy, especially if blisters form. Weight monitoring is important, especially with gabapentin.

Patient Education

Patients must be informed of the risks and benefits of these drugs as well as the possible side effects. Patients taking topiramate need to be advised to drink plenty of water owing to the risk of kidney stones. Advise patients of the potential for Stevens–Johnson syndrome and what to do if a rash appears.

MUSCLE RELAXANTS AND ANTISPASMOTICS

Muscle relaxants and antispasmotic drugs are used to treat severe muscle spasms and the associated pain. The two categories of muscle relaxants are those that act in the CNS and the direct-acting drugs or antispasmotics. The commonly used centrally acting muscle relaxants include baclofen (Lioresal), carisoprodol (Soma), chloraxazone (Paraflex, Parafon Forte), cyclobenzaprine (Flexeril), methocarbamol (Robaxin), orphenadrine (Banflex, Norflex), and tizanidine (Zanaflex). The benzodiazepines (diazepam) that are centrally acting muscle relaxants have been previously discussed. The direct-acting antispasmotics include dantrolene (Dantrium) and botulinum toxin type A (Botox). Muscle relaxants and antispasmotics are often combined with nonpharmacological measures such as stretching, massage, and heat or cold to relieve muscle spasms and pain.

CENTRALLY ACTING MUSCLE RELAXANTS

Pharmacodynamics

The exact mechanism whereby the centrally acting muscle relaxants relieve muscle spasms is not well understood. The centrally acting medications appear to act on the monosynaptic and polysynaptic spinal reflexes, rather than on the muscles themselves. Inhibiting the synaptic reflex arcs impacts the messages that are producing and maintaining the skeletal muscle spasm. Centrally acting muscle relaxants also have a sedative effect, which causes drowsiness and may enable a patient with muscle spasms to relax and sleep. Tizanidine is a centrally acting alpha$_2$-adrenergic agonist that produces presynaptic inhibition of motor neurons in the spinal cord, reducing muscle spasticity.

Pharmacokinetics

Absorption and Distribution

The centrally acting muscle relaxants baclofen, carisoprodol, chloraxazone, cyclobenzaprine, methocarbamol, and tizanidine are rapidly absorbed after oral administration. Metaxalone is more slowly absorbed and has an onset of 3 hours after oral dose on an empty stomach. The centrally acting muscle relaxants are distributed into the CNS (site of action). The pharmacokinetics of orphenadrine is not described.

Metabolism and Excretion

Most of the centrally acting muscle relaxants are metabolized in the liver and excreted in the urine. Carisoprodol is metabolized in the liver by CYP2C19 into the active metabolite meprobamate, which has antianxiety properties. Cyclobenzaprine is subject to enterohepatic circulation and will accumulate if dosed 3 times a day, with steady-state plasma levels significantly higher than when given in a single dose. Tizanidine is metabolized via CYPO 1A2 into inactive metabolites, which are excreted in the urine.

Pharmacotherapeutics

Precautions and Contraindications

The centrally acting muscle relaxants may cause CNS sedation and increase the risk of falls and injury. Patients should not drive or use any other CNS sedating drug while taking muscle relaxants. Many of the centrally acting muscle relaxants (carisoprodol, chlorzoxazone, cyclobenzaprine, methocarbamol, and orphenadrine) are on the Beer's list of medications to be avoided in the elderly.

Baclofen's only true contraindication is hypersensitivity to baclofen. Baclofen should be used cautiously in patients with decreased renal function, as it is excreted primarily via the kidneys. Patients with seizure disorder should be prescribed baclofen carefully, with seizure control and EEG monitored because of a deterioration in seizure control associated with baclofen use. Baclofen is Pregnancy Category C and should be avoided in pregnancy due to increased incidence of omphaloceles in fetal rats and unossified forelimbs and hindlimbs in rabbits. Case reports of neonatal withdrawal have been reported. Limited information on use of baclofen during lactation indicates there are low levels of baclofen in breast milk, but not enough to cause adverse effects in the infant (LactMed, 2014). Breastfed infants should be monitored for sedation.

Carisoprodol is contraindicated in patients with porphyria or hypersensitivity to carisoprodol or its active metabolite meprobamate. Carisoprodol (Soma) may cause physical dependence and abuse or result in criminal diversion. Abuse of carisoprodol may lead to overdose, CNS and respiratory depression, and death. Carisoprodol is Pregnancy Category C. It is known to cross the placenta, and animal studies indicate adverse effects on fetal growth but no clear teratogen effects. Carisoprodol and its metabolite meprobamate can be measured in human breast milk, with mild sedation noted in breastfed newborns of women taking the drug (LactMed, 2014). Carisoprodol is not approved for use in children younger than age 16 years.

Rare reports of hepatoxocity have been noted with chlorzoxazone use. Chlorzaxone is Pregnancy Category C. Safety in lactation or in children has not been established.

Cyclobenzaprine is contraindicated in patients with hyperthyroidism or in the acute recovery phase of a myocardial infarction or who have heart failure, dysrhythmias, or conduction disturbances. Serotonin syndrome has been reported with cyclobenzaprine use. Owing to its anticholinergic effects, cyclobenzaprine should be used cautiously in patients with urinary retention, angle-closure glaucoma, or increased intraocular pressure. Patients with hepatic impairment are not able to metabolize cyclobenzaprine well; therefore, those with mild liver dysfunction should be prescribed small doses (5 mg) and those with moderate to severe liver dysfunction should not be prescribed cyclobenzaprine. Cyclobenzaprine is Pregnancy Category B, with no impact on pregnancy or the fetus recorded. There is no available information regarding the use of cyclobenzaprine while breastfeeding; therefore, it should be used with caution and the infant monitored for sedation. The safety and efficacy of cyclobenzaprine in children younger than age 15 years have not been established.

Metaxalone is contraindicated in patients with known hypersensitivity and those with significantly impaired renal or hepatic function. If administered to a patient with liver dysfunction, serial liver function studies should be performed. Metaxalone does not have a pregnancy category assigned, and safe use in pregnancy has not been determined. It is not known whether metaxalone is excreted in breast milk. The safety and effectiveness in children younger than age 12 years have not been established.

Methocarbamol is contraindicated in patients who are hypersensitive to the drug. Patients with renal or hepatic dysfunction should be prescribed methocarbamol with caution. Methocarbamol is Pregnancy Category C. Rare reports of fetal malformations have been recorded following in utero exposure. It is not known whether methocarbamol is excreted in human breast milk, although it has been measured in dog milk. The safety and efficacy in children younger than age 16 years have not been established.

Orphenadrine has significant anticholinergic effects and therefore should not be used in patients with urinary retention, prostatic hypertrophy, glaucoma, or achalasia. Orphenadrine is Pregancy Category C. Safety during lactation or in children has not been established.

Tizanidine is contraindicated in patients who are hypersensitive or who are taking CYP1A2 inhibitors (fluvoxamine or ciprofloxacin). Anaphylaxis and angioedema has been reported with tizanidine use. Tizanidine is hepatotoxic and should be used cautiously in patients with liver dysfunction. Liver function should be monitored during use. Older adults or patients with renal dysfunction should be prescribed tizanidine cautiously due to increased adverse effects. Tizanidine is an alpha$_2$-adrenergic agonist and patients who abruptly stop taking the medication may experience hypertension or tachycardia. Tizanidine is Pregnancy Category C. There are no human studies, but animal studies have noted developmental retardation and fetal loss. Safety and efficacy in children or during lactation have not been established.

Adverse Drug Reactions

As previously noted, all the muscle relaxants cause CNS sedation to some extent, with some causing significant sedation, drowsiness, and dizziness. Baclofen may cause neuropsychiatric effects, including confusion, headache, insomnia, and seizures.

Carisoprodol causes significant CNS and respiratory depression, which is worsened by coadministration of other CNS depressants. Carisoprodol may cause headache, tachycardia, vertigo, atazia, syncope, insomnia, and seizures. Physical dependence on carisoprodol may occur, as well as leukopenia or pancytopenia.

Chlorzaxazone may be hepatotoxic and may rarely cause angioedema or anaphylaxis. Gastrointestinal effects of chlorzaxazone include nausea, vomiting, diarrhea or constipation, heartburn, or gastrointestinal bleeding.

Patients taking cyclobenzaprine may experience dry mouth, fatigue, nausea and vomiting, constipation, hallucinations, and blurred vision. Cyclobenzaprine may cause dysrhythmias or prolonged QT syndrome.

The adverse effects of metaxalone include confusion, headache, anxiety, nausea, dry mouth, or gastrointestinal upset. Metaxalone may also cause leukopenia or hemolytic anemia.

Methocarbamol may cause significant sedation and dizziness. Anaphylaxis, urticaria, and rash may occur. Blurred vision, headache, leukopenia, jaundice, nausea, and vomiting have also been reported in patients taking methocarbamol.

Orphenadrine may cause CNS excitation, agitation and hallucinations, dry mouth, tachycardia, syncope, palpitation, blurred vision, nausea and vomiting, and abdominal cramps. Anaphylaxis may occur with orphenadrine use.

Tizanidine may cause dry mouth (49% in clinical trials), asthenia (weakness), fatigue, constipation, hypotension, and bradycardia. Tizanidine may be hepatotoxic and liver function should be monitored.

Drug Interactions

All of the muscle relaxants have additive sedation with other CNS depressants and patients should be warned not to consume alcohol or antihistamines while taking these medications.

Coadministration of carisoprodol and CYP2C19 inhibitors (omeprazole, fluvoxamine, aspirin) may result in increased carisoprodol levels.

Cyclobenzaprine may have a life-threatening interaction with MAO inhibitors. Coadministration of cyclobenzaprine with serotinergic drugs (SSRIs, SNRIs, TCAs, bupropion, MAOIs) may cause serotonin syndrome.

Methocarbamol decreases the effect of pyridostigmine. Use cautiously in patients taking anticholinesterase medications, such as those with myasthenia gravis.

Tizanidine's effects may be increased if taken concurrently with fluvoxamine, ciprofloxacin, or alpha$_2$-adrenergic antihypertensives, leading to hypotension, increased drowsiness, and increased impairment. Concurrent use with CYP 1A2 inhibitors is contraindicated—including zileuton, fluroquinolones, amiodoarone, mexiletine, propafenone, verapamil, cimetidine, famotidine, oral contraceptives, acyclovir, and ticlopidine—due to increased levels of tizanidine that lead to increased risk of hypotension and sedation. Alcohol increases tizanidine blood levels and additionally causes additive sedation.

Clinical Use and Dosing

Baclofen is prescribed to relieve spasticity associated with multiple sclerosis, spinal cord injuries, and occasionally cerebral palsy. Baclofen dosage is individualized to the patients, with slow titration to desired effect. Adult patients are started at 5 mg TID and increased every 3 days until desired effect to a maximum of 80 mg/day. Baclofen is also delivered intrathecally via pump to treat spasticity in both children and adults.

Carisoprodol (Soma) is dosed at 250 to 350 mg 3 times a day for a maximum of 2 to 3 weeks. Limiting the length of treatment to 3 weeks helps avoid dependence and abuse.

Chlorzoxazone (Parafon Forte) in addition to rest and physical therapy is indicated for the treatment of painful musculoskeletal conditions. The usual adult dose is 500 mg 3 to 4 times a day. The dose may be increased to 750 mg 3 to 4 times a day if needed, but the dose should be reduced as soon as improvement occurs.

Cyclobenzaprine (Flexeril) is used for the short-term treatment of painful muscle spasms that impact activities of daily living. The recommended dose of cyclobenzaprine is 5 mg 3 times a day for 2 to 3 weeks. The dosage may be increased to 10 mg 3 times a day if indicated. Lowered or less frequent doses are recommended for the elderly or patients with hepatic impairment. Cyclobenzaprine should not be prescribed for longer than 3 weeks.

Metaxalone (Skelaxin) is indicated for the short-term treatment of acute, painful musculoskeletal conditions. It is to be used in conjuction with rest and other measures to relieve muscle pain. The recommended adult dose is 800 mg 3 to 4 times a day.

Methocarbamol (Robaxin) is prescribed for short-term treatment of acute painful musculoskeletal conditions in adults or adolescents age 16 years or older. The initial dose of methocarbamol for muscle spasms is 1.5 g 4 times a day for 2 to 3 days. The maintenance dose is 1.0 g 4 times a day or 1.5 g 3 times a day. Dosage should be adjusted downward in patients with renal or hepatic impairment. Intravenous methocarbamol is used to treat tetanus.

Orphenadrine (Norgesic or Norgesic Forte) is used for short-term relief of moderate pain associated with musculoskeletal disorders in conjunction with rest and other measures to relieve muscle pain. The dose of Norgesic (orphenadrine 25 mg with aspirin 385 mg and caffeine 30 mg) is one to two tablets 3 to 4 times a day. The dose of Norgesic Forte (orphenadrine 50 mg with aspirin 770 mg and caffeine 60 mg) is one-half to one tablet 3 to 4 times daily.

Tizanidine (Zanaflex) is used for spasticity and is recommended only when spasticity is affecting activities of daily living. Tizanidine may be taken with or without food, but once a patient decides it should be taken consistently with or without food because pharmacokinetics differ depending on food intake. The recommended initial dose of tizanidine is 2 mg every 6 to 8 hours, for a maximum of three doses in 24 hours. The dose may be increased by 2 mg per dose every 1 to 4 days to a maximum of 36 mg per 24 hours. Lower doses should be prescribed for patients with renal or hepatic impairment. Patients are at risk for rebound when discontinuing tizanidine; therefore, they should be tapered slowly (2 to 4 mg per day taper) to prevent rebound hypertension, tachycardia, and hypertonia.

Rational Drug Selection

Drug selection is dependent on the patient's underlying condition and health status. The evidence for the use of muscle relaxants is lacking, and they have not been proven to be more effective than acetaminophen or NSAIDS for low back pain. Elderly patients and those with hepatic impairment should be prescribed the antispasmotics with caution. Tizanidine and cyclobenzaprine are sedating and may be helpful if muscle spasms cause insomnia. Methocarbamol is less sedating if patients need to take it during the day, but the patient should not drive while using the drug.

Monitoring

It is important to monitor for adverse reactions to muscle relaxants, as discussed previously. The clinician should monitor that the amount of drug used is consistent with the amounts prescribed and dispensed.

Patient Education

Patients being prescribed muscle relaxants should be educated on the appropriate use and adverse effects. All of the muscle relaxant drugs are sedating, and patients should be cautioned not to drive or combine them with other sedating medications or alcohol. Muscle relaxants are for short-term use; therefore nonpharmacological therapies should be addressed, including heat/cold, physical therapy, and back exercises.

DIRECT-ACTING ANTISPASMOTICS

Pharmacodynamics

The direct-acting antispasmotics dantrolene (Dantrium) and botulinum toxin type A (Botox) have unique uses based on their pharmacodynamics. Dantrolene is administered orally or via IV and is used to treat spasticity associated with upper neuron disorders, including spinal cord injury, stroke, cerebral palsy, and multiple sclerosis. Botulinum toxin type A is injected to provide localized reduction in muscle activitiy.

Dantrolene causes muscle relaxation by interfering with the release of calcium from the sarcoplasmic reticulum, affecting the fast muscle fibers more than the slow fibers. The intensity of the skeletal muscle relaxation is dose-related. Botulinum toxin type A acts locally to block neuromuscular transmission by binding to receptor sites on the motor or sympathetic nerves, depending on site of injection. At the nerve terminal, botulinum toxin type A works to inhibit the release of acetylcholine. When injected intradermally, botulinum toxin type A causes temporary denervation of the sweat glands, causing decreased production of sweat locally. When injected into the detrusor muscle, botulinum toxin type A affects the afferent pathways of the detrusor muscle by inhibiting acetylcholine release.

Pharmacokinetics

Absorption and Distribution

Absorption of dantrolene after oral administration is incomplete but not well described. The half-life of dantrolene is 8.7 hours after a 100 mg dose, with the duration of action related to dosage. Botulinum toxin type A is not absorbed and is not detected in the blood after intramuscular injection.

Metabolism and Excretion

Dantrolene is metabolized into a 5-hydroxy analog and an acetamido analog and excreted in the urine.

Pharmacotherapeutics

Precautions and Contraindications

Dantrolene is contraindicated in patients with active liver disease such as hepatitis or cirrhosis. Dantrolene may induce potentially fatal hepatocellular disease, with a higher risk noted in female patients and those over age 35. The elderly may have an increased likelihood of fatal hepatoticity, possibly due to concomitant illness or interacting medications.

Botulinum toxin type A may spread from the site of injection to produce effects similar to botulinum toxin. Symptoms may appear hours to weeks after injection and include muscle weakness, dysphagia, dysphonia, urinary incontinence, and breathing difficulties. If muscles of the respiratory system are involved, the patient may need intubation and mechanical ventilation. If the muscles of the oropharynx or esophagus are affected, patients may aspirate. Antitoxin is available for overdose from the Centers for Disease Control and Prevention. Intradetrusor injection with botulinum toxin type A is contraindicated in patients with a urinary tract infection or urinary retention.

Dantrolene is Pregnancy Category C. There is no long-term data on use during lactation; therefore it should not be used during breastfeeding (LactMed, 2014). Botulinum toxin type A is Pregnancy Catetory C.

Adverse Drug Reactions

Although dantrolene is a direct-acting antispasmotic, the major ADRs involve CNS sedation, including drowsiness, dizziness, weakness, fatigue, and malaise. These adverse effects can be reduced by starting at a low dose and slowing the increase to the target dose. Other CNS effects include mental depression, confusion, nervousness, headache, insomnia, drooling, and alteration in taste. Patients may experience diarrhea that may be severe and require the temporary cessation of therapy. If diarrhea recurs when dantrolene is restarted, the patient may not be able to tolerate the medication. Less common GI adverse effects include constipation, abdominal cramps, anorexia, nausea, and vomiting. Patients may also experience hepatitis, tachycardia, heart failure, urinary frequency, hematuria, erectile dysfunction, or urinary incontinence or retention. Hematologic adverse effects are not common but include aplastic anemia, anemia, leukopenia, and thrombocytopenia.

Adverse effects of injected botulinum toxin type A are mostly related to the effects of the spread of the toxin, including dysphagia and breathing difficulties when treating cervical dystonia and bronchitis and upper respiratory tract infections in patients treated for spasticity. Patients being treated with intradetruser injections for bladder dysfunction experienced urinary tract infection (18%), urinary tract retention (6%), and residual urine volume (3%). Patients with diabetes who were treated with 100 units of intradetruser botulinum toxin type A injections had a 31% incidence of urinary tract infections. Patients being treated for chronic migraines reported neck pain (9%), eyelid ptosis (4%), muscular weakness (4%), and musculoskeletal stiffness (4%).

Drug Interactions

Administration of dantrolene and other CNS depressants will lead to additive sedation. Estrogen may increase risk of hepatotoxicity, so dantrolene should be used concomitantly with caution. Combining IV dantrolene and verapamil has led to ventricular fibrillation and cardiovascular collapse in anesthetized pigs; therefore, the combination of dantrolene and calcium channel blockers is not recommended during the management of malignant hyperthermia.

Aminoglycosides and anticholinergic drugs may potentiate the effects of botulinum toxin type A. Muscle relaxants may lead to exaggerated weakness when given before or after administration of botulinum toxin type A. A second dose or type of botulinum toxin should not be administered until the effects of the first dose resolve because excessive neuromuscular weakness may occur.

Clinical Use and Dosing

Dantrolene is gradually titrated to optimum dose to decrease adverse effects. Adult patients are started on 25 mg daily for 7 days then increased to 25 mg 3 times a day for 7 days. If the patient tolerates that dose, it is increased to 50 mg 3 times a day for 7 days and can be increased to a maxiumum of 100 mg 3 to 4 times daily if necessary. The maximum dose is 100 mg 4 times a day. In children over age 5, the patient is started on 0.5 mg/kg dantrolene daily for 7 days, then increased to 0.5 mg/kg 3 times a day for 7 days. If the patient is tolerating the dose, the dantrolene is increased to 1 mg/kg 3 times a day. The patient may take 2 mg/kg 3 or 4 times a day, with a maximum dose of 100 mg 4 times a day.

The dantrolene dose for malignant hyperthermia is 4 to 8 mg/kg/day (divided in three or four doses) for 1 or 2 days prior to surgery. The dose of dantrolene after a malignant hyperthermia crisis is 4 to 8 mg/kg/day (divided in three to four doses) for 1 to 3 days to prevent recurrence.

Botulinum toxin type A (Botox) injections require providers skilled in proper technique to prevent accidental paralysis. The use of Botox is reserved for specialty practice and is outside the scope of this text.

Rational Drug Selection

Dantrolene and botulinum toxin type A are unique drugs with specific, unique uses and are the only drugs for their respective uses.

Monitoring

Patients who are taking dantrolene should be monitored for effectivess of the medication as seen by decreasesd spasticity and for adverse effects, including excessive drowsiness, dizziness, and fatigue. Diarrhea may occur and requires dantrolene be stopped and restarted once symptoms resolve.

Patients who have received botulinum toxin type A injections should be monitored for the effects of toxin spread and hypersensitivity.

Patient Education

The titration schedule for dantrolene needs to be explained to patients carefully and written down. They should be advised of the adverse effects and to not drive or participate in hazardous activities. Patients should avoid CNS sedating drugs and alcohol.

Patients being injected with botulinum toxin type A (Botox) should be educated on the expected effects of the medication and the adverse effects. Patients should be warned of life-threatening adverse effects, including respiratory paralysis and problems swallowing. The effects of botulinum toxin type A may last for several months and may occur hours or weeks after injection.

OPIOID ANALGESICS AND THEIR ANTAGONISTS

When nonopioid agents are ineffective for pain relief, opioids are a next logical step in the treatment of pain. These agents alter the perception of and response to painful stimuli. This group of drugs includes natural opium alkaloids, synthetic agents, and a combination of the two. Most of these drugs are Schedule II narcotics under federal law. And although many states allow prescription of these agents by nurse practitioners, state laws may vary.

Opioids are generally classified as agonists, mixed agonist-antagonists, or partial agonists. Agonists include codeine (Tylenol #3 or #4), fentanyl (Sublimaze, Duragesic), hydrocodone (Vicodin, Lortab), hydromorphone (Dilaudid), levorphanol (Levo-Dromoran), meperidine (Demerol), methadone (Dolophine), morphine (MSIR, Roxanol, MS Contin, Oramorph, Kadian), oxycodone (Percocet, Percodan, Roxicodone, OxyContin), and propoxyphene (Darvon, Darvocet). Propoxyphene (Darvon, Darvocet) was removed from the U.S. and European markets in 2010 owing to its role in altering cardiac conduction, which can result in serious adverse effects including sudden cardiac death. Some of these agents, such as hydrocodone and codeine, are typically combined with acetaminophen or an NSAID. Opiate antagonists include naloxone HCL (Narcan), naltrexone HCL (Revia), and nalmefene HCL (Revex).

Mixed agonist-antagonists include butorphanol (Stadol), nalbuphine (Nubain), and pentazocine (Talwin). Partial agonists include buprenorphine (Buprenex) and dezocine (Dalgan). Suboxone is a combination of a partial opioid agonist, buprenorphine and an antagonist, naloxone.

Pharmacodynamics

Narcotic analgesics are active at various opioid receptor sites and act as agonists, partial agonists, or mixed agonist-antagonists of endogenously occurring opioid peptides (eukephalins, endorphins). Opioids interact with mu, kappa, delta, or sigma receptors, producing both the desired and adverse effects of opioids. The primary receptors associated with analgesia are the mu and kappa receptors. Activation of these receptors is thought to create an analgesic effect by inhibiting adenyl cyclase activity, which results in a reduction in intracellular cyclic adenosine monophosphate. In addition to an analgesic effect, activation of mu receptors may cause euphoria, physical dependence, and respiratory depression. Activation of kappa receptors may cause miosis, sedation, and respiratory depression. Activation of delta and sigma receptors accounts for many of the adverse effects of opioids, such as dysphoria, hallucinations, and respiratory and vasomotor stimulation. Mixed agonist-antagonists can cause withdrawal symptoms when given to narcotic-dependent individuals because of their preference at specific opioid receptor sites.

Narcotic antagonists block or reverse opioids by competing at their receptor sites and reverse respiratory depression, hypotension, and sedation. Indications for use are narcotic overdose and prolonged surgical use of narcotics.

Pharmacokinetics

Absorption and Distribution

Opioid analgesics may be administered via oral, parenteral, rectal, sublingual, and transdermal routes. The rate of absorption depends on the route used. Oral drugs are convenient and have a slower onset of action, delayed peak time, and a longer duration of action than drugs administered parenterally. Overall, the onset of action of opioid analgesics is rapid and varies from 2 or 3 minutes up to 60 minutes, depending on the route of administration. Half-life is generally up to 6 hours, although some are longer, for example, levorphanol with a half-life of 12 to 16 hours and methadone with a half-life

of 15 to 30 hours. Meperidine has an active metabolite, normeperidine, with a half-life of 15 to 30 hours.

The opioid antagonists nalmefene HCL, naloxone HCL, and naltrexone HCL are indicated for acute crises and are given parenterally. Their onset of action is within 2 to 15 minutes, with duration of action of 1 to 4 hours. Because their half-lives can be shorter than the narcotic they are reversing, patients must be closely monitored for symptoms of a recurrence of respiratory depression.

Metabolism and Excretion

Opioid analgesics and antagonists are metabolized in the liver and excreted in urine. Codeine is metabolized into morphine, which is metabolized and excreted in the urine. Table 15-36 presents the pharmacokinetics.

Pharmacotherapeutics

Precautions and Contraindications

Because of the respiratory depressant effect of these drugs, compromised pulmonary function is a contraindication. Cautious use is indicated in the case of head injury, increased intracranial pressure, and acute abdominal conditions because of the drugs' capacity to mask symptoms of pain and to increase cerebrospinal fluid pressure.

Table 15–36 ✚ Pharmacokinetics: Opioid Analgesics and Antagonists

Drug	Onset	Peak	Duration	Half-Life	Excretion
Alfentanil	Immediate	—	—	1–2 h	Urine
Codeine	10–30 min	0.5–1 h	4–6 h	3 h	Urine
Fentanyl IM transdermal	7–15 min; 6 h	20–30 min; 12–24 h	1–2 h; 72 h	1.5–6 h	Urine
Hydromorphone	15–30 min	0.5–1 h	4–5 h	2–3 h	Urine
Levorphanol	30–90 min	0.5–1 h	6–8 h	1–16 h	Urine
Meperidine	10–45 min	0.5–1 h	2–4 h	3–4 h	Urine
Methadone	30–60 min	0.5–1 h	4–6 h	15–30 h	Urine
Morphine	15–60 min	0.5–1 h	3–7 h	1.5–2 h	Urine
Oxycodone	15–30 min	1 h	4–6 h	—	Urine
Oxymorphone	5–10 min	0.5–1 h	3–6 h	—	Urine
Propoxyphene	30–60 min	2–2.5 h	4–6 h	6–12 h	Urine
Sufentanil	1.3–3 min	—	—	2.5 h	Urine
Nalmefene	5–15 min	1.5–2.3 h	—	1–10.8 h	Urine
Naloxone	2 min	—	1–4 h	30–81 min	Urine
Naltrexone	Rapid	Within 1 h	—	4–13 h	Urine
Buprenorphine	15 min	60 min	6 h	2.2–3.5 h	Urine
Butorphanol	<10 min	30–60 min	3–4 h	2.5–4 h	Urine
Dezocine	<15–30 min	30–150 min	2–4 h	2.4 h	Urine
Nalbuphine	15–30 min	30–60 min	3–6 h	5 h	Urine
Pentazocine	15–30 min	15–60 min	3 h	2.2–3.5 h	Urine

Safety of use in pregnant and nursing women is not established, and they are classified as Pregnancy Category C. Infants born to addicted mothers suffer sedation, respiratory depression, and withdrawal. Oxycodone, methadone, oxymorphone, and hydromorphone should not be used in children.

Narcotic analgesics carry the risk of physical tolerance and dependence, as well as having street value. Thus, the prescribing clinician needs to obtain a clear history of current substance use because of the dangers of cross-tolerance and additive CNS depression. These agents have been implicated in suicide or accidental death, particularly in combination with alcohol. As indicated previously, mixed agonist-antagonists should not be prescribed for narcotic-addicted individuals because of the risk of physical withdrawal. Patients wishing treatment of narcotic addiction with methadone should be referred to an appropriate treatment facility.

Careful titration of opioid antagonists is required, because the blockade of opioids by antagonistic action means that the individual may experience withdrawal symptoms, called *acute abstinence syndrome*, at about the time the next narcotic dose would be due. Achieving a balance between reversing CNS depression and preventing acute withdrawal is delicate and requires careful titration in small increments. This situation applies equally to the drug-affected neonate. In addition to these concerns, attention is also needed in post-operative situations in which the antagonist's action may leave the patient in severe, acute pain.

The FDA issued a Safety Alert regarding the use of codeine in children, particularly after tonsillectomy and/or adenoidectomy because of reports of respiratory depression. Codeine is metabolized in the liver to morphine via CYP 2D6 and ultrametabolizers may be at risk of toxicity. Lactating women who are ultrametabolizers and take codeine may have increased levels of morphine in the breast milk.

Adverse Drug Reactions

Adverse reactions to opioids include respiratory depression, hypotension, confusion, sedation, nausea, vomiting, dizziness, visual disturbances, hallucinations, euphoria, lethargy, uncoordinated movements, constipation, agitation, depression of cough reflexes, and paresthesias. Most patients experience constipation when taking an opioid agonist.

Adverse reactions to antagonists include nausea, vomiting, tachycardia, hypertension, fever, and dizziness. Naltrexone is

particularly hepatotoxic and can be injurious to the liver when used in high doses. Individuals with impaired liver function should be assessed carefully for signs of further damage.

Drug Interactions

Some interacting drugs, such as alcohol, sedative-hypnotics, barbiturates, antihistamines, and antipsychotics, can create additive CNS-depressant effects. Others, such as cimetidine, hydantoins, nicotine, and droperidol, can interfere with narcotic effects. Other drug interactions, for example, with carbamazepine and warfarin, may decrease the effect of the interacting drug. Use with extreme caution with MAOIs because severe, even fatal, reactions may occur. Table 15-37 presents drug interactions.

Clinical Use and Dosing

Table 15-38 presents the indications and dosage schedules of opioid analgesics and antagonists.

Rational Drug Selection

Indications for the use of opioid analgesics are the control of pain, primarily acute pain as in the case of post-operative situations, cancer, and obstetric pain. Opioid analgesics are also used in the treatment of chronic pain, which is not alleviated with nonopioid agents. In selecting among available agents, the degree and duration of pain must be considered as well as the patient variables of subjective therapeutic response to an agent and adverse effects experienced. Morphine is the standard against which other opioids are measured and is considered the drug of choice for cancer pain.

For the treatment of mild to moderate pain not alleviated by nonopioids, treatment can start with a lower-potency opioid, such as codeine, often given in combination with acetaminophen. If pain is not alleviated by codeine, the derivatives of codeine, oxycodone and hydrocodone, are approximately 8 times more potent. These drugs are available in combination with aspirin and acetaminophen, which limit the overall dose of the opioid that can be given. Caution should be taken to instruct patients regarding proper dosing to avoid acetaminophen toxicity.

For patients with moderate to severe pain who have not been treated with opioids, treatment can begin with a short half-life agonist (morphine, hydromorphone, oxycodone).

Table 15–37 ⦙⦙⦙ Drug Interactions: Opioid Analgesics and Antagonists

Drug	Interacting Drug	Possible Effect	Implications
Opioids	CNS depressants, alcohol, hypnotics, barbiturates, benzodiazepines, antipsychotics	Additive CNS depression	
	Cimetidine, hydantoins, rifampin, droperidol, charcoal, nicotine	Decreased effect of opioid	Increased doses of opioid may be required
	Carbamazepine, warfarin, MAOIs, furazolidone, nitrous oxide	Decreased effect of interacting drug	Monitor blood levels when possible
Nalmefene	Flumazenil	Seizures	Use with caution
Naltrexone	Thioridazine	Decreased effect of thioridazine	Higher dose may be required

Table 15–38 ⊗ Dosage Schedule: Opioid Analgesics and Antagonists

Drug	Indications	Dosage	Available Dosage Forms
Alfentanil HCl (Alfenta)	Anesthetic adjunct only	—	*Injection:* 500 mcg/mL
Codeine	Mild to moderate pain; coughing	*Adults:* PO, IM, IV, SC: 15–60 mg every 4 h to maximum of 360 mg/24 h; usual dose is 30 mg *Children >1 yr:* PO, IM, SC: 0.5 mg/kg every 4–6 h	*Tablet:* 15, 30, 60 mg *Acetaminophen and No. 3 codeine tablet:* 300 mg acetaminophen and 30 mg codeine *Acetaminophen and codeine solution:* Acetaminophen 120 mg and codeine 12 mg per 5 mL *Aspirin and codeine:* Aspirin 325 mg/codeine 30 mg, aspirin 325 mg/codeine 60 mg
Fentanyl (Sublimaze, Duragesic, Oralet)	Anesthesia; post-operative analgesia; management of chronic pain	*Adults:* Post-operative analgesia: 0.05–0.1 mg IM every 1–2 h Transdermal: 25, 50, 75, 100, 125, 150, 175, 200, 225, 250, 275, and 300 mcg/h system; change once every 72 h Titrate dose upward first time only in 3 d, thereafter at 6 d intervals	*Injection:* 0.05 mg/mL *Film for buccal application:* 200, 400, 800, 1,200 mcg *Patch:* 12, 25, 50, 75, 100 mcg/h *Tablet, sublingual:* 100, 200, 300, 400, 800 mcg
Hydromorphone HCl (Dilaudid)	Moderate to severe pain	*Adults:* PO: 2–4 mg every 4–6 h Parenteral: 1–4 mg every 4–6 h; slow IV over 1–5 min Rectal: 3 mg every 6–8 h	*Liquid:* 1 mg/mL *Tablet:* 2, 4, 8 mg *Injection:* 10 mg/mL
Levorphanol tartrate (Levo-Dromoran)	Management of opioid dependence	*Adults:* PO, SC: 2–3 mg	*Tablets:* 2 mg
Meperidine (Demerol)	Moderate to severe pain; pre-operative sedation	*Adults:* PO, IM, SC: 50–150 mg every 3–4 h *Children:* PO, IM, SC: 1–1.8 mg/kg (0.5–0.8 mg/lb) every 3–4 h	*Tablets:* 50, 100 mg *Oral solution:* 50 mg/5mL *Injection:* 25 mg/mL
Methadone (Dolophine)	Severe pain; management of opioid dependence	*Adults:* PO, IM, SC: 2.5–10 mg every 3–4 h; oral dose is half of parenteral	*Oral concentrate:* 10 mg/mL *Oral solution:* 5 mg/5 mL *Tablet:* 5 mg, 10 mg
Morphine sulfate (Astramorph PF, Duramorph, Infumorph, MSIR, MS Contin, Oramorph SR, Roxanol, OMS concentrate, MS/L, RMS)	Moderate to severe acute and chronic pain; preanesthetic sedation	*Adults:* PO: 10–30 mg every 4 h Controlled-release: 30 mg every 8 h; do not crush or chew SC/IM: 5–20 mg/70 kg every 4 h IV: 2.5–15 mg/70 kg in 4–5 mL water for injection over 4–5 min Continuous IV pump infusion: 0.1–1 mg/mL in 5% dextrose Rectal: 10–20 mg every 4 h *Children:* SC, IM: 0.1–0.2 mg/kg to maximum of 15 mg every 4 h	*Capsule:* 30, 45, 60, 75, 90, 120 mg *Oral solution:* 1 mg/mL *Tablet:* 15, 30 mg *Extended-release tablet:* 15, 30, 60, 100, 200 mg *Injection:* 0.5 mg/mL
Oxycodone (Roxicodone, OxyContin)	Moderate to moderately severe pain	*Adults:* 2.5 to 5 mg *Children:* 0.1-0.2 mg/kg/dose q 4–6 h prn	*Tablet:* 5, 7.5 mg *Oral solution:* 5 mg/5 mL
Oxymorphone (Numorphan)	Moderate to severe pain; preanesthetic sedation; relief of anxiety/dyspnea in pulmonary edema and left ventricular failure	*Adults:* SC, IM: 1–1.5 mg every 4–6 h IV: 0.5 mg Rectal: 5 mg every 4–6 h	*Injection:* 1 mg/mL
Buprenorphine (Buprenex, Subutex, Zubsolv) Buprenorphine/naloxone (Suboxone)	Moderate to severe pain Maintenance of opioid dependence	*Adults and children >13 yr:* IM, IV: 0.3 mg every 6 h; may repeat once 30–60 min later if needed; compatible with most IV solutions	*Tablet:* 2, 8, 12, 16 mg *Injection solution:* 0.3 mg/mL *Sublingual film:* Buprenorphine/naloxone 2 mg/0.5 mg, buprenorphine/naloxone 4 mg/1 mg, buprenorphine/naloxone 8 mg/2 mg, buprenorphine/naloxone 12 mg/3 mg *Sublingual tablet:* 2 mg/0.5 mg, 8 mg/2 mg

Table 15–38 ⊗ Dosage Schedule: Opioid Analgesics and Antagonists—cont'd

Drug	Indications	Available Dosage Forms	Dosage
Butorphanol tartrate (Stadol)	Pain; preanesthesia sedation	*Adults:* IM: 1–4 mg every 3–4 h to nonambulatory patients IV: 0.5–2 mg every 3–4 h Nasal: 1 mg = 1 spray in each nostril; may repeat if needed in 60–90 min; may repeat 2 dose sequences in 3–4 h	*Injection:* 1 mg/mL, 2 mg/mL
Nalbuphine (Nubain)	Moderate to severe pain; preoperative sedation	*Adults:* SC, IM, IV: 10 mg/70 kg every 3–6 h to maximum of 20 mg/dose or 160 mg/24 h	*Injection:* 10, 20 mg/mL
Pentazocine (Talwin, Talwin NX)	Moderate to severe pain; pre-operative sedation	*Adults:* PO: 50–100 mg every 3–4 h to maximum of 600 mg/24 h; initial dose 50 mg IM, SC, IV: 30 mg every 3–4 h to maximum of 360 mg/24 h	*Injection:* 30 mg/mL
Pentazocine combinations	Mild to moderate pain	*Adults:* 12.5 mg with 325 ASA (Talwin compound caplets): 2 tabs tid qid 25 mg with acetaminophen 650 mg (Talacen caplets): 1 tab every 4 h to maximum of 6 tabs/24 h	
Nalmefene	Reversal of opioid effects	Opioid-dependent patients: Initial challenge dose of 0.1 mg/70 kg. If no signs or symptoms of withdrawal within 2 min, use following guidelines: Non–opioid-dependent patients: Initial dose of 0.25 mg/kg followed by 0.25 mcg/kg doses at 2–5 min intervals until degree of opioid reversal is attained Give IV; if no IV access is available, give 1 mg SC or IM as single dose	Injection: 100 mcg/mL, 1 mg/mL
Naloxone (Narcan)	Reversal of opioid depression	*Adults:* IV, IM, SC For overdose: 0.4–2 mg IV; may repeat at 2–3 min intervals Post-operative: 0.1–0.2 mg IV at 2–3 min intervals; may repeat in 1–2 h intervals if needed *Children:* For overdose: 0.01 mg/kg IV; may follow with 0.1 mg if needed; if no IV access, give IM or SC in divided doses Post-operative: Initial dose of 0.005–0.01 mg IV repeated at 2–3 min increments if needed	*Injection:* 0.02, 0.4, 1 mg/mL
Naltrexone (ReVia)	Blocks effects of opioids; treatment of alcohol dependence	Alcoholism: 100 mg PO once daily Opioid dependence: do not give until patient has been abstinent for 10 d, then give challenge dose of 25 mg once; if no withdrawal signs and symptoms occur, continue with maintenance dose; if signs and symptoms occur, repeat challenge in 24 h Maintenance: 50 mg every 24 h; dosing may be flexible (e.g., 100 mg on Mon and Wed; 150 mg on Fri)	Tablets: 50 mg

These drugs are easier to titrate than those with a longer half-life, such as methadone or levorphanol. Morphine is the drug of choice for severe pain. Sustained-release preparations such as MS Contin and Oramorph SR provide pain relief for 8 to 12 hours. Morphine has the advantage of a wide range and flexibility of dosing.

Chronic stable pain may be managed with sustained-release morphine, oxycodone, methadone, or transdermal fentanyl. Methadone has the advantage of low cost and oral efficacy, but it can cause excessive sedation. Methadone has the ability to antagonize NMDA (*N*-methyl-D-aspartate) receptors and is particularly useful in the treatment of chronic and neuropathic pain. Fentanyl is a potent opioid, available as a transdermal patch that provides up to 3 days of continuous analgesia. Fentanyl must be titrated carefully, however, to avoid oversedation. Meperidine is not recommended for chronic pain because it has a short half-life and has a toxic metabolite, normeperidine, that causes CNS excitability as manifested by dysphoria, tremors, seizures, and irritability.

Partial agonists and mixed agonist-antagonists are limited by a dose-related ceiling effect, but they are effective in treating moderate to severe pain. These agents are useful for patients who are intolerant of morphine or meperidine. Mixed agonist-antagonists are contraindicated in patients receiving full agonist opioids because they reverse some of the pain control provided by the full agonist. These agents may cause less respiratory depression than morphine, however, which is a consideration for patients with compromised pulmonary function.

In addition to pain relief, some of these opioids may be utilized for other purposes, such as antitussive or antidiarrheal effects. For example, camphorated tincture of opium (paregoric) is used in the treatment of diarrhea. Codeine possesses both antitussive and antidiarrheal properties.

Further discussion of pain management is found in Chapter 52.

Monitoring

It is important to monitor for adverse reactions, as discussed previously. It is also important to monitor for opioid withdrawal. Symptoms of opioid withdrawal resemble a flu-like syndrome manifested by muscle cramps, dilated pupils, lacrimation, rhinorrhea, yawning, sneezing, anxiety, anorexia, nausea, vomiting, diarrhea, and gooseflesh.

Patient Education

Patients should be warned about the potential for physical dependence and advised that these agents should primarily be used for relief of acute, severe pain. Long-term use for chronic pain can result in tolerance and hypersensitivity to pain. Patients should be instructed to avoid the concurrent use of alcohol and other CNS depressants. To prevent overdose patients should also avoid using acetaminophen with acetaminophen/opioid combinations. Opioid analgesics may cause drowsiness and, for safety reasons, should not be used when mental or physical alertness is required. Advise the patient to change position slowly to minimize postural hypotension. Because these agents may cause constipation, patients should be advised to increase daily intake of fluid and fiber. Opioids may be taken with food to prevent nausea. Because opioids are controlled substances, patients should be cautioned to prevent use or theft of these agents by unauthorized persons.

STIMULANTS

The FDA approved the use of stimulants in treating attention deficit-hyperactivity disorder (ADHD), narcolepsy, and weight reduction. In therapeutic ranges, these drugs improve alertness, mood, attention, wakefulness, vigilance, and psychomotor performance and have an anorexiant effect. The prototype stimulant drug is amphetamine, which was developed more than 100 years ago. It has been used to treat depression, obesity, narcolepsy, and respiratory depression and as an energizer during World War II. Because of these same foci, amphetamines are notorious street drugs of abuse.

The stimulants amphetamine, dextroamphetamine, methylphenidate, and, less commonly, methamphetamine (Desoxyn) are used in the treatment of ADHD and narcolepsy. Primarily, methylphenidate (Ritalin, Methylin, Metadate, Concerta, Focalin, Daytrana patch) and Adderall, a combination of dextroamphetamine (Dexedrine) and amphetamine salts, are used. In addition, atomoxetine (Strattera), a norepinephrine reuptake inhibitor, is available as an alternative to stimulants for ADHD. Other stimulants such as caffeine found in over-the-counter cold medicines are significant because of the additive stimulant effects they have in combination with other stimulants.

Pharmacodynamics

The CNS stimulants are sympathomimetic amines that act as dopamine agonists and indirectly release and prevent the reuptake of dopamine, serotonin, and norepinephrine in presynaptic nerve endings. This action stimulates the cerebral cortex, brainstem, and reticular activating system and appears to stimulate the reward center in the brain that consists of the nucleus accumbens, the amygdala, and the ventral tegmentum. The dopamine and norepinephrine (and to a lesser extent the serotonin) nerve fibers connect these regions of the brain to the prefrontal cortex to coordinate thinking, feeling, and responding to emotional stimuli. When receptors in the reward center are occupied, there is a sense of well-being; it is because of this response that these drugs have considerable potential for abuse.

Pharmacokinetics
Absorption and Distribution

Taken orally, these drugs are quickly and thoroughly absorbed, with a rapid onset of action. Depending on the formulation, peak plasma levels occur in fewer than 1 to 4 hours. Their half-lives are from 1 to 12 hours. Although biodistribution is unknown for methylphenidate, atomoxetine is highly protein bound.

Metabolism and Excretion

Dextroamphetamine and methylphenidate are metabolized in the liver by de-esterification without the influence of the P450 system, whereas atomoxetine is predominantly metabolized by 2D6 and 2C19. In addition, atomoxetine has an equally potent metabolite that circulates in a lower concentration. All three are excreted by the kidneys. Urine acidity affects the rate of excretion of amphetamine in that increased alkalinity increases its half-life, a fact that can be important in drug overdose. Table 15-39 presents the pharmacokinetics of these stimulants.

Pharmacotherapeutics

Precautions and Contraindications

Contraindications to use include arteriosclerotic and symptomatic heart disease, hypertension, hyperthyroidism hypersensitivity to sympathomimetic amines, glaucoma, motor tics, agitation, history of drug abuse, and during or within 14 days of use of an MAOI.

Stimulants are contraindicated for pregnant (Pregnancy Category C) and lactating women. Methylphenidate is found in high concentrations in breast milk. Stimulants may cause insomnia and should therefore be taken no closer than 6 hours before bedtime. Concerta should be used cautiously in patients with esophageal motility disorders, as there is an increased risk of obstruction.

Adverse Drug Reactions

Undesirable effects include insomnia, undesired weight loss, growth retardation in children, tachycardia, palpitations, restlessness, irritability, euphoria, headache, blurred vision, tremor, increased libido with impaired ability, hypertension, and arrhythmias. Some individuals may experience a paradoxical drowsiness.

Drug Interactions

Various undesirable drug interactions may occur, perhaps the most significant being the risk of hypertensive crisis if stimulants are taken within 14 days of an MAOI. Additive sympathomimetic effects occur if these agents are taken concurrently with other adrenergics, including vasoconstrictors and decongestants. Metabolism of warfarin, anticonvulsants, and tricyclic antidepressants may be decreased and their effects increased.

Due to the P450 involvement, atomoxetine has a different interaction profile than methylphenidate or dextroamphetamine. CY2D6 inhibitors (e.g., fluoxetine) will increase the plasma levels of atomoxetine, and pressor agents will contribute to increased effects on blood pressure. Atomoxetine needs to be used with caution with albuterol due to the potentiation of the cardiovascular effects of albuterol. Table 15-40 presents drug interactions.

Clinical Use and Dosing

Table 15-41 presents the indications, dosage schedules, and available dosage forms of stimulants.

Rational Drug Selection

With the exception of atomoxetine, stimulants are on the Drug Enforcement Agency's (DEA) Schedule II and can be

Table 15–39 ⊞ Pharmacokinetics: Stimulants

Drug	Onset	Peak	Duration	Half-Life	Excretion
Dextroamphetamine	30 min	1–3 h	4–20 h	10–30 h	Urine
Methamphetamine HCl	30 min	1–3 h	3–6 h	4–5 h	Urine
Methylphenidate HCl	30–60 min	1.9–4.7 h	4–6 h	1–3 h	Urine
Atomoxetine	—	1–2 h		5–22 h	Urine

Table 15–40 ⊞ Drug Interactions: Stimulants

Drug	Interacting Drug	Possible Effect	Implications
All stimulants	MAOIs	Increased risk of hypertensive crisis and stroke	Avoid
	CNS depressants, alkalinizing agents	Decreased effect of stimulant	Dosage may need adjustment
	Antidepressants	Increased effect of antidepressant, especially with TCAs; increased risk of cardiotoxicity in children	Avoid use of TCAs
	Guanethidine	Increased hypotensive effect	Warn patient about dizziness and syncope
	Hypoglycemic agents	Increased glucose lability and decreased control	Monitor blood glucose
	Acidifying agents	Decreased effect of stimulant	Dosage adjustment may be required
	Phenytoin	Increased plasma level of phenytoin	Monitor plasma level
Atomoxetine	Fluoxetine, paroxetine, and quinidine	Increased plasma level of atomoxetine	Increase dosage only after 4 wk

Table 15–41 ⊗ **Dosage Schedule: Stimulants**

Drug	Indications	Dosage	Available Dosage Forms
Dextroamphetamine (DextroStat, Dexedrine ER)	ADHD, narcolepsy, exogenous obesity	*Adults:* 10 mg daily; may increase by 10 mg increments every week to maximum of 30 mg/d; give individual doses at 4–6 h intervals *Children age 3–5:* 2.5 mg/d; increase by 2.5 mg daily at weekly intervals to range of 0.1–0.5 mg/kg/d; give in morning *Children >5 yr:* 5 mg 1–2 times/d; may increase in 5 mg increments weekly to maximum of 40 mg/d; usual range 0.1–0.5 mg/kg/d *Extended-release: Adult and child 6 and older:* 5 mg qam, increase by 5 mg/d qwk Max 40 mg/d	Tablets: 5, 10 mg Sustained-release spansules: 5, 10, 15 mg
Methamphetamine HCl (generic)	ADHD, narcolepsy, exogenous obesity	*Adults and children >12 yr:* 5 mg 1–2 times/d; may increase at 5 mg increments weekly to maximum of 25 mg/d, may be twice-daily dosing	5, 10, 20 mg tab
Amphetamine and dextroamphetamine (Adderall, Adderall XR)	ADHD Narcolepsy XR for ADHD only	*Age 3–5:* 2.5 mg qd, increase by 2.5 mg/wk *Age 6 and up:* 5 mg qd or bid, then increase by 5 mg q wk. Not to exceed 40 mg *Narcolepsy: Children 6–12 yr:* 5 mg daily up to 60 mg/d max *Sustained-release for age 6 and up only:* 6–12, 10–30 mg qd *Age 12–18:* 10–20 mg qd *Adults:* 20 mg qd	Adderall: 5, 7.5, 10, 12.5, 15, 20, 30 mg tabs Adderall XR: 5, 10, 15, 20, 25, 30 mg caps
Lisdexamfetamine (Vyvanse)	ADHD	*Age 6 and up:* 30 mg qam, increase by 10–20 mg/d every 7 days. Not to exceed 70 mg total qd for any patient May dissolve contents in water, drink immediately, do not subdivide caps	20, 30, 40, 50, 60, 70 mg caps
Methylphenidate HCl (Ritalin, Ritalin SR, Ritalin LA, Methylin, Methylin ER, Daytrana patch)	ADHD, narcolepsy (Ritalin and Ritalin SR)	*Ritalin and Methylin: Adults:* 10–30 mg/d in 2–3 divided doses; maximum 60 mg/d in divided doses. *Children >6 yr:* 5 mg bid before breakfast and lunch, with increase of 5–10 mg at weekly intervals; maximum 60 mg/d in divided doses. Stop drug if no improvement in 4 wk. *All ages:* Ritalin SR tabs taken in morning may be supplemented with afternoon regular tablets, if needed, no later than 6 p.m. *Ritalin LA: age 6 and up:* Whole or sprinkled in applesauce, 20 mg qam, increase by 10 mg weekly to max 60 mg/d *Methylin ER:* *Child age 6 and up:* 10 mg qam, increase weekly by 10 mg/d to max 60 mg in divided doses. *Adults:* 10–20 mg qam, increase by 10 mg weekly to max of 60 mg in divided doses. *Daytrana patch: 6–12 yr:* 10 mg patch to hips 2 h before desired effect. Remove 9 h after application, earlier if shorter duration needed. Titrate dose q week. Rotate application site.	Ritalin tablets: 5, 10, 20 mg Methylin tabs: 5, 10, 20 mg Methylin chews: 2.5, 5, 10 mg Methylin oral solution: 5 mg/ 5ml, 10 mg/5 ml. Ritalin SR Sustained-release tablets: 20 mg Ritalin LA: Extended-release caps:10, 20, 30, 40 mg (half immediate-release, half extended-release beads) Methylin ER: 10, 20 mg tabs Daytrana patch: 10, 15, 20, 30 mg delivered over 9 h
Methylphenidate (Concerta)	ADHD	*Age 6-12:* Start at 18 mg qd, max 54 mg/d *Age 13–17:* Start at 18 mg/d, max 72 mg/d *Adults:* 18–36 mg/d, max 72 mg/d For patients already on methylphenidate: 5 mg bid/tid = 18 mg 10 mg bid/tid = 36 mg 15 mg bid/tid = 54 mg 20 mg bid/tid = 72 mg/d	18, 27, 36, 54 mg extended-release

Table 15–41 ⊗ **Dosage Schedule: Stimulants—cont'd**

Drug	Indications	Dosage	Available Dosage Forms
Metadate ER	ADHD, Narcolepsy	*Metadate ER: Age 6 and up:* swallow whole, 10 mg qam, increase by 10 mg q week. Max 60 mg/d in divided doses.	Metadate ER:10, 20 mg tabs
Metadate CD	ADHD	*Metadate CD: Age 6 and up:* swallow whole or sprinkle on applesauce: 20 mg before breakfast, increase weekly by 10–20 mg/d. Max 60 mg once daily.	Metadate CD: 10, 20, 30, 40, 50, 60 mg caps (immediate-release and extended-release beads)
Dexmethylphenidate (Focalin, Focalin XR)	ADHD	*Age 6 and up:* 2.5 mg bid, increase by 2.5 mg at weekly intervals. Max 20 mg/d. *Extended-release:* Once daily in a.m. Swallow whole or sprinkle onto applesauce. *Age 6 and up:* 5 mg/d, may increase by 5 mg/wk. *Adults:* Start at 10 mg/d, increase by 10 mg weekly. Max dose for adults and children 20 mg/d.	2.5, 5, 10 mg tablets XR: 5, 10, 15, 20 mg caps. (contains immediate- and extended-delayed release beads)
Atomoxetine (Strattera)	Drug-resistant depression	*PO Adults and Children >70 kg:* Start w/40 mg/d and increase dose every 3 days to target 80 mg. After 2–4 wk dose may be increased to 100 mg/d.	Capsules: 10, 18, 20, 25, 40, 60, 80, 100 mg
Modafinil (Provigil)	ADHD Narcolepsy, and excessive sleepiness due to sleep apnea and shift work	*Age 16 and up:* 200 mg qd in a.m. Max 400 mg/d in divided doses. For shift work, take dose 1 h before work.	100, 200 mg tabs

ER, XR = extended release,
CD = continuous release, SR = sustained release.

prescribed only by nurse practitioners whose state permits Schedule II prescribing. Because they are Schedule II drugs, the pharmacy requires a new hard copy of the prescription every month. Stimulants can be prescribed only without refills, although states may have a mechanism for providing more than 1 month's prescription at a time. Providers should check with the state's regulatory authorities.

To prevent anorexia and slowed growth in children, providers should maintain records of growth and weight and consider drug holidays to permit the child to catch up on growth. Some children may exhibit symptoms of ADHD as the drug begins to wear off and may do better on a sustained-release formulation, especially if they must complete homework in the afternoon or early evening. If symptom coverage with extended release is not adequate, a short-acting formulation after school may be needed.

CNS stimulants are indicated for the treatment of ADHD, narcolepsy, and exogenous obesity refractive to other forms of treatment. The use of stimulants in the treatment of adolescent and residual adult ADHD is a matter of some controversy, given the street value of these drugs, the increase in societal abuse of these drugs, and the association of these agents with violent behavior. Because atomoxetine seems to stimulate the reward center less than do other agents and has a delayed onset of action, it is less useful as a drug of abuse but may also be less effective therapeutically. These agents should be given cautiously to emotionally unstable patients, including those with a history of drug or alcohol abuse, because such patients may be more likely to increase their doses unnecessarily.

Monitoring

It is important to monitor for adverse reactions, as discussed previously. The clinician should monitor that the amount of drug used is consistent with the amounts prescribed and dispensed.

Patient Education

Stimulant agents may cause insomnia, so patients should not take them within 6 hours of bedtime. Abrupt cessation of stimulants may cause extreme fatigue and mental depression. These agents may cause dizziness or blurred vision, so caution patients to avoid driving or other hazardous activities until their response to the medication is known. To reduce anorexia and growth retardation in children, these agents should be given with or after meals. Parents should notify the school nurse of the medication regimen and need to be aware that these drugs have street value and should be stored safely in the home. Children and teens require an explanation of why these drugs are appropriate for their disorder as distinct from drugs of abuse and assistance in handling peers' responses to their use of these medications.

REFERENCES

Borders-Hemphill, V. (2012). Drug utilization trends of anti-obesity products in the outpatient setting Y1991-Y2011. U.S. Food and Drug

Administration Division of Epidemiology. Retrieved from http://www.fda.gov/downloads/advisorycommittees/committeesmeetingmaterials/drugs/endocrinologicandmetabolicdrugsadvisorycommittee/ucm299133.pdf

Detke, M. J., Lu, Y., Goldstein, D. J., Hayes, J. R., & Demitrack, M. A. (2002). Duloxetine, 60 mg once daily, for major depressive disorder: A randomized double-blind placebo-controlled trial. *Journal of Clinical Psychiatry, 63*(4), 308–315.

Drug facts and comparisons. (2010). Philadelphia: Wolters Kluwer Health.

Dubovsky, S. (2005). *Clinical guide to psychotropic medications.* New York: W. W. Norton.

Forest Laboratories. (2013). Savella. Retrieved from http://www.frx.com/pi/savella_pi.pdf

Janicak, P. G., Davis, J. M., Preskorn, S. H., & Ayd, F. J. (2006). *Principles and practice of psychopharmacology* (4th ed.). Philadelphia: Lippincott Williams & Wilkins.

Keltner, N. L., & Folk, D. G. (2005). *Psychotropic drugs* (4th ed.). Philadelphia: Elsevier.

LactMed. (2014). Drugs and lactation database. Toxnet. Toxicology Data Network. National Institute of Medicine. Retrieved from http://toxnet.nlm.nih.gov/

Meltzer, H. Y., Arvanitis, L., Bauer, D., & Rein, W., Meta-Trial Study Group. (2004). Placebo-controlled evaluation of four novel compounds for the treatment of schizophrenia and schizoaffective disorder. *American Journal of Psychiatry, 161*, 975–984.

Schatzberg, A., Cole, J., & DeBattista, C. (2007). *Manual of clinical psychopharmacology* (6th ed.). Washington, DC: American Psychiatric Publishing.

Schatzberg, A. F., & Nemeroff, C. B. (2009). *The American Psychiatric Press textbook of psychopharmacology* (4th ed.). Washington, DC: American Psychiatric Publishing.

Stahl, S. (2009). *Essential psychopharmacology: The prescriber's guide.* New York: Cambridge University Press.

Toxnet (2014). *Topiramate.* LactMed National Library of Medicine: Bethesda MD. http://toxnet.nlm.nih.gov/

Williams, K., & Oke, S. (2000). Lithium and pregnancy. *The Psychiatrist, 24*, 229–231.

CHAPTER 16

DRUGS AFFECTING THE CARDIOVASCULAR AND RENAL SYSTEMS

Marylou V. Robinson

ANGIOTENSIN-CONVERTING ENZYME INHIBITORS, ANGIOTENSIN II RECEPTOR BLOCKERS, AND DIRECT RENIN INHIBITORS

Angiotensin-converting enzyme inhibitors (ACEIs), angiotensin II receptor blockers (ARBs), and direct renin inhibitors (DRI) have multiple uses related to the cardiovascular system. Their action on the renin-angiotensin-aldosterone (RAA) system lowers blood pressure (BP) and reduces the adverse affects of diabetes on the kidney. The DRIs are related but act uniquely by direct blocking of renin itself, not on its genesis or on the angiotensin components of the RAA. ACEIs improve oxygenation to heart muscle and decrease inappropriate remodeling of heart muscle after myocardial infarction (MI) or with heart failure (HF). Their mild and usually transient adverse effects and their ease of dosing make them popular drugs. ARBs have similar roles and profiles in hypertension (HTN). The DRIs and most ARBs do not have HF indications except candesartan and valsartan.

Pharmacodynamics

As shown in Figure 16-1, inhibition of ACE activity (ACEIs) results in decreased production of both angiotensin II (AT II) and aldosterone. AT II has multiple roles in the cardiovascular system. It increases vasomotor tone by direct stimulation of vascular smooth muscle contraction and through the inhibition of endothelial nitric oxide and prostaglandin release, raising BP and decreasing blood flow through arteries, including the coronary arteries. AT II increases intravascular volume through its stimulation of sodium and water retention (with aldosterone), shifting of the pressure-natriuresis relationship, and altering glomerular hemodynamics. It is also produced in response to tissue injury. This latter action results in stimulation of smooth muscle cell and fibroblast proliferation with thickening of the vessel wall (remodeling). This action, combined with its inhibition of the endothelium's ability to resist monocyte and platelet adhesion, promotes intravascular inflammation and clotting and contributes to the atherosclerotic process. Finally, in the heart, AT II also causes remodeling, resulting in hypertrophy and fibrosis of myocardial tissue after ischemic injury or in response to persistent afterload. This is a primary mechanism in HF.

ACE also has a role in the kinin-kallikrein-bradykinin system. Bradykinin in low doses causes dilation of vessels and acts with prostaglandin to produce pain and cause extravascular smooth muscle contraction, increased vascular permeability, and increased leukocyte chemostaxis. Bradykinin has a primary role in inflammation. ACE facilitates the breakdown of bradykinin into inactive fragments, thus reducing these actions. High levels of bradykinin are thought to be a factor in the cough associated with ACEI use.

ARBs do not affect ACE activity but rather act by blocking the AT II receptor. They have similar action to ACEIs on vasoconstriction and aldosterone secretion, but no activity related to bradykinin. ACEIs and ARBs do not affect cardiac output and so do not produce reflex tachycardia. DRIs directly impact renin levels with subsequent AT I and AT II reductions. The suppression of AT II levels actually triggers a feedback mechanism that increases renin production. The drug effect is more than adequate to offset this rise.

ACEI are reno-protective for individuals with proteinuria but is not as protective in renal patients without proteinuria (Kent et al., 2007). The effectiveness of ACEIs in preventing diabetic nephropathy probably results from decreased glomerular efferent arteriolar resistance and a reduction in intraglomerular capillary pressure, which causes improved renal hemodynamics, diminished proteinuria, retarded glomerular hypertrophy, and a slower rate of decline in glomerular filtration rate (GFR). These drugs do not affect glucose metabolism or raise serum lipid levels, but they do

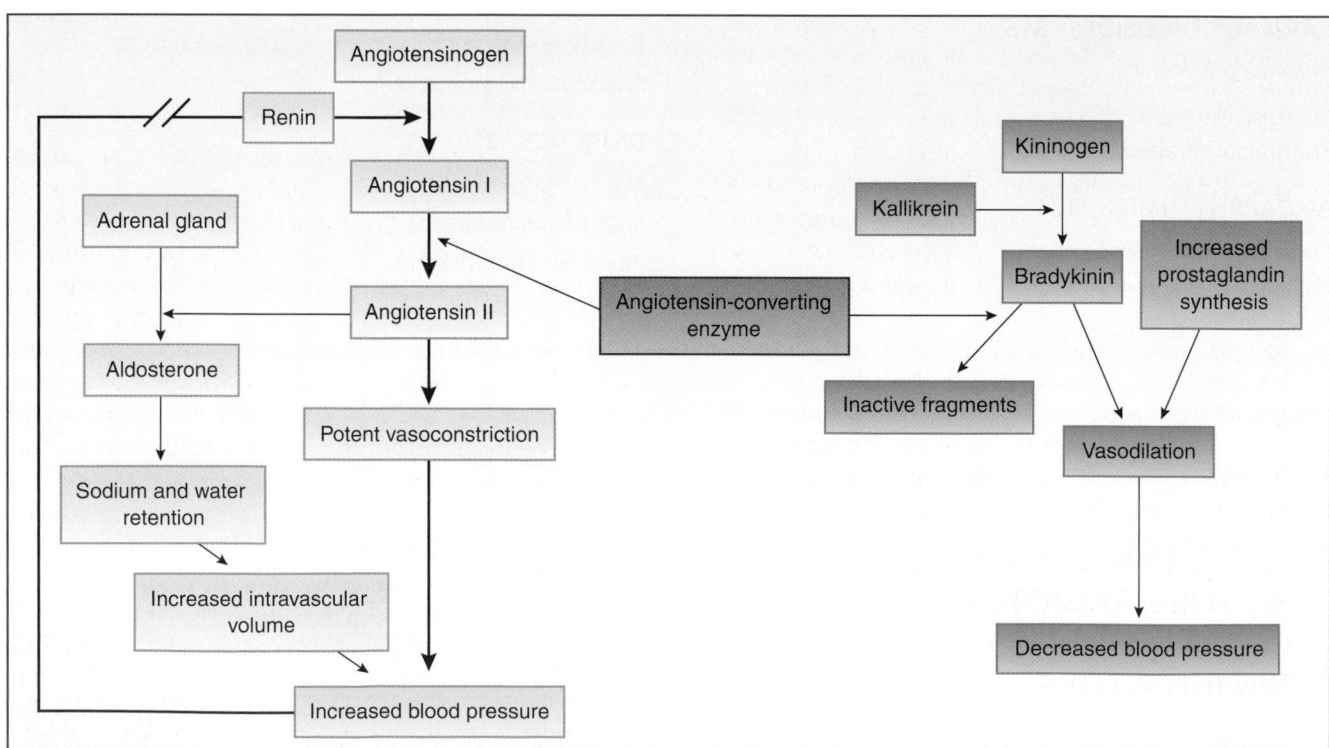

Figure 16–1. Renin-angiotensin-aldosterone system. Renin acts on angiotensinogen to create the inactive decapeptide angiotensin I. Angiotensin I is then converted, primarily in the lung, to angiotensin II, a potent vasoconstrictor, through the activity of angiotensin-converting enzyme (ACE). Angiotensin II stimulates aldosterone secretion, causing retention of sodium and water and loss of potassium by the kidney. ACE is also involved in the inactivation of bradykinin, a vasodilator. Together, these systems help to control blood pressure.

improve insulin sensitivity; all of these are important issues in type 2 diabetes mellitus. ARBs do not prevent diabetic nephropathy but do suppress the rate of progression (ADA, 2015). DRIs in diabetic (DM) patients who already have nephropathy do not preserve renal function (Parving et al, 2012). DRIs are not to be used in diabetic patients with renal function of less than 60 mL/min.

Pharmacokinetics

Absorption and Distribution

The ACEIs and ARBs are well absorbed orally, with some variation in bioavailability based on the presence of food in the gut (Table 16-1). Captopril (Capoten), the prototype drug for the ACEI class, is rapidly absorbed, with a bioavailability of about 70% when taken on an empty stomach. Bioavailability is decreased to 30% to 40% if taken with food. Losartan (Cozaar), the prototype drug for the ARB class, undergoes extensive first-pass metabolism, resulting in 33% bioavailability. It may be taken without regard to food. Distribution is to most body tissues except the central nervous system (CNS). ACEIs and ARBs cross the placenta and are found in breast milk. Alsikren, the only DRI at this time, is poorly absorbed, which is made worse by high-fat meals. Bioavailability is 55%. Its presence in breast milk is yet to be determined.

Metabolism and Excretion

Except for captopril and lisinopril (Zestril, Prinivil), all ACEIs are prodrugs converted to active metabolites by hydrolysis, primarily in the liver. Losartan has both an active drug and an active metabolite (5-carboxylic acid) hydrolyzed by the liver. Captopril is metabolized by the liver to inactive compounds. The kidney is the primary organ of excretion for all ACEIs except fosinopril (Monopril) and moexipril (Univasc), and impaired renal function can significantly prolong their half-lives. ARBs have significant excretion in feces. The percentage excreted in feces varies from 50% to more than 97%. Alsikren is not a prodrug and is mostly eliminated via the feces. Mild to moderate renal impairment does not require dose changes.

Captopril, with a half-life of less than 2 hours, is the only short-acting ACEI. It requires two or three doses daily with steady state achieved in 2 to 3 days. All other members of the class have 6 to12 hour half-lives and require more time to achieve steady state but can be given daily. Losartan has a 2 hour half-life, and its active metabolite has a 6 to 9 hour half-life. Dosing may be daily or in two divided doses. Steady state is achieved in 3 to 6 weeks. Alsikren has a 24 hour half-life with full therapeutic effect seen in 2 weeks.

Pharmacotherapeutics

Precautions and Contraindications

There are only three absolute contraindications to the use of these three drug classes: bilateral renal artery stenosis, angioedema, and pregnancy. In bilateral renal artery stenosis, increased vascular pressure and vasoconstriction appear to

be required to sufficiently overcome the stenotic blood flow to perfuse the kidney. The vasodilating effect of these meds prevents the kidney from maintaining its perfusion, and ischemic renal failure may develop; therefore, ACEIs, ARBs, and DRIs should be used cautiously with patients who have impaired renal function, *especially older adults.* Hypovolemic or hyponatremic states also require cautious use of all three. Adequate hydration is required to maintain an appropriate GFR and must be adequate before starting these drugs to prevent renal dysfunction. Hyperkalemia contraindicates use because reduced aldosterone secretion may worsen this electrolyte imbalance. Hyperkalemia risk increases for patients with chronic heart failure (HF) because of the reduced blood flow to the kidneys. Patients should have their serum potassium level checked prior to initiating therapy and within one week to note trends.

Hepatic impairment also requires cautious use. For ACEIs, fosinopril metabolism is cut in half; the maximum concentration (C_{max}) is cut in half and the area under the curve (AUC) is increased 300% for moexipril; plasma concentrations are 50% higher for perindopril; and plasma concentrations are reduced for quinapril. For ARBs, losartan total plasma clearance is about 50% lower and bioavailability is twice as high; the AUC is increased 60% for olmesartan; the AUC is twice that for valsartan and increased 40% for eprosartan. DRIs are not significantly impacted by hepatic issues.

Because ACEIs, ARBs, and DRIs can cause fetal and neonatal morbidity and mortality, they are Pregnancy Category C in the first trimester of pregnancy and Pregnancy Category D in the second and third trimesters and during lactation. Safety and efficacy in children have been established for some drugs, as indicated in Table 16-2.

Adverse Drug Reactions

Angioedema occurs in approximately 0.2% of patients taking ACEIs and DRIs. It can be life-threatening. The physiological reason for this adverse response appears to be related to an increase in bradykinin level associated with inhibition of ACE. It is not known if DRIs interact with bradykinin, but they have caused angioedema. It usually occurs with the first dose or within the first month of therapy and is more common in the longer-acting ACEI agents. Because this is a class phenomenon, the ACEI or DRI must be discontinued, and no other drug in this class may be used. ARBs do not affect the bradykinin system and should not cause this adverse response; however, administration of an ARB in a patient who exhibited angioedema with an ACEI is to be done with close observation.

Adverse reactions for ACEIs, ARBs, and DRIs are usually transient, mild, and more common in longer-acting agents. Most common are those associated with hypotension (dizziness, headache, fatigue, orthostatic hypotension). Tachyphylaxis frequently occurs with continued therapy. Also common and often cited as the reason for discontinuance of ACEIs is a dry, hacking cough that usually occurs in the first week of therapy. This is a class phenomenon, but changing to a newer-generation ACEI has been associated with less cough.

Table 16-1 ✚ Pharmacokinetics: Angiotensin-Converting-Enzyme Inhibitors Angiotensin II Receptor Blockers, and Direct Renin Inhibitors

Drug	Onset(h)	Peak (h)	Duration (h)	Protein Binding	Bioavailability (BA)	Effect of Food on Absorption	Active Metabolite	Half-Life (h)	Elimination
ACE Inhibitors									
Benazepril	1	2–4	24	95%	37%	Slows	Benazeprilat	NRF: 10–11 IRF: prolonged	20% in urine; 11%–12% in bile
Captopril	0.25	0.5–1.5	6–12	25%–30%	75%	Reduced by 30%–40%	—	NRF: <2 IRF: 3.5–32	>90% in urine
Enalapril	1	4–6	24	50%–60%	60%	None	Enalaprilat	NRF: 1.3 IRF: nd	Total: 94% in urine and feces Unchanged: 54% in urine
Enalaprilat	0.25	1–4	6	UK	NA	NA	NA	UK	>90% in urine
Fosinopril	1	2–6	24	95%	36%	Slows	Fosinoprilat	NRF: 12 IRF: prolonged	Total: 50% in urine and feces Unchanged: 54% in urine
Lisinopril	1	6	24	none	25%	None	—	NRF: 12 IRF: prolonged	Total: nd Unchanged: 100% in urine
Moexipril	1	3–6	24	50%	15%	Markedly reduced	Moexiprilat	NRF: 2–9 IRF: prolonged	Total: 13% in urine; 50% in feces Unchanged: negligible
Perindopril	UK	3–7	24	60%	75%	Reduced BA of metabolite	Perindoprilat	0.8–1	In urine
Quinapril	1	2–4	24	97%	60%	Reduced	Quinaprilat	NRF: 2 IRF: prolonged	Total: 60% in urine; 37% in feces Unchanged: trace
Ramipril	1–2	4–6.5	24	73%	50%–60%	Reduced	Ramiprilat	NRF: 13–17 IRF: prolonged	Total: 60% in urine; 40% in feces Unchanged: <2%
Trandolapril	1	4–8	24	80%	10% (70%) metabolite	Slows	Trandolaprilat	6	33% in urine; 66% in feces

ARBs

Candesartan	2–4	6–8	24	99%	15%	None	Inactive metabolite	9	33% in urine; 66% in feces
Eprosartan	1	2	24	98%	13%	Decreased by 25%	Inactive	5–9	7% in urine; 90% in feces
Irbesartan	2	3–14	24	90%	60%–80%	None	Inactive metabolite	11%–15%	20% in urine; 80% in feces
Losartan	Varies	1 parent; 6 metabolites	24	98%	33%	Decreased by 10%	5-carboxylic acid	1 parent; 6–9 metabolites	35% in urine; 60% in feces
Olmesartan	1	2	24	99%	26%	None	None	13	35% in urine; 65% in feces
Telmisartan	3	UK	24	99.5%	42% (40 mg)/58% (160 mg)	Reduced 6% (40 mg)/20% (160 mg)	Active; less potent	24	0.5% in urine; >97% in feces
Valsartan	2	4–6	24	95%	25%	Decreased by 40%–50%	Metabolite significantly less potent	6	13% in urine; 83% in feces

Direct Renin Inhibitor

Aliskiren	UK	1–3	UK	UK	3%	Reduced by fat	UK	24	Feces

NRF = normal renal function; IRF = impaired renal function; nd = no data; UK = unknown.

Table 16–2 ⊗ **Dosage Schedules: Angiotensin-Converting-Enzyme Inhibitors and Angiotensin II Receptor Blockers and Direct Renin Inhibitors**

Drug	Indication	Dose Form	Initial Dose	Maintenance Dose
ACEI				
Benazapril (Lotensin) (G)	HTN (not recommended for children <6 years of age)	Tablets: 5 mg (not Lotensin); 10, 20, 40 mg	10 mg daily (if not on a diuretic; 5 mg if on diuretic or older adult) 5 mg daily (for Ccr <30 mL/min) *Children:* 0.2 mg/kg once daily (up to 10 mg)	20–40 mg daily in a single or divided dose *Max Dose:* 80 mg/d 40 mg/d *Children:* 0.1–0.6 mg/kg (up to 40 mg)
Captopril (no brand name) (G)	HTN (adult)	Tablets: 12.5, 25, 50, 100 mg	25 mg 2 or 3 times daily (6.25–12.5 mg twice a day if older adult)	Increase to 50 mg twice daily to 3 times daily after 2 weeks if BP not controlled. If BP still not controlled, add 25 mg/d HCTZ. *Max Dose:* 450 mg/d (300 mg if older adult).
	Heart failure		6.25–12.5 mg 3 times daily (if previous or concurrent diuretic or older adult) 25 mg 3 times daily (adult)	Titrate every 2 wk Increase to 50 mg 3 times daily in 2 wk if no improvement *Max:* 450 mg/d
	Diabetic nephropathy		25 mg 3 times daily	25 mg 3 times daily *Max:* 450 mg/d
	LVD/post-MI		6.25 mg for one dose (3 d post-MI)	12.5 mg 3 times daily, then increase to 25 mg 3 times daily with a target of 50 mg 3 times daily over several weeks *Max:* 450 mg/d
	HTN in children		Infant: 0.15–3 mg/kg/dose Child: 0.3–0.5 mg/kg/dose Older child: 6.25–12.5 mg/kg/dose every 12–25 hours Teen: 12.5–25 mg/dose	Infant: titrate to *Max:* 6 mg/kg/d in 1–4 divided doses Child: same *Max* as infant Older child: *Max* as infant Teen *Max:* 450 mg/day
Enalapril (Vasotec) (G)	HTN (may use for children 1 month–16 yr)	Tablets: 2.5, 5, 10, 20 mg	2.5–5 mg daily *Children:* 0.08 mg/kg (up to 5 mg) once daily	Increase at 4 d intervals to 10–40 mg/d as single or two divided doses. *Max:* 40 mg/d *Children:* 0.58 mg/kg (upto 40 mg)
			2.5 mg daily (if serum creatinine >1.6 mg/dL **or** on a diuretic)	Increase by 2.5 mg/d at 4 d intervals. *Max:* 40 mg/d
	Heart failure (unlabeled for children)		2.5 mg once or twice daily	Increase to 40 mg/d over wks
	LVD (no symptoms)		2.5 mg two doses daily	Increase over wk to 20 mg/d in divided doses

Table 16–2 ✂ **Dosage Schedules: Angiotensin-Converting-Enzyme Inhibitors and Angiotensin II Receptor Blockers and Direct Renin Inhibitors—cont'd**

Drug	Indication	Dose Form	Initial Dose	Maintenance Dose
Fosinopril (Monopril) (G)	HTN *Children:* Not recommended for children <6 yr or <50 kg	Tablet: 10, 20, 40 mg	10 mg daily *Children:* 5–10 mg/d	20–40 mg/d Can divide dose if not adequate to control BP *Max:* 80 mg/d *Child Max:* 40 mg/d
	Heart failure		10 mg daily (5 mg with renal issues)	Increase over wk to 20–40 mg/d *Max:* 40 mg/d
Lisinopril (Prinivil or Zesteril) (G)	HTN *Peds:* Not recommended for children <6 yr	Tablets: 2.5 mg (not Prinivil); 5, 10, 20, 30 mg (not Prinivil); 40 mg (not Prinivil)	10 mg daily 5 mg daily (if Ccr ≥10 <30 mL/min **or** on diuretic) 2.5 mg daily (if Ccr <10 mL/min or older adult) *Children: ≥6 yr old:* 0.07 mg/kg/d (up to 5 mg)	20–40 mg/d to max of 80 mg/d *Max:* 40 mg/d *Max:* 40 mg/d *Max Children:* 0.61 mg/kg/d (up to 40 mg/d)
	Heart failure (decrease afterload)		2.5–5 mg daily	Titrate over 2 wk no more than 10 mg at a time up to 5–40 mg *Max:* 40 mg;
	24 h post-MI survival and/or post-MI LV dysfunction		5 mg at time of MI followed by 5 mg 24 h later, then 10 mg after 48 h	*Max:* 10 mg daily Continue for 6 wk
Moexipril (Univasc) (G)	HTN	Tablets: 7.5, 15 mg	7.5 mg prior to meal once daily or 3.5 mg if taking diuretics	7.5–30 mg/d in single or divided doses; 1 h prior to meal *Max:* 60 mg/d
			3.75 mg (if Ccr <40 mL/min)	7.5–15 mg/d *Max:* 15 mg/d
Perindopril (Aceon) (G)	HTN	Tablets: 2, 4, 8 mg	4 mg daily	4–8 mg in single or divided doses titrated weekly *Max:* 8 mg/d
Quinapril (Accupril) (G)	HTN	Tablets: 5, 10, 20, 40 mg	10–20 mg/d (5 mg if on diuretic)	20–80 mg/d Increase at 2 wk intervals based on peak and trough levels *Max:* 80 g/d
	Heart failure		5 mg once or twice daily	20–40 mg in divided doses. Increase at weekly intervals. *Max:* 40 mg/d
Ramipril (Altace) (G)	HTN	Tablets: 1.25, 2.5, 5, 10 mg	2.5–5mg daily	2.5–20 mg/d in single or divided doses *Max:* 20mg/d
			1.25 mg daily (if Ccr <40 mL/min)	1.25 mg in two doses daily *Max:* 5 mg/d
	LV dysfunction post-MI		2.5 mg twice daily 1.25 mg in two doses daily (if Ccr <40 mL/min)	Increase in 1 wk to 5 mg in two doses daily; *Max:* 10 mg/d 1.25 mg in two doses daily *Max:* 2.5 mg in two doses daily

Continued

Table 16–2 ⊗ **Dosage Schedules: Angiotensin-Converting-Enzyme Inhibitors and Angiotensin II Receptor Blockers and Direct Renin Inhibitors—cont'd**

Drug	Indication	Dose Form	Initial Dose	Maintenance Dose
	Reduce risk MI, stroke, and CV death		2.5 mg daily for 1 wk, then 5 mg for next 3 wk	Titrate to 10 mg (if on diuretic, reduce dose of diuretic)
Trandolapril (Mavik) (G)	HTN	Tablets: 1, 2, 4 mg	1 mg/d (2 mg/d in blacks) 0.5 mg/d (if Ccr <40 mL/min)	Increase dose at 1 wk intervals to 2–4 mg/d *Max:* 8 mg/d
	Heart failure, post-MI or LVD		1 mg/d	Increase dose at 1 wk intervals to 4 mg/d *Max:* 8 mg/d
Candesartan (Atacand) (B)	HTN	Tablets: 4, 8, 16, 32 mg	16 mg daily *Children: 1-6 yr:* 0.2 mg/kg/d in 1–2 divided doses *Children: 6-16 (<50 kg) yr:* 4–8 mg/kg in 1–2 divided doses; >50 kg 8–16mg/d in 1–2 divided doses	8–32 mg Increase dose at 2 wk intervals *Max:* 32 mg/d *Child range:* 0.05 mg– 0.4 mg/kg/d *Max:*0.4 mg/kg/d *Child 6–16:* titrate in 2 wk to range 2–16 mg/day • *50 kg:* titrate in 2 wk to 4–32 mg/d • *Max:* 32 mg/d
	Heart failure NYHA II–IV		4 mg daily	Double dose at 2 wk intervals; target 32 mg daily
Eprosartan (Teveten) (B)	HTN	Tablets: 400 mg (B) 600 mg (G, B)	600 mg daily	400–800 mg. Increase dose at 2 wk intervals *Max:* 800 mg/d
Irbesartan (Avapro) (G)	HTN diabetic nephropathy in type II not taking insulin	Tablets: 75, 150, 300 mg	150 mg daily	300 mg/d in single dose *Max:* 300 mg/d
	HTN		150 mg daily *Children: 6– 12 yr:* 75 mg daily; over age 13 use adult dosing	As above *Children:* Titrated to *Max* of 150 mg
Losartan Cozaar) (G)	HTN *Children:* Not recommended for children <6 yr of age	Tablets: 25, 50, 100 mg	50 mg daily *Children:* 0.7 mg/kg (up to 50 mg) once daily	25–100 mg in single or divided doses *Max:* 100 mg/d *Max Children:* 1.4 mg/kg (up to 100 mg)
			25 mg/d (if volume depleted or diuretics)	Increase dose at 1 wk intervals
	Stroke risk reduction in HTN with LVD		50 mg/d	Add HCTZ 12.5 mg/d and increase dose at 1 wk intervals to *Max* of 100 mg/d
	Diabetic nephropathy		50 mg/d	Increase at 1 wk intervals to *Max* of 100 mg/d
Olmesartan (Benicar) (B)	HTN	Tablets: 5, 20, 40 mg	20 mg/d *Children: 6–16 yr:* 10 mg daily	20–40 mg/d. Increase dose at 2 wk intervals *Max:* 40 mg/d *Children:* Titrate after 2 wk *Max:* 20 mg/d
Telmisartan (Micardis) (B)	HTN	Tablets: 20, 40, 80 mg	40 mg/d (lower if volume depletion)	20–80 mg/d. Increase dose at 2 wk intervals *Max:* 80 mg/d

Table 16–2 ⊗ **Dosage Schedules: Angiotensin-Converting-Enzyme Inhibitors and Angiotensin II Receptor Blockers and Direct Renin Inhibitors—cont'd**

Drug	Indication	Dose Form	Initial Dose	Maintenance Dose
	CV risk reduction	Tablets: 20, 40, 80 mg	80 mg daily	80 mg daily
Valsartan (Diovan) (B)	HTN *Children:* Not recommended for children <6 yr of age	Tablets: 40, 80, 160, 320 mg	80 mg/d *Children:* 1.3 mg/kg (up to 40 mg) once daily	80–160 mg/d. Increase dose at 2 wk intervals. *Max* 320 mg/d. Adding diuretic has greater effect than doses above 80 mg/d. *Max Children:* 2.7 mg/kg (up to 160 mg)
DRI				
Aliskiren (Tekturna) (B)	HTN	150 mg and 300 mg	150 mg daily	150–300 mg/day *Max:* 300 mg/day

LVD = left ventricular dysfunction; (G) = generic available; (B) brand-name only. All maintenance doses are titrated to target blood pressure. Lowest dose that meets target is used.

Because the action of bradykinin may be responsible for the adverse reactions of cough, changing to an ARB provides benefits similar to those of the ACEI with less likelihood of cough. DRIs sometimes produce this cough. Less common adverse reactions with ACEIs include a rash that is most common with captopril and neutropenia that increases with high doses, renal impairment, and concomitant collagen diseases. Enalipril, quinapril, and ramipril can cause photosensitivity reactions. Valsartan is the only ARB noted to also do this (Drucker & Rosen, 2011).

Drug Interactions

Losartan levels are significantly lowered by inhibitors of cytochrome P450 (CYP450) 3A4 and 2C9. Irebesartan has a similar problem with CYP450 2C9. Drugs that inhibit this system (e.g., cimetidine) may cause increased levels of free drug. The clinical significance of these inhibitions is negligible, however, because the active metabolite is unaffected. Alsikren has minor issues in the CYP 3A4 system but greater ones in other meds with *P*-glycoprotein (e.g., cyclosporine and itraconazole).

Typically, additive hypotensive effects occur with diuretics, but the DRIs make furosemide less effective. Additive hypotension may also occur with other antihypertensives, nitrates, phenothiazines, and acute alcohol ingestion. Due to the interference with aldosterone secretion, the concurrent use of potassium supplements, potassium-sparing diuretics, or cyclosporine may result in hyperkalemia. The antihypertensive response is reduced by NSAIDs because of their effect on prostaglandins. Other specific drug interactions and the appropriate actions to prevent them are given in Table 16-3.

Table 16–3 ▦ **Drug Interactions: Angiotensin-Converting-Enzyme Inhibitors, Angiotensin II Receptor Antagonists, and Direct Renin Inhibitors**

Drug	Interacting Drug	Possible Effect	Implications
All ACEIs	Lithium	Increased serum lithium levels and symptoms of toxicity	Monitor lithium levels more closely.
Captopril	Diuretics	Hypotension and renal dysfunction	Discontinue 2–3 days before initiating therapy with ACEI or initiate with low dose. Ensure adequate hydration prior to first dose and warn about potential for dizziness.
Enalapril	Antihypertensives, nitrates, alcohol, phenothiazines	Hypotension	Warn patient. Avoid concurrent use if possible. Avoid or reduce alcohol use.
Losartan	Potassium supplements, potassium-sparing diuretics	Hyperkalemia	Avoid concurrent use. Teach patient that salt substitutes often are high in potassium. Read label and check with provider before using.
Telmisartan	NSAIDs	Blunted antihypertensive effects	Avoid concurrent use or monitor for need to increase ACEI dose. Teach patient not to take over-the-counter drugs (OTCs) without informing provider.
All ARBs	Antacids	Decreased absorption of ACEI; increased risk for digoxin or lithium toxicity	Avoid use or separate doses by at least 1 h.

Continued

Table 16–3 ::: Drug Interactions: Angiotensin-Converting-Enzyme Inhibitors, Angiotensin II Receptor Antagonists, and Direct Renin Inhibitors—cont'd

Drug	Interacting Drug	Possible Effect	Implications
	Allopurinol	Increased risk of hypersensitivity reactions	Avoid concurrent use.
	Capsaicin	Increased incidence of cough	Avoid concurrent use.
	Probenecid	Decreased elimination and increased levels of captopril	Monitor for need to increase dose of enalapril or select a different ACEI.
	Rifampin	Decreased effectiveness of enalapril	Fluconazole does not affect eprosartan. Select different antifungal or use eprosartan.
	Fluconazole	May inhibit metabolism of losartan causing increased antihypertensive and adverse effects	Avoid concurrent use. Select different ARB.
	Indomethacin	Reduced hypotensive effects of losartan	Avoid concurrent use. Select different ARB.
	Digoxin	Median increase in digoxin peak concentration (49%) and trough concentration (20%)	Select different histamine$_2$ blocking agent.
	Cimetidine	Increased effects of ARB	If use is necessary, monitor for need to change ARB dose.
	Phenobarbital	May decrease effects of ARB	Same as for ARBs.
	Diuretics, especially thiazide diuretics	Hypotension	
DRI meds	Furosemide	Less effective diuresis	Use other loop or thiazide diuretic.
	Atorvastatin, cyclosporine, ketoconazole	Increased level of aliskiren	Avoid concurrent use if possible.
	Ibesartan	Decreased DRI effect	HTN is less controlled.

Clinical Use and Dosing

Hypertension

Primary HTN has no identifiable cause; therefore, the treatment depends on interfering with normal physiological mechanisms that regulate BP. ACEIs, ARBs, and DRIs act on the RAA system to reduce pressure by decreasing sodium and water retention (aldosterone action), by decreasing vasoconstriction (angiotensin direct action), and by increasing vasodilation (bradykinin action). ACEIs and ARBs are the drugs of choice for patients who are younger and white and for patients with diabetes, HF, or MI, for whom they are most effective and have the lowest incidence of adverse reactions. They are generally not as effective for black patients; however, the interracial differences in BP-lowering observed with any drug class are mitigated when the drugs are combined with a diuretic. Despite noted differences in BP response at the population level, race alone is a poor predictor of BP response to any particular class of drugs if they are given in adequate doses and with sufficient time to work. Literature on the DRIs has not mentioned altered ethnic group responses of significance.

Racial differences in adverse responses may occur. African Americans and Asians, for example, have a 3- to 4-fold higher risk of angioedema (Wright et al, 2009), and more cough in these groups has been attributed to ACE than in whites (Elliot, 1996). Unfortunately, insufficient numbers of Hispanics, Native Americans, or Asian/Pacific Islanders have been included in most of the major clinical trials to make strong recommendations about adverse response patterns.

No specific difference related to gender has been shown (National High Blood Pressure Education Program [NHBPEP], 2003). Doses for HTN vary with each drug, but adverse reactions increase with higher doses. The first dose may cause a steep drop in BP, especially for patients taking diuretics. Diuretics should be stopped for 2 to 3 days to allow rehydration before starting an ACEI, ARB, or DRI. All three drug classes increase in effectiveness when given with a diuretic. Diuretics should be reintroduced after the monotherapy dose has been stabilized. Because reduced aldosterone secretion may result in potassium retention, thiazide diuretics make an excellent combination owing to their tendency to foster potassium loss. The best approach is to start low and go slow. Begin with the lowest dose recommended and increase the dose at 1 to 2 week intervals until BP is controlled. Table 16-4 provides dosage schedules for each of the combination drugs based on their indications. For further information, see Chapter 40 on HTN.

Hypertensive Proteinuric Diabetes

To prevent diabetic nephropathy or slow its progression, ACEIs or ARBs should be selected to treat the HTN (AACE Hypertension Task Force, 2006; American Diabetes Association, 2015). The use of DRIs for proteinuria is still

Table 16–4 ❀ **Indication and Dosage Forms: Selected ACEI and ARB Combinations**

Drug	Indication	Dosage Form	Initial Dosing	Maintenance Dosing
ACEI				
Benazepril + HCTZ (Lotensin HCT) (G)	HTN (not for initial tx)	Tablets: 5 mg/6.2.5 mg (not brand); 10/12.5 mg; 20/12.5mg; 20/25 mg	10–20/12.5 mg daily. For those s BP on 25 mg HCTZ, but K loss: 5 mg/6.25 mg	Titrate 2–3 wk intervals
			Cr <30 not recommended	Give loop
Amlodipine + Benazapril (Lotrel) (G)		Caps: 2.5/10 mg; 5/10 mg; 5/20 mg; 5/40 mg; 10/40 mg	2.5–10 mg amlodipine and 10–40 mg benazapril daily	*Max:* amlodipine 10 mg and 80 mg Benazapril
		Cr <30 not recommended		
Captopril +HCTZ (no longer brand name)	HTN	Tablets: 25 mg/15 mg; 25 mg/25 mg; 50 mg/15 mg; 50 mg/25 mg	25 mg/15 mg daily	*Max dose* of captopril is 150 mg and *Max dose* of HCTZ is 50 mg
Enalapril + HCTZ (Vaseretic) (G)	HTN	Tablets: 5 mg/12.5 mg (not vaseretic); 10 mg/25 mg	5–10 mg enalapril + HCTZ	*Max:* 40 mg/d enalapril and 50 mg/d HCTZ
Lisinopril+ HCTZ (Prinzide or Zestoretic) (G)	HTN	Tablets: 10 mg/12.5 mg; 20 mg/12.5 mg (not available as prinzide brand); 20 mg/25 mg	10 mg/12.5 mg	Increases of either or both drugs per BP response *Max:* 80 mg lisinopril or 50 mg HCTZ
Moexipril + HCTZ (Uniretic) (G)	HTN (not for initial tx)	Tablets: 7.5 mg/12.5 mg; 15 mg/12.5 mg; 15 mg/25 mg	7.5–30 mg of moexipril in one to two divided doses with HCTZ dose less than 50 mg	
Quinapril + HCTZ (Accuretic)	HTN (not for initial tx)	Tablets: 10 mg/12.5 mg; 20 mg/12.5 mg; 20 mg/25 mg	10 mg/12.5 mg	20 mg/12.5 mg daily
Trandolapril + Verapamil (Tarka) (G)	HTN (not initial tx)	Tablets: 1 mg/240 mg; 2 mg/180 mg; 2 mg/240 mg; 4 mg/240 mg	Start at equivalent dose of monotherapy daily	Individualize dose
ARB				
Candesartan + (Atacand HCT) (B)	HTN (not of initial tx)	Tablets: 16 mg/12.5 mg; 32 mg/12.5 mg; 32 mg/25 mg	Substitute dose for original agents in one to two divided doses	Max effect in 4 wk at 16–32 mg/d for the candesartan and at 12.5–25 mg for the HCTZ
Eprosartan + HCTZ (Teveten HCT) (B)	HTN (not initial tx)	600 mg/12.5 mg; 600 mg/25 mg	600 mg/12.5 mg daily	*Max:* 600 mg/25 mg daily
Irbesartan + HCTZ (Avalide) (G)	HTN	Tablets: 150 mg/12.5 mg; 300 mg/12.5 mg	Initial Tx: 150 mg/12.5 mg Add-on Tx: 150 mg/12.5 mg	Can titrate as soon as 1 wk; max effect seen in 2 wk *Max:* 300 mg/25 mg
Losartan + HCTZ (Hyzaar) (G)	HTN	50 mg/12.5 mg; 100 mg/12.5 mg; 100 mg/25 mg	Individualized based on individual drug impact	May be titrated after 2–4 wk
	Stroke risk reduction HTN + LVD		50 mg daily	
Olmesartan + HCTZ (Benicar HCT) (B)	HTN (not initial tx)	Tablets: 20 mg/12.5 mg; 40 mg/12.5 mg; 40 mg/25 mg	Substitute for previously effective doses For noncontrolled: Lowest available dose	Titrate at 2–4 wk *Max:* 40 mg/25 mg
Telmisartan + HCTZ (Micardis HCT) (B)	HTN (not for initial tx)	Tablets: 40 mg/12.5 mg; 80 mg/12.5 mg; 80 mg/25 mg	*Currently only on Telmisartan* 80 mg: 80 mg/12.5 mg *Currently only on HCTZ* 25 mg: 80 mg/12.5mg	Titrate to 160 mg/25mg prn Titrate to 160 mg/25 mg after 2–4 wk

Continued

Table 16–4 ✿ **Indication and Dosage Forms: Selected ACEI and ARB Combinations—cont'd**

Drug	Indication	Dosage Form	Initial Dosing	Maintenance Dosing
Telmisartan + Amlodipine (Twynsta) (B)	HTN	40 mg/5 mg; 40 mg/10 mg; 80 mg/5 mg; 80 mg/10 mg	*Initial tx:* 40 mg/5 mg daily *Replacement dosing:* 40–80 mg/5–10 mg daily	*Initial tx:* Titrate 2 wk to 80 mg/10 mg *Max:* 80 mg/10 mg Titrate after 2 wk *Max:* 80 mg/10 mg
Valsartan + HCTZ (Diovan HCT) (B)	HTN	Tablets: 80 mg/12.5 mg; 160 mg/12.5 mg; 160 mg/25 mg; 320 mg/12.5 mg; 320 mg/25 mg	Initial Rx: 160 mg/12.5 mg daily Add-on RX; 80–160 mg valsartan and 12.5–25mg HCTZ	Titrate after 1–2 wk *Max:* 320 mg/25 mg Titrate after 3–4 wk *Max:* 320 mg/25 mg
Amlodipine + Valsartan + HCTZ (Exforge HCT) (B)	HTN (not initial tx)	5 mg/160 mg/12.5 mg; 5 mg/160 mg/25 mg; 10 mg/160 mg/12.5 mg; 10 mg/160 mg/25 mg; 10 mg/320 mg/25 mg	Add-on or replacement dose: 5–10 mg/ 160–320 mg/ 12.5–25 mg daily	*Max:* 10 mg/320 mg/25 mg
Amlodipine +Valsartan (Exforge) (B)	HTN	5 mg/160 mg; 5 mg/320 mg; 10 mg/160 mg;10 mg/ 320 mg	5 mg/160 mg daily	Titrate after 1–2 wk *Max:* 10 mg/320 mg

(G) = generic; (B) = brand; (P) = Prinivil; (Z) = Zestril; tx = treatment

off-label. In patients with type 1 diabetes, with or without HTN, ACEIs have been demonstrated to significantly delay the progression of diabetic nephropathy. In patients with type 2 diabetes, HTN, and microalbuminuria, ACEIs and ARBs have been shown to delay the progression to macroalbuminuria. In diabetic patients with macroalbuminuria and renal insufficiency, ARBs have been shown to delay the progression to nephropathy (American Diabetes Association, 2015). Though dual blockade by combining an ACEI and an ARB has been shown to provide statistically significant reduction in albuminuria and BP, this combination is not recommended. (Remuzzi, Schieppati, & Ruggenenti, 2003; Wade & Gleason, 2004). Dosages generally used for HTN are appropriate for this indication. DRIs are typically not mixed with ACEIs or ARBs due to significant risks of hyperkalemia.

Angina and Ischemic Heart Disease

Angina is largely a problem of imbalance between myocardial oxygen supply (MOS) and myocardial oxygen demand (MOD). ACEIs affect both the MOS and the MOD sides of the equation. Their prevention of formation of AT II decreases peripheral-vascular resistance (PVR) and, thereby, MOD; decreases the thickening of coronary artery walls, resulting in increased MOS; and decreases the thickening of ventricular walls, resulting in decreased MOD. Their reduced secretion of aldosterone decreases the retention of sodium and water, thereby reducing extracellular fluid (ECF) volume and preload.

ACEIs are recommended for all symptomatic patients with chronic stable angina to prevent MI or death and to reduce symptoms (American College of Cardiology Foundation/American Heart Association [ACCF/AHA], 2009). They are also recommended to limit coronary artery disease (CAD) patients who also have diabetes or left ventricular

(LV) dysfunction. The ACCF/AHA recommend that ACEIs be considered in CAD patients even without LV dysfunction. The Institute for Clinical Symptoms Improvement (ICSI, 2011a) also states that ACEIs and ARBs are appropriate treatment options for stable CAD. Ample evidence exists for basing the use of both ACEIs and ARBs for long-term use in patients with CAD even without other comorbidities. Doses are found in Table 16-4. DRIs do not have this indication.

Postmyocardial Infarction

Survivors of acute MI have a risk for subsequent morbidity and mortality that is 1.5 to 15 times greater than that of the general population. A combination of an ACEI, a non-ISA beta blocker (BB), antiplatelet therapy, and lipid-lowering therapy after MI is appropriate. The reduced morbidity and mortality owing to the use of ACEIs results from: reduced AT II after myocardial injury, prevention of ventricular remodeling in noninfarcted myocytes, alteration of ventricular mass, and positive hemodynamic effects on BP and fluid and electrolyte balance. ARBs are also extremely effective here because they affect not only AT II but also AT I receptors. In addition, bradykinin has cardioprotective effects, and a combination of an ACEI and an ARB provides complete inhibition of AT II and increased levels of bradykinin, which may be more beneficial than either class alone

ACEIs, with or without ARBs, should be started early after MI in stable high-risk patients (anterior MI, previous MI, Killip class II). They should be continued indefinitely for all patients with LV dysfunction (ejection fractions less than 40%) or symptoms of HF and used as needed to manage BP or symptoms in all other patients. Dosages usual for treating HTN are used unless HF is present (see Table 16-4). DRIs do not have this post-MI indication because they do not contribute to positive outcomes more than standard care.

Heart Failure

CAD is the underlying cause in about two-thirds of patients with LV dysfunction, which begins with some injury to the myocardium and progresses even in the absence of additional myocardial insults. The principal mechanism relates to remodeling. ACEIs and ARBs are useful in treating heart failure related to CAD, primarily for their role in reducing remodeling. Another underlying cause for HF is chronic HTN. ACEIs and ARBs are also effective in treating this underlying cause. DRIs do not carry an indication for HF.

ACEIs are a cornerstone of therapy for HF and are recommended for patients with a history of atherosclerotic vascular disease, diabetes mellitus, or HTN. They have been shown to improve symptoms, decrease morbidity, and increase life expectancy. Because they are the only drugs that address all of the pathological mechanisms that produce HF, they are appropriate for all subsets of patients unless these patients have an absolute contraindication. They are also useful for preventing the development of HF in patients with ventricular dysfunction but no overt symptoms. ACEIs are superior to all other drugs and drug combinations used to treat HF. They should be started immediately without waiting for symptoms to become overt.

For symptomatic HF, the dose is about half that used for HTN. Start low and go slow also applies here. In patients with congestive heart failure (CHF) and low ejection fractions (less than 40%), the vasodilating effect of ACEIs provides adequate perfusion even with SBP below 90 mm Hg. For patients who cannot tolerate an ACEI, hydralazine, in combination with a long-acting nitrate (ISDN), BiDil has been shown to be equally effective in reducing morbidity and mortality from HF. This is especially noted in African Americans (see Chap. 36).

Rational Drug Selection

Short-Acting versus Long-Acting

Adverse reactions such as angioedema and renal dysfunction usually occur within the first few doses. Instituting therapy with captopril, a short-acting form, enables rapid onset of action, assessment of patient tolerance, and the ability to clear the drug quickly should an adverse reaction occur. Captopril requires frequent dosing, and adherence is less likely with this treatment regimen in the long term. Other ACEIs have the advantage of once-daily dosing, and as soon as patient tolerance is determined, patients should be converted to these other agents to improve adherence. ARBs and DRIs also allow once-daily dosing.

Cost

Brand-name ACEIs and ARBs are expensive. Most have become generic, which has reduced costs. Combination drug formulations, if needed for control, can additionally reduce these costs. Initiate therapy with captopril for the reasons given previously and then change to the least-expensive long-acting form or to an ARB. DRIs are expensive brand names.

Difficulty in Swallowing

For patients who have difficulty in swallowing, ramipril (Altace) may be a good choice. The capsules may be opened and sprinkled on applesauce, added to apple juice, or dissolved in 4 oz water with no change in the effectiveness of the drug. Captopril may be crushed but may have a sulfurous odor and requires two or three doses daily. Available dosage forms are listed in Table 16-4.

Monitoring

Baseline BP and a pulse reading should be taken before initiating therapy and with each change in dosage. Weight and other indicators of fluid status should also be monitored. See Chapter 40 for further BP monitoring guidelines and other related chapters for monitoring guidelines for the various disease processes for which these drugs are used.

During administration of ACEIs, ARBs, and DRIs, monitoring renal function is important. Serum creatinine levels should be drawn before beginning therapy, after the first week of therapy, monthly during the first 3 months, and when increasing the dose. The ACEI dose should be reduced if serum creatinine is more than 2.5 mg/dL. Potassium levels are also obtained at baseline and with the other labs suggested.

CLINICAL PEARL

Many brand-name **ACEIs** have the same cost for different strengths. It is possible to prescribe a high strength of the drug and have the patient halve it to achieve the desired dose, resulting in considerable cost savings.

CLINICAL PEARL

If you hear an abdominal bruit in a patient known to have vascular disease, give **captopril**, a short-acting **ACEI**, and measure serum creatinine prior to the dose and within 1 or 2 days after the dose. A rapid rise in the creatinine level suggests renal artery stenosis. A slower rise probably indicates a problem with poor hydration that can be corrected by rehydrating the patient and discontinuing or lowering the dose of any **diuretics** the patient is taking.

For patients with renal impairment or receiving an ACEI or ARB that requires dosage adjustments for renal impairment, assess urine protein prior to initiation, every 2 to 4 weeks for the first 3 months of therapy, and regularly thereafter for up to 1 year. Increased proteinuria suggests reevaluation of ACEI therapy. For patients on ARBs, no change in dosage is required based on renal impairment. Initial ARB doses may be lower for patients with impaired hepatic function. Liver function tests (LFTs) should be performed prior to initiating therapy. The dose may be increased as tolerated. According to drug company literature, no patient has had to discontinue an ARB because of increased LFT values. DRIs need renal and potassium monitoring.

For ACEIs, the white blood cell (WBC) count with differential should be monitored prior to initiation of therapy, monthly for the first 3 to 6 months, and periodically for up to 1 year for patients at risk for neutropenia (renal impairment, collagen vascular disease, high doses). Therapy should be discontinued if the neutrophil count is less than 1,000/mm³.

Patient Education

Patient education focuses on administration of the drug, adverse reactions to expect and appropriate responses to each, and concomitant lifestyle management.

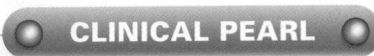

CLINICAL PEARL

Patients should be monitored for indications of angioedema. Suspect angioedema in any patient who calls the next morning after taking the first dose and complains of voice changes or swollen lips or tongue. Stop the drug immediately. The symptoms recede as the drug is eliminated. Protection of the airway is rarely needed, but careful assessment of airway status is required.

Administration

The drug should be taken exactly as prescribed, at the same time each day. Missed doses should be taken as soon as remembered unless it is almost time for the next dose. Doses should not be doubled. The ACEIs vary on whether food alters absorption (see Table 16-1). ARBs may be administered without regard to food intake. DRIs do not have a long enough use pattern for a definitive statement, except to avoid high-fat meals.

The patient should be educated to consult the health-care provider before taking any OTC drugs, especially cold remedies. NSAIDs should be avoided because they may counteract the effects of all three drug classes. Salt substitutes often contain potassium and should be avoided unless approved by the health-care provider.

Adverse Reactions

Education concerning hypotensive reactions can reduce the risk of falls. Changing position slowly, not exercising in hot weather, and keeping fluid intake at more than 2 L/day (noncaffeinated) will decrease these reactions. Fluid intake at this level may not be practical in patients with HF who need to limit their fluid intake, but ACEIs are not contraindicated in this situation (see Chap. 36). There is no effective treatment to date for ACEI-related cough. Changing to another ACEI or to an ARB may help. For the few patients who experience impairment in taste, this generally resolves in 8 to 12 weeks, even with continued therapy. Rash is rare and mostly occurs with captopril. It should be reported, and a different ACEI may be prescribed. DRI effects mirror the other two drugs in the group.

Patients also need to be aware of the serious adverse reactions, including angioedema and renal failure. If flushing or pallor of the face; hoarseness; swelling of the face, eyes, lips, or tongue; or difficulty in swallowing or breathing occurs, the patient should discontinue the drug and notify the health-care provider immediately. Swelling of the feet and ankles and decreased urine output should also be reported. Childbearing women need to understand that ACEIs, ARBs, and DRIs are contraindicated in pregnancy. This topic should be discussed and effective contraception instituted prior to prescription.

Lifestyle Management

Patients are directed toward a cardiac-healthy lifestyle that includes weight loss, aerobic exercise, tobacco avoidance, decreased dietary saturated fats, and moderation in alcohol and dietary sodium. Stress management is also important. They must be made aware that potassium-rich foods and supplements touted as being important for some of the other medications they might be taking should not be increased without provider direction.

CALCIUM CHANNEL BLOCKERS

Calcium is a vital component in the excitation-contraction process in muscles, in electrical excitation, and in facilitating myocardial relaxation. Calcium enters cells via three types of voltage-dependent calcium channels (L-type, N-type, and T-type). The L-type, or long-lasting, channels are predominant in cardiac and smooth muscle and are the ones blocked by most calcium channel blockers (CCBs). CCBs have multiple indications, including angina, HTN, and selected tachyarrhythmias. Unlabeled indications include migraine headache prophylaxis, Raynaud's syndrome, cardiomyopathy, and esophageal spasm. Laboratory evidence indicates that CCBs may interfere with platelet aggregation and reduce the development of atherosclerotic lesions.

Pharmacodynamics

As shown in Figure 16-2, contraction of smooth muscles is triggered by an influx of calcium through transmembrane calcium channels. CCBs directly block the influx of calcium at the onset of the cycle, like the sodium channel blockade in local anesthetics. The drugs act from the inner side of the membrane and bind to channels in depolarized membranes, converting the mode of operation of the channel from frequent openings to rare openings. The result is a marked decrease in transmembrane calcium content and prolonged vascular smooth muscle relaxation.

The blocking action of CCBs occurs via three different receptors: diphenylalkylamine-based and benzothiazepine-based (both type 1 receptors) and dihydropyridine-based (type 2 receptors). The physiological response in the calcium channel is different for these two receptor types, and these differences are important in the clinical choice of CCB. All CCBs relax arterial smooth muscle but have little effect on venous beds. This results in significant reduction in afterload but limited effect on cardiac preload. In cardiac

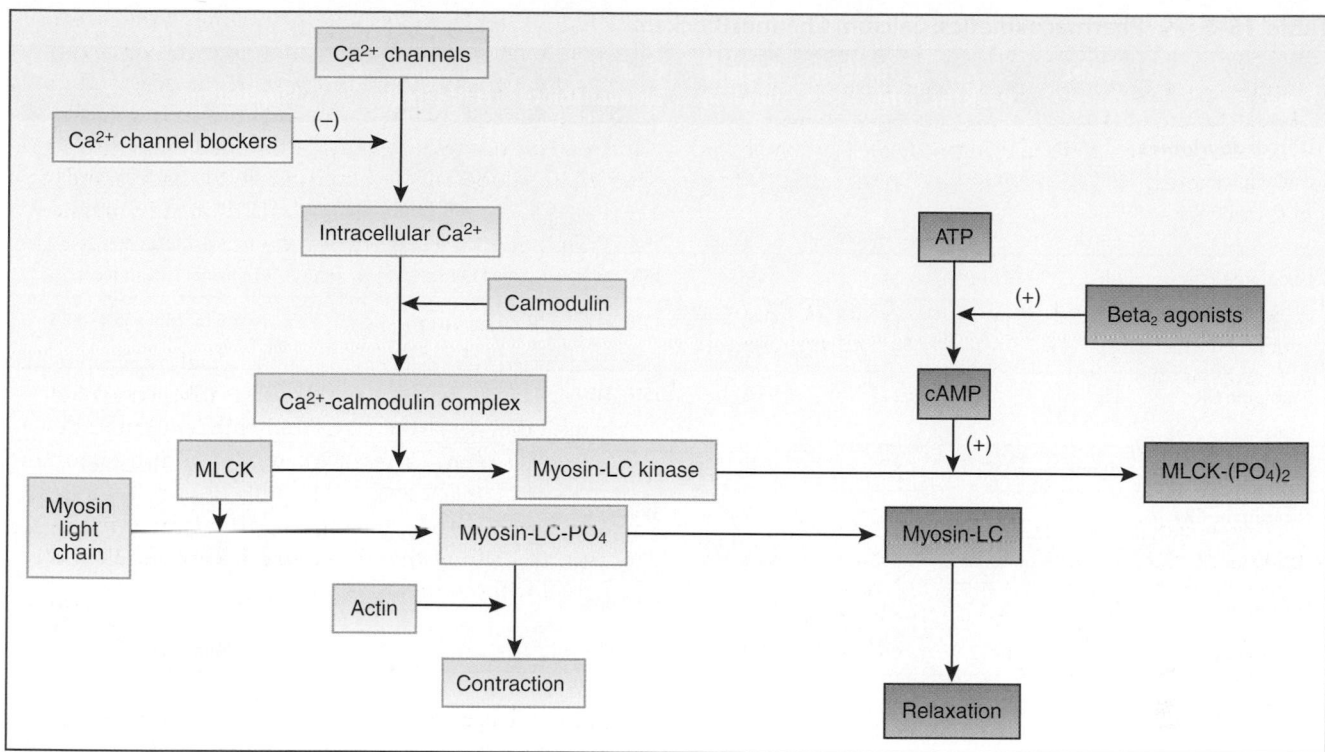

Figure 16–2. Control of smooth muscle contraction. Contraction is triggered by the influx of calcium (Ca) through transmembrane calcium channels. The calcium combines with calmodulin to form a complex that converts the enzyme myosin light-chain kinase (MLCK) to its active form. The latter phosphorylates the myosin light chains, initiating the interaction of myosin with actin that produces contraction. Relaxation begins with the reabsorption of calcium, removing it from interaction with the myosin system. Substances that increase cyclic adenosine monophosphate (cAMP), including beta agonists, may cause relaxation in smooth muscle by accelerating the inactivation of MLCK.

muscle, reduction in contractility (negative inotropism) and decreases in sinoatrial (SA) and atrioventricular (AV) nodal conduction velocity also occur. Although this is true of all classes of CCBs, the greater degree of vasodilation seen in the dihydropyridines causes sufficient reflex increase in sympathetic tone to overcome the negative inotropic effects.

The effect of a CCB on nodal conduction depends on whether it delays slow calcium channel recovery. Nifedipine (Adalat, Procardia) and the other dihydropyridines do not affect the rate of recovery of these channels. At doses used clinically, they do not affect conduction through the AV node. In contrast, verapamil (Calan, Isoptin) not only affects openings of calcium channels but also decreases the rate of recovery, resulting in depression of the SA node firing rate and slowing of AV nodal conduction. This is the basis of its use in treating supraventricular tachycardia. Verapamil is also a direct negative inotrope.

Pharmacokinetics

Absorption and Distribution

All CCBs are well absorbed orally, but there is variance in bioavailability among them (Table 16-5). Verapamil and diltiazem (Cardizem), prototype type 1 CCBs, are rapidly absorbed but rapidly metabolized to yield bioavailabilities of 20% to 35% and 40% to 65%, respectively. The dihydropyridines (type 2 CCBs) are absorbed at varying rates,

and their bioavailabilities vary from 65% to 90% for amlodipine (Norvasc) and to 15% for isradipine (DynaCirc). The presence of food in the gut does not affect bioavailability in any of these drugs. IV forms are available for some CCBs. This latter form is not used in primary care and is not discussed in this chapter.

Distribution is to most body tissues, with only nimodipine (Nimotop) crossing the blood–brain barrier. Because nimodipine has only one very restricted application in the acute care setting, it is not discussed further. All cross the placenta. Verapamil, diltiazem, and nicardipine (Cardene) are excreted extensively in breast milk. Nifedipine is excreted at less than 5% in breast milk, making it the drug of choice during lactation if a CCB is required.

Metabolism and Excretion

All CCBs are extensively metabolized by the liver via the CYP 3A4 channel. Inducers and inhibitors of that isoenzyme system can affect CCB metabolism. This is more of a problem for type 1 CCBs than for dihydropyridines. Many CCBs have elimination routes in both the urine and the feces (see Table 16-5). Dosage reduction based on renal impairment is recommended only for nicardipine.

Most CCBs have short-acting forms with half-lives between 2 and 8 hours and sustained-release forms with half-lives of 12 to 24 hours. Amlodipine is the exception, with a half-life of 30 to 50 hours. Reduced adverse reactions are seen with the use of sustained-release forms.

Table 16–5 ✂ Pharmacokinetics: Calcium Channel Blockers

Drug	Onset (h)	Peak (h)	Duration (h)	Protein Binding	Oral Bioavailability	Half-Life (h)	Elimination
Dihydropyridines							
Amlodipine	1 h	6–12	24+	>93%	65%–90%	30–50 (56 in hepatic impairment)	10% drug and 60% metabolite in urine
Felodipine	1 h	2.5–5	24	>99%	15%–20%	11–16	70% in urine; 10% in feces
Isradipine	<2 h	1.5	12	95%	15%–24%	8	60%–65% in urine; 25%–30% in feces
Isradipine CR	2 h	7–18	24	95%	15%–24%	8	60%–65% in urine; 25%–30% in feces
Nicardipine IR	20 min	1–2	8	95%	35%	2–4	<1% unchanged in urine
Nicardipine SR	UK	1–4	12	>95%	35%	2–4	60% in urine; 35% in feces
Nifedipine IR	20 min	0.5–1	6–8	90%	45%–70%	2–5	60%–80% in urine; 15% in feces
Nifedipine XL	20 min	6–8	24	92%–98%	85%–90%	2–5	60%–80% in urine; 15% in feces
Nisoldipine	UK	6–12	24	99%	5%	7–12	60%–80% in urine
Type 1 CCB							
Diltiazem IR	30 min	2–3	6–8	70%–80%	40%–65%	4.5	2%–4% unchanged in urine
Diltiazem ER	UK	10–14	24	70%–80%	40%	4–9.5	2%–4% unchanged in urine
Diltiazem SR/CD	30–60 min	6–11	24	70%–80%	67%	5–7	2%–4% unchanged in urine
Verapimil IR	30 min	0.5–1	3–7	90%	20%–35%	4.5–12	70% in urine; 16% in feces
Verapamil SR	1.2	5–7	24	88%–92%	20%–35%	4–12	70% in urine; 16% in feces
Verapamil ER	UK	11	24	>90%		4.5–12	70% in urine; 16% in feces

IR = immediate release; UK = unknown; SR = sustained release; CR = controlled release; ER = extended released; CD = continuous dosing.

Pharmacotherapeutics

Precautions and Contraindications

Verapamil has the strongest negative inotropic effect and should be avoided in HF, in which this effect can worsen the disorder. It also has the strongest effect on nodal conduction and can significantly worsen bradycardia. Diltiazem also affects nodal conduction and can worsen or cause bradycardia, although less than verapamil. None of the CCBs are drugs of choice immediately after MI, but diltiazem has shown some benefit in reducing mortality in non–Q-wave MI for a selected group of patients whose ejection fractions are above 40%. For those with ejection fractions below 40% and for all other patients early after MI, type 1 CCBs are contraindicated because of their negative inotropic and bradycardic effects. Patients with ventricular dysfunction, SA or AV nodal conduction disturbances, and SBPs below 90 mm Hg should not be treated with type 1 CCBs because of the high risk for induction of HF and significant hypotension.

The dihydropyridines are less dependent on the heart for their effects, but they are still not the drugs of choice after MI. Dihydropyridines should also be avoided for patients with significant peripheral edema. Their strong peripheral vasodilating effects result in peripheral pooling of blood and may lead to reflex tachycardia. They are also contraindicated in unstable angina because of their potential to cause tachycardia. If it is necessary to give a dihydropyridine to a patient who has peripheral edema or a tachyarrhythmia disturbance, the sustained-release forms are preferred. All CCBs should be used cautiously in severe hepatic impairment, with dosage reduction recommended for most agents.

Teratogenic and embryotoxic effects have been demonstrated in small animals. There are no adequate and well-controlled studies in pregnant women. These drugs are Pregnancy Category C. Female patients capable of childbearing should be made aware of the risks of these drugs, and contraception should be instituted before CCBs are prescribed. They should be used only when benefits clearly outweigh risks.

Verapamil, diltiazem, nifedipine, and nicardipine are all found in breast milk. They should not be given to nursing mothers. It is not known if amlodipine, isradipine, nislodipine (Sular), or felodipine (Plendil) are excreted in breast milk. For these drugs, the determination to continue nursing is based on the importance of the drug for the mother and the presence or absence of acceptable alternatives. Safety and efficacy of these drugs have not been established in children.

Adverse Drug Reactions

The more common adverse reactions of CCBs are extensions of their actions. Reduction in BP secondary to vasodilation may result in dizziness, headache, hypotension, and syncope. These lead to HF with congestion, shortness of breath, cough, and palpitations; though a potential class effect, HF is worse with verapamil, diltiazem, and nifedipine. Gastrointestinal (GI) symptoms can include dry mouth, nausea, vomiting, reflux, and constipation. Although not common, sexual dysfunction and gynecomastia may occur. Hyperglycemia is also uncommon but may affect the choice of the drug in patients with diabetes, especially with nifedipine, verapamil, and diltiazem at high doses. Photosensitivity and facial telangiectasia can occur with amlodipine, nifedipine, and diltiazem. These drugs are also associated with hyperpigmentation (Drucker & Rosen, 2011).

The highest rate of adverse reactions is found in the short-acting dihydropyridines (17%), with the lowest rate for this group being in amlodipine (less than 4%). All adverse drug reactions for CCBs are less common with sustained-release forms because the amount of drug in the system at any given time is more stable.

Drug Interactions

Additive hypotensive effects are major concerns with all CCBs given concurrently with other antihypertensives, nitrates, quinidine, or alcohol. Antihypertensive effects may be decreased with concurrent use of NSAIDs. Verapamil, diltiazem, and some dihydropyridines have an additive bradycardic effect with BBs or digoxin. Serum digoxin levels may be increased with risk of toxicity when it is concurrently used with verapamil, diltiazem, or nifedipine. Verapamil may decrease the effectiveness of rifampin, and the effectiveness of verapamil may be decreased by concurrent administration of vitamin D and calcium. Verapamil may also alter serum lithium levels.

CYP3A4 isoenzymes are involved in the metabolism of all CCBs. Drugs that inhibit this system, including grapefruit juice, may increase free drug levels. Both verapamil and diltiazem increase the risk of myalgia in simvastatin. Food interactions also occur for several of the CCBs. Specific drug and food interactions and appropriate actions to prevent them are found in Table 16-6.

Table 16–6 ⠿ Drug Interactions: Selected Calcium Channel Blockers

Drug	Interacting Drug	Possible Effect	Implications
All CCBs	Histamine$_2$ blockers	Serum concentrations of CCB may increase	Monitor cardiovascular status closely. May need to adjust dose.
	Fentanyl, nitrates, antihypertensives, acute alcohol ingestion, quinidine	Additive hypotension	Monitor for orthostatic changes. Warn patient. Reduce or avoid alcohol use.
	NSAIDs	Decreased antihypertensive effects	Warn patient. Avoid concurrent use or monitor therapeutic response and adjust CCB dose.
Diltiazem and verapamil	Benzodiazepines, buspirone, carbamazepine	Serum concentrations of psychotropics increased	Monitor serum levels closely and adjust dose as needed.
	HMG-Co-A reductase inhibitors	Serum concentrations of statin may be elevated, except lovastatin, which may be reduced	Monitor clinical response and adjust dose as needed if concurrent use cannot be avoided. Lovastatin limited to 20 mg daily.
Verapamil, diltiazem, nifedipine	Digoxin	Increased serum digoxin levels	Monitor for digoxin toxicity. Teach signs and symptoms to report to provider.
	CYP-450 3A4 inhibitors (including grapefruit juice)	Decreased hepatic clearance of CCB with increased risk of toxicity to CCB	Monitor for orthostatic changes, rate and rhythm changes.
	Calcium salts, vitamin D	Reduced response to CCB	Avoid concurrent use. If use is necessary, monitor therapeutic response and adjust CCB dose.
	Cyclosporine, prazosin, quinidine, theophylline, carbamazepine	Decreased metabolism of these drugs and increased toxicity risk	Monitor therapeutic levels and signs and symptoms of toxicity.
Verapamil, diltiazem, felodipine, isradipine, nicardipine, nifedipine, nimodipine	Beta-adrenergic blockers, digoxin, disopyramide, phenytoin	Myocardial depression, bradycardia, conduction defects, CHF	Do not administer within 24 h of each other. If you must give both, monitor for heart failure and decreased peripheral perfusion.

Continued

Table 16–6 ⣿ **Drug Interactions: Selected Calcium Channel Blockers—cont'd**

Drug	Interacting Drug	Possible Effect	Implications
Diltiazem	Phenobarbital, phenytoin	Increased metabolism and decreased effect of diltiazem	Avoid concurrent use. Select different anticonvulsant.
	Cyclosporine	Enhanced action of cyclosporine	Monitor renal function with blood urea nitrogen (BUN) and creatinine levels. Monitor cyclosporine levels.
Verapamil	Rifampin	Decreased effect of rifampin	Avoid concurrent use. Select different CCB if rifampin is needed to treat tuberculosis.
	Lithium	Altered serum lithium levels with increased toxicity risk	Avoid concurrent use. Select different CCB.
	Statins	Toxicity risk	Do not exceed simvastatin 10 mg; lovastatin 20 mg
Dihydropyridines	Azole antifungals	Increased concentrations of CCB	Monitor cardiovascular effects and adjust dose if concurrent use cannot be avoided.
Food Interactions			
Felodipine, nifedipine, nislodipine, verapamil, amlodipine	Grapefruit juice	Increased serum concentrations of CCB	Avoid concurrent use.
Diltiazem, felodipine, nislodipine	High-fat or high-carbohydrate meal	Drug taken with this kind of meal has increased AUC and C_{max} of CCB	Avoid taking drug and eating this type of meal concurrently.
Nicardipine	High-fat meal	Taken together results in decreased AUC and C_{max} for CCB	Avoid taking drug and eating this type of meal concurrently.

Clinical Use and Dosing

Chronic Angina

Both type 1 and type 2 CCBs are effective in the treatment of stable and exertional angina (Table 16-7). They act on both sides of the supply–demand equation: peripheral vasodilation and negative inotropism reduce oxygen demand; dilation of coronary arteries increases oxygen supply.

Among the dihydropyridines, nifedipine, nicardipine, and amlodipine are drugs of choice. The long-acting form of nifedipine (Procardia XL) is the most often prescribed. Combining this drug with propranolol (Inderal), a BB, has proved more effective than either agent given alone, possibly because the BB suppresses the reflex tachycardia that may occur with type 2 CCBs.

Nicardipine is structurally similar to nifedipine but less likely to cause hypotension and LV dysfunction. It is useful for patients with angina who also have mild HF or borderline HTN. Amlodipine is well tolerated, with less venous pooling and minimum reflex tachycardia. It is safe to use for patients with significant ventricular dysfunction. Its long half-life means it acts like a sustained-release form. Although sustained-release forms of the other drugs cannot be crushed, amlodipine can be crushed so that patients who have difficulty in swallowing or who have nasogastric (NG) tubes can use this drug and still benefit from the reduced adverse effects

associated with sustained release. The dose is 5 mg initially. Doses higher than 10 mg have not demonstrated any increase in benefit. Amlodipine has been used in combination with several BBs to produce improved response. The long-acting form of each of these drugs offers once-daily dosing, which improves adherence.

CLINICAL PEARL

Amlodipine can be crushed and put down a nasogastric (NG) tube, which is not possible with sustained-release preparations. This provides the clinical advantage of allowing amlodipine to act as if it were sustained-release with less venous pooling, less reflex tachycardia, and once-daily dosing.

CLINICAL PEARL

Constipation is especially common with verapamil, with almost 100% of patients experiencing significant issues. Patients taking this drug should be encouraged to increase the fiber in their diet and may need to use a stool softener.

Table 16–7 ✂ Dosage Schedule: Selected Calcium Channel Blockers

Drug	Indication	Dosage Forms	Starting Dose	Maintenance Dose
Amlodipine (Norvasc) (G)	HTN *Peds:* Not recommended for children <6 yr of age	Tablets: 2.5, 5, 10 mg	5 mg daily *Children:* 2.5–5 mg	5–10 mg daily; titrate over 7–14 d *Max:* 10 mg daily
	Angina		5–10 mg	10 mg
Diltiazem (Cardizem) (G)	Angina	Tablets: 30; 60, 90, 120 mg	30 mg 4 times/d	Titrate dose 1–2 d, 12–320 mg in divided doses
Diltiazem CD (Cardizem CD; Cartia XT) (G)	Angina	Capsule (CD): 120, 180, 240, 300, 360 mg	120 mg daily	120–180 mg daily Titrate over 1–2 wk *Max:* 480 mg/d
	HTN		180 mg	180–240 mg/d titrate *Max:* 480 mg/d
Diltiazem ER (Cardizem LA) (G)	Angina	Capsules (ER): 60, 90, 120, 180, 240, 300 mg Tablets: All as above except no 60 mg	Tab: 180 mg/d Caps: 120 mg/d	Tab:120–320 mg/d titrate every 1–2 wk *Max:* 360 mg/d Caps: 120–320mg/d *Max:* 480 mg/d
	HTN		Caps: 180–240 mg/d or 60–120 mg twice daily Tabs: 180 mg/d	Tabs: 120–540 mg/d Caps:180–480 mg/d Adjust after 2 wk *Max:* 480 mg/d
Felodipine (Plendil) (G)	HTN	Tablets: 2.5, 5, 10 mg (G)	2.5 mg daily	2.5–5 mg daily *Max:* 20 mg/d
Isradipine (DynaCirc CR) (G)	HTN	Capsules: 2.5, 5 mg Tablets: 5, 10 mg	Caps: 2.5 mg q12h Tabs: 5 mg daily	Increase caps 2.5–5 mg every 2–4 wk; increase tabs 5 mg every 2–4 wk 2.5–5 mg q12h *Max:* 20 mg/d
			Cr 30–80 has only 45% bioavailability Cr <10 drops to 20%–50% bioavail.	
Nicardipine (Cardene) (G)	Angina	Capsules: 20, 30 mg	20 mg 3 times/d	60–120 mg/d Increase every 3 d *Max:* 120 mg/d
	HTN		20 mg 3 times/d	20–40 mg 3 times daily
Nicardipine SR (Cardene SR) (G)	HTN	Capsules (SR): 30, 45, 60 mg	30 mg q12h	Titrate up to 60 mg q12h *Max:* 120 mg/d
Nifedipine (Procardia) (G)	Angina	Cap:	10 mg 3 times/d	10–20 mg 3 times daily; spasm may require 20–30 mg 4 times daily *Max:* 180 mg/d
Nifedipine (Procardia XL; Adalat CC)	HTN	Tablets ER: 30, 60, 90 mg (only Adalat, Procardia)	30 or 60 mg daily	Max 9–120 mg/d
	Angina		30 or 60 mg	30–60 mg daily *Max:* 120 mg/d
Nislodipine (Sular) (G) Sular Geomatrix is not = to generic extended release	HTN	Tablets: 8.5, 17, 20, 25.5 mg 30, 34, 40 mg	Tabs: 20 mg daily	Increase by 10 mg per wk; range 10–40 mg daily *Max:* 60 mg

Continued

Table 16–7 ⊗ **Dosage Schedule: Selected Calcium Channel Blockers—cont'd**

Drug	Indication	Dosage Forms	Starting Dose	Maintenance Dose
		GeoMatrix form: 8.5, 17, 25.5, 34 mg	GeoMatrix: 17 mg	Increase 8.5 mg weekly; range 17–34 mg *Max:* 34 mg
Verapamil (Calan) (G)	Angina	Immediate release oral tab: 40 (not Calan), 80, 120 mg	40–80 mg 3 times daily	80–160 mg 3 times daily *Max:* 480 mg/d
	HTN		80 mg 3 times/d	80–320 mg/d in 2 divided doses
	AFib rate control		240–480 mg/d in divided doses	Range 120–360 mg/d in divided doses
Verapamil SR (Calan SR) (G except SR Caplet	HTN	Caplet (Calan SR): 120, 180, 240 mg Capsule (Verelan): 120, 180, 240, 360 mg Tablet SR (Isoptin SR): 120, 180, 240 mg	120–180 mg daily in the a.m.	120–480 mg daily or q12h *Max:* 240 mg/twice daily of Calan SR and Isoptin SR *Max:* 480 mg Verelan
Verapamil ER (G except ER controlled onset)	Angina	ER: Capsule:120, 180, 240 mg Tablet: 120, 180, 240 mg Controlled onset: Capsule (Verelan PM): 100, 200, 300 mg Tablet (Covera HS): 180, 240 mg	180 mg at bedtime (Covera HS)	Increase in weekly intervals to 240 mg daily, then 360 mg *Max:* 480 mg/d
	HTN		180 mg at bedtime (Covera Hs) or 200 mg (Verelan PM)	Increase weekly doses *Max* dose of 480 mg (Covera HS) or 400 mg (Verelan PM)

(G) = generic; (B) = brand; (ER), (CD), (HS), (XL), (XT), and (XR) = extended release forms are not interchangeable even within same brand.
(SR) = sustained release; (CR) = controlled release.

Diltiazem, also effective in angina therapy, is less likely to cause hypotension and other adverse responses associated with peripheral vasodilation (reflex tachycardia) than nifedipine. It has less negative inotropic activity than verapamil. The reduction in average daily heart rate improves coronary artery filling time and myocardial oxygen supply. Diltiazem is a good choice for patients who need to reduce their heart rate. Verapamil is more often prescribed for treatment of arrhythmias because it has the most potent negative inotropic effect and significantly slows AV nodal conduction. It is not used for patients with compromised LV function, bradycardia, or AV block. Verapamil might be chosen for patients with supraventricular tachycardia who also have angina.

Vasospastic (Variant, Prinzmetal's) Angina

CCBs that produce more coronary artery vasodilation and reduce vasospasm are the drugs of choice. Diltiazem, long-acting nifedipine, and amlodipine are the most commonly used.

Unstable Angina

Medical therapy for unstable angina involves nitrates, BBs, and heparin, which are effective in controlling pain, and aspirin, which reduces mortality. When vasospasm is a component of this angina, CCBs may offer an additional treatment. There is insufficient evidence whether this addition decreases mortality. Verapamil is the CCB of choice. Type 2 CCBs are contraindicated because they tend to increase heart rate and have less vasospastic protection. Because verapamil is often given in combination with other drugs that lower BP, hypotension is a serious potential adverse response.

Hypertension

Initial drug therapy for HTN is monotherapy. Because ACEIs, ARBs, and diuretics have been shown to reduce cardiovascular morbidity and mortality in controlled trials, all are considered first-line medications in the new "JNC-8" guidelines (James et al, 2013). BBs are no longer used as first-line treatment for reducing BP. They are used in the post-MI population or added to the plan if the first-line drugs have proved ineffective.

The guidelines indicate black patients as a group are more responsive to diuretics and CCBs than they are to RAAS medications. CCBs are also indicated for both severe (BP greater than 160/110) and nonsevere hypertension (BP 140 to 159/90 to 109) in pregnancy. Nifedipine capsules and Peripheral Arterial Dilator drugs are useful for both disorders (ACOG, 2012). CCBs would also be appropriate for patients with certain concomitant pathologies (such as unstable asthma) in which BBs are contraindicated.

Amlodipine is especially good for HTN patients with LV dysfunction and CHF. Long-acting nifedipine, diltiazem, or verapamil may be used for patients with CAD. Long-acting nifedipine is a good choice as well for patients who also have peripheral-vascular disease (PVD) because of its peripheral vasodilating effect. For all CCBs, older adults should be started on half the usual dose, and increases in dosage should be gradual to reduce adverse drug responses. (See Chap. 40 for further discussion.)

Supraventricular Tachycardia and Atrial Fibrillation

Type 1 CCBs are useful in treating selected supraventricular tachycardias because they slow AV nodal conduction. Verapamil (80 to 120 mg orally) can be used to terminate the rhythm. Conversion usually occurs in about 1 hour. Diltiazem (40 to 80 mg orally) can also be tried. Prophylaxis with verapamil (240 to 480 mg/d) is effective for patients with paroxysmal supraventricular tachycardia (PSVT). It is important to be certain that the rhythm is not ventricular; verapamil may worsen ventricular rhythm disturbances because of its negative inotropic effects. Verapamil is also used as an alternative to digoxin to slow a rapid ventricular response in the treatment of atrial fibrillation through its direct effect on the AV node, prolonging its refractory period and conduction time. Doses are similar to those used for PSVT. If it must be used concurrently with digoxin, then the digoxin level must be evaluated frequently because verapamil slows the clearance of digoxin and may increase the risk of toxicity.

Patients with Wolff–Parkinson–White (WPW) syndrome can have ventricular responses that are dangerously rapid. Drugs commonly used to control ventricular response such as diltiazem, verapamil, and digoxin are ineffective in this situation and can facilitate conduction through the accessory pathway, increasing the risk for ventricular fibrillation (ACCF/AHA, 2012). The move away from only pharmaceutical intervention and toward physiologic ablation methods has diminished the risks somewhat in this population. In cases of second- and third-degree block, drugs with the rate and conduction alterations are typically contraindicated.

Migraine Headache Prophylaxis

Migraine prophylaxis is an unlabeled indication for CCBs. Of patients with frequent migraines for whom CCBs are prescribed, 30% report a 30% reduction in migraines. The CCB used most often is verapamil (240 to 480 mg/d). To facilitate adherence, it is best to use the sustained-release form to permit once-daily dosing. The trial to determine effectiveness should last at least 3 months. Failure to give an adequate dose or an adequate trial time with a sustained-release form is a common reason for failure of migraine prophylaxis.

Raynaud's Syndrome

Raynaud's syndrome is also an unlabeled indication. Type 2 CCBs are the choice for this disorder because of their peripheral vasodilating effects and some platelet inhibition. The drug most studied and the first choice is long-acting nifedipine. The initial dose is 10 mg orally given in the office to assess the effect on BP. If the patient does not experience a drop in SBP more than 20 mm Hg below baseline or a drop below 90 mm Hg, then 10 mg orally 3 times daily is prescribed. The dose may be increased by 10 mg/d every 3 to 4 days to a maximum of 30 mg 3 times daily to achieve the desired effect. Monitoring every 2 to 4 months is necessary because the initial response may be transient. If nifedipine does not work, diltiazem may be tried, beginning at 30 mg given four doses daily and increasing every 3 to 4 days until a maximum of four 120 mg doses daily is reached. Felodipine and isradipine are also powerful vasodilators and may be tried. Raynaud's syndrome symptoms are often present only during exposure to cold temperatures. Drugs may be stopped during the summer months in some patients.

Esophageal Spasm

Although this is an unlabeled indication, CCBs may offer transient improvement for patients with mild spasm. Diltiazem (90 mg, four doses daily) has been used. Because this drug makes GERD worse, this disorder might cause a CCB to be discontinued.

Rational Drug Selection

Short-Acting Versus Long-Acting Forms

Short-acting forms of CCBs have been associated with more adverse drug reactions. In several trials, the short-acting form of nifedipine was associated with increased mortality in post-MI patients. All type 2 CCBs cause vasodilation that results in reflex tachycardia and peripheral pooling of blood. These actions are greatly reduced in the long-acting forms. To reduce adverse drug reactions and improve adherence, long-acting forms are suggested.

Cost

Branded CCBs are expensive; the generics are less so. Verapamil is the least costly, but its adverse reaction profile includes significant constipation in almost 100% of patients. Although this reaction can be mitigated by the concurrent prescription of a stool softener, the cost advantage is lost by the additional cost of the stool softener. The sustained-release forms of diltiazem are the most expensive CCBs and must be given twice daily. The remaining drugs fall between these two. Cost may be a factor in choosing to use a CCB, but it is not a major factor in choosing among them.

Indication

Specific drugs are more appropriate for specific indications previously discussed. Any CCB should be chosen with these indications clearly in mind.

Difficulty in Swallowing or Nasogastric Tube Placement

Only amlodipine can be crushed and mixed with food for patients who have difficulty swallowing; it can also be put down an NG tube. The longer half-life allows daily dosing.

Monitoring

Liver function should be evaluated prior to initiating therapy. Dosage reductions for most CCBs are recommended with severe hepatic impairment because of the extensive metabolism of these drugs by the liver. Monitoring HR, peripheral edema, and for HF symptoms is critical as well.

Patient Education

Administration

The drug should be taken exactly as prescribed, at the same time each day. Sustained-release drugs taken once daily are best taken in the morning for therapeutic effect. Missed doses should be taken as soon as remembered unless it is almost the time for the next dose. Doses should not be doubled. Sudden withdrawal may precipitate myocardial ischemia, so withdrawal is gradual. CCBs cannot relieve acute anginal attacks; they only have a role in prevention. For patients taking isradipine or nifedipine, anginal attacks sometimes occur 30 minutes after administration because of reflex tachycardia. This is usually temporary and not necessarily an indication for stopping the drug, but this symptom should be reported to the health-care provider who needs to consider if other therapy is warranted.

Several of the CCBs come in more than one form, from short-acting drugs requiring multiple doses daily to long-acting drugs with once-daily dosing (see Table 16-7). The patient has to read the label carefully and follow the appropriate dosing schedule. This is especially important if a different form or a different CCB is prescribed and patients have old bottles at home.

Some CCBs have food interactions, especially with high-fat or high-carbohydrate meals and with grapefruit juice. The patient should be informed so that the interactions can be avoided. Drug interactions also occur with some OTC and prescription drugs and with alcohol. CCB can be taken safely with calcium supplements; the extra calcium does not impair drug effect.

Adverse Reactions

Hypotensive reactions are the most common. Orthostatic precautions, such as changing position slowly, not exercising in hot weather, and keeping intake of noncaffeinated fluids above 2 L/d, will decrease these reactions. Patients who must limit their fluid intake must have a lower dose if hypotensive reactions occur. Bradycardia is also possible, especially for patients on type 2 CCBs. Patients should learn how to monitor their own pulse rate and contact the health-care provider if the rate is less than 50 beats per minute (bpm) or if they have irregular beats. HF symptoms such as dyspnea, pronounced dizziness, or nausea, or more than the usual swelling of hands, feet, or ankles and/or decreased urine output should generate provider contact because CCB can increase HF risk.

Preventive action is required to alleviate the expected constipation. The patient should increase dietary fiber and fluid (if allowed). Stool softeners are prescribed prophylactically with verapamil and as needed with other CCBs.

Lifestyle Management

See the section "Angiotensin-Converting Enzyme Inhibitors and Angiotensin II Receptor Blockers." The cautions about K+ do not pertain. Wearing protective clothing, using sunscreen, and other sun-smart measures will reduce photosensitivity reactions.

CARDIAC GLYCOSIDES

Cardiac glycosides (CGs) are among the oldest known drugs. They have been medically recognized in the treatment of HF since 1785. Although there are three main glycosides available, digoxin is by far the most commonly prescribed because of its convenient pharmacokinetics, the alternative routes of administration, and the techniques for monitoring its serum level. It has lost the preeminence it once held but is still a major cardiac medication.

Pharmacodynamics

Mechanical Effects on Heart Muscle

All CGs are strong and highly selective inhibitors of the sodium-potassium-adenosine triphosphatase (ATPase) system: the "sodium pump." The preferential binding of CGs to ATPase occurs following phosphorylation of the alpha subunit of the enzyme. Extracellular potassium promotes dephosphorylation of the enzyme and decreases the affinity of the enzyme for the CG. This may explain why increased extracellular potassium reverses some of the toxic effects of these drugs.

The sodium pump is the major determinant of the concentration of sodium in the cell. As shown in Figure 16-3, inhibition of this pump results in sodium and calcium buildup inside the cell. The combination of the changes in sodium and calcium results in increased velocity of the shortening of cardiac muscle, with a shift upward and to the left in the ventricular function curve, causing an increase in stroke work for a given filling volume or pressure (positive inotropism).

Electrical Effects on Heart Muscle

A mixture of direct and autonomic actions produces the electrical effects (negative chronotropism) seen with CGs. At therapeutic levels, CGs decrease automaticity and conduction velocity (negative dromotropism) through the AV node via central vagal stimulation and facilitation of muscarinic transmission at the cardiac muscle cell. Because cholinergic innervation is more prevalent in the atria, these actions affect atrial and AV nodal response more than in the Purkinje fibers or ventricular system.

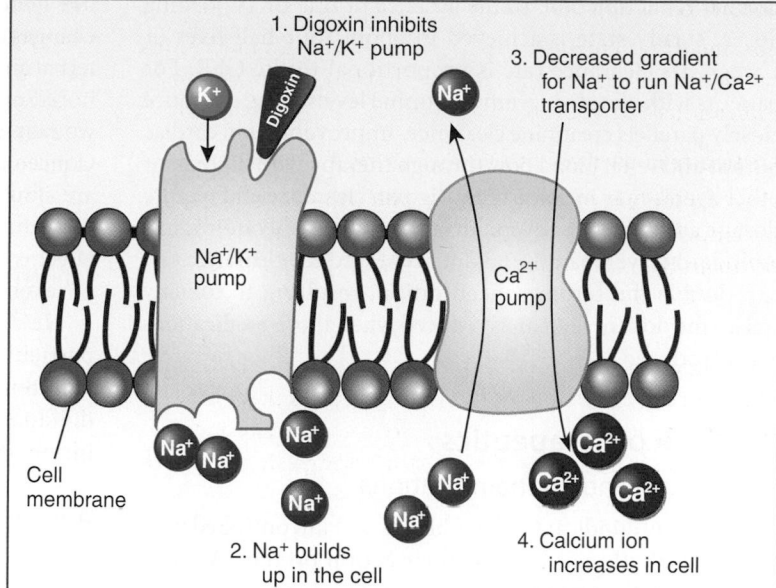

Figure 16–3. Effects of digoxin on the sodium–potassium pump. The sodium pump is the major determinant of the concentration of sodium in the cell. Inhibition of this pump results in sodium buildup inside the cell. The resultant decrease in sodium gradient reduces the sodium–calcium transport mechanism, and calcium ions also increase inside the cell. The influx of sodium through voltage-gated channels is a major determinant in cardiac action potentials. This influx is reduced when the sodium gradient is decreased. Ultimately, contraction of cardiac muscle results from the interaction of calcium with the actin–myosin system. Reduced extracellular calcium levels decrease this contraction.

Other Effects

Several studies suggest that digoxin may also decrease plasma renin activity, reduce plasma norepinephrine levels, and restore baroreceptor sensitivity, all of which are factors in HF pathology. CGs affect all smooth excitable tissues, including smooth muscle and the CNS. These actions on other tissues explain many of their adverse responses.

Pharmacokinetics

Absorption and Distribution

Digoxin is well absorbed orally (Table 16-8). Taking digoxin with food, fiber, or after meals results in slower absorption. Approximately 10% of individuals have intestinal bacteria that inactivate digoxin in the gut, greatly reducing bioavailability and requiring higher-than-average doses to produce a therapeutic response. Treatment of these individuals with antibiotics can cause a sudden increase in bioavailability, which results in toxicity. Product formulation may also be a factor in bioavailability. Generic tablet preparations have a bioavailability of 70% to 80%; the bioavailability is 90% to 100% for digoxin elixir and encapsulated gel. The narrow safety margin between therapeutic effect, loss of effect, and toxicity means that even small variations in bioavailability can have serious consequences. It is best to prescribe using the same manufacturer.

Once absorbed, CGs are widely distributed to tissues, including the CNS. Digoxin's volume of distribution is large (4 to 7 L/kg) and dependent on plasma protein-binding capacity. Its highest tissue concentration (10 to 50 times that in plasma) is found in the heart, kidney, and liver. Digoxin crosses the placenta, and drug levels in maternal and umbilical vein blood are similar. The principal tissue reservoir is skeletal muscle, so dosing is based on lean muscle mass. Neonates and infants require higher doses to achieve a therapeutic effect than do older children and adults. When skeletal mass reduces with cachexia or advancing age, dose adjustments are needed.

Metabolism and Excretion

Digoxin is not extensively metabolized and is excreted largely unchanged by the kidneys. Its half-life is 36 to 48 hours with

Table 16–8 ⠿ Pharmacokinetics: Cardiac Glycosides

Drug	Onset	Peak	Duration	Protein Binding	Oral Bioavailability	Half-Life	Time to Steady State	Volume of Distribution	Elimination
Digoxin	1–2 h	6–8 h	2–4 d	20%–40%	Tablets: 60%–80% Capsules: 90%–100% Elixir: 75%–85%	NRF: 36–48 h IRF: prolonged	1 wk or 4 doses	6.3 L/kg	Unchanged PO by kidney
Digoxin IM	30 min	4–6 h	2–4 d	20%–40%	50%–75%	NRF: 36–48 h IRF: prolonged	1 wk or 4 doses	6.3 L/kg	Unchanged by kidney

NRF = normal renal function; IRF = impaired renal function.

normal renal function. In the absence of oral or IV loading doses, steady state is achieved in about four half-lives or 1 week. Its clearance rate is proportional to the GFR. For patients with elevated serum creatinine levels, drug clearance closely parallels creatinine clearance. Improvement in cardiac output and renal blood flow through therapy with digoxin or other agents may increase renal digoxin clearance and require dosage adjustments. Several drugs (most notably quinidine, amiodarone, verapamil, and diltiazem) reduce clearance and can double the serum concentration, resulting in toxicity unless the dose of digoxin is reduced when those medications are introduced.

Pharmacotherapeutics

Precautions and Contraindications

CGs are contraindicated in AV blocks and uncontrolled ventricular arrhythmias because their action on the AV node may worsen the arrhythmia. They are used for rate control only after BB; verapamil or diltiazem cannot be used or are inadequate to achieve the desired rate range. Patients with idiopathic hypertrophic subaortic stenosis (IHSS) may develop worsening outflow tract obstruction with CG use owing to the action on myocardial contractility. CG use in cor pulmonale is questionable. Toxicity risk increases in the presence of hypoxia from any cause.

Because digoxin is excreted essentially unchanged by the kidneys, severe renal impairment effectively contraindicates its use. Patients with chronic kidney disease (CKD) have very labile creatinine levels, which can be easily disturbed, so it becomes very difficult to monitor these patients in primary care without frequent visits and constant lab testing. Hypothyroidism and CKD decrease digoxin's volume of distribution, necessitating a decrease in both loading and maintenance doses. Digoxin may be used safely in renal impairment as long as necessary dosage adjustments are made.

CGs are used cautiously for patients with electrolyte abnormalities because the concentrations of potassium, calcium, and magnesium in the extracellular compartment affect sensitivity to CGs and may result in toxicity. Digoxin may exacerbate atrial fibrillation due to WPW syndrome by facilitating conduction through the bypass tract and shortening its refractory period. It should not be used to treat this disorder (ACCF/AHA, 2012).

Because 20% to 30% of digoxin is bound to plasma proteins, diseases that lower serum albumin may require alterations in loading doses. Older adults are particularly at risk for toxic effects because of protein levels and chronically altered renal clearance; they require slower digitalization and careful monitoring. Most of the time loading doses are safely eliminated in this group.

Digoxin is a Pregnancy Category C drug. Although safety has not been formally established, digoxin has been used for many years without adverse effects to the fetus. The volume of distribution (Vd) of this drug, however, suggests that it will use fetal tissue as a distribution site. Blood volume also changes throughout pregnancy, and this may affect both maternal and fetal levels of digoxin. Blood levels should be monitored carefully during this time to avoid toxicity. Pregnant women who require digoxin are best managed by a specialist. Concentrations of digoxin in the mother's serum and milk are similar. However, the actual amount of drug the infant gets while nursing is relatively small, so no pharmacological effect is usually seen in the infant. Nonetheless, care should be taken in this case.

Newborns and premature and immature infants are particularly sensitive to the effects of digoxin. There are children's doses for this drug, but they must be highly individualized. Consultation or referral is suggested in these instances.

Adverse Drug Reactions

The GI tract is the most common site of adverse drug reactions, including anorexia, nausea, vomiting, and diarrhea. These result from CNS actions, including chemoreceptor trigger zone stimulation. Other CNS-based adverse responses include fatigue, disorientation, and hallucinations, especially in older adults, and visual disturbances, including yellow vision and green halos around lights. The visual disturbances are considered classic signs of toxicity but actually occur rarely. Atrial arrhythmias and atrial tachycardia with AV block are the most common signs of toxicity in children. Cardiac adverse reactions are extensions of the therapeutic action of these drugs (bradycardia, junctional and AV block arrhythmias, premature ventricular contractions [PVCs], and bigeminy). Gynecomastia is a rare adverse reaction.

Toxicity

Toxicity typically occurs with serum levels greater than 2 ng/mL. Toxicity is commonly caused by excessive administration of a CG, too much diuresis resulting in hypokalemia, concurrent development of renal insufficiency, or by administration of drugs that interfere with excretion of digoxin (see the section "Drug Interactions"). This is especially common in older adults who have polypharmacy changes. Each of these common etiologies and the patient's calcium and magnesium levels should be considered in the differential diagnosis.

Diagnosis of toxicity is based on both clinical and laboratory data. Serum levels alone are insufficient to diagnose toxicity. Patient tolerance plus cardiac output and vital sign outcomes are important considerations to determine if individuals actually need levels above or below common ranges. Providers are cautioned that a faster heart rate in a patient previously controlled on a CG may be a sign of toxicity, not the need for increasing the dose! Incorrect timing of lab draws can be a factor (see the Monitoring section for times to draw serum levels). Toxicity is an important differential diagnosis of arrhythmias and neurological and GI symptoms for patients taking CGs.

> **CLINICAL PEARL**
>
> A full neutralizing dose of **Digibind** is expensive (up to 20 vials at $750 per vial). This cost should be considered in deciding to treat patients with suspected or non–life-threatening toxicity. It should also be remembered that Digibind has a half-life of 2 to 6 hours, and during that time the rhythm disturbance for which the CG was given may recur and cannot be treated with a CG.

Treatment of toxicity depends on the problem. AV junctional and first-degree block rhythms, ventricular ectopic beats, or an excessively slow ventricular response to atrial fibrillation often requires CG dosage adjustment and careful monitoring. Potassium administration should be considered to reduce automaticity, even when serum potassium is in the normal range, unless a high-grade AV block is also present. Lidocaine has minimum effects on the AV node and may be used to treat ventricular ectopic beats that threaten hemodynamics. Bradycardia and second- or third-degree AV block usually respond to atropine. When toxicity is severe or life-threatening, the antidote for CG toxicity is antidigoxin immunotherapy, digoxin immune fab (Digibind). Patients who require this medication are hospitalized so that cardiopulmonary resuscitation equipment and medications are available when it is administered. A short holding of the next dose or two may be sufficient to return to normal values without using Digibind.

Any patient who becomes toxic on a CG should have the indications for that drug carefully reviewed. In some cases, it is possible to stop the drug altogether. There is new recognition that women fare worse on CG, so as a group they should be evaluated for treatment with other meds. Several studies, however, have shown negative consequences for withdrawal of digoxin, so the decision should be carefully made in consultation with cardiology.

Drug Interactions

Any drug that may cause hypokalemia, hypercalcemia, or hypomagnesemia increases the risk of toxicity. Several antiarrhythmic drugs (quinidine, amiodarone, verapamil, diltiazem, and propafenone) increase serum CG levels and toxicity risk. Drugs that induce bradycardia can exhibit additive bradycardia when given with CGs. This is especially a concern with BBs.

Interactions with Potassium, Calcium, and Magnesium

Potassium and CGs interact by inhibiting each other's binding to sodium-potassium-ATPase. Hyperkalemia reduces the enzyme-inhibiting actions of CGs, and hypokalemia facilitates these actions. Hyperkalemia, however, inhibits the abnormal cardiac automaticity seen in excessive doses of CGs so that moderately increased extracellular potassium reduces toxic effects of CGs. Calcium facilitates the toxic actions of CGs by overloading the intracellular calcium stores. Hypercalcemia increases the risk of CG-induced arrhythmias. Magnesium has the opposite effects to calcium. Hypomagnesemia is a risk factor for arrhythmias. Specific drug interactions and the appropriate actions to prevent them are given in Table 16-9.

Table 16–9 ⠿ Drug Interactions: Cardiac Glycosides

Drug	Interacting Drug	Possible Effect	Implications
CGs	Phenobarbital, phenytoin, rifampin	Decreases the effect of digoxin	Increase dose of digoxin or change to digoxin
	Thiazide and loop diuretics, mezlocillin, piperacillin, ticarcillin, amphotericin B, glucocorticoids	May cause hypokalemia and increase risk of CG toxicity	Monitor serum potassium levels and teach patient signs and symptoms of hypokalemia to monitor for and report. Administer potassium supplement prn and encourage diet high in potassium. Where possible, choose alternative drug, especially antibiotic.
	Calcium preparations	Facilitates toxicity by accelerating overloading of intracellular calcium stores	Monitor for indications of toxicity. Avoid concurrent administration. Separate administration of CG and milk intake by at least 30 min.
	Spironolactone	Increases digoxin half-life	Reduce dose of digoxin or increase dosing interval
	Beta-adrenergic blockers, quinidine, disopyramide	Additive bradycardia	Avoid concurrent use or teach patient to monitor pulse rate and report pulse <60 bpm. Monitor electrocardiogram (ECG) regularly.
	Antacids, colestipol, kaolin pectin, cholestyramine	Decreases absorption of CG if given concurrently	Separate administration by at least 1 h and give CG first
	Thyroid hormones	May decrease therapeutic effects and cause arrhythmias	Monitor for effectiveness. Monitor ECG at regular intervals.

Continued

Table 16–9 ⚏ Drug Interactions: Cardiac Glycosides—cont'd

Drug	Interacting Drug	Possible Effect	Implications
Digoxin	Quinidine, cyclosporine, amiodarone, verapamil, diltiazem, propafenone, diflunisal	Increases serum levels of digitalis and risk of toxicity	Avoid concurrent use or monitor serum levels 5–7 d after adding one of these drugs. Consider reducing digitalis dose by half if patient has signs of toxicity or a high normal digitalis level at initiation of interacting drug.
	Aminoglycosides (oral), colestipol, rifampin, St. John's wort, sulfasalazine	Decreases digitalis serum levels	Avoid concomitant use
	Benzodiazepines, clarithromycin, diphenoxylate, erythromycin, indomethasone, itraconazole, tetracycline, verapamil	Increases serum levels of digitalis and risk of toxicity	Avoid concurrent use or monitor serum levels 5–7 d after adding one of these drugs. Consider reducing digitalis dose by half if patient has signs of toxicity or a high normal digitalis level at initiation of interacting drug.
	Calcium channel blockers	Additive effects on AV node may result in complete heart block	Monitor patient carefully if both are chosen with HF
Food Interactions	High-bran meal	Taking with this meal results in reduced absorption of digitalis	Take 30 min prior to meal

Clinical Use and Dosing

Atrial Fibrillation, Paroxysmal Supraventricular Tachycardia

Asymptomatic or mildly symptomatic patients with a rapid ventricular response can be treated with a CG. Treatment is aimed at slowing the rate and converting to sinus rhythm if possible. The goal is a resting ventricular rate between 70 and 80 bpm (Table 16-10). Digoxin is preferred because it slows AV nodal conduction, resulting in a slower ventricular rate. It does not convert the rhythm directly. Slowing heart rate yields greater diastolic filling time, permitting improved myocardial oxygenation. Cardiac muscle with an improved supply-demand ratio may then return to sinus rhythm. Digoxin is less effective at slowing heart rate when vagal tone is low and adrenergic stimulation is high, such as during exercise, and in maintaining sinus rhythm or reducing the incidence of PSVT. Additional antiarrhythmic drugs may be needed.

Table 16–10 ⚘ Dosage Schedule: Cardiac Glycosides

Drug Form	Indication	Patient Status	Digitalizing or Loading Dose	Maintenance
Digoxin (G)	Atrial fibrillation with ventricular response <120 bpm or stable CHF	Young adult or normal renal function	None	0.25–0.5 mg/d for atrial fibrillation; 0.25 mg/d for CHF
		Older adult or impaired renal function	None	0.125 mg/d
	Atrial fibrillation with ventricular response 120–150 bpm or less stable CHF	Young adult or normal renal function	1–1.5 mg/d in 4 divided doses 6 h apart	0.25–0.5 mg/d for atrial fibrillation; 0.25 mg/d for CHF
		Older adult or impaired renal function	If creatinine clearance <20 mL/min, give half the loading dose in 4 divided doses 6 h apart	0.125 mg/d
	Atrial fibrillation with rapid ventricular response or heart failure	Adult with normal renal function	0.75–1.25 mg (10–15 mcg/kg) given as 50% of dose initially and additional fractions at 4–8 h intervals	0.063–0.5 mg/d as tablets or 0.035–0.5 mg/d as gelatin capsules. Dose is based on lean body mass and Ccr.* Usual dose is 0.25 mg/d in morning.

Table 16–10 ⊗ **Dosage Schedule: Cardiac Glycosides—cont'd**

Drug Form	Indication	Patient Status	Digitalizing or Loading Dose	Maintenance
		Older adult or impaired renal function	Same as adult	Same calculation. Usual dose is 0.125 mg in morning.
		Children with normal renal function based on lean body weight: 2–5 yr	25–35 mcg/kg given as 50% of dose initially and additional fractions at 4–8 h intervals	25%–35% of digitalizing dose given daily in 2 divided doses
		5–10 yr	15–30 mcg/kg given as above	Same as above
		>10 yr	8–12 mcg/kg given as above	Same as above except in single dose
Digoxin (elixir50 mcg/mL)	Heart failure	Children with normal renal function based on lean body weight: Premature infant Full-term 1–24 mo 2–5 yr 5–10 yr >10 yr	20–30 mcg/kg given as 50% of dose initially and additional fractions at 4–8 h intervals 25–35 mcg/kg given as above 35–60 mcg/kg given as above 30–40 mcg/kg given as above 20–35 mcg/kg given as above 10–15 mcg/kg given as above	20%–30% of oral digitalizing dose given daily in 2 divided doses 25%–35% of oral digitalizing dose for full term to >10 yr All in 2 divided doses except for >10 yr

Oral tablet forms: 0.125 mcg = 125 mg; 0.25 mcg = 250 mg; capsules: 0.05 mg, 0.1 mg, 0.2 mg. Also available tablets of 0.625 mg and 0.1875mg.
*Maintenance dose = loading dose × (14 + Ccr/5). Ccr should be corrected to 70 kg body weight.
Therapeutic serum level of digoxin: atrial fibrillation, 1.5–2 ng/mL; CHF, 0.8–1.2 ng/mL.

Digoxin is classically presented as a medication requiring loading dose schedules. For elders and mildly symptomatic patients, a loading dose is rarely required. Treatment is started with a maintenance dose if the ventricular response is less than 120 bpm. For young patients and those with normal renal function, the maintenance dose is 0.25 mg to 0.5 mg daily. For older adults and those with renal impairment, the maintenance dose is 0.125 mg daily. Drug levels may be drawn at steady state (5 to 7 days), but the best indication of appropriate dosing is an acceptable heart rate.

If the ventricular rate is 120 to 150 bpm and still well tolerated, outpatient digitalization with an oral loading dose is reasonable. The dose is 10 to 15 mcg/kg in divided doses over 24 hours. The usual pattern is 50% of the total digitalizing dose and the remainder in divided doses over 4 to 8 hours. If creatinine clearance is less than 20 mL/min, give one-half the loading dose and start with 0.125 mg daily for maintenance. Patients who are not hemodynamically stable require rapid digitalization in a hospital.

Heart Failure

Although no longer the first-line drug for treatment of HF, digoxin is still central to treatment for patients with severe systolic dysfunction (ejection fractions less than 40% and with an audible S_3 heart sound). In fact, the resolution of S_3 is a potent predictor of response to CG therapy. The primary mechanism of action in HF is through its positive inotropic action, increasing ejection fraction at a given preload and afterload. Digoxin is also beneficial in HF resulting from uncontrolled HTN or severe aortic stenosis, although BP reduction and valve surgery are the mainstays of therapy in these disorders. CGs are less beneficial with ejection fractions more than 40% or in

HF secondary to hypertrophic cardiomyopathies. They have no benefit in HF due to recurrent transient ischemia. An adequately digitalized HF patient has a serum level of 0.8 to 1.2 ng/mL, lower than that needed to treat atrial fibrillation, because it is only add-on therapy.

The American College of Cardiology/American Heart Association (ACCF/AHA, 2009) and ICSI (2011b) guidelines suggest that patients with mild-to-moderate HF often become asymptomatic on optimal doses of ACEIs and diuretics and usually do not require digoxin. It is added only after ACE/ARB and diruetics are already on board. For less stable patients, the treatment regimen includes a digoxin loading dose similar to that used to treat atrial fibrillation and a usual maintenance dose of 0.25 to 0.5 mg/d. (See Chap. 36 for further discussion.)

Rational Drug Selection

Formulation

Digoxin is well absorbed orally, with a bioavailability of 60% to 80% for tablets. Digoxin elixir in capsules and encapsulated gel form (Lanoxicaps) has a 90% to 100% bioavailability and may be useful when careful titration of the dose is important. Pediatric elixir has a bioavailability of 70% to 85%. Tablets are not generally used for children, but children's digitalizing and maintenance doses are provided for both the capsule and the elixir (see Table 16-10).

Brand and Cost

The best choice of CG is the purified glycoside, digoxin. It is well absorbed, can be used parenterally if needed, and has an intermediate duration of action, with a half-life of 36 to 48 hours. Even in the presence of renal failure, it can be used if the dose is adjusted. Digoxin is available in a generic form that reduces the cost. Using the same generic manufacturer will reduce the impact of FDA allowable variance in bioavailability for generics.

Monitoring

Routine monitoring of digoxin levels is generally overdone. Monitoring should occur in addition to clinical judgment, rather than as a substitute for it. In general, testing should be done when any of the following occurs:

1. The patient is taking other drugs that may alter the pharmacokinetics of digoxin.
2. Steady state has been achieved (4 to 5 half-lives or 1 to 2 weeks) after starting a new dose.
3. Toxicity is suspected.
4. Confirmation of adequacy of maintenance dose is needed in situations of poor therapeutic response or patient adherence.
5. A reference point is needed in adjusting a dose.
6. The patient has progressive renal function decline.

To avoid sampling during the distribution phase of the drug response curve, levels should be drawn at least 6 hours after the last dose. Because of their critical role in sensitivity to toxicity, serum electrolytes (potassium, calcium, magnesium) and renal status should be monitored concurrently, especially for patients who are also taking diuretics. Levels should be evaluated periodically and prior to any dosage change.

Patient Education

Administration

The patient should take the drug exactly as prescribed, at the same time each day. The long half-life means that taking it at different times each day would be permissible, but the narrow therapeutic range means that missing a dose or doubling a dose could result in toxicity. Taking the drug at the same time each day lessens the likelihood of nonadherence to the appropriate regimen. When the drug is prescribed on an eccentric schedule (e.g., 0.25 mg Monday, Wednesday, Friday and 0.125 mg Tuesday, Thursday, Saturday, Sunday), taking a dose at the same time each day reduces the complexity of the schedule. Placing the appropriate dose in a pill container with compartments for each day of the week also reduces the chance of nonadherence and dosing mishap. If one dose is missed but remembered within 12 hours, it should be taken. If two doses are missed, the health-care provider should be contacted for instructions. The drug should not be stopped or the dosage altered without first contacting the health-care provider.

Although the presence of food in the gut does not alter absorption of CGs, the ingestion of a high-fiber meal may decrease absorption. Tablets can be crushed and administered with food for patients who have difficulty swallowing. Patients should eat a diet high in potassium (bananas, orange juice, tomato juice, spinach, melons, dates, raisins, soybeans, prunes, potatoes, and molasses), unless also taking a potassium-sparing diuretic or an ACEI, and eat moderate amounts of calcium (800 to 1,000 mg/d). Milk may have some effect on absorption, so doses should be separated by 1 hour.

CLINICAL PEARL

Heart failure treatment

1. CGs should not be used unless there is clear evidence of severe chronic systolic dysfunction or atrial fibrillation. In older adults, ankle edema is more often due to venous insufficiency than to heart failure. Even if it is related to heart failure, it is more often caused by diastolic dysfunction and better treated with diuretics or ACEIs.
2. Digoxin should not be discontinued unless a reversible cause of the heart failure has been completely corrected or there was no basis for the drug in the first place.
3. ST-T wave changes on the ECG do not correlate directly with serum drug levels and should not be used as an indication of toxicity. Serum drug levels are needed.

Do not alternate between dosage forms (see Table 16-10) such as liquids and capsules. Each form has a different bioavailability, and changing forms may result in toxicity. Store the drug in its original, tightly covered, light-resistant container. The patient who uses a pillbox for weekly dosing should not mix the digoxin with other drugs in the same compartment. Drugs often look alike and can be mistaken for one another. This allows for easier withholding of a dose if the HR is too low. Patients should also avoid concurrent use of OTC drugs and should not take antacids or antidiarrheal drugs within 1 hour of taking the CG.

Adverse Reactions

Patients should learn to take their own carotid pulse and then contact the health-care provider before taking the drug if the pulse rate is less than 60 or more than 100 bpm. Relying on a peripheral pulse counter may not accurately identify a pulse deficit. This may trigger an inaccurate withholding of a dose due to a low reading when dosing was still indicated.

Patients are also typically educated on signs and symptoms of toxicity, including nausea, vomiting, diarrhea, confusion, irregular pulse, yellow vision, and green halos around lights. Pulse changes and these symptoms should be reported to the health-care provider immediately. Some patients can tolerate pulses as low as 50 bpm without other symptoms and can be taught mainly to report symptoms of worsening HF. These signs and symptoms include persistent cough; shortness of breath; weight gain of more than 2 lb in 1 day or 5 lb in one week; swelling of ankles, legs, or hands; and a sensation of fullness in the abdomen. Follow-up appointments are also critical to evaluate the effectiveness of these drugs and to monitor for toxicity.

Lifestyle Management

A cardiac-healthy lifestyle is discussed in the drug class sections above. At all times, patients should carry identification or wear a medical information bracelet or necklace that describes the disease process and drug regimen.

ANTIARRHYTHMICS

Cardiac rhythm disturbances can range from benign and asymptomatic to malignant and life-threatening. For some arrhythmias, definitive drug therapy has research support; for others, selection of a specific drug is largely based on expert opinion, adverse responses, potential interactions with other drugs being taken, and concurrent clinical problems. Antiarrhythmic drugs are understood to be pro-arrhythmic; they can paradoxically correct one issue, but then cause another lethal arrhythmia. Deciding not to treat may be a better choice, especially in asymptomatic or minimally symptomatic patients.

Debate continues about the relative merits of invasive versus noninvasive testing to assist in the selection of a specific antiarrhythmic. Given these variables, it is best to refer to a cardiologist any patients with new rhythm disturbances or for whom rhythm control is difficult. When the drug is chosen by the specialist, management in the primary care setting requires understanding both the beneficial effects and the adverse effects of these drugs, the monitoring required, and appropriate patient education. The six classes of antiarrhythmics are discussed here with that management approach in mind. To be practical in a primary care setting, the drug must be available in oral form and have an effective half-life of at least 6 hours. Drugs that do not meet these criteria are not discussed.

Pharmacodynamics

Arrhythmias are caused either by abnormal pacemaker activity or by abnormal impulse conduction. The goal of therapy with an antiarrhythmic is to reduce ectopic pacemaker activity or alter abnormal conduction. The major mechanisms by which antiarrhythmics act to do this are (1) sodium channel blockade, (2) blockade of sympathetic nervous system (SNS) effects on the heart, (3) prolongation of the effective refractory period, and (4) blockade of the calcium channel. Different classes of antiarrhythmics act in one or more of these ways. Drugs in one class may have significant actions more commonly associated with a different class. Placement in a given class is based on predominant action.

All pacemakers in the heart, normal and ectopic, depend on appropriate phase 4 diastolic depolarization. Increasing the phase 4 slope may result in accelerated pacemaker discharge. Figure 16-4 depicts the cardiac action potential with slope phases. Potential causes of this increased slope include hypokalemia, beta-adrenergic stimulation, fiber stretch, acidosis, and partial depolarization by currents of injury. Blockade of sodium channels (class I drugs) or calcium channels (class IV) reduces the permeability ratio of these ions to potassium, making the threshold more negative and reducing the phase 4 slope. BBs (class II) indirectly reduce the slope by blocking the chronotropic impact of

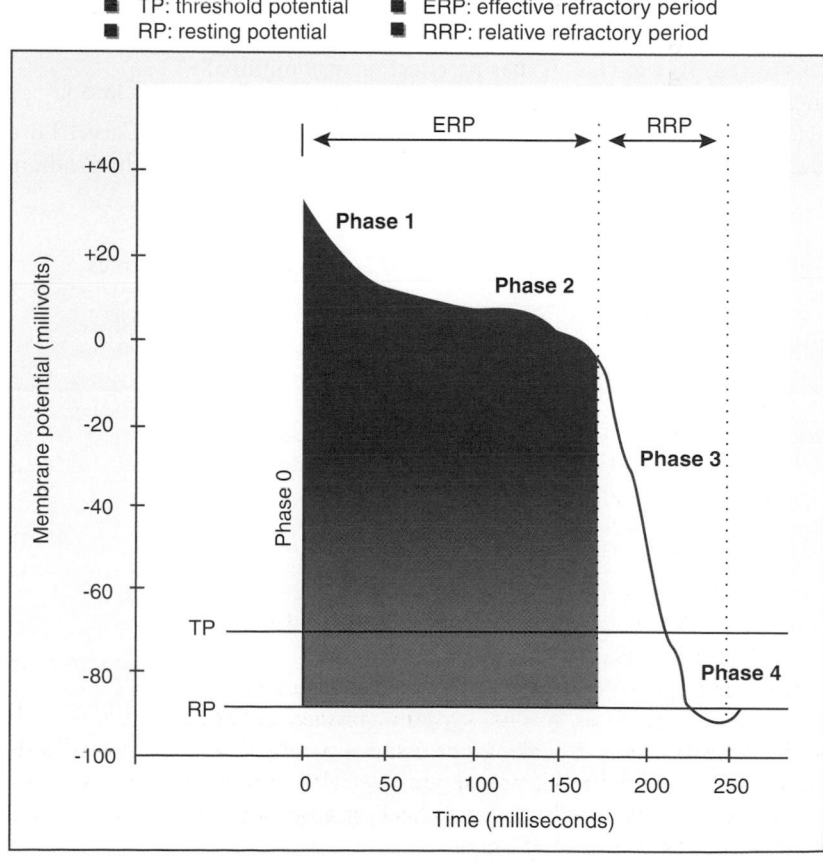

■ TP: threshold potential   ■ ERP: effective refractory period
■ RP: resting potential   ■ RRP: relative refractory period

Figure 16–4. Cardiac action potential: ventricles.

norepinephrine. Hyperkalemia raises the membrane potential, which reduces the rate of pacemaker firing. Vagal discharge also reduces phase 4 slope and makes the potential more negative (CG activity).

Disturbances in impulse conduction are either (1) simple blocks related to depressed conduction that may be relieved by the parasympathetic action of atropine or (2) reentry conduction, in which one impulse excites areas of the heart more than once. Reentry requires (1) an obstacle to normal conduction, (2) a unidirectional block in the circuit, and (3) conduction flow around the circuit timed so that the impulse does not enter refractory tissue. Too slow an impulse results in bidirectional block or the impulse colliding with the next normal impulse; too fast results in bidirectional conduction or the impulse reaching tissue that is still refractory. Slowing conduction by depressing the sodium current (class I) or calcium current (class IV) abolishes reentry arrhythmias. Lengthening or shortening the refractory period also makes reentry less likely. Converting unidirectional block to bidirectional block (class III) also decreases reentry. See Table 16-11 for the mechanism of action.

Safer antiarrhythmics act more on cardiac tissue being abnormally stimulated than on normal cardiac tissue. These drugs decrease the automaticity of ectopic pacemakers more than the SA node, and they reduce conduction or increase the refractory period more in depolarized tissue than in normally polarized tissue.

Class I

Class I antiarrhythmic drugs are sodium channel blockers. Class IA lengthens the duration of the action potential, class IB shortens it, and class IC has no effect or may minimally increase the duration of the action potential. Class IB interacts rapidly with sodium channels, class IC acts slowly, and class IA is intermediate.

Class IA drugs reduce the rate of firing of ectopic foci, increase the effective refractory period (ERP), and reduce the speed of conduction. They also block parasympathetic nervous discharge, resulting in an increased conduction rate at the AV node. This anticholinergic activity can produce serious increases in ventricular rate in the presence of rapid atrial activity, such as that found in atrial fibrillation. Class IB drugs block both activated and inactivated sodium channels. The effect is extremely limited in normally polarized tissue but highly effective in depolarized and injured tissue. Class IB drugs do not affect the automaticity of the SA node or conductivity through the AV node. Their shortening effect on the ERP eliminates unidirectional block and may trigger reentry arrhythmias. Class IC drugs primarily block the sodium fast channel during phase 0 of the action potential. Because of their propensity for severe exacerbation of arrhythmias, even in normal doses with post-MI patients, they are reserved for patients with severe ventricular tachycardias for whom other drugs have not worked.

Class II

Class II drugs (BBs) reduce adrenergic activity in the heart. Blockade by these drugs increases threshold potential and prolongs ERP, thereby decreasing heart rate and conduction velocity. These effects probably convert unidirectional block to bidirectional. They also exert a significant negative inotropic effect, reducing force of contraction. This class includes beta$_1$ selective drugs that act mainly on cardiac muscle and nonselective beta$_1$ and beta$_2$ drugs that also act on lung, arteriole, pancreatic, kidney, adipose, and liver tissues, resulting in a range of adverse responses. BBs are also discussed in Chapters 14 and 40.

Class III

Class III drugs prolong the ERP by some mechanism other than sodium channel blockade, often by blocking potassium

Table 16–11   Mechanism of Action of Selected Antiarrhythmics

Drug	Effect on Sinoatrial Rate	Effect on Atrioventricular Node Refractory Period	Effect on PR Interval	Effect on QRS Duration	Effect on QT Interval	Sinoatrial Node Automaticity
Amiodarone	−	+	+	+	++	−
Disopyramide	± (2)	± (2)	± (2)	+	++	±
Flecainide	0	0	+	++	0	−
Mexiletine	0 (1)	±	0	0	0	−
Procainamide	±	± (2)	± (2)	+	+	±
Propafenone	0	+	+	+	0	0
Quinidine	± (2)	± (2)	± (2)	+	+	±
Sotalol	−	++	++	0	++	−
Tocainide	0 (1)	−	0	0	0	0/−

− = suppresses or slows; + = stimulates or increases speed or duration; (1) = may suppress diseased sinus nodes; (2) = anticholinergic effect and direct depressant action.

channels, which results in a decreased rate of automaticity of ventricular ectopic beats. They may also convert unidirectional block to bidirectional block in reentry arrhythmias but have little effect on depolarization. Most of the drugs in this class have significant actions associated with other classes.

Class IV

CCBs constitute class IV. They were discussed in more detail, including their role in arrhythmia management, earlier in this chapter. They are good for rate control, increasing O_2 supply via vasodilation and afterload reduction. The reduced workload helps depress abnormal function.

Pharmacokinetics

Absorption and Distribution

All classes of antiarrhythmics are well absorbed orally, with sustained-release forms and amiodarone (Cordarone) having slower absorption times (Table 16-12). Bioavailabilities vary greatly depending on protein binding, with propafenone (Rhythmol) having the lowest at 3% bioavailability, with 97% protein binding, and sotalol (Betapace) having the highest (90%), with no protein binding. The presence of food in the gut does not negatively affect bioavailability except for sotalol; food may reduce its absorption by as much as 20%. Fatty food increases dronedarone availability.

Distribution is to most body tissues. Amiodarone exhibits high levels of drug in fat, muscle, lung, and spleen tissues. Cardiac tissue concentration is about 30 times higher than plasma concentration. Amiodarone and quinidine easily cross the placenta. Quinidine and sotalol are found in breast milk, and mexiletine (Mexitil) is found in breast milk in concentrations similar to those found in plasma.

Metabolism and Excretion

All antiarrhythmics are metabolized by the liver. Half-lives of these drugs vary from 3 to 4 hours for procainamide to 26 or more days for amiodarone. As the only short-acting

Table 16–12 ⊞ Pharmacokinetics: Selected Antiarrhythmics

Drug	Onset	Peak	Duration	Bioavailability	Protein Binding	Half-Life	Active Metabolite	Elimination
Amiodarone	1–3 wk	UK	wk–mo	35%–65%	95%	26–107 d	Yes (DEA)	99% in bile
Dronedarone	UK	3–6 h	UK	98%	4% w food; 15% high-fat	13–19 h	Yes (1/10th) potency	Feces 84%; urine 6%
Flecainide	Days	d–wk	12 h	>80%	40%	20 h	No	30% unchanged in urine
Mexiletine	0.5–2 h	2–3 h	8–12 h	>80%	60%–75%	12 h	No	10% unchanged in urine
Propafenone	UK	4–5 d	UK	3%–11%	97%	7 h (90% of patients); 10–32 h in slow metabolizers (10%)	Yes	<1% excreted unchanged
Quinidine PO (sulfate)	0.5 h	1–1.5 h	6–8 h		80%	6–8 h; increased in CHF and severe liver impairment	Yes	20% unchanged in urine; urinary excretion enhanced in acid urine
Quinidine PO (sulfate-ER)	0.5 h	4 h	8–12 h		80%	6–8 h; increased in CHF and severe liver impairment	Yes	20% unchanged in urine; urinary excretion enhanced in acid urine
Quinidine PO (gluconate)	0.5 h	3–5 h	6–8 h		80%	6–8 h; increased in CHF and severe liver impairment	Yes	20%% unchanged in urine; urinary excretion enhanced in acid urine
Sotalol	Hours	2–3 d	UK	90%	Not bound	7–12 h	No	90% unchanged in urine

UK = unknown; CHF = congestive heart failure.

Class II (beta blockers) are covered in Chapter 14; class IV (CCBs) are covered earlier in this chapter.

antiarrhythmic, procainamide requires frequent dosing administration, with steady state achieved in 2 to 3 days. Other antiarrhythmics have longer half-lives and require more time to achieve steady state. Hepatic impairment increases half-life in those drugs eliminated totally or partially in feces. Renal impairment significantly increases half-life in those drugs eliminated all or largely in the urine. Reduced dosages of procainamide and quinidine are required for patients with CHF or renal impairment that decreases volumes of distribution of these drugs. Many cardiac patients who need antiarrythmics have either decreased systolic function or renal impairment. Because of these concerns, quinidine and procainamide are infrequently used for such patients. Approximately 10% of patients are slow metabolizers of propafenone, resulting in an increase in half-life from 7 hours to 10 to 32 hours. Because this drug has been associated with pro-arrhythmia and increased mortality post-MI, the trend is away from its use.

Pharmacotherapeutics

Precautions and Contraindications

Because their mechanisms of action differ, the various classes also have different precautions and contraindications.

Class IA

Antimuscarinic actions in the heart common to this class inhibit vagal effects and may lead to increased sinus rate and AV conduction. Use cautiously for patients with cardiac problems for whom increased heart rate might worsen the condition. Quinidine comes in a gluconate and sulfate form that has different dosing regimens.

Class IB

Use cautiously for patients with HF related to the potential for hypotension secondary to decreased myocardial contractility. This occurs mainly with large doses and in fewer than 10% of patients. The major extra cardiac adverse effects of these drugs are neurological and occur most frequently in older adults, so patients with neurological conditions and older adults should be carefully monitored for these adverse responses.

Class IC

No muscarinic effects are present with this class, but severe exacerbations of arrhythmia have occurred in patients with preexisting ventricular tachyarrhythmias and previous MI, even with normal doses of the drugs. These drugs should be reserved for patients unresponsive to less toxic drugs, especially if these patients have CHF, sinus nodal dysfunction, or heart block.

Class II

BBs are generally contraindicated for patients with unstable bronchospastic disorders such as asthma. They are used with caution for patients with diabetes who have major sugar variation ranges because they decrease insulin secretion and may mask many of the signs of hypoglycemia. BBs are the gold standard to help reduce the second cardiac event post-MI.

This recommendation is based on older data collected prior to the advent of stents and "clot busters" (Bangalore et al, 2014). More recent data puts this indoubt following modern intervention. DM is considered a cardiac risk equivalent. The protective impact of a BB holds greater import in most DM patients than the fear of hypoglycemia. Because of their peripheral vasoconstrictive effects, they are a poor choice for patients with PVD and Raynaud's syndrome. Chronic use is linked with age-related macular degeneration (Klein, Myers, & Klein, 2014) and psoriasis (Wu, Han, Li, & Quershi, 2014).

Abrupt withdrawal of BBs may result in rebound beta stimulation resulting in tachycardia; therefore, they should be tapered by half every 4 hours. Patients at high risk for serious exacerbation of their disease related to abrupt withdrawal include those with angina, CAD with ventricular arrhythmias, and migraines. Hypertensive patients are at lower risk.

Asian patients have a higher probability of lacking an enzyme to handle propranolol, causing toxic profiles that surface early in therapy. BBs are also discussed in Chapters 14 and 40.

Class III

Sotalol is the major class III drug used in primary care. It is a nonselective BB that also prolongs action potential. Its precautions are similar to those for class II. Amiodarone, also a class III drug, has significant properties of several other classes as well. The muscarinic effects associated with sodium channel blockade suggest cautious use for patients with SA or AV nodal dysfunction, bradycardia, or HF. Amiodarone inhibits the enzyme that converts T4 to T3, and iodine is a major component of this drug; therefore, about 5% of patients with underlying predisposition to thyroid disease may develop thyrotoxicosis or hypothyroidism. If this drug must be used to treat the rhythm disturbance, careful monitoring and treatment of the thyroid disorder must be undertaken. Potentially fatal pulmonary fibrosis occurs in 5% to 15% of patients, but preexisting pulmonary disorders do not make the risk more likely. Patients with known risk at baseline should have thyroid and pulmonary function studies done before amiodarone therapy is initiated.

Class III drugs are potassium channel blockers, but they also have effects found in other classes. Amiodarone, quinidine, and sotalol also have effects on sodium channels or beta receptors. "Pure" potassium channel-blocking drugs are currently entering clinical trials. Potassium channel blockade would result in increased action potential duration, increased refractoriness, and reduced automaticity. They should be effective in treating reentry problems, in inhibiting ventricular fibrillation that is due to myocardial ischemia, and in improving contractility.

> **CLINICAL PEARL**
>
> For patients with diabetes who must take a beta blocker, the diaphoresis associated with hypoglycemia is not masked by these drugs, and diabetics should be taught to recognize this indication of hypoglycemia.

Class IV

CCBs have been discussed earlier in this chapter. Worsening HF can trigger more rhythm issues. Only diltiazem and verapamil have FDA-approved rhythm indications.

Adverse Drug Reactions

The more common adverse reactions of antiarrhythmics are extensions of their actions. Reduction in BP may result in dizziness, hypotension, fatigue, and syncope. Decreased myocardial contractility may result in HF. Each class has the potential to produce rhythm disturbances, often exaggerations of or the reverse of the one being treated. Class IC drugs are especially pro-arrhythmic. GI symptoms that are especially disturbing to patients include nausea, vomiting, diarrhea, and constipation and can trigger nonadherence. GI symptoms are especially prevalent in class IA drugs, occurring in 33% to 50% of patients. Although not common, sexual dysfunction and urinary retention may occur in classes I and III. The atropine-like activity of disopyramide (urinary retention, dry mouth, and constipation) may require discontinuance of the drug. Adverse neurological reactions of antiarrhythmics include tremor, blurred vision, and nervousness. Amiodarone has several adverse drug effects not common to other antiarrhythmics, including extrapyramidal syndrome (EPS) effects, hepatitis, epididymitis, corneal deposits, peripheral neuropathy, and extreme burning photosensitivity that can result in a blue-grey skin tone (Drucker & Rosen, 2011). These effects increase with cumulative doses and limit its utility for long-term therapy. Adverse effects associated with beta blockade in class II drugs and sotalol are discussed in Chapter 14. Those relevant to CCBs have been discussed earlier in this chapter. All antiarrhythmics are Pregnancy Category C, except amiodarone, which is Pregnancy Category D.

Drug Interactions

Cross-class and intraclass increases in cardiac effects are common between antiarrhythmics, increasing serum levels and toxicity risks. Several drugs increase or decrease the metabolism of antiarrhythmics: cimetidine (Tagamet), phenobarbital, and rifampin (Rifadin). Phenytoin (Dilantin), which also has class IB antiarrhythmic activity, results in alterations in effectiveness and increases toxicity risk. The anticoagulation effects of warfarin (Coumadin) are increased by many antiarrhythmics, particularly amiodarone.

Additive anticholinergic effects occur as an interaction between several antiarrhythmics and other drugs that have anticholinergic properties. The metabolism and excretions of several class I drugs are significantly affected by urine pH, resulting in altered serum levels and toxicity risk. The CYP 3A4 system is involved in the metabolism of quinidine. Drugs that inhibit this system, including grapefruit juice, may increase free drug levels. CYP 2D6 is involved in flecainide (Tambocor) and propafenone metabolism. Drugs that inhibit this system may similarly increase free drug levels. Selected antiarrhythmics may potentiate the hypotensive effects of antihypertensives, nitrates, and alcohol. BBs may alter the effectiveness of insulin and oral hypoglycemics. Specific drug interactions and the appropriate actions to prevent them are given in Table 16-13.

Table 16–13 ⁝⁝⁝ Drug and Food Interactions: Selected Antiarrhythmics

Drug	Interacting Drug/Food	Possible Effect	Implications
Amiodarone*	Digoxin	Increases blood levels and toxicity risk	Decrease dose of digoxin by 50%. Monitor for toxicity.
	Class I antiarrhythmics	Increase blood levels and toxicity risk	Decrease these drugs by 30%–50%.
	Phenytoin	Increases blood levels of phenytoin; may decrease amiodarone blood levels	Avoid concurrent use. If they must be given together, monitor serum levels of both drugs.
	BBs, CCBs	Increases risk for bradyrhythms, sinus arrest, and AV block	Monitor for dizziness and orthostatic and mental status change. Safety issues.
	Cholestyramine	May decrease amiodarone blood levels	Separate doses by 1 h and give amiodarone first.
	Lovastatin		Limit statin to 40 mg/d (simvastatin 20 mg/d).
	Antihypertensives	May produce profound hypotension	Monitor BP. Safety issues.
Dronedarone	CCB, digoxin, BB, ciprofloxacin, CYP 3A4 inhibitors like grapefruit juice, topical lidocaine, other QT-prolonging agents	Increase dronedarone levels	Toxicity, cardiac suppression Decrease dose or avoid use altogether.
	CYP3A inducers (carbamazepine, phenobar, phenytoin, rifampin	Decrease dronedarone levels	

Continued

Table 16–13 ▦ Drug and Food Interactions: Selected Antiarrhythmics—cont'd

Drug	Interacting Drug/Food	Possible Effect	Implications
	Some statins, BB, CCB (non-dyp), colchicine, dabigatran, tamoxifen	May increase the levels of these drugs	Toxicity of the interacting drugs
	P-glycoproteins (digoxin)	Increase dronedarone	Decrease digoxin dose by 50%
	Phenothiazines, TCA	Both drugs are increased in levels	Contraindicated
	SSRI, midazolam tacrolimus	Increase dronedarone levels	Adjust doses of each
Flecainide[†]	CCBs, disopyramide	Increase arrhythmia risk	
	BBs, verapamil	Additive myocardial depression	Combination should be avoided or given cautiously
	Amiodarone	Doubles serum flecainide levels	Decrease flecainide dose by 50%
	Digoxin	Increases serum digoxin levels by small amount	Monitor serum digoxin level and indications of toxicity
	Alkalinizing agents, foods that increase urine pH to >7,[§] strict vegetarian diet	Promote reabsorption, increase blood levels, increase toxicity risk	Monitor serum levels
	Acidifying agents, foods that decrease urine pH to <5,[§] acidic juices	Increase renal elimination, decrease effectiveness	Monitor serum levels and clinical indicators of effectiveness
Mexiletine	Opioid analgesics, atropine, antacids	Slows absorption of mexiletine	Separate administration of antacids by at least 1 h
	Metoclopramide	Speeds absorption	
	Phenytoin; phenobarbital, cigarette smoking	Increase metabolism and decrease effectiveness of mexiletine	Avoid concurrent use
	Alkalinizing and acidifying agents[§]	Same as with flecainide	Same as with flecainide
Quinidine[†, ‡]	Digoxin	Increases serum levels and toxicity risk	Dosage reduction recommended
	Amiodarone	See amiodarone	See amiodarone
	Phenytoin, phenobarbital	Increase metabolism and decrease effectiveness of quinidine	Monitor therapeutic effects
	Verapamil	Decreases metabolism and increases serum levels of quinidine	Monitor for toxicity
	Antihypertensives, nitrates, alcohol	Additive hypotension	
	Procainamide, propafenone, tricyclic antidepressants (TCAs)	Increase serum levels and risk for toxicity for each of these drugs	
	Drugs with anticholinergic properties	Additive anticholinergic effects	Monitor for dry mouth, wheezing, urinary retention, orthostatic hypotension
	Alkalinizing and acidifying foods and drugs[§]	See flecainide	
Sotalol	General anesthetics, IV phenytoin, CCBs	Additive myocardial depression	
	Digoxin	Additive bradycardia	
	Antihypertensives, nitrates, alcohol	Additive hypotension	
	Amphetamines, ephedrine, epinephrine, norepinephrine, phenylephrine, pseudoephedrine	Unopposed alpha-adrenergic stimulation, leading to excessive HTN and bradycardia	Avoid concurrent use. Teach patient not to use OTCs without contacting health-care provider.
	Amiodarone, disopyramide, procainamide, quinidine	Increase pro-arrhythmia risk	Avoid concurrent use

Table 16–13 ⠿ Drug and Food Interactions: Selected Antiarrhythmics—cont'd

Drug	Interacting Drug/Food	Possible Effect	Implications
	Clonidine	Potentiates rebound HTN when clonidine discontinued	Use caution and monitor BP closely when discontinuing clonidine
	Insulin, oral hypoglycemics	May alter effectiveness of diabetic drugs	Dosage adjustment of diabetic drugs may be required
	Monoamine oxidase inhibitors (MAOIs)	May result in increased HTN	Use cautiously within 14 d of MAOI

*Interacts with warfarin to increase anticoagulation. Monitor prothrombin time. Dosage of warfarin may need to be decreased. For amiodarone, the decrease may be 33%–50%.

†Interacts with cimetidine to increase serum levels of the antiarrhythmic. Choose different histamine$_2$ blocker. Monitor for toxicity if cimetidine must be used.

‡Interacts with rifampin to decrease serum levels and effectiveness of antiarrhythmic. If they must be used together, monitor for decreased therapeutic effect of antiarrhythmic, and adjust dosage as needed.

§Foods that alkalinize urine: all fruits except cranberries, prunes, plums; all vegetables; milk. Foods that acidify urine: cheeses, cranberries, eggs, fish, grains, meats, plums, poultry, prunes.

Clinical Use and Dosing

Atrial Arrhythmias (Atrial Fibrillation/Flutter, Atrioventricular Nodal Reentrant Tachycardia, Wolff–Parkinson–White Tachycardias)

All antiarrhythmics have some use in these disorders. Class IA drugs (quinidine, procainamide) are especially useful. Quinidine has a short-acting form that is given every 4 to 6 hours, a long-acting form for every 8-hour administration, and Quinidex Extentabs, which can be given twice daily (see Table 16-2). It has been combined with mexiletine to enhance effectiveness and reduce adverse effects.

Procainamide can be used in a hemodynamically stable patient for the acute treatment of focal atrial tachycardia and the acute management of stable atrial flutter (American College of Cardiology/American Heart Association/European Society of Cardiology [ACC/AHA/ESC], 2003; ACCF/AHA 2011). It can also be used in the long-term management of recurrent, well-tolerated atrial flutter if combined with an AV node-blocking agent and if no significant structural cardiac disease is present.

Amirodarone is very effective against supraventricular arrhythmias, especially in children, in whom it appears to be quite safe. The wide range of adverse reactions seen in adults and its many drug interactions make it a second-line drug choice. Dronedarone is possibly better for acute atrial fib (AF) conversion but should not be used for persistent AF suppression, because over 65% of patients return to the rhythm in less than 1 year (Connolly et al, 2011).

Reentrant supraventricular tachycardia is a major indication for verapamil; however, it can increase the risk for ventricular fibrillation in patients with reexcitation. It can also be used to decrease the rate in atrial fibrillation/flutter with rapid ventricular response. The long-acting form has the advantage of once-daily administration. The high risk for clot formation associated with atrial fibrillation requires concurrent anticoagulation therapy with warfarin.

Ventricular Arrhythmias (Ventricular Ectopic Beats, Ventricular Tachycardia, Ventricular Fibrillation)

Simple ventricular rhythm disturbances such as occasional PVCs are rarely treated in primary care. Complex ventricular irritability demonstrated with ventricular rhythm disturbances is associated with increased risk for MI and sudden death. Despite this fact, only symptomatic patients with underlying heart disease, malignant forms of arrhythmia such as recurrent ventricular tachycardia, and poor LV function seem to benefit from prophylactic antiarrhythmic therapy. Controlled trials of antiarrhythmic therapy in minimally symptomatic post-MI patients with reduced ejection fractions actually showed increased rates of arrhythmia-associated death in those treated.

Class IA agents have moderate efficacy in treating ventricular arrhythmias and are sometimes prescribed. Disopyramide has a pronounced negative inotropic effect, however, which limits its usefulness. For patients with HF, discontinuation of most antiarrythmics, CCBs, and NSAIDs is recommended (ACCF/AHA, 2009). Class IA agents in patients with reduced left ventricular ejection fraction especially increase the risk of serious arrhythmias. This is also true for class IC flecainide and propafenone and class III sotalol (ACC/AHA, 2003). These drugs are both cardiodepressant and pro-arrhythmic in HF patients. Class IB drugs are fairly weak antiarrhythmics for these problems and are either second-line drugs or used with class IA drugs. Their relatively long half-lives allow two doses daily or three times daily dosing. They are well tolerated in HF, having little negative inotropic effect, with mexiletine more negatively inotropic than tocainide. Class IC drugs are moderately effective but are reserved for very refractory cases because of their pro-arrhythmic qualities.

Class II drugs are useful in exercise-induced ventricular tachycardia but should be monitored with serial exercise testing to check efficacy. They are safe and especially useful in arrhythmias caused by ischemic heart disease because they are among the few drugs proven to reduce CAD mortality. Selection for beta$_1$ receptors reduces many of their adverse reactions. Atenolol (Tenormin) has strong beta$_1$ selectivity, resulting in a low adverse-effect profile, and is used for post-MI arrhythmia prophylaxis. Propranolol (Inderal), a nonselective BB, is used for several arrhythmias. Class III drugs are the best choice for monomorphic ventricular tachycardia.

A common noncardiac cause of tachyarrhythmias is hyperthyroidism. Propranolol, a class II drug, slows the heart rate by its beta-blocking action and has the added effect of preventing peripheral conversion of T4 to T3, thereby reducing the serum levels of the more active form of thyroid hormone. (See hyperthyroid indication in Chap. 41)

Rational Drug Selection

Risk Versus Benefit

The choice of antiarrhythmic drugs is usually based not only on benefit (correction or prevention of the rhythm) but also on risks (adverse effects and toxicity). Benefits may be assessed and drugs chosen by electrophysiological studies. When no agent meets electrophysiological study criteria for choice, empiric amiodarone may be prescribed because of its effects in all classes and because it has been shown to reduce mortality in cardiac arrest survivors from 50% to 20% at 2 years' post-cardiac arrest. The more potentially lethal the arrhythmia is, the more acceptable the risks become. In terms of prevention, only BBs have been definitively shown by research to reduce mortality in relatively asymptomatic patients. Risks related to adverse reactions are present in all antiarrhythmics and increase with higher doses and longer times of administration.

Concurrent Diseases

The presence of diseases in other organ systems may dictate the choice of drug, based on the effects of the antiarrhythmic on that system (bronchospasm in asthma, urinary retention in benign prostatic hyperplasia).

Cost

Many antiarrhythmics are expensive. Those medications requiring frequent monitoring by diagnostic tests need to have the cost of this monitoring factored into final price. For example, amiodarone may require a chest x-ray every 3 to 6 months, pulmonary function tests, and ophthalmic examinations, as well as thyroid-stimulating hormone (TSH) and free thyroxine (T4) levels. This significantly raises the cost of this drug. Generic procainamide requires dosing every 6 to 8 hours; its cost is increased when switched to the sustained-release form, but adherence is improved.

Decision Steps

Because the margin between therapeutic efficacy and toxicity is narrow and the knowledge needed to prescribe these drugs is extensive, it is best to refer patients to a cardiologist for initiation of therapy. Phone consultation may also be required during therapy unless the provider has extensive experience with antiarrhythmic therapy. Several important steps are used in deciding on therapy:

1. Any factor that might be precipitating the arrhythmia should be determined and eliminated. Especially relevant are adverse drug reactions, underlying disease states such as thyroid disorders, and electrolyte disturbances.
2. A firm arrhythmia diagnosis should be established. Use of inappropriate drugs because of a misdiagnosis of the arrhythmia can be catastrophic in some cases.
3. Establish a reliable baseline on which to judge the efficacy of any subsequent dose change or new antiarrhythmic therapy. Methods include ambulatory monitoring, electrophysiological studies, and treadmill exercises.
4. The mere identification of an arrhythmia does not necessarily require its treatment. Evaluation of risk, symptomatology, and a risk/benefit analysis is imperative.

Monitoring

Laboratory Data

Potassium concentration in the extracellular space is the major determinant of resting membrane potential and membrane stability. Levels should always be checked and kept midrange (more than 4 mEq/L) for patients with rhythm disturbances. Renal and hepatic functions (blood urea nitrogen [BUN], creatinine, transaminases) are watched because they are the principal routes of excretion for antiarrhythmic drugs. Antiarrhythmics tend to have narrow therapeutic ranges and are often given to patients who are taking other drugs with which they may interact, increasing the risk of toxicity or lack of efficacy. Serum drug levels should be monitored at regular intervals after steady state is achieved. Timing of the blood draw is critical. The sample is usually drawn 4 to 6 hours after the last oral dose so that a peak serum level is not mistaken for a steady-state level. Anticoagulation studies (prothrombin time [PT], international normalized ratio [INR], activated partial thromboplastin time [apt]) are discussed in Chapter 18. Laboratory studies related to the underlying disease that may be causing the arrhythmia are not discussed here.

Electrocardiogram

Monitoring 12-lead electrocardiograms (ECGs) for indications of efficacy and toxicity is essential, especially concerning drugs for which ECG changes are the primary indicators of such problems. The frequency of monitoring depends on the stability of the patient's drug regimen and the presence of symptoms; however, potential asymptomatic issues with QT changes and development of conduction defects suggest at least yearly recordings.

Other Studies

Electrophysiological studies, echocardiography, and exercise stress testing are best done in consultation with a cardiologist. Monitoring for BBs is discussed in Chapter 14 and for CCBs earlier in this chapter. Monitoring parameters are further delineated in Table 16-14.

Table 16–14   Monitoring Parameters for Selected Antiarrhythmics

Drug	Parameters	Timing	Comments
Amiodarone	Chest x-ray, pulmonary function studies	Every 3–6 mo	High risk for pulmonary fibrosis. Risk of sudden cardiac death may outweigh risk associated with pulmonary dysfunction. Every effort should be made to rule out other treatable cause of pulmonary problem. Some providers schedule tests based on symptoms after 1 yr without problems.
	Thyroid-stimulating hormone (TSH), free T_4	Every 6 mo	Monitor closely for other indications of thyroid dysfunction as well
	Ophthalmic exam (slit lamp and fundoscopy)	Every 6 mo	Although rare, visual impairment may progress to permanent blindness. Any symptoms of impairment should result in prompt ophthalmic exam. Corneal microdeposits are reversible with reduction in dose and no reason to stop treatment.
Flecainide*	ECG Liver function studies Serum drug levels		Watch for sinus node problems and AV block. Highly metabolized in liver. Liver disease may significantly increase free drug level. Keep trough <1 mcg/mL.
Mexiletine*	Liver function studies		Aspartate aminotransferase (AST) elevations >3 times upper limit of normal (ULN) have been observed. Assess for other treatable causes such as CHF or acute MI before stopping drug.
Procainamide†	Complete blood count (CBC) Antinuclear antibody (ANA) titer		At initiation of therapy to assess for blood dyscrasias At initiation of therapy and at any indication of lupus-like syndrome
Propafenone	Liver function studies		Highly metabolized by liver. Liver disease may increase bioavailability to 70%.
Quinidine†	CBC, renal and liver function studies		Discontinue drug if blood dyscrasias or hepatic or renal dysfunction occurs.
Sotalol	Fasting blood glucose		May affect insulin secretion and glucose metabolism. May mask indications of hypoglycemia in patients with diabetes.

All require monitoring of potassium level and 12-lead ECG. Most require serum drug levels. Monitoring of renal function is prudent in all.

   *Changes in urine pH can alter drug excretion. Monitor urinalysis on annual visits.

   †ECG changes are the primary indicators of toxicity in these drugs. QRS >25% above normal or prolonged QT intervals suggest reduction in dose by as much as 50%.

Patient Education

Cardiac rhythm disturbances tend to engender fear. A thin line exists between enough information to have the patient appreciate the seriousness of the disorder (or the lack of seriousness in benign forms of arrhythmia) and, therefore, adhere to the treatment regimen, and so much information that fear or denial takes over and adherence suffers. Most patients and their families appreciate an honest discussion of the disorder and the requirements for frequent monitoring that allow safer and effective treatment. Most antiarrhythmics have annoying side effects that patients are more likely to tolerate when the importance of the drug is explained.

Administration

The patient should take the drug exactly as prescribed. For doses taken more than once daily, the doses should be evenly spaced. Abrupt withdrawal of these drugs may result in life-threatening arrhythmias, HTN, or myocardial ischemia. The patient should keep enough medication on hand for weekends, holidays, and vacations. For amiodarone, if a dose is missed at its usual time, it should not be taken at all that day; the patient should simply take the next day's dose. Its very long half-life maintains a stable level. For disopyramide, mexiletine, procainamide sustained-release, propafenone, and tocainide, a dose that is missed should be taken as soon as it is remembered, unless the next dose is due in 4 hours or less. For flecainide, the missed dose should be taken unless the next dose is due in 6 hours, and for sotalol, 8 hours. For quinidine and standard formulations of procainamide, the separation is 2 hours.

Several drugs come in more than one formulation, from standard to sustained-release (Table 16-15). The patient should read the label carefully and follow the appropriate dosing schedule, especially if the drug is changed to a different form or a different drug. For sustained-release formulations, the tablets should not be crushed or chewed but must be swallowed whole. Patients who have difficulty in swallowing should be placed on standard formulations that can be crushed.

Food intake is a concern with some of the antiarrhythmics. Sotalol absorption is significantly decreased when it is taken with food, so it should always be taken on an empty stomach. Mexiletine, tocainide, and quinidine, however, have uncomfortable GI adverse effects unless they are taken

Table 16–15 ⊗ Dosage Schedule for Selected Outpatient Labeled Uses: Selected Antiarrhythmics

Drug	Indication/Plasma Concentration	Dosage Forms	Starting Dose	Maintenance Dose
Amiodarone (Cordarone, Pacerone) (G)	Ventricular arrhythmias Level: 1–2 mcg/mL	Tablets: 100 mg (Pacerone only); 200, 400 mg	800–1,600 mg/d in 1–2 divided doses for 1–3 wk; then 600–800 mg in divided doses for a month	Maint: 400 mg/d
Atenolol (Tenormin) (G)	Prevent primary arrhythmic event post-MI	Tablets: 25, 50, 100 mg	100 mg daily or 50 mg 2 doses daily	100 mg daily or 50 mg 2 doses daily for at least 9 d: post-MI
	Insufficient control of atrial fibrillation with digoxin		25–50 mg/d added to digoxin dose	100 mg/d; 50 mg/d if severe renal impairment
Flecainide* (Tambocor) (G)	Sustained ventricular tachycardia, PSVT	Tablets: 50, 100, 150 mg	100 mg q12 h for ventricular tachycardia; 50 mg q12h for PSVT	100–150 mg q12h for ventricular tachycardia; 50–100 q12h for PSVT MAX Adjusted Dose: Ventricular tachycardia: 400 mg/d; PSVT: 300 mg/d; adjust doses by 50 mg increments; minimum 4 d between adjustments
Mexiletine (Mexitil) (G)	Ventricular arrhythmias Level: 0.5–2 mcg/mL	Capsules: 150, 200, 250 mg	200 mg q8h (if rapid control of arrhythmia is essential, load with 400 mg)	200–300 mg q8h MAX Adjusted Dose: 1, 200 mg/d: adjust doses by 50–100 mg increments; minimum 2–3 d between adjustments.
Propafenone* Rythmol (G)	Ventricular arrhythmias (unlabeled use in PSVT associated with WPW) Level: 0.2–1.5 mcg/mL (nonlinear change in plasma level related to dose increase)	Tablet: 150, 225, 300 mg	150 mg q8h	225–300 mg q8h MAX Adjusted Dose: 300 mg per dose Increases doses at minimum of 34 d intervals:
Propafenone SR (Rythmol SR)		Capsule SR	225 mg every 12 hours	325 mg Max: 425 mg Increase dose in 5 d intervals
Propranolol (Inderal, (G)	PSVT: atrial fibrillation; tachycardias associated with digitalis toxicity, excessive catecholamines; thyroid disorders	Tablets: 10, 20, 40, 60, 80 mg Solution (500 mL): 4 mg/mL, 8 mg/mL	10–30 mg 3 times daily–4 doses daily given ac and hs; for atrial fibrillation uncontrolled by digoxin, add 40–80 mg of propranolol to digoxin dose	Max Adjusted Dose: 240 mg/d
Quinidine Sulfate (G) Quinidine Gluconate (G)	Conversion/prevention atrial fibrillation, atrial flutter, atrioventricular nodal reentry; suppress ventricular rhythms not associated with complete heart block	Tablets: 200, 300 mg; Tablet XR: 300, 324 mg Dose of 267 gluconate = to 200 mg sulfate	Single-dose 200 mg to assess for idiosyncratic reaction. Then 300 mg of gluconate or 324 mg sulfate every 8–12 h.	200–300 mg 3 times daily or 4 doses daily immed. release; 300 mg–600 mg q8h for sustained release†*
Sotalol (Betapace)(G)	Ventricular arrhythmias	Tablets: 80, 120, 160, 240 mg	80 mg 2 doses daily	240–320 mg/d in 2 divided doses; Max Adjusted Dose: 640 mg; adjust doses at minimum 3 d interval
(Betapacce AF) (G)	Suppression AF	Tablets: 80, 120, 160 mg. Cannot substitute regular Betapace	80 mg 2 doses daily	120 mg twice daily Max: 160 mg twice daily

PSVT = paroxysmal supraventricular tachycardia; MI = myocardial infarction; WPW = Wolff–Parkinson–White syndrome.

*Because of pro-arrhythmic effects, use with lesser arrhythmias is not recommended.

†Because the rate of absorption from various sustained-release formulations may be markedly different, they are not interchangeable.

with food. Foods that alter urine pH affect the excretion of flecainide, mexiletine, and quinidine and should be avoided or taken in consistent amounts. (See Table 16-13 for a list of such foods.)

Drug interactions are frequent with both prescription and OTC drugs. The patient should consult a health-care provider before taking any other drugs, including OTC cold remedies.

Adverse Reactions

Dizziness is the most common adverse response. Changing position slowly, especially when arising from a lying position, decreases this reaction. Caution should be taken in driving or other activities that require alertness until any sedating response is known. Monitoring of pulse rate and rhythm and BP provides early indications of efficacy and toxicity. Patients should learn to take their own pulse and BP and check them whenever symptoms occur. Hypotension and slow, rapid, or irregular heart rates should be reported promptly. Bone marrow is affected in some classes. Patients should report fever, chills, sore throat, or unusual bruising. Photosensitivity may occur through window glass, thin clothing, and low-value sunscreens for patients who are taking amiodarone, disopyramide, or quinidine. Protective clothing and high SPF sunblock are recommended during therapy and for 4 months following it. Some find wearing dark glasses helpful for photosensitivity in the eyes. With amiodarone, a bluish discoloration of the skin in areas exposed to sunlight may occur. It is usually reversible and fades over several months. This drug is also associated with epididymitis and pulmonary fibrosis. Patients should report scrotal pain or swelling and decreased exercise tolerance. Procainamide occasionally is associated with a lupus-like syndrome. Joint swelling and rashes should be reported. Frequently using mouthwashes, practicing good oral hygiene, chewing sugarless gum, or sucking on hard candy may relieve the dry mouth commonly found with disopyramide. The patient should notify the health-care provider if dry mouth, constipation, difficulty in urinating, or blurred vision persist with this drug. Tremors are an early indication of excessive doses of mexiletine and should be reported promptly.

For all of these drugs, the importance of keeping follow-up appointments to monitor efficacy and adverse reactions cannot be overstated. Failure to discover problems early can result in permanent adverse changes and include life-threatening events.

Because these drugs are Pregnancy Category C or D, female patients capable of childbearing should be made aware of the risks of these drugs, and contraception should be instituted before prescribing them.

Lifestyle Management

Lifestyle management is similar to that discussed for ACEIs and general cardiovascular health. The patient should carry a medical identification card that states the name of the drug and the disorder for which it is being taken. Patient education related to BBs is discussed in Chapter 14. CG and CCB issues were covered earlier.

NITRATES

Nitrates were first introduced for the treatment of angina in the 19th century. Their ability to affect both oxygen supply and demand and their effectiveness in rapid relief of acute angina has made them one important part of the treatment for this disorder. They are joined by other drug groups to control this pain syndrome. A newer drug not part of the nitrate, CCB, or ACE/ARB drug classes is ranolazine (Renexa). This medication is not indicated in acute angina. It is covered in more detail in Chapter 28 on angina management, not in the section below.

Pharmacodynamics

Nitroglycerin (NTG) and its analogues act largely by providing more nitric oxide (NO) to vascular endothelium and arterial smooth muscle, resulting in vasodilation (Fig. 16-5). All parts of the vascular system, from larger arteries to large veins, relax in response to nitrates. Nitrates affect the supply–demand equation on both sides. Dilation of venous capacitance vessels results in decreased systemic vascular resistance (afterload), venous pooling, and decreased venous return to the heart, which leads to decreased preload. Arterial dilation, which occurs more commonly with higher doses, decreases systemic arterial pressure, resulting in decreased afterload. MOD is reduced by the reduced cardiac workload.

The decreased venous return decreases LV end-diastolic pressure (preload), resulting in decreased wall tension and an increased transmyocardial gradient. This increased gradient improves perfusion between the coronary arteries and the subendocardium and increases oxygen supply to the myocardium. Their coronary artery vasodilating effect—originally thought to be their primary role in improving MOD—is now thought to play a limited role because of atherosclerotic changes in the coronary arteries. They have little effect on angina associated with longer-duration atherosclerotic CAD.

Indirect actions include reflex responses of baroreceptors and hormonal mechanisms to decreased arterial pressure. The primary mechanism is sympathetic discharge, resulting in tachycardia and increased myocardial contractility. Another action of clinical significance is on platelet aggregation. NO released from NTG increases cyclic guanosine monophosphate (cGMP), resulting in decreased platelet aggregation. This action is believed to play a role in reduction of infarct size and mortality post-MI for patients given IV NTG and may also exist for other forms of NTG. Relaxation of smooth muscle of the bronchi, GI tract, and genitourinary tract also occurs but so briefly that this action is not considered clinically significant.

Pharmacokinetics

Absorption and Distribution

Nitrates are well absorbed by oral, buccal, sublingual, and transdermal routes (Table 16-16). Sublingual absorption is dependent on salivary secretion. Dry mouth (including drug-induced) decreases absorption. Amyl nitrite is available

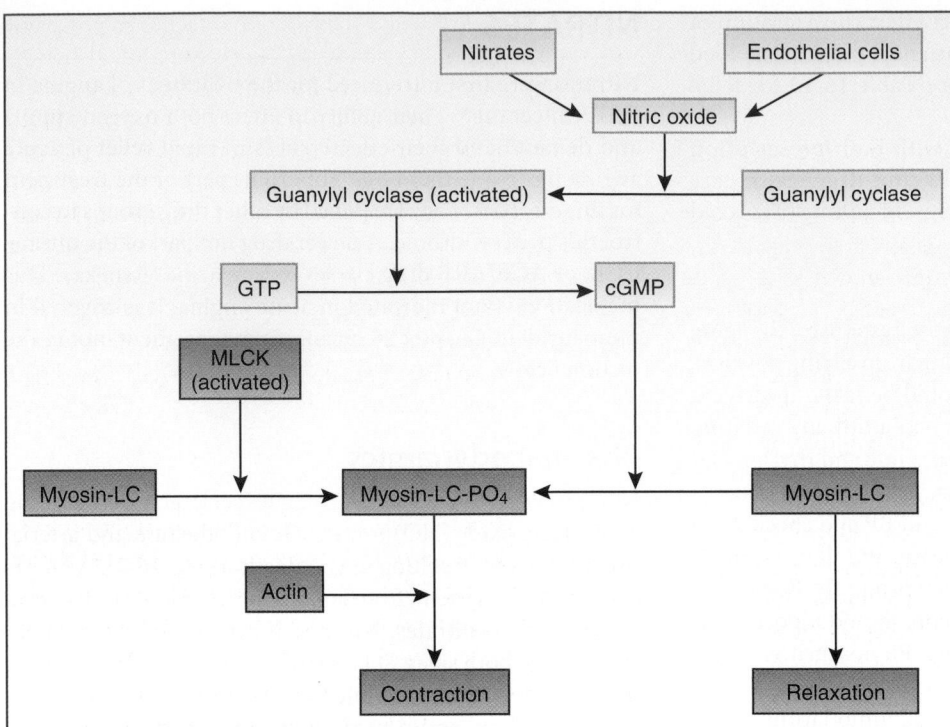

Figure 16–5. Action of substances that increase nitric oxide concentration in smooth muscle cells. Nitrates, nitrites, and other substances that increase nitric oxide concentration in smooth muscle cells potentiate the activation of guanylyl cyclase. Activated guanylyl cyclase then facilitates the production of cyclic guanosine monophosphate (cGMP). Through a series of not clearly known intermediate steps, the cGMP facilitates the dephosphorylation of the myosin light chain, resulting in muscle relaxation.

Table 16–16 ✚ Pharmacokinetics: Selected Nitrates

Drug	Onset	Peak	Duration	Metabolite	Half-Life	Excretion
Amyl nitrate inhalant	0.5 min		3–5 min	None	UK	1/3 in urine
Isosorbide dinitrate, sublingual	2–5 min	6 min	1–3 h	Mononitrate	Drug 45 min Metabolite: 2–5 h	In urine
Isosorbide dinitrate, Oral	20–40 min	6 min	4–6 h	Isosorbide mononitrate	Drug: 45 min Metabolite: 2–5 h	In urine
Isosorbide dinitrate, oral (SR)	Up to 4 h	6 min	6–8 h	Isosorbide mononitrate	Drug: 45 min Metabolite: 2–5 h	In urine
Isosorbide mononitrate, oral	30–60 min	UK	7 h	Metabolized to glycerol and CO_2	UK	In urine and lung
Isosorbide mononitrate, oral (SR)	Slow	3–4 h	>12 h	Metabolized to glycerol and CO_2	UK	In urine and lung
NTG, sublingual	1–3 min	4 min	30–60 min	1,2-dinitroglycerol and 1,3-dinitroglycerol	Drug: 1–3 min Metabolites: approx. 40 min	In urine
NTG, translingual spray	2 min	4 min	30–69 min	1,2-dinitroglycerol and 1,3-dinitroglycerol	Drug: 1–3 min Metabolites: approx. 40 min	In urine
NTG oral (SR)	20–45 min	UK	3–8 h	1,2-dinitroglycerol and 1,3-dinitroglycerol	Drug: 1–3 min Metabolites: approx. 40 min	In urine
NTG transdermal patch	30–60 min	UK	Up to 24 h	1,2-dinitroglycerol and 1,3-dinitroglycerol	Drug: 1–3 min Metabolites: approx. 40 min	In urine

UK = unknown. All have approximately 60% protein binding. Half-life of NTG is 1–4 min; others have longer half-lives, with SR preparations up to 12 h.

in an inhaled form ("popper"), providing for very rapid absorption, but its use is not common clinically.

Metabolism and Excretion

Oral nitrates have a significant hepatic first-pass effect. Hepatic organic nitrate reductase removes nitrate groups from the parent molecule, yielding less potent vasodilators than the parent drug and resulting in low bioavailability for most products. Oral nitrates must be given in sufficiently high doses to sustain blood levels despite the first-pass effect. NTG has a short half-life (1 to 4 min), but the two major metabolites (1,2 and 1,3 dinitrates) have longer half-lives and appear in substantial concentrations, making them responsible for some of the pharmacological activity. The dinitrates are further metabolized to mononitrates. Isosorbide dinitrate is metabolized to active metabolites that accumulate more than the parent drug with long-term therapy. Because isosorbide mononitrate is the major active metabolite of isosorbide dinitrate and most of the clinical activity is attributed to this metabolite, it is now available as a single-entity product with a bioavailability of nearly 100%.

The sublingual route avoids hepatic first-pass effect and is preferred for achieving a rapid blood level. The buccal and transdermal routes also avoid the first-pass problems but have slower onsets of action. Total duration of effect by these routes is brief. When longer duration of action is needed, oral or topical preparations are given.

Metabolism of nitrates leads to glucuronide derivatives and carbon dioxide excreted by the kidneys and the lungs. Table 16-16 includes the pharmacokinetics of all formulations.

Pharmacotherapeutics

Precautions and Contraindications

Precautions and contraindications are largely related to the actions of these drugs. Vasodilation can result in increased intracranial pressure, so nitrates are contraindicated in head trauma or cerebral hemorrhage. Vasodilation can also result in postural hypotension. Patients with volume depletion and anemia should avoid using nitrates. *Drug Facts and Comparisons* (Wolters Kluwer Health, 2011) states that closed-angle glaucoma is also a contraindication because intraocular pressure (IOP) may be increased. Some individuals have hypersensitivity or idiosyncratic responses to nitrates and must avoid them. For the transdermal patches, allergy to their adhesive may limit their use.

Because the activity of these drugs may compromise maternal-to-fetal circulation, they are Pregnancy Category C. Amyl nitrite is Pregnancy Category X because it markedly reduces system BP and blood flow on the maternal side of the placenta. It is not known if nitrates are excreted in breast milk. The importance of the drug for the mother and possible risks to the infant should be taken into consideration when deciding on nitrate use in nursing mothers. Safety and efficacy in children have not been established.

Adverse Drug Reactions

The major adverse reactions are direct extensions of therapeutic vasodilation: orthostatic hypotension with potential for syncope, tachycardia, and throbbing headache. Hypotension may result in decreased diastolic filling pressure, and the tachycardia may result in decreased diastolic filling time, leading to myocardial ischemia, arrhythmias, and rebound HTN. Headache may be severe and persists in up to 50% of patients. For patients with severe, persistent headache, it may be necessary to use a different drug group to treat the disease process.

Less common adverse reactions include nausea, vomiting, incontinence of urine and feces, dysuria, impotence, and urinary frequency. Nonallergic rash and cutaneous vasodilation with flushing may occur with transdermal applications. This can be reduced by rotating sites. The vasodilating effect is linked with an increased risk of age-related macular degeneration (Klein et al, 2014).

Tolerance

With continuous exposure, smooth muscle develops clinically significant tolerance (tachyphylaxis). In well-controlled clinical trials, nitrates were no more effective than placebo after 18 to 24 hours of continuous therapy, particularly for long-acting/sustained-release preparations. The mechanisms by which this occurs are not fully understood. One mechanism proposed is that, over time, decreased substrate (sulfhydryl) results in decreased cGMP, leading to decreased vasodilation. Orally bioavailable compounds containing sulfhydryl groups, such as *N*-acetylcysteine, may also diminish tolerance to the hemodynamic effects of nitrates in HF. Attempts to overcome nitrate tolerance by increasing dosage have failed. Only after nitrates have been absent from the body for 10 to 12 hours does their effectiveness return. See the section "Clinical Use and Dosing" for recommendations to overcome this problem.

Drug Interactions

Additive hypotension is possible with other drug classes that have actions or adverse effects of hypotension (i.e., antihypertensives, BBs, CCBs, haloperidol, or phenothiazines). Drugs with anticholinergic effects may decrease absorption of sublingual or buccal NTG. Aspirin increases nitrate serum concentrations and may potentiate their action. Nitrates may decrease the pharmacological effects of heparin. Specific drug interactions and the appropriate actions to prevent them are given in Table 16-17.

Clinical Use and Dosing

Angina

Oxygen extracted from the coronary arteries is at maximum efficiency at all times, so there is no oxygen reserve during periods of increased oxygen demand. Ischemia occurs when demand exceeds supply. Increased oxygen supply is created by dilating the arteries to bring more blood flow to the myocardium. Unfortunately, atherosclerosis and plaque formation makes dilation of these arteries difficult, if not impossible. Although they have some ability to dilate the coronary arteries, nitrates are also able to facilitate movement of oxygen across the arterial–myocardial membrane. Their use in CAD relates as much to this action as it does to vasodilation. Ischemia caused by the imbalance between MOS and MOD produces pain (angina).

Table 16–17 ⠿ Drug Interactions: Nitrates

Drug	Interacting Drug	Possible Effect	Implications
Isosorbide dinitrate	Antihypertensives, alcohol, BBs, phenothiazines	Additive hypotension	Monitor BP closely. Isosorbide mononitrate Teach home BP monitoring.
NTG	Antihypertensives, alcohol, BBs, CCBs, haloperidol, phenothiazines	Additive hypotension	Monitor BP closely. Teach home BP monitoring.
	Agents with anticholinergic properties	May decrease absorption of SL and buccal formulations	Use other formulation if possible

There are three types of angina: chronic stable angina, unstable angina, and Prinzmetal's angina. Chronic stable angina (exertional angina) is caused by narrowing of the arterial lumen and hardening of the arterial walls so that the affected vessels cannot dilate in response to the increased MOD associated with physical exertion or emotional stress. For many patients with stable, predictable angina, nitrates are sufficient to control symptoms. Dosage depends on formulation, with sublingual doses used to treat acute attacks and long-acting forms used for chronic prevention (Table 16-18). In exertional angina, short-acting forms taken within 5 or 10 minutes of exercise may prevent the anginal episode. For an angina episode, sublingual dosing is 0.4 to 0.6 mg every 5 minutes for up to three doses. If the angina is not relieved by the second dose, the recommendation is to take the third dose and call 911. Dosing for isosorbide dinitrate, a long-acting form, is 10 to 40 mg orally twice or three times daily; the sustained-release form is 40 to 80 mg daily. Isosorbide mononitrate dosing is 20 mg twice daily. For both long-acting forms, twice-daily dosing on an eccentric schedule, with doses separated by 7 hours, is preferred to reduce problems with tolerance.

For variant (Prinzmetal's) angina, in which the mechanism may be largely related to vasospasm, long-acting nitrates

Table 16–18 ⠿ Dosage Schedule: Selected Nitrates

Clinical Use	Dosage Form	Starting Dose	Maintenance Dose
Treatment of acute angina (if NTG not effective)	Tablets SL: 2.5, 5, 10 mg	2.5–5 mg SL every 5–10 min	Titrate upward until angina relieved or adverse reactions limit. *Max* of 3 doses in 15–30 min
Treatment and prevention of angina; not for acute attack	Tablets: 5, 10, 20, 30, 40 mg (B) SR Caps (B): 40 mg	Tablets: 5–20 mg 2–3 times/d; SR Caps: 40–160 mg/d or 40 mg twice daily	10–40 mg bid (eccentric schedule 8 a.m. and 2 p.m.)
Treatment and prevention of angina; not for acute attack	Tablets: 10, 20 mg	5–10 mg 2 doses daily (eccentric schedule)	20 mg 2 doses daily (eccentric schedule)
Same as above	Tablets ER: 30, 60, 120 mg	30–60 mg daily	120 mg daily after several days on initial dose *Max*: 240 mg/d
Prophylaxis	Tablets: 0.3, 0.4, 0.6 mg	5–10 min prior to activities that might precipitate attack	N/A
Treatment of acute anginal attacks		0.4–0.6 mg tab under tongue every 5 min 3 times	Max: 3 tabs in 15 min
Prophylaxis	Spray: 0.4 mg/spray in 4.9 or 12 g	5–10 min prior to activities that might precipitate attack. Do not inhale spray.	
Treatment of acute anginal attacks		1–2 metered sprays onto or under tongue	3 metered sprays in 15 min
Prophylaxis or treatment of angina	Capsule: 2.5, 6.5, 9 mg	2.5–2.6 mg 3 times daily or 4 doses daily	Increase by 2.6/2.6 mg increments over a period of days or weeks until adverse reactions limit or reach 2.6 mg 4 doses/d
Prevention of angina	0.1., 0.2, 0.4, 0.6, 0.8 mg/h	0.2–0.4 mg/h on 12–14 h, then off 10–12 h	0.4–0.8 mg/h on 12–14 h, then off 10–12 h

(I) = Isordil brand; (S) = Sorbitrate brand; (M) = IMSO; (Mo) = Monoket; (Im) = Imdur. Patches: (M) = Minitran; (N) = NitroDur; (T) = Transderm-Nitro. Patch.

are occasionally sufficient to control symptoms, although CCBs are often added to the treatment regimen. Dosing is similar. For unstable angina, the prophylactic value of long-acting nitrates is uncertain, depending on the underlying pathology.

Angina nonresponding to initial therapy suggests serious progression of illness and the need for immediate assessment in a monitored area of an emergency room. Early therapy for such patients includes aspirin, nitroglycerine, and morphine. Long-acting nitrates appear to reduce mortality in trials that did not include thrombolysis. Optimal therapy for post-infarction angina is with BBs and long-acting nitrates. Isosorbide dinitrate is effective for this indication.

Heart Failure

With the advent of ACEIs and ARBs and the redefined role of BBs in HF, the newer guidelines no longer present an early role for nitrates in the management of HF (see Chap. 36). Their role in reducing ventricular filling pressure and pulmonary and system vascular resistance is sometimes useful. Isosorbide dinitrate administered chronically has been shown to be effective in improving exercise capacity and in reducing symptoms. Its limited effect on systemic vascular resistance and the problem of tolerance means that it is rarely single-drug therapy. Combining this drug with hydralazine has produced a more sustained improvement than either drug alone.

Initiation of Therapy

Start low and go slow are the appropriate steps if chronic therapy is indicated. Advancing low doses slowly over a period of 1 to 2 weeks usually results in the desired effects without the headaches or severe orthostasis. Headache or its absence is not a reliable variable by which to judge therapy because tachyphylaxis for this adverse effect is common within 1 to 4 weeks. Dosage increases should be made against the following parameters:

1. Reduced angina or lack of angina occurs with usual activity.
2. Heart rate at rest increases by no more than 15 bpm.
3. BP does not fall to the point of causing orthostatic hypotension.

Prevention of Tolerance

To prevent or reduce the development of tolerance, a nitrate-free interval of 10 to 12 hours/day is required. This is why nitro patches are applied and removed within a set period of time. Sustained-release preparations are more likely to lead to tolerance and should be avoided unless used daily. Short-acting products with two or three doses daily are less likely to lead to tolerance. For twice-daily dosing, use an eccentric dosing schedule separated by 7 hours (e.g., 7 a.m., 2 p.m.). Patients whose anginal symptoms occur at night may do best with a daytime nitrate-free interval, and the reverse holds for those whose symptoms occur during the daytime. If around-the-clock coverage is necessary for anginal symptoms, using a BB or CCB during the nitrate-free interval may be needed.

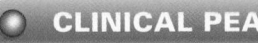 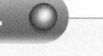

CLINICAL PEARL

Patients with migraine headaches are especially at risk for **nitrate headaches**. Start them first on a beta blocker for migraine prophylaxis, and then add the nitrate to prevent the problem with chronic use.

Rational Drug Selection

Formulation and Cost

Sublingual NTG has rapid action, long-established efficacy, easy use, and low cost. A disadvantage is its short duration of action. It is also volatile and must be kept in a tightly capped, amber container and stored in a cool place. Once a bottle is opened, it is generally effective for only about 6 months. Onset and duration of action of a single metered dose of translingual spray is about the same as for sublingual NTG. Each canister contains 200 doses and retains efficacy for up to 3 years. Some skill is required to use it; however, patients with advanced arthritis may prefer it to opening tightly closed bottles. Cost per dose is substantially higher than for the sublingual form, but the prolonged shelf-life helps reduce total cost for those patients who rarely need a dose. It is also a good alternative for patients who wear dentures or have dry mucosa.

Transdermal delivery systems offer easy use and release NTG at a constant rate to maintain steady-state plasma levels. Bioavailability varies significantly from patient to patient. Physical exercise and ambient temperatures may increase absorption.

Oral NTG has questionable efficacy and is available only in sustained release, a form associated with increased incidence of tolerance. Among the oral nitrates, isosorbide dinitrate provides sustained nitrate activity and better anginal prophylaxis. Single doses significantly improve hemodynamic parameters and exercise tolerance for up to 4 hours. Its action is not as rapid as sublingual NTG but does occur in 15 to 30 minutes, which is appropriate for angina prevention but not emergency intervention.

In generic form, the cost of NTG is low. Chewable forms provide more rapid onset of action, but the duration of action falls to about 2 hours. Because there appears to be no clear benefit over sublingual NTG, the higher cost may not justify chewable forms. Isosorbide dinitrate is also available in a sustained-release form that requires only one to two doses daily, but it has highly variable intestinal absorption, and the risk of nitrate tolerance is higher unless it is used only once daily.

Isosorbide mononitrate offers 100% bioavailability and the convenience of once-daily dosing, but otherwise appears to have no significant clinical advantage over isosorbide dinitrate. Nitrate tolerance occurs less often for the regular formulation. The sustained-release form has the same problems with tolerance as other sustained-release formulations, and the cost is higher.

Monitoring

No specific laboratory monitoring parameters exist for nitrates. Taking the history of efficacy and the number of tablets to get pain relief is key. Trends of increased use can be tolerance, use of expired meds, or progression of the disease state.

Patient Education

Administration

Patients should take the drug exactly as prescribed. For oral doses taken more than once daily, a nitrate-free interval of 10 to 12 hours is necessary to prevent nitrate tolerance. An eccentric dosing schedule separated by 7 hours (e.g., 7 a.m., 2 p.m.) must be explained to help adherence.

Several drugs come in more than one formulation, from standard to sustained release (see Table 16-18). The patient should read the label if the drug is changed to a different form or a different drug. For sustained-release formulations, the tablets should not be crushed or chewed but must be swallowed whole, and they should be stored in tightly closed amber glass containers. Tablets lose potency when exposed to air, heat, or moisture or when mixed with other tablets. The bottle should not be opened frequently or kept next to the body (e.g., in a shirt pocket) or in an automobile glove compartment. A burning sensation under the tongue is not a reliable method of testing potency. When first opened, the bottle should be dated. It should be replaced within 6 months.

At the first sign of an angina attack, the patient should sit down and place one sublingual tablet under the tongue and allow it to dissolve. It should not be swallowed. If the pain is not relieved, repeat every 5 minutes for up to three doses. If the angina is not relieved by the second dose, the patient should take the third dose and call 911. Dry mouth may reduce the effectiveness of sublingual NTG. Dry-mouth problems should be discussed with the health-care provider. Sublingual spray, which is useful even with dry mouth, may be used in the same manner as the tablet. Lift the tongue and spray the dose under the tongue.

Transdermal patches also require a nitrate-free interval of 10 to 12 hours. The site of application should be changed each time, with the best sites being the anterior chest and the upper arms in areas not covered with hair. Before applying, the clear plastic cover over the medication side of the patch should be removed. A firm pressure should be applied over the patch to ensure contact with the skin. Physical exercise and ambient temperatures may increase absorption by this route. Caregivers should avoid touching the active portion of the patch to avoid getting a HA. Gloves are recommended.

For all forms, doses should not be doubled and should not be discontinued abruptly, which may result in rebound angina. Concurrent use of alcohol should be avoided with these drugs. Because some OTC drugs interact with nitrates or contain alcohol, no new OTC drugs should be taken, including cold remedies, without first discussing this with the health-care provider.

Adverse Reactions

The major adverse reactions are throbbing headaches, rapid heart rates, and decreased BP when arising from a sitting or lying position, with the potential for fainting. Headache may be severe; it is best treated with acetaminophen (Tylenol).

Unremitting headaches should be reported to the health-care provider. Rapid heart rate reactions post-dose should also be reported right away. They may worsen the condition for which the nitrate is prescribed. The chronic background headaches with newly prescribed daily dose formulations abate over a few weeks.

Incontinence of urine and bowel movements, pain on urination, frequent urination, and impotence are rare adverse responses. They should be reported so that a potential cause other than the nitrate can be ruled out or alterations in the drug regimen can be undertaken.

Lifestyle Management

See the previous drug class sections for general information. Orthostatic changes should be anticipated. Slowly making position changes minimizes the BP changes. When arising from lying down, the patient should sit on the edge of the bed for a few minutes before standing to allow the body to adjust to this different position.

PERIPHERAL VASODILATORS (PADs)

Peripheral vasodilators (PADs) are used to treat resistant HTN and PVD, although significant clinical improvement of PVD rarely occurs with these drugs alone. Peripheral alpha$_1$ antagonists and central alpha$_2$ agonists can be used for these purposes. They are discussed in Chapter 14. The focus of the discussion here is on the two remaining PAD drugs, hydralazine (Apresoline) and minoxidil (Loniten). Both are seldom-used add-on therapies, not first-line HTN medications.

Pharmacodynamics

Peripheral vasodilators useful in the treatment of HTN act by direct relaxation and dilation of arteriolar smooth muscle, thereby decreasing PVR. They do not dilate the epicardial coronary arteries and do not relax venous smooth muscle. Minoxidil is considered the more potent.

Pharmacokinetics

Absorption and Distribution

Hydralazine is well absorbed orally. Taking it with food increases absorption. It is widely distributed and crosses the placenta but enters breast milk in minimal amounts. It is compatible with breastfeeding, according to the American Academy of Pediatrics. Minoxidil is also well absorbed orally and widely distributed. It enters breast milk in larger amounts and should not be used while breastfeeding (see Table 16-19).

Metabolism and Excretion

With hydralazine, bioavailability is low and variable among patients, based on their genetics. Rapid acetylators have greater hepatic first-pass metabolism, lower bioavailability, and less antihypertensive benefit than do slow acetylators. Although hydralazine's half-life is short, vascular effects persist longer than blood concentrations would suggest, based on

Table 16–19 ⊞ **Pharmacokinetics: Selected Peripheral Vasodilators**

Drug	Onset	Peak	Duration	Protein Binding	Bioavailability	Half-Life	Elimination
Hydralazine PO	45 min	1–2 h	6–12 h	87%	30%–50%	3–7 h	12%–14% in urine
Minoxidil	30 min	2–3 h	24+ h	None	UK	4.2 h	20% in urine

UK = unknown.

the avid binding of this drug to vascular tissue. Minoxidil is not protein bound and has a higher bioavailability. Its half-life is also short, but it also has a longer antihypertensive effect because of the persistence of its active metabolite, minoxidil sulfate.

Pharmacotherapeutics

Precautions and Contraindications

Use cautiously in patients with cardiovascular disease. Myocardial ischemia may result from the increased oxygen demand associated with SNS stimulation. Because these drugs do not dilate the epicardial coronary arteries, the peripheral arterial vasodilation may "steal" blood flow from any ischemic region of the heart. If used alone, sodium and water retention may precipitate high-output HF, especially in elders. Cautious use is also recommended for patients with pulmonary HTN related to the potential for severe hypotension in the pulmonary circuit.

Adverse Drug Reactions

Decreased peripheral resistance secondary to peripheral vasodilation triggers compensatory responses in the SNS and in the RAA system. These responses prevent the orthostatic hypotension and sexual dysfunction caused by many other antihypertensives, but they precipitate added tachycardia, increased cardiac contractility and output, sodium and water retention, headache, and tachyphylaxis to the antihypertensive effects. Hydralazine sometimes induces a lupus-like syndrome. It appears to be dose-related in that it occurs almost exclusively with doses above 50 mg. The incidence is highest in white women. A positive antinuclear antibody (ANA) test is found

in these patients, but no renal impairment is seen. Discontinuing the drug reverses the syndrome, but the ANA does not return to normal until 6 to 8 months after the drug is stopped. Minoxidil has been associated with elongation, thickening, and enhanced pigmentation of fine body hair. This effect has resulted in its use in treating male pattern baldness.

Both drugs are Pregnancy Category C and should be used only when benefits clearly outweigh risks. Hydralazine is acceptable with breastfeeding, but minoxidil is not. The safety and efficacy of both drugs have not been established by clinical trials with children, but children's doses are listed in the drug literature.

Drug Interactions

Additive effects may occur with other antihypertensives. NSAIDs may decrease their antihypertensive effects. Interactions with BBs and loop diuretics are positive in that they prevent the adverse effects common to the PADs. Specific drug interactions and the appropriate actions to prevent them are given in Table 16-20.

Clinical Use and Dosing

Hypertension

The usual oral dose of hydralazine is four doses daily of 25 to 100 mg, which provides smooth control of BP regardless of acetylator type. The maximum dose recommended is 200 mg/day to minimize the risk of the lupus-like syndrome. Minoxidil is usually started at 5 mg daily and increased at 3-day intervals to 10 mg, then 20 mg, and then 40 mg, each in two divided doses. Effective control of BP may occur at any of these doses. Adult's and children's doses are provided in Table 16-21.

Table 16–20 ⊞ **Drug Interactions: Peripheral Vasodilators**

Drug	Interacting Drug	Possible Effect	Implications
Hydralazine	Antihypertensives, alcohol, nitrates*	Additive hypotension	Avoid concurrent use or monitor BP closely
	MAOIs	Severe hypotension	Avoid concurrent use
	NSAIDs	Reduced antihypertensive effects	Choose different analgesic or anti-inflammatory
	Beta blockers	Increased blood levels of hydralazine	Used concurrently to treat adverse reactions. May require reduction of hydralazine dose.
Minoxidil	Antihypertensives, alcohol, nitrates, guanethidine	Additive hypotension	Avoid concurrent use or monitor BP closely
	NSAIDs	Reduced antihypertensive effects	Choose different analgesic or anti-inflammatory

*Hydralazine may be prescribed with isosorbide dinitrate to treat CHF.

Table 16–21 ⊗ **Dosage Schedule and Available Dosage Forms: Peripheral Vasodilators**

Drug	Indication	Available Dosage Form	Starting Dose	Maintenance Dose
Hydralazine (Apresoline) (G)	Add on for HTN or primary in pregnancy	Tablets: 10, 25, 50, 100 mg	10 mg 4 doses daily. After 2–4 d, may increase to 25 mg 4 doses daily for the rest of the first week, then increase to 50 mg 4 doses daily.	25–100 mg 4 doses daily. Once maintenance dose is achieved, may go to 2 doses daily dosing *Max*: 400 mg/d; to min risk of lupus syndrome 200 mg/d
	Children:		*Children:* 0.75 mg/kg/d in four divided doses	Increase over next 3–4 wk to BP control (see adult dose for protocol).
Minoxidil (G)	Add-on for severe HTN	Tablets: 2.5, 10 mg	5 mg/d increased at 3 d intervals to 10 mg/d then 20 mg/d then 40 mg/d; each in 2 divided doses	5–40 mg/d in two divided doses
			Children <12 yr: 0.2 mg/kg/d in single dose	Increase dose in 50%–100% increments in 3 d intervals until BP control. Usual dose: 0.25–1 mg/kg/d

The SNS stimulation and sodium and water retention problems associated with both of these drugs require the concurrent administration of a BB and a loop diuretic. BBs prevent tachycardia, increased cardiac output, and increased renin release; diuretics prevent the salt and water retention caused by decreased renal sodium excretion.

Heart Failure

Hydralazine with concurrent administration of isosorbide dinitrate has been used to treat HF. This combination has been demonstrated to reduce mortality in HF but is not a primary recommendation in current guidelines. The dosage is up to 800 mg three times daily to reduce afterload. This is not usually a long-term management solution unless the effects of an ACEI are desired in a patient with renal dysfunction. ACEIs, ARBs, BBs, CGs (digoxin), and diuretics are the drugs generally used to treat HF, not PAD drugs.

Rational Drug Selection

These drugs are third-line therapy for moderate to severe HTN. If the individual cannot tolerate the addition of a BB to counter the SNS stimulation of these PAD medications, a nondihydropride CCB (diltiazem, verapamil) might adequately substitute.

Monitoring

These drugs have no specific monitoring requirements beyond those used for patients with HTN. HTN is discussed in Chapter 40 and HF in Chapter 36.

Patient Education

Administration

Patients should take the drug exactly as prescribed at the same time each day. A missed dose should be taken as soon as it is remembered; doses should not be doubled. If more than two doses in a row are missed, the patient should consult the health-care provider. The patient should not stop or alter the dose without first contacting the health-care provider. Hydralazine should be taken with meals to enhance absorption. Minoxidil may be taken without regard to meals.

Adverse Reactions

Hypotensive reactions are the most common. Changing position slowly and avoiding exercise in hot weather can decrease these reactions. The patient should learn home BP and pulse monitoring and report decreases in BP by more than 20 mm Hg or increases in pulse of more than 20 bpm above baseline. Dyspnea, pronounced dizziness, or nausea should be reported. Because fluid retention may occur, patients should weigh themselves daily and report weight gain of more than 5 lb in 1 week or more than 1 lb in 1 day, as well as swelling of hands, feet, or ankles or decreased urine output.

Drug interactions occur with NSAIDs and some OTC drugs, especially cough, cold, and allergy remedies. Because these drugs are Pregnancy Category C, female patients capable of childbearing should be made aware of the risks of these drugs, and contraception should be instituted before they are prescribed.

Lifestyle Management

Adherence with other interventions for HTN, such as weight reduction, low-sodium diet, smoking cessation, moderation of alcohol intake, regular exercise, and stress management, is as important as in the other drug classes.

ANTILIPIDEMICS

Atherosclerosis is the major cause of CVD. It is characterized by deposits of cholesterol and other lipoproteins on the walls of arteries. Four major classes of lipoproteins are found in the serum of fasting individuals: low-density lipoproteins (LDLs), high-density lipoproteins (HDLs), very-low-density lipoproteins

(VLDLs), and triglycerides. The risk for CVD is associated with serum cholesterol levels greater than 200 mg/dL, fasting triglyceride levels greater than 150 mg/dL, LDL levels greater than 100 mg/dL, and HDL levels less than 45 for men and 55 for women. Lifestyle and pharmacological therapies are directed toward bringing elevated levels of these lipoproteins down to specific levels associated with reduced cardiovascular disease risk. The "lower the better" mantra has stronger evidence as the decades extend past the first use of statins (Boekholdt et al, 2014). Raising HDL levels is also theorized as important, but not yet a major part of the treatment protocol because evidence that raising this level has a real impact does not yet exist. Drugs differentially affect LDLs, HDLs, VLDLs, and triglyceride levels. The choice of drug is based on how that drug affects each of these.

This section focuses on the drugs used to lower plasma lipoprotein levels. The pathophysiology of atherosclerosis, the relationship of hyperlipidemia to atherosclerosis development, and the management of hyperlipidemia based on the National Cholesterol Education Program guidelines are discussed in Chapter 39.

Pharmacodynamics

Two pathways are involved in the metabolism of lipoproteins. The *exogenous pathway* is central to the lifestyle modifications that are the core of hyperlipidemia therapy. Drugs that affect absorption of fat and cholesterol in the intestine (bile-acid sequestrants and ezetimibe) and drugs that increase lipolysis of triglycerides via lipoprotein lipase (fibric-acid derivatives) also have some of their mechanism of action through this pathway. VLDLs are synthesized and secreted by the liver into the circulation in the endogenous pathway. They are triglyceride-rich, with some cholesterol present. VLDL interacts with lipoprotein lipase in the capillary endothelium to hydrolyze triglycerides into free fatty acids and glycerol, which are then absorbed by fat and muscle cells. About 50% of the VLDL remnants stay in the circulation and become intermediate-density lipoproteins (IDLs). IDLs are then enriched with cholesterol by hepatic triglyceride lipase to become LDLs, which carry about 75% of the circulating cholesterol.

LDL receptors in the liver are down-regulated by the presence of LDL; therefore, one mechanism for lowering LDL is drug therapy that increases the number of LDL receptors in the liver (bile-acid–binding resins, 3-hydroxy-3-methylglutaryl coenzyme A [HMG-CoA] reductase inhibitors). Drugs that

inhibit VLDL synthesis in the liver (niacin, fibric-acid derivatives) also reduce LDL via the endogenous pathway.

Elevated lipoproteins, especially LDLs, have been associated with serious and potentially lethal cardiovascular disorders associated with atherosclerosis. HDLs, by contrast, exert antiatherogenic effects. Lowering LDL levels and raising HDL levels through diet, exercise, and drugs have been shown to decrease the progression of atherosclerosis.

Drugs differentially affect LDL, HDL, and triglyceride levels. Their clinical application is based on how they affect each of these. There are four general classes of lipid-lowering drugs: niacin, fibric-acid derivatives, bile-acid sequestrants, and competitive inhibitors of HMG-CoA reductase (Fig. 16-6). Each is discussed separately.

Niacin decreases VLDL and LDL levels. The primary mechanism of action is probably inhibition of VLDL secretion, which, in turn, decreases production of LDL levels by 10% to 15%. Clearance of VLDL via the lipoprotein lipase pathway also results in lowering of triglyceride levels by 20% to 80%. HDL catabolism is concurrently decreased, resulting in elevations of HDL levels by 20 to 30 mg/dL. The drug has no effect on bile-acid production. Reduction in circulating fibrinogen levels and increases in tissue plasminogen levels also decrease the risk for thrombogenesis. In theory, adding it to a statin should bolster the CV risk reduction, but evidence is not there; in fact CV events and strokes increase (Boden et al, 2011). It has fallen out of favor (The HPS2-THRIVE Collaborative Group, 2014).

Fibric acid derivatives (gemfibrozil [Lopid] and fenofibrate [Tricor]) increase lipolysis of triglycerides via lipoprotein lipase, resulting in a decrease of 50% or more in triglyceride

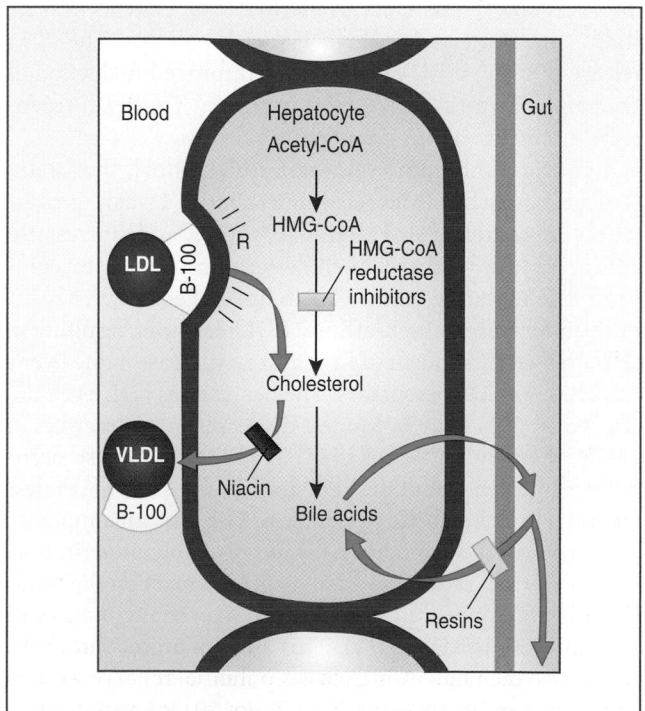

Figure 16–6. Sites of action of antihyperlipidemics.

levels. A decrease in VLDL is also related to decreased secretion by the liver. Only modest reductions in LDL levels (15% to 20%) occur in most patients. Patients with combined hyperlipidemia may actually increase their LDL levels. HDL levels increase by 15% to 25% as a direct consequence of decreasing triglycerides, not by direct action. The reduction of triglycerides (TG) by fenofibric acid does not independently benefit the CV outcomes of the patient but dramatically reduces the risk for pancreatitis that occurs with TG levels over 400 to 500 (Preiss et al, 2012).

A new omega 3 carboxylic acid drug group has added another alternative for high trigylcerdies. Eiscosapentaneoic acid (EPA) + docosahexcienoic acid (DHA) (Epanova) is indicated for triglyceride levels greater than 500mg/dL. The impact on pancreatitis and CV events is not yet known. Icosapentethyl (Vascepa) was marketed in 2012 for the same indication.

Bile acid sequestrants (colestipol [Colestid] and cholestyramine [Questran]) exchange chloride ions for negatively charged bile acids, promoting a 10-fold increase in bile-acid excretion. The increased clearance results in enhanced conversion of cholesterol to bile acids by the liver. Increased uptake of LDL from plasma results from the upregulation of high-affinity LDL receptors on cell membranes, especially in the liver. The net result is decreased LDL levels by 10% to 35%. HDL levels increase about 5%. Triglycerides may also rise initially, but they return to baseline within a few weeks.

Ezetimbe (Zetia) blocks the absorption of cholesterol across the intestinal border. This results in a 12% reduction in LDL; however, it is not considered a first-line therapy. In combination with a statin (e.g., Vytorin), it should increase LDL reduction, but this boosting benefit was not originally reported in a study that used an atypical endpoint not used in other studies for efficacy. This dramatically dropped the use of ezetimbe. It remains an alternative for patients who are statin intolerant and in high CV risk patients. The 2015 release of the IMPROVE—IT data (Improved Reduction of Outcomes: Vytorin Efficacy International Trial) will regenerate discussion of this combination therapy.

Reductase inhibitors (atorvastatin [Lipitor], fluvastatin [Lescol], lovastatin [Mevacor], pitivastatin [Livalo], pravastatin [Pravachol], rosuvastatin [Crestor], and simvastatin [Zocor]) block synthesis of cholesterol in the liver by competitively inhibiting HMG-CoA reductase activity. They induce an increase in high-affinity LDL receptors, resulting in an increased catabolism of LDL and an increase in the liver's extraction of LDL precursors. The net result is LDL levels decreased by 25% to 63%. Modest decreases in triglycerides of 12% to 43% and increases in HDL of 8% to 17% also occur that are independent of the LDL drop, but this response is less vigorous in the diabetic population. The anti-inflammatory properties of these medications are probably more important in CV risk reduction than just the impact on the lipids themselves. Some are associated with reversing the size of atheromas (Nicholls, 2011). This anti-inflammatory property is also being investigated as a potential renal protective agent from radio-contrast dyes (Toso, 2013; Leoncini et al, 2014)).

On The Horizon — PROPROTEIN CONVERTASE SUBTILISIN/ KESIN TYPE 9 INHIBITORS

A new biological drug class called proprotein convertase subtilisin/kesin type 9 inhibitors helps clear LDL. Studies done on statin-intolerant patients demonstrated over 50% of LDL reduction in just 12 weeks. These monoclonal antibodies do appear to have a neurological adverse side effect profile. Because they are just coming to market, they are not further covered in this chapter.

Pharmacokinetics

Absorption and Distribution

Absorption and distribution vary greatly among antilipidemics (Table 16-22). Atorvastatin, niacin, fenofibrate, fluvastatin, gemfibrozil, and simvastatin are all well absorbed. Lovastatin, pravastatin, and rosuvastatin are poorly absorbed. The latter are dosed to enable them to have efficacy. Food decreases the rate of absorption of most reductase inhibitors. Food intake increases the rate of absorption of lovastatin and fenofibrate. It does not affect absorption of the other antilipidemics.

Most are widely distributed and enter breast milk in variable amounts. Cholestyramine and colestipol are not absorbed at all and have no distribution. Their action is entirely related to binding bile acids in the gut. Ezetimbe is also not absorbed.

On The Horizon — PHARMACOMETABOLICS

The new field of pharmacometabolics uses genetic and environmental data to inform treatment choices. The microbiome of the gut is being studied as the reason why some patients respond to statins and others do not. Bacteria modify the drug into its active metabolites. Poor responders do not have good levels of bile acids mediated by gut flora (Kaddurah-Daouk et al, 2011).

Metabolism and Excretion

Niacin, fenofibrate, and gemfibrozil have some metabolism by the liver but are excreted mostly unchanged in the urine. These drugs are affected by impaired renal function (Bonds et al, 2012). The reductase inhibitors are extensively metabolized by the liver, often employing CYP 2C6 and 3A4 enzyme systems, and usually on first pass. This explains the universally low bioavailabilities for the immediate-release formulations from less than 5% for simvastatin to 24% for fluvastatin. The extended-release formulation of lovastatin, however, has a bioavailability of 190%. Because reductase inhibitors are largely excreted in bile and feces, with only small amounts excreted unchanged in the urine, plasma levels are not significantly affected by renal function but may increase markedly with hepatic failure and chronic alcoholic cirrhosis. Plasma half-lives are generally short (45 min to 3 h), with

Table 16–22 ⚏ Pharmacokinetics: Selected Antilipidemics

Drug	Onset	Peak	Duration	Protein Binding	Bioavailability	Half-Life	Elimination
Atorvastatin	Rapid	1–2 h	20–30 h	>98%	14%. First pass (CYP3A4)	14 h	<2% in urine
Cholestyramine	24–48 h	1–3 wk	2–4 wk	NA	0%	UK	Insoluble complex in feces
Colestipol	24–48 h	1 mo	1 mo	NA	0%	UK	Insoluble complex in feces
Fluvastatin	1–2 wk*	4–6 wk*	UK	>98%	24% (IR); 29% (XR). Saturable first pass (CYP2C9)	<1 h	5% in urine, 90% in feces
Gemfibrozil	2–5 d*	4 wk*	Months	95%	UK	1.5 h	70% in urine; 6% in feces
Lovastatin	2 wk*	4–6 wk	6 wk	>95%	<5% (IR); 190% (XR). Extensive first pass (CYP3A4)	3–4 h	10% in urine; 83% in feces
Niacin		45 min	UK	UK	UK	45 min	88% unchanged in urine
Pitivastin	UK	1 hour	UK	>99%	51%	12 h	79% feces; 20% urine
Pravastatin	1–2 wk*	4–6 wk*	UK	50%	17%. Extensive first pass	1.8 h	20% in urine; 70% in feces
Rosuvastatin	UK	2–4 wk	UK	88%	20%. 10% metabolized by CYP2C9	19 h	90% in feces
Simvastatin	1–2 wk*	4–6 wk*	UK	95%	<5%. Extensive first pass (CYP3A4)	3 h	13% in urine; 60% in feces

NA = not applicable; UK = unknown.
*Effect on plasma lipids.

the exception of atorvastatin, whose half-life is 14 hours. Bile-acid sequestrants and ezetimibe bind with cholesterol in the intestine and are not metabolized by the liver. They are excreted in bound form in the feces.

Pharmacotherapeutics

Precautions and Contraindications

Active liver disease is a contraindication for all antilipidemics except the bile-acid sequestrants. Marked persistent increases in serum transaminases and drug-induced hepatitis have occurred with reductase inhibitors, and they should be used with caution in any patient who consumes substantial quantities of alcohol or who has a history of liver disease. Routine monitoring of liver function is no longer recommended by the FDA after an intial baseline assessment is normal. Cautious use of the bile-acid sequestrants is suggested for patients with a history of constipation. Phenylketonuria (PKU) is a contraindication for cholestyramine. Severe renal impairment warrants cautious use of those drugs excreted largely unchanged in the urine (niacin, fenofibrate, and gemfibrozil). Some niacin products contain tartrazine (FDC yellow dye #5) and should be avoided for patients with an aspirin allergy. Because of its tendency to GI irritation, niacin should also be

used cautiously for patients with a history of peptic ulcer disease. The extended-release form is linked with hepatitis.

Niacin, fenofibrate, and gemfibrozil are Pregnancy Category C. Risks and benefits should be weighed. All the reductase inhibitors are Pregnancy Category X and should not be given to women who have the potential to become pregnant. No pregnancy category has been assigned to the bile-acid sequestrants because they are not absorbed systemically. All antilipidemics should be avoided during breastfeeding.

The FDA has required that all reductase inhibitors carry a warning about possible blood sugar increases along with concentration and memory issues (FDA, 2012). The JUPITER trial uncovered a 27% increase in new diabetic diagnoses for otherwise "healthy" participants using rosuvastatin, but the warning applies to the entire drug class. There is a small risk of developing more than glucose intolerance (OR, 1.09) (Naci, Brugts, & Ades, 2013). The risk of a major CV event is far greater, so the use of statins should continue.

The low cost of lovastatin has made it a popular generic medication. In 2012, the FDA placed new labeling changes on this statin restricting its use with many classes of medications. These issues did not come to light until its broad use with individuals with polypharmacy resulted in adverse events (Table 16-23).

Table 16–23 ▓ Drug Interactions: Selected Antilipidemics

Drug	Interacting Drug	Possible Effect	Implications
All reductase inhibitors	Digoxin	Slight elevation in digoxin levels. Concurrent administration with atorvastatin may increase steady-state levels by 20%.	If unable to choose alternative drug, monitor for digoxin toxicity. Avoid concurrent use of atorvastatin.
	Warfarin	Increased anticoagulant effect	Monitor PT/INR closely
	Itraconazole and other azole antifungals	Coadministration increases reductase inhibitor levels 20-fold	Temporarily interrupt reductase inhibitor if systemic azole antifungals needed or reduce dose
	Propranolol	Decreases antilipidemic activity	Choose alternative beta blocker
	Erythromycin, HIV protease inhibitors, nefazodone	Potent inhibitors of CYP3A4; may increase risk of myopathy	If must coadminister, monitor closely for myopathy
Atorvastatin*	Maalox TC	Coadministration decreases atorvastatin level by 35%; LDL reduction is not altered	Separate doses by at least 1 h
	Norethindrone, ethinyl estradiol	Increases contraceptive levels by 30% and 20%, respectively	Choose alternative contraceptive or antilipidemic
	Colestipol	Coadministration decreases atorvastatin levels by 25%; LDL reduction greater than either alone	May be therapeutic choice
	Erythromycin	Atorvastatin levels increased by 40%; increased myopathy risk	Choose alternative antibiotic (not clarithromycin)
	Cyclosporine, gemfibrozil, niacin	Increased myopathy and rhabdomyolysis risk	Avoid concurrent use
Cholestyramine	Mycophenolate	Decreases area under curve (AUC) by 40%	Monitor for indications of rejection
	Piroxicam	Elimination enhanced	Choose alternative NSAID
	Thyroid hormones	Possible loss of efficacy with potential hypothyroidism	Choose alternative antilipidemic
	Vitamins A, D, E, K, and folic acid	May interfere with vitamin absorption, with resultant bleeding tendencies	With long-term therapy vitamins A and D may be given in water-miscible form; vitamin K can be supplemented parenterally or orally
	Warfarin	Decreased anticoagulant effect	Choose alternative antilipidemic, or monitor PT/INR more closely
Fluvastatin	Alcohol	Daily intake of 20 g more than 2 h after evening meal or within 1 h of fluvastatin dose increases AUC by 30%	Avoid daily alcohol intake
	Niacin, propranolol, digoxin	Decreases fluvastatin bioavailability	Avoid concurrent administration
	Rifampin	May cause decrease in fluvastatin AUC and plasma clearance	Choose alternative antilipidemic
Gemfibrozil	Warfarin	Enhances anticoagulant effect	Choose alternative antilipidemic or monitor PT/INR closely
	Colestipol	Bioavailability of gemfibrozil reduced	Avoid concurrent use
	Lovastatin, Fluvastatin, Pitavastin, Rosuvastatin	Severe myopathy or rhabdomyolysis	Avoid concurrent use
	Pravastatin	Urinary excretion and protein binding reduced	Avoid concurrent use
Lovastatin	Isradipine	Increased lovastatin clearance with reduced effect	Choose alternative CCB
	Food	Taking on empty stomach decreases absorption by 30%	Take consistently with food
	Grapefruit	Large quantities may increase risk of myopathy	

Table 16–23 ⠿ **Drug Interactions: Selected Antilipidemics—cont'd**

Drug	Interacting Drug	Possible Effect	Implications
	Itraconazole, ketoconazole, posaconazole		
	Erythromycin, clarithromycin, teliothromycin		
	HIV protease inhibitors, boceprevir, telaprevir		
	Nefazodone		
Pravastatin†	Cholestyramine, colestipol	Decreases pravastatin levels by 40%–50%	Take pravastatin 1 h before or 4 h after bile-acid–binding resins
	Cyclosporine	Coadministration increases pravastatin level 7-fold	Separate doses as above

*Atorvastatin, lovastatin, simvastatin: avoid potent CYP 3A4 inhibitors and do dose reduction with CYP3A4.
†In seniors on clarithromycin avoid rosuvastatin, atorvastatin and fluvastatin.

Adverse Drug Reactions

Cutaneous flushing, especially of the face and upper body, has been associated with niacin. Gradually increasing initial low doses over a few weeks helps to reduce this adverse reaction. Niaspan, an extended-release form of niacin, can be administered at bedtime, with the smaller amount of cutaneous flushing occurring while the patient is sleeping to make the drug more easily tolerated. Taking an ASA 30 minutes prior to niacin, is touted as reducing the hot flashing; however, research does not support this claim. Combining niacin with the antiflushing agent laropiprant generated more adverse outcomes in the HPS2-THRIVE study (2014). Debate exists whether it was the previously untested laropiprant or the niacin at fault. Therefore more research is required.

Fenofibrate and gemfibrozil have a few GI symptoms, including dyspepsia, abdominal pain, and diarrhea. They may also produce cholelithiasis secondary to their increased cholesterol excretion into the bile. They are discontinued if gallstones are found. Both of these drugs have also been associated with mild to moderate decreases in hemoglobin, hematocrit, and WBCs. These levels tend to stabilize, however, with long-term use.

The bile-acid sequestrants' major problems are GI effects, including constipation that may be severe and result in impaction. Constipation is more common in older adults. A laxative or stool softener may be helpful. Other GI symptoms include flatulence, nausea, vomiting, and abdominal pain. Headache is also common. Reduced folate levels have been reported with long-term use, so supplementation with folic acid is suggested. A fairly rare symptom is a burnt odor to the urine.

The reductase inhibitors all have mild headache as a common adverse reaction. A recent concern of increases in intracerebral hemorrhage (ICH) has not been substantiated, but appears to be more common in those with the very lowest of LDL values (Boekholdt et al, 2014). Even patients already with ICH should benefit from statin use. Only those with a lobular bleed appear to have higher risk; however, those types of bleeds have a high re-bleed rate with or without statins (Bustamonte & Montaner, 2013).

Atorvastatin and simvastatin have the lowest adverse reaction profiles, with myalgia reported more at higher doses and more frequently with simvastatin. The water-soluble forms (rosuvastin, pravastin, and pitivastatin [Lovalo]) are reputed to have fewer myalgias than the other lipid-soluble forms (Parker et al, 2012). Fluvastatin, lovastatin, and pravastatin all have GI-associated adverse reactions (dyspepsia, abdominal pain, flatulence, constipation, or diarrhea). Generally, these reactions are mild and transient.

Rhabdomyolysis with renal dysfunction secondary to myoglobinuria has occurred with reductase inhibitors and fibric-acid derivatives. Although it occurs in only 0.1% to 0.5% of patients, when it does occur, it is serious with a fatality rate of 10%. The mechanism for the muscle disruption may be mediated by coenzyme Q10 depletion, among other things (Scordo, 2012). Studies to co-treat with CoQ10 supplementation are mixed. Generally 100 mg twice a day appears to reduce muscle issues (Parker et al, 2012). Pitivastatin does not change CQ10 levels (Parker et al, 2012). Myopathy should be considered in any patient with diffuse myalgias, muscle tenderness and weakness, and elevations in creatine kinase (CK) values more than 10 times the upper limit of normal. Consider temporarily withholding or discontinuing drug therapy in patients with a risk factor predisposing them to the development of renal failure secondary to rhabdomyolysis, including hypotension; major surgery or trauma; severe metabolic, endocrine, or electrolyte disorder; or uncontrolled seizures. Reactions tend to run in families. There are no tests to predetermine who is at risk. Myalgias with one drug might be alleviated by switching to another reductase inhibitor. Interestingly, myalgias are not linked with true muscle weakness (Parker et al, 2012). In 2012, a maximum dose reduction of simvastatin was required owing to higher levels of muscle problems related to its dosing above 40 mg.

Long-term, higher doses of reductase inhibitors were once theorized as being linked with cancer. The 11-year Heart Protection Study did not find any significant differences in cancer rates or incidence (Nicholls, 2011). This finding was repeated in the Cholesteral Treatment Trialist's (CTT) Collaboration meta-analysis of 2015.

Drug Interactions

All antilipidemics except niacin affect warfarin activity: bile acid sequestrants decrease its effect, and the other classes increase its effect. Gemfibrozil and fenofibrate interact with several other antilipidemics. All reductase inhibitors—atorvastatin most of all—increase digoxin levels. Systemic imidazole and triazole therapies increase reductase inhibitor levels by 20-fold. Propranolol decreases the antilipidemic activity of reductase inhibitors. Niacin, erythromycin, and cyclosporine all increase the risk of rhabdomyolysis when given with reductase inhibitors. Combining reductase inhibitors and fibric-acid derivatives also increases the risk for rhabdomyolysis. Taking lovastatin with food enhances its blood levels. Grapefruit ingestion should be avoided with simvastatin, lovastatin and atorvastatin. Specific drug interactions and the appropriate actions to prevent them are given in Table 16-23.

Clinical Use and Dosing

Increased Low-Density Lipoproteins

Niacin, bile-acid sequestrants, and reductase inhibitors all reduce LDL. Reductase inhibitors are first-line drugs in monotherapy and in combinations. Because of the diurnal pattern of cholesterol synthesis, reductase inhibitors are traditionally given in the evening in a single daily dose.

Rosuvastatin is considered the most potent drug in the class with an adverse reactions profile similar to that of atorvastatin, but considered higher risk. The usual starting dose is 5 to 20 mg/d with a maximum of 40 mg/d. Atorvastatin is the next most potent and has the best adverse reaction profile. The usual dose is 10 mg/d initially, increased at 2 to 4 week intervals to up to 80 mg/d.

If costs or other issues prevent using the new lipid drugs for heterozygous familial hyperlipidemia (FH) in children 10 to 17 year olds, reductase inhibitors can be used with the same starting dose, but the maximum dose recommended is 20 mg/d. Simvastatin also has an excellent research profile. It is twice as potent on a weight basis as lovastatin and pravastatin, but less so than atorvastatin. The initial dose is 20 to 40 mg/d, with a maximum of 40 mg/d. For adolescents (10 to 17 yr) with FH, the starting dose is 10 mg/d, with a maximum of 40 mg/d. Lovastatin has a midrange adverse reactions profile. It must be taken with food. The initial dose is 20 mg/d in immediate-release (IR) form or 20, 40, or 60 mg daily of the extended-release form (XR), with dosage increases at 6 to 8 week intervals to a maximum dose of 80 mg/d. For adolescents with FH, the starting dose is 10 mg/d, with a maximum dose of 40 mg.

Pravastatin is similar in potency and its adverse effects profile to lovastatin. The initial dose is 40 mg/d, with a maximum of 80 mg. Pediatric doses for this drug are available for children as young as 8 years of age. For 8- to 13-year-olds, the dose is 20 mg/d, for both initial and maximum doses. For 14- to 18-year-olds, the starting and maximum dose is 40 mg/d. Fluvastatin is about one-half as potent as lovastatin and has a midrange adverse reactions profile. The initial dose is 40 mg/d, with a maximum dose of 80 mg/d. Splitting the dose into two daily doses slightly improves its LDL-lowering ability (Table 16-24).

Table 16–24 ⚸ Dosage Schedule: Selected Antilipidemics Labeled Uses

Drug	Indication	Dosage Form	Starting Dose	Maintenance Dose
Atorvastatin (Lipitor) (G)	Hypercholesterolemia	Tablets: 10, 20, 40, 80 mg	10–20 mg daily. If >45% LDL reduction needed, 40 mg daily	10–80 mg daily. Dosage adjust 2–4 wk intervals *Max:* 80 mg/day
	Intensive LDL reduction post-MI		80 mg	Taper only if LDL levels reached
	Elevated TG		10 mg	10–40 mg/d
			Children: 10 mg	10–20 mg *Max:* 20 mg/d
Cholestryamine (Questran or Questran Light) (G)	Hyperlipidemia	Powder for suspension: 4 g/5 g; 4 g/5.7 g; 4 g/9 g	1 pkt (4 g) mixed in 6–8 oz juice slurry taken 30 min before, during, or 30 min after breakfast and dinner	2–4 pkt (8–16 g) mixed and taken as before *Max:* 24 g/d
			Children: Same as adults	Same as adults
Colesevelam (WelChol) (B)	Hyperlipidemia	Packet for suspension 3.75 mg Tablet: 625 mg	3.75 mg or 6 ts daily with meals and divided doses	3.75 mg/d
Colestipol (Colestid) (G)	Hyperlipidemia	Tablet: 1 g Granules: 5 g per scoop	Granules: 5 g/d in 1–2 divided doses. ts: 2 g/d in 1–2 divided doses	5–30 g/d. Dosage adjust at 1–2 mo intervals

Table 16–24 ✂ **Dosage Schedule: Selected Antilipidemics Labeled Uses—cont'd**

Drug	Indication	Dosage Form	Starting Dose	Maintenance Dose
Fenofibrate (Antara micronized), Fenoglide, Lipofen, Lofibra Tricor; Triglide) (G)	Hyperlipidemia	Tablet: by market brand (F): 40, 120mg (G): 54, 160 mg (Lo): 54, 160 mg (T) 48, 145 mg (Tg): 50, 160 mg Capsules (A): 43, 130 mg (G): 67, 134, 200 mg (L) 50, 150 mg (Lo) 67, 134, 200 mg	(A): 130 mg/d; (F) 120 mg/d; (Li) 150 mg/d (Lo) 200 mg/d cap or 150 mg tab (T) 145 mg/d (Tgd) 160 mg/d If renal <30 mL/min contraindicated. If mild impairment, refer to package insert by brand.	If started at lowest levels increase dose at 4–8 wk intervals to target lipid levels
	Triglycerides		(A) 43–130 mg/d (F) 40–120 mg/d (Li) 50–150 mg/d (Lo) 54–160 mg/d (Lo micronized) 67–200 mg/d (T) 48–145 mg/d (Tg) 50–160 mg/d	*Max:* 130 mg/d *Max:* 120 mg/d *Max:* 150 mg/d *Max:* 160 mg/d *Max:* 200 mg/d *Max:* 145 mg/d *Max:* 160 mg/d
Fenofibric acid (Trilipix, Fibricor) (G)	Dyslipidemia	Tablet; 35, 105 mg Capsule delayed release: 45, 135 mg	Tablet: 105 mg daily or capsule: 135 mg daily Renal 30–80 mL/min; 35 or 45 mg daily	*Max:* 105 mg or 135 mg daily
	Triglycerides		Tablet: 35–105 mg daily Capsule: 45–135 mg daily	*Max:* Tablet 105 mg or capsule 135 mg daily
Fluvastain (Lescol and Lescol XL) (G)	Hyperlipidemia	Capsules: 20, 40 mg Tablets XL: 80 mg	40 mg/d	40 mg/d or 40 mg 2 doses daily or 80 mg XR/d *Max:* 80 mg/d
	10–16 yr and at 1 yr post-menarche		*Children:* 20 mg/d	Increase as tolerated
Gemfibrozil (Lopid) (G)	Hypertriglyceridemia, adjunct	Tablets: 600 mg	1,200 mg/d in 2 divided doses, 30 min before morning and evening meals	600–1,200 mg 2 doses daily *Max:* 2,400 mg/d
Lovastatin (Mevacor) (G) Extended release (Brand Altoprev)	Hyperlipidemia and primary prevention from CHD	Tablets: 10, 20, 40 mg ER 20 mg (B) 40 mg (B); 60 mg (B)	Adults: (IR) 20 mg/d with evening meal (XR) 20, 40, or 60 mg at bedtime	20–40 mg/d. Dosage adjustments at 4-wk intervals 10–40 mg/d *New Max:* 40 mg/day
	10–17 yr	(IR only) 10–20 mg/d	*Children:* 10 mg/d with evening meal	
			Renal: < 30 mL/min caution	
Niacin (IR = Nicor; XR = Niaspan) (G)	Hyperlipidemia, adjunct for high triglycerides or low HDL	Tablets: 500 mg (Nicor) Tablets (XR): 500, 750, 1,000 mg (Niaspan) Time-release OTC forms are not equal substitute for XL	(IR): 250 mg following the evening meal (XR): 500 mg at bedtime for 1–4 wk	1.5–2 g/d in 2–3 divided doses. Adjust at 4–7 d intervals; may increase to 3 g/d *Max:* 6 g/d Increase to 1 g at bedtime during wk 5–8. If target not met, increase to 1,500 mg at bedtime. *Max:* 2 g/d
Pitivastatin (Livalo brand only)	Hyperlipidemia	Tablets: 1, 2, 4 mg	2 mg daily	2–4 mg day *Max:* 4 mg/day Renal start 1 mg and *max* 2 mg
Pravastatin (Pravachol) (G)	Hyperlipidemia and primary prevention of CHD	Tablets: 10, 20, 40, 80 mg	40 mg once daily	40–80 mg once daily *Max:* 80 mg/d Signf. renal: 10 mg/d

Continued

Table 16–24 ⊗ Dosage Schedule: Selected Antilipidemics Labeled Uses—cont'd

Drug	Indication	Dosage Form	Starting Dose	Maintenance Dose
			Children: 8–13 yr: 20 mg once daily. Children: *14–18 yr:* 40 mg once daily	20 mg once daily *Max:* 20 mg/d 40 mg once daily *Max:* 40 mg/d
Rosuvastatin (Crestor brand only)	Hypercholesterolemia	Tablets: 5, 10, 20, 40 mg	5–10 mg once daily Renal: < 30 mL/min 5 mg max	5–40 mg once daily. Dosage adjustments at 2–4 wk intervals *Max:* 40 mg/d
		10–17 yrs	*Children:* individualized per LDL need	*Max:* 20 mg/d
Simvastatin (Zocor) (G)	Hypercholesterolemia	Tablets: 5, 10, 20, 40 mg	20–40 mg daily in the evening. 10 mg/d for older adults or renal impairment (Ccr <30 mL/min)	20–40 mg/d. 20 mg/d for older adults and renal impairment *New Max:* 40 mg unless on 80 mg prior to 2010 without myalgias
		Girls 10–17 yr at least 1 yr post-menarche	*Children:* 10 mg/d	10–40 mg once daily or in 3 divided doses: *Max:* 40 mg

FH = familial hyperlipidemia; TG = triglycerides; BAS = bile-acid sequestrants; (IR) immediate release; (XR) = extended release.

Chapter 39 presents further discussion on the use of statins. Recent clinical trials have shown that LDL lipid-lowering therapy can now be used in persons in categories near but below the level required for the diagnosis of hyperlipidemia. In general, these new trials strongly reinforce prior recommendations and add a newer imperative of reducing C-reactive protein levels. The emphasis on diet and exercise remains the key, with patients on statins who do active exercise having up to 70% reduction in mortality events. The statin and the lifestyle changes were independent in their impact on outcomes (Kokkinos, Faselis, Myers, Pangiotakos, & Doumas, 2012).

Niacin is touted as lowering LDL cholesterol (20%) and triglyceride levels (30% to 40%) and raising HDL levels (30%); these claims are now suspect. As a B-complex vitamin, it is available OTC, but OTC doses are not sufficient to lower LDL. In prescription strength, niacin has been shown to reduce all-cause mortality for patients with CVD, when given as monotherapy. It failed to positively increase any CV outcomes when mixed with statins in both the AIM-HIGH (Boden, et al, 2011) and HPS2-THRIVE studies (2014). Because of its many adverse reactions, if used at all, it is most frequently given as adjunctive therapy with a bile acid sequestrant or a reductase inhibitor for patients with very high triglyceride and/or low HDL levels. For hyperlipidemia, a dose of 1.5 to 2 g/d is usually enough. The daily dose should be divided and given with meals, starting at 250 mg at bedtime and gradually increased at 4 to 7 day intervals (see Table 16-24).

Bile-acid sequestrants are best for patients with a low CV risk profile and moderately elevated LDL levels but who are unable to reduce their LDL by diet alone. Their biggest drawback is their GI adverse effect profile. Cholestyramine and colestipol come in powdered form. The initial dose is one packet mixed with juice in a slurry. They are never swallowed in dry form. Colestipol and colesevelam come in tablet form and require a large glass of water to follow. The dose is taken one-half hour before or during a meal or one-half hour after a meal for several days. Doses are increased gradually, based largely on GI adverse reactions. A common dose is 2 to 4 packets or 3 tablets at breakfast and supper.

Elevated Very-Low-Density Lipoproteins and Elevated Triglycerides

Fenofibrate and gemfibrozil are the most potent triglyceride-lowering agents because of their effect on VLDL. To prevent pancreatitis in patients with marked hypertriglyceridemia, niacin in large doses may be used for patients who do not respond to fibric-acid derivatives. Doses vary not only by drug but also by brand of fenofibrate. Data from the Helsinki Heart Study resulted in the recommendation that this drug not be used for patients with combined hyperlipidemia who have CVD symptoms. Bile-acid sequestrants and reductase inhibitors also produce marked reduction in triglyceride levels.

Omega-3 fatty acids can also be used for triglyceride care. EPA and DHA are found in fish and ALA is found in plants and flax seed oil; only the first two lower TG (American Academy of Nurse Practitioners [AANP], 2012). Prescription strength (Lovanza) and OTC omega-3 are also available. The prescription drug can drop TG by 14% to 30% and increase HDL by 15%. The highly reported "fish burp" side effect is actually only documented in 6% of research subjects. Evidence has not yet been established that fish oils impact mortality and the hope that they will reduce atrial arrthymias has been discounted (Mozffarian et al, 2012). They have also lost luster as good lipid therapy alternatives.

Decreased High-Density Lipoproteins

Niacin is an effective agent in increasing levels of HDL, with the percentage of increase near 30%. Gemfibrozil and fenofibrate are the next best at increasing HDL, followed by some reductase inhibitors. Rosuvastatin, atorvastatin, and simvastatin also have an ability to raise HDL 15%. Now recognized as a risk factor in heart disease, isolated low HDL levels are now addressed. Any increase in HDL is a bonus effect when choosing a drug to treat elevated LDL or VLDL levels. Currently there are no specific HDL-raising agents that reflect the same success as found in the statin impact on LDL (Parker et al, 2012).

Rational Drug Selection

In addition to the nature of the lipoprotein abnormality and the mechanism of action and adverse reaction profile of the drug, as discussed previously, factors taken into account in selecting the appropriate drug or drug combination include degree of CVD risk, age of the patient, and cost.

Degree of Coronary Vascular Disease Risk

For all risk groups, dietary reduction in saturated fat and cholesterol along with increased fiber intake is first-line therapy. For the highest-risk patient, these lifestyle changes are concurrently initiated with medications. For low-risk patients, diet might be adequate to control LDL levels.

For high-risk patients, reductase inhibitors are the most cost-effective and should be tried first. Absolute cut points of LDL values are no longer used with the new guidelines. However, the old ATP III values help new providers quantify what is a high or low benchmark for consideration when drawing up individualized therapeutic plans. When baseline LDL is greater than 130 mg/dL, relatively high doses or combination with other antilipidemics may be needed to achieve desired outcomes (Gibson et al, 2009; Nicholls et al, 2011). Commonly, achieving a individualized LDL goal is difficult with only one drug class. If patient response is inadequate after 4 months, switching to a more potent drug or trying a combination of drugs is standard step therapy. Combinations of reductase inhibitors with bile-acid sequestrants or niacin logically should increase impact, but the AIM-HIGH and HPS-THRIVE studies have dampened this expectation. The combination of a reductase inhibitor with fibric-acid derivatives is risky because of the increased risk for rhabdomyolysis. Patients whose response is still inadequate should be referred to a lipid disorder specialist. Aiming for the lowest LDL is indicated for the highest risk patients (Boekholdt et al, 2014).

For moderate-risk patients, drug therapy is based on 10-year CV risk. If that risk is greater than 7% to 10 %, reductase inhibitors are appropriate per the 2013 guidelines. Now, almost 1 of 3 Americans possibly qualify for statin therapy. For lower levels of risk, drugs generally are not needed if dietary modifications are followed. For isolated low-HDL patients, aerobic exercise, smoking cessation, and weight loss if they are obese are added to the dietary therapy. There is to date no evidence that drug treatment to increase HDL levels reduces CVD risk or mortality. Further discussion occurs in Chapter 40.

Elevated triglycerides are recognized as an independent risk factor for CVD, especially in women. Fibric-acid derivatives are the drugs of choice when treatment is chosen. It is also the drug of choice for patients with very high triglyceride levels (greater than 800 mg/dL) who are at risk for pancreatitis because of this high level. Attention to LDL reduction remains paramount, because TG reduction typically comes with LDL reduction.

Age

The prevalence of hypercholesterolemia and CVD risk is greatest among people older than age 65 years. Because dietary therapy alone often fails to achieve the LDL goal in older adults, drug therapy is used as an adjunct. Reductase inhibitors are the first-line choice. These drugs are well tolerated in the older adult, with minor diarrhea and occasional sleep disturbances being the most common problems. Monitoring of LFTs is no longer required for the general population. Because of the polypharmacy of elders and the fact these drugs are processed in the liver, it is prudent to monitor LFTs in selected older patients. Seniors on the antibiotic clarithromycin have a slight increased risk of acute renal injury and potassium levels with rosuvastatin, pravastatin, and fluvastatin (Li et al, 2014).

Niacin is not suggested in elders because it triggers hypotension and arrhythmias. Multiple daily dosing is also required, which may increase the complexity of a drug regimen often already complex. Bile-acid sequestrants are safe for older adults, but their GI problems, especially the risk of constipation and impaction, and their effect on the absorption of many of the drugs that older adults are often also taking make them less desirable than reductase inhibitors. Fibrates are known to increase creatinine levels in elders with DM but paradoxically may also slow down renal functional loss over time (Bonds et al, 2012).

Some reductase inhibitors (see current dosing circulars) have been approved for children with heterozygous or homozygous familial hypercholesterolemias with some residual receptor activity. The safety of most other antilipidemics has not been established for those under age 18.

Cost

Brand-name drugs are always more expensive than generic. Currently rosuvastin does not come in generic form; nor do the fibrates.

Monotherapy Versus Multiple Drugs

Few patients can achieve lipid targets on one drug class alone. The high doses required to do so result in unacceptable adverse responses. Combinations of drugs are the rule to achieve target levels. Specific combinations are discussed in Chapter 39.

Monitoring

Reduction of the LDL cholesterol level is the top priority, but the other lipid levels are gaining in importance. Labs should be measured beginning about 4 to 6 weeks after initiation of therapy and then every 3 to 4 months until control is established. After that, every 6 to 12 months is usually enough.

Monitoring protocols for specific drugs in addition to the standard lipid levels are as follows. For niacin, LFTs, uric-acid levels, and blood glucose levels are done initially at 4 to 6 week intervals until a stable dose is determined, and thereafter at 3 to 4 month intervals. For reductase inhibitors, LFTs are done prior to initiating therapy, after the first 3 months of therapy, and then only as indicated. If aspartate aminotransferase (AST) or alanine aminotransferase (ALT) levels increase to 3 times normal, reduce the dose or discontinue therapy. CK levels are monitored if muscle tenderness is exhibited. Statins may raise fasting blood sugars; however, the low glucose levels drawn in fasting patients can give a false sense of security. Longer-term glucose monitoring (i.e., HgA1C) will give a clearer picture of the impact of glucose metabolism for individual patients. For fibric-acid derivatives, LFTs should be assessed prior to initiating therapy and with the same protocol as reductase inhibitors.

Patient Education

The importance of patient education in the treatment of hyperlipidemia cannot be overemphasized because lifestyle management is the key to success (Kokkinos et al, 2012). This is also discussed in Chapter 39.

Administration

The patient should take the drug exactly as prescribed and not skip doses or double up on missed doses. Bile-acid sequestrants are taken before meals, mixed and vigorously shaken with 4 to 6 oz water, milk, fruit juice, or other noncarbonated beverage. Rinsing the glass with a small amount of additional liquid ensures that the entire dose is taken. For patients who require thick liquids, these drugs can also be mixed with cereals or pulpy fruits such as applesauce. The powder cannot be taken dry. If other drugs are to be taken, administer them 1 hour before or 4 hours after the bile-acid sequestrant. Reductase inhibitors are traditionally taken in the evening because of their action on cholesterol synthesis; however, this is not clinically significant except for lovastatin. Lovastatin is the only reductase inhibitor that should be taken with the evening meal to improve its absorption. Atorvastatin can be taken at any time of the day and without regard to food.

Adverse Reactions

Cutaneous flushing, especially of the face and upper body, has been associated with niacin. Hot fluids taken near the time of the dose make the flushing worse. Taking niacin with meals reduces the incidence of this reaction. A high-fiber diet or psyllium supplement just before a meal usually ameliorates the flatulence, constipation, or abdominal pain associated with bile-acid sequestrants. Natural laxatives such as prunes or stool softeners can also be helpful. For these drugs and for fibric-acid derivatives, the provider should be notified of persistent constipation. For all reductase inhibitors, muscle tenderness or pain may indicate a serious problem that may require discontinuance of the drug. Fluvastatin, lovastatin, and pravastatin all have GI-associated adverse reactions (dyspepsia, abdominal pain, flatulence, constipation, or diarrhea) and headache. Generally, these effects are mild and transient.

Suggestions to try a CQ10 supplement may be helpful, but the evidence on its usefulness is not well established (Scordo, 2012).Because the reductase inhibitors are Pregnancy Category D or X, female patients capable of childbearing should not take these drugs, or contraception should be instituted before prescribing them. The health-care provider should be notified if pregnancy is planned or suspected.

A meta-anlysis has put to rest the idea that women do not benefit as much as men from statin therapy. The positive effect is the same for each gender with a proportional reduction in major CV events no matter the level of risk (CTT, 2015).

Lifestyle Management

For a cardiac-healthy lifestyle, it is important to stress the need for regular aerobic exercise and smoking cessation. Medication helps to control hyperlipidemia, but it does not cure it. Lifestyle management is discussed in more detail in Chapter 39.

DIURETICS

Diuretics are first-line therapy in the treatment of HF and HTN through their reduction in ECF volume. Of the several classes of diuretics, the ones most commonly used in primary care are the distal tubular (thiazides and aldosterone antagonists) and loop diuretics. These drugs are the focus of this discussion. Amiloride (Midamor) is not an aldosterone antagonist, but is also a potassium sparing diuretic. It is covered tangentially as an adjunct medication.

Pharmacodynamics

Disease processes that increase renal sodium and water retention result in increased ECF volume. This increased volume increases capillary hydrostatic pressure. Taken together, the result is increased afterload, which leads to increased myocardial workload. Increased ECF volume also contributes to HTN. Diuretics act to reduce this volume in different ways (Fig. 16-7). The loop diuretics inhibit sodium reabsorption in the ascending loop of Henle. These drugs are short-acting and cause a large natriuresis. The thiazide-type diuretics act on the distal renal tubule to inhibit sodium reabsorption. Their effect is generally longer-lasting, and they cause less brisk diuresis. Both of these classes increase potassium excretion. The potassium-sparing diuretics include aldosterone antagonists and agents like amiloride that inhibit excretion of potassium distally. These agents are weak diuretics, often used in combination with thiazides to reduce potassium loss.

Initially, diuretics promote natriuresis, decrease plasma volume, and reduce cardiac output. With time, these effects return to baseline, but total peripheral resistance remains decreased. The mechanism behind this additional long-term effect of diuretics is not clearly known but may be related to the amount of sodium in the vessel walls themselves. Theoretically, sodium in vessel walls contributes to the ability of the vessels to constrict, and loss of sodium from the vessel walls may contribute to vasodilation, leading to decreased

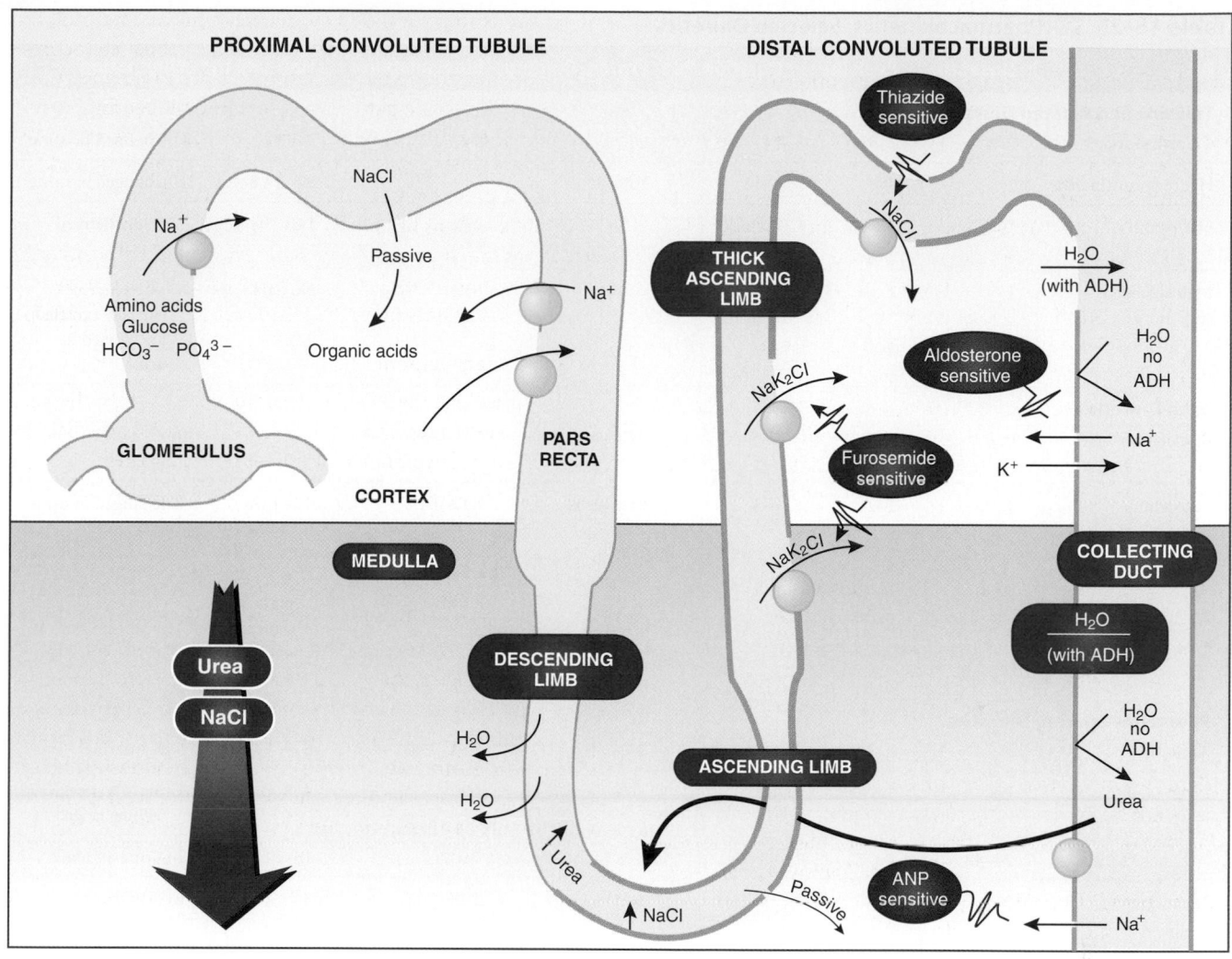

Figure 16–7. Sites of action of diuretics.

PVR. Decreased PVR reduces afterload to improve cardiac functioning and reduce BP.

Diuretics may also be used as adjunct therapy for disease processes in which the treatment itself may contribute to fluid retention—for example, use of some CCBs and antiarrhythmics. Spironolactone blocks the mineral corticosteroid receptor that aldosterone binds to. This could be a useful action for aldosteronism. It is also useful in ventricular remodeling and decreasing the inflammatory cascade that can occur in the days following an MI; however, evidence is not yet there to demonstrate any long-term outcomes of HF symptoms or QOL measures (Edelmann et al, 2013). Amiloride's potassium-sparing characteristics are used to counter any chronic potassium losses that cannot be reliably corrected with diet or supplements.

Pharmacokinetics

Absorption and Distribution

Absorption and distribution vary among the diuretics (Table 16-25). Thiazide and loop diuretics are all well absorbed orally. Among the potassium-sparing diuretics, spironolactone (Aldactone) is well absorbed, amiloride (Midamor) is poorly absorbed, and triamterene (Dyrenium) has an absorption rate somewhere between the two. Food enhances the absorption of metolazone (Zaroxolyn). All are widely distributed, cross the placenta, and enter breast milk. The thiazides enter intracellular spaces as well, which may explain their preferential use in refractory edema.

Metabolism and Excretion

The liver is the primary site of metabolism for most diuretics. Furosemide (Lasix) has nonhepatic and hepatic metabolism. Amiloride is not metabolized by the liver. All diuretics are excreted mostly unchanged in the urine. Metolazone, amiloride, bumetanide (Bumex), and spironolactone have some excretion in feces and bile. Plasma half-lives vary from 30 to 60 minutes for furosemide to 35 to 50 hours for chlorthalidone. Impaired renal or hepatic function increases the half-life of furosemide.

The Kidney Disease Outcomes Quality Initiative (KDO-QI) guidelines encourage replacing thiazide diuretics with loop medications when GFR drops to 30 mL/min. Amiloride

Table 16–25 ✂ **Pharmacokinetics: Selected Diuretics**

Drug	Onset (h)	Peak (h)	Duration (h)	Protein Binding	Bioavailability	Half-Life (h)	Elimination
Thiazide and Related Diuretics							
Chlorthalidone	2–3	2–6	24–72	UK	64%	35–50	Unchanged in urine
Hydrochlorothiazide	2	4–6	6–12	20%–80%	65%–75%	5.6–14.8	Unchanged in urine
Indapamide	1–2	2	up to 36	71%–79%	93%	14	–7%; unchanged in urine
Metolazone	1	2	12–24	<20%	65%	No data	6%–15% in feces, partially excreted; unchanged in urine
Loop Diuretics							
Bumetanide	0.5–1	1–2	4–6	94%–96%	72%–96%	1–1.5	50% in urine; 20% in feces
Furosemide	1	1–2	6–8	91%–97%	60%–64%	0.5–1 (increased in renal and hepatic impairment and in neonates)	Unchanged in urine
Potassium-Sparing Diuretics							
Amiloride	2	6–10	24	23%	15%–25%	6–9	50% in urine
Eplerenone	UK	1.5 hr	UK	50%	69%	4–6	Urine 67%; feces 32%; 5% unchanged
Spironolactone	24–48	48–72	48–72	>98%	>90%	13–24	In urine and bile
Triamterene	2–4	6–8	12–16	50%–67%	30%–70%	3	21% in urine

UK = unknown.

is contraindicated in diabetic nephropathy patients, and others with BUN levels over 30 mg/100 mL or creatinine levels over 1.5 mg. Metolazone is the only thiazide effective in stage 3 or 4 CKD (Zuber & Davis, 2012).

Pharmacotherapeutics

Precautions and Contradictions

All diuretics affect electrolytes. They should be used cautiously for patients with preexisting electrolyte abnormalities. Potassium-sparing diuretics have an absolute contraindication for patients with severely impaired renal function because they can produce hyperkalemia. Creatinine clearances less than 25 to 30 mL/min suggest careful monitoring of electrolytes and cautious use with all diuretic classes. Hepatic dysfunction suggests cautious use with all diuretics, especially those with some excretion in feces or bile.

For patients with a history of gout or renal calculi, cautious use of diuretics is suggested because of the potential for hyperuricemia. Diuretics should be used cautiously for patients with diabetes, who may require alterations in their hypoglycemic regimen related to glucose intolerance. The glucose issues with thiazides may turn out to be transient and not

clinically significant in the long term. There are fewer issues with metolazone and indapamide.

Older adults are at increased risk for hypotension with these drugs. They require careful BP monitoring and patient teaching about mobility with the background of possible orthostasis. The use of thiazide and loop diuretics has been associated with increased risk of falls in older adults. Any tinnitus or hearing loss should not be dismissed as age-related but be considered significant side effects.

Diuretics decrease plasma volume and may decrease placental perfusion. Several thiazide and loop diuretics are Pregnancy Category C and should be used only when benefits clearly outweigh risks. Jaundice and thrombocytopenia may be seen in neonates. Spironolactone, amiloride, hydrochlorothiazide, and chlorthalidone are Pregnancy Category B. Spironolactone appears to be the best choice for pregnant women when a diuretic must be used. Safety has been established in children only for furosemide, hydrochlorothiazide, and spironolactone.

Adverse Drug Reactions

Electrolyte imbalances are common in all diuretic classes. Thiazide and loop diuretics cause hypokalemia and may cause hypercalcemia, hyponatremia, and hypomagnesemia. When it occurs, the hypomagnesemia must be corrected first to permit successful treatment of the hypokalemia. The average potassium loss is 0.6 mEq/L and is dose-related. High sodium intake as is found in many American diets exacerbates the potassium loss. Metabolic alkalosis may be associated with the hypokalemia. Potassium-sparing diuretics cause hyperkalemia especially when combined with ACE or ARB medications. High levels of uric acid may occur with all diuretics; thiazide and loop diuretics and spironolactone are the most likely to cause it, and indapamide (Lozol) is the least likely. The hyperuricemia itself is usually not treated unless gout or renal calculi develop.

Glucose intolerance can be a problem with all diuretic groups; thiazide and loop diuretics cause the most difficulty. This intolerance is directly linked to the serum potassium level. Correcting hypokalemia often relieves the problem. Hyperlipidemia with increases in cholesterol, LDL, and triglycerides has been seen with thiazide diuretics. The elevations are transient and tend to return to baseline in about 6 months. It is unknown what, if any, CV implications this transient rise has for diabetics who are already considered high-CV risk.

Hypotension secondary to fluid volume deficits can also occur with all diuretics. Starting with a low dose and increasing the dose gradually can reduce this problem. Instructing patients that oral fluid reduction is not indicated with these medications can help in this regard.

Gynecomastia occurs in 50% of patients receiving spironolactone. Impotence occurs in a smaller number. This can be distressing to men and their significant other. The next generation of this drug class, eplerenone (Inspra), has more affinity for the mineral corticoid receptor, but the reputed decrease in menstrual irregularity, acne, and gynecomastia is not considered significant enough to replace the older, generic spironolactone with this costly alternative (Chatterjee et al, 2012). The positive impact of eplerenone on HF outcomes during ACS is due to the reduction in BNP, a fact not previously researched with this drug class (Montalescot, 2013). Thiazide is known to have photosensitive reactions that can last years after discontinuation (Drucker & Rosen, 2011).

Drug Interactions

All diuretics have potential additive hypotensive effects with other drugs that lower BP. Synergistic hypokalemia is probable between thiazide and loop diuretics, and additive hypokalemia may occur between these classes and mezlocillin, piperacillin, ticarcillin, amphotericin B, and glucocorticoids. Hypokalemia may increase the risk of CG toxicity. Concurrent administration of potassium-sparing diuretics and ACEIs may lead to significant hyperkalemia. Potassium preparations, including nonsodium salt substitutes, may also result in significant hyperkalemia.

Thiazide and loop diuretics decrease the renal excretion of lithium and may induce lithium toxicity. These two classes may decrease the action of sulfonylureas and insulin. Thiazide diuretics and spironolactone diminish the anticoagulant effects of warfarin, whereas loop diuretics enhance its anticoagulant effects. Additive ototoxicity occurs between loop diuretics and aminoglycosides and cisplatin. NSAIDs and salicylates may decrease the diuretic effectiveness of all classes. Specific drug interactions and the appropriate actions to prevent them are given in Table 16-26.

Table 16–26 ⠿ Drug Interactions: Selected Diuretics

Drug	Interacting Drug	Possible Effect	Implications
Thiazide diuretics	Allopurinol	Concurrent use may increase incidence of hypersensitivity reactions	Avoid concurrent use
	Anticholinergics	Increased diuretic absorption	Monitor diuretic effect
	Anticoagulants	Diminished anticoagulant effect	Monitor PT/INR. Adjust anticoagulant dose prn.
	Antigout agents	Diuretic may increase uric acid levels	Choose different diuretic or adjust antigout agent dose
	Antineoplastics	Diuretic may prolong antineoplastic-induced leukopenia	Monitor WBC. Choose alternative diuretic.
	Bile-acid–binding resins	Resins bind thiazides and reduce absorption by up to 85%	Give thiazide 2 h before or 4 h after bile-acid–binding resin
	Calcium salts	Hypercalcemia may be worsened	Avoid concurrent use
	Diazoxide	Hyperglycemia, often with symptoms of frank diabetes	Choose alternative antihypertensive
	Digitalis glycosides	Digitalis toxicity and toxicity-induced arrhythmias	Monitor potassium level and administer supplement as needed
	Lithium	Decreased renal excretion of lithium, resulting in toxicity	Monitor lithium level closely, or choose alternative diuretic
	Loop diuretics	Synergistic diuresis and hypokalemic effects	Reduce doses of both or one of these unless planned for therapeutic reasons. Monitor electrolytes closely.

Continued

Table 16–26 ⠿ **Drug Interactions: Selected Diuretics—cont'd**

Drug	Interacting Drug	Possible Effect	Implications
	NSAIDs	Some may reduce diuretic effect; concurrent administration of indomethacin has been associated with renal failure	Monitor diuresis. Avoid concurrent administration of indomethacin.
	Sulfonylureas, insulin	Diuretics induce hyperglycemia and may decrease hypoglycemic effects	Monitor serum glucose. Adjust dose of hypoglycemic.
	Vitamin D	Biologic actions of vitamin D enhanced, resulting in hypercalcemia	Monitor serum calcium levels
Loop diuretics	Aminoglycosides, cisplatin	Increased risk for ototoxicity	Avoid concurrent use. If you must use aminoglycoside, use different diuretic during time it is administered.
	Anticoagulants	Enhanced anticoagulant activity	Monitor PT/INR. Adjust dose prn.
	Digitalis glycosides	Digitalis toxicity and toxicity-induced arrhythmias	Monitor potassium levels and administer potassium supplement prn
	Hydantoins	Reduces diuretic effect of furosemide	Monitor diuretic effect and adjust dose prn
	Lithium	Decreased renal excretion of lithium, resulting in toxicity	Monitor lithium levels closely or choose different diuretic
	NSAIDs, salicylates	Reduces effects of diuretic	Monitor diuretic effect and adjust dose
	Sulfonylureas	Diuretic-induced hyperglycemia may reduce hypoglycemic effect	Monitor serum glucose and adjust dose of sulfonylurea, or choose different diuretic
	Theophylline	Actions of theophylline may be enhanced or inhibited	Monitor theophylline levels closely, or choose different bronchodilator
Potassium-sparing diuretics	ACE inhibitors, potassium preparations	Concurrent use may result in hyperkalemia	Avoid concurrent use. Choose different diuretic.
	Anticoagulants	Decreased anticoagulant effects	Monitor PT/INR and adjust dose prn
	Cimetidine	May increase bioavailability and decrease renal clearance of triamterene only	Choose alternative histamine$_2$ blocker
	Digitalis glycosides	Interaction complex and difficult to predict risk of toxicity	Monitor digitalis level closely or avoid concurrent use
	NSAIDs salicylates	Decreased diuretic effect; interaction with indomethacin has resulted in renal failure	Monitor diuretic effect. Avoid concurrent use with indomethacin.

Clinical Use and Dosing

Regardless of the clinical use, start with the lowest effective dose, increase the dose gradually to reduce the likelihood of adverse reactions, consider reducing doses where appropriate, and consider potassium supplementation or combination with a potassium-sparing diuretic when laboratory studies indicate it is appropriate. Supplementation with potassium chloride of 20 mEq daily is sufficient for prevention of hypokalemia in most patients. Those with additional potassium losses will need 40 mEq/daily or more (Cohn, Kowey, Whelton, & Prisant, 2000).

Hypertension

Initial drug therapy for HTN is monotherapy, although rarely is one drug sufficient to achieve target BP. When the decision is made to begin drug therapy and there are no clear indications for another type of drug, a thiazide-type diuretic should be chosen because, in randomized controlled trials (RCTs) comparing diuretics with other classes of antihypertensive

drugs, diuretics have been unsurpassed in preventing cardiovascular complications of HTN (Wright et al, 2009). The choice of diuretic should be based on level of kidney function and possibly weight. For estimated GFR rates higher than the mid-40 mL/min range, a thiazide diuretic should be used because loop diuretics are not as effective as thiazides in this setting. For GFRs less than the mid-40 mL/min range, loop diuretics, sometimes in combination with metolazone, are more appropriate. They are most effective when dosed twice daily.

Diuretics are preferred as initial therapy for sodium-sensitive patients such as blacks, older adults, the obese, and those with renal insufficiency. Thiazide diuretics are generally not the first drugs of choice for patients with hyperlipidemia because of their potential for worsening the hyperlipidemia; however, lipid disorders do not contraindicate the use of thiazide diuretics. Newer interpretation of the evidence implies nonobese patients are not good candidates for diuretics as first-line drugs. The ACCOMPLISH trial demonstrated a 30+% difference in therapeutic impact based on weight with a recommendation that nonobese patients without another compelling reason for volume control be started on a different class of medications (Weber et al, 2012).

All classes of diuretics have been used to treat HTN, but the best results are with thiazide-type diuretics. The dose–response curve of diuretics is fairly flat. Increasing the dose produces more adverse reactions with little change in therapeutic benefit. Dosage should be increased no sooner than 4 weeks, which is the length of time usually required to achieve optimal therapeutic effect. When a thiazide diuretic is added to an existing antihypertensive regimen, reduce the dosage of the other antihypertensives to prevent excessive hypotension and orthostasis.

Edema Associated With Congestive Heart Failure, Hepatic Cirrhosis, and Renal Disease

First-line therapy in treating HF is with ACEIs, depending on the stage of failure. Chapter 36 discusses the most appropriate drug for initiation of therapy based on stage. Drugs are often introduced in combinations. The role of diuretics is supplemental and only part of a treatment regimen. The most effective class for this indication is the loop diuretics. Torsemide is a very good long-acting loop diuretic that is especially useful in HF management.

Loop diuretics are effective in moderate to severe disease and can be used when Ccr is less than 25 mL/min. Indapamide is also indicated for edema associated with HF and is effective with these low Ccr levels. Thiazide diuretics may be used to treat the edema associated with mild HF, corticosteroid and estrogen therapy, premenstrual syndrome, and limited renal dysfunction. They are not useful if the Ccr is less than 25 mL/min. Among the thiazides, hydrochlorothiazide and chlorthalidone are the first choices for this indication. Intermittent dosing may be advantageous and reduce the incidence of adverse reactions. With premenstrual syndrome, the drug should be taken 3 to 5 days before menstruation and discontinued when menstruation begins. Frequent dosage adjustments may be necessary in edematous patients. Dosages for both indications for each drug are indicated in Table 16-27.

Table 16–27 ⊗ Dosage Schedule: Selected Diuretics Labeled Use

Drug	Indication	Dosage Forms	Starting Dose	Maintenance Dose
Amiloride (Midamore) (G)	K$^+$ sparing. Adjunct Rx edema of CHF and HTN	Tablets: 5 mg	5 mg daily	10 mg daily or 5 mg 2 doses daily *Max:* 20 mg/d
Bumetanide (Bumex) (G)	Edema of CHF, hepatic and renal disease; alt for Lasix allergy	Tablets: 0.5, 1, 2 mg	0.5 mg daily	2 mg/d; or dosing every other day or 3–4 d with 1–2 d between is safe and most effective *Max:* 20 mg/d
			Children: 0.015– 0.1 mg/kg/d every 6–24 h *Max:* 10 mg	
Chlorthalidone (Hygroten and Thalitone) (G)	Edema	Tablets: 15 mg (T only) 25, 50, 100 mg	50–100 mg/d	150–200 mg/d *Max:* 200 mg/d *Renal:* 40 mL/min probably ineffective
	Edema from HF		12.5 mg	12.5–25 mg/d *Max:* 100 mg/d
	HTN	<None>	25 mg/d	25–50 mg/d *Max:* 100 mg/d
Eplerenone (Inspra) (G)	HTN	Tablets: 25, 50 mg	50 mg/d (make take 4 wk for full effect)	Up to 50 mg twice daily
	HF post-MI		25 mg/d	Titrate to 50 mg in 4 wk
	High K$^+$ dosing in HF		5.5–5.9 mEq/L decrease from 50 mg to 25 mg/d or every other day 6.0+ withhold	
Furosemide (Lasix) (G)	Refractory edema of CHF, hepatic and renal disease	Solution: 40 mg/5 mL; 10 mg/mL Tablets: 20, 40, 80 mg	20–80 mg daily or 2 doses daily	Titrate in increments of 20–40 mg q6–8h until desired diuresis; give 2 doses daily 8 a.m. and 2 p.m. *Max:* 600 mg/d in divided doses

Continued

Table 16–27 🔀 **Dosage Schedule: Selected Diuretics Labeled Use—cont'd**

Drug	Indication	Dosage Forms	Starting Dose	Maintenance Dose
	HTN		40 mg 2 doses daily	Titrate up or down to control HTN
	Edema in infants and children		*Children:* 2 mg/kg/d	Titrate in increments of 1 mg/kg q6–8h until desired diuresis *Max:* 6 mg/kg/d
Hydrochlorothiazide (HydroDiurilMicrozide)	HTN	Capsules: 12.5 mg Tablets: 12.5, 25, 50 mg Micronized capsules: 12.5 mg (Minzide only)	12.5 mg/d	12.5–50 mg daily or in two divided doses Rarely need more than 50 mg/d *Max:* 100 mg/d
	Edema		25–100 mg/d in 1–2 divided doses	*Max:* 200 mg/d
	Edema or HTN: Infants <6 mo Infants 6 mo–2 yr Children 2–17 yr		1–3 mg/kg/d in 2 divided doses Same 3 mg/kg/d	*Max:* 37.5 mg age 6 mo–2 yr *Max:* 50 mg/d until age 17
Indapamide (Lozol) (G)	HTN	Tablets: 1.25 mg (B) 2.5 mg (B) 2.5 mg (G)	1.25 mg daily	2.5–5 mg d; increase at 4-wk intervals *Max:* 5 mg/d
	Edema of CHF		2.5 mg daily	If inadequate in 1 wk, up to *max* 5 mg/d
Metolazone (Zaroxolyn) (G)	Adjunct therapy for HTN	Tablets: 2.5, 5, 10 mg (G only)	2.5 mg daily	2–5 mg daily *Max:* 20 mg daily
	Edema		5 mg daily	10 mg daily *Max:* 20 mg daily
Spironolactone (Aldactone) (G)	HTN	Tablets: 25, 50, 100 mg	25–50 mg/d in divided dose	50–100 mg in 1–2 doses daily *Max:* 100 mg/d
	Edema of CHF (not severe), hepatic and nephrotic syndrome		25–100 mg/d; 3 times loading dose for fast effect	25–200 mg/d in divided doses; if inadequate after 5 d, change diuretics *Max:* >100 mg/d;
Triamterene/HCTZ (Dyazide, Maxzide) (G)	HTN add on RX and/or edema	HCTZ/Triamterne Capsules: 25 mg/37.5 mg Tablets: 25 mg/37.5 mg; 50 mg/75mg	25 mg/37.5 mg daily	Titrate to 50/75 mg in 2 doses daily *Max:* 300 mg/d

CHF = congestive heart failure; HTN = hypertension.

(G) = generic (*Note:* HCTZ is the generic hydrochlorothiazide); (B) = brand. Where more than one brand exists, the initial of the brand is used to differentiate them.

Rational Drug Selection

Indications

When HTN is mild, diuretic therapy can be initiated with 12.5 mg hydrochlorothiazide and increased to 25 mg. Due to the flat dosing impact, greater than 25 to 50 mg is generally unnecessary. Chlorthalidone (Thalitone) initiated at 15 mg and increased as needed to a maximum of 50 mg, was superior to all other drugs in the ALLHAT trial in treating hypertension with no change in subsequent trials and meta-analysis even 10 years later (Wright et al, 2009). For patients with renal impairment, the addition of 2.5 to 5 mg of metolazone is helpful. When these conditions are moderate to severe, 20 to 40 mg of furosemide is necessary. Potassium-sparing diuretics are relatively weak agents and are used mainly in conjunction with thiazide or loop diuretics to prevent hypokalemia. Some experts believe the hypertension guidelines will soon recommend more use of chlorthalidone in lieu of the thiazides.

Concurrent Disease Processes

Increasing glucose levels can be a problem for patients with diabetes, and hyperuricemia can be a problem for patients with gout. In the order of most likely to least likely to have these adverse effects, the drugs are thiazides, loop diuretics, potassium-sparing diuretics, metolazone, and indapamide. Drug choices for patients with diabetes or gout are in the reverse order of this list. Low doses of thiazide diuretics can be used for patients with these disorders.

Hypokalemia can be a significant problem for patients with cardiac disorders. Drugs likely to have this adverse reaction are mostly the loop and then the thiazide diuretics. These drugs are still often chosen for their effects on the edema associated with HF. Careful monitoring of potassium levels must accompany their use with these patients. Hyperkalemia can be lethal for patients with renal failure and problematic for those with reduced renal function. Potassium-sparing diuretics are contraindicated in the former and rarely chosen in the latter. Both potassium-sparing diuretics and thiazides should be avoided for patients with Ccr less than 25 to 30 mL/min. Loop diuretics, metolazone, and indapamide are safe alternatives for these patients.

Hyperlipidemia is usually a transient phenomenon, and there is no consensus on the restriction of a drug class because of it. Indapamide effectively controls mild to moderate HTN, with no adverse reaction of lipids and minimum impact on potassium, glucose, and uric acid. It appears to address most concerns.

Combinations

Metolazone by itself is not a strong diuretic, but as an adjunct to loop diuretics its synergistic effect frequently overcomes refractory cases or enables dosage reduction of the loop diuretic, resulting in fewer adverse reactions. Combining a potassium-wasting diuretic with a potassium-sparing diuretic can prevent hypokalemia. Some drugs come in this combination (triamterene and hydrochlorothiazide [Maxzide], spironolactone and hydrochlorothiazide [Aldactazide]), making it possible to take only one tablet. Thiazides are typically the diuretic combined with other antihypertensives for dual therapy. (See Table 16-4.)

Cost

The generic form of each of these drugs is less expensive than the brand name and the combination tablets. The value of generic diuretics is quite clear.

Monitoring

In addition to monitoring the clinical indicators (BP, heart rate, edema, weight gain, dyspnea, cough, urine output), it is also critical to monitor renal function, glucose level, and electrolytes. Prior to initiating therapy, BUN, creatinine, electrolytes (sodium, potassium, calcium, and magnesium), uric acid, and glucose levels should be drawn. The patient should return to the clinic 4 weeks after initial prescription for a follow-up visit to check the clinical indicators and their electrolytes. Potassium levels of 3.5 to 4 mEq/L are usually not an indication for prescription supplementation in a noncardiac patient. Patients with cardiac disorders should have their potassium levels maintained at 4 to 4.5 mEq/L. Supplements need to be started even on asymptomatic patients with levels less than 3.5 mEq/L (Cohn et al, 2000). Spacing of monitoring after the first visit depends on lability of symptoms and dosage adjustments. Specific indicators to monitor depend on the common adverse effects of the specific drug(s) being used. This topic is discussed further in Chapters 36 and 40.

Patient Education

Administration

Patients should take the drug exactly as prescribed and not skip or double doses. For drugs given twice daily, the morning dose should be taken at breakfast and the evening dose no later in the day than 4 p.m. These drugs increase urine output, and taking the drug later may make the patient get up at night to urinate. Some of these drugs come alone or in combination. Check with the pharmacist with each refill to make certain the drug is in the correct form. For patients experiencing extreme diarrheal illness and dehydration, a call to the provider is indicated to help manage a temporary change in dosing.

Patients needing potassium supplements typically find the liquid forms unpalatable. They need precautions about tooth staining and the need for oral care after taking them. The medications can create gastric distress. Adherence is best with microencapsulated formulas due to no taste and fewer GI issues (Cohn et al, 2000).

Adverse Reactions

Hypotensive reactions are the most common. Changing position slowly, not using alcohol, not standing for long periods, and avoiding exercise in hot weather can decrease these reactions. These drugs are used to reduce fluid volume in the body in HF patients. Weighing daily helps to monitor that fluid. The patient should notify the health-care provider if weight loss of more than 1 lb per day or 5 lb per week, excessive thirst, dry skin or mucous membranes, dizziness, muscle pain, weakness or cramps, nausea, vomiting, increased heart rate, or diarrhea occurs. These may indicate an abnormal potassium level.

Potassium-wasting diuretics may cause potassium loss from the body. The health-care provider monitors this loss with laboratory work. If instructed by the health-care provider, a diet high in potassium may be needed. Foods high in potassium include bananas, dates, figs, fish, citrus juices, melons, molasses, baked potatoes, prunes, soybeans, and tomatoes. If an oral potassium supplement is prescribed, powders or liquids can be diluted in at least 4 oz fruit juice to improve the taste. Tablets taken with meals reduce GI irritation.

Potassium-sparing diuretics cause the body to hold potassium. The health-care provider monitors this gain with laboratory work. Patients should not take potassium supplements or use salt substitutes that have potassium in them.

Occasionally, these drugs cause GI upset, which may be reduced by taking them with meals. Use of a sunscreen prevents photosensitivity reactions, although these are rare. Changes in blood sugar and other body chemicals may occur. Follow-up appointments that allow the health-care provider to assess levels of these chemicals and progression of the disease process are important.

Lifestyle Management

If diuretics are taken for HTN, it is important to continue with the other therapies for HTN, including weight loss, sensible sodium intake, stress reduction, regular aerobic exercise, not using tobacco products, and moderation in alcohol intake. These drugs help to control HTN but do not cure it. Patients should not use OTC preparations without first checking with the health-care provider. They may interact with these drugs or make the disease process worse.

Lifestyle management for the specific disorders managed in whole or part with diuretics is covered in Chapters 36 and 40.

REFERENCES

AACE Hypertension Task Force. (2006). American Association of Clinical Endocrinologists medical guidelines for clinical practice for the diagnosis and treatment of hypertension. *Endocrinology Practice, 12*(2), 193–222.

American Academy of Nurse Practitioners [AANP]. (2012). A roadmap for managing your triglycerides and protecting your heart. Educational Flip Chart.

American College of Cardiology Foundation, American Heart Association Task Force on Practice Guidelines, American College of Physicians, American Association for Thoracic Surgery, Preventative Cardiovascular Nurses Association, Society for Cardiovascular Angiography and Interventions, & Society of Thoracic Surgeons [ACCF/AHA+]. (2012). Chronic angina focused update of the ACC/AHA guideline update for the management of patients with chronic angina. *Journal of the American College of Cardiology, 60*(24), 2564–2603.

American College of Cardiology Foundation/American Heart Association [ACCF/AHA]. (2009). ACC/AHA guidelines for the diagnosis and management of heart failure in adults: A report of the American College of Cardiology Foundation/American Heart Association Task Force on Practice Guidelines developed in collaboration with the International Society for Heart and Lung Transplantation. *Journal of the American College of Cardiology, 53*(15), 1343–1382.

American College of Cardiology Foundation/American Heart Association [ACCF/AHA]. (2011). Focused update on management of patients with atrial fibrillation—(Updating the 2006 guideline) : *Journal of the American College of Cardiology, 57*(2), 223–242.

American College of Cardiology Foundation/American Heart Association [ACCF/AHA]. (2013). Guideline on the treatment of blood cholesterol to reduce atherosclerotic cardiovascular risk in adults: Circulation. http://circ.ahajournals.org/content/early/2013/11/01/cir.0000437738.638 53.7a.citation

American College of Cardiology/American Heart Association/European Society of Cardiology (ACC/AHA/ESC). (2003). ACC/AHA/ESC guidelines for the management of patients with supraventricular arrhythmias—executive summary: A report of the American College of Cardiology/American Heart Association Task Force on Practice Guidelines and the European Society of Cardiology Committee for Practice Guidelines. *Journal of the American College of Cardiology, 42*(8), 1493–1531.

American College of Obstetricians and Gynecologists [ACOG]. (2012). ACOG Practice Bulletin No 125. Chronic hypertension in pregnancy. *Obstetrics & Gynecology, 119*, 396–407.

American Diabetes Association. (2015). Standards of medical care in diabetes. *Diabetes Care, 38*(1), S1–S94.

Bangalore, S., Makani, H., Radford, M., Thakur, K., Toklu, B., Katz, S., et.al. (2014). Clinical outcomes with beta-blockers for myocardial infarction: A meta-anlysis of randomized trials. *American Journal of Medicine, 127*(10), 939–953.

Boden, W., Probstfield, J. Anderson, T., Chaitman, B., Desvignes-Nickens, P., Koprowicz, K., et al. (2011). Niacin in patient with low HDL cholesterol levels receiving intensive statin therapy. AIM-HIGH study. *New England Journal of Medicine, 365*(24), 2255–2265.

Boekholdt, S., Hovingh, G., Mora, S., Arsenault, B., Amerenco, P., Pedersen, T., et al. (2014). Very low levels of atherogenic lipoproteins and the risk

for cardiovascular events: A meta-analysis of statin trials. *Journal of the American College of Cardiology, 64*(5),485–494.

Bonds, D., Craven, T., Buse, J., Crouse, J., Cuddihy, R., Elam, M., et al. (2012). Fenofibrate-associated changes in renal function and relationship to clinical outcomes among individuals with type 2 diabetes: The action to control cardiovascular risk in diabetics (ACCORD) experience. *Diabetologia, 55*, 1641–1650. doi: 10.1007/s00125-012-2524-2.

Brenner, B., Cooper, M., DeZeeuw, D., Keane, W., Mitch, W., Parving, H., et al, RENAAL Study Investigators. (2001). Effects of losartan on renal and cardiovascular outcomes in patients with type 2 diabetes and nephropathy. *New England Journal of Medicine, 345*(12), 861–869.

Bustamonte, A.& Montaner, J., (2013). Statin therapy should not be discontinued in patients with intra-cerebral hemorrhage. *Stroke, 44*(7) 2060-2061.

Chatterjee, S., Moeller, C., Shah, N., Bolorunduro, O., Lichstein, E., Moskovitz, N., et al. (2012, Aug 12). Eplerenone is not superior to older and less expensive aldosterone antagonist. *American Journal of Medicine, 125*(8), 817–825.

Cohn, J., Kowey, P., Whelton, P., & Prisant, M. (2000, Sept 11). New guidelines for potassium replacement in clinical practice. *Archives of Internal Medicine, 160*(16), 2429–2436.

Connolly, S., Camm, A. J., Halperin, J., Joyner, C., Alings, M., Amerena, J., Atar, D., et al. (2011). *New England Journal of Medicine, 365*(24), 2268–2276.

Daniels, S., Greer, F., & Committee on Nutrition. (2008). Lipid screening and cardiovascular health in childhood. *Pediatrics, 122*(1), 198–208.

Digitalis Investigation Group. (1997). The effect of digoxin on mortality and morbidity in patients with heart failure. *New England Journal of Medicine, 336*(8), 525–533.

Drucker, A., & Rosen, C. (2011). Drug-induced photosensitivity culprit drugs, management and prevention. *Drug Safety, 34*(10), 821–837.

Edelmann, F., Wachter, R., Schmidt, A., Karugher-Krainer, D., Colantonio, C., Kamke, W., et al. (2013, 27 Feb). Effect of spironolactone on diastolic function and exercise capacity in patients with heart failure and preserved ejection fraction: The Aldo-DHF RCT. *Journal of the American Medical Association, 309*(8), 781–791.

Elliot, W. (1996). Higher incidence of discontinuance of angiotensin converting enzyme inhibitors due to cough in black subjects. *Clinical Pharmacology and Therapy, 60*, 582–588.

Federal Drug Administration. (2012, 28 Feb). FDA announces safety changes in labeling for some cholesterol-lowering drugs. *FDA News Release.* www.FDA.gov

Gibson, C., Pride, Y., Hochberg, C., Sloan, S., Sabatine, M., & Cannon, C. (2009, 8 Dec). PROVE-IT Effect of intensive statin therapy on clinical outcomes among patients undergoing percutaneous coronary intervention for ACS. *Journal of the American College of Cardiologists, 54*(2), 2290–2295.

Grundy, S., Cleeman, J., Merz, C., Brewer, H., Jr., Clark, L., Hunninghake, D., et al. (2004). Implications of recent clinical trials for the National Cholesterol Education Program Adult Treatment Panel III guidelines. *Circulation, 110*(2), 227–239.

Hecht, H., & Harman, M. (2003a). Comparison of effectiveness of statin monotherapy versus statin and niacin combination therapy in primary prevention and effects on calcified plaque burden. *American Journal of Cardiology, 91*, 348–350.

Hecht, H., & Harman, M. (2003b). Comparisons of the effects of atorvastatin versus simvastatin on subclinical atherosclerosis in primary prevention as determined by electron beam tomography. *American Journal of Cardiology, 91*, 42–45.

Institute for Clinical Symptoms Improvement. (2011a, April). *S coronary artery disease* (14th ed.) Institute for Clinical Symptoms Improvement, 59 pp. www.icsi.org

Institute for Clinical Systems Improvement (ICSI). (2011b, Aug). *Heart failure in adults* (12th ed.). Institute for Clinical Systems Improvement, 112 pp. www.ICSI.org http://www.guideline.gov/summary/summary.aspx

Institute for Clinical Symptoms Improvement (ICSI). (2012, Nov). *Diagnosis and treatment of chest pain and acute coronary syndrome (ACS).* Institute for Clinical Symptoms Improvement. 92 pp. www.icsi.org

JNC-8 (James et al). (2013). Evidence based guideline for the management of high blood pressure in adults: Report from the panel members appointed to the eighth joint national committee. Published online 18 Dec 2013. doi: 10.1001/jama.2013.284427

Kaddurah-Daouk, R., Baillie, R., Zhu, H., Zeng, A., Wiest, M., Nguyen, U., et al. (2011, 13 Oct). Enteric microbiome metabolites correlate with response to simvastatin treatment. *PLoS ONE, 6*(10) e25482. doi: 10.1371/journal.pone.0025482

Kent, D., Jafar, T., Hayward R., Tighiouart, H., Landa, M., de Jong, P., et al. (2007). Progression risk, urinary protein excretion and treatment effects of angiotensin-converting enzyme inhibitors in nondiabetic kidney disease. *Journal of the American Society of Nephrology, 18*(6), 1959–1965.

Klein, R., Myers, C.& Klein, B. (2014). Vasodilators, blood pressure-lowering medications, and age-related macular degeneration. The Beaver Dam Study. *Opthalmology 121*(8), 1604-1611.

Kokkinos, P., Faselis, C., Myers, J., Pangiotakos, D., & Doumas, M. (2012). Interactive effects of fitness and statin treatment on mortality risk in veterans with dyslipidemia. *The Lancet, 381*(9864), 394–399. doi: 10.1016/S0140-6736(12)61426-3

Leoncini, M., Toso, A., Maioli, M., Tropeano, F., Villani, S., Bellandi, F. (2014) Early High-Dose Rosuvastatin for Contrast-Induced Nephropathy Prevention in Acute Coronary Syndrome: Results From the PRATO-ACS Study (Protective Effect of Rosuvastatin and Antiplatelet Therapy On Contrast-Induced Acute Kidney Injury and Myocardial Damage in Patients With Acute Coronary Syndrome). *Journal of the American College of Cardiology, 63*(1), 71–79. doi:10.1016/j.jacc.2013.04.105. Retrieved from http://content.onlinejacc.org/article.aspx?articleID=1748222

Li, D., Kim, R., McArthur, E., Fleet, J., Bailey, D., Juurlink, D., et al. (2014). Risk of adverse events among older adults following co-prescrition of clarithromycin and statins not metabolized by cytochrome P450 3A4. *Canadian Medical Journal. Epub ahead of print* doi 10.1503/cmaj.140950.

McCrindle, B., Urbina, E., Dennison, B., Jacobson, M., Steinberger, J., Rocchini, A., et al, American Heart Association Atherosclerosis, Hypertension and Obesity in Youth Committee, American Heart Association Council of Cardiovascular Disease in the Young, American Heart Association Council on Cardiovascular Nursing. (2007). Drug therapy of high-risk lipid abnormalities in children and adolescents. *Circulation, 115*(14), 1948–1967.

Mente, A., deKoning, L., Shannon, H., & Anand, S. (2009). A systematic review of the evidence supporting a causal link between dietary factors and coronary heart disease. *Archives of Internal Medicine, 169*(7), 659–669.

Montalescot, G. (2013). Early administration of eplerenone in patients with acute myocardial infarction without heart failure: Results of the randomized, double-blind controlled REMINDER trial. Podium presentation at ACC March 2013, San Francisco, CA.

Mozaffarian, D., Marchioli, R., Macchia, A., Silletta, M., Ferrazi, P., Gardner, T., et al. (2012) Fish oil and post-operative atrial fibrillation: The omega-3 fatty acids for prevention of post-operative atrial fibrillation (OPERA) randomized trial. *Journal of the American Medical Association, 308*(19), 2001–2011. doi: 10.1001/jama2012.28733

Naci, H., Brugts, J., & Ades, T. (2013). Comparative tolerability and harms of individual statins: A study-level network meta-analysis of 245,955 participants from 135 randomized controlled trials. *Circulation Quality and Outcomes.* 6(4) 390–399.

National Cholesterol Education Program (NCEP). (2001). *Third report of the Expert Panel on Detection, Evaluation, and Treatment of High Blood Cholesterol in Adults (Adult Treatment Panel III).* Rockville, MD: National Institutes of Health, National Heart, Lung, and Blood Institute.

National Collaborating Centre for Chronic Conditions (NCCC). (2003). *Chronic heart failure: National clinical guideline for diagnosis and management in primary and secondary care.* Salisbury, Wiltshire, England: Sarum Colour View Group.

National High Blood Pressure Education Program (NHBPEP). (2003). *The seventh report of the Joint National Committee on Prevention, Detection, Evaluation, and Treatment of High Blood Pressure.* Rockville, MD: National Institutes of Health, National Heart, Lung, and Blood Institute.

Nicholls, S., Ballantyne, C., Barter, P., Chapman, M., Erbel, R., Libby, P., et al. (2011). Effect of two intensive statin regimens on progression of coronary disease. *New England Journal of Medicine, 365* (22), 2078–2087.

Packer, M., Gheorghiade, M., Young, J., Constantini, P., Adams, K., Cody, R., et al. (1993). Withdrawal of digoxin from patients with chronic heart failure treated with angiotensin-converting enzyme inhibitors. RADIANCE Study. *New England Journal of Medicine, 329,* 1–7.

Parker, B., Capizzi, J., Grimaldi, A., Clarkson, P., Cole, S., Keadle, J., et al. (2012, 26 Nov). The effects of statins on skeletal muscle function. STOMP. *Circulation online.* doi: 10.1161/CirculationAHA.112.136101

Parving, H., Brenner, B., McMurray, J., deZeeuw, D., Haffner, S., Solomen, S., et al. (2012). Cardiorenal end points in trial of aliskiren for type 2 diabetes. (ALTITUDE). *New England Journal of Medicine, 367*(23), 2204–2213.

Preiss, D. Tikkanen, M., Welsh, P., Ford, I., Lovato, L., Elam, M., et al. (2012). Lipid-modifying therapies and risk of pancreatitis; A metaanalysis. *Clinical Review, 308*(8), 804–811.

Remuzzi, G., Schieppati, A., & Ruggenenti, P. (2003). Nephropathy in patients with type 2 diabetes. *New England Journal of Medicine, 346*(15), 1145–1151.

Scordo, K. (2012). Statin intolerance: Management strategies. *The American Journal for Nurse Practitioners, 16*(3/4), 20–24.

The HPS2-THRIVE Collaborative Group. (2014). Effects of extended release niacin with laropiprant in high risk patients. *New England Journal of Medicine.* 371(3), 203-212.

Toso, A. (2013). Early high dose rosuvastin for contrast-induced nephropathy prevention in acute coronary syndrome PRAT0-ACS study. Presentation at ACC March 2013. San Francisco, CA.

Uretsky, B., Young, J., Shahidi, F., Yellen, L., Harrison, M., & Joily, M. (1993). Randomized study assessing the effect of digoxin withdrawal in patients with mild to moderate chronic congestive heart failure: Results of the PROVED trial. *Journal of the American College of Cardiology, 22,* 955–962.

Wade, V., & Gleason, B. (2004). Dual blockade of the renin-angiotensin system in diabetic nephropathy. *Annals of Pharmacotherapy, 38*(7), 1278–1282.

Weber, M., Jamerson K., Bakris, G., Weir, M., Zappe, D., & Zhang, Y. (2012). Effects of body size and hypertension treatments on cardiovascular event rates: Sub analysis of the ACCOMPLISH randomized controlled trial. *The Lancet, 381*(9866), 537–545. doi: pii: S0140-6736(12)61343-1349

Wolters Kluwer Health. (2011). *Drug facts and comparisons.* St. Louis, MO: Wolters Kluwer Health.

Wright, J., Probstfield, J., Cushman, W., Pressel, S., Cutler, J., Davis, B., et al. for the ALLHAT Collaborative Research Group. (2009). ALLHAT findings revisited in the context of subsequent analyses, other trials, and metaanalyses. *Archives of Internal Medicine, 169*(9), 832–842.

Wu, S., Han, J., Li, W-Q., & Quereshi, A. (2014). Hypertension, antihypensive medication use, and risk of psoriasis. *Journal of the American Medical Association: Dermatology, 154*(9) 957-963.

Zuber, D., & Davis, J. (2012). Loop diuretics and kidney classes. *Clinician Reviews, 22*(10), 11–12.

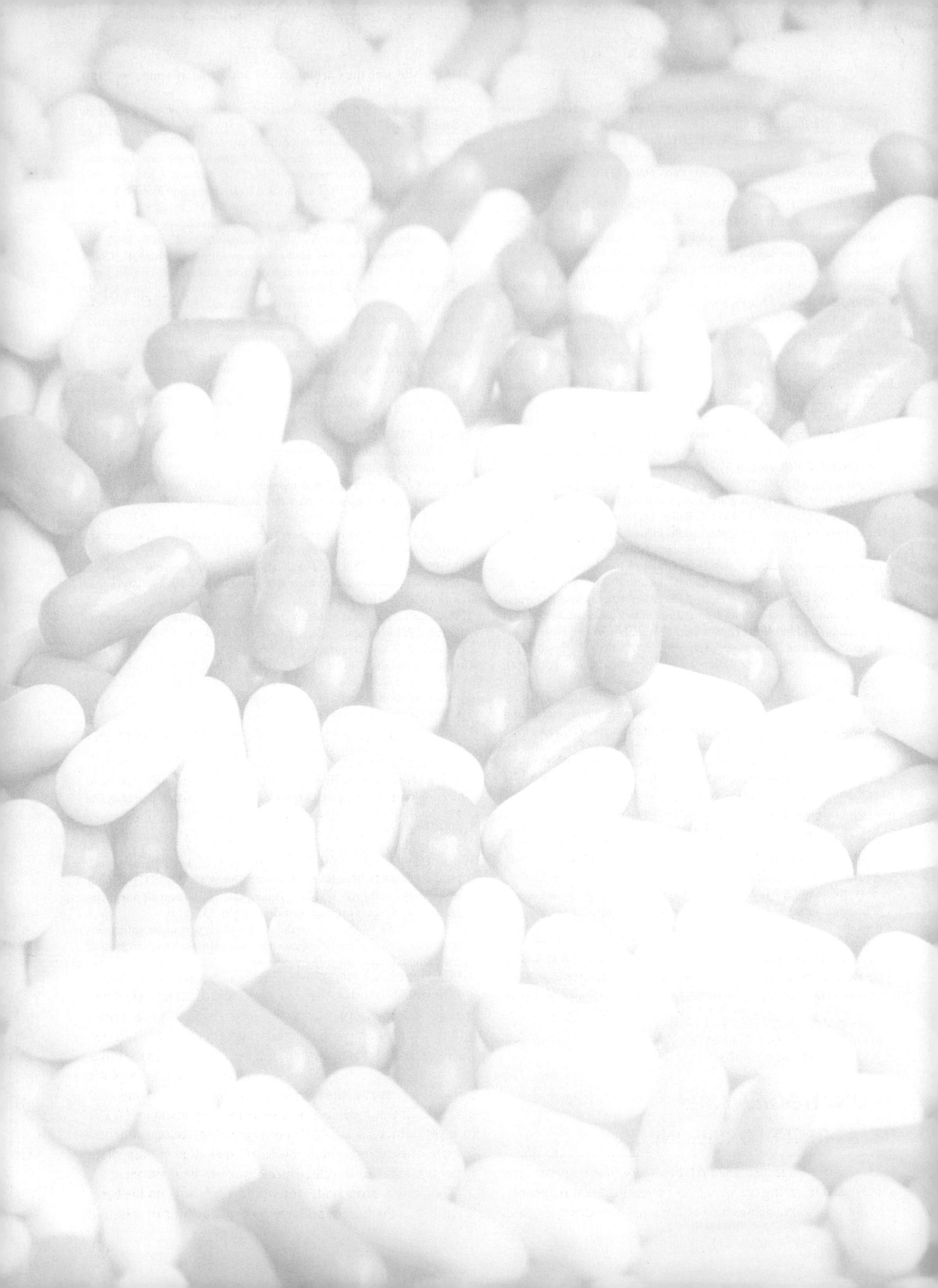

CHAPTER 17

DRUGS AFFECTING THE RESPIRATORY SYSTEM

Teri Moser Woo

Numerous medications are available to treat disorders of the respiratory system. Those discussed in this chapter include bronchodilators, which act on the bronchial smooth muscle to reverse bronchospasm, and leukotriene-receptor agents, which act to decrease the inflammation in the lungs of patients with asthma. Included in this chapter are antihistamines, decongestants, expectorants, and antitussive over-the-counter (OTC) medications. Inhaled anti-inflammatory medications used for asthma and intranasal steroids used for the treatment of seasonal or perennial rhinitis are also discussed. Prescribing recommendations for the multiple medications used in the treatment of asthma or chronic obstructive pulmonary disease (COPD) are provided in Chapter 31; prescribing recommendations for decongestants for upper respiratory infections are also found in Chapter 47. IV forms of respiratory medications, which are rarely used in primary care, are not discussed here.

BRONCHODILATORS

BETA$_2$-RECEPTOR AGONISTS

Beta$_2$-receptor-agonist (B2RA) bronchodilator agents are widely used in caring for all ages of patients to treat reversible bronchoconstriction caused by asthma, reactive airway disease

(RAD), or COPD. A variety of beta-agonist bronchodilators are available, and the medications come in multiple forms and delivery systems. Albuterol (ProAir, Ventolin, Proventil) is the most commonly prescribed drug in this class. Other sympathomimetic bronchodilator medications used in primary care are the short-acting B2RAs metaproterenol (Alupent), terbutaline (Brethine, Brethaire), bitolterol (Tornalate), pirbuterol (Maxair), and levalbuterol (Xopenex). The long-acting B2RAs include arformoterol (Brovana), formoterol (Foradil), indacaterol (Arcapta), and salmeterol (Serevent).

Pharmacodynamics

Bronchodilators act on the smooth muscle of the bronchial tree to reverse bronchospasm, thereby decreasing airway resistance and residual volume and increasing vital capacity and airflow. Beta agonists stimulate beta$_2$ adrenergic receptors in the lungs to increase production of cyclic adenosine monophosphate (cAMP) by activation of adenyl cyclase, the enzyme that catalyzes the conversion of adenosine triphosphate (ATP) to cAMP. Increased cAMP concentrations relax bronchial smooth muscle and inhibit release of mediators of immediate hypersensitivity from cells, especially from the mast cells.

The perfect bronchodilator would work only on the beta$_2$ receptors in the lungs and have no other actions or systemic effects. Unfortunately, all of the currently available preparations have some effects on other body systems, such as the cardiovascular system, skeletal muscles, and the central nervous system (CNS).

Albuterol is a selective $beta_2$ agonist with some minor $beta_1$ activity. Albuterol's International Nonproprietary Name is salbutamol. It can increase heart rate by directly stimulating $beta_2$ receptors in the heart and by stimulating $beta_2$ receptors in vascular smooth muscle. The effect on cardiac $beta_2$ receptors is of consequence only at high serum levels of albuterol because it has a low affinity for these receptors and there are fewer $beta_2$ receptors than $beta_1$ receptors in the heart. Stimulation of the $beta_2$ receptors in the vascular smooth muscle leads to vasodilation, a decrease in diastolic blood pressure, and therefore a reflex increase in heart rate. Albuterol causes $beta_2$-receptor stimulation of skeletal muscle that leads to tremors. Albuterol has fewer cardiac and CNS effects than some of the other beta agonists and is, therefore, often the drug of choice for first-line therapy. Levalbuterol is similar to albuterol, where the (S)-isomer from racemic albuterol is removed, leaving the (R)-isomer, which has less adverse effects. Pirbuterol is a selective $beta_2$ agonist that is structurally identical to albuterol, except for the substitution of a pyridine ring for the benzene ring in its chemical makeup.

Terbutaline has a pharmacodynamic profile similar to that of albuterol, in that it is a selective $beta_2$ agonist with minor $beta_1$ activity. Terbutaline is also known to inhibit uterine contractions via its beta receptor–mediated action on uterine smooth muscle. Metaproterenol is also a selective $beta_2$ agonist with some $beta_1$ activity, although it is less selective than albuterol or terbutaline. Bitolterol is hydrolyzed by the esterases in the lung to colterol, or terbutylnorepinephrine, which is a selective $beta_2$ agonist.

Salmeterol, formoterol, indacaterol, and aformoterol are long-acting inhaled bronchodilators with a half-life ranging from 10 hours (formoterol) to more than 40 hours (indacaterol). Salmeterol is more selective for $beta_2$ receptors than is albuterol and has minor $beta_1$ activity. Formoterol has a 200-fold greater agonist activity at $beta_2$ receptors than at $beta_1$ receptors. Aformoterol is the (R, R)-enantiomer of formoterol and has twice the potency of formoterol. Indacaterol has a 24-fold greater agonist activity at $beta_2$ receptors than to $beta_1$ receptors. Salmeterol and formoterol exert long-lasting bronchoprotection effects against allergen-, exercise-, histamine-, and methacholine-caused bronchospasm.

Pharmacokinetics

Absorption and Distribution

Albuterol is most commonly inhaled and gradually absorbed from the bronchi. The overall systemic concentration remains low following recommended doses. The low systemic concentration is because of the need to use only 5% of the dose required orally to achieve the desired effects. Oral forms of albuterol are well absorbed from the gastrointestinal (GI) tract, rapidly enter the bloodstream, and are widely distributed in the body fluids and tissues. Extended-release oral albuterol is formulated to be absorbed from the stomach more slowly. Breast milk excretion is not known.

Levalbuterol is minimally absorbed from the respiratory tract and its distribution is unknown.

Pirbuterol is minimally absorbed from the respiratory tract, with amounts below the limits of serum assay detected after administration via inhalation. Its distribution is unknown.

Terbutaline is available in inhaled, oral, and subcutaneous (SC) forms. The inhaled form of terbutaline is minimally absorbed from the respiratory tract. Approximately 33% to 50% of the oral form is absorbed from the GI tract and is widely distributed. If administered SC, terbutaline is almost completely absorbed and is widely distributed. It crosses the placenta and is excreted in breast milk.

Metaproterenol may be administered via the inhaled route or orally. Approximately 3% of the inhaled metaproterenol dose is absorbed intact through the lungs. Oral dosing results in approximately 10% of the dose being absorbed intact. Distribution of metaproterenol is unknown.

Bitolterol absorption is too low to be measured by serum assay; distribution is unknown.

Salmeterol administered via inhaler is absorbed via the lungs in small amounts; undetectable amounts are found in the serum with recommended doses. With chronic administration, salmeterol is detected in the serum at very low levels. Salmeterol is excreted in breast milk in small amounts, approximately equal to plasma levels.

Formoterol is an inhaled dry powder capsule administered via a unique Aerolizer Inhaler. The powdered medication is quickly absorbed in the lungs, with an onset of 1 to 3 minutes. There are no human studies of distribution of formoterol into breast milk; in rat studies, the drug could be measured in milk.

Aformoterol inhalation solution is administered via standard jet nebulizer. Approximately 75% of an aformoterol dose is absorbed via the lungs and reaches peak levels in 30 minutes. Aformoterol has been measured in rat milk, but it is not known whether it is excreted in human milk.

Indacaterol is a dry powder packaged in gelatin capsules and is administered via the Arcapta Neohaler. Indacaterol reaches peak levels 15 minutes after inhalation. It is not known whether indacaterol is distributed in human breast milk.

Metabolism and Excretion

Most of the common bronchodilators are metabolized in the liver and excreted primarily in the urine.

Albuterol is metabolized into albuterol 49-O-sulfate, which has little or no beta adrenergic–stimulating effect and no beta adrenergic–blocking effect. Approximately 72% of inhaled albuterol is excreted in the urine within 24 hours of inhalation, 28% of this as unchanged drug and 44% as the metabolite. Another 10% of the inhaled albuterol is excreted in the feces. Oral administration of albuterol results in 65% to 90% of the dose being excreted in the urine over 3 days, the majority in the first 24 hours. About 4% of the oral albuterol dose is excreted in feces.

Levalbuterol is metabolized and excreted in the same fashion as albuterol.

Pirbuterol is not metabolized extensively, with 51% of the dose excreted in the urine as pirbuterol plus its sulfate conjugate. Terbutaline is partially metabolized in the liver, primarily to inactive sulfate conjugate, and is excreted in the urine. Metaproterenol is metabolized by the liver into its sulfate conjugate and excreted in the urine. Bitolterol is a prodrug that is hydrolyzed by esterases in tissue and blood to the active moiety colterol. Within 24 hours, 83% of the dose is excreted in the urine. After 72 hours, 85.6% of the dose has been excreted in the urine and 8% in the feces, as conjugated colterol.

Salmeterol xinafoate, an ionic salt, dissociates so that the salmeterol and 1-hydroxy-2-naphthoic acid (xinafoate) are metabolized and excreted independently. Salmeterol base is extensively metabolized by hydroxylation in the liver. Urinary elimination accounts for 25% of the drug, and 60% is eliminated in the feces over a period of 7 days. The xinafoate moiety has no apparent pharmacological activity, is extensively protein bound, and has a long elimination half-life of 11 days.

Formoterol fumarate is metabolized by glucuronidation in the liver. Renal elimination accounts for 59% to 62% of elimination; 32% to 34% is eliminated in the feces.

Aformoterol is almost completely metabolized in the liver, primarily by CYP2D6 and CYP2C19. Aformoterol is primarily excreted by the kidneys, with 67% excreted in the urine and 22% excreted in the feces.

Indacaterol is metabolized predominantly by CYP3A4 and is eliminated in the feces (54% unchanged, 23% hydroxylated metabolite) and urine (less than 2% unchanged).

Table 17-1 shows the pharmacokinetic properties of selected bronchodilators.

Pharmacotherapeutics
Precautions and Contraindications

Sympathomimetic bronchodilators have relatively few contraindications to use. Cardiac arrhythmias associated with tachycardia or heart block caused by digitalis intoxication, angina, narrow-angle glaucoma, organic brain damage (epinephrine only), and shock during general anesthesia with halogenated agents are all contraindications to beta$_2$ agonists. Because of these drugs' effects on the cardiovascular system, patients with hypertension, ischemic heart disease, coronary insufficiency, congestive heart failure, and a history of stroke and/or cardiac arrhythmias should be monitored closely for adverse effects during administration of any of the sympathomimetic bronchodilators. For patients with diabetes mellitus, there is a potential drug-induced hyperglycemia that may result in loss of diabetic control when using any of the beta$_2$ agonists, and their insulin dosage may need to be increased. For patients with hyperthyroidism, adverse reactions are more likely to occur with the use of bronchodilators. Patients taking digoxin require close monitoring when albuterol is started because albuterol increases the volume of distribution of digoxin and can cause up to a 30% decrease in blood digoxin levels. Patients with diagnosed or suspected pheochromocytoma should avoid the beta-adrenergic antagonists because severe hypertension may occur.

Table 17–1 ⠿ Pharmacokinetics: Selected Bronchodilators

Drug	Onset	Peak	Duration	Half-Life	Metabolism	Elimination
Beta$_2$ Agonists						
Aformeterol Inhalation	5 min	30 min		10 h	Hepatic	Renal 67%; fecal 22%
Albuterol					Hepatic	Renal 90%; fecal 10%
Inhalation	5–15 min	0.5–2 h	2–6 h	3.8 h		
Oral short-acting	15–30 min	2–3 h	4–6 h	2.7–5 h		
Oral extended-release			8–12 h			
Bitolterol				UK	Hydrolyzed by esterases in tissues and blood to colterol	Renal
Inhalation	3–4 min	0.5–1	5–8 h			
Indacaterol		15 min		~40–56 hours	Hydroxylation predominantly by CYP3A4	Feces (54% unchanged, 23% hydroxylated metabolite); urine (<2% unchange)
Formoterol	1–3 min	15 min	12 h	10–14 h	Hepatic	Renal
Levalbuterol	10–17 min	1.5 h	5–6 h	3.3–4.0 h	Hepatic	Renal

Continued

Table 17–1 ✂ **Pharmacokinetics: Selected Bronchodilators—cont'd**

Drug	Onset	Peak	Duration	Half-Life	Metabolism	Elimination
Metaproterenol				UK	Hepatic	Renal
Inhalation	1 min	1 h	1–2.5 h			
Nebulization	5–30 min	1 h	4 h			
Oral	15–30 min	1 h	4 h			
Pirbuterol	5 min	0.5–1 h	5 h	2 h	Hepatic	Renal
Inhalation	5 min	0.5–1 h	5 h			
Salmeterol	14 min	3–4 h	12 h	2.5 h	Hydroxylation	Feces
Inhalation						
Terbutaline				UK	Liver (partial)	Renal; small amount in bile, feces
Inhalation	5–30 min	—	3–6 h			
Oral	30 min	—	4–8 h			
Anticholinergic						
Aclidinium		5–10 min		1–4 h	Hydrolysis	54%–65% renal; 20%–33% feces
Ipratropium Inhalation	15–30 min	1–2 h	4–5 h	2 h	Ester hydrolysis	Renal
Tiotropium		5 min	24 h		Liver	Renal
Xanthine Derivatives						

Theophylline
  Immediate-release
  Extended-release
  Liquid
		2 h
		4–7 h
		1 h
			—	*Children <6 mo: >*
				  24 h; >6 mo:
				  1.1–3.7 h
				Adult nonsmokers:
				  8.7–2.2 h
				Adult smokers:
				  4–5 h
				Adults with COPD,
				  congestive heart
				  failure (CHF), cor
				  pulmonale, or liver
				  disease may
				  exceed 24 h
					Liver	Renal

UK = unknown.

Lower doses of bronchodilators may be necessary in older adults because of increased sympathomimetic sensitivity.

In the Salmeterol Multicenter Asthma Research Trial (SMART), there was a small but statistically significant increase in respiratory-related and asthma-related deaths in the study population receiving salmeterol versus placebo (Nelson et al, 2006). The study was terminated early owing to these findings. Further analysis indicates that the risk may be greater for African Americans than for white subjects (Nelson et al, 2006). The U.S. Food and Drug Administration (FDA) subsequently issued a Black-Box Warning for salmeterol and formoterol in 2005, and in December 2008 a follow-up FDA advisory was issued stating that the risks of salmeterol (Serevent) and formoterol (Foradil) outweighed the benefits and that they should not be used singly in asthma for all ages. Aformoterol and indacaterol were subsequently issued Black-Box Warnings when they became FDA-approved.

The safety and risks of the long-acting beta agonists (LABAs) continued to be studied with an emphasis on examining the risk for intubation and death in patients who use LABAs. Salpeter, Wall, and Buckley (2010) conducted a meta-analysis of pooled data of randomized controlled trials (RCTs) totaling 36,588 patients and found a 2-fold increase in catastrophic events (asthma-related intubations and death) in patients who were treated with LABAs. In February 2010, the FDA released a safety announcement regarding LABAs:

To ensure the safe use of these products:

• The use of LABAs is contraindicated without the use of an asthma controller medication such as an inhaled corticosteroid. Single-ingredient LABAs should only be used in combination with an asthma controller medication; they should not be used alone.

- LABAs should only be used long-term in patients whose asthma cannot be adequately controlled on asthma controller medications.
- LABAs should be used for the shortest duration of time required to achieve control of asthma symptoms and discontinued, if possible, once asthma control is achieved. Patients should then be maintained on an asthma controller medication.
- Pediatric and adolescent patients who require the addition of a LABA to an inhaled corticosteroid should use a combination product containing both an inhaled corticosteroid and a LABA, to ensure compliance with both medications (http://www. fda.gov/Safety/MedWatch/SafetyInformation/SafetyAlertsforHumanMedical Products/ucm201003.htm).

Providers should use caution when prescribing LABAs and provide close follow-up to ensure patient safety.

Terbutaline is Pregnancy Category B; the rest of the beta-agonist bronchodilators are Pregnancy Category C. No reports linking the use of albuterol with human congenital anomalies have been published. Terbutaline is used during pregnancy to prevent contractions related to preterm labor. This is not an FDA-approved use; therefore, oral forms of the beta agonists should be used selectively in patients in labor. Inhaled forms of the beta agonists are less likely to affect uterine contractions.

Small amounts of terbutaline and salmeterol can be measured in breast milk. The other inhaled beta-agonist bronchodilators cannot be measured in breast milk, probably because of the small amount of drug that is used and absorbed. The use of inhaled bronchodilators during lactation is most likely safe, with careful monitoring of the infant.

Albuterol is used extensively in infants and children with minimal adverse effects. Metaproterenol may also be used in young children, although albuterol is generally the first-choice medication. Dosing guidelines are provided on the label by the manufacturer of levalbuterol for children down to age 6, although a study of safety and efficacy in 2- to 5-year-olds indicated that the drug was effective and well tolerated by younger children (Skoner et al, 2005). Terbutaline may be safely prescribed to children, although it is not a first-line beta agonist for asthma. The safety of pirbuterol and bitolterol for use in children aged 12 years and under has not been established.

As previously mentioned, the FDA has issued a warning that LABA should not be prescribed as monotherapy to children or adolescents. Salmeterol should not be prescribed to children younger than age 4 and formoterol is not recommended for children age 5 years or younger. Indacaterol and aformeterol are indicated for chronic obstructive pulmonary disease (COPD), which is an adult disease and are not indicated for use in children or adolescents.

Adverse Drug Reactions

Adverse reactions to the beta-agonist bronchodilators are usually transient, and discontinuing the medication is not usually necessary, but a temporary reduction in the dose may alleviate some of the side effects. Slowly increase the dose after the reaction to the optimal dosing has subsided.

Supraventricular and ventricular ectopic beats have occurred with beta-agonist inhalation, but the incidence is low (bitolterol 0.5%, terbutaline about 4%, pirbuterol less than 1%). Tachycardia and palpitations are reported in 14% of patients who use these sympathomimetic bronchodilators.

The beta-agonist bronchodilators exhibit some CNS excitation effects, with tremors, dizziness, shakiness, nervousness, and restlessness reported in some patients. Headaches may occur with bronchodilator use in 2% to 28% of patients. Insomnia is rare, reported in 1% to 3% of patients. Patients (up to 26%) may exhibit a post-inhalation cough after using indacaterol.

Salmeterol has a documented increased risk of exacerbation of severe asthma symptoms if the patient is deteriorating. To avoid this risk, none of the LABAs should be started in patients with acutely deteriorating asthma and are best used in combination with an inhaled steroid.

Drug Interactions

Because of the cardiovascular effects of the bronchodilators, careful monitoring for drug interactions is necessary. If any of the beta agonists are prescribed with digitalis glycosides, caution and careful monitoring of the patient's electrocardiogram (ECG) is necessary because there is an increased risk of cardiac arrhythmia.

Beta agonists used with beta-adrenergic blocking agents (including ophthalmic preparations) may result in mutual inhibition of therapeutic effects. Tricyclic antidepressants and monoamine oxidase inhibitors (MAOIs) used with albuterol, metaproterenol, or terbutaline may potentiate the effects of the bronchodilator on the vascular system.

Hypokalemia or electrocardiogram changes may be seen with coadministration of the beta agonists with drugs that lower the potassium level, such as diuretics.

Table 17-2 shows drug interaction information.

Clinical Use and Dosing

Bronchospasm

The bronchodilators are used primarily in the treatment of bronchospasm associated with asthma, bronchitis (acute or chronic), and COPD.

The dose of albuterol metered-dose inhaler (MDI) in children over age 4 years and adults is two puffs every 4 to 6 hours. The dose of albuterol (Ventolin, Proventil) delivered via nebulizer for children over age 12 years as well as for adults is 2.5 mg (0.5 mL) in 2 mL normal saline; for younger children up to 15 kg, the dose is 0.1 to 0.15 mg/kg per dose. For children over 15 kg, the dose is the same as it is for adults, 2.5 mg/dose. Inhaled forms of albuterol may be repeated once after 5 to 10 minutes, up to 2 times (three doses total) during exacerbations. The oral albuterol dose in adults is 2 to 4 mg 3 or 4 times a day, up to a maximum of 32 mg/day. For children aged 6 to 12, 2 mg albuterol 3 or 4 times a day may be prescribed, although oral albuterol is rarely used in children.

Table 17–2 ▓ Drug Interactions: Selected Bronchodilators

Drug	Interacting Drug	Possible Effect	Implications
Beta₂ Agonists			
Aformoterol	Adrenergics	Sympathetic effects of aformoterol may be potentiated	Monitor HR and BP, use with caution in patients with cardiovascular disorders
	Beta blockers (including ophthalmic agents)	Mutual inhibition of therapeutic effects	Should not be used together
	Xanthine derivatives	May potentiate hypokalemia	Monitor potassium levels
	Steroids	May potentiate hypokalemic effect	Monitor potassium levels
	Diuretics	May potentiate hypokalemic effects ECG changes	Monitor potassium
	MAOIs	Potentiates adrenergic effects of aformoterol	Severe hypertension, headache, hyperpyrexia, and possible hypertensive crisis; do not use concurrently
	Tricyclic antidepressants	Potentiate andrenergic effects	Monitor HR and BP
	QTc prolonging drugs	Prolong QTc interval	Avoid concurrent use
Albuterol	Digoxin	Digoxin serum levels may be decreased	Decreased dose of albuterol may be needed
	Other sympathomimetics	Additive effects	Serious adverse cardiac effects; do not use concurrently
	MAOIs	Potentiates albuterol	Severe hypertension, headache, hyperpyrexia, and possible hypertensive crisis; do not use concurrently
	Tricyclic antidepressants	Potentiates the pressor response of sympathomimetics	Arrhythmias if used concurrently
	Beta blockers (including ophthalmic agents)	Mutual inhibition of therapeutic effects	Should not be used together
	Cocaine	Increased CNS stimulation	Observe patients for cardiac and CNS effects
	Thyroid hormones	Cardiac effects of both drugs enhanced	Increased risk of coronary insufficiency from combined use of these drugs; avoid this combination in patients with preexisting cardiac disease
	Ritodrine	Increased CNS stimulation	Avoid concurrent use
Bitolterol	Other sympathomimetics	Additive effects	Serious adverse cardiac effects; avoid concurrent use of sympathomimetics
	MAOIs	Potentiates bitolterol	Severe hypertension, headache, hyperpyrexia, and possible hypertensive crisis; do not use together
	Tricyclic antidepressants	Potentiates the pressor response of sympathomimetics	May cause arrhythmias; do not use together
	Beta blockers (including ophthalmic agents)	Mutual inhibition of therapeutic effects	Should not be used together
Indacaterol	Adrenergic drugs	↑ sympathetic effects	Monitor
	Xanthine derivatives	May potentiate hypokalemia	Monitor potassium levels
	Steroids	May potentiate hypokalemic effect	Monitor potassium levels
	Diuretics	May potentiate hypokalemic effects ECG changes	Monitor potassium

Table 17–2 ▦ Drug Interactions: Selected Bronchodilators—cont'd

Drug	Interacting Drug	Possible Effect	Implications
	MAOIs	Potentiates adrenergic effects of aformoterol	Severe hypertension, headache, hyperpyrexia, and possible hypertensive crisis; do not use concurrently
	Tricyclic andidepressants	Potentiate andrenergic effects	Monitor HR and BP
	QTc prolonging drugs	Prolong QTc interval	Avoid concurrent use
	Beta blockers (including ophthalmic agents)	Mutual inhibition of therapeutic effects	Should not be used together
Levalbuterol	Beta blockers	Mutual inhibition of therapeutic effects	Should not be used together
	MAOIs	Potentiates albuterol	Severe hypertension, headache, hyperpyrexia, and possible hypertensive crisis; do not use concurrently
	Tricyclic antidepressants	Potentiates the pressor response of sympathomimetics	Arrhythmias if used concurrently
	Digoxin	Digoxin serum levels may be decreased	Decreased dose of albuterol may be needed
	Other sympathomimetics	Additive effects	Serious adverse cardiac effects; do not use concurrently
Metaproterenol	Other sympathomimetics	Additive effects	Serious adverse cardiac effects; avoid concurrent use
	MAOIs	Potentiates metaproterenol	Severe hypertension, headache, hyperpyrexia, and possible hypertensive crisis; do not use together
	Tricyclic antidepressants	Potentiates the pressor response of sympathomimetics	May cause arrhythmias; do not use together
	Beta blockers (including ophthalmic agents)	Mutual inhibition of therapeutic effects	Should not be used together
	Inhalation anesthetics	Sensitizes the myocardium to the effects of metaproterenol	May cause arrhythmias; use with caution and, if possible, avoid concurrent use
	Theophylline or caffeine	Additive toxic effects	CNS stimulation or toxicity a concern; use with caution and close monitoring
	Thyroid hormones	Cardiac effects of both drugs enhanced	Increased risk of coronary insufficiency from the combined use of these drugs; use with caution in patients with preexisting cardiac disease
Pirbuterol	Other beta agonists	Additive effects	Increased adverse effects; avoid concurrent use
	MAOIs, tricyclic antidepressants	Potentiates pirbuterol	Severe hypertension, headache, hyperpyrexia, and possible hypertensive crisis; do not use within 14 d of each other
Salmeterol	Beta blockers (including ophthalmic agents)	Mutual inhibition	Avoid concurrent use
	MAOIs, tricyclic antidepressants	Potentiates vascular effects of salmeterol	Severe hypertension, headache, hyperpyrexia, and possible hypertensive crisis; do not use concurrently

Continued

Table 17–2 ⚏ Drug Interactions: Selected Bronchodilators—cont'd

Drug	Interacting Drug	Possible Effect	Implications
Terbutaline	Halogenated anesthetics	Sensitizes the myocardium to the effects of terbutaline	Ventricular arrhythmias; do not use concurrently
	MAOIs, tricyclic antidepressants, maprotiline	Potentiates vascular effects of terbutaline	Severe hypertension, headache, hyperpyrexia, and possible hypertensive crisis; do not use concurrently Decreased antihypertensive effect; should not be used together
	Beta blockers and other antihypertensive agents	Mutual inhibition	Do not use together
	Cocaine	Increased CNS and cardiac stimulation	Observe patients for arrhythmias
	Cardiac glycosides, levodopa	Increased potential for cardiac arrhythmias	Dosage of cardiac glycoside or levodopa should be decreased and the patient closely monitored
Anticholinergics			
Aclidinium	Anticholinergics	Additive anticholinergic effects	Avoid concurrent use
Ipratropium	Cromolyn inhalation solution	Forms a precipitate when mixed together	Do not mix
Tiotropium	Anticholinergics	Additive anticholinergic effects	Avoid concurrent use
Xanthine Derivatives			
Theophylline	Allopurinol, beta blockers, calcium channel blockers, cimetidine, ciprofloxacin oral contraceptives, corticosteroids, disulfiram, ephedrine, influenza virus vaccine, interferon, macrolides, mexiletine, quinolones, thiabendazole, thyroid hormones, carbamazepine, isoniazid, loop diuretics, fluvoxamine, ticlopidine, propafenone	Increased serum theophylline levels if taken concurrently	Lower doses of theophylline may be necessary; monitor theophylline level closely when starting, stopping, or changing the dose of these medications; doses of theophylline may need to be temporarily decreased after administration of influenza vaccine
	Aminoglutethimide, barbiturates, charcoal, hydantoins, ketoconazole, rifampin, smoking (cigarettes, marijuana), sulfinpyrazone, beta agonists, thioamines, carbamazepine, isoniazid, loop diuretics, lansoprazole, primidone, ritonavir	Decreased serum theophylline levels if taken concurrently	Increased doses of theophylline may be necessary; monitor theophylline level closely when starting, stopping, or changing the dose of these medications; theophylline toxicity may occur if these medications are stopped suddenly
	Inhalation anesthetics	Increased risk of cardiac arrhythmias	Avoid or use with caution
	Sympathomimetics	May cause excessive stimulation, nervousness, irritability, and insomnia	Avoid concurrent use or use with caution
	Lithium	Theophylline may increase renal clearance of lithium	Monitor lithium clinical effectiveness if theophylline is prescribed
	Zafirlukast	May increase theophylline levels if added to an existing theophylline regimen	Monitor theophylline levels closely after adding zafirlukast to the treatment regimen

If prescribing to children under age 6, albuterol syrup is dosed at 0.1 mg/kg 3 times a day. Albuterol syrup is rarely used because the inhaled form is more effective and has less adverse effects.

Aformoterol (Brovana) is administered via nebulizer, dosed at 15 mcg by inhalation twice a day. Aformoterol is not approved for use in children and should not be used for acute asthma exacerbation.

Indacaterol (Arcapta Neohaler) is available as an inhalation powder that is administered by the Neohaler device. Indacaterol (Acarpta) dosing for adults with COPD is one capsule administered once a day using the Neohaler device. Capsules are not to be swallowed and should be used immediately after removing from the blister pack.

The recommended dose of levalbuterol (Xopenex) inhalation solution in adolescents over age 12 years and adults is 0.63 mg 3 times a day, every 6 to 8 hours. Dosing for children aged 6 to 11 is 0.31 mg 3 times a day per the manufacturer's label, with routine dosing not to exceed 0.63 mg 3 times a day. In the Skoner and colleagues (2005) study, children aged 2 to 5 years were dosed at both 0.31 mg and 0.63 mg 3 times a day without regard to weight; both doses were tolerated by the children, although they had less variation in heart rate when dosed at 0.31 mg. The authors recommend dosing young children at 0.31 mg 3 times a day, but note that 0.63 mg may be indicated for some patients. *Expert Panel Report 3: Guidelines for the Diagnosis and Management of Asthma* (National Asthma Education and Prevention Program [NAEPP], 2007) recommends dosing levalbuterol via nebulizer, administering 0.31 to 1.25 mg in 3 mL of normal saline every 4 to 6 hours to children 4 years of age or younger, although the NAEPP notes that levalbuterol is not FDA-approved for children younger than 6 years. Levalbuterol (Xopenex HFA) inhaler is FDA-approved for use in adults and children age 4 and older; with a dose of one to two puffs repeated every 4 to 6 hours for wheezing appropriate for all patients.

Metaproterenol (Alupent) comes in MDI, inhalation solution, and syrup forms. The dose of metaproterenol MDI in children over age 12 and adults is two to three inhalations every 3 to 4 hours, not to exceed 12 inhalations per day. The dose of metaproterenol delivered via nebulizer in children age 12 and older and adults is 0.1 to 0.2 mL of 5% solution diluted in 2.5 mL normal saline up to every 4 hours. Metaproterenol is also available in nebulizer solution. The dose for infants and children of metaproterenol nebulizer solution is 5 to 15 mg diluted in 2 to 3 mL of normal saline every 4 to 6 hours. For adolescents and adults, the dose of metaproterenol nebulizer solution is 10 to 15 mg every 4 to 6 hours. Metaproterenol MDI is not recommended for children under age 12 years; oral syrup or nebulizer solution is the suggested therapy in this age group. Metaproterenol syrup dose in children over age 9 years is 20 mg (10 mL) 3 or 4 times a day. For children aged 6 to 9, the dose of metaproterenol syrup is 10 mg (5 mL) 3 or 4 times a day. The dose of metaproterenol in children aged 2 to 6 is 1.3 to 2.6 mg/kg per day in doses divided to take 3 or 4 times a day. Children under age 2 are dosed at 0.4 mg/kg per dose given 3 to 4 times a day; infants should be dosed every 8 to 12 hours.

Terbutaline is available in MDI (Brethaire), oral tablets (Brethine), or parenteral form for SC injection. The dose of terbutaline MDI in children age 12 and older and adults is two puffs every 4 to 6 hours. The dose of oral terbutaline for bronchospasm in adolescents age 15 or older and adults is 5 mg 3 times a day, with a maximum of 15 mg in 24 hours. For children aged 12 to 15 years, the dose of terbutaline is 2.5 mg 3 times a day, with a maximum dose of 7.5 mg in 24 hours. Children less than age 12 are dosed at 0.5 mg/kg every 8 hours, which may be gradually increased up to 0.15 mg/kg per dose, with a maximum daily dose of 5 mg. The dose of parenteral terbutaline (Brethine injection) in adults is 0.25 mg SC in the lateral deltoid. The dose may be repeated in 15 to 30 minutes. The maximum dose is 0.75 mg in 4 hours.

Pirbuterol is available only in MDI form (Maxair Autohaler). The dose of pirbuterol in children over age 12 and adults is one to two inhalations every 4 to 6 hours for a maximum of 12 inhalations in 24 hours. Younger children are dosed at 4 to 8 inhalations every 20 minutes for a total of three doses, then every 1 to 4 hours. Maintenance therapy for children and adults is two inhalations 3 to 4 times a day.

Bitolterol (Tornalate) is available in MDI form. The adult dose to treat acute bronchospasm is two puffs, 1 to 3 minutes apart, followed by a third puff if needed. For prevention of bronchospasm, the adult dose is two puffs every 8 hours. Bitolterol is not recommended for use in children younger than 12 years.

Salmeterol (Serevent DISKUS) is a long-acting bronchodilator available in powder for oral inhalation, packaged in a specially designed plastic delivery device that delivers 50 mcg per inhalation. The dose for children aged 4 and older and adults to control asthma and to prevent bronchospasm is one actuation/puff twice a day. Salmeterol is not to be used for short-term bronchospasm relief. If prescribing salmeterol for persistent asthma, the drug must be prescribed in conjunction with an inhaled corticosteroid or other asthma controller medication. LABAs should be prescribed for as short a time as possible to get the asthma under control, and then patients are maintained on their controller medication. To prevent exercise-induced bronchospasm, the dose of one actuation/puff (50 mcg) is inhaled 30 minutes before exercise. Patients who are using salmeterol twice a day for asthma control should not use an additional dose before exercise. Frequent use of LABAs for exercise-induced asthma is discouraged by the *Expert Panel 3* guidelines because it may be masking persistent asthma. Patients also need to have a short-acting bronchodilator prescribed for them to use for short-term relief, and they need to be educated not to use salmeterol for acute exacerbations. Salmeterol is packaged in combination with fluticasone (Advair DISKUS) with differing dosages of fluticasone (100 mcg, 250 mcg, 500 mcg per actuation) combined with 50 mcg of salmeterol (Advair DISKUS 100/50, Advair DISKUS 250/50, Advair DISKUS 500/50). The FDA recommends pediatric and adolescent patients who require the addition of a LABA to an inhaled corticosteroid be prescribed a combination product to increase compliance and ensure patient safety (U.S. Food and Drug Administration, 2010). Dosing is covered in the "Inhaled Corticosteroid" section of this chapter.

Formoterol is packaged as a 12 mcg, single-use dry powder capsule. Dosing for children older than age 5 or adults is one capsule every 12 hours. Children younger than age 4 cannot generate enough inspiratory flow to administer the dry powder capsules.

Ipratropium is an inhaled anticholinergic that may be used in combination with albuterol to treat asthma exacerbation in the emergency department (NAEPP, 2007). Hospital admission may be avoided by the addition of ipratropium to the treatment regimen in cases of exacerbation seen in the clinic or emergency department. Ipratropium is the bronchodilator of choice in patients who are taking beta blockers or who do not tolerate beta$_2$ agonists.

Exercise-Induced Bronchospasm

Bronchodilators used just before exercise can prevent exercise-induced bronchospasm (EIB). The medications recommended by the *Expert Panel Report 3: Guidelines for the Diagnosis and Management of Asthma* (NAEPP, 2007) are inhaled albuterol or other short-acting beta$_2$ agonist and salmeterol. The dose of albuterol MDI to prevent EIB is two puffs 15 minutes prior to exercise, which should prevent EIB for 2 to 3 hours. The dose of salmeterol is two puffs 30 to 60 minutes prior to exercise. Salmeterol should prevent EIB for 10 to 12 hours. Salmeterol and other long-acting beta$_2$ agonists have a shortened duration of action if used on a daily basis (NAEPP, 2007). Cromolyn or nedocromyl may be used before exercise, but they are not as effective as short-acting beta$_2$ agonists. Leukotriene modifiers may improve EIB in up to 50% of patients (NAEPP, 2007). Table 17-3 presents dosage recommendations.

Rational Drug Selection

The *Expert Panel Report 3* (NAEPP, 2007) does not differentiate or recommend a specific short-acting beta$_2$ agonist for use in asthma. Therefore, the practitioner who is prescribing

Table 17–3 ⊗ Dosage Schedule: Selected Bronchodilators

Drug	Indication	Dosage Form	Dose	Comments
Beta$_2$ Agonists				
Aformoterol Brovana	Long-term management of bronchoconstriction associated with COPD	Inhalation solution 15 mcg/2 mL	15 mcg/2 mL vial q 12 hr	
Albuterol **INHALER** ProAir HFA Proventil HFA Ventolin HFA Generic **INHALATION SOLUTION** Accuneb Generic **ORAL** Vospire ER tablets Generic	Bronchospasm associated with asthma or COPD	*Inhaler* 17 g (about 200 inhalations) *Accuneb inhalation solution* 0.63 mg/3 mL 1.25 mg/3 mL *Albuterol generic* Solution for nebulizer: 0.5% (5 mg/mL) Solution for nebulizer: 0.083% in unit-dose vial *Vospire ER Tablets* Extended-release tablets: 4 mg, 8 mg *Oral generic* Tablets: 2 mg, 4 mg Syrup: 2 mg/5 mL	*Inhaled:* 2 puffs q 4–6 h *Nebulizer* (run over 10–15 min) *Adults:* dilute 0.5 mL of 0.5% solution in 3 mL normal saline OR give 1 unit dose *Children:* 0.01–0.05 mL/kg of 0.5% solution diluted in 2 mL normal saline *Oral* *Adults:* 2–4 mg tid or qid up to a max of 32 mg/day *Children 6–12 yr:* 2 mg tid or qid *Children <6 yr:* 0.1 mg/kg divided tid	May repeat dose in 20 min × 3 during exacerbations; check proper inhaler technique with every clinic visit *Min:* 0.25 mL *Max:* 1.0 mL
	Exercise-induced asthma		*Inhaled:* 2 puffs 5 min prior to exercise	
Bitolterol Tornalate	Acute bronchospasm	Inhaler: 15 mL (about 300 inhalations)	*Inhaled* *Children >12 yr and adults:* 2 puffs 1–3 min apart, followed by a third puff if needed	Not recommended for children <12 yr
	Bronchospasm prevention		*Inhaled:* 2 puffs every 8 h	
Formoterol Foradil Aerolizer Oxeze Turbuhaler (Canada)	Long-acting bronchodilator for preventing bronchospasm	*Inhalation powder* 12 mcg capsule for inhalation	*Children >5 yr and adults:* 12 mg (contents of one capsule) q 12h	Should not be used as monotherapy for asthma

Table 17–3 ⊗ Dosage Schedule: Selected Bronchodilators—cont'd

Drug	Indication	Dosage Form	Dose	Comments
Perforomist Inhalation solution		*Inhalation solution* 20 mcg twice daily (morning and evening) by nebulization (max: 40 mcg/day)		
	Prevention of exercise-induced asthma		*Children >5 yr and adults:* 12 mg (contents of one capsule) 15 min before exercise	Should not use a second dose within 12 h
Indacaterol Arcapta Neohaler	Long-term mainte-nance of patients with COPD	75 mcg dry powder capsule for use in Neohaler device	75 mcg once daily via Neohaler	Not approved for use in children
Levalbuterol Xopenex	Bronchospasm in patients with reversible obstructive airway disease	HFA inhaler 45 mcg/inhalation Unit dose solution for nebulizer: 0.31 mg/3 mL 0.63 mg/3 mL 1.25 mg/3 mL Concentrated solu-tion for inhalation: 1.25 mg/0.5 mL	HFA MDI: ≥4 yr: 1–2 puffs every 4–6 h *Nebulizer* *Children ≥4 yr and adults:* 0.63 mg 3 times a day every 6–8 h; may be increased to 1.25 mg 3 times a day *Children 6–11 yr:* 0.31 mg 3 times a day every 6–8 h; not to exceed 0.63 mg 3 times a day *Children 2–6 yr:* Not labeled for use in this age. See comments.	*Children 2–5 yr:* 0.31–0.63 mg every 6–8 h; 0.31 mg well tolerated (Skoner et al, 2005)
Metaproterenol Alupent Metaprel Generic	Bronchospasm associated with asthma or COPD	Tablets: 10 mg, 20 mg Syrup: 10 mg/5 mL Metered-dose inhaler: 0.65 mg/puff Solution for inhala-tion: 0.4%, 0.6% Solution for inhalation: 5%	*Inhaler* *Children >12 yr and adults:* 2–3 inhalations every 3–4 h; do not exceed 12 inhalations/d *Nebulizer* *Children >6 yr and adults:* 0.1–0.2 mL of 5% solution diluted in 2.5 mL normal saline up to every 4 h *Hand bulb nebulizer* *Children >12 yr and adults:* 5–15 (usually 10) inhalations every 4 h or 3–4 times/d (chronic use) *Syrup* *Children >9 yr or who weigh >60 lb:* 20 mg (10 mL) tid or qid *Children 6–9 yr who weigh <60 lb:* 10 mg (5 mL) tid or qid *Children <6 yr:* 1.3–2.6 mg/kg/d in doses divided tid or qid	Metaproterenol MDI not recommended in children <12 yr Nebulizer solution not recommended in children <6 yr; oral syrup is the suggested therapy in this age group
Pirbuterol Maxair Autoinhaler	Bronchospasm associated with asthma	14 g MDI (about 400 inhalations; 0.2 mg/puff)	*Inhaled* *Children >4 yr and adults:* 2 puffs every 6–8 h (NIH guidelines)	Not recommended for children <4 yr
Salmeterol Serevent Diskus	Long-acting bronchodilator for preventing bronchospasm	Diskus Inhaler: (60 inhalations, 50 mcg/inhalation)	*Inhaled DISKUS* *Children >4 yr and adults:* 1 actuation/puff bid, 12 h apart	Not to be used for short-term relief or acute exacerba-tions; patients need to have a short-acting bronchodila-tor also prescribed for them. If using salmeterol for asthma control, patients should not use another dose for exercise-induced asthma; a short-acting bronchodilator or cromolyn should be used
	Exercise-induced asthma		*Inhaled Diskus* 1 puff/actuation 30–60 min before exercise	

Continued

Table 17–3 ⊗ Dosage Schedule: Selected Bronchodilators—cont'd

Drug	Indication	Dosage Form	Dose	Comments
Terbutaline Generic Brethine Bricanyl	Bronchospasm associated with asthma or COPD	10.5 g MDI (about 300 inhalations, 0.2 mcg/puff) Tablets: 2.5 mg, 5 mg Parenteral: 1 mg/mL	*Inhaled* 2 puffs every 4–6 h; do not repeat more often than every 4–6 h *Oral* *Children >15 yr and adults:* 5 mg tid; max 15 mg/24 h *Children 12–15 yr:* 2.5 mg tid; max 7.5 mg/24 h *Parenteral* *Adults:* 0.5 mg SC in the lateral deltoid; may repeat in 15–30 min; maximum dose is 0.5 mg in 4 h *Children <12 yr:* 0.05 mg/kg every 8 hr. May increase to 0.15 mg/kg dose. Maximum 5 mg/d.	Not recommended in children <12 yr Terbutaline is used to control premature contractions in pregnant women, so use with care in the patient in the third trimester nearing due date because it may affect labor
Anticholinergics				
Ipratropium Atrovent	Bronchospasm associated with asthma or COPD	12.9 g MDI (200 inhalations, 17 mcg/puff) 25 unit-dose vials (2.5 mL each, 500 mcg per unit-dose vial) per foil pouch	*Acute Exacerbation of Asthma* (NIH guidelines) *Children:* Nebulization: 250 mcg of 20 min × 3 doses then every 2–4 h MDI: 4–8 puffs as needed *Children >12 yr and adults:* Nebulization 500 mcg of 30 min × 3 then every 2–4 h MDI: 4–8 puffs as needed *Asthma Maintenance* (NIH Guidelines) *Children:* Nebulization: 250–500 mcg of 6 h MDI: 1–2 inhalations of 6 h; max 12 puffs/day *Children >12 yr and adults:* Nebulization: 250 mcg of 6 h MDI: 2–3 inhalations of 6 h; max 12 puffs/day *COPD MDI:* *Adults:* 2 puffs qid, may increase to 12 puffs/day Nebulizer: One unit-dose vial 500 mcg 3–4 times a day via nebulizer	Contraindicated in patients with soybean or peanut allergy. Ipratropium can be mixed with albuterol 0.5% solution for nebulizer use if used within 1 h.
Aclidinium bromide Tudorza	brochospasm associated with COPD	Inhalation powder (400 mcg/ inhalation) 30 dose, 60 dose	*Inhaled* *Adults:* 400 mcg bid	Not approved in children.
Tiotropium Spiriva	brochospasm associated with COPD	Handi Haler Inhalation: 18 mcg/inhalation	*Inhaled* *Adults:* 18 mcg qid	Not approved in children.
Combination Medications				
Albuterol/ ipratropium (Combivent)	Bronchospasm associated with COPD, not controlled with one bronchodilator alone	14.7 g MDI (200 inhalations, ipratropium 18 mcg/ puff combined with albuterol 90 mcg/puff)	*Inhaled* *Adults:* 2 puffs qid *Children <12 yr:* 1–2 puffs qid *Nebulizer* *Adults:* 3 mL q4–6h *Children:* 1.5 to 3 mL q 8h	Primarily used for COPD patients; simplifies medication regimen by combining two commonly prescribed medications
Xanthine Derivatives				
Theophylline IMMEDIATE-RELEASE Slo-Phyllin Theolair Generic	Bronchospasm associated with asthma, COPD, and bronchitis	Tablets: 100, 200 mg Syrup: 80 mg/5 mL Tablets: 125, 250 mg Solution: 80 mg/15 mL Tablets: 100, 200, 300 mg	The dose for asthma and COPD is variable with the patient's weight and serum theophylline levels *Adults (>16):* Initially: 6 mg/kg/24 h or 400 mg/ 24 h tid or qid; the dose is increased	Dosing adjustments are made based on the serum theophylline level: If the level is 5–10 mcg/mL, the dose is increased by 25% every 3 d until desired serum concentrations of theophylline

Table 17–3 ⊗ **Dosage Schedule: Selected Bronchodilators—cont'd**

Drug	Indication	Dosage Form	Dose	Comments
TIMED-RELEASE Generic Theophylline CR Slo-bid Gyrocaps Slo-Phyllin Theo-24 Theo-Dur Sprinkles Theo-Dur Uni-Dur Uniphyl Generic		Elixir: 80 mg/15 mL Timed-release 12 h capsule: 125, 200, 300 mg Timed-release capsules (8–12 h): 50, 75, 100, 125, 200, 300 mg Timed-release capsules (8–12 h): 60, 125, 250 mg Timed-release capsules (24 h): 100, 200, 300 mg Timed-release capsules (12 h): 50, 75, 125, 200 mg Timed-release tablets (8–24 h): 100, 200, 300, 400 mg Timed-release scored tablets (24 h): 400, 600 mg Timed-release tablets (24 h): 400, 600 mg Timed-release tablets (24 h): 400 mg	every 3 d in 25% increments until desired serum theophylline levels are achieved (ideally between 10 and 20 mcg/mL); max dose: 13 mg/kg/d *Children 1–9 yr:* Initially: 16 mg/kg/24 h; max 400 mg/d; dosage may be increased by 25% every 3 d to a maximum based on age (1–9 yr, max 24 mg/kg/d; 9–12 yr, max 20 mg/kg/d; 12–16 yr, max daily dose is 18 mg/kg) Monitoring for serum theophylline levels is the same in children as for adults, with a steady-state theophylline level of 5–15 mcg/mL the goal	are reached; if the serum concentration is between 10 and 15 mcg/mL, maintain dosage if tolerated and recheck at 6 to 12 mo intervals; if level is 15–19.9 mcg/mL, consider decreasing dose by 10% to provide a greater margin of safety; if the level is 20–25 mcg/mL, then decrease dose by 10% and recheck level in 3 d; if serum level is 25–30 mcg/mL, then decrease subsequent doses by 25%, and redraw level in 3 d; if theophylline level is > 30 mcg/mL, then skip next 2 doses, decrease dose by 50%, and recheck in 3 d
Caffeine citrate Cafcit	Apnea of prematurity	Oral solution: 20 mg/mL	Loading dose: 10–20 mg/kg Maintenance: 5 mg/kg/d	If theophylline has been given in last 3 d, decrease loading dose by 50%–75%

for adults may choose any of the short-acting bronchodilators. Choosing an appropriate bronchodilator is a matter of the age of the patient and the cost.

Patient Age

The only short-acting bronchodilators that can be prescribed for children under age 4 are albuterol and metaproterenol. Levalbuterol is labeled to be used in children older than age 4, and the *Expert Panel 3* (NAEPP, 2007) guidelines indicate that it should not be used in children younger than age 4. Albuterol is by far the most often used medication in clinical practice and is safe to use even in infants.

Cost

Of the short-acting bronchodilators, albuterol is the least expensive, especially if a generic formula is prescribed.

Monitoring

There is no specific monitoring required for bronchodilators. As a part of overall asthma management, pulmonary function and response to bronchodilators should be monitored with a peak flowmeter. If a patient is on digitalis, an ECG should be done prior to starting a beta agonist and routinely during therapy to detect cardiac arrhythmias that may occur. Patients who are concurrently taking diuretics or anything that affects potassium levels should be monitored for dysrhythmias.

Patient Education

Administration

The bronchodilator should be used as prescribed. Overuse of bronchodilators will lead to increased adverse effects, and using the bronchodilator less than prescribed may lead to increased bronchospasm and decreased pulmonary function.

The administration of bronchodilators via MDI can be difficult for most adults and all children. Learning to coordinate the release of the medication from the inhaler with a deep breath is difficult. Written and pictorial instructions are available with the inhaler, but the provider must not assume that the patient understands the proper method of administering inhaled medications. It is recommended that a spacer device be used with MDIs (Aerochamber, InspirEase) to increase deposition of medication into the lungs, rather than just in the mouth. Use verbal instructions as well as actual demonstration with a placebo inhaler to reinforce the written instructions. These instructions and demonstrations should be repeated at follow-up visits.

To use an inhaler properly, the patient should first exhale and then tilt the head slightly back and place the inhaler mouthpiece either about 2 inches from the open mouth or between the open lips. While inhaling, the patient should press down on the canister, breathe in slowly and deeply, and hold his or her breath for 10 seconds (count of 10) or as long as comfortable. If two puffs are prescribed, then the patient should wait at least 1 full minute between inhalations.

CLINICAL PEARL

Administering a medication via a nebulizer to an infant or toddler is, at times, a challenge. A pediatric mask may be used if the child tolerates it. One trick is to "blow" the nebulized medication into the patient's face near the nose and mouth. This is achieved by occluding the mouthpiece end of the unit and aiming the "tail" end toward the patient's nose and mouth. This is especially effective if the child is sleeping and needs the medication. Another suggestion to parents of young children is to read a book to the child during the treatment or play an appropriate short video to make the time pass more quickly.

To assist with the delivery of inhaled medications, a spacer can be prescribed. The Global Initiative for Asthma Web site has instructions with diagrams for using all the different types of spacers, inhalers, and asthma medication delivery systems (www.ginasthma.org/documents/11). The Aerochamber is a tube-like device that has pictures drawn on the outside to remind the patient of the proper technique for using the inhaler. For younger children and older adults, the InspirEase spacer gives a visual cue of the spacer bag deflating to help in taking a deep-enough breath, or an Aerochamber with the appropriate-size mask can be used. Both of these devices emit a whistling sound if the patient is taking too rapid a breath, giving a cue to breathe more slowly.

The use of a nebulizer should be demonstrated to the patient either in the clinic or by the home health agency that is providing the device. Specific instructions vary slightly with the manufacturer. The key points that should be covered with nebulizer use are accurate measurement of the medication (if using nebulizer solution) and appropriate cleaning of the equipment. Many nebulizer medications are available in unit-dose packaging, which, although more expensive, is helpful if patients have difficulty accurately measuring their medication.

Instructions for salmeterol dry powder DISKUS (Serevent DISKUS, Advair DISKUS) administration say that the patient should use the medication as prescribed and should not exceed the prescribed dose. Patients should not exhale or blow into the DISKUS. The DISKUS should not be washed or taken apart.

Formoterol (Foradil AEROLIZER) is a dry powder capsule administered via a patented aerolizer. The Foradil capsule is placed into the aerolizer, then the aerolizer is squeezed to break the capsule. The patient inhales the medication. Patients should receive clear instructions not to swallow the capsule.

Indacaterol (Arcapta Neohaler) is a dry powder capsule administered via a patented inhalation device (Neohaler). Patients inhale the dry powder from the Neohaler device. The capsule must be removed from a blister pack immediately before inserting into the Neohaler, and Arcapta capsules that are exposed to air for prolonged periods should be discarded. Capsules should not be swallowed.

Adverse Reactions

The patient should be instructed not to exceed the recommended dosage of the medication because excessive use may lead to increased adverse effects. Overuse of the beta$_2$-agonist bronchodilators can lead to seizures, hypokalemia, anginal pain, and hypertension. Patients should understand that they may have some stimulant-like effects (e.g., increased heart rate, tremors) when they initially begin the medication, but these effects should lessen if they use it correctly. Some patients may get a headache with the use of bronchodilators. Patients who experience GI upset when taking oral medications should take the medications with food. The patient should inform the provider if palpitations, tachycardia, chest pain, muscle tremors, dizziness, headache, or flushing occurs.

Lifestyle Management

Lifestyle management issues related to the disease process being treated should be discussed. They often include the following:

1. The patient needs to self-monitor respiratory status with a peak flowmeter to determine the effectiveness of the prescribed medication.
2. The patient should avoid or quit smoking.
3. The patient should avoid environmental triggers for asthma at home, work, and school.

XANTHINE DERIVATIVES

Methylxanthines have declined in importance in the treatment of asthma, but some patients may still benefit from the use of theophylline. The other methylxanthines include aminophylline and caffeine. Theophylline and caffeine are closely related chemically in that theophylline is 1,3-dimethylxanthine and caffeine is 1,3,7-triethylxanthine, and they share many of the same effects on the body. Because many patients throughout the world consume caffeine in tea, coffee, and cola beverages and because many OTC preparations for analgesia contain caffeine, caffeine pharmacodynamics is discussed briefly here.

Pharmacodynamics

Theophylline and the other methylxanthines work directly by an unknown mechanism believed to be mediated by selective inhibition of specific phosphodiesterases (PDEs). This, in turn, produces an increase in cAMP, which then leads to bronchial smooth muscle and pulmonary vessel relaxation.

Theophylline and caffeine have an impact on most of the major body systems. They are powerful CNS stimulants, often causing insomnia and excitability. Although both drugs have cardiovascular effects, theophylline has a greater effect on the cardiovascular system. Theophylline directly stimulates the myocardium and increases myocardial contractility and heart rate. By relaxing vascular smooth muscle, theophylline dilates the coronary, pulmonary, and systemic blood vessels. Both theophylline and caffeine increase gastric acid secretion and may produce nausea and vomiting, although this reaction is probably due to CNS effects. Both methylxanthines stimulate skeletal muscle, causing tremors. Theophylline acts directly on the renal tubules to cause increased sodium and chloride excretion. By increasing renal blood flow (from increased heart rate) and the glomerular filtration rate, theophylline and caffeine also cause diuresis. Often, these effects occur even when theophylline is within the therapeutic range.

Pharmacokinetics
Absorption and Distribution
Methylxanthines, such as theophylline, are most commonly used in an oral form that is rapidly and completely absorbed from the GI tract. Delayed-release and extended-release tablets are also available, and their rate of absorption varies among the various formulations. The absorption of slow-release forms of theophylline can be significantly altered by gastric pH and food ingestion; therefore, patient education regarding the timing of these medications is important to the success of the medication. Theophylline distributes rapidly in nonadipose tissue and body water, including breast milk and cerebral spinal fluid. Theophylline crosses the placenta. The volume of distribution (V_D) for theophylline averages 0.45 L per kg of body weight (L/kg) and ranges from 0.3 to 0.7 L/kg from infants to adults. The volume of distribution may be altered in premature neonates, elderly patients, adults with cirrhosis, pregnant women during the third trimester, and critically ill patients, probably because of altered protein binding. Serum theophylline levels should be monitored closely in these patients. Theophylline distributes readily into breast milk with milk levels at 70% of maternal serum levels.

Metabolism and Excretion
Theophylline is metabolized primarily in the liver, with very little or no first-pass effect. Metabolism is believed to occur over multiple parallel pathways, mediated by cytochrome P450 (CYP450) isoenzyme. Medications that induce CYP 450 can significantly increase clearance of theophylline. In neonates, several of these pathways are undeveloped but mature slowly over the first year of life. Caffeine is a minor active metabolite of theophylline in older children and adults. In premature neonates and children younger than 6 months, caffeine has a long half-life because of their immature livers, which results in significant accumulation. As the liver matures, the half-life of caffeine shortens and, therefore, does not accumulate in older children and adults. Table 17-1 outlines the half-life of theophylline in various ages of patients with a variety of diseases. Patients with congestive heart failure, cor pulmonale, pulmonary edema, and prolonged fever can have decreased metabolism of theophylline and, therefore, need to be closely monitored. Smoking and high-protein diets can increase the theophylline excretion rate, and high-carbohydrate diets can decrease it.

Pharmacotherapeutics
Precautions and Contraindications
The only true contraindications to theophylline are hypersensitivity to any xanthine, peptic ulcer disease, and underlying seizure disorder. Contraindications to caffeine include hypersensitivity to caffeine and use of caffeine sodium benzoate formulation in neonates.

Because of its effects on the cardiovascular system, patients with hypertension, ischemic heart disease, coronary insufficiency, congestive heart failure, or a history of stroke and cardiac arrhythmias should be monitored closely for adverse effects while taking theophylline.

Excessive doses may lead to toxicity. Incidence of toxicity increases when serum theophylline levels are above 20 mcg/mL. Toxicity is found if serum theophylline levels reach 25 mcg/mL in 75% of patients. Toxicity should not occur at recommended dosages but may occur if theophylline clearance is decreased (hepatic impairment, chronic lung disease, cardiac failure, patients older than age 55, and infants under age 1 year). Theophylline clearance may be decreased in patients over age 55.

Caffeine has a prolonged half-life of 72 to 96 hours in the neonate, whereas in infants over 9 months, children, and adults, the half-life is 5 hours.

Theophylline is Pregnancy Category C. There are no published reports linking theophylline with congenital defects. Theophylline crosses the placenta, and newborn infants may have therapeutic serum levels if maternal serum theophylline levels are in the high-normal range. Transient tachycardia, irritability, and vomiting can be found in newborns of women consuming theophylline.

With close monitoring, theophylline may be used in children. Infants younger than 1 year have decreased theophylline clearance and should have close monitoring of serum theophylline levels. Theophylline is used to treat apnea in preterm infants, with a therapeutic serum theophylline range of 5 to 10 mcg/mL. If levels are kept in this range, the neonate should not have signs of toxicity. Caffeine citrate is also commonly used to treat apnea of prematurity.

Adverse Drug Reactions
Adverse drug reactions are uncommon with serum theophylline levels below 20 mcg/mL, although some patients may show toxic effects between 15 and 20 mcg/mL, especially during initiation of therapy. The CNS adverse effects that may be seen include irritability, restlessness, seizures, and insomnia. Gastroesophageal reflux may occur. The cardiovascular adverse effects that may occur include palpitations, tachycardia, hypotension, and life-threatening arrhythmias. Other adverse effects include rash, diuresis, and tachypnea.

At serum theophylline levels above 20 mcg/mL, patients may experience nausea, vomiting, diarrhea, headache, insomnia, and irritability. At levels above 35 mcg/mL, the patient may have hyperglycemia, hypotension, cardiac arrhythmias, tachycardia, seizures, brain damage, and death.

Adverse effects of caffeine include cardiac arrhythmias, tachycardia, insomnia, agitation, irritability, headache, nausea, vomiting, and gastric irritation.

Drug and Food Interactions
Many medications act to either increase or decrease theophylline clearance due to metabolism via CYP450 isoenzyme CYP1A2, CYP2E1, and CYP3A3/4 substrate. These medications

are shown in Table 17-2. Of significance is smoking tobacco, which increases theophylline clearance. Theophylline levels should be monitored closely if the patient begins or quits smoking while on theophylline. Nicotine replacement products (gum or patch) also affect theophylline clearance. Theophylline clearance may not return to normal for 3 months to 2 years after smoking cessation.

The sedative effects of benzodiazepines may be antagonized by theophylline. Concurrent use of theophylline with beta$_2$-agonist bronchodilators may result in additive toxicity. Lithium levels may be reduced by theophylline. The concurrent use of tetracyclines with theophylline may lead to an increased incidence of theophylline adverse reactions. See Table 17-2 for other drugs that affect theophylline levels or interact with theophylline.

Theophylline elimination may be influenced by the patient's diet. A diet that is low in carbohydrates and high in protein increases the elimination (shortens the half-life) of theophylline. A diet high in carbohydrates and low in protein decreases the elimination (lengthens the half-life) of theophylline. A diet that contains a lot of charcoal-broiled foods accelerates the hepatic metabolism of theophylline because of the high polycyclic hydrocarbon content.

Caffeine is metabolized via the CYP450 isoenzyme CYP1A2, CYP2E1, and CYP3A3/4 substrate; therefore, other drugs metabolized via these isoenzymes will possibly interact. Cimetidine, ketoconazole, fluconazole, mexiletine, and phenylpropanolamine may impair caffeine metabolism, leading to increased serum levels. Caffeine elimination may be increased by coadministration of phenobarbital and phenytoin (FDA, 2005).

Clinical Use and Dosing

Theophylline and Chronic Obstructive Pulmonary Disease

The National Heart, Lung, and Blood Institute (NHLBI) *Expert Panel Report 3* (NAEPP, 2007), which provides guidelines for the management of asthma, recommends reserving theophylline for long-term control of asthma and an "alternative, not preferred" therapy in step 2 of asthma care. The *Expert Panel Report 3* recommends using theophylline as an alternative treatment in combination with inhaled corticosteroids (NAEPP, 2007). The guidelines recommend that long-acting beta$_2$ agonists (in combination with inhaled corticosteroids) be tried before theophylline because of toxicity issues with theophylline. Theophylline is not recommended for first-line therapy in the COPD patient, although if the patient has been stable on theophylline, there is no reason to discontinue the medication as long as serum theophylline levels are monitored.

The dose of theophylline for asthma and COPD varies with the patient's weight and serum theophylline levels. The adult patient (older than age 16 years) is started on a dose of 6 mg/kg per 24 hours or 400 mg/24 hours, whichever is less, divided at 6 to 8 hour intervals. The dose is increased every 3 days in 25% increments until the desired serum theophylline levels are achieved (ideally between 10 and 20 mcg/mL). The maximum dose for patients age 12 to 16 years is 13 mg/kg per day, and 10 mg/kg/day in healthy adolescents

older than age 16 and adults. Dosing adjustments are made based on the serum theophylline level. If the level is 5 to 10 mcg/mL, then the dose of theophylline is increased by 25% every 3 days until desired serum concentrations of theophylline are reached. If the serum concentration is between 10 and 15 mcg/mL, maintain dosage if tolerated and recheck at 6 to 12 month intervals. If the serum theophylline level is 15 to 19.9 mcg/mL, consider decreasing the dose by 10% to provide a greater margin of safety. If the serum theophylline level is 20 to 25 mcg/mL, then decrease the dose by 10% and recheck the level in 3 days. If the serum level is 25 to 30 mcg/mL, skip the next dose and decrease subsequent doses by 25%; redraw the theophylline level in 3 days. If the theophylline level is above 30 mcg/mL, then skip the next two doses and decrease the dose by 50%; recheck in 3 days. If the patient has a serum theophylline level above 20 mcg/mL, consultation with a physician is indicated to determine if hospitalization for theophylline toxicity is warranted, based on clinical status.

The *Expert Panel Report 3* (NAEPP, 2007) for the management of asthma in children indicates theophylline as alternative therapy in moderate persistent asthma, in combination with low-dose inhaled corticosteroid in children aged 5 years or older. The initial dose of theophylline in children is 16 mg/kg per 24 hours up to a maximum of 400 mg per day. The dosage may be increased by 25% every 3 days to a maximum that is based on age. For children aged 1 to 9 years, the maximum is 24 mg/kg per day; for 9 to 12 years, the maximum dose is 20 mg/kg per day; for 12- to 16-year-old patients, the maximum daily dose is 18 mg/kg. If the patient is over age 16, then the dosing is the same as it is for adults—maximum 13 mg/kg per day. Monitoring for serum theophylline levels is the same in children as for adults, with a steady-state theophylline level of 5 to 15 mcg/mL the goal. Theophylline is not recommended for use in children with asthma who are younger than age 5 because of altered metabolism during viral or febrile illnesses affecting serum concentration (NAEPP, 2007).

Apnea of Prematurity

A loading dose of caffeine citrate 10 to 20 mg/kg is given in the treatment of apnea of prematurity, with a maintenance dose of 5 mg/kg per day. If theophylline has been given to the patient in the previous 3 days, the loading dose is decreased by 50% to 70%. The maintenance dose is adjusted based on clinical response and serum caffeine levels (8 to 20 mcg/mL). If theophylline is used to treat apnea of prematurity, the patient is given a loading dose of 4 mg/kg per dose, with a maintenance dose of 4 mg/kg per day in the premature infant or newborn up to age 6 weeks. The total daily dose is divided and administered every 12 hours. A recent RCT comparing caffeine and theophylline for the treatment of apnea of prematurity found both drugs are equally effective in decreasing apnea spells in infants less than 33 weeks' gestation, but caffeine is significantly more effective as prophylaxis against apnea in infants at risk (Skouroliakou, Bacopoulou, & Markantonis, 2009). The Skouroliakau and colleagues study found no sustained benefit of one drug over the other after the first week of therapy.

Rational Drug Selection

Because theophylline is the only xanthine derivative that is commonly used in asthma and COPD, the selection process basically involves choosing between the different forms of theophylline that are available on the basis of their cost and convenience. There are immediate-release, timed-release, and liquid formulas. Capsules that can be opened and sprinkled on soft foods are convenient for some patients.

Immediate Release

When therapy is initiated, the daily dose may be changing frequently based on serum theophylline levels, and immediate-release tablets or capsules should be prescribed. The variety of dosage tablets available (100 mg, 125 mg, 200 mg, 250 mg, 300 mg) makes titrating the dose easier if incremental increases or decreases are required. Immediate-release theophylline requires dosing every 6 to 8 hours. Children younger than age 12 usually require every-6-hour dosing, whereas adolescents and adults usually require every-8-hour dosing, although this timing may vary by individual. The cost of immediate-release theophylline is slightly higher than that of most of the timed-release formulas because more doses are taken and, therefore, more tablets need to be dispensed in a month. Many patients are stabilized to a set dose per 24 hours and then switched to a timed-release formula.

Timed Release

The variety of available timed-release theophylline products are described in Table 17-3. The formulas range from 8 to 24 hour release. It is recommended that patients be stabilized on immediate-release formulas to determine the total 24-hour dose that is required and then switched to a timed-release formula of choice. With some timed-release theophylline formulas offering once-daily dosing, there is a definite improvement in convenience with the timed-release products. One caution for the patient is that the dose must be taken at the same time every day to have steady serum theophylline levels.

Liquid

The liquid forms of theophylline may be used for children or patients who have difficulty in swallowing pills or capsules. The liquid is available in 80 mg/15 mL.

Monitoring

The patient who is taking theophylline needs to be monitored closely for signs of toxicity. When therapy is initiated, theophylline levels should be drawn frequently as the dosage is titrated. If the patient is demonstrating any signs of toxicity, a serum theophylline level should be drawn. Once the patient is stabilized and has a steady theophylline level, then monitoring should be done every 6 to 12 months. More frequent levels may need to be done if a new medication is added to the patient's regimen (see Table 17-2) or if the patient has a change in overall health that may affect the ability to metabolize or excrete theophylline. Theophylline levels need to be timed to measure peak levels of the drug. A serum theophylline level should be drawn 1 to 2 hours after immediate-release formulas and 5 to 9 hours after the morning dose of sustained-release formulas. The patient should have a theophylline level drawn when changing brands of theophylline because the bioavailability varies among brands.

Patient Education

Administration

The patient should be instructed to take the medication exactly as prescribed. Missed doses or irregular timing of doses can cause wide variations in the serum theophylline level, resulting in either subtherapeutic or toxic levels. The patient may take the medication either with or without food, but consistency is important because food can alter the absorption of the medication. The patient should not chew or crush enteric-coated, sustained-release tablets or capsules.

Adverse Reactions

Toxicity should be discussed with any patient who is taking theophylline. Patients who are having signs of toxicity may mistakenly think they have a viral illness. Instead, patients with any unusual symptoms should contact their provider. The symptoms to report include nausea, vomiting, insomnia, jitteriness, headache, rash, severe GI pain, restlessness, convulsions, or irregular heartbeat.

The patient should avoid large amounts of caffeine-containing beverages, which can increase the adverse effects of theophylline. Explain that theophylline elimination may be influenced by the patient's diet. A diet that is low in carbohydrates and high in protein increases the elimination of theophylline, a diet that is high in carbohydrates and low in protein decreases the elimination of theophylline, and a diet that contains a lot of charcoal-broiled foods accelerates the hepatic metabolism of theophylline. Any drastic changes in patients' diets should be discussed with the provider and a plan for monitoring developed.

The impact on serum theophylline levels that different drugs may have should be discussed with the patient. Any change in the patient's overall medication regimen should warrant a status review and possibly the drawing of serum theophylline levels. The impact of smoking on theophylline levels should be discussed and patients advised to notify their provider if they start or stop smoking.

Lifestyle Management

Lifestyle management issues related to the disease process should be discussed. They often include the following:

1. The patient needs to self-monitor respiratory status with a peak flowmeter to determine the effectiveness of the medication prescribed.
2. The patient should avoid or quit smoking.
3. The patient should avoid environmental triggers for asthma at home, work, and school.

ANTICHOLINERGICS

Inhaled anticholinergics are used primarily to treat COPD, although ipratropium may be used in combination with albuterol as the emergent treatment of an asthma exacerbation or when a patient is intolerant to beta$_2$ agonists (NAEPP,

2007). Ipratropium bromide (Atrovent) is a quaternary amine anticholinergic that is structurally similar to atropine. It is available as a single medication (Atrovent) or combined with albuterol (Combivent). Tiotropium bromide (Spiriva) and aclidinium bromide (Tadorza Pressair) are inhaled anticholinergics available to treat COPD.

Pharmacodynamics

The action of each of the inhaled anticholinergics is similar. Ipratropium acts to block the muscarinic cholinergic receptors by antagonizing the action of acetylcholine. Blocking the cholinergic receptors decreases the formation of cyclic guanosine monophosphate (cGMP), which leads to decreased contractility of the smooth muscle of the lungs, probably because of the actions of cGMP on intracellular calcium. The amount of bronchodilation caused by ipratropium inhalation is thought to reflect the level of parasympathetic tone. When inhaled, ipratropium's actions are confined to the mouth and airways. Tiotropium and aclidinium bromide exhibit their pharmacological action by inhibiting the muscarinic M_3 receptors in the lungs, causing smooth muscle bronchodilation.

Pharmacokinetics

Absorption and Distribution

Ipratropium, when inhaled, is poorly absorbed from both the lungs and the GI tract. Only 1% to 2% of a dose is systemically absorbed. Ipratropium penetrates the CNS poorly. It is unknown whether ipratropium crosses the placenta. Ipratropium is excreted into breast milk in minimal amounts.

Tiotropium is administered via dry powder inhaler, has a bioavailability of 19.5%, and is 72% protein bound in human plasma. Similar to ipratropium, tiotropium demonstrates poor GI absorption when administered orally with an absolute bioavailability of 2% to 3%. Tiotropium does not cross the blood–brain barrier. Tiotropium is distributed in breast milk of rats; it is unknown whether it is excreted in human milk or whether it crosses the placenta.

Aclidinium bromide is a dry powder administered via inhalation. Aclidinium is absorbed via the lungs and has a bioavailability of 6%. Peak onset of aclindinium is 10 minutes after inhalation. Aclidinium bromide is excreted into the milk of lactating female rats; it is not known if it is excreted in human milk.

Metabolism and Excretion

Most of the dose (90%) of ipratropium is swallowed and excreted in the feces unchanged. The portion of the dose that is absorbed is partially metabolized by ester hydrolysis to inactive metabolites. Approximately 50% of the absorbed drug is excreted unchanged in the urine. Tiotropium that is absorbed is eliminated unchanged in the urine. Aclidinium bromide is rapidly and extensively metabolized by hydrolysis, with 54% to 65% excreted in the urine and 20% to 33% excreted in feces.

Pharmacotherapeutics

Precautions and Contraindications

Ipratropium is contraindicated in patients with hypersensitivity to atropine or atropine derivatives and for those with bromide sensitivity. Tiotropium is contraindicated in patients with hypersensitivity to ipratropium or tiotropium.

The inhaled anticholinergics (aclidinium, ipratropium, and tiotropium) should not be used for the treatment of acute bronchospasm. The exception is if ipratropium is combined with albuterol in emergency room treatment of acute bronchospasm (NAEPP, 2007).

Inhaled anticholinergics (aclidinium, ipratropium, and tiotropium), even though poorly absorbed systemically, should be avoided for patients with urinary retention, bladder neck obstruction, or prostatic hypertrophy because of the anticholinergic effects. A systematic review found an increased risk of acute urinary retention associated with the use of inhaled anticholinergics, with older patients with benign prostatic hyperplasia at the greatest risk, particularly at the beginning of therapy (Loke & Singh, 2013). All three inhaled anticholinergic drugs may increase intraocular pressure in patients with closed-angle glaucoma.

Ipratropium bromide is Pregnancy Category B; aclidinium and tiotropium are Pregnancy Category C. Their safety in pregnancy has had limited study; therefore, inhaled anticholinergics should be used in pregnancy only if clearly indicated. Ipratropium is excreted in breast milk in minimal amounts. Atropine, a chemically related drug, is considered safe during lactation. Because such small amounts of drug reach the breast milk, ipratropium is probably safe for use if needed during breastfeeding.

The safety and effectiveness of ipratropium have not been established in children under age 12. Providers may use ipratropium in younger children as an adjunct to beta-agonist (albuterol) therapy in acute exacerbations of asthma per the *NAEPP Expert Panel Report 3* (2007). Aclidinium and tiotropium are approved only for COPD, which does not normally occur in children. Safety and effectiveness of aclidinium and tiotropium in children have not been established.

Adverse Drug Reactions

The most common adverse drug reaction reported with ipratropium is cough. Also reported are the related symptoms of hoarseness, throat irritation, and dysgeusia. Nausea, vomiting, and dyspepsia are thought to be related to the local anticholinergic effects that ipratropium has on the GI system. Xerostomia (dry mouth) is reported in 2% of patients.

Dry mouth is the most commonly reported adverse reaction to inhaled tiotropium (Spiriva HandiHaler), reported in 16% of patients in the manufacturer's clinical trials. Mouth irritation, pharyngitis, nasal congestion, sinusitis, headache, and upper respiratory infections occurred at slightly higher rates in patients using Spiriva than in those using a placebo in the initial clinical trials (Boehringer-Ingelheim, 2009).

Headache was the most common adverse reaction reported in premarketing studies of aclidinium, with 6.6% of patients reporting headache compared to 5% who were using placebo (Forest Pharmaceuticals, 2012). Nasopharyngitis, cough, and rhinitis were all reported more frequently in inhaled aclidinium users than in placebo users.

Other anticholinergic effects that are reported in premarketing trials (in less than 2% of patients) include urinary retention, dizziness, drowsiness, and constipation. Prostate disorders may also be noted (less than 2% reported) in patients using ipratropium. In a 4-year trial of tiotropium (Spiriva HandiHaler) constipation occurred at a slightly higher rate than it did in those using a placebo (5.1% versus 3.7% in placebo patients). Urinary retention is increased with the use of inhaled anticholinergics, particularly in patients with benign prostatic hyperplasia (Loke & Singh, 2013).

If ipratropium is accidentally sprayed in the eyes, the patient may experience temporary eye irritation, pain, mydriasis, blurred vision, cycloplegia (paralysis of the ciliary muscle), irritant conjunctivitis, and visual disturbances.

Rare allergic and anaphylactoid reactions may occur. Reactions include urticaria; maculopapular rash; bronchospasm; pruritus; laryngospasm; oropharyngeal edema; and angioedema of the tongue, lips, and face. The patient's history usually includes sensitivity to other drugs and foods. Patients with milk protein hypersensitivity should not be prescribed aclidinium bromide (Tudorza Pressair).

Drug Interactions

Ipratropium and tiotropium are minimally absorbed into the systemic circulation after inhalation; therefore, there are no major drug interactions. Patients who are concurrently using cromolyn sodium and ipratropium bromide via nebulizer should be cautioned not to mix the two, because a precipitate will form.

Clinical Use and Dosage

Chronic Obstructive Pulmonary Disease

The dose of ipratropium from an MDI is 18 mcg per spray. The dose of ipratropium for adults with COPD is two inhalations (36 mcg) 4 times a day, for a total of eight puffs per day. If needed, the patient may take up to 12 puffs per day (maximum of 216 mcg /24 h). If using a nebulizer, the dose of ipratropium is one unit-dose vial (500 mcg) 3 to 4 times a day via nebulizer, with doses 6 to 8 hours apart. Ipratropium may be mixed with albuterol if used within 1 hour.

Aclidinium bromide (Tudorza Pressair) is an inhalation powder administered via inhaler, with 400 mcg delivered via each actuation of the inhaler. Dosing for COPD is one inhalation twice a day.

Tiotropium (Spiriva) is a dry powder capsule administered via a patented HandiHaler device. The dosage for COPD is two inhalations of a single 18-mcg capsule once daily.

The ipratropium-albuterol combination (Combivent) is indicated for second-line use for patients with COPD. It should be prescribed for patients already on a bronchodilator who continue to have bronchospasms that may benefit from a second bronchodilator. Each inhalation of Combivent administers 103 mcg of albuterol sulfate and 18 mcg of ipratropium bromide. The dose of Combivent is two inhalations 4 times a day. The patient may take additional inhalations but must not exceed 12 inhalations per 24 hours.

Asthma

The adult dose of ipratropium for asthma maintenance is two to three inhalations 4 times a day. It should not be used for exercise-induced asthma. For children under age 12 years, the dose is one or two inhalations every 6 hours. The dose of ipratropium solution in adults is 250 mcg administered via a nebulizer 4 times a day. The dose for children under age 12 is 250 to 500 mcg every 8 hours. Infants are dosed at 125 to 250 mcg 3 times a day. Dosing for acute exacerbation of asthma per the National Institutes of Health (NIH) guidelines is found in Table 17-3. Ipratropium may be mixed with albuterol if the combination is used within 1 hour.

The ipratropium-albuterol combination (Combivent) is a second-line quick-relief medication in the treatment of asthma. Each inhalation of Combivent administers 103 mcg of albuterol sulfate and 18 mcg of ipratropium bromide. The dose of Combivent in adults is two to three inhalations 4 times a day, and in children under age 12, one to two inhalations every 6 hours. The dose of nebulizer solution of albuterol (2.5 mg/3 mL) and ipratropium (0.5 mg/3 mL) is 3 mL every 4 to 6 hours for adults and 1.5 to 3 mL every 8 hours in children under age 12.

Tiotropium is not indicated for the treatment of asthma. The dosing for the treatment of COPD is one 18-mcg capsule daily via HandiHaler.

Rational Drug Selection

Ipratropium is a second-line bronchodilator in the treatment of asthma and COPD. For the practitioner considering prescribing both ipratropium and albuterol, an appropriate choice would be the combination product Combivent. Tiotropium (Spiriva) is for use in COPD; cost and ease of use (dry powder versus inhaler) may be the deciding factor.

Cost

The cost of a month's supply of Atrovent HFA MDI is $237 at multiple retail pharmacies (Walmart, K-Mart, Kroger, Costco). Generic ipratropium inhaler is no longer available. The cost of Atrovent inhalation solution is more than $200 for 150 unit-dose vials, and generic ipratropium inhalation solution is $57 for 150 unit-dose vials. The cost of the combination product Combivent is $307 (Costco.com) or $76.19 for Duoneb (ipratropium and albuterol nebulizer solution) per 30 vials, a significant cost savings over prescribing the two products individually. The generic combination product is even less expensive at $13.97 for ipratropium/albuterol nebulizer solution (http://www.costco.com). The provider needs to be familiar with the cost to the patient for each medication when making decisions regarding prescribing. It may be less expensive to prescribe the combined medication for COPD, or, depending on the patient's prescription drug coverage, it may be less expensive to prescribe each product individually.

Tiotropium (Spriva) is available only as a dry powder capsule for use with the HandiHaler. The cost of 1 month's worth of capsules (30) is $223.07.

Aclidinium bromide (Tudorza Pressair) inhaler costs $234 for 60 doses, or 1 month's supply.

Monitoring

There is no specific laboratory monitoring necessary with the use of the inhaled anticholinergics, other than monitoring the disease process.

Patient Education

Administration

Ipratropium, aclidinium, and tiotropium should be used as prescribed. Overuse of bronchodilators leads to increased adverse effects, and using the bronchodilator less than prescribed may lead to increased bronchospasm and decreased pulmonary function.

The administration of medication via an MDI can be difficult for most adults and all children. Learning to coordinate the release of the medication from the inhaler with a deep breath is difficult. Written and pictorial instructions are available with the inhaler, but the provider must not assume that the patient understands the proper method of administering inhaled medications. Use verbal instructions as well as actual demonstration with a placebo inhaler to reinforce the written instructions. These instructions and demonstrations should be repeated at follow-up visits.

To use an inhaler properly, the patient should first exhale and then tilt the head slightly back and place the inhaler mouthpiece either about 2 inches from the open mouth or between the open lips. While inhaling, the patient should press down on the canister, breathe in slowly and deeply, and hold her or his breath for 10 seconds (count of 10) or as long as comfortable. If two puffs are prescribed, then the patient should wait at least 1 full minute between inhalations. If the patient is prescribed other inhalers, advise the patient to use the ipratropium first and wait 5 minutes before using the other inhalers as directed.

To assist with the delivery of inhaled medications, a spacer can be prescribed. The Aerochamber is a tube-like device that has pictures drawn on the outside to remind the patient of the proper technique to use in administering the inhaler. For younger children and older adults, the InspirEase spacer gives a visual cue of the spacer bag deflating to help in taking a deep-enough breath. If the patient is taking too rapid a breath, both of these devices emit a whistling sound as a cue to breathe more slowly.

Administration of ipratropium via nebulizer is per the manufacturer's directions. One unit dose of ipratropium is administered every 6 to 8 hours. Albuterol can be added to the ipratropium if the mixture is used within 1 hour. Cromolyn will precipitate if added to ipratropium solution; the patient should be advised of this if both medications are prescribed. The nebulizer medication cup should be rinsed well between drugs if these two medications are to be used concurrently via nebulizer. Regardless of administration method, patients should rinse their mouth with water after inhaling ipratropium or tiotropium to minimize dry mouth.

To prime the MDI, patients using Combivent are recommended to "test-spray" the oral inhalation aerosol 3 times into the air before using it the first time. The patient should also prime the MDI in this manner if the medication has not been used in more than 24 hours.

Spiriva should be administered via the patented HandiHaler device only. Capsules of tiotropium (Spiriva) dry powder are inserted into the HandiHaler, and the medication is administered via breath actuation. The Spiriva package insert has step-by-step pictures and text explaining how to administer the medication.

Adverse Reactions

The patient should be advised that a cough may develop with either inhaled anticholinergic and that less common complaints of throat irritation, hoarseness, or dry mouth may occur. Using a spacer device and rinsing the mouth with water after administration will decrease the incidence of these adverse effects. Other adverse effects occur less often, but patients should be aware of the possible adverse effects and be instructed to notify their provider if they begin to have adverse effects from the inhaled anticholinergics, particularly urinary retention.

Lifestyle Management

Lifestyle management issues related to the disease process should be discussed. They often include the following:

1. Patients need to self-monitor their respiratory status with a peak flowmeter to determine the effectiveness of the medication prescribed.
2. The patient should avoid or quit smoking.
3. The patient should avoid environmental triggers for asthma at home, work, and school.
4. Patients with COPD should avoid unnecessary exposure to viral respiratory infections.

LEUKOTRIENE MODIFIERS

Leukotriene-receptor agonists (LTRAs) and 5-lipoxygenase pathway inhibitors were developed under the theory that cysteinyl leukotrienes play a significant role in the chronic inflammation associated with asthma and allergy. Leukotrienes are substances that induce numerous effects that contribute to the inflammatory process, including smooth muscle contractility; neutrophil aggregation, degranulation, and chemotaxis; vascular permeability; and on lymphocytes. There are two LTRAs available for use in asthma, zafirlukast (Accolate) and montelukast (Singulair), and one 5-lipoxygenase pathway inhibitor, zileuton (Zyflo).

Pharmacodynamics

Leukotriene-Receptor Agonists

Zafirlukast is a synthetic, selective, and competitive LTRA of leukotriene D4 and E4 (LTD4 and LTE4). These leukotrienes have been identified as components of slow-reacting substance of anaphylaxis. Montelukast is a selective LTRA that inhibits the cysteinyl leukotriene (CysLT1) receptor. It binds with high affinity and selectivity to the CysLT1 receptor. Montelukast inhibits the actions of LTD4 at the CysLT1 receptor. There is evidence that the cysteinyl leukotrienes contribute to the pathophysiology of asthma and allergy, including airway edema, smooth muscle constriction, and cellular changes associated with the inflammatory process. In vitro studies demonstrated that zafirlukast antagonized the contractile activity of three leukotrienes (LTC4, LTD4, and LTE4) in the conducting airway smooth muscle. Montelukast may also inhibit symptoms of allergic rhinitis, as leukotrienes are also released from the nasal mucosa during allergen exposure.

5-Lipoxygenase Pathway Inhibitors

Zileuton is an inhibitor of 5-lipoxygenase, the enzyme that catalyzes the formation of leukotrienes from arachidonic acid. By inhibiting 5-lipoxygenase, zileuton inhibits the formation of leukotrienes LTB_4, LTC_4, and LTE_4, identified as components of slow-reacting substance of anaphylaxis.

Pharmacokinetics

Absorption and Distribution

Zafirlukast is rapidly absorbed from the GI tract following oral administration. Peak plasma concentrations are reached in 3 hours. The bioavailability of zafirlukast may be decreased when taken with food, and it should be taken on an empty stomach. Zafirlukast is greater than 99% protein bound, primarily to albumin. Zafirlukast is excreted in breast milk in measurable amounts (50 ng/mL) compared with 255 ng/mL in plasma, when administered in healthy women in 40 mg/day dosages.

Montelukast is rapidly absorbed following oral administration, with peak plasma concentration achieved in 3 to 4 hours for the film-coated tablet and in 2 to 2.5 hours after administration of the chewable tablet. Montelukast is more than 99% protein bound. There is minimal distribution across the blood–brain barrier in rats; no human studies are available. Montelukast crosses the placenta in rats and is excreted in rat milk; there are no human studies available.

Zileuton is rapidly absorbed after oral administration, with a peak time of 1.7 hours. Food increases the maximum concentration (C_{max}) of zileuton up to 27%. Zileuton is 93% protein bound. It crosses the placental barrier in rats and is excreted in rat's milk. There are no controlled studies in pregnant women.

Metabolism and Excretion

Zafirlukast is extensively metabolized. In vitro studies using human liver microsomes showed that the hydroxylated metabolites of zafirlukast are formed through the CYP450 2C9 (CYP2C9) enzyme pathway. Additional studies using human liver microsomes show that zafirlukast inhibits

CYP3A4 and CYP2C9 isoenzymes at concentrations close to the clinically achieved plasma concentrations. The metabolites of zafirlukast found in plasma are at least 90 times less potent LTD4 receptor antagonists than zafirlukast. Following oral administration of zafirlukast, urinary excretion accounts for approximately 10% of the dose, and the remainder is excreted in the feces. Unmetabolized zafirlukast is not found in the urine.

Montelukast is extensively metabolized by the liver, with no detectable amounts of metabolites found in the plasma. CYP3A4 and CYP2C9 are the liver enzymes involved with the metabolism of montelukast. Montelukast and its metabolites are excreted almost exclusively via the bile, with less than 0.2% excreted in the urine.

Zileuton is metabolized in the liver via CYP1A2, CYP2C9, and CYP3A4. Renal elimination is the primary method of elimination, with 94.5% eliminated in the urine.

Table 17-4 presents the pharmacokinetics of the leukotriene modifiers.

Pharmacotherapeutics

Precautions and Contraindications

The leukotriene modifiers are not to be used for primary treatment of an acute asthma attack. The only true contraindication to the leukotriene modifiers zafirlukast and montelukast is hypersensitivity to any of the components of the medication. Chewable montelukast tablets are contraindicated in patients with phenylketonuria because the product contains phenylalanine. Zileuton is contraindicated in patients with active liver disease.

Zafirlukast should be used with caution in patients with hepatic dysfunction because it is extensively metabolized by the liver. If a patient has alcoholic cirrhosis, the clearance of zafirlukast is reduced about 50% to 60%. There is no need to adjust the dose of montelukast in the patient with mild to moderate hepatic insufficiency because the elimination is only slightly prolonged, although use should be avoided in patients with severe liver disease.

Leukotriene modifiers should not be abruptly substituted for inhaled or oral steroids. Caution is advised as systemic corticosteroids are reduced. There have been reports that the reduction of oral steroid dose in some patients on zafirlukast has been followed by eosinophilia, vasculitic rash, worsening pulmonary symptoms, cardiac complications, and/or neuropathy sometimes presenting as Churg–Strauss syndrome, a systemic eosinophilic rash.

Table 17–4 ⬛ Pharmacokinetics: Leukotriene Modifiers

Drug	Onset	Peak	Duration	Protein Binding	Bioavailability	Half-Life	Metabolism	Elimination
Montelukast	—	3–4 h	—	>99%	64%	2.7–5.5 h	Extensive hepatic	Bile
Zafirlukast	3–14 d	2–4 h	—	>99%	Unknown	About 10 h	Extensive hepatic	Feces: 90%; urine: 10%
Zileutin		1.7 h		93%	UK	2.5 h	Hepatic	Urine: 95%

Neuropsychiatric events have been reported in postmarketing surveillance of adult, adolescent, and pediatric patients taking leukotriene modifiers. The reported neuropsychiatric events include agitation, aggression, anxiousness, dream abnormalities and hallucinations, depression, insomnia, irritability, restlessness, suicidal thinking and behavior (including suicide), and tremor (FDA, 2009). Sleep disorders were more frequent in all three products than in placebo in the original clinical trials (FDA, 2009). The FDA (2009) recommends that patients be informed of the potential for neuropsychiatric events with these medications and should consider discontinuing leukotriene modifiers if the patient develops neuropsychiatric problems.

Zafirlukast and montelukast are Pregnancy Category B. Zileuton is Pregnancy Category C.

The safety and efficacy of zafirlukast have been established in children aged 5 and older. Montelukast may be prescribed for children as young as age 12 months for chronic asthma. The safety and effectiveness of Zileuton in pediatric patients younger than age 12 years have not been established.

Caution should be used in prescribing any of the leukotriene modifiers to lactating women because the effects on infants are unknown.

Adverse Reactions

The most common adverse reaction reported with zafirlukast use is headache. GI upset, myalgias, and fever are reported in a small percentage of patients. There is a reported increase in respiratory infections in patients older than age 55 years who are taking zafirlukast. The respiratory infections were usually mild to moderate and associated with coadministration of inhaled corticosteroids.

The reported adverse reactions of those taking montelukast are similar to placebo.

Zileuton has similar effects to placebo in clinical trials, except for a significant increase in dyspepsia (8.2% versus 2.9%) in patients treated with zileuton. Hepatic injury, including hepatitis and death, is reported, with 1.9% of patients exhibiting elevated ALT in the clinical trials.

Drug Interactions

Zafirlukast should be used with caution with any drug that is metabolized by CYP2C9 and CYP3A3/4 isoenzymes. Coadministration of aspirin with zafirlukast results in about a 45% increase in plasma zafirlukast level. Erythromycin coadministered with zafirlukast results in a 40% decrease in plasma zafirlukast level. Concurrent terfenadine use leads to decreased plasma zafirlukast levels, and theophylline use has a similar profile. When warfarin is prescribed to the patient taking zafirlukast, there is a clinically significant increase in prothrombin time (PT).

Monitor closely the patient who is taking drugs that are metabolized by CYP450 isoenzymes CYP2A6, CYP2C9, and CYP3A3/4 (phenobarbital, rifampin) concurrently with montelukast. Coadministration with drugs metabolized by CYP3A4 and zileuton should be monitored closely as there is a theoretical interaction. Coadministration of zileuton and theophylline may elevate serum theophylline levels. A reduction of theophylline dose by 50% is recommended by the manufacturer of Zyflo. Terfenadine plasma levels are increased by up to 35% and clearance is reduced by 22% when administered with zileuton. Coadministration with warfarin may theoretically increase prothrombin time; monitoring closely is warranted.

Table 17-5 presents drug interactions between the leukotriene modifiers and other medications.

Table 17–5 ⣿ Drug Interactions: Leukotriene Modifiers

Drug	Interacting Drug	Possible Effect	Implications
Montelukast	Phenobarbital	Decreases area under curve (AUC) of dose by about 40%	Monitor patient closely
	Rifampin	Decreased metabolism of montelukast	Monitor
Zafirlukast	Aspirin	Increased plasma levels of zafirlukast	Monitor
	Erythromycin	Decreased plasma levels of zafirlukast	Use together with caution
	Theophylline	Decreased plasma levels of zafirlukast	Use cautiously
	Warfarin	Increased PT/INR	Closely monitor PT/INR
	Drugs metabolized by CYP2C9: amitriptyline, diclofenac, ibuprofen, imipramine, phenytoin, tolbutamide	Possible interactions	Until more data known, zafirlukast should be used cautiously in patients stabilized on these medications
	Drugs metabolized by CYP3A4: alprazolam, astemizole, carbamazepine, cisapride, some corticosteroids, cyclosporine, diazepam, calcium channel blockers (felodipine, isradipine, nicardipine, nifedipine, nimodipine), diltiazem, erythromycin, lidocaine, lovastatin, midazolam, quinidine, simvastatin, triazolam, verapamil	Possible interactions	Until more data known, zafirlukast should be used cautiously in patients stabilized on these medications

Table 17–5 ⚏ Drug Interactions: Leukotriene Modifiers—cont'd

Drug	Interacting Drug	Possible Effect	Implications
Zileutin			
	Theophylline	Increased half-life of theophylline. More theophylline ADRs	Use cautiously
	Warfarin	Increased AUC of warfarin	Closely monitor PT/INR
	Proproanolol	Increased propranolol concentration	Monitor HR closely. Decrease dose of propranolol if needed.

Clinical Use and Dosing

Zafirlukast is indicated in the treatment of chronic asthma in children aged 5 years or older and adults. Montelukast is indicated for use in the treatment of persistent asthma for patients aged 12 months or older. Montelukast may be prescribed for the prevention of exercise-induced bronchoconstriction in adolescents age 15 years or older and adults. Montelukast may also be used to treat seasonal allergic rhinitis in patients 2 years or older and perennial allergic rhinitis in patients 6 months and older. Zileuton is indicated for the treatment of persistent asthma in children aged 12 years and older and adults.

The dose for zafirlukast is 20 mg twice daily in children aged 12 years or older and adults, and 10 mg twice a day for children aged 5 to 11 years. Because food reduces the bioavailability of zafirlukast, it must be taken on an empty stomach.

The adult dosage (patients aged 15 years or older) of montelukast is 10 mg once a day in the evening. The dose of montelukast in children aged 6 to 14 years is 5 mg once a day in the evening. Children aged 2 to 5 years are dosed with 4 mg of montelukast before bed; children aged 12 to 24 months are prescribed 4 mg of oral granules. Montelukast may be taken without regard to meals. Montelukast is dosed the same for allergy as for asthma.

The dose of zileuton is 600 mg 4 times a day or two 600 mg extended-release tablets twice a day, 1 hour after meals. Table 17-6 shows the dosage schedule.

Rational Drug Selection

Drug selection is based on the age of the patient and convenience in dosing. Children under age 5 years may be prescribed only montelukast. Montelukast offers once-a-day dosing without regard to meals, which may make it more convenient than zafirlukast. Zileuton is dosed 4 times a day or extended-release twice a day. Singulair (montelukast) costs $170 for a 30-day supply (30 tablets), generic montelukast costs $40 for a 30 day supply. Accolate (zafirlukast) costs $135 for 60 tablets, a 30-day supply and generic zafirlukast $63 for 60 tablets. A 30-day supply of zileuton (Zyflo) costs$525.

Monitoring

Monitoring of improving or worsening asthmatic symptoms, bronchodilator use, and pulmonary function is necessary to determine the efficacy of the leukotriene modifiers. Patients should be monitored for new onset of neuropsychiatric symptoms, including depression or behavior change.

Patient Education

Patient education focuses on proper dosing of the medication, adverse reactions, and the general asthma management plan. The incorporation of the leukotriene medications into the asthma treatment plan is covered in Chapter 31.

Administration

The patient must take the medication as prescribed, even if symptom-free. These medications are not for acute episodes

Table 17–6 ⚏ Dosage Schedule: Leukotriene Modifiers

Drug	Indication	Dosage Form	Dose	Comments
Montelukast Singulair Generic	Prophylaxis and treatment of chronic asthma	Tablets: 10 mg Chewable tablets: 5, 4 mg Granules: 4 mg/packet	*Adults:* 10 mg once daily in p.m. *Children 6–14 yr:* 5 mg at bedtime *Children 2–5 yr:* 4 mg at bedtime *Children 12–24 mo:* 4 mg granules at bedtime	Not recommended for children <12 mo
Zafirlukast Accolate Generic	Prophylaxis and treatment of chronic asthma	Tablets: 20 mg Tablets: 10 mg	*Adults:* 20 mg bid *Children 5–11 yr:* 10 mg bid	Not recommended for children <5 yr; must be taken on an empty stomach
Zileutin Zyflo Zyflo CR Generic	Prophylaxis and treatment of chronic asthma	600 mg tablet Zyflo CR: 600 mg extended-release tablet	Adults: 600 mg qid	Not recommended for children

of asthma. Patients must continue to use the bronchodilator inhaler for acute episodes of bronchospasm. They are not to decrease or discontinue any of their other asthma medications unless instructed to do so by their health-care provider.

Zafirlukast must be taken on an empty stomach, whereas montelukast may be taken without regard to meals. Zileuton may be taken with or without food.

Pregnant or nursing women should not take these medications.

Patients should be aware of significant drug interactions with leukotriene modifiers because of the way these drugs are metabolized by the liver. Patients should be advised to discuss with their health-care provider any new medications that are prescribed or discontinued.

Adverse Reactions

Patients and parents of pediatric patients should be informed of the potential for neuropsychiatric events, including agitation, aggression, anxiousness, dream abnormalities and hallucinations, depression, insomnia, irritability, restlessness, suicidal thinking and behavior (including suicide), and tremor. Any new neuropsychiatric symptoms should be reported to the provider.

Lifestyle Management

Lifestyle management issues related to the disease process should be discussed. They often include the following:

1. The patient needs to self-monitor respiratory status with a peak flowmeter to determine the effectiveness of the medication prescribed.
2. The patient should avoid or quit smoking.
3. The patient should avoid environmental triggers for asthma at home, work, and school.

Table 17-6 presents the available dosage forms.

RESPIRATORY INHALANTS

CORTICOSTEROIDS

The *Expert Panel Report 3* states that corticosteroids are the "most potent and effective anti-inflammatory medication currently available" (NAEPP, 2007, p 213). Their anti-inflammatory effects lead to reduction in the severity of asthma symptoms, increased peak flow readings, and decreased airway hyperresponsiveness. In general, inhaled steroids are safe and well tolerated at recommended dosages and can be used by both children and adults. Corticosteroids are also used intranasally for the treatment of allergic rhinitis.

The commonly prescribed inhaled corticosteroids for asthma are beclomethasone dipropionate (QVAR), triamcinolone acetonide (Azmacort), budesonide (Pulmicort), flunisolide (AeroBid), mometasone furoate (Asmanex Twisthaler), fluticasone (Flovent), and ciclesonide (Alvesco). There are significant differences among the different formulations in the amount of steroid delivered per inhalation, and they are not interchangeable without adjusting the inhalations per day.

The corticosteroids that are available for intranasal use are beclomethasone (Beconase), triamcinolone (Nasacort AQ), budesonide (Rhinocort Aqua), flunisolide (Nasalide, Nasarel), mometasone (Nasonex), fluticasone (Flonase), and ciclesonide (Omnaris).

Pharmacodynamics

In the treatment of asthma and allergic rhinitis, the primary actions of orally inhaled corticosteroids are anti-inflammatory. The inhaled adrenocorticosteroids inhibit the immunoglobulin E (IgE) and mast cell–mediated migration of inflammatory cells into the bronchial tissue (late-phase allergic reaction). The exact mechanism of action by which the inhaled corticosteroids inhibit bronchoconstrictor mechanisms and produce smooth muscle relaxation is unknown. The exact mechanism of action of corticosteroids on the nasal mucosa is unknown. Intranasal corticosteroids applied topically to the nasal tissues exert local anti-inflammatory effects without any systemic glucocorticoid effects.

Pharmacokinetics

Absorption and Distribution

Absorption of inhaled corticosteroids occurs from the lungs and from the GI tract. Approximately 10% to 30% of the dose from an MDI is delivered to the lungs. If a spacer device is not used, approximately 80% of the dose from an MDI is swallowed, with the oral bioavailability differing from drug to drug.

Beclomethasone is rapidly absorbed from the nasal and pulmonary tissues and GI tract. Upon inhalation, 10% to 25% of the drug is deposited in the tissues of the mouth, trachea, and lungs, where it is completely absorbed. The remainder of the dose is swallowed. The oral bioavailability of inhaled beclomethasone is 20%. Beclomethasone is highly protein bound. It and its metabolites do not appear to distribute into the tissues, but beclomethasone does cross the placenta. With systemic administration, steroids are excreted in breast milk; it is unknown whether inhaled beclomethasone is found in breast milk.

Triamcinolone (Azmacort) MDI is packaged with a built-in spacer to enhance the delivery of the medication to the lungs. Triamcinolone (Nasacort) for intranasal use is delivered via intranasal metered-dose pump. Triamcinolone is rapidly and completely absorbed from lung tissues and nasal mucosa. It is distributed throughout the hilar areas of the lungs. The oral bioavailability of the swallowed portion of the dose is 10.6%. Triamcinolone is weakly protein bound and crosses the placenta. It is unknown whether inhaled triamcinolone is excreted in breast milk.

Approximately 20% of the inhaled dose of budesonide reaches the systemic circulation. Once absorbed from the nasal tissues or lungs, the distribution of budesonide is extensive. Budesonide is 88% protein bound. It is unknown if budesonide is excreted in breast milk, but it passes through the placenta.

Flunisolide is rapidly absorbed from the bronchial tree, with 10% to 20% of the inhaled dose distributing into the lungs. Fifty percent of an intranasal dose of flunisolide is absorbed into the systemic circulation. The oral bioavailability of the dose is 20% to 40%. Flunisolide crosses the placental barrier. Breast milk excretion is unknown.

Less than 1% of mometasone oral powder for inhalation is absorbed. With nasal administration, the medication that is swallowed is absorbed, although plasma concentrations are near or below the level of quantification. Breast milk excretion is unknown.

Fluticasone is primarily absorbed in the lungs, resulting in systemic bioavailability of 30% of the dose. Intranasal fluticasone has a systemic bioavailability of less than 2%. It is highly lipid-soluble, is rapidly distributed into the tissues, and is 91% protein bound. Fluticasone crosses the placenta. Breast milk excretion is unknown.

Ciclesonide is minimally absorbed and what is absorbed is 99% protein bound in distribution.

Metabolism and Excretion

Some portion of the dose of all inhaled corticosteroids is swallowed. After GI absorption, they all undergo high first-pass liver metabolism.

In the lung, beclomethasone is rapidly metabolized to beclomethasone 17-monopropionate and more slowly to free beclomethasone. Metabolites of beclomethasone are excreted mainly in the feces, with a small portion excreted in the urine.

Triamcinolone is metabolized into three less-active ingredients: 6-β-hydroxy triamcinolone acetonide, 21-carboxytriamcinolone, and 21-carboxy-6-β-hydroxytriamcinolone acetonide. All of the metabolites of triamcinolone are eliminated in the feces.

Budesonide undergoes extensive first-pass metabolism into two main metabolites: 16-α-hydroxyprednisolone (24%) and 6-β-hydroxybudesonide (5%). The metabolites are excreted in the urine (66%) and the feces.

The part of the flunisolide dose that is swallowed is absorbed and metabolized by the liver into several metabolites. One of the metabolites has minor glucocorticoid activity. The drug is further metabolized into inactive metabolites. Excretion of inhaled flunisolide is not described, but oral doses are excreted equally in the feces and the urine.

Mometasone is extensively metabolized in the liver via CYP3A4 isoenzyme. It is excreted primarily via the bile; 74% of metabolites is excreted in feces.

Fluticasone is metabolized in the liver primarily by CYP3A4. The only detectable metabolite is a 1-β-carboxylic acid derivative. Excretion is primarily in the feces; less than 5% is excreted in the urine.

Ciclesonide is metabolized by CYP3A4 into an active metabolite, des-ciclesonide. Sixty-six percent of ciclesonide is excreted in the feces and approximately 20% in the urine.

Pharmacokinetics is presented in Table 17-7.

Pharmacotherapeutics

Precautions and Contraindications

All of the inhaled corticosteroid preparations are contraindicated in acute status asthmaticus or when intensive, acute therapy is warranted. They should not be used for relief of acute bronchospasm.

Care should be used when substituting any of the inhaled corticosteroids for oral corticosteroid therapy. There have

Table 17–7 ❖ Pharmacokinetics: Respiratory Inhalants

Drug	Onset	Peak	Protein Binding	Bioavailability	Half-Life	Metabolism	Elimination
Corticosteroids							
Beclomethasone	Few days to 3 wk	—	—	<5%	15 h	Hepatic	Feces
Budesonide	—	—	88%	10%	2 h	Hepatic	Renal
Flunisolide	Few days to 4 wk	10–30 min	—	20%	1.8–2 h	Hepatic	Renal, feces
Fluticasone	—	—	91%	30%	—	Hepatic	Feces
Mometasone	11 h	1–2 wk	98%	—	5.8 h	Hepatic	Bile, renal
Triamcinolone	—	—	Weak	10%	0.5–1 h	Hepatic	Feces
Inhaled Antihistamine							
Azelastine	30 min–1 h	2–3 h	88%	40%	22 h	Hepatic	Feces
Anti-Inflammatory Agents							
Cromolyn sodium	—	—	—	<1%	—	Not metabolized	Bile, renal
Nedocromil	—	20 min	—	6–9%	1.5–2.3 h	Not metabolized	Renal: 64%; feces: 36%

been deaths due to adrenal insufficiency in asthmatic patients who were switched from oral to inhaled corticosteroids.

The risk for hypothalamic-pituitary-adrenal (HPA) suppression is low with inhaled corticosteroids, but the risk increases when inhaled corticosteroids are administered while the patient is taking oral steroids.

Inhaled corticosteroids should be avoided in patients with Cushing's syndrome. They should be used with caution in patients with ocular herpes simplex infections, tuberculosis, oral or nasal surgery or trauma, healing nasal septal ulcers, and untreated respiratory infection (viral, fungal, or bacterial).

All of the inhaled corticosteroids are Pregnancy Category C. There have been no well-controlled studies of the effects of inhaled corticosteroids during pregnancy.

The use of high-dose inhaled steroids in children may inhibit growth, but so can poorly controlled asthma. A large ($N = 943$) long-term study of the effects of inhaled corticosteroids on children followed for more than 12 years, to an average age of 25 years, observed a 0.47 inch difference in average height for the subjects in the budesonide group (NHLBI, 2012). Doses higher than 400 mcg/day in younger children warrant close monitoring of growth. Triamcinolone inhalant therapy should not be prescribed to children under age 6 years because the safety and efficacy have not been established. Budesonide safety has been determined for children as young as 6 months. Inhibition of growth has been noted in children on high-dose inhaled fluticasone. Fluticasone must be prescribed with caution to children under age 4 years. Mometasone nasal spray may be prescribed for children as young as age 2 years, but the safety of mometasone oral inhalation powder for asthma management has not been established for children younger than age 12. The safety of inhaled flunisolide in children under age 6 has not been established. Studies were conducted in children aged 6 to 11 years regarding the safety of nasal ciclesonide; nasal ciclesonide (Omnaris) is considered safe and effective in children aged 6 or older. During clinical trials the safety and efficacy of inhaled ciclesonide (Alvesco) was studied in children aged 4 to 11 years with asthma. To control asthma symptoms, ciclesonide (Alvesco) was determined to be safe, but not effective, in children younger than 12.

Adverse Reactions

All of the inhaled corticosteroids have associated xerostomia, hoarseness (5% to 50% of patients), tongue and mouth irritation, flushing, and dysgeusia (altered taste sensation). Rash and urticaria have been reported with the use of flunisolide, beclomethasone, and fluticasone. Dysmenorrhea has been reported in 1% to 3% of patients using inhaled fluticasone and 4% to 9% using mometasone oral inhalation powder.

Local immunosuppression can lead to oral candidiasis with any of the inhaled corticosteroids. Cataracts can be induced with corticosteroid use, even with inhaled corticosteroids. Bronchospasm may occur with any of the inhaled

corticosteroids. With high-dose inhaled corticosteroid use, HPA suppression is theoretically possible. Concurrent use of systemic corticosteroids with inhaled corticosteroids increases the likelihood of HPA suppression, compared with the use of either one alone.

Pulmonary infiltrates with eosinophilia may occur with inhaled flunisolide, usually when inhalation corticosteroid therapy replaces systemic corticosteroid therapy. The cause is unknown.

Intranasal corticosteroid use may cause nasal irritation, itching, sneezing, and nasal dryness. The patient may experience bloody nasal mucus or epistaxis.

Drug Interactions

There are no known drug interactions with inhaled triamcinolone, flunisolide, mometasone, beclomethasone, or ciclesonide.

Ritonavir significantly increases fluticasone serum concentrations and may lead to increased corticosteroid effects of fluticasone. Ketoconazole increases plasma concentration of fluticasone and budesonide when coadministered. The interaction is due to inhibition of CYP3A4 isoenzyme, the enzyme that metabolizes fluticasone and budesonide. There are no other known drug interactions, but close monitoring for corticosteroid-related side effects is advisable if coadministered with other drugs that are known to inhibit CYP3A4. Those drugs include anastrozole (Arimidex) in high doses, delavirdine (Rescriptor), erythromycin, fluconazole (Diflucan), fluoxetine (Prozac), itraconazole (Sporanox), mibefradil (Posicor), nefazodone (Serzone), nelfinavir (Viracept), ritonavir (Norvir), and zileuton (Zyflo). Drug interactions are presented in Table 17-8.

Clinical Use and Dosing

Asthma

The inhaled corticosteroids are the preferred long-term control medications for managing the inflammatory process associated with asthma (NAEPP, 2007). Dosages for the inhaled corticosteroids vary with the specific product and the delivery method. The patient with persistent asthma is started on inhaled corticosteroids according to the *Expert Panel Report 3* guidelines for the management of asthma discussed in detail in Chapter 30 (NAEPP, 2007). All patients with mild persistent asthma are started on a low dose of inhaled corticosteroids. Children older than age 12 and adults may be treated with cromolyn, nedocromil, leukotriene modifiers, or theophylline as alternative therapy. If the patient has moderate persistent asthma, then the patient is prescribed daily low- to medium-dose inhaled corticosteroids combined with a long-acting beta agonist. Alternatively, the patient can be prescribed medium-dose inhaled corticosteroids or a combination of low- to medium-dose inhaled corticosteroids and a leukotriene modifier. Severe persistent asthma requires daily high-dose inhaled corticosteroids and long-acting beta agonists. See Table 17-9 for dosing inhaled corticosteroids for children over age 5 and adults.

Table 17–8 ▦ Drug Interactions: Respiratory Inhalants

Drug	Interacting Drug	Possible Effect	Implications
Corticosteroids			
Beclomethasone	None known	—	—
Budesonide	Ketoconazole*	Increased budesonide concentrations and suppression of plasma cortisol levels	Observe the patient for increased corticosteroid-related side effects
Flunisolide	None known	—	—
Fluticasone	Ketoconazole* Ritonavir	Increased fluticasone concentrations and suppression of plasma cortisol levels	Observe the patient for increased corticosteroid-related side effects
Mometasone	None known	—	—
Triamcinolone	None known	—	—
Inhaled Antihistamines			
Azelastine	Cimetidine	The mean maximum concentration (C_{max}) and area under the curve (AUC) of azelastine is increased when coadministered with cimetidine	Monitor closely if coadministering
	Ethanol or other CNS depressants	Reduced mental alertness and impairment of CNS performance may occur	Use concurrently with caution
Anti-Inflammatory Agents			
Cromolyn	None known	—	—
Nedocromil	None known	—	—

*There are no other known drug interactions, but close monitoring is advisable if coadministered with other drugs that are known to inhibit CYP3A4. Those drugs include anastrozole in high doses, delavirdine, erythromycin, fluconazole, fluoxetine, itraconazole, mibefradil, nefazodone, nelfinavir, ritonavir, and zileuton.

Table 17–9 ✂ Dosage Schedule: Respiratory Inhalants

Drug	Indication	Dosage Form	Dose	Comments
Corticosteroids				
Beclomethasone QVAR	Asthma	40 mcg/puff 80 mcg/puff	*Children >12 yrs and adults:* Low dose: 80–240 mcg daily in divided doses either bid, tid, or qid Medium dose: 240–480 mcg daily in divided doses High dose: >480 mcg daily in divided doses *Children 5 yrs to 11 yrs:* Low dose: 80–160 mcg daily in divided doses (2–4 puffs 40 mcg/puff; 1–2 puffs 80 mcg/puff) Medium dose: 160–320 mcg daily in divided doses (4–8 puffs 40 mcg/puff; 2–4 puffs 80 mcg/puff) High dose: >320 mcg daily in divided doses (>8 puffs 40 mcg/puff; >4 puffs 80 mcg/puff)	Patients should rinse their mouth with water after use; if needed, use inhaled bronchodilator first
Qnasl Beconase AQ	Allergic rhinitis	80 mcg/inhalation 42 mcg/inhalation	*Children >6 yr and adults:* 42 mcg/spray nasal inhaler: 1 spray each nostril bid times/d 80 mcg/spray aqueous nasal spray: 1–2 sprays each nostril once a day	Not recommended for use in children <6 yr
Budesonide Pulmicort Flexihaler Pulmicort Respules Generic	Asthma	Power inhalation: 90 mcg/inhalation 180 mg/inhalation Nebulizer suspension 0.25 mg/2mL	*NIH Asthma Guidelines (2007):* *>age 12 yr and adults:* Low dose: 180–600 mcg daily Medium dose: 600–1,200 mcg daily High dose: >1,200 mcg daily	Rinse mouth after use Has rapid onset for an inhaled steroid Improvement can occur within 24 h of beginning treatment,

Continued

Table 17–9 ⊗ **Dosage Schedule: Respiratory Inhalants—cont'd**

Drug	Indication	Dosage Form	Dose	Comments

			Children 5–11 yr:
			Low dose: 180–400 mcg/d
			Medium dose: 400–800 mcg/d
			High dose: > 800 mcg/d
			Children 12 mo–8 yr:
			Pulmicort respules or generic nebulizer solution:
			Previously treated with bronchodilators alone:
			   0.25 mg twice daily or 0.5 mg daily, max 0.5 mg/d
			Previously treated with inhaled corticosteroids:
			   0.25 mg bid or 0.5 mg daily, max 2 mg/d
			Previously treated with oral corticosteroids: 0.5 mg
			   or 1 mg daily, max 1 mg daily
			Children >6 yr previously treated with bronchodilators:
			Low dose: 200 mcg daily (1 inhalation daily)
			Medium dose: 200–400 mcg daily (2–3 inhalations
			   daily)
			High dose: >400 mcg/d (>2 inhalations daily)
			NIH Asthma Guidelines:
			Nebulization
			Children ≤ 4 yr:
			Low dose: 0.25–0.5 mg/d
			Medium dose: 0.5–1.0 mg/d
			High dose: > 1 mg/d
			Children 5–11 yr:
			Low dose: 0.5 mg/d
			Medium dose: 1 mg/d
			High dose: 2 mg/d
				although maximum benefit may not be achieved for 1–2 wk
				Dose should be titrated to the lowest effective dose once asthma is controlled

Rhinocort Tubohaler Rhinocort Aqua	Allergic rhinitis	100 mcg/inhalation 64 mcg/inhalation	*Children >6 yr and adults:* Initially 2 sprays in each nostril bid or 4 sprays once daily in the a.m. (max 4 sprays/nostril/d)	Blow nose prior to using For perennial rhinitis, gradually reduce over 2–4 wk to lowest effective dose

Flunisolide	Allergic rhinitis		*Adults:*
			Initially 2 sprays each nostril bid, maximum
			   8 sprays each nostril/d
			Children 6–14 yr:
			Initially 1 spray each nostril tid or 2 sprays each
			   nostril bid; maximum 4 sprays/nostril/d
				Blow nose prior to using
				Safety in children <6 yr has not been established

Fluticasone Flovent Diskus Flovent HFA	Asthma	Oral dry powder inhaler (60):
		50, 100, 260 mcg
		Inhaler (120 puffs):
		44, 110, 220 mcg/
		inhalation
			Dry powder inhaler:
			Children >12 yr and adults:
			Low dose: 100–300 mcg daily
			Medium dose: 300–500 mcg daily
			High dose: >500 mcg daily
			Children 5–11 yr:
			Low dose: 100–200 mcg daily
			Medium dose: 200–400 mcg daily
			High dose: >400 mcg daily
			Inhaler:
			Children >12 yr and adults:
			Low dose: 88–264 mcg daily (2–6 puffs
			   44 mcg/puff divided bid)
			Medium dose: 264–660 mcg daily (2–6 puffs
			   110 mcg/puff daily divided bid)
			High dose: >660 mcg (>6 puffs 110 mcg/puff or
			   >3 puffs 220 mcg/puff)
			Children 5–11 yr:
			Low dose: 88–176 mcg daily (2–4 puffs
			   44 mcg/puff divided bid)
			Medium dose: 176–352 mcg daily (2–4 puffs
			   110 mcg/puff divided bid)
			High dose: >264–440 mcg (>4 puffs 110 mcg/puff or
			   >2 puffs 220 mcg/puff)
				Safety in children <4 yr has not been established

Table 17–9 ⊗ **Dosage Schedule: Respiratory Inhalants—cont'd**

Drug	Indication	Dosage Form	Dose			Comments
			Children 0–4 yrs: Low dose: 176 mcg Medium dose: >176–352 mcg High dose: >352			
Veramyst Flonase Generic	Allergic rhinitis	27.5 mcg/ inhalation 50 mcg/inhalation	*Children >11 yr and adults:* Initially 2 sprays each nostril once a day or 1 spray in each nostril bid; for maintenance, reduce dose to 1 spray each nostril daily *Children 4–11 yr:* Initially 1 spray in each nostril once daily; may increase to 2 sprays in each nostril once daily if needed; for maintenance: 1 spray in each nostril once daily			Safety in children <4 yr has not been established
Fluticasone and Salmeterol Advair HFA Advair Diskus	Persistent asthma	Inhaler: ADVAIR HFA 45/21 Inhalation Aerosol (fluticasone propionate 45 mcg and salmeterol 21 mcg) ADVAIR HFA 115/21 Inhalation Aerosol (fluticasone propionate 115 mcg and salmeterol 21 mcg), and ADVAIR HFA 230/21 Inhalation Aerosol (fluticasone propionate 230 mcg and salmeterol 21 mcg) Oral inhalation powder: ADVAIR DISKUS 100/50 (fluticasone propionate 100 mcg and salmeterol 50 mcg) Inhalation Powder ADVAIR DISKUS 250/50 (fluticasone propionate 250 mcg and salmeterol 50 mcg) Inhalation Powder ADVAIR DISKUS 500/50 (fluticasone propionate 500 mcg and salmeterol 50 mcg) Inhalation Powder	*No prior inhaled corticosteroid:* *Children 4–11 yr:* Fluticasone 100 mcg/salmeterol 50 mcg 1 inhalation bid *Children ≥12 yr and adults:* Fluticasone 100 mcg/salmeterol 50 mcg 1 inhalation bid *COPD: Adults:* Fluticasone 250 mcg/salmeterol 50 mcg 1 inhalation bid			Titrate dose to lowest effective strength that maintains control of asthma
Mometasone Nasonex	Allergic rhinitis	50 mcg/spray	*Children 2–11 yr:* 1 spray each nostril once a day *Children ≥12 yr and adults:* 2 sprays each nostril twice a day			
Asmanex Twisthaler	Asthma	200 mcg, 400 mcg	*Children ≥12 yr and adults:*			Contains lactose. If administered once a day, dose should be taken in the p.m. Safety not established in children <12 yr.
			Previous therapy	Recommended starting dose	Highest recommended daily dose	
			Bronchodilators alone	220 mcg daily p.m.	440 mcg	
			Inhaled corticosteroids	220 mcg daily p.m.	440 mcg	
			Oral corticosteroids	440 mcg bid	880 mcg	

Continued

Table 17–9 ⨉ **Dosage Schedule: Respiratory Inhalants—cont'd**

Drug	Indication	Dosage Form	Dose	Comments
Mometasone and formoterol Dulera	Chronic asthma	**DULERA 100 mcg/ 5 mcg** (mometasone furoate 100 mcg and formoterol fumarate dihydrate 5 mcg) **DULERA 200 mcg/ 5 mcg** (mometasone furoate 200 mcg and formoterol fumarate dihydrate 5 mcg)	Previously on medium dose inhaled corticosteroids: DULERA 100 mcg/5 mcg, 2 inhalations twice daily, maximum 400 mcg daily Previously on high dose inhaled corticosteroids: DULERA 200 mcg/5 mcg, 2 inhalations twice daily, max 800 mcg/daily	Rinse mouth after use Safety in children <6 yr has not been established
Triamcinolone Nasacort AQ	Allergic rhinitis	55 mcg/inhalation	*Children >12 yr and adults:* 2 sprays in each nostril once daily; may increase if needed to a maximum of 8 sprays/d; reduce dose as condition improves *Children 6–12 yr:* 2 sprays each nostril once daily; may reduce as condition improves	Safety in children <6 yr has not been established
Inhaled Antihistamine				
Azelastine Astelin Astepro	Allergic rhinitis	0.1% solution: 137 mcg/ inhalation 0.15% solution: 205 mcg/ inhalation	*Children >12 yr and adults:* 2 sprays (137 mcg/spray) per nostril bid *Children 5–11 yr:* 1 spray per nostril bid	Safety in children <5 yr has not been established The unit must be primed before using for the first time by pumping the activator 4 times, until a fine mist occurs
Anti-Inflammatory Agents				
Cromolyn Generic	Asthma	20 mg/2 mL solution	*Nebulizer* *Children >2 yr and adults:* 1 unit dose qid, weaning down to bid	Cromolyn must be used continuously 3–4 wk before maximum effect is achieved Cromolyn is very safe to use in children, with fewer side effects than inhaled steroids
Cromolyn NasalCrom	Allergic rhinitis	40 mg/mL solution	*Children >6 yr and adults:* 1 spray in each nostril 3–4 times a day; may increase dosage to 6/d if needed	Begin therapy 1 wk before known exposure; for allergic rhinitis; 2–4 wk of therapy may be needed to produce relief; blow nose prior to administering Once control is established, the dose can be reduced to 3 times a day; after several weeks the dose can be further decreased to bid

Chapter 31 should be referred to for comprehensive asthma management.

Children with persistent asthma require daily anti-inflammatory therapy. Young children with mild persistent asthma are usually started on step 2 therapy, a low-dose inhaled corticosteroid (via nebulizer or MDI and mask), with an alternative therapy being cromolyn or montelukast. If the child has moderate persistent asthma, low-dose inhaled corticosteroids combined with montelukast or a long-acting inhaled beta agonist are begun. Because salmeterol is not approved for children younger than age 4, an alternative treatment would be medium-dose inhaled corticosteroids, or low-dose inhaled corticosteroids combined with a leukotriene modifier (montelukast). High-dose inhaled steroids combined with a long-acting inhaled beta agonist or montelukast are prescribed for severe persistent asthma. The provider should be familiar with the differences in dosing young children and adults. The full *Expert Panel Report 3* guidelines for step-wise management of asthma are available in Chapter 31.

Allergic Rhinitis

Allergic rhinitis results when allergens come in contact with the nasal mucosa, causing a hypersensitivity reaction. Nasal corticosteroids are used to manage the inflammatory response associated with seasonal or perennial allergies. Intranasal corticosteroids may be used once or twice a day, depending on the drug chosen. Once clinical improvement occurs, usually in 3 to 7 days, the dose can be decreased. See Table 17-9 for dosing information.

Rational Drug Selection

The *Expert Panel Report 3* and update (NAEPP, 2007) do not recommend one inhaled corticosteroid over another; therefore, the choice is mostly based on ease of dosing and the adverse drug interactions and indications previously addressed. There are no generic equivalent formulas for the inhaled corticosteroids but there is generic fluticasone nasal spray, which may make cost a factor as more generic formulas are available.

Dosing

If a patient requires a high dose of inhaled steroid, the beclomethasone 42 mcg/puff dose would be more than 20 puffs per day, whereas the dose of budesonide would be 8 or more puffs per day. High-dose triamcinolone would also be 20 puffs per day. Fluticasone and flunisolide have the highest steroid anti-inflammatory effect per puff, which makes dosing high-dose inhaled steroids more convenient (see Table 17-9 for dosing). If the patient requires a low dose or if trying to wean the dose, beclomethasone or triamcinolone would be the first choice.

Monitoring

The patient who is using inhaled corticosteroids needs to be monitored for adverse effects of the medication, effectiveness of the medication, and the asthma disease process. If high-dose inhaled corticosteroids are used for a long time, blood glucose and potassium should be monitored, as well as growth in young children.

Patient Education

Administration

Patients who are concurrently using an inhaled bronchodilator should administer the bronchodilator first and wait several minutes before using the inhaled corticosteroid. This procedure enhances the absorption of the steroid in the bronchial tree.

The administration of inhaled corticosteroids via an MDI can be difficult for most adults and all children. Learning to coordinate the release of the medication from the inhaler with a deep breath is difficult. Written and pictorial instructions

are available with the inhaler, but the provider must not assume that the patient understands the proper method of administering inhaled medications. Use verbal instructions as well as actual demonstration with a placebo inhaler to reinforce the written instructions. These instructions and demonstrations should be repeated at follow-up visits.

To use an inhaler properly, the patient should first exhale and then tilt the head slightly back and place the inhaler mouthpiece either about 2 inches from the open mouth or between the open lips. While inhaling, the patient should press down on the canister, breathe in slowly and deeply, and hold his or her breath for 10 seconds (count of 10) or as long as comfortable. If multiple puffs are prescribed, then the patient should wait at least 1 full minute between inhalations.

To assist with the delivery of inhaled medications, spacers can be prescribed to ensure the medication is deposited in the lungs, not the mouth. The Aerochamber is a tube-like device that has pictures drawn on the outside to remind the patient of the proper techniques. For younger children and older adults, the InspirEase spacer gives a visual cue of the spacer bag deflating to help in taking a deep-enough breath. Both of these devices cue the patient to breathe slowly by emitting a whistling sound if the patient is taking too rapid a breath. The Global Initiative for Asthma Web site has extensive information and diagrams on the use of the different types of spacers and inhalation delivery devices (www.ginasthma.org/documents/11).

Dry powder, breath-actuated inhalers require adequate inspiratory effort to deliver the medication into the bronchial tree. Patient self-administration should be observed to determine whether the medication is being used appropriately.

Patients should rinse their mouth with water after each use to help reduce dry mouth, hoarseness, and candidiasis infection.

The patient should clear the nasal passages of mucus prior to using intranasal corticosteroids. If the nasal passages are swollen and blocked, the patient should administer a topical decongestant prior to using intranasal corticosteroids. The medication is sprayed into the nasal passages. The patient does not need to inhale the medication. The patient should understand that the effects are not immediate and that clinical improvement may take 3 to 7 days. Rinsing the mouth with water after use will reduce the rare chance of candidiasis infection associated with intranasal corticosteroid use.

Inhaled steroids are not to be used as abortive asthma medications; they are for preventive therapy only. The provider should have patients bring in all their inhalers and review which are to be used for abortive therapy (short-acting beta agonists) and which are for preventive therapy. The patient should be advised to continue to use the inhaled corticosteroid even when not having asthma symptoms.

Adverse Reactions

The patient should be advised to notify the provider if sore mouth or throat occurs. Oral *Candida* infections are possible, and the patient should get prompt treatment. The patient should be aware of the possibility of dysphonia developing. Rinsing the mouth with water and using a spacer device will decrease its incidence. Other adverse effects occur less often, but the patient should be aware of them and be instructed to notify the provider if adverse effects begin to develop from the inhaled medication.

Relatively few medications interact with the inhaled corticosteroids. Ketoconazole should be avoided for patients who are prescribed fluticasone, ciclesonide, and budesonide. Patients should be instructed to notify all providers that they are on inhaled corticosteroids to avoid possible interactions.

Lifestyle Management

Lifestyle management issues related to the disease process should be discussed. They often include the following:

1. Patients need to self-monitor their respiratory status with a peak flowmeter to determine the effectiveness of the medication prescribed.
2. The patient should avoid or quit smoking.
3. The patient should avoid environmental triggers for asthma at home, work, and school.

Available dosage forms are presented in Table 17-9.

INHALED ANTI-INFLAMMATORY AGENTS

Cromolyn sodium and nedocromil are synthetic compounds that inhibit antigen-induced bronchospasm. Cromolyn was originally produced to be used as a bronchodilator but was found to have no bronchodilator activity. Nevertheless, cromolyn inhibits antigen-induced bronchospasm, blocks the release of histamine, and is a mast cell stabilizer. Nedocromil is similar to cromolyn in many ways but is now only available in ophthalmic solution, which is discussed in Chapter 27. Cromolyn is used in the treatment of asthma; it (Nasalcrom) is also used in treating allergic rhinitis.

Pharmacodynamics

Cromolyn acts to inhibit mast cell degranulation, which prevents the release of histamine and slow-reacting substance of anaphylaxis (SRS-A). Neither drug prevents the binding of IgE to the mast cell or the binding of antigen to IgE. Cromolyn also prevents the release of leukotrienes, which induce numerous effects that contribute to the inflammatory process in the lungs. With continued use, cromolyn reduces bronchi hyperreactivity to stimuli such as cold air, allergens, and environmental irritants. Cromolyn does not have bronchodilator, antihistamine, or vasoconstrictor activity, and at therapeutic doses, does not have systemic activity.

Pharmacokinetics

Absorption and Distribution

Inhaled cromolyn is poorly absorbed systemically; only 8% of the dose is absorbed. Approximately 5% to 10% of the inhaled dose reaches the lungs, with the amount affected by the degree of bronchoconstriction present. Intranasal cromolyn is minimally absorbed. Distribution of the absorbed amount of the drug is unknown. Minimal amounts of cromolyn cross the placenta and distribute into breast milk.

Metabolism and Excretion

The portion of the dose of cromolyn that is absorbed from the lung is rapidly excreted unchanged in the urine and bile. The remaining portion of the dose is exhaled or swallowed and excreted unchanged in the feces.

Pharmacotherapeutics

Precautions and Contraindications

Cromolyn is not a bronchodilator, and it is contraindicated in the treatment of acute bronchospasm or status asthmaticus. Hypersensitivity to cromolyn is a contraindication to its use.

Cromolyn is Pregnancy Category B and should be used with caution in the lactating mother because safety has not been established. Cromolyn is safe for use in children as young as 2 years (nebulizer solution).

Adverse Reactions

Cromolyn is generally well tolerated. Inhaled cromolyn may cause bronchospasm, which can be avoided by preadministering a beta-agonist bronchodilator. Throat irritation and cough are also reported. Intranasal cromolyn may produce nasal irritation and cause sneezing.

Drug Interactions

There are no clinically significant drug interactions with cromolyn. Cromolyn solution for nebulizer use will form a precipitate if mixed with ipratropium solution.

Clinical Use and Dosing

Asthma

Cromolyn is considered an alternative long-term control drug for the treatment of mild persistent asthma. It is available in inhaled form and nebulizer solution. The dosage of cromolyn MDI for children older than 5 years and adults is two sprays (800 mcg/spray) inhaled 4 times a day at regular intervals. The dose of nebulizer solution of cromolyn is one ampule (20 mg) 4 times a day at regular intervals. The dose of cromolyn may be decreased after the patient is stabilized (usually after 4 weeks) to two or three doses a day. If used concurrently with bronchodilators, the bronchodilator should be administered first. Cromolyn may be mixed with albuterol in a nebulizer cup to simplify dosing. The patient should understand that the effectiveness of cromolyn depends on using it regularly.

Oral cromolyn is also used for systemic mast-cell disease (mastocytosis) and inflammatory bowel disease. Dosing for mastocytosis is 200 mg of Gastrocrom oral concentrate 4 times a day in adults and 100 mg 4 times a day in children aged 2 to 12 years. Initial adult dosing for inflammatory bowel disease is 200 mg 4 times a day of Gastrocrom oral concentrate, which may be doubled if not responding after 2 to 3 weeks to 400 mg 4 times a day. Children aged 2 to 12 with inflammatory bowel disease are dosed at 100 mg 4 times a day. The dose may be doubled but should not exceed 40 mg/kg/day (Takemoto et al, 2009).

Bronchospasm Prophylaxis

Cromolyn is indicated for patients with exercise-induced bronchospasm or individuals who have bronchospasm with known precipitating factors (e.g., pet exposure). The dose of cromolyn MDI for children aged 5 years or older and adults is two inhalations 10 to 15 minutes before exercise. If exercise is prolonged, the dose may be repeated. Nebulizer dosing in children aged 2 years or older and adults is one ampule administered via nebulized solution not more than 1 hour prior to exercise. For maximum effectiveness, the time between the use of inhaled cromolyn sodium and exercise should be as brief as possible.

Allergic Rhinitis

The dosage of cromolyn sodium nasal inhalation spray in children aged 6 years and older and adults is one spray in each nostril 3 to 4 times a day. The dose may be increased to 6 times a day if needed. The dose is administered while the patient is inhaling, and the nostrils should first be cleared of mucus. Two to four weeks of therapy may be needed to produce relief from perennial rhinitis.

Rational Drug Selection

The decision regarding which inhaled anti-inflammatory to use is often based on cost, availability, and patient variables such as age or ease of dosing.

Patient Variables

Cromolyn has dosage forms available for use in children as young as 2 years.

Administration

Cromolyn comes in multiple formulations that allow the provider to match the patient's age and lifestyle with an administration form. Cromolyn MDI (Intal) has been discontinued in the United States, but generic inhalation solution for nebulizer use is available.

Cost

Cromolyn is available in generic nebulizer solution; the cost of 96 ampules is $212.

Monitoring

No specific monitoring is required other than monitoring associated with the disease process.

Patient Education

Administration

The administration of inhaled anti-inflammatory agents requires the patient to use the medication as prescribed. Cromolyn is not effective if not used at regular intervals. Clarification regarding the use of inhaled bronchodilators that can be used as needed and the inhaled anti-inflammatory agents will enable the patient to use the medication appropriately, as will a written plan.

The use of cromolyn via nebulizer must be demonstrated to the patient in the clinic or by the home health agency that is providing the nebulizer. Because the vials are premeasured, there is no concern about dosing error.

Adverse Reactions

At therapeutic dosages, minimal adverse reactions are reported. The patient should be instructed not to exceed the recommended dosage of the medication.

Lifestyle Management

Lifestyle management issues related to the disease process being treated should be discussed. They often include the following:

1. The patient needs to self-monitor respiratory status with a peak flowmeter to determine the effectiveness of the medication prescribed.
2. The patient should avoid or quit smoking.
3. The patient should avoid environmental triggers for the asthma at home, work, and school.

INHALED ANTIHISTAMINES

Azelastine (Astelin, Astepro) and olopatadine (Patanase) are the intranasal H_1 blockers currently available in the United States. They are used for the treatment of seasonal allergic rhinitis and vasomotor rhinitis.

Pharmacodynamics

Azelastine is an H_1 agonist and a potent inhibitor of histamine release from the mast cells. Azelastine and its metabolite desmethylazelastine inhibit the effects of histamine by competing with histamine for H_1 binding sites. Azelastine may also interfere with histamine- and leukotriene-induced bronchospasm. Olopatadine is a selective H_1 receptor antagonist.

Pharmacokinetics

Absorption and Distribution

Azelastine, administered intranasally, has a systemic oral bioavailability of 40%. Protein binding of azelastine is 88% and for the active metabolite desmethylazelastine, it is 97%. Peak serum concentrations are reached in 2 to 3 hours. Exact absorption information is unknown. Distribution is unknown, but because somnolence is a reported adverse effect, azelastine is assumed to enter the CNS. It is unknown whether azelastine crosses the placenta or is distributed in breast milk.

Olopatadine is absorbed from nasal mucosa and peaks in 15 minutes to 2 hours after administration. The portion of olopatadine absorbed is 55% protein bound.

Metabolism and Excretion

Azelastine is metabolized into the principal active metabolite desmethylazelastine. Following intranasal dosing of azelastine to steady state, plasma concentration of desmethylazelastine is 20% to 30% of azelastine. Excretion of azelastine and desmethylazelastine is via the feces. Olopatadine is not extensively metabolized and is eliminated in the urine.

Pharmacotherapeutics

Precautions and Contraindications

Some patients using intranasal azelastine may experience somnolence and should be cautioned not to drive or operate heavy equipment while using it. Patients should not use alcohol or other CNS depressants while using azelastine. Olopatadine is contraindicated only in patients with nasal diseases other than allergies. Spraying into the eyes should be avoided.

It is unknown whether azelastine is excreted in breast milk. Use during lactation with caution. Olopatadine has been measured in the milk of nursing rats; no studies of use in lactating women have been done. Because seasonal allergic rhinitis is not generally a life-threatening disease, the benefits do not outweigh the unknown risks to the infant.

Azelastine and olopatadine are Pregnancy Category C. It should be used in pregnancy only if the potential benefits outweigh the risks to the fetus. There are no adequate studies in pregnant women. In animals receiving more than 240 times the normal dose, external and skeletal abnormalities have been noted.

The safety of azelastine in children under age 5 years and of olopatadine in children younger than age 12 years has not been established.

Adverse Reactions

The most commonly reported adverse reaction to azelastine is bitter taste (19%). Other reported adverse reactions are somnolence (11%), headache, weight gain (2%), and myalgia (1.5%). Local effects such as nasal irritation, epistaxis, sneezing, and rhinitis are also reported. Bitter taste (12.8%), headache (4.4%), and epitaxis (3.2%) are also reported in patients using intranasal olopatadine.

Drug Interactions

There is an additive impairment of CNS function when azelastine is used with ethanol or other CNS depressants. When azelastine is coadministered orally with cimetidine, the area under the curve (AUC) and C_{max} are increased by 65%. Data regarding interactions with intranasal azelastine and cimetidine are not available. Azelastine should be used cautiously with other antihistamines. There is theoretical additive CNS depression when olopatadine is administered with other CNS depressants or alcohol.

Clinical Use and Dosing

Allergic Rhinitis

Azelastine is approved for use in seasonal allergic rhinitis. It is used to treat the specific symptoms of rhinorrhea, sneezing, and nasal pruritus. The dose for children older than age 12 years and adults is two sprays (137 mcg/spray) per nostril twice a day. Children age 5 to 12 years should use one spray in each nostril twice a day. Dosing for olopatadine is two sprays in each nostril twice a day in children older than age 12 years and in adults.

Rational Drug Selection

Oral Versus Intranasal Antihistamine

The provider may choose to use intranasal azelastine or olopatadine rather than a systemic antihistamine because of decreased adverse effects or fewer drug interactions noted with the intranasal product.

Cost

The cost of azelastine (Astelin) is $146 for a 30 mL bottle, with the generic costing $77 for a 30 mL bottle. Olopatadine (Patanase) costs $175 for a 30.5 g bottle.

Patient Variables

Azelastine should not be prescribed to children under age 5 years and olopatadine should not be prescribed to children younger than age 12. Both drugs should be used with caution in pregnant and lactating patients.

Monitoring

There is no specific monitoring required with the use of azelastine or olopatadine other than symptoms of allergic rhinitis to determine efficacy.

Patient Education

Administration

The patient should be instructed to prime the medication unit before use by pumping the activator 4 times, or until a fine mist appears. The patient should keep the sprayer pointed away from the face, other people, and pets when priming the medication. The patient should wipe the tip of the sprayer with a clean tissue after using and replace the cap between uses. To prevent the spread of infection, the sprayer should be used by only one person.

Adverse Reactions

The patient should be instructed about the most common adverse reactions. Caution regarding driving or operating heavy equipment while using azelastine should be stressed. The bitter taste that some patients experience may be decreased by drinking water or another fluid after administration. The patient should report any unusual adverse reactions to the provider.

The patient should be cautioned not to drink alcohol or take any other CNS depressants while using intranasal azelastine. The patient may not be aware that an intranasal medication can have an interaction with an orally administered medication, and therefore, the provider must give careful instructions before prescribing azelastine.

Lifestyle Management

Lifestyle management related to the disease process needs to be discussed with the patient. Points to discuss often include avoidance of known allergens and using environmental methods to control dust mites and other common allergens.

OXYGEN

Oxygen is a basic element essential for human life; oxygen deprivation leads to rapid death. Therapy with oxygen is necessary for life in several diseases that interfere with normal oxygenation of blood and tissues. Oxygen as a therapeutic gas is delivered from steel containers and is 99% pure.

Pharmacodynamics

Oxygen is prescribed to treat hypoxia, or tissue deprivation of oxygen. Hypoxia can be caused by an inadequate supply of oxygen to the lungs, which can be due to poor ventilation or inadequate partial pressure of inspired oxygen. Inadequate pulmonary function can lead to hypoxia, as in a mismatch between ventilation and perfusion. Tissue hypoxia may occur with inadequate delivery of oxygen to the tissues, such as occurs in low cardiac output. Tissue hypoxia may also occur if the oxygen concentration of the blood is low, as occurs in anemia.

The effects of hypoxia can be observed in all major organ systems. The respiratory system increases the ventilatory rate and depth as a result of stimulation of carotid and aortic chemoreceptors. The heart increases cardiac output by increasing the heart rate. With severe hypoxia, bradycardia develops and ultimately leads to circulatory failure. The CNS is the most sensitive to hypoxia, with initial impaired judgment and psychomotor ability, leading to confusion; restlessness; and ultimately stupor, coma, and death.

Pharmacokinetics

The oxygen content of inhaled air is normally 20.9%, equivalent to a partial pressure of 159 mm Hg. As oxygen is inhaled, it enters the pulmonary airways and travels to the distal airways and alveoli. In the distal airways, the partial pressure of oxygen (PO_2) is decreased by dilution with carbon dioxide and water vapor and by uptake into the blood. The diffusion of oxygen into the pulmonary capillary blood is driven by the gradient between the PO_2 in mixed venous blood and that in the alveolar gas. The pressure gradient increases when 100% oxygen is administered, causing increased oxygen diffusion into the pulmonary capillary blood. Oxygen is delivered via the circulation to the tissue capillary beds, where it is diffused by its higher partial pressure out of the blood and into the cells.

Oxygen in the blood is carried by the hemoglobin, with a small amount in physical solution in the plasma. The amount of oxygen carried by the hemoglobin depends on the partial pressure of carbon dioxide ($PaCO_2$) and is usually illustrated with the oxyhemoglobin dissociation curve.

Pharmacotherapeutics

Precautions and Contraindications

The only contraindication to oxygen use is concurrent smoking while the oxygen is running. Oxygen is a flammable gas that will ignite if a flame is too near. This has implications for chronic smokers, who should turn off their oxygen to smoke.

Oxygen should be prescribed to patients with chronic carbon dioxide retention with extreme caution and close monitoring. Because hypoxemia may be the primary stimulus for respiration in these patients, the lowest possible concentration of oxygen to avoid serious tissue hypoxia should be used. In patients with hypercapnia, the sudden increases in $PaCO_2$ produced by oxygen may result in cessation of respiration.

Adverse Drug Reactions

Dry Nasal Passages

The most common adverse drug reaction reported in patients who are administered oxygen is dry nasal passages from the flow of gas through the nasal cannula (NC). This can be prevented by administering humidified oxygen by mask or by keeping the flow rate low (less than 5 to 6 L/min).

Toxicity

Oxygen toxicity occurs when inspired concentrations of oxygen exceed those of air for prolonged periods of time. Cell membrane damage and death are thought to be caused by increased production of reactive species such as superoxide anion, singlet oxygen, hydroxyl radical, and hydrogen peroxide. Some tissues, including the respiratory tract, the CNS, and the retina, are more sensitive to high oxygen concentration.

In the respiratory tract, inhalation of 100% oxygen for 6 to 8 hours can lead to decreased movement of tracheal mucus. In as little as 12 hours of 100% oxygen, the patient may experience tracheobronchial irritation and complain of chest tightness. After 17 hours, there is increased alveolar permeability and inflammation. Overall pulmonary function decreases after 18 to 24 hours of continuous 100% oxygen. After 24 hours of 100% oxygen, the patient usually has symptoms of nausea, vomiting, and anorexia. The patient may survive 1 week on toxic levels of oxygen. Death occurs from pulmonary edema. Oxygen toxicity of the CNS does not occur until the partial pressure of inspired oxygen (PIO_2) is greater than 2 atm, which usually occurs in a hyperbaric chamber.

The retina of a premature neonate can be damaged by exposure to high levels of oxygen for prolonged periods. The development of retrolental fibroplasia is thought to be related to high levels of partial pressure of oxygen in arterial blood (PaO_2) administered to the neonate. Adults rarely have oxygen-induced retinopathy, even with hyperbaric levels.

Drug Interactions

There are no drug interactions with oxygen.

Clinical Use and Dosing

Oxygen is administered to treat hypoxia as determined by pulse oximetry or arterial or mixed venous blood gases. Hypoxia is usually a symptom or manifestation of an underlying disease, and therefore, oxygen therapy is not curative, but it does provide symptomatic and temporary improvement in the patient's status. The underlying cause of hypoxia needs to be treated.

Correction of Hypoxia

To correct hypoxia, oxygen is administered to the patient via a variety of oxygen-delivery systems. The provider chooses a delivery system based on the fraction or percentage of oxygen (FIO_2) that is desired for treatment. The goal of treatment is to maintain oxygen saturation above 90%.

An NC will deliver an FIO_2 of 0.24 to 0.35 if the flow of oxygen is at 5 to 6 L/min. Higher flow rates via NC dry out the nasal mucosa and will not achieve higher FIO_2 because the oxygen is mixed with ambient air. Humidified oxygen can be delivered to decrease nasal passage dryness. The percentage of oxygen that can be delivered via NC is 22% to 44%.

Masks cover the mouth and nose and allow for a higher concentration of oxygen to be delivered. Oxygen delivery via mask requires a flow rate above 5 L/min to avoid accumulation of exhaled air in the mask. A flow rate of 8 to 10 L/min is recommended. A simple face mask, which allows room air to dilute the oxygen, delivers 40% to 60% oxygen to the patient. A face mask with an oxygen reservoir provides a constant flow of oxygen at above 60% concentration. If the flow rate of oxygen is 6 L/min, then the oxygen concentration is 60%. The oxygen concentration increases by 10% for every liter per minute increase in flow. When 10 L/min of oxygen is delivered via a mask with an oxygen reservoir, the percentage of oxygen delivered reaches 100%. A Venturi mask allows for controlled percentages of oxygen to be delivered to patients. The mask can be adjusted to deliver 24%, 28%, 35%, and 40%. This type of mask is used on patients with chronic hypercapnia (e.g., COPD patients) to tightly control the amount of oxygen delivered and avoid respiratory depression associated with high oxygen concentrations in these patients.

Oxygen may also be delivered by hood or tent to provide a known concentration to the patient, with little cooperation required from the patient. Flow rates must be high enough to prevent accumulation of carbon dioxide.

Monitoring

Monitoring the patient on oxygen is necessary to treat hypoxia and to avoid toxicity. The most accurate yet invasive method to monitor blood oxygenation is by arterial or mixed venous blood gas sampling. This procedure can be painful for the patient and requires rapid transport of the specimen to the laboratory. Blood gases have the advantage of providing additional information, besides oxygenation, regarding the patient's status that may assist in the treatment of the underlying cause of hypoxemia. Pulse oximetry is a noninvasive method of monitoring the patient receiving oxygen therapy. It measures the difference in absorption of light by oxyhemoglobin and deoxyhemoglobin in an accessible location, such as the finger, toe (in children), or ear. Pulse oximetry measures the hemoglobin saturation and not PO_2.

The need for continuing oxygen therapy should be monitored by drawing arterial blood gases after 1, 3, and 6 months of therapy.

Patient Education

Administration

The patient who is receiving home oxygen therapy requires knowledge of the appropriate use of oxygen, as well as education about safe administration. The patient should use the oxygen as prescribed by the provider. Increasing or decreasing the flow rate of oxygen may have adverse effects. Using oxygen for fewer hours than prescribed will increase hypoxia and will have detrimental effects.

The patient should understand that oxygen is a flammable gas that should be kept away from open flame. Patients who smoke should be cautioned not to smoke while their oxygen is running.

Adverse Reactions

There are minimal adverse reactions with the use of oxygen. The patient should be advised of the potential of developing dry nasal passages. Increasing hydration and increasing the humidity of the home will help somewhat.

Oxygen toxicity should be discussed and the patient advised to use the oxygen only as directed. Patients who begin to exhibit symptoms that may be related to toxicity should contact their health-care provider.

Lifestyle Management

Lifestyle management issues related to the disease process being treated should be discussed. They often include the following:

1. The patient should avoid or quit smoking.
2. COPD patients should avoid unnecessary exposure to viral respiratory infections.
3. Patients with COPD or other chronic respiratory diseases should avoid high altitudes.
4. Before traveling by air, the patient should contact the provider to formulate a plan of care.

ALLERGY MEDICATIONS
ANTIHISTAMINES

Antihistamines are used in primary care to treat a variety of allergic conditions. This chapter addresses the antihistamines used to treat allergic symptoms specific to the respiratory tract. Antihistamines are also called H_1 receptor antagonists, which describes the action the medication has at the cellular level. This text uses *antihistamine*, the more commonly used name in clinical practice.

The first antihistamines became available in the 1940s, with the still widely used diphenhydramine first available in the 1950s. They are referred to as the first-generation antihistamines. The 1980s brought a new generation of nonsedating antihistamines that provided relief to allergy sufferers without causing the drowsiness of the earlier medications. They are referred to as second-generation antihistamines. New antihistamines that are longer acting and have better adverse-effect profiles continue to be developed.

Pharmacodynamics

Antihistamines are H_1 receptor antagonists that reduce or prevent most of the physiological effects of histamine at the H_1 receptor site. Antihistamines compete with histamine for H_1 receptor sites on the effector cells. They do not prevent histamine release or bind with histamine that has already been released. They prevent, but do not reverse, responses mediated by histamine. The effects of antihistamines include inhibition of respiratory, vascular, and GI smooth muscle constriction by antagonism of the constrictor action on smooth muscle. Antihistamines strongly block the action of histamine that results in increased capillary permeability and formation of edema and wheal. They also decrease the flare and itch responses of histamine on peripheral nerve endings. Histamine-activated exocrine secretions (salivary, lacrimal) are decreased with the use of systemic antihistamines. Antihistamines with strong anticholinergic (atropine-like) properties may have an increased drying effect by decreasing secretions from cholinergically innervated glands.

The first-generation antihistamines competitively antagonize the effects of histamine at the peripheral H_1 receptor sites in the GI tract, uterus, large blood vessels, and bronchial muscle. First-generation antihistamines bind nonselectively to the central H_1 receptors and can cause both CNS stimulation and depression. CNS depression is found even with therapeutic doses of the first-generation antihistamines. Some of them are more likely than others to depress the CNS, and patients vary in their sensitivity to the different preparations. Commonly prescribed first-generation antihistamines include the ethanolamine drugs diphenhydramine (Benadryl) and clemastine (Tavist), the alkylamines brompheniramine (Dimetane) and chlorpheniramine (Chlor-Trimeton), the piperazine hydroxyzine (Atarax, Vistaril), the piperidine cyproheptadine (Periactin), and carbinoxamine maleate (Arbinoxa).

Second-generation antihistamines are selective for peripheral H_1 receptors and therefore as a group are less sedating. They do not cross the blood–brain barrier in appreciable amounts; consequently, very little of the second-generation antihistamines gets into the brain. Their effects on performance and on objective measures of sedation vary little from those of a placebo. Second-generation antihistamines that are commonly prescribed include the piperazine drug cetirizine (Zyrtec) and the piperidines desloratadine (Clarinex), fexofenadine (Allegra), and loratadine (Claritin).

Antihistamines have other pharmacodynamic properties related to their central action rather than their histamine-receptor blockade action. Several first-generation antihistamines have significant antiemetic and antinausea properties owing to strong anticholinergic properties caused by the antihistamine's binding to the muscarinic receptors. Diphenhydramine can be used to reverse the extrapyramidal adverse effects caused by phenothiazines. Probably because of their anticholinergic actions, some of the antihistamines (diphenhydramine) have effects on Parkinson's symptoms and may be effective in the early stages of treatment.

Pharmacokinetics

Absorption and Distribution

The first-generation antihistamines are stable, lipid-soluble amines that are well absorbed from the GI tract. Diphenhydramine is widely distributed throughout the body tissues and fluids, including the CNS. It crosses the placenta and is found in breast milk. The distribution of clemastine is unknown, but the drug does cross the placenta and is distributed in breast milk. Chlorpheniramine is approximately 72% protein bound and is widely distributed in body tissue and fluids. Chlorpheniramine crosses the placenta and is found in breast milk. Distribution of hydroxyzine has not been fully described, and it is unknown whether it crosses the placenta or is distributed in breast milk. The distribution of cyproheptadine, dimenhydrinate, and brompheniramine is unknown.

The second-generation antihistamines are rapidly absorbed from the GI tract, although concurrent food ingestion can decrease or delay absorption. Fexofenadine is rapidly absorbed, and absorption is not affected by food intake. Administration

of loratadine with food decreases absorption up to 40% for the syrup or tablet and 48% for the rapid-disintegrating tablet. Desloratadine is well absorbed, and food intake dose not affect absorption. Absorption of cetirizine is slightly reduced by food intake. Cetirizine is widely distributed, except in the CNS, where concentrations are less than 10% of the peak serum concentration. It is unknown whether cetirizine crosses the placenta, but it has been measured in breast milk. Fexofenadine distribution is unknown. Loratadine is 97% protein bound and is excreted in breast milk. It is not known if loratadine crosses the placenta. Desloratadine is highly (82% to 87%) protein bound, it is not known whether it crosses the placenta, and only minimal amounts are excreted in breast milk.

Metabolism and Excretion

The first-generation antihistamines are metabolized primarily in the liver. Diphenhydramine is metabolized in the liver, with the unchanged portion of the dose and metabolites excreted in the urine in 24 to 48 hours. Clemastine is extensively metabolized by an unknown mechanism. Clemastine and its metabolites are excreted primarily in the urine. Metabolism of chlorpheniramine is extensive, occurring first in the gastric mucosa and then on the first pass through the liver. Metabolites of chlorpheniramine are excreted in the urine, with the excretion rate dependent on the pH of the urine and urinary flow. Cyproheptadine is metabolized in the liver into several conjugated metabolites, with excretion in the urine and feces. Hydroxyzine is completely metabolized by the liver. Metabolism and excretion of brompheniramine and dimenhydrinate are unknown.

Most of the second-generation antihistamines are metabolized by the liver to active metabolites by the hepatic microsomal P450 system. Consequently, metabolism of these drugs can be affected by competition for the P450 enzymes by other drugs. Cetirizine is minimally metabolized by the P450 enzymes and is primarily excreted unchanged in the urine. Approximately 5% of the dose of fexofenadine is metabolized, with 80% excreted in the feces and 11% excreted in the urine. Loratadine has a high first-pass effect and is metabolized in the liver to the active metabolite descarboethoxyloratadine. Patients with chronic liver disease have higher peak plasma concentrations (double the normal levels) of loratadine than do healthy patients. Elimination of loratadine is through the urine and feces.

See Table 17-10 for the pharmacokinetics.

Pharmacotherapeutics

Precautions and Contraindications

The precautions and contraindications differ between the first-generation and second-generation antihistamines.

First-Generation Antihistamines

Although first-generation antihistamines are available without prescription and all antihistamines are widely prescribed, the provider must be aware of the precautions and absolute contraindications to the antihistamines.

Table 17–10 ⋮⋮ **Pharmacokinetics: Selected Antihistamines**

Drug	Onset	Peak	Duration	Protein Binding	Half-Life	Metabolism	Elimination
First-Generation Antihistamines							
Brompheniramine	15–30 min	2–5 h	4–6 h	—	25 h	Hepatic	Renal
Clemastine	15–30 min	2–5 h	10–12 h (up to 24 h)	—	—	Probably hepatic	Renal
Chlorpheniramine	30–60 min	2–6 h	4–8 h	72%	*Adults:* 20–24 h *Children:* 10–13 h	Gastric mucosa and hepatic	Renal
Cyproheptadine	—	6–9 h	8 h	—	1–4 h	Hepatic	Primary renal; some in feces
Diphenhydramine	15–30 min	2–4 h	4–6 h	98%–99%	1–4 h	Hepatic	Renal
Hydroxyzine	15–60 min	—	4–6 h	—	3–20 h	Hepatic	Renal
Second-Generation Antihistamines							
Cetirizine	Rapid	1 h	—	93%	8.3 h	Minimal 60% excreted unchanged	Renal, feces (10%)
Desloratadine	1 h	3 h	24 h	82%–87%	27 h	Hepatic	Renal, fecal
Fexofenadine	1 h	2.6 h	12 h	60%–70%	14.4 h	95% excreted unchanged	Fecal (80%); renal (11%)
Loratadine	1–3 h	8–12 h	>24 h	97%	8.4 h	Hepatic CYP3A4 and CYP2D6	Fecal, renal

The first-generation antihistamines are generally safe and effective. Antihistamines are contraindicated in patients with narrow-angle glaucoma, lower respiratory tract symptoms (they thicken secretions and impair expectoration), stenosing peptic ulcer, symptomatic prostatic hypertrophy, bladder neck obstruction, pyloroduodenal obstruction, and MAOI use.

There are few but significant precautions to the first-generation antihistamines. Because of the anticholinergic effects, caution is required for patients with a predisposition to urinary retention, history of bronchial asthma, increased intraocular pressure, hyperthyroidism, cardiovascular disease, or hypertension. Antihistamines cause varying degrees of sedation and drowsiness and reduce mental alertness; therefore, patients should not drive or perform other tasks requiring mental alertness while taking the first-generation antihistamines. Children should be supervised when they are taking these medications and performing potentially unsafe activities such as swimming or bicycling.

The first-generation antihistamines—chlorpheniramine, brompheniramine, diphenhydramine, clemastine, and cyproheptadine—are Pregnancy Category B. Hydroxyzine and carbinoxamine are the only first-generation antihistamines classified as Pregnancy Category C.

First-generation antihistamines are contraindicated in newborns and premature infants, who may have severe reactions (convulsions). Breastfeeding is also a contraindication for the use of first-generation antihistamines because all of the medications are excreted in breast milk and they may decrease milk production.

Caution should be exercised with the use of first-generation antihistamines in young children because a paradoxical CNS stimulation can occur. Do not exceed recommended dosages for each age group of children. Chlorpheniramine, brompheniramine, cyproheptadine, dimenhydrinate, and diphenhydramine are all labeled to be used in children over the age of 2 years. Hydroxyzine syrup may be prescribed for infants and children for pruritus, although cetirizine may be a safer choice. Carbinoxamine is not recommended for children younger than 2 years of age.

The first-generation antihistamines—carbinoxamine, chlorpheniramine, diphenhydramine, clemastine, and cyproheptadine—are all on the Beers criteria list of medications that should be avoided in geriatric patients.

Second-Generation Antihistamines

The second-generation antihistamines have only a few contraindications. Two second-generation antihistamines, astemizole (Hismanal) and terfenadine (Seldane), have been voluntarily removed from the market because of potentially life-threatening drug interactions and increased prolonged QT interval associated with their use.

The second-generation antihistamines are generally not recommended during pregnancy, especially during the third trimester, because of a seizure risk to the fetus. Loratadine and cetirizine are classified Pregnancy Category B. The other second-generation antihistamines—loratadine, desloratadine, and fexofenadine—are Pregnancy Category C, and their use should be avoided.

Fexofenadine are not recommended for children under age 6. Loratadine may be prescribed to children as young as age 2. Cetirizine syrup and desloratadine syrup may be used in children as young as 6 months.

Adverse Drug Reactions

As described previously, the major adverse reaction to first-generation antihistamines is sedation, which can interfere with a patient's ability to function at work or school. Other central adverse effects include dizziness, tinnitus, lassitude, disturbed coordination, fatigue, headache, irritability, nervousness, blurred vision, diplopia, and tremors. The next most common adverse effects are GI and include increased or decreased appetite, nausea, epigastric distress, vomiting, constipation, and diarrhea. Dry mouth, urinary retention, and dysuria are also adverse effects reported in patients taking first-generation antihistamines. The concurrent ingestion of alcohol or other CNS depressants produces an additive effect that further impairs function.

The second-generation antihistamines have few central adverse effects. The major improvement in the second-generation antihistamines is that the incidence of drowsiness is greatly reduced. They are well tolerated by the GI system and have a minimal incidence of dry mouth (less than or equal to 5%). Overall, when patients have adverse reactions to the first-generation antihistamines, a change to a second-generation drug often alleviates the problem.

Drug Interactions

The first-generation antihistamines should be used with caution concurrently with any medication that has CNS depressant effects. All of the first-generation antihistamines exhibit additive CNS sedation effects if coadministered with ethanol, anxiolytics, sedatives, hypnotics, and barbiturates. The anticholinergic effects of antihistamines may be enhanced if coadministered with tricyclic antidepressants and phenothiazines.It is recommended that H_1 agonists not be used within 2 weeks of MAOIs because of increased anticholinergic effects. Cyproheptadine may reverse the antidepressant effects of selective serotonin reuptake inhibitors (SSRIs). Two antihistamines should not be prescribed at the same time to avoid additive anticholinergic and sedative effects.

The second-generation antihistamines, although not sedating when used singly, may have additive CNS sedation effects if used with other CNS depressants (barbiturates, anxiolytics, sedatives, hypnotics, ethanol, and benzodiazepines). Concurrent use with another H_1 blocker may cause sedation.

Desloratadine and loratadine are extensively metabolized by the CYP450 enzymes, and coadministration of other medications that are also metabolized by these enzymes should be avoided, such as are erythromycin, cimetidine, and ketoconazole.

Table 17-11 presents drug interactions.

Table 17–11 ⚏ Drug Interactions: Selected Antihistamines

Drug	Interacting	Drug Possible Effect	Implications
First-Generation Antihistamines			
Brompheniramine	MAOIs	MAOIs can prolong and intensify the effects of antihistamines	Avoid concurrent use
	Ethanol and other CNS depressants	Additive CNS depression	Use with caution
Clemastine	MAOIs	Additive anticholinergic effects	Concurrent use contraindicated
	Antimuscarinics: Tricyclic antidepressants, phenothiazines, ethanolamine-derivative H_1 blockers (clemastine, carbinoxamine, promethazine, trimeprazine) clozapine, cyclobenzaprine, disopyramide	Additive anticholinergic effects	Avoid concurrent use
	CNS depressants: Ethanol, antipsychotics, sedatives, hypnotics, opiate agonists, barbiturates	Enhanced CNS-depressant effect	Avoid concurrent use
Chlorpheniramine	MAOIs	Additive anticholinergic effects	Avoid concurrent use
	Antimuscarinics: Tricyclic antidepressants, phenothiazines, benztropine	Enhanced anticholinergic effects of chlorpheniramine	Chlorpheniramine has moderate anticholinergic effects and is preferable to other H_1 blockers when an H_1 blocker must be used

Continued

Table 17–11 ⠿ Drug Interactions: Selected Antihistamines—cont'd

Drug	Interacting	Drug Possible Effect	Implications
	CNS depressants	Enhanced CNS-depressant effect	Avoid concurrent use
Cyproheptadine	*Antimuscarinics:* Tricyclic antidepressants, phenothiazines, ethanolamine-derivative H₁ blockers (clemastine, diphenhydramine), benztropine	Increased anticholinergic effects of cyproheptadine	Avoid concurrent use
	CNS depressants: Barbiturates, ethanol, benzodiazepines, tricyclic antidepressants, opiate agonists	Enhanced CNS-depressant effect	Avoid concurrent use
	SSRIs	Reversal of antidepressant effects of SSRIs	Use cyproheptadine only if needed
Diphenhydramine	MAOIs	Additive anticholinergic effects	Do not use within 2 wk of each other
	Antimuscarinics: Tricyclic antidepressants, phenothiazines, ethanolamine-derivative H₁ blockers (clemastine, carbinoxamine, promethazine, trimeprazine) clozapine, cyclobenzaprine, disopyramide	Additive anticholinergic effects	Avoid or use with caution; monitor closely if coadministration is necessary
	CNS depressants: Ethanol, antipsychotics, sedatives, hypnotics, opiate agonists, barbiturates	Enhanced CNS-depressant effect	Avoid concurrent use
Hydroxyzine	MAOIs	May prolong and intensify the anticholinergic effects of antihistamines	Concurrent use contraindicated; avoid use within 2 wk of each other
	Antimuscarinics: Tricyclic antidepressants, phenothiazines, ethanolamine-derivative H₁ blockers (clemastine, carbinoxamine, promethazine, trimeprazine) atropine, benztropine	Additive anticholinergic effects	Avoid concurrent use
	CNS depressants: Ethanol, antipsychotics, sedatives, hypnotics, opiate agonists, barbiturates	Additive CNS-depressant effects	Avoid concurrent use
Second-Generation Antihistamines			
Cetirizine	Theophylline	May ↓ cetirizine clearance	Avoid concurrent use
	CNS depressants: Barbiturates, ethanol, benzodiazepines, tricyclic antidepressants, opiate agonists	Additive CNS-depressant effects and drowsiness	Use with caution
Desloratadine	Ketoconazole, erythromycin, CNS depressants	Increases plasma concentrations of desloratadine Additive CNS depression	Does not cause cardiac toxicity, but coadminister with caution Avoid or minimize concurrent use
Loratadine	Macrolide antibiotics (clarithromycin, erythromycin, troleandomycin)	Interferes with the metabolism of loratadine, resulting in increased serum concentrations of loratadine	Does not cause cardiac toxicity, but coadminister with caution
	CNS depressants: Barbiturates, ethanol, benzodiazepines, tricyclic antidepressants, opiate agonists	Additive CNS-depressant effects and drowsiness	Avoid or minimize concurrent use

Table 17–11 ▦ **Drug Interactions: Selected Antihistamines—cont'd**

Drug	Interacting	Drug Possible Effect	Implications
Fexofenadine	Ketoconazole	↑ fexofenadine plasma levels	Avoid concurrent use
	Erythromycin	↑ fexofenadine levels	Avoid concurrent use
	Aluminum- and magnesium-containing antacids	↓ fexofenadine absorption	Administer fexofenadine 1 h before antacids
	Alcohol	CNS depression	Avoid concurrent use

Clinical Use and Dosing

Respiratory Allergies

Most of the antihistamines are effective in the treatment of seasonal allergic rhinitis and conjunctivitis. Antihistamines effectively treat the sneezing, rhinorrhea, watery eyes, and itching of eyes, nose, and throat associated with seasonal allergies or hay fever. The treatment decision is often made according to the adverse-effect profile and cost. Although the first-generation drugs diphenhydramine, chlorpheniramine, brompheniramine, and clemastine are effective, inexpensive, and available without prescription, their adverse effect of drowsiness often prevents patients from being able to continue their daily activities. The usual adult dose of diphenhydramine for respiratory allergies is 25 to 50 mg every 4 to 6 hours. The adult dose of chlorpheniramine is 4 mg every 4 to 6 hours or 8 to 12 mg of the extended-release form every 8 to 12 hours. Brompheniramine is dosed at 4 mg every 4 to 6 hours in adults with respiratory allergies. Carbinoxamine dosing for adults is 4 mg to 8 mg 3 to 4 times a day. Pediatric doses for these medications are given in Table 17-12.

If a patient cannot tolerate the first-generation antihistamines, a second-generation medication can be prescribed to treat respiratory allergies. The dose of cetirizine that should be prescribed for children over 12 years and adults is 5 to 10 mg/day given once a day. In children aged 6 to 11 years, the dose of cetirizine is 5 to 10 mg once daily. For cetirizine syrup prescribed to children aged 2 to 5 years, the dose is 2.5 mg (half tsp of 5 mg/5mL syrup) once daily. The dose of cetirizine may be increased to 5 mg/day, delivered as 5 mg once daily or 2.5 mg twice a day. Children aged 6 to 12 months are dosed at 2.5 mg once a day. Children aged 12 to 23 months are also prescribed 2.5 mg once a day, with an increase to 2.5 mg twice a day if needed. The dose of fexofenadine in healthy children aged 12 years or older and adults is 60 mg twice a day. Children aged 6 to 11 years should be prescribed 30 mg twice a day of fexofenadine. If a patient has renal impairment (creatinine clearance [CCr] less than 80 mL/min), the dose of fexofenadine is 60 mg once daily. The dose of loratadine in healthy children over age 6 years and adults is 10 mg once a day, with children aged 2 to 5 prescribed 5 mg once a day. If an adult has renal or liver disease, the dose of

Table 17–12 ⚗ **Dosage Schedule: Selected Antihistamines**

Drug	Indication	Dosage Form	Dose	Comments
First-Generation Antihistamines				
Brompheniramine Dimetapp Allergy Bromfed Children's Dimetapp Cold & Allergy	Allergic and vasomotor rhinitis, pruritus, conjunctivitis	Capsules: 4 mg Scored tablets: 4 mg Brompheniramine 4 mg Pseudoephedrine 60 mg Per 5 mL: Brompheniramine 1 mg; phenylephrine 2.5 mg	*Adults:* 4 mg PO q 4–6 h *or* 8–12 mg of sustained-release form 2 to 3 times/d; Maximum dose: 12 mg/24 h *Children 6–12 yr:* 2 mg q 4–6 h; max 12 mg/24 h *Children <6 yr:* 0.125 mg/ kg/d in divided doses every 6–8 h	May be administered with or without food Cough and cold medications are not recommended for use in children younger than 4 years of age
Clemastine Tavist Generic	Allergic rhinitis	Scored tablets: 1.34 mg (1 mg clemastine) Scored tablets: 2.68 mg (2 mg clemastine) Syrup: 0.67 mg (0.5 mg clemastine)/5 mL	*Children >12 yr and adults:* 1 mg bid *Children 6–12 yr:* 0.5 mg bid	May be administered without regard to meals
	Pruritus, mild urticaria, angioedema		*Children >12 and adults:* 2 mg bid *Children 6–12 yr:* 1 mg bid	May be administered without regard to meals
Chlorpheniramine Chlor-Trimeton Allergy 4 hour	Allergic rhinitis, conjunctivitis, pruritus, urticaria	4 mg tablets 8 mg sustained-release tablet	*Children >12 yr and adults:* 4 mg every 4–6 h; max 24 mg/d	Administer with food or milk to minimize gastric irritation

Continued

Table 17–12 ⊗ Dosage Schedule: Selected Antihistamines—cont'd

Drug	Indication	Dosage Form	Dose	Comments
Chlor-Trimeton Allergy 8 hour Chlor-Trimeton Allergy 12 hour Chlor-Trimeton syrup Generic		12 mg sustained-release tablet Syrup: 2 mg/5 mL	*Children 6–12 yr:* 2 mg every 4–6 hr; max 12 mg/d *Children 2–5 yr:* 1 mg every 4–6 h; max 4 mg/d *Extended-release form:* *Children >12 yr and adults:* 8–12 mg bid or tid; max 24 mg/d *Children 6–12 yr:* 8 mg once daily; max 12 mg/d *Children 2–5 yr:* use other forms	Do not crush or chew extended-release tablets
Cyproheptadine Periactin Periactin syrup Generic	Allergic rhinitis, conjunctivitis, pruritus, urticaria	Tablets: 4 mg Syrup: 2 mg/5 mL	*Children >14 yr and adults:* 4 mg q 8–12 h; usual range 12–16 mg/d; max dose 0.5 mg/kg/d *Children 7–14 yr:* 4 mg q 8–12 h; max 16 mg/d *Children 2–6 yr:* 2 mg q 8–12 h; max 12 mg/d	Administered without regard to meals
Diphenhydramine Benadryl Allergy Benadryl Dye-Free Allergy Softgels Benadryl Allergy liquid Benadryl Allergy Dye-Free liquid Benadryl Allergy Chewables Generic	Upper respiratory allergies	25 mg capsules 25 mg tablets 12.5 mg/5 mL 6.25 mg/5 mL 12.5 mg chewable tablet	*Children >12 yr and adults:* 25–50 mg every 4–6 h; max 300 mg/d *Children 6–12 yr:* 12.5–25 mg q 4–6 h; max 150 mg/24 h *Children 2–6 yr:* 6.25 mg; max 37.5 mg/24 h	May cause drowsiness; may cause excitability in young children
Hydroxyzine Atarax Vistaril	Allergic and vasomotor rhinitis, pruritus Nausea/ vomiting	Tablets: 10, 25, 50, 100 mg Syrup: 10 mg/5 mL Tablets: 25, 50, 100 mg Suspension: 25 mg/5 mL	*Adults:* 25 mg 3–4 times/d *Children >6 yr:* 12.5–25 mg 3–4 times/d; max 50–100 mg/24 h *Children <6 yr:* 1–2 mg/kg every 6–8 h *Adults:* 25–100 mg 3–4 times/d *Children 6–12 yr:* 12.5 mg every 6 h or 1–2 mg /kg/d/ in divided doses *Children <6 yr:* 12.5 mg every 6 h or 1–2 mg/kg/d in divided doses	May cause drowsiness
	Insomnia		*Adults:* 50–100 mg PO 30–60 min before bedtime	May cause drowsiness
Second-Generation Antihistamines				
Cetirizine Zyrtec Generic	Seasonal or perennial rhinitis, chronic urticaria, pruritus	5 mg tablet 10 mg tablet Syrup: 1 mg/mL	*Children >12 yr and adults:* 5–10 mg once a day *Children >6–11 yr:* 5–10 mg once a day *Children 2–5 yr:* 2.5 mg initially; can increase dose to 5 mg/d (either as one 5 mg dose or 2.5 mg q 12 h) *Children 6–12 mo:* 2.5 mg once daily *Children 12–23 mo:* 2.5 mg once daily; may be increased to 2.5 mg twice daily	May be administered without regard to food, but food may delay absorption by up to 1 h; patients with renal impairment (CCr <31 mL/min) decrease dose to 5 mg once daily

Table 17–12 ⊗ **Dosage Schedule: Selected Antihistamines—cont'd**

Drug	Indication	Dosage Form	Dose	Comments
Desloratadine Clarinex	Allergic rhinitis, chronic urticaria	5 mg tablet 2.5 mg, 5 mg disintegrating tablet Syrup: 0.5 mg/mL	*Children >12 yr and adults:* 5 mg once a day *Children 6–11 yr:* 2.5 mg once a day *Children 1–5 yr:* 1.25 mg once a day Children 6–12 mo: 1 mg once a day	
Fexofenadine Allegra Generic	Allergic rhinitis	Tablets: 180, 60, 30 mg 30 mg/mL suspension	*Children >12 yr and adults:* 60 mg PO bid *Children 6–11 yr:* 30 mg PO bid	Dose without regard to meals; not recommended in children <12; patients with renal impairment (CCr <80 mL/min) reduce starting dose to 60 mg once daily
Loratadine Claritin Generic Allegra	Allergic rhinitis, chronic urticaria	Tablets: 10 mg Syrup: 1 mg/mL Rapidly disintegrating tablets: 10 mg (Claritin Reditabs) Rapidly disintegrating tablets: 10 mg	*Children >6 yr and adults:* 10 mg once daily *Children 2–5 yr:* 5 mg once daily	Dose without regard to meals; patients with renal impairment (CCr <30 mL/min) reduce starting dosage to 10 mg every other day

loratadine is 10 mg every other day. Desloratadine is dosed at 5 mg once daily in children 12 and older and adults. In patients with renal or hepatic impairment, desloratadine is given every other day. Pediatric dosing for the second-generation antihistamines is found in Table 17-12.

Hypersensitivity Reactions

The first-generation antihistamine diphenhydramine is usually the drug of choice for patients with acute hypersensitivity reactions. It is available in oral tablet, capsule, and liquid forms without prescription and in parenteral form for acute IM or IV use. The adult oral dose of diphenhydramine is 25 to 50 mg every 4 to 6 hours for hypersensitivity reactions. In children 6 to 12 years with hypersensitivity reactions, the dose of diphenhydramine is 12.5 to 25 mg every 4 hours. Children aged 2 to 6 are prescribed diphenhydramine syrup, at a dose of 6.25 mg every 4 hours. In an acute hypersensitivity reaction, IM administration of diphenhydramine may be necessary. The adult dose of diphenhydramine is 10 to 50 mg deep IM or IV, with a maximum of 400 mg/day. In children, the dose is 1.25 mg/kg per dose IV or given deep IM every 4 hours, or 5 mg/kg/day divided every 6 to 8 hours, with a maximum daily diphenhydramine dose of 300 mg. Cyproheptadine is also indicated for use in hypersensitivity reactions. The adult dose of cyproheptadine is 4 mg 3 times a day. No second-generation antihistamines are indicated for use in hypersensitivity reactions.

Urticaria and Angioedema

In urticaria, histamine is the primary mediator and therefore the antihistamines are the drugs of choice and quite effective. Clemastine, a very effective treatment for urticaria, is available in both tablet and liquid form for use with children (older than 6 years) and adults. Hydroxyzine is effective in the management of pruritus due to allergic conditions such as chronic urticaria and in histamine-mediated pruritus. It is also available

in tablet and liquid form. Hydroxyzine may be used safely in children younger than age 6 and therefore may be a better choice than clemastine in younger children with urticaria. Cetirizine, desloratadine, and loratadine may be prescribed for urticaria. See Table 17-12 for dosing information.

Nighttime Sleep Aid

Diphenhydramine is available without prescription as a sleep aid and is a safe treatment for occasional insomnia. The recommended dose for adults is 50 mg at bedtime. Table 17-12 presents dosing information.

Motion Sickness/Antiemetic

Dimenhydrinate (Dramamine) is used in the treatment and prevention of nausea, vertigo, and vomiting associated with motion sickness. Dosing for children aged 2 to 5 years is 12.4 to 25 mg every 6 to 8 hours, to a maximum of 75 mg/day. Children aged 6 to 12 are given 25 to 50 mg of dimenhydrinate every 6 to 8 hours, with a maximum of 150 mg/day. An alternative dose is 5 mg/kg per day divided into four doses. Children 12 years and older and adults are given 50 to 100 mg every 4 to 6 hours, not to exceed 400 mg/day. The onset of action of dimenhydrinate is 15 to 30 minutes, so predosing for motion sickness would require that the medication be taken with food or water at least 15 minutes before needed.

Rational Drug Selection

First- Versus Second-Generation Antihistamines

Although many of the first-generation antihistamines are readily available without prescription, the common adverse effect of sedation prevents their use during the day by patients who need to be alert for work or school. The second-generation antihistamines are well tolerated and do not impair daytime functioning. They are also longer acting, allowing for convenient once- or twice-a-day dosing.

Cost

The second-generation antihistamines used to be more expensive than the first-generation antihistamines, but with many second-generation drugs now available in generic form, cost has less impact on decision making. Most insurance companies will not pay for the cost of the more expensive, brand-name, second-generation antihistamines. For the patient, the cost is offset by the ability to perform daily functions more easily when taking the second-generation medications.

Monitoring

No specific laboratory monitoring is necessary with antihistamines.

Patient Education

Patient education focuses on proper use of the medication, adverse reactions, and safety precautions while using the medications.

Administration

Patients should be instructed regarding the proper dosing of the drug. Especially if patients are switching from a shorter-acting first-generation to a longer-acting second-generation antihistamine, they need to be aware of the dosing schedule. Doses should not be doubled or increased unless prescribed by the health-care provider. The long-acting second-generation antihistamines should not be taken closer together than prescribed, so missed doses need to be held until the time of the next dose (every 12 or 24 hours).

Some antihistamines cause GI upset and need to be taken with food. Loratadine should be taken on an empty stomach because absorption may be decreased by as much as 60%.

Patients should be instructed not to crush or chew sustained-release tablets.

Adverse Reactions

Some antihistamines (first generation) may cause drowsiness, and patients should observe caution while driving or performing other tasks requiring alertness. Patients should avoid alcohol and other CNS depressants while taking antihistamines and should be instructed to report excessive drowsiness to their health-care provider to determine whether another medication would provide therapeutic effects without sedation.

Patients taking loratadine should be aware of the serious interaction between the antihistamines and macrolide antibiotics and the oral azol antifungals. Written instructions regarding the specific medications to avoid are the most effective and safest method of ensuring that patients do not accidentally get placed on any new medication that would cause a serious adverse reaction. The additive CNS depression that occurs with the antihistamine and other CNS depressants (e.g., alcohol) should be addressed and the patient cautioned regarding driving or operating heavy machinery.

Lifestyle Management

Lifestyle management related to the disease process needs to be discussed with the patient. Points to discuss often include avoidance of known allergens and using environmental methods to control dust mites and other common allergens. Available dosage forms are presented in Table 17-12.

COUGH AND COLD MEDICATIONS
DECONGESTANTS

Decongestants are widely used for congestion associated with the common cold and allergic rhinitis. Many preparations are available without a prescription, and they are available in many formulations. They come in liquid, tablet, capsule, nasal spray, or drops, providing a variety of methods of administration. Although patients may self-treat with decongestants and the health-care provider may rarely prescribe them, they are included here for the provider to learn about the proper dosing and potential adverse effects or drug interactions that may occur with these medications.

Pharmacodynamics

The decongestants are alpha-adrenergic–receptor agonists (sympathomimetic) that produce vasoconstriction by stimulating alpha receptors within the mucosa of the respiratory tract, which temporarily reduces the swelling associated with inflammation of the mucous membranes. These sympathomimetic amines act on the alpha receptors of the vascular smooth muscle, causing vasoconstriction, pressor effects, and nasal decongestion. Other alpha effects include constriction of the GI and urinary sphincters, mydriasis, and decreased pancreatic beta cell secretion. Pseudoephedrine (Sudafed), the most commonly used systemic decongestant, is noted to have mild CNS stimulant effects, especially in patients sensitive to sympathomimetic drugs. Phenylpropanolamine, which was often combined with an antihistamine in OTC cold medications, was removed from the market in 2005 after a public health advisory found an increased risk for hemorrhagic stroke in women. Other effects of the systemic decongestants are increased heart rate, force of contraction, and cardiac output. These effects are usually mild in healthy patients, and at appropriate dosages, decongestion occurs without dramatic blood pressure changes.

Pseudoephedrine is being replaced in some decongestant products with phenylephrine hydrochloride to deter the manufacture of methamphetamine, which uses pseudoephedrine as an ingredient. In 2006, the Combat Methamphetamine Epidemic Act was added to the USA Patriot Act. The Combat act applies to all cough and cold products (including combination products) that contain the methamphetamine precursor chemicals ephedrine, pseudoephedrine, or phenylpropanolamine. The law includes a daily and 30-day limit on purchases of known methamphetamine precursors whether at a retail store or via the Internet. All potential precursors are to be stored behind the counter in retail stores and retailers are required to ask for identification and keep a log of who is purchasing the drugs. Some states (Oregon) have made pseudoephedrine a Schedule III drug, requiring a prescription to be written by a provider who is licensed to prescribe controlled substances.

Topical decongestants are sympathomimetic amines that cause intense vasoconstriction when applied directly to swollen mucous membranes of the nasal passage. This shrinks the swollen membranes, causing almost immediate relief from nasal congestion. There are minimal systemic effects from topical use of nasal decongestants.

Pharmacokinetics

Absorption and Distribution

The oral decongestants are well absorbed from the GI tract and widely distributed. Pseudoephedrine is widely distributed and presumed to cross the blood–brain barrier and placenta. Small amounts of pseudoephedrine are excreted in breast milk. Absorption and distribution of the topical decongestants have not been described.

Metabolism and Excretion

Pseudoephedrine is partially metabolized in the liver into norpseudoephedrine, an active metabolite. Pseudoephedrine and its metabolite are excreted in the urine, with 50% to 75% of the dose excreted as unchanged drug. Excretion of pseudoephedrine is highly dependent on the pH of the urine. If the urine is acidic (pH near 5), the rate of urinary excretion is increased. If the urine is alkaline (pH of 8), the rate of excretion is slowed, as some of the drug is reabsorbed into the renal tubule.

Metabolism of phenylephrine is via the enzyme monoamine oxidase in the liver. Excretion of phenylephrine or its metabolites has not been described. Metabolism and excretion of the topical decongestants are not available.

Table 17-13 presents the pharmacokinetics of selected decongestant.

Pharmacotherapeutics

Precautions and Contraindications

There are only a few absolute contraindications to taking decongestants. The oral decongestants are absolutely contraindicated for patients on concurrent MAOI therapy. Concurrent use of these medications may result in severe headache, hypertension and hyperpyrexia, and possibly hypertensive crisis. Oral decongestants are also contraindicated for patients with severe hypertension or coronary artery disease.

Safety and efficacy of decongestant medications have been questioned after a number of reports of deaths of infants taking cold medications (Centers for Disease Control and Prevention, 2007). In October 2007, an FDA panel met and recommended all pediatric cough and cold medications be relabeled as not indicated for use in children under age 4 years. In October 2007, manufacturers voluntarily removed all infant drop formulas of cough and cold medications from the market. After decongestants were relabeled in 2007, the American Association of Poison Control Centers reported 54% fewer reports of therapeutic errors involving OTC cough and cold medications in children younger than 2 years of age (Klein-Schwartz, Sorkin, & Doyon, 2010).

Topical imidazolines (oxymetazoline) are to be used with caution in children under age 6 years. Topical naphazoline is contraindicated for patients with glaucoma.

Adverse Drug Reactions

Adverse effects are minimal at recommended doses, unless a patient is sensitive to sympathomimetics. CNS effects may include anxiety, tenseness, restlessness, headache, lightheadedness, dizziness, drowsiness, tremor, insomnia, hallucinations, psychological disturbances, CNS depression, and weakness. Of these CNS effects, the most common adverse effects are restlessness and tremors. Cardiovascular adverse effects include transient hypertension, arrhythmia, and cardiovascular collapse, with hypotension, palpitations, tachycardia, and bradycardia. These adverse reactions are rare at recommended doses in healthy individuals. Other adverse effects are nausea, vomiting, pallor, and, rarely, shortness of breath or respiratory difficulty (at higher doses).

Topical decongestants have adverse reactions related to the intense vasoconstrictor effect of the nasal spray or sensitivity to additives such as sulfites. Transient stinging is the most common adverse effect reported. Burning, sneezing, dryness, and local irritation are all reported with topical

Table 17–13 ⸬ Pharmacokinetics: Selected Decongestants

Drug	Onset	Peak	Duration	Protein Binding	Half-Life	Metabolism	Elimination
Systemic							
Pseudoephedrine	30 min	—	4–8 h 12 h (extended release)	—	9–16 h	Hepatic	Renal 55%–75% as unchanged drug; affected by urine pH
Phenylephrine	15–20 min	—	2–4 h	—	2.5 h	—	—
Topical							
Phenylephrine	—	—	0.5–4 h	—		Hepatic, intestinal	Unknown
Oxymetazoline	—	—	—	—	—	—	—
Tetrahydrozoline		3 h		—	—	—	—

drugs. The most significant adverse reaction with topical decongestants is rebound congestion (rhinitis medicamentosa) with prolonged or chronic use. This does not occur with short-term (3 to 5 day) use.

Drug Interactions

The MAOIs and beta-adrenergic blockers increase the effects of sympathomimetics; therefore, patients taking these medications should avoid decongestants. Phenothiazines and tricyclic antidepressants potentiate the pressor effects of pseudoephedrine. See Table 17-14 for further drug interactions.

Clinical Use and Dosing

Nasal Congestion

Oral decongestants are used for the temporary relief of nasal congestion due to the common cold, sinus infection, and allergic rhinitis. They may be used to promote nasal or sinus drainage and are also indicated in the relief of eustachian tube congestion. The adult dose of pseudoephedrine for nasal congestion is 60 mg every 4 to 6 hours. In children aged 6 to 12 years, the dose is 30 mg every 4 to 6 hours, and in children aged 2 to 6, the dose of pseudoephedrine is 15 mg every 4 to 6 hours. Pseudoephedrine is no longer recommended for use in children younger than 4 years, but if prescribing, the dose of pseudoephedrine is 4 mg/kg per day divided in four-times-a-day doses. Phenylephrine (Sudafed PE) is dosed at 10 mg every 4 hours in children over age 12 and adults (maximum 60 mg in 24 hours). Dosing of phenylephrine for children aged 6 to 12 years is 7.5 mg every 4 to 6 hours up to 30 mg per day. In children aged 2 to 6 the dose of phenylephrine is 3.75 mg every 4 to 6 hours, up to 15 mg per day. Phenylephrine is not recommended for use in children younger than 2 years. Complete dosing of the different forms of the oral decongestants is found in Table 17-15.

Table 17–14 ⣿ Drug Interactions: Selected Decongestants

Drug	Interacting Drug	Possible Effect	Implications
Systemic			
Phenylephrine	MAOIs	Hypertensive crisis	Do not use within 14 d of each other
Pseudoephedrine	Caffeine, cocaine, and other sympathomimetic drugs	Additive sympathomimetic activity	Use concurrently with caution
	MAOIs, furazolidone, procarbazine	Concurrent use can prolong and intensify the cardiac stimulation and vasopressor effects; may lead to severe cardiovascular and cerebrovascular response	Avoid use within 14 d of each other
	Ergot alkaloids	Peripheral vasoconstriction, additive vasoconstriction	Avoid concurrent use
	Methyldopa, reserpine	Decreased antihypertensive effects	Monitor BP closely if using concurrently
	Thyroid hormones	Increased effects of both agents on the cardiovascular system	Use concurrently with caution
	Urinary alkalinizers: Sodium bicarbonate, sodium citrate, potassium citrate, sodium lactate, sodium acetate	Increased alkalinization of the urine leads to tubular reabsorption of pseudoephedrine	Observe for increased adverse effects; use together with caution
Topical			
Phenylephrine	MAOIs, tricyclic antidepressants	Hypertensive crisis	Do not use within 14 d of each other
	Beta blockers	May increase vasopressor effects of sympathomimetics	Monitor closely for adverse reaction
Oxymetazoline	MAOIs, tricyclic antidepressants	Hypertensive crisis	Do not use within 14 d of each other
	Beta blockers *Anesthetics:* Cyclopropane, halothane	May increase vasopressor effects of sympathomimetics May sensitize the myocardium to sympathomimetics	Monitor closely for adverse reaction Discontinue oxymetazoline prior to use
Tetrahydrozoline	None reported	—	—

Table 17–15 ⊗ **Dosage Schedule: Selected Decongestants**

Drug	Indication	Dosage Form	Dose	Comments
Systemic				
Phenylephrine	Nasal congestion		*Children >12 yr and adults:* 10 mg every 4 h	Maximum of 6 doses Not recommended for children <12 yr
Pseudoephedrine Sudafed PE Sudogest Pediacare Children's Decongestant Sudafed PE Children's Generic	Nasal congestion	Tablet: 5, 10 mg Liquid: 2.5 mg/mL	*Children >12 yr and adults:* 60 mg every 4–6 hr (20 mL of 15 mg/5 mL liquid); max 240 mg/d *Children 6–12 yr:* 30 mg every 4–6 h (10 mL of 15 mg/5 mL liquid); max 120 mg/d *Children 2–6 yr:* 15 mg every 4–6 h (5 mL of 15 mg/5 mL liquid); max 60 mg/d *Children <2 yr:* 1 mg/kg/dose every 4–6 h, max 4 doses or *Extended-release (12-h formula):* *Children >12 yr and adults:* 120 mg every 12 h: max 240 mg/d *Children <12 yr:* Not recommended *Extended release (24-h formula):* *Children >12 yr and adults:* 1 tablet; max 240 mg/d *Children <12 yr:* Not recommended	Note: Use of pseudoephedrine in children <2 yr is not recommended as standard practice.
Topical				
Phenylephrine Little Noses Rhinal 4 Way Fast Acting Neo-Synephrine Mild Formula Neo-Synephrine Regular Forumla Neo-Synephrine Extra Strength Vicks Sinex VapoSpray Generic	Nasal congestion and eustachian tube congestion	0.125% drops 0.25% drops 1% solution 0.25% solution 0.5% solution 1% solution 0.5% solution	*Children >12 yr and adults:* 1–2 sprays of 0.25% or 0.5% solution in each nostril every 4 h prn congestion; 1% solution can be used in adults with severe congestion *Children 6–12 yr:* 1–2 sprays of 0.25% solution in each nostril every 4 h prn congestion *Children 2–6 yr:* 2 drops or sprays of 0.125% or 0.16% solution to each nostril every 4 h as needed *Children 6 mo–2 yr:* 1–2 drops of 0.16% solution in each nostril every 3–4 h prn	Advise patients to use nasal decongestant spray for a maximum of 2–3 d in a row to avoid rebound congestion
Oxymetazoline Afrin 12-hour Nasal Relief 4-Way 12 Hour Dristan Neo-Synephrine Nightime 12-Hour Nostrilla Vicks Sinex Vapo Spray 12-Hour	Nasal congestion	0.05% solution	*Children >6 yr and adults:* use 1–2 drops or sprays of 0.05% solution in each nostril bid *Children 2–5 yr:* 1–2 drops of 0.025% solution in each nostril bid; do not use 0.05% solution in young children *Children <2 yr:* Not recommended	Advise patients to use nasal decongestant spray for a maximum of 2–3 d in a row to avoid rebound congestion
Tetrahydrozoline Tyzine Tyzine Pediatric Drops Generic	Nasal congestion	Solution: 0.1% Solution: 0.05%	*Children >6 yr and adults:* 2–4 drops or 3–4 sprays of 0.1% solution in each nostril every 3–4 h prn *Children <6 yr:* 2–3 drops of 0.05% solution in each nostril every 3–4 h prn	Advise patients to use nasal decongestant spray for a maximum of 2–3 d in a row to avoid rebound congestion

Topical decongestants are indicated in the symptomatic relief of nasal congestion due to the common cold, sinus infection, and allergic rhinitis. As previously mentioned, topical decongestants are only for short-term (3 to 5 day) use because of the rebound congestion of long-term use. Nasal decongestants may also relieve ear block and pressure pain in air travel, especially if a patient is suffering from a common cold or sinus infection. The adult dose of oxymetazoline topical nasal spray is one or two drops or sprays of 0.05% solution in each nostril twice a day or up to every 6 hours if needed. Children aged 2 to 5 years should use two to three drops of the 0.025% solution in each nostril. The use of 0.05% oxymetazoline should be avoided in children. The dose of topical phenylephrine nasal solution in adults is one to two sprays or drops of 0.25% or 0.5% solution every 4 hours as needed for congestion. Adults with severe congestion can use phenylephrine 1% solution. Children aged 6 to 12 years should use 0.25% solution, two sprays in each nostril every 4 hours. If the child is between age 6 months and 6 years, the 0.16% solution should be prescribed. The dose of phenylephrine in young children (younger than age 6 years) and infants is 1 to 2 drops or sprays every 4 hours. Use topical nasal decongestants sparingly in young children.

Table 17-15 presents dosing information.

Rational Drug Selection

Topical Versus Systemic

Topical decongestants are effective and have few adverse effects. Many health-care providers recommend them for short-term use for the common cold and sinusitis. A concern is the significant rebound congestion that occurs if the topical decongestants are used long term. It can occur in as little as a week of constant use. Therefore, topical decongestants for allergic rhinitis, although safe, must be accompanied with strict patient education to prevent rebound congestion. In patients who are sensitive to the drying effects of the topical decongestants, the oral form may be better tolerated. The reverse is also true; in patients sensitive to sympathomimetics, the topical decongestants are usually tolerated.

Short- Versus Long-Acting

There are short- and long-acting forms of both oral and topical decongestants. In general, the short-acting forms are better tolerated and have fewer adverse effects. The longer-acting forms are useful for patients who require all-day or all-night relief, if the patients can tolerate them.

Cost

Cost is usually not a major factor in prescribing decongestants, which are available OTC, and generic forms of all the medications are available.

Monitoring

There is no specific monitoring required with the decongestants.

Patient Education

Administration

The first concern that the health-care provider should address is self-prescribing and dosing of the nonprescription decongestants. Whether a drug interaction is a concern or a patient may be taking an inappropriate dose, it is important for the health-care provider to be aware that the patient may be taking a decongestant. A thorough history should include any self-prescribed medications and the amount and timing of these medications. Patient teaching should include proper dosing, especially in pediatric patients. Patients with cardiovascular disease, hyperthyroidism, diabetes mellitus, or prostatic hypertrophy should use these products sparingly and only on the advice of their health-care provider.

When topical decongestants are recommended, it is imperative that the patient be warned about rebound congestion and cautioned to use the medication for only 3 to 5 days or, for chronic allergic rhinitis use, only 2 of every 7 days.

Parents should be cautioned not to use adult-formula nasal sprays in children. Children's strength oxymetazoline (0.025%) and phenylephrine HCl (0.125%) are available.

Adverse Reactions

Patients should notify their health-care provider if insomnia, dizziness, weakness, tremor, or irregular heartbeat occurs with topical decongestants. Patients should be cautioned not to exceed the recommended dosage because higher doses cause nervousness, dizziness, or sleeplessness.

Lifestyle Management

Patients should maintain adequate hydration while taking decongestants to keep mucus mobile. They should also refrain from smoking when they are congested. Caffeine-containing products may cause tachycardia if ingested with decongestants.

Table 17-15 presents available dosage forms.

ANTITUSSIVES

Antitussives are widely used by patients to self-treat coughs. It is essential for the health-care provider to educate the patient on the useful physiological mechanism a cough provides by clearing the airway of secretions and foreign material. Therefore, a cough should not be suppressed if it is protecting the airway. There are times when an antitussive is necessary to provide rest or sleep. The cough reflex is complicated, involving both the CNS and peripheral nervous system, as well as the smooth muscle of the bronchial tree. The drugs that can affect this complex mechanism are diverse, ranging from bronchodilators to drugs that act centrally or peripherally to suppress cough. This section discusses the nonprescription antitussives dextromethorphan and benzonatate. Codeine, which is also used as an antitussive, is covered in Chapter 16 with the other opioids. Dosing of codeine for antitussive use is included here.

Pharmacodynamics

Cough results when sensory stimuli or irritation in the bronchial tree stimulates cough receptors, probably located in the bronchial smooth muscle. A message is sent via the afferent nervous system to the cough centers in the medulla. Antitussives work either centrally or peripherally to affect the cough. The exact mechanism of action of antitussives is poorly understood. Dextromethorphan, the d-isomer of the codeine analogue levorphanol, acts centrally in the cough center in the medulla to elevate the threshold for coughing. Codeine works as an antitussive through direct action on receptors in the cough center of the medulla, at lower doses than is required for analgesia. Benzonatate (Tessalon) is related to tetracaine and is thought to anesthetize the stretch receptors in the respiratory passages, thereby decreasing their activity and calming the cough peripherally at its source.

Pharmacokinetics

Absorption and Distribution

Dextromethorphan, codeine, and benzonatate are absorbed well from the GI tract. The distribution of dextromethorphan and benzonatate is unknown. Codeine is 7% protein bound and widely distributed, including in the CNS. Codeine freely crosses the placenta and is distributed into breast milk.

Metabolism and Excretion

Dextromethorphan is extensively metabolized by the liver and excreted in the urine, mostly as metabolites. Codeine is metabolized in the liver by glucuronidation into morphine and norcodeine. The metabolism of codeine into morphine is mediated by CYP450 2D6. Codeine is eliminated in the urine as unchanged drug, norcodeine, and free and conjugated morphine. The metabolism and excretion of benzonatate is unknown. See Table 17-16 for the pharmacokinetics of selected preparations.

Pharmacotherapeutics

Precautions and Contraindications

Antitussives are not to be used for persistent or chronic cough caused by smoking, asthma, or emphysema. In asthma, antitussives may impair expectoration and thus cause increased airway resistance. Expectorants must not be used by patients with excessive respiratory secretions for the same reason. Patients must be cautioned not to self-medicate their cough for long periods (more than 7 days) without seeking the care of their health-care provider. If high fever or rash accompanies a cough, patients must be seen by their health-care provider.

Benzonatate is contraindicated for patients allergic to tetracaine, procaine, or related compounds.

Dextromethorphan, codeine, and benzonatate can cause drowsiness, dizziness, nausea, and GI upset. In addition, patients taking benzonatate may experience headache, constipation, pruritus, skin eruptions, a sensation of burning eyes, a vague "chilly" sensation, chest numbness, and hypersensitivity. Patients with hepatic function impairment should be monitored if dextromethorphan is prescribed because metabolism of the drug may be impaired. The metabolism of codeine can be affected by deficiency of CYP450D or by medications that may inhibit CYP2D6.

Codeine may cause dependence and should be used with caution in a patient with a history of substance abuse. Although dextromethorphan is not addictive, there have been reports of abuse of dextromethorphan-containing products, especially among teenagers. The FDA issued a Talk Paper in 2005 to warn the public, providers, and law enforcement of the potential for dextromethorphan abuse and has begun exploring whether dextromethorphan should become a scheduled drug.

Codeine causes decreased gastric motility and therefore should be used cautiously by patients with GI obstruction, ileus, or preexisting constipation. Patients with acute ulcerative colitis may be more sensitive to the constipating effects of codeine.

Dextromethorphan and codeine are Pregnancy Category C, but no teratogenic effects have been demonstrated. Codeine should be used with caution near term in pregnancy. Benzonatate is Pregnancy Category C and is to be given to pregnant women only if clearly needed. There are better-studied choices for antitussives in pregnancy, such as dextromethorphan or short-term codeine.

Drug Interactions

Use of antitussives with any CNS depressant may cause increased CNS depression. Concurrent use of dextromethorphan and MAOIs is contraindicated.

Codeine should be used with caution concurrently with medications that are metabolized by CYP2D6 isoenzymes. Quinidine has been shown to interfere with the metabolism of codeine. Other medications that inhibit CYP2D6 are amiodarone (Cordarone), tricyclic antidepressants, metoclopramide (Reglan), selective serotonin reuptake inhibitors (SSRIs), cimetidine (Tagamet), thioridazine (Mellaril), propafenone (Rythmol), and haloperidol (Haldol).

Drugs interactions are shown in Table 17-17.

Table 17–16 ❖ Pharmacokinetics: Selected Cough Preparations

Drug	Onset	Peak	Duration	Protein Binding	Half-Life	Metabolism	Elimination
Dextromethorphan	15–30 min	—	5–6 h	—	11 h	Extensive hepatic	Renal
Codeine (used as an antitussive)	30–60 min	1–2 h	4–6 h	7%	3–4 h	Primarily hepatic (CYP2D6)	Renal
Benzonatate	15–20 min	—	3 8 h	—	—	—	—
Expectorants							
Guaifenesin	Rapid	—	—	—	1 h	—	Renal

Table 17–17 ▦ **Drug Interactions: Selected Cough Preparations**

Drug	Interacting Drug	Possible Effect	Implications
Antitussives			
Dextromethorphan	MAOIs	Dextromethorphan can block neuronal uptake of serotonin and can increase concentrations of serotonin if combined with MAOIs; hypertensive or hyperpyretic crisis is possible	Use concurrently with caution, if at all; avoid use within 14 d
	SSRIs	SSRIs interfere with dextromethorphan metabolism, leading to toxicity	Use lower doses of dextromethorphan
	CNS depressants	Additive CNS depression	Use with caution
	Amiodarone, quinidine	These drugs inhibit CYP2D6; dextromethorphan toxicity may occur	Monitor for toxicity if prescribed concurrently
Codeine (used as an antitussive)	CNS depressants, alcohol	Additive CNS depression	Use cautiously and reduce dose to avoid additive effects
	Antihypertensive agents	Antagonizes antihypertensives	Monitor patients closely
	Antidiarrheals	Can lead to severe constipation	Use with caution; monitor the patient
Benzonatate	None known	—	—
Expectorants			
Guaifenesin	None known	—	—

Clinical Use and Dosing

Cough

Dextromethorphan, codeine, and benzonatate are used to control nonproductive cough. Antitussives should be used only for the nonproductive, irritant-like cough, after other pathology has been ruled out, specifically asthma or pneumonia. Antitussives are not to be used for asthmatic cough or for coughs accompanied by excessive respiratory secretions.

Dextromethorphan is available in many forms and either singly or in combination with expectorants. As it is available without prescription, it is widely used by patients to self-medicate their cough, not always appropriately. The adult dose of dextromethorphan is 10 to 30 mg every 4 to 8 hours. Children aged 6 to 12 years are given a dose of 5 to 10 mg every 4 hours or 15 mg every 6 to 8 hours. The dose of dextromethorphan in children aged 2 to 6 years is 2.5 to 7.5 mg every 4 to 8 hours, although current guidelines recommend not using cough medication in children with cough (Chang & Glomb, 2006).

Benzonatate is available only by prescription and is effective in controlling dry, irritant-like coughs. The dose for children aged 10 years and older and adults is 100 mg 3 times a day. Benzonatate does not cause CNS sedation and may be preferred over dextromethorphan or codeine in patients who need to remain alert or who have a history of substance abuse and want to avoid opioids.

Codeine, a Schedule III, IV, or V medication (depending on combination with other medications), may be administered alone or in combination with another agent such as guaifenesin for cough suppression. The adult dose of codeine for cough suppression is 10 to 20 mg every 4 to 6 hours, with the maximum daily dose not exceeding 120 mg. Children aged 6 to 12 years can be prescribed 5 to 10 mg every 4 to 6 hours (maximum 60 mg/d). Guidelines recommend against the use of antitussives in children (Chang & Glomb, 2006). Table 17-18 presents dosing information.

Rational Drug Selection

Patients may self-medicate their cough with a nonprescription form of dextromethorphan, and the health-care provider has little to do with the choice of the medication. (Advertising has the largest impact.) The health-care provider becomes involved when the patient asks for a recommended formula or if nonprescription products are not effective.

Cost

Although nonprescription dextromethorphan is less expensive than benzonatate- or codeine-containing preparations, patients with good prescriptive coverage may actually pay less out of pocket for the prescription product. Cost must therefore be evaluated on an individual basis.

Effectiveness

Patients might feel that a prescription medication is more effective than nonprescription, but dextromethorphan has been found to be as effective as codeine in the treatment of cough.

Monitoring

There is no specific monitoring required when prescribing antitussive medications.

Table 17–18 ⊗ **Dosage Schedule: Selected Cough Preparations**

Drug	Indication	Dosage Form	Dose	Comments
Antitussives				
Dextromethorphan Scot-Tussen DM Cough Chasers Hold DM Robitussin Cough Calmers Supress Cough Robitussin Pediatric Vicks Formula 44 Vicks Formula 44 Pediatric Delsym Generic	Cough	Lozenges: 2.5 mg Lozenges: 5 mg Lozenges: 5 mg Lozenges: 7.5 mg Liquid: 7.5 mg/5 mL Liquid: 15 mg/5 mL Liquid: 15 mg/15 mL (1 mg/mL) Sustained-action liquid: 30 mg/5 mL	*Children >12 yr and adults:* 10–30 mg every 4 h or 30 mg every 6–8 h *Children 6–12 yr:* 5–10 mg every 4 h or 15 mg every 6–8 h *Children 2–6 yr:* 2.5–5 mg every 4 h or 7.5 mg every 6–8 h *Children 7 mo–2 yr:* 2–4 mg every 6–8 h	Do not exceed 120 mg in 24 h. Do not exceed 60 mg in 24 h. Do not exceed 30 mg in 24 h. Dosage in children younger than 4 yr is not well established. Evidence suggests lack of efficacy in children.
Codeine (used as an antitussive) Generic	Cough	Tablets: 15, 30, 60 mg	*Adults:* 10–20 mg every 4 h *Children 6–12 yr:* 5–10 mg every 4 h *Children 2–6 yr:* 2.5–5 mg every 4 h	Do not exceed 120 mg in 24 h. Do not exceed 60 mg in 24 h. Do not exceed 30 mg in 24 h. Not recommended for acute or chronic cough in children. Educate parents to monitor closely for respiratory depression.
Benzonatate Tessalon Perles	Cough	Capsules: 100 mg	*Children >10 yr and adults:* 100 mg tid, up to 600 mg per day	Do not chew or crush capsules.
Expectorants				
Guaifenesin Robitussin Generic Mucinex Kids Mucinex Kid's Mini-Melts Mucinex Mucinex Maximum Strength	Cough	Syrup: 100 mg/5 mL Liquid: 100 mg/5 mL 50 mg/packet, 100 mg/packet Extended-release tablet: 600 mg Extended-release tablet: 1,200 mg	*Children >12 yr and adults:* 200–400 mg every 4 h, or as extended release 600–1,200 mg every 12 h *Children 6–11 yr:* 100–200 mg every 4 h *Children 2–5 yr:* 50–100 mg every 4 h	*Children > 12 yrs and adult:* Maximum 2.4 g/24 h *Children 6–11 yr:* Maximum 1.2 g/24 h *Children 2–5 yr:* Maximum 600 mg/24 h

Patient Education

Patient education centers on proper administration, adverse reactions, and drug interactions with the antitussive agents.

Administration

Patients should be aware of the proper dosing of antitussive medication. When they are self-medicating, they are often not following the recommended dosing schedule. The health-care provider needs to determine if the patient is taking the proper amount, measured with a calibrated measuring spoon (not a flatware teaspoon or tablespoon), and spacing the dosage appropriately. The medications may be taken without regard to food but may be better tolerated if taken with food or milk.

Adverse Reactions

CNS depression is the major concern. Some of the antitussives are in alcohol-containing syrup form, and others may cause sedation. Driving or operating hazardous machinery should be undertaken with caution, and not at all if the patient is sensitive to the sedating effects of the antitussives.

Patients should also be aware that if they have long-term cough (occurring for more than 7 days) or cough accompanied by fever, they should be seen by their health-care provider.

Patients concurrently taking MAOIs should not take antitussives. Antitussives should be taken with caution if the patient is concurrently taking any other CNS-sedating medications.

Lifestyle Management

The patient with a cough should be encouraged to increase fluid intake to improve the viscosity of the respiratory secretions. The patient should refrain from smoking and, if possible, stop smoking. Avoidance of respiratory irritants and people with respiratory infections will decrease the incidence of cough.

Table 17-18 presents available dosage forms.

EXPECTORANTS

Guaifenesin is the only expectorant ingredient listed by the FDA panel as having scientific evidence of safety and efficacy.

Guaifenesin is indicated as an expectorant in the symptomatic treatment of cough due to the common cold and mild upper respiratory infections.

Pharmacodynamics

Guaifenesin's main mechanism of action is to increase the output of the respiratory tract by decreasing adhesiveness and surface tension. The increased flow of the thinned secretions promotes ciliary action and facilitates the removal of respiratory mucus. This changes a dry, nonproductive cough into a more productive cough.

Pharmacokinetics

Absorption and Distribution

Guaifenesin is rapidly absorbed from the GI tract after oral administration. Distribution is unknown. It is not known whether guaifenesin crosses the placenta or is distributed in breast milk.

Metabolism and Excretion

The exact mechanism of metabolism of guaifenesin is unknown. Its major metabolite, beta (2-methoxyphenoxy) lactic acid, is excreted in the urine.

Pharmacotherapeutics

Precautions and Contraindications

Guaifenesin is not to be used for persistent cough, such as that found with smoking, asthma, or emphysema. Cough related to heart failure or angiotensin-converting enzyme (ACE) inhibitor therapy should not be treated with guaifenesin. A cough accompanied by high fever or lasting longer than 7 days should be evaluated by a health-care provider.

Guaifenesin is Pregnancy Category C. There have been no problems documented in breastfeeding women taking this medication. Use in children as young as age 2 years is considered safe.

Adverse Drug Effects

GI upset, nausea, and vomiting are the most commonly reported adverse effects of guaifenesin. Drowsiness, diarrhea, dizziness, rash, and headache have also been reported. Guaifenesin is contraindicated only if the patient is hypersensitive to guaifenesin.

Drug Interactions

There are no drug interactions of significance with guaifenesin; however, guaifenesin may cause false readings in certain laboratory determinations of 5-hydroxyindoleacetic acid (5-HIAA) and vanillylmandelic acid (VMA).

Clinical Use and Dosing

Dry, Nonproductive Cough

Guaifenesin is indicated in the symptomatic relief of dry, nonproductive cough, with mucus in the respiratory tract.

The dose of guaifenesin for children over age 12 years and adults is 200 to 400 mg every 4 hours. The guaifenesin dose in children aged 6 to 11 years is 100 to 200 mg every 4 hours. Children aged 2 to 5 years should be dosed with 50 to 100 mg of guaifenesin every 4 hours.

Monitoring

There is no specific laboratory monitoring required with the use of guaifenesin.

Patient Education

Administration

The patient should be aware of the proper dose of guaifenesin. The patient should be using a calibrated medication spoon and taking the appropriate dose per age.

Guaifenesin is an OTC product, and patients may self-medicate, often without proper understanding of the medication. The provider may assist the patient in making the proper choice of cough medication by explaining the difference between the OTC products guaifenesin and dextromethorphan. An explanation of the many combination products that are available and some guidance about appropriate use will assist the patient in making an informed choice.

Adverse Reactions

Although the adverse drug reactions of guaifenesin are mild, patients should be instructed regarding the mild gastrointestinal upset that may occur.

Lifestyle Management

Patients should be instructed to remain well hydrated while taking guaifenesin, and they should refrain from smoking.

REFERENCES

Berger, W. E. (2003). Levalbuterol: Pharmacologic properties and use in the treatment of pediatric and adult asthma. *Annals of Allergy, Asthma, and Immunology, 90*(6), 583–592.

Centers for Disease Control and Prevention. (2007). Infant deaths associated with cough and cold medications—two states, 2005. *Mortality and Morbidity Weekly Report, 56*(1), 104.

Chang, A. B., & Glomb, W. B. (2006). Guidelines for evaluating chronic cough in pediatrics: ACCP evidence-based clinical practice guidelines. *Chest, 129,* 260S–283S.

Food and Drug Administration (2005). Caficit: Caffeine citrate injection label. Retrieved from http://www.accessdata.fda.gov/drugsatfda_docs/nda/99/020793_000_CafcitTOC.cfm

Klein-Schwartz, W., Sorkin, J., & Doyon, S. (2010). Impact of the voluntary withdrawal of over-the-counter cough and cold medications on pediatric ingestions reported to poison centers. *Pharmacoepidemiology and Drug Safety, 19*(8), 819–824.

Loke, Y. K., & Singh, L. (2013). Risk of acute urinary retention associated with inhaled anticholinergics in patients with chronic obstructive lung disease: Systematic review. *Therapeutic Advances in Drug Safety, 4*(1), 19–26.

Man, S. E. P., & Sin, D. D. (2005). Inhaled corticosteroids in chronic obstructive pulmonary disease. *Drugs, 65*(5), 579–591.

National Asthma Education and Prevention Program (NAEPP). (2007). *The Expert Panel Report 3: Guidelines for the diagnosis and management of asthma.* Bethesda, MD: National Heart, Lung, and Blood Institute, National Institutes of Health. Retrieved from http://www.nhlbi.nih.gov/guidelines/asthma/

National Heart, Lung, and Blood Institute. (2012). Inhaled corticosteroids for childhood asthma may affect adult height. National Institutes of Health. Retrieved from http://www.nhlbi.nih.gov/news/press-releases/2012/inhaled-corticosteroids-for-childhood-asthma-may-affect-adult-height.html

Nelson, H. S., Weiss, S. T., Bleecker, E. R., Yancey, S. W., Dorinsky, P. M., & the SMART Study Group. (2006). The Salmeterol Multicenter Asthma Research Trial: A comparison of usual pharmacotherapy for asthma or usual pharmacotherapy plus salmeterol. *Chest, 129*(1), 15–26.

Parsons, J. P., & Mastronarde, J. G. (2005). Exercise-induced bronchoconstriction in athletes. *Chest, 128*(6), 3966–3974.

Salpeter, S. R., Wall, A. J., & Buckley, N. S. (2010). Long-acting beta-agonists with and without inhaled corticosteroids and catastrophic asthma events. *American Journal of Medicine, 123,* 322–328.

Skoner, D. P., Greos, L. S., Kim, K. T., Roach, J. M., Parsey, M., & Baumgartner, R. A. (2005). Evaluation of the safety and efficacy of levalbuterol in 2- to 5-year-old patients with asthma. *Pediatric Pulmonology, 40*(6), 477–486.

Skouroliakou, M., Bacopoulou, F., & Markantonis, S. L. (2009). Caffeine versus theophylline of apnea of prematurity: A randomized controlled trial. *Journal of Paediatrics and Child Health, 45*(10), 587–592.

U.S. Food and Drug Administration (2009). Updated information on leukotriene inhibitors: Montelukast (marketed as Singulair), zafirlukast (marketed as Accolate), and zileuton (marketed as Zyflo and Zyflo CR). Retrieved from http://www.fda.gov/Drugs/DrugSafety/PostmarketDrugSafetyInformationforPatientsandProviders/DrugSafetyInformationforHeathcareProfessionals/ucm165489.htm

U.S. Food and Drug Administration. (2010). FDA Drug Safety Communication: New safety requirements for long-acting inhaled asthma medications called long-acting beta-agonists (LABAs). Retrieved from http://www.fda.gov/Drugs/DrugSafety/PostmarketDrugSafetyInformationforPatientsandProviders/ucm200776.htm

Zieger, R. S., Szefler, S. J., Phillips, B. R., Schatz, M., Martinez, F. D., Chinchilli, V. M., et al. (2006). Response to fluticasone and montelukast in mild-to-moderate persistent childhood asthma. *Journal of Allergy and Clinical Immunology, 117*(1), 45–52.

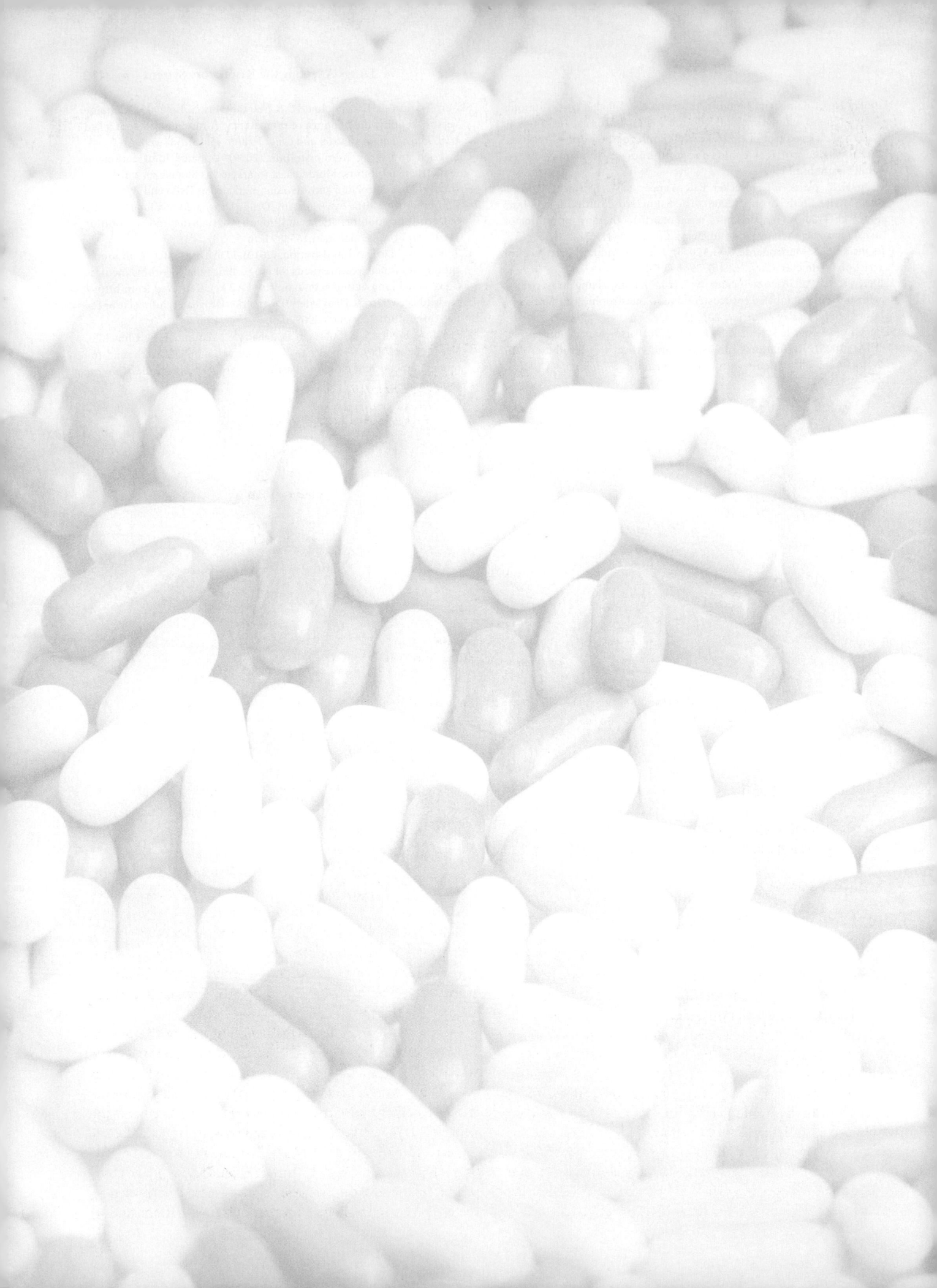

CHAPTER 18

DRUGS AFFECTING THE HEMATOPOIETIC SYSTEM

Teri Moser Woo • Kristen Osborne

There are multiple classes of medications that affect the hematopoietic system, including anticoagulants and antiplatelet drugs that affect clotting, hematopoietic growth factors, and the supplements, iron, folic acid, and vitamin B$_{12}$.

ANTICOAGULANTS AND ANTIPLATELETS

Thromboemboli are a common cause of morbidity and mortality. Venous thromboembolism occurs in approximately 108 of every 100,000 persons in the United States each year (American Heart Association Writing Group Members et al, 2012). Pulmonary embolism is a common complication of deep vein thrombosis (DVT), with silent pulmonary embolism occurring in up to one-third of patients with DVT (Stein, Matta, Musani, & Diaczok, 2010). The morbidity and mortality associated with these emboli could be significantly reduced by timely use of anticoagulation therapy. Oral anticoagulation therapy has been used in primary care for over 50 years, and the number of indications for its use has steadily increased. The introduction of low-molecular-weight heparin (LMWH) with less bleeding risk has allowed the outpatient use of injectable anticoagulation therapy as well. With more selective and reliable laboratory tests to monitor blood levels, the management of anticoagulation therapy has become a major tool in the prevention of thrombus formation in primary care.

Thrombi tend to develop whenever intravascular conditions promote activation of the clotting cascade. These conditions include injury to the intimal lining of the artery; roughing of this surface such as occurs in atherosclerosis; inflammation, which is a cardinal part of atherogenesis; traumatic injury; infection; alteration in the normal laminar blood flow; low blood pressure; or obstructions that cause blood stasis and pooling within the vessels.

Although the exact details of the clotting mechanism are not fully understood, it is generally accepted that clotting occurs when several circulating proteins interact in a cascading series of limited proteolytic actions (Fig. 18-1). At each step, a precursor protein is converted to an active protease that activates the next clotting factor, and finally, a solid clot is formed. The key regulatory protein in this cascade that initiates blood coagulation is likely factor VII (McCance & Huether, 2010). The components involved at each stage are a protease from the preceding stage, a precursor protein, a protein activator, calcium, and an

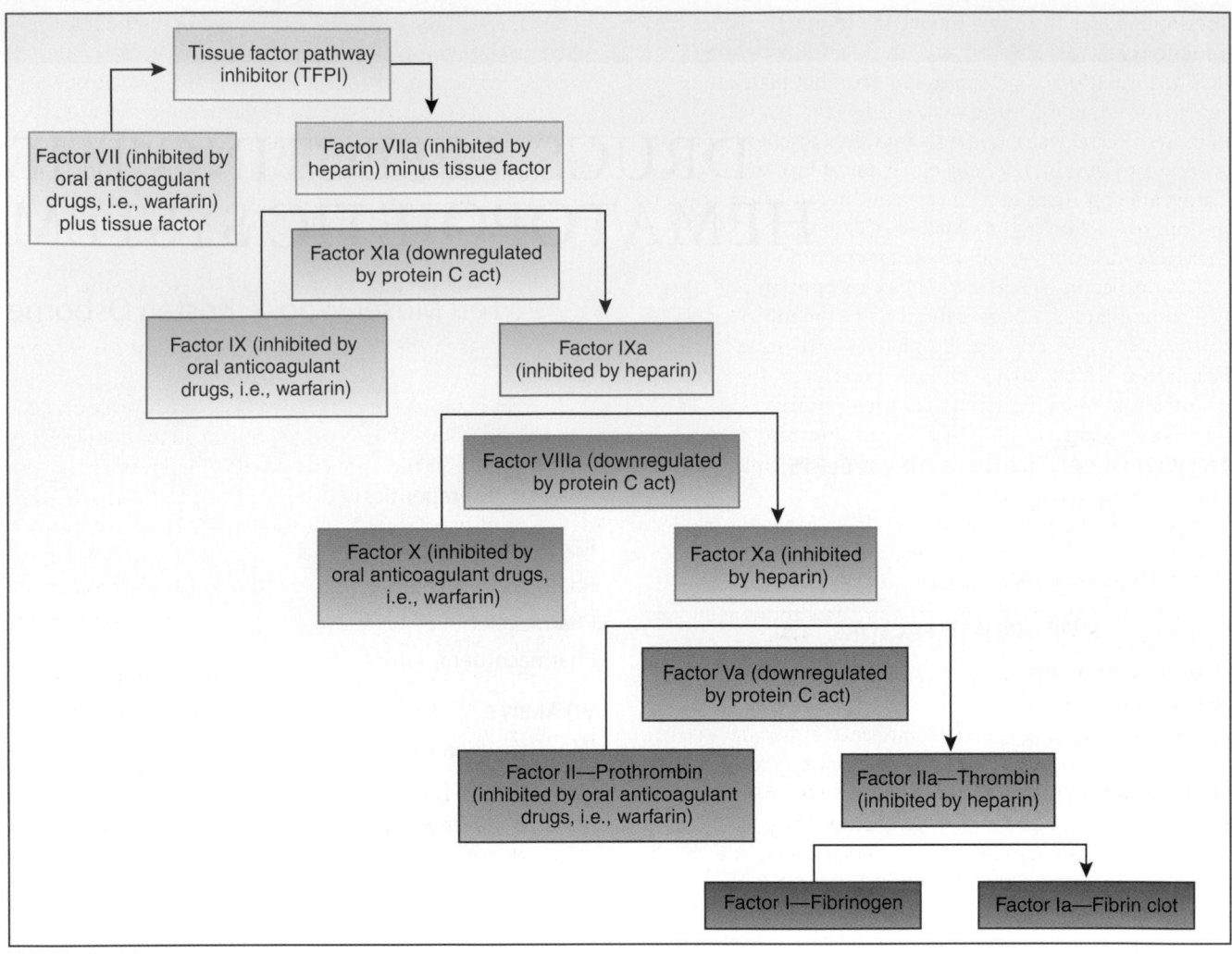

Figure 18–1. The clotting cascade.

organizing surface provided by platelets. Fibrinogen is the substrate for the enzyme thrombin (factor IIa). This protease is formed by activation of its precursor protein, prothrombin. Prothrombin is bound by calcium to a platelet surface, where activated factor X (Xa), in the presence of factor V (Va), converts it to circulating thrombin. Thrombin then converts fibrinogen to fibrin to form the clot. Venous thrombi are mainly fibrin and red blood cells (RBCs) and occur when the balance of the clotting pathway is altered by thrombophilic abnormalities, vessel wall damage, or stasis (Weitz, Hirsh, & Samama, 2004). Arterial thrombosis occurs when an atherosclerotic plaque is disrupted and a thrombus forms at the site of disruption (Weitz et al, 2004).

Pharmacodynamics

Oral anticoagulants such as warfarin (Coumadin) inhibit the hepatic synthesis of several clotting factors, including factor X. The decline in clotting factors is a function of the half-life of each factor, which varies from 5 hours for factor VII to 72 hours for factor II. Plasma also contains protease inhibitors that inactivate coagulation proteins. One of these factors is antithrombin III. Heparin inhibits the activity of several activated clotting factors by accelerating the activity of antithrombin III. LMWH enoxaparin (Lovenox) potentiates the activity of antithrombin III and inactivates factors Xa and IIa (thrombin). Dabigatran (Pradaxa) is a direct thrombin inhibitor. Thrombin is required for the conversion of fibrinogen to fibrin in the clotting cascade, thus dabigatran's inhibition of thrombin prevents thrombi from forming. Fondaparinux (Arixtra) is a selective inhibitor of antithrombin III and a factor Xa inhibitor. An anticoagulant, rivaroxaban (Xarelto), is a highly selective factor Xa inhibitor that inhibits thrombin formation and the

On The Horizon — IDRABIOTAPARINUX

Idraparinux is an analog of fondaparinux given once a week, but trials were discontinued due to excessive bleeding. Idrabiotaparinux is a biotinylated version of idraparinux that is currently being studied for treatment of pulmonary embolism and is as effective as warfarin with less bleeding (Büller et al. 2012). Idrabiotaparinux is also being studied for prophylaxis treatment of DVT (Equinox Investigators, 2011).

development of thrombi. Apixaban (Eliquis) is a selective inhibitor of factor Xa.

The formation of a clot also requires that platelets aggregate to form the organizing base for the clot. Platelets adhere to injured vessel walls, undergo granulate discharge, and aggregate into clumps, releasing biochemical mediators. Several factors affect platelet adherence, including sufficient concentrations of calcium in the platelet so that it can change shape, aggregate, degranulate, and activate arachidonic pathways. Adhesion occurs when the platelet receptor binds to von Willebrand factor, bridging the plate to the injury site. Two of the mediators released by platelets are serotonin and histamine, which affect smooth muscle in the vascular endothelium causing an immediate temporary vasoconstriction. Vasoconstriction reduces blood flow and diminishes bleeding. Vasodilation follows to permit the inflammatory process to occur.

The arachidonic pathway uses cyclooxygenase to produce thromboxane A_2 (TXA$_2$), a prostaglandin, and prostacyclin I_2 (PGI$_2$). TXA$_2$ causes vasoconstriction and promotes degranulation of other platelets, which then release more adenosine diphosphate (ADP) to promote adherence. PGI$_2$ inhibits the effect of TXA$_2$ by promoting vasodilation and inhibiting platelet degranulation. The net effect is to permit platelet aggregation at the injury site but to prevent adherence to normal vascular endothelium. Aspirin antagonizes the cyclooxygenase pathway and interferes with platelet aggregation. NSAIDs have this same action. NSAIDs are not used as antiplatelet drugs, but this explains why concurrent use with anticoagulants is contraindicated (Kniff-Dutmer, Schut, & van der Laar, 2003). Ticlopidine (Ticlid) and clopidogrel (Plavix) reduce platelet aggregation by inhibiting the ADP pathway of platelets. Unlike aspirin, they have no effect on prostaglandin metabolism. Ticagrelor (Brilinta) reversibly interacts with the platelet P2Y$_{12}$ ADP-receptor to prevent platelet activation. Vorapaxar (Zontivity) is a protease-activated receptor-1 (PAR-1) antagonist, inhibiting thrombin-induced and thrombin receptor agonist peptide-induced platelet aggregation.

Aspirin and ibuprofen also have analgesic, antipyretic, and anti-inflammatory actions related to their cyclooxygenase (COX) activity. These actions are discussed in Chapter 25.

Pharmacokinetics

Absorption and Distribution

Heparin, including the low-molecular-weight drugs dalteparin (Fragmin), enoxaparin (Lovenox), fondaparinux (Arixtra), and tinzaparin (Innohep), are not absorbed in the gastrointestinal (GI) tract and must be given IV or SC. The IV route is used in acute care. SC injection of heparin results in considerable individual variation in bioavailability. LMWHs have less variation, but bioavailability between drugs is not consistent, and these drugs are not interchangeable. Once absorbed, heparin is distributed in plasma and extensively protein bound. The LMWHs are distributed in plasma and have limited to no protein binding (Table 18-1). Volume of distribution (V_d) is different between the

LMWHs and may factor into choosing among them for specific populations.

The coumarin derivative most commonly used is warfarin (Coumadin). Warfarin is rapidly and completely absorbed orally. Although serum levels are found in 1 to 2 hours, the anticoagulation effect is dependent on depletion of clotting factors. Because factor II has a life of 72 hours, the full effect does not occur for 3 to 4 days. Warfarin is highly bound to plasma protein.

Rivaroxaban is rapidly absorbed when given orally, is 80% to 100% bioavailable, and is highly protein bound. Rivaroxaban effects protime (PT) in 2 to 4 hours after the first tablet is ingested.

Aspirin is rapidly and completely absorbed after oral administration. Bioavailability is dependent on the dosage form, the presence of food, gastric emptying time, gastric pH, presence of antacids or buffering agents, and particle size. Bioavailability of enteric-coated forms is erratic. Aspirin is partially hydrolyzed during absorption and distributed to all body tissues and fluids, including fetal tissues and breast milk. Protein binding is highest with low plasma concentrations and lower with high concentrations.

Ticlopidine is rapidly absorbed after oral administration. Administration after meals increases the area under the curve (AUC) by 20%.

Clopidogrel is rapidly absorbed after oral administration. Bioavailability is not affected by food.

Ticagrelor is absorbed from the GI tract with a bioavailability of 36% and with peak serum levels 1.5 hours after ingestion. Ticagrelor is extensively protein bound (greater than 99% bound).

Dabigatran is absorbed slowly from the GI tract with peak serum levels in 1 hour. High-fat foods delay peak to 2 hours. Food intake does not affect bioavailability. Dabigatran is 35% bound to plasma proteins.

Vorapaxar peaks 1 to 2 hours after a single oral dose and is 100% bioavailable. A high fat meal delays peak time by approximately 45 minutes. Vorapaxar is 99% protein bound.

Apixaban reaches maximum concentrations 3 to 4 hours after oral administration. Apixaban is 87% protein bound.

Metabolism and Excretion

Heparins are metabolized by the liver and the reticuloendothelial system. A secondary site of metabolism may be in the kidney. Clearance is nonlinear, and the half-life may be prolonged at higher doses and in liver disease.

In patients with severe renal insufficiency, the mean dalteparin terminal half-life of anti-factor Xa may be considerably longer, with greater accumulation than in other patients. The AUC for anti-factor Xa is marginally increased with enoxaparin for mild to moderate renal insufficiency but significantly increased with creatinine clearance (Ccr) less than 30 mL. Tinzaparin has a similar problem with a 24% reduction in clearance in severe renal insufficiency.

The risk of fondaparinux-associated major bleeding increases with age, from 1.8% for those under age 65 to 2.7% for those older than 75. This drug should be used cautiously

Table 18–1 ⚓ **Pharmacokinetics: Selected Anticoagulants and Antiplatelets**

Drug	Onset	Peak	Duration	Protein Binding	Bioavailability/ Volume of Distribution	Half-Life	Elimination
Anticoagulants							
Dalteparin	—	4 h	Up to 24 h	—	87%/40–60 mL	3–5 h (increased in renal insufficiency)	In urine
Dabigatran		1 h		35%	50 to 70 L	12–17 h	In urine
Enoxaparin	—	3–5 h	12 h	—	100%/4.3 L	4.5 h	In urine
Heparin (SC only)	20–60 min	2–4 h	8–12 h	Extensive	—	1–3 h (nonlinear and dose-dependent; 30 min for doses of 25 mcg/ kg vs. 150 min for doses of 400 mcg/kg); half-life shorter for patients with deep vein thrombosis (DVT) than those with pulmonary embolism; half-life may be prolonged in liver disease	50% unchanged in urine; some urine degradation products have anticoagulant activity; also eliminated by reticuloendothelial system (lymph nodes and spleen)
Fondaparinux	—	2 h	—	None	100%/7–11 L	11–21 h	In urine
Tinzaparin	—	—	—	None	87%/3.1–5 L	3–4 h	In urine
Warfarin	—	3–5 d	2–5 d	99%	100%/0.14 L	40 h	92% in urine as metabolites
Antiplatelets							
Aspirin	5–30 min	1–3 h	3–6 h	Concentration-dependent low doses: (100 mcg/mL) = 90% high doses: (400 mcg/mL) = 76%	—	15–20 min	Renal excretion depends on urine pH; as pH increases from 5 to 8, renal clearance increases from 2%–3% to more than 80%
Clopidogrel	—	1 h	3–7 d	98%	50%	8 h	50% in urine; 46% in feces
Ticagrelor		1.5 h		99%		7 h	58% in feces, 26% in urine
Ticlopidine	2 h	8–11 d	2 wk	98%	—	12.6 h for single dose; 4–5 d with repeated dosing	60% in urine, 23% in feces; clearance decreases with age
Rivaroxaban		2–4 h		92%–95%		5–9 h	urine (30%), feces (21%)

in the elderly. It also has increased terminal half-life in renal impairment.

Warfarin is metabolized by hepatic microsomal enzymes cyproheptadine (CYP) 1A2 and 2C9 and is excreted primarily in the urine as inactive metabolites.

Rivaroxaban is metabolized by CYP 3A4 and 2J2 and is eliminated renally with a half-life of 7 to 11 hours.

Apixaban is primarily metabolized by CYP3A4 and excreted in the urine and feces.

Aspirin is extensively metabolized by the liver and excreted by the kidney. The amount excreted depends on urine pH. As pH increases, the amount excreted as unchanged drug increases from 2% or 3% to 80%.

Ticlopidine is extensively metabolized by the liver. Because of its nonlinear pharmacokinetics, clearance decreases markedly with repeated administration. In older adults, half-lives of 12.6 hours after the first dose increased to 4 to 5 days with repeated dosing. Steady-state levels occur in about 14 to

21 days. Trace amounts of intact drug are found in the urine, and one-third of the dose is excreted in feces and bile as intact drug. Clearance decreases with age. Renal impairment alters plasma levels but does not seem to affect platelet aggregation or bleeding times, except in moderately impaired patients.

Clopidogrel is a prodrug and the liver rapidly converts it to a metabolite that is the active antiplatelet compound. Plasma levels are significantly higher in the elderly but are not associated with differences in platelet aggregation and bleeding time, so no dosage adjustment is needed for this population. Steady state occurs in 3 to 7 days. It is excreted almost equally in urine and in feces, making it safer for patients with renal insufficiency.

Ticagrelor is metabolized in the liver by CYP3A4 into an active metabolite, which also has antiplatelet activity. Ticagrelor and its active metabolite are extensively metabolized into inactive metabolites and excreted in the bile.

After oral administration, dabigatran etexilate is converted to dabigatran via conjugation. Dabigatran is renally eliminated.

Vorapaxar is metabolized via CYP3A4 and CYP2J2, with metabolites excreted 58% in the feces and 25% in the urine. The half-life for vorapaxar is 8 days (range 5 to 13 days).

Pharmacotherapeutics

Precautions and Contraindications

All anticoagulants are contraindicated for patients who are hypersensitive to the drug or actively bleeding or who have hemophilia, thrombocytopenia, severe hypertension (HTN), intracranial hemorrhage, infective endocarditis, active tuberculosis, or ulcerative lesions of the GI tract.

Heparins are contraindicated in advanced hepatic or renal disease. They may be used in patients who are actively bleeding to treat disseminated intravascular coagulation (DIC). Heparin is Pregnancy Category C. Although it does not cross the placenta, its use during pregnancy has been associated with unfavorable outcomes, including stillbirth and prematurity. It should be used only when clearly indicated. Safety has not been established in neonates. Some heparin preparations contain benzyl alcohol, which is known to cause "gasping syndrome," a fatal toxicity in neonates. Hyperkalemia may develop, and use for patients with diabetes or renal insufficiency requires care and frequent monitoring of activated partial thromboplastin time (aPTT). Heparin has been associated with fatal medication errors because of the different strengths of preparations available, including a highly concentrated 10,000 units in 1 mL. The Joint Commission has listed anticoagulant therapy as a National Patient Safety Goal requiring each facility to have a plan in place to reduce patient harm (Joint Commission, 2015).

LMWHs are contraindicated for patients with allergies to pork, sulfites, or benzyl alcohol; uncontrolled bleeding; and in patients who have antiplatelet antibodies. Renal impairment requires cautious use and is discussed in the metabolism and excretion section. Body weight less than 50 kg is also associated with markedly increased risk for bleeding; however, it is possible to adjust the dose of enoxaparin for patients who weigh less than 45 kg. Cautious use is also indicated in untreated HTN, retinopathy (hypertensive or diabetic), severe liver disease, recent history of ulcer, or malignancy. LMWH should not be used for thromboprophylaxis in patients with mechanical prosthetic heart valves, especially pregnant women, as prosthetic heart valve thrombosis may occur.

Enoxaparin is Pregnancy Category B. Teratogenicity and fetal death have been reported as well for tinzaparin, although a clear cause-and-effect relationship was not established. Fondaparinux is also listed as Pregnancy Category B but without adequate or well-controlled studies in pregnancy. LMWHs do not cross the placenta and do not cause teratogenicity or fetal bleeding (Bates et al, 2012). The American College of Chest Physicians recommends LMWH as the first-line drug for women who require antithrombotic therapy during pregnancy (Guyatt et al, 2012). The pharmacokinetics of LMWHs are altered during pregnancy. LMWH passes in small amounts into breast milk but has low oral bioavailability and may be safely used during breastfeeding (Bates et al, 2012).

Hepatic dysfunction potentiates the response to warfarin through impaired synthesis of coagulation factors. Hypermetabolic states produced by fever or hyperthyroidism also increase responsiveness to warfarin, probably by increasing the catabolism of vitamin K–dependent coagulation factors. Warfarin should be used cautiously with these patients. Increased risk for bleeding is also an issue with older adults. Cautious use based on a balance between the potential for decreased risk of thromboembolism and the risk for bleeding is necessary for older adults with dementia or severe cognitive impairment; history of three falls within the previous year or recurrent, injurious falls; uncontrolled HTN; or who are nonadherent or unreliable (Sebastian & Tresch, 2000). Warfarin crosses the placenta and can cause hemorrhagic disorders in the fetus and serious birth defects. It is Pregnancy Category X and should not be administered during pregnancy. The Institute for Clinical Improvements ([ICSI], 2010) states that the amount of warfarin in breast milk is too small to affect the baby. Warfarin is considered safe during lactation, because a minimal amount is excreted in breast milk (LactMed, 2010).

Rivaroxaban (Xarelto) was given a Black-Box Warning in August 2013 indicating the premature discontinuation of anticoagulants including rivaroxaban may lead to thrombotic events. An increased risk of stroke is seen in patients with atrial fibrillation when transitioning to warfarin. Rivaroxaban is Pregnancy Category C and is not recommended for use in pregnant women. Apixaban (Eliquis) was given a similar Black Box warning regarding premature discontinuation leading to thrombotic events when it was approved. Although there are no well-controlled studies, apixaban is Pregnancy Category B.

Hypersensitivity to aspirin and cross-sensitivity with NSAIDs may occur, contraindicating the drug. Aspirin hypersensitivity is more prevalent in patients with asthma, nasal polyps, or chronic urticaria. Reye syndrome has been associated with its use in children and teenagers who have influenza or chickenpox. Reversible hepatotoxicity has occurred.

Use aspirin cautiously in patients who have liver damage, preexisting hypoprothrombinemia, or vitamin K deficiency. Aspirin is Pregnancy Category C and Pregnancy Category D in the third trimester. Aspirin should be avoided during lactation, especially in young infants (LactMed, 2010). If a woman is on chronic high-dose aspirin therapy, salicylates levels should be monitored in the infant (LactMed, 2010).

Patients with severe hepatic disease may have bleeding disorders; neither clopidogrel nor ticlopidine is recommended for these patients. They are also not recommended for patients with GI ulcers. Both drugs are Pregnancy Category B. Despite the lack of evidence of teratogenic potential with this drug, it should be used in pregnancy only when clearly indicated. Safety and efficacy in children under age 18 have not been established. Clearance of ticlopidine increases with age, and older adults' increased sensitivity to this drug requires close monitoring for adverse effects. Older adults have increased plasma levels of clopidogrel, but no dosage adjustments are needed. In older adults, clopidogrel is a safer drug. See the discussion in the Metabolism and Excretion sections for more detail. Ticlopidine causes elevations in serum cholesterol (8% to 10%) and triglycerides within 1 month of therapy, and the higher levels persist. The ratios of subfractions of cholesterol remain unchanged. This may be a factor in choosing a drug for patients with dyslipidemias.

Ticagrelor has a Black-Box Warning to not use in a patient with active pathological bleeding or history of intracranial hemorrhage. Ticagrelor should be discontinued 5 days prior to any surgery.

Dabigatran has a Black-Box Warning concerning discontinuation increasing risk of thrombotic events. There is no reversal agent available for dabigatron if excessive bleeding occurs.

Vorapaxar has a Black-Box Warning to not use in patients with a history of stroke, transient ischemic attack (TIA), intracranial hemorrhage, or active pathological bleeding. Vorapaxar is Pregnancy Category B, with no congenital malformations found in animal studies, but no studies conducted in pregnant women. Safety and effectiveness in children has not been established.

Adverse Drug Reactions

All anticoagulants can cause excessive bleeding. Several studies have shown that the incidence of bleeding severe enough to require hospitalization or transfusion is less than 5%. Risk of this complication is higher early in the initiation of therapy, with wide fluctuations in aPTT or international normalized ratio (INR) and in older adults, especially women above age 60. Patients with laboratory studies within the therapeutic range who exhibit this adverse reaction should be evaluated for underlying pathological processes that may be the source of the bleeding before implication of the anticoagulant.

Heparins can also cause thrombocytopenia and anemia. The incidence of thrombocytopenia is up to 30% and is more likely with bovine than with porcine heparin. Early thrombocytopenia occurs 2 to 3 days after initiating therapy, and a delayed form occurs 7 to 12 days after initiation. If the platelet count falls below 100,000/mm^3, the heparin should be discontinued. The antidote for enoxaparin overdose is protamine sulfate 1 mg for each mg of enoxaparin; for dalteparin and tinzaparin, it is 1 mg for each 100 anti-Xa international units (IU) of dalteparin. Both are given by slow IV injection. There is no known antidote for fondaparinux. Because of heparin's short half-life, heparin overdose is usually treated by withdrawal of the drug. If treatment is required, protamine sulfate is also the antidote for heparin overdose.

Toxicity and overdose of warfarin are usually treated by withholding one or more doses. If it must be treated, 1 to 10 mg of vitamin K is the antidote for warfarin overdose with minor bleeding; 5 to 50 mg may be used for frank bleeding.

Hemorrhagic skin necrosis in women and cyanotic toes in men have been observed in patients taking warfarin with therapeutic INR levels (Maddali et al, 2013). The mechanism appears to be related to a transient inhibition in proteins S and C in patients in whom these clotting factors are congenitally absent and in patients with heparin-induced thrombocytopenia (Maddali et al, 2013).

Although rare, allergic reactions do occur with warfarin, they are characterized by symmetrical, maculopapular, erythematous lesions. Some are isolated and some confluent. They tend to occur on the face, neck, and torso. Because of the length of time to therapeutic dose for warfarin, the drug reaction does not occur until the patient has been on the drug for 8 to 10 days.

Bleeding is the major adverse effect of ribaroxaban, with 5.6% of patients experiencing major bleeding during clinical trials. There is no reversal agent for ribaroxaban. Other adverse effects seen more commonly in patients taking ribaroxaban than placebo include back pain (3.7%), upper abdominal pain (1.7%), osteoarthritis (1.7%), dyspepsia (1.3%), and fatigue (1.0%).

The major adverse effect seen with apixaban is bleeding with major bleeding occurring in 2.13% of patients who used it for a year. There is no reversal agent for apixaban.

Aspirin can produce gastric erosions that increase the risk of serious upper GI bleeding. This adverse effect is more likely when it is used in combination with other anticoagulants such as warfarin. Salicylism (tinnitus) associated with the use of aspirin occurs at serum levels above 200 mcg/mL. In addition to tinnitus, indications of aspirin toxicity are headache, hyperventilation, agitation, mental confusion, lethargy, diarrhea, and sweating. Severe toxic effects may occur at levels above 400 mcg/mL that occur with high doses. Such high doses are not used for antiplatelet therapy, so the management of severe toxicity is discussed in Chapter 25, which covers the use of aspirin for anti-inflammatory therapy.

The major adverse effect of ticagrelor is bleeding, with 4.5% of patients experiencing major bleeding in clinical trials and 2.1% experiencing life-threatening bleeding. Dyspnea is the major nonbleeding-related adverse effect seen with ticagrelor, with 13.8% of patients reporting symptoms. The dyspnea was mild to moderate in intensity and usually resolved with continued use but occasionally required discontinuation of therapy (0.9% of patients). Headache (6.5%), cough (4.9%), dizziness (4.5%), and nausea (4.3%) were other common adverse effects of ticagrelor.

Reversible neutropenia has occurred 3 weeks to 3 months after the initiation of therapy with ticlopidine. Severe neutropenia (less than 450 neutrophils/mm³) or thrombocytopenia (less than 80,000 platelets/mm³) is an indication to discontinue the drug.

Clopidogrel has been evaluated for safety in a very large number of patients and its tolerability is similar to that of aspirin, with approximately the same number of patients withdrawing from treatment because of adverse reactions.

Adverse effects of dabigatran include bleeding, with 16.6% of patients experiencing any bleeding during clinical trials and 3.3% experiencing a major bleed. Gastrointestinal side effects of dabigatran include dyspepsia and gastritis-like symptoms. Angioedema and thrombocytopenia have been reported in post-marketing surveillance of dabigatran (Pradaxa).

Vorapaxar adverse effects measured during clinical trials include bleeding, with 27.5% experiencing any bleeding and 1.3% of study subjects experiencing severe bleeding. GI bleeding was experienced by 4.7% of subjects in clinical trials. Other adverse reactions observed during clinical trials include anemia (5%), depression (2.4% vs 2.1% for placebo) and rashes or eruptions (2.2%).

Drug Interactions

Cephalosporins and penicillins given parenterally have both been associated with coagulopathies, increasing the risk of bleeding when given with heparin. Although not reported for these drugs when they are given orally, there is a theoretical increased risk for bleeding. Second- and third-generation cephalosporins and high doses of penicillins, regardless of route of administration, have also been associated with an increased bleeding risk with warfarin because they inhibit the cyclic interconversion of vitamin K.

Drugs that affect platelet functioning or cause hypoprothrombinemia—including aspirin, NSAIDs, dipyridamole, quinidine, and valproic acid—increase the risk of bleeding when used with any anticoagulant. Others are listed in Table 18-2.

Table 18–2 ▦ Drug Interactions: Selected Anticoagulants and Antiplatelets

Drug	Interacting Drug	Possible Effect	Implications
Anticoagulants			
Dalteparin, Enoxaparin	Salicylates, NSAIDs, dipyridamole sulfinpyrazone, ticlopidine	Increased risk of bleeding	
Fondaparinux, Tinzaparin	Thrombolytics, dextran, clopidogrel, some penicillins Natural products: anise, arnica, chamomile, clove, feverfew, garlic, ginger, ginkgo, and panax ginseng	Increased risk of bleeding Increased risk of bleeding	Avoid concurrent use Some are used as spices in cooking. Warn patients about this interaction and to avoid their concurrent use.
Heparin	Cephalosporins and penicillins	Altered platelet aggregation and other coagulopathies with increased risk of bleeding	Mainly related to parenteral administration of these drugs; close monitoring required regardless of route of administration if used concurrently
	Nitroglycerin	Effect of heparin may be decreased	Reports are conflicting; monitor drug effects closely
	Platelet inhibitors: aspirin, salicylates, NSAIDs, dipyridamole, hydroxychloroquine, phenylbutazone, ticlopidine	Increased risk of bleeding	Avoid concurrent use
	Digitalis, tetracycline, nicotine, antihistamines	May partially counteract anticoagulant action	Avoid concurrent use
Warfarin	Alcohol (if concomitant liver disease), amiodarone, anabolic steroids, cimetidine, clofibrate, cotrimoxazole, erythromycin, fluconazole, isoniazid, metronidazole, omeprazole, phenylbutazone, piroxicam, propafenone, propranolol, sulfinpyrazone, citalopram, entacapone, sertraline, zileuton,	Evidence indicates it is highly probable that these drugs potentiate action with increased risk of bleeding	Avoid concurrent use; if necessary, dosage adjustment of warfarin may be required. Draw INR within 4–7 d of starting concerning drug.
	Food/supplement: fish oil, mango		

Continued

Table 18–2 ▓▓ Drug Interactions: Selected Anticoagulants and Antiplatelets—cont'd

Drug	Interacting Drug	Possible Effect	Implications
	Acetaminophen, chloral hydrate, ciprofloxacin, celecoxib, disulfiram, itraconazole, quinidine, phenytoin, tamoxifen, pachitaxel, tolterodine, tetracycline, amoxicillin/clavulanate, azithromycin, levofloxacin, ritonavir, simvastatin, ropinirole, interferon, tramadol Food: grapefruit	Evidence indicates these drugs probably potentiate action with increased risk of bleeding	Close monitoring of INR. Draw INR within 4–7 d of starting drug with possible interaction.
	Herbal supplements: dashen, dong quai, lycium barbarum, PC-SPES		
	Aspirin	Increases risk of bleeding with higher doses; even low doses of aspirin (100 mg/d) have been associated with increased risk of minor bleeding	Avoid concurrent use
	Oral contraceptives Barbiturates, carbamazepine, chlordiazepoxide, cholestyramine, dicloxacillin, griseofulvin, nafcillin, rifampin, flu vaccine Foods: foods high in vitamin K,* large amounts of avocado, soy milk Herbs: ginseng	May decrease the anticoagulant effect Inhibits anticoagulant action	Use other birth control method Avoid concurrent use of drugs. Maintain stable intake of foods high in vitamin K so that diet is balanced.
Dabigatran	Rifampin P-gp inhibitors ketoconazole, amiodarone, verapamil, and quinidine	Decreased dabigatran levels Increased dabigatran levels	Avoid concurrent use If renal function normal, no dosage adjustment needed. The concomitant use of P-gp inhibitors in patients with severe renal impairment (CrCl 15–30 mL/min) should be avoided.
	Platelet inhibitors: aspirin, salicylates, NSAIDs, dipyridamole, hydroxychloroquine, phenylbutazone, ticlopidine Heparin	Increased risk of bleeding Increased risk of bleeding	
Apixaban	Dual inhibitors of CYP3A4 andP-gp (ketoconazole, itraconazole, ritonavir, clarithromycin)	Increased bleeding risk	Decrease apixaban dose by 50%
	Strong dual inducers of CYP3A4 and P-gp (rifampin, carbamazepine, pheyntoin, St. John's Wort)	Decreased apixaban and increased risk of stroke and other thrombotic events	Avoid concomitant use
Antiplatelets			
Clopidogrel	Platelet inhibitors: aspirin, NSAIDs, dipyridamole, ticlopidine Anticoagulants: heparin and warfarin	Increased risk of bleeding	Avoid concurrent use except with aspirin in selected cases (see ACCP recommendations)
	Proton pump inhibitors Cimetidine, esomeprazole, fluoxetine, fluconazole, ketoconazole	Significant interaction that lowers antiplatelet effect of clopidogrel due to competitive inhibition of CYP2C19	The FDA recommends PPIs and other drugs that inhibit CYP2C19 be avoided in patients taking clopidogrel
	Phenytoin, tolbutamide, tamoxifen, torsemide, fluvastatin, and NSAIDs Natural products: see LMWHs above	May decrease metabolism and increase effects of interacting drugs	With high doses and based on data related to CYP450 2C9 inhibition. No data to predict level of interaction. Use with caution.
Ticagrelor	Strong CYP3A inhibitors (e.g., ketoconazole, itraconazole, and clarithromycin)	Increased ticagrelor exposure	
	CYP3A inducers (e.g., rifampin)	Substantially reduces ticagrelor blood levels	
	P-gp inhibitors (e.g., cyclosporine)	Increase ticagrelor exposure	

Table 18–2 ⊞ Drug Interactions: Selected Anticoagulants and Antiplatelets—cont'd

Drug	Interacting Drug	Possible Effect	Implications
Ticlopidine	Platelet inhibitors: aspirin, NSAIDs, dipyridamole, clopidogrel Anticoagulants: heparin, LMWHs, and warfarin	Increased risk of bleeding	Avoid concurrent use
	Antacids	Concurrent administration results in 18% decrease in ticlopidine plasma levels	Separate drug administration; give ticlopidine first and antacids 1 h later
	Cimetidine	Chronic use of cimetidine reduced ticlopidine clearance by 50%	Use different histamine₂ blocker if reducing gastric acid is required
	Digoxin	Digoxin plasma levels decreased 15%	Avoid concurrent use
	Phenytoin	Elevated phenytoin plasma levels associated with somnolence and lethargy	Use with caution and remeasure phenytoin levels
	Theophylline	Significantly increased theophylline elimination half-life with comparable reduction in total plasma clearance	Avoid concurrent use
Rivaroxaban	Combined P-gp and strong CYP3A4 inhibitors (e.g., ketoconazole, itraconazole, lopinavir/ritonavir, ritonavir, indinavir/ritonavir, and conivaptan)	Increases in rivaroxaban exposure and pharmacodynamic effects	Avoid concomitant use
	Combined P-gp and strong CYP3A4 inducers (e.g., carbamazepine, phenytoin, rifampin, St. John's wort)	Decreased rivaroxaban exposure by up to 50%	Avoid concomitant use

*Foods high in vitamin K: asparagus, beans, broccoli, Brussels sprouts, cabbage, cauliflower, cheese, collards, fish, milk, mustard greens, pork, rice, spinach, turnips, yogurt.

Heparin and LMWHs have similar drug interactions but also interact with antiplatelets (including NSAIDs) and dextran. Some natural products are also associated with increased risk for bleeding (see Table 18-2). Some of these are used as spices in cooking, and patients should be warned about their use. Clopidogrel has increased risk for bleeding from this same group of natural products.

Warfarin has many drug interactions and increased INR monitoring (within 4 to 7 days) is recommended when other drugs are started or stopped, even short-term drugs such as antibiotics. Vitamin K has an antagonistic interaction with warfarin, decreasing warfarin's effectiveness. Inhibitors of CYP 1A2, 2C9, or 3A4 isoenzymes increase the effect of warfarin. Inhibitors of CYP 1A2, 2C9, or 3A4 decrease the effectiveness of warfarin. Drugs inducing and inhibiting warfarin are shown in Table 18-2. Warfarin interacts with any other drug that increases bleeding, including anticoagulants, antiplatelets, NSAIDs, and SSRIs. Antibiotics and antifungals may affect INR levels in patients taking warfarin. Herbal products that may increase bleeding include ginkgo biloba, and garlic. Herbal therapies that may decrease effectiveness of warfarin include St. John's wort, ginseng, and coenzyme Q10. Herbal therapies and foods that may influence the metabolism of warfarin include St. John's wort, echinacea, ginkgo, goldenseal, and grapefruit juice.

Rifampin interacts with dabigatran, leading to decreased levels of dabigatran (66% of expected). Dronedarone increases

dabigatran levels by 70% to 150%. The calcium channel blocker verapamil increases dabigatran levels with levels dependent on verapamil dose and time of administration. Amiodarone increases dabigatran levels by 50% and clopidogrel increases dibigatran levels by 40%.

Ticagrelor is metabolized by CYP3A4; therefore, use of strong inhibitors of CYP3A should be avoided, including ketoconazole, itraconazole, voriconazole, clarithromycin, nefazodone, ritonavir, saquinavir, nelfinavir, indinavir, atazinavir, and telithromycin. Inducers of CYP3A should be avoided, including rifampin, dexamethasone, phenytoin, carbamazepine, and phenobarbital.

Avoid use of vorapaxar with inhibitors of CYP3A, including ketoconazole, itraconazole, posconazole, clarithromycin, nefazodone, ritonavir, saquinavir, nelfinavir, indinavir, boceprevir, telaprevir, telithromycin and conivaptan. Use of strong inducers of CYP3A should also be avoided (rifampin, carbamazepine, St. John's Wort and phenytoin).

Clinical Use and Dosing

Prevention and Treatment of Thromboembolism

Warfarin is the drug of choice for the prevention of venous thrombosis, systemic thrombosis, and pulmonary embolism. For prevention, warfarin should be given in a dose sufficient to maintain an INR between 2 and 3 (Guyatt et al, 2012). The beginning dose is 10 mg daily for the first 2 days, with a recheck of INR in two to three doses (Guyatt et al, 2012).

The ICSI antithrombotic guidelines recommend starting warfarin at 5 mg per day with a range of 2.5 mg to 7.5 mg daily (Maddali et al, 2013). Further dosing is based on INR ICSI recommends lower initiation doses be considered for patients with any of the following (Maddali et al, 2013):

- Older than 75 years
- Multiple comorbid conditions
- Poor nutrition (low albumin)
- Elevated INR when off warfarin
- Elevated liver function tests
- Changing thyroid status

If the INR is greater than 2 after the first three doses, consider decreasing the dose by one-half. If INR rises rapidly, search for reasons, such as drug interactions, poor nutritional status, infection, or systemic disease process. Monitoring is discussed later.

Patients with acute pulmonary emboli (PE), DVT, or acute systemic embolization are admitted to the hospital for parenteral anticoagulation therapy with heparin, LMWH, or SC fondaparinux and then placed on oral anticoagulation. If PE is highly suspected, the American College of Chest Physicians (ACCP) recommends treatment with anticoagulants while awaiting diagnostic tests. In patients with acute PE, initial treatment is heparin, LMWH, or fondaparinux for at least 5 days and until INR is greater than or equal to 2.0 for at least 24 hours (Guyatt et al, 2012). The ACCP recommends starting warfarin on the first day of treatment in conjunction with heparin, LMWH, or fondaparinux, with LMWH and fondaparinux favored over IV or SX heparin (Guyatt et al, 2012). Treatment for PE due to a transient (reversible) risk factor is warfarin for 3 months (Guyatt et al, 2012).

Superficial Vein Thrombosis

The ACCP recommends 45 days of prophylaxis with fondaparinux or LMWH in patients with superficial vein thrombosis of the lower limb of at least 5 cm in length (Guyatt et al, 2012). The ACCP recommends fondaparinux 2.5 mg daily over prophylactic LMWH.

Deep Vein Thrombosis

The ACCP divides the treatment of acute DVT into acute treatment of DVT of the leg and treatment of upper extremity DVT. The initial treatment of acute DVT of the leg or upper extremity is short-term treatment with SC LMWHs, SC fondaparinux, or IV or SC heparin for at least 5 days and until the INR is 2.0 for at least 24 hours (Guyatt et al, 2012). LMWH and SC fondaparinux are preferred over heparin (Guyatt et al, 2012). Warfarin should be initiated on the first treatment day, as for PE. For a patient with an idiopathic DVT, the patient is maintained on warfarin with a target of 2.5 (range 2.0 to 3.0) for 3 months (Guyatt et al, 2012).

Patients with an indwelling central line catheter are at risk for developing a DVT. In most patients with an indwelling central venous catheter, the catheter is not removed if it is functional and is needed for therapy (i.e., chemotherapy). Treatment is the same as for leg DVT. If the catheter is removed, the patient should still receive at least 3 months of anticoagulant therapy (Guyatt et al, 2012).

All other patients requiring anticoagulant therapy can be safely started on warfarin as outpatients. Therapy is initiated with 10 mg daily (ACCP Guidelines) or 5 mg daily (ICHI Guidelines) unless the patient weighs less than 110 lb, is over age 75, or is at increased risk of bleeding. Patients with these weight, age, and risk parameters are started on 2.5 mg daily. Steady state is achieved in 5 to 7 days, at which time dosage adjustments are made, based on INR laboratory results. The goal of therapy is an INR of 2 to 3 for all treatment durations. Therapy is usually continued for 3 months for patients with a transient (reversible) DVT risk factor. Although not in the ACCP guidelines, the dose of apixaban to treat DVT and PE is 10 mg twice daily for 7 days then 5 mg twice daily. The maintenance dose of apixaban to reduce the risk of further DVT and PE is 2.5 mg twice daily.

For patients with DVT or PE and cancer, the ACCP guideline recommends LMWH for the first 3 to 6 months of long-term anticoagulant therapy (Guyatt et al, 2012). Patients who have coagulopathies should be referred for management.

Air travel time longer than 8 hours places patients at risk of developing a DVT. The ACCP (Guyatt et al, 2012) recommends the following measures to prevent thrombus formation: wearing loose clothing, avoiding tight clothing around the waistline or lower extremities, achieving good hydration, and performing frequent calf muscle exercises. If patients have a high risk of developing a DVT, the ACCP recommends that they wear compression stockings providing 15 to 30 mm Hg of pressure during air travel. For all patients, the ACCP stresses that immobility (bedrest) is counterproductive. They recommend ambulation as tolerated and the use of elastic compression stockings with a pressure of 30 to 40 mm Hg at the ankle for 2 years after an episode of DVT.

Dosage recommendations for anticoagulants are given in Table 18-3.

Prevention of Embolic Stroke in Atrial Fibrillation

Atrial fibrillation (AF) is a common cardiac arrhythmia, with up to 1 in 4 persons experiencing AF during their lifetime. The turbulence associated with AF places the patient at risk for stroke if not on antithrombotic therapy. For patients at low risk of stroke or with a $CHADS_2$ (congestive heart failure, hypertension, age equal to or greater than 75 years, diabetes mellitus, prior stroke or TIA or thromboembolism) score of 0, the ACCP guidelines recommend no therapy. If a patient chooses antithrombotic therapy, then aspirin dosed at 75 mg to 325 mg daily is prescribed (You et al, 2012). Patients with intermediate risk of stroke (a $CHADS_2$ score of 1) should be treated with oral anticoagulation therapy. If intermediate-risk patients refuse to take anticoagulants, a combination of aspirin (75 mg to 325 mg once daily) and clopidrogrel (You et al, 2012) may be prescribed. Patients at high risk of stroke ($CHADS_2$ score of 2 or greater) require oral anticoagulation therapy. The 2012 ACCP guidelines recommend 150 mg of dabigatran twice daily as the anticoagulant therapy of choice rather than warfarin (You et al, 2012). For patients with persistent or paroxysmal AF at high risk for stroke, the recommendation is warfarin with a target INR between 2 and 3. For patients with AF and mitral stenosis, the recommendations

Table 18–3 ⊗ Dosage Schedule: Selected Anticoagulants and Antiplatelets

Drug	Indication	Dosage Form	Initial Dose	Maintenance Dose
Aspirin	MI and stroke prevention	81 mg chewable (orange flavor) 81 mg tablet 165 mg enteric-coated 325 mg tablet	75–325 mg daily	75–325 mg daily
Clopidogrel (Plavix)	Prevention of new ischemic event (CVA or MI) in patients with recent CVA, MI, or established PAD	75 mg tablets	75 mg once (may need 150 mg in some patients)	75 mg daily
	Acute coronary syndromes		300 mg once	75 mg daily. Aspirin 75–325 mg given concurrently
Dalteparin* (Fragmin)	Prevention of DVT after abdominal surgery	2,500, 5,000, 7,500, 10,000, 12,500, 15,000, or 18,000 anti-factor Xa international units (IU)	2,500–5,000 IU on day of surgery	2,500–5,000 IU daily for 5–10 d post-operatively
	Hip replacement		2,500 2 h pre-op	2,500 IU evening post-op, then 5,000 IU daily for 5–9 d
Enoxaparin* (Lovenox)	DVT and/or PE	Prefilled syringes: 30 mg/0.3 mL 40 mg/0.4 mL 60 mg/0.6 mL 80 mg/0.8 mL 100 mg/1 mL	1 mg/kg q 12 h	Transition to warfarin
	Hip replacement and knee replacement		30 mg 12–24 h post-op or 40 mg 12 h pre-op	or 40 mg daily for 3 weeks
	Abdominal surgery		40 mg 2 h pre-op	40 mg daily for 7–10 d
Fondaparinux† (Arixtra)	Hip-fracture surgery and hip or knee replacement	2.5 mg in 0.5 mL single-dose prefilled syringe with needle	2.5 mg 6–8 h after surgery	2.5 mg for 24 d following hip-fracture surgery or 5–9 d for hip or knee replacement
	Therapy for DVT		Patients <50 kg: 5.0 mg daily Patients 50–100 kg: 7.5 mg daily Patients >100 kg: 10 mg daily	Continue same dose
Heparin	Preventive of post-operative thromboembolism	In multidose vials: 1,000 U/mL 5,000 U/mL 10,000 U/mL	5,000 IU 2 h pre-op	5,000 U q 8–12 h for 7 d after surgery
Ticlopidine (Ticlid)	Preventive of stroke in patients intolerant of aspirin	250 mg tablets	250 mg bid with food	250 mg bid with food
Tinzaparin* (Innohep)	DVT and/or PE	20,000 U/mL in 2 mL multidose vials	175 anti-Xa IU/kg	175 anti-Xa IU/kg daily for 6 d with transition to warfarin
Warfarin (Coumadin)	Prevention and treatment of venous thrombosis, systemic embolism, and pulmonary embolism; prevention of embolic stroke in atrial fibrillation	Scored tablets: 1 mg pink 2 mg lavender 2.5 mg green 3 mg tan 4 mg blue 5 mg peach 6 mg teal 7.5 mg yellow 10 mg white	5 mg–10 mg daily; for patients <50 kg; >age 75, or at increased risk of bleeding: 2.5 mg daily	Measure INR at 5–7 d and adjust to INR of 2–3

Continued

Table 18–3 ⚗ **Dosage Schedule: Selected Anticoagulants and Antiplatelets—cont'd**

Drug	Indication	Dosage Form	Initial Dose	Maintenance Dose
	Recurrent systemic embolism and mechanical heart valves			Measure INR at 5–7 d and adjust to INR of 3 (2.5–3.5)
	Total hip replacement or hip-fracture surgery*		5 mg daily for patients <110 lb; >age 75, or at increased risk of bleeding: 2.5 mg daily	Measure INR at 5–7 d and adjust to INR of 2–3
Dabigatran* (Pradaxa)	Reduce the risk of stroke and systemic embolism in patients with non-valvular atrial fibrillation	150 mg capsule	150 mg bid Severe renal impairment (CrCl 15–30 mL/min): 75 mg twice daily	
Ticagrelor (Brilinta)	Acute coronary syndrome	90 mg tablet	180 mg (two 90 mg tablets) loading dose	
Vorapaxar (Zontivity)	Reduction of thrombotic cardiovascular events in patients with a history of myocardial infarction or with peripheral arterial disease	Tablet: 2.08 mg	One tablet daily	
Apixaban (Eliquis)	Reduction of risk of stroke and systemic embolism in non-valvular atrial fibrillation.	2.5 mg, 5 mg tablet	5 mg bid	5 mg bid
	prophylaxis of DVT following knee replacement surgery		2.5 mg twice daily	
	Treatment of DVT and PE		10 mg bid for 7 days, followed by 5 mg bid	2.5 mg bid

*Doses reduced for severe renal impairment (Ccr <30 mL/min). Only outpatient indications are covered.
†Recommendation of the American College of Chest Physicians. The ACCP also states that low-molecular-weight heparin may be used for hip-fracture surgery, ischemic stroke with paralysis of lower extremities, and medical patients with clinical risk factors. Specific doses are not given for these indications, but fixed dose bid started post-operatively is recommended for surgical patients.

follow those for patients at high risk. If the valvular heart disease has resulted in valve replacement, the recommendations follow those for patients with heart valves, regardless of the presence or absence of AF.

Apixaban dose to reduce risk of stroke and systemic embolism in nonvalvular atrial fibrillation is 5 mg orally twice daily. Patients who are older than age 80 years, weigh less than 60 kg, or have serum creatinine greater than 1.5 mg/dL should be dosed at 2.5 mg twice daily.

Mitral Valve Disease

For patients with rheumatic mitral valve disease but no AF and a left atrial diameter of less than 55 mm, the ACCP recommends no antithrombotic therapy (Guyatt et al, 2012). Patients with rheumatic mitral valve disease with a left atrial diameter of greater than 55 mm or left atrial thrombus or atrial fibrillation or previous embolism are all managed with warfarin to a target INR of 2.5 (range 2.0 to 3.0). Therapy is continued indefinitely in all these cases.

Antithrombotic Therapy for Ischemic Stroke

The ACCP recommendation for patients with an acute ischemic stroke or transient ischemic attack (TIA) is early (within 48 hours) aspirin therapy at a dose of 160 to 325 mg; with aspirin preferred over parenteral anticoagulant therapy

(Guyatt et al, 2012). ACCP recommends three options for long-term therapy after a noncardioembolic ischemic stroke or TIA: 75 to 100 mg aspirin daily, the combination of aspirin (25 mg) and extended-release dipyridamole (200 mg bid), 75 mg clopidogrel daily, or 100 mg cilostazol twice daily (Guyatt et al, 2012). The ACCP guidelines recommend the combination of aspirin and extended-release dipyridamole or clopidogrel over aspirin alone be used as preventive therapy for TIA or stroke. Patients with a history of ischemic stroke or TIA with AF should be prescribed anticoagulants with 150 mg dabigatran twice daily preferred over warfarin in these patients (Guyatt et al, 2012).

Recurrent Embolism or Prosthetic Heart Valves

Warfarin is the drug of choice for patients with recurrent embolism or a prosthetic heart valve. Therapy is initiated and maintained the same as for prevention of venous thrombosis, except that the target INR depends on the type of valve. The targets are shown in Table 18-4. Of note, for patients who have mechanical valves and additional risk factors such as AF, myocardial infarction (MI), left atrial enlargement, endocardial damage, and low ejection fraction, 75 to 100 mg/day of aspirin should be added to their warfarin protocol. The same is true for patients with caged ball or caged disc valves. Long-term management of patients with bioprosthetic valves who are in sinus

Table 18–4 Recommended INR Values Based on Reason for Warfarin Use

Reason for Use	INR range
Prevention of DVT, pulmonary embolism, or systemic embolism	2.0–3.0
Prevention of embolic stroke in patients with atrial fibrillation	2.0–3.0
Patients with St. Jude Medical bileaflet prosthetic heart valve	2.0–3.0
Patients with tilting disk valves and bileaflet prosthetic heart valves in aortic position	2.5–3.5
Patients with CarboMedics bileaflet valve or Medtronic Hall tilting disk prosthetic heart valve	2.0–3.0
Patients with mechanical valves and high risk (e.g., atrial thrombus, AF, hypercoagulable state, low ejection fraction)*	2.5–3.5
Patients with caged ball or caged disk prosthetic heart valves*	2.5–3.5
Patients with bioprosthetic valve in mitral position	2.0–3.0
Patients with bioprosthetic valve in aortic position	2.0–3.0

*In addition to warfarin, these patients should also receive aspirin 75–100 mg/d.

rhythm may be managed on 75 to 100 mg/day of aspirin alone (Guyatt et al, 2012). Therapy is continued indefinitely for mechanical heart valves. For systemic embolization that recurs after 6 months of therapy, therapy is usually continued for an additional 12 months.

Pregnant patients with a mechanical heart valve require anticoagulant therapy that places the fetus and mother at lowest risk of complications. The ACCP guidelines for use of anticoagulants in pregnancy recommend women with a mechanical heart valve be treated with one of three regimens: (1) LMWH twice daily during pregnancy; (2) SC heparin every 12 hours; or (3) SX heparin or LMWH until the 13th week of pregnancy, then warfarin until close to delivery when LMWH or heparin is resumed (Bates et al, 2013). Warfarin is a known teratogen and may cause fetal hemorrhage, whereas heparin and LMWH do not cross the placenta and therefore do not cause teratogenicity or fetal bleeding, though bleeding at the uteroplacental junction is possible (Maddali et al, 2013). Women with mechanical heart valves at high risk of thromboembolism should have low-dose aspirin (75 to 100 mg daily) added to the anticoagulant regimen (Bates et al, 2012). Women on warfarin who are planning a pregnancy should have frequent pregnancy tests and substitution of heparin or LMWH when pregnancy is achieved (Bates et al, 2012). Despite the ACCP presenting guidelines for the use of thrombotic agents during pregnancy, in general, pregnant patients with prosthetic heart valves should be managed by an anticoagulation specialist and perinatologist (Bates et al, 2012).

Prevention of Myocardial Infarction

Results of clinical trials have shown that several protocols are effective in prevention of MI in patients with and without chronic coronary artery disease. The ACCP presents a number of options for treatment in its guidelines (Guyatt et al, 2012). Patients over age 50 without symptomatic cardiovascular disease should be prescribed low-dose aspirin therapy (75 to 100 mg daily). Patients with established coronary artery disease, including those with 1-year post-acute coronary syndrome, with prior revascularization, coronary stenoses greater than 50% by coronary angiogram, and/or evidence for cardiac

ischemia on diagnostic testing, may be treated with aspirin (75 to 100 mg/day) or clopidogrel (75 mg/day) (Vandvik et al, 2012). Patients with acute coronary syndrome who have undergone percutaneous coronary intervention (PCI) with or without stent placement should be placed on dual antiplatelet therapy with 90 mg ticagrelor twice daily plus 75 to 100 mg aspirin daily (Vandvik et al, 2012). Clopidogrel 75 mg and low-dose aspirin may be used for patients who have undergone PCI, but the ACCP guidelines recommend the use of ticagrelor over clopidogrel (Vandvik et al, 2012).

Patients who have already experienced an acute MI (AMI) also need to be maintained on anticlot therapy. Patients who have AMI with ST-segment elevation (STEMI) are often treated acutely with fibrinolytics, then with ongoing therapy after hospital discharge. A number of options are available for post-AMI treatment. Patients with anterior AMI with risk for left ventricular thrombus (ejection fraction less than 40% or anteroapical wall motion abnormality) who do not get a stent are treated with warfarin (INR target 2.0 to 3.0) and 75 to 100 mg aspirin daily (Vandvik et al, 2012). Patients with an acute MI who have a bare-metal stent placed are treated with triple therapy consisting of warfarin (INR target 2.0 to 3.0), low-dose aspirin and 75 mg daily clopidogrel for a month after stent placement, then warfarin and one antiplatelet drug for months 2 and 3 after stent placement (Vandivik et al, 2012). After 3 months, warfarin can be discontinued and replaced with dual antiplatelet therapy (90 mg ticagrelor twice daily plus 75 to 100 mg aspirin daily or 75 mg clopidogrel daily plus low-dose aspirin) for up to 12 months. The appropriate dose of medication for prevention of cardiovascular disease in diabetic patients is not yet clearly determined by evidence. The increased prevalence of cardiovascular morbidity and mortality and disturbances in coagulation in diabetes patients leads to a recommendation of 75 to 162 mg/day aspirin in a joint statement by the American Heart Association, American Diabetes Association, and the American College of Cardiology (Pignone et al, 2010).

Vorapaxar received FDA approval in 2014, after the ACCP guidelines were published. Vorapaxar is approved for reduction of thrombotic cardiovascular events in patients with a history of myocardial infarction or with peripheral arterial disease. The patient takes one 2.08 mg tablet daily in addition to aspirin or clopidogrel.

Prevention of Post-Operative Thromboembolism

All hospitals are required by the Joint Commission to have a formal, active strategy to prevent venous thrombosis. The ACCP recommends the use of LMWH, low-dose heparin, or fondaparinux as thromboprophylaxis in the following surgical procedures: moderate-risk major general surgery, higher-risk patients who are having a major procedure for cancer, major vascular surgery, major gynecological surgery, major urological procedures, bariatric surgery, thoracic surgery, and many orthopedic surgeries (Guyatt et al, 2012). The length of treatment is determined by the type of surgery, ranging from a single dose with minor procedures to 10 days for most orthopedic procedures, to 28 days in high-risk patients, patients undergoing major gynecological surgery, and patients having major surgery for cancer (Guyatt et al, 2012). Apixaban dose following hip or knee replacement surgery is 2.5 mg twice daily.

Perioperative Therapy of Patients on Warfarin or Antiplatelet Therapy

Patients who are having surgery should stop warfarin 5 days before surgery and resume 12 to 24 hours after surgery (Guyatt et al, 2012; Maddali et al, 2013). Patients on warfarin therapy for prevention of thromboembolism (mechanical heart valve, atrial fibrillation) who need an invasive procedure may require parenteral anticoagulation perioperatively. The decision to take a patient off warfarin and "bridge" with heparin is determined by balancing bleeding risk due to the surgical procedure and clotting risk due to the underlying disorder (Maddali et al, 2013). Patients who have procedures with a low bleeding risk (for example, skin biopsies, cataract eye surgery, and most dental procedures) can remain on warfarin. For patients undergoing dental procedures, tranexamic acid mouthwash can be used without interrupting anticoagulant therapy (Maddali et al, 2013). If a patient is at low thromboembolic risk (for example, atrial fibrillation without prior stroke or remote history of venous thrombosis), warfarin may be stopped 5 days prior to surgery and resumed the evening of surgery. If the patient is at high thromboembolic risk (for example, prosthetic heart valves), bridging with a therapeutic dose of LMWH or unfractionated heparin may be indicated (Guyatt et al, 2012).

In the hospital, patients can be placed on IV heparin that can be discontinued 4 to 6 hours before surgery; the SC route is stopped 24 hours before surgery (Guyatt et al, 2012). The ACCP recommends that antiplatelets not be discontinued before surgery, which is a change from previous recommendations to stop antiplatelet therapy a week before surgery (Guyatt et al, 2012).

Rational Drug Selection

Cost

Although SC administration of an anticoagulant (heparin) is usually a short-term measure, cost is still a significant factor. The difference in cost between heparin and the newer LMWHs is significant; the newer drugs are much more expensive. Enoxaparin (Lovenox) is $442 for ten 30 mg syringes ($206 for generic enoxaparin) and fondaparinux (Arixtra) is $905 for ten 2.5 mg syringes, whereas heparin is $26 for a 5 mL vial of 10,000 unit/mL solution, a 10-day supply at 5,000 units per dose. When the cost of laboratory monitoring is factored into the equation, the difference in cost between the LMWHs and regular heparin is less dramatic. Of all the drugs used to prevent clotting, aspirin is by far the cheapest.

Routes of Administration

Oral anticoagulation is preferred because it does not require specialized equipment or skills to administer, and it is less expensive. For patients who cannot swallow or for other reasons cannot take an oral anticoagulant, SC injections of heparin in either standard or low-molecular-weight formulation can be used. Patients or their family members must be taught correct techniques for SC administration.

Brand

Anticoagulant effects may vary slightly by brand. Because even small variances can cause significant differences in anticoagulation, brands should not be interchanged. Warfarin comes in a variety of tablet strengths, making it possible to be exact in dosing, and it is the preferred oral anticoagulant. The tablets are color coded by dose, which also makes it easier to be certain the patient takes the correct dose, especially if the dose is prescribed over the telephone. LMWHs are not interchangeable. There is only one brand name for each, but the patient cannot be changed from one drug to another, as their actions and indications vary. The same is true for the antiplatelets.

Monitoring

Monitoring for dosage adjustments of warfarin is by INR blood tests. Daily INRs are done initially to guard against excessive anticoagulation in unusually sensitive patients and are continued until the therapeutic range is achieved and maintained for at least 2 consecutive days. The testing interval is then lengthened to 2 or 3 times weekly for 1 or 2 weeks, then less often, depending on the stability of the INR results. If the INR results remain stable, testing is reduced to as seldom as every 6 weeks. Drawing the blood in the morning with the patient taking the drug in the evening provides more stable results and allows rapid dosage changes if necessary.

Point-of-care patient self-testing is now possible with a variety of machines. The feasibility and accuracy of patient self-testing at home has been evaluated in several small studies with promising results. Such self-testing with associated self-management provides increased freedom for the patient, especially if they travel. The ACCP guidelines recommend patients who are on warfarin may use self-testing for monitoring INR if the patient can demonstrate competency in using the equipment (Guyatt et al, 2012).

Computer-assisted, validated, decision-support tools for warfarin dose regulation has been shown to be more effective than traditional dosing at maintaining therapeutic INR values (Holbrook et al, 2012). A systematic approach that includes evidence-based dosing tools, patient education, follow-up, and optimal patient communication have the best patient outcomes. Many health systems have anticoagulant clinics that manage patients on anticoagulant therapy, leading to optimal outcomes for the patient.

Protocols for dosage adjustments vary, but to maximize safety and avoid wide swings in anticoagulation, 10% changes in weekly doses are best unless the INR is widely out of range. If the INR is too low, the total weekly dose is adjusted upward by 10% and the INR is rechecked in 2 weeks. If the INR is too high, the daily dose is held for 1 day and then the weekly dose is adjusted downward by 10% and the INR is rechecked in 2 weeks. If the INR is above therapeutic range but less than 5, the patient is not bleeding, and rapid reversal is not indicated for surgical intervention, then one dose can be omitted and daily INRs are drawn. Warfarin is then resumed at a lower dose when the INR is within therapeutic range. If the INR is greater than 4.5 but less than 10 and the patient is not bleeding, routing use of vitamin K is no longer recommended (Holbrook et al, 2012). When INR results are greater than 10 but with no serious bleeding, then 3 to 5 mg of vitamin K may be given orally, anticipating that the INR will fall within 24 to 48 hours. For serious bleeding, vitamin K should be given by slow IV infusion in a dose of 5 to 10 mg, supplemented with four-factor prothrombin complex concentrate (Holbrook et al, 2012). If the INR has frequent variability, external reasons, such as dietary changes, undisclosed drug use, poor adherence, and intermittent alcohol consumption, are evaluated, and the INR is drawn daily or weekly until a stable INR is reached. Once a stable dose is reached, monitoring may be done every 3 months.

Pharmacogenetic testing is not routinely recommended when starting warfarin therapy (Holbrook et al, 2012). If the patient's genotype is known, those with a CYP 2C9 or VKORC1 gene variant may require 2 to 4 weeks longer to reach target INR.

Monitoring for dosage adjustment of heparin is by aPTT blood tests. The goal of therapy is 1.5 to 2.5 times the control. Platelet counts and hematocrit (Hct) are done every 2 or 3 days initially. Thrombocytopenia tends to occur about the fourth day and resolves despite continued heparin therapy. Thrombocytopenia severe enough to require discontinuing therapy may occur about the eighth day of therapy. After this time, periodic testing of platelet and Hct levels and testing for occult blood in the stool are done during the course of heparin therapy regardless of the route of administration. Low doses of SC heparin (5,000 U bid) do not require monitoring because this regimen does not prolong the aPTT.

For the LMWHs, the same periodic monitoring of platelet and Hct levels is required, but the likelihood of thrombocytopenia is much less. The recommended test for monitoring these drugs is anti-factor Xa assay. A standard curve is constructed for each different LMWH preparation. Although the aPTT may be prolonged in patients on LMWH, it does not reliably reflect their activity. In general, routine monitoring of factor Xa is not recommended, except in pregnant patients.

The dose of aspirin for antiplatelet therapy is low to moderate. The serum salicylate level is approximately 100 mcg/mL. At low doses, no specific monitoring is required, although aspirin will prolong bleeding time. Clopidogrel has a safety profile similar to that of aspirin and no routine monitoring is required.

Severe neutropenia and thrombocytopenia have occurred with the administration of ticlopidine. The onset of these problems occurred 3 weeks to 3 months after the start of therapy, with no documented cases beyond that time. It is essential that complete blood counts (CBCs) and white blood cell (WBC) differential counts be performed every 2 weeks, starting from the second week to the end of the third month of therapy. More frequent monitoring is necessary for patients whose absolute neutrophil counts consistently decline or are 30% lower than baseline counts. After the first 3 months of therapy, CBCs are needed only for patients with signs or symptoms suggesting an infection.

Patient Education: Anticoagulants

Administration

Anticoagulants should be taken exactly as prescribed, at the same time each day, even if the patient is feeling well. Missed doses should be taken as soon as remembered the same day. Doses should not be doubled. The health-care provider should be informed of missed doses at the time of checkup or laboratory tests. Doses are highly individualized and are determined by the results of laboratory tests (INR for oral anticoagulants; aPTT, platelet counts, and Hct for heparin; and anti-factor Xa assays for LMWHs). Patients should not change the dose unless directed to do so by the health-care provider and should have the laboratory tests drawn each time they are ordered. If self-testing of INR is warranted, patients should be taught and demonstrate competence in accurately self-monitoring.

Differences in anticoagulation effect can occur between brands. The drug is prescribed by brand name and should be consistently filled that way. Warfarin tablets are color coded by dose, and patients should learn the color code for the brand used. For the heparins, which are injectable, the patient or a family member must be taught correct SC injection technique.

Oral anticoagulants may be taken without regard to timing of food intake. The type of food, however, is important. Ingestion of large quantities of foods high in vitamin K may antagonize the anticoagulant effect. This does not mean that these foods must be avoided entirely. They are part of a well-balanced diet. They should be eaten in consistent amounts so that anticoagulation levels can be maintained at a consistent level. Patients should be given written information regarding vitamin K content of common foods. The U.S. Department of Agriculture (USDA) has an extensive handout on vitamin K content in many common foods that is available on the Internet (www.nal.usda.gov/fnic/foodcomp/Data/SR17/wtrank/sr17w 430.pdf). Some patients may need a nutrition consultation to manage their diet. Drug interactions may also occur with some over-the-counter (OTC) drugs, particularly aspirin, NSAIDs, and cold remedies that contain these products, and with alcohol. Many drugs are also prepared in an alcohol base. Some multivitamins contain vitamin K and should not be taken. The patient should consult with the primary care provider or pharmacist before taking any OTC medications or new prescription medications.

Some natural products, including some used as spices in cooking, have interactions with LMWHs and clopidogrel (see Table 18-2). Patients should be taught to avoid use of these products or to use them in consistent amounts. They should also inform their health-care provider if they use them, because that may affect monitoring test results.

Clopidogrel should not be taken with proton pump inhibitors (PPI), such as OTC omeprazole (Prilosec OTC), because the PPI decreases the effectiveness of the clopidogrel.

Adverse Reactions

Unusual bleeding is the most common adverse effect for all anticoagulants. To prevent bleeding, the patient should use a soft toothbrush, avoid flossing, shave with an electric razor, and if cut, apply pressure for 5 to 10 minutes. If the bleeding does not stop, the patient should continue the pressure and contact the health-care provider. Whenever possible, IM injections should be avoided. If they must be given, apply pressure to the injection site for 2 to 5 minutes to prevent bleeding or hematoma formation. Applying ice to the site of an SC injection for about 30 seconds prior to injecting the heparin reduces the chances of bleeding and hematoma formation. The following should be reported to the health-care provider:

1. Any bleeding that does not stop within 5 minutes
2. Nosebleeds and bleeding gums
3. Red- or pink-tinged urine
4. Faintness or weakness
5. Headaches
6. Stomach pains
7. Skin rash or unusual bruising
8. Red, black, or tarry stools or diarrhea

Warfarin is contraindicated in pregnancy. This topic should be discussed with women who are capable of becoming pregnant, and contraception should be instituted before prescribing this drug.

To reduce the risk of adverse reactions, the patient should wear an identification bracelet that states the anticoagulant being taken. Inform all health-care providers about the anticoagulation therapy so that new prescriptions and any treatments can take it into account. The patient should consult the health-care provider before undergoing dental work or elective surgery.

Patient Education: Antiplatelets

Administration

Daily dosing is the usual way aspirin is taken for antiplatelet effects. Taking it with a full glass of water reduces the risk of the drug dissolving in the esophagus, causing irritation. If aspirin causes GI upset, it should be taken with food or after meals. Enteric-coated forms of aspirin are available and may be better tolerated by some patients. Patients taking enteric-coated aspirin require instruction that tablets should not be crushed or chewed. Aspirin is also available in a buffered form (Bufferin), which is aspirin buffered with calcium carbonate, magnesium carbonate, and magnesium oxide for those who have GI upset. For patients who have difficulty in swallowing, liquid forms are available. Aspirin that has a strong vinegar-like odor should not be used.

Ticlopidine may also cause GI upset and ought to be taken with a full glass of water and with food or after meals.

Adverse Reactions

In some patients toxicity to aspirin may occur even with small doses; they should immediately report to the health-care provider ringing in the ears (tinnitus), unusual headache, hyperventilation, agitation, mental confusion, lethargy, diarrhea, or sweating.

For ticlopidine, a decrease in the number of WBCs can occur, especially during the first 3 months of therapy. A severe decrease can increase risk for infection. Patients should obtain scheduled blood tests to detect reduced WBCs and report to the health-care provider any indications of infection, such as fever, chills, or sore throat. Ticlopidine can also affect liver function. Patients should promptly report severe or persistent diarrhea, skin rashes, yellow skin or sclerae, dark urine, or light-colored stools.

Unusual bleeding is the most common adverse effect of drugs that inhibit platelets, including aspirin, clopidogrel, ticlodipine, and ticagrelor. To prevent bleeding, the patient should use a soft toothbrush, avoid flossing, shave with an electric razor, and if cut, apply pressure for 5 to 10 minutes. They should also inform health-care providers, including dentists, that they are taking these drugs before any surgery or procedure is scheduled or any new drug is prescribed.

HEMATOPOIETIC GROWTH FACTORS

Hematopoietic growth factors are glycoprotein hormones that regulate the proliferation and differentiation of hematopoietic progenitor cells in bone marrow. Produced by recombinant DNA technology, these factors include erythropoietin, granulocyte colony–stimulating factor (G-CSF), granulocyte-macrophage colony–stimulating factor (GM-CSF), and thrombopoietic growth factor. Anemias due to deficiency in erythropoietin, such as those found in patients with end-stage renal disease or AIDS or patients undergoing chemotherapy; infections associated with myelosuppressive chemotherapy, myeloid cancers, and AIDS; and thrombocytopenia associated with all of these are among the most refractory to treatment. The introduction of these growth factors has made effective treatment possible. Erythropoietin is indicated for anemic patients (hemoglobin greater than 10 to less than or equal to 13 g/dL) with normal erythropoietin levels who wish to donate their own blood before high-risk, elective, noncardiac, nonvascular surgery for allogenic transfusions. G-CSF is used for neutropenic patients, particularly those with neutropenia caused by bone marrow transplant and some blood cancers (Sieff, 2012).

Pharmacodynamics

Stem cells in the hematopoietic bone marrow respond to various colony-stimulating factors; megakaryocyte stimulators; and erythropoietin to produce mature WBCs, platelets, and erythrocytes. Erythrocyte differentiation proceeds from erythroblasts through normoblasts to reticulocytes and finally to mature erythrocytes, based on stimulation from erythropoietin, with additional support from GM-CSF and interleukin-3 (IL-3). Granulocytes (neutrophils, eosinophils, and basophils/mast cells) are fully matured in the bone marrow by stimulation from G-CSF, GM-CSF, and IL-3. The agranulocytes (monocytes and lymphocytes) are produced by the stimulation from GM-CSF, IL-3, and macrophage colony–stimulating factor (M-CSF) and are released into the bloodstream before they mature. Monocytes become mature macrophages within 1 or 2 days, and lymphocytes travel to the lymphoid tissues, where they are stimulated to differentiate into T cells or B cells. Platelets develop from megakaryocytes by a unique process of proliferations termed endomitosis. In this process, the megakaryocyte undergoes the nuclear phase of cellular division but fails to undergo the cytoplasmic phase. Without cytokinesis, the cell does not divide into two daughter cells. Rather, the megakaryocyte expands to accommodate the doubling of its DNA content and breaks up into platelets. Optimal numbers of platelets and their precursors in the bone marrow are maintained by the actions of thrombopoietin, GM-CSF, and IL-11 (McCance & Huether, 2010). The development of these blood cells is shown in Figure 18-2 with the controlling factor indicated.

Endogenous erythropoietin is produced by the normal kidney in response to tissue hypoxia. In anemia, more erythropoietin is produced, signaling the bone marrow to produce more erythrocytes. Unless a patient has an iron deficiency, a primary bone marrow disorder, or bone marrow suppression from drugs and chronic disease, this stimulation of erythrocyte production corrects the anemia. In addition to iron, erythropoiesis is dependent on sufficient amounts of vitamin B_{12} and folic acid. In end-stage renal disease, the kidney is unable to produce the erythropoietin necessary for the stimulation of erythrocyte growth. Epoetin alfa (Epogen, Eprex, Procrit) and darbepoetin alfa (Aranesp) have the same biological effects as erythropoietin. Endogenous colony-stimulating factors respond to decreased leukocyte counts or the presence of infection to signal the production of leukocytes. G-CSF is lineage specific, supporting the proliferation and differentiation of neutrophils. GM-CSF is multipotential, stimulating proliferation and differentiation of early and late granulocyte progenitor cells, as well as erythroid and megakaryocyte progenitors. Filgrastim (Neupogen) and pegfilgrastim (Neulasta) have the same biological effects as G-CSF. Sargramostim (Leukine) has the same biological effect as GM-CSF.

Low platelet mass activates thrombopoietin (TPO), a human growth factor, increasing the number of megakaryocytes. IL-11 is a thrombopoietic growth factor that directly stimulates the maturation of megakaryocytes. The biological effects of oprelvekin (Neumega) are the same as those of thrombopoietin and IL-11.

Pharmacokinetics

Absorption and Distribution

All hematopoietic growth factors are well absorbed following SC injection. Some can be given IV. Their distribution is similar to that of their endogenous equivalents (Table 18-5).

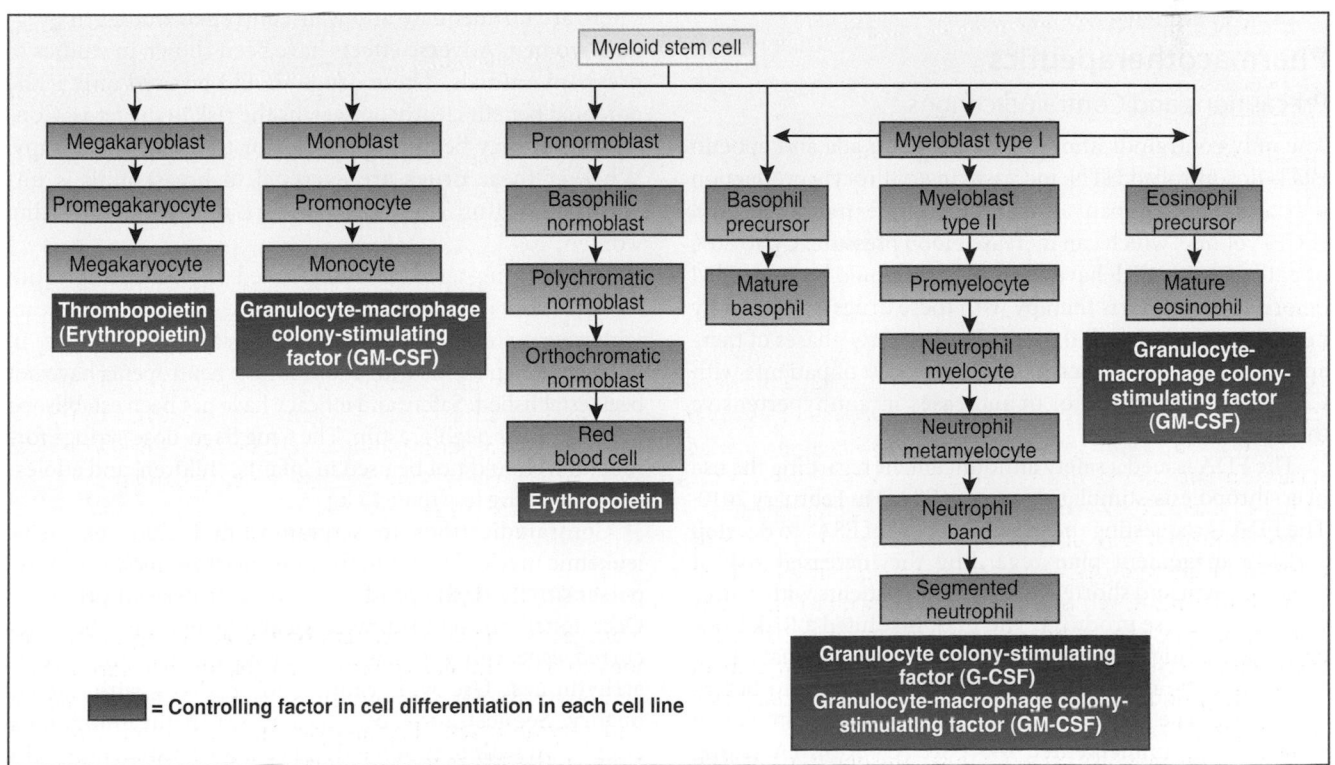

Figure 18–2. Development of blood cells.

Table 18–5 ✂ Pharmacokinetics: Hematopoietic Growth Factors

Drug	Onset	Peak	Duration	Half-Life
Darbepoetin	2–6 wk (increase in reticulocytes)	34–90 h	UK	49 h (SC); 21 h (IV)
Epoetin alfa	7–10 d (increase in reticulocytes)	5–24 h	>24 h	4–13 h in chronic renal failure (about 20% shorter in healthy patients)
Filgrastim	–	2–8 h	–	3.5 h
Oprelvekin	5–9 d (increase in platelets)	3.2 h	7–14 d	6.9 h
Pegfilgrastim	–	2–8 h	–	15–80 h (SC)
Sargramostim	–	1–3 h	12 h	1.6–2.6 h

*Increase in reticulocytes.

Metabolism and Excretion

Darbepoetin alfa has a circulating half-life of about 49 hours post-SC injection. Following IV administration, the serum concentration is biphasic, with a distribution half-life of 1.4 hours and a mean terminal half-life of 21 hours. Epoetin alfa has a circulating half-life of 4 to 13 hours in patients with chronic renal failure (CRF). There is no apparent difference in half-life for patients on or not on dialysis. The half-life is about 20% shorter in healthy patients. Filgrastim has an elimination half-life of 3.5 hours in healthy patients and those with cancer. Oprelvekin has a half-life of 6.9 hours. Pegfilgrastim has a half-life of 15 to 80 hours. Sargramostim has a half-life after SC injection of 2.6 hours. All are eliminated by first-order kinetics. The exact method of metabolism and excretion is unknown in most of these drugs, with some elimination thought to occur in the kidneys.

Pharmacotherapeutics

Precautions and Contraindications

The only contraindication for darbepoetin alfa and epoetin alfa is uncontrolled HTN; increases in erythrocyte production may also be accompanied by increases in extracellular fluid (ECF) volume, which can increase blood pressure. Up to 80% of patients with CRF have HTN, which should be controlled before a patient starts therapy with these drugs and carefully monitored during such therapy. During early phases of therapy, when the Hct is increasing, about 25% of patients with CRF require initiation of or increases in antihypertensive therapy.

The FDA issued a safety announcement regarding the use of erythropoiesis-stimulating agents (ESAs) in February 2010. The FDA is requesting the manufacturers of ESAs to develop a risk-management plan regarding the increased risk of tumor growth and shortened survival in patients with cancer who receive these products. The FDA instituted a Risk Evaluation and Mitigation Strategy (REMS) requiring that all patients have the risk and benefits of ESAs explained before prescribing. The manufacturers of erythropoiesis-stimulating drugs (ESAs) implemented the ESA APPRISE (Assisting Providers and cancer Patients with Risk Information for the Safe use of ESAs) Oncology Program for health-care providers to use to inform patients of the risks associated with ESAs (www.esa-apprise.com).

Darbepoetin and epoetin alfa are Pregnancy Category C. Adverse effects have occurred in rats, and no adequate and well-controlled studies have been conducted in pregnant women. The drugs should be used only if the potential benefit clearly outweighs the risk to the fetus. Contraception may be appropriate prior to initiating therapy. Some women's menses have resumed after therapy with these drugs. Whether the drugs are excreted in breast milk is unknown. Caution is advised in prescribing to lactating women. Safety and efficacy have not been established in children.

The only contraindication for filgrastim and pegfilgrastim is hypersensitivity to *Escherichia coli*–derived proteins because this drug is derived from DNA manipulation of *E. coli.* Filgrastim and pegfilgrastim are Pregnancy Category C. There are no adequate and well-controlled studies in pregnant women. Adverse effects have been shown in studies of pregnant animals. These drugs should be used only if the potential benefit clearly outweighs the risk to the fetus. Contraception may be appropriate prior to initiating therapy. Whether these drugs are excreted in breast milk is unknown. Caution is advised in prescribing to lactating women.

Serious long-term risks associated with daily filgrastim have not been identified in children aged 4 months to 17 years with severe chronic neutropenia. The safety and efficacy in neonates and patients with autoimmune neutropenia have not been established. Safety and efficacy have not been established in children for pegfilgrastim. The 6 mg fixed-dose syringe formulation should not be used in infants, children, and adolescents weighing less than 45 kg.

Contraindications to sargramostim include excessive leukemic myeloid blasts in the bone marrow and known hypersensitivity to the product or to yeast-derived products. Occasional transient supraventricular arrhythmias have occurred, especially with patients who have a history of cardiac arrhythmias. Use with caution for patients with such a history. Sequestration of granulocytes in the pulmonary circulation with occasional dyspnea has occurred, especially in patients with preexisting lung diseases. Administer with caution to patients with hypoxia. Fluid retention has occurred in a few patients. Use with caution for patients with preexisting fluid retention, pulmonary infiltrates, or congestive heart failure.

The only contraindication to oprelvekin is hypersensitivity to that drug. Fluid retention has occurred with this drug and a diuretic may be needed. Use with caution in patients with clinically evident congestive heart failure, patients receiving aggressive hydration, and patients who have a history of heart failure. In clinical trials, atrial arrhythmias occurred in 15% of the patients, especially with patients who have a history of cardiac arrhythmias. The rhythm stopped when the drug was stopped but recurred on rechallenge. This adverse effect may be related to fluid retention. Use with caution for patients with such a history.

Oprelvekin is Pregnancy Category C. Adverse effects were noted in animal studies and there are no adequate, well-controlled studies in pregnant women. Use only if the potential benefit clearly outweighs the risk to the fetus. Contraception may be appropriate prior to initiating therapy. It is not known whether this drug is excreted in breast milk. Caution is advised in prescribing to lactating women.

There are no controlled trials that have established a safe and effective dose of oprelvekin in children. The administration of this drug to children, particularly under age 12, should be reserved for clinical trials with closely monitored safety assessments. Limited data are available from one clinical trial for pediatric patients receiving 50 mcg/kg per day. Adverse effects in this study were the same as for adults. No studies have been done to assess the long-term effects of its use on growth and development. Animal studies have shown bone and joint changes.

Sargramostim is Pregnancy Category C. There are no adequate and well-controlled studies in pregnant women. This drug should be used only if the potential benefit clearly outweighs the risk to the fetus. Contraception may be appropriate prior to initiating therapy. Whether this drug is excreted in breast milk is unknown. Caution is advised in prescribing to lactating women. Safety and efficacy in children have not been established.

Adverse Drug Reactions

Seizures have been observed in some patients being treated with darbepoetin alfa and epoetin alfa (2.5% of patients undergoing dialysis during the first 90 days of therapy). The relationship with seizure is uncertain, and the risk appears to lessen when the rate of increase in Hct is slower. Recommendations are that the dose be decreased if the hemoglobin (Hgb) increase exceeds 1 g/dL in any 2-week period.

The major adverse reaction is HTN. The risk is higher in patients with CRF, and the reaction is discussed in the Precautions and Contraindications section. Both of these drugs may increase the risk for cardiovascular events, especially thrombogenesis. The higher risk has, once again, been associated with rates of rise in Hgb, and the target level of Hgb should be less than 12 g/dL.

As mentioned above, the FDA has issued a safety warning regarding the use of ESAs, and decreased overall survival and/or increased risk of tumor progression has been reported in patients with breast, non–small-cell lung, head and neck, lymphoid, and cervical cancers. The FDA is requiring that all patients have the risk and benefits of ESAs explained to them before the provider prescribes. Updates on the FDA warning can be found at the FDA Web site (www.fda.gov).

Allergic-type reactions have developed with filgrastim on initial and subsequent treatment in fewer than 1 in 4,000 patients. Skin, respiratory, and cardiovascular systems common to most hypersensitivity reactions are typical. Administration of antihistamines, steroids, bronchodilators, or epinephrine resulted in resolution. Symptoms recurred in more than 50% of the patients who were rechallenged with this drug. Such allergic reactions have not occurred in clinical trials of pegfilgrastim. Adult respiratory distress syndrome (ARDS) has been reported in neutropenic patients with sepsis receiving filgrastim and is postulated to be related to an influx of neutrophils to the sites of inflammation in the lungs. Patients receiving pegfilgrastim are also at risk. If ARDS develops, these drugs should be discontinued.

The adverse reactions with oprelvekin were mild to moderate in severity, reversible with discontinuance, and mainly similar to those of placebo groups when the dose was 50 mcg/kg. Tachycardia, edema, dizziness, conjunctival hemorrhage, and neutropenic fever were observed.

Adverse reactions to sargramostim include headache and transient pruritic rashes. Hypersensitivity reactions are rare. Cardiovascular, respiratory, and fluid retention problems are discussed in the Precautions and Contraindications section.

All of the hematopoietic growth factors can produce bone pain from the stimulation of the bone marrow. This may require analgesia.

Drug Interactions

Drug interactions for all the hematopoietic growth factors are minimal (Table 18-6). Only those drugs such as lithium that may potentiate myeloproliferative effects require avoidance of concurrent use or cautious use. There are no drug interactions reported with darbepoetin alfa or oprelvekin.

Clinical Use and Dosing

Anemia Associated With Chronic Renal Failure

Darbepoetin alfa and epoetin alfa are the drugs of choice to elevate and maintain erythrocyte levels and decrease the need for transfusions. Patients both on dialysis and not on dialysis benefit equally. They are not intended for immediate correction of severe anemia because it takes 7 to 10 days to see increases in reticulocyte counts. The starting dose for epoetin alfa is 50 to 100 U/kg given SC 3 times weekly. Maintenance doses are based on individual responses, and adjustments are based on Hct levels. The starting dose for darbepoetin alfa is 0.45 mcg/kg SC once weekly. Dosage adjustments are made no more frequently than once a month, because it takes that long to see increases in blood values. Table 18-7 shows guidelines for dosage adjustments for both drugs. Dosage

Table 18–6 ⠿ **Drug Interactions: Hematopoietic Growth Factors**

Drug	Interacting Drug	Possible Effect	Implications
Epoetin alfa	Heparin	May increase requirement for heparin anticoagulation during dialysis	Monitor aPTT carefully in dialysis patients
Filgrastim	Lithium	May potentiate the release of neutrophils	Drug interaction not fully studied; no recommendations at this time
Pegfilgrastim	Antineoplastic agents	Simultaneous use may have adverse effect on rapidly proliferating neutrophils	Avoid use 24 h before or 24 h after chemotherapy
Sargramostim	Lithium	May potentiate myeloproliferative effects of sargramostim	Avoid concurrent use or use cautiously

Table 18–7 ⠿ **Dosage Schedule: Hematopoietic Growth Factors**

Drug	Indication	Initial Dose	Maintenance Dose
Darbepoetin alfa	Anemia in chronic renal failure	0.45 mcg/kg SC once weekly	Individualized; goal Hgb is 12 g/dL; as goal is approached the dose is reduced by 25%. If Hgb continues to increase, doses are withheld until it begins to drop. Then drug is restarted at a dose about 25% below previous dose. If Hgb increase is <1 g/dL over 4 wk, and iron stores are adequate, dose may be increased by 25%. Further increases made at 4 wk intervals.
	Cancer patients receiving chemotherapy	2.25 mcg/kg SC once weekly	Individualized to target Hgb. If <1 g/dL increase in Hgb after 6 wk of therapy, increase dose to 4.5 mcg/kg. If Hgb exceeds 12 g/dL, reduce dose by 25%. If Hgb exceeds 13 g/dL, withhold dose until Hgb ≤12 g/dL. Restart at dose 25% below previous dose.
Epoetin alfa	Anemia in chronic renal failure	50–100 U/kg 3 times weekly	Individualized; reduced dose when hematocrit (Hct) approaches 36% or increases >4 points in any 2 wk period. Increase dose if Hct does not increase by 5–6 points after 8 wk of therapy and remains below target range of 30%–36%.
	Zidovudine-treated HIV-infected patients	100 U/kg 3 times weekly for 8 wk	Individualized; when the desired response is attained, titrate to maintain it. If response is too low, increase by 50–100 U/kg 3 times weekly. Evaluate response every 4–8 wk and adjust by 50–100 U/kg increments. If response is too low at 300 U/kg, response is unlikely. If Hct exceeds 40%, stop dose until Hct is 36%, then resume treatment with a dose reduced by 25%.
	Cancer patients on chemotherapy	150 U/kg 3 times weekly	If response is too low after 8 wk, increase dose up to 300 U/kg 3 times weekly; higher doses are not likely to produce a response. If Hct exceeds 40%, or increases >4% in any 2 wk period, stop dose until Hct is 36%, then resume treatment with a dose reduced by 25%.
	Presurgery	300 U/kg/d or	Given 10 d prior to surgery, day of surgery, and for 4 d after surgery
		600 U/kg once weekly	Given 21, 14, and 7 d prior to surgery and then day of surgery
Filgrastim	Myelosuppressive chemotherapy	5 mcg/kg/d no earlier than 24 h after or 24 h before next dose of chemotherapy	Dose given daily for up to 2 wk. Discontinue therapy if ANC >10,000 mm³ after expected nadir of chemotherapy
	Severe chronic neutropenia: Congenital cyclic/idiopathic	6 mcg/kg twice daily 5 mcg/kg daily	Individualized; reduce dose if ANC persistently >10,000 mm³
Oprelvekin	Myelosuppressive chemotherapy	50 mcg/kg SC once daily; 6–24 hours after completion of chemotherapy	Continue dosing until the postnadir platelet count is ≥50,000 mcL. Dosing beyond 21 d is not recommended
Pegfilgrastim	Myelosuppressive chemotherapy	Single injection of 6 mg SC administered once per chemotherapy cycle	Do not give between 14 d before and 24 h after administration of cytotoxic chemotherapy

adjustments are not to be made more than once monthly, based on the time it takes for erythroid progenitors to mature and red blood cell (RBC) survival time.

Anemia Related to Zidovudine Therapy

Epoetin alfa is the drug of choice to elevate and maintain erythrocyte levels and decrease the need for transfusions when the endogenous erythropoietin level is 500 mU/mL or less and the dose of zidovudine is 4,200 mg/week or less. The initial dose is 100 U/kg SC 3 times weekly for 8 weeks. Maintenance doses are based on individual responses, and adjustments are based on Hct levels. Table 18-7 shows the general guidelines for dosage adjustments. Dosage adjustments are timed as noted previously.

Anemia in Patients With Cancer on Chemotherapy

Darbepoetin alfa and epoetin alfa are drugs used to elevate and maintain erythrocyte levels and decrease the need for transfusions. The initial dose of darbepoetin is 2.25 mcg/kg SC once weekly for darbepoetin alfa or 500 mcg once every 3 weeks; and of epoetin alfa it is 150 U/kg given SC 3 times weekly or 40,000 U weekly for epoetin alfa. Patients with lower baseline serum erythropoietin levels tend to respond more vigorously to this drug. Treatment is not recommended for patients with serum erythropoietin levels below 200 mU/mL. Dosage adjustments are made after 6 weeks for darbepoetin alfa and after 8 weeks of therapy for epoetin alfa. Table 18-7 shows the general guidelines for dosage adjustments. Dosage adjustments are timed as noted previously.

Decreasing Blood Transfusions in Surgery Patients

Anemic patients (hemoglobin greater than 10 g/dL and less than 13 g/dL) scheduled to undergo elective, noncardiac, nonvascular surgery, with anticipated significant blood loss, benefit from epoetin alfa therapy to reduce the need for allogeneic blood transfusions. The recommended dose is 300 U/kg a day SC for 10 days prior to surgery, on the day of surgery, and for 4 days after surgery. An alternative dosing schedule is 600 U/kg once weekly at 21, 14, and 7 days before surgery, plus a fourth dose on the day of surgery. All patients on these regimens must receive adequate iron supplementation, beginning no later than the start of the epoetin therapy and continuing throughout the therapy. Prophylactic anticoagulant therapy is recommended for patients receiving epoetin alpha perioperatively.

Patients on Myelosuppressive Therapy

Filgrastim, pegfilgrastim, and sargramostim have been used for this indication. It is an off-labeled use for sargramostim. The recommended starting dose for filgrastim is 5 to 10 mcg/kg a day given as a single dose SC. Dosage adjustments are based on CBC and platelet data and are done in increments of 5 mcg/kg per day, according to the duration and severity of the absolute neutrophil count (ANC) nadir. It is given daily for up to 2 weeks until the ANC has reached 10,000 mm³. Clinical trials have shown effective doses to be 4 to 8 mcg/kg a day. Pegfilgrastim is given as a once-only dose of 6 mg beginning 24 to 72 hours after completion of each chemotherapy cycle. Sargramostim is started at least 24 hours after chemotherapy, dosed lower when starting therapy and gradually increased to avoid first-dose reaction (respiratory distress, hypoxia, flushing, syncope, and tachycardia). The initial dose is 125 to 250 mcg/m²/day daily for 21 days.

Severe Chronic Neutropenia

Severe chronic neutropenia (SCN) can be congenital, cyclic, or idiopathic. Chronic administration of filgrastim reduces the incidence and duration of sequelae of neutropenia, such as fever, infection, and oropharyngeal ulcers. The initial dose for congenital SCN is 6 mcg/kg twice daily SC. For cyclic or idiopathic SCN, the initial dose is 5 mcg/kg every day. Dosage adjustments are based on the patient's clinical course and ANC.

Prevention of Severe Thrombocytopenia

Oprelvekin is used for prevention of severe thrombocytopenia and reduced need for platelet transfusion post-myelosuppressive therapy. Adults are prescribed a dose of 50 mcg given as one dose 6 to 24 hours after the completion of chemotherapy and continued on a daily basis until the postnadir platelet count is above 50,000. Dosing duration is between 10 and 21 days and dosing beyond 21 days is not recommended.

Other indications for the use of these drugs, including bone marrow transplant, are beyond the scope of this book.

Rational Drug Selection

The drug choice is based on its indication because each drug has very specific uses.

Monitoring

Monitoring parameters are different for each drug and are discussed specific to that drug.

Darbepoetin Alfa

Hgb levels are determined weekly until they have stabilized and the maintenance dose has been established. After dosage adjustments, weekly Hgb levels are also drawn for at least 4 weeks until it has been determined that the Hgb has stabilized in response to the new dose. Hgb is then monitored at regular intervals. Iron status should also be evaluated before and during treatment, because the majority of patients will require supplemental iron. Supplemental iron is recommended when the serum ferritin is less than 100 mcg/L or the serum transferrin is less than 20%.

Epoetin Alfa

Patients with CRF not on dialysis require monitoring of blood pressure and Hct no less frequently than patients maintained on dialysis. Hct is monitored twice weekly until it is stabilized in the target zone and the maintenance dose has been established and then for at least 2 to 6 weeks after each dosage adjustment. Maintenance monitoring is individualized, based on patient stability. In some patients, increases in blood urea nitrogen (BUN), creatinine, uric acid, phosphorus, and potassium have been noted. These values are routinely monitored in patients with CRF and require no additional monitoring.

Patients on zidovudine therapy for HIV infection require monitoring of Hct weekly until it is stabilized. Periodic monitoring thereafter is based on the progression of the disease.

During therapy with epoetin alfa, absolute and functional iron deficiency may develop. Functional iron deficiency is presumed to be based on inability to mobilize iron stores rapidly enough to support increased erythropoiesis. Transferrin saturation should be at least 20%, and ferritin should be at least 100 mcg/mL. Prior to initiating therapy and at regular intervals during therapy, determine transferrin and ferritin levels. Virtually all patients at some point require supplemental iron. Delayed or diminished responses suggest referral to a hematologist. Possible common etiologies for patients who fail to respond or to maintain a response to doses within the recommended range for both darbepoetin alfa and epoetin alfa include the following:

1. Functional iron deficiency
2. Underlying infectious, inflammatory, or malignant disease
3. Occult blood loss
4. Underlying hematological diseases, such as thalassemia, refractory anemia, or myelodysplastic disorder
5. Vitamin B_{12} or folic acid deficiency
6. Hemolysis
7. Aluminum intoxication

Filgrastim

For patients on myelosuppressive chemotherapy, CBCs and platelet counts are done prior to initiating therapy and twice weekly during therapy. Following therapy, the same indicators are monitored around the time of the nadir of the chemotherapy. Filgrastim or pegfilgrastim therapy may be terminated when the ANC is 10,000 mm³ or greater. For patients with SCN treated with filgrastim, CBCs with differential, platelet counts, and evaluation of bone marrow morphology and karyotype are done prior to initiating therapy. During the initial 4 weeks of therapy and for 2 weeks after any dosage adjustment, CBCs with differential and platelet counts are done. Once the patient is stable, monthly CBCs with differential and platelet counts are sufficient.

For oprelvekin, fluid balance needs to be monitored during dosing. If a diuretic is used, electrolyte balance may also need to be monitored. A CBC is drawn prior to chemotherapy and at regular intervals during therapy to monitor platelet counts. Monitoring continues during the time of expected nadir for the chemotherapy and until platelet counts are 50,000 or higher postnadir.

Patient Education

Administration

If the patient can safely and effectively self-administer these drugs, instruction is provided in correct SC injection technique and proper dosage (Table 18-8). Self-administration is common in patients with CRF. Detailed instructions on dilution and storage stability are included in the package insert.

Adverse Drug Reactions

HTN and allergic reactions are the two most common adverse reactions. Self-monitoring of blood pressure and signs and symptoms of an allergic reaction are taught.

IRON PREPARATIONS

Iron is an essential mineral in the production of Hgb, myoglobin, and a number of enzymes. Iron deficiency anemia results in problems with oxygen transport that affect the energy

Table 18–8 ❀ Available Dosage Forms: Hematopoietic Growth Factors

Drug	Dosage Form	Other Forms	Cost	
Darbepoetin alfa (Aranesp)	Solution for SC injection (in 1 mL single-dose vial): 25, 40, 60, 100, 150, 200, 300, and 500 mcg/mL		25 mcg = $124.69/vial 40 mcg = $199.50/vial 60 mcg = $299.25/vial 100 mcg = $498.75/vial 150 mcg = $748.13/vial 200 mcg = $997.50/vial	
Epoetin alfa (Epogen, Procrit)	Subcutaneous (in 1 mL single-dose vials): 2,000, 3,000, 4,000, 10,000, 20,000, 40,000 U/mL	—	*Epogen* $125.20/vial $269/vial $527.73/vial	*Procrit* $129.69/vial $259/vial $517/vial
Filgrastim (Neupogen)	Subcutaneous (in 1 and 1.6 mL single-dose vials; preservative-free): 300 mcg/mL	—	$202.50/1 mL vial $322.50/1.6 mL vial	
Oprelvekin (Neumega)	Powder for injection (in single-dose vial with diluent): 5 mg		No cost data	
Pegfilgrastim (Neulasta)	Solution for injection (in single-dose syringe with needle): 10 mg/mL		$2,850.56 for 6 mg/0.6 mL	
Sargramostim (Leukine)	Powder for injection (in vials): 250 mcg		No cost data	
	Liquid (in multidose vials): 500 mcg/mL			

metabolism of every cell in the body. Iron deficiency anemia is commonly seen in infants, particularly premature infants; in children during rapid growth periods; and in pregnant and lactating women. It may also occur after gastrectomy and with malabsorption disorders, particularly those of the small bowel. The most common cause in adults is blood loss. Menstruation may cause the loss of more than 30 mg of iron with each period. Occult blood loss may occur from GI bleeding and from cancer. In an attempt to replace blood lost, erythropoiesis may occur at an increased rate and increased iron may be used and drawn from storage. Prevention and treatment of iron deficiency anemia are accomplished by administration of supplemental iron.

Pharmacodynamics

Approximately 67% of total body iron is bound to heme in RBCs and muscle cells, and approximately 30% is stored bound to ferritin or hemosiderin mononuclear phagocytes and hepatic parenchymal cells. The remaining 3% is lost daily

On The Horizon | **INTERLEUKIN-3, STEM CELL FACTOR, AND MONOCYTE-MACROPHAGE COLONY–STIMULATING FACTOR**

IL-3, stem cell factor, and monocyte-macrophage colony–stimulating factor are currently in clinical trials. **IL-3** would provide broad-based therapy because it is involved in the generation and stimulation of all progenitor cells. Stem cell factor would provide therapy at an even earlier stage in blood cell development. Monocyte-macrophage colony–stimulating factor would provide a targeted approach to patients who do not require such a broad stimulation of blood cell growth.

in urine, sweat, bile, and epithelial cells shed from the GI tract. Iron not lost is continuously recycled, as shown in Figure 18-3. Recycling is made possible by transferrin.

As iron deficiency develops, storage iron decreases and then disappears, followed by decreased serum ferritin and then serum iron. Finally, iron-binding capacity increases,

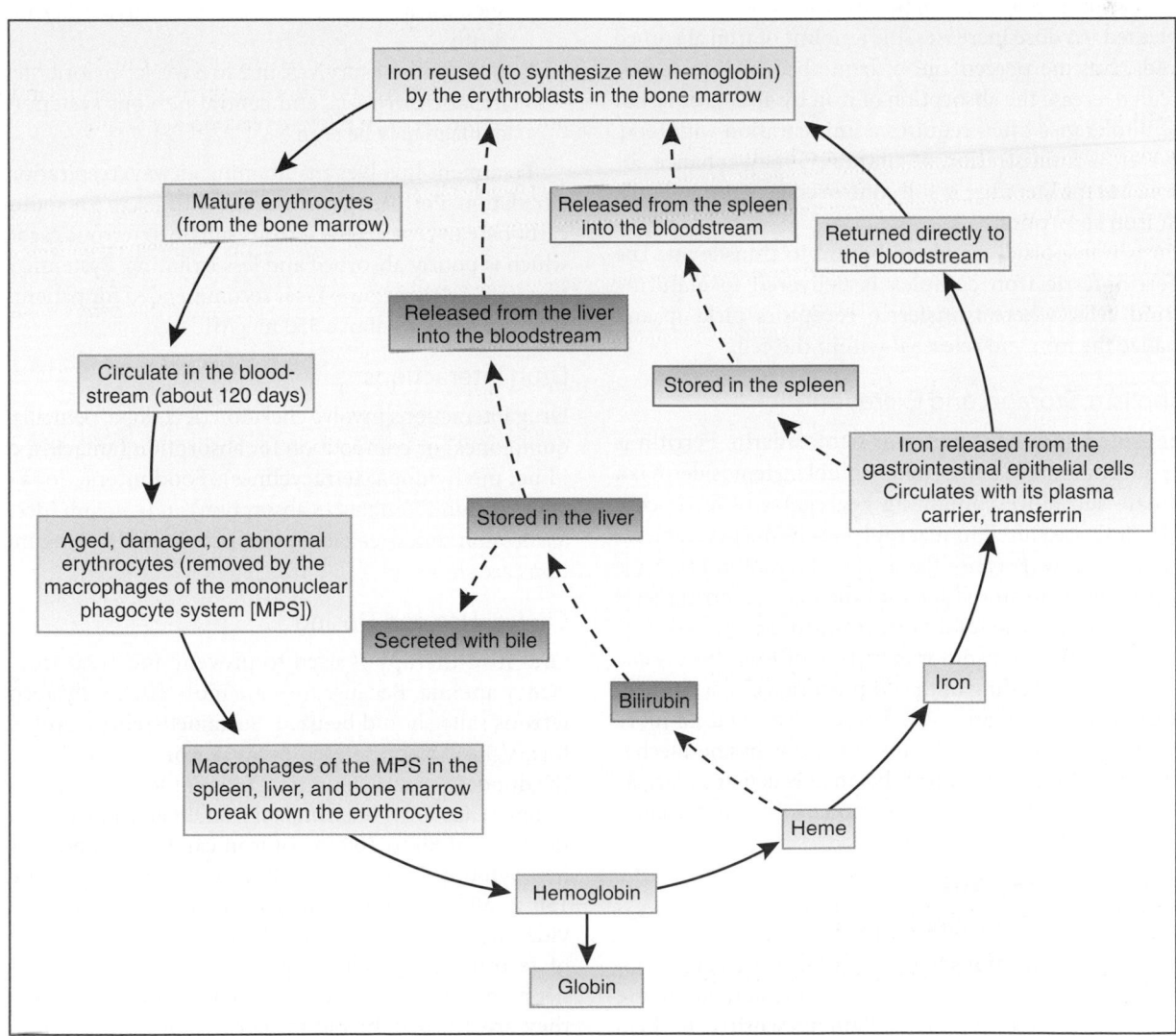

Figure 18–3. The iron cycle.

resulting in a decrease in transferrin saturation. At this point, anemia develops. Administration of iron reverses the process so that eventually not only is serum iron improved but also iron storage is replenished. Management of anemia is discussed in Chapter 27.

Pharmacokinetics

Absorption and Distribution

Only about 10% of the average daily dietary intake of iron is absorbed (1 to 2 mg/day) in patients with adequate iron stores. Absorption is enhanced in the presence of depleted iron stores and when erythropoiesis is increased. Iron is primarily absorbed in the duodenum and upper jejunum by an active transport mechanism. The ferrous form is absorbed 3 times more readily than the ferric form. The common ferrous forms (sulfate, gluconate, and fumarate) are absorbed almost on a milligram-for-milligram basis but differ in the amount of elemental iron each contains.

Factors that significantly affect absorption include sustained-release forms, dose, and the presence of food. Sustained-release or enteric-coated forms have less available iron because they transport the iron beyond the duodenum before it is released. As dose increases, the amount of iron absorbed increases, but the percentage of iron absorbed decreases. Food can decrease the absorption of iron by 40% to 66%, but gastric intolerance often requires administration with food. Concurrent administration of vitamin C may enhance absorption, but the literature is still controversial. Eggs and milk inhibit iron absorption.

Iron is transported via blood bound to transferrin. The transferrin–ferric iron complex is delivered to maturing erythroid cells, where transferrin receptors pick up and internalize the iron and release it within the cell.

Metabolism, Storage, and Excretion

Iron is stored as either ferritin or hemosiderin. Ferritin is more readily available and is water soluble. Hemosiderin is a particulate substance containing aggregates of ferric core crystals. Both are stored in macrophages in the liver, spleen, and bone marrow. Because the ferritin present in plasma is in equilibrium with stored ferritin, the plasma ferritin level can be used to estimate total-body iron stores.

There is no mechanism for excretion of iron. Iron is lost mainly through shedding of the GI mucosal cells, with small losses in urine, sweat, and bile. These losses total no more than 1 mg of iron per day. Because the body has no mechanism for excretion of iron, iron balance is achieved largely through control of the amount of iron absorbed in the gut.

Pharmacotherapeutics

Precautions and Contraindications

The only contraindications to the use of iron are hemochromatosis and hemolytic anemia. Tartrazine and sulfite are found in some iron formulations. Patients sensitive to them should not take these formulations.

Adverse Drug Reactions

GI symptoms are the most common adverse reactions and are usually mild. Irritation, anorexia, nausea and vomiting, constipation, or diarrhea may occur. Administering the iron with food reduces most of these problems. Stools may appear darker in color, which can present a problem in assessing GI bleeding. Iron-containing preparations may cause temporary staining of the teeth. Dilution of the drug reduces this problem.

Acute Toxicity

Acute iron toxicity is seen almost exclusively in children who have ingested many iron tablets. As few as 10 tablets of common oral iron preparations can be lethal in young children. Symptoms of iron toxicity occur in four stages:

1. Within 1 to 6 hours, lethargy, nausea, vomiting, abdominal pain, tarry stools, weak and rapid pulse, hypotension, acidosis, and coma occur.
2. If not immediately fatal, symptoms may subside for about 24 hours.
3. Symptoms return in 12 to 48 hours and may also include diffuse vascular congestion, pulmonary edema, shock, acidosis, convulsions, anuria, hyperthermia, and death.
4. If the patient survives, in 2 to 6 weeks, pyloric stenosis, hepatic cirrhosis, and central nervous system (CNS) damage may be seen.

Treatment involves maintaining airway, respiration, and circulation. Perform gastric lavage with 1% to 5% sodium bicarbonate to convert the ferrous sulfate to ferrous carbonate, which is poorly absorbed and less irritating. Systemic chelation with deferoxamine IM is recommended for patients with serum iron levels above 350 mcg/dL.

Drug Interactions

Drug interactions involve chelation (levodopa, penicillamine, quinolones) or competition for absorption (antacids, cimetidine, methyldopa, tetracyclines). Food interactions occur with vitamin C (enhances absorption) and calcium (decreases absorption unless calcium carbonate is used). Drug interactions are shown in Table 18-9.

Clinical Use and Dosing

Oral iron therapy is used to prevent and treat iron deficiency anemia. Because they are more efficiently absorbed, ferrous salts should be used. Sustained-release and enteric forms should not be used because iron is best absorbed in the duodenum and jejunum. Different ferrous salts provide different amounts of elemental iron. In an iron-deficient patient, about 50 to 100 mg of iron can be incorporated into hemoglobin daily. The adult dose for iron replacement is 150 to 300 mg of elemental iron daily in two or three divided doses to correct iron deficiency rapidly. About 25% of ferrous salt given orally can be absorbed. Premature neonates require 2 mg of elemental iron/kg/day orally until they are 12 months old (Baker, Greer, & the Committee on Nutrition, 2010). The American Academy of Pediatrics

Table 18–9 ⠿ **Drug Interactions: Iron**

Drug	Interacting Drug	Possible Effect	Implications
Iron	Antacids	Absorption reduced	Separate administration by at least 2 h
	Ascorbic acid	Absorption enhanced	Increase may not be significant; must be given concurrently
	Calcium	Coadministration decreases absorption of both; calcium carbonate does not decrease iron absorption	Separate administration by at least 2 h or use calcium carbonate for calcium supplementation and take between meals
	Chloramphenicol	Serum iron levels may be increased	—
	Cimetidine	Absorption reduced	Separate administration by at least 2 h
	Levodopa	Forms chelates with iron salts, decreasing levodopa levels by up to 90%	Avoid concurrent use
	Methyldopa	Methyldopa absorption decreased	Avoid concurrent use
	Penicillamine	Marked reduction in penicillamine absorption	Avoid concurrent use
	Quinolones	Decreased absorption of quinolones by up to 90%	Choose different antibiotic
	Tetracyclines	Coadministration decreases absorption and serum levels of both by up to 90%	Separate administration by at least 2 h
	Vitamin C	Absorption enhanced	May not be significant and requires concurrent administration

recommends all breastfed infants receive 1 mg/kg/day of elemental iron beginning at age 4 months and continuing until the infant is consuming adequate iron-containing foods (Baker et al, 2010). Formula-fed infants do not need iron supplementation. Toddlers age 1 to 3 years need 7 mg/day ideally from iron-fortified foods. Toddlers who do not or are not able to ingest adequate iron in their diet can be supplemented with liquid or chewable iron (combined with multivitamins). Infants and young children require 4 to 6 mg/kg/day divided in three doses to treat severe iron deficiency and 3 mg/kg/day to treat mild to moderate iron deficiency. Doses for infants, children, and adults are provided in Table 18-10. If the patient cannot tolerate large doses, lower doses may be given, but resolving the deficiency takes longer. Treatment continues for 3 to 4 months after hemoglobin/hematocrit return to normal to correct the anemia and replenish iron stores.

Rational Drug Selection

Cost

Iron supplements are available OTC in generic form and are not very expensive. The most expensive ferrous sulfate is Fer-In-Sol, a liquid form used mostly for infants and small children.

Formulation

Ferrous salts come in tablets, capsules, suspensions, drops, and chewable formulations. Unless a patient's age or disease process makes swallowing difficult or impossible, the tablets are the cheapest, and they are easily digested and absorbed.

Monitoring

The reticulocyte count is measured 7 to 10 days after initiation of therapy because it is the first measurable response to iron therapy. A significant rise should be noted toward the normal 0.5% to 1.5% of the body's RBCs. Hemoglobin levels drawn at 2 weeks from initiation of therapy should indicate a rise in Hgb concentration of 0.1 to 0.2 g/100 mL per day of therapy. Normal Hgb levels of 14 to 18 g/dL in men and 12 to 16 g/dL in women should be reached in 1 to 3 months. Monitoring of RBC and Hgb levels thereafter is based on individual patient risk, response, and symptoms.

Patient Education

Prevention

Prevention of iron deficiency is the most important issue. The average American diet contains about 12 mg of iron daily. Twenty percent of this is absorbed in markedly deficient patients, but only 10% is absorbed in normal patients. This means that 0.6 to 1.2 mg of elemental iron is taken up under normal circumstances. This is an adequate requirement for men and postmenopausal women; however, menstruating women need 1.5 mg/day, and pregnant and lactating women need 2.5 mg/day. Eating iron-rich foods can prevent the need for iron supplements, especially in adults. Red meat is the best source of iron, but fish and iron-enriched breads and cereals are also good sources. The iron in eggs and green vegetables is not absorbed because it is bound to phosphates and phytates in these foods. Nutrition should be discussed, including iron-rich foods that are reasonable in cost. Most people who eat a balanced diet do not need iron supplements. Pregnant

Table 18–10 ⚕ **Dosage Schedule: Iron**

Drug	Indication	Dosage Form	Maintenance Dose
Iron	Replacement in iron-deficiency anemia		*Adults:*
Ferrous sulfate (20% elemental iron)		Ferrous sulfate: Tablets: 325 mg (65 mg elemental iron) Elixir: 220 mg/5 mL (44 mg iron/5 mL) Drops: 75 mg/0.6 mL (15 mg iron/0.6 mL) Feosol: Capsules: 325 mg (65 mg iron) FeroSul: Capsules: 325 mg (65 mg iron) Fer-In-Sol: Drops: 75 mg/0.6 mL (15 mg iron/0.6 mL) Fer-Gen-Sol: Drops: 75 mg/0.6 mL (15 mg iron/0.6 mL)	Ferrous sulfate 300–325 mg (60–65 mg of elemental iron) tid-qid Ferrous gluconate 300–325 mg (34–38 mg of elemental iron) qid Ferrous fumarate 200 mg (66 mg of elemental iron) tid-qid Ferrous fumarate 325 mg (106 mg elemental iron) bid-tid *Note:* Goal is 150–250 mg of elemental iron/d RDA: Male >18 yr: 10 mg/d Female 11–50 yr: 15 mg/d Female >50 yr: 10 mg/d
Ferrous sulfate (Dried)		Feosol: Tablet: 200 mg (65 mg iron) Feratab: Tablet: 300 mg (60 mg iron) Ferrous sulfate: Slow-release tablet: 160 mg (50 mg iron) Slow Fe: Slow-release tablet: 160 mg (50 mg iron)	*Children:* 2–12 yr: goal is 4 to 6 mg/kg/d of elemental iron in 3 divided doses. 6 mo–2 yr: goal is up to 6 mg/kg/d of elemental iron in 3 divided doses. RDA: <5 months: 5 mg/d 5 mo to 10 yr: 10 mg/d Males: 11 to 18 yr: 12 mg/d Females: 11 to 18 yr: 15 mg/d
Ferrous gluconate (12% elemental iron)		Ferrous gluconate: Tablet: 225 mg (28 mg iron) Fergon: Tablet: 225 mg (27 mg iron) Ferrous gluconate: Tablet: 300 mg (35 mg of iron); 324 mg (38 mg iron) Tablet: 325 mg (36 mg iron)	
Ferrous fumarate (33% elemental iron		Ferrous fumarate: Tablet: 90 mg (29.5 mg iron) Ferrous fumarate: Tablet: 324 mg (106 mg iron) Femiron: 63 mg (20 mg iron) Hemocyte: Tablet: 324 mg (106 mg iron) Ferrets: Tablet: 325 mg (106 mg iron) Nephro-Fer: Tablet: 350 mg (115 mg iron) Feostat: Chewable tablet: 100 mg (33 mg iron) Ferro-Sequels: Timed-release tablet: 150 mg (50 mg iron)	
Carbonyl iron (pure iron microparticles)		Feosol: Tablet: 45 mg iron Sundown tablet: 50 mg iron Ircon: Tablet: 66 mg iron Icar: Chewable tablet: 15 mg iron Suspension: 15 mg iron/1.25 mL	
	Iron supplement in pregnancy and lactation		30 mg elemental iron daily (not taken with meals)

women, infants, and children during rapid growth periods usually need iron supplementation.

Administration

Patients should take iron as directed. If a dose is missed, they should take it as soon as it is remembered within 12 hours but not double doses. Iron should be taken on an empty stomach. If GI upset occurs, iron can be taken with food, but the amount absorbed will be less. Taking it with vitamin C or citrus juice may enhance absorption. Patients should avoid taking iron at the same time as milk, antacids, tetracycline, or quinolones, which decrease absorption, and drink liquid iron preparations in water or citrus juice or through a straw to prevent discoloration of teeth. Do not use sustained-release preparations.

Adverse Responses

Constipation is the most common problem in patients taking iron. Increase fluids and fiber in the diet, especially iron-rich cereals. Stools may turn dark green or black. This color change is harmless. A stool softener may be used if needed to treat constipation.

Acute iron toxicity/poisoning can occur with an overdose. This is especially a problem with children, in whom as few as 10 of the commonly available iron tablets can be fatal. Patients should keep iron preparations in childproof containers and in a locked medicine cabinet and not refer to vitamins or drugs as candy. The local Poison Control Center should be contacted immediately if overdose is suspected.

Detailed discussion of the management of iron deficiency anemia as well as other forms of anemia is presented in Chapter 27.

FOLIC ACID

Folic acid deficiency is most often related to inadequate dietary intake of green vegetables or excessive boiling of these vegetables in cooking. Other sources of folic acid deficiency include impaired absorption because of ileal disease or phenytoin use; increased demand during pregnancy, hyperthyroidism, hemolytic anemia, or malignancy; and impaired utilization for patients taking methotrexate, triamterene, and trimethoprim.

Pharmacodynamics

Exogenous folate is required for nucleoprotein synthesis and maintenance of normal erythropoiesis. Folic acid stimulates the production of erythrocytes, WBCs, and platelets. Folic acid undergoes a series of oxidative-reductive changes that result in the formation of tetrahydrofolic acid, a cofactor in transformation reactions in the biosynthesis of purines and thymidylates. Impaired thymidylate synthesis is thought to be the mechanism behind neural tube defects in the offspring of pregnant women with folic acid deficiency. Within 3 months of inadequate intake of folates, megaloblastic changes and anemia can develop. Supplemental folic acid is useful in preventing folic acid deficiency in high-risk patients with high folate requirements, such as pregnant women, and in alcoholics and patients with liver disease, who may have deficient storage of folate.

Pharmacokinetics

Absorption and Distribution

Only about 50 to 200 mcg of folate are absorbed from the daily intake of 500 to 700 mcg in the average diet. Pregnant women may absorb as much as 300 to 400 mcg of folate daily. Oral folic acid supplements are well absorbed from the proximal jejunum, and IM or SC administration also results in excellent absorption.

Metabolism, Storage, and Excretion

Folic acid is converted by the liver to its active metabolite (dihydrofolate reductase). Approximately 5 to 20 mg of folate extensively bound to plasma proteins are stored in the liver and other tissues. Folates are excreted in the urine and stool and destroyed by catabolism so that serum levels fall within days when intake is inadequate.

Pharmacotherapeutics

Precautions and Contraindications

The only contraindication is administration when vitamin B_{12} is deficient. Folic acid in doses greater than 0.1 mg/day may mask the indications of pernicious anemia in that the hematological symptoms are gone, but the neurological symptoms continue to progress. Except in pregnancy and lactation, daily doses of folic acid should not exceed 0.4 mg/day until pernicious anemia has been ruled out.

Folic acid is Pregnancy Category A. Pregnant women are more prone to develop folic acid deficiencies, and their diet should be supplemented. The recommended dietary allowance (RDA) for folate during pregnancy is 0.4 mg/day.

Adverse Drug Reactions

Rare transient rashes are the only adverse drug reaction.

Drug Interactions

Sulfonamides, methotrexate, and triamterene interfere with the activity of folate reductase and prevent the activation of folic acid (Table 18-11). Absorption is decreased if it is given concurrently with sulfasalazine. Folic acid requirements are increased in the presence of estrogens, phenytoin, and glucocorticoids.

Clinical Use and Dosing

Anemia Due to Folic Acid Deficiency

After pernicious anemia has been ruled out, the initial dose is up to 1 mg/day in adults and children. When clinical symptoms have subsided and the laboratory studies have normalized, maintenance doses range from 0.1 mg/day for infants to 0.8 mg/day for pregnant and lactating patients. Table 18-12 shows these dosages by age group. Chapter 27 discusses the management of pernicious anemia.

Prevention of Folic Acid Deficiency

Maintenance doses of folic acid may be sufficient to prevent folic acid deficiency in these patients if the upper limit for each age is used. Doses of 0.4 mg prior to conception and throughout pregnancy have been associated with risk reductions of up to 50% for neural tube defects in the offspring. The U.S. Public Health Service recommends that all women of childbearing age who are capable of becoming pregnant consume 0.4 mg of folic acid daily. Because of the risks with higher doses of folic acid that B_{12} deficiency may be overlooked, total folate intake should not exceed 1 mg/day. Chapter 27 discusses the management of folic acid deficiency anemia with pregnancy considerations.

Folic Acid During Lactation

During lactation, folic acid requirements are markedly increased. Mothers who are breastfeeding and have folic acid deficiency require doses of 0.8 mg/day to prevent folic acid deficiency in their infants.

Table 18–11 ▦ Drug Interactions: Folic Acid

Drug	Interacting Drug	Possible Effect	Implications
Folic Acid	Aminosalicylic acid	Decreased serum folate levels	Avoid concurrent use
	Oral contraceptives	May impair folate metabolism and produce folate depletion, but the effect is mild and not likely to cause anemia	Monitor for clinical indications of anemia
	Sulfonamides	Prevent the activation of folic acid by causing a dihydrofolate reductase deficiency	Avoid concurrent use
	Methotrexate	Signs of folate deficiency have been reported	Monitor for indications of anemia
	Triamterene		
	Sulfasalazine		
	Hydantoins	An increase in seizure activity and a decrease in serum concentrations of the hydantoin to subtherapeutic levels Phenytoin may cause a decrease in serum folate levels, but clinically important anemia occurs in <1% of patients on long-term therapy	If folic acid is administered, a higher dose of phenytoin may be needed

Table 18–12 ✂ Dosage Schedule: Folic Acid

Drug	Indication	Initial Dose	Maintenance Dose
Folic acid	Treatment of megaloblastic anemia	Up to 1 mg/d until laboratory studies are normal	*Infants:* 0.1 mg/d *Children <4 yr:* 0.3 mg/d *Adults and children >4 yr:* 0.4 mg/d Pregnant and lactating women, patients who are alcoholic, and patients with liver disease: 0.8 mg/d
	Prevention of folic acid deficiency		*Infants:* 0.1 mg/d *Children <4 yr:* 0.3 mg/d *Adults and children >4 yr:* 0.4 mg/d Pregnant and lactating women, patients who are alcoholic, and patients with liver disease: 0.4 mg/d

Rational Drug Selection

Folic acid is available OTC at less cost than in prescription form (Table 18-13).

Monitoring

The only specific monitoring parameters are those associated with managing the anemia that is being treated.

Patient Education

Although folic acid is part of a normal diet, supplemental folic acid should be taken only after consultation with a health-care provider. In particular, pregnant women and those who may become pregnant should discuss the need for folic acid with their provider. Foods high in folate include green vegetables (especially asparagus, lettuce, spinach, and broccoli), liver, yeast, and mushrooms, which should be included in a balanced diet.

VITAMIN B$_{12}$

Vitamin B$_{12}$ deficiency can be caused by poor intake, impaired absorption, increased demand, or faulty utilization.

Poor intake is rare, except in strict vegetarians who do not eat eggs or use dairy products. Impaired absorption is most often related to the lack of intrinsic factor found in pernicious anemia. Absorption can also be impaired by diseases of the ileum, by bacterial overgrowth from stasis such as occurs with severe constipation, and by altered digestive enzymes associated with gastrectomy. Faulty utilization is associated with rare genetic defects.

Pharmacodynamics

Vitamin B$_{12}$ is critical to two essential enzyme systems. In one system, it is the cofactor in metabolism of methylmalonyl-CoA. When this metabolism does not take place, methylmalonyl-CoA accumulates, and abnormal fatty acids are synthesized. It is believed that these abnormal fatty acids in cell membranes of the CNS are responsible for the neurological manifestations of vitamin B$_{12}$ deficiency. The other system involves folate metabolism. In the presence of vitamin B$_{12}$ deficiency, the final steps in folate metabolism cannot occur, which explains why the megaloblastic anemia found in vitamin B$_{12}$ deficiency can be partially corrected by folic acid administration. Management of anemia is discussed in Chapter 27.

Table 18–13 ❀ **Available Dosage Forms: Folic Acid**

Drug	Dosage Form	Other Forms	Cost
Folic acid (OTC)	Tablets: 0.4, 0.8 mg		0.4 mg = \$4.59/250 0.8 mg = \$4.99/100
Folic acid (prescription)	Tablets: 1 mg	Multidose vial for injection (Folvite); 5 mg/mL	1 mg = \$4.99/90 tablets

OTC = over the counter.

Pharmacokinetics

Absorption and Distribution

Approximately 1 to 5 mcg of the daily dietary intake of 5 to 30 mcg is absorbed. In the stomach and duodenum, vitamin B_{12} complexes with intrinsic factor are secreted by the parietal cells of the gastric mucosa. This complex is then separated in the terminal ileum in the presence of calcium and absorbed by a highly specific receptor-mediated transport system. Patients with intrinsic factor deficits require parenteral administration of vitamin B_{12} to bypass this absorption problem. Vitamin B_{12} is well absorbed following IM and SC injection or intranasal administration. Plasma level peaks within 1 hour after injection. Once absorbed, vitamin B_{12} is distributed throughout the body, bound to a plasma protein, transcobalamin II.

Metabolism, Storage, and Excretion

Excess vitamin B_{12} is stored mainly in the liver and released when needed to carry out normal cellular functions. Because the normal daily requirement of vitamin B_{12} is only about 2 mcg, it would take approximately 5 years for all the stored vitamin B_{12} to be exhausted and megaloblastic anemia to develop if vitamin B_{12} absorption stopped. After injection, vitamin B_{12} is stored in the liver for approximately 400 days. Within 48 hours after injection, 50% to 98% of the dose appears in the urine. The major portion is excreted within the first 8 hours.

Pharmacotherapeutics

Precautions and Contraindications

The only contraindications to injectable vitamin B_{12} are hypersensitivity to cobalt, B_{12}, or any component of these and the presence of Leber's disease, a hereditary optic nerve atrophy. Severe and swift optic nerve atrophy occurs in patients with this disease who are treated with cyanocobalamin.

Pulmonary edema, peripheral vascular thrombosis, and congestive heart failure may occur early in treatment with vitamin B_{12}. Cautious use and careful monitoring are suggested. Blunted or impeded therapeutic response may occur in the presence of uremia, folic acid deficiency, concurrent infection, or iron deficiency.

Vitamin B_{12} (parenteral) is Pregnancy Category C. Adequate and well-controlled studies have not been done with pregnant women.

Adverse Drug Reactions

Hypokalemia and sudden death have occurred in severe megaloblastic anemia treated intensely. Serum potassium levels should be carefully monitored, and supplementation provided as needed. Anaphylactic shock and death have occurred after parenteral administration. An interdermal test dose is given to patients sensitive to the cobalamins. Transient diarrhea, urticaria, and pruritus may occur but are not common. Pain is common at the injection site.

Drug Interactions

Injectable vitamin B_{12} has few drug interactions. Several drugs, extended-release potassium, and excessive intake of alcohol or vitamin C may decrease absorption of oral vitamin B_{12}. Table 18-14 shows these drug interactions.

Clinical Use and Dosing

Prevention of Vitamin B_{12} Deficiency

Vitamin B_{12} is an essential vitamin, and needs increase during pregnancy. The National Academy of Sciences recommends oral doses of 2.2 mcg/day during pregnancy. Vitamin B_{12} is excreted in breast milk in concentrations that approximate the mother's vitamin B_{12} blood level. The Food and Nutrition Board of the National Academy of Sciences—National Research Council recommends 2.6 mcg/day during lactation, 0.3 to 0.5 mcg/day for infants under age 1, and 0.7 to 1.4 mcg/day for children aged 1 to 10 (Table 18-15).

Pernicious Anemia

Because the underlying problem in almost all cases of pernicious anemia is malabsorption, therapy with vitamin B_{12} is required for life. Oral, IM, and intranasal replacement is available. Oral vitamin B_{12} is useful only for patients who cannot take the parenteral form. Initial dosing is 1,000 mcg daily for 7 days by IM or deep SC injection. The hematological response to injected vitamin B_{12} is usually rapid. Reticulocytosis begins on the second or third day and is usually maximal by the fifth to tenth day. If there is clinical improvement and an appropriate reticulocyte response has occurred after 7 days of therapy, then 100 to 1,000 mcg IM are given weekly for a month. Doses of 1,000 mcg may be used, as excess vitamin B_{12} is excreted in the urine. By this time, the hematological values should be normal. Hgb and Hct levels should return to normal within 1 to 2 months. It may take up to 6 months to resolve neurological symptoms. If neurological symptoms are present, a twice-monthly dose is recommended for

Table 18–14 ⊞ **Drug Interactions: Vitamin B₁₂**

Drug	Interacting Drug	Possible Effect	Implications
Vitamin B₁₂	Aminosalicylic acid	Reduced biological and therapeutic action of B₁₂ Abnormal Schilling test and symptoms of B₁₂ deficiency	Avoid concomitant administration
	Chloramphenicol	Hematological effects of B₁₂ may be decreased in patients with pernicious anemia	Choose a different antimicrobial
	Colchicine	May cause malabsorption of B₁₂ (oral)	If unable to avoid concomitant use, administer B₁₂ parenterally
	Aminoglycosides Extended-release potassium supplements Cimetidine Excessive intake of alcohol or vitamin C		

Table 18–15 ⊗ **Dosage Schedule: Vitamin B₁₂**

Drug	Indication	Initial Dose	Maintenance Dose
Vitamin B₁₂	Pernicious anemia	1,000 mcg/d for 7 d IM or deep SC	If clinical improvement and reticulocyte response, give 100 to 1,000 mcg IM weekly for a month. Then give 1,000 mcg monthly for life of patient. If neurological symptoms are present, a twice-monthly dose is recommended for 6 mo prior to beginning the monthly dose Nasal therapy would consist of 500 mcg cyanocobalamin weekly Oral therapy consists of 1,000 mcg daily for life
	Vitamin B₁₂ deficiency without pernicious anemia	Cyanocobalamin: Parenteral *Adults:* 30 mcg/d for 5–10 d *Children:* For hematological signs: 10–50 mcg/d for 5–10 d For neurological signs: 100 mcg/d for 10–15 d Oral 1,000 mcg/d Hydroxocobalamin: *Adults:* 30 mcg/d for 5–10 d *Children:* 100 mcg doses to equal 1–5 mg over 2 wk	Parenteral *Adults:* 100–200 mcg monthly *Children:* For hematological signs: 100–250 mcg/d every 2–4 wk For neurological signs: 100 mcg once or twice weekly for several months, then taper to 250–1,000 mcg monthly by 1 yr *Adults:* 100–200 mcg/mo *Children:* 30–50 mcg every 4 wk

6 months prior to beginning the monthly dose. Because pernicious anemia is not correctable, vitamin B₁₂ must be taken once monthly for the life of the patient. Parenteral, nasal, or oral therapy may be used once a patient's B₁₂ levels return to normal. Parenteral therapy consists of 1,000 mcg of vitamin B₁₂ monthly. Nasal therapy would consist of 500 mcg of cyanocobalamin weekly. Oral therapy consists of 1,000 mcg daily for life. Oral therapy should be tried because of ease of administration and cost. Further discussion is found in Chapter 27.

Patients With Vitamin B₁₂ Deficiency

For adults with vitamin B₁₂ deficiency that is not pernicious anemia, 1,000 mcg of oral cobalamin are given until normal B₁₂ levels are achieved—usually 6 to 12 weeks. In seriously ill patients, both vitamin B₁₂ and folic acid may need to be administered. Dosages for children vary, based on the presence of hematological versus neurological signs. Oral doses up to 1,000 mcg have been used; however, oral therapy is not usually recommended for deficiency states in children.

Unnecessary Vitamin B₁₂ Therapy

Some well-meaning health-care providers have given parenteral vitamin B₁₂ to patients with fatigue or other vague symptoms. Sometimes these patients report feeling better, in all probability related to a placebo effect. There is no indication that vitamin B₁₂ is useful for patients who do not have a deficiency state. Although the risk in giving this drug is low, a better approach is to determine the patient's underlying problem, such as depression, anxiety, or the presence of an inflammatory disease or other disorder that may inhibit erythropoiesis.

Rational Drug Selection

Of the two main parenteral forms of vitamin B_{12}, cyanocobalamin (Crystamine, Cyanoject, Cyomin) is less protein bound and has a shorter duration of action than hydroxocobalamin (Hydrobexan, Hydro-Cobex, Hydro-Crysti-12) (Table 18-16). The latter form may mean less frequent injections, but antibody reactions are more common; either one works as well.

For patients with pernicious anemia, dietary deficiency, or inadequate secretion of intrinsic factor, intranasal cyanocobalamin (Nascobal) has been approved by the FDA for maintenance therapy of patients with hematological remission after initial treatment. Once-weekly dosing of cyanocobalamin gives a 500 mcg dose.

Oral replacement may be used once the patient has reached normal vitamin B_{12} levels via parenteral administration. Oral cyanocobalamin offers ease of administration and is inexpensive ($5.99 for 60 tablets at http://www.drugstore.com).

Monitoring

Sudden drops in serum potassium levels have been reported with vitamin B_{12} therapy. Serum potassium levels should be monitored closely for the first 48 hours and supplemental oral potassium given if needed. Reticulocyte counts, Hct, iron, folic acid, and vitamin B_{12} serum levels are obtained prior to treatment, between the fifth and the seventh day of therapy, at 1 month, then every 3 to 6 months. If folate levels are also low, folic acid may need to be administered. Monitoring for folic acid is discussed in the section on that drug. Relapse of symptoms is not uncommon in the presence of continuing therapy. Hematological evaluations should continue at regular intervals throughout the patient's lifetime, based on the individual's response to therapy.

Patient Education

Administration

Orally administered vitamin B_{12} should be taken with meals to increase absorption. It may be taken with fruit juices, but ascorbic acid alters the stability of the drug. Expensive vitamin preparations are no more efficacious than are less costly ones. Vitamins are not a substitute for a well-balanced diet.

Treating pernicious anemia requires administrating vitamin B_{12} for the rest of the patient's life. Failure to do so leads to the return of anemia and the development of incapacitating and irreversible damage to spinal cord nerves. IM injections should be given in large muscles such as the buttock or thigh, and SC injections should be given deeply in these same areas.

Adverse Drug Reactions

Diarrhea, itching, and urticaria may sometimes temporarily occur. Hypokalemia has occurred early in the treatment of severe anemia. Health-care providers should monitor for this problem. Diets high in potassium may help. Rare cardiac and pulmonary symptoms have occurred. Patients should report shortness of breath, swelling in the lower legs or ankles, and pain or redness in the calves.

Table 18–16 ❈ Available Dosage Forms: Vitamin B_{12}

Drug	Dosage Form	How Supplied	Cost
Vitamin B_{12}	Tablet: 100, 500, and 1,000-mcg	In bottles of 100	500 mcg = $5.99/100 tablets 1,000 mcg = $10.79/100 tablets
Big-Shot B_{12}	Tablet: 5,000 mcg	In bottles of 30 and 60	5,000 mcg = $34.99/120 tablets
Vitamin B_{12}	Lozenges: 100, 250, and 500 mcg	In bottles of 100 In bottles of 100 and 250	2,500 mcg = $6.49/50 lozenges 5,000 mcg = $6.49/30 lozenges
Nascobal	Intranasal: 500 mcg/0.1 mL (500 mcg in each activation)	In 2.3 mL bottle In 5 mL bottle	$277.97/2.3 mL
Hydroxocobalamin, crystalline (Hydro Cobex, Hydro-Crysti 12, LA-12)	Injection: 1,000 mcg/mL	In 30 mL multidose vial	
Cyanocobalamin, crystalline (vitamin B_{12})	Tablet: 500 mcg and 1,000 mcg	In bottle of 100	
Cyanocobalamin, crystalline (vitamin B_{12}, Crystamine, Crysti 1000 Cyanojet, Cyomin, Rubesol-1000)	Injection: 1,000 mcg/mL	In 1 mL vial In 10 and 30 mL multidose vials	1 mL vial = $35.99/25 vials $19.99/30 mL $13.99/10 mL

REFERENCES

American Heart Association Writing Group Members, et al. (2012). Heart disease and stroke statistics—2012 update: A report from the American Heart Association. *Circulation, 125,* e2–e220.

Baker, R. D., Greer, F. R., & The Committee on Nutrition. (2010). Diagnosis and prevention of iron deficiency and iron-deficiency anemia in infants and young children (0–3 years of age). *Pediatrics, 126*(5), 1040–1050.

Bates, S. M., Greer, I. A., Middeldorp, S., Veenstra, D. L., Prabulos, A. M., & Vandvik, P.O. (2012). VTE, thrombophilia, antithrombotic therapy, and pregnancy: American College of Chest Physicians Evidence-Based Clinical Practice Guidelines (9th ed.). *Chest, 141*(62 Suppl), e691S–e736S.

Büller, H. R., Gallus, A. S., Pillion, G., Prins, M. H., Raskob, G. E., & Cassiopea Investigators (2012). Enoxaparin followed by once-weekly idrabiotaparinux versus enoxaparin plus warfarin for patients with acute symptomatic pulmonary embolism: A randomised, double-blind, double-dummy, non-inferiority trial. *The Lancet, 379,* 123–129.

Guyatt, G. H., Akl, E. A., Crowther, M., Gutterman, D. D., Schuunemann, H, J., & American College of Chest Physicians Antithrombotic Therapy and Prevention of Thrombosis Panel (2012). Antithrombotic therapy and prevention of thrombosis, 9th ed.: American College of Chest Physicians Evidence-based Clinical Practice Guidelines. *Chest, 141* (2 Suppl), 7S–47S.

Holbrook, H., Schulman, S., Witt, D. M., Vandvik, P. O., Fish, J., Kovacs, M. J., et al. (2012). Evidenced-based management of anticoagulant therapy. *Chest, 141*(2 Suppl), e152S-184S.

Institute for Clinical Systems Improvement (ICSI). (2013). *Antithrombolic therapy supplement* (8th ed.). Bloomington, MN: ICSI Health Care Guideline. Retrieved from http://www.icsi.org

LactMed (2013). Warfarin. LactMed. National Library of Medicine: Bethesda, MD. Retrieved from http://toxnet.nlm.nih.gov/cgi-bin/sis/search/f?./temp/~HQpIfb:1

Maddali, S., Biring, T., Bluhm, J., Kopecky, S., Krueger, K., Larson, T., et al. (2013). Antithrombotic Therapy Supplement. Institute for Clinical Systems Improvement. Retrieved from www.icsi.org

McCance, K., & Huether, S. (2010). *Pathophysiology: The biological basis for disease in adults and children* (6th ed.). St. Louis, MO: Mosby.

Pignone, M., Alberts, M. J., Colwell, J. A., Cushman, S. E., Mukherjee, D., Rosenson, R. S., et al. (2010). Aspirin for primary prevention of cardiovascular events in people with diabetes: A position statement from the American Diabetes Association, a scientific statement of the American Heart Association, and an expert consensus document of the American College of Cardiology Foundation. *Diabetes Care, 33*(6), 1395–1402.

Sebastian, J., & Tresch, D. (2000). Use of oral anticoagulants in older patients. *Drugs and Aging, 16,* 409–435.

Sieff, C. A. (2012). Introduction to recombinant hematopoietic growth factors. *UpToDate online.* Retrieved from http://www.uptodate.com/contents/introduction-to-recombinant-hematopoietic-growth-factors

Stein, P. D., Matta, F., Masani, M. H., & Diaczok, B. (2010). Silent pulmonary embolism in patients with deep venous thrombosis: A systemic review. *American Journal of Medicine, 123,* 426–431.

The Joint Commission. (2015). 2015 Hospital National Patient Safety Goals. Retrieved from http://www.jointcommission.org/assets/1/6/2015_HAP_NPSG_ER.pdf

Vandvik, P. O., Lincoff, A. M., Gore, J. M., Gutterman, D. D., Sonnenberg, F. A., Alonso-Coello, P., et al. (2012). Primary and secondary prevention of cardiovascular disease: Antithrombotic therapy and prevention of thrombosis, 9th ed: American College of Chest Physicians Evidence-Based Clinical Practice Guidelines. *Chest, 141*(2 Suppl), 363TS–e668S.

You, J. J., Singer, D. E., Howard, P. A., Lane, D. A., Eckman, M. H., Fang, M. C., et al. (2012). Antithrombotic therapy for atrial fibrillation: Antithrombotic therapy and prevention of thrombosis, 9th ed: American College of Chest Physicians Evidenced-based Clinical Practice Guidelines. *Chest, 141*(2 Suppl), e531S–e575S.

CHAPTER 19

DRUGS AFFECTING THE IMMUNE SYSTEM

Teri Moser Woo

Primary care providers prescribe immunizations frequently, with pediatric providers prescribing many vaccines daily. Although vaccination is typically associated with children, the Centers for Disease Control and Prevention (CDC) recommends a number of vaccines for adolescents and adults. A dramatic decrease is seen in vaccine-preventable diseases when mass campaigns are implemented, with cases of diphtheria decreasing 100%, invasive *Haemophilus influenzae* decreasing 99%, pertussis decreasing 86%, and hepatitis A dropping 93% (Hinman, Orenstein, & Schuchat, 2011). A recent study reviewing weekly reports of infectious diseases in

the United States from 1888 to 2011 estimates 103.1 million cases of infectious disease have been prevented since 1924 due to vaccines (van Panhuis et al, 2013).

The immunization schedules may change, but the underlying premise of preventing the spread of infectious disease through mass immunization of susceptible populations does not change. The success of mass vaccination is measured not only in decreased numbers of vaccine-preventable illnesses but also in the resurgence of diseases such as polio and measles when programs are halted (Andre et al, 2008; Hinman et al, 2011). This chapter discusses immunizations, immune globulin (IG) serums, and the diagnostic drugs used in primary care, such as purified protein derivative (PPD) for tuberculosis (TB) screening. The immunomodulators cyclosporine and azathioprine are addressed. The use of interferon is not discussed here because it is usually prescribed by specialty care providers.

IMMUNIZATIONS

Vaccination is the single best technique for preventing infectious disease. Vaccines exist for many diseases that affect adults and children. This section of the chapter discusses active immunization with either attenuated or inactivated infective agents, the recommended schedule of immunizations for adults and children, and the true precautions and contraindications to immunization. Issues such as barriers surrounding immunization are discussed, as well as immunization of special populations and travel immunizations.

Vaccines are divided into two different types: those that are made from attenuated ("modified-live") or inactivated ("killed") infective agents. Attenuated vaccines include measles, mumps, and rubella (MMR); oral polio (OPV); varicella virus (Varivax, ProQuad); yellow fever (YF-Vax); live, attenuated virus influenza vaccine (Flumist); rotavirus (Rotarix, RotaTeq); varicella zoster (Zostavax); and bacilli Calmette–Guérin (BCG). Inactivated vaccines include diphtheria, tetanus, and pertussis (DTP, DTaP, DT, Td, Tdap), *H. influenzae* type B (HIB), hepatitis A and B, influenza (Fluzone), meningococcal (Menactra, Menomune, Trumenba, Bexsero), inactivated polio vaccine (IPV), human papillomavirus vaccine (Gardasil, Cervarix), pneumococcal polysaccharide (PPV23), and pneumococcal conjugate vaccine (PCV13). Cholera, Japanese encephalitis virus, and plague vaccines are other inactivated vaccines. Typhoid vaccine is available in an inactivated form and an oral live, attenuated form. The pharmacodynamics of each vaccine is discussed according to its category.

ATTENUATED VACCINES

INFLUENZA LIVE, ATTENUATED INFLUENZA VACCINE

Pharmacodynamics

Influenza reaches epidemic levels in the winter months in temperate areas and was responsible for 23,607 deaths per year in the United States between 1976 and 2007 (Thompson et al, 2010). Influenza live, attenuated influenza vaccine (LAIV3) (Flumist) was a trivalent vaccine containing two strains of influenza A and one of influenza B, the strains depending on the predicted circulating influenza virus strains. In 2013, a quadravalent vaccine became available. The quadravalent attenuated influenza vaccine (LAIV4) (Flumist Quadravalent) contains two strains of influenza A and two strains of influenza B, strains of which vary by season. The vaccine is cold-adapted, meaning the virus replicates easily in the mucosa of the nasopharynx, and temperature-sensitive so it does not replicate effectively at core body temperature (38°C to 39°C).

Pharmacokinetics

LAIV4 (Flumist Quadravalent) vaccine is administered intranasally, with half of the dose administered in each nostril. In radiolabeled studies 89.7% of the vaccine remains in the nasal cavity. After administration of LAIV4, viral shedding measured at 11 days was present in 0.9% of 19- to 49-year-olds and 7% of children 6 to 23 months of age (MedImmune, 2013).

Pharmacotherapeutics

Precautions and Contraindications

LAIV is contraindicated in patients with egg or egg product hypersensitivity. LAIV is contraindicated in persons with asthma, reactive airways disease, or other chronic disorders of the pulmonary or cardiovascular systems; persons with other underlying medical conditions, including such metabolic diseases as diabetes, renal dysfunction, and hemoglobinopathies; and persons with known or suspected immunodeficiency diseases or who are receiving immunosuppressive therapies (MedImmune, 2013). Patients who are immunocompromised or who have HIV should not be vaccinated with LAIV. LAIV should not be administered to patients who have had Guillain–Barré syndrome.

LAIV is Pregnancy Category C, and pregnant women should not be vaccinated with influenza LAIV.

Use of live influenza vaccine is contraindicated in children under age 2 years owing to significant increased incidence of reactive airway disease and asthma. The vaccine is also contraindicated in children or adolescents receiving aspirin or other salicylates because of the association of Reye syndrome with wild-type influenza infection.

Adverse Drug Reactions

LAIV is usually well tolerated with generally mild and transient adverse effects. Adults in clinical trials of LAIV4 (Flumist Quadravalent) reported respiratory symptoms at the same rate as LAIF3 (Flumist), with 44% reporting runny nose or nasal congestion, 28% headache, 19% sore throat, 14% cough, and 10% reporting muscle aches (MedImmune, 2013). No serious adverse reactions have been reported in either children (older than age 2 years) or adult vaccine recipients.

Drug Interactions

The administration of LAIV and concurrent use of antivirals active against influenza A and/or B viruses have not been studied. The manufacturer recommends waiting 48 hours after discontinuing antivirals before administering LAIV.

LAIV should not be administered to children under age 17 years on aspirin therapy owing to the theoretical increased risk for Reye syndrome.

LAIV may be concurrently administered with measles, mumps, rubella (MMR), and varicella with no problems noted in developing an immune response. LAIV may be simultaneously administered with any of the inactivated vaccines. Inactivated or live vaccines may be administered the same day as LAIV, but if not administered the same day, the two live vaccines need to be separated by 4 weeks.

Clinical Use and Dosing

Children and adults aged 9 through 49 years should receive 0.2 mL of LAIV as soon as it becomes available in the fall. Children aged 5 to 8 who have not had previous influenza vaccination should receive two doses (0.2 mL each) separated by 4 weeks (Grohskopf et al, 2013). Children 8 years and younger who have previously received two doses of influenza vaccine in the same year need only one dose (0.2 mL) annually.

LAIV (FluMist Quadravalent) comes prepackaged in pre-filled single-use sprayers. The vaccine is thawed by holding the sprayer in the palm of the hand. It may also be thawed in the refrigerator and stored for up to 24 hours before use. Half of the dose is administered in one nostril while the patient is in an upright position; then the second half is administered in the second nostril.

Monitoring

Laboratory monitoring is not necessary after LAIV administration.

Patient Education

Because LAIV is a live-virus vaccine, recipients should be advised to stay away from close contact with immunocompromised persons for 7 days after administration, although the risk is theoretical. Patients should report serious or moderate reactions, such as difficulty breathing, wheezing, hives, swelling, unusual weakness, and temperature 38.9°C or higher to their health-care provider.

MEASLES, MUMPS, AND RUBELLA VACCINE

Pharmacodynamics

Immunization with MMR or measles vaccine alone stimulates the immune system to produce disease-specific antibodies by inducing a subclinical infection with attenuated virus particles. This subclinical infection is not contagious. The vaccine-induced antibodies are capable of virus neutralization by complement activation, induction of cell-mediated immunity, and opsonization. Measles and measles and rubella live-virus vaccine (M-R-Vax II) is the commonly used combined vaccine. In 2009 Merck discontinued production of single-agent vaccines based on input from the Advisory Committee on Immunization Practices (ACIP), professional societies, scientific leaders, including measles virus vaccine (Attenuvax), mumps live-virus vaccine (Mumpsvax), rubella (Meruvax II). In 2005, a vaccine (ProQuad) that added varicella to MMR (MMRV) received licensing; it is discussed in the next section.

Pharmacokinetics

The MMR vaccine is administered SC. Following SC injection, antibodies are detectable in 2 weeks (rubella may take 2 to 6 wk) in 95% of patients vaccinated, and immunity occurs in about 10 days. Immunity persists for 15 years or more, with permanent immunity developing in most patients. More than 99% of people who receive two doses of MMR separated by at least 1 month develop evidence of immunity to measles, which is why the current recommendation is for two doses. Mumps outbreaks in New York in 2005 and Iowa in late 2005 and early 2006 indicate that the effectiveness of MMR against mumps is 80% after one dose and 90% after two doses, based on limited data (CDC, 2006a). An outbreak of 3,502 cases of mumps that occurred in 2009–2010 among a well-vaccinated population in the Northeast United States (85% of those infected had had two doses of MMR) demonstrated 94.8% protection against mumps after two doses of MMR (Fiebelkorn, Lawler, Curns, Brandeburg, & Wallace, 2013). Outbreaks of mumps on college campuses in California in 2011 and in Virginia and Maryland in 2013 indicated two doses of MMR are 80% to 92% effective in preventing clinical disease (CDC, 2013a). Mumps antibodies are present in 74% to 95% of persons 12 years after the second dose of MMR vaccine (CDC, 2013a).

Pharmacotherapeutics

Precautions and Contraindications

MMR contains live, attenuated virus, and virus has been detected for 1 to 4 weeks after vaccination in the pharynx or nose of most patients who receive the vaccine; however, this does not appear to cause virus transmission.

According to the CDC (2013a), there are relatively few true contraindications to administering MMR vaccine. They include previous anaphylactic reaction to the MMR vaccine or any component of the vaccine, including neomycin (topically or systemically administered) or gelatin. A history of contact dermatitis to neomycin is not a contraindication to MMR. Anaphylactic reaction or hypersensitivity to eggs is no longer a contraindication to MMR.

Immunosuppression can potentiate virus production, and therefore, MMR vaccination is not recommended for immunocompromised patients. In patients with HIV infection, MMR vaccine can be administered if the patient is asymptomatic or without evidence of severe immunosuppression (CDC, 2013a). MMR should not be given to patients who are severely immunocompromised because of cancer, leukemia, or lymphoma or who are on immunosuppressive drug therapy, including high-dose steroids (prednisone greater than 2 mg/kg/day or 20 mg/day in patients weighing more than 10 kg) or radiation therapy (American Academy of Pediatrics [AAP], 2012a; CDC, 2013a). MMR may be given to close contacts of immunosuppressed patients, including health-care workers.

MMR vaccination is generally deferred if a patient has a moderate or severe febrile illness and is given when the patient recovers from the acute phase of the illness. Minor illnesses, with or without fever (diarrhea, upper respiratory infection, or otitis media), are not contraindications to MMR vaccination, and vaccination should not be postponed (AAP, 2012).

Patients who receive blood products should wait 3 months before being administered MMR (CDC, 2013a). MMR should be given at least 2 weeks before IG. Patients who receive IG should wait 3 to 11 months before being administered MMR (AAP, 2012).

MMR vaccine should not be given to pregnant women or women who may become pregnant within 3 months after administration. There is a theoretical possibility of congenital rubella syndrome in the infant if the mother is given rubella vaccine when pregnant. Women should be asked if they are pregnant before administration of MMR and advised to avoid pregnancy for 3 months after administration of the vaccine. Pregnancy in the mother of a patient receiving MMR is not a contraindication. MMR may be administered to breastfeeding women.

The MMR vaccine may be safely administered to children of all ages, although it may not be immunogenic in infants under age 12 months. If MMR vaccine is administered to a child under age 12 months, then the child should be revaccinated with MMR at 12 to 15 months of age and receive a third dose of MMR at age 4 to 6 years.

Adverse Drug Reactions

Approximately 5% to 15% of children develop a fever of at least 103°F (39.5°C) after vaccination with MMR. The fever usually occurs 7 to 12 days after MMR vaccination (CDC, 2013a). The fever usually lasts 1 to 2 days, and the patient is otherwise asymptomatic. MMR may cause a transient maculopapular rash 7 to 10 days after vaccination in 5% of patients. MMR vaccine may cause a febrile seizure with the fever that occurs post-vaccination, with the highest risk of febrile seizure 6 to 14 days after administration. The risk of febrile seizure is 1 per 3,000 to 4,000 doses of MMR. The risk of febrile seizures is higher if the patient receives MMRV as their first dose of MMR (CDC, 2013a).

Thrombocytopenia is a rare adverse reaction that may occur within 2 months of administration of MMR vaccine. The incidence of thrombocytopenia is 1 case per 1 million doses upon passive surveillance in the United States and 1 case per 30,000 to 40,000 doses in prospective studies. The clinical course of thrombocytopenia is generally benign and transient.

In times of mumps outbreak a third dose of MMR has been administered with minimal adverse effects, including injection site pain, redness and swelling (2% to 4%), muscle or joint aches (2% to 3%), and dizziness or light-headedness (2%) (CDC, 2013a).

Drug Interactions

MMR should not be administered to patients receiving immunosuppressants, including high-dose corticosteroids, interferon, and antineoplastic drugs, because they may have insufficient response to immunization. Patients may remain susceptible despite immunization. The AAP states, "Children receiving <2 mg/kg per day of prednisone or its equivalent, or <20 mg/day if they weigh more than 10 kg, can receive attenuated live-virus vaccines during corticosteroid treatment" (AAP, 2013a).

The MMR vaccine may be inactivated by IG. To avoid inactivation of the attenuated virus, administer the MMR vaccine at least 14 to 30 days before or 3 months after the IG. If IG is being given in preparation for international travel, the MMR vaccine should be administered at least 2 weeks before IG (AAP, 2012b).

MMR is not contraindicated if a PPD was done recently. PPD should be delayed for 4 to 6 weeks after an MMR has been given because it may interfere with the tuberculin skin test, causing a temporary decrease in tuberculin skin sensitivity (CDC, 2013a).

Administration of the MMR and varicella vaccines is compatible if done on the same day, with different needles and at separate sites. If the two live vaccines are not given at the same time, an interval of 1 month between MMR and varicella vaccine is indicated. MMRV (ProQuad) is indicated for simultaneous vaccination against measles, mumps, rubella, and varicella in children 12 months to 12 years of age, although for the first dose separate MMR and varicella vaccines are recommended due to increased risk of febrile seizures with MMRV (CDC, 2013a). MMR may be administered with LAIV (Flumist Quadravalent) vaccine on the same day (Grohskopf et al, 2013). Administration of two live vaccines should be separated by 4 weeks if not given the same day.

Clinical Use and Dosing

MMR is routinely given SC at 12 to 15 months of age with a repeat dose at age 4 to 6 years (CDC, 2013a). The second dose of MMR may be given as soon as 4 weeks after the first dose, which is indicated during an epidemic or before international travel. The CDC recommends the second dose be administered as MMRV (CDC, 2013a). Those children who have not received their second dose of MMR by age 12 should have it at that time. Adults born in 1957 or later who are at least age 18 (including those born outside the United States) should receive at least one dose of MMR if there is no serological proof of immunity or documentation of a dose given on or after the patient's first birthday. Health-care workers and other adults in high-risk groups, such as students entering college, military recruits, and international travelers, should receive a total of two doses of MMR. Adults born before 1957 are considered immune, but proof of immunity may be desirable for health-care workers. See Table 19-1 for further information on routine dosing. The catch-up schedule for dosing children who are behind in the routine vaccine schedule is found in Table 19-2.

Monitoring

Laboratory monitoring is not necessary after MMR administration if the patient received two age-appropriate doses of MMR. Rubella titer may be drawn to determine if a patient is immune. Health-care providers born after 1957 who cannot provide documented evidence of two doses of MMR require serologic testing to determine immunity (Shefer et al, 2011).

Patient Education

All patients or the parents or guardians of the patients are required by law to receive Vaccine Information Statements (VISs) that are developed by the CDC. They are available in a variety of languages, and every effort to provide adequate information to the patient or parent before immunization

Table 19–1 ⊗ Recommended Immunization Schedule for Persons Aged 0 Through 18 Years—United States, 2015

Figure 1. Recommended immunization schedule for persons aged 0 through 18 years – United States, 2015.

(FOR THOSE WHO FALL BEHIND OR START LATE, SEE THE CATCH-UP SCHEDULE [FIGURE 2]).

These recommendations must be read with the footnotes that follow. For those who fall behind or start late, provide catch-up vaccination at the earliest opportunity as indicated by the green bars in Figure 1. To determine minimum intervals between doses, see the catch-up schedule (Figure 2). School entry and adolescent vaccine age groups are shaded.

Vaccine	Birth	1 mo	2 mos	4 mos	6 mos	9 mos	12 mos	15 mos	18 mos	19–23 mos	2-3 yrs	4-6 yrs	7-10 yrs	11-12 yrs	13-15 yrs	16–18 yrs
Hepatitis B[1] (HepB)	1st dose	2nd dose			←——— 3rd dose ———→											
Rotavirus[2] (RV) RV1 (2-dose series); RV5 (3-dose series)			1st dose	2nd dose	See footnote 2											
Diphtheria, tetanus, & acellular pertussis[3] (DTaP: <7 yrs)			1st dose	2nd dose	3rd dose			←——— 4th dose ———→				5th dose				
Tetanus, diphtheria, & acellular pertussis[4] (Tdap: ≥7 yrs)														(Tdap)		
Haemophilus influenzae type b[5] (Hib)			1st dose	2nd dose	See footnote 5		←— 3rd or 4th dose, See footnote 5 —→									
Pneumococcal conjugate[6] (PCV13)			1st dose	2nd dose	3rd dose		←——— 4th dose ———→									
Pneumococcal polysaccharide[6] (PPSV23)																
Inactivated poliovirus[7] (IPV: <18 yrs)			1st dose	2nd dose	←——— 3rd dose ———→							4th dose				
Influenza[8] (IIV; LAIV) 2 doses for some: See footnote 8					Annual vaccination (IIV only) 1 or 2 doses						Annual vaccination (LAIV or IIV) 1 or 2 doses		Annual vaccination (LAIV or IIV) 1 dose only			
Measles, mumps, rubella[9] (MMR)					See footnote 9		←——— 1st dose ———→					2nd dose				
Varicella[10] (VAR)							←——— 1st dose ———→					2nd dose				
Hepatitis A[11] (HepA)							←———— 2-dose series, See footnote 11 ————→									
Human papillomavirus[12] (HPV2: females only; HPV4: males and females)														(3-dose series)		
Meningococcal[13] (Hib-MenCY ≥ 6 weeks; MenACWY-D ≥9 mos; MenACWY-CRM ≥ 2 mos)			←———————————————— See footnote 13 ————————————————→											1st dose		Booster

Legend:

| | Range of recommended ages for all children | | Range of recommended ages for catch-up immunization | | Range of recommended ages for certain high-risk groups | | Range of recommended ages during which catch-up is encouraged and for certain high-risk groups | | Not routinely recommended |

This schedule includes recommendations in effect as of January 1, 2015. Any dose not administered at the recommended age should be administered at a subsequent visit, when indicated and feasible. The use of a combination vaccine generally is preferred over separate injections of its equivalent component vaccines. Vaccination providers should consult the relevant Advisory Committee on Immunization Practices (ACIP) statement for detailed recommendations, availab e online at http://www.cdc.gov/vaccines/hcp/acip-recs/index.html. Clinically significant adverse events that follow vaccination should be reported to the Vaccine Adverse Event Reporting System (VAERS) online (http://www.vaers.hhs.gov) or by telephone (800-822-7967). Suspected cases of vaccine-preventable diseases should be reported to the state or local health department. Additional information, including precautions and contraindications for vaccination, is available from CDC online (http://www.cdc.gov/vaccines/recs/vac-admin/contraindications.htm) or by telephone (800-CDC-INFO [800-232-4636]).

This schedule is approved by the Advisory Committee on Immunization Practices (http://www.cdc.gov/vaccines/acip/), the American Academy of Pediatrics (http://www.aap.org), the American Academy of Family Physicians (http://www.aafp.org), and the American College of Obstetricians and Gynecologists (http://www.acog.org).

NOTE: The above recommendations must be read along with the footnotes of this schedule.

Continued

Table 19-1 ⊗ Recommended Immunization Schedule for Persons Aged 0 Through 18 Years—United States, 2015—cont'd

Footnotes — Recommended immunization schedule for persons aged 0 through 18 years—United States, 2015

For further guidance on the use of the vaccines mentioned below, see: http://www.cdc.gov/vaccines/hcp/acip-recs/index.html.
For vaccine recommendations for persons 19 years of age and older, see the Adult Immunization Schedule.

Additional information

- For contraindications and precautions to use of a vaccine and for additional information regarding that vaccine, vaccination providers should consult the relevant ACIP statement available online at http://www.cdc.gov/vaccines/hcp/acip-recs/index.html.
- For purposes of calculating intervals between doses, 4 weeks = 28 days. Intervals of 4 months or greater are determined by calendar months.
- Vaccine doses administered 4 days or less before the minimum interval are considered valid. Doses of any vaccine administered ≥5 days earlier than the minimum interval or minimum age should not be counted as valid doses and should be repeated as age-appropriate. The repeat dose should be spaced after the invalid dose by the recommended minimum interval. For further details, see *MMWR, General Recommendations on Immunization and Reports / Vol. 60 / No. 2; Table 1. Recommended and minimum ages and intervals between vaccine doses* available online at http://www.cdc.gov/mmwr/pdf/rr/rr6002.pdf.
- Information on travel vaccine requirements and recommendations is available at http://wwwnc.cdc.gov/travel/destinations/list.
- For vaccination of persons with primary and secondary immunodeficiencies, see Table 13, *"Vaccination of persons with primary and secondary immunodeficiencies,"* in *General Recommendations on Immunization* (ACIP), available at http://www.cdc.gov/mmwr/pdf/rr/rr6002.pdf.; and American Academy of Pediatrics. "Immunization in Special Clinical Circumstances," in Pickering LK, Baker CJ, Kimberlin DW, Long SS eds. *Red Book: 2012 report of the Committee on Infectious Diseases. 29th ed.* Elk Grove Village, IL: American Academy of Pediatrics.

1. Hepatitis B (HepB) vaccine. (Minimum age: birth)
Routine vaccination:
At birth:

- Administer monovalent HepB vaccine to all newborns before hospital discharge.
- For infants born to hepatitis B surface antigen (HBsAg)-positive mothers, administer HepB vaccine and 0.5 mL of hepatitis B immune globulin (HBIG) within 12 hours of birth. These infants should be tested for HBsAg and antibody to HBsAg (anti-HBs) 1 to 2 months after completion of the HepB series at age 9 through 18 months (preferably at the next well-child visit).
- If mother's HBsAg status is unknown, within 12 hours of birth administer HepB vaccine regardless of birth-weight. For infants weighing less than 2,000 grams, administer HBIG in addition to HepB vaccine within 12 hours of birth. Determine mother's HBsAg status as soon as possible and, if mother is HBsAg-positive, also administer HBIG for infants weighing 2,000 grams or more as soon as possible, but no later than age 7 days.

Doses following the birth dose:

- The second dose should be administered at age 1 or 2 months. Monovalent HepB vaccine should be used for doses administered before age 6 weeks.
- Infants who did not receive a birth dose should receive 3 doses of a HepB-containing vaccine on a schedule of 0, 1 to 2 months, and 6 months starting as soon as feasible. See Figure 2.
- Administer the second dose 1 to 2 months after the first dose (minimum interval of 4 weeks), administer the third dose at least 8 weeks after the second dose AND at least 16 weeks after the **first** dose. The final (third or fourth) dose in the HepB vaccine series should be administered **no earlier than age 24 weeks**.
- Administration of a total of 4 doses of HepB vaccine is permitted when a combination vaccine containing HepB is administered after the birth dose.

Catch-up vaccination:

- Unvaccinated persons should complete a 3-dose series.
- A 2-dose series (doses separated by at least 4 months) of adult formulation Recombivax HB is licensed for use in children aged 11 through 15 years.
- For other catch-up guidance, see Figure 2.

2. Rotavirus (RV) vaccines. (Minimum age: 6 weeks for both RV1 [Rotarix] and RV5 [RotaTeq])
Routine vaccination:

Administer a series of RV vaccine to all infants as follows:
1. If Rotarix is used, administer a 2-dose series at 2 and 4 months of age.
2. If RotaTeq is used, administer a 3-dose series at ages 2, 4, and 6 months.
3. If any dose in the series was RotaTeq or vaccine product is unknown for any dose in the series, a total of 3 doses of RV vaccine should be administered.

Catch-up vaccination:

- The maximum age for the first dose in the series is 14 weeks, 6 days; vaccination should not be initiated for infants aged 15 weeks, 0 days or older.
- The maximum age for the final dose in the series is 8 months, 0 days.
- For other catch-up guidance, see Figure 2.

3. Diphtheria and tetanus toxoids and acellular pertussis (DTaP) vaccine. (Minimum age: 6 weeks. Exception: DTaP-IPV [Kinrix]: 4 years)
Routine vaccination:

- Administer a 5-dose series of DTaP vaccine at ages 2, 4, 6, 15 through 18 months, and 4 through 6 years. The fourth dose may be administered as early as age 12 months, provided at least 6 months have elapsed since the third dose. However, the fourth dose of DTaP need not be repeated if it was administered at least 4 months after the third dose of DTaP.

3. Diphtheria and tetanus toxoids and acellular pertussis (DTaP) vaccine (cont'd)
Catch-up vaccination:

- The fifth dose of DTaP vaccine is not necessary if the fourth dose was administered at age 4 years or older.
- For other catch-up guidance, see Figure 2.

4. Tetanus and diphtheria toxoids and acellular pertussis (Tdap) vaccine. (Minimum age: 10 years for both Boostrix and Adacel)
Routine vaccination:

- Administer 1 dose of Tdap vaccine to all adolescents aged 11 through 12 years.
- Tdap may be administered regardless of the interval since the last tetanus and diphtheria toxoid-containing vaccine.
- Administer 1 dose of Tdap vaccine to pregnant adolescents during each pregnancy (preferred during 27 through 36 weeks' gestation) regardless of time since prior Td or Tdap vaccination.

Catch-up vaccination:

- Persons aged 7 years and older who are not fully immunized with DTaP vaccine should receive Tdap vaccine as 1 dose (preferably the first) in the catch-up series; if additional doses are needed, use Td vaccine. For children 7 through 10 years who receive a dose of Tdap as part of the catch-up series, an adolescent Tdap vaccine dose at age 11 through 12 years should NOT be administered. Td should be administered instead 10 years after the Tdap dose.
- Persons aged 11 through 18 years who have not received Tdap vaccine should receive a dose followed by tetanus and diphtheria toxoid (Td) booster doses every 10 years thereafter.
- Inadvertent doses of DTaP vaccine:
  - If administered inadvertently to a child aged 7 through 10 years may count as part of the catch-up series. This dose may count as the adolescent Tdap dose, or the child can later receive a Tdap booster dose at age 11 through 12 years.
  - If administered inadvertently to an adolescent aged 11 through 18 years, the dose should be counted as the adolescent Tdap booster.
- For other catch-up guidance, see Figure 2.

5. *Haemophilus influenzae* type b (Hib) conjugate vaccine. (Minimum age: 6 weeks for PRP-T [ACTHIB, DTaP-IPV/Hib (Pentacel) and Hib-MenCY (MenHibrix)], PRP-OMP [PedvaxHIB or COMVAX], 12 months for PRP-T [Hiberix])
Routine vaccination:

- Administer a 2- or 3-dose Hib vaccine primary series and a booster dose (dose 3 or 4 depending on vaccine used in primary series) at age 12 through 15 months to complete a full Hib vaccine series.
- The primary series with ActHIB, MenHibrix, or Pentacel consists of 3 doses and should be administered at 2, 4, and 6 months of age. The primary series with PedvaxHib or COMVAX consists of 2 doses and should be administered at 2 and 4 months of age; a dose at age 6 months is not indicated.
- One booster dose (dose 3 or 4 depending on vaccine used in primary series) of any Hib vaccine should be administered at age 12 through 15 months. An exception is Hiberix vaccine. Hiberix should only be used for the booster (final) dose in children aged 12 months through 4 years who have received at least 1 prior dose of Hib-containing vaccine.
- For recommendations on the use of MenHibrix in patients at increased risk for meningococcal disease, please refer to the meningococcal vaccine footnotes and also to *MMWR* February 28, 2014 / 63(RR01):1-13, available at http://www.cdc.gov/mmwr/PDF/rr/rr6301.pdf.

For further guidance on the use of the vaccines mentioned below, see: http://www.cdc.gov/vaccines/hcp/acip-recs/index.html.

5. Haemophilus influenzae type b (Hib) conjugate vaccine (cont'd)

Catch-up vaccination:

- If dose 1 was administered at ages 12 through 14 months, administer a second (final) dose at least 8 weeks after dose 1, regardless of Hib vaccine used in the primary series.
- If both doses were PRP-OMP (PedvaxHIB or COMVAX), and were administered before the first birthday, the third (and final) dose should be administered at age 12 through 59 months and at least 8 weeks after the second dose.
- If the first dose was administered at age 7 through 11 months, administer the second dose at least 4 weeks later and a third (and final) dose at age 12 through 15 months or 8 weeks after second dose, whichever is later.
- If first dose is administered before the first birthday and second dose administered at younger than 15 months, a third (and final) dose should be given 8 weeks later.
- For unvaccinated children aged 15 months or older, administer only 1 dose.
- For other catch-up guidance, see Figure 2. For catch-up guidance related to MenHibrix, please see the meningococcal vaccine footnotes and also MMWR February 28, 2014 / 63(RR01);1-13, available at http://www.cdc.gov/mmwr/PDF/rr/rr6301.pdf.

Vaccination of persons with high-risk conditions:

- Children aged 12 through 59 months who are at increased risk for Hib disease, including chemotherapy recipients and those with anatomic or functional asplenia (including sickle cell disease), human immunodeficiency virus (HIV) infection, immunoglobulin deficiency, or early component complement deficiency, who have received either no doses or only 1 dose of Hib vaccine before 12 months of age, should receive 2 additional doses of Hib vaccine 8 weeks apart; children who received 2 or more doses of Hib vaccine before 12 months of age should receive 1 additional dose.
- For patients younger than 5 years of age undergoing chemotherapy or radiation treatment who received a Hib vaccine dose(s) within 14 days of starting therapy or during therapy, repeat the dose(s) at least 3 months following therapy completion.
- Recipients of hematopoietic stem cell transplant (HSCT) should be revaccinated with a 3-dose regimen of Hib vaccine starting 6 to 12 months after successful transplant, regardless of vaccination history; doses should be administered at least 4 weeks apart.
- A single dose of any Hib-containing vaccine should be administered to unimmunized* children and adolescents 15 months of age and older undergoing an elective splenectomy; if possible, vaccine should be administered at least 14 days before procedure.
- Hib vaccine is not routinely recommended for patients 5 years or older. However, 1 dose of Hib vaccine should be administered to unimmunized* persons aged 5 years or older who have anatomic or functional asplenia (including sickle cell disease) and unvaccinated persons 5 through 18 years of age with human immunodeficiency virus (HIV) infection.

*Patients who have not received a primary series and booster dose or at least 1 dose of Hib vaccine after 14 months of age are considered unimmunized.

6. Pneumococcal vaccines. (Minimum age: 6 weeks for PCV13, 2 years for PPSV23)

Routine vaccination with PCV13:

- Administer a 4-dose series of PCV13 vaccine at ages 2, 4, and 6 months and at age 12 through 15 months.
- For children aged 14 through 59 months who have received an age-appropriate series of 7-valent PCV (PCV7), administer a single supplemental dose of 13-valent PCV (PCV13).

Catch-up vaccination with PCV13:

- Administer 1 dose of PCV13 to all healthy children aged 24 through 59 months who are not completely vaccinated for their age.
- For other catch-up guidance, see Figure 2.

Vaccination of persons with high-risk conditions with PCV13 and PPSV23:

- All recommended PCV13 doses should be administered prior to PPSV23 vaccination if possible.
- For children 2 through 5 years of age with any of the following conditions: chronic heart disease (particularly cyanotic congenital heart disease and cardiac failure); chronic lung disease (including asthma if treated with high-dose oral corticosteroid therapy); diabetes mellitus; cerebrospinal fluid leak; cochlear implant; sickle cell disease and other hemoglobinopathies; anatomic or functional asplenia; HIV infection; chronic renal failure; nephrotic syndrome; diseases associated with treatment with immunosuppressive drugs or radiation therapy, including malignant neoplasms, leukemias, lymphomas, and Hodgkin's disease; solid organ transplantation; or congenital immunodeficiency:
  1. Administer 1 dose of PCV13 if any incomplete schedule of 3 doses of PCV (PCV7 and/or PCV13) were received previously.
  2. Administer 2 doses of PCV13 at least 8 weeks apart if unvaccinated or any incomplete schedule of fewer than 3 doses of PCV (PCV7 and/or PCV13) were received previously.
  3. Administer 1 supplemental dose of PCV13 if 4 doses of PCV7 or other age-appropriate complete PCV7 series was received previously.
  4. The minimum interval between doses of PPSV23 is 8 weeks.
  5. For children with no history of PPSV23 vaccination, administer PPSV23 at least 8 weeks after the most recent dose of PCV13.

6. Pneumococcal vaccines (cont'd)

- For children aged 6 through 18 years who have cerebrospinal fluid leak; cochlear implant; sickle cell disease and other hemoglobinopathies; anatomic or functional asplenia; congenital or acquired immunodeficiencies; HIV infection; chronic renal failure; nephrotic syndrome; diseases associated with treatment with immunosuppressive drugs or radiation therapy, including malignant neoplasms, leukemias, lymphomas, and Hodgkin's disease; generalized malignancy; solid organ transplantation; or multiple myeloma:
  1. If neither PCV13 nor PPSV23 has been received previously, administer 1 dose of PCV13 now and 1 dose of PPSV23 at least 8 weeks later.
  2. If PCV13 has been received previously but PPSV23 has not, administer 1 dose of PPSV23 at least 8 weeks after the most recent dose of PCV13.
  3. If PPSV23 has been received but PCV13 has not, administer 1 dose of PCV13 at least 8 weeks after the most recent dose of PPSV23.
- For children aged 6 through 18 years with chronic heart disease (particularly cyanotic congenital heart disease and cardiac failure), chronic lung disease (including asthma if treated with high-dose oral corticosteroid therapy), diabetes mellitus, alcoholism, or chronic liver disease, who have not received PPSV23, administer 1 dose of PPSV23. If PCV13 has been received previously, then PPSV23 should be administered at least 8 weeks after any prior PCV13 dose.
- A single revaccination with PPSV23 should be administered 5 years after the first dose to children with sickle cell disease or other hemoglobinopathies; anatomic or functional asplenia; congenital or acquired immunodeficiencies; HIV infection; chronic renal failure; nephrotic syndrome; diseases associated with treatment with immunosuppressive drugs or radiation therapy, including malignant neoplasms, leukemias, lymphomas, and Hodgkin's disease; generalizec malignancy; solid organ transplantation; or multiple myeloma.

7. Inactivated poliovirus vaccine (IPV). (Minimum age: 6 weeks)

Routine vaccination:

- Administer a 4-dose series of IPV at ages 2, 4, 6 through 18 months, and 4 through 6 years. The final dose in the series should be administered on or after the fourth birthday and at least 6 months after the previous dose.

Catch-up vaccination:

- In the first 6 months of life, minimum age and minimum intervals are only recommended if the person is at risk of imminent exposure to circulating poliovirus (i.e., travel to a polio-endemic region or during an outbreak).
- If 4 or more doses are administered before age 4 years, an additional dose should be administered at age 4 through 6 years and at least 6 month's after the previous dose.
- A fourth dose is not necessary if the third dose was administered at age 4 years or older and at least 6 months after the previous dose.
- If both OPV and IPV were administered as part of a series, a total of 4 doses should be administered, regardless of the child's current age. IPV is not routinely recommended for U.S. residents aged 18 years or older.
- For catch-up guidance, see Figure 2.

8. Influenza vaccines. (Minimum age: 6 months for inactivated influenza vaccine [IIV], 2 years for live, attenuated influenza vaccine [LAIV])

Routine vaccination:

- Administer influenza vaccine annually to all children beginning at age 6 months. For most healthy, nonpregnant persons aged 2 through 49 years, either LAIV or IIV may be used. However, LAIV should NOT be administered to some persons, including 1) persons who have experienced severe allergic reactions to LAIV, any of its components, or tc a previous dose of any other influenza vaccine; 2) children 2 through 17 years receiving aspirin or aspirin-containing products; 3) persons who are allergic to eggs; 4) pregnant women; 5) immunosuppressed persons; 6) children 2 through 4 years of age with asthma or who had wheezing in the past 12 months; or 7) persons who have taken influenza antiviral medications in the previous 48 hours. For all other contraindications and precautions to use of LAIV, see MMWR August 15, 2014 / 63(32);691-697 [40 pages] available at http://www.cdc.gov/mmwr/pdf/wk/mm6332.pdf.

For children aged 6 months through 8 years:

- For the 2014-15 season, administer 2 doses (separated by at east 4 weeks) to children who are receiving influenza vaccine for the first time. Some children in this age group who have been vaccinated previously will also need 2 doses. For additiona guidance, follow dosing guidelines in the 2014-15 ACIP influenza vaccine recommendations, MMWR August 15, 2014 / 63(32);691-697 [40 pages] available at http://www.cdc.gov/mmwr/pdf/wk/mm6332.pdf.
- For the 2015-16 season, follow dosing guidelines in the 2015 ACIP influenza vaccine recommendations.

For persons aged 9 years and older:

- Administer 1 dose.

Continued

Table 19-1 ⊗ Recommended Immunization Schedule for Persons Aged 0 Through 18 Years—United States, 2015—cont'd

For further guidance on the use of the vaccines mentioned below, see: http://www.cdc.gov/vaccines/hcp/acip-recs/index.html.

9. Measles, mumps, and rubella (MMR) vaccine. (Minimum age: 12 months for routine vaccination)

Routine vaccination:

- Administer a 2-dose series of MMR vaccine at ages 12 through 15 months and 4 through 6 years. The second dose may be administered before age 4 years, provided at least 4 weeks have elapsed since the first dose.
- Administer 1 dose of MMR vaccine to infants aged 6 through 11 months before departure from the United States for international travel. These children should be revaccinated with 2 doses of MMR vaccine, the first at age 12 through 15 months (12 months if the child remains in an area where disease risk is high), and the second dose at least 4 weeks later.
- Administer 2 doses of MMR vaccine to children aged 12 months and older before departure from the United States for international travel. The first dose should be administered on or after age 12 months and the second dose at least 4 weeks later.

Catch-up vaccination:

- Ensure that all school-aged children and adolescents have had 2 doses of MMR vaccine; the minimum interval between the 2 doses is 4 weeks.

10. Varicella (VAR) vaccine. (Minimum age: 12 months)

Routine vaccination:

- Administer a 2-dose series of VAR vaccine at ages 12 through 15 months and 4 through 6 years. The second dose may be administered before age 4 years, provided at least 3 months have elapsed since the first dose. If the second dose was administered at least 4 weeks after the first dose, it can be accepted as valid.

Catch-up vaccination:

- Ensure that all persons aged 7 through 18 years without evidence of immunity (see *MMWR* 2007 / 56 [No. RR-4], available at http://www.cdc.gov/mmwr/pdf/rr/rr5604.pdf) have 2 doses of varicella vaccine. For children aged 7 through 12 years, the recommended minimum interval between doses is 3 months (if the second dose was administered at least 4 weeks after the first dose, it can be accepted as valid); for persons aged 13 years and older, the minimum interval between doses is 4 weeks.

11. Hepatitis A (HepA) vaccine. (Minimum age: 12 months)

Routine vaccination:

- Initiate the 2-dose HepA vaccine series at 12 through 23 months; separate the 2 doses by 6 to 18 months.
- Children who have received 1 dose of HepA vaccine before age 24 months should receive a second dose 6 to 18 months after the first dose.
- For any person aged 2 years and older who has not already received the HepA vaccine series, 2 doses of HepA vaccine separated by 6 to 18 months may be administered if immunity against hepatitis A virus infection is desired.

Catch-up vaccination:

- The minimum interval between the two doses is 6 months.

Special populations:

- Administer 2 doses of HepA vaccine at least 6 months apart to previously unvaccinated persons who live in areas where vaccination programs target older children, or who are at increased risk for infection. This includes persons traveling to or working in countries that have high or intermediate endemicity of infection; men having sex with men; users of injection and non-injection illicit drugs; persons who work with HAV-infected primates or with HAV in a research laboratory; persons with clotting-factor disorders; persons with chronic liver disease; and persons who anticipate close personal contact (e.g., household or regular babysitting) with an international adoptee during the first 60 days after arrival in the United States from a country with high or intermediate endemicity. The first dose should be administered as soon as the adoption is planned, ideally 2 or more weeks before the arrival of the adoptee.

12. Human papillomavirus (HPV) vaccines. (Minimum age: 9 years for HPV2 [Cervarix] and HPV4 [Gardasil])

Routine vaccination:

- Administer a 3-dose series of HPV vaccine on a schedule of 0, 1–2, and 6 months to all adolescents aged 11 through 12 years. Either HPV4 or HPV2 may be used for females, and only HPV4 may be used for males.
- The vaccine series may be started at age 9 years.
- Administer the second dose 1 to 2 months after the first dose (minimum interval of 4 weeks); administer the third dose 24 weeks after the first dose and 16 weeks after the second dose (minimum interval of 12 weeks).

Catch-up vaccination:

- Administer the vaccine series to females (either HPV2 or HPV4) and males (HPV4) at age 13 through 18 years if not previously vaccinated.
- Use recommended routine dosing intervals (see Routine vaccination above) for vaccine series catch-up.

13. Meningococcal conjugate vaccines. (Minimum age: 6 weeks for Hib-MenCY [MenHibrix], 9 months for MenACWY-D [Menactra], 2 months for MenACWY-CRM [Menveo])

Routine vaccination:

- Administer a single dose of Menactra or Menveo vaccine at age 11 through 12 years, with a booster dose at age 16 years.
- Adolescents aged 11 through 18 years with human immunodeficiency virus (HIV) infection should receive a 2-dose primary series of Menactra or Menveo with at least 8 weeks between doses.
- For children aged 2 months through 18 years with high-risk conditions, see below.

Catch-up vaccination:

- Administer Menactra or Menveo vaccine at age 13 through 18 years if not previously vaccinated.
- If the first dose is administered at age 13 through 15 years, a booster dose should be administered at age 16 through 18 years with a minimum interval of at least 8 weeks between doses.
- If the first dose is administered at age 16 years or older, a booster dose is not needed.
- For other catch-up guidance, see Figure 2.

Vaccination of persons with high-risk conditions and other persons at increased risk of disease:

- Children with anatomic or functional asplenia (including sickle cell disease):

  1. Menveo
     - *Children who initiate vaccination at 8 weeks through 6 months:* Administer doses at 2, 4, 6, and 12 months of age.
     - *Unvaccinated children 7 through 23 months:* Administer 2 doses, with the second dose at least 12 weeks after the first dose AND after the first birthday.
     - *Children 24 months and older who have not received a complete series:* Administer 2 primary doses at least 8 weeks apart.
  2. MenHibrix
     - *Children 6 weeks through 18 months:* Administer doses at 2, 4, 6, and 12 through 15 months of age.
     - If the first dose of MenHibrix is given at or after 12 months of age, a total of 2 doses should be given at least 8 weeks apart to ensure protection against serogroups C and Y meningococcal disease.
  3. Menactra
     - *Children 24 months and older who have not received a complete series:* Administer 2 primary doses at least 8 weeks apart. If Menactra is administered to a child with asplenia (including sickle cell disease), do not administer Menactra until 2 years of age and at least 4 weeks after the completion of all PCV13 doses.

- Children with persistent complement component deficiency:

  1. Menveo
     - *Children who initiate vaccination at 8 weeks through 6 months:* Administer doses at 2, 4, 6, and 12 months of age.
     - *Unvaccinated children 7 through 23 months:* Administer 2 doses, with the second dose at least 12 weeks after the first dose AND after the first birthday.
     - *Children 24 months and older who have not received a complete series:* Administer 2 primary doses at least 8 weeks apart.
  2. MenHibrix
     - *Children 6 weeks through 18 months:* Administer doses at 2, 4, 6, and 12 through 15 months of age.
     - If the first dose of MenHibrix is given at or after 12 months of age, a total of 2 doses should be given at least 8 weeks apart to ensure protection against serogroups C and Y meningococcal disease.
  3. Menactra
     - *Children 9 through 23 months:* Administer 2 primary doses at least 12 weeks apart.
     - *Children 24 months and older who have not received a complete series:* Administer 2 primary doses at least 8 weeks apart.

- For children who travel to or reside in countries in which meningococcal disease is hyperendemic or epidemic, including countries in the African meningitis belt or the Hajj, administer an age-appropriate formulation and series of Menactra or Menveo for protection against serogroups A and W meningococcal disease. Prior receipt of MenHibrix is not sufficient for children traveling to the meningitis belt or the Hajj because it does not contain serogroups A or W.
- For children at risk during a community outbreak attributable to a vaccine serogroup, administer or complete an age- and formulation-appropriate series of MenHibrix, Menactra, or Menveo.
- For booster doses among persons with high-risk conditions, refer to *MMWR* 2013 / 62(RR02):1-22, available at http://www.cdc.gov/mmwr/preview/mmwrhtml/rr6202a1.htm.

For other catch-up recommendations for these persons, and complete information on use of meningococcal vaccines, including guidance related to vaccination of persons at increased risk of infection, see MMWR March 22, 2013 / 62(RR02) / 62(RR02);1-22, available at http://www.cdc.gov/mmwr/pdf/rr/rr6202.pdf.

CS 244083-B

Table 19–2 ⊗ Catch-Up Immunization Schedule for Persons Aged 4 Months Through 18 Years Who Start Late or Who Are More Than 1 Month Behind – United States, 2015

FIGURE 2. Catch-up immunization schedule for persons aged 4 months through 18 years who start late or who are more than 1 month behind —United States, 2015.
The figure below provides catch-up schedules and minimum intervals between doses for children whose vaccinations have been delayed. A vaccine series does not need to be restarted, regardless of the time that has elapsed between doses. Use the section appropriate for the child's age. Always use this table in conjunction with Figure 1 and the footnotes that follow.

Vaccine	Minimum Age for Dose 1	Minimum Interval Between Doses			
		Dose 1 to Dose 2	Dose 2 to Dose 3	Dose 3 to Dose 4	Dose 4 to Dose 5
Children age 4 months through 6 years					
Hepatitis B[1]	Birth	4 weeks	8 weeks and at least 16 weeks after first dose. Minimum age for the final dose is 24 weeks.		
Rotavirus[2]	6 weeks	4 weeks	4 weeks[2]		
Diphtheria, tetanus, and acellular pertussis[3]	6 weeks	4 weeks	4 weeks	6 months	6 months[3]
Haemophilus influenzae type b[5]	6 weeks	4 weeks if first dose was administered before the 1st birthday. / 8 weeks (as final dose) if first dose was administered at age 12 through 14 months. / No further doses needed if first dose was administered at age 15 months or older.	4 weeks[5] if current age is younger than 12 months and first dose was administered at younger than age 7 months, and at least 1 previous dose was PRP-T (ActHib, Pentacel) or unknown. / 8 weeks and age 12 through 59 months (as final dose)[5] • if current age is younger than 12 months and first dose was administered at age 7 through 11 months; OR • if current age is 12 through 59 months and first dose was administered before the 1st birthday, and second dose administered at younger than 15 months; OR • if both doses were PRP-OMP (PedvaxHIB; Comvax) and were administered before the 1st birthday. / No further doses needed if previous dose was administered at age 15 months or older.	8 weeks (as final dose) This dose only necessary for children age 12 through 59 months who received 3 doses before the 1st birthday.	
Pneumococcal[6]	6 weeks	4 weeks if first dose administered before the 1st birthday. / 8 weeks (as final dose for healthy children) if first dose was administered at the 1st birthday or after. / No further doses needed for healthy children if first dose administered at age 24 months or older.	4 weeks if current age is younger than 12 months and previous dose given at <7months old. / 8 weeks (as final dose for healthy children) if previous dose given between 7-11 months (wait until at least 12 months old); OR if current age is 12 months or older and at least 1 dose was given before age 12 months. / No further doses needed for healthy children if previous dose administered at age 24 months or older.	8 weeks (as final dose) This dose only necessary for children aged 12 through 59 months who received 3 doses before age 12 months or for children at high risk who received 3 doses at any age.	
Inactivated poliovirus[7]	6 weeks	4 weeks[7]	4 weeks[7]	6 months[7] (minimum age 4 years for final dose).	
Meningococcal[13]	6 weeks	8 weeks[13]	See footnote 13	See Footnote 13	
Measles, mumps, rubella[9]	12 months	4 weeks			
Varicella[10]	12 months	3 months			
Hepatitis A[11]	12 months	6 months			
Children and adolescents age 7 through 18 years					
Tetanus, diphtheria; tetanus, diphtheria, and acellular pertussis[4]	7 years[4]	4 weeks	4 weeks if first dose of DTaP/DT was administered before the 1st birthday. / 6 months if first dose of DTaP/DT was administered at or after the 1st birthday.	6 months if first dose of DTaP/DT was administered before the 1st birthday.	
Human papillomavirus[12]	9 years	Routine dosing intervals are recommended.[12]			
Hepatitis A[11]	Not applicable (N/A)	6 months			
Hepatitis B[1]	N/A	4 weeks	8 weeks and at least 16 weeks after first dose.		
Inactivated poliovirus[7]	N/A	4 weeks	4 weeks[7]	6 months[7]	
Meningococcal[13]	N/A	8 weeks[13]	6 months[7]		
Measles, mumps, rubella[9]	N/A	4 weeks			
Varicella[10]	N/A	3 months if younger than age 13 years. / 4 weeks if age 13 years or older.			

NOTE: The above recommendations must be read along with the footnotes of this schedule.

Continued

Table 19–2 ⊗ Catch-Up Immunization Schedule for Persons Aged 4 Months Through 18 Years Who Start Late or Who Are More Than 1 Month Behind – United States, 2015—cont'd

Footnotes — Recommended immunization schedule for persons aged 0 through 18 years—United States, 2015

For further guidance on the use of the vaccines mentioned below, see: http://www.cdc.gov/vaccines/hcp/acip-recs/index.html.
For vaccine recommendations for persons 19 years of age and older, see the Adult Immunization Schedule.

Additional information

- For contraindications and precautions to use of a vaccine and for additional information regarding that vaccine, vaccination providers should consult the relevant ACIP statement available online at http://www.cdc.gov/vaccines/hcp/acip-recs/index.html.
- For purposes of calculating intervals between doses, 4 weeks = 28 days. Intervals of 4 months or greater are determined by calendar months.
- Vaccine doses administered 4 days or less before the minimum interval are considered valid. Doses of any vaccine administered ≥5 days earlier than the minimum interval or minimum age should not be counted as valid doses and should be repeated as age-appropriate. The repeat dose should be spaced after the invalid dose by the recommended minimum interval. For further details, see *MMWR, General Recommendations on Immunization and Reports / Vol. 60 / No. 2; Table 1. Recommended and minimum ages and intervals between vaccine doses* available online at http://www.cdc.gov/mmwr/pdf/rr/rr6002.pdf.
- Information on travel vaccine requirements and recommendations is available at http://wwwnc.cdc.gov/travel/destinations/list.
- For vaccination of persons with primary and secondary immunodeficiencies, see Table 13, *"Vaccination of persons with primary and secondary immunodeficiencies,"* in *General Recommendations on Immunization* (ACIP), available at http://www.cdc.gov/mmwr/pdf/rr/rr6002.pdf; and American Academy of Pediatrics. *"Immunization in Special Clinical Circumstances,"* in Pickering LK, Baker CJ, Kimberlin DW, Long SS eds. *Red Book: 2012 report of the Committee on Infectious Diseases. 29th ed.* Elk Grove Village, IL: American Academy of Pediatrics.

1. Hepatitis B (HepB) vaccine. (Minimum age: birth)

Routine vaccination:

At birth:

- Administer monovalent HepB vaccine to all newborns before hospital discharge.
- For infants born to hepatitis B surface antigen (HBsAg)-positive mothers, administer HepB vaccine and 0.5 mL of hepatitis B immune globulin (HBIG) within 12 hours of birth. These infants should be tested for HBsAg and antibody to HBsAg (anti-HBs) 1 to 2 months after completion of the HepB series at age 9 through 18 months (preferably at the next well-child visit).
- If mother's HBsAg status is unknown, within 12 hours of birth administer HepB vaccine regardless of birth-weight. For infants weighing less than 2,000 grams, administer HBIG in addition to HepB vaccine within 12 hours of birth. Determine mother's HBsAg status as soon as possible and, if mother is HBsAg-positive, also administer HBIG for infants weighing 2,000 grams or more as soon as possible, but no later than age 7 days.

Doses following the birth dose:

- The second dose should be administered at age 1 or 2 months. Monovalent HepB vaccine should be used for doses administered before age 6 weeks.
- Infants who did not receive a birth dose should receive 3 doses of a HepB-containing vaccine on a schedule of 0, 1 to 2 months, and 6 months starting as soon as feasible. See Figure 2.
- Administer the second dose 1 to 2 months after the first dose (minimum interval of 4 weeks), administer the third dose at least 8 weeks after the second dose AND at least 16 weeks after the **first** dose. The final (third or fourth) dose in the HepB vaccine series should be administered **no earlier than age 24 weeks.**
- Administration of a total of 4 doses of HepB vaccine is permitted when a combination vaccine containing HepB is administered after the birth dose.

Catch-up vaccination:

- Unvaccinated persons should complete a 3-dose series.
- A 2-dose series (doses separated by at least 4 months) of adult formulation Recombivax HB is licensed for use in children aged 11 through 15 years.
- For other catch-up guidance, see Figure 2.

2. Rotavirus (RV) vaccines. (Minimum age: 6 weeks for both RV1 [Rotarix] and RV5 [RotaTeq])

Routine vaccination:

Administer a series of RV vaccine to all infants as follows:

1. If Rotarix is used, administer a 2-dose series at 2 and 4 months of age.
2. If RotaTeq is used, administer a 3-dose series at ages 2, 4, and 6 months.
3. If any dose in the series was RotaTeq or vaccine product is unknown for any dose in the series, a total of 3 doses of RV vaccine should be administered.

Catch-up vaccination:

- The maximum age for the first dose in the series is 14 weeks, 6 days; vaccination should not be initiated for infants aged 15 weeks, 0 days or older.
- The maximum age for the final dose in the series is 8 months, 0 days.
- For other catch-up guidance, see Figure 2.

3. Diphtheria and tetanus toxoids and acellular pertussis (DTaP) vaccine. (Minimum age: 6 weeks. Exception: DTaP-IPV [Kinrix]: 4 years)

Routine vaccination:

- Administer a 5-dose series of DTaP vaccine at ages 2, 4, 6, 15 through 18 months, and 4 through 6 years. The fourth dose may be administered as early as age 12 months, provided at least 6 months have elapsed since the third dose. However, the fourth dose of DTaP need not be repeated if it was administered at least 4 months after the third dose of DTaP.

3. Diphtheria and tetanus toxoids and acellular pertussis (DTaP) vaccine (cont'd)

Catch-up vaccination:

- The fifth dose of DTaP vaccine is not necessary if the fourth dose was administered at age 4 years or older.
- For other catch-up guidance, see Figure 2.

4. Tetanus and diphtheria toxoids and acellular pertussis (Tdap) vaccine. (Minimum age: 10 years for both Boostrix and Adacel)

Routine vaccination:

- Administer 1 dose of Tdap vaccine to all adolescents aged 11 through 12 years.
- Tdap may be administered regardless of the interval since the last tetanus and diphtheria toxoid-containing vaccine.
- Administer 1 dose of Tdap vaccine to pregnant adolescents during each pregnancy (preferred during 27 through 36 weeks' gestation) regardless of time since prior Td or Tdap vaccination.

Catch-up vaccination:

- Persons aged 7 years and older who are not fully immunized with DTaP vaccine should receive Tdap vaccine as 1 dose (preferably the first) in the catch-up series; if additional doses are needed, use Td vaccine. For children 7 through 10 years who receive a dose of Tdap as part of the catch-up series, an adolescent Tdap vaccine dose at age 11 through 12 years should NOT be administered. Td should be administered instead 10 years after the Tdap dose.
- Persons aged 11 through 18 years who have not received Tdap vaccine should receive a dose followed by tetanus and diphtheria toxoid (Td) booster doses every 10 years thereafter.
- Inadvertent doses of DTaP vaccine:
  - If administered inadvertently to a child aged 7 through 10 years may count as part of the catch-up series. This dose may count as the adolescent Tdap dose, or the child can later receive a Tdap booster dose at age 11 through 12 years.
  - If administered inadvertently to an adolescent aged 11 through 18 years, the dose should be counted as the adolescent Tdap booster.
- For other catch-up guidance, see Figure 2.

5. _Haemophilus influenzae_ type b (Hib) conjugate vaccine. (Minimum age: 6 weeks for PRP-T [ACTHIB, DTaP-IPV/Hib (Pentacel) and Hib-MenCY (MenHibrix)], PRP-OMP [PedvaxHIB or COMVAX], 12 months for PRP-T [Hiberix])

Routine vaccination:

- Administer a 2- or 3-dose Hib vaccine primary series and a booster dose (dose 3 or 4 depending on vaccine used in primary series) at age 12 through 15 months to complete a full Hib vaccine series.
- The primary series with ActHIB, MenHibrix, or Pentacel consists of 3 doses and should be administered at 2, 4, and 6 months of age. The primary series with PedvaxHib or COMVAX consists of 2 doses and should be administered at 2 and 4 months of age; a dose at age 6 months is not indicated.
- One booster dose (dose 3 or 4 depending on vaccine used in primary series) of any Hib vaccine should be administered at age 12 through 15 months. An exception is Hiberix vaccine. Hiberix should only be used for the booster (final) dose in children aged 12 months through 4 years who have received at least 1 prior dose of Hib-containing vaccine.
- For recommendations on the use of MenHibrix in patients at increased risk for meningococcal disease, please refer to the meningococcal vaccine footnotes and also to *MMWR* February 28, 2014 / 63(RR01);1-13, available at http://www.cdc.gov/mmwr/PDF/rr/rr6301.pdf.

For further guidance on the use of the vaccines mentioned below, see: http://www.cdc.gov/vaccines/hcp/acip-recs/index.html.

5. **Haemophilus influenzae type b (Hib) conjugate vaccine (cont'd)**

Catch-up vaccination:
- If dose 1 was administered at ages 12 through 14 months, administer a second (final) dose at least 8 weeks after dose 1, regardless of Hib vaccine used in the primary series.
- If both doses were PRP-OMP (PedvaxHIB or COMVAX), and were administered before the first birthday, the third (and final) dose should be administered at age 12 through 59 months and at least 8 weeks after the second dose.
- If the first dose was administered at age 7 through 11 months, administer the second dose at least 4 weeks later and a third (and final) dose at age 12 through 15 months or 8 weeks after second dose, whichever is later.
- If first dose is administered before the first birthday and second dose administered at younger than 15 months, a third (and final) dose should be given 8 weeks later.
- For unvaccinated children aged 15 months or older, administer only 1 dose.
- For catch-up guidance, see Figure 2. For catch-up guidance related to MenHibrix, please see the meningococcal vaccine footnotes and also MMWR February 28, 2014 / 63(RR01);1–13, available at http://www.cdc.gov/mmwr/PDF/rr/rr6301.pdf.

Vaccination of persons with high-risk conditions:
- Children aged 12 through 59 months who are at increased risk for Hib disease, including chemotherapy recipients and those with anatomic or functional asplenia (including sickle cell disease), human immunodeficiency virus (HIV) infection, immunoglobulin deficiency, or early component complement deficiency, who have received either no doses or only 1 dose of Hib vaccine before 12 months of age, should receive 2 additional doses of Hib vaccine 8 weeks apart; children who received 2 or more doses of Hib vaccine before 12 months of age should receive 1 additional dose.
- For patients younger than 5 years of age undergoing chemotherapy or radiation treatment who received a Hib vaccine dose(s) within 14 days of starting therapy or during therapy, repeat the dose(s) at least 3 months following therapy completion.
- Recipients of hematopoietic stem cell transplant (HSCT) should be revaccinated with a 3-dose regimen of Hib vaccine starting 6 to 12 months after successful transplant, regardless of vaccination history; doses should be administered at least 4 weeks apart.
- A single dose of any Hib-containing vaccine should be administered to unimmunized* children and adolescents 15 months of age and older undergoing an elective splenectomy; if possible, vaccine should be administered at least 14 days before procedure.
- Hib vaccine is not routinely recommended for patients 5 years or older. However, 1 dose of Hib vaccine should be administered to unimmunized* persons aged 5 years or older who have anatomic or functional asplenia (including sickle cell disease) and unvaccinated persons 5 through 18 years of age with human immunodeficiency virus (HIV) infection.

*Patients who have not received a primary series and booster dose or at least 1 dose of Hib vaccine after 14 months of age are considered unimmunized.

6. **Pneumococcal vaccines. (Minimum age: 6 weeks for PCV13, 2 years for PPSV23)**

Routine vaccination with PCV13:
- Administer a 4-dose series of PCV13 vaccine at ages 2, 4, and 6 months and at age 12 through 15 months.
- For children aged 14 through 59 months who have received an age-appropriate series of 7-valent PCV (PCV7), administer a single supplemental dose of 13-valent PCV (PCV13).

Catch-up vaccination with PCV13:
- Administer 1 dose of PCV13 to all healthy children aged 24 through 59 months who are not completely vaccinated for their age.
- For other catch-up guidance, see Figure 2.

Vaccination of persons with high-risk conditions with PCV13 and PPSV23:
- All recommended PCV13 doses should be administered prior to PPSV23 vaccination if possible.
- For children 2 through 5 years of age with any of the following conditions: chronic heart disease (particularly cyanotic congenital heart disease and cardiac failure); chronic lung disease (including asthma if treated with high-dose oral corticosteroid therapy); diabetes mellitus; cerebrospinal fluid leak; cochlear implant; sickle cell disease and other hemoglobinopathies; anatomic or functional asplenia; HIV infection; chronic renal failure; nephrotic syndrome; diseases associated with treatment with immunosuppressive drugs or radiation therapy, including malignant neoplasms, leukemias, lymphomas, and Hodgkin's disease; solid organ transplantation; or congenital immunodeficiency:
1. Administer 1 dose of PCV13 if any incomplete schedule of 3 doses of PCV (PCV7 and/or PCV13) were received previously.
2. Administer 2 doses of PCV13 at least 8 weeks apart if unvaccinated or any incomplete schedule of fewer than 3 doses of PCV (PCV7 and/or PCV13) were received previously.
3. Administer 1 supplemental dose of PCV13 if 4 doses of PCV7 or other age-appropriate complete PCV7 series was received previously.
4. The minimum interval between doses of PCV (PCV7 or PCV13) is 8 weeks.
5. For children with no history of PPSV23 vaccination, administer PPSV23 at least 8 weeks after the most recent dose of PCV13.

6. **Pneumococcal vaccines (cont'd)**
- For children aged 6 through 18 years who have cerebrospinal fluid leak; cochlear implant; sickle cell disease and other hemoglobinopathies; anatomic or functional asplenia; congenital or acquired immunodeficiencies; HIV infection; chronic renal failure; nephrotic syndrome; diseases associated with treatment with immunosuppressive drugs or radiation therapy, including malignant neoplasms, leukemias, lymphomas, and Hodgkin's disease; generalized malignancy; solid organ transplantation; or multiple myeloma:
1. If neither PCV13 nor PPSV23 has been received previously, administer 1 dose of PCV13 now and 1 dose of PPSV23 at least 8 weeks later.
2. If PCV13 has been received previously but PPSV23 has not, administer 1 dose of PPSV23 at least 8 weeks after the most recent dose of PCV13.
3. If PPSV23 has been received but PCV13 has not, administer 1 dose of PCV13 at least 8 weeks after the most recent dose of PPSV23.
- For children aged 6 through 18 years with chronic heart disease (particularly cyanotic congenital heart disease and cardiac failure), chronic lung disease (including asthma if treated with high-dose oral corticosteroid therapy), diabetes mellitus, alcoholism, or chronic liver disease, who have not received PPSV23, administer 1 dose of PPSV23. If PCV13 has been received previously, then PPSV23 should be administered at least 8 weeks after any prior PCV13 dose.
- A single revaccination with PPSV23 should be administered 5 years after the first dose to children with sickle cell disease or other hemoglobinopathies; anatomic or functional asplenia; congenital or acquired immunodeficiencies; HIV infection; chronic renal failure; nephrotic syndrome; diseases associated with treatment with immunosuppressive drugs or radiation therapy, including malignant neoplasms, leukemias, lymphomas, and Hodgkin's disease; generalized malignancy; solid organ transplantation; or multiple myeloma.

7. **Inactivated poliovirus vaccine (IPV). (Minimum age: 6 weeks)**

Routine vaccination:
- Administer a 4-dose series of IPV at ages 2, 4, 6 through 18 months, and 4 through 6 years. The final dose in the series should be administered on or after the fourth birthday and at least 6 months after the previous dose.

Catch-up vaccination:
- In the first 6 months of life, minimum age and minimum intervals are only recommended if the person is at risk of imminent exposure to circulating poliovirus (i.e., travel to a polio-endemic region or during an outbreak).
- If 4 or more doses are administered before age 4 years, an additional dose should be administered at age 4 through 6 years and at least 6 months after the previous dose.
- A fourth dose is not necessary if the third dose was administered at age 4 years or older and at least 6 months after the previous dose.
- If both OPV and IPV were administered as part of a series, a total of 4 doses should be administered, regardless of the child's current age. IPV is not routinely recommended for U.S. residents aged 18 years or older.
- For other catch-up guidance, see Figure 2.

8. **Influenza vaccines. (Minimum age: 6 months for inactivated influenza vaccine [IIV], 2 years for live, attenuated influenza vaccine [LAIV])**

Routine vaccination:
- Administer influenza vaccine annually to all children beginning at age 6 months. For most healthy, nonpregnant persons aged 2 through 49 years, either LAIV or IIV may be used. However, LAIV should NOT be administered to some persons, including 1) persons who have experienced severe allergic reactions to LAIV, any of its components, or to a previous dose of any influenza vaccine; 2) children 2 through 17 years receiving aspirin or aspirin-containing products; 3) persons who are allergic to eggs; 4) pregnant women; 5) immunosuppressed persons; 6) children 2 through 4 years of age with asthma or who had wheezing in the past 12 months; or 7) persons who have taken influenza antiviral medications in the previous 48 hours. For all other contraindications and precautions to use of LAIV, see MMWR August 15, 2014 / 63(32);691–697 [40 pages] available at http://www.cdc.gov/mmwr/pdf/wk/mm6332.pdf.

For children aged 6 months through 8 years:
- For the 2014-15 season, administer 2 doses (separated by at least 4 weeks) to children who are receiving influenza vaccine for the first time. Some children in this age group who have been vaccinated previously will also need 2 doses. For additional guidance, follow dosing guidelines in the 2014-15 ACIP influenza vaccine recommendations, MMWR August 15, 2014 / 63(32);591–697 [40 pages] available at http://www.cdc.gov/mmwr/pdf/wk/mm6332.pdf.
- For the 2015-16 season, follow dosing guidelines in the 2015 ACIP influenza vaccine recommendations.

For persons aged 9 years and older:
- Administer 1 dose.

Continued

Table 19–2 ⊗ Catch-Up Immunization Schedule for Persons Aged 4 Months Through 18 Years Who Start Late or Who Are More Than 1 Month Behind – United States, 2015—cont'd

For further guidance on the use of the vaccines mentioned below, see: http://www.cdc.gov/vaccines/hcp/acip-recs/index.html.

9. Measles, mumps, and rubella (MMR) vaccine. (Minimum age: 12 months for routine vaccination)

Routine vaccination:

- Administer a 2-dose series of MMR vaccine at ages 12 through 15 months and 4 through 6 years. The second dose may be administered before age 4 years, provided at least 4 weeks have elapsed since the first dose.
- Administer 1 dose of MMR vaccine to infants aged 6 through 11 months before departure from the United States for international travel. These children should be revaccinated with 2 doses of MMR vaccine, the first at age 12 through 15 months (12 months if the child remains in an area where disease risk is high), and the second dose at least 4 weeks later.
- Administer 2 doses of MMR vaccine to children aged 12 months and older before departure from the United States for international travel. The first dose should be administered on or after age 12 months and the second dose at least 4 weeks later.

Catch-up vaccination:

- Ensure that all school-aged children and adolescents have had 2 doses of MMR vaccine; the minimum interval between the 2 doses is 4 weeks.

10. Varicella (VAR) vaccine. (Minimum age: 12 months)

Routine vaccination:

- Administer a 2-dose series of VAR vaccine at ages 12 through 15 months and 4 through 6 years. The second dose may be administered before age 4 years, provided at least 3 months have elapsed since the first dose. If the second dose was administered at least 4 weeks after the first dose, it can be accepted as valid.

Catch-up vaccination:

- Ensure that all persons aged 7 through 18 years without evidence of immunity (see *MMWR 2007 / 56* [No. RR-4], available at http://www.cdc.gov/mmwr/pdf/rr/rr5604.pdf] have 2 doses of varicella vaccine. For children aged 7 through 12 years, the recommended minimum interval between doses is 3 months (if the second dose was administered at least 4 weeks after the first dose, it can be accepted as valid); for persons aged 13 years and older, the minimum interval between doses is 4 weeks.

11. Hepatitis A (HepA) vaccine. (Minimum age: 12 months)

Routine vaccination:

- Initiate the 2-dose HepA vaccine series at 12 through 23 months; separate the 2 doses by 6 to 18 months.
- Children who have received 1 dose of HepA vaccine before age 24 months should receive a second dose 6 to 18 months after the first dose.
- For any person aged 2 years and older who has not already received the HepA vaccine series, 2 doses of HepA vaccine separated by 6 to 18 months may be administered if immunity against hepatitis A virus infection is desired.

Catch-up vaccination:

- The minimum interval between the two doses is 6 months.

Special populations:

- Administer 2 doses of HepA vaccine at least 6 months apart to previously unvaccinated persons who live in areas where vaccination programs target older children, or who are at increased risk for infection. This includes persons traveling to or working in countries that have high or intermediate endemicity of infection; men having sex with men; users of injection and non-injection illicit drugs; persons who work with HAV-infected primates or with HAV in a research laboratory; persons with clotting-factor disorders; persons with chronic liver disease; and persons who anticipate close personal contact (e.g., household or regular babysitting) with an international adoptee during the first 60 days after arrival in the United States from a country with high or intermediate endemicity. The first dose should be administered as soon as the adoption is planned, ideally 2 or more weeks before the arrival of the adoptee.

12. Human papillomavirus (HPV) vaccines. (Minimum age: 9 years for HPV2 [Cervarix] and HPV4 [Gardasil])

Routine vaccination:

- Administer a 3-dose series of HPV vaccine on a schedule of 0, 1-2, and 6 months to all adolescents aged 11 through 12 years. Either HPV4 or HPV2 may be used for females, and only HPV4 may be used for males.
- The vaccine series may be started at age 9 years.
- Administer the second dose 1 to 2 months after the first dose (minimum interval of 4 weeks); administer the third dose 24 weeks after the first dose and 16 weeks after the second dose (minimum interval of 12 weeks).

Catch-up vaccination:

- Administer the vaccine series to females (either HPV2 or HPV4) and males (HPV4) at age 13 through 18 years if not previously vaccinated.
- Use recommended routine dosing intervals (see Routine vaccination above) for vaccine series catch-up.

13. Meningococcal conjugate vaccines. (Minimum age: 6 weeks for Hib-MenCY [MenHibrix], 9 months for MenACWY-D [Menactra], 2 months for MenACWY-CRM [Menveo])

Routine vaccination:

- Administer a single dose of Menactra or Menveo vaccine at age 11 through 12 years, with a booster dose at age 16 years.
- Adolescents aged 11 through 18 years with human immunodeficiency virus (HIV) infection should receive a 2-dose primary series of Menactra or Menveo with at least 8 weeks between doses.
- For children aged 2 months through 18 years with high-risk conditions, see below.

Catch-up vaccination:

- Administer Menactra or Menveo vaccine at age 13 through 18 years if not previously vaccinated.
- If the first dose is administered at age 13 through 15 years, a booster dose should be administered at age 16 through 18 years with a minimum interval of at least 8 weeks between doses.
- If the first dose is administered at age 16 years or older, a booster dose is not needed.
- For other catch-up guidance, see Figure 2.

Vaccination of persons with high-risk conditions and other persons at increased risk of disease:

- Children with anatomic or functional asplenia (including sickle cell disease):

1. Menveo
   - *Children who initiate vaccination at 8 weeks through 6 months:* Administer doses at 2, 4, 6, and 12 months of age.
   - *Unvaccinated children 7 through 23 months:* Administer 2 doses, with the second dose at least 12 weeks after the first dose AND after the first birthday.
   - *Children 24 months and older who have not received a complete series:* Administer 2 primary doses at least 8 weeks apart.
2. MenHibrix
   - *Children 6 weeks through 18 months:* Administer doses at 2, 4, 6, and 12 through 15 months of age.
   - If the first dose of MenHibrix is given at or after 12 months of age, a total of 2 doses should be given at least 8 weeks apart to ensure protection against serogroups C and Y meningococcal disease.
3. Menactra
   - *Children 24 months and older who have not received a complete series:* Administer 2 primary doses at least 8 weeks apart. If Menactra is administered to a child with asplenia (including sickle cell disease), do not administer Menactra until 2 years of age and at least 4 weeks after the completion of all PCV13 doses.

- Children with persistent complement component deficiency:

1. Menveo
   - *Children who initiate vaccination at 8 weeks through 6 months:* Administer doses at 2, 4, 6, and 12 months of age.
   - *Unvaccinated children 7 through 23 months:* Administer 2 doses, with the second dose at least 12 weeks after the first dose AND after the first birthday.
   - *Children 24 months and older who have not received a complete series:* Administer 2 primary doses at least 8 weeks apart.
2. MenHibrix
   - *Children 6 weeks through 18 months:* Administer doses at 2, 4, 6, and 12 through 15 months of age.
   - If the first dose of MenHibrix is given at or after 12 months of age, a total of 2 doses should be given at least 8 weeks apart to ensure protection against serogroups C and Y meningococcal disease.
3. Menactra
   - *Children 9 through 23 months:* Administer 2 primary doses at least 12 weeks apart.
   - *Children 24 months and older who have not received a complete series:* Administer 2 primary doses at least 8 weeks apart.

- For children who travel to or reside in countries in which meningococcal disease is hyperendemic or epidemic, including countries in the African meningitis belt or the Hajj, administer an age-appropriate formulation and series of Menactra or Menveo for protection against serogroups A and W meningococcal disease. Prior receipt of MenHibrix is not sufficient for children traveling to the meningitis belt or the Hajj because it does not contain serogroups A or W.
- For children at risk during a community outbreak attributable to a vaccine serogroup, administer or complete an age- and formulation-appropriate series of MenHibrix, Menactra, or Menveo.
- For booster doses among persons with high-risk conditions, refer to *MMWR 2013 / 62(RR02):1-22*, available at http://www.cdc.gov/mmwr/preview/mmwrhtml/rr6202a1.htm.

For other catch-up recommendations for these persons, and complete information on use of meningococcal vaccines, including guidance related to vaccination of persons at increased risk of infection, see MMWR March 22, 2013 / 62(RR02):1-22, available at http://www.cdc.gov/mmwr/pdf/rr/rr6202.pdf.

CS 244083-B

should be made. These statements are available at the CDC Web site or at www.immunize.org in multiple languages (Table 19-3).

The SC injection of MMR may sting the patient, who may have post-injection discomfort. The VIS states that 5% to 15% of patients may experience a fever of up to 103°F (39.5°C) approximately 7 to 12 days after administration of MMR. The patient may also experience rash, malaise, or sore throat.

Table 19–3   Vaccine Information Statements

Vaccine Information Statements (VISs) are available from the Centers for Disease Control and Prevention (CDC) or your local health department for the following vaccines. They have also been translated into the languages listed below. A PDF version of these VISs (English and other languages) can be found at www.immunize.org.

Vaccines	
Anthrax	Meningococcal
Chickenpox	Measles, mumps, and rubella
Diphtheria, tetanus, and pertussis	Pneumococcus
HIB	Polio (oral and inactivated)
Hepatitis A	Rabies
Hepatitis B	Rotavirus
Influenza	Smallpox
Japanese encephalitis	Td, Tdap
Lyme disease	Typhoid
Varicella	Yellow fever

Languages	
Arabic	Korean
Armenian	Laotian
Bosnian	Marshallese
Burmese	Portuguese
Cambodian	Polish
Chinese	Punjabi
Croatian	Romanian
Farsi	Russian
French	Samoan
German	Serbo-Croatian
Haitian	Somali
Hindi	Spanish
Hmong	Tagalog
Ilokano	Thai
Italian	Turkish
Japanese	Vietnamese

MEASLES, MUMPS, RUBELLA, AND VARICELLA VACCINE

Pharmacodynamics

Similar to MMR, the MMRV (ProQuad) vaccine is a live, attenuated virus vaccine that produces a subclinical infection, creating active immunity to measles, mumps, rubella, and varicella viruses.

Pharmacokinetics

The MMRV vaccine is administered SC. Following SC injection of the first dose, the response rate at 6 weeks for patients is 91.2% for varicella, 97.4% for measles, 98.8% for mumps, and 98.5% for rubella (Merck, 2013). More than 99% of people who receive two doses of MMRV separated by at least 3 months develop evidence of immunity to all four covered viruses; for that reason, the current recommendation is for two doses.

Pharmacotherapeutics

Precautions and Contraindications

The contraindications for MMRV are the same as for MMR, including a history of anaphylactic reaction to neomycin or gelatin or any other component of the vaccine. Immediate treatment for anaphylaxis reaction should be available when administering MMRV.

MMRV is contraindicated in patients with primary or acquired immunodeficiency, including patients with immunosuppression associated with HIV/AIDS and patients with blood dyscrasias, leukemia, lymphomas of any type, or other malignant neoplasms affecting the bone marrow or lymphatic system. Immunosuppressive therapy, including high-dose steroids, may result in a more extensive vaccine-associated rash or disseminated disease. Low-dose, replacement, or short-burst therapy for asthma, are not contraindications for MMRV administration.

MMRV is Pregnancy Category C and MMRV (ProQuad) should not be administered to a pregnant patient. The manufacturer recommends pregnancy should be avoided for at least 3 months following vaccination (Merck, 2013). Merck Sharp & Dohme maintains a registry to monitor fetal outcomes if a woman is administered ProQuad during pregnancy. Inadvertent exposure during pregnancy should be reported to Merck & Co., Inc., at 1-877-888-4231 or VAERS at 1-800-822-7967, or www.vaers.hhs.gov.

If a patient has untreated tuberculosis or a febrile illness with temperature greater than 101.3°F (38.5°C), then vaccination with MMRV should be deferred until the patient is well. Because of the increased risk of fever and febrile seizures with MMRV, it should be used with caution in patients with a history of cerebral injury, seizures, or other conditions in which physiological stress due to fever should be avoided.

No data is available on the development of thrombocytopenia in patients vaccinated with MMRV (ProQuad). Because of the known risk for thrombocytopenia with MMR, use caution when administering MMRV.

Vaccination with MMRV should be avoided for 3 months after a blood transfusion or immune globulin administration.

Adverse Drug Reactions

The adverse drug reactions seen in MMRV are similar to those for MMR, except patients are more likely to develop fever and rash. There is a risk for developing a fever 7 to 12 days after MMR administration. In pre-licensure studies MMRV fever (equal to or greater than 102°F; equal to or greater than 39°C) was seen in 21.5% of patients, compared to 14.9% of patients receiving MMR (CDC, 2013a). Post-licensure studies of febrile seizures post-MMRV vaccination indicate one additional febrile seizure occurred 5 to 12 days after vaccination per 2,300 to 2,600 children aged 12 to 23 months who had received the first dose of MMRV vaccine compared with children who had received the first dose of MMR vaccine and varicella vaccine administered as separate injections at the same visit (CDC, 2013a). This increased risk of febrile seizure is not seen after the second dose of MMRV administered at the 4- to 6-year visit.

There is a slightly increased risk of developing a measles-like rash from 2.1% with MMR alone to 3% with MMRV. Additional adverse reactions include pain at injection site (22%), erythema (14.4%), and swelling (8.4%), similar to what is seen in patients receiving MMR (Merck, 2013).

Drug Interactions

Drug interactions with MMRV are the same as for MMR: immunosuppressants, IG, tuberculin skin tests, and salicylates.

Clinical Use and Dosing

MMRV is given SC at 12 to 15 months of age. The first dose may be given any time before age 12 years. Use of MMRV for the repeat dose at 4 to 6 years is well tolerated and results in higher levels of varicella antibodies (Reisinger et al, 2006). Three months should elapse before a second dose of MMRV is administered. MMRV may be administered 1 month after a dose of MMR.

Patient Education

The CDC recommends providers administering MMRV to children have a conversation with parents regarding the increased risk of fever and febrile seizures with the combination vaccine (CDC, 2013a). Parents of children should be informed about the slightly increased risk of febrile seizures 5 to 12 days after receiving the MMRV combination (Marin, Broder, Temte, Snider, & Seward, 2010). This risk will need to be weighed against the discomfort of two injections.

ORAL POLIOVIRUS VACCINE

Although oral polio vaccine (OPV) is no longer used in the United States, it is still used in other countries because of administrative ease and low cost.

Pharmacodynamics

OPV stimulates the immune system to produce antipoliovirus antibodies against Sabin poliovirus types 1, 2, and 3.

After oral administration, the live, attenuated virus enters the small intestine, where it replicates in the villous epithelial cells. These specialized epithelial cells transport the viral antigens to the B cells and macrophages, which process and produce antipoliovirus antibodies. In 1 to 2 weeks after a dose of OPV, antibodies are present. The live, attenuated poliovirus lingers in the gastrointestinal (GI) tract for 4 to 6 weeks, inducing both mucosal and serum antipoliovirus antibodies. The local secretory (intestinal) immune responses to OPV are greater than those induced by IPV. OPV induces intestinal immunity against wild strains of poliovirus; IPV does not. At least two doses of OPV are necessary for intestinal immunity. OPV may induce a herd-type of immunity because of the spread of live, attenuated viruses to susceptible contacts during the viral shedding period of 4 to 6 weeks after dosing. Three doses of OPV result in sustained, lifelong immunity.

Pharmacokinetics

After oral administration of OPV, antibody stimulation occurs within 7 to 10 days. Poliovirus antibodies have been found in serum, nasal secretions, saliva, duodenal fluids, urine, and feces. Poliovirus antibodies are distributed into breast milk.

Pharmacotherapeutics

Precautions and Contraindications

An anaphylactic reaction to any previous dose of OPV is a contraindication to its use. Patients with neomycin or streptomycin hypersensitivity also should not receive OPV because these agents are contained in OPV in small quantities.

OPV should be delayed if a patient has a moderate or severe febrile illness or severe respiratory infection. Administration of OPV with current viral GI infection, ongoing diarrhea, or vomiting is contraindicated. Vomiting may prevent the vaccine from reaching the stomach and small intestine. Diarrhea may increase transit time, preventing proper contact of the vaccine viruses with villous intestinal cells, and lead to decreased immune response. Vaccine administration should be delayed until the vomiting and diarrhea have been resolved.

There is a risk that immunocompromised individuals may develop poliomyelitis from use of live poliovirus, which is in OPV. Cancer, leukemia, lymphoma, radiation therapy, and immunodeficiency, including HIV or AIDS, are contraindications to OPV use. Drugs that affect the immune system, including high-dose steroids, are also a contraindication to OPV use. There is a chance that immunosuppressed individuals may contract OPV-associated poliomyelitis from coming in contact with a patient who is shedding the virus. IPV is the drug of choice in immunocompromised patients. IPV should also be used if household members are immunocompromised.

Vaccination of pregnant women with OPV should be avoided. OPV is Pregnancy Category C. If exposure to poliomyelitis is imminent and immediate protection is needed, vaccinate with OPV or IPV according to the adult dosing schedule. OPV is safe during breastfeeding and is routinely given during infancy.

Adverse Drug Reactions

The administration of OPV is associated with a low incidence (1 case/2.6 million doses) of paralytic poliomyelitis in patients who receive the vaccine and in household contacts. Vaccine-associated paralytic poliomyelitis (VAPP) is most likely to occur after the first dose of OPV. Household contacts are put at risk of developing VAPP because poliovirus is shed in the feces for 6 to 8 weeks after a dose of OPV. There is no risk of VAPP with the use of IPV, which is why, as of January 2000, IPV is the drug of choice for routine childhood immunization against polio in the United States.

Drug Interactions

OPV should not be administered to patients receiving immunosuppressants, including corticosteroids, interferon, and antineoplastic drugs, because there may be insufficient response to immunization. Patients may remain susceptible despite immunization. IPV is the recommended drug to use in these patients.

The CDC recommends that administration of live-virus vaccines be separated by intervals of at least 1 month, unless data are available regarding simultaneous vaccination (MMR, MMRV, hepatitis B vaccine [HBV], DTP, DTaP, influenza, and HIB may be given with OPV). Concurrent administration of OPV and cholera vaccine, parenteral typhoid vaccine, or plague vaccine should generally be avoided because of increased adverse effects. Concurrent administration of live oral typhoid vaccine may result in decreased immune responses to OPV. IG may be given with OPV.

Clinical Use and Dosing

To eliminate the risk of VAPP, the CDC recommended in January 2000 an all-IPV schedule for childhood immunizations. OPV may be used only for special circumstances, such as mass vaccination campaigns to control outbreaks of paralytic polio and in unvaccinated children who will be traveling in less than 4 weeks to areas where polio is endemic or epidemic. OPV may be used in children who have received at least two doses of IPV and whose parents do not accept the recommended number of vaccine injections. VAPP should be discussed with these parents before administering OPV. See Tables 19-1, 19-2, and 19-3 for dosing schedules.

Patient Education

All patients or their parents or guardians are required by law to receive CDC VISs, which are available in a variety of languages. Every effort should be made to provide adequate information to patients and parents before immunization. If a patient receives OPV, the patient and family should be instructed that virus is shed in the stools for 6 to 8 weeks and that good hand washing is crucial to preventing the small chance of contracting VAPP from the infected feces. As previously mentioned, VAPP should be discussed with the parent or, if applicable, the patient before administering OPV.

ROTAVIRUS VACCINE

Pharmacodynamics

Rotavirus is the leading cause of gastroenteritis in infants and young children worldwide. Almost every child in the United States will become infected with rotavirus by age 5 years, causing 400,000 doctor visits, and 55,000 to 70,000 hospital admissions (Cortese & Parashar, 2009). RotaTeq is a live oral vaccine that contains five strains of rotavirus (G1, G2, G3 or G4, P7). Rotarix is indicated for the prevention of rotavirus gastroenteritis caused by G1, G3, G4, and G9. Both vaccines are live vaccines that replicate in the small intestine and induce active immunity against rotavirus.

Pharmacokinetics

Pharmacokinetic information regarding rotavirus vaccine is not available.

Pharmacotherapeutics

Precautions and Contraindications

Because rotavirus vaccine is a live-virus vaccine, it should not be administered to infants who are or may be potentially immunocompromised, including infants with blood dyscrasias, leukemia, lymphomas, or other malignant neoplasms; infants on immunosuppressive therapy; infants with primary and acquired immunodeficiency states including HIV/AIDS; and infants who have received blood transfusions or blood products in the past 42 days.

Infants who have a febrile illness should have the vaccine delayed, except when withholding the vaccine creates greater risk to the patient. A minor upper respiratory infection with low-grade fever (under 100.5°F) is not a reason for withholding rotavirus vaccine. The virus should not be administered to infants with acute gastroenteritis until it improves.

Rotavirus may be shed in the stools of patients receiving the vaccine (8.9% of patients in clinical trials); therefore, it is prudent to use caution if the infant will have close contact with persons with malignancies or who are otherwise immunocompromised and contacts who are receiving immunosuppressive therapy.

A history of intussusception is a contraindication for the rotavirus vaccine because there may be an increased risk of intussusception following the first dose of rotavirus vaccine (CDC, 2011a).

Adverse Drug Reactions

A previous live rhesus rotavirus–based vaccine (RotaShield) was withdrawn from the market after it was found to be associated with intussusception. The risk for intussusception was evaluated in a large preclinical trials of more than 70,000 infants, which found no association with intussusception and administration of RotaTeq or Rotarix (Cortese & Parashar, 2009). Postmarketing studies in Mexico found a slight increased risk (0 to 4 cases per 100,000 vaccinated infants) of developing intussusception in the 31 days after administration of the first dose of rotavirus vaccine, with highest risk in the first 7 days after vaccine dose (Food and Drug Administration [FDA], 2012).

GI symptoms are the major reported adverse effects in the clinical trials of RotaTeq. There was a slight increased incidence of vomiting in the RotaTeq patients (6.7% versus 5.4% for placebo after dose 1, 5.0% versus 4.4% for placebo after dose 2, and 3.6% versus 3.2% for placebo after dose 3), as well as a slight increase in reports of diarrhea in the RotaTeq group (10.4% versus 9.1% in placebo after dose 1, 8.6% versus 6.4% in placebo group after dose 2, and 6.1% versus 5.4% in placebo after dose 3). Symptoms of irritability did not differ between RotaTeq and placebo infants in all three doses.

Rotarix clinical trials found no increase in fever, diarrhea, or fussiness in patients who received Rotarix over placebo. Patients who received Rotarix had a slightly increased (13% versus 11%) incidence of vomiting in the week after administration.

Drug Interactions

During clinical trials, RotaTeq and Rotarix were routinely administered concurrently with DTaP, IPV, HIB, HBV, and pneumococcal conjugate vaccine. There was no evidence of reduced antibody response to these vaccines when administered with RotaTeq or Rotarix (Cortese & Parashar, 2009).

Clinical Use and Dosing

RotaTeq vaccination consists of a series of three ready-to-use oral liquid doses. The vaccine is administered orally beginning at 6 to 12 weeks of age with the second and third doses delivered in 4- to 10-week intervals. All doses of the vaccine should be delivered by age 32 weeks. RotaTeq was administered to preterm infants (25- to 36-weeks' gestation) according to their age in weeks, and there was no difference in adverse effects between the vaccine and the placebo. There are insufficient data on safety and efficacy outside of these age ranges.

Rotarix is a two-dose schedule of 1 mL per dose given at 2 to 4 months of age. The two doses may be administered between 6 and 24 weeks of age. The two doses should be administered at least 4 weeks apart.

The CDC has recommendations for both rotavirus vaccines, including the maximum age for the first dose, which is 14 weeks 6 days (Cortese & Parashar, 2009). If a child is inadvertently given the first dose after 15 weeks and 0 days, then the series should be continued and completed by 8 months 0 days (Cortese & Parashar, 2009). Rotavirus vaccine may be administered before, after, or concurrently with any blood product or antibody-containing product (IG). Ideally, the series should all be the same rotavirus product, but if it is unknown whether the patient received RotaTeq or Rotarix, then the series should be completed with the product available to the clinic (Cortese & Parashar, 2009). If the patient regurgitates, spits out, or vomits the rotavirus vaccine, it should not be readministered. Children who have had rotavirus gastroenteritis before completing the series should start or complete the series according to the standard schedule.

Patient Education

All patients or their parents or guardians are required by law to receive CDC VISs, which are available in a variety of languages.

Every effort should be made to provide adequate information to patients and their parents before immunization. Because rotavirus vaccine is a live vaccine shed in the stool, caregivers should encourage strict hand-washing practices.

Parents should be instructed to report any adverse reactions to their health-care provider. Providers should fill out a Vaccine Adverse Event Reporting System (VAERS) form, available at www.vaers.hhs.gov/.

VARICELLA VIRUS VACCINE

Pharmacodynamics

Varicella virus vaccine (Varivax) is a live vaccine that produces an IgG antibody humoral immune response to varicella zoster virus (VZV). Vaccinated patients also have a cell-mediated immune response, with activation of both CD41 helper T cells and CD81 T lymphocytes. Efficacy of varicella vaccine is measured by protection against disease and by protection against severe disease. The efficacy of one dose of varicella vaccine is 94.4% over a 10-year period, with protection against household exposure of 90.2% (CDC, 2007). The two-dose regimen is 98.3% effective against any disease and 96.4% effective against household exposure (CDC, 2007). Vaccination appears to prevent serious disease even in patients who do not seroconvert. Post-vaccination cases of varicella are mild (less than 50 lesions, frequently not vesicular, mild or no fever) and patients recover quicker than when infected with wild virus (CDC, 2007).

Pharmacokinetics

A single SC dose of varicella virus vaccine given to children aged 12 months to 12 years stimulates IgG antibody production and results in seroconversion rates of 85.7% 6 weeks after the first dose (CDC, 2007). According to the CDC (2007), in children aged 12 months to 12 years who are administered a second dose with 3 months between doses, there is a 99.6% seroconversion response rate. When the second dose is given at age 4 to 6 years, the response is a 99.4% seroconversion rate. In patients, aged 13 and older, seroconversion rates are 78% to 82%; a second dose results in 99% seroconversion in adolescents and adults. Waning immunity has not been demonstrated, with high antibody levels measured for at least 10 years after vaccination.

Post-exposure prophylaxis with varicella vaccine is effective in preventing varicella disease. Administration to unvaccinated children within 3 days of exposure to varicella rash is 90% effective in preventing varicella and 70% effective if administered within 5 days of exposure (CDC, 2007). Post-exposure prophylaxis is 100% effective in decreasing the severity of disease.

Pharmacotherapeutics

Precautions and Contraindications

Patients with neomycin or gelatin hypersensitivity should not receive varicella vaccine because there are small quantities of each in the vaccine. Varicella vaccine should be delayed if a patient has a moderate or severe illness, with or without fever.

There is a risk that immunocompromised individuals will develop varicella from use of live virus for vaccination. Cancer, leukemia, lymphoma, radiation therapy, and immunodeficiency are contraindications to varicella vaccine use. Patients with symptomatic HIV infection should not receive varicella vaccine. Regarding asymptomatic HIV-infected children, the CDC states, "HIV-infected children with CD4+ T-lymphocyte percentage >15 percent should be considered for vaccination with the single antigen varicella vaccine" (CDC, 2007, p 24).

Drugs that affect the immune system, including high-dose steroids, also contraindicate varicella vaccine use. Patients who are on systemic steroids (e.g., for asthma) may be vaccinated if they are receiving less than 2 mg/kg or less than 20 mg per day of prednisone and are not otherwise immunocompromised (CDC, 2007). Varicella vaccine may be given to a patient if an immunocompromised person is in the household. The patient who develops a rash after vaccination should avoid contact with the immunocompromised person for the duration of the rash, although there has been no evidence of transmission of virus to an immunocompromised person in post-licensure monitoring of more than 55 million doses (CDC, 2007).

Vaccination of pregnant women should be avoided. Varicella vaccine is Pregnancy Category C. Pregnancy should be avoided for 1 to 3 months after vaccination. The manufacturer of Varivax has established a pregnancy registry to monitor maternal–fetal outcomes of pregnant women inadvertently administered the live varicella virus vaccine 3 months before or during pregnancy. For information about the registry, call 1-800-986-8999. In 10 years of monitoring via the pregnancy registry, no cases of congenital varicella syndrome or congenital varicella birth defects have been documented (CDC, 2007). Varicella vaccine may be given if there is a pregnant household contact, such as the patient's mother. Varicella vaccine may be given to a nursing mother if the risk of exposure to natural VZV is high. It is not known if it is excreted in breast milk.

Adverse Drug Reactions

The reactions reported most frequently in children and adults that can be attributed to varicella vaccine include fever, injection site reaction, and a vesicular rash. In healthy children, fever of 102°F or higher is reported in 14.7% of vaccine recipients. Pain or discomfort at the injection site is reported in 19.3%, with 3.4% of patients developing a vesicular rash at the injection site. A generalized vesicular rash developed in 3.8% of patients, with the median number of five or fewer lesions in healthy children. The vesicular rash occurs within 26 days of injection with varicella vaccine.

Adult and adolescent patients require two injections and have similar adverse reactions. Fever in vaccine recipients aged 12 years and older was defined as a temperature of 100°F or higher. After the first dose of varicella vaccine, 10.2% reported fever, and 9.5% reported fever after the second dose. Localized reaction at the injection site was reported in 3% of adolescent and adult patients after the first dose and in 1% after the second dose. A generalized vesicular rash was reported by 5.5% after the first dose and 0.9% after the second dose.

Drug Interactions

Varicella vaccine should not be administered to patients receiving immunosuppressants, including high-dose corticosteroids, interferon, and antineoplastic drugs, because response to immunization may be insufficient, that is, patients may remain susceptible despite immunization. Patients receiving prednisone up to 20 mg per day or less than 2 mg/kg per day for less than 2 weeks may receive varicella vaccine (CDC, 2007).

Whether varicella vaccine may be inactivated by IG is unknown, although other live-virus vaccines may be inactivated. Varicella vaccine should not be given for 3 to 11 months after IG is administered depending on the IG produced (CDC, 2007). The CDC recommends that IG preparations should not be administered for 2 weeks after varicella vaccine is given; the manufacturer recommends waiting 2 months. If IG is given in the interval after vaccination, the recipient should be either revaccinated in 5 months or tested for varicella immunity 6 months later and revaccinated if indicated.

The MMR and varicella vaccines are compatible if they are administered on the same day, with different needles, and at separate sites, or in the form of MMRV. If the two live vaccines are not given at the same time, an interval of 1 month between MMR and varicella vaccine is indicated. Varicella vaccine may be given simultaneously with DTaP, DT, Td, HIB, IPV, OPV, PCV13, or HBV, using separate sites of injection.

Although no adverse effects from the use of salicylates or aspirin (ASA) have been reported, the manufacturer recommends avoidance of ASA for 6 weeks after vaccination. Reye syndrome, which affects children younger than age 15 exclusively, has been associated with aspirin use following active varicella infection. Children who are on therapeutic ASA therapy may be vaccinated with the varicella vaccine, with close clinical monitoring. According to the CDC (2007), vaccination is thought to present less risk than natural varicella vaccine in these children.

Clinical Use and Dosing

The CDC and the AAP recommend that all healthy children who lack a reliable history of varicella infection be routinely vaccinated at age 12 to 15 months. A second dose of varicella vaccine is recommended at age 4 to 6 years (before entering kindergarten). The second dose may be administered earlier, as long as the interval between the two doses is more than 3 months. Healthy adolescents age 13 and older, who have no history of varicella infection and who have not previously received varicella vaccine, should be administered two doses 4 to 8 weeks apart.

Administration error: If a child is accidentally administered zoster vaccine (Zostavax) instead of varicella vaccine (Varivax), then it should be counted as a valid vaccine and reported to the VAERS whether or not an adverse reaction occurs. The child will still require two doses of varicella vaccine.

The ACIP of the CDC recommends that all healthy adults be screened for varicella immunity and adults without immunity should receive varicella vaccine. Attention should be given to those adults at high risk of exposure or transmission of varicella disease. They include adults who live in households with children, live or work in an environment in which varicella transmission is likely (teachers, health-care workers, day-care workers) or could occur (college dorm, correctional institution, military), or have household contact with an immunocompromised person; nonpregnant women of childbearing age; and international travelers. Performing serological testing of adults before administering is optional and may be cost-effective. The varicella vaccine dose for adults is two doses separated by 4 to 8 weeks.

Monitoring

There is no need to do post-vaccination titers after patients receive the varicella vaccine. At this time there is no commercially available test to determine immunity from varicella vaccine, just disease-induced immunity; therefore, the test may detect a false-positive outcome (CDC, 2007).

Patient Education

All patients or their parents or guardians are required by law to receive CDC VISs, which are available in a variety of languages. Every effort should be made to provide adequate information to patients and their parents before immunization.

There may be transient burning or stinging at administration. Patients should be informed that there is a small chance that they may develop a fever, reaction at the injection site, or vesicular rash after administration of varicella vaccine.

ZOSTER VACCINE

Pharmacodynamics

Shingles is a localized and painful cutaneous eruption caused by the reactivation of varicella zoster virus, the same virus that causes chickenpox in children. The varicella virus becomes latent in the neuronal cell bodies and when reactivated causes shingles. The triggers for reactivation are not well understood, but it is known that cell-mediated immunity may prevent reactivation. The lifetime incidence of shingles is 1 in 3 and it affects approximately 1 million patients in the United States annually (CDC, 2008).

Zoster vaccine (Zostavax) is a live, attenuated varicella zoster vaccine from the same strain used to develop the varicella vaccine (Varivax, ProQuad). The zoster vaccine reduced the risk of developing zoster by 51.3% in pre-licensure trials and was 66.5% effective in preventing post-herpetic neuralgia in the study group that was followed for 3 years. The vaccine also reduces severity of zoster by 57% in the vaccine recipients who developed post-herpetic neuralgia.

The zoster vaccine has been studied and approved by the U.S. Food and Drug Administration (FDA) for adults aged 50 years and older (CDC, 2011b). The vaccine is most effective in patients aged 60 to 69 years and least effective in patients over age 80 years (CDC, 2008).

> ### ● CLINICAL PEARL ●
>
> **Administering Multiple Vaccines**
>
> Currently a child from age 12 to 18 months should receive six possible injections. This can be traumatic for patient and parent. Most public health officials recommend giving all the recommended vaccines at one visit; therefore, the child who is 15 months old could be getting as many as all six injections at that visit. Using combined vaccines is best (Pediarix, Pentacel) to decrease the number of injections or spread the administration of the vaccines over two or three visits. If it is necessary to give all the vaccines in one visit, as in the case of upcoming international travel or a history of unreliable attendance at well-child examinations, two people can administer the vaccines simultaneously. Giving the vaccines simultaneously makes the process faster and simpler for the patient and the person administering the vaccine. The CDC guidelines for administering multiple injections to infants are located in Appendix D of the *Pink Book* at www.cdc.gov/vaccines/pubs/pinkbook/index.html.

Pharmacokinetics

A single SC 0.65-mL dose of zoster vaccine produces a peak in cell-mediated response to varicella zoster in 1 to 3 weeks. Patients in the 60-to-69 age group demonstrated a better immune response to the vaccine than patients over age 70.

Pharmacotherapeutics

Precautions and Contraindications

Zoster vaccine should not be administered to patients with a history of anaphylactic reaction to neomycin, gelatin, or any other component of the vaccine. Patients with primary immunodeficiency states should not be administered zoster vaccine. As zoster vaccine is a live, attenuated virus, patients with leukemia, lymphoma, cancer of the bone marrow or lymphatic system, or AIDS should not be given the vaccine, because they may develop disseminated disease. Patients receiving high-dose corticosteroids (greater than 20 mg/day of prednisone) for more than 2 weeks should wait at least a month after prednisone is stopped to get the zoster vaccine.

Zoster vaccine (Zostavax) is not approved for women of childbearing age and should not be administered to pregnant women. Zoster vaccine should not be administered to patients with active tuberculosis or acute illness, or with fever.

Adverse Drug Reactions

The most common adverse drug reactions to zoster vaccine reported during the clinical trials were related to the injection site. Pain/tenderness (33.4%), erythema (33.7%), swelling (24.9%), and pruritus (6.6%) are all reported by patients receiving zoster vaccine. Headache was reported by 1.4% of patients who received the zoster vaccine versus 0.8% of patients who received a placebo.

Drug Interactions

Antiviral drugs (acyclovir, famciclovir, and valacyclovir) should be stopped at least 24 hours before zoster vaccine is administered. Antivirals should not be used for at least 14 days after vaccination (CDC, 2008).

Zoster vaccine can be administered before, after, or at the same time as blood product or antibody-containing products.

Patients who are taking high-dose corticosteroids (greater than 20 mg/d prednisone) should not be vaccinated and need to be off prednisone for a month before vaccination. Patients on short-term corticosteroids (less than 14 d) or low-dose (less than 20 mg/d) prednisone may be vaccinated with zoster virus.

Patients taking low-doses of methotrexate (less than or equal to 0.4 mg/kg/wk), azathioprine (less than or equal to 3.0 mg/kg/d), or 6-mercaptopurine (less than or equal to 1.5 mg/kg/d) for treatment of rheumatoid arthritis, psoriasis, polymyositis, sarcoidosis, or inflammatory bowel disease may be vaccinated with zoster vaccine (CDC, 2008).

Clinical Use and Dosing

A single dose of zoster vaccine is recommended by the ACIP for all adults aged 60 years or older. The zoster vaccine may be administered to adults age 50 years or older who request the vaccine or who are at risk of poor outcomes if they contract herpes zoster or post-herpetic neuralgia (CDC, 2011b). The dose is 0.65 mL administered in the SC tissue of the deltoid region. The vaccine is given even if a patient has a history of herpes zoster (CDC, 2008). It is not necessary to screen for history of varicella disease or vaccine, nor is it necessary to test for varicella immunity prior to immunization. Zoster vaccine may be administered with other common vaccines in this age group: Td, Tdap, and pneumococcal. Administration of zoster vaccine and other live-virus vaccines should be separated by 4 weeks. Zoster vaccine is not recommended for patients who have received the varicella vaccine, although patients in the approved age range have most likely had wild varicella infection.

Patients with chronic medical conditions (e.g., chronic renal failure, diabetes mellitus, rheumatoid arthritis, and chronic pulmonary disease) may be vaccinated (CDC, 2008). Zoster vaccine should be deferred in patients with severe illness or with fever. It may be administered if the patient has a minor acute illness without fever (that is, an upper respiratory infection).

Patients who are immunosuppressed have greater morbidity and mortality from herpes zoster. If patients will be initiating immunosuppressive therapy or have diseases that might lead to immunodeficiency, zoster vaccine should be administered as soon as possible while their immunity is still intact. Zoster vaccine should be administered at least 14 days before immunosuppressive therapy is started. Zoster vaccine should be avoided for at least 24 months after stem cell transplant (CDC, 2008).

Antiviral medications should be avoided for 14 days after zoster vaccine.

Administration error: If a child is accidentally administered zoster vaccine (Zostavax) instead of varicella vaccine (Varivax), then it should be counted as a valid vaccine and reported to the VAERS whether or not an adverse reaction occurs. If an adult over age 60 is administered the varicella vaccine (Varivax), it is not considered a valid dose and the patient is administered zoster vaccine (Zostavax) the same day (CDC, 2008). If the zoster vaccine is not administered the same day, then a dose of zoster vaccine should be administered at least 28 days later.

Monitoring

There is no specific monitoring of patients after receiving the zoster vaccine.

Patient Education

All patients who receive vaccines are required by law to receive a VIS in the appropriate language. Patients should be informed they may have discomfort at the injection site, including pain, swelling, erythema, and pruritus. See Table 19-4.

ORAL TYPHOID VACCINE

Pharmacodynamics

Typhoid vaccines are used to increase resistance to enteric fever caused by *Salmonella typhi*. Typhoid fever is spread by ingesting water contaminated by feces from infected persons. Worldwide, an estimated 22 million cases of typhoid fever occur annually (Newton & Mintz, 2014). The risk is greatest in travelers to South Asia, although the disease can be seen in East and Southeast Asia, Africa, the Caribbean, and Central and South America (Newton & Mintz, 2014). Oral typhoid vaccine (Vivotif Berna) is a live, attenuated vaccine, Ty21a. The oral vaccine is ingested and works in the small intestine to synthesize a lipopolysaccharide that evokes a protective immune response. The vaccine is estimated to be 50% to 80% effective in preventing typhoid fever. The efficacy of protective immunity depends on the size of the bacterial inoculum consumed.

Pharmacokinetics

The absorption, distribution, and metabolism of oral typhoid vaccine are unknown.

Pharmacotherapeutics
Precautions and Contraindications

Hypersensitivity to typhoid vaccine is a contraindication to its use. Because oral typhoid vaccine is a live, attenuated virus, it should not be administered to immunocompromised patients, including those who are HIV-infected. Do not administer it to a patient with acute febrile illness or an acute GI illness (diarrhea).

Oral typhoid vaccine is Pregnancy Category C. It is not known if the vaccine is harmful to the fetus. If it is necessary to vaccinate a pregnant patient, inactivated vaccine is recommended.

Oral typhoid vaccine is not recommended for use in children younger than age 6 years. Use inactivated vaccine in young children.

Table 19–4 🔀 **Recommended Adult Immunization Schedule – United States, 2015**

Recommended Adult Immunization Schedule—United States - 2015

Note: These recommendations must be read with the footnotes that follow containing number of doses, intervals between doses, and other important information.

Figure 1. Recommended adult immunization schedule, by vaccine and age group[1]

VACCINE ▼ AGE GROUP ►	19-21 years	22-26 years	27-49 years	50-59 years	60-64 years	≥ 65 years
Influenza[*,2]	1 dose annually					
Tetanus, diphtheria, pertussis (Td/Tdap)[*,3]	Substitute 1-time dose of Tdap for Td booster; then boost with Td every 10 yrs					
Varicella[*,4]	2 doses					
Human papillomavirus (HPV) Female[*,5]	3 doses					
Human papillomavirus (HPV) Male[*,5]	3 doses					
Zoster[6]					1 dose	
Measles, mumps, rubella (MMR)[*,7]	1 or 2 doses					
Pneumococcal 13-valent conjugate (PCV13)[*,8]					1-time dose	
Pneumococcal polysaccharide (PPSV23)[8]	1 or 2 doses					1 dose
Meningococcal[*,9]	1 or more doses					
Hepatitis A[*,10]	2 doses					
Hepatitis B[*,11]	3 doses					
Haemophilus influenzae type b (Hib)[*,12]	1 or 3 doses					

*Covered by the Vaccine Injury Compensation Program

▨	For all persons in this category who meet the age requirements and who lack documentation of vaccination or have no evidence of previous infection; zoster vaccine recommended regardless of prior episode of zoster
▨	Recommended if some other risk factor is present (e.g., on the basis of medical, occupational, lifestyle, or other indication)
▢	No recommendation

Report all clinically significant postvaccination reactions to the Vaccine Adverse Event Reporting System (VAERS). Reporting forms and instructions on filing a VAERS report are available at www.vaers.hhs.gov or by telephone, 800-822-7967.

Information on how to file a Vaccine Injury Compensation Program claim is available at www.hrsa.gov/vaccinecompensation or by telephone, 800-338-2382. To file a claim for vaccine injury, contact the U.S. Court of Federal Claims, 717 Madison Place, N.W., Washington, D.C. 20005; telephone, 202-357-6400.

Additional information about the vaccines in this schedule, extent of available data, and contraindications for vaccination is also available at www.cdc.gov/vaccines or from the CDC-INFO Contact Center at 800-CDC-INFO (800-232-4636) in English and Spanish, 8:00 a.m. - 8:00 p.m. Eastern Time, Monday - Friday, excluding holidays.

Use of trade names and commercial sources is for identification only and does not imply endorsement by the U.S. Department of Health and Human Services.

The recommendations in this schedule were approved by the Centers for Disease Control and Prevention's (CDC) Advisory Committee on Immunization Practices (ACIP), the American Academy of Family Physicians (AAFP), the America College of Physicians (ACP), American College of Obstetricians and Gynecologists (ACOG) and American College of Nurse-Midwives (ACNM).

Figure 2. Vaccines that might be indicated for adults based on medical and other indications[1]

VACCINE ▼ INDICATION ►	Pregnancy	Immuno-compromising conditions (excluding human immunodeficiency virus [HIV])[4,6,7,8,13]	HIV infection CD4+ T lymphocyte count[4,6,7,8,13] < 200 cells/μL	HIV infection CD4+ T lymphocyte count ≥ 200 cells/μL	Men who have sex with men (MSM)	Kidney failure, end-stage renal disease, receipt of hemodialysis	Heart disease, chronic lung disease, chronic alcoholism	Asplenia (including elective splenectomy and persistent complement component deficiencies)[8,12]	Chronic liver disease	Diabetes	Healthcare personnel
Influenza[*,2]	1 dose IIV annually		1 dose IIV or LAIV annually	1 dose IIV annually							1 does IIV or LAIV annually
Tetanus, diphtheria, pertussis (Td/Tdap)[*,3]	1 dose Tdap each pregnancy	Substitute 1-time dose of Tdap for Td booster; then boost with Td every 10 yrs									
Varicella[*,4]	Contraindicated			2 doses							
Human papillomavirus (HPV) Female[*,5]		3 doses through age 26 yrs				3 doses through age 26 yrs					
Human papillomavirus (HPV) Male[*,5]		3 doses through age 26 yrs				3 doses through age 21 yrs					
Zoster[6]	Contraindicated			1 dose							
Measles, mumps, rubella (MMR)[*,7]	Contraindicated			1 or 2 doses							
Pneumococcal 13-valent conjugate (PCV13)[*,8]			1 dose								
Pneumococcal polysaccharide (PPSV23)[8]			1 or 2 doses								
Meningococcal[*,9]			1 or more doses								
Hepatitis A[*,10]			2 doses								
Hepatitis B[*,11]			3 doses								
Haemophilus influenzae type b (Hib)[*,12]		post-HSCT recipients only	1 or 3 doses								

*Covered by the Vaccine Injury Compensation Program

▨ For all persons in this category who meet the age requirements and who lack documentation of vaccination or have no evidence of previous infection; zoster vaccine recommended regardless of prior episode of zoster	▨ Recommended if some other risk factor is present (e.g., on the basis of medical, occupational, lifestyle, or other indications)
	▢ No recommendation

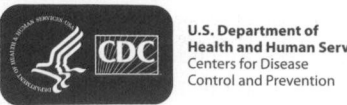

U.S. Department of Health and Human Services
Centers for Disease Control and Prevention

These schedules indicate the recommended age groups and medical indications for which administration of currently licensed vaccines is commonly recommended for adults ages 19 years and older, as of February 1, 2015. For all vaccines being recommended on the Adult Immunization Schedule: a vaccine series does not need to be restarted, regardless of the time that has elapsed between doses. Licensed combination vaccines may be used whenever any components of the combination are indicated and when the vaccine's other components are not contraindicated. For detailed recommendations on all vaccines, including those used primarily for travelers or that are issued during the year, consult the manufacturers' package inserts and the complete statements from the Advisory Committee on Immunization Practices (www.cdc.gov/vaccines/hcp/acip-recs/index.html). Use of trade names and commercial sources is for identification only and does not imply endorsement by the U.S. Department of Health and Human Services.

Table 19–4 ⊗ **Recommended Adult Immunization Schedule – United States, 2015—cont'd**

Footnotes—Recommended Immunization Schedule for Adults Aged 19 Years or Older: United States, 2015

1. Additional information
- Additional guidance for the use of the vaccines described in this supplement is available at www.cdc.gov/vaccines/hcp/acip-recs/index.html.
- Information on vaccination recommendations when vaccination status is unknown and other general immunization information can be found in the General Recommendations on Immunization at www.cdc.gov/mmwr/preview/mmwrhtml/rr6002a1.htm.
- Information on travel vaccine requirements and recommendations (e.g., for hepatitis A and B, meningococcal, and other vaccines) is available at wwwnc.cdc.gov/travel/destinations/list.
- Additional information and resources regarding vaccination of pregnant women can be found at www.cdc.gov/vaccines/adults/rec-vac/pregnant.html.

2. Influenza vaccination
- Annual vaccination against influenza is recommended for all persons aged 6 months or older.
- Persons aged 6 months or older, including pregnant women and persons with hives-only allergy to eggs can receive the inactivated influenza vaccine (IIV). An age-appropriate IIV formulation should be used.
- Adults aged 18 years or older can receive the recombinant influenza vaccine (RIV) (FluBlok). RIV does not contain any egg protein and can be given to age-appropriate persons with egg allergy of any severity.
- Healthy, nonpregnant persons aged 2 to 49 years without high-risk medical conditions can receive either intranasally administered live, attenuated influenza vaccine (LAIV) (FluMist) or IIV.
- Health care personnel who care for severely immunocompromised persons who require care in a protected environment should receive IIV or RIV; health care personnel who receive LAIV should avoid providing care for severely immunosuppressed persons for 7 days after vaccination.
- The intramuscularly or intradermally administered IIV are options for adults aged 18 through 64 years.
- Adults aged 65 years or older can receive the standard-dose IIV or the high-dose IIV (Fluzone High-Dose).
- A list of currently available influenza vaccines can be found at www.cdc.gov/flu/protect/vaccine/vaccines.htm.

3. Tetanus, diphtheria, and acellular pertussis (Td/Tdap) vaccination
- Administer 1 dose of Tdap vaccine to pregnant women during each pregnancy (preferably during 27 to 36 weeks' gestation) regardless of interval since prior Td or Tdap vaccination.
- Persons aged 11 years or older who have not received Tdap vaccine or for whom vaccine status is unknown should receive a dose of Tdap followed by tetanus and diphtheria toxoids (Td) booster doses every 10 years thereafter. Tdap can be administered regardless of interval since the most recent tetanus or diphtheria-toxoid containing vaccine.
- Adults with an unknown or incomplete history of completing a 3-dose primary vaccination series with Td-containing vaccines should begin or complete a primary vaccination series including a Tdap dose.
- For unvaccinated adults, administer the first 2 doses at least 4 weeks apart and the third dose 6 to 12 months after the second.
- For incompletely vaccinated (i.e., less than 3 doses) adults, administer remaining doses.
- Refer to the ACIP statement for recommendations for administering Td/Tdap as prophylaxis in wound management (see footnote 1).

4. Varicella vaccination
- All adults without evidence of immunity to varicella (as defined below) should receive 2 doses of single-antigen varicella vaccine or a second dose if they have received only 1 dose.
- Vaccination should be emphasized for those who have close contact with persons at high risk for severe disease (e.g., health care personnel and family contacts of persons with immunocompromising conditions) or are at high risk for exposure or transmission (e.g., teachers; child care employees; residents and staff members of institutional settings, including correctional institutions; college students; military personnel; adolescents and adults living in households with children; nonpregnant women of childbearing age; and international travelers).
- Pregnant women should be assessed for evidence of varicella immunity. Women who do not have evidence of immunity should receive the first dose of varicella vaccine upon completion or termination of pregnancy and before discharge from the health care facility. The second dose should be administered 4 to 8 weeks after the first dose.
- Evidence of immunity to varicella in adults includes any of the following:
  - documentation of 2 doses of varicella vaccine at least 4 weeks apart;
  - U.S.-born before 1980, except health care personnel and pregnant women;
  - history of varicella based on diagnosis or verification of varicella disease by a health care provider;
  - history of herpes zoster based on diagnosis or verification of herpes zoster disease by a health care provider; or
  - laboratory evidence of immunity or laboratory confirmation of disease.

5. Human papillomavirus (HPV) vaccination
- Two vaccines are licensed for use in females, bivalent HPV vaccine (HPV2) and quadrivalent HPV vaccine (HPV4), and one HPV vaccine for use in males (HPV4).
- For females, either HPV4 or HPV2 is recommended in a 3-dose series for routine vaccination at age 11 or 12 years and for those aged 13 through 26 years, if not previously vaccinated.

- For males, HPV4 is recommended in a 3-dose series for routine vaccination at age 11 or 12 years and for those aged 13 through 21 years, if not previously vaccinated. Males aged 22 through 26 years may be vaccinated.
- HPV4 is recommended for men who have sex with men through age 26 years for those who did not get any or all doses when they were younger.
- Vaccination is recommended for immunocompromised persons (including those with HIV infection) through age 26 years for those who did not get any or all doses when they were younger.
- A complete series for either HPV4 or HPV2 consists of 3 doses. The second dose should be administered 4 to 8 weeks (minimum interval of 4 weeks) after the first dose; the third dose should be administered 24 weeks after the first dose and 16 weeks after the second dose (minimum interval of at least 12 weeks).
- HPV vaccines are not recommended for use in pregnant women. However, pregnancy testing is not needed before vaccination. If a woman is found to be pregnant after initiating the vaccination series, no intervention is needed; the remainder of the 3-dose series should be delayed until completion or termination of pregnancy.

6. Zoster vaccination
- A single dose of zoster vaccine is recommended for adults aged 60 years or older regardless of whether they report a prior episode of herpes zoster. Although the vaccine is licensed by the U.S. Food and Drug Administration for use among and can be administered to persons aged 50 years or older, ACIP recommends that vaccination begin at age 60 years.
- Persons aged 60 years or older with chronic medical conditions may be vaccinated unless their condition constitutes a contraindication, such as pregnancy or severe immunodeficiency.

7. Measles, mumps, rubella (MMR) vaccination
- Adults born before 1957 are generally considered immune to measles and mumps. All adults born in 1957 or later should have documentation of 1 or more doses of MMR vaccine unless they have a medical contraindication to the vaccine or laboratory evidence of immunity to each of the three diseases. Documentation of provider-diagnosed disease is not considered acceptable evidence of immunity for measles, mumps, or rubella.

Measles component:
- A routine second dose of MMR vaccine, administered a minimum of 28 days after the first dose, is recommended for adults who:
  - are students in postsecondary educational institutions,
  - work in a health care facility, or
  - plan to travel internationally.
- Persons who received inactivated (killed) measles vaccine or measles vaccine of unknown type during 1963–1967 should be revaccinated with 2 doses of MMR vaccine.

Mumps component:
- A routine second dose of MMR vaccine, administered a minimum of 28 days after the first dose, is recommended for adults who:
  - are students in a postsecondary educational institution,
  - work in a health care facility, or
  - plan to travel internationally.
- Persons vaccinated before 1979 with either killed mumps vaccine or mumps vaccine of unknown type who are at high risk for mumps infection (e.g., persons who are working in a health care facility) should be considered for revaccination with 2 doses of MMR vaccine.

Rubella component:
- For women of childbearing age, regardless of birth year, rubella immunity should be determined. If there is no evidence of immunity, women who are not pregnant should be vaccinated. Pregnant women who do not have evidence of immunity should receive MMR vaccine upon completion or termination of pregnancy and before discharge from the health care facility.

Health care personnel born before 1957:
- For unvaccinated health care personnel born before 1957 who lack laboratory evidence of measles, mumps, and/or rubella immunity or laboratory confirmation of disease, health care facilities should consider vaccinating personnel with 2 doses of MMR vaccine at the appropriate interval for measles and mumps or 1 dose of MMR vaccine for rubella.

8. Pneumococcal (13-valent pneumococcal conjugate vaccine [PCV13] and 23-valent pneumococcal polysaccharide vaccine [PPSV23]) vaccination
- General information
  - When indicated, only a single dose of PCV13 is recommended for adults.
  - No additional dose of PPSV23 is indicated for adults vaccinated with PPSV23 at or after age 65 years.
  - When both PCV13 and PPSV23 are indicated, PCV13 should be administered first; PCV13 and PPSV23 should not be administered during the same visit.
  - When indicated, PCV13 and PPSV23 should be administered to adults whose pneumococcal vaccination history is incomplete or unknown.
- Adults aged 65 years or older who
  - Have not received PCV13 or PPSV23: Administer PCV13 followed by PPSV23 in 6 to 12 months.
  - Have not received PCV13 but have received a dose of PPSV23 at age 65 years or older: Administer PCV13 at least 1 year after the dose of PPSV23 received at age 65 years or older.

Continued

Table 19–4 ⚕ **Recommended Adult Immunization Schedule – United States, 2015—cont'd**

Footnotes—Recommended Immunization Schedule for Adults Aged 19 Years or Older: United States, 2015

8. Pneumococcal vaccination (continued)
— Have not received PCV13 but have received 1 or more doses of PPSV23 before age 65: Administer PCV13 at least 1 year after the most recent dose of PPSV23; administer a dose of PPSV23 6 to 12 months after PCV13, or as soon as possible if this time window has passed, and at least 5 years after the most recent dose of PPSV23.
— Have received PCV13 but not PPSV23 before age 65 years: Administer PPSV23 6 to 12 months after PCV13 or as soon as possible if this time window has passed.
— Have received PCV13 and 1 or more doses of PPSV23 before age 65 years: Administer PPSV23 6 to 12 months after PCV13, or as soon as possible if this time window has passed, and at least 5 years after the most recent dose of PPSV23.
• Adults aged 19 through 64 years with immunocompromising conditions or anatomical or functional asplenia (defined below) who
— Have not received PCV13 or PPSV23: Administer PCV13 followed by PPSV23 at least 8 weeks after PCV13; administer a second dose of PPSV23 at least 5 years after the first dose of PPSV23.
— Have not received PCV13 but have received 1 dose of PPSV23: Administer PCV13 at least 1 year after the PPSV23; administer a second dose of PPSV23 at least 8 weeks after PCV13 and at least 5 years after the first dose of PPSV23.
— Have not received PCV13 but have received 2 doses of PPSV23: Administer PCV13 at least 1 year after the most recent dose of PPSV23.
— Have received PCV13 but not PPSV23: Administer PPSV23 at least 8 weeks after PCV13; administer a second dose of PPSV23 at least 5 years after the first dose of PPSV23.
— Have received PCV13 and 1 dose of PPSV23: Administer a second dose of PPSV23 at least 5 years after the first dose of PPSV23.
• Adults aged 19 through 64 years with cerebrospinal fluid leaks or cochlear implants: Administer PCV13 followed by PPSV23 at least 8 weeks after PCV13.
• Adults aged 19 through 64 years with chronic heart disease (including congestive heart failure and cardiomyopathies, excluding hypertension), chronic lung disease (including chronic obstructive lung disease, emphysema, and asthma), chronic liver disease (including cirrhosis), alcoholism, or diabetes mellitus: Administer PPSV23.
• Adults aged 19 through 64 years who smoke cigarettes or reside in nursing home or long-term care facilities: Administer PPSV23.
• Routine pneumococcal vaccination is not recommended for American Indian/Alaska Native or other adults unless they have the indications as above; however, public health authorities may consider recommending the use of pneumococcal vaccines for American Indians/Alaska Natives or other adults who live in areas with increased risk for invasive pneumococcal disease.
• Immunocompromising conditions that are indications for pneumococcal vaccination are: Congenital or acquired immunodeficiency (including B- or T-lymphocyte deficiency, complement deficiencies, and phagocytic disorders excluding chronic granulomatous disease), HIV infection, chronic renal failure, nephrotic syndrome, leukemia, lymphoma, Hodgkin disease, generalized malignancy, multiple myeloma, solid organ transplant, and iatrogenic immunosuppression (including long-term systemic corticosteroids and radiation therapy).
• Anatomical or functional asplenia that are indications for pneumococcal vaccination are: Sickle cell disease and other hemoglobinopathies, congenital or acquired asplenia, splenic dysfunction, and splenectomy. Administer pneumococcal vaccines at least 2 weeks before immunosuppressive therapy or an elective splenectomy, and as soon as possible to adults who are newly diagnosed with asymptomatic or symptomatic HIV infection.

9. Meningococcal vaccination
• Administer 2 doses of quadrivalent meningococcal conjugate vaccine (MenACWY [Menactra, Menveo]) at least 2 months apart to adults of all ages with anatomical or functional asplenia or persistent complement component deficiencies. HIV infection is not an indication for routine vaccination with MenACWY. If an HIV-infected person of any age is vaccinated, 2 doses of MenACWY should be administered at least 2 months apart.
• Administer a single dose of meningococcal vaccine to microbiologists routinely exposed to isolates of *Neisseria meningitidis*, military recruits, persons at risk during an outbreak attributable to a vaccine serogroup, and persons who travel to or live in countries in which meningococcal disease is hyperendemic or epidemic.
• First-year college students up through age 21 years who are living in residence halls should be vaccinated if they have not received a dose on or after their 16th birthday.
• MenACWY is preferred for adults with any of the preceding indications who are aged 55 years or younger as well as for adults aged 56 years or older who a) were vaccinated previously with MenACWY and are recommended for revaccination, or b) for whom multiple doses are anticipated. Meningococcal polysaccharide vaccine (MPSV4 [Menomune]) is preferred for adults aged 56 years or older who have not received MenACWY previously and who require a single dose only (e.g., travelers).
• Revaccination with MenACWY every 5 years is recommended for adults previously vaccinated with MenACWY or MPSV4 who remain at increased risk for infection (e.g., adults with anatomical or functional asplenia, persistent complement component deficiencies, or microbiologists).

10. Hepatitis A vaccination
• Vaccinate any person seeking protection from hepatitis A virus (HAV) infection and persons with any of the following indications:
— men who have sex with men and persons who use injection or noninjection illicit drugs;
— persons working with HAV-infected primates or with HAV in a research laboratory setting;
— persons with chronic liver disease and persons who receive clotting factor concentrates;
— persons traveling to or working in countries that have high or intermediate endemicity of hepatitis A; and
— unvaccinated persons who anticipate close personal contact (e.g., household or regular babysitting) with an international adoptee during the first 60 days after arrival in the United States from a country with high or intermediate endemicity. (See footnote 1 for more information on travel recommendations.) The first dose of the 2-dose hepatitis A vaccine series should be administered as soon as adoption is planned, ideally 2 or more weeks before the arrival of the adoptee.
• Single-antigen vaccine formulations should be administered in a 2-dose schedule at either 0 and 6 to 12 months (Havrix), or 0 and 6 to 18 months (Vaqta). If the combined hepatitis A and hepatitis B vaccine (Twinrix) is used, administer 3 doses at 0, 1, and 6 months; alternatively, a 4-dose schedule may be used, administered on days 0, 7, and 21 to 30 followed by a booster dose at month 12.

11. Hepatitis B vaccination
• Vaccinate persons with any of the following indications and any person seeking protection from hepatitis B virus (HBV) infection:
— sexually active persons who are not in a long-term, mutually monogamous relationship (e.g., persons with more than 1 sex partner during the previous 6 months); persons seeking evaluation or treatment for a sexually transmitted disease (STD); current or recent injection drug users; and men who have sex with men;
— health care personnel and public safety workers who are potentially exposed to blood or other infectious body fluids;
— persons with diabetes who are younger than age 60 years as soon as feasible after diagnosis; persons with diabetes who are age 60 years or older at the discretion of the treating clinician based on the likelihood of acquiring HBV infection, including the risk posed by an increased need for assisted blood glucose monitoring in long-term care facilities, the likelihood of experiencing chronic sequelae if infected with HBV, and the likelihood of immune response to vaccination;
— persons with end-stage renal disease, including patients receiving hemodialysis, persons with HIV infection, and persons with chronic liver disease;
— household contacts and sex partners of hepatitis B surface antigen–positive persons, clients and staff members of institutions for persons with developmental disabilities, and international travelers to countries with high or intermediate prevalence of chronic HBV infection; and
— all adults in the following settings: STD treatment facilities, HIV testing and treatment facilities, facilities providing drug abuse treatment and prevention services, health care settings targeting services to injection drug users or men who have sex with men, correctional facilities, end-stage renal disease programs and facilities for chronic hemodialysis patients, and institutions and nonresidential day care facilities for persons with developmental disabilities.
• Administer missing doses to complete a 3-dose series of hepatitis B vaccine to those persons not vaccinated or not completely vaccinated. The second dose should be administered 1 month after the first dose; the third dose should be given at least 2 months after the second dose (and at least 4 months after the first dose). If the combined hepatitis A and hepatitis B vaccine (Twinrix) is used, give 3 doses at 0, 1, and 6 months; alternatively, a 4-dose Twinrix schedule, administered on days 0, 7, and 21 to 30 followed by a booster dose at month 12 may be used.
• Adult patients receiving hemodialysis or with other immunocompromising conditions should receive 1 dose of 40 mcg/mL (Recombivax HB) administered on a 3-dose schedule at 0, 1, and 6 months or 2 doses of 20 mcg/mL (Engerix-B) administered simultaneously on a 4-dose schedule at 0, 1, 2, and 6 months.

12. *Haemophilus influenzae* type b (Hib) vaccination
• One dose of Hib vaccine should be administered to persons who have anatomical or functional asplenia or sickle cell disease or are undergoing elective splenectomy if they have not previously received Hib vaccine. Hib vaccination 14 or more days before splenectomy is suggested.
• Recipients of a hematopoietic stem cell transplant (HSCT) should be vaccinated with a 3-dose regimen 6 to 12 months after a successful transplant, regardless of vaccination history; at least 4 weeks should separate doses.
• Hib vaccine is not recommended for adults with HIV infection since their risk for Hib infection is low.

13. Immunocompromising conditions
• Inactivated vaccines generally are acceptable (e.g., pneumococcal, meningococcal, and inactivated influenza vaccine) and live vaccines generally are avoided in persons with immune deficiencies or immunocompromising conditions. Information on specific conditions is available at www.cdc.gov/vaccines/hcp/acip-recs/index.html.

Adverse Drug Reactions

Adverse effects of oral typhoid vaccine are infrequent and transient and resolve with intervention. Abdominal pain, diarrhea, vomiting, fever, headache, and rash have been reported.

Drug Interactions

The antimalarial drug mefloquine (Lariam) can inhibit the growth of the live Ty21a strain in vitro. It is recommended that oral typhoid vaccine be given either 24 hours before or 24 hours after mefloquine. Immunosuppressants may cause insufficient response to the vaccine.

The manufacturer recommends that oral typhoid vaccine not be administered to individuals receiving sulfonamides and antibiotics, which may be active against the vaccine strains and prevent a sufficient degree of multiplication to induce a protective immune response.

Clinical Use and Dosing

Oral typhoid vaccine is used for primary immunization against *S. typhi* infection in the following:

1. Travelers to areas where a risk of exposure to *S. typhi* is recognized
2. People who have household contact with a documented typhoid fever carrier
3. Laboratory workers who have frequent contact with *S. typhi*

For primary immunization of patients over age 6 years, the dose is one capsule on alternate days (every 48 hours; days 1, 3, 5, 7) for a total of four doses (Newton & Mintz, 2014). The capsule needs to be taken 1 hour before meals with a glass of cold water (not warmer than body temperature). The vaccine capsule should be swallowed whole. Ideally, the patient should finish the four doses at least 1 week prior to exposure or travel. A booster dose of four capsules, given every other day, is recommended every 5 years under conditions of repeated exposure (Newton & Mintz, 2014).

Monitoring

There is no specific monitoring of patients after receiving oral typhoid vaccine.

Patient Education

The oral typhoid vaccine should be taken exactly as prescribed. It must be taken on an empty stomach with cold water. Every-other-day dosing should be explained. The patient must understand that all four doses must be taken, at least 1 week prior to travel, to provide the best protection.

Although the possible adverse effects of the vaccine are mild and usually transient, the patient should be informed about them. The best protection against typhoid fever is food and water precautions to prevent contracting *S. typhi*.

YELLOW FEVER VACCINE

Pharmacodynamics

Yellow fever is a viral illness spread by some species of mosquitoes in Central and South America and in tropical regions of Africa. Yellow fever is endemic in sub-Saharan Africa and tropical South America (Gershman & Staples, 2014). The CDC estimates the risk of an unvaccinated traveler contracting yellow fever during a 2-week visit to West Africa as 10 cases per 100,000 and in travelers to South America 1 case per 100,000 (Gershman & Staples, 2014). Yellow fever produces a hemorrhagic fever and is fatal in 20% to 50% of severe cases (Staples, Gershman, & Fischer, 2010). All travelers should use personal protective measures to avoid mosquito bites to prevent yellow fever transmission.

Vaccination is recommended for travel to endemic areas. Endemic regions may change, therefore, travelers and healthcare providers should refer to the current CDC *Yellow Book* (www.cdc.gov/travel) to determine the need for vaccination. Certification of yellow fever vaccine may be required for all persons aged 9 months or older to enter certain countries in endemic areas. Current recommendations are listed at the CDC Travel Web site: *Yellow Book* (www.cdc.gov/travel). Yellow fever vaccine (YF-Vax) is a live, attenuated virus that is prepared by culturing the 17D strain virus in a living chick embryo.

Pharmacokinetics

After SC administration of the vaccine, active immunity to yellow fever occurs in 7 to 10 days and lasts for 10 years or more. The World Health Organization publishes international health regulations requiring revaccination at 10-year intervals for those at high risk.

Pharmacotherapeutics

Precautions and Contraindications

Yellow fever vaccine should be avoided in any patient with a history of egg hypersensitivity or sensitivity to chicken protein or gelatin (Gershman & Staples, 2014). Because yellow fever vaccine is a live, attenuated virus, it is contraindicated in immunocompromised patients, including those who are HIV-infected with a CD4 T-lymphocyte less than 15%, patients with primary immunodeficiencies, malignant neoplasms, transplant patients, or other patients on immunosuppressive therapies (Gershman & Staples, 2014). The vaccine should be used with caution in HIV-infected patients with CD4 counts of 15% to 24%. Yellow fever vaccine is contraindicated in patients with a thymus disorder that affects immune function. Defer vaccination with yellow fever vaccine for 8 weeks following blood or plasma transfusion.

Yellow fever vaccine is Pregnancy Category C. It is not known if the vaccine is harmful to the fetus. Vaccinate only those pregnant women who are at high risk of contracting the disease. Use with caution in breastfeeding women.

Yellow fever vaccine is contraindicated in infants younger than 6 months due to increased risk for vaccine-associated neurologic disease (Gershman & Staples, 2014). Use with caution in infants aged 6 to 8 months. Rare cases of encephalitis have occurred in infants of this age who have received yellow fever vaccine.

Yellow fever vaccine should be used with caution in patients who are aged 60 years or older. VAERS reports indicate an increase in serious adverse events after vaccination of patients in this age group. If patients are traveling to endemic areas, vaccination risks need to be weighed against the risk of exposure to the yellow fever virus.

Adverse Drug Reactions

Up to 10% of patients experience fever or malaise, usually 7 to 14 days after administration of yellow fever vaccine. Myalgia or headache is reported in 2% to 5% of vaccine recipients. Incidence of mild adverse events has been 25% or less in clinical trials (Gershman & Staples, 2014). Anaphylaxis may occur and epinephrine should be on hand when administering the vaccine.

A very rare reaction is yellow fever vaccine–associated viscerotropic disease, with symptoms of fever and multiple organ failure (Gershman & Staples, 2014). The rate is higher among persons 60 years or older, 1/100,000 in 60- to 69-year-olds and 2.3/100,000 in persons aged 70 or older (Brunette et al, 2010). The case-fatality ratio for yellow fever vaccine–associated viscerotropic disease is 53%. The onset of illness is an average of 3.5 days after vaccination.

Yellow fever vaccine–associated neurological disease is a conglomerate of clinical syndromes, including meningoencephalitis, Guillain–Barré syndrome, encephalomyelitis, bulbar palsy, and Bell's palsy. Adverse neurological outcomes are usually seen among infants as encephalitis but may occur at any age.

Drug Interactions

Concurrent vaccination with yellow fever vaccine and hepatitis A vaccine (HAV) and hepatitis B vaccine (HBV), meningococcal vaccine (Menomune), typhoid fever vaccine (Typhim Vi), diphtheria, tetanus and pertussis (DTaP, Tdap), and measles vaccine does not appear to affect response to yellow fever vaccine (Staples et al, 2010).

Immunosuppressants may cause insufficient response to the yellow fever vaccine. Yellow fever vaccine should be reconstituted with the diluent supplied with the vaccine. Preservatives in diluent of other vaccines may kill the live virus in the yellow fever vaccine.

Clinical Use and Dosing

Immunization against yellow fever is recommended for all people over age 9 months who are living in or traveling to endemic areas. Vaccination is required by international regulations for travel to certain countries. The dose is a single 0.5 mL dose given SC. The vaccine should be repeated every 10 years (Gershman & Staples, 2014).

Monitoring

There is no specific monitoring of patients needed after receiving yellow fever vaccine other than for the rare adverse drug reactions listed previously.

Patient Education

Patients should be educated about the mild transient adverse effects that can occur from vaccine administration. Patients should be instructed about protecting themselves against mosquitoes. Insect repellent and proper protective clothing and netting provide the best defense against insect-borne diseases.

BACILLUS CALMETTE–GUÉRIN VACCINE

Pharmacodynamics

Immunization with bacillus Calmette–Guérin (BCG) vaccine lowers the risk of serious complications of primary TB in children. It is not widely used in the United States but is given to infants and young children in countries where TB is endemic (CDC, 2012a). Vaccination with BCG stimulates natural infection with *Mycobacterium tuberculosis* and results in a T-cell–mediated immune reaction and immunity against TB, but with variable degrees of protection. The protective effect of BCG use in children against miliary and meningeal TB is about 80%; it is less effective in adults.

Pharmacokinetics

BCG is administered percutaneously (CDC, 1996a). Specific pharmacokinetic information is not available. The duration of protection against TB varies according to the potency of the strain of BCG used. TB sensitivity may last up to 10 years.

Pharmacotherapeutics

Precautions and Contraindications

Patients with active TB should not receive BCG. PPD skin testing should be performed on all patients over 2 months of age who are receiving BCG. Cancer, leukemia, lymphoma, radiation therapy, and immunodeficiency are contraindications to BCG use. Patients with symptomatic or asymptomatic HIV infection should not receive BCG. Drugs that affect the immune system, including high-dose steroids, are also a contraindication to BCG use.

Precautions should be taken to avoid accidental exposure to BCG solutions during preparation and administration because these solutions contain live, attenuated *M. tuberculosis*.

BCG is Pregnancy Category C. The CDC does not recommend the use of BCG in pregnant women.

The World Health Organization recommends that HIV-infected infants not receive BCG even in areas of high TB activity because of the risk of disseminated BCG disease (WHO, 2010).

Adverse Drug Reactions

A normal reaction to the BCG vaccine is skin lesions that appear within 10 to 14 days after the multiple-puncture disc application of BCG. The lesions consist of small red papules at the site of administration. The papules reach maximum diameter (3 mm) after 4 to 6 weeks and then scale away and slowly subside. Six months after vaccination, there is usually no visible sign of vaccination, although faint disc marks may be noted.

Lymphadenopathy may occur in a regional lymph node and resolves spontaneously. Osteomyelitis is a rare occurrence (1/1 million doses). BCG-induced osteomyelitis affects the epiphyses of the long bones and can occur from 4 months to 2 years after administration. Rarely, lupoid-like skin reactions have occurred. It has been recommended that patients who experience lupus-like symptoms after BCG administration be treated with isoniazid (INH) for 3 months. Disseminated BCG infection and death are very rare (about 0.06 to 1.56 cases/ 1 million doses) and usually occur in patients with impaired immune systems (CDC, 1996a).

Drug Interactions

Antituberculosis agents (rifampin, INH, streptomycin) and immunosuppressives may interfere with the development of an appropriate immune response to BCG administration. BCG administration will cause PPD skin tests to give false-positive readings for up to 10 years after administration. After 10 years, a positive PPD usually indicates infection with *M. tuberculosis*.

Clinical Use and Dosing

In the United States, BCG is administered only in very special circumstances, such as unavoidable risk of exposure to *M. tuberculosis* and failure of other methods of prevention and control of TB (CDC, 2012a). The ACIP has set clear criteria for the use of BCG in the United States: "BCG vaccination should be considered for infants and children who reside in settings in which the likelihood of *M. tuberculosis* transmission and subsequent infection is high provided no other measures can be implemented (e.g., removing child from the source of infection). In addition, BCG vaccination may be considered for health-care workers who are employed in settings in which the likelihood of transmission and subsequent infection with *M. tuberculosis* strains resistant to INH and rifampin is high" (CDC, 1996a, 2012a).

BCG is given to healthy infants from birth to 2 months without TB skin testing. After that, BCG is given only to children with negative Mantoux skin tests.

The administration of BCG must be exactly as the manufacturer directs. The vaccine is dropped onto clean, dry skin over the deltoid muscle and spread over the area to be punctured, using the edge of the multipuncture disc. The prongs of the disc are coated with the virus by lightly dipping them into the spread vaccine. The prongs of the disc are pressed into the skin and held for 5 to 10 seconds. After the disc is removed, the vaccine is respread to fill all the puncture areas. Additional vaccine may be applied to ensure a "wet" vaccine site. The vaccinated area needs to be kept dry for 24 hours. No dressing is required. The person administering the vaccine should take precautions against coming into contact with the live virus.

The dose for infants 1 month or younger is diluted to 50% by adding 2 mL of sterile water to the vaccine.

Monitoring

There is no specific monitoring of patients who receive BCG, although providers are reminded it may affect TB test results.

Patient Education

The patient or parent should be instructed that the vaccine contains live virus and that the site should not be touched. The vaccine site should be kept clean until the local reaction has resolved. Clear instructions regarding the normal skin reaction should be given to the patient or parent prior to administration.

INACTIVATED VACCINES

DIPHTHERIA, TETANUS, AND PERTUSSIS VACCINE

Pharmacodynamics

Various combinations of diphtheria, tetanus, and pertussis vaccines are available on the market. Regardless of the combination of vaccines, the basic pharmacodynamic principles are the same.

Diphtheria toxoid induces the production of antibodies against the exotoxin excreted by *Corynebacterium diphtheriae*. Complete immunization (four doses, then boosters every 10 years) induces specific antibodies and reduces the incidence of diphtheria by more than 95%. Immunized persons who develop diphtheria have milder illness. Infection with *C. diphtheriae* does not confer immunity, and previously infected persons should still receive toxoid.

Adsorbed tetanus toxoid contains antigens that induce the production of antibodies against the exotoxin excreted by *Clostridium tetani*. The duration of immunity against *C. tetani* is about 10 years. Natural immunity to *C. tetani* does not occur in the United States, and even patients with previous *C. tetani* infection should receive the tetanus toxoid.

Pertussis vaccine contains inactivated pertussis antigens. Acellular pertussis vaccine contains one or more immunogens derived from *Bordetella pertussis* and, unlike whole-cell vaccine, contains little or no endotoxin. Immunization with pertussis vaccine produces antibodies against *B. pertussis*. The efficacy of whole-cell pertussis vaccine for children exposed to pertussis who received at least three doses of DPT is estimated at 59% to 90%. Whole-cell pertussis vaccine, DPT, is no longer available in the United States. Acellular pertussis vaccine has a clinical efficacy of 79% to 93% in protecting against clinical pertussis after household exposure. Vaccinated patients who do contract pertussis usually have a milder case. Pertussis vaccine is always given in combination with diphtheria and tetanus vaccines (DTaP, Tdap, Tdap).

Pharmacokinetics

The DTaP and Tdap vaccines are given IM. Ninety percent of patients who receive three doses of DTaP develop protective immunity against diphtheria and tetanus. Patients who receive four doses of DTaP have immunity that persists for 10 years or more. In patients who receive four doses of DTaP, immunity to pertussis begins to wane after 4 to 6 years (Tartof et al, 2013). Ten years after immunization, fewer than 50% of vaccine recipients have protective antibodies against *B. pertussis*, which is why a booster dose of Tdap is recommended in adolescents (CDC, 2006d). Vaccination is also recommended for all adults, including health-care workers and caregivers of infants younger than 12 months of age (CDC, 2006c).

Pharmacotherapeutics

Precautions and Contraindications

In the United States, it is currently recommended that DTaP be used for primary immunization of infants and children.

Therefore, the precautions and contraindications to DTaP are discussed here, and DTP is not discussed, although the contraindications are the same for each vaccine. Tdap is discussed later in this section.

The true contraindication to DTaP vaccination is a patient who experienced an immediate anaphylactic reaction with a previous dose. Encephalopathy that occurred within 7 days of a previous dose, unexplained by another cause, is a possible contraindication to further pertussis vaccine use (CDC, 2006c). In this case, DT should be substituted for DTaP. Patients with unstable, progressive, neurological problems may have the vaccine deferred until the neurologic status is clarified.

Precautions associated with DTaP include a previous temperature of 105°F (40.5°C) or higher within 48 hours after a dose, history of continuous crying (more than 3 hours) within 48 hours of a dose, convulsions within 3 days of a previous dose, and collapse or shock-like state (hypotonic-hyporesponsive episode) within 48 hours of a previous dose. Although these precautions were once considered contraindications, they are now considered precautions because they have not been proved to cause permanent sequelae.

Additional precautions include seizures 3 days or less after a previous dose of DTaP, persistent or inconsolable crying lasting more than 3 hours within 48 hours of a previous dose, Guillain–Barré syndrome (GBS) less than 6 weeks after a previous dose of tetanus toxoid–containing vaccine, or moderate or severe acute illness with or without fever (CDC, 2006c). A temperature less than 104°F (less than 40.5°C), fussiness, or mild drowsiness after a previous dose of DTaP, family history of seizures, family history of an adverse event after a DTP vaccine, or a stable neurological condition are not contraindications to vaccinating with DTaP.

DTaP may be given to immunocompromised patients or patients on immunosuppressive therapy, although the immune response to the vaccine may be less than optimal. Patients with HIV infection may be immunized. Patients with a minor acute or febrile illness, including otitis media, may be immunized. Immunization should be delayed in cases of moderate or severe illnesses, with or without fever.

Infants born prematurely should begin the vaccine series based on their date of birth, with the first vaccine given routinely at age 2 months.

The ACIP has recommended that pregnant women, including pregnant adolescents, receive a booster of Tdap with each pregnancy, ideally between 27 and 36 weeks' gestation to provide passive pertussis immunity to the infant (CDC, 2013b). Infants born to women given pertussis vaccine during the third trimester have measurable antibodies that protect them from pertussis during the first 2 to 3 months of life (Vilajeliu et al, 2015). Td and Tdap are Pregnancy Category C, but they have been used extensively worldwide in pregnant women with no adverse effects reported.

The contraindications to DT include patients older than age 7 years, who should be given Td or Tdap, as appropriate. The contraindications to DT or Td include hypersensitivity to any component of the vaccine and moderate-to-severe illness, with or without fever. Do not postpone for minor illness, including otitis media.

The contraindications to Tdap include Guillain–Barré syndrome 6 weeks or sooner after previous use of tetanus toxoid–containing vaccine, previous arthus reaction after receiving tetanus or diphtheria vaccine, or a progressive neurological disorder (CDC, 2006c). Tdap or Td should be deferred in a patient with moderate or severe illness, with or without fever. Fever with previous DTaP vaccine is not a reason to withhold DTaP or Tdap vaccine (CDC, 2006c).

Adverse Drug Reactions

Injection site reactions of mild to moderate pain, erythema, swelling, and induration may last for a few days after injection. Transient low-grade fever, chills, malaise, generalized aches and pains, and headache may occur. Fever was common after DPT and less common after DTaP. Drowsiness, fretfulness, and GI upset may occur. Pain at the injection site is the most frequent adverse event reported for Tdap (CDC, 2006b, 2006c).

Seizures may occur and are more likely in children with a history of seizures, although less common now that DPT is no longer used in the United States. Seizures may be related to fever, and antipyretic prophylaxis is recommended after DTaP administration every 4 to 6 hours in children with a history of febrile seizures to decrease the incidence of febrile seizure after vaccination.

Drug Interactions

Coadministration of radiation therapy, antineoplastic agents, or immunosuppressives can decrease the immunological response to the DTaP vaccine. DTaP, DT, and Td should not be administered concurrently with cholera vaccine, typhoid vaccine, or plague vaccine because there may be accentuated adverse effects. DTaP, DT, Tdap, or Td may be coadministered with HBV, HIB, meningococcal, influenza, hepatitis A, and pneumococcal vaccines.

Clinical Use and Dosing

DTaP is routinely given at age 2, 4, 6, and 15 to 18 months and 4 to 6 years. DT, if used, is given on the same schedule.

As a booster, Tdap is recommended at age 11 to 12 years. Tdap (ADACEL) is labeled for use in persons aged 11 to 64 years. Tdap (BOOSTRIX) is labeled for persons 10 to 64 years. Patients should receive a booster dose of Td or Tdap every 10 years. If a patient older than age 7 has never been immunized, the primary series is one dose of Tdap followed by 2 doses of Td. The first dose of Tdap is followed by the second dose 4 weeks later. The third dose is given 6 to 12 months after the second dose. Every adult needs a booster every 10 years after completion of the primary series of three doses.

Pregnant women and adolescents should receive a dose of Tdap, ideally between 27 and 36 weeks' gestation, with every pregnancy to provide passive immunity for the infant (CDC, 2013b). If Tdap is not administered during pregnancy, it should be administered immediately postpartum.

The ACIP recommends "cocooning," where parents, siblings, grandparents, child-care providers, and health-care personnel who care for infants younger than 12 months receive Tdap vaccine to protect the infant against exposure to pertussis (CDC, 2013b).

Monitoring

There is no laboratory monitoring needed with DTaP, DT, Tdap, or Td vaccine.

Patient Education

The parent or patient should receive a VIS prior to administration of vaccine. Any questions or concerns regarding the vaccine should be addressed. The most common adverse reaction after DTaP, Tdap, or Td injection is pain and erythema at the injection site. Advise the patient to take acetaminophen for discomfort for the first 24 hours after injection. Post-vaccination fever, myalgia, and headache can be treated with acetaminophen or ibuprofen prophylaxis. Premedicating with antipyretics before vaccination is not routinely recommended.

HAEMOPHILUS B CONJUGATE VACCINE

Pharmacodynamics

HIB conjugate vaccine consists of the HIB capsular polysaccharide covalently linked to another antigen to increase immunogenicity. HIB conjugate vaccine exposure stimulates the immune system to produce HIB capsule–specific antibodies that destroy the capsule. This makes the organism vulnerable to antibody- and cell-mediated immunity. Unconjugated capsule polysaccharide vaccines cause B-cell stimulation only. By conjugating the capsule polysaccharide, T-cell stimulation occurs as well. HIB conjugate vaccine comes singly (ActHIB, Hiberix) and in combination with other vaccines (HBV/HIB [Comvax], DTaP/HIB [TriHibit], DTaP/IPV/HIB [Pentacel], meningococcal/HIB [MenHibrix]).

Pharmacokinetics

HIB is administered IM. Antibodies are detected approximately 1 to 2 weeks after administration. The HIB is more immunogenic in older children; therefore, only one dose is needed for children receiving their first dose at age 15 months or older.

Ideally, the patient should receive the same conjugate vaccine product for all of the primary series of immunizations. However, when different products are given for the series, serum antibodies are similar to those of patients who received all the same formula.

The anticapsular antibodies may cross the placenta and are distributed in breast milk.

Pharmacotherapeutics

Precautions and Contraindications

Anaphylactic reaction to the vaccine or any component is a contraindication to HIB. Moderate to severe illness, with or without fever, may be a reason to delay vaccination. Minor illness, including otitis media, is not a reason to delay administration. HIB vaccine should be administered only to children under the age of 6.

Adverse Drug Reactions

The most common adverse reaction following HIB is pain, redness, and swelling at the injection site. These symptoms are mild and usually last less than 24 hours. Systemic reactions are infrequent, and when HIB is given with DTaP, there is no increased incidence of systemic reaction over DTaP given alone.

Drug Interactions

There are no known interactions.

Clinical Use and Dosing

Dosing of HIB depends on the vaccine used. HibTITER (HbOC) and ActHib (PRP-T) are given at 2, 4, and 6 months and a booster at 12 to 15 months. PedvaxHIB (PRP-OMP) is given at 2 and 4 months and a booster at 12 to 15 months. HIB/HBV (Combax) is given at 2, 4 and 12 to 15 months. Pentacel (DTaP/OPV/HIB) can be administered at 2, 4, 5 and 15 to 18 months. TriHIBit (DTaP/HIB) can be administered as the booster DTaP dose at 12 to 18 months if the primary HIB series was completed at least 6 months before. The first dose of HIB can be given at age 6 weeks but no earlier. Any HIB vaccine, including Hiberix (HIB), can be used for the booster dose at age 12 to 15 months. If a child receives the first dose at age 15 months or older but younger than 5 years, only one dose of HIB is needed. MenHibrix is administered at 2, 4, 6, and 12 to 15 months of age.

Monitoring

No laboratory monitoring is necessary.

Patient Education

Parents should receive a VIS prior to administration of the vaccine. Any questions or concerns regarding the vaccine should be addressed. The most common adverse reaction after HIB injection is pain and erythema at the injection site. Advise the parent to give acetaminophen for discomfort for the first 24 hours after injection.

INACTIVATED POLIOVIRUS VACCINE

Pharmacodynamics

IPV is a parenteral noninfectious suspension of three types of inactivated poliovirus. The IPV available in the United States since the late 1980s is of enhanced potency and is highly immunogenic. In 1999, the ACIP recommended that all polio virus in the United States be administered as inactivated polio

---

CLINICAL PEARL

Patients With Shot Phobia

In older children and adults who have a true phobia of injections, use **EMLA** cream to anesthetize the injection area. Have the patient apply the disk or cream 1 hour prior to the scheduled administration time, or the cream can be applied in the clinic and the injection administered after 1 hour.

vaccine to eliminate the risk of vaccine-associated polio (CDC, 2009a). IPV inhibits pharyngeal acquisition of poliovirus and, to a lesser extent, provides gut immunity. IPV is available in combination with diphtheria, tetanus, pertussis, and hepatitis B (Pediarix) or in combination with DTaP and HIB (Pentacel).

Pharmacokinetics

After IM administration of two doses, approximately 95% of patients have antibodies to polio. After three doses, 99% to 100% of patients have high antibody titers.

Pharmacotherapeutics

Precautions and Contraindications

A history of immediate hypersensitivity reaction after receiving IPV is a contraindication. Patients with neomycin, streptomycin, or polymyxin B hypersensitivity should not receive the vaccine because there are small amounts of these substances in the vaccine.

IPV is the preferred drug (over OPV) in immunosuppressed patients, although a protective immune response cannot be guaranteed. IPV can be administered to patients with HIV disease. If it is needed to protect the patient, IPV may be administered during pregnancy. IPV is Pregnancy Category C. IPV can be used in infants as young as 6 weeks of age.

Adverse Drug Reactions

Injection site reaction is reported in 13% of patients. Systemic reactions are infrequent, and when IPV is given with DTaP, there is no increased incidence of systemic reaction over DTaP given alone.

Drug Interactions

The immune response to IPV may be diminished if the patient is taking immunosuppressant medication. Revaccinate 3 months after discontinuing immunosuppressants. IPV can be coadministered with all other childhood vaccines.

Clinical Use and Dosing

The primary series of IPV is four doses administered at 2, 4, and 6 to 18 months and 4 to 6 years (CDC, 2009a). The minimum age for the first dose is 6 weeks. The final dose of IPV should be administered after the fourth birthday regardless of the number of previous doses. The minimal interval between doses 1 and 2 and doses 2 to 3 is 4 weeks. The minimal interval between dose 3 and dose 4 is 6 months (CDC, 2009a).

Monitoring

There is no need for laboratory monitoring after administration of IPV.

Patient Education

Parents should receive a VIS prior to administration of the vaccine. Any questions or concerns regarding the vaccine should be addressed. The most common adverse reaction after IPV injection is pain and erythema at the injection site. Advise the parent to give acetaminophen for discomfort.

HEPATITIS B VIRUS VACCINE

Pharmacodynamics

HBV is produced by recombinant DNA technology from common baker's yeast that is genetically modified to synthesize HbsAg. Active immunization with HBV stimulates the immune system to produce antihepatitis B surface antigen antibodies (anti-HBs). HBV is available in combination with diphtheria, tetanus, acellular pertussis, and inactivated polio vaccine (Pediarix), in combination with HAV (Twinrix), and in combination with HIB (Comvax).

Pharmacokinetics

Three doses of HBV induce protective antibody response in more than 95% of infants, children, and adolescents and in more than 90% of adults. Anti-HBs appear in the serum 2 weeks after IM administration. The minimum anti-HB titer needed to provide protection against hepatitis B is 10 milli-international units (mIU)/mL.

Pharmacotherapeutics

Precautions and Contraindications

The only true contraindication to HBV is hypersensitivity to yeast or other components of the vaccine. Moderate or severe illness, with or without fever, is a contraindication to HBV. Patients with renal disease requiring hemodialysis or patients with immunosuppression may require larger doses to achieve adequate serum levels of anti-HBs.

HBV is Pregnancy Category C. The CDC (2013c) has stated that pregnancy is not a contraindication to HBV and it may be given in pregnancy if indicated.

Adverse Drug Reactions

Localized reaction at the injection site is reported by 17% of HBV vaccine recipients. Approximately 15% of patients report systemic complaints, including fatigue, weakness, malaise, fever, headache, nausea or vomiting, diarrhea, and pharyngitis. Serum sickness has occurred days to weeks after administration of HBV. A very rare side effect is alopecia (occurs 5/1 billion doses).

Drug Interactions

Patients who are taking immunosuppressants or antineoplastic agents may require larger doses or additional doses of HBV to achieve adequate anti-HB titers.

Clinical Use and Dosing

Vaccination with HBV is recommended for all ages, particularly patients at high risk of contracting hepatitis B. Those at high risk include IV drug users, infants born to mothers who are HbsAg-positive, hemodialysis patients, sexually active people with multiple partners, incarcerated people, international travelers, household contacts of hepatitis B carriers, and sexual contacts of hepatitis B carriers. Patients who are getting tattoos or who share razors, toothbrushes, or body-piercing jewelry are

---

CLINICAL PEARL

Administering Injections

A technique to help older children, adolescents, or adults who are anxious about receiving injections is to encourage them to take slow, deep breaths. Younger children (5-year-olds) can be told to pretend they are blowing up a balloon. Have the patient inhale and exhale two or three times, and then, on the third or fourth exhalation, administer the injection.

---

also at risk of contracting hepatitis B. Health-care workers, day-care staff, and other people who may have exposure to body fluids also have a greater risk of contracting hepatitis B. Patients with diabetes are at increased risk of contracting HBV and it is recommended they receive the HBV series (CDC, 2011c).

The ACIP and the AAP recommend universal vaccination of all infants as a comprehensive strategy to control hepatitis B. The current recommendations for childhood immunizations include administering the three-dose HBV series to newborns or at age 11 to 12 years to children not previously vaccinated. The series can be started at any age, although it is recommended that preterm infants be at least 1 month of age before starting HPV series (CDC, 2005a). Some states are requiring proof of HBV series completion for entry to the seventh grade.

Vaccination with HBV is recommended for all adults who are at high risk of contracting hepatitis B infection. The ACIP has issued a recommendation that HBV be offered to unvaccinated adults assumed to be at risk, including patients of sexually transmitted disease treatment clinics, HIV treatment facilities, drug abuse treatment programs, correctional facilities, chronic hemodialysis treatment centers, and services providing care to developmentally delayed adults (CDC, 2005a).

The recommended schedule for vaccinating infants with HBV is to give the first dose at birth or before age 2 months. The second dose is given at age 1 to 4 months. Dose 3 is given at age 6 to 18 months. The rules regarding minimum HBV dose spacing in older children and adults are that there must be 4 weeks between doses 1 and 2, 2 months between doses 2 and 3, and 4 months between doses 1 and 3, allowing the series to be completed in as little as 4 months. The series is never restarted, no matter how long it has been since the previous dose. The recommended dosing of HBV is provided in Table 19-5.

Table 19–5 ⊗ Recommended Doses of Currently Licensed Formulations of Hepatitis B Vaccine by Age Group and Vaccine Type

Age Group	Single-Antigen Vaccine Recombivax HB Dose (mcg)	Volume (mL)	Engerix-B Dose (mcg)	Volume (mL)	Combination Vaccine †Comvax* Dose (mcg)	x§ Volume (mL)	Pediarix Dose (mcg)	Volume (mL)	Twinri Dose (mcg)	Volume (mL)
>6 wk to 4 yr* or 6 yr†	NA	NA	NA	NA	5	0.5	0	0.5	NA**	NA
Children (0–19 yr)	5	0.5	10	0.5	5*	0.5	10†	0.5	NA	NA
Adolescents										
11–15 yr	10‡	1.0‡	10	0.5	NA	NA	NA	NA	NA	NA
11–19 yr	5	0.5	10	0.5	NA	NA	NA	NA	NA	NA
Adults (= 20 yr)	10	1.0	20	1.0	NA	NA	NA	NA	20§	1.0
Hemodialysis Patients and Other Immunocompromised Persons										
<20 yr§§	5	0.5	10	0.5	NA	NA	NA	NA	NA	NA
= 20 yr	40§§	1.0	40***	2.0	NA	NA	NA	NA	NA	NA

*Combined hepatitis B–*Haemophilus influenzae* type b conjugate vaccine. This vaccine cannot be administered at birth, before age 6 wk, or after age 71 mo.

†Combined hepatitis B–diphtheria, tetanus, and acellular pertussis-inactivated poliovirus vaccine. This vaccine cannot be administered at birth, before age 6 wk, or at age = 7 yr.

§Combined hepatitis A and hepatitis B vaccines. This vaccine is recommended for persons aged =18 yr who are at increased risk for both hepatitis B virus and hepatitis A virus infections.

¶Recombinant hepatitis B surface antigen protein dose.

**Not applicable.

‡Adult formulation administered on a two-dose schedule.

§§Higher doses might be more immunogenic, but no specific recommendations have been made.

¶¶Dialysis formulation administered on a three-dose schedule at age 0, 1, and 6 mo.

***Two 1.0 mL doses administered at one site, on a four-dose schedule, at ages 0, 1, 2, and 6 mo.

(Centers for Disease Control, 2005a).

HBV is generally given IM but may be given SC if IM injections are contraindicated (as in hemophiliacs). HBV should be given IM in the deltoid or anterolateral thigh. The immunogenicity of HBV is decreased when given in the buttock. HBV should not be given with the same syringe or at the same site as hepatitis B immune globulin (H-BIG).

Patients who do not develop a serum anti-HB antibody response (greater than or equal to 10 mIU/mL) after three doses of HBV should be revaccinated with one to three doses. If the patient does not respond after three additional doses, he or she is unlikely to respond to any additional doses.

Monitoring

Susceptibility testing before HBV vaccination is not routinely indicated for children or adolescents. Testing for previous infection may be considered in adults in high-risk groups with high rates of hepatitis B infection, such as users of IV drugs, men who have sex with men, and household contacts of hepatitis B carriers.

Routine post-vaccination testing for anti-HBs is not necessary. Post-vaccination testing is advised 1 to 2 months after the third dose of HBV for those whose subsequent management is determined by their anti-HB status: (1) those at risk for occupational exposure risk from sharp injuries, (2) those with HIV infection, (3) hemodialysis patients, (4) immunocompromised patients at risk of contracting hepatitis B, (5) regular sexual contact of hepatitis carriers, and (6) infants born to HbsAg-positive mothers.

Patient Education

Parents should receive a VIS prior to administration of the vaccine. Any questions or concerns regarding the vaccine should be addressed. The most common adverse reaction after HBV injection is pain and erythema at the injection site. Advise the parent to give acetaminophen for discomfort for the first 24 hours after injection.

HEPATITIS A VIRUS VACCINE

Pharmacodynamics

HAV vaccine is used to confer immunity to hepatitis A in people at risk of contracting the disease. With HAV administration, stimulation of specific antibodies takes place without producing disease symptoms. Serum antibody titers after HAV are lower than those resulting from hepatitis A infection. Serum antibody titer of 20 mIU/mL is considered protective. There are two HAV products available; both provide immunity with a two-dose schedule.

Pharmacokinetics

HAV is administered IM. One dose of HAV can induce seroconversion in 88% of patients by 15 days and 99% of patients by 1 month. This rapid seroconversion from a single dose can provide protection for at least 12 months (CDC, 2006d). Administration of a second dose at 6 to 12 months after the first dose provides 100% protection. The duration of the vaccine protection has not been determined yet, as long-term efficacy has not been established. Theoretically, antibody levels should last 20 years or more. The CDC does not recommend any post-vaccination monitoring of serological response because of the high vaccine response in children and adults (CDC, 2006d).

Pharmacotherapeutics

Precautions and Contraindications

HAV should not be administered to patients with a previous history of severe reaction to HAV. Moderate or severe illness, with or without fever, is a contraindication to HAV. Patients with immunosuppression may be given HAV, but they may have lower antibody titers than immunocompetent people.

HAV is Pregnancy Category C. The CDC (2013c) has stated HAV may be given in pregnancy if indicated and that it poses no risk to the fetus. The safety and effectiveness of HAV in children under age 12 months has not been established.

Adverse Drug Reactions

The most frequently reported adverse reaction to HAV is soreness at the injection site (56% in adults and 15% in children). Headache and malaise are other minor adverse reactions that have been reported.

Drug Interactions

Patients who are taking immunosuppressants or antineoplastic agents may have a decreased immunological response to HAV.

Clinical Use and Dosing

HAV vaccine provides pre-exposure protection from hepatitis A infection in adults and children. HAV is recommended for people who are at increased risk for infection and for any person wishing to obtain immunity. The ACIP, AAP, and American Academy of Family Physicians (AAFP) recommend that all children begin HAV series at age 12 months. People at increased risk for hepatitis A infection who should be routinely vaccinated include the following:

1. People over age 1 year who are traveling or working in countries that have high or intermediate endemic infection. All of South America, Africa, Greenland, and Asia have a high incidence of hepatitis A infection. Russia and eastern Europe are areas of intermediate prevalence. IG is recommended for children under age 1 who are traveling to these areas.
2. Men who have sex with men.
3. Illegal drug users.
4. People who have an occupational risk for infection, including those who work with hepatitis A–infected primates or with hepatitis A in a research laboratory setting.
5. People with clotting factor disorders.
6. People with chronic liver disease.
7. Household members and close personal contacts of internationally adopted children from countries with high or intermediate hepatitis A endemicity.

The ACIP recommends administering the first dose of HAV as soon as the adoption planning process begins, ideally at least 2 weeks before the arrival of the adoptee (CDC, 2009b).

Two different HAV products are currently available, HAVrix and VAQTA, as well as a combination product that combines HAV and HBV, Twinrix. HAVrix is available in two strengths: 1,440 enzyme-linked immunoassay units (EL.U) and 720 EL.U. The adult (age 19 years and older) dose is 1,440 EL.U administered in a two-dose schedule, 6 to 12 months apart. The pediatric (age 1 to 18 years) dose of HAVrix is 720 EL.U, administered in a two-dose schedule 6 to 12 months apart. VAQTA is available in two strengths: adult, which has 50 antigen U/1 mL dose, and pediatric-adolescent strength, which has 25 U/0.5 mL dose. The dose for adults is 50 U administered 6 months apart. The dose for children aged 1 to 18 years is 25 U administered 6 to 18 months apart. Twinrix is HAVrix (720 EL.U) combined with Engerix-B (20 mcg) and is approved for persons 18 years and older. The dosing schedule of Twinrix is 1.0 mL in three doses, at 0, 1, and 6 months.

HAV is injected IM into the deltoid muscle in adults and children age 3 years or older and in the vastus lateralis muscle (anterolateral thigh) in children age 12 months to 36 months. Injection in the gluteal region results in suboptimal response. Patients with an impaired immune system may require additional doses to obtain an adequate anti–hepatitis A response.

> ### CLINICAL PEARL
>
> **Bioterrorism**
> Providers need to have a basic understanding of vaccines available against possible biological weapons. The CDC Web site has an area dedicated to bioterrorism located at www.bt.cdc.gov/bioterrorism/. There are vaccines available for anthrax and smallpox, although this chapter does not discuss them because they are not currently recommended. Full prescribing information for both the anthrax and the smallpox vaccines are available at the CDC National Immunization Web site at www.cdc.gov/nip/publications/acip-list.htm.

Monitoring

Pre-immunization testing of children for hepatitis A antibodies is generally not recommended. Pretesting may be cost-effective in adults who have a high likelihood of immunity from prior infection, such as those who have lived in areas of high hepatitis incidence, those older than 40, and those with a history of jaundice that potentially may have been hepatitis A infection (CDC, 2006d).

Post-immunization testing is not indicated in immunocompetent persons because of the high seroconversion rates in children and adults who receive HAV. Post-immunization testing is warranted in immunocompromised patients who may have suboptimal response to the vaccine.

Patient Education

Parents should receive a VIS prior to administration of the vaccine. Any questions or concerns regarding the vaccine should be addressed. The most common adverse reaction after HAV injection is pain and erythema at the injection site. Advise the patient to take acetaminophen for discomfort for the first 24 hours after injection.

HUMAN PAPILLOMAVIRUS VACCINE

Pharmacodynamics

Human papillomavirus (HPV) causes cervical cancer, the second-biggest cause of female cancer mortality worldwide, with an estimated 288,000 deaths yearly (WHO, 2011). "Genital HPV infection is extremely common and most often remains subclinical, but a proportion of the infected individuals with low-risk HPV types such as HPV-6 or HPV-11 will develop genital warts, whereas a subset of women with high-risk HPVs such as HPV-16 or HPV-18 will develop preneoplastic lesions of cervical intraepithelial neoplasia (CIN)" (WHO, 2005, p 85). Approximately 500,000 cases of genital warts occur in men and women in the United States annually (CDC, 2010a, 2010b). Two vaccines to treat HPV are currently available: Gardisil is a quadrivalent human papillomavirus recombinant vaccine that provides immunity against types 6, 11, 16, and 18; Gardisil 9 provides immunity against types 16, 18, 31, 33, 45, 52 and 58. and Cervarix, a bivalent vaccine against HPV strains 16 and 18.

Pharmacokinetics

Cervarix (HPV2) is well tolerated after IM injection at 0, 1, and 6 months with a 99.8% antibody response, providing 100% efficacy against HPV 16 cervical infections and 89.6% efficacy against HPV 16 plus HPV 18 cervical infections (Pagliusi & Aguado, 2004; Markowitz et al, 2014). Gardasil (HPV4) has also demonstrated 100% efficacy in women against HPV 16 infection (median follow-up 17.4 months) using a 0-, 2-, and 6-month schedule of vaccination (Markowitz et al, 2014). Gardasil (HPV4) is 89.4% effective in preventing genital warts in males caused by HPV 6, 11, 16, and/or 18 strains (CDC, 2010b; Markowitz et al, 2014).

Pharmacotherapeutics

Precautions and Contraindications

The only true contraindication to HPV vaccine is severe allergic reactions to any component of the vaccine. Gardasil should not be administered to patients allergic to yeast. Both vaccines have a reported adverse effect of syncope. Patients should be observed for 15 minutes after administration and put in a supine or Trendelenburg position if they become symptomatic.

Both HPV vaccines are rated Pregnancy Category B. They are not recommended for use in pregnancy. No causally associated adverse pregnancy outcome has been reported in preclinical or post-licensure studies. If a patient is administered

HPV vaccine during pregnancy, a registry has been set up by both manufacturers to report exposure (Gardasil: Merck & Co. at 800-986-8999; Cervarix: GlaxoSmithKline at 888-452-9622). Pregnancy testing is not needed before vaccination.

Adverse Drug Reactions

Pain, redness, and swelling at the injection site were the most commonly reported local adverse reaction, reported in over 20% of subjects receiving the vaccines. The most common general adverse events were fatigue, headache, myalgias, and arthalgias. The most common serious reaction to HPV vaccine is syncopal episodes. Reports of falling with injury due to syncope after receiving HPV have been recorded; recommendations are that all patients who receive the HPV vaccine be observed for 15 minutes after administration.

Drug Interactions

No known drug interactions occur with HPV vaccine. Immunosuppressants may reduce the immune response to the vaccine.

Clinical Use and Dosing

Dosing of the HPV vaccines varies with the drug and the gender of the patient. HPV4 (Gardasil) is approved for use in girls and women ages 9 to 26 years to prevent cervical, vulvar, and vaginal cancer caused by HPV types 16 and 18 and genital warts (condyloma acuminata) caused by HPV types 6 and 11. HPV9 (Gardasil 9) is approved for use in girls and women ages 9 to 26 years to prevent cervical, vulvar, and vaginal cancer caused by HPV types 16, 18, 33, 45, 52 and 58; and genital warts (condyloma acuminata) caused by HPV types 6 and 11. HPV4/HPV9 is recommended for all girls starting at age 11 to 12 years but may be started as young as age 9 years. The dosing schedule is three doses of 0.5 mL given IM at 0, 2, and 6 months.

HPV4 (Gardasil) is approved for the prevention of genital warts caused by HPV types 6 and 11 in males. HPV9 (Gardasil 9) is approved for anal warts caused by HPV types 16, 18, 31, 33, 45, 52 and 58; and genital warts (condyloma acuminata) caused by HPV types 6 and 11. The dosing schedule for HPV4/HPV9 in males is 0.5 mL given IM at 0, 2, and 6 months.

HPV2 (Cervarix) is approved to prevent cervical cancer caused by HPV types 16 and 18 in females aged 10 to 25 years. HPV2 is recommended by the ACIP as one of the two HPV vaccines for routine vaccination of females beginning at age 11 to 12 (CDC, 2010a). The dose of HPV2 (Cervarix) is three 0.5 mL doses at 0, 1, and 6 months.

After patients receive HPV vaccine, they should be monitored for 15 minutes because of the risk for syncope after the vaccine.

Monitoring

No ongoing monitoring of patients is needed after vaccination with HPV vaccine.

Patient Education

Parents should receive a VIS prior to administration of the vaccine. Any questions or concerns regarding the vaccine should be addressed. Patients should be informed of the risk for syncope and why they need to be monitored after administration of HPV. The most common adverse reactions after HPV injection are pain, erythema, and swelling at the injection site. Advise the patient to take acetaminophen for discomfort for the first 24 hours after injection.

INFLUENZA VACCINE

Pharmacodynamics

Influenza vaccine (Afluria, Fluarix, Flucelvax, FluLaval, Fluvirin, Fluzone, Fluzone Intradermal, Fluzone High-dose) is a multivalent vaccine that contains three different viral subtypes. It is available as a trivalent or quadravalent vaccine (Fluarix Quadrivalent, Flulaval Quadrivalent, Fluzone Quadrivalent). Flucelvax, a trivalent vaccine, is the first cell-based influenza vaccine. FluBlok is a trivalent recombinant hemagluten (HA) influenza vaccine containing purified HA proteins, which uses cell-based technology.

Each year, the World Health Organization recommends to the FDA's Vaccines and Related Biologic Products Advisory Committee what strains will be included in the following year's vaccine. Data from the WHO Influenza Surveillance Network are used to determine the composition of the Northern and Southern Hemisphere influenza vaccine for the following season. Because influenza viruses are constantly changing and immunity wanes over time, annual immunization is required. The previous year's vaccine cannot be used for the current year. Influenza virus vaccine imparts immunity by stimulating production of antibodies that are specific to the disease strain. Patients who receive the vaccine are immune only to the strains included in the vaccine for that year.

Pharmacokinetics

The influenza vaccine is administered IM. The vaccine produces protective antibodies within 10 to 14 days. The duration of immunity generally lasts from 6 months to 1 year.

Pharmacotherapeutics

Precautions and Contraindications

Anaphylactic reaction to the influenza vaccine, eggs, or egg products is a contraindication to the use of influenza vaccine. The CDC has developed an algorithm to be used with patients who report an allergy to eggs (Grohskopf et al, 2013). The recommendation includes administering the inactivated influenza vaccine to patients who can eat lightly cooked eggs without a reaction. If patients age 18 to 49 only experience hives from eating eggs, the recommendations are to administer recombinant influenza vaccine (Flucelvax, FluBlok) or inactivated influenza vaccine and observe the patient for at least 30 minutes following vaccination (Grohskopf et al, 2013). Patients who have severe hypersensitivity to eggs should only be administered the recombinant influenza vaccine (Flucelvax, FluBlok), which is produced using non-egg technologies.

Thimerosal is used as a preservative in the vaccine; therefore, patients with hypersensitivity to thimerosal should not receive the influenza vaccine. Some of the influenza vaccines contain sulfites; care should be taken to check the ingredients listed on the packaging prior to administering vaccine to a patient with sulfite hypersensitivity.

Patients with an active neurological disorder should defer the vaccine until the condition stabilizes. Any patient with a history of Guillain–Barré syndrome (GBS) less than 6 weeks after a previous dose of influenza vaccine should not receive the vaccine. Patients with HIV disease may be immunized with influenza vaccine, but they may have lower vaccine-induced antibody levels. Patients with an acute febrile illness should defer the vaccine until their symptoms subside.

Influenza vaccine is Pregnancy Category C, but according to the CDC (2013c) influenza vaccine may be safely administered to pregnant women. Influenza vaccine may be administered to lactating women with no effect on the infant.

The safety of influenza vaccine has not been established in children younger than 6 months of age.

Administration error: The dosing schedules for children and adults for injectable influenza vaccine are different. If an adult is accidentally administered a pediatric dose (0.25 mL), the adult should receive an additional pediatric dose (0.25 mL) the same day. If the mistake is not discovered until later, a full adult dose is administered. If a child is administered an adult dose, no action needs to be taken.

Adverse Drug Reactions

Adverse reactions to the influenza vaccine are usually mild and more common in children than in adults. Local injection site reaction occurs in about 23% percent of patients. In addition, 5% to 10% of patients experience mild adverse systemic effects, including low-grade fever, malaise, and myalgia.

Rarely, a patient has an immediate hypersensitivity reaction to the vaccine, including urticaria, angioedema, bronchospasm, and/or anaphylactic shock. These reactions are most likely the result of hypersensitivity to residual egg protein.

Drug Interactions

Patients who are taking immunosuppressants or antineoplastic agents may have a decreased immunological response to influenza vaccine. Medications that may have inhibited clearance after administration of influenza vaccine include theophylline, phenytoin, and warfarin. Reports concerning impaired drug clearance are conflicting, and the concurrent administration of influenza vaccine to patients taking these medications is not contraindicated.

Clinical Use and Dosing

The influenza vaccine should be administered annually to all persons aged 6 months and older, including pregnant women. The optimal time for organized vaccination programs is October through mid-November. Travelers to areas in which influenza is endemic should be vaccinated 2 to 4 weeks prior to travel. The dosing of influenza vaccine is as follows:

1. Patients aged 9 years or older are given one 0.5 mL dose of influenza vaccine annually.
2. Adults aged 65 years or older may receive high-dose influenza vaccine (Fluzone High-Dose).
3. Previously vaccinated children aged 3 to 8 are given one 0.5 mL dose.
4. Children aged 3 to 8 who have never been vaccinated receive 0.5 mL, with a repeat dose in 4 weeks.
5. Children aged 6 to 35 months who have been previously vaccinated receive 0.25 mL of vaccine.
6. Children aged 6 to 35 months who have not been previously vaccinated with influenza vaccine receive 0.25 mL, with a second dose in 4 weeks.

Patients who experience only hives when eating eggs or egg-containing foods can be administered FluBlok or Flucelvax and observed for 30 minutes. Patients who have symptoms of anaphylaxis when eating eggs may be administered FluBlok or referred to an allergist.

Monitoring

There is no laboratory monitoring needed after patients receive the influenza vaccine.

Patient Education

Parents should receive a VIS prior to administration of vaccine. Any questions or concerns regarding the vaccine should be addressed. The most common adverse reaction after influenza vaccine injection is pain and erythema at the injection site. Some patients may also experience low-grade fever and malaise. Advise the patient to take acetaminophen for discomfort for the first 24 hours after injection.

PNEUMOCOCCAL VACCINE

Pharmacodynamics

There are two types of pneumococcal vaccine currently available (Pneumovax 23, Prevnar). Polyvalent pneumococcal polysaccharide vaccine (PPV) contains 23 highly purified capsular polysaccharides from *Streptococcus pneumoniae*. These are the 23 most prevalent or invasive pneumococcal types, accounting for at least 90% of all blood isolates associated with clinical infection. PPV stimulates the immune system to produce pneumococcus capsule–specific antibodies. These antibodies presumably destroy the capsule, making the pneumococcus vulnerable to antibody- and cell-mediated immunity. Clinical trials suggest a protective efficacy of 60% to 90%. The 23-valent PPV has limited immunogenicity in children younger than 2 years. The 23-valent vaccine was approved by the FDA in 1977.

In February 2000, the FDA approved the first vaccine to prevent invasive pneumococcal disease in infants and children, pneumococcal 7-valent conjugate vaccine (Prevnar). The vaccine targeted the seven most common strains of pneumococcus, which accounted for 80% of invasive disease in infants. With universal vaccination of children under the age of 5 years with PCV7, invasive pneumococcol disease decreased by 76% over 10 years of use (CDC, 2010c). In spite of this reduction, there were still cases of invasive pneumococcal disease in children caused by strains not in the PCV7 vaccine.

In 2010, the FDA approved a 13-valent conjugate vaccine (Prevnar13; PCV13), which is active against six additional strains of pneumococcus, responsible for 64% of invasive pneumococcal disease in children vaccinated with PCV7 (CDC, 2010c). In 2011 PCV13 was approved for use in adults age 50 and older; and in 2012 PCV13 was approved for age 19 and older with immunocompromising conditions, functional or anatomic asplenia, cerebrospinal fluid leak, or cochlear implants. PCV13 not meant to replace the 23-valent vaccine.

Pharmacokinetics

PPV is administered either SC or IM. Immunity after SC or IM injection occurs in 2 to 3 weeks. Serotype-specific antibodies decline after 5 to 10 years. Children may decline to pre-vaccination levels in 3 to 5 years, especially asplenic children and children with sickle cell disease.

PCV13 is administered IM, with measurable titers present 1 month after the fourth dose in children. Antibodies were measured in adults one month after a dose of PCV13 was administered.

Pharmacotherapeutics

Precautions and Contraindications

Previous anaphylactic reaction to the vaccine or any component is a contraindication to its use. Moderate to severe illness, with or without fever, is a reason to defer the vaccine until the patient has improved.

Pneumococcal vaccine should be given at least 10 to 14 days before elective splenectomy, organ transplant, immunosuppressive therapy, or chemotherapy. Patients with Hodgkin's disease and immunosuppressed patients have suboptimal antibody response to vaccination.

Use PPV cautiously in patients with idiopathic thrombocytopenic purpura (ITP), as PPV has been associated with relapse of ITP.

PPV is Pregnancy Category C. Use of the vaccine during the first trimester should be avoided. It is not known if the vaccine is excreted in breast milk.

PCV13 is Pregnancy Category B. There are no adequate, well-controlled studies in pregnant women.

PPV 23-valent vaccine is not recommended in children under 2 years. PCV13 is not for use in adults.

Adverse Drug Reactions

Seventy-two percent of PPV recipients report local injection site reactions of erythema, induration, and soreness that last up to 48 hours. Occasionally, low-grade fever and arthralgia have been reported. High fever is rare.

During clinical trials of Prevnar, adverse effects were generally mild and included local injection site reaction,

irritability, drowsiness, and decreased appetite. Approximately 21% of children in the vaccine group had a fever of 100.8°F or higher, compared with 14% of the control group. During clinical trials of PCV13 (Prevnar 13) infants had redness (24.3%), swelling (20.1%), and tenderness (62.5%) at the injection site and experienced fever (24.3%), irritability (85.6%), and increased sleep (71.5%) after the first dose at approximately the same rate as infants who received PCV7 (CDC, 2010e).

Drug Interactions

No known drug interactions have occurred.

Clinical Use and Dosing

Dosing of PPV is based on the age and medical condition of the patient:

1. PPV is recommended for all adults aged 65 or older. The dose is 0.5 mL IM or SC. Revaccinate (a second dose) if the original vaccination was 5 years or more ago *and* the patient was under age 65 when the dose was given.
2. People aged 2 to 65 years who have chronic illness and who are at increased risk of morbidity or mortality from pneumococcal disease should receive PPV. These risk factors include chronic cardiac or pulmonary disease, chronic liver disease or alcoholism, diabetes mellitus, and cerebrospinal fluid leaks. The dose of PPV is 0.5 mL given IM or SC once. Revaccination is not recommended in these populations.
3. Immunocompetent patients aged 2 to 65 years with functional or anatomic asplenia (including sickle cell anemia) should receive 0.5 mL IM or SC. Revaccination is recommended 5 years or more after the first dose; if the patient is under 10 years old, revaccination should be considered 5 years after the first dose.
4. Immunocompromised patients (including HIV infection); those with chronic renal failure, hematological malignancy, Hodgkin's disease, lymphoma, or multiple myeloma; patients receiving immunosuppressive therapy; and patients who have received an organ or bone marrow transplant should receive a dose of 0.5 mL IM or SC. Revaccination should be considered if the first vaccine was 5 years or more ago; in children under age 10, revaccination is considered 5 years after the first dose.
5. Adult smokers between the ages of 19 and 64 years should be given one dose of PPV.
6. Patients with asthma between the ages of 19 and 64 years should receive one dose of PPV.
7. One dose of PPV should be administered at 12 and 24 months following bone marrow transplant.
8. A dose of PPV is administered 2 or more months after last dose of PCV13 to children age 2 years or older.

The dosing schedule for PCV13 is:

1. Infants and toddlers: four doses given at 2, 4, 6, and 12 to 15 months of age.

2. Children up to age 59 months who are not vaccinated with PCV 13 at the routine infant vaccine times should be dosed following the Catch-Up schedule with a minimum dosing (see Table 19-2).

3. Children age 6 to 18 years with anatomic or functional asplenia (including SCD), HIV infection, cochlear implant, CSF leak, or other immunocompromising conditions who have not previously received PCV13 should receive one dose of PCV13, followed by PPV 8 weeks later.

4. Immunocompromised adults age 19 years or older who have not received pneumococcal vaccine should receive a dose of PCV13, followed by a dose of PPV at least 8 weeks later.

5. Immunocompromised adults age 19 years or older who have received PPV should receive a dose of PCV13 at least one year after last PPV dose.

6. All adults age 65 or older should receive a dose of PCV13. If they have not had any doses of pneumococcal vaccine they should receive a dose of PCV13, followed by a dose of PPV in 6 to 12 months.

7. Persons age 65 or older who have previously received PPV should be administered a dose of PCV13 at least a year after the last dose of PPV.

Monitoring

No laboratory monitoring is necessary.

Patient Education

Parents should receive a VIS prior to administration of the vaccine. Any questions or concerns regarding the vaccine should be addressed. The most common adverse reaction after pneumococcal vaccine injection is pain and erythema at the injection site. Advise the patient to take acetaminophen for discomfort for the first 24 hours after injection.

MENINGOCOCCAL VACCINE

Pharmacodynamics

Meningococcal polysaccharide vaccine (MPSV) for groups A, C, Y, and W-135 (Menomune A/C/Y/W-135) is currently approved in the United States for use against meningococcemia and meningitis caused by *Neisseria meningitidis* serogroups A, C, Y, and W-135. MCV4 (Menactra, Menveo) is a tetravalent meningococcal conjugate vaccine that also provides protection against serogroups A, C, Y, and W-135. In 2012, Hib-MenCY (MenHibrix) was approved and provides coverage against *Neisseria meningitidis* serogroups C and Y and *Haemophilus influenzae* type b. In 2014 the FDA approved a serogroup B meningococcal vaccine Trumemba for use in 10- to 25-year-olds. A second meningococcal serotype B vaccine Bexero was approved in 2015 for use in 10- to 25-year-olds.

In the United States, *N. meningitidis* serogroup C, Y, and W accounts for 73% of meningococcal disease in persons 11 years of age or older and serogroup B for 60% of cases in children 0 to 59 months (Cohn et al, 2013). Serogroup A is rare in the United States but is the most common cause of epidemics in Africa and Asia. There were two major outbreaks of serotype B disease on college campuses in 2013 and 2014 (CDC, 2015).

All of the meningococcal vaccines induce the formation of bactericidal antibodies to meningococcal antigens. Post-immunization seroconversion rates for Menomune A/C/Y/W-135 reported by the manufacturer in children aged 2 to 12 years were group A, 72%; group C, 58%; group Y, 90%; and group W-135, 82%. Among 20,000 military recruits under epidemic conditions, the vaccine demonstrated 90% efficacy against serogroup C. MCV4 (Menactra, Menveo) demonstrated similar efficacy in patients age 11 to 55 years in clinical trials (Cohn et al, 2013). Two doses of Hib-MenCY demonstrated 94% efficacy for serotype C and 83% for serotype Y (Cohn et al, 2013). Two doses of serotype B vaccine demonstrate efficacy, with Bexsero demonstrating 62% to 88% efficacy against three serotype B strains, and 82% demonstrate antibodies to four serotype B strains after receiving Trumenba.

Limitations of the meningococcal polysaccharide vaccine (Menomune) include the following. Serogroup C polysaccharide is poorly immunogenic among children aged less than 2 years, it does not confer long-lasting immunity, and it does not cause a sustainable reduction of nasopharyngeal carriage of *N. meningitidis* (Cohn et al, 2013). Conjugation of polysaccharide (as in MCV4) to a protein carrier changes the immune response from T-cell independent to T-cell dependent, leading to stronger response to the vaccine and reduction of the asymptomatic carrier state (CDC, 2006b).

Pharmacokinetics

Protective antibody levels may be achieved within 7 to 10 days after vaccination. The measurable levels of antibodies to serogroups A and C are measured 3 to 5 years following vaccination (Cohn et al, 2013). This decrease occurs more rapidly in infants and young children than it does in adults.

Pharmacotherapeutics

Precautions and Contraindications

Previous anaphylactic reaction to any component of the vaccine is a contraindication to its use. Moderate to severe illness, with or without fever, is a reason to defer the vaccine until the patient has improved.

A history of Guillain–Barré Syndrome (GBS) is listed as a precaution for MCV4 in the package insert, although the ACIP removed GBS as a precaution in 2010 because the benefits of meningococcal vaccination outweigh the risk for recurrent GBS (Cohn et al, 2013).

The expected immune response may not be obtained if the vaccine is used in patients on immunosuppressive therapy.

Menomune A/C/Y/W-135 should not be given to pregnant women. It is not recommended for children under age 2 years. MCV4 (Menactra) is approved for use in children aged 9 months or older and in adults; it is not recommended in adults older than 55 years. MCV4 (Menveo) is not recommended for children younger than 2 years or adults older than 55 years.

HibMenCY is approved for children aged 6 weeks to 18 months and is not approved in older children or adults.

MPSV (Menomune) is the only vaccine approved for adults older than age 55 years.

Both serotype B vaccines (Bexsero, Trumenba) are Pregnancy Category B. Neither serotype B vaccine is approved for children younger than age 10 years.

Adverse Drug Reactions

Adverse reactions to either vaccine are mild and consist of pain and tenderness at the injection site for 1 to 2 days.

Drug Interactions

There are no known drug interactions to this vaccine.

Clinical Use and Dosing

The ACIP (Cohn et al, 2013) recommends routine vaccination of young adolescents (defined as aged 11 to 12 years) with MCV4 at the preadolescent health-care visit or on entering high school (age 15). One booster dose of MCV4 is administered between age 16 and 18 years to adolescents who receive the first dose before age 16 years. While MCV4 is not routinely recommended for those older than 19 years, a catch-up dose can be administered to those aged 19 to 21 years who have not received a dose after their 16th birthday.

HibMenCY is recommended for routine vaccination of infants aged 2 to 18 months with persistent complement deficiencies or functional or anatomic asplenia (Cohn et al, 2013). HibMenCY may also be used to vaccinate infants aged 2 to 18 months during an outbreak of meningitis covered by the vaccine.

The ACIP also recommends that the following high-risk groups receive meningococcal vaccine:

1. Patients with deficiencies in late complement components (C3, C5, to C9).
2. Persons with functional or actual asplenia.
3. Research, industrial, and clinical laboratory personnel who routinely are exposed to *N. meningitidis* in solutions that may be aerosolized.
4. Travelers to, and residents of, hyperendemic areas such as sub-Saharan Africa. Epidemics have occurred recently in Saudi Arabia, Kenya, Tanzania, Burundi, and Mongolia.
5. College freshmen living in dorms.
6. Military recruits.

HibMenCY is administered as a primary series IM at age 2, 4, 6, and 12 through 15 months. MCV4 is administered IM as a single 0.5 mL dose with a second dose in 12 weeks in children aged 9 to 23 months and at 8 to 12 weeks in patients aged 2 to 55 years The dose of Menomune for all ages is a single SC 0.5 mL dose. In patients aged 9 months to 10 years, MCV4 (Menactra) is the preferred vaccine. Adults over age 55 years should receive MPSV.

Revaccination may be indicated for persons at high risk for infection (travel to or living in epidemic areas) who were previously vaccinated with MPSV or MCV4. Children who were vaccinated between age 2 months and 6 years old should be revaccinated with Menactra in 3 years if they remain at high risk. If a previous dose was given at age 7 years or older, either brand of MCV4 may be given after 5 years. Revaccination with MCV4 of high-risk older children and adults is recommended every 5 years after the first dose of MPSV or MCV4.

A booster dose of MCV4 is recommended at age 16 years in children who received their first dose of MCV4 at age 11 to 12 years. Adolescents who receive their first dose of MCV4 at age 13 to 15 years should receive a booster dose at age 16 to 18 years. The minimum interval between doses of MCV4 is 8 weeks (Cohn et al, 2013).

Serotype B vaccine is administered to 10- to 25-year-olds during an outbreak, or to those at increased risk for meningococcal disease, including those with persistent complement component deficiencies, with anatomic or functional asplenia, and microbiologists routinely exposed to isolates of *N. meningitides*. Bexsero is administered in two doses 1 month apart. Trumenba is administered in three doses at 1, 2, and 6 months.

Monitoring

Laboratory monitoring is not necessary with this vaccine.

Patient Education

Parents should receive information regarding the benefits and risks of the vaccine prior to administration. Any questions or concerns regarding the vaccine should be addressed. The most common adverse reaction after vaccine injection is pain and erythema at the injection site. Advise the patient to take acetaminophen for discomfort for the first 24 hours after injection.

LYME DISEASE VACCINE

Pharmacodynamics

Lyme disease is a vector-borne illness caused by ticks infested with *Borrelia burgdorferi*. Recombinant Lyme disease vaccine (LYMErix, Immulyme) imparts immunity against *B. burgdorferi* by stimulating production of antibodies to the lipoprotein OspA. OspA is a lipoprotein of the *B. burgdorferi* spirochete. The mechanism by which Lyme disease vaccine works is thought to be by antibody killing of the spirochete in the tick. Transmission of the OspA antibody occurs while the tick is feeding on the blood of an immunized host, and the antibodies kill the spirochete even before transmission occurs. In February 2002, SmithKline Beecham, the maker of the only approved Lyme disease vaccine, LYMErix, discontinued its production after there were concerns about the side effects of the vaccine, although an FDA investigation did not find the vaccine to be dangerous. The long-term immunity for patients who previously received the vaccine is unknown. A new vaccine active against *B. burgdorferi* is undergoing clinical trials in Austria and Germany, with promising early results (Wressnigg et al, 2013).

TYPHOID VACCINE

Pharmacodynamics

Typhoid vaccines (Typhoid Vaccine, Typhim Vi) are used to increase resistance to enteric fever caused by *S. typhi*. The efficacy of protective immunity depends on the size of the bacterial inoculum consumed.

There are two parenteral typhoid vaccines available, a heat- and phenol-inactivated vaccine (Typhoid Vaccine) and a purified Vi polysaccharide (Typhim Vi). The efficacy of Typhoid Vaccine is 71% to 77%. The efficacy of Typhim Vi is 49% to 87% in reducing disease incidence. Typhim Vi is used in the United States, and a second brand of Vi polysaccharide, Typherix, is used in Canada.

Pharmacokinetics

The absorption, distribution, and metabolism of typhoid vaccine are unknown.

Pharmacotherapeutics

Precautions and Contraindications

Hypersensitivity to typhoid vaccine is a contraindication to its use. Do not administer to a patient with acute febrile illness.

Typhoid vaccine is Pregnancy Category C. It is not known if the vaccine is harmful to the fetus. If vaccinating a pregnant patient is necessary, inactivated vaccine is recommended.

Typhim Vi and Typherix are not recommended for children under age 2.

Adverse Drug Reactions

Vaccine recipients report local injection site reactions of erythema, induration, and soreness that begin within 24 hours and last 1 to 2 days. Systemic symptoms including low-grade fever, headache, and myalgias have been reported. High fever is rare.

Drug Interactions

If possible, plague vaccine should not be given at the same time as typhoid vaccine to avoid the possibility of accentuated adverse effects. Immunosuppressants may cause insufficient response to the vaccine.

Clinical Use and Dosing

Typhoid vaccine is used for primary immunization against *S. typhi* infection in the following:

1. Travelers to areas where a risk of exposure to *S. typhi* is recognized
2. Persons with household contact with a documented typhoid fever carrier
3. Laboratory workers with frequent contact with *S. typhi*

The dose of Typhim Vi and Typherix in children older than age 2 years and adults is 0.5 mL SC. A booster dose should be administered every 2 years to patients at continued risk of contracting typhoid.

Monitoring

There is no laboratory monitoring needed after typhoid vaccine.

Patient Education

Parents should receive information regarding the benefits and risks of the vaccine prior to administration. Any questions or concerns regarding the vaccine should be addressed. The most common adverse reaction after typhoid vaccination injection is pain and erythema at the injection site. Advise the patient to take acetaminophen for discomfort for the first 24 hours after injection.

The best protection against typhoid fever is food and water precautions to prevent contracting *S. typhi*.

CHOLERA VACCINE

Pharmacodynamics

Cholera vaccine is a suspension of equal parts inactivated Ogawa and Inuba serotypes of killed *Vibrio cholerae* and provides active immunity against cholera. The vaccine is 50% effective in reducing disease in endemic areas. The manufacture and sale of the only licensed cholera vaccine in the United States (Wyeth-Ayerst) has been discontinued. It has not been recommended for travelers because of the brief and incomplete immunity it offers. No cholera vaccination requirements exist for entry or exit in any country (CDC, 2005b).

JAPANESE ENCEPHALITIS VIRUS VACCINE

Pharmacodynamics

Japanese encephalitis (JE) is the most common form of viral encephalitis in Asia and is spread by mosquitoes. An estimated 35,000 to 50,000 cases occur annually. JE is usually severe, resulting in death in 20% to 30% of cases, miscarriage in pregnant women, and serious neurological outcomes in 30% to 50% of infected patients (CDC, 2010d). Currently the only vaccine in production in the United States for JE is an inactivated Vero cell culture–derived vaccine (JE-VC) or IXIARO.

Pharmacokinetics

JE-VC is administered via a two-dose schedule at 0 and 28 days; 96% of vaccine recipients demonstrated an adequate level of immunity against JE. The length of full protection against JE is unknown

Pharmacotherapeutics

Precautions and Contraindications

Previous anaphylactic reaction to any component of the vaccine, including thimerosal, is a contraindication to its use. Pregnancy is a contraindication to JE-VC use. There are no adequate trials investigating safety during pregnancy. IXIARO was approved for children age 2 months through 16 years in 2013 (CDC, 2013d).

Adverse Drug Reactions

IXIARO appears to have the same reported adverse reactions as placebo or comparison vaccine (PCV7 or HAV). Injection site tenderness is reported in approximately 10% to 37% of children receiving the vaccine and fever is reported in 2% to 7% of children (CDC, 2013d). Report any significant adverse effects to the VAERS.

Drug Interactions

There are no known drug interactions.

Clinical Use and Dosing

The best way to avoid JE is to prevent mosquito bites (Hills, Weber, & Fischer, 2013). The ACIP recommends that JE-VC be administered to those who plan on residing for more than a month in areas in which JE is endemic or epidemic. The probability of JE viral infection and illness increases with the duration of the stay in rural endemic areas. Current information on locations of JE virus transmission can be obtained from the CDC *Yellow Book* or Travel Web site (www.cdc.gov/travel).

JE-VC is not recommended for all travelers to Asia. The vaccine should be offered to people spending a month or longer in endemic areas during the transmission season, especially if they are traveling to rural areas (Hills et al, 2013). It should also be offered to those who will be spending extensive time outdoors during their travel.

The dose of JE-VC in adults is two 0.5 mL doses administered IM 28 days apart. For children aged 2 months through 2 years, each dose is 0.25 mL (CDC, 2013d). The series should be completed at least 1 week before potential exposure to Japanese encephalitis virus. The need for a booster is not known because the vaccine is newly approved. Providers are referred to the CDC Travel Web site for dosing information (www.cdc.gov/travel).

Monitoring

There is no monitoring needed after the vaccine.

Patient Education

Patients should receive information regarding the benefits and risks of the vaccine prior to administration. Any questions or concerns regarding the vaccine should be addressed. The most common adverse reactions after vaccination are pain and erythema at the injection site and low-grade systemic symptoms. Adverse reactions may occur up to 10 days after immunization. Patients are advised not to travel outside the United States for 10 days after administration in case of adverse reaction.

Personal protection against mosquitoes is essential for all travelers to endemic areas. Patients should be advised to protect themselves by wearing long-sleeved shirts and long pants. Use of insect repellent should be encouraged. Permethrin should be applied to clothing.

PLAGUE VACCINE

Pharmacodynamics

Plague vaccine, a whole-cell vaccine consisting of a suspension of inactivated plague bacilli (*Yersinia pestis*), is no longer available in the United States. Vaccination against plague is not required by any country as a condition for entry. Travelers who may be exposed to plague should carry prophylactic antibiotics (doxycycline, or trimethoprim-sulfamethoxazole for children under 8 years of age) and use them according to the CDC guidelines for plague, which can be found at the CDC Traveler's Health Web site, www.cdc.gov/travel.

RABIES VACCINE

Pharmacodynamics

Rabies vaccine (Imovax, RabAvert) is a preparation of inactivated rabies virus that induces active immunity. The two products available differ only in the cell culture used to develop the vaccine. Imovax uses human diploid cell (HDC) culture, and RabAvert uses purified chick embryo cell culture.

Pharmacokinetics

An antibody response to rabies vaccine can be measured in 7 to 10 days after administration. Antibodies persist for 2 years.

Pharmacotherapeutics

Precautions and Contraindications

Previous anaphylactic reaction to any component of the vaccine, including neomycin, is a contraindication to its use. Moderate to severe illness, with or without fever, is a reason to defer the vaccine until the patient has improved. The expected immune response may not be obtained if the vaccine is used in patients on immunosuppressive therapy.

Rabies vaccine is Pregnancy Category C. Pregnancy is not a contraindication to post-exposure vaccination of pregnant women. Safety in children under age 6 has not been established.

Adverse Drug Reactions

Local reactions, including pain, erythema, and swelling of the injection site, have been reported by 30% to 70% of vaccine recipients. Systemic reactions have been reported by 5% to 40% of recipients. Systemic reactions include headache, nausea, abdominal pain, muscle aches, and dizziness. Three cases of a neurological illness resembling Guillain–Barré syndrome have been reported. A serum sickness–like reaction has been reported among about 6% of patients who received booster doses of Imovax.

Drug Interactions

Long-term therapy with chloroquine (Aralen) can interfere with the active antibody response to rabies vaccine. Patients who are taking immunosuppressants or antineoplastic agents may have a decreased immunological response to rabies vaccine.

Rabies IG (RIG) can partially suppress the antibody response to rabies vaccine. Follow the CDC recommendations for simultaneous administration exactly, and give no more than the recommended dose of RIG.

Clinical Use and Dosing

Rabies vaccine can be given for primary or pre-exposure vaccination or as part of post-exposure prophylaxis. Pre-exposure vaccination is recommended to high-risk groups, such as veterinarians, animal handlers, and certain laboratory workers. Post-exposure prophylaxis is recommended if the patient has a bite from a rabid animal that penetrates the skin. Post-exposure vaccine administration should always be accompanied by the use of RIG.

Pre-exposure vaccine dosing consists of three 1 mL IM injections of vaccine in the deltoid muscle. The doses are given on day 0, day 7, and either day 21 or day 28. A booster dose of 1 mL is given every 2 years to those considered at frequent risk if their serum antibody titer is less than 1:5. Persons considered at frequent risk include veterinarians, animal control officers, wildlife officers, and staff where rabies is enzootic. In very high-risk patients, those who work in research laboratories or vaccine production facilities, a serum rabies antibody test should be done every 6 months and vaccine administered if levels are less than 1:5.

Post-exposure prophylaxis always includes administration of both passive antibody and vaccine, with the exception of those who have previously received complete vaccination (pre-exposure or post-exposure). For post-exposure vaccination, the ACIP recommends four doses of rabies vaccine. The dose is 1 mL given IM on days 0, 3, 7, and 14, with RIG given on day 0 (Rupprecht et al, 2010). For those who have previously been vaccinated, two doses of rabies vaccine are given on days 0 and 3, with no RIG needed.

Monitoring

Patients who receive a four-dose schedule of rabies vaccine do not need post-vaccination serological testing (Rupprecht et al, 2010).

Patient Education

Patients should receive information regarding the benefits and risks of the vaccine prior to administration. Any questions or concerns regarding the vaccine should be addressed. The need for repeated doses should be discussed. The most common adverse reactions after rabies vaccination injection are pain and erythema at the injection site and systemic symptoms including headache, nausea, abdominal pain, muscle aches, and dizziness. Advise the patient to take acetaminophen for discomfort.

Table 19-6 presents issues concerning immunizations.

Table 19–6 Issues in Immunization

Childhood Immunization

Ideally, immunizations should be given as a part of comprehensive child health care. It is widely recognized that childhood immunizations are the most cost-effective way of preventing infectious diseases in children. Identified barriers to childhood immunization include the following:
1. Financial, with low socioeconomic status placing a child at risk of underimmunization
2. Family structure issues, such as single or teen parenthood
3. Perceived attitudes regarding the benefit of immunization
4. Provider policies and practices that lead to missed vaccine opportunities during clinic visits

Standards for Child and Adolescent Immunization Practices (National Vaccine Advisory Committee, 2009)

AVAILABILITY OF VACCINES
1. Vaccination services are readily available.
2. Vaccinations are coordinated with other health-care services and provided in a medical home when possible.
3. Barriers to vaccination are identified and minimized.
4. Patient costs are minimized.

ASSESSMENT OF VACCINATION STATUS
1. Health-care professionals review the vaccination and health status of patients at every encounter to determine which vaccines are indicated.
2. Health-care professionals assess for and follow only medically indicated contraindications.

EFFECTIVE COMMUNICATION ABOUT VACCINE BENEFITS AND RISKS
1. Parents/guardians and patients are educated about the benefits and risks of vaccination in a culturally appropriate manner and in easy-to-understand language.

PROPER STORAGE AND ADMINISTRATION OF VACCINES AND DOCUMENTATION OF VACCINATIONS
1. Health-care professionals follow appropriate procedures for vaccine storage and handling.
2. Up-to-date, written vaccination protocols are accessible at all locations where vaccines are administered.
3. Persons who administer vaccines and staff who manage or support vaccine administration are knowledgeable and receive ongoing education.
4. Health-care professionals simultaneously administer as many indicated vaccine doses as possible.
5. Vaccination records for patients are accurate, complete, and easily accessible.
6. Health-care professionals report adverse events following vaccination promptly and accurately to the Vaccine Adverse Events Reporting System (VAERS) and are aware of a separate program, the National Vaccine Injury Compensation Program (NVICP).
7. All personnel who have contact with patients are appropriately vaccinated.

IMPLEMENTATION OF STRATEGIES TO IMPROVE VACCINATION COVERAGE
1. Systems are used to remind parents/guardians, patients, and health-care professionals when vaccinations are due and to recall those who are overdue.
2. Office- or clinic-based patient record reviews and vaccination coverage assessments are performed annually.
3. Health-care professionals practice community-based approaches.

Continued

Table 19–6   Issues in Immunization—cont'd

Standards for Adult Immunization Practices (National Vaccine Advisory Committee, 2013)

MAKE VACCINATIONS AVAILABLE.

1. Adult vaccination services are readily available.
2. Barriers to receiving vaccines are identified and minimized.
3. Patient "out-of-pocket" vaccination costs are minimized.

ASSESS PATIENTS' VACCINATION STANDARDS.

1. Health-care professionals routinely review the vaccination status of patients.
2. Health-care professionals assess for valid contraindications.

COMMUNICATE EFFECTIVELY WITH PATIENTS.

1. Patients are educated about risks and benefits of vaccination in easy-to-understand language.

ADMINISTER AND DOCUMENT VACCINATIONS PROPERLY.

1. Written vaccination protocols are available at all locations where vaccines are administered.
2. Persons who administer vaccines are properly trained.
3. Health-care professionals recommend simultaneous administration of indicated vaccine doses.
4. Vaccination records for patients are accurate and easily accessible.
5. All personnel who have contact with patients are appropriately vaccinated.

IMPLEMENT STRATEGIES TO IMPROVE VACCINATION RATES.

1. Systems are developed and used to remind patients and health-care professionals when vaccinations are due and to recall patients who are overdue.
2. Standing orders for vaccinations are employed.
3. Regular assessments of vaccination coverage levels are conducted in a provider's practice.

PARTNER WITH THE COMMUNITY.

1. Patient-oriented and community-based approaches are used to reach the target.

Immunization in Special Populations

PREGNANT PATIENTS

The ACIP has published guidelines for vaccinating pregnant women (CDC, 2013c): "The risk from vaccination during pregnancy is largely theoretical. The benefit of vaccination among pregnant women usually outweighs the potential risk for disease when (a) the risk for disease exposure is high, (b) infections would pose a special risk for the mother or fetus, and (c) the vaccine is unlikely to cause harm."

Generally, live-virus vaccines are contraindicated in pregnant women because of the possible risk of transmission to the fetus. If a woman is inadvertently given live-virus vaccine while pregnant, she should be counseled about the potential effects on the fetus. It is not normally an indication to terminate pregnancy.

Recommendations for Vaccination During Pregnancy Include the Following:			
Vaccine	May Be Given if Indicated	Contraindicated During Pregnancy	Comments
Routine			
Hepatitis A	X		
Hepatitis B	X		The theoretical risk to the fetus is low from the inactivated vaccine.
Human papillomavirus			Not recommended during pregnancy.
Influenza (Inactivated)	X		Recommended for all women pregnant during flu season
Influenza (LAIV)		X	
MMR		X	
Meningococcal	X		Safety has not been evaluated in pregnant women.
PCV13			Inadequate data available
PPSV23	X		Inadequate data available
Polio	X		
Td	X		
Tdap	X		Pregnancy is not a contraindication for Tdap administration. ACIP recommends pregnant women receive the Tdap vaccine with every pregnancy.

Table 19–6   Issues in Immunization—cont'd

Vaccine	May Be Given if Indicated	Contraindicated During Pregnancy	Comments
Varicella		X	
Pneumococcal	X		The safety of the pneumococcal vaccine in the first trimester of pregnancy has not been determined.
Travel and Others			
Anthrax			Vaccinate only if benefits outweigh risks to fetus.
BCG		X	
Japanese encephalitis (JE)			The vaccine should not be routinely administered during pregnancy. If a pregnant woman will be moving to an area of high risk of JE, then vaccination should be considered.
Meningococcal (MPSV)	X		
Rabies	X		
Typhoid (parenteral and oral)			It is not known if the vaccine is harmful to the fetus. If necessary to vaccinate a pregnant patient, inactivated vaccine is recommended.
Vaccinia (smallpox)			Vaccinia vaccine should not be administered to pregnant women for routine nonemergency indications. Pregnant women who have had a definite exposure to smallpox virus (i.e., face-to-face, household, or close-proximity contact with a smallpox patient) and are, therefore, at high risk for contracting the disease, should be vaccinated.
Yellow fever			It is not known if the vaccine is harmful to the fetus. Only vaccinate pregnant women who are at high risk of contracting disease.
Zoster		X	

Immunocompromised Patients

For practical considerations, persons with immunocompromising conditions may be divided into three groups:

1. Persons who are severely immunocompromised not as a result of HIV infection
2. Persons with HIV infection
3. Persons with conditions that cause limited immune deficits (e.g., asplenia, renal failure) that may require use of special vaccines or higher doses of vaccines but that do not contraindicate use of any particular vaccine

   ACIP recommendation for vaccinations is based on where the patient falls within these three groups.

1. Persons who are severely immunocompromised not as a result of HIV infection: In general, these patients should not be administered live vaccines. Measles, mumps, and rubella (MMR) vaccine is not contraindicated for the close contacts. Passive immunization with immune globulin should be considered for immunocompromised persons instead of or in addition to vaccination.
2. In general, persons known to be HIV-infected should not receive live-virus or live-bacteria vaccines. MMR vaccination is recommended for all children and for adults when otherwise indicated, regardless of their HIV status. Enhanced inactivated polio vaccine (eIPV) is the preferred polio vaccine for persons known to have HIV infection. Pneumococcal vaccine is indicated for all HIV-infected persons ≥2 yr of age.
3. Persons with conditions that cause limited immune deficits (e.g., asplenia, renal failure) that may require use of special vaccines or higher doses of vaccines but that do not contraindicate use of any particular vaccine. Persons with these conditions are generally not considered immunosuppressed for the purposes of vaccination and should receive routine vaccinations with both live and inactivated vaccines according to the usual schedules.

Travel Immunization

International travel is becoming more common, with jet travel allowing people to travel great distances in a few hours. With international travel comes exposure to infectious diseases not common in the United States. Patients should be advised to begin to prepare for their trip at least 8 wk prior to departure. To determine what vaccines the traveling patient will need, the provider can consult with a local travel clinic or the CDC. The CDC Web site has a travel information section, maintained by the National Center for Infectious Disease (http://www.cdc.gov/travel/). The Web site allows the provider or patient to inquire into recommendations based on the region the patient will be traveling to. Information on traveling with children, outbreaks, and special needs travelers is also located at this site. The CDC also publishes an annual guide, *The Yellow Book: Health Information for International Travel.*

In addition to special immunizations required by travel, patients should also have all of the recommended routine immunizations for their age, including influenza vaccine. Patients should have a copy of their current immunizations included with their travel documents.

IMMUNE GLOBULIN SERUMS

IG serums provide passive immunity to infectious diseases. The choice of IG is determined by the types of products available, the type of antibody desired, route of administration, timing, and other considerations. IG products that may be used in primary care include immune globulin IM (IGIM, BayGam; GamaSTAN S/D), hepatitis B immune globulin (H-BIG, HepaGam B), tetanus immune globulin (TIG, HyperTET S/D), respiratory syncytial virus immune globulin (RSV-IGIV, RespiGam), varicella-zoster immune globulin (VZIG, VariZIG), rabies immune globulin (RIG, HyperRab S/D, Imogam), $Rh_o(D)$ immune globulin (RhoGAM, HyperRHO-S/D), and vaccinia immune globulin (VIG).

Pharmacodynamics

IGs are derived from the pooled plasma of adults, processed by cold ethanol fractionation. It consists primarily of immunoglobulin fraction (95% IgG) and is not known to transmit hepatitis, HIV, or other infectious diseases. The concentrated protein solution contains specific antibodies in proportion to the infectious and immunization experience of the donor population from which the plasma was derived. IG serums undergo processing to remove and inactivate viruses, including hepatitis A, B, and C; parvovirus B-19; and HIV. Specific IGs differ from IGIM, which is sometimes referred to as gamma globulin, in that they have high levels of a specific IG.

IGIM (BayGam; GamaSTAN S/D) is a sterile preparation of concentrated antibodies. IGIM provides protection against hepatitis A and measles through passive transfer of antibody. It may be used for pre-exposure prophylaxis or post-exposure prevention in the treatment of hepatitis A; it is used post-exposure in measles.

Hepatitis B immune globulin (HBIG, HepaGam B) is a sterile solution of IGs (10% to 18%) against HbsAg. Anti-HBsAg antibodies are collected from donors with high titers of anti-HBsAg. HBIG is used to provide passive immunity to patients following exposure to blood infected with hepatitis B, sexual and household contacts with people infected with hepatitis B virus, and infants born to HbsAg-positive mothers.

Tetanus immune globulin (TIG, HyperTET S/D) is prepared from the plasma of adults who are hyperimmunized with tetanus toxoid. TIG contains antibodies that neutralize the exotoxin produced by *C. tetani*. The passive immunity bestowed by TIG is capable of attenuating or preventing tetanus infection by binding free exotoxin.

Respiratory syncytial virus immune globulin (RSV-IGIV) is a polyclonal human hyperimmune globulin. The product is prepared by extracting IgG antibodies from the plasma of humans who have high titers of antibodies against respiratory syncytial virus (RSV). Resistance to RSV disease is via cellular and humoral immunity. RSV-IGIV does not protect the nasal mucosa from RSV and thus does not prevent acquired immunity to RSV.

Varicella-zoster immune globulin (VZIG) was approved in 2013 and is derived from human plasma and consists of IgG that contains antibodies to varicella-zoster virus. VZIG is used primarily for passive immunization of high-risk susceptible patients after exposure to chickenpox or herpes zoster. High-risk groups include pregnant women, newborns of women with varicella shortly before or after delivery, immunocompromised children and adults, neonates and infants younger than 12 months, and adults without evidence of immunity. The administration of VZIG has shown to significantly reduce the mortality in untreated patients.

Rabies immune globulin (RIG, HyperRab S/D, Imogam) is primarily gamma globulin. RIG is used to provide passive immunity to rabies in patients exposed to the virus. Rabies antibodies neutralize the rabies virus to retard its spread and to inhibit its effectiveness.

$Rh_o(D)$ immune globulin (RhoGAM, HyperRHO S/D) is used to prevent isoimmunization in $Rh_o(D)$-negative women exposed to $Rh_o(D)$-positive blood. $Rh_o(D)$ immune globulin is a solution containing IgG antibodies against erythrocyte antigen $Rh_o(D)$, collected from the plasma of human donors. It is believed that the anti-$Rh_o(D)$ antibodies in $Rh_o(D)$ immune globulin interact directly with the $Rh_o(D)$ antigens, preventing interaction between the antigens and the maternal immune system. $Rh_o(D)$ immune globulin prevents the development of erythroblastosis fetalis in current or subsequent pregnancies.

Vaccinia immune globulin intravenous (VIGIV) provides passive immunity for smallpox-associated eczema vaccinatum, severe or progressive vaccinia, and vaccinia infections in patients with skin conditions (impetigo, poison ivy, eczema, varicella zoster) that would lead to severe rash with smallpox infection.

Pharmacokinetics

IGIM, when used for pre-exposure prophylaxis for hepatitis A, confers protection for less than 3 months. It is greater than 85% effective in preventing hepatitis A if given within 2 weeks after exposure. IGIM can be given to prevent or modify measles in susceptible persons if used within 6 days of exposure.

HBIG is slowly absorbed, with antibodies appearing in 1 to 6 days and peak levels reached in 3 to 9 days. The antibodies remain in the serum for up to 2 months. HBIG probably crosses the placenta and may be distributed in breast milk.

TIG is given IM, with peak levels of IgG noted 2 days after administration. The half-life of IgG in circulation is 3.5 to 4.5 weeks.

RSV-IGIV is administered IV on a monthly basis. The serum half-life of RSV-IGIV is 22 to 28 days.

VZIG is administered IM, with peak IgG levels obtained in 2 days after administration. It is the most effective if administered within 4 days of exposure to VZV. Antibody protection lasts 3 weeks.

RIG is administered by infiltrating the wound with half of the dose and giving the other half of the dose IM in a separate limb from the injury.

$Rh_o(D)$ immune globulin pharmacokinetics is not well described. Peak antibody levels are reached in 5 to 10 days after

IM administration. Anti-Rh$_0$(D) antibodies are not detectable 6 months after administration of Rh$_0$(D) immune globulin.

VIGIV peaks in 2 hours and has a half-life of 30 days.

Pharmacotherapeutics

Precautions and Contraindications

An allergic response to IGIM or anti-IGA antibodies is a contraindication to IG serum use, as is thimerosal allergy. Patients with IgA deficiency often develop antibodies against IgA and are more likely to have anaphylactic or immune-mediated adverse reaction to pooled IG products.

RSV-IGIV is contraindicated in patients with cyanotic congenital heart disease.

Live-virus vaccines should not be administered within 3 months of an IG serum.

Pregnancy is not a contraindication to most IG serums.

VIGIV is contraindicated in patients with vaccinia keratitis. VIGIV may cause falsely high blood glucose readings on some test systems due to the maltose in the preparation. Blood glucose testing should be done with a glucose-specific method.

Adverse Drug Reactions

Local reactions include tenderness and pain in the injection site that may last for several hours. Systemic reactions include urticaria and angioedema. Less frequently reported adverse reactions include emesis, chills, fever, myalgia, lethargy, and nausea.

Drug Interactions

IG serums interfere with the immune response to live-virus vaccines. Live virus vaccines should not be administered within 3 months of an IG serum.

Clinical Use and Dosing

IG serums are used to prevent disease by either pre-exposure or post-exposure administration. The clinical use and dosing of the IG serums are detailed in Table 19-7.

Table 19–7 ⊗ Dosage Schedule: Immune Globulins

Drug	Indication	Dose	Comments
I/gamma globulin	Hepatitis A prophylaxis	Length of stay: <3 mo, give 0.02 mL/kg IM. Prolonged (>3 mo), give 0.06 mL/kg and repeat every 4 to 6 mo.	Effective if given before exposure or within 2 wk of exposure
	Measles	Give 0.25 mL/kg IM. If child is also immunocompromised, give 0.5 mL/kg IM.	Must be given within 6 d of exposure to measles
	Immunoglobulin	Deficiency 0.66 mL/kg every 3–4 wk	
Hepatitis B immune globulin (HBIG)	After exposure to blood infected with hepatitis B (HBV)	*Children ≥12 mo and adults:* Administer 0.06 mL/kg IM within 24 h; repeat in 28–30 d *Children <12 mo:* 0.5 mL × 1	Give hepatitis B vaccine within 7 d and repeat at 1 and 6 mo
	Sexual contacts of HBV-infected people	Administer 0.06 mL/kg IM within 14 d of sexual contact	Give hepatitis B vaccine within 7 d and repeat at 1 and 6 mo
	Infants born to HbsAg-positive mothers	Administer 0.5 mL IM within 12 h of birth	Give hepatitis B vaccine within 12 h of birth and repeat at 1 or 2 and at 6 mo
Tetanus immune globulin (TIG)	Passive immunization against tetanus	Clean minor wounds: No TIG necessary. Give Td/DTaP if indicated. All other wounds (may be contaminated with dirt, feces, soil, saliva, and puncture wounds): Unknown or <3 doses of DTaP/Td: Give adults 250 U TIG, children 4 U/kg of TIG, give a booster dose of TD/DTaP. History of >3 doses of tetanus toxoid: No TIG, no Td/DTaP booster.	
Respiratory syncytial virus immune globulin (RSV-IGIV)	RSV prophylaxis in high-risk children	*Children <24 mo with bronchopulmonary dysplasia or chronic lung disease:* Give 750 mg/kg IV once monthly throughout RSV season *Infants <6 mo born at 32 wk gestation or earlier or infants <12 mo of age if less than 28 wk gestation:* Give 750 mg/kg IV once monthly throughout RSV season	Medication should be infused at a rate of 1.5 mL/kg/h for the first 15 min, then increase to 3 mL/kg/h for 15 min; maximum rate of 6 mL/kg/h

Continued

Table 19–7 ⊗ **Dosage Schedule: Immune Globulins—cont'd**

Drug	Indication	Dose	Comments
Varicella-zoster immune globulin (VZIG)	Passive immunization for high-risk patients exposed to varicella	Administer VZIG within 96 h of exposure *Adults and adolescents:* 125 U/10 kg, up to 625 U maximum	VZIG administration is recommended in the following groups: Immunocompromised patients (patients with HIV, cancer, or receiving immunosuppressive therapy), neonates of women who have symptoms of varicella at delivery, premature neonates exposed postnatally, pregnant women
		Children and infants: 125 U/10 kg, rounded to nearest 125 U >40 kg: 625 U IM 30.1–40 kg: 500 U 20.1–30 kg: 375 U 10.1–20 kg: 250 U <10 kg: 125 U	Patients should meet the additional requirements: 1. Not immune to varicella 2. Significant exposure <96 h prior to VZIG administration; significant exposure defined as household contact, playmate contact (>1 h contact), hospital contact (in same room)
Rabies immune globulin (RIG)	Provides passive immunity to rabies	Previously unvaccinated against rabies: Administer 20 IU/kg up to 7 d after the first dose of rabies vaccine	Post-exposure prophylaxis always includes administration of both passive antibody and vaccine, with the exception of those who have previously received complete vaccination. For post-exposure vaccination, the ACIP recommends that 4 doses of rabies vaccine be given, with RIG given at the same time as the first vaccine dose
Rh$_o$ (D) immune globulin (RhoGAM)	Rh isoimmunization prophylaxis	Administer 300 mcg IM at 28 wk gestation and/or within 72 h of an Rh-incompatible delivery, miscarriage, abortion, or transfusion accident Administer 50 mcg IM if pregnancy terminated prior to 13 wk gestation	Each vial or syringe (~300 mcg) prevents sensitization to a volume of up to 15 mL of Rh-positive red blood cells

Monitoring

Laboratory monitoring is not necessary. The patient's Rh status should be determined prior to administering Rh$_o$(D) immune globulin.

Patient Education

Patients should receive information regarding the benefits and risks of the IG prior to administration. Any questions or concerns regarding the vaccine should be addressed. The most common adverse reactions after IG administration are pain and erythema at the injection site.

DIAGNOSTIC BIOLOGICALS

TUBERCULIN PURIFIED PROTEIN DERIVATIVE

The diagnostic biological agent that is commonly used in primary care is tuberculin PPD. PPD is used to screen asymptomatic individuals for infection with *M. tuberculosis.*

Pharmacodynamics

PPD is administered intradermally to asymptomatic individuals. Once a person has become sensitized to mycobacterial antigens, a hypersensitivity reaction occurs to the administration of the intradermal PPD. In sensitive people, the reaction includes induration and erythema at the site of administration. A positive reaction to PPD indicates that the person at some time has had a TB infection. A positive test does not indicate an active infection but rather that further testing is indicated. See Chapter 45 for more information regarding TB evaluation.

Pharmacotherapeutics

Precautions and Contraindications

Do not administer PPD to known tuberculin-positive reactors because they may have a severe reaction, including ulceration and necrosis at the site of administration. SC administration should be avoided, as a general febrile reaction or acute inflammation may occur.

Skin testing of immunodeficient people may not be accurate because skin-test responsiveness may be suppressed. Skin test responsiveness may be delayed in the older adult patient.

PPD testing is safe in pregnancy, during lactation, and in children of all ages, including infants.

Adverse Drug Reactions

In highly sensitive people, vesiculation, ulceration, and necrosis can occur at the administration site. A normal adverse reaction is a minimal amount of bleeding at the administration site.

Drug Interactions

Live-virus vaccines (MMR, varicella) can suppress the reaction to PPD if given within 4 to 6 weeks prior to the PPD. PPD can be administered at the time that MMR and varicella vaccines are administered. Patients who have been vaccinated with BCG generally are sensitive to PPD. Immunosuppressant medications can suppress the reaction to PPD testing.

Clinical Use and Dosing

The Mantoux PPD test containing 5 tuberculin units (TU) is the preferred test because the interpretation of the reaction has been standardized. Previously, multiple puncture tests were used, and there were many problems with interpretation. The test consists of injecting 5 TU of PPD intradermally. A small white bleb should appear at the injection site if it is done correctly. Reactions are read in 48 to 72 hours after administration. For patients who may be highly sensitized, a test dose of 1 TU is used.

Determining the results of the skin test is based on the likelihood of infection and the risk of active TB if infection has occurred. If the patient is HIV-positive or has fibrotic lesions on chest x-ray, a reaction of 5 mm or more induration is considered positive. A reaction of 10 mm or more induration is considered positive in other at-risk patients, including infants and children. In patients who are not in any high-risk category or high-risk environment, a result of 15 mm or more induration is considered positive.

Patients are considered high risk if they have any of the following: (1) diabetes mellitus; (2) prolonged therapy with adrenocorticosteroids; (3) immunosuppressive therapy; (4) hematological and/or reticuloendothelial diseases, such as leukemia or Hodgkin's disease; (5) injection drug users known to be HIV-seronegative; (6) end-stage renal disease; or (6) any clinical presentation that includes substantial rapid weight loss or chronic malnutrition.

People who are in a high-incidence group with a skin test reaction of 10 mm or more induration are candidates for preventive therapy, even if they do not have any of the risk factors. High-incidence groups include the following: (1) foreign-born persons from high-prevalence countries, (2) medically underserved low-income populations, and (3) residents of facilities for long-term care.

Monitoring

The PPD should be read by an experienced health-care professional who has been trained in the proper method of interpreting the results.

Patient Education

Patients must have an understanding of the reason for PPD testing and why the test must be read in 48 to 72 hours. Adverse reactions are rare in patients who are not already sensitized to TB.

IMMUNOMODULATORS

Although not generally prescribed by primary care providers, two immunomodulator medications commonly prescribed to patients by specialty providers are covered in this chapter—cyclosporine and azathioprine. Cyclosporine (Sandimmune) is prescribed to organ transplant patients and is used for severe rheumatoid arthritis. Azathioprine (Imuran) is also prescribed for transplant patients and patients with severe rheumatoid arthritis. The topical immunomodulators pimecrolimus (Elidel) and tacrolimus (Protopic) are discussed in the chapter on integumentary medications (Chap. 23).

Pharmacodynamics

Cyclosporine is an oral and parenteral immunosuppressive agent. It is believed to act by inhibiting the production or release of various lymphokines. The actions of the T-helper cell, the mediators of cellular immunity and tissue rejection, are impaired. Cyclosporine may inhibit T-suppressor cells. Cyclosporine also inhibits the synthesis of gamma-interferon. Cyclosporine does not cause myelosuppression.

Azathioprine is an oral and parenteral immunosuppressive that decreases the metabolism of purines and may inhibit DNA and RNA synthesis. It may interfere with coenzyme functioning, decreasing cellular metabolism. Azathioprine has the ability to inhibit the delayed hypersensitivity reaction and cellular cytotoxic activity that occur during renal transplantation.

Pharmacokinetics
Absorption and Distribution

After oral administration, approximately 20% to 50% of cyclosporine is absorbed. Absorption from the GI tract is highly variable. It is widely distributed throughout the body, crosses the placenta, and is excreted in breast milk. Azathioprine is well absorbed following oral administration. It is widely distributed and crosses the placenta.

Metabolism and Excretion

Cyclosporine undergoes extensive first-pass metabolism. It is metabolized extensively by the liver cytochrome P450 3A (CYP450 3A) enzyme system. Elimination of cyclosporine and its metabolites is primarily through the bile and feces, with only 6% excreted renally. Azathioprine is metabolized in the liver to its active metabolite, mercaptopurine. The metabolites and some unchanged azathioprine are excreted in the urine.

Pharmacotherapeutics

Precautions and Contraindications

Hypersensitivity to the medication or components of the product is a contraindication to its use. Cyclosporine has a Black-Box Warning regarding anaphylaxis with IV administration. Oral cyclosporine preparations contain corn, castor oil, and/or olive oil, and patients with hypersensitivity to these food products should avoid its use. Patients with renal dysfunction should be monitored for worsening renal function while taking cyclosporine. Azathioprine can accumulate in patients with renal impairment, possibly causing toxicity. Hepatic dysfunction can affect the metabolism of both drugs.

Both cyclosporine and azathioprine are contraindicated in pregnancy and breastfeeding.

Cyclosporine has a Black-Box Warning regarding increased susceptibility for severe, even fatal infections. Azathioprine has a Black-Box Warning regarding increased risk of developing neoplasms.

Adverse Drug Reactions

Nephrotoxicity is the most common adverse effect of cyclosporine therapy. Cyclosporine may also cause hypertension; headaches; GI upset; hirsutism (50% of patients); gingival hyperplasia (4% to 16%); hypercholesterolemia; and neurological effects such as seizures, tremor, paresthesias, and mood changes.

Hepatic failure can occur with azathioprine use. Nausea and vomiting occurred in 12% of patients. Patients taking azathioprine should be monitored for bone marrow suppression. Other adverse effects reported are fever, rash, pancreatitis, alopecia, and retinopathy.

Drug Interactions

Cyclosporine interacts with many drugs, especially those metabolized by the hepatic enzymes. Azathioprine suppresses the immune system; therefore, live or inactivated vaccines should not be given to patients receiving this drug. OPV should not be administered to household contacts of patients taking azathioprine. It may take the immune system 3 to 12 months to return to normal after administration of azathioprine. Other drug interactions are shown in Table 19-8.

Clinical Use and Dosing

Cyclosporine and azathioprine are usually prescribed by specialty providers. If in consultation with a specialist, the primary care provider is prescribing these products for

Table 19–8 ⠿ Drug Interactions: Immunomodulators

Drug	Interacting Drug	Possible Effect	Implications
Azathioprine	Live vaccines (MMR, varicella)	Decreased antibody response to vaccine	Wait 3 mo to 1 yr after stopping azathioprine before administering live vaccines
	Allopurinol	Increased pharmacological and toxic effects of azathioprine	Avoid concurrent use, or reduce dose of azathioprine by one-third to one-half
	Angiotensin-converting enzyme (ACE) inhibitors	May induce severe leukopenia or anemia	
	Methotrexate	May increase plasma levels of azathioprine metabolite 6-MP	Avoid concurrent use
	Anticoagulants	Decreased effectiveness of anticoagulants	Avoid concurrent use
	Alkylating agents/antineoplastic agents	Prior treatment with alkylating agents puts patient at higher risk of developing neoplasms or infection	
	Cyclosporine	Cyclosporine plasma levels might be decreased	
Cyclosporine	*Nephrotoxic drugs:* amphotericin B, acyclovir, aminoglycosides, foscarnet, NSAIDs, vancomycin, ganciclovir	Additive nephrotoxicity	
	Immunosuppressants	Increased risk of lymphoma and infection	
	Potassium-sparing diuretics: amiloride, spironolactone, triamterene	Hyperkalemia	Monitor potassium levels
	Drug metabolized by CYP450 3A isoenzyme inhibitors: calcium channel blockers, androgens, clarithromycin, azole antifungals, methylprednisolone,	Increased cyclosporine levels, leading to cyclosporine toxicity	Monitor cyclosporine levels

Table 19–8 ▓ Drug Interactions: Immunomodulators—cont'd

Drug	Interacting Drug	Possible Effect	Implications
	allopurinol, bromocriptine, danazol, erythromycin, dalfopristin, metoclopramide		
	Drugs metabolized by CYP450 3A isoenzyme inducers: nafcillin, modanil, troglitazone, rifampin, carbamazepine, pentobarbital, phenytoin, octreotide, ticlopidine, primidone	Decreased cyclosporine levels	Monitor cyclosporine levels if any of these drugs are added or deleted from medication regimen
	Vaccines	Decreased effectiveness of vaccines	Wait at least 3 mo after therapy with cyclosporine is completed to administer live vaccines
	Digoxin	Increased digoxin levels	Monitor digoxin levels
	Prednisolone	Increased prednisolone levels	
	Lovastatin	Increased lovastatin levels	
	Grapefruit juice	Increased cyclosporine levels	
	Protease inhibitors	Cyclosporine toxicity	
	SMX/TMP	Decreased blood levels of cyclosporine	
	Clonidine	Interferes with clonidine pharmacokinetics	
	Metoclopramide (oral)	Increases oral bioavailability of cyclosporine by 30%	Monitor cyclosporine concentrations
	Colchicine	Nephrotoxicity and azotemia	Avoid concurrent use
	Orlistat	Altered bioavailability of cyclosporine	Monitor if using concurrently

rheumatoid arthritis, the dosing is as follows: Cyclosporine is started at 1.25 mg/kg twice daily and may increase by 0.5 to 0.75 mg/kg/day at 8 weeks and at 12 weeks, if indicated. The maximum dose is 4 mg/kg/day. Decrease the dose by 25% to 50% if adverse effects occur. Azathioprine is begun at 1 mg/kg/day in one to two divided doses. The dose can be increased in 6 to 8 weeks, by 0.5 mg/kg/day. The dose can be increased every 4 weeks to a maximum of 2.5 mg/kg/day.

Monitoring

Patients prescribed these medications need monitoring of their blood pressure, renal function, and hepatic function. Patients taking cyclosporine also need to have serum cyclosporine levels checked periodically. Patients taking azathioprine need a complete blood count (CBC) and serum amylase drawn periodically.

Patient Education

Patients should be instructed to take the medication exactly as prescribed. Any symptoms of adverse reactions should be reported to the provider immediately. The patient should be cautioned to report any flu-like symptoms, which may be a sign of hepatic or renal dysfunction.

REFERENCES

American Academy of Pediatrics. (2012a). Immunocompromised children. In L. K. Pickering (Ed.), *Red book: 2012 Report of the Committee on Infectious Diseases* (29th ed., p 74). Elk Grove Village, IL: American Academy of Pediatrics. Retrieved from http://aapredbook.aappublications.org/content/1/SEC8/SEC56/SEC59.body

American Academy of Pediatrics. Measles. (2012b) In L. K. Pickering (Ed.), *Red book: 2012 Report of the Committee on Infectious Diseases* (29th ed., pp 514–518). Elk Grove Village, IL: American Academy of Pediatrics. Retrieved from http://aapredbook.aappublications.org/content/1/SEC131/SEC222.body

American College Health Association (ACHA). (2000). *Recommendations for institutional prematriculation guidelines.* Baltimore: ACHA. Retrieved from http://www.acha.org

Andre, F. E., Booy, R., Bock, H. L., Clemens, J., Datta, S. K., John, T. J., et al. (2008). Vaccination greatly reduces disease, disability, death and inequity worldwide. *Bulletin of the World Health Organization, 86*(2), 81––160. Retrieved from http://www.who.int/bulletin/volumes/86/2/07-040089/en/.

Brady, M. T. (2011). Changes in MCV4 use include booster dose for adolescents. *AAP News, 32*(1), 1.

Centers for Disease Control and Prevention (CDC). (1996a). The role of BCG vaccine in the prevention and control of tuberculosis in the United States: A joint statement by the advisory council of the elimination of tuberculosis and the ACIP. *Morbidity and Mortality Weekly Report, 45*(RR-4), 1–18.

Centers for Disease Control and Prevention (CDC). (1997b). Pertussis vaccination: Use of acellular pertussis vaccines among infants and young children:

Recommendations of the ACIP. *Morbidity and Mortality Weekly Report, 46*(RR-7), 1–25.

Centers for Disease Control and Prevention (CDC). (1997c). Poliomyelitis prevention in the United States: Introduction of a sequential vaccination schedule of inactivated poliovirus vaccine followed by oral poliovirus vaccine: Recommendations of the ACIP. *Morbidity and Mortality Weekly Report, 46*(RR-3), 1–25.

Centers for Disease Control and Prevention (CDC). (1999). Human rabies prevention—United States, 1999: Recommendations of the ACIP. *Morbidity and Mortality Weekly Report, 48*(RR-1), 1–33.

Centers for Disease Control and Prevention (CDC). (2002). Yellow fever vaccine: Recommendations of the Advisory Committee on Immunization Practices (ACIP). *Morbidity and Mortality Weekly Report, 51*(RR-17), 1–11.

Centers for Disease Control and Prevention (CDC). (2005a). A comprehensive immunization strategy to eliminate transmission of hepatitis B virus infection in the United States. *Morbidity and Mortality Weekly Report, 54*(RR-16), 1–23.

Centers for Disease Control and Prevention (CDC). (2006a). CDC Health Advisory: Multi-state mumps outbreak. *Centers for Disease Control Health Alert Network.* Retrieved April 15, 2006, from http://www.phppo.cdc.gov/HAN/ArchiveSys/ViewMsgV.asp?AlertNum=00243

Centers for Disease Control and Prevention (CDC). (2006b). Preventing tetanus, diphtheria, and pertussis among adolescents: Use of tetanus toxoid, reduced diphtheria toxoid and acellular pertussis vaccines: Recommendations of the Advisory Committee on Immunization Practices (ACIP). *Morbidity and Mortality Weekly Report, 55*(RR-3), 1–43.

Centers for Disease Control and Prevention (CDC). (2006c). Preventing tetanus, diphtheria, and pertussis among adults: Use of tetanus toxoid, reduced diphtheria toxoid and acellular pertussis vaccines: Recommendations of the Advisory Committee on Immunization Practices (ACIP). *Morbidity and Mortality Weekly Report, 55*(RR17), 1–33.

Centers for Disease Control and Prevention (CDC). (2006d). Prevention of hepatitis A through active or passive immunization: Recommendations of the Advisory Committee on Immunization Practices (ACIP). *Morbidity and Mortality Weekly Report, 55*(RR07), 1–23.

Centers for Disease Control and Prevention (CDC). (2007). Prevention of varicella: Recommendations of the Advisory Committee on Immunization Practices. *Morbidity and Mortality Weekly Report, 56*(RR4), 1–40.

Centers for Disease Control and Prevention (CDC). (2008). Prevention of herpes zoster: Recommendations of the Advisory Committee on Immunization Practices. *Morbidity and Mortality Weekly Report, 57*(RR-5), 1–30.

Centers for Disease Control and Prevention (CDC). (2009a). Updated recommendations of the Advisory Committee on Immunization Practices (ACIP) regarding routine poliovirus vaccination. *Morbidity and Mortality Weekly Report, 58*(30), 829–830.

Centers for Disease Control and Prevention (CDC). (2009b). Updated recommendations from the Advisory Committee on Immunization Practices (ACIP) for use of hepatitis A vaccine in close contacts of newly arriving international adoptees. *Morbidity and Mortality Weekly Report, 58*(36), 1006–1007.

Centers for Disease Control and Prevention (CDC). (2010a). FDA licensure of bivalent human papillomavirus vaccine (HPV2, Cervarix) for use in females: Updated HPV vaccination recommendations from the Advisory Committee on Immunization Practices (ACIP). *Morbidity and Mortality Weekly Report, 59*(20), 626–629.

Centers for Disease Control and Prevention (CDC). (2010b). FDA licensure of quadrivalent human papillomavirus vaccine (HPV4, Gardasil) for use in males and guidance from the Advisory Committee on Immunization Practices (ACIP). *Morbidity and Mortality Weekly Report, 59*(20), 630–632.

Centers for Disease Control and Prevention (CDC). (2010c). Invasive pneumococcal disease in young children before licensure of 13-valent pneumococcal conjugate vaccine—United States, 2007. *Morbidity and Mortality Weekly Report, 59*(09), 253–257.

Centers for Disease Control and Prevention (CDC). (2010d). Japanese encephalitis vaccines: Recommendations of the Advisory Committee on Immunization Practices (ACIP). *Morbidity and Mortality Weekly Report, 59*(RR-1), 1–27.

Centers for Disease Control and Prevention (CDC). (2010e). Licensure of a 13-valent pneumococcal conjugate vaccine (PCV13) and recommendations for use among children—Advisory Committee on Immunization Practices (ACIP). *Morbidity and Mortality Weekly Report, 59*(09), 258–261.

Centers for Disease Control and Prevention (CDC). (2011a). Addition of history of intussusception as a contraindication for rotavirus vaccination. *Morbidity and Mortality Weekly Report, 60*(41), 1427.

Centers for Disease Control and Prevention (CDC). (2011b). Update on herpes zoster vaccine: Licensure for persons aged 50 through 59 years. *Morbidity and Mortality Weekly Report, 60*(44), 1528.

Centers for Disease Control and Prevention (CDC). (2011c). Use of hepatitis B vaccination for adults with diabetes mellitus: Recommendations of the Advisory Committee on Immunizations Practices (ACIP). *Morbidity and Mortality Weekly Report, 60*(50), 1709–1711.

Centers for Disease Control and Prevention (2012a). Tuberculosis: Vaccines and immunizations. Retrieved from www.cdc.gov/tb/topic/vaccines/default.htm

Centers for Disease Control and Prevention (2013a). Prevention of measles, rubella, congenital rubella syndrome, and mumps, 2013: Summary recommendations of the Advisory Committee on Immunization Practices (ACIP). *Morbidity and Mortality Weekly Report, 62*(4), 1–34.

Centers for Disease Control and Prevention (2013b). Updated recommendation for use of tetanus toxoid, reduced diptherial toxoid, and acellular pertussis vaccine (Tdap) in pregnant women—Advisory Committee on Immunizations Practices (ACIP), 2012. *Morbidity and Mortality Weekly Report, 62*(07), 131–135.

Centers for Disease Control and Prevention. (2013c). Guidelines for vaccinating pregnant women. Retrieved from http://www.cdc.gov/vaccines/pubs/downloads/b_preg_guide.pdf

Centers for Disease Control and Prevention. (2013d). Use of Japanese encephalitis vaccine in children: Recommendations of the Advisory Committee on Immunization Practice. *Morbidity and Mortality Weekly Report, 62*(45), 898–890. Retrieved from www.cdc.gov/mmwr/preview/mmwrhtml/mm6245a3.htm

Centers for Disease Control (2015). Serotype B meningococcal vaccine and outbreaks. Retrieved from http://www.cdc.gov/meningococcal/outbreaks/vaccine-serogroupb.html

Cohn, A. C., MacNeil, J. R., Clark, T. A., Ortega-Sanchez, I. R., Briere, E. Z., Meissner, H. C., et al. (2013). Prevention and control of meningococcal disease: Recommendations of the Advisory Committee on Immunization Practices (ACIP). *Morbidity and Mortality Weekly Report, 62*(RR02), 1–22.

Cortese, M. M., & Parashar, U. D. (2009). Prevention of rotavirus gastroenteritis among infants and children: Recommendations of the Advisory Committee on Immunization Practices (ACIP). *MMWR Recommendations and Reports, 58*(RR02), 1–25.

Fiebelkorn, A. P., Lawler, J., Curns, A, T., Brandeburg, C., & Wallace, G. S. (2013). Mumps postexposure prophylaxis with a third dose of measles-mumps-rubella vaccine, Orange County, New York, USA. *Emerging Infectious Diseases, 19*(9), 1411–1417.

Fiore, A. E., Shay, D. K., Broder, K., Isakander, J. K., Uyeki, T. M., Mootrey, G., et al. (2009). Prevention and control of seasonal influenza with vaccines: Recommendations of the Advisory Committee on Immunization Practices (ACIP). *Morbidity and Mortality Weekly Report, 58*(RR08), 1–52.

Food and Drug Administration (FDA). (2012). Update: Information on Rotarix—Labeling revision pertaining to intussusception. Retrieved from http://www.fda.gov/BiologicsBloodVaccines/Vaccines/ApprovedProducts/ucm226690.htm

Franco, E. L., & Harper, D. M. (2005). Vaccination against human papillomavirus infection: A new paradigm in cervical cancer control. *Vaccine, 23,* 2388–2394.

Gershman, M. D., & Staples, J. E. (2014). Yellow fever. In Centers for Disease Control and Prevention. *CDC health information for international travel.* New York: Oxford University Press. Retrieved from http://wwwnc.cdc.gov/travel/yellowbook/2014/chapter-3-infectious-diseases-related-to-travel/yellow-fever

Grohskopf, L. A., Shay, D. K., Shimabukuro, T. T., Sokolow, L. Z., Keitel, W. A., Bresee, J. S., et al. (2013). Prevention and control of seasonal influenza with vaccines: Recommendations of the Advisory Committee on Immunization Practices—United States, 2013–2014. *Morbidity and Mortality Weekly Report, 62*(RR07), 1–43.

Hills, S. L., Weber, I. B., & Fischer, M. (2013). Japanese encephalitis. *CDC health information for international travel*. Retrieved from http://wwwnc.cdc.gov/travel/yellowbook/2014/chapter-3-infectious-diseases-related-to-travel/japanese-encephalitis

Hinman, A. R, Orenstein, W, A., & Schuchat, A. (2011). Vaccine-preventable diseases, immunizations, and the epidemic intelligence service. *American Journal of Epidemiology, 174*(11), S16–S22.

Immunization Action Coalition. (2010). Vaccines work! CDC statistics demonstrate dramatic declines in vaccine-preventable diseases when compared with pre-vaccine era. Immunization Action Coalition. Retrieved from http://www.immunize.org/catg.d/p4037.pdf

Koutsky, L. A., Ault, K. A., Wheeler, C. M., Brown, D. R., Barr, E., Alvarez, F. B., et al. (2002). A controlled trial of a human papillomavirus type 16 vaccine. *New England Journal of Medicine, 347*(21), 1645–1651.

Markowitz, L. E., Dunne, E. F., Saraiya, M., Chesson, H. W., Curtis, C. R., Gee, J., et al. (2014). Human papillomavirus vaccination: Recommendations of the Advisory Committee on Immunization Practices (ACIP). *Morbidity and Mortality Weekly Report, 63*(RR05), 1–30.

Marin, M., Broder, K. R., Ternte, J. L., Snider, D. E., & Seward, J. F. (2010). Use of combination measles, mumps, rubella, and varicella vaccine: Recommendations of the Advisory Committee on Immunization Practices (ACIP). *Morbidity and Mortality Weekly Report, 59*(RR-3), 1–11.

MedImmune (2013). FluMist Quadrivalent (Influenza Vaccine Live, Intranasal) Prescribing information. Retrieved from www.medimmune.com/docs/default-source/default-document-library/product-and-patient-information-for-flumist-quadrivalent.pdf?sfvrsn=0

Merck & Co. (2010). M-M-R II (Measles, mumps and rubella virus vaccine live). Whitehouse Station, NJ: Merck. Retrieved from http://www.merck.com/product/usa/pi_circulars/m/mmr_ii/mmr_ii_pi.pdf

Newton, A, E., & Mintz, E. (2014). Typhoid & paratyphoid fever. In Centers for Disease Control and Prevention. *CDC health information for international travel*. New York: Oxford University Press. Retrieved from http://wwwnc.cdc.gov/travel/yellowbook/2014/chapter-3-infectious-diseases-related-to-travel/typhoid-and-paratyphoid-fever

Pagliusi, S. R., & Aguado, M. T. (2004). Efficacy and other milestones for human papillomavirus vaccine introduction. *Vaccine, 23*, 569–578.

Reisinger, K. S., Brown, M. L., Xu, J., Sullivan, B. J., Marshall, G. S., Nauert, B., et al. (2006). A combination measles, mumps, rubella, and varicella vaccine (ProQuad) given to 4- to 6-year-old healthy children vaccinated previously with M-M-RII and Varivax. *Pediatrics, 117*(2), 265–272.

Roush, S. W., Murphy, T. V., & the Vaccine-Preventable Disease Table Working Group. (2007). Historical comparisons of morbidity and mortality for vaccine-preventable diseases in the United States. *Journal of the American Medical Association, 298*(18), 2155–2163.

Rupprecht, C. E., Briggs, D., Brown, C. M., Franka, R., Katz, S. L., Kerr, H. D., et al. (2010). Use of a reduced (4-dose) vaccine schedule for postexposure prophylaxis to prevent human rabies. *Morbidity and Mortality Weekly Report, 59*(RR-02), 1–9.

Shefer, A., Atkinson, W., Friedman, C., Kuhar, D. T., Mootrey, G., Bialek, S. R., et al. (2011). Immunization of health-care personnel: Recommendations of the Advisory Committee on Immunization Practices (ACIP). *Morbidity and Mortality Weekly Report, 60*(RR07), 1–45.

Shinefield, H., Black, S., Digilio, L., Reisinger, K., Blatter, M., Gress, J. O., et al. (2005). Evaluation of a quadrivalent measles, mumps, rubella and varicella vaccine in healthy children. *Pediatric Infectious Disease Journal, 24*(8), 665–669.

Staples, J. E., Gershman, M., & Fischer, M. (2010). Yellow fever vaccine: Recommendations of the Advisory Committee on Immunization Practices (ACIP). *Morbidity and Mortality Weekly Report, 59*(RR07), 1–27.

Tartof, S. Y., Lewis, M., Kenyon, C., White, K., Osborn, A., Liko, J., et al. (2013). Waning immunity to pertussis following 5 doses of DTaP. *Pediatrics, 131*(4), e1047–e1052.

Thompson, M. G., Shay, D. K., Zhou, H., Bridges, C. B., Cheng, P. Y., Burns, E., et al. (2010). Estimates of deaths associated with seasonal influenza—United States, 1976–2007. *Morbidity and Mortality Weekly Report, 59*(33), 1057–1062.

Tyring, S. K., Diaz-Mitoma, F., Padget, L. G., Nunez, M., Poland, G., Cassidy, W. M., et al. (2007). Safety and tolerability of a high-potency zoster vaccine in adults >/= 50 years of age. *Vaccine, 25*(10), 1877–1883.

van Panhuis, W. G., Grefenstette, J., Jung. S. Y., Chok, N. S., Cross, A., Eng, H., et al. (2013). Contagious diseases in the United States from 1888 to the present. *New England Journal of Medicine, 369*, 2152–2158.

Vesikari, T., Karvonen, A., Korhonen, T., Edelman, K., Vainionpaa, R., & Salmi, A. (2006). A randomized, double-blind study of the safety, transmissibility and phenotypic and genotypic stability of cold-adapted influenza virus vaccine. *Pediatric Infectious Diseases Journal, 25*(7), 590–595.

Vilajeliu, A., Gonce, A., Lopez, M., Costa, J., Rocamora, L., Rios, J. et al. (2015). Combined tetanus-diptheria and pertussis vaccine during pregnancy: Transfer of maternal pertussis antibodies to the newborn. *Vaccine, 33*(8), 1056–1062.

World Health Organization (WHO). (2005). Viral cancers. *In state of the art of vaccine research and development*. (Publication No. WHO/IVB/05). Geneva, Switzerland: World Health Organization.

World Health Organization (WHO). (2010). Use of BCG vaccine in HIV-infected infants. *WHO Weekly Epidemiological Record, 85*(5), 32–33. Retrieved from www.who.int/wer/2010/wer8505.pdf

World Health Organization (WHO). (2011). Human papillomavirus infection and cervical cancer. Retrieved from www.who.int/vaccine_research/diseases/hpv/en/

Wressnigg, N., Pollabauer, E. M., Aichinger, G., Portsmouth, D., Low-Baselli, A., Fritsch, S., et al. (2013). Safety and immunogenicity of a novel multivalent OspA vaccine against Lyme borreliosis in healthy adults: A double-blind, randomized, dose-escalation phase 1/2 trial. *The Lancet Infectious Diseases, 13*(8), 680–689.

CHAPTER 20

DRUGS AFFECTING THE GASTROINTESTINAL SYSTEM

Teri Moser Woo

There is a wide variety of drugs used to treat disorders affecting the gastrointestinal (GI) tract. Cholinergic drugs increase gastric acid secretion and increase peristalsis; anticholinergic drugs inhibit gastric acid secretion and decrease peristalsis. These drugs are discussed in Chapter 15. Phenothiazines have antiemetic properties; some narcotic analgesics or their derivatives are used to treat diarrhea and are discussed in Chapter 16. Several groups of drugs are used almost exclusively to treat GI disorders, such as antacids, antidiarrheals, antiemetics, laxatives, and drugs used to decrease gastric acid production. These drugs are discussed in this chapter. IV forms of GI drugs not used in primary care are not discussed in this chapter.

ANTACIDS

Antacids are weak bases that react with hydrochloric acid (HCl) to form a salt and water. They are used to reduce gastric acidity in the treatment of gastroesophageal reflux and peptic ulcer disease. Antacids contain various combinations of metallic cation (aluminum, calcium, magnesium, and sodium) and basic anion (hydroxide, bicarbonate, carbonate, citrate, and trisilicate). Most in current use have as their cation aluminum, calcium, or magnesium, and their anion is usually hydroxide (OH), bicarbonate (HCO_3), or carbonate (CO_3). The buffering capacity of the other two anions is too limited to be clinically effective.

Pharmacodynamics

Antacids neutralize gastric acidity, which causes an increase in the pH of the stomach and duodenal bulb. They also inhibit the proteolytic activity of pepsin and increase lower esophageal sphincter tone. Aluminum-based products inhibit smooth muscle contraction and thus slow gastric emptying. Calcium-based antacids are also used to treat calcium-deficiency states, such as those that occur postmenopause and in chronic renal failure. They are also used to bind phosphates in chronic renal failure, as are aluminum-based antacids. Magnesium-based antacids are used to treat magnesium deficiencies from malnutrition, alcoholism, or magnesium-depleting drugs. The use of drugs as nutrient therapy is discussed in Chapter 9.

Acid-neutralizing capacity (ANC) varies between products and is expressed in milliequivalents (mEq) of HCl required to keep an antacid suspension at pH 3.5 for 10 minutes in vitro. Antacids must neutralize at least 5 mEq per dose. Those with higher ANC values are more likely to be effective in vivo. Sodium bicarbonate and calcium carbonate have the highest ANC but are not used for chronic therapy because of their systemic effects. Suspensions have greater ANC than do powders or tablets.

Pharmacokinetics

Absorption and Distribution

Aluminum- and magnesium-based antacids are not absorbable with routine use. With chronic use, 5% to 20% of magnesium and smaller amounts of aluminum may be absorbed. These small absorbed amounts are widely distributed, cross the placenta, and appear in breast milk. Aluminum concentrates in the central nervous system. Calcium-based antacids require vitamin D for absorption from the GI tract. The small amount that is absorbed enters the extracellular fluid, crosses the placenta, and enters breast milk.

If ingested in a fasting state, antacids reduce acidity for approximately 20 to 40 minutes. If taken 1 hour after a meal,

acidity is reduced for 2 to 3 hours. A second dose given 3 hours after a meal maintains the reduced acidity for more than 4 hours after the meal.

Metabolism and Excretion

The action of antacids occurs locally in the GI tract with minimal absorption, and so there is minimal metabolism. Magnesium-based antacids are excreted in the urine. Aluminum-based antacids bind with phosphate ions in the intestine to form insoluble aluminum phosphate, which is excreted in the feces. Calcium-based antacids are excreted mainly in feces, with 20% eliminated in urine. Table 20-1 shows the pharmacokinetic properties of selected antacids.

Pharmacotherapeutics

Precautions and Contraindications

All antacids are contraindicated in the presence of severe abdominal pain of unknown cause, especially if accompanied by fever. Calcium-based antacids are contraindicated in the presence of hypercalcemia and renal calculi.

Renal impairment presents several issues for patients who take antacids. Magnesium-based antacids are contraindicated in patients with renal failure and used with caution for patients with any degree of renal insufficiency because the malfunctioning kidney is unable to excrete magnesium and hypermagnesemia may result. Prolonged use of aluminum-based antacids for patients with renal failure may result in or worsen dialysis osteomalacia. Aluminum is not easily removed by dialysis because it is bound to albumin and transferrin, which do not cross the dialysis membrane. As a result, aluminum is deposited in bone and osteomalacia occurs. Elevated tissue aluminum levels also contribute to the development of dialysis encephalopathy.

Many antacids have high sodium content. Patients with hypertension (HTN), congestive heart failure (CHF), marked renal failure, or on low-sodium diets should use a low-sodium preparation.

Table 20–1 ⋮⋮ Pharmacokinetics: Selected Antacids

Drug	Onset	Peak	Duration	Acid-Neutralizing Capacity (ANC)	Half-Life	Elimination
Aluminum hydroxide	Slightly delayed	30 min	30 min–1 h on empty stomach; 3 h after meals	3.2 (AlternaGEL) 2.0 (Amphojel) 10.6	Unknown	As aluminum phosphate in feces
Magnesium hydroxide	Immediate	30 min	30 min–1 h on empty stomach; 3 h after meals	11.4	Unknown	In urine
Aluminum hydroxide-magnesium hydroxide combinations	Immediate	30 min	30 min–1 h on empty stomach; 3 h after meals	2.7 (Maalox) 5.7 (Maalox HRF) 5.1 (Mylanta)	Unknown	In urine and feces
Calcium carbonate	Slightly delayed	30 min	30 min–1 h on empty stomach; 3 h after meals	10	Unknown	Mostly in feces; 20% in urine

Adverse Drug Reactions

Aluminum- and calcium-based antacids cause constipation; magnesium-based antacids cause diarrhea. Alkalosis may occur but tends to be a clinically significant problem only for patients with renal impairment.

Drug Interactions

All antacids have drug interactions with orally administered weakly acidic and weakly basic drugs, decreasing or increasing their absorption and, therefore, their effects. Enteric coating on drugs is used to protect them from the acid of the stomach, and the coating dissolves in the more basic medium of the duodenum. Concurrent administration of antacids with enteric-coated drugs destroys the coating, alters their absorption, and increases the risk for adverse reactions. Some antacids adsorb or bind to the surface of other drugs, resulting in decreased bioavailability. Magnesium hydroxide (Milk of Magnesia, Maalox, Mylanta) has the greatest ability to adsorb, and calcium carbonate and aluminum hydroxide (AlternaGEL, Amphojel) have intermediate ability to adsorb certain drugs.

Increasing urinary pH affects the rate of elimination by inhibiting the excretion of weakly basic drugs and increasing the elimination of weakly acidic ones. Separating the administration of the antacid and the interacting drug by at least 2 hours and giving the interacting drug first in this sequence often can avoid these problems. Table 20-2 provides specific information on drug interactions with selected antacids.

Clinical Use and Dosing

Hyperacidity

Antacids are used for symptomatic relief of stomach upset associated with the hyperacidity of heartburn, acid indigestion, and "sour stomach." Because they are sold over the counter (OTC), doses may vary, as patients choose the amount they think they need to relieve symptoms. Generally, dosing is one to two tablets or 1 to 2 tablespoons of suspension taken intermittently. Dosing of common antacids is found in Table 20-3.

Peptic Ulcer Disease

Although the main factor in most duodenal ulcers and many gastric ulcers is infection with *Helicobacter pylori,* hyperacidity

Table 20–2 ⠿ Drug Interactions: Selected Antacids

Drug	Interacting Drug	Possible Effect	Implications
All antacids	Weakly acidic drugs (e.g., digoxin, phenytoin, chlorpromazine, isoniazid, ketoconazole)	Decreased absorption with possible decreased drug effects	Separate administration by at least 2 h, giving the antacid after the drug
	Weakly basic drugs (e.g., pseudoephedrine, levodopa)	Increased absorption with possible toxicity or adverse reactions	Separate administration by at least 2 h, giving the antacid after the drug
	Drugs acidic at the time of excretion (e.g., salicylates)	Enhanced excretion	May be used therapeutically to treat salicylate toxicity. Otherwise, avoid concurrent use or alter dosage of drug.
	Drugs basic at the time of excretion (e.g., quinidine, amphetamines)	Decreased excretion	Avoid concurrent use or alter dosage of drug
	Drugs with enteric coating	Antacids may destroy the coating, resulting in altered absorption or adverse reactions	Avoid concurrent use or separate administration by at least 2 h, giving the antacid after the drug
	Buffered aspirin products	Alkalinization of urine accelerates aspirin excretion, and systemic alkalosis and increased sodium load may occur	Caution against use of these antacid-analgesic combinations in chronic pain syndromes. Not an issue if used only intermittently.
Aluminum-based antacids	Allopurinol, chloroquine, corticosteroids, ethambutol, histamine₂ blockers, iron salts, phenothiazines, tetracyclines, thyroid hormones, ticlopidine	Decreased pharmacological effect of the drug	Avoid concurrent use or separate administration by at least 2 h, giving the antacid after the drug
	Benzodiazepines	Increased pharmacological effect of the drug	Avoid concurrent use

Continued

Table 20–2 ⚏ **Drug Interactions: Selected Antacids—cont'd**

Drug	Interacting Drug	Possible Effect	Implications
Calcium-based antacids	Fluoroquinolones, hydantoins, iron salts, salicylates, tetracyclines	Decreased pharmacological effect of the drug	Avoid concurrent administration
	Quinidine	Increased pharmacological effect of the drug	Avoid concurrent administration
Magnesium-based antacids	Benzodiazepines, cortico-steroids, histamine$_2$ blockers, hydantoins, iron salts, nitrofu-rantoin, phenothiazines, tetra-cyclines, ticlopidine	Decreased pharmacological effect of the drug	Avoid concurrent administration
	Quinidine, sulfonylureas	Increased pharmacological effect of the drug	Avoid concurrent administration

Table 20–3 ⚯ **Dosage Schedule: Selected Antacids**

Drug	Indication	Dosage Form	Dosage Schedule
Aluminum hydroxide	Hyperphosphatemia		*Adolescents or adults:* 300–600 mg 3 or 4 times a day, max 3,000 mg/day *Children:* 30 mg/kg/day
AlternaGEL Amphojel Alu-Tab Alu-Cap Generic	Hyperacidity	Liquid: 600 mg/5 mL Tablets: 300 mg, 600 mg Tablets: 500 mg Capsules: 500 mg (sodium content <1.2 mg) Suspension: 320 mg/5 mL Concentrated suspension: 450 mg/5 mL Concentrated suspension: 675 mg/5 mL Concentrated liquid: 600 mg/5 mL	*Adults:* Tablets or capsules: 500–1,500 mg 3–6 times daily between meals and at bedtime Suspension: 5–30 mL prn between meals and at bedtime *Children:* 300–900 mg per dose between meals and at bedtime
Calcium carbonate	Calcium deficiency in chronic renal failure		*Adults:* 1–2 g/day in divided doses *Children:* 45–65 mg/kg/day in 4 divided doses Adjust dose based on serum calcium concentration
Alka-Mints Tums Maalox Chewables Generic	Postmenopause or osteoporosis Hyperacidity	Tablets, chewable: 850 mg (sodium content <5 mg) Tablets, chewable: 500 mg (sodium content <2 mg) Extra-strength, chewable: 750 mg (sodium content <4 mg) Ultra, chewable: 1,000 mg (sodium content <4 mg) Tablets: 600 mg Tablets: 500, 600, 650, 1,250 mg	*Adults:* 1,000–1,500 mg elemental calcium/d *Children >11 yr and adults:* TUMS (500 mg calcium carbonate) chew 2–4 tablets for symptoms, not to exceed 15 tablets/d; TUMS E-X (750 mg calcium carbonate) chew 2–4 tablets for symptoms, not to exceed 10 tablets/d *Children 5 yr to 11 yr:* 800 mg calcium carbonate for symptoms; do not exceed 4,800 mg/d *Children 2–5 yr:* 400 mg as needed; do not exceed 1,200 mg/d
Magnesium hydroxide Phillips' Chewables Phillips' Milk of Magnesia Generic	Hyperacidity	Tablets: 311 mg Liquid: 400 mg/5 mL Concentrated liquid: 800 mg/5 mL Liquid: 400 mg/5 mL	*Children >12 yr and adults:* Tablets: 622–1,244 mg up to qid Liquid: 5–15 mL up to qid with water Liquid concentrate: 2.5–7.5 mL up to qid with water
Phillips' Caplets Phillips' Milk of Magnesia	Laxative	Caplets: 500 mg Liquid: 400 mg/5 mL	*Adults:* 30–60 mL at bedtime with water *Adults and children ≥ 12 yrs:* 2 to 4 caplets daily

Table 20–3 ⚗ Dosage Schedule: Selected Antacids—cont'd

Drug	Indication	Dosage Form	Dosage Schedule
Generic		Liquid: 400 mg/5 mL	*Children:* 2–5 yr: 5–15 mL/d at bedtime 6–11 yr: 15–30 mL/d at bedtime
Aluminum hydroxide-magnesium hydroxide combinations Maalox Maalox Advanced Extra Strength Mylanta Regular Strength Mylanta Ultimate Strength Generic	Hyperacidity	Aluminum hydroxide 200 mg and magnesium hydroxide 200 mg and simethicone 20 mg per 5 mL Aluminum hydroxide 400 mg and magnesium hydroxide 400 mg and simethicone 40 mg per 5 mL Aluminum hydroxide 200 mg and magnesium hydroxide 200 mg and simethicone 20 mg per 5 mL Aluminum hydroxide 500 mg and magnesium hydroxide 500 mg per 5 mL	Tablets: 1 or 2 prn *Adults and children >12 yr:* 2–4 tsp bid, max *Adults and children >12 yr:* 2–4 tsp bid, max 8 tsp /24 h *Adults and children >12 yr:* 2–4 tsp between meals and at bedtime, max 24 tsp/24 h *Adults and children >12 yr:* 2–4 tsp between meals and at bedtime, max 9 tsp/24 h
Maalox Mylanta Regular Strength	Peptic ulcer disease	Aluminum hydroxide 200 mg and magnesium hydroxide 200 mg and simethicone 20 mg per 5 mL	Suspension: 15–30 mL prn Suspension: 15–30 mL 1 h and 3 h after meals and at bedtime
	Gastroesophageal reflux disease		*Children >12 yr and adults:* Suspension: 5–30 mL every 30–60 min for acute management; 5–30 mL 1 h and 3 h after meals and at bedtime for maintenance *Infants and children <12 yr:* Suspension: 0.5 mL/kg (average dose 2–15 mL) 1–2 h after meals or feedings; max 15 mL/dose

is also a factor in peptic ulcer disease (PUD). Antacids were formerly considered step 1 in PUD management, but the current guidelines follow a stepped-down approach and treatment is begun with a proton pump inhibitor. Patients with uncomplicated PUD can benefit from 15 to 30 mL of antacid suspension 1 to 3 hours after meals and at bedtime and often select to do this before consulting a health-care provider. Additional doses may be used for recurring symptoms. Because ANC is higher in patients with uncomplicated PUD, combined antacids with both aluminum hydroxide and magnesium hydroxide are best unless the patient also has renal insufficiency or failure. Further discussion of PUD occurs in Chapter 34.

Gastroesophageal Reflux Disease

Lifestyle management and drugs to increase lower esophageal sphincter tone are central to the management of gastroesophageal reflux disease (GERD), but there is a role for antacids in mild disease. Antacids (calcium carbonate, aluminum hydroxide) and antacids/alginic acid (Gaviscon) are more effective than placebo for daytime GERD symptoms, with up to 20% of patients with mild symptoms responding to OTC antacids (Heidelbaugh, Harrison, McQuillan, & Nostrant, 2012). For acute management, antacid doses may be given every 30 to 60 minutes until symptoms are relieved; for maintenance, doses are given 1 and 3 hours after meals and at bedtime. Additional doses may be given for recurring symptoms. Dosing of antacids is found in Table 20-3. Further discussion of GERD occurs in Chapter 35.

Hyperphosphatemia

Aluminum carbonate (Basalgel) and aluminum hydroxide have been used, along with a low-phosphate diet, to treat hyperphosphatemia in patients with chronic renal failure. They have also been used to prevent the formation of phosphate urinary stones. The dose is 30 mL of suspension with each meal.

Calcium Deficiency

Calcium carbonate (Tums) is routinely used to treat calcium deficiency states associated with chronic renal failure, postmenopause, and osteoporosis. Tablets, often in chewable form, are commonly used. A dose of 1,000 mg/day of calcium carbonate is sufficient to provide adequate calcium for patients with chronic renal failure. Higher doses are needed for osteoporosis prevention: 1,000 mg daily for men and for premenopausal women and 1,500 mg/day of calcium for postmenopausal women. Doses higher than 2,000 mg/day are not advised because of increased adverse effects. Patients with osteoporosis require a combination of calcium, vitamin D, and another bone density–building medication such as a bisphosphonate.

Rational Drug Selection

In addition to consideration of adverse drug reactions and the indications discussed previously, other major factors used to choose among antacids are ANC, sodium content, and cost.

Acid-Neutralizing Capacity

Combination products that contain aluminum hydroxide and magnesium hydroxide have the highest ANC (see Table 20-1). When moderate to severe hyperacidity is a factor in the disease process under treatment, these drugs are chosen over other antacids.

Sodium Content

The sodium content of antacids may be significant. Patients who must restrict sodium intake (e.g., those with HTN, CHF, or marked renal failure) should use a low-sodium antacid. The sodium content is listed on the product label.

Cost

Antacids are sold OTC. In general, they are inexpensive, but the cost of a high-dose regimen varies significantly. Costs of OTC antacids may vary and "shopping" different stores and using generic forms of the drug may yield cost savings.

Monitoring

No specific monitoring is required beyond that related to the disease process for which the patient is being treated. Serum phosphate, potassium, and calcium levels may be monitored periodically during chronic use. These drugs may cause increased serum calcium and decreased serum phosphate. Chronic magnesium hydroxide use may cause elevated magnesium levels in patients with renal failure or the elderly with decreased renal function.

Patient Education

Administration

Antacids should be taken as prescribed, especially related to mealtimes. For best effects, they should be taken 1 to 3 hours after meals and at bedtime. To prevent chewable tablets from entering the small intestine in undissolved form, they must be chewed thoroughly before they are swallowed and followed with half a glass of water. Suspensions should be shaken before administration (see Table 20-3).

Antacids have many drug interactions when taken concurrently with other drugs because the altered acidity of the stomach affects acid-labile drugs. Antacids bind with many drugs affecting their absorption. The dose of antacid may need to be separated from the dose of another drug by as much as 2 hours. Health-care providers should instruct the patient in timing the administration of such drugs. Patients should be told not to begin taking OTC antacids on their own without first consulting their health-care provider or the pharmacist to discuss any potential drug interactions.

Calcium-based antacids should not be administered with food containing large amounts of oxalic acid (e.g., spinach, rhubarb) or phytic acid (e.g., bran, cereals). These foods decrease the absorption of calcium. Taking these antacids with food that contains phosphorus (milk or other dairy products) may lead to milk-alkali syndrome (nausea, vomiting, confusion, and headache). Taking calcium-based antacids with an acidic fruit juice may improve absorption.

Adverse Reactions

Patients should be told to consult their health-care provider before taking antacids for more than 2 weeks if a problem recurs, if relief is not obtained, or if symptoms of GI bleeding (black, tarry stools; coffee-ground emesis) occur.

Aluminum- and calcium-based antacids may cause constipation. Methods of preventing constipation such as increased bulk in the diet, greater fluid intake, and more mobility should be recommended. A stool softener may be needed to treat constipation related to antacid use. Magnesium-based antacids may cause diarrhea. Increased fiber in the diet may help this problem.

Lifestyle Management

Lifestyle management issues related to the disease process should be discussed. They often include avoiding: smoking, flat-lying body position while sleeping, foods that irritate the gastric mucosa (e.g., spicy foods) or stimulate acid production (e.g., alcohol), and foods that decrease lower esophageal sphincter tone (e.g., fatty food, chocolate, and caffeine).

ANTIDIARRHEALS

Diarrhea is a common reason for self-treatment and for patients to seek treatment from a health-care provider. Much of the diarrhea seen in a primary care setting has an infectious etiology, is food- or drug-induced, or is the result of inflammatory bowel disease. Diarrhea that lasts for less than 2 weeks is considered acute; if it lasts more than 2 weeks, it is considered chronic. Most episodes are acute and self-limiting, with few serious consequences. The exception is diarrhea in children, for whom dehydration can occur rather quickly, even with short-term diarrhea. Chronic diarrhea can result in weight loss, dehydration, perianal skin breakdown, and nutritional deficits.

Diarrhea that is drug-induced may be treated simply by removal of the offending drug. Food-induced diarrhea related to food poisoning and other diarrheas of an infectious etiology may require antimicrobial therapy, depending on the pathogen. Drugs used to treat infectious diseases are the subject of Chapter 25. The focus of this chapter is drugs used for symptomatic relief. Some drugs used to treat diarrhea are chemically related to opioids. Opioids are discussed further in Chapter 16. Anticholinergic agents are also sometimes used to treat diarrhea and are discussed in Chapter 15. This chapter does not discuss the diagnosis of diarrhea.

Pharmacodynamics

Three main classes of drugs used to treat diarrhea are absorbent preparations (kaolin and pectin [Kapectolin] and bismuth subsalicylate [Pepto-Bismol, Kaopectate Liquid]), opiates (diphenoxylate with atropine [Lomotil], diphenoxin with atropine [Motofen], and loperamide [Imodium]), and anticholinergics. Anticholinergics are useful only for inflammatory bowel disease. In 2012, a new antidiarrheal drug, crofelemer (Fulyzaq), was approved by the U.S. Food and Drug

Administration (FDA) to treat diarrhea in patients with HIV/AIDS taking antiretroviral therapy.

Kaolin is a clay-like powder that attracts and holds onto bacteria, and pectin thickens the stool by absorbing moisture in the stool. The combination product does not affect total water loss, however. Commonly used to treat simple diarrhea, the combination was rated by the FDA in 1986 as "safe and effective"; however, there are no specific trials to demonstrate this.

Bismuth subsalicylate appears to have antisecretory and antimicrobial effects in vitro and may have some anti-inflammatory effects. The salicylate moiety provides the antisecretory effect, and the bismuth moiety may exert direct antimicrobial effects against bacterial and viral enteropathogens. Because of these effects, it is also used as part of a multidrug regimen for the eradication of *H. pylori*.

Diphenoxylate with atropine is a constipating meperidine congener that lacks analgesic activity. High doses (4 to 60 mg), however, can cause opioid activity, including euphoria, and physical dependence with chronic use. The addition of atropine provides anticholinergic effects that decrease secretion in the bowel and slow peristalsis.

Loperamide binds to the opiate receptors of the intestinal wall, leading to slowed gastric motility. It also reduces fecal volume, increases viscosity and bulk, and diminishes the loss of fluid and electrolytes.

Crofelemer (Fulyzaq) is a botanical blocking chloride secretion from the epithelial cells in the intestinal lumen, decreasing water loss in diarrhea and normalizing the flow of chloride and water in the intestinal tract.

Pharmacokinetics

Absorption and Distribution

Kaolin and pectin act locally in the bowel and are not systemically absorbed (Table 20-4). Bismuth subsalicylate undergoes chemical dissociation in the GI tract; the salicylate moiety is absorbed, with plasma levels similar to those of aspirin. There is only negligible absorption of the bismuth moiety. Diphenoxylate with atropine and difenoxin with atropine are both well absorbed from the GI tract. Their distribution is unknown, but they do enter breast milk. The atropine in the drug readily crosses the blood–brain barrier and the placenta and enters breast milk. It also produces mild to moderate anticholinergic effects. Forty percent of loperamide is absorbed after oral administration, but it does not cross the blood–brain barrier well, so there are limited central nervous system (CNS) effects. Minimal amounts of crofelemer are absorbed after oral administration.

Metabolism and Excretion

The salicylate portion of bismuth subsalicylate is metabolized in the liver and more than 90% is excreted in urine. Diphenoxylate with atropine is rapidly and extensively metabolized to diphenoxylic acid, which is biologically active and its main metabolite. It is excreted in urine and feces. Difenoxin with atropine is rapidly metabolized to an inactive hydroxylated metabolite. Both the drug and its metabolite are excreted, mainly as conjugates, in the urine and feces. Loperamide is partially metabolized by the liver and undergoes enterohepatic recirculation to be completely metabolized. Most is eliminated in feces, with a minimal amount excreted in urine. Metabolism and excretion of crofelemer are not known.

Pharmacotherapeutics

Precautions and Contraindications

Drugs that reduce intestinal motility or delay intestinal transit time have induced toxic megacolon, especially in patients with inflammatory bowel disease. Diphenoxylate with atropine, difenoxin with atropine, and loperamide should be used cautiously for these patients and promptly discontinued if abdominal distention occurs. Because of their hepatic metabolism and renal excretion, these drugs should also be used with extreme caution in patients with advanced hepatorenal disease and in all patients with abnormal liver function studies because hepatic coma may occur.

The atropine component of diphenoxylate and difenoxin contraindicates their use in narrow-angle glaucoma and requires cautious use in prostatic hyperplasia. Children, especially

Table 20–4 ⁙ Pharmacokinetics: Selected Antidiarrheals

Drug	Onset	Peak	Duration	Half-Life	Elimination
Bismuth subsalicylate	—	—	—	2–3 h for low doses; 15–30 h for larger doses	>90% of salicylate in urine
Crofelemer	—	—	—	Unknown	Unknown
Difenoxin with atropine		20–40 min	3–4 h	24–72 h	Excreted as conjugates in urine and feces
Diphenoxylate with atropine	45–60 m	2 h	3–4 h	2.5 h (12–14 h for the metabolite)	14% of drug and metabolites in urine; 49% in feces
Loperamide	1 h	2.5–5 h	10 h	10.8 h (range 9.1–14.4 h)	25% unchanged in feces; 1.3% in urine as free drug and glucuronic acid conjugate

those with Down syndrome, have increased sensitivity to atropine. This drug should be avoided or used with extreme caution in children. It is not recommended for use in children younger than 12 years. This drug may prolong or aggravate diarrhea associated with organisms that penetrate the intestinal mucosa, such as *Escherichia coli, Salmonella,* and *Shigella,* or in pseudomembranous colitis associated with broad-spectrum antimicrobial therapy. It should not be used in these conditions.

The salicylate component of bismuth subsalicylate contraindicates its use in children or teenagers during or after recovery from chickenpox or flu-like illness. It is also contraindicated for patients with aspirin hypersensitivity.

All antidiarrheals (except crofelemer) require cautious use in older adults and others in whom impaction is a high risk. Older adults are especially sensitive to diphenoxylate or difenoxin because of the atropine content and anticholinergic properties.

There are no contraindications for the use of crofelemer in patients with HIV/AIDS–associated diarrhea.

Pregnancy categories vary among the antidiarrheal drugs. Kaolin and pectin are Pregnancy Category B. All others are Pregnancy Category C except loperamide, which is Pregnancy Category B. Crofelemer is Pregnancy Category C. However, there are no adequate and well-controlled studies in pregnant women for any of these drugs, and safety during pregnancy has not been established. Some of the drugs are excreted in breast milk, and the safety of any of the antidiarrheals has not been established in lactating women. They should be avoided or used with caution.

None of the antidiarrheals has established safety for children younger than age 2 years. All except crofelemer have published children's doses. It is important to keep in mind that dehydration may influence younger children's response to these drugs. Antidiarrheals are contraindicated in the treatment of diarrhea in most children; the standard of care is oral rehydration therapy (ORT) to treat the electrolyte and fluid loss of diarrhea. The safety and effectiveness of crofelemer in children with or without HIV/AIDS have not been established.

Adverse Drug Reactions

The main adverse drug reaction for all traditional antidiarrheals is rebound constipation. For bismuth subsalicylate, additional reactions that all patients should be warned about are gray/black stools and black tongue, the results of the bismuth. Patients should be told to expect this reaction and that it does not indicate GI bleeding.

The adverse reactions associated with the diphenoxylate and difenoxin drugs are related to their anticholinergic and opioid-like effects. Diphenoxylate and difenoxin (both with atropine) may exhibit anticholinergic adverse reactions such as dry mouth and mucous membranes, flushing, tachycardia, and urinary retention, especially in children. Loperamide also exhibits these reactions, but to a lesser degree. Both drugs have CNS reactions of dizziness and drowsiness, loperamide less so than diphenoxylate or difenoxin (both with atropine). Because they cross the blood–brain barrier better,

diphenoxylate and difenoxin (both with atropine) also exhibit sedation, headache, and, in higher doses or with chronic use, euphoria or depression, although difenoxin exhibits these slightly less so than diphenoxylate.

Patients treated with crofelemer in clinical trials were more likely to have upper respiratory infections (5.7%), bronchitis (3.9%), and cough (3.5%) than those taking placebo (Salix Pharmaceuticals, 2013). Patients treated with crofelemer also experienced GI adverse effects including flatulence (3.1%), increased bilirubin (3.1%), and nausea (2.6%).

Drug Interactions

Bismuth subsalicylate may potentiate the risk for toxicity if taken with aspirin, and the risk for hypoglycemia if given in large doses with insulin or oral hypoglycemics. Diphenoxylate with atropine, difenoxin with atropine, and loperamide all have additive or potentiating CNS effects with other CNS depressants and additive anticholinergic effects with other drugs that share these effects. There are few other drug interactions (Table 20-5).

Crofelemer has a theoretical potential to inhibit CYP 3A isoenzyme but is not absorbed enough to inhibit CYP isoenzymes. Crofelemer does not interact with the antiretrovirals nelfinavir, zidovudine, or lamivudine.

Clinical Use and Dosing

Simple, Acute Diarrhea

After the cause of the diarrhea has been determined and, if possible, eliminated, absorbent preparations are commonly used for relief of symptoms in adults. Kaolin-pectin or bismuth subsalicylate taken after each loose stool may be effective. The majority of acute diarrheal illnesses are self-limiting, and the main concern is to maintain hydration.

Hydration can usually be maintained in adults, even with profuse diarrhea, by the use of oral fluids. Commercial hydrating fluids (Pedialyte, Rehydralyte) or powdered salts are available; adding a pinch of table salt and a half-teaspoon of honey to an 8 ounce glass of fruit juice also makes a hydrating solution for older children and adults. Nondiet colas that have been allowed to lose their carbonation may also be used in older children and adults. Alternate these solutions with 8 ounce glasses of water to which has been added one-quarter teaspoon of baking soda to replenish the electrolytes commonly lost in acute, infectious diarrhea (sodium, potassium, bicarbonate, and chloride).

Children with severe diarrhea need oral rehydrating solutions (ORS) to prevent dehydration. Examples include Infalyte, Kao-Lectrolyte, and Pedialyte. These OTC products are available in pharmacies or supermarkets. If the child does not like the flavor, one-quarter teaspoon of sugar-free Kool-Aid powder may be added. Jell-O, water, or sports drinks should be avoided because they do not contain enough sodium. For infants, a homemade recipe includes one-half cup infant rice cereal mixed with 16 ounces of water and one-quarter teaspoon of salt. Children should be given ORS to satisfy their thirst for at least 6 hours and often

Table 20–5 ⠿ **Drug Interactions: Selected Antidiarrheals**

Drug	Interacting Drug	Possible Effect	Implications
Bismuth subsalicylate	Aspirin	May potentiate salicylate toxicity	Avoid concurrent use
	Tetracycline	May decrease GL absorption	Separate administration by 2 h
	Thrombolytics, warfarin, heparin	Large doses may increase risk for bleeding	Avoid concurrent use or use small doses; monitor clotting studies closely
	Insulin, oral hypoglycemics	Large doses increase risk of hypoglycemia	Avoid concurrent use or use small doses
Crofelemer	Potential to inhibit CYP450 3A		Monitor patient if given concurrently
Diphenoxylate with atropine	CNS depressants, including alcohol, antihistamines, opioids, sedative hypnotics	Additive/potentiating CNS depression	Monitor patient closely if these drugs must be given concurrently
	Monoamine oxidase inhibitors (MAOIs)	Because chemical structure is similar, concurrent use may precipitate hypertensive crisis	Avoid concurrent use or within 14 d of use of MAOIs
	Drugs that have anticholinergic properties	Additive anticholinergic effect	Monitor for toxicity; treat symptoms with good oral hygiene, hard candy, sugarless gum
Kaolin-pectin	Digoxin, chloroquine	Decreases GL absorption	Avoid concurrent use or separate doses by at least 2 h, giving kaolin-pectin last
Loperamide	CNS depressants, including alcohol, antihistamines, opioids, sedative hypnotics Drugs that have anticholinergic properties	Additive/potentiating CNS depression Additive anticholinergic effect	Monitor patient closely if these drugs must be given concurrently Monitor for toxicity; treat symptoms with good oral hygiene, hard candy, sugarless gum

for 24 hours. Infants and young children need electrolyte replacement with their fluids, whereas older children and adults may be able to be rehydrated with fluids alone. Full management of acute diarrhea is not within the scope of this chapter.

If the absorbents do not resolve the diarrhea, diphenoxylate or difenoxin (both with atropine) or loperamide may be added. Diphenoxylate with atropine is given 3 to 4 times daily rather than after each loose stool. Difenoxin with atropine is dosed both after each stool or every 3 to 4 hours as needed to avoid exceeding the maximum 24-hour dose. Antidiarrheals are generally not recommended in children.

Oral Rehydration Therapy
Evaluation of the effectiveness of oral rehydration is based on at least three wet diapers per 24 hours in infants. For children older than 1 year, avoid all fruit juices and other drinks that contain fructose because they usually make the diarrhea worse. If the infant or child is drinking milk or lactose-based formula, try withholding milk or lactose products. Probiotics may decrease the duration of diarrhea. Resolution of the diarrhea suggests lactose intolerance.

Unlike acute diarrhea, chronic diarrhea requires etiological diagnosis and specific therapy for that diagnosis. Simply suppressing symptoms is not sufficient.

Chronic Diarrhea Associated With Inflammatory Bowel Disease

Steroids and sulfasalazine are needed to control diarrhea exacerbated by inflammatory bowel disease. Loperamide, 4 mg initially followed by doses of 2 to 4 mg 4 times a day, may be used as adjunct therapy, and it may lead to substantial clinical improvement, especially if combined with added fiber in the diet and anticholinergics. If clinical improvement is not observed with doses of 16 mg/day for at least 10 days, symptoms are unlikely to be controlled by further use of this drug.

Chronic Diarrhea Associated With Pancreatic Insufficiency

Malabsorption due to pancreatic insufficiency requires use of enzyme supplements. Antidiarrheal medications are not generally used for this indication.

Chronic Infantile Diarrhea

Bismuth subsalicylate has been used to treat chronic infantile diarrhea. The dose is 2.5 mL every 4 hours for children 2 to 24 months; 5 mL for children 24 to 48 months; and 10 mL for children 48 to 70 months (Taketomo, Hodding, & Kraus, 2009).

Diarrhea in HIV/AIDS Patients Taking Antiretroviral Drugs

Crofelemer (Fulyzaq) is indicated for the symptomatic relief of noninfectious diarrhea in adult patients with HIV/AIDS on antiretroviral therapy. Dosing is one 125 mg tablet twice a day, without regard for food. The mean duration of therapy during clinical trials was 141 days (Salix Pharmaceuticals, 2013).

Traveler's Diarrhea

Bismuth subsalicylate appears to have antibacterial and antisecretory properties and is used to treat traveler's diarrhea in doses of two tablets or 2 fluid oz before each meal and at bedtime (4 times/d) for up to 3 weeks during brief periods of high risk (Centers for Disease Control and Prevention [CDC], 2014). The management of traveler's diarrhea can be divided into prevention and treatment. The most important risk factor for acquiring this disorder is the patient's destination. High-risk areas include Central and South America, Africa, the Middle East, Mexico, and Asia. Intermittent-risk areas include Eastern Europe, South Africa, and a number of the Caribbean islands. Enterotoxigenic *E. coli* is the most common causative organism found in traveler's diarrhea,

followed by *Campylobacter, Shigella,* and *Salmonella.* Oral antimicrobials are also used for both prevention and treatment of this disorder; the provider should refer to the CDC Travel Web site (www.cdc.gov/travel) for current antimicrobial recommendations. Table 20-6 provides adults' and children's doses of selected antidiarrheals.

Rational Drug Selection

Indication

For acute diarrhea, any of the antidiarrheals is appropriate. The more severe the diarrhea is, the less likely it will be that absorbent agents will help. Bismuth subsalicylate and loperamide are the only drugs indicated for traveler's diarrhea. Loperamide is the only drug with an indication for use with inflammatory bowel disease.

Cost

Brand names are more expensive than generic formulations, and there is no significant clinical difference between the two. Diphenoxylate with atropine generic is $13.99 for 30 tablets, whereas the brand Lomotil is $41.99 (http://drugstore.com). Loperamide (Imodium) is available OTC and is $9.99 for 24 tablets, or the generic loperamide at $5.99

Table 20–6 ⚛ Dosage Schedule: Selected Antidiarrheals

Drug	Indication	Dosage Form	Initial Dose	Additional Doses
Bismuth subsalicylate*† Pepto-Bismol Kaopectate	Acute diarrhea	Tablets/chewable: 262 mg Liquid: 262 mg/15 mL Liquid: 524 mg/15 mL	*Adults:* 524 mg every 30 min or 1,048–1,200 mg every 60 min as needed *Children 9–12 yr:* 262–300 mg every 30–60 min as needed *Children 6–9 yr:* 176 mg every 30–60 min as needed *Children 3–6 yr:* 88 mg every 30–60 min as needed *Children <3 yr weighing >13 kg:* 88 mg *Children <3 yr weighing 6.4–8 kg:* 44 mg May repeat q4h; not to exceed 6 doses/24 h	Not to exceed 4.2 g/24 h Not to exceed 2.4 g/24 h Not to exceed 1.4 g/24 h Not to exceed 704 mg/24 h May repeat q4h; not to exceed 6 doses/24 h
	Traveler's diarrhea		524 mg (2 tablets or 30 mL of 262 mg/15 mL liquid) every 30 min for up to 8 doses	Not to be used for more than 48 h
Crofelemer (Fulyzaq)	Symptomatic relief of noninfectious diarrhea in adult patients with HIV/AIDS on antiretroviral therapy	125 mg delayed-release tablet	1 tablet bid, with or without food	
Difenoxin with atropine Motofen	Acute diarrhea	Tablets: 1 mg difenoxin and 0.025 mg atropine sulfate	*Adults:* 2 mg	1 mg after each loose stool or 1 mg every 3–4 h as needed. Total 24 h dose not to exceed 8 mg
Diphenoxylate with atropine Lomotil	Acute diarrhea	Tablets: 2.5 mg diphenoxylate, 0.025 mg atropine sulfate	*Adults:* 5 mg tid to qid initially	5 mg daily as needed; not to exceed 20 mg/d

Table 20–6 ⊗ **Dosage Schedule: Selected Antidiarrheals—cont'd**

Drug	Indication	Dosage Form	Initial Dose	Additional Doses
		Liquid: 2.5 mg diphenoxy-late, 0.025 mg atropine sulfate/5 mL	*Children 2–12 yr:* all doses qid and in liquid form *2 yr/11–14 kg:* 1.5–3 mL *3 yr/12–16 kg:* 2–3 mL *4 yr/14–20 kg:* 2–4 mL *5 yr/16–23 kg:* 2.5–4.5 mL *6–8 yr/17–32 kg:* 2.5–5.5 mL *9–12 yr/23–55 kg:* 3.5–5 mL	Not recommended for children <2 yr Reduce dosage as soon as control of symptoms is achieved; maintenance dosage may be as low as one-fourth of initial daily dose; maximum daily dose 20 mg Overdosage may result in respiratory depression
Kaolin-pectin Kapectolin Kao-Spen	Acute diarrhea	Suspension: 5.2 g kaolin plus 260 mg pectin/30 mL; 5.85 mg kaolin plus 130 mg pectin/30 mL Also comes in combinations with paregoric, bismuth, carboxy-methylcellulose, and others	*Adults:* 60–120 mL after each loose stool *Children >12 yr:* 40–60 mL after each loose stool *Children 6–12 yr:* 30–60 mL after each loose stool *Children 3–6 yr:* 15–30 mL after each loose stool	
Loperamide Imodium A-D Imodium Generic	Acute diarrhea, traveler's diarrhea	Tablets/capsule: 2 mg Liquid: 1 mg/5 mL	*Adults:* 4 mg initially *Children 9–11 yr or 30–47 kg:* 2 mg initially *Children 6–8 yr or 24–30 kg:* 1 mg initially	2 mg after each loose stool; not to exceed 8 mg/d for OTC use or 16 mg/d for prescription use 1 mg after each loose stool; not to exceed 6 mg/24 h; OTC use not to exceed 48 h 1 mg after each loose stool; not to exceed 4 mg/24 h; OTC use not to exceed 48 h
	Chronic diarrhea associated with inflammatory bowel disease		*Adults only:* 4 mg initially	2 mg after each loose stool until symptoms resolved; maintenance dose is usually 4–8 mg/d in divided doses; not to exceed 16 mg/d

*The dosage schedule for eradication of *H. pylori* is discussed in Chapter 34.

†Avoid bismuth subsalicylate in pediatric patients with influenza or chicken pox because of the risk of Reye syndrome.

(http://drugstore.com). Crofelemer (Fulyzaq) costs $290 for 30 tablets or 15 days of therapy (goodrx.com).

Monitoring

There is no specific monitoring beyond that required for the disease process being treated. Patients with chronic diarrhea may benefit from monitoring of hydration status and electrolyte studies.

Patient Education

Administration

Despite the fact that many of these drugs are available OTC, they are not innocuous. Patients need to be informed that they should take the antidiarrheal exactly as directed; to not make up missed doses or double the doses, and to not exceed the maximum number of doses recommended for 24 hours. The health-care

provider should be notified if the diarrhea continues beyond 48 hours or if abdominal pain, fever, or distention occurs.

Tablets may be administered with food if GI irritation occurs (see Table 20-6). They may also be crushed and taken with fluid. Chewable tablets may be chewed or allowed to dissolve. Calibrated measuring devices should be used for liquid preparations. Suspensions should be shaken before they are measured and administered.

Drug interactions may occur, especially with diphenoxylate with atropine and loperamide. Patients should be told not to take any OTC antidiarrheal if they are taking other drugs, especially digoxin, cephalosporin antimicrobials, warfarin or heparin, or CNS depressants (including alcohol) without first contacting their health-care provider. Patients concurrently taking aspirin and bismuth subsalicylate are at risk for salicylate poisoning.

Adverse Reactions

All antidiarrheals have the potential for rebound constipation. As soon as symptoms of diarrhea are reduced, the dosage of the antidiarrheal drug should be reduced; it should be stopped as soon as symptoms resolve.

Bismuth subsalicylate can turn the tongue and stools gray/black. Patients should be told that this reaction can be expected and that it does not indicate GI bleeding.

Diphenoxylate and difenoxin (both with atropine) can cause dry mouth and mucous membranes. These symptoms can be improved by good oral hygiene, sucking hard candy, or chewing sugarless gum. Flushing, tachycardia, and urinary retention may also occur. These symptoms are especially notable in children and in older men. They may necessitate stopping the drug. Loperamide also exhibits these reactions but to a lesser degree. Both drugs can produce CNS reactions of dizziness and drowsiness, loperamide less so than diphenoxylate or difenoxin (both with atropine). Driving or other activities requiring mental alertness should be avoided until the patient's response to the drug is known.

Crofelemer (Fulyzaq) may cause upper respiratory infection or cough, as well as GI symptoms such as nausea and flatulence.

Lifestyle Management

Adding fiber to the diet and using oral rehydrating solutions were discussed previously. The importance of washing one's hands after each bowel movement should be stressed. Education about maintaining nutritional intake is also important. Sometimes patients think that they can stop their diarrhea by stopping their food intake. Resting the GI tract briefly (e.g., for 24 hours) may be appropriate, but reducing fluid intake is never appropriate, and food intake should be restarted after the GI rest.

A bland food diet can assist in maintaining nutrition and is also helpful in reducing the diarrhea. Stopping milk or other lactose-based food products for a few days may give an indication whether the diarrhea is associated with lactose intolerance.

CYTOPROTECTIVE AGENTS

Peptic ulceration can be caused by a variety of conditions, some of which are iatrogenic. The administration of NSAIDs, for example, has been associated with gastric mucosal damage and ulcer formation. Ulcer formation and GI bleeding related to NSAID use often occur without warning.

Patients at high risk are those with a previous history of ulcers; also those on steroids, on high doses of NSAIDS, concurrently taking anticoagulants, or older than 75 years. Among the agents used to treat or prevent ulcer formation are two cytoprotective agents, sucralfate (Carafate) and misoprostol (Cytotec). These drugs are the focus of this section.

Pharmacodynamics

Sucralfate is a basic aluminum salt of a sulfated disaccharide, which is believed to act by polymerization and selective binding to necrotic ulcer tissue, where it covers the ulcer site and acts as a barrier to acid, pepsin, and bile salts. It has no acid-neutralizing activity, and little is absorbed, although some aluminum salts are released. In addition, the drug may directly absorb bile salts and stimulate endogenous prostaglandin synthesis. Prostaglandins are central to the formation and maintenance of the protective mucosa of the GI tract.

Misoprostol is a methyl analogue of prostaglandin E_1. The principal mechanism of action of this drug appears to be inhibition of gastric secretion through inhibition of histamine-stimulated cyclic adenosine monophosphate (AMP) production. Over a dosage range of 50 to 200 mcg, it inhibits basal and nocturnal gastric acid secretion and acid secretion in response to a variety of stimuli, including meals, histamine, and coffee by binding to prostaglandin E receptors. It has no significant effect on fasting or postprandial gastrin or on intrinsic factor output; however, it produces a moderate decrease in pepsin concentration during basal conditions.

Misoprostol also has mucosal protective qualities. Prostaglandin E receptors have a high affinity for misoprostol and for its acid metabolite. These receptors facilitate the production of mucus and bicarbonate. They also allow the drug taken with food to be effective, despite the lower serum concentration. Misoprostol also produces uterine contractions that may endanger pregnancy. See the discussion below.

Pharmacokinetics

Absorption and Distribution

Sucralfate is minimally absorbed (Table 20-7). Its action is largely topical. Misoprostol is rapidly and extensively absorbed after oral administration. Distribution of this drug is unknown.

Table 20–7 ⠿ **Pharmacokinetics: Cytoprotective Agents**

Drug	Onset	Peak	Duration	Protein Binding	Half-Life	Elimination
Misoprostol	Minutes	12–15 min	3–6 h	<90%	20–40 min (doubles in renal impairment)	80% in urine
Sucralfate	30 min	UK	5 h	UK	6–20 h	90% in feces

UK = unknown.

Metabolism and Excretion

Sucralfate is essentially not absorbed; more than 90% is excreted in feces. Misoprostol is rapidly converted to its free acid, which is responsible for its clinical activity. It does not affect the cytochrome P450 (CYP450) enzyme systems. The half-life of this drug is 20 to 40 minutes, but renal impairment results in a doubling of this half-life. The metabolite is excreted in urine.

Pharmacotherapeutics

Precautions and Contraindications

Sucralfate's action is topical; there are no specific precautions or contraindications. It is Pregnancy Category B. Its safety and efficacy have not been established in children.

Misoprostol must be used with caution in renal impairment. Its half-life, maximum concentration, and the area under the curve (AUC) double with renal insufficiency. No routine dosage adjustments have been recommended, but dosage may need to be reduced if the usual dose is not tolerated. In older adults (older than 64 years), the AUC for the acid metabolite of misoprostol is increased. The cause may be decreased renal functioning associated with aging, and recommendations are the same as for renal impairment.

Misoprostol is Pregnancy Category X. It may cause abortion, premature birth, or birth defects. Uterine rupture has been reported in women who were administered misoprostol to induce labor. It should not be administered to pregnant women to treat NSAID induced ulcers. Patients should be warned of the abortifacient properties of the drug and be advised not to give it to others (www.drugs.com). Misoprostol is metabolized in the mother to misoprostol acid that is excreted in breast milk. Caution is advised when administered to a nursing woman.

Safety and efficacy in children younger than 18 years have not been established.

Adverse Drug Reactions

Adverse reactions in clinical trials with sucralfate were minor and rarely led to discontinuance of the drug. Constipation, the most frequent complaint, occurs in only 2% of patients. Other adverse reactions, including dizziness and gastric discomfort, occurred in less than 0.5% of patients.

Adverse reactions with misoprostol were largely GI or gynecological. Diarrhea is the most common complaint (13% to 40% of patients). Abdominal pain, nausea, and flatulence occur in small numbers of patients and are difficult to separate from the symptoms of the disorder for which the drug was prescribed. Postmenopausal bleeding, spotting (0.7%), cramps (0.6%), hypermenorrhea (0.5%), menstrual disorder (0.3%), and dysmenorrhea (0.1%) occur in women. Reactions related to pregnancy were discussed previously.

Drug Interactions

Sucralfate may decrease the absorption of several drugs when given concurrently or prior to their administration (Table 20-8). Separating the administration of the interacting drug by at least 2 hours and giving the interacting drug first can often solve the problem. Sucralfate and antacids should be separated by at least 2 hours.

The only drug of concern with misoprostol is the potential for increased diarrhea risk with magnesium-based antacids. Food can decrease maximum plasma concentrations, but this has little clinical significance.

Clinical Use and Dosing

Prophylaxis and Treatment of Duodenal Ulcers Associated With NSAID Use

NSAIDs inhibit prostaglandin synthesis and damage the mucosal lining of the stomach, which may result in ulcer formation. The first choice is to discontinue the NSAID. Misoprostol is approved by the FDA for prophylaxis or treatment of duodenal ulcers that are due to use of NSAIDs for those

Table 20–8 ⚏ Drug Interactions: Cytoprotective Agents

Drug	Interacting Drug	Possible Effect	Implications
Misoprostol	Magnesium-based antacids	Increased risk for diarrhea	Choose different antacid
	Food	Maximum plasma concentrations of acid metabolite are diminished when taken with food	Little clinical significance, but best taken on empty stomach
Sucralfate	Aluminum-based antacids	Increased constipation risk; increase in total body burden of aluminum	Choose different antacid
	Anticoagulants	Decrease in effect of warfarin	Avoid concurrent use
	Digoxin	Reduced serum levels of digoxin; reduced effects	Avoid concurrent use
	Hydantoins	Absorption may be decreased	Separate administration by 2 h and give hydantoin first
	Ketoconazole, quinolones	Bioavailability decreased	Separate administration by 2 h and give drugs first
	Quinidine	Reduced serum levels of quinidine; reduced effects	Separate administration by 2 h and give quinidine first

patients who must continue NSAID use. Dosage is 200 mcg 4 times a day with food (Table 20-9). If this dose cannot be tolerated, 100 mcg can be used. Misoprostol should be taken with meals and at bedtime. The drug is taken for the duration of NSAID therapy.

Because misoprostol commonly causes a dose-dependent diarrhea and other GI symptoms, and because its stimulant effect on the uterus contraindicates its use for women with childbearing potential, its use as prophylaxis is reserved for those with high risk for and little tolerance of the GI hazards of NSAIDs.

In a *Cochrane Review* of the literature regarding prevention of NSAID-induced gastroduodenal ulcers, misoprostol significantly reduced the risk of endoscopic ulcers. In gastric ulcers, 800 mg/day of misoprostol was more effective than 400 mg/day but not in duodenal ulcers (Rostom et al, 2002).

Treatment of Duodenal Ulcers From Other Causes

Sucralfate can be used for short-term (up to 8 weeks) treatment of active duodenal ulcer. Dosage is 1 g 4 times a day on an empty stomach, 1 hour before meals and at bedtime. Healing usually occurs within 2 weeks. Maintenance therapy after the ulcer has healed is 1 g twice a day. Sucralfate has off-labeled uses in treating gastric and esophageal ulcers, with the same dosing schedule. It appears to have some advantage over antacids and H_2RAs in stress ulcer prophylaxis.

Although more effective than placebo, misoprostol is less effective than H_2RAs or PPIs for treatment of duodenal ulcers from other causes. In doses greater than 400 mcg/day, it has an off-labeled use for treatment of duodenal ulcers not responsive to H_2RAs.

Rational Drug Selection

Drug selection is based on indications cited previously (see Table 20-9). Sucralfate is preferred over misoprostol for treatment of active duodenal ulcers not caused by NSAIDs. Sucralfate is also the cytoprotective drug of choice for women of childbearing age.

Monitoring

No specific monitoring parameters exist for these drugs. Monitoring should relate to the disease process being treated. Women of childbearing age should have a negative pregnancy test before misoprostol is prescribed to them.

Patient Education

Administration

Patients should be taught to take the drug exactly as prescribed. Sucralfate is taken on an empty stomach; misoprostol with food. Patients should not take antacids while taking sucralfate. Advise the patient to continue the therapy even if feeling better. Sucralfate is given for 4 to 8 weeks to ensure ulcer healing; misoprostol is given for the duration of NSAID therapy. Missed doses should be taken as soon as remembered unless it is almost time for the next dose. Doses should not be doubled. Women of childbearing age should have a negative pregnancy test and start misoprostol on day 2 or 3 of their menstrual period.

Adverse Reactions

Increased fluid intake, dietary bulk, and exercise may reduce the incidence of constipation associated with sucralfate. Diarrhea may occur with misoprostol. If it continues for more than 1 week, the health-care provider should be notified. The patient should also report onset of black, tarry stools or severe abdominal pain, which may indicate treatment failure and the onset of GI bleeding.

Women of childbearing age should be informed that misoprostol will cause spontaneous abortion. The drug should not be prescribed until contraceptive therapy is established and the patient has a negative serum pregnancy test within 2 weeks of starting therapy. If pregnancy is suspected, the drug should be immediately stopped and the health-care provider notified so that pregnancy testing can be performed.

Lifestyle Management

Lifestyle management related to peptic ulcers is discussed in Chapter 35.

ANTIEMETICS

Nausea and vomiting are common complaints in primary care and have a multitude of causes. Treatment is often nonpharmacological, but antiemetics may also be used to provide symptom relief and prevent fluid and electrolyte disturbances. This section discusses drugs used for these purposes.

Drug classes with antiemetic properties commonly used include antihistamines, phenothiazines, sedative hypnotics, cannabinoids, 5-HT_3 receptor antagonists, anticholinergics,

Table 20–9 ✂ Dosage Schedule: Cytoprotective Agents

Drug	Indication	Dosage Forms	Dosage Schedule
Misoprostol Cytotec	Prophylaxis and treatment of duodenal ulcers due to NSAID use	Tablets: 100, 200 mcg	200 mcg qid with food. Last dose usually at bedtime. Taken for duration of NSAID therapy. If this dose is not tolerated, 100 mcg qid may be used.
Sucralfate Carafate	Active duodenal ulcer Maintenance after healing of duodenal ulcer	Tablets: 1 g Suspension: 1 g/10 mL	1 g qid taken 1 h before meals and at bedtime 1 g bid taken on empty stomach

and a substance P/neurokinin 1 (NK1) receptor antagonist. The antihistamines most commonly used for these antiemetic properties are dimenhydrinate (Dramamine), diphenhydramine (Benadryl), hydroxyzine (Vistaril), and meclizine (Antivert). The phenothiazines include prochlorperazine (Compazine), perphenazine, and promethazine (Phenergan). The cannabinoid dronabinol (Marinol) is used for nausea and vomiting associated with cancer. The 5-HT$_3$ receptor antagonists include palonosetron (Aloxi), dolasetron mesylate (Anzemet), granisetron (Kytril, Sancuso), and ondansetron (Zofran). Scopolamine (Transderm Scop) is an anticholinergic. Aprepitant (Emend) is a substance P/neurokinin 1 (NK1) receptor antagonist. A miscellaneous antiemetic not from the previous classes of drugs is trimethobenzamide (Tigan). Each of these drugs is discussed in this section.

Pharmacodynamics

Antihistamines that possess significant antiemetic activity have strong anticholinergic effects as well as histamine$_1$-blocking effects. Blockade of histamine$_1$ receptors results in decreased exocrine gland secretion (e.g., salivary and lacrimal). First-generation antihistamines with strong anticholinergic properties bind to central cholinergic receptors and produce antiemetic effects, decreasing nausea and vomiting. They are especially helpful in the nausea associated with motion sickness because of their depression of conduction in the vestibulocerebellar pathway. The antiemetic drugs in this class are dimenhydrinate, diphenhydramine, hydroxyzine, and meclizine.

Phenothiazines block dopamine receptors in the chemoreceptor trigger zone (CTZ). They also bind to and block cholinergic, alpha$_1$-adrenergic, and histamine$_1$ receptors. Although all phenothiazines have these actions to some degree, their use as antiemetics is limited by their sedating and extrapyramidal effects. The antiemetic drugs in this class are prochlorperazine and promethazine. They are less sedating and have antiemetic effects at lower doses than some other phenothiazines. Metoclopramide also blocks dopamine receptors and has been used as an antiemetic. Its main use, however, is as a prokinetic, and it is discussed in that section of this chapter.

Cannabinoids work in the CNS similar to cannabis (marijuana) to prevent nausea and vomiting associated with cancer chemotherapy and as an appetite stimulant, especially in HIV patients.

The 5-HT$_3$ receptor antagonists block serotonin both peripherally on vagal nerve terminals and centrally in the CTZ. Chemotherapy causes the release of serotonin from the enterochromaffin cells; pretreatment with a 5-HT$_3$ receptor antagonist decreases emesis.

Transdermal scopolamine is a belladonna alkaloid anticholinergic that acts as a competitive inhibitor of muscarinic receptors in the parasympathetic nervous system. Scopolamine may also work to block cholinergic transmission from the reticular center to the vomiting center in the brain. Anticholinergics also decrease secretion of saliva and decrease gastrointestinal motility.

Aprepitant (Emend) is a highly selective antagonist of substance P/neurokinin 1 (NK1) receptors. Aprepitant crosses the blood–brain barrier and occupies the NK$_1$ receptors. It has no affinity for 5-HT$_3$ or dopamine receptors. Aprepitant augments the activity of the 5-HT$_3$ receptor antagonists such as ondansetron and the corticosteroid dexamethasone to prevent nausea and vomiting in patients receiving chemotherapy.

Trimethobenzamide inhibits emetic stimulation of the CTZ.

Pharmacokinetics

Absorption and Distribution

All of the antiemetic drugs (except for transdermal scopolamine) are well absorbed after oral administration (Table 20-10). Oral liquid formulations provide the most reliable absorption. The antihistamines, phenothiazines, 5-HT$_3$ receptor antagonists, and aprepitant come in IV form. Prochlorperazine, promethazine, and trimethobenzamide have formulations for administration by the rectal route. The IM and rectal routes are commonly used when vomiting is present. Scopolamine is available as a transdermal patch and is well absorbed through the skin behind the ear.

Distribution of antihistamines is not clearly known, but phenothiazines are widely distributed, cross the blood–brain barrier and placenta, and enter breast milk. As a result, they are associated with more adverse reactions. Scopolamine crosses the blood–brain barrier and the placenta. Aprepitant crosses the blood–brain barrier in humans, and in animal studies it crosses the placenta.

Metabolism and Excretion

Dimenhydrinate, diphenhydramine, and hydroxyzine are extensively metabolized by the liver and eliminated in feces by biliary excretion. The cannabinoid dronabinol undergoes extensive first-pass hepatic metabolism and is eliminated as active and inactive metabolite in the feces and urine; as well, the 5-HT$_3$ receptor antagonists undergo extensive first-pass metabolism and are eliminated in the urine and feces. Trimethobenzamide is metabolized by the liver and is excreted in urine. The phenothiazines are metabolized by the liver into active compounds that persist for prolonged periods. Phenothiazines are eliminated half by the kidney in urine and half through enterohepatic circulation. The fetus, infants, and older adults have decreased ability to metabolize and excrete the phenothiazines. Scopolomine is extensively metabolized with less than 5% of active drug excreted in the urine. Aprepitant is extensively metabolized primarily by CYP 3A4 into seven weakly active metabolites. Aprepitant is not renally excreted; it is primarily eliminated via metabolism.

Pharmacotherapeutics

Precautions and Contraindications

The drug class determines the precautions and contraindications. Antihistamines have anticholinergic properties and

Table 20–10 ✂ Pharmacokinetics: Selected Antiemetics

Drug	Onset	Peak	Duration	Protein Binding	Half-Life	Elimination
Aprepitant						
		3 h	24 h	95%	9–13 h	
Dimenhydrinate						
PO	15–60 min	1–2 h	3–6 h	UK	UK	In feces via biliary excretion
PO ER	UK	UK	12 h	UK	UK	
IM	20–30 min	1–2 h	3–6 h	UK	UK	
PR	30–45 min	UK	6–12 h	UK	UK	
Diphenhydramine						
PO	15–60 min	1–4 h	4–8 h	98%–99%	2.4–7 h	In feces via biliary excretion
IM	20–30 min	1–4 h	4–8 h	98%–99%	2.4–7 h	
Dolasetron						
PO		1 h			8 h	Urine and feces
IV		0.6 h			10 min	Urine and feces
Dronabinol						
PO	0.5–1 h	2–4 hr	4–6 hr	97%	4 h	Feces and urine
Ondansetron						
		2 hr			3 hr	Urine and feces
PO	10 min	UK	4–12 h	65%–90%	UK	Half in urine; half by enterohepatic circulation
PR	20 min	UK	12 h	65%–90%	UK	
IM	20 min	UK	12 h	65%–90%	UK	
Prochlorperazine						
PO	30–40 min	UK	10–12 h	>90%	UK	Half in urine; half by enterohepatic circulation
PR	60 min	UK	3–4 h	>90%	UK	
IM	10–20 min	10–30 min	3–4 h	>90%	UK	
Scopolamine						
Transdermal	4 h	24 h		UK	9.5 h	Renal
Trimethobenzamide						
PO	10–40 m	UK	3–4 h	UK	UK	In urine
PR	10–40 m	UK	3–4 h	UK	UK	
IM	15–35 m	UK	2–3 h	UK	UK	

ER = extended release; PR = per rectum; UK = unknown.

have precautions and contraindications similar to anticholinergics. Cautious use in narrow-angle glaucoma, seizure disorders, pyloric obstruction, hyperthyroidism, cardiovascular disease, and prostatic hypertrophy is in order. Because they are metabolized so extensively by the liver, they are contraindicated in severe liver disease. Cautious use is also suggested for older adults, and dosage reductions may be required.

Dimenhydrinate and diphenhydramine are Pregnancy Category B, and they are safe for use in children. Meclizine is also Pregnancy Category B. Safety and efficacy of meclizine has not been established in children less than 12 years or during lactation. Hydroxyzine is Pregnancy Category C but has been used safely during labor. Safety in lactation and in children has not been established, but it has been used for both, and children's doses are published.

Phenothiazines produce extrapyramidal reactions and are contraindicated in Parkinson's disease. They are also contraindicated in narrow-angle glaucoma, bone marrow depression, and severe cardiovascular or hepatic disease because of their serious adverse reactions. Cautious use is suggested in respiratory impairment caused by acute pulmonary infection or chronic respiratory disorders, such as severe asthma or emphysema. "Silent pneumonia" may develop in these patients when they are treated with phenothiazines. Because these drugs suppress the cough reflex, aspiration of vomitus is possible, and they should be used cautiously where aspiration is a risk. Although all of these points are important to consider, they are less likely to be a problem in very short-term use as an antiemetic.

The phenothiazines are Pregnancy Category C. Children of all ages are more prone to develop extrapyramidal reactions. Prochlorperazine should be avoided in children younger than age 5 years due to high incidence of extrapyramidal reactions. Promethazine is contraindicated in children younger than 2 years of age due to severe and potentially fatal respiratory depression. Promethazine is also associated with respiratory depression and sudden death in children 2 years of age or older and should be used with caution and at the lowest effective dose.

Dronabinol contains cannabinoid and sesame oil and should not be used by anyone sensitive to these ingredients.

Dronabinol should be used with caution in patients with a history of seizure disorder because it may lower the seizure threshold. Patients with cardiac disorders should be monitored for hypotension, possible hypertension, syncope, or tachycardia. Dronabinol has a high potential for abuse. Dronabinol is Pregnancy Category C.

The 5-HT$_3$ receptor antagonists may mask progressive ileus. Zofran ODT disintegrating tablets contain aspartame and should be used with caution in patients with phenylketonuria. Dolasetron, granisetron, and palonosetron are Pregnancy Category B.

Anticholinergics such as transdermal scopolomaine should be used cautiously in patients with open-angle glaucoma or gastrointestinal or bladder neck obstruction and is contraindicated in narrow-angle glaucoma. Transdermal scopolamine should be used cautiously in the elderly due to the increased likelihood of CNS effects. Transdermal scopolamine is Pregnancy Category C and is not approved for use in children.

Aprepitant is contraindicated in patients who are hypersensitive to any component of the product. Aprepitant inhibits CYP 3A4, and patients taking medications concurrently that are metabolized by CYP 3A4 may have elevated plasma concentrations leading to significant adverse effects (Table 20-11). Aprepitant is Pregnancy Category C and is not approved for use in children.

Table 20–11 ⠿ Drug Interactions: Selected Antiemetics

Drug	Interacting Drug	Possible Effect	Implications
Aprepitant	Dexamethasone	Increased plasma dexamethasone levels	Decrease dexamethasone dose by 50% when coadministering
	Methylprednisolone	Increased methylprednisolone levels	Decrease IV methylprednisolone dose by 25% and oral methylprednisolone level by 50%
	CYP 2C9 substrates (warfarin, tolbutamide)	May result in lower plasma concentrations of drugs metabolized by CYP 2C9	Warfarin: monitor INR levels Tolbutamide: monitor for adverse effects
	Oral contraceptive containing ethinyl estradiol and norgestimate or norethindrone	May reduce efficacy of hormonal contraceptives	Use alternative or back-up method for birth control
	Benzodiazepines (alprazolam, midazolam, triazolam)	Increased plasma concentrations of benzodiazepine	Dosage adjustment may be necessary if IV benzodiazepines are given concurrently
	Ketoconazole	Increased ketoconazole levels 5-fold	Avoid concurrent use
	Rifampin	Decreased aprepitant levels	Avoid concurrent use
	Diltiazem	Increased diltiazem and aprepitant levels	Monitor for adverse effects
	Paroxetine	Decreased paroxetine levels	Monitor if coadministering
Dimenhydrinate, diphenhydramine, hydroxyzine, meclizine	Alcohol, other antihistamines, opioids, sedative hypnotics, other CNS depressants	Additive CNS depression	Avoid concurrent use or warn patient of drowsiness and its consequences
	Aminoglycosides, ethacrynic acid, other ototoxic drugs	May mask indications of ototoxicity of these drugs	Avoid concurrent use

Continued

Table 20–11 ⊞ Drug Interactions: Selected Antiemetics—cont'd

Drug	Interacting Drug	Possible Effect	Implications
	Tricyclic antidepressants (TCAs), monoamine oxidase inhibitors, quinidine, and other drugs with anticholinergic properties	Additive anticholinergic effects	Avoid concurrent use or provide patient education about ways to reduce or treat anticholinergic effects
	Azole antifungals	Plasma levels (including metabolites) may be increased	Choose different antiemetic
	Macrolide antibiotics	Plasma levels (including metabolites) may be increased	Choose different antiemetic
	Serotonin reuptake inhibitors	Plasma levels (including metabolites) may be increased	Choose different antiemetic
Perphenazine	CYP 2D6 inhibitors tricyclic antidepressants and selective serotonin reuptake inhibitors	Concomitant administration of other drugs that inhibit the activity of P450 2D6 may acutely increase plasma concentrations	Close monitoring and dosage reduction may be necessary
Prochlorperazine, promethazine	Antihypertensives, nitrates, and acute ingestion of alcohol	Additive hypotensive effects	Avoid concurrent administration or monitor blood pressure closely
	Alcohol, antihistamines, antidepressants, opioids, sedative hypnotics, and other CNS depressants	Additive CNS depression May increase TCA serum levels	Avoid concurrent administration or warn about drowsiness and its risks; select different antiemetic or antidepressant other than TCA
	Antihistamines, antidepressants, atropine, haloperidol, other phenothiazines, and other drugs with anticholinergic properties	Additive anticholinergic effects	Avoid concurrent use or provide patient education about ways to reduce or treat anticholinergic effects
	Lithium	Lithium increases risk of extrapyramidal symptom (EPS) reactions; prochlorperazine may mask indications of lithium toxicity	Avoid concurrent use
	Antithyroid agents	Increased risk for agranulocytosis	Choose different antiemetic
	Antacids	Concurrent administration may decrease absorption	Separate administration or give antiemetic by IM or rectal route
Scopolamine	CNS sedatives	Increased sedation	Use concurrently with care
Trimethobenzamide	Alcohol, antihistamines, antidepressants, opioids, sedative hypnotics, and other CNS depressants	Additive CNS depression	Avoid concurrent use or warn patient of drowsiness and its consequences
Dronabinol	Alcohol, benzodiazepines, barbiturates, CNS depressants	Additive CNS depression	Write for smallest practical amount of dronabinol
	Tricyclic antidepressants (amitriptyline, amoxapine, desipramine,)	Additive tachycardia, hypertension, drowsiness	Avoid concurrent administration if possible
	Theophylline	antagonizes	
Dolasetron	Drugs that prolong QT interval		
Ondansetron	Potent inducers of CYP3A4 (i.e., phenytoin, carbamazepine, and rifampicin)	Clearance of ondansetron was significantly increased and ondansetron blood concentrations were decreased	No dosage adjustment necessary
	Apomorphine	Increased apomorphine levels	Avoid concomitant use
	P-glycoprotein inhibitors	Ondansetron levels increased	

Adverse Drug Reactions

The most common adverse reactions for antihistamines are drowsiness and the common anticholinergic effects of dry mouth, blurred vision, and urinary retention. Paradoxical excitation may occur in children. Pain at the injection site occurs in IM injections.

Phenothiazines produce drowsiness as well, but they also produce serious adverse reactions that sometimes occur even with short-term use and low doses. These reactions include extrapyramidal reactions such as dystonia, akathisia, and tardive dyskinesia. Other serious concerns are their ability to mask acute symptoms of surgical and neurological conditions and the potential for agranulocytosis 4 to 10 weeks after initiation of therapy.

Promethazine has been known to cause fatal respiratory depression in children younger than 2 years of age and has a Black-Box Warning regarding its use in children. In children older than age 2 years, the lowest effective dose should be used and coadministration of respiratory depressants should be avoided.

Other adverse reactions are associated with the anticholinergic effects of phenothiazines and include dry mouth, dry eyes, blurred vision, constipation, and urinary retention. They also discolor urine pink to reddish brown, and patients should be told that this reaction does not indicate hematuria.

The cannabinoid dronabinol may cause euphoria, depression, dizziness, paranoid thoughts, somnolence, and abnormal thoughts. Cardiac effects include palpitations, tachycardia, and hypotension. Seizures and seizure-like activity have been reported in patients receiving Marinol capsules in post-marketing surveillance.

The 5-HT$_3$ receptor antagonists have the common side effects of constipation, headache, fatigue, dizziness, and diarrhea. Less common but concerning are rare cases of tachycardia, bradycardia, hypotension, and QT prolongation.

The most frequently reported adverse effect of transdermal scopolamine is dry mouth. Some patients experience drowsiness, blurred vision, and dilated pupils. Patients have reported a withdrawal syndrome that occurs 24 hours or more after the patch has been removed, including symptoms of dizziness, nausea, vomiting, and headache.

Patients taking aprepitant for highly emetogenic chemotherapy reported greater fatigue (17.8% versus 11.8%), dizziness (6.6% versus 4.4%), and hiccups (10.8% versus 5.6%) than patients receiving standard therapy. Patients taking aprepitant were slightly more likely to experience elevated ALT/AST and BUN than patients receiving standard antiemetic therapy during clinical trials.

Drug Interactions

Antihistamines and phenothiazines have additive CNS depression with other drugs that produce CNS depression and additive anticholinergic effects with other drugs that have anticholinergic effects or adverse reactions.

Phenothiazines also have additive hypotensive effects with antihypertensive agents or acute ingestion of alcohol. Concurrent administration of lithium increases the risk for extrapyramidal reactions, and phenothiazines may mask the signs of lithium toxicity. Antithyroid agents increase the risk for agranulocytosis.

The cannabinoid dronabinol interacts with other CNS depressants, causing additive CNS depression with benzodiazepines, barbiturates, alcohol, opioids, antihistamines, muscle relaxants, and other CNS depressants. Dronabinol has been studied and administered with cytotoxic agents, anti-infective agents, sedatives, or opioid analgesics without significant adverse effects.

Aprepitant is an inducer of CYP 3A4 and can increase plasma concentrations of drugs that are metabolized via CYP 3A4, including hormonal contraceptives and some chemotherapy agents. Concurrent use of aprepitant and pimozide, terfenadine, astemizole, or cisapride is contraindicated due to potentially life-threatening reactions. These and additional drug interactions are listed in Table 20-11.

Clinical Use and Dosing

The only clinical use presented here is to treat nausea and vomiting. Table 20-12 shows the dosing schedules for each of the drugs for this purpose. Other uses for these drugs are discussed in Chapter 16.

Rational Drug Selection

Treatment of Nausea and Vomiting Due to Drugs or Gastroenteritis

Nausea and vomiting as an adverse effect of medication or gastroenteritis often improve with treatment using an antiemetic. Because of their low side-effect profile and tolerance, the 5-HT$_3$ receptor antagonists are being used extensively to treat nausea and vomiting. The phenothiazines are also a good choice for initial and short-term treatment of nausea, except in children. Trimethobenzamide is also effective. The antihistamines can also be used and, because they have less serious adverse reactions, are better for longer-term applications. All are available in a variety of dosage forms so that they need not be taken orally by a patient who is nauseated. Dronabinol is approved only for use in chemotherapy-associated nausea and vomiting and appetite stimulation. Aprepitant is approved for post-operative nausea and vomiting and in conjunction with other antiemetic agents for prevention of acute and delayed nausea and vomiting associated with initial and repeated doses of emetogenic cancer chemotherapy.

Motion Sickness

Antihistamines are useful for this indication because they act on the vestibular system and the CTZ to help control the nausea and vomiting associated with vestibular dysfunction. They also provide rapid onset of action and have a prolonged effect. Dimenhydrinate and meclizine are the most commonly used. Meclizine is also used to treat vertigo. The phenothiazines are not effective for motion sickness or vestibular disease because their site of action does not involve the vestibular system. Transdermal scopolamine is indicated for prevention of nausea and vomiting associated with motion

Table 20–12 ⊗ Dosage Schedule: Selected Antiemetics

Drug	Indications	Dosage Form	Dosage Schedule	Notes
Aprepitant Emend	Prevention of chemotherapy-induced nausea and vomiting Prevention of post-operative nausea and vomiting	Capsules: 40, 80, 125 mg	Prevention of chemotherapy-induced nausea and vomiting: Day 1: 125 mg PO Day 2: 80 mg PO Day 3: 80 mg PO Post-operative nausea and vomiting: 40 mg PO within 3 h of anesthesia	For chemotherapy-induced nausea and vomiting, patients are coadministered dexamethasone 12 mg day 1 and 8 mg days 2–4
Dimenhydrinate Dramamine Generic	Antiemetic	Tablets: 50 mg Chewable tablets: 50 mg Liquid: 12.5 mg/5 mL	*Children >12 yr and adults:* 50 mg PO/IM or 25 mg ER capsules q4h; not to exceed 400 mg/d; PR = 50–100 mg q6–8h	For motion sickness, give dose 1–2 h prior to departure or ER dose 12 h prior to departure
Dramamine Gravol		Chewable tablets: 50 mg Liquid: 12.5 mg/5 mL Quick-dissolve tablets: 15 mg Liquid: 15 mg/5 mL	*Children 6–12 yr:* 25–50 mg (PO/IM) q6–8h; not to exceed 150 mg/d *Children 2 to 5 yrs:* 12.5–25 mg (PO/IM) q 6–8 h, maximum dose 75 mg/day	Use calibrated measuring device when giving liquid doses
Gravol Generic		Rectal suppositories: 25, 50, 100 mg	*Children 8–12 yr:* PR = 25–50 mg q8–12 h *Children 6–8 yr:* 12.5–25 PR q8–12 h *Children 2–6 yr:* Up to 12.5–25 mg q6–8 h; not to exceed 75 mg/d	
Diphenhydramine Benadryl Generic	Antiemetic	Soft gels: 25 mg Tablets: 25 mg	*Adults:* 25–50 mg q6h PO; 10–50 mg q2–3h IM; not to exceed 300 mg/d	For motion sickness, give dose 1–2 h prior to departure or ER dose 12 h prior to departure
		Chewable tablets: 12.5 mg	*Children >20 lb (9.1 kg):* 12.5–25 mg 3–4 times daily (5 mg/kg) not to exceed 300 mg/d	
		Liquid: 6.25 mg/ 5mL	*Children:* 1–1.5 mg/kg q4–6h PO; not to exceed 300 mg/d	Use calibrated measuring device when giving liquid doses.
		Injection: 50 mg/mL	IM = 1.25 mg/kg qid; not to exceed 300 mg/d	Give IM into deep, well-developed muscle; avoid SC administration
Hydroxyzine Atarax Vistaril	Antiemetic	Tablets: 10, 25, 50 mg Tablets: 100 mg Capsules: 25, 50, 100 mg Injection: 25 mg/mL, 50 mg/mL	*Children >12 yr and adults:* 25–100 mg PO/IM tid or qid	Tablets may be crushed and capsules opened and administered with food or fluid for patients with difficulty in swallowing
		Syrup: 10 mg/5 mL	*Children 6–12 yr:* 12.5–25 mg PO/IM q6h *Children <6 yr:* 12.5 mg q6h (General calculation for children: 0.5 mg/kg q6h)	Give IM into deep, well-developed muscle using Z track. Do not use deltoid. Injection is painful. Rotate sites frequently. Avoid SC or IV administration.
Meclizine Dramamine Less Drowsy Antivert Generic	Motion sickness	Tablets: 12.5, 25, 50 mg Chewable tablets: 25 mg Capsules: 25 mg	*Children >12 yr and adults:* 25–50 mg	Take 1 h prior to travel. May repeat dose every 24 h for duration of journey

Table 20–12 ⊗ **Dosage Schedule: Selected Antiemetics—cont'd**

Drug	Indications	Dosage Form	Dosage Schedule	Notes
	Vertigo		Adults: 25–100 mg daily in divided doses	
	Nausea and vomiting in pregnancy		Lowest dose that relieves nausea	Pregnancy Category B
Prochlorperazine Compazine Generic	Antiemetic	Tablets: 5, 10, 25 mg Spansules (SR): 10, 15, 30 mg Syrup: 5 mg/5 mL Injection: 5 mg/mL Suppositories: 2.5, 5, 25 mg	*Children >12 yr and adults:* 5–10 mg PO/IM tid or qid; not to exceed 40 mg/d *Children 19–39 kg:* 2.5 mg PO/PR tid or 5 mg bid; not to exceed 15 mg/d *Children 15-18 kg:* 2.5 mg PO/PR bid or tid; not to exceed 10 mg/d *Children >2 yr or 10-14 kg:* 2.5 mg PO/PR qd or bid; not to exceed 7.5 mg/d	Do not crush or chew ER capsules. Administer with food or milk or a full glass of water to minimize GI distress. Dilute syrup in citrus or chocolate-flavored drinks. Give IM into deep, well-developed muscle. Keep patient recumbent for at least 30 min following injection to avoid hypotensive effects. Do not use in pediatric patients under 2 yr of age or under 20 lb.
Promethazine Phenergan Generic	Antiemetic	Tablets: 12.5, 25, 50 mg Syrup: 6.25 mg/5 mL Suppositories: 12.5, 25, 50 mg Injection: 25 mg/mL, 50 mg/mL	*Adults:* 25 mg PO/IM/PR q4h *Children >2 yr:* 0.25–0.5 mg/kg q4–6h PO/IM/PR. Do not exceed 25 mg/dose.	For motion sickness, give dose 1–2 h prior to departure. Administer with food, water, or milk to minimize GI distress. Tablets may be crushed and mixed with food or fluids for patients with difficulty in swallowing. Use calibrated measuring device when giving liquid doses. Give IM into deep, well-developed muscle; SC administration may cause tissue necrosis. Do not administer to children <2 yr. Use with extreme caution in children using the lowest, most-effective dose.
Trimethobenzamide Tigan Generic	Antiemetic	Capsules: 100, 250, 300 mg Injection: 100 mg/mL	*Adults:* 300 mg PO tid/qid; IM = 200 mg tid/qid *Children:* 15–20 mg/kg/day PO divided tid/qid OR *Children > 40 kg:* 300 mg tid/qid *Children 15–40 kg:* 100–200 mg PO tid/qid or 15 mg/kg/d in 3–4 divided doses *Children <15 kg:* 100 mg PR tid/qid	Capsules can be opened and contents mixed with food or fluid for patients with difficulty in swallowing. Inject deep into well-developed muscle to minimize tissue irritation.
Dronabinol Marinol	Refractory nausea and vomiting associated with cancer chemotherapy	Capsules: 2.5 mg, 5 mg, 10 mg	*Adults and children:* 5 mg/m² 1–3 h before chemotherapy. Then every 2–4 h after chemo. May increase as needed by increments of 2.5 mg/m² to a max of 15 mg/m²	Individualize the dosing

Continued

Table 20–12 ⊗ Dosage Schedule: Selected Antiemetics—cont'd

Drug	Indications	Dosage Form	Dosage Schedule	Notes
	Anorexia associated with weight loss in patients with AIDS		*Adults:* 2.5 mg bid before lunch and supper; dosage can be reduced to 2.5 qhs	
Dolasetron Anzemet	Prevention of nausea and vomiting after chemotherapy or surgery	Tablets: 50, 100 mg Injection solution: 20 mg/mL	*Children ≥16 yr and adults:* 100 mg within 1 h before chemotherapy or 2 h before surgery *Children 2 yr–16 yr:* 1.8 mg within 1 h of chemotherapy or 1.2 mg within 2 h before surgery	Dolasetron injection solution may be diluted in apple juice and taken orally. This solution is stable for 2 h.
Ondansetron Zofran Generic	Prevention of nausea and vomiting associated with chemotherapy Post-operative nausea and vomiting Gastroenteritis	Tablets: 4, 8 mg ODT (disintegrating tab): 4, 8 mg Solution: 4 mg/5 mL	*Adults:* 24 mg administered 30 min before the start of chemotherapy or 8 mg tid *Children 4–11 yr:* 4 mg tid *Infants and children < 40 kg:* 0.1 mg/kg/dose before induction of anesthesia *Children > 12 yr:* 4 mg *Adults:* 16 mg PO 1 h before induction of anesthesia, OR 4 mg IV *Infants and children 6 mo to 10 yr:* 8–15 kg: 2 mg/dose × 1 15–30 kg: 4 mg/dose × 1 > 30 kg: 8 mg/dose × 1	Routine use of ondasetron is not recommended in most cases of acute gastroenteritis.
Scopolamine Transderm Scop	Prevention of nausea and vomiting associated with motion sickness	Transdermal patch: 1.5 mg	*Adults:* Apply patch to hairless area behind one ear and leave in place for 3 days	Transdermal patch is programmed to deliver 1 mg over 3 days.

ER = extended release; PR = per rectum.

sickness in adults and is commonly used in patients who are cruising in large or small ships.

Vomiting Due to Gastroparesis

For this indication, prokinetic drugs are best. They are discussed later in this chapter.

Monitoring

When antiemetic drugs are used for a single dose or very short-term, no specific monitoring is required beyond that associated with the disease process and the potential fluid and electrolyte shifts that may result from vomiting. If treatment is needed for longer than a few days, the following monitoring parameters are suggested. Promethazine has been associated with bone marrow depression. A complete blood count (CBC) prior to initiation of therapy is appropriate. Phenothiazines have also been associated with blood dyscrasias that tend to occur between week 4 and week 10 of therapy. A CBC may be done prior to initiation and after 4 weeks of therapy.

Patient Education

Administration

These drugs should be taken as prescribed (Table 20-12). Each of them has special considerations related to administration,

which are presented in Table 20-12. All of the drugs used to treat motion sickness should be taken 1 to 2 hours prior to departure, except for extended-release dimenhydrinate, which is taken 12 hours before departure. For all liquid formulations, a calibrated measuring device should be used to attain an accurate dose. All injections should be administered deep into well-developed muscle, avoiding the deltoid and subcutaneous (SC) injections. A Z-track method of injection should also be used for hydroxyzine. All tablets except extended-release ones can be crushed or mixed with food, water, or milk to minimize GI distress and for patients who have difficulty with swallowing. Capsules can be opened and emptied to allow mixing for the same reasons. Transdermal scopolamine is applied to the hairless area behind one ear at least 4 hours before the antiemetic effect is needed and may be left in place for up to 3 days. If therapy is required for longer than 3 days, the patch should be removed and a new patch placed behind the other ear.

Adverse Reactions

Single-dose or short-term use have relatively few adverse reactions. All are associated with drowsiness, dry mouth, dry eyes, constipation, and urinary retention. Phenothiazines turn the urine pink to reddish brown. Patients need to be told that this effect does not constitute hematuria.

Longer-term administration of phenothiazines is not recommended because of potentially serious adverse reactions. Patients should be told the indications of dystonia, akathisia, and tardive dyskinesia and to stop the drug and report these immediately.

Phenergan should not be administered with other respiratory depressants in children.

Dronabinol (Marinol) may cause euphoria and behavior changes. Patients should not drive until they know how they will respond to the medication.

Scopolamine may cause dry mouth and, less frequently, drowsiness. Patients should wash their hands with soap and water after handling transdermal scopolamine (Transderm Scop) patches to avoid getting medication in their eyes. Temporary blurring of vision and pupil dilation may occur if unwashed hands come in contact with the eyes.

Lifestyle Management

Nausea and vomiting are often self-limiting disorders. Before drug therapy begins, unless there is clear indication of fluid or electrolyte disturbances, nonpharmacological interventions can be tried. Resting the GI tract for a brief time (8 hours) by taking only clear liquids in small amounts is often helpful. Clear liquids are those that can be held up to light and seen through. For infants, ORS (discussed in the Antidiarrheals section) such as Pedialyte may be used instead of other clear liquids. Formula and milk should be withheld for these 8 hours. For breastfed babies, continue breastfeeding, but nurse on only one side at each feeding during the first 8 hours. Older children and adults can take any clear liquid and require ORS only if they appear dehydrated. Remember, this treatment does not mean as much clear liquid as the patient can hold. Start with small amounts and gradually increase the intake.

After 8 hours without vomiting, start with bland food such as saltine crackers, honey on white bread, bland soup, rice, or mashed potatoes. For babies, start with applesauce, strained bananas, and rice cereal. If the baby takes only formula, give 1 or 2 oz less than usual with each feeding. Breastfed babies can return to regular breastfeeding after 1 hour without vomiting. Most patients will be back on a regular diet within 24 hours.

EMETICS

Poisoning is a serious problem in the United States, despite extensive prevention programs. According to the American Association of Poison Control Centers, 2.3 million poisoning cases are documented each year (Bronstein, Spyker, Cantilena, Rumack, & Dart, 2012). In the past, vomiting to remove a poison was advised in some circumstances. However, problems occurred with use of emetics, so they are no longer recommended. Poisoning is now treated with antidotes or gastric lavage. For this reason, emetics are not discussed in this book.

HISTAMINE₂ RECEPTOR ANTAGONISTS

Histamine₂ blockers (also known as histamine₂ antagonists [H₂RAs]) inhibit acid secretion by gastric parietal cells through a reversible blockade of histamine at histamine₂ receptors. They are used to reduce gastric acid in patients who are temporarily not taking anything by mouth and for prophylaxis and management of duodenal and gastric ulcers and GERD. They are also used to treat heartburn, acid indigestion, and "sour stomach."

Pharmacodynamics

Gastric parietal cells have three receptors that can be stimulated to cause the parietal cell to produce H^+: acetylcholine, gastrin, and histamine₂. H₂RAs are reversible competitive blockers of histamine at histamine₂ receptors. They are highly selective, do not affect histamine₁ receptors, and are not anticholinergic agents. They are potent inhibitors of all phases of gastric acid secretion, including that caused by muscarinic agonists and gastrin. Fasting and nocturnal secretions and those stimulated by food, insulin, caffeine, pentagastrin, and betazole are all inhibited. Because they do not inhibit acetylcholine, they reduce gastric acid secretion by only 35% to 50%.

The volume and hydrogen ion concentration of gastric juice, gastric emptying, and the lower esophageal sphincter pressure are all affected to varying degrees by different drugs in this class. Cimetidine (Tagamet), ranitidine (Zantac), and famotidine (Pepcid) have no effect on gastric emptying. Cimetidine and famotidine have no effect on lower esophageal sphincter pressure. Ranitidine, nizatidine (Axid), and famotidine have little or no effect on fasting or postprandial serum gastrin. Ranitidine does not affect pepsin secretion or pentagastrin-stimulated intrinsic factor secretion.

Ranitidine is 5 to 12 times more potent and famotidine is 30 to 60 times more potent than cimetidine in controlling gastric acid secretion, but there is no clear evidence that greater potency has any clinical advantage. Treatment failures have occurred with each of these drugs, and it is doubtful that treatment failure with one drug in the class can be corrected by changing drugs within the class.

Pharmacokinetics

Absorption and Distribution

All drugs in the class are well absorbed following oral administration (Table 20-13). The absorption of cimetidine, famotidine, and ranitidine may be decreased by antacids but is unaffected by food. The absorption of nizatidine is decreased by 10% by aluminum and magnesium hydroxides. With food, AUC and maximum concentration of nizatidine increases by 10%. Cimetidine and ranitidine also have IM routes of absorption. All agents enter breast milk and cerebrospinal fluid.

Metabolism and Excretion

All agents are metabolized to differing degrees by the CYP450 enzyme system of the liver and excreted in differing percentages as unchanged drug in the urine. Nizatidine has at least one metabolite that has histamine-blocking activity. All others are metabolized to inactive compounds.

Table 20–13 ▪▪ Pharmacokinetics: Histamine₂ Blockers

Drug	Onset	Peak	Duration	Protein Binding	Bioavailability	Half-Life	Metabolized	Elimination
Cimetidine	30 min	45–90 min	4–5 h	13%–25%	60%–70%	2 h	30%–40%	48% unchanged in urine
Famotidine	60 min	1–4 h	1–4 h	15%–20%	40%–45%	2.5–3.5 h	30%–35%	25%–30% unchanged in urine
Nizatidine	60 min	0.5–3 h	UK	35%	>90%	1–2 h	<18%	60% unchanged in urine, <6% in feces
Ranitidine	60 min	1–3 h	1–3 h	15%	50%–60%	2–3 h	<10%	30%–35% unchanged in urine

UK = unknown.

Pharmacotherapeutics

Precautions and Contraindications

Renal impairment requires cautious use of the H₂RAs and dosage adjustments. Patients with renal impairment are more subject to the CNS adverse reactions. Older adults may have reduced renal function, and these drugs should be used cautiously with this age group. Cimetidine seems to have the most problems with decreased renal clearance, and ranitidine the fewest.

Hepatocellular injury may occur with nizatidine, as evidenced by elevated liver enzymes (alanine transaminase [ALT], aspartate aminotransferase [AST], or alkaline phosphatase). These abnormalities are reversible with discontinuation of the drug. Because of this risk, it should not be used for patients with a history of liver disease.

Occasional reversible hepatitis or hepatocellular disorders have occurred with ranitidine. It is contraindicated for patients with a history of liver disease.

H₂RAs are Pregnancy Category B; however, there are no adequate and well-controlled studies of these agents in pregnant women. They should be used only when the potential benefits outweigh the potential risks to the fetus.

These drugs vary in their excretion in breast milk. Cimetidine is excreted in breast milk in milk:plasma ratios of 5:1 to 12:1. The potential daily dose to the infant is 6 mg; nursing should be avoided. Famotidine is excreted in the breast milk of rats. It is not known whether it is excreted in human breast milk. The decision to discontinue the drug is made based on the need of the mother for the drug. Nizatidine is excreted in breast milk in a concentration of 0.1% of the oral dose in proportion to plasma concentrations. Once again, the decision to discontinue the drug is made based on the need of the mother for the drug. Ranitidine is excreted in breast milk with milk:plasma ratios of 1:1 to 6.7:1. Exercise caution when giving to a nursing mother.

There has been extensive study of the H₂RAs in the past few years as a part of the Best Pharmaceuticals for Children Act. The safety and efficacy of ranitidine have been established in children aged 1 month to 16 years. Famotidine is labeled safe for infants and children as young as neonates, although children younger than 1 year have experienced agitation that stopped when famotidine was stopped (FDA, 2010).

Adverse Drug Reactions

All of these drugs have similar adverse reaction profiles. Cimetidine appears to have the greatest degree of antiandrogenic reactions (e.g., gynecomastia and impotence). Reversible CNS adverse reactions (e.g., mental confusion, agitation, psychosis, depression, and disorientation) have also occurred with this drug.

Hematological adverse reactions include agranulocytosis, granulocytopenia, thrombocytopenia, and aplastic anemia. These reactions are rare but should be monitored. Other less common adverse drug reactions include drowsiness, dizziness, constipation or diarrhea, and nausea. Adverse drug reactions related to liver function are discussed in the Precautions and Contraindications section.

Drug Interactions

Many of the drug interactions with this class of drugs are related to their metabolism by the CYPP450 enzyme system of the liver. Cimetidine is the most problematic because it uses several isoenzymes (CYP1A2, CYP2C9, and CYP2D6). Any drug metabolized extensively by these isoenzymes will have its metabolism inhibited by cimetidine, with a risk for increased plasma levels and toxicity for that drug. Famotidine, nizatidine, and ranitidine have less effect on the CYP system and use a narrower number of isoenzymes in their metabolism. Although they still have drug interactions, they are fewer than with cimetidine. Table 20-14 provides a list of drug interactions for the various histamine₂ blockers.

Clinical Use and Dosing

Gastroesophageal Reflux Disease

Histamine₂ receptor antagonists are available OTC and are a popular self-treatment for heartburn and GERD. They are most effective if used as on-demand therapy for relief of GERD symptoms (Hershcovici & Fass, 2011). Owing to development of tachyphylaxis, H₂RAs are not recommended for first-line continuous treatment of GERD, but a dose before bed may help patients on PPIs with nighttime reflux (Katz, Gerson, & Vela, 2013). If no esophageal erosive disease is present, H₂RAs may be used as maintenance therapy after PPI treatment (Katz et al, 2013). Once-daily dosing of H₂RAs is not effective in treating GERD.

Table 20–14 ▦ Drug Interactions: Histamine₂ Blockers

Drug	Interacting Drug	Possible Effect	Implications
Cimetidine	Benzodiazepines, caffeine, calcium channel blockers, carbamazepine, labetalol, metoprolol, metronidazole, pentoxifylline, propafenone, propranolol, quinidine, quinine, sulfonylureas, tacrine, theophylline, triamterene, tricyclic antidepressants, valproic acid, warfarin*	Decreased hepatic metabolism of these drugs	Select different histamine₂ blocker Monitor drug levels of those with narrow therapeutic range or potential for cardiac rhythm disturbances
	Ferrous salts, indomethacin, ketoconazole, tetracyclines	Action of these drugs decreased because of decreased absorption	Avoid concurrent administration; separate doses or select different histamine₂ blocker
	Digoxin	Decreased serum digoxin concentrations during coadministration	Select different histamine₂ blocker
	Flecainide	Increased drug effects of flecainide	Select different histamine₂ blocker
	Narcotic analgesics	Toxic effects (e.g., respiratory depression) may be increased	Select different histamine₂ blocker
	Procainamide	Increased plasma levels of procainamide and its cardioactive metabolite by decreasing renal tubular secretion	Select different histamine₂ blocker; ranitidine was shown to have similar action in only one study, so best not to choose that drug
	Tocainide	Decreased drug effects of tocainide	Select different histamine₂ blocker
	Cigarette smoking	Smoking reverses cimetidine-induced inhibition of nocturnal gastric secretion, hindering ulcer healing	Avoid cigarette smoking
Famotidine	Ketoconazole	Action of drug decreased by reduced absorption	Separate administration by at least 1 h and give ketoconazole first
	Food	May increase bioavailability of famotidine	No clinical significance
Nizatidine	Salicylates	Increased serum salicylate levels when given to patients receiving high doses (3.9 g/d) of salicylate	Monitor salicylate levels or select different histamine₂ blocker
	Food	May increase bioavailability of nizatidine	No clinical significance
Ranitidine	Diazepam	Decreased drug effects of diazepam due to decreased drug absorption	Separate doses by at least 1 h and give diazepam first
	Sulfonylureas	Increased hypoglycemic effects of glipizide or glyburide	Dosage adjustments may be needed
	Warfarin	May interfere with warfarin clearance; data conflicting	Monitor PT/INR more closely; may need dosage adjustment
All histamine₂ blockers	Alcohol	May increase blood alcohol levels	Avoid use of alcohol
	Antacids, anticholinergics, metoclopramide	May decrease absorption of cimetidine, ranitidine; less effect on nizatidine and famotidine	Separate dose by at least 1 h for cimetidine and ranitidine; no special precautions needed for nizatidine and famotidine

INR = international normalized ratio; PT = prothrombin time.

*Although interactions with these drugs are not listed for other histamine₂ blockers, some effect is probable, even though it is not to the same extent.

Infants and children with GERD have also been successfully treated with histamine$_2$ blockers for several years with good response and few adverse reactions. The international consensus on the diagnosis and management of gastroesophageal reflux (GER) and GERD reached by the North American Society for Pediatric Gastroenterology, Hepatology, and Nutrition (NASPGHAN) and European Society for Pediatric Gastroenterology, Hepatology, and Nutrition (ESPGHAN) no longer recommends empiric treatment with H$_2$RAs in infants (Vandenplas et al, 2009). Dosing of histamine$_2$ blockers for infants and children is shown in Table 20-15. Once again, twice-daily dosing is required.

Table 20–15 ⊗ Dosage Schedule: Histamine$_2$ Blockers

Drug	Indication	Dosage Form	Initial Dose	Maintenance Dose
Cimetidine Tagamet Tagamet HB 200	Short-term treatment of active duodenal ulcer	Tablets: 200, 300, 400, 800 mg Liquid: 300 mg/5 mL Injection: 300 mg/2 mL	*Adults:* 800 mg at bedtime or 300 mg qid with meals and at bedtime or 400 mg bid *Infants:* 10–20 mg/kg/d divided q 6 to 12 h *Children:* 20–40 mg/kg/d in 4 divided doses	*Adults:* 400 mg at bedtime; dosage not to exceed 2.4 g/d. In severe renal impairment, use 300 mg every 8–12 h. *Children:* 20 mg/kg/d; 10–15 mg/kg/d in renal impairment
	Duodenal ulcer prophylaxis		*Adults:* 800 mg at bedtime	Same
	Treatment of active benign gastric ulcer		*Adults:* 800 mg at bedtime or 300 mg qid with meals and at bedtime	800 mg at bedtime. In severe renal impairment, use 300 mg every 8–12 h. No information concerning usefulness of treatment periods >8 wk.
	GERD		*Adults:* 800 mg bid in morning and at bedtime or 400 mg qid with meals and at bedtime *Children:* 20–40 mg/kg/d in 4 divided doses	*Adults:* Same dose for up to 12 wk. Use >12 wk has not been established. May go as high as 600 mg qid if needed. In severe renal impairment, use 300 mg every 8–12 h.
	Pathological hypersecretory conditions		*Adults:* 300 mg to 600 mg qid with meals and at bedtime	*Children:* 20 mg/kg/d; 10–15 mg/kg/d if renal impairment Individualize dose. Do not exceed 2,400 mg/d. Continue as long as clinically indicated.
	Heartburn, indigestion, sour stomach		*Adults:* 200 mg (OTC) 30 min before a meal. Max 2 tablets/24 h.	Take up to 400 mg bid. Do not take maximum dose for more than 2 wk without consulting health-care provider.
Famotidine Pepcid Generic	Short-term treatment of active duodenal ulcer	Tablets: 10, 20, 40 mg Powder for oral suspension: 40 mg/5 mL when reconstituted Injection: 10 mg/mL	*Adults:* 40 mg/d at bedtime or ≤20 mg bid (in morning and at bedtime) *Children:* 1–2 mg/kg/d in 1 or 2 divided doses	*Adults:* 20 mg at bedtime for up to 8 wk. Most heal in 4 wk. If CCr <10 mL/min, give 20 mg at bedtime or increase dosing interval to 36–48 h. *Children:* Same dose for up to 8 wk. Most heal in 4 wk.
	Duodenal ulcer prophylaxis		*Adults:* 20 mg at bedtime	Same

Table 20–15 ✂ Dosage Schedule: Histamine₂ Blockers—cont'd

Drug	Indication	Dosage Form	Initial Dose	Maintenance Dose
	Treatment of benign active gastric ulcer		*Adults:* 40 mg at bedtime	Same dose. If CCr <10 mL/min, give 20 mg at bedtime or increase dosing interval to 36–48 h. No data to support treatment beyond 8 wk.
	GERD		*Adults:* 20 mg bid (in morning and at bedtime) *Children:* 1–2 mg/kg/d in 1 or 2 divided doses	*Adults:* 20 mg for up to 6 wk. If erosive disease, 20–40 mg bid for up to 12 wk. *Children:* Same dose. Treatment trial for 2–4 wk.
Pepcid Complete	Heartburn, acid indigestion, and sour stomach	Chewable tablet: Famotidine 10 mg, calcium carbonate 800 mg, magnesium hydroxide 165 mg	*Adults:* Relief: 10 mg (1 tablet) with water Prophylaxis: 10 mg 1 h prior to meal that is expected to cause symptoms *Adults and children >12 yr:* Chew and swallow 1 tablet prn; do not exceed 2 tablets in 24 h.	Can be used up to bid for <2 wk
Nizatidine Axid	Short-term treatment of active duodenal ulcer	Capsule: 150, 300 mg Solution: 15 mg/ mL	*Adults:* 300 mg at bedtime or 150 mg bid (in morning and at bedtime) *Infants 6 mo to Children 11 yr:* 5–10 mg/kg/d divided bid	300 mg at bedtime. If CCr 20–50 mL/min, give 150 mg at bedtime. If CCr <20 mL/min, give 150 mg every 2 or 3 d.
	Maintenance of healed duodenal ulcer		*Adults:* 150 mg at bedtime	150 mg at bedtime
	GERD		*Adults and children >12 yr:* 150 mg bid (in morning and at bedtime)	150 mg bid
Ranitidine Zantac Generic	Short-term treatment of active duodenal ulcer	Tablets: 75, 150, 300 mg Effervescent tablets: 150 mg Geldose: capsules: 150 mg Syrup: 15 mg/mL Efferdose: granules: 150 mg	*Adults:* 100–150 mg bid (in morning and at bedtime) or 300 mg at bedtime *Infants and children <16 yr:* 4–8 mg/kg/day, max 300 mg/day	150 mg at bedtime. If CCr <50 mL/min, give 150 mg at bedtime.
	Duodenal ulcer prophylaxis		*Adults:* 150 mg at bedtime	150 mg at bedtime
	Treatment of benign active gastric ulcer		*Adults:* 150 mg bid (in morning and at bedtime)	150 mg at bedtime
	GERD		*Adults:* 150 mg bid (in morning and at bedtime); if erosive disease, give 150 mg qid *Infants and children < 6 yr:* 4–10 mg/kg/d, max 300 mg/d	*Adults:* 150 mg bid. If CCr <50 mL/min, give 150 mg at bedtime. If erosive disease, give 150 mg bid.
	Pathologic hypersecretory conditions Heartburn, acid indigestion, and sour stomach		*Children:* 2–4 mg/kg/d in 2 divided doses *Adults:* 150 mg bid (in morning and at bedtime) *Adults:* Relief: 75 mg up to bid	*Children:* 2 mg/kg/d in 2 divided doses Individualize dose; doses up to 6 g/d have been used Can be used up to bid for <2 wk

GERD = gastroesophageal reflux disease.

For all children <12 years of age, consultation with pediatric specialist is advised.

A more detailed discussion of the management of GERD is found in Chapter 35.

Peptic Ulcer Disease

With the advent of the discovery that the cause of PUD is usually an infection rather than excessive acid due to stress, diet, smoking, alcohol consumption, and NSAIDs, the treatment pattern has changed. Most patients will have tried an OTC H$_2$RA before they present with peptic ulcer symptoms. There is no treatment protocol that includes histamine$_2$ blockers when eradication of *H. pylori* as the source of the ulcer is required. Continued acid suppression may be accomplished with H$_2$RAs after the peptic ulcer has healed. A more detailed discussion of the management of PUD is found in Chapter 35.

Heartburn, Acid Indigestion, and "Sour Stomach"

Relief of symptoms may be provided by OTC use of H$_2$RAs. However, it is important for patients to be informed about the potential for drug interactions.

All Uses

Regardless of the reason for which the H$_2$RA is prescribed, consideration of renal function is important in determining dosage. In the presence of renal impairment, dosage intervals need to be increased. For cimetidine, the interval is increased if the renal impairment is severe; for famotidine, it is increased if creatinine clearance (CCr) is less than 10 mL/min; and for nizatidine and ranitidine, if CCr is less than 50 mL/min.

Rational Drug Selection

No specific H$_2$RA is preferred over another for effectiveness. Choice is based on cost and whether the patient is taking other drugs that might have interactions with the specific H$_2$RA.

Cost

Generic formulations are always less expensive than brand names. OTC drugs are usually less expensive than prescriptions, but because their dose is lower, the cost difference is lost in the increased number of pills required.

Other Drugs

Cimetidine has the most drug interaction potential. Other histamine$_2$ blockers have fewer listed drug interactions.

Monitoring

Because of the potential for hepatocellular damage, patients who require higher doses or more than short-term use of this class of drugs should have laboratory testing of liver function prior to initiation of therapy and at regular intervals throughout therapy.

Renal impairment influences drug dosing for all drugs in this class. Patients who require higher doses or more than short-term therapy or for whom renal impairment is a likely risk (e.g., older adults) should have renal function assessment done prior to initiation of therapy.

Patient Education

Administration

Instruct patients to take the drug as prescribed for the full course of therapy, even if they are feeling better. If a dose is missed, it should be taken as soon as remembered but not if it is almost time for the next dose. They should not double doses.

H$_2$RA should be taken with meals or immediately afterward and at bedtime to achieve the best effects. Doses taken once daily are best taken at bedtime. Oral suspensions are shaken prior to administration, and unused portions are discarded after 30 days. The foil is removed from ranitidine effervescent tablets or granules, and they are dissolved in 6 to 8 oz of water before they are taken. The available dosage forms of H$_2$RAs are found in Table 20-15.

If the patient is also taking antacids or other drugs whose interaction with H$_2$RA produces interference with absorption, the drugs' administration should be separated by at least 30 minutes to 1 hour. Sucralfate should be taken 2 hours after the H$_2$RA.

Patients taking OTC preparations are not to take the maximum doses continuously for more than 2 weeks without consulting their health-care provider. A diagnostic work-up is in order under these circumstances.

Adverse Reactions

H$_2$RA may cause drowsiness or dizziness. Caution patients to avoid driving or other activities requiring alertness until their response to the drug is known.

For male patients taking cimetidine, warn about the potential for gynecomastia and impotence. Because other drugs in the class are less likely to cause these problems, a different drug may be selected.

Advise patients to report the onset of black, tarry stools. They are not adverse reactions to the drug but may indicate GI bleeding. Sore throat, diarrhea, rash, confusion, or hallucinations should also be reported promptly. These adverse reactions may require dosage alteration or discontinuation of the drug. Increasing the fluid and fiber in the diet may minimize constipation.

Lifestyle Management

Smoking interferes with the absorption of H$_2$RA and increases gastric acid secretion. Advise the patient to stop smoking. Alcohol and products containing aspirin or NSAIDs and some foods may also increase gastric acid secretion; they should be avoided. Other lifestyle modifications are discussed in Chapter 35.

PROKINETICS

Prokinetic drugs, also known as gastrointestinal stimulants, stimulate the motility of the GI tract without stimulating gastric, biliary, or pancreatic secretions. These drugs are used in the management of a wide range of disorders in which reduced GI motility is a problem, including gastroparesis associated with diabetes mellitus, GERD, and emesis associated with cancer chemotherapy. Only one drug, metoclopramide (Reglan, Metalov ODT), remains in this class since the removal of cisapride (Propulsid) from the market in 2004; metoclopramide will be discussed in this section.

Pharmacodynamics

Metoclopramide stimulates motility in the upper GI tract. Its mode of action is unclear but appears to be related to sensitizing tissues to the action of acetylcholine. The action does not depend on an intact vagal innervation system, but anticholinergic drugs can reverse the action. This drug increases the tone and amplitude of gastric contractions, relaxes the pyloric sphincter and duodenal bulb, and increases peristalsis of the duodenum and jejunum, resulting in accelerated gastric emptying and increased speed of gastric transit. It has almost no effect on the colon or gallbladder, nor does it stimulate gastric, biliary, or pancreatic secretions. For patients with GERD secondary to decreased lower esophageal sphincter pressure (LESP), metoclopramide produces dose-related increases in LESP. These effects begin at doses as low as 5 mg and continue through 20 mg doses.

Metoclopramide is a dopamine receptor antagonist in the CNS, including the chemoreceptor trigger zone leading to prevention of emesis (Taketomo et al, 2012). Metoclopramide has actions similar to the phenothiazines and other dopamine antagonists and produces sedation and may cause tardive dyskinesia or EPS. It also induces release of prolactin and transiently increases circulating aldosterone levels.

Pharmacokinetics

Absorption and Distribution

Metoclopramide is well absorbed after oral administration (Table 20-16) and has an injectable formulation. It has low protein binding and high bioavailability.

Metoclopramide is widely distributed throughout body tissues, crosses the blood–brain barrier and the placenta, and enters breast milk in concentrations greater than in plasma.

Metabolism and Excretion

Metoclopramide is partially metabolized by the liver. Because it is excreted in urine, clearance is affected by renal function. In patients whose creatinine clearance is less than 40 mL/min, the recommended dose is cut in half.

Pharmacotherapeutics

Precautions and Contraindications

Metoclopramide has a Black-Box Warning because of the risk of developing tardive dyskinesia. The risk for tardive dyskinesia increases with the length of treatment. Metoclopramide should be discontinued if patients develop signs of movement disorder. Treatment should not exceed 12 weeks, except in rare cases.

Metoclopramide is contraindicated in the presence of disorders in which stimulation of GI motility might be dangerous (GI hemorrhage, mechanical obstruction, new surgery on the GI tract, or perforation). Its dopamine-associated activity affects the CNS, and the drug is used cautiously with patients who have a history of depression. Depression with symptoms ranging from mild to severe, including suicide ideation, have been reported. Caution for patients who are at risk for EPS is also required. Metoclopramide is contraindicated in patients with known hypersensitivity to the drug and patients with pheochromocytoma, because the drug may cause a hypertensive crisis. Because metoclopramide is excreted primarily through the kidneys, it should be used with caution for patients with renal impairment. Dosage adjustments are mentioned above. It undergoes minimal hepatic metabolism and is safe to administer to patients with impaired hepatic function as long as their renal function is normal.

Metoclopramide is Pregnancy Category B; however, there are no adequate and well-controlled studies in pregnant women. Case reports to date have not been associated with fetal harm, but the drug should be prescribed only when the benefits clearly outweigh the risks to the fetus.

Metoclopramide is excreted in breast milk and concentrates at about twice the plasma level at 2 hours after taking the dose. However, in a mother taking 30 mg/day, the infant would receive less than 45 mg/day, which is still much less than the recommended maximum dose for infants. Exercise caution when giving to a nursing mother, but recognize that there appears to be little, if any, risk to the infant.

The safety and effectiveness of metoclopramide have not been established in infants and children. Caution should be used in neonates due to decreased clearance of metoclopramide and are more susceptible to methemoglobinemia. Movement disorders and EPS are more frequent in children than in adults taking metoclopramide.

Adverse Drug Reactions

The most serious adverse reaction are EPS, including acute dystonic reactions and the development of tardive dyskinesia

Table 20–16 Pharmacokinetics: Prokinetic Agents

	Onset	Peak	Duration	Protein Binding	Bioavailability	Half-Life	Elimination
Metoclopramide	30–60 m	1–2 h	1–2 h	30%	65%–95%	2.5–5 h	85% in urine after
PO IM	10–15 m	1–2 h	1–2 h	30%	65%–95%	2.5–5 h	72 h (25% as unchanged drug); clearance affected by renal function

and parkinsonian-like symptoms. Children and young adults more frequently develop EPS with metoclopromide use. Metoclopromide should be discontinued in any patient exhibiting movement disorders. There have been rare reports of neuroleptic malignant syndrome in patients taking metoclopramide. Other adverse reactions associated with metoclopramide include depression, dizziness, diarrhea, and hypoglycemia in patients with diabetes. Less common adverse reactions include galactorrhea, amenorrhea, gynecomastia, impotence secondary to hyperprolactinemia, and fluid retention secondary to transient elevations in aldosterone. Approximately 20% to 30% of all patients taking this drug experience some adverse reaction. The incidence correlates with the dose and duration of therapy.

Drug Interactions

Drug interactions with metoclopramide are largely related to its cholinergic and dopaminergic activities. Additive CNS depression occurs with other CNS depressants, and increased risk of EPS occurs with other drugs that have the potential for EPS. Drugs with anticholinergic effects reverse the action of metoclopramide, and the reverse is also true. There is a potential for hypertensive crisis if administered with MAOIs. Table 20-17 provides a more detailed list of these drug interactions.

Clinical Use and Dosing

Gastroesophageal Reflux Disease

The principal effect of metoclopramide in the management of GERD is on symptoms of postprandial and daytime heartburn. For adults, if symptoms occur throughout the day, a dose of 10 mg taken 30 minutes prior to each meal and at bedtime is recommended (Table 20-18). When symptoms are confined to specific situations, such as after the evening meal, a single 10 to 20 mg dose 30 minutes prior to that meal or at bedtime is effective in preventing the symptoms.

Occasionally, patients who are more sensitive to the therapeutic dose (e.g., older adults) require only 5 mg per dose. Neonatal dosing of metoclopramide (oral or IV) for GERD is 0.1 to 0.15 mg/kg/dose every 6 hours; avoid doses greater than 0.15 mg/kg/dose. Metoclopramide doses for gastroesophageal reflux in infants and children are 0.4 to 0.8 mg/kg/day divided in four doses (30 minutes prior to each meal). For patients whose CCr is less than 40 mL/min, doses are reduced (see above).

Nausea and Vomiting

Metoclopramide's action in the chemoreceptor trigger zone prevents nausea and vomiting. Post-operative nausea and vomiting in children 14 years of age or younger may be treated with 0.1 to 0.2 mg/kg IV metoclopramide with a maximum dose of 10 mg. Adults and children older than age 14 years are dosed at 10 mg every 6 to 8 hours to treat postoperative nausea and vomiting. Chemotherapy-induced emesis in adults and children is treated with 1 to 2 mg/kg/dose every 2 to 4 hours, with a maximum of 5 doses per day. If higher doses are used, such as with chemotherapy, the patient should be pretreated with diphenhydramine to prevent EPS (Taketomo et al, 2012).

Diabetic Gastroparesis

Metoclopramide has an indication for treatment of diabetic gastroparesis. Dosage is 10 mg 30 minutes before meals and

Table 20–17 ⚏ Drug Interactions: Prokinetic Agents

Drug	Interacting Drug	Possible Effect	Implications
Metoclopramide	Alcohol, antidepressants, antihistamines, opioids, and sedative hypnotics	Additive CNS depression; increases rate of absorption of alcohol	Avoid concurrent use or warn of potential CNS depression
	Haloperidol, phenothiazines, other drugs with EPS effects	Increased risk of extrapyramidal reactions	Avoid concurrent use; select different prokinetic
	Anticholinergics and opioids	Effects of metoclopramide on GL motility may antagonize these drugs	If not used therapeutically, avoid concurrent use
	Cimetidine	Reduced bioavailability of cimetidine	Select different histamine$_2$ blocker
	Digoxin	Decreased absorption, plasma levels, and therapeutic effects	Capsules, elixir, and tablets with high dissolution rate are least affected; use these formulations if both drugs must be given
	Levodopa	These drugs have opposite effects on dopamine receptors: bioavailability of levodopa increased; effects of metoclopramide decreased	Avoid concurrent use; metoclopramide is relatively contraindicated for patients with Parkinson's disease
	Monoamine oxidase inhibitors (MAOIs)	Metoclopramide releases catecholamines that may produce hypertension in patients taking MAOIs	Use cautiously concurrently, if at all; monitor blood pressure closely

Table 20–18 ⊗ Dosage Schedule: Prokinetic Agents

Drug	Indication	Available Dosage	Dosage Schedule	Notes
Metoclopramide Reglan Generic	GERD	Tablets: 5 mg Tablets: 10 mg Syrup: 5 mg/5 mL Injection: 5 mg/mL	*Adults:* Treatment: 10–15 mg qid (30 min before meals and at bedtime) Prophylaxis: 20 mg at bedtime *Children:* 0.4–0.8 mg/kg/d in 4 divided doses (30 min before meals and at bedtime)	Some patients respond to doses as low as 5 mg. Dose not to exceed 0.5 mg/kg/d. Therapy not to exceed 8 wk. Patients with CCr <40 mL/min, initiate therapy with half the recommended dose.
	Diabetic gastroparesis		*Adults:* 10 mg qid (30 min before meals and at bedtime)	

GERD = gastroesophageal reflux disease.

at bedtime for 2 to 8 weeks. The route of administration is based on the severity of symptoms. If only the earliest manifestation of gastroparesis is present, oral administration is adequate. If the symptoms are more severe, parenteral therapy with 10 mg IV over 1 to 2 minutes for up to 10 days may be needed before oral therapy can be initiated. Rectal formulations can be made by a pharmacist to avoid the IV route. The suppositories each contain 25 mg of metoclopramide in polyethylene glycol. One suppository is administered 30 to 60 minutes before each meal and at bedtime. After symptoms are resolved (no more than 8 weeks of therapy), the drug is stopped and reinstituted at the earliest indications of symptom return.

Diabetics often experience renal impairment. Because metoclopramide is excreted principally by the kidney, those patients with CCr below 40 mL/min should have their therapy initiated at approximately half the recommended dosage. Depending on clinical efficacy and safety considerations, the dosage may be increased or decreased as appropriate.

Rational Drug Selection

Efficacy

Metoclopramide has demonstrated limited symptomatic improvement and endoscopically demonstrated esophageal healing for patients with GERD. Given its significantly higher cost and increased adverse effects, it is difficult to justify its use in place of H_2RAs or PPIs.

Length of Therapy

Metoclopramide is not used for management of GERD if treatment must be long-term. With longer than 8 weeks of therapy, there is a much higher risk for adverse reactions, including EPS.

Concomitant Diseases

Metoclopramide should be used cautiously for patients with diseases that place them at risk for EPS disorders or for patients taking drugs that place them at risk for these

disorders. Other considerations based on concomitant disorders are discussed in the Precautions and Contraindications section.

Monitoring

Because of the need to adjust dosage in the presence of renal impairment, renal function should be assessed before therapy with metoclopramide is begun. Patients should be educated about and monitored for movement disorders or EPS. No other monitoring is required except that for the disease process being treated.

Patient Education

Administration

Advise the patient to take the drug exactly as prescribed (see Table 20-18). Metoclopramide is taken 30 minutes before each meal and at bedtime. If a dose is missed, it should be taken as soon as the patient remembers unless it is almost time for the next dose. Patients should not double doses or exceed the recommended dose.

Adverse Reactions

Metoclopramide may cause drowsiness. Caution patients to avoid driving or other activities that require alertness until their response to the drug is known. Concurrent use of other CNS depressants, including alcohol, makes this problem worse and causes additive CNS depression.

Warn patients taking metoclopramide to notify their health-care provider immediately if involuntary movement of the eyes, face, or limbs occurs, which may be EPS-related. Depression may occur, and any change in mood should be reported to their providers.

Lifestyle Management

Lifestyle modifications are tried before any drug in the management of both GERD and diabetic gastroparesis. First, patients should try to avoid alcohol, NSAIDs, large meals, fatty foods, chocolate, caffeine, citrus, and food or fluid intake within 3 hours of going to bed at night. They should also attempt smoking cessation, weight loss, and sleeping with the head of the bed elevated. These modifications are discussed in more detail in Chapter 35.

PROTON PUMP INHIBITORS

PPIs are antisecretory drugs used to treat gastric conditions characterized by hyperacidity. They are used for erosive gastritis, GERD, and Zollinger–Ellison syndrome and as part of a multidrug regimen for short-term treatment of active PUD, especially duodenal ulcers caused by *H. pylori*.

Pharmacodynamics

PPIs do not exhibit anticholinergic or histamine$_2$-blockade properties but suppress gastric acid secretion These drugs reduce H^+ secretion by inhibition of the $H^+/K^+/ATPase$ enzyme system at the secretory surface of the parietal cell itself to block the final step in H^+ secretion. The effect is dose-related and inhibits basal and stimulated acid secretion regardless of the stimulus. They reduce gastric acid by more than 90% and frequently produce achlorhydria. Serum gastrin levels increase parallel with inhibition of the acid secretion. The decrease in acid secretion lasts for up to 72 hours after each dose. Gastric acid secretion begins within 3 to 5 days after the drug is discontinued and returns to pretreatment levels within 1 to 2 weeks with omeprazole (Prilosec), 4 weeks with esomeprazole (Nexium) and lansoprazole (Prevacid), or 3 months with pantoprazole (Protonix).

Normal physiological effects related to suppression of gastric acid secretion result in decreased blood flow to the antrum, pylorus, and duodenal bulb. Increased serum pepsinogen levels and decreased pepsin activity also occur. As with other drugs that increase gastric pH, related increases in nitrate-reducing bacteria and elevation of nitrate

concentration in gastric juice occur in patients with gastric ulcer. Compensatory increases in serum gastrin levels develop initially, but no further increase occurs with continued treatment, and there are no apparent ill effects from this increase.

Pharmacokinetics

Absorption and Distribution

All of the PPIs are acid labile and so most are formulated as enteric-coated tablets or granules (Table 20-19). Absorption is rapid and begins after the granules leave the stomach and reach the less acidic duodenum. Peak plasma concentrations are approximately proportional, but because of a saturable first-pass effect, omeprazole has a greater-than-linear response when given in doses above 40 mg. Esomeprazole peak increases proportionally when the dose is increased, and there is a three-fold increase in the AUC from 20 to 40 mg. The AUC is decreased by 43% to 53% after food intake compared to fasting conditions for this drug. Esomeprazole should be taken at least 1 hour before meals.

The peak and AUC of lansoprazole are diminished by 50% to 70% if the drug is given after food as opposed to the fasting state. It should be given on an empty stomach. When pantoprazole is given with food, absorption may be delayed by 2 hours or longer. Taking rabeprazole (Aciphex) with a

---

On The Horizon | **ILAPRAZOLE**

Ilaprazole is a proton pump inhibitor developed by Il-Yang Pharmaceutical (Korea) and is approved for use in Korea and China. It has completed phase II trials in the United States.

Table 20–19 ⊞ Pharmacokinetics: Proton Pump Inhibitors

Drug	Onset	Peak	Duration	Protein Binding	Bioavailability	Half-Life	Elimination
Esomeprazole	UK	1.5 h	UK	97%	64% (single dose); 90% (multiple doses)	1–1.5 h	80% in urine as metabolite; <1% unchanged drug
Lansoprazole	1 h	1.7 h	>24 h	97%	>80%	1.5 h; increases to 3.2–7.2 h in hepatic impairment	33% in urine; remainder in feces
Omeprazole	1 h	0.5–3.5 h	>72 h	95%	30%–40%; increases to 100% in hepatic impairment	30–60 min; increases to 3 h in hepatic impairment	77% in urine; remainder in feces
Pantoprazole	UK	2.5 h	>24 h	98%	77%	1 h	71% in urine as metabolite; 18% in feces
Rabeprazole	<1 h	2–5 h	UK	96.3%	52%	1–2 h	90% in urine as metabolites; 10% in feces
Dexlansoprazole		4–5 h		96.1%		1–2 h	50.7% is excreted in the urine and 47.6% in the feces

high-fat meal may delay its absorption by up to 4 hours. In each case, the peak and AUC are not altered.

All drugs are distributed to the parietal cells of the stomach. They all cross the placenta. Omeprazole has been measured in human breast milk; the other PPIs have been found in breast milk in animal studies.

Metabolism and Excretion

These drugs are extensively metabolized by CYP450 2C19 and CYP450 3A4, and several metabolites have been identified that appear to have little or no antisecretory activity. Omeprazole is metabolized by the CYP450 system and may interact with other drugs also metabolized by this system. Lansoprazole and dexlansoprazole are metabolized by the CYP450 3A4 and CYP450 2C19 isoenzyme systems; however, they do not have clinically significant drug interactions related to this metabolic site.

In patients with varying degrees of hepatic disease, the mean plasma half-life of each of these drugs increases from a low of 3 hours with omeprazole to a high of 9 hours for pantoprazole. The plasma elimination half-life of these drugs does not reflect the duration of suppression of gastric acid secretion, apparently because of prolonged binding to the parietal $H^+/K^+/ATPase$ enzyme.

Little unchanged drug is excreted in the urine, but 33% to 90% of the metabolites is excreted in the urine. The rest is excreted in feces. A significant biliary excretion route is implied, especially for omeprazole and lansoprazole. Older adults have somewhat decreased elimination rates of all of these drugs, perhaps related to the decreased renal function associated with aging.

Pharmacotherapeutics

Precautions and Contraindications

The only true contraindication to the PPIs are hypersensitivity to the ingredients. The PPIs are extensively metabolized in the liver; therefore, they should be used cautiously in patients with hepatic dysfunction and in the elderly. No dosage adjustments are recommended for these patients, however.

Omeprazole is Pregnancy Category C. Multiple studies have followed women exposed to omeprazole during pregnancy and found no increase in congenital malformations, perinatal mortality, or morbidity (Arnon et al, 2003; Matok et al, 2012). Guidelines for treatment of GERD state, "PPIs are safe in pregnant patients if clinically indicated" (Katz et al, 2013). Lansoprazole, esomeprazole, pantoprazole, and rabeprazole are Pregnancy Category B, but there have been no adequate and well-controlled studies in pregnant women for these drugs, either. Use in pregnancy only if the potential benefits outweigh the potential risks to the fetus.

Omeprazole is excreted in low levels in human breast milk and the other drugs in this class have been found in breast milk in animal studies. Omeprazole (20 mg/day), esomeprazole (20 mg/day), or pantoprazole (40 mg/day) do not cause any adverse effects in breastfed infants (LactMed, 2013).

There is little information on the use of lansoprazole, dexlansoprazole, or rabeprazole during lactation (LactMed, 2013). The decision to discontinue the drug or discontinue nursing should take into account the importance of the drug to the mother.

The safety and efficacy of pantoprazole and rabeprazole have not been established in children younger than age 12 years. Esomeprazole, omeprazole, and lansoprazole have been found safe and efficacious for short-term treatment of GERD and erosive esophagitis in pediatric patients and are FDA-approved for use in children as young as 1 year of age. There have been no large-scale long-term safety studies of PPI use in growing children, but there is a concern for increased respiratory and gastrointestinal infections found in a few small studies (Tjon, Pe, Soscia, & Mahant, 2013).

Adverse Drug Reactions

These drugs are generally well tolerated when used for short-term treatment, and the adverse reactions that did occur in more than 1% of patients in clinical trials included dizziness, drowsiness, abdominal pain, constipation, diarrhea, and flatulence. It is difficult to determine if the GI-related symptoms were associated with the disease or the drug.

PPIs have now been on the market long enough to have a large body of long-term safety data. In an extensive review of the literature to determine the long-term safety of PPIs, Ali, Roberts, and Tierney (2009) suggest the combined body of knowledge raises concerns. There is evidence for significant nutrient deficiencies in patients taking PPIs long-term. Iron, vitamin B_{12}, and calcium all need an acid environment for optimal absorption. The PPIs are so effective in reducing acid production that patients are at risk for iron deficiency anemia, vitamin B_{12} deficiency, and calcium deficiency (Ali et al, 2009; Lodato et al, 2010). Patients on long-term PPIs may be at risk for osteoporosis and increased hip fractures, especially when combined with other risk factors for fracture such as age and female gender (Ali et al, 2009; Corley, Kubo, Zhao, & Quesenberry, 2010; Lodato et al, 2010; Thomson, Sauve, Kassam, & Kamitakahara, 2010).

Stomach acid provides a natural defense against microbial pathogens. Patients on long-term PPI therapy have an increased risk of *Clostridium difficile*, salmonella, and camphylobacter infections (Ali et al, 2009). Short-term use of PPIs increases the risk of pneumonia (Katz et al, 2013).

There are cellular level changes that occur with long-term PPI therapy, including hyperplasia of enterochromaffin-like cells, leading to a concern about the development of gastric cancers (Ali et al, 2009; Lodato et al, 2010; Vandenplas et al, 2009). Atrophic gastritis has been noted in patients taking omeprazole long-term, and chronic atrophic gastritis is a risk factor for developing gastric carcinoid tumors (Lodato et al, 2010). In spite of these cellular changes, at this time there is not strong evidence for the development of gastric cancers from long-term PPI use (Lodato et al, 2010; Thomson et al, 2010; Brunner, Athmann, & Schneider, 2012).

Drug Interactions

Drug interactions with PPIs relate to their use of the CYP450 enzyme system for metabolism and the change in bioavailability of concurrently administered drugs requiring an acid environment for absorption. PPIs may decrease the effects of atazanavir, indinavir, and nelfinavir, and coadministration is not recommended. All PPIs may interfere with absorption of drugs given orally that depend on an acidic gastric pH to be effective. These drugs include ketoconazole, esters of ampicillin, digoxin, and iron salts. Increased monitoring of INR is required if warfarin is administered with PPIs.

Clopidogrel (Plavix) has a Black-Box Warning regarding poor metabolizers of CYP2C19 and concurrent administration of medications that interfere with CYP2C19. Coadministration of clopidogrel and omeprazole has been shown to decrease the active metabolite of clopidogrel by 46%, leading to decreased effectiveness. Clinically, a decrease in the antiplatelet effect of clopidogrel may lead to increased clot formation. The FDA issued a warning in November 2009 to avoid concurrent use of PPIs and clopidogrel, followed by a labeling update for clopidogrel in December 2011 that recommends avoiding concomitant use with the PPIs omeprazole or esomeprazole due to reduced antiplatelet activity of clopidogrel caused by impaired CYP2C19 function (FDA, 2012). The American College of Gastroenterology GERD guidelines continue to recommend using PPIs with clopidogrel due to lack of clinical data to support that concomitant use increases cardiovascular events (Katz et al, 2013). Given the conflicting expert opinion, choose a PPI with less CYP2C19 activity (dexlansoprazole, lansoprazole, and pantoprazole) and monitor patients carefully who are taking clopidrogrel with any PPI. These and other interactions are shown in Table 20-19.

Clinical Use and Dosing

Duodenal and Gastric Ulcers

Treatment for patients with uncomplicated gastric ulcers includes testing and treating for *H. pylori* and acid-suppressive therapy with PPIs. Lansoprazole, omeprazole, esomeprazole, and rabeprazole are used for treatment of active duodenal ulcer and active benign gastric ulcer. The once-daily dose is taken before a meal, preferably in the morning (Table 20-20). Treatment is for 12 weeks.

Table 20–20 ▦ Drug Interactions: Proton Pump Inhibitors

Drug	Interacting Drug	Possible Effect	Implications
Esomeprazole	Benzodiazepines	Oxidative metabolism of BDZ decreased Reduced clearance and increased half-life	Reduce dose of BDZ or increase dose interval
	Clarithromycin	Increased concentrations of both drugs	No action required
Lansoprazole	Theophylline	10% increase in theophylline clearance	Additional titration of theophylline dosage may be required
Omeprazole	Clarithromycin	Coadministration may result in increased plasma levels of both drugs	This combination is among the FDA-approved treatment options for *H.pylori* eradication
	Benzodiazepines, phenytoin	103% increase in diazepam half-life; 15% reduced clearance of phenytoin	Use lansoprazole or select a treatment regimen that does not require a proton pump inhibitor if the interacting drugs must be given
	Sulfonylureas	Concurrent use may increase serum sulfonylurea concentration, increasing hypoglycemic effects	No specific action beyond monitoring blood glucose
Rabeprazole	Clarithromycin	Increased concentrations of both drugs	No action required; may be part of *H. pylori* protocol
All PPIs	Sucralfate	Decreased absorption of proton pump inhibitor	Take proton pump inhibitor 30 min prior to sucralfate
	Ketoconazole, esters of ampicillin, digoxin, iron salts	Proton pump inhibitors decrease absorption of these drugs	Avoid concurrent administration; for digoxin, monitor serum levels closely
	Azole antifungals (itraconazole, ketoconazole, etc.)	Bioavailability of azole decreased due to high gastric pH interference with tablet dissolving	Avoid concomitant administration
	Digoxin	Increased serum digoxin levels	Magnitude of change may not be clinically significant, but need to monitor
	Salicylates	Enteric-coated salicylates may dissolve more rapidly, increasing gastric adverse response	Separate administration by at least one h and give salicylate first
	Warfarin	Prolonged elimination of warfarin; increased INR	Increase monitoring frequency

More than 90% of duodenal ulcers and 80% of gastric ulcers are thought to be related to infection with *H. pylori*. Multiple treatment regimens are available for *H. pylori* eradication; triple regimens combine a PPI with two antibiotics for 14 days and the quadruple regimen combines a PPI with two antibiotics and bismuth subsalicylate (Lew, 2009). Acid suppression by the PPI in conjunction with the antimicrobial helps alleviate the ulcer-related symptoms, heals gastric mucosal inflammation, and may enhance the efficacy of the antimicrobial agent against *H. pylori* at the mucosal surface. Eradication of *H. pylori* significantly affects healing and recurrence rates. The recurrence rate of peptic ulcers is 6% to 15% for patients taking antimicrobial therapy versus 80% recurrence for those on conventional antisecretory therapy (Chey & Wong, 2007). Chapter 35 discusses the treatment of peptic ulcer disease in depth and Table 35-6 discusses triple and quadruple therapy for gastric ulcers. Any of the PPIs can be used in these protocols. See Table 20-20.

Gastroesophageal Reflux Disease

For most patients, GERD is treated with stepped therapy. The steps are based on symptom relief and degree of esophageal damage. Either the step-up approach or the step-down approach may be used. There is evidence supporting both and the provider may select either. Regardless of the approach chosen, lifestyle modifications occur throughout therapy. They are discussed in detail in Chapter 35.

GERD treatment begins with lifestyle modifications and OTC antacids or H$_2$RAs, which patients have often tried before seeking care from a provider. The American College of Gastroenterology GERD guidelines recommend 8 weeks of PPIs for symptom relief and healing of erosive esophagitis associated with GERD (Katz et al, 2013). Standard once-a-day therapy is started and tailored to symptom relief. If night-time symptoms are an issue, dosing can be adjusted or twice-a-day dosing can be used for the traditional PPIs. Another option would be to add an H$_2$RA before bed to address night-time symptoms (Katz et al, 2013).

Failure to achieve symptom relief after 3 months or the presence of symptoms that suggest complications should be referred to a gastroenterologist. PPIs may mask the symptoms of gastric cancers, and the provider should keep this in mind. The presence of alarm symptoms (dysphagia, painful swallowing, noncardiac chest pain, weight loss, hematemesis, and choking) suggests endoscopy as part of the initial evaluation.

All PPIs are approved for the treatment of GERD. The once-daily dosing is taken 30 to 60 minutes before breakfast. The length of therapy is 8 weeks. In the rare patient whose healing does not occur by then, an additional 4 weeks may be needed. Nonresponsive patients require referral to a gastroenterology specialist. Patients may need long-term intermittent therapy for GERD. Dosage schedules for GERD are found in Table 20-21.

Table 20–21 ⊗ Dosage Schedule: Proton Pump Inhibitors

Drug	Indication	Dosage Form	Initial Dose	Maintenance Dose
Esomeprazole Nexium	GERD with erosive esophagitis	Capsules: delayed-release: 20, 40 mg Granules for suspension: 10, 20, 40 mg/packet	*Adolescents and adults:* 20 or 40 mg daily for 4–8 wk. Maintenance: 20 mg daily for 4 wk. *Children:* <20 kg: 10 mg daily for 8 wk; >20 kg: 10–20 mg daily for 8 wk	20 mg/d
	Symptomatic GERD *H. pylori* eradication/ prevent duodenal ulcer		*Adults:* 20 mg daily for 8 wk *Children 1–11 yr:* 10 mg daily for 8 wk Triple therapy: Esomeprazole 40 mg daily + amoxicillin 1 g bid + clarithromycin 500 mg bid for 7–10 d	
Lansoprazole Prevacid	Duodenal ulcer *H. pylori* eradication/ prevent duodenal ulcer	Capsules, delayed-release: 15, 30 mg Tablet: 15, 30 mg Suspension: 3 mg/mL	*Children 12 yr and adults:* 15 mg qd for 4 wk *H. pylori:* Triple therapy: Lansoprazole 30 mg bid + amoxicillin 1 g bid + clarithromycin 500 mg tid for 10 d Double therapy: Lansoprazole 30 mg tid + amoxicillin 1 g tid for 14 d	15 mg qd
	Benign gastric ulcer		30 mg daily for <8 wk	
	Erosive esophagitis		30 mg daily for <8 wk	15 mg qd
	Hypersecretory disorders		60 mg daily	Up to 90 mg bid; doses >120 mg/d must be divided
	Erosive esophagitis		*Adults:* 30 mg once daily for up to 8 wk *Children 12–17 yr and adults:* 30 mg once daily for up to 8 wk *Children 1–11 yr:* ≤30 kg: 15 mg daily for up to 12 wk >30 kg: 30 mg daily for up to 12 wk	If not healed, repeat dose for additional 8 wk Increase to 30 mg bid in patients who remain symptomatic after 2 wk of therapy

Continued

Table 20–21 ⊗ Dosage Schedule: Proton Pump Inhibitors—cont'd

Drug	Indication	Dosage Form	Initial Dose	Maintenance Dose
	Gastric ulcer associated with NSAID therapy		*Adults:* 30 mg daily for up to 8 wk	15 mg/d for up to 12 wk
	GERD	Prevacid OTC: Capsules, delayed-release: 15 mg	*Children 12–17 yr and adults:* 15 mg daily for up to 8 wk *Children 1–11 yr:* ≤30 kg: 15 mg daily for up to 12 wk >30 kg: 30 mg daily for up to 12 wk	
Omeprazole Prilosec Generic	Duodenal ulcer	Capsules, delayed-release: 10, 20, 40 mg Granules for suspension: 2.5, 10 mg/packet	*Adults:* 20 mg daily for 4–8 wk *Infants and children:* 15–30 kg: 10 mg bid, >30 kg: 20 mg bid *H. pylori:* Triple therapy: Omeprazole 20 mg bid + clarithromycin 500 mg bid + amoxicillin 1 g bid for 10 d Double therapy: Omeprazole 40 daily + clarithromycin 500 mg tid for 14 d; then omeprazole 20 mg daily for 14 additional d	
	Benign gastric ulcer		40 mg daily for 4–8 wk	
	Erosive esophagitis		20 mg daily for 4–8 wk	20 mg qid
	GERD		*Children 2–18 yr:* ≤20 kg: 10 mg daily for 4–8 wk >20 kg: 20 mg daily for 4–8 wk	Note: On a per kg basis doses are higher for children than adults.
	Hypersecretory disorders		*Adolescents > 16 yr and adults:* 60 mg daily	Up to 120 mg tid; doses >80 mg/d must be divided
Pantoprazole Protonix	Symptomatic GERD	Tablets: delayed-release: 20 40 mg Granules for suspension: 40 mg/packet	20–40 mg daily for 7–10 d	20 mg/d
	GERD with erosive esophagitis		40 mg daily for up to 8 wk	40 mg/d If not healed, repeat same dose for additional 8 wk
	Hypersecretory disorders		Individualized. 40 mg bid; may treat for up to 2 yr	Doses up to 240 mg/d have been used
Rabeprazole Aciphex	Duodenal ulcers	Tablets, delayed-release: 20 mg	*Adults and adolescents >12 yr:* 20 mg daily after the morning meal for up to 4 wk	If not healed, repeat dose for 4 wk
	GERD		*Adults and adolescents >12 yr:* 20 mg daily for 4 wk	If symptoms, repeat dose for 4 wk
	Erosive esophagitis		20 mg daily for 4–8 wk	If not healed, repeat dose for 4 wk
	H. pylori eradication/ prevent duodenal ulcer		Triple therapy: Rabeprazole 20 mg bid + amoxicillin 1 g bid + clarithromycin 500 mg bid for 7 d	
	Hypersecretory disorders		Individualized: 60 mg daily; may treat for up to 1 yr	Dose up to 100 mg/d or 60 mg bid have been used
Dexlansoprazole Dexilant Kapidex	Erosive esophagitis	Delayed-release capsules: 30, 60 mg 60 mg capsule	Treatment: 60 mg daily for 8 wk Maintenance for healed EE: 30 mg daily for up to 6 mo	Moderate hepatic dysfunction: 30 mg/d Not recommended for children <18 yr
	GERD		30 mg daily for 4 wk	

Further discussion of multidrug treatment for *H. pylori* is found in Chapter 34.

Hypersecretory Conditions (Including Zollinger–Ellison Syndrome)

All PPIs can be used to treat hypersecretory conditions such as Zollinger–Ellison syndrome. These disorders usually require higher dosing than does GERD or PUD and vary depending on the drug used. Some patients with Zollinger–Ellison syndrome have been treated continuously for more than 5 years.

Rational Drug Selection

Drug Interactions

For patients taking drugs metabolized by the CYP450 system, lansoprazole is the best choice. Although all PPIs are metabolized by CYP450 enzymes, lansoprazole appears to have no clinically significant drug interactions with warfarin or other drugs metabolized by CYP450. All the PPIs interact with atazanavir equally.

Difficulty in Swallowing

For patients with difficulty in swallowing, omeprazole, esomeprazole, and lansoprazole capsules can be opened and the intact granules sprinkled on 1 tablespoon of applesauce and swallowed immediately. Patients should not chew or crush the granules. Lansoprazole comes as a quick-dissolve tablet (Prevacid SoluTab) or as granules for suspension (Prevacid for Oral Suspension) that are mixed in 30 mL of water. Omeprazole (Prilosec for Delayed-Release Oral Suspension) comes as granules for suspension that are mixed with water and left to thicken for 2 to 3 minutes before administration. Pantoprazole (Protonix) comes as granules for delayed-release suspension that are mixed in applesauce or apple juice. The instructions for rabeprazole specifically state not to crush the tablet. All the PPIs have an enteric coating, even the granules; therefore, none of them should be crushed or chewed.

Patients being tube fed require a formulation that will not clog the tube. Omeprazole capsules or granules may be used with these patients. An omeprazole capsule may be opened and mixed with an acidic juice or omeprazole granules may be mixed with water in a catheter-tip syringe and administered after waiting 2 to 3 minutes for the mixture to thicken. Pantoprazole granules are emptied into the barrel of a syringe and 10 mL of apple juice is added; additional apple juice may be needed to rinse the syringe of granules. Lansoprazole granules for suspension or quick-dissolve tablets should not be used for nasogastric feedings. A lansoprazole capsule may be opened and mixed with 40 mL of apple, cranberry, grape, orange, tomato, or V-8 juice and administered via nasogastric tube.

H. Pylori Treatment

To increase adherence, choose the least complex regimen with the fewest adverse reactions that still has a high eradication rate. Chapter 35 has more discussion of this treatment.

Monitoring

The only monitoring relates to the disease process being treated. However, patients taking proton pump inhibitors to treat ulcers should be tested for *H. pylori* infection. Patients taking PPIs should stop therapy for 2 weeks before undergoing urea breath testing to diagnose this infection or be tested via stool antigen testing. PPIs alone rarely eradicate *H. pylori* infection, but they can suppress it so that testing during antisecretory therapy may lead to false-negative results.

Patient Education

Administration

Patients should take the drug exactly as prescribed, even if they are feeling better. If a dose is missed, it should be taken as soon as the patient remembers it, unless it is almost time for the next dose. Patients should not double up on doses. All of these drugs are taken before a meal. Drugs taken once daily are preferably taken in the morning. These drugs may safely be taken with antacids. Patients who have difficulty swallowing should be instructed not to chew or crush tablets or granules. Patients or caregivers should have clear instructions on how to administer PPIs to those with swallowing problems or tube feedings.

Adverse Reactions

PPIs may occasionally cause drowsiness or dizziness. Patients should avoid activities that require mental alertness until their response to the drug is known. Advise patients to promptly report to their health-care provider the onset of black, tarry stool; diarrhea; abdominal pain; or persistent headache, which may indicate progression of the disease or adverse drug effects.

Lifestyle Management

Lifestyle modifications are always attempted before drugs are used to treat GERD. They are also often used prior to treatment of the other indications for PPIs. These modifications are discussed in more detail in Chapter 35.

LAXATIVES

Constipation is a common affliction caused by everything from lack of sufficient fluids, fiber, and exercise to serious GI diseases to iatrogenic causes secondary to adverse reactions to drugs. It is among the most frequent reasons for self-medication and is particularly troublesome to older adults.

Treatment often takes the form of laxative use. More than $500 million is spent annually in the United States on laxatives. The pathophysiology of constipation varies with its cause, and the action of the drug chosen to treat the constipation must also vary to match the cause. In light of these differences, six main classes of drugs are used to promote evacuation of the bowel: stimulants, osmotics, bulk-producing laxatives, lubricants, surfactants, and hyperosmolar laxatives. Each class is discussed in this section. Because each laxative has several brand names, only the generic name is used.

A newer treatment for opioid-induced constipation is methylnaltrexone (Relistor), a mu-opioid receptor antagonist.

Pharmacodynamics

Stimulants

The stimulant laxatives have a direct action on intestinal mucosa by stimulating the myenteric plexus. Stimulants facilitate the release of prostaglandins and increase cyclic adenosine monophosphate (cAMP) concentration. This increase in cAMP increases the secretion of electrolytes and stimulates peristalsis. Drugs in the stimulant class include cascara, senna, bisacodyl, and castor oil.

The stimulants are used most often for treatment of constipation associated with reduced mobility, constipating drugs, reduced motility, neurogenic bowel secondary to spinal cord injury, and irritable bowel syndrome. They are also used to prepare the bowel for radiological or surgical procedures.

Osmotics

The class of osmotics exerts its effects mainly by drawing water into the intestinal lumen to increase intraluminal pressure. These drugs are hypertonic salt-based solutions that cause the diffusion of fluid from the plasma into the intestine to dilute the solution to an isotonic state. The magnesium salts also cause an increase in the release of cholecystokinin by the duodenum. Sulfate salts are considered the most powerful. Drugs in this class include magnesium hydroxide, magnesium citrate, sodium phosphate, polyethylene glycol electrolyte solution, and polyethylene glycol (PEG) 3350.

Polyethylene glycol electrolyte solution is used to cleanse the entire GI tract for diagnostic purposes, to flush poisons from the system, and to remove parasites. PEG 3350 powder is used for constipation.

Bulk-Producing Laxatives

The bulk-producing laxatives are the safest and most physiological because their action is similar to that achieved by increasing fiber in the diet. They do not hinder absorption of nutrients and are less likely to be habit-forming. The bulk-producing laxatives consist of natural and semisynthetic polysaccharides and cellulose. When combined with water in the intestine, they produce mechanical distention resulting in an increase in peristalsis. Drugs in this class include psyllium, methylcellulose, and polycarbophil.

The bulk-producing laxatives may be used for long-term management of simple, chronic constipation, especially if it is related to low fiber intake in the diet. They are also useful in situations in which straining at stool is to be avoided and in the management of chronic, watery diarrhea.

Lubricants

Mineral oil is the main ingredient in lubricant laxatives. Its action is to retard colonic absorption of fecal water and soften the stool. It does not stimulate peristalsis. It is used to soften stool associated with fecal impaction. Mineral oil also lubricates the intestine to facilitate the passage of stool. Major concerns with the use of mineral oil are that it may decrease absorption of fat-soluble vitamins, and there is concern for aspiration in children younger than 4 years of age if given orally.

Surfactants

Surfactants are often referred to as "stool softeners" because they reduce the surface tension of the oil–water interface on the stool and facilitate admixture of fat and water into the stool, producing an emollient action. Drugs in this class are the docusate compounds: docusate sodium, docusate calcium, and docusate potassium.

Surfactants are most beneficial when feces are hard or dry, in anorectal conditions in which passage for firm stool is painful, and in situations when straining at stool is to be avoided. Docusate sodium can be safely administered to all ages from infants to the elderly.

Hyperosmolar Laxatives

Hyperosmolar laxatives are often listed as "miscellaneous," but they share a similar mechanism of action. Glycerin produces local irritation and, as a hyperosmotic compound, draws water from the extravascular spaces into the lumen of the intestine, resulting in more liquid stool. Lactulose is a hyperosmotic disaccharide. In the colon, resident bacteria transform the drug into lactic acid and acetic and formic acids. These acids exert an osmotic effect by drawing water from the extravascular spaces into the intestinal lumen.

Glycerin is used to treat fecal impaction and patients with neurogenic bowel, in which the bowel is filled with feces that cannot be evacuated. Lactulose is used to treat chronic constipation in older adults, but it also is the only laxative used to treat hepatic encephalopathy. It lowers the pH of the colon, which in turn inhibits the diffusion of ammonia across colonic membranes.

Chloride Channel Activators

Lubiprostone (Amitiza) acts by activating CIC-2 chloride channels in the gastrointestinal epithelial lining, producing chloride-rich secretions that soften the stool and increase gastrointestinal motility. Lubiprostone does not affect serum sodium or potassium concentrations. Lubiprostone is used to treat chronic idiopathic constipation, irritable bowel syndrome with constipation in women aged 18 years or older, and chronic opioid-induced constipation in adults with chronic noncancer pain.

Opioid-Receptor Antagonists

Methylnaltrexone works as an antagonist to the mu-receptor in the GI track and treats the constipation patients experience when taking opioids. Methylnaltrexone does not cross the blood–brain barrier; therefore, it does not affect the kappa receptor analgesic effect of opioids.

Pharmacokinetics

Absorption and Distribution

Absorption is highly variable between classes, from no absorption for the bulk-forming laxatives to 3% or less for all other classes except the magnesium salts, of which up to 30% may be absorbed (Table 20-22). Magnesium salts are widely

Table 20–22 ⚬ Pharmacokinetics: Selected Laxatives

Drug Class	Onset	Peak	Site of Action	Elimination
Stimulants	6–10 h 0.25–1 h bisacodyl PR 2–6 h castor oil	UK	Colon Colon Small intestine	Mostly in feces
Osmotics (magnesium salts)	0.5–3 h	UK	Small and large intestine	Primarily in urine
Bulk-forming	12–24 h	2–3 d	Small and large intestine	In feces
Lubricants	6–8 h PO 2–15 min PR	UK	Colon Colon	In feces
Surfactants	24–48 h PO 2–15 min PR	UK	Small and large intestine	Small amount absorbed is eliminated in bile
Hyperosmolar	0.25–0.5 h glycerin 24–48 h lactulose	UK UK	Colon Colon	UK Small amount absorbed is excreted unchanged in urine

PR = per rectum; UK = unknown.

distributed, cross the placenta, and enter breast milk. Small amounts of metabolites of bisacodyl have been found in breast milk. The remaining drugs in each class have no distribution, with their action being localized in the intestine. Methylnaltrexone is administered subcutaneous and peaks in 30 minutes.

Metabolism and Excretion

Locally acting drugs have no specific metabolism and are excreted in feces. The liver metabolizes small amounts of bisacodyl. Glycerin is 80% metabolized by the liver and 10% to 20% by the kidney. Magnesium salts are metabolized by the liver and excreted primarily by the kidney.

Methylnaltrexone is metabolized in the liver into five metabolites including o methyl-6-naltrexol isomers and methylnaltrexone sulfate. The half-life of methylnaltrexone is 8 hours and it is renally excreted.

Pharmacotherapeutics

Precautions and Contraindications

Precautions and contraindications vary by class of laxative, but all share the contraindication of use in the presence of nausea, vomiting, or undiagnosed abdominal pain or if bowel obstruction is suspected or diagnosed. Other precautions and contraindications are specific to a class or a drug.

Stimulants

Bisacodyl is to be used with caution in the presence of severe cardiovascular disease. The extract of cascara sagrada contains alcohol and should be avoided by people with alcohol intolerance.

Castor oil is contraindicated in pregnancy because it has been associated with induction of uterine contractions. Cascara derivatives are Pregnancy Category C. Bisacodyl is safe to use in pregnancy and is listed as Pregnancy Category B.

Cascara sagrada is excreted in breast milk and may increase the incidence of diarrhea in the nursing infant.

Osmotics

Magnesium hydroxide is contraindicated in the presence of any degree of renal insufficiency because the kidney may be unable to excrete excessive magnesium ions. Hypermagnesemia, hypocalcemia, and heart block also contraindicate their use. Because large quantities of polyethylene glycol electrolyte solution must be taken, these salts are used cautiously for patients with diminished gag reflex unless it is being administered by nasogastric tube. Osmotics should be avoided in patients with bowel obstruction or ileus.

Magnesium hydroxide is Pregnancy Category B. Polyethylene glycol electrolyte solution is Pregnancy Category C, as is PEG 3350 (Miralax).

PEG 3350 should not be used in children younger than 4 years of age. The use of polyethylene glycol electrolyte solution to treat constipation in children is contraindicated because of concerns about electrolyte disturbance.

Bulk-Forming Laxatives

Bulk-forming laxatives are used with caution for patients with a narrowed esophageal or intestinal lumen. Some dosage forms contain sugar or salt and should be avoided by patients who must restrict these substances. Bulk-forming laxatives should be avoided in patients who are impacted. Bulk-forming agents are not given a specific pregnancy category but have been safely used during pregnancy.

Lubricants

Lipid pneumonia has occurred in patients who aspirated mineral oil. The very young, older adults, people with dysphagia, and debilitated patients are at highest risk.

Although no specific pregnancy category is listed for mineral oil, it should be avoided during pregnancy because chronic use decreases the absorption of fat-soluble vitamins and causes hypoprothrombinemia in the newborn.

Surfactants

Docusate compounds have no specific contraindications or precautions. They have not been given a specific pregnancy category but have been safely used during pregnancy.

Hyperosmolar Agents

Hyperosmolar agents are used with caution in the presence of volume depletion. Older adults are especially at risk for dehydration. Hyperglycemia has been noted in some patients taking lactulose, and it is used with caution in the presence of diabetes mellitus.

Glycerin is Pregnancy Category C; lactulose is Pregnancy Category B. It is not known if lactulose is excreted in breast milk.

Sodium Channel Activators

Nausea is the most common adverse effect of lubiprosone, with 29% of patients in clinical trials experiencing nausea that may be relieved by administration with food (Sucampo Pharma Americas, 2013). Dyspnea has been reported in patients taking 24 mcg twice daily, with the onset of chest tightness and shortness of breath 30 to 60 minutes after taking the first dose. The dyspnea generally resolves after a few hours but may recur with subsequent doses; some patients have discontinued treatment due to dyspnea (Sucampo Pharma Americas, 2013). Diarrhea occurred in 13% of patients during clinical trials.

Lubiprosone is Pregnancy Category C. There are no adequate, well-controlled studies of lubiprosone in pregnant women. There was a dose-dependent fetal loss noted in guinea pig studies of lubiprosone.

Opioid-Receptor Antagonists

Methylnaltrexone may cause opioid withdrawal particularly if the blood–brain barrier is disturbed. Patients should be monitored closely. Patients with constipation are at risk for bowel rupture and methylnaltrexone should be used with care and the patient monitored for severe abdominal pain.

Precautions for All Laxatives

Other general laxative precautions include the following:

1. Abuse and dependency: Chronic use of laxatives, particularly stimulants, may lead to laxative dependency, which in turn may result in fluid and electrolyte imbalances, steatorrhea, osteomalacia, and vitamin and mineral deficiencies. The "laxative abuse syndrome" is most commonly seen in women with depression, personality disorders, or anorexia nervosa. Cathartic colon can also result. The pathology resembles ulcerative colitis.
2. Tartrazine sensitivity: Some of these products contain tartrazine, which may cause allergic types of reactions, including asthma, in susceptible individuals. Although the incidence of this sensitivity in the general population is low, it is frequently seen in patients who also have aspirin sensitivity.

Adverse Drug Reactions

Adverse drug reactions are most commonly extensions of the drug's action and include excessive bowel activity, cramping, flatulence, and bloating. Perianal irritation may also develop. Allergic reactions such as urticaria, dermatitis, rhinitis, and bronchospasm have occurred when patients accidentally inhaled bulk-forming laxatives. Phenolphthalein may cause a skin hypersensitivity characterized by a fixed drug eruption. Discontinue the drug if this occurs.

In clinical trials of methylnaltrexone 21% of patients reported abdominal pain versus 9% of those taking a placebo. Other adverse effects of methylnaltrexone that occurred more frequently than placebo were nausea (9% versus 6% taking placebo), diarrhea (6% versus 4%), and hyperhidrosis (6% versus 1%).

Drug Interactions

Because most laxatives have local activity and limited absorption, few drug interactions occur. Methylnaltrexone should not be taken with other opioid antagonists because of the potential for additive effects. Table 20-23 lists drug interactions with laxatives.

Clinical Use and Dosing

All laxatives are used to treat constipation or to prepare the bowel for a procedure. Specific uses for each class are discussed in the Pharmacodynamics section. Table 20-24 lists the dosing schedules for each indication.

Rational Drug Selection

The choice of drug to treat constipation depends on the severity of the constipation, the reason for it, and the speed with which resolution is needed. Drugs are used only after the reason for the constipation has been corrected if possible (stop or decrease the dose of the drug that induced the constipation). Indications for the use of each class of drug are presented in the Pharmacodynamics section.

Rapid Response and Short Term

Stimulants are the drug of choice when rapid response is needed. All are equally effective. They should be used only for the short term. Safer drugs can be used for long-term management when speed is not the main issue. The choice of drug depends largely on cost.

Osmotic laxatives work quickly as well. Magnesium hydroxide produces evacuation in 6 to 8 hours and is generally administered before bedtime. PEG 3350 produces a bowel movement in 1 to 3 days. Docusate sodium is the preferred surfactant.

Slower Response and Long Term

Bulk-forming laxatives are the drug of choice when rapid response is not needed and long-term management with the least adverse reactions is desired. They are especially suited to older adults. The choice of product depends upon the patient's acceptance of texture and taste. Lactulose can be used if the bulk-forming laxatives do not work or are not well tolerated. It works well in older adults and children.

Table 20–23 ▓ Drug Interactions: Selected Laxatives

Drug	Interacting Drug	Possible Effect	Implications
All laxatives	Other orally administered drugs	May decrease absorption of other orally administered drugs because of increased motility and decreased transit time	Separate administration by at least 1 h
Bisacodyl	Antacids, histamine$_2$ blockers, proton pump inhibitors	May remove enteric coating of tablets	Separate administration or select different laxative
Lactulose	Antimicrobials	Concurrent use may decrease effectiveness of lactulose used in hepatic encephalopathy	If concurrent use cannot be avoided, dosage adjustments of lactulose may be required
	Antacids	May decrease the effect of lactulose on colon pH	Separate doses by at least 1 h
Magnesium salts	Fluoroquinolones, nitrofurantoin, tetracycline	May decrease absorption of these drugs	Avoid concurrent administration
Mineral oil	Docusate compounds	Concurrent use may increase mineral oil absorption	Avoid concurrent use
	Foods	May decrease absorption of vitamins A, D, E, K	
Psyllium	Digoxin, salicylates, warfarin	May decrease absorption of these drugs	Separate administration by at least 1 h and give drug before psyllium

Table 20–24 ⊗ Dosage Schedule: Selected Laxatives

Drug	Indication	Dosage Form	Dose	Notes
Bisacodyl Dulcolax	Constipation	Tablets: 5 mg Suppositories: 10 mg	*Children >12 yr and adults:* Tablets: 10–15 mg once daily PR: 10 mg once daily *Children 2–11 yr:* Tablets: 5 mg (0.3 mg/kg) once daily PR: 5 mg once daily *Children <2 yr:* PR: 5 mg single dose	Up to 30 mg have been used as preparation for bowel procedure
Cascara sagrada	Constipation	Tablets: 325 mg	*Children >12 yr and adults:* Tablets: 300 mg–1 g once daily Extract tablet: 200–400 mg daily	Tablets and liquids come in combinations with docusate and milk of magnesia
Castor oil Generic	Constipation	Oil	*Children >12 yr and adults:* 15–60 mL in a single dose *Children 2–11 yr:* 5–15 mL in a single dose	
Docusate calcium Surfak	Constipation	Capsules: 50, 240 mg	*Calcium* *Adults:* 240 mg once daily *Children >6 yr:* 50–150 mg once daily	
Docusate potassium (Diocto-K, Dialose, Kasof)		Capsules: 100, 240 mg	*Potassium* *Adults:* 100–300 mg once daily *Children >6 yr:* 100 mg once daily at bedtime	
Docusate sodium (Colace)		Capsules: 50, 100 mg Syrup: 60 mg/15 mL Liquid: 150 mg/15 mL	*Sodium* *Children >12 yr and adults:* 50–500 mg once daily *Children 6–11 yr:* 40–120 mg once daily *Children 3–6 yr:* 20–60 mg once daily *Children <3 yr:* 10–40 mg Suppository: *Adults:* 50–100 mg or 1 suppository	
Glycerin PR	Constipation	Suppositories: Adult, Pediatric	*Children >6 yr and adults:* 2–3 g as suppository or 5–15 mg as enema *Children <6 yr:* 1–1.7 g as a suppository or 2–5 mL as enema	

Continued

Table 20–24 ✄ **Dosage Schedule: Selected Laxatives—cont'd**

Drug	Indication	Dosage Form	Dose	Notes
Lactulose (Cephulac, Chronulac, Enulose) Generic	Constipation	Syrup: 10 g lactulose/ 15 mL	*Adults:* 15–30 mL once daily *Children:* 7.5 mL once daily	May use up to 60 mg/d; unlabeled use
	Hepatic encephalopathy		*Adults:* 30–45 mL tid–qid *Children and adolescents:* 40–90 mL daily in divided doses *Infants:* 2.5–10 mL daily in divided doses	May be given q1–2 h initially; goal is 2–3 soft stools/d; discontinue if diarrhea develops
Magnesium salts Epsom salts Magnesium hydroxide Milk of magnesia Magnesium citrate	Constipation	Granules: 40 mEq Mg²⁺ per 5g Chewable tablets: 300 and 600 mg Liquid: 80 mEq Mg²⁺ per 30 mL Liquid: 77 mEq Mg²⁺ per 100 mL	*Hydroxide (milk of magnesia)* *Children >12 yr and adults:* 30–60 mL once daily (in concentrate: 10–20 mL once daily) *Children 6–11 yr:* 15–30 mL in single or divided doses *Children 2–5 yr:* 5–15 mg in divided doses	
	Bowel prep or bowel cleanout if impacted		*Citrate* *Children >12 yr and adults:* 240 mL *Children 6–11 yr:* 100 mL	
Polyethylene glycol/ electrolyte solution (Colyte, GoLYTEly)	Bowel prep	In oral solution or powder for oral solution	*Adults:* 240 mL every 10 min (up to 4 L) until fecal discharge is clear with no solid material *Children:* 25–40 mg/kg/h until fecal discharge is clear with no solid material	Tastes salty, making it difficult to take. Ice it. May suck on hard candy or breath mints to make more palatable.
PEG 3350 (Miralax)	Constipation	Powder for solution: 17 g/dose	*Adults:* oral 17 g daily *Children >4 yr:* 0.7–1.5 g/kg daily, do not exceed 17 g	Mix with 4 to 8 oz of beverage
Psyllium (Fiberall, Konsyl, Metamucil)	Constipation	Powder: 3.4 g psyllium/5 mL, 6 g psyllium/5 mL Wafers: 1.7 g psyllium, 3.4 g psyllium Effervescent powder: 3.4 g/5 mL	*Adults:* 1–2 tsp/packet/wafer (3–6 g psyllium) in or with a full glass of liquid bid–tid *Children >6 yr:* 1 tsp/packet/wafer (1.5–3 g psyllium) in or with ½–1 glass of liquid bid–tid	Up to 30 g/d in divided doses Up to 15 g/d in divided doses
Senna (Senokot, Fletcher's Castoria)	Constipation	Tablets: 187 mg Granules: 326 mg Syrup: 218 mg/5 mL Liquid: 33.3 mg/mL	*Children >12 yr and adults:* 360 mg–2 g at bedtime *Children 6–11 yr:* 50% of adult dose *Children 1–5 yr:* 33% of adult dose Rectal: *Children >12 yr and adults:* 30 mg qid–bid	Fletcher's Castoria lists a children's dose of 10–15 mL (6–15 yr) and 5–10 mL (2–5 yr)

PR = per rectum.

Special Indications

Polyethylene glycol electrolyte solution is the best drug for cleansing the bowel in preparation for radiological or surgical procedures. It is very effective and does not produce electrolyte disturbances.

Lactulose is effective in reducing ammonia levels in the blood and brain with patients who have hepatic encephalopathy. It prevents absorption of ammonia from the intestine and produces diarrhea that flushes the ammonia out. Dietary adjustments to reduce ammonia production are simultaneously implemented.

Lubiprostone is indicated for the treatment of constipation associated with irritable bowel syndrome in women aged 18 years or older or chronic idiopathic constipation. It may also be used for opioid-induced constipation in patients with chronic noncancer pain. Methylnaltrexone is indicated for constipation associated with chronic opioid use.

Pregnancy

For pregnant women, bulk-forming laxatives and surfactants are safe and effective for regular use throughout pregnancy and for lactating women. Magnesium hydroxide is Pregnancy

Category B and can be used intermittently. Lubiprostone should not be prescribed for pregnant women unless the risk outweighs the benefit.

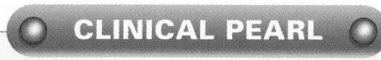

CLINICAL PEARL

Polyethylene Glycol/Electrolyte Solution
The taste of polyethylene glycol/electrolyte solution is quite salty, and many patients find it difficult to consume the required volume in the required amount of time. Place the container of solution in ice in a basin. Do not pour it over ice, which will melt and increase the volume the patient must consume. Have the patient drink 240 mL of fluid each 10 minutes and give a Tic-Tac or similar small mint-flavored hard candy to suck on between glasses of the drug. This reduces the salty taste in the mouth and makes the drug more palatable.

The Precautions and Contraindications section lists the pregnancy categories for other drugs, including those that should not be used during pregnancy.

Monitoring

In general, the monitoring for patients taking laxatives for more than 6 months includes laboratory assessment of fluid and electrolyte status, especially potassium and in the case of magnesium hydroxide use, magnesium level. For patients taking lactulose for hepatic encephalopathy, the overall management of this disorder requires careful monitoring because it is a serious disease with a high potential for complications. Monitoring includes serum electrolytes for hypokalemia and hypernatremia. For older adults taking lactulose for more than 6 months to manage their constipation, laboratory assessment of potassium, chloride, and carbon dioxide should be done periodically or with any indication of fluid or electrolyte disturbance.

Patient Education

Laxatives should not be taken in the presence of nausea, vomiting, or abdominal pain. These symptoms may indicate serious disorders that may be the cause of the constipation and that require a work-up. Patients should not take a laxative but instead contact their health-care provider.

Administration

Rapid-acting laxatives are best taken in the morning; slower-acting ones are best taken at bedtime. Taking a laxative on an empty stomach and with a full glass of water will produce more rapid results. Do not crush or chew enteric-coated tablets. Liquids can be given with fruit juice. For infants, taking liquids with fruit juice may mask any unpleasant taste. Suspensions are shaken before they are taken. Effervescent tablets are dissolved in a full glass of water before they are taken.

Suppositories are usually given close to the time that a bowel movement is desired. Lubricate them with a water-soluble lubricant and insert far enough into the rectum to pass the internal rectal sphincter. Encourage the patient to retain the suppository for 15 to 30 minutes before expelling.

Some liquid laxatives have special storage requirements and manufacturers' recommendations should be followed.

Adverse Reactions

The most common adverse drug reactions are excessive bowel activity, cramping, flatulence, and bloating. Perianal irritation may also occur. Allergic reactions such as a rash, rhinitis, and bronchospasm have occurred when patients accidentally inhaled bulk-forming laxatives. Be careful when pouring the powder to avoid this possibility. Phenolphthalein may cause a skin hypersensitivity rash. Advise the patient to notify the health-care provider if this occurs. The drug is discontinued and a different laxative chosen if the need for a laxative continues. Teach patients the indications of a fluid or electrolyte disturbance and have them report these symptoms promptly.

Lifestyle Management

Prevention is the key with regard to constipation. Lifestyle management should be a major focus. Stress the need for adequate fluids, fiber, and exercise. Laxatives are last-resort and temporary measures. They are not intended for long-term management in most cases.

Misconceptions about bowel function should be corrected. Different people have different bowel patterns, all of which may be normal and not signal pathology. Stressing this point is especially important for older adults, who were often taught in their youth that maintenance of health depended on having one bowel movement every day.

Constipation in children may be a control issue or signal pathology. Discuss this topic with the parents. A trial of a laxative concurrently with behavior modification is appropriate, but the child needs to be monitored for the need for referral for a GI work-up.

REFERENCES

Ali, T., Roberts, D. N., & Tierney, W. M. (2009). Long-term safety concerns with proton pump inhibitors. *American Journal of Medicine, 122*, 896–903.

American Gastroenterological Association (AGA) Institute Medical Position Panel. (2008). American Gastroenterological Association medical position statement on the management of gastroesophageal reflux disease. *Gastroenterology, 135,* 1383–1391.

Arnon, J. Shechtman, S., Diav-Citrin, O., Schaefer, C., van Tonningen, M. R., Clementi, M., et al. (2003, Jul-Aug). The safety of proton pump inhibotors in pregnancy: A multicenter prospective controlled study. *Reproductive Toxicology, 17*(4), 485–486.

Bronstein, A. C., Spyker, D. A., Cantilena, L. R., Rumack, B. H., & Dart, R. C. (2012). 2011 annual report of the American Association of Poison Control Centers National Poison Data System (NPDS), 29th annual report. *Clinical Toxicology, 50,* 911–1164. Retrieved from https://aapcc.s3.amazonaws.com/pdfs/annual_reports/2011_NPDS_Annual_Report.pdf

Brunner, G., Athmann, C., & Schneider, A. (2012). Long-term, open-label trial: Safety and efficacy of continuous maintenance treatment with pantoprazole for up to 15 years in severe acid-peptic disease. *Alimentary Pharmacology & Therapeutics, 36,* 37–47.

Centers for Disease Control and Prevention (CDC). (2014). *Traveler's diarrhea. CDC Health Information for International Travel 2014: The Yellow*

Book. Retrieved from http://wwwnc.cdc.gov/travel/yellowbook/2014/chapter-2-the-pre-travel-consultation/travelers-diarrhea

Chey, W. D., & Wong, B. C. Y. (2007). American College of Gastroenterology guideline on the management of *Helicobacter pylori* infection. *American Journal of Gastroenterology, 102*, 1808–1825.

Corley, D. A., Kubo, A., Zhao, W., & Quesenberry, C. (2010). Proton pump inhibitors and histamine-2 receptor antagonists are associated with hip fractures among at-risk patients. *Gastroenterology,* March 27, 2010. Epub ahead of print.

Food and Drug Administration (2012). Safety: Plavix (clopidogrel bisulfate) tablet. Retrieved from http://www.fda.gov/safety/medwatch/safetyinformation/ucm225843.htm

Heidelbaugh, J. J., Harrison R. V., McQuillan, M. A., & Nostrant, T. T. (2012). Guidelines for clinical care: Gastroesophageal reflux disease (GERD). University of Michigan Health System. Retrieved from http://www.med.umich.edu/1info/fhp/practiceguides/gerd/gerd.12.pdf

Katz, P. O., Gerson, L. B., & Vela, M. F. (2013). Guidelines for the diagnosis and management of gastroesophageal reflux disease. *American Journal of Gastroenterology, 108*(308–328).

LactMed: Drugs and Lactation Database. (2013). National Library of Medicine. http://toxnet.nlm.nih.gov

Lew, E. (2009). Peptic ulcer disease. In N. J. Greenberger (Ed.), *Current diagnosis & treatment gastroenterology, hepatology, & endoscopy* (3rd ed.). New York: McGraw Hill.

Lodato, F., Azzaroli, F., Turco, L., Mazzella, N., Buonfiglioli, F., Zoli, M., et al. (2010). Adverse effects of proton pump inhibitors. *Best Practices in Research and Clinical Gastroenterology, 24*(2), 193–201.

Matok, I., Levy, A., Wiznitzer, A., Uziel, E., Koren, G., & Gorodischer, R. (2012). The safety of fetal exposure to proton-pump inhibitors during pregnancy. *Digestive Diseases and Sciences, 57*(3), 699–705.

Rostom, A., Dube, C., Wells, G. A., Tugwell, T., Welch, V., Jolicoeur, E., et al. (2002). Prevention of NSAID-induced gastroduodenal ulcers. *Cochrane Database of Systematic Reviews*, 4. Art. No.: CD002296. DOI: 10.1002/14651858.CD002296.

Salix Pharmaceuticals (2013). Fulyzaq. Retrieved from http://cdn.salix.com/shared/pi/fulyzaq-pi.pdf

Sucampo Pharma Americas. (2013). Amitiza. Retrieved from http://www.amitizahcp.com/

Thomson, A. B. R., Sauve, M. D., Kassam, N., & Kamitakahara, H. (2010). Safety of the long-term use of proton pump inhibitors. *World Journal of Gastroenterology, 16*(19), 2323–2330.

Tjon, J. A., Pe, M., Soscia, J., & Mahant, S. (2013). Efficacy and safety of proton pump inhibitors in the management of pediatric gastroesophageal reflux disease. *Pharmacotherapy, 33*(9), 956–971.

Vandenplas, Y., Rudolph, C. D., DiLorenzo, C., Hassall, E., Liptak, G., Mazur, L., et al. (2009). Pediatric gastroesophageal reflux clinical practice guidelines: Joint recommendations of the North American Society for Pediatric Gastroenterology, Hepatology, and Nutrition (NASPGHAN) and the European Society for Pediatric Gastroenterology, Hepatology, and Nutrition (ESPGHAN). *Journal of Pediatric Gastroenterology and Nutrition, 49*, 498–547.

CHAPTER 21

DRUGS AFFECTING THE ENDOCRINE SYSTEM

Marylou Robinson • Kathy Shaw

BISPHOSPHONATES

Bone is dynamic tissue that undergoes a continuous process of resorption (osteoclastic activity) and formation (osteoblastic activity) throughout life. Under normal physiological states, the two processes are about equal. Skeletal mass is usually maximal at about age 35 and declines in women after age 40 and men after age 50. The rate of decline becomes most rapid in women within 2 years of menopause, with one-third to one-half of all bone that will be lost going during the first 5 years after menopause.

The cycle of bone remodeling takes longer to complete and the rate of mineralization slows with aging. As the life expectancy of women reaches the mid-80s, osteopenia in perimenopausal women takes on epidemic proportions (50%), especially among white and Asian women in industrial societies (International Osteoporosis Foundation [IOF], 2012). Men experience bone loss as well, but at later ages and slower rates than women. Initial bone mass is also about 30% higher in men than it is in women, so the loss is less disabling (McCance & Huether, 2014). The femoral neck and lumbar vertebrae lose the most. Cortical (compact) bone, which is 80% of the skeleton, is lost less rapidly than is cancellous (spongy) bone. Bone loss is related to smoking, calcium deficiency, magnesium deficiency, vitamin D deficiency, high-protein intake, excess phosphorus intake, overly vigorous exercise, certain prescription and over-the-counter (OTC) drugs, alcohol intake, and reduced physical activity. There are 5,500 osteoporosis-related fractures in the United States daily, of which 80% are in women (IOF, 2012). Chapters 38 and 48 discuss this concern as it relates to women's health.

In addition to normal aging, pathophysiological conditions can also alter the balance between resorption and formation. Even a minor imbalance can have devastating effects. For example, if bone resorption exceeds formation by only 2% per year, in 20 years 40% of skeletal mass will be lost. Malignancy, syndromes of ectopic calcification, and Paget's disease are examples of pathological conditions associated with altered bone remodeling.

Longitudinal reevaluation of the risks versus benefits of osteoporosis prevention is shifting the primary clinical use of bone remodeling drugs toward those patients with the highest risk of fracture development. FRAX (Fracture Risk Assessment Tool) scores estimate the 10-year probability for major bone fractures of the hip, wrist, and shoulder. Revised guidelines using FRAX scores and BMD (bone mass density) T scores of less than 2.5 are the major focus of any prefracture treatment. Those patients with BMD T scores between −1.0 and −2.5 with other factors that increase fracture risk to more than 20% in 10 years are also considered for drug interventions. There is no consensus as to how often BMD is measured after the start of therapy, though 2 years is the time line most often cited (Rosen & Drezner, 2012).

The IOF (2012) estimates that only 17% of patients who have sustained an osteoporotic fracture get bone support medications even after a second fracture. Men are less likely to be treated than women and less likely to be screened for the disease. Concerns about the rare, atypical fractures and osteonecrosis should be mitigated by considering the reported incidents are about 10 per 10,000 patients, or 0.1%; however, some experts believe the incidences are underreported (Hellier & Ross, 2012). This said, the very low incidence rate of these rare events should not overshadow the benefit gained from therapy (Black et al, 2010; U.S. Food and Drug Administration [FDA], 2010a; Rizzoli et al, 2011).

Pharmacodynamics

The remodeling cycle is initiated by osteoclastic activity. In response to microfractures and other damage associated with normal wear and tear, osteoclasts are drawn to the damaged area of the trabecula, attach to its surface, and resorb the damaged and surrounding bone, creating a resorption pit (Fig. 21-1). Resorption is accomplished by

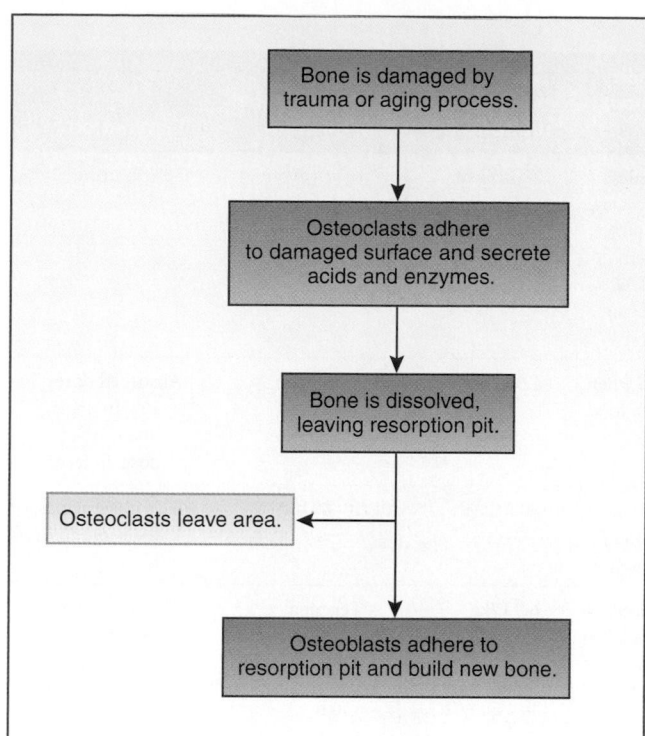

Figure 21–1. Bone remodeling. Damaged bone sections are removed by osteoclasts that use pseudopods to attach to bone surface. Bone is dissolved, leaving a resorption pit. The osteoclasts then leave the site of damage. Osteoblasts enter the resorption pit and build new bone. The process takes 4 to 5 months.

pseudopodia, which attach tightly to the bone surface and secrete acids and enzymes that dissolve bone. The osteoclasts then leave the area and osteoblasts move in, line up to cover the surface of the pit, and form new bone. RANKL, one component of the TNF-associated ligands and receptors, facilitates osteoclast formation. The newest monoclonal antibody approaches to modifying bone remodeling (like demosumab) reduces RANKL action. These meds are covered further in Chapter 38.

Several medication groups, including estrogens, SERMS, and parathyroid hormone agents, can be used to support bone health. Bisphosphonates remain the most commonly used agents and are the focus of this section.

Bisphosphonates adhere tightly to bone and, by inhibiting osteoclastic activity, are potent inhibitors of both normal and abnormal bone resorption. Among this group of drugs, etidronate (Didronel) reduces both bone resorption and bone formation because formation is coupled with resorption. Pamidronate (Aredia) and risedronate (Actonel) inhibit bone resorption without inhibiting bone formation and mineralization. Alendronate (Fosamax) is a highly selective inhibitor of bone resorption and is 100 to 500 times more potent than the other drugs. It does not interfere with osteoclast recruitment or attachment, but it does inhibit osteoclastic activity. Tiludronate (Skelid) inhibits osteoclastic activity through two different mechanisms. It inhibits protein-tyrosine-phosphatase, resulting in detachment of osteoclasts from the bone surface, and it inhibits the osteoclastic proton pump.

Zoledronic acid (Zometa) inhibits osteoclastic activity and induces osteoclast apoptosis. It also inhibits the increased osteoclastic activity and skeletal calcium release induced by various stimulatory factors released by tumors. Ibandronate (Boniva) inhibits osteoclast activity and reduces bone resorption and turnover based on its affinity for hydroxyapatite, which is part of the mineral matrix of the bone. All reduce vertebral fractures, only aldendronate, risedronate, and zoledronic acid have demonstrated nonvertebral fracture reductions; it cannot be assumed the others can achieve the same endpoint (*Drug Facts and Comparisons [DF & C]*, 2011). Alendronate, risedronate, and zolendronic acid have been studied in men, but transferability of results with other medications is considered a safe assumption. Because pamidronate and zoledronic acid are available only for parenteral use, they are not discussed in detail except to alert the primary care provider about monitoring the drug and its place in the total treatment regimen of the patient.

Pharmacokinetics

Absorption and Distribution

All oral bisphosphonates potentially cause esophagitis and gastric irritation. Absorption and bioavailability of oral doses are significantly reduced by the presence of food in the gut or other preparations containing divalent cations. To enhance absorption, the patient takes the drug with 8 oz of water. No other food or drink should be ingested, and the patient must remain upright for at least half an hour (1 hour with ibandronate). Table 21-1 shows the effect of food, coffee, and juice on bioavailability.

These drugs are all mainly distributed to bone. Their terminal half-life in bone is exceedingly long, varying from more than 10 years for alendronate to more than 90 days for etidronate. The half-life of risedronate is much shorter, at 480 hours; ibandronate is 220 hours; zoledronic acid is 167 hours; and tiludronate is 150 hours, but these times are thought to represent the dissociation of the drug from the bone surface, rather than its time within the bone. Their volumes of distribution exclusive of bone vary significantly from 90 L/kg for ibandronate to 1.3 L/kg for etidronate.

Most bisphosphonates are Pregnancy Category C. Pamidronate and zoledronic acid are Category D. *Drug Facts and Comparisons* (2011) states that fetal anomalies have occurred in animal studies. There are no adequate and well-controlled studies in pregnant women. Bisphosphonates should be prescribed only when they are clearly needed and the benefits to the mother outweigh the potential hazards to the fetus. All bisphosphonates are used with extreme caution during breastfeeding; zoledronic acid binds to bone for long periods so is never used in lactating mothers.

Safety and efficacy in children have not been fully established, but children have been treated with etidronate (Pregnancy Category B) at doses recommended for adults to prevent heterotopic ossifications or soft tissue calcifications. The epiphyseal changes that occurred were reversible with discontinuation of the drug. In children with low bone

Table 21–1 ✂ **Pharmacokinetics: Bisphosphonates**

Drug	Onset of Effect	Peak	Duration	Bioavailability (With/Without Food)	Steady-State V_d Exclusive of Bone	Half-Life Normal Renal (Function)	Elimination
Alendronate	1 mo	3–6 mo	7 mo (following after discontinuation of the drug)	0.7% in females; 0.59% in males. Reduced 40% when taken with food; 60% with coffee or juice.	28 L/kg or more	10 yr (in bone)	50% in urine
Etidronate	1 mo	UK	1 yr (following after discontinuation of the drug)	1%; reduced when taken with food or juice	1.37 L/kg	More than 90 d (in bone	Absorbed dose: 50% in urine; unabsorbed dose: in feces
Ibandronate	UK	0.5–2 h	Up to 1 mo	0.6% absorbed; less with food	90 L	10–60 h	50%–60% urine; unabsorbed in feces
Risedronate	Days	1 h	16 mo (following after discontinuance of drug)	0.63%; reduced by 55% when taken with food	6.3 L/kg	Terminal half-life 480 h	50% absorbed drug in urine; rest in feces
Tiludronate	UK	2 h	UK	6%; reduced when taken with food	1–4.6 mg/L	150 h	60% in urine

UK = unknown; V_d = volume/density.

density due to malabsorption syndromes such as cystic fibrosis, alendronate was shown to increase BMD to normal levels after only 1 year of therapy; the impact was greatest in children who also achieved puberty during the clinical trial (Bianchi et al., 2013).

Metabolism and Excretion

There is no evidence that any of the bisphosphonates are systemically metabolized. Drug that is not distributed to bone is largely excreted in the urine. Because of the fairly exclusive renal excretion and the high volumes of distribution exclusive of bone, these drugs are not recommended for patients with moderate to severe renal impairment (serum creatinine greater than 4.9; creatinine clearance (CCr) less than 30 to 35 mL/min). Dosage adjustments may be necessary if the drug must be given (FDA, 2011a).

Pharmacotherapeutics

Precautions and Contraindications

There are no absolute contraindications except uncorrected hypocalcemia, documented Barrett's esophagus, and renal insufficiency (*DF&C*, 2011; FDA, 2010a, 2011a). Cautious use is recommended for patients with gastrointestinal (GI) disorders. The risk for severe esophageal adverse reactions is greater in patients who lie down after taking these drugs or who fail to swallow them with a full glass (8 oz) of water. Etidronate has been withheld from patients with enterocolitis because diarrhea has occurred in some patients, particularly at high doses.

Etidronate has also been associated with fractures in patients with Paget's disease when they are given high doses or when therapy lasted longer than 6 months. These patients must be carefully monitored with x-rays and laboratory work to assess for these lesions. The development of a rare form of subtrochanteric femur fracture in non-Paget's patients using bisphosphonates is under close scrutiny and has contributed to movement away from osteopenia prevention care to only osteoporosis therapy (FDA, 2010a). The personal and economic impact of a patient sustaining a preventable hip fracture overshadows these risks (Black et al., 2010; Rizzoli et al., 2011).

IV formulations are associated with higher renal toxicity risk, especially with rapid infusion. Checking serum creatinine prior to every dose is required. Forcing fluids before and after infusion is also recommended (FDA, 2011).

Adverse Drug Reactions

An adverse drug reaction for all bisphosphonates is musculoskeletal pain. It is more common for patients with Paget's disease and in those taking risedronate and higher doses of etidronate. Musculoskeletal pain occurred in about 6% of patients taking alendronate and ibandronate.

Rare reports of osteonecrosis of the jaw have been associated with active dental disease or invasive procedures, especially in cancer patients, but it can occur without dental issues in those receiving frequent high IV doses. Earlier onset is associated with the IV forms of bisphosphonates, but oral medications may also carry the risk after 3 years of use (Fleisha et al, 2013; Zhang, Saag, & Curtis, 2011). If elective dental procedures are planned, drug cessation for 3 months pre- and post-procedure may decrease the risk, but there is no evidence to support this plan (*DF & C*, 2011; McClung et al., 2013; Ruggiero et al, 2009).

Some concerns have arisen about increased risk of atrial fibrillation. A systematic review has shown a 27% increased risk to develop the rhythm, but no associated increase in stroke or cardiovascular related deaths (Sharma et al, 2013). Risk is increased with both oral and IV drug forms. Recommendations to halt use have not been made in those with pre-treatment atrial fib or for those at risk for other reasons (FDA, 2011; Institute for Clinical Systems Improvement [ICSI], 2011; Kim, Kim, Cadarette, & Solomon, 2010).

Drug Interactions

Because of these drugs' adverse reactions on the GI tract, drug interactions are most common with other drugs that also affect the GI tract. Histamine$_2$ blocking agents double alendronate bioavailability, but the impact is unknown (*DF & C*, 2011). Calcium supplements and antacids interfere with bisphosphonate absorption when taken within 1 hour of each other. The risk of GI bleeding is increased when aspirin and NSAIDs are concomitantly taken. Aspirin may decrease the bioavailability of tiludronate by up to 50% when taken 2 hours after the tiludronate. Although

indomethacin increases the bioavailability of tiludronate by 2- to 4-fold, the bioavailability is not significantly altered by diclofenac; therefore, each NSAID must be considered individually. Table 21-2 presents these and other drug interactions.

Concurrent use of bisphosphonates and other drugs known to build bone density, such as estrogens and SERMs, prove to have additive bone density, but fracture reduction potential is unknown. The safety of combination therapy appears to be the same as the use of each drug separately (*DF & C*, 2011). It is reserved for extreme cases where one drug is inadequate.

Clinical Use and Dosing

Osteoporosis

Clinical trial data support the use of bisphosphonates for prevention and treatment of osteoporosis and its risk for fractures in men and postmenopausal women, especially vertebral fractures. The best trials have been done with alendronate, risedronate, and zoledronic acid with hip fracture reductions (ICSI, 2011) and have received FDA approval for this indication. Ibandronate is considered a second-line drug (Watts et al, 2010). Ibandronate and zoledronic acid come in an IV form and alendronate has an oral solution (Binosto) for those patients unable to take tablets. Among

Table 21–2 ⁜ Drug and Food Interactions: Bisphosphonates

Drug	Interacting Drugs and Food	Possible Effect	Implications
Alendronate	Ranitidine, aspirin, NSAIDs	Bioavailability doubled Increases risk of GI bleeding with doses more than 10 mg/d	Clinical significance unknown Avoid concurrent use
	Any food	Bioavailability decreased by 40%	Take 30 min or more before any food intake
	Coffee, orange juice	Bioavailability decreased by 60%	Take 30 min or more before intake
Etidronate	Warfarin	INR may increase when added to regimen that includes warfarin	Increase INR monitoring
Ibandronate	Ca^{++}, aluminum, Mg^{++}, and iron products Food and milk products	Decreased absorption	Take 60 min prior to food or mineral products
Risedronate	Any food	Bioavailability decreased	Take 30 min or more before any food intake
Tiludronate	Aspirin	Tiludronate bioavailability decreased by up to 50% when aspirin taken 2 h after the tiludronate	Avoid concurrent use or give aspirin more than 2 h after tiludronate
	Indomethacin	Increases tiludronate bioavailability 2- to 4-fold	Clinical significance unknown
	Any food	Bioavailability decreased by 90%	Take after overnight fast and 4 h before standard breakfast
Zoledronic acid	Concurrent use loop diuretics or aminoglycosides	Increases hypocalcemia risk	Check Ca^{++} levels before
All bisphosphonates	Calcium supplements, antacids	Interferes with bisphosphonate absorption Bioavailability may be decreased by 60% when given within 1 h	Take most bisphosphonates at least 30 min before; ibandronate requires 1 h before

these alternative forms, only the zoledronic acid shows evidence of hip fracture reduction.

Practitioners should consider prophylactic use of bisphosphonates in patients with early osteopenia related to long-term use of medications that contribute to bone loss, such as thyroid hormone, aromatase inhibitors, and glucocorticoids (Watts et al, 2010). The use of proton-pump inhibitors (PPI) and serontonin-receptor inhibitors (SSRIs) are newly linked with significant bone loss at a level equal to that of glucocorticoids (Adachi, 2013).

It is recommended that all adults taking more than 7.5 mg of prednisone or its equivalent for more than 3 weeks be given alendronate or risedronate (*DF &C*, 2011; Watts et al, 2010). In very high-risk patients, a maximum 2-year use of teriparatide (Forteo), a parathyroid hormone, may be more efficacious (ICSI, 2011). The bone mass benefit disappears after teriparatide discontinuance, a decline not seen with the

bisphosphonates for 5 years. Concerns about a cancer link (osteosarcoma) need to be considered with the use of teriparatide. There is currently an ongoing 15-year surveillance study of post-marketing incidence of osteosarcoma in patients taking teriparatide which started in 2003, with no pattern indicative of causal association at the 7-year mark in the study (Andrews et al, 2012).

Initial doses for prevention of bone loss for alendronate and risedronate are 5 mg/day or 35 mg/week. For treatment of existing osteoporosis, the dose of alendronate doubles to 10 mg/day or 70 mg/week, and the dose of risedronate increases to 75 mg for 2 consecutive days or 150 mg once a month. Therapy with 10 mg daily can increase bone density by up to 10% after 3 years and can decrease vertebral and hip fractures by 50% (Table 21-3). Use for more than 4 years is currently under review concerning its efficacy or safety. A "drug holiday" for up to 3 years may be considered for lower-risk

Table 21–3 ⊗ Dosage Schedule: Selected Bisphosphonates

Drug	Indication	Dosage Forms	Initial Dose	Maintenance Dose
Alendronate	Osteoporosis: men, post-menopausal women, glucocorticoid-induced	Tablets: 5, 10, 35, 40, 70 mg Oral solution: 70 mg	Prevention: 5 mg/d or 35 mg/wk Treatment: 10 mg/d or 70 mg/wk	5 mg/d or 35 mg/wk 10 mg/d or 70 mg/wk Renal parameters: CCr 35–60: no dosage adjustment CCr 35: use not recommended
	Paget's disease		40 mg/d for 6 mo	Re-treat if needed with same dose only after 6 mo post-treatment evaluation Renal dose as above
Etidronate (Didronel)	Paget's disease	Tablets: 200. 400 mg	5 mg/kg/d	5–10 mg/kg/d not to exceed 6 mo or 11–20 mg/kg/d not to exceed 3 mo; re-treat if needed with same dose only after 3–6 mo post-treatment evaluation Renal dose: serum creatinine 2.5–4.9, reduce dose Creatinine more than 5: use not recommended
	Heterotropic ossification: hip replacement		20 mg/kg/d for 1 mo pre-operatively	20 mg/kg/d for 3 mo post-operatively Renal dose as above
	Spinal cord injury		20 mg/kg/d for 2 wk	10 mg/kg/d for 10 wk Renal dose as above
Ibandronate (Boniva)	Osteoporosis prevention and treatment	Tablets: 150 mg 1 mg/mL prefilled syringe for IV is brand only	2.5 mg daily or 150 mg monthly; IV 3 mg over 30 sec bolus	Same Renal dose: CCr <30 contraindicated
Pamidronate (Aredia)	Paget's disease	Powder for injection 30 mg and 90 mg; injection 3, 6, 9 mg	30 mg IV over 4 hon 3 consec days	Evaluate in 6–9 mo if repeated dose required
Risedronate (Actonel)	Osteoporosis prevention and treatment: men, postmenopausal women, and glucocorticoid-induced osteoporosis	Tablets: 5, 30, 35, 75, 150 mg	5 mg/d or 35 mg/wk or 75 mg on two consecutive dates monthly or 150 mg/mo	Not to exceed 10 mg/kg/d for 6 mo or 11–20 mg/kg/d for 3 mo Renal dose: CCr less than 30: use not recommended

Table 21–3 ⊗ **Dosage Schedule: Selected Bisphosphonates—cont'd**

Drug	Indication	Dosage Forms	Initial Dose	Maintenance Dose
	Paget's disease		30 mg/d for 2 mo	Re-treat if needed with same dose only after 2 mo post-treatment evaluation Renal dose: as above
Tiludronate (Skelid)	Paget's disease	Tablet: 240 mg in foil strips of 56	Two 240 mg tabs give 400 mg of actual medication	400 mg/d for 3 mo; re-treat if needed with same dose only after 3 mo post-treatment evaluation Renal dose: CCr less than 30: use not recommended
Zoledronic acid (Reclast and Zometa)	Osteoporosis Paget's disease Treatment and prevention	5 mg/100 mL IV dose	5 mg IV infusion yearly	Renal dose: If serum Cr greater than 4.5, consider risks

patients; higher-risk patients are encouraged to remain on therapy due to a better risk versus harm profile (McClure, et al, 2013).

The initial and maintenance dosage of ibandronate for both prevention and treatment is one 2.5 mg tablet taken daily or one 150 mg tablet taken once monthly on the same date of each month. The IV dose is 3 mg given over 30 seconds and repeated every 3 months, a schedule that must be closely maintained for best results. Another IV osteoporosis treatment and fracture prevention medication is zoledronic acid (5 mg), which is taken only yearly. The 4 mg dosing is typically reserved for monthly cancer metastasis prevention and treatment.

Although its labeled use is for treatment of Paget's disease, etidronate has been prescribed off-label to treat post-menopausal osteoporosis and prevent further bone loss in early postmenopausal women. Dosage is 400 mg daily for 14 days, followed by 76 days of elemental calcium, 500 mg daily. This drug also has an off-labeled use in the treatment of glucocorticoid-induced bone loss in postmenopausal women. Dosage is 400 mg daily for 1 month and then 400 mg daily for 2 weeks every third month, plus calcium and ergocalciferol. None of the major guidelines mentions etidronate for this indication.

The antiresorptive property of raloxifene (a SERM) as a bone supplement is less dramatic. Post menopausal estrogen replacement is covered elsewhere. The combination of estrogens with an atypical SERM, bazedoxifene (Duavee), is a limited impact medication for bone health. (See Chap. 38.) The RANKL drugs such as teriparatide have some cancer concerns that are dose and treatment duration dependent (Forteo Package Insert, 2012). Alternative agents such as phytoestrogens, synthetic isoflavones, natural progesterone cream, magnesium, vitamin K, and eicosapentaenoic acid have also been subjected to limited randomized clinical trials. Findings from these trials have been inconsistent in their support of these alternative agents (Whelen, Jurgens, Bowles, & Doyle, 2009). Fluoride is of no help (Grey et al, 2013). Vitamin D alone is not an effective alternative.

The costs for bisphosphonates are high for the branded and IV-delivered products. The advent of generic tablets has significantly changed prices from several hundred dollars a month to about a hundred dollars per month. The lowest cost drug tends to be aldendronate generic.

Paget's Disease *(Osteitis Deformans)*

All bisphosphonates are used to treat Paget's disease when the alkaline phosphatase is at least twice the upper limit of normal. They may also be used for those who are asymptomatic or at risk for future complications from their disease. Symptomatic Paget's disease is best treated with etidronate. Editronate slows accelerated bone turnover in pagetic lesions and, to a lesser extent, in normal bone. This reduced turnover is accompanied by symptomatic improvement, including less bone pain and decreased bone fractures. The initial dose is 5 to 10 mg/kg daily for up to, but not exceeding, 6 months, or 11 to 20 mg/kg daily, not to exceed 3 months. The higher doses are reserved for times when lower doses are ineffective or when there is an overriding need for suppression of increased bone turnover. Doses greater than 20 mg/kg daily are not recommended. Retreatment for relapse is acceptable only after more than 90 drug-free days and when there is evidence of active disease. Dosage is the same as for initial treatment.

Treatment with alendronate using doses of 40 mg daily for 6 months has produced highly significant decreases in serum alkaline phosphatase as well as in urinary markers of bone collagen degradation (*DF & C*, 2011). Retreatment may be considered after a 6-month post-treatment evaluation period. Risedronate treatment is 30 mg daily for 2 months. In patients with this treatment protocol, bone turnover returned to normal in a majority of the patients and no evidence of new fractures was found (*DF & C*, 2011). Retreatment requires a post-treatment evaluation time of 2 months. Tiludronate treatment is 400 mg daily for 3 months. Patients on this protocol had a reduction toward normal in the rate of bone turnover and a reduced number of osteoclasts. Retreatment occurs only after a 3-month post-treatment evaluation. Pamidronate IV is useful in patients with moderate to severe Paget's disease. For all of these drugs, indications for retreatment are evidence of active disease or failure to normalize alkaline phosphatase levels.

Patients with Paget's disease benefit from supplemental calcium and vitamin D if their dietary intake is not adequate. Consideration must be given to spacing the administration of the calcium supplement and the bisphosphonate to prevent reduction in bioavailability.

Heterotopic Ossification

When heterotopic ossification is a complication of total hip replacement, etidronate may be used at 20 mg/kg daily for 1 month pre-operatively and 20 mg/kg daily for 3 months post-operatively. Etidronate is also used when heterotopic ossification occurs secondary to spinal cord injury. The dosage then is 20 mg/kg daily for 2 weeks, followed by 10 mg/kg daily for 10 weeks, begun as soon as possible after the injury and prior to evidence of heterotopic ossification.

Other uses of bisphosphonates to treat the hypercalcemia of malignancy are with parenteral dosage forms and are usually reserved for use by specialists. These uses are not discussed here.

Rational Drug Selection

Alendronate, ibandronate, risedonrate, and zoledronic acid are approved by the FDA for prevention and treatment of osteoporosis in postmenopausal women, but some health-care providers have used etidronate. There have been no randomized, controlled studies comparing the FDA-approved drugs with etidronate, but the same bone mineral density has not been achieved by cyclic use of etidronate as has been achieved by the use of the other drugs. In addition, 3- to 4-year studies of etidronate are inconclusive with regard to fracture prevention.

For the treatment of Paget's disease, bisphosphonates may be used, but ibandronate does not have approval for this indication. Etidronate has been used longer for this indication and has midrange adverse drug reactions. Clinical trials reported in *Drug Facts and Comparisons* (2011), however, showed increased efficacy of alendronate over etidronate in suppression of alkaline phosphatase, with a response rate of 85% for alendronate as compared with 30% for etidronate and 0% for placebo. In addition, alendronate produced mild, transient, and asymptomatic decreases in serum calcium and phosphate as compared with etidronate. *Drug Facts and Comparisons* also reported a positive-controlled study conducted in Europe, with treatment groups taking 400 mg/day of tiludronate versus 400 mg/day of etidronate for 6 months. Tiludronate was more efficacious than etidronate in that trial. Risedronate has the highest adverse drug reaction profile. With consideration of all these factors, the drugs of choice appear to be alendronate and tiludronate.

Monitoring

Before beginning treatment, rule out common treatable disorders that can also cause low bone density. These include hyperparathyroidism, vitamin D deficiency, hyperthyroidism, and renal disease. Tests for these disorders are serum calcium and albumin, 25-hydroxy vitamin D, thyroid-stimulating hormone (TSH), and serum creatinine levels, respectively. Serum creatinine levels are drawn prior to initiating therapy. Dosage alterations or contraindications to using specific bisphosphonates occur with serum creatinine levels above 2.5 mg/dL. Because bisphosphonates inhibit intestinal calcium transport, careful monitoring of serum calcium should be done during therapy. Phosphate, magnesium, and potassium should also be monitored because these electrolytes may be altered by bisphosphonate administration.

Elevation of alkaline phosphatase is a major indicator of Paget's disease and its reduction is an indicator of the efficacy of treatment. Alkaline phosphatase should be monitored prior to initiating therapy, at the end of each cycle of therapy, and prior to initiating any retreatment.

Measurement of bone mineral density is the most accurate predictor of fracture risk and the efficacy of these drugs. Each 10% change below peak bone mass is associated with a doubling of the fracture risk for patients with osteoporosis. Dual-energy x-ray absorptiometry (DEXA) is the gold standard by which bone mineral density and therapy are monitored. Initial evaluation with DEXA can also suggest when a disease process other than aging is the probable cause of the bone loss. Once therapy has been established, DEXA is repeated 1 to 2 years later to determine progress. Whether to repeat DEXA again at later dates is controversial (Watts et al, 2010). The use of DEXA and other bone risk factors are also covered in Chapter 38.

Patient Education

Administration

The oral drugs should be taken first thing in the morning, at least 30 minutes prior to other medications, beverages, or food (60 min for ibandronate). Etidronate and tiludronate should be taken 2 hours before any food. Alendronate, ibandronate, risedronate, and tiludronate should be taken with 8 oz of plain water. Mineral water, coffee, orange juice, and other beverages greatly reduce absorption. If supplemental calcium or antacids are taken, the bisphosphonate must be administered at least 1 hour before these other drugs. If a daily dose is missed, that dose should be skipped and the patient should resume taking the drug the next morning. For ibandronate, if the once-monthly dose is missed, and the next scheduled dose is more than 7 days away, the patient should take one 150 mg tablet in the morning following the date that it is remembered and then return to the every month dosing on the original schedule. Double doses should not be taken nor should the patient take doses later in the day. Remaining upright for at least 30 minutes after taking the oral medications (60 min for ibandronate) facilitates passage out of the stomach and minimizes the risk for esophageal irritation. The IV forms of zoledronic acid and ibandronate can be taken without regard for food but must be administered by health-care professionals.

Adverse Reactions

GI distress and dyspepsia are the most common adverse reactions. If needed, aluminum- or magnesium-containing antacids may be taken more than 2 hours after the bisphosphonate. If diarrhea occurs with etidronate, the health-care provider may divide the dose throughout the day to control the diarrhea. Female patients should advise their health-care provider if pregnancy is planned or suspected or if they are breastfeeding. The drug may have to be changed or stopped.

Lifestyle Management

The patient should eat a balanced diet with adequate amounts of calcium and vitamin D. Supplemental calcium and vitamin D are typically needed. Regular exercise is beneficial for cardiovascular fitness as well as preserving bone mass. Behaviors such as smoking and alcohol intake that increase the risk of osteoporosis should be reduced or stopped. Because relapse is not uncommon, keeping follow-up appointments to monitor progress, even after the drug is discontinued, is important.

HYPOTHALAMIC AND PITUITARY HORMONES

A combination of neural and endocrine systems located in the hypothalamus and the pituitary gland mediates control of metabolism, growth, and certain aspects of reproduction. The hormones involved in these hypothalamus-pituitary-hormone axes are adrenocorticotropic hormone, corticotropin-releasing hormone, follicle-stimulating hormone, growth hormone, growth hormone–binding protein, growth hormone–releasing hormone, gonadotropin-releasing hormone, insulin-like growth factor 1, luteinizing hormone, luteinizing hormone–releasing factor, prolactin-releasing factor, prolactin, somatotropin-releasing factor, thyrotropin-releasing hormone, and thyroid-stimulating hormone.

The reproductive hormones are covered in Chapter 22, the corticosteroid-related hormones are covered in Chapter 25, and the thyroid-related hormones are discussed later in this chapter. This section discusses the growth-hormone axis. Drugs affecting this axis are prescribed by specialists; the role of the primary care provider is largely to monitor the drug and its place in the total treatment regimen of the patient. The predominant use is in children with short stature; however, some adults with pan-pituitary failure may also benefit (Molitch, Clemmons, Malozowski, Merriam, & Vance, 2011).

Pharmacodynamics

The hypothalamus-pituitary–growth hormone axis (Fig. 21-2) begins with growth hormone–releasing hormone (GHRH), which is secreted by the hypothalamus in response to decreased serum glucose levels in the body (hypoglycemia stimulates secretion, and hyperglycemia inhibits it). GHRH then binds to receptors in the anterior pituitary, resulting in the secretion by that gland of growth hormone (GH) (also called somatotropin). GH is a single peptide that attaches to receptors that allow it to pass through the cell membrane. Once inside cells, GH fosters protein synthesis, fat breakdown, and tissue growth. GH also causes hyperglycemia by decreasing glucose utilization by cells and increasing the rate by which

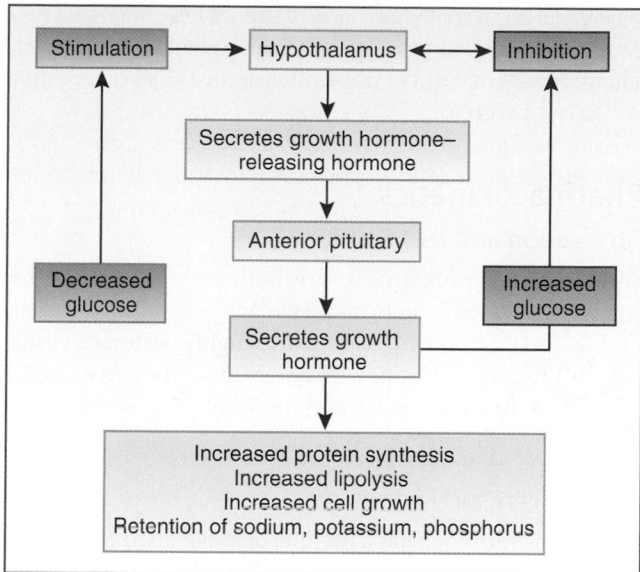

Figure 21–2. Hypothalamus-pituitary–growth hormone axis.

glycogen is broken down into glucose. Both GHRH and GH have now been synthesized by recombinant DNA technology and are available in drug form. They produce the same actions as the natural hormones.

The primary role of GHRH is as a diagnostic tool for evaluation of children of short stature in order to assess for dysfunction of the hypothalamus or the pituitary. It will not be discussed further.

Administration of synthetic GH somatropin (191 amino acids) and somatrem (somatropin plus the amino acid methionine), results in an initial insulin-like effect, with increased tissue uptake of both glucose and amino acids and decreased lipolysis. Within a few hours, there is a peripheral insulin antagonistic effect, with impaired glucose uptake and increased lipolysis. These drugs also stimulate synthesis of somatomedins in the growth plate cartilage and the liver, resulting in increased linear, organ, and skeletal growth and increased cellular protein synthesis. Children with GH deficiency sometimes experience hypoglycemia that is improved by administration of these drugs. Patients may also experience reduction in fat stores, increased lean muscle mass, and decreased mean cholesterol levels. Conflicting results are reported for adult patients (Molitch et al, 2011). Tesamorelin (Egrifta—a synthetic growth hormone–releasing factor) has been approved by the FDA to treat the lipodystrophy of HIV patients (FDA, 2010c). Reduction of wasting and cachexia are desired effects when used in AIDS patients (Serostim somatropin [rDNA origin] only) (FDA, 2003).

In cases of overabundance of growth axis hormones (acromegaly), pituitary surgical interventions are primary interventions, but the recurrence rate sometimes requires the use of somatostatin analogues such as octreotide or lancreotide (Katznelson et al, 2011). These GH suppressant agents are also used in GI bleeds and cases of severe diarrhea in AIDS patients. The benefit of using GH for AIDS wasting is reversed if the analogues are also used. These high-cost parenteral medications are not further discussed in this chapter. The supplemental use of dopamine agonists like cabergoline is also not covered.

Pharmacokinetics

Absorption and Distribution

Somatrem and somatropin are both well absorbed after subcutaneous (SC) or intramuscular (IM) administration (Table 21-4). They tend to localize to highly perfused organs, such as the liver and kidney. The area under the curve (AUC) of the two drugs is similar and does not vary based on the injection type or site.

Metabolism and Excretion

Circulating hormone has a half-life of about 20 to 25 minutes and is predominantly cleared by the liver. In the kidney, both drugs are filtered by the glomerulus, reabsorbed in the proximal tubule, and broken down within the renal cells into amino acids that return to the circulation. The total mean half-life of both drugs from administration to elimination is 3.8 to 4.9 hours. Active blood levels persist for up to 36 hours. This factor is the basis for every-other-day treatment plans; however, daily dosing produces more consistent growth (Rogel, 2012).There is a reduction in hormone clearance in patients with hepatic or renal dysfunction.

Pharmacotherapeutics

Precautions and Contraindications

Growth hormone supplements are generally contraindicated in patients with closed epiphyses and those with evidence of active tumor growth. GH is used cautiously in patients with intracranial tumors because it can increase the tumor growth. Patients with coexisting adrenocorticotropic hormone deficiency may experience increased symptoms of this disorder. Serum levels of inorganic phosphorus, alkaline phosphatase, and parathyroid hormone may increase with GH therapy. Changes in thyroid hormone levels have also occurred. This makes management of thyroid disorders more difficult. In addition, untreated hypothyroidism prevents optimal response to GH therapy.

Insulin resistance may be induced by GH. The drugs are used cautiously with diabetic patients and those with glucose intolerance or risk of metabolic syndrome. The potential lipid benefits may make the risk worthwhile. The safety and efficacy of synthetic GH have not been established in pregnancy

and lactation. They are Pregnancy Category C and should be used only if clearly needed.

Adverse Drug Reactions

Approximately 30% to 40% of patients on somatrem and 2% to 4.7% of patients on somatropin develop persistent antibodies, making them less likely to respond to the drug. Other adverse reactions are rare and include pain at the injection site, hyperglycemia, hypothyroidism, and edema secondary to retained sodium. Rare instances of death have been reported (FDA, 2011). Evidence is not available on longer-term issues of carbohydrate, protein, and fat metabolism.

Drug Interactions

Glucocorticoid therapy and estrogens may inhibit the growth-promoting effect of GH. Anticonvulsants may have more severe side effects. Insulin may lose its effectiveness.

Clinical Use and Dosing

Growth Failure Associated With Chronic Renal Insufficiency

Growth hormone is used to treat children with growth failure up to the time of renal transplantation (National Institute for Health and Clinical Excellence [NICE], 2010). The dosages used are higher than normal due to a relative hormone resistance. Use after transplantation is typically restricted to children 2 standard deviations below the mean for their gender if they have not experienced epiphyseal closure. Growth hormone is known to increase the side effects of cyclosporine, so it is typically evaluated 1 year after transplant for continued use. To optimize therapy for patients receiving hemodialysis, injections are given at night, just prior to going to sleep, or at least 3 to 4 hours after dialysis to prevent hematoma formation caused by the heparin. Patients undergoing chronic cycling peritoneal dialysis (CCPD) receive their injections in the morning after they have completed dialysis. Patients undergoing chronic ambulatory peritoneal dialysis (CAPD) receive their injections in the evening at the time of the overnight exchange.

Long-Term Treatment of Growth Failure in Children Who Lack Adequate Endogenous GH

Somatrem and all forms of somatropin (except Serostim) have been used for this indication. Dosing is started at 40 mcg/kg day and titrated to individual patient response. Younger children respond better than prepubertal adolescents. Doses in excess of 0.3 mg/kg have resulted in risks of known effects of excess human GH. Dosage of the various

---

Table 21–4 ⁘ Pharmacokinetics: Growth Hormones

Drug	Onset of Effect	Peak (Drug in Plasma)	Duration (Drug in Plasma)	Bioavailability	Half-Life (Normal Renal Function)	Elimination
Somatrem, somatropin	Within 3 mo	7.5 h	36 h	75% (SC) 63% (IM)	3.8 h (SC) 4.9 h (IM)	By liver and kidney

forms of somatropin varies by manufacturer; selected forms shown in Table 21-5. Nocturnal administration is based on expert opinion to mimic native GH secretion patterns, not on evidence establishing circadian efficacy (Rogel, 2012).

Turner's Syndrome

Somatropin is approved for long-term treatment of short stature associated with Turner's syndrome. Specific dosing scheduling is individualized. A relative hormone resistance

Table 21–5 ✂ Dosage Schedule: Selected Growth Hormones

Drug*	Indication	Dosage Form	Initial Dose	Maintenance Dose
Somatropin (Nutropin and Nutropin AQ)	Growth failure related to chronic renal failure	Powder: 5 mg and 10 mg vial Depot: 13.5, 18, and 22.5 mg AQ: 10 mg vial	Not more than 0.0006 mg/kg daily	0.35 mg/kg/wk (see note in text regarding hemodialysis and transplant)
Somatrem (Protropin)	Growth failure due to inadequate endogenous growth hormone (kids)	Powder for injection: 5 mg per vial, 10 mg per vial	0.1 mg/kg	0.1–0.3 mg/kg 3 times/wk; not to exceed 0.3 mg/kg
Somatropin (Gentropin)	Growth failure due to inadequate endogenous growth hormone	10 mg (30 IU) in 3mL cartridges	*Children:* 0.07 mg/kg/d *Adults:* 0.3 mg/d	*Children:* 0.16–0.24 mg/kg/wk in equal doses divided into 6–7 injections *Adults:* Increase every 1–2 mo by 0.15 mg/d
	Turner's syndrome		0.375 mg/kg in divided 6–7 doses per wk	
Somatropin (Humatrope)	Growth failure due to inadequate endogenous growth hormone or somatropin deficiency	Powder for injection: 5, 6, or 24 mg In vial with 5 mL of diluents In cartridge with prefilled syringe and diluent	*Children:* 0.18 mg/kg/wk *Adults:* 0.006 mg/kg/d	*Children :* 0.18–0.3 mg/kg/wk divided into equal doses, given on 3 alternate days or 6 d/wk *Adults:* 0.006 mg/kg/d
Somatropin (Norditropin)	Growth failure due to inadequate endogenous growth hormone	Powder for injection: 4 and 8 mg Injection: 5, 10, and 15 mg/ 1.5 mL In vials with diluents or cartridges	0.024 mg/kg	0.024–0.034 mg/kg, given 6–7 times weekly
Somatropin (Nutropin)	Growth failure due to inadequate endogenous growth hormone	Powder for injection: 5 and 10 mg vial in cartons of 2 vials with 10 mL multidose vial of diluent Depot: 13.5,18, and 22.5 mg in single-use vials with 1.5 mL diluent and needles AQ: 10 mg multidose vial	0.3 mg/kg	0.3 mg/kg/wk
Somatropin (Accretropin)	Growth failure due to inadequate endogenous growth hormone	15 IU/mL vial	0.18mg/kg in divided doses	Up to 0.3mg/kg divided over 6–7 times/wk
	Turner's syndrome		0.36 mg/kg in divided doses given 6–7 times/wk	
Somatropin (Saizen)	Growth failure due to inadequate endogenous growth hormone	Powder: 5 and 8.8 mg vials Easy Click System: 8.8 mg drug + 1 cartridge diluent	*Children:* 0.18 mg/kg/wk in equal divided doses in 3 alternate or 6 times/wk or daily dosing *Adults:* 0.2 mg/day	*Adults:* increase every 1–2 months by increments of 0.1–0.2 mg/d Max of 0.01 kg/d

Continued

Table 21–5 ⊗ **Dosage Schedule: Selected Growth Hormones—cont'd**

Drug*	Indication	Dosage Form	Initial Dose	Maintenance Dose
Somatropin (Serostim)	Treatment of HIV patients with wasting and cachexia	4, 5, or 6 mg vial needing to mix with sterile water for injection	*Adults:* 0.1 mg/daily at bedtime	*Adults:* Increase up to 6 mg total

Many additional formulations available with unique dosing patterns.

is common, requiring higher doses to obtain growth. Traditionally, introduction of estrogen to stimulate puberty has been delayed as long as possible for best terminal height achievement. Small studies introducing very-low-dose estrogen around normal menarche indicate improved outcomes. This might influence practice in the future in combination with the known positive effects of estrogen on other body systems (Ross et al, 2011).

Somatropin Deficiency

Patients must meet strict criteria before growth hormone is prescribed by the endocrinology team. For children, the recommended weekly dose of Humatrope is 0.18 mg/kg, divided into equal doses and given either on 3 alternate days or 6 times per week SC. For adults, the recommended SC dose is started at 0.006 mg/kg given daily and increased to a maximum of 0.0125 mg/kg daily, based on patient response. Practitioners are cautioned to reference the dosing schedules of each individual brand, as they all vary. This is not an independent primary care decision.

Rational Drug Selection

Choice of drug is based on indication and multiple variables considered by the endocrinology team. Costs are significant and coordination with patient assistance and prior authorization of insurance programs is typically needed. There are no evidence-based indications growth hormone will stop aging (Molitch et al, 2011). Inappropriate use is akin to anabolic steroid abuse. It results in similar issues of insulin resistance, fluid resistance, liver damage, and organ hypertrophy.

Monitoring

Prior to initiating and throughout therapy, hepatic and renal function studies are done. Patients with thyroid dysfunction, diabetes mellitus, or glucose intolerance have their disease processes more carefully monitored, as discussed in the Precautions and Contraindications section.

Growth responses are not linearly associated with dosing. A target height goal is set at the 75th percentile for other children of similar parental heritage or at a calculated genetic target height calculated from the parents (Box 21-1). Monitoring of bone age by x-ray is done to evaluate growth and to determine epiphyseal closure (typically age 14 or 15 in girls, 15 or 16 in boys). The schedule for this assessment is determined by the endocrinology team and may be influenced by IGF-1–level monitoring and Tanner stages. Dosing is typically

---

BOX 21–1 CALCULATING TARGET HEIGHT GOAL

The average expected growth with hormone therapy can be estimated. For girls, subtract 13 cm from the father's height and average this number with the mother's height. For boys, add 13 cm to the mother's height and average the sum with the father's height (Albert, 2012). Conversion from inches to cm is achieved by using the formula 1 in. = 2.54 cm. A mother who is 65 in. tall would be 165.1 cm. A father who is 68 in. tall would be 172.72 cm. For their daughter, the calculation would be 172.72 – 13 cm, or 159.72, which averaged with the mother's 165.1 cm would yield a 162.41 cm expected height.

---

halted when growth is less than 2 cm over the previous year (NICE, 2010). The majority of children do not need dosing into adulthood. They should be monitored for increasing alkaline phosphate, hypertension, and acromegalic changes (in adults), which are indicative of excessive dosing. Abuse of all of these drug formulations exists for illegal athletic performance enhancement and non-FDA-approved antiaging properties. Excessive requests for refills should be monitored.

Patient Education

These drugs are usually injected at home by a family member or self-administered. Education is directed to both the patient and the person who will administer the drug. Information about proper use and disposal of needles and syringes and cautions against reuse of needles is important. Consistent dosing yields consistent results; however, stopping the drug for financial or supply considerations does not induce any major adverse issues. Caution that one drug dosing is not the same as another and reconstitution requirements differ between brands.

Administration

These drugs have specific reconstitution and storage requirements. Storage for all of them is at temperatures from 2°C to 8°C (36°F to 46°F). They are not to be frozen. Each brand has a specific reconstitution formula. Reconstituted vials are stable in refrigeration for 14 to 28 days, depending on the brand (except for Serostim, which is stable for only 24 hours). Newer formulations do not always require reconstitution.

The techniques for injection and site selection must be taught to the patient or caregiver. The dosage schedule must be reviewed because it can vary on a weekly basis. A calendar marked with the days of the week when the drug is to be given and the appropriate dose may be helpful to children assuming self-management of their therapy.

Adverse Reactions

Adverse reactions are typically minimal. Patients and their parents should be taught to report persistent pain at the injection site and edema. Because of the potential for hyperglycemia, patients should also be taught the signs and symptoms of this disorder and what to do should it occur. Growing pains are to be anticipated. Development of cancer requires discontinuation. Growth of pseudo-tumor cerebrii has been reported, so headache and neurological changes must be evaluated.

Lifestyle Management

Emphasize the need for regular follow-up visits with the endocrinology team to ensure appropriate growth rate, laboratory work, and determination of bone age by x-ray. Bone health nutrition tips to include active exercise with calcium and vitamin D supplementation also applies to this population.

EXOCRINE PANCREATIC ENZYMES

The exocrine functions of the pancreas are related to secretion of enzymes into the gut for digestion. Disorders that decrease pancreatic function impair the production and secretion of these enzymes and, therefore, impair digestion. Two major disorders that are characterized by decreased pancreatic functioning are cystic fibrosis and pancreatitis. Some bariatric procedures may also induce need for enzymatic supplementation. Pancreatic cancer and short bowel syndrome patients may also benefit. The prescriber is cautioned that pancreatic endocrine insufficiency can coexist with pancreatic exocrine issues.

Cystic fibrosis (CF) affects approximately 30,000 people in the United States (Cystic Fibrosis Foundation, 2014). Once a disease of childhood, improved and aggressive management has resulted in survival into adulthood and middle age with approximately half of CF patients over age 18 years. Initially, this disorder is an obstructive lung disease, but plugging of the pancreatic ducts eventually results in pancreatic insufficiency, with resultant malabsorption of protein, fat, and carbohydrates. This potentially results in failure to thrive and growth impairment as well.

Acute pancreatitis and chronic pancreatitis are both characterized by inflammation that results in swelling and obstruction of the pancreatic ducts. This obstruction leads not only to activated enzymes digesting the pancreas itself but also to failure of the enzymes to reach the duodenum; thus, the same malabsorption problems as occur in CF. Only bariatric surgery patients exhibiting malabsorption issues need enzyme supplementation.

Pharmacodynamics

The enzymes secreted by the exocrine pancreas are trypsinogen (protein digestion), chymotrypsin (protein digestion), amylase (carbohydrate digestion), and lipase (fat digestion). These enzymes are secreted into the bowel distal to the stomach. Pancrelipase contains principally lipase with some amylase and protease. This drug family substitutes for pancreatic enzymes and hydrolyzes fats to glycerol and fatty acids, changes proteins into peptides and amino acids, and converts starch into dextrins and sugars.

Pharmacokinetics
Absorption and Distribution

These agents exert most of their effects in the duodenum and upper jejunum with limited if any systemic distribution. Because they are inactivated by gastric acid pH of 4 or less and pepsin secretion, problems in drug delivery by the oral route may occur. Enteric coating may prevent destruction or inactivation by gastric acid but inhibits enzyme delivery to the duodenum. For this reason, it is important to synchronize the delivery of the drug with gastric emptying; therefore, the drug is taken immediately before or with a meal. Current FDA-approved products are not formally approved for use with GI tubes but are being tested. Safe, long-term experience with earlier formulations did not reveal any particular issue of concern (FDA, 2012).

Metabolism and Excretion

There is limited if any systemic distribution. There is no metabolism or excretion beyond that which would normally occur in the body with the natural secretion of these enzymes.

Pharmacotherapeutics
Precautions and Contraindications

Pancrelipase is derived from a porcine source. The enzymes increase uric acid levels, which may be an issue for those with gout or renal impairment. Pancreatin products are not FDA-approved at this time. They are derived from porcine, bovine, or vegetable sources, depending on the brand that patients might purchase internationally on the Internet. These drugs are contraindicated during acute exacerbations of chronic pancreatitis. During this time, patients receive nothing by mouth in order to rest the GI tract and have no need for these enzymes. The presence of these enzymes would exacerbate the pancreatic disorder.

It is not known whether these drugs can cause fetal harm when administered to a pregnant woman. Most are considered Pregnancy Category C. Because there are no well-controlled studies on pregnant women, supplements should be given only if the benefit to the mother outweighs any risk to the fetus. It is also not known whether these drugs are excreted in breast milk and so should be used cautiously by nursing mothers.

Adverse Drug Reactions

High doses have been associated with GI symptoms, such as nausea, cramping, abdominal pain, diarrhea, and colonic strictures. One brand (Viokase) must be administered with a proton pump inhibitor (PPI) to help protect the gastric lining.

Irritation of the skin and mucous membranes occurs less commonly. Powder from inside capsules spilled on the hands may cause local irritation or irritate the nasal mucosa and respiratory tract. Inhalation of airborne powder can precipitate an asthma attack.

Drug and Food Interactions

Calcium- and magnesium-based antacids will decrease the effectiveness of the enzymes (Table 21-6). The ability of oral iron to increase serum iron levels may be reduced by concomitant administration. Alkaline foods destroy the coating of enteric-coated products, resulting in destruction of the enzymes by gastric acids.

Clinical Use and Dosing

Enzyme Replacement in Patients With Deficient Exocrine Pancreatic Secretions, Cystic Fibrosis, Chronic Pancreatitis, Pancreatic Insufficiency and Steatorrhea of Malabsorption Syndromes, and Post-Gastrectomy

The dosing and schedule for cystic fibrosis is the same for each of the FDA-approved enzymes. Adult dosing for pancreatic insufficiency is individualized and based on stool output and consistency. Although each drug is specified in lipase, protease, and amylase units, the drugs are prescribed in units of lipase. Infants under 1 year initiate therapy with 3,000 units of lipase per bottle or breast feed (Table 21-7). Some brands do not have infant dosing because dose formulations are

Table 21–6 ▦ Drug and Food Interactions: Pancreatic Enzymes

Drug	Interacting Drug	Possible Effect	Implications
Pancreatin, pancrelipase	Calcium carbonate, magnesium hydroxide	Decreases effectiveness of pancreatin and pancrelipase	Avoid concurrent administration
	Oral iron	Decreases the serum iron response	Avoid concurrent administration
	Alkaline foods	Destroys coating on enteric-coated products	Give enzymes first and separate administration by at least 1 h

Table 21–7 ⌘ Dosage Schedule: Pancreatic Enzymes

Drug	Indication	Dosage in USP Units	Initial Dose	Maintenance Dose
Pancrelipase (Creon delayed-release caps)	Enzyme replacement in patients with deficient exocrine pancreatic secretions, cystic fibrosis,	L: 3,000 P: 15,000 A: 30,000 L: 6,000 P: 19,000 A: 30,000 L: 12,000 P: 38,000 A: 60,000 L: 24,000 P: 76,000 A: 120,000	*Infants <12 months:* 3,000 USP units of lipase per 120 mL formula or one breast feed	*Infants <12 months:* Alter downward per response
			Children 1–4 yr: 1,000 units of lipase/ kg per meal	*Children 1–4 yr:* Max 2,500 units/kg per meal or <10,000 units/kg/d OR <4,000 units/g fat ingested per day
			4 yr–Adults: Begin 500 units lipase/kg per meal	*4 yr–Adults:* Max as above
	Chronic pancreatitis, pancreatectomy		*Adults only:* Individualized per response	Same

Table 21–7 ⊗ **Dosage Schedule: Pancreatic Enzymes—cont'd**

Drug	Indication	Dosage in USP Units	Initial Dose	Maintenance Dose
Pancrelipase (Pancreaze Delayed-Release Caps)	Cystic fibrosis	L: 4,200 P: 10,000 A: 17,500 L: 10,500 P: 25,000 A: 43,750 L: 16,800 P: 40,000 A: 70,000 L: 21,000 P: 37,000 A: 61,000	Dosing as above for Creon	As above for Creon
Pancrelipase (Pertzye Delayed-Release Caps)	Cystic fibrosis	L: 8,000 P: 28,700 A: 30, 250 L: 16,000 P: 57,500 A: 60,500	No infant dosing less than 12 months *Children and adults:* As for Creon	Same as Creon
Pancrelipase (Ultressa Delayed-Release Caps)	Cystic fibrosis	L: 13,800 P: 27,600 A: 27,600 L: 20,700 P: 41,400 A: 41,400	No infant dosing less than 12 mo *Children 1–4 yr:* Must be at least 14 kg to use Dosing same as Creon *Children 4 yr to adults:* Must be at least 28 kg to use Dosing same as Creon adults	Same as Creon
Pancrelipase (Viokase)	Adult pancreatic insufficiency, chronic pancreatitis, pancretectomy	L: 10,440 P: 39,150 A: 39,150 L: 20,880 P: 78,300 A: 78,300	*Adults only:* Same as Creon adults dosing Must be taken with concurrent PPI	Same as Creon
Pancrelipase (ZEN-pep Delayed-Release Capsules)	Cystic fibrosis	L: 3,000 P: 10,000 A: 16,000 L: 5,000 P: 17,000 A: 27,000 L: 10,000 P: 34, 000 A: 55,000 L: 15,000 P: 51,000 A: 82,000 L: 20,000 P: 68,000 A: 109,000	*Infants <12 mo:* Same as for Creon *Children 1–4 yr:* Same as for Creon *Children 4yr–Adult:* Same as for Creon	Same as Creon

For dosage forms: L = lipase USP units; P = protease USP units; A = amylase.

not small enough to accurately dose infants. Capsules must be opened and sprinkled directly into the infant's mouth or on applesauce; the medication cannot be dissolved in milk or formula. Children 1 to 4 years old initiate therapy with 4,000 to 8,000 units of lipase sprinkled on acidic foods such as applesauce or commercially prepared bananas or pears. Several brands have dosage forms that can deliver this dose. Initial doses for children over 4 are listed the same as for adults because actual dosing is titrated to stool response. There are no studies using weight as an outcome, only this subjective steatorrhea response (Fieker, Philpott, & Armand, 2011).

Post-Pancreatectomy and Ductal Obstructions Caused by Cancer of the Pancreas or Common Bile Duct

The dosing and schedule for these indications starts with low values and can be taken at 2-hour intervals. In severe deficiencies, the dose may be increased to a larger number of units of lipase with meals. The frequency of administration may be increased to hourly intervals unless nausea, cramps, or diarrhea occurs.

Rational Drug Selection

Cost

Historically, there have been many available dosages and brands of these drugs. Now with only six FDA-approved products, costs have become unpredictable as insurance companies adjust to FDA recommendations. Cash prices for one approved med (ZenPop) runs around $140.00 for a month's supply. Traditionally, pancrealipase drugs with higher lipase units are more expensive but are about as expensive as it would be to take enough of the lower-dose tablets to gain the higher dose. Given this fact, the dose per unit of lipase is about the same across brands. Many formulas available online have not completed the newest FDA approval process (FDA, 2010). The Cystic Fibrosis Foundation (CFF) only endorses FDA-approved medications (CFF, 2009). Table 21-7 reflects only the FDA-approved meds as of this publication.

Brand

It is important to remember that the various brands are not bioequivalent. Each drug varies in the number of units of lipase, protease, and amylase present. When it is necessary to change brands to obtain a more rational dosing amount, the health-care provider should monitor the effect of the new drug on endpoints. Treatment failures have been reported in CF patients when brand-name products were replaced by a generic or when one product was switched for another (*DF & C*, 2011). Variability in manufacturing standards and bioavailability prompted the FDA to require all pancreatic enzymes to apply for approval from the FDA or to be eventually removed from the market (FDA, 2012).

Monitoring

Assessment of the efficacy of pancreatic enzyme replacement and the dosage of drug required is accomplished by determining which dose minimizes steatorrhea and maintains good nutritional status. The assessment of the endpoints in children is aided by charting growth curves. Other data include skinfold thickness, arm muscle circumference, and laboratory values such as albumin, cholesterol, glucose, hemoglobin, hematocrit, transferrin, and electrolytes. Because these drugs may produce elevated uric acid levels, serum and urine are tested for uric acid at regular intervals. Stools are monitored for fat content (steatorrhea), and the patient is told to report foul-smelling and frothy stools.

CF patients are originally diagnosed using a fecal elastase test to determine the need for pancreatic enzyme replacement. This test is not a quantitative measure; therefore, it is not used to monitor enzyme effect (CFF, 2009). In infants, fecal fat up to 15% of of total fat intake is normal, but this drops to less than 7% in childhood (CFF, 2009). Because fat malabsorption pathologies can render patients at risk for deficiencies in the fat soluble vitamins (A, C, E, and K), suspicion of hypovitaminosis and osteopenia should trigger monitoring of these key factors.

Patient Education

Administration

All doses are taken immediately before or with meals or snacks with a fatty component. Fruit, hard candy, fruit juice-like drinks, tea or coffee, or popsicles do not require enzymes (CFF, 2009). Capsules may be opened and sprinkled on food. Capsules with enteric-coated beads should not be chewed. They may be sprinkled on soft acidic food that is not hot and that can be swallowed without chewing, such as applesauce or gelatin. Swallow immediately because the proteolytic enzymes may irritate the mucosa. Following with a glass of water or juice or eating immediately after taking the drug helps to ensure that the medication is swallowed and does not remain in contact with the mouth and esophagus for long periods. Pancrelipase is destroyed by acid. Proton pump inhibitors, sodium bicarbonate, or aluminum-based antacids may be used with preparations without enteric coating to neutralize gastric pH. Calcium- and magnesium-based antacids should not be used for this purpose because they interfere with drug action. Enteric-coated beads are designed to withstand the acid pH of the stomach. Enteric-coated formulations should not be mixed with alkaline food or the coating will be destroyed.

Adverse Reactions

Adverse reactions are usually GI in nature. The lowest effective dose should be used to minimize nausea, stomach cramps, abdominal pain, or diarrhea. Dosages or brands may need to be changed if symptoms persist. Washing off powder in contact with the skin is the only treatment required for any irritation. The dust of finely powdered concentrates may irritate the nasal mucosa and respiratory tract. Super-sensitive patients may need to mask during dose preparation.

Lifestyle Management

Pancreatic enzyme replacement is only part of the treatment regimen. It will not be successful without adherence to the rest of the treatment regimen. Dietary recommendations depend on the reason enzyme replacement is needed, but generally the diet is high calorie, high protein, and low fat. For children with CF, the diet is high calorie, high protein, and high fat. The dosage of the enzyme replacement is based on fat content of the diet, so the amount of fat in each meal should be fairly consistent. Small, frequent meals are often better tolerated than three large meals, especially when the reason for the enzyme replacement is CF, post-operative gastrectomy, or bariatric procedure. Use the same brand consistently. Enzymes should not be refrigerated, nor stored in hot places, and must be checked for expiration dates. The lid should be replaced tightly to avoid air and humidity interactions as needed.

ENDOCRINE PANCREATIC HORMONES (INSULIN)

Insulin is a small protein molecule secreted by the beta cells of the pancreas. It is essential to the utilization of glucose by all body cells. Disorders of insulin secretion and utilization are found in diabetes mellitus, and the primary use of insulin as a drug is the treatment for this disorder.

Type 1 diabetes accounts for 5% to 10% of total diabetes and results from an autoimmune destruction of the beta cells of the islet of Langerhans leading to complete insulin deficiency. Before hyperglycemia occurs, 80% to 90% of the function of insulin-secreting beta cells must be lost. Beta cell abnormalities are present long before the acute clinical onset of type 1 diabetes. Regardless of the cause, the pathology is probably disequilibrium between the relative excess production of glucagon by the pancreatic A cells and the lack of insulin produced by the B cells. Treatment requires insulin replacement. If the disease progresses without treatment, diabetic ketoacidosis (DKA), weight loss, muscle wasting, and death may occur. Chapter 33 discusses the treatment of both type 1 and type 2 diabetes, including the use of insulin. Figure 33-1 depicts the pathological cause of the various symptoms of type 1 diabetes.

Pharmacodynamics

Insulin is normally released from pancreatic beta cells at a constant low basal rate with intermittent bursts in response to a variety of stimuli, including stress, vagal activity, and high blood glucose levels. Figure 21-3 shows one mechanism for the stimulation of insulin release from beta cells. Once the insulin has arrived at an insulin-sensitive cell, it is bound to specialized receptors that are found on the cell membrane. These receptors foster changes within the cell membrane that result in translocation of certain proteins, such as glucose transporters, from sequestered sites within the cell to the cell surface. Once on the cell surface, the transporter facilitates the intake of glucose by the cell. Several hormonal agents such as corticosteroids lower the affinity of the insulin receptor, and others such as GH increase this affinity. Insulin promotes the storage of fat as well as glucose and influences cell growth and metabolic functions in a wide variety of tissues.

Action on Glucose Transporters

The GLUT 1 insulin transporter is found in all tissue, especially in red blood cells and in the brain. It is associated with basal uptake of glucose and transport of glucose across the blood–brain barrier. The GLUT 2 transporter is found in the beta cells of the pancreas and in the liver, kidney, and gut. It regulates insulin release and glucose homeostasis. Defects in this receptor are thought to contribute to the reduced insulin secretion seen in type 2 diabetes. The GLUT 3 transporter is located in the brain, kidney, and placenta and is related to uptake of glucose in neurons and some other tissues. The GLUT 4 transporter is located in muscle and adipose tissue. It is the transporter most associated with lowering blood glucose (BG) levels and is the primary influence in glucose uptake, especially during exercise. It is also the one most associated with insulin resistance in type 2 diabetes. GLUT 5 transporters are found in the gut and the kidney. They are associated with intestinal absorption of fructose.

The total number of insulin receptors can be suppressed by such factors as obesity and long-standing hyperglycemia. This may explain why weight loss can be a significant factor in diabetes management.

Action on the Liver

Insulin acts on the liver to increase storage of glucose as glycogen and resets the liver after food intake by reversing the amount of catabolic activity. Insulin also decreases urea production, protein catabolism, and cyclic adenosine monophosphate (cAMP) in the liver; promotes triglyceride synthesis; and increases potassium and phosphate uptake by the liver.

Action on Muscle Cells

Insulin promotes protein synthesis by increasing amino acid transport and by stimulating ribosomal activity. It also promotes glycogen synthesis to replace glycogen stores used during muscle activity.

Action on Adipose Tissue

Finally, insulin reduces the circulation of free fatty acids and promotes the storage of triglycerides in adipose tissue. This process is accomplished, in part, by suppression of cAMP production and dephosphorylation of the lipases in fat cells.

Administration of insulin acts on each of these receptors to produce the same effect as the naturally occurring hormone. Although it is given largely to control blood glucose (BG) in patients with diabetes, that is not its only effect on the body.

Pharmacokinetics

Absorption and Distribution

Insulin is absorbed from SC or IM injection sites because it would be destroyed by proteolytic enzymes in the stomach if given orally. The absorption rate is determined by type of insulin, injection site, and volume injected. Inhaled forms are faster onset than the most rapid standard forms due to the capillary network of the lung. Insulin may also be given via IV and goes directly into circulation without the need for absorption. Insulin preparations are divided into types based on onset, duration, and peak intensity of action and whether inhaled or parenteral. Table 21-8 presents each type. Because human insulin has a more rapid onset and shorter duration of action than pork or beef insulin, and because it is less antigenic, it has replaced animal insulin. Injection sites in the abdomen have as much as 50% more absorption than the arm, followed by the thighs and buttocks.

Types of Insulin

Rapid-Acting (RAI)

Lispro is an insulin analogue produced by recombinant DNA technology. It is created by reversing two amino acids on the insulin B chain. This rapid-acting insulin (RAI) has the same method of binding to insulin receptors, the same circulating half-life, and the same immunogenicity as regular insulin. Its onset of action, however, is much shorter—15 minutes—and it reaches its peak within 1 hour. Clinical trials have demonstrated that the optimal time for preprandial injection of this insulin is 15 minutes rather than the 30-minute interval used for regular insulin. The duration of action of this insulin is not increased with a larger dose. It is compatible with neutral protamine Hagedorn (NPH). Insulin aspart, homologous with regular human insulin except for one amino acid, has a rapid onset of action similar to that of insulin lispro. Insulin glulisine is created by replacing lysine and glutamic acid on the insulin B chain. Its profile is similar to that of lispro. The RAIs are used as bolus doses to correct hyperglycemia or to cover food eaten at meals, specifically carbohydrate (CHO).

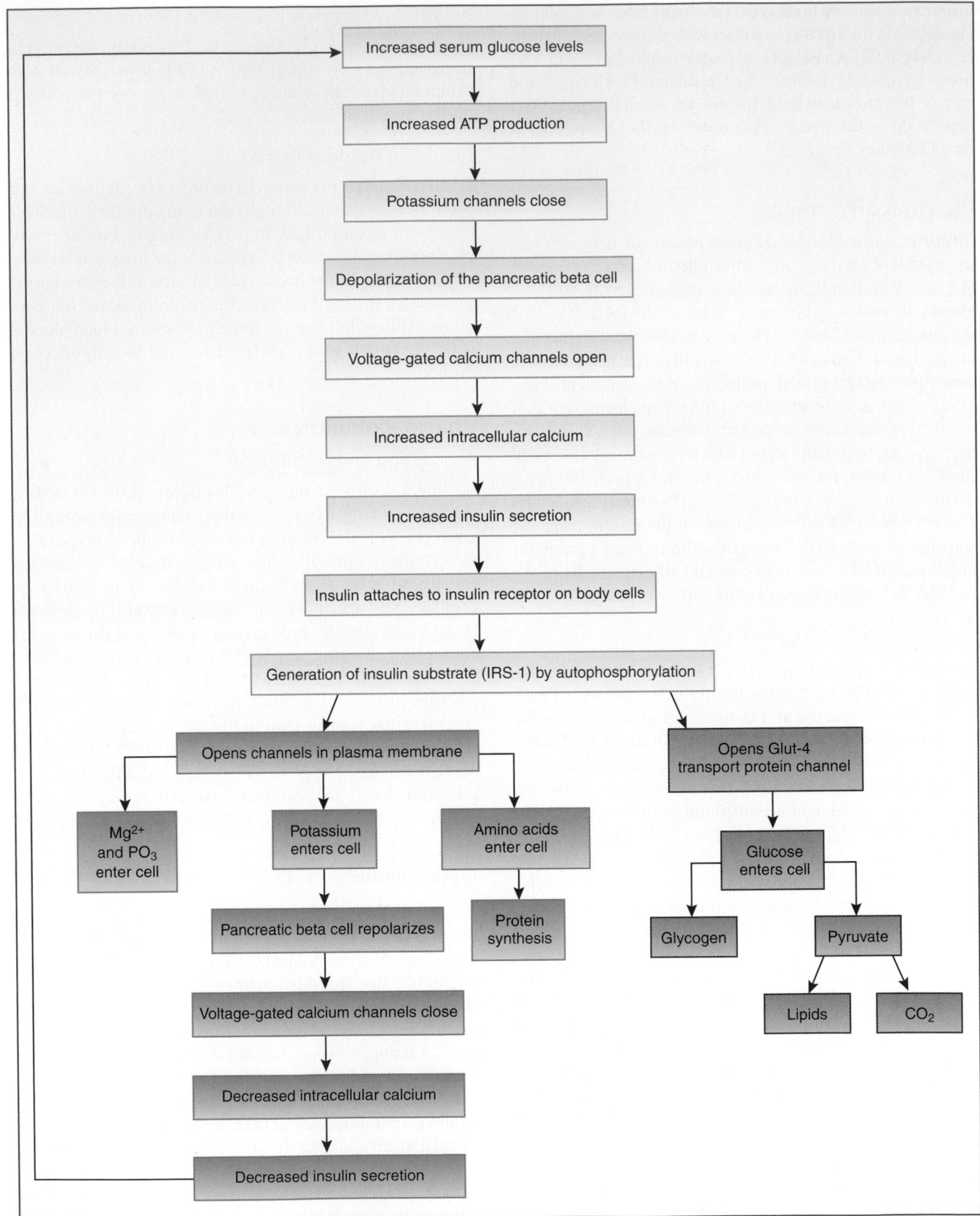

Figure 21–3. Mechanism of insulin release from beta cells.

Table 21–8 ▦ **Pharmacokinetics: Insulins**

	Onset (m)	Peak (h)	Duration (h)*	Elimination	Compatibility
Rapid-Acting					
Insulin aspart	0–15	0.5–2	3–5	Urine	NPH
Insulin glulisine	0–15	0.5–2	3–5	Urine	NPH
Lispro	0–15	0.5-1.5	3–5	Urine	NPH
Short-Acting					
Regular	30–60	2–3	3–7	Very little unchanged insulin is excreted in the urine	NPH
Regular U-500	30–45	2-4	8–24 hr*	Same	Not recommended
Intermediate-Acting					
NPH	30–60	4–10	10–16	Very little unchanged insulin is excreted in the urine	Regular, Glulisine, Lipro, Aspart
Long-Acting					
Insulin glargine	60	—	24	Urine	No other insulin
Insulin detemir	60	—	Up to 24	Urine	No other insulin
Inhaled					
Inhaled Human Insulin (Afrezza)	0-12**	1	2-3	Urine	N/A

*Duration of U 500 dependent on volume injected.

**Afrezza has rapid absoption, but its actual onset of action is not faster than regular.

Short-Acting (SAI)

Regular insulin is a short-acting insulin (SAI) whose effect appears within 30 minutes of injection and generally lasts for 8 to 12 hours. The clinically significant duration of action is slightly less, at 4 to 6 hours. It is used as bolus insulin to correct hyperglycemia or to cover food eaten at meals.

Intermediate-Acting (IAI)

Neutral protamine Hagedorn (NPH) or isophane is an intermediate-acting insulin. The onset of action is delayed by combining the insulin with protamine. After SC injection, proteolytic enzymes degrade the protamine in NPH to permit absorption of the insulin. Its onset of action is 1 to 1.5 hours, and its duration is 12 to 24 hours, although the duration is usually no longer than 16 hours in actual clinical effect. NPH is used as basal insulin in both types 1 and 2 diabetes.

Long-Acting (LAI)

Insulin glargine is created by substituting glycine and arginine for other amino acids in human insulin. It has a unique AUC profile that has no pronounced peak, as small amounts of insulin are released slowly, resulting in a constant concentration/time profile over 24 hours. This profile has resulted in improved glycemic control in large, diverse populations with long-standing type 2 diabetes. White and colleagues (2009) found greater reductions in glucose variability for insulin glargine when compared with NPH insulin. Because variability in blood glucose has been associated with an increased incidence of diabetic complications, this is an important finding (Kilpatrick, Rigby, & Atkin, 2008; Marfella et al, 2009).

Insulin detemir is an insulin analogue that differs from human insulin by a single amino acid deletion and the acylation of myristic acid to the B terminus of the molecule. These changes prolong absorption from the subcutaneous depot, resulting in a more prolonged, less peaked absorption compared to that of NPH insulin. It has a pharmacokinetic profile similar to insulin. Insulin is widely distributed to most body tissues.

Both LAIs are used in types 1 and 2 as basal insulin and are typically given at bedtime, although they can be given at other times of the day.

On The Horizon **INSULIN DEGLUDEC**

The ultra–long-acting basal insulin analogue degludec (Tresiba) has been placed on a more extended roll-out by Novo-Nordisk in the United States. It is used for both type 1 and type 2 patients, especially those who need to overcome nocturnal hypoglycemia. The 42 hour action time may allow a staggered administration plan. Due to limited post-marketing experience, it is not fully described in this edition.

PIPELINE DRUGS

There are many drugs currently in the pipeline to treat DM. Insulin degludec (Tresiba) has a longer duration of action than insulin glargine. Insulin degludec/liraglutide (Xultopy) is an insulin/GLP-1 agonist combination in phase 3 trials. Other diabetes drugs in phase III trials include exenatice subcutaneous implant (ITCA 650, Intarcia Therapeutics); semaglutide (Novo Nordisk) is a once-weekly GLP-1 analog; omariglipin (Merck) is a once-weekly DPP-4 inhibitor similar to once daily Januvia; Oral-Lyn (Generex) is an investigational liquid regular recombinant human insulin that is delivered to the buccal mucosa using a trademarked RapidMist device; and insulin peglispro (Eli Lilly) is a new long-acting basal insulin.

Lixisenatide (Lyxumia), a once-daily prandial GLP-1 receptor agonist approved in Europe, was denied FDA approval in June 2014 due to pronounced after meal hypoglycemia.

Inhaled Insulin

A new inhaled human insulin (Afrezza Inhalation Powder) was approved by the FDA in 2014. It is the most rapid acting of any type of insulin. It has a short time to peak (12 to 15 minutes) with a short duration of action (2 to 3 hours). This short duration of action is thought to be one reason why this forumulation has less weight gain impact than other forms of insulin. It is given with meals. It has no indication for treating diabetic emergencies. If it is used in Type I DM, a long-acting insulin must also be part of the therapeutic plan.

Metabolism and Excretion

Insulin is metabolized by the liver, the kidney, and muscle cells. Almost all of it is metabolized, and a very small amount is excreted unchanged in the urine. For inhaled insulin, 39% is excreted in the urine and 7% is swallowed and not absorbed in the intestines.

Pharmacotherapeutics

Precautions and Contraindications

The only contraindications to insulin are hypoglycemia and hypersensitivity to any of the ingredients in the product. Human insulin derived by recombinant DNA technology from *Escherichia coli* bacteria or yeast rarely poses hypersensitivity problems.

Some studies with human insulin have shown increased circulating levels of insulin in patients with renal failure (*DF & C*, 2011). Because renal insufficiency and failure are common complications of diabetes, careful glucose monitoring and dose adjustments are needed for patients with renal dysfunction.

Studies have also shown increased circulating levels of insulin in patients with hepatic function impairment. Hepatic failure is uncommon in diabetes, but careful glucose monitoring and dose adjustments are needed for these patients as well.

Pregnancy requires careful diabetes management. Human insulin does not cross the placenta and is the drug of choice for pregnant women and those considering pregnancy. Most insulin is Pregnancy Category B; however, insulin aspart, insulin glargine, insulin glulisine, insulin detemir, and inhaled insulin formulations have not been studied in pregnant women and use during pregnancy is on a risk/benefit basis. They are listed as Pregnancy Category C. Although human insulin is excreted in breast milk, because it is given by injection, it is not absorbed intact by the breastfeeding infant. Inadequate or excessive insulin treatment of mothers with diabetes, however, reduces milk production. It is not known if insulin aspart, insulin glargine, insulin glulisine, and insulin detemir are excreted in breast milk and so caution should be exercised in administering these drugs to nursing mothers. In rat studies 10% of inhaled insulin (Afrezza) is measured in breast milk. Insulin can be used safely in infants and children.

Hypothyroidism may delay insulin turnover, requiring less insulin to treat diabetes. Hyperthyroidism may cause an increase in the renal clearance of insulin. Patients with either of these concurrent diseases require more frequent monitoring of glucose levels than other patients with diabetes when insulin management is required.

Insulin resistance, a suboptimal response of insulin-sensitive tissues to insulin (especially in the liver, muscle, and adipose tissue) occurs in patients with type 2 diabetes. The result is an increased rate of endogenous glucose production secondary to increased glucagon levels because liver cells do not receive feedback messages about the amount of insulin being secreted or the amount of glucose already in the bloodstream. Type 2 diabetes is also associated with down-regulation of insulin receptors in skeletal muscle, resulting in insulin resistance. Patients who have this problem may require more than 1.5 units/kg/day in the absence of ketoacidosis or acute infection. Patients who may exhibit this resistance include obese patients; patients with acanthosis nigricans, ketoacidosis, or endocrinopathies; and patients with insulin receptor defects who may need to have their diabetes managed by an endocrinologist. They typically need to use a concentrated form of insulin U-500, to keep volumes of injections down.

Adverse Drug Reactions

Two life-threatening adverse reactions are central to patient management with insulin: hypoglycemia and diabetic ketoacidosis. One is associated with too much insulin or not enough food and the other with too little insulin. Bronchospasm can occur with inhaled insulin especially in those with COPD and asthma. Spirometry is indicated at baseline and 6 months, then annually for all patients, even if not symptomatic. Inhaled insulin should not be prescribed to a patient with lung cancer or a history of lung cancer.

Hypoglycemia

Hypoglycemia may result from an excessive insulin dose, excessive work or exercise without eating, food that is not absorbed in the usual manner because of a postponed or omitted meal, not eating enough food, or an illness that results in vomiting or diarrhea. It may also be associated with concurrent administration of another drug that increases the hypoglycemic effects of insulin. Alcohol is especially risky in this regard because it not only induces hypoglycemia but also masks the signs and symptoms of the disorder. Table 21-9 shows these drug interactions. Signs and symptoms of hypoglycemia include decreased levels of consciousness, hunger, diaphoresis, weakness, dizziness, and tachycardia. The peak of action for each type of insulin is the most likely time for a hypoglycemic reaction. This is especially important when more than one type of insulin is being used and the peaks of the different types of insulin coincide. It also occurs when a change in dose occurs or when a provider "over-corrects" a reported high sugar value.

Hypoglycemia is defined as BG less than 70 mg/dL. The treatment that should be used is known as "The Rule of 15": when symptoms occur, consume 15 gr of fast-acting carbohydrate (CHO), wait 15 minutes, and check BG. Examples of fast-acting CHO are 4 oz juice, 8 oz milk, one-half can of a regular soft drink, 1 tbsp honey, or four to five hard or soft candies. Commercial glucose tablets and gel may also be used. It is important to emphasize chocolate candy is not effective in treating hypoglycemia due to the fat content, which delays glucose absorption. A snack or small meal should be eaten within a few hours of the hypoglycemic episode. Adjustments in insulin dosage, meal patterns, or exercise may be needed to prevent further episodes. More severe episodes, with coma, seizure activity, or neurological impairment, require treatment with IM or SC glucagon or concentrated IV glucose.

Diabetic Ketoacidosis (DKA)

Diabetic ketoacidosis (DKA) may result from stress, illness, infection, or insulin omission. It may also develop slowly after a long period of adequate control of BG. Children with undiagnosed type 1 diabetes may present with DKA at the time of diagnosis. Signs and symptoms of DKA include drowsiness, dim vision, and Kussmaul respiration.

Indications of hyperglycemia that may precede DKA and give warning of its impending occurrence include polyuria, polydipsia, polyphagia, weight loss and fatigue, vomiting, dehydration, ketone odor to the breath, and abdominal pain. Treatment requires hospitalization and is directed at the acid–base and fluid imbalances that result, as well as the elevated BG. IV fluids, correction of the acidosis and hypotension, and low-dose regular insulin by SC or IV are required. There is no role for U-500 or inhaled insulin with DKA.

Drug Interactions

Many drugs either decrease or increase the effects of insulin because of their effects on BG. Table 21-9 shows these interactions. Beta blockers are especially problematic because they can increase insulin resistance, producing hyperglycemia, but can also mask most of the signs and symptoms of hypoglycemia. The one indication of hypoglycemia that beta blockers do not mask is diaphoresis, and people with diabetes who must take beta blockers for a concurrent disease or condition should be taught to test their blood sugar level whenever they experience diaphoresis. Inhaled insulin has he same potential drug interactions as injectable insulin, something most patients do not anticipate because it is perceived as not being "injected" into the body.

Clinical Use and Dosing

Type 1 Diabetes Mellitus

Patients with type 1 diabetes mellitus do not produce insulin, therefore they must receive insulin replacement. A wide variety of regimens are used in this treatment, including regular insulin delivered only via insulin pump, split-mix regimens, and intensive insulin therapy. Mixtures of SAI and IAI or SAI or RAI and LAI are given in multiple doses from 2 to 4 times daily (see Table 21-10). Table 33-6 discusses in more detail the various insulin regimens that are used for management of type 1 diabetes mellitus. Now inhaled insulin can be part of the plan.

Table 21–9 ⠿ Drug Interactions With Insulin

Interacting Drug	Possible Effects	Implications
Acetazolamide, AIDS antivirals, asparaginase, calcitonin, corticosteroids, cyclophosphamide, dextrothyroxine, diazoxide, diltiazem, dobutamine, epinephrine, estrogens, ethacrynic acid, isoniazid, lithium carbonate, morphine sulfate, niacin, phenothiazines, phenytoin, nicotine, thiazide diuretics, thyroid hormones	Decreases hypoglycemic effect of insulin, including inhaled forms	Close monitoring of blood glucose levels is required if concurrent administration
Alcohol, anabolic steroids, beta-adrenergic blockers,* chloroquine, guanethidine, lithium carbonate, monoamine oxidase inhibitors, mebendazole, octreotide, pentamidine, phenylbutazone, pyridoxine, salicylates, sulfinpyrazone, sulfonamides, tetracyclines	Increases hypoglycemic effect of insulin, including inhaled forms	Close monitoring of blood glucose levels is required if concurrent administration

*Cardioselective beta-adrenergic blockers (those affecting only or mainly beta$_1$ receptors) are less likely to affect insulin's hypoglycemic effect and may be acceptable alternatives for patients who must take beta-adrenergic blockers.

Table 21–10 ⚗ Dosage Schedule: Insulin

Drug	Dosage Form	Schedule	Initial Dose	Comments
Insulin aspart* (Novolog) and Insulin glulisine (Apidra)	Vial Disposable pen Cartridge	Use in combination with IA or LA due to rapid onset and short duration. *Start meal within 5–10 min of injection.* Also used in pumps.	50%–70% of TDD requirement as aspart. Remainder as IA or LA insulin.	May need increased basal insulin or more total daily insulin to prevent premeal hyperglycemia
Insulin lispro* (Humalog)	Vial Disposable pen Cartridge U 100	Use in combination with IA or LA insulin due to rapid onset and short duration of action. Also used in pumps.	50%–70% of TDD before meals. Remainder as IA given 2/3 in morning and 1/3 in evening or as LA given in morning.	Draw lispro into the syringe first if mixing with IA insulin. Inject immediately after mixing. Concentrations higher, duration shorter if given in abdomen
Regular (Humulin, Novolin)	Vial Cartridge U 100	Used in combination with IA or LA insulin due to short onset and short duration of action	50%–70% of TDD as regular given 30–60 min before meals. Remainder as IA given 2/3 in morning and 1/3 in evening or as LA given in morning.	Also comes in U 500 for patients who need high doses. See Chap. 33 for more information
NPH (Lilly) (Novolog)	Lilly: Vial Disposable pen Novolog: Vial Cartridge	Often used in combination with RA or SA insulin 2:1 ratio in a.m., 1:1 ratio in p.m. If using for basal: Start with 6–10 units or 0.1–0.2 unit/kg body weight/d at breakfast or HS to initiate therapy.	Give twice daily with 2/3 of daily dose in morning and 1/3 in evening. Same protocol with 70/30 or 50/50.	See text related to mixing
		With oral agent for type 2 patients who cannot control with oral agent and lifestyle modifications alone	10 units of NPH at bedtime with oral agent in morning	Individualized
Insulin glargine (Lantus)	Vial, disposable pen	Use as single dose (once daily) at bedtime. May be given at other times of day. RA can be given at meals.	Glargine to = 50% of TDD at bedtime, then split remainder of TDD with RAI at breakfast and evening meal.	Calculate total daily insulin requirement at 0.3 units /kg/d
		As single dose at bedtime given with 70/30 mixed insulin	Glargine to = 50% of TDD at bedtime; 70/30 mixed insulin at bedtime and morning for remainder of TDD	
		As single dose with oral agent	As single dose in morning with oral agent	See text for notes on use
Insulin detemir (Levemir)	Vial, disposable pen	Use as single dose (once daily) at bedtime. Given with RAI at meals.	Detemir to = 50% TDD at bedtime, then split remainder of TDD insulin dose with RAI at meal times. Initiate at 0.1–0.2 units/kg in the evening.	Calculate TDD at 0.3–0.5 Units/kg/d
		As a single dose with oral agent Twice daily	0.1–0.2 units/kg or 10 units	Dosage adjusted to achieve glycemic goals
Human Inhaled Insulin (Afrezza)	Single use cartridge 4 or 8 units each.	As a single dose with meals or as needed	Can be adjunct to injectable; multiple cartridges required in multiples of 4 or 8 units	Typically reserved for those with severe fear of needles
Humulin or Novolin 70/30	Vial, disposable pen 70% Isophane suspension 30% Regular			

Table 21-10 ⊗ **Dosage Schedule: Insulin—cont'd**

Drug	Dosage Form	Schedule	Initial Dose	Comments
Humulin 50/50	Vial 50% Isophane suspension 30% Regular			
Humalog Mix 50/50	Vial, disposable pen 50% Lispro Protamine Suspension (IA) 50% Humalog			
Humalog Mix 75/25	75% Lispro Protamine Suspension (IA) 25% Humalog Vial, disposable pen, cartridge			
Novolog Mix 70/30	70% Aspart Protamine Suspension (IA) 30% Novolog Vial, disposable pen, cartridge			

RA = rapid-acting; IA = intermediate-acing; LA = long-acting.

   NOTE: Usual daily insulin requirement is 0.6–0.8 U/kg/d for adults and 0.8–1.2 U/kg/d for children during rapid growth. For drugs with*, daily insulin requirement is 0.05–1 U/kg/d. These do not represent all possible combinations or scheduling protocols.

Type 2 Diabetes Mellitus

Patients with type 2 diabetes produce insulin, but they may not produce enough to meet the body's needs. They also have insulin receptor defects, insulin resistance, and altered hepatic glucose metabolism. Insulin is prescribed when the disease process cannot be adequately controlled by diet, exercise, weight reduction, and oral agents. Chapter 33 and Table 33-6 discusses in more detail insulin regimens used for the management of type 2 diabetes mellitus. Insulin may be used alone or in conjunction with oral agents, and several regimens may be used, as in type 1.

Dosing

Average insulin doses are 0.6 to 0.8 units/kg/d. Starting doses are 0.3 to 0.5 units/kg/d. Obese patients may require more than 100 units per day. Volumes approaching 200 units per injection triggers a switch to the concentrated U-500 formulation. How the doses are dispersed throughout the day depends on the pharmacokinetics of the type of insulin used. For example, for twice-daily dosing for IAI and SAI, two-thirds of the total daily dose is given in the morning and one-third in the evening in most cases. One way to give insulin glargine is to calculate the daily dose of insulin at 0.3 units/kg/d and start bedtime glargine at 50% of the total dose and split the remaining 50% with short-acting insulin before meals. In type 2, LAI can be initiated at a dose of approximately 0.1 unit/kg/d while simultaneously starting an oral agent. A third possibility is to calculate the daily dose of insulin at 0.3 units/kg/d and use premixed 70/30 insulin with two-thirds of the total daily dose in the morning and one-third of the dose in the evening. Basal plus meal time dosing regimens are becoming more populuar. Inhaled insulin in 4 or 8 unit inhalations is used with meals. Table 33-6 lists the commonly used insulin regimens. The use of a sliding scale with regular insulin is no longer used for long-term management; however, it may be used for short-term management in an acute care setting.

   If persons with type 1 or type 2 diabetes mellitus who are on insulin are NPO (i.e., for a procedure), it is advisable to schedule the procedure in the morning to avoid disruption of the insulin regimen. BG levels should be monitored before, during, and after the procedure. Persons with type 1 diabetes require insulin even when NPO because ketosis can occur within 12 to 24 hours. For either type 1 or 2, one-half of IAI can be administered on the morning of the procedure. For patient on bedtime glargine or detemir, the usual dose can be given the night before or the dose can be reduced from 20% to 50%, depending on the level of glycemic control. RAI and SAI should not be given unless the BG level is greater than 200, and if that is the case, insulin is given in small doses of 1 to 4 units to achieve a BG level less than 200 mg/dL (Duncan, 2012; Inzucchi, 2011).

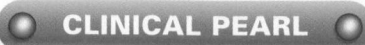

CLINICAL PEARL

For patients on insulin pumps, be attentive to daylight saving time changes. Many pump computers are not GPS enabled or time zone adjusting. This is not an issue with basal insulin provision, but could be significant for rapid-acting forms. Verify date and time settings during appointments (Aldasouqui & Reed, 2014).

Mixing

Mixing insulin is common practice in diabetic regimens, but not all insulin is compatible. LAI insulin cannot be mixed with other insulin, which requires an additional injection. It is recommended that when mixing two different types of insulin to always draw clear insulin into the syringe first. Patients will have a consistent response if the method of mixing is standardized. "Clear to cloudy" is a good way to remember and teach this. Do not suggest mixing of U-500 insulin with other types due to the confusing variance of mixing insulin in units and TB syringe measurements in mL.

All premixed formulations of insulin (70/30 Novolin, 70/30 Humulin, and 50/50 Humulin) contain NPH (the first number) and regular (SAI) or aspart or lispro (RAI) (the second number). These premixed insulins remain stable at room temperature for 1 month or for 3 months under refrigeration. NPH and regular insulin mixed in plastic or glass syringes may be stored for 1 week at room temperature and 14 days if refrigerated. RAIs can be mixed with NPH immediately before injection without affecting its rapid absorption. Regardless of the insulin mixture used, the patient should standardize the interval between mixing the insulins and injecting them.

Switching Insulins

Every insulin has unique characteristics and neither brand of insulin nor type of syringe nor needle should be changed without monitoring by the health-care provider. The provider may want, however, to switch from an insulin formulation that has peaks in its action to one that does not. If changing from a treatment regimen with an IAI to a regimen with LAI, the amount and timing of the RAI or oral antihyperglycemic may need to be adjusted. This is especially true for patients who have developed insulin antibodies and require high doses of insulin. In one clinical study with insulin-naïve patients with type 2 diabetes and already being treated with oral antihyperglycemic agents, insulin glargine was started at 10 units once daily and subsequently adjusted based on the patient's response to a total daily dose between 2 units and 100 units. In other clinical studies, when patients were switched from once-daily NPH to once-daily insulin glargine, the initial dose was usually not changed. If the change was from twice-daily NPH to insulin glargine, to avoid hypoglycemia the initial dose of insulin glargine was reduced by 20% and then adjusted based on patient response (*DF & C*, 2011). Regardless of the drugs

involved in the switch, careful monitoring of BG is required during the transition period. Monitoring for respiratory issues is required if inhaled insulin is added to a regimen. A one to one substitution of inhaled units with short-acting SQ units is a common switch; rounding up to the closest 4 or 8 unit cartridge dosing is required.

Switching patients to U-500 insulin because they take large doses of U-100 insulin is not a simple division of dose by 5. Due to the significant risks of using concentrated insulin, providers who are not fully familiar with dosing this medication are advised to consult with an expert endocrinologist or Certified Diabetes Educator. See Chapter 33 for specifics of switching.

Hyperkalemia

IV infusions of glucose and insulin produce a shift of potassium into cells and lower serum potassium levels. This treatment is usually reserved for hospitalized patients with very high potassium levels or those at risk for cardiac arrhythmias.

Severe Ketoacidosis or Diabetic Coma

Regular insulin given IV is used for rapid effect in severe ketoacidosis or diabetic coma. Because there is a high risk for inducing hyperosmolar coma with this therapy, these patients are also hospitalized.

Pregnancy

For treatment of gestational diabetes and management of patients with diabetes who become pregnant, insulin is usually the drug of choice. Most oral hypoglycemic agents are contraindicated in pregnancy; the exceptions are metformin and glyburide. Any of the insulin treatment regimens may be used during pregnancy. Special care must be taken to avoid hypoglycemic episodes. Coordination with a provider versed in obstetrical implications is strongly suggested. Inhaled insulin is Category C.

Rational Drug Selection

Level of Intensity of Control

Results of the Diabetes Control and Complications Trial (DCCT, 1993) indicate that BG levels closer to target range can significantly reduce the risk of complications associated with diabetes. This trial conclusively demonstrated, in patients with type 1 diabetes, that the risk for development or progression of retinopathy was reduced by 76%, for nephropathy by 50%, for neuropathy by 60%, and for cardiovascular disease by 35%. These benefits were observed with an average Hb A1c of less than 7%. This has been further supported in other studies (Kilpatrick et al, 2008; Marfella et al, 2009). The American Diabetic Association [ADA], Canadian Diabetic Association, and the European Association for the Study of Diabetes [EASD] recommend that A1C levels of less than 7% are desirable for most patients with diabetes. More latitude is recommended for senior patients as the risk of hypoglycemia has many more consequences for elders than adults.

The reduction in risk in the DCCT correlated continuously with reduction in Hb A1c. This relationship implies that complete normalization of glycemic levels may prevent complications. These benefits have also been demonstrated for patients with type 2 diabetes. DCCT patients on tight control used combinations of SAI and IAI given 3 to 4 times per day. Those on intensive insulin therapy used LAI at night and RAI before each meal or more frequently, based on self-monitored glucose measurements. A third group used an insulin pump.

Presence of Complications Such as Retinopathy and Neuropathy

Patients with complications such as retinopathy and neuropathy may find it difficult to draw up their own insulin. Premixed insulin may assist with this problem. Choice of insulin is based on the commercial availability of premixed insulin or those that can be safely stored for some time after mixing. To ensure safety in patients with visual or dexterity problems, pens that click to indicate number of units, magnifiers, and other aids should be considered.

Type 2 Diabetes Mellitus Unable to Control

About 28% of patients with type 2 diabetes use some form of insulin to control blood glucose levels and limit complication risks (Agency for Healthcare Research and Quality [AHRQ], 2008). Because type 2 diabetes is a chronic disease, most patients will need insulin when oral agents fail.

Patients with type 2 diabetes who are not controlled on oral agents and have postprandial hyperglycemia may benefit from an RAI added immediately prior to meals. Patients who have fasting hyperglycemia may have bedtime NPH added. If they have overall poor control, intensive insulin therapy or the split-mix regimen is used. Initially, therapy is started with the use of once- or twice-daily injections of either IAI or LAI.

A systematic review of 45 research studies comparing the newer premixed insulins and the newer insulin analogues with other diabetic medicines for type 2 diabetes (AHRQ, 2008) have indicated risks and benefits for each choice:

- The premixed insulin analogues are better at lowering Hb A1c and preprandial blood glucose than are the oral antihyperglycemic agents; however, they have more risk for hypoglycemia.
- The premixed insulin analogues and the newer premixed insulins are associated with less weight gain than all of the oral antihyperglycemic agents except metformin and the gliptins.
- Long-acting insulin analogues appear to be more effective than premixed insulin analogues in lowering fasting blood glucose levels, but the reverse is true for lowering blood glucose levels after a meal with high sugar content.
- The newer premixed insulins are better at lowering Hb A1c and postprandial glucose than long-acting insulin; however, they carry a higher risk for hypoglycemia.

- Cost is a major factor with all the newer insulin analogues, regardless of formulation; they are more expensive than either regular or NPH insulin. Inhaled insulins are cost consistent with the newer agents.

The number of times the drug must be administered (complexity) was not discussed in this article, but the more complex the regimen, the greater is the risk for nonadherence. These data are further supported by other studies (Buse et al, 2009; Umpierrez et al, 2009). Chapter 33 provides more information on dosing.

Monitoring

Two categories of monitoring are needed for persons with diabetes: (1) BG within target range and (2) signs of complications.

Control of Blood Glucose

For patients with type 1 and 2 diabetes, the goals of therapy are preprandial BG levels of 70 to 130 mg/dL, postprandial BG levels less than 180 mg/dL, bedtime glucose levels of 100 to 140 mg/dL, and Hb A1c levels of less than 7% (ADA, 2012). See Table 33-7 for recommendations. Patients with comorbid diseases, the very young, older adults, and others with unusual conditions or circumstances may warrant different treatment goals. Every 1% change in Hb A1c equals a change in BG of about 30 mg/dL. Hb A1c values can be increased by iron-deficiency anemia, alcohol use, and lead toxicity and can be decreased by chronic blood loss, chronic renal failure, and pregnancy when performed by some techniques. These potential confounding variables should be considered in assessing changes in Hb A1c levels.

Pre- and postprandial and/or bedtime BG levels can be assessed by self-monitoring blood glucose (SMBG). All patients on insulin therapy should be taught and routinely assessed for accurate SMBG. The frequency and pattern of SMBG should be based on level of control, episodes of both hypo- and hyperglycemia, medication regimen, activity, and meal patterns. Both SMBG and Hb A1c should be monitored; the SMBG reflects day-to-day control and trends, while the Hb A1c reflects the average BG level over a period of 90 to 120 days. Current recommendations for patients with type 1 diabetes are quarterly Hb A1c levels, and at least every 6 months for patients with type 2 diabetes if treatment goals are being met (ADA, 2012). More frequent testing is needed every 3 months if treatment goals are not being met or if therapy has changed. Chapter 33 includes more discussion of this monitoring.

Signs of Complications

Acute Complications

Acute complications include DKA in patients with type 1 and hyperosmolar hyperglycemic nonketotic syndrome (HHNKS) in patients with type 2. All patients with diabetes may experience hypoglycemic episodes; therefore, all patients with diabetes who are on medication should be taught how to prevent, monitor, and treat hypoglycemia.

Chronic Complications

The most common chronic complications of diabetes are nephropathy, retinopathy, peripheral and GI neuropathies, hypertension, cardiovascular disease, and dyslipidemia. Progressive weight gain also occurs. Providers need to be aware of the physical examination and laboratory evaluations that are appropriate to determine the degree of glycemic control and associated complications and risks. Pharmacological therapies are discussed in the ADA clinical practice recommendations that are updated and published annually.

Patient Education

Administration

The number, type, and amount of daily insulin administrations depend on numerous factors, including BG, diet, and activity levels. The provider must work with the patient to establish the diet-exercise-insulin-glucose monitoring regimen with active patient participation.

Patients and/or caregivers should be educated on the onset, peak, and duration of the type of insulin being used. See Table 21-8. For insulin suspensions such as NPH, ensure uniform dispersion of insulin by rolling the vial gently between the hands until the color is even. Avoid vigorous shaking, which produces air bubbles or foam. Lispro and regular insulins are clear solutions and do not require dispersion of suspended particles. Do not use them if they are cloudy, discolored, or unusually viscous, which may indicate loss of potency.

Vials of insulin not in use should be refrigerated in temperatures from 36°F to 46°F. Extreme temperatures (greater than 86°F or less than 28°F) and excessive agitation should be avoided to prevent loss of potency, clumping, frosting, or precipitation. Insulin in use may be kept at a room temperature lower than 86°F. Most insulin, including premixed types, is stable at room temperature for 1 month and for 3 months if refrigerated between 2°C and 8°C (36°F to 46°F). Mixtures involving lispro that patients mix themselves must be given immediately after they are mixed. Regular and NPH are stable for 7 days at room temperature and 14 days if refrigerated. Patients should be taught storage requirements for their specific insulin.

Parenteral insulin is available in either disposable or reusable pens. Disposable pens are prefilled with insulin and are discarded when empty. They should be stored in the refrigerator before use, then stored at room temperature once opened. Reusable pens have cartridges that are purchased separately. While the cartridges can be stored in the refrigerator prior to use, the reusable pens should not be put in the refrigerator at any time. Either type of pen requires a special pen needle. Some pens come in half-unit dosages and others in whole-unit dosages. The amount of insulin delivered at one time depends on the pen and ranges from 30 to 80 units.

The patient must be taught the technique for drawing up the correct dose, SC injection, site selection and rotation, disposal of syringes, and mixing if required. Only insulin syringes should be used to draw up U-100 insulin dosages. U-500 insulin uses a standard 1cc tuberculin (TB) syringe. Sites should be rotated, but because the abdomen, arm, and leg have different absorption rates, rotation should occur within one general area (e.g., the abdomen). As a general rule, do not administer within 1 inch of the same site for 1 month. Exercise increases the rate of absorption from injection sites and increases glucose recycling, both of which may result in increased risk for hypoglycemia if the dose of insulin is unchanged. Exercise should be planned and consistent within a treatment regimen.

When different types of insulin are mixed, always draw clear insulin into the syringe first. The order of mixing and the procedure used, including the model or brand of syringe and needle, should not be changed from dose to dose. Patients stabilized on a mixture of insulins should have a consistent response if the procedure is the same each time. Premixed insulin is available commercially and may be used if the type and concentration mix fit the patient. Some formulations cannot be mixed.

Different brands of insulin are not bioequivalent. The patient should not change brands without first consulting the provider, who will arrange for close monitoring if the change is appropriate.

Inhaled insulin comes in single dose cartridges, placed into a special inhaler. Only one inhalation is required to deliver the full dose from the cartridge. The delivery system is much less cumbersome than the original forumulation (Exubura) that was removed from the market by the manufacturer. Afrezza is easier to deliver, but requires hand and breath coordination akin to other inhaled medications. No special oral care after inhalation is required. Baseline spirometry is recommended for all patients before starting inhaled insulin, at 6 months and annually, regardless of respiratory symptoms.

Adverse Reactions

Common adverse drug reactions are related to altered insulin effects. Hypoglycemia can be life-threatening and has a higher risk of occurrence as the intensity of therapy increases. The patient should be taught the signs and symptoms of hypoglycemia and the appropriate treatment for it, based on whether it is mild, moderate, or severe. Decreased food intake, skipping meals, and increased activity may decrease insulin requirements and increase the risk for hypoglycemia.

Alcohol intake is especially dangerous for patients with diabetes. The effect of alcohol on BG is dependent on the amount ingested and the relationship to food intake. Alcohol is not metabolized to glucose and inhibits gluconeogenesis. If it is ingested without food, hypoglycemia can result, even at levels that do not exceed mild intoxication. Not only can it cause hypoglycemia but it also can mask the signs and symptoms of the disorder. For patients using insulin, no more than two alcoholic beverages a day for men, one per day for women, are recommended with and in addition to the regular meal plan. One alcoholic beverage equals 12 oz beer, 5 oz wine, or 1.5 oz distilled spirits. The calories from this alcohol must be calculated as part of the total caloric intake and substituted as one alcoholic beverage that equals two fat exchanges. Reduction of or abstinence from alcohol is preferable.

Hyperglycemia is less immediately life-threatening than hypoglycemia but is an indication of poor BG control and may be life-threatening if it is high enough to produce ketosis and/or hyperosmolar state. Patients should be taught to recognize early indications of hyperglycemia and the treatment.

Site reactions and lipodystrophy are skin issues that can generate future problems if not limited at the first sign of development. Progression to an infection and/or issues with dosage absorption will contribute to glucose imbalances. For inhaled insulin, an adverse reaction can be cough and sore throat. For respiratory patients with COPD or asthma, and for indviduals who are sensitive to particles in the air with reactive airways, this form of insulin is not recommended.

Lifestyle Modification

Management of type 1 or type 2 diabetes involves diet, exercise, weight control, stress management, SMBG, administration of medication, and preventive care. Patient teaching related to management of diabetes is discussed in Chapter 33 .

ORAL AGENTS

Ninety percent of patients with diabetes mellitus have type 2 diabetes. The main physiological alteration in type 2 diabetes is insulin resistance, a suboptimal response of insulin-sensitive tissues (especially in the liver, muscle, and adipose tissue) to insulin. The result is four primary alterations in glucose metabolism: (1) insufficient production of endogenous insulin by the beta cells of the pancreas, (2) tissue insensitivity to insulin, (3) impaired response of the beta cells to BG levels, and (4) excessive production of glucose by the liver secondary to increased glucagon levels. Glucagon-like peptide 1 (GLP-1), an incretin hormone released by the intestine throughout the day and increased in response to a meal, stimulates insulin secretion by the beta cells and suppresses glucagon secretion. GLP-1 levels are decreased in type 2 diabetes.

These patients do not have an absence of insulin secretion, although some may eventually develop absence of insulin. If the pancreas is the major organ involved in type 1diabetes, the liver and the incretin hormone system are the major organs in type 2. Patients with type 2 have few and nonspecific pancreatic changes. Many years of compensatory hyperinsulinemia may occur before the onset of clinical symptoms of diabetes. Eventually, the beta cell responsiveness to glucose stimulus diminishes and hyperglycemia prevails.

Adipose tissue also does not take up glucose in response to insulin, resulting in obesity. Increased visceral fat shows an inverse relationship with insulin. Because the link between obesity and type 2 diabetes is firmly established, oral hypoglycemic agents and other oral antihyperglycemic agents should be considered in relation to their tendency to contribute to weight gain, to their being weight neutral, or to contribute to weight loss.

Because there is endogenous insulin production in type 2, insulin may not be required initially but may be required later in the disease process or during acute illness or stress. Oral hypoglycemic agents and other oral antihyperglycemic agents are effective in addressing one or more of the metabolic defects in type 2 diabetes; insulin is added during episodes when glycemic control is not possible with oral agents alone.

BIGUANIDES

The biguanides are oral antihyperglycemic drugs used in the treatment of type 2 diabetes mellitus. To date, metformin (Glucophage) is the only drug in this class used clinically. Because its actions directly address the major pathological defects in type 2 diabetes, it is first-line therapy in adults and children older than 10 years of age. Monotherapy with metformin is effective as initial drug therapy. If monotherapy with metformin is not effective, it is used as combination therapy with a variety of drugs from other antihyperglycemic agent classes or insulin. It is commonly used with significant effect for those with "pre-diabetes" or glucose intolerance; however, this is not an FDA-approved indication.

Pharmacodynamics

Metformin increases peripheral glucose uptake and utilization (insulin sensitivity), decreases hepatic glucose production, and decreases intestinal absorption of glucose. Together, these actions address the primary pathological defects of type 2 diabetes to improve glucose tolerance and lower both basal and postprandial plasma glucose levels. Metformin does not stimulate insulin release from the pancreatic beta cells, nor does it produce hypoglycemia except in specific circumstances. Metformin does not cause hyperinsulinemia. Metformin also does not cause weight gain; often patients lose weight. Because obesity is a major factor in the pathogenesis of type 2 diabetes, this is an important drug action. Metformin also inhibits platelet aggregation and reduces blood viscosity. This property is a factor in its use in metabolic syndrome, which is discussed below.

The magnitude of decline in FPG (fasting plasma glucose) concentrations with metformin therapy is directly proportional to the level of fasting hyperglycemia. Patients with higher BG levels experience a greater percentage of decrease in BG and A1C levels than those with lower BG levels. This is a significant factor because those with higher BG levels for longer periods of time have more complications. African Americans with diabetes tend to have higher BG levels; the recent study that metformin may work almost twice as well in this population than in whites is very good news indeed.

Metformin also has a modestly favorable impact on lipids because of its actions in the liver. In clinical studies, metformin alone lowered mean fasting serum triglycerides by 16%, total cholesterol by 5%, and low-density lipids (LDL) by 8%, and increased high-density lipids (HDL) by 2%. The same was true when metformin was combined with a sulfonylurea or other antihyperglycemic, but the magnitude of the changes was less for the combination (*DF & C*, 2011).

Pharmacokinetics

Absorption and Distribution

Metformin is 50% to 60% absorbed after oral administration under fasting conditions. The extended-release form of the drug has a different absorption profile from the immediate-release form (Table 21-11). Food decreases the extent and slightly delays the absorption in the immediate-release form, with an approximately 40% decrease in C_{max} and a 25% decrease in AUC. It is not known if these are clinically relevant. The extent of absorption from the extended-release form (Fortamet) was increased by approximately 60% when given with food. Glumetza must be administered immediately after a meal to maximize absorption. The rate and extent of absorption with metformin solution is comparable with that of the tablets under fasting or fed conditions (*DF & C*, 2011). Absorption is not linearly related to dose. The higher the dose the patient takes, the lower the percentage that is absorbed. Increased doses do not result in proportionally increased amounts of drug in the body.

Metformin is negligibly bound to plasma proteins. Plasma half-life is 6.2 hours, but the half-life in the blood is

Table 21–11 Pharmacokinetics: Selected Antihyperglycemic Agents

Drug	Onset*	Peak*	Duration*	Protein Binding	Bioavailability	Half-Life	Excretion
Metformin IR and solution	Days	1–8 h	UK	Minimal	50%–60% if taken fasting; nonlinear; reduced by food intake	6.2 h (plasma) 17.6 h (blood)	100% excreted unchanged in urine
Metformin ER (Fortamet, Glumetza)	Days	3–10 h	UK	Minimal	Increased by 60% with food for Fortamet and Glumetza	UK	In urine
Acarbose (Precose)	0.5–1 h	1 h	2–3 h		Less than 2% in plasma	2 h	51% in feces as unabsorbed drug; 34% in urine
Miglitol (Glyset)	0.5–1 h	2 h	3h		100% in extra-cellular fluids at 25 mg; 50%–70% at higher doses	Normal renal function: 2 h; renal impairment: CCr <25: 4 h	95% in urine as unchanged drug
Nateglinide (Starlix)	20 min	1 h	4 h	98%	73%	1.5 h	83% in urine; 10% in feces
Pioglitazone (Actos)	UA	2–4 h	UA		99%	3–7 h	15%–30% in urine
Repaglinide (Prandin)	0.5 h	1 h	1.4 h		100%	1–1.4 h	90% in feces; 8% in urine
Rosiglitazone (Avandia)	UA	1–3 h	UA		99%	3–4 h	64% in urine; 23% in feces
Sitagliptin (Januvia) (B)	UK	1–4 h	24 h	38%	87%	12.4 h	87% in urine; 13% in feces
Linagliptin Tradjenta (B)	UK	1.5 h	UA	75%–99%	30%	12 h	Enterohepatic 80%, urine 5%
Alogliptin Nesina (B)	UK	1–2 h	UA	20%	100%	21 h	Urine 76%; feces 13%

Table 21–11 ⊞ **Pharmacokinetics: Selected Antihyperglycemic Agents—cont'd**

Drug	Onset*	Peak*	Duration*	Protein Binding	Bioavailability	Half-Life	Excretion
Saxagliptin (Onglyza) (B)	UK	2 h	12–24 h	UK	75%	2.2–3.8 h	70% in urine
Exenatide (Byetta) (B)	UK	2.1 h	10 h	UK	UK	2.4 h	Mainly in urine
Liraglutide (Victoza)(B)	UK	9–12 h	UK	UK	51%	11–15 h	As metabolites in urine and feces
Pramlintide (Symlin)(B)	UK	19–21 min	UK	40%	30%–40%	48 min	As metabolites in urine
Canagliflozin (Invokana)(B)	Within 24 h	1–2 h	UA	99%	65%	10–13 h dose-dependent	Feces 41%, metabolites in urine 31%
Dapagliflozin (Farxiga) (B)	UA	2h	UA	91%	78%	12.9 h	75% urine; 21% feces
Empagliflozin (Jardiance) (B)	UA	1.5h	UA	86.2%	UA	10-19h	41% urine; 55% feces

UA = data unavailable; UK = unknown.
*Of antihyperglycemic effect.

17.6 hours, suggesting that RBCs may be a compartment of distribution. The apparent volume of distribution is very high and averages 654 L following single doses of 850 mg.

Metabolism and Excretion

There is no hepatic metabolism for metformin, and it is excreted unchanged in the urine. There is no biliary excretion. Renal clearance is 3.5 times that of CCr, indicating that renal tubular secretion is the major route of elimination. Data suggest a trend toward higher C_{max} and AUC values for Glumetza in Asian subjects when compared with white, Hispanic, and African American subjects. This difference does not appear to be clinically significant.

Pharmacotherapeutics

Precautions and Contraindications

There are two major contraindications to metformin use: (1) renal disease or dysfunction and (2) metabolic acidosis.Current standards state males with serum creatinine levels 1.5 or higher, females with levels 1.4 or higher, and patients of either gender with abnormal CCr rates should not receive metformin because of its heavy dependence on renal function for elimination. The ADA is recommending using eGFR above 30 mL/min as the cut point, which is moderate kidney disease. This is would allow many more DM patients to use this effective medication under cautious supervision (Inzucchi, Lipska, Mayo, Bailey, & McGuire, 2014). The FDA has yet to respond to the ADA recommendation. Patients with acute or chronic metabolic

acidosis and patients at high risk for lactic acidosis because of tissue hypoperfusion or hypoxia (e.g., severe dehydration, heart failure, respiratory failure, and chronic alcoholism with severe liver damage) also should not receive this drug when being managed solely by primary care providers.

Lactic acidosis is a rare, but serious, complication that can occur with metformin because of its accumulation during treatment. When it occurs, it is fatal 50% of the time. The risk for lactic acidosis increases in the presence of renal and hepatic dysfunction, making the interaction of these two contraindications more serious than either one alone. Metformin also should not be used for patients with clinical and laboratory evidence of hepatic disease.

Cautious use is suggested with patients over age 80 due to the probability of decreased renal function. Limited data suggest that total plasma clearance is decreased and half-life is prolonged in healthy older adults as compared with healthy young subjects (*DF & C*, 2011). These data suggest that the change in pharmacokinetics is primarily accounted for by change in renal function. For older adults, CCr should be tested before beginning therapy and at least annually during therapy.

Metformin should also be temporarily withheld 48 hours before to 48 hours after undergoing radiological studies that involve an iodine-based contrast medium because such materials may result in altered renal function and have been associated with lactic acidosis in patients receiving metformin. Metformin should be reinstituted only after renal function has been reevaluated and found to be normal. It should also be temporarily withheld from patients undergoing surgical procedures in which fluid will be withheld because of the risk for dehydration and hypoperfusion that may result in lactic acidosis. The time frame for withholding the drug is the same.

A decrease in vitamin B_{12} levels to subnormal without clinical manifestations has been observed in about 7% of patients receiving metformin. This decrease is probably due to interference with vitamin B_{12} absorption from the intrinsic factor–vitamin B_{12} complex. Patients with or at risk for anemia associated with altered vitamin B_{12} utilization should have the disorder treated and under control before beginning metformin therapy. The low levels may be the reason why some studies have found a dementia link with the medication.

There is evidence that metformin increases the risk of developing low TSH levels. This occurs more frequently within the first 6 months of use. This does not occur in persons with normal thyroid function, but is increased 55% for those with hypothyroid issues (Duntas, Orgiazzi, & Brabant, 2011). Metformin is listed as Pregnancy Category B, and has been studied for safety during pregnancy, but its use during pregnancy requires obstetric or endocrinology consultation (Feig & Moses, 2011; Kumar & Kahn, 2012). Studies in rats indicate that metformin is excreted in breast milk in levels approximately the same as in the plasma. Similar studies have not been conducted in nursing mothers. Because the potential for hypoglycemia in nursing infants may exist, decide whether the patient should discontinue nursing or discontinue metformin based on the importance of the drug to the mother.

Use of metformin in 10- to 16-year-old children is supported by evidence from adequate and well-controlled clinical trials with children of this age with type 2 diabetes; the trials demonstrated a similar response in glycemic control and adverse reactions to those seen in adults. Studies in children younger than 10 years have not been conducted.

African Americans, a group that is at higher risk of diabetes and faster onset of complications, appear to be more responsive to metformin than European Americans. There is a clinically important average decrease in Hb A1c levels when the two groups are compared (Williams et. al, 2014); the minority group has more benefit.

Adverse Drug Reactions

The most common adverse reaction involves GI disturbances (e.g., abdominal bloating, diarrhea, nausea, vomiting, and an unpleasant metallic taste). These adverse reactions are usually transient and resolve in about 2 weeks without a change in dose. They may be reduced by initiating therapy with a low dose and titrating the dose slowly.

Lactic acidosis is rare. Hypoglycemia is also rare unless there is a concurrent reduction in caloric intake, an increase in strenuous exercise not compensated for with increased caloric intake, or concurrent use of another glucose-lowering drug or alcohol. Older adults, debilitated and malnourished patients, and those with adrenal or pituitary insufficiency are also at increased risk for hypoglycemia. It is safe in most populations.

Drug Interactions

There are many drug interactions with metformin (Table 21-12). Carbonic anhydrase inhibitors may increase the risk for lactic acidosis and should be used cautiously. Cationic drugs that are eliminated by renal secretion (e.g., amiloride, digoxin, morphine, procainamide, quinidine, ranitidine, triamterene, trimethoprim, and vancomycin) may compete with metformin for its elimination pathway. Dosage adjustments may be needed in metformin or the interacting drugs. Cimetidine increases the peak metformin plasma level by 60%, with an increase of 40% in its AUC. Furosemide increases these levels by 15% without any significant change in renal clearance. Both of these

Table 21–12 ⊞ Drug Interactions With Metformin

Interacting Drug	Possible Effects	Implications
Alcohol	Potentiates the effect of metformin on lactate metabolism	Warn patients against excessive alcohol intake while taking metformin
Amiloride, digoxin, morphine, procainamide, quinidine, ranitidine, triamterene, trimethoprim, vancomycin	May compete for elimination pathway	Dosage adjustments may be needed for metformin or interacting drug
Beta-adrenergic blockers	May mask signs and symptoms of hypoglycemia	Does not affect diaphoresis as indicator of hypoglycemia; teach patient to check blood glucose level if experiencing diaphoresis
Cimetidine, furosemide	Increases plasma levels of metformin without concurrent increase in renal excretion	Dosage adjustments of metformin may be needed
Iodine-based contrast media	May affect renal function and increase the risk for lactic acidosis	Withhold metformin for 48 h before and after procedure in which contrast is used
Nifedipine	Enhances absorption of metformin and may increase effects	Dosage adjustments of metformin may be needed

drugs may increase the effects of metformin because of these alterations. Dosage adjustment for metformin may be necessary. Alcohol should be avoided when metformin is used.

Clinical Use and Dosing

Type 2 Diabetes Mellitus

Metformin is indicated as monotherapy and in multidrug therapy for patients with type 2 diabetes who cannot achieve adequate BG control on healthy eating, increased activity, and weight loss. It is the first-line drug therapy for patients with type 2 diabetes (ADA, 2012). The Hb A1c reduction commonly achieved with this drug alone is approximately 1.5% (Nathan et al, 2006). It is especially useful for obese patients because it is not associated with weight gain and may produce some weight loss. Its positive effect on lipids creates a clear advantage for patients with hyperlipidemia.

The pharmacodynamics of metformin are different from those of sulfonylureas so that the two drugs taken together potentiate each other's actions. In clinical trials, both the fasting and the postprandial BG levels of patients decreased by 20% to 30%. Because this drop is so dramatic, it is important to monitor BG levels closely when metformin is added to the treatment regimen of a drug that can produce hypoglycemia.

Metformin is available in intermediate- and extended-release formulations and in an oral solution of 500 mg/5 mL. Begin therapy with 500 mg bid with the morning and evening meal or 850 mg bid with the morning and evening meal for adults (Table 21-13). For children, the starting dose is 500 mg bid with the morning and evening meals. The dose is increased in increments of 500 mg at weekly intervals for both adults and children or 850 mg every other week for adults. The most common adverse reactions are GI disturbances. If they occur, the starting dose can be lowered or

Table 21–13 ⚗ Dosage Schedule: Selected Metformin Formulations

Drug	Initial Dose	Dosage Form	Maintenance Dose	Maximum Dose
Metformin IR (G) Glucophage IR (B) Riomet 500 mg/5 mL solution (B)	*Adults ≥17 yr:* Initial: 500 mg twice daily **or** 850 mg once daily; titrate in increments of 500 mg weekly or 850 mg every other week; may also titrate from 500 mg twice a day to 850 mg twice a day after 2 wk *Children 10 to 16 yrs:* 500 mg twice daily, dosage increases weekly, in increments of 500 mg/day, up to a maximum of 2000 mg/day	500, 850, 1,000 mg tablets		Maximum dose 2,550 mg *Children 10–16 yr:* 2,000 mg
Extended-Release				
Metformin ER (G), Glucophage XR (B), Fortamet (B), Glumetza (B)	*Adults and children >17 yr:* Fortamet: Initial: 500–1,000 mg once daily; dosage may be increased by 500 mg weekly Glucophage XR: Initial: 500 mg once daily; dosage may be increased by 500 mg weekly Glumetza: Initial: 1,000 mg once daily; dosage may be increased by 500 mg weekly	500 mg or 1,000 mg tablets		Maximum dose: 2,500 mg once daily for Fortamet Maximum dose: 2,000 mg daily for both Glucophage XR and Glumetza
Combination Drugs				
Glipizide/ metformin (G), Metaglip (B)	2.5 mg/250 mg glipizide/metformin daily with food **If FPG = 280–320 mg/dL:** 2.5/500 mg every 12 h Titrate every 2 wk to no more than 10/2,000 mg per day in divided doses **Second-line treatment if not controlled on metformin and/or sulfonylurea:** 2.5/ 500 mg or 5/500 mg every 12 h with food Titrate to no more than 20/2,000 mg daily in divided doses **Older adults:** Use conservatively; do not titrate to max dose	2.5 mg/500 mg tablets 5 mg/500 mg tablets		20 mg glipizide/ 2,000 mg metformin
Glyburide/ metformin (G), Glucovance (B)	1.25 mg/250 mg once daily or every 12 h Titrate up in 2 wk intervals **Older adults:** 1.25 mg/250 mg daily or every 12 h; use conservative dosing. Assess renal function if using in adults >80 yr; do not titrate to max dose	1.25 mg/250 mg 2.5 mg/500 mg 5 mg/500 mg		20/2,000 mg daily

IR = immediate release; ER = extended release.

the current dose can be held at that level and not increased. The symptoms will most likely resolve in about 2 weeks, at which time the dosage can be increased again until target BG levels are reached. The maximum dose recommended is 2,550 mg/d for adults or 2,000 mg/d for children. The maximum dose should be divided and given 3 times daily to reduce GI reactions.

Conversion of Immediate-Release Formulation to Extended-Release Formulation

Clinical trials have shown that patients treated with the immediate-release (IR) formulation of metformin who were switched to the extended-release (ER) formulation could safely be transferred with the same total daily dose. Close monitoring of glucose levels is recommended during the transition; the understanding that metformin typically does not cause hypoglycemia does not apply to this transition period.

Concomitant Metformin and Sulfonylurea Therapy in Adults

If a patient is not responsive to metformin monotherapy after 3 months, addition of another drug, including insulin, should be considered (see Table 33-3). There are combination formulations that include metformin plus glipizide (Metaglip) and metformin plus glyburide (Glucovance). These combination drugs are administered similarly to metformin IR and carry the precautions/contraindications, adverse effects, and drug interactions of both drugs. If a patient has not met BG and Hb A1c targets by 3 months of combination therapy, consider adding a third drug to the regimen. This patient may benefit from referral to an endocrinologist.

Concomitant Metformin and Thiazolidinediones

Thiazolidinediones can also be added to a treatment regimen when the patient has not achieved BG targets on metformin alone or in combination with other drugs. The starting dose is based on the patient's current regimen of each of the drugs. The starting doses of these drugs are discussed in their section below. There are combination formulations that include metformin plus pioglitazone (ActoPlus Met and ActoPlus Met XR) and metformin plus rosiglitazone (Avandamet). The same issues related to administration and combining that are stated with sulfonylureas apply, as does the information about achieving target Hb A1c goals.

Concomitant Metformin and Meglitinides

These drugs can be added to a treatment regimen when the patient has not achieved BG targets on metformin alone or in combination with other drugs. The starting dose is based on the patient's current regimen of each of the drugs. The starting doses of these drugs are discussed in their section below. There is a combination formulation of metformin plus repaglinde (PrandiMet). The same data apply to the combination as stated above.

Concomitant Metformin and Gliptins

All of the gliptins have been approved for this combination. The starting doses of these drugs are discussed in their section below. There is a combination formulation of sitagliptin plus metformin (Janumet). It is given twice daily with meals with a gradual dose escalation to reduce the adverse GI reaction caused by metformin (*DF & C*, 2011; Reynolds, 2009). This combination is purported to have fewer hypoglycemic risks than the combination of a glypizide (Metaglip) and metformin but is under scrutiny for worsening renal impairment (most likely the impact of the sitagliptin) and pancreatitis (Olansky, 2010).

Concomitant Metformin and Insulin Therapy

Initiate metformin IR or ER at 500 mg once daily in patients on insulin therapy. For patients who do not respond adequately, increase the dose of metformin by 500 mg daily after 1 week and by 500 mg daily every week thereafter until adequate glycemic control is achieved. The maximum daily dose is the same as for metformin alone for both adults and children. The insulin dose should then be decreased by 10% to 25% when the fasting blood glucose (FBG) decreases to less than 120 mg/dL.

Concomitant Metformin and SGLT2 medications

There is no long-term experience with this combination of medications. At least one combination tablet is on the market as of this time, dapagliflozin/metforminin extended release (Xigduo XR). As with any other combination tablet, it may be prudent to start one, then the other to determine tolerance prior to ordering a combination tablet. The side effects of both medications are important to monitor; therefore, lactic acidosis, renal response, and genital infections become important things to monitor. The starting dose would be consistent with the current dosing of each medication and increased to a max of 10 mg of the SGLT2 and 2,000 mg of the metformin. The duplication of hypoglycemic effect increases the risk of hypoglycemia if it is started without an initial trial period of dual prescriptions. It is taken in the a.m. with food to reduce the GI side effects. This medication cannot be crushed.

Metabolic Syndrome

Metformin inhibits platelet aggregation and decreases blood viscosity. It is recommended along with angiotensin converting enzyme (ACE) inhibitors or angiotensin II receptor blockers (ARBs) and statins in the treatment of insulin resistance syndromes including metabolic syndrome (Bloomgarden, 2003). Other chapters have more discussion of this syndrome, which includes obesity, hypertension, hyperlipidemia, and insulin resistance.

Prevention of Conversion of Prediabetes to Diabetes

The Diabetes Prevention Program Research Group (2002) tested metformin and lifestyle modifications as methods for preventing the conversion of prediabetes to type 2 diabetes. This group also found that both of these interventions were cost-effective across subjects regardless of age, ethnicity, or gender and affordable in routine clinical practice. Because prevention of movement from prediabetes to diabetes is a primary goal of treatment directed at children who may develop type 2 diabetes, metformin has become first-line therapy for this indication. This is discussed further in Chapter 33. Table 21-13 lists the available dosage forms of metformin, including the ER and oral solution formulations.

Monitoring

Before initiating therapy and at least annually thereafter, assess renal function. Assessment is by serum creatinine and CCr initially and then by serum creatinine annually. For patients with increased risk for developing altered renal function, the assessment should be made more often. Patients who have been previously well controlled on metformin who are no longer controlled or who develop illnesses that place them at risk for metabolic acidosis should be assessed for evidence of ketoacidosis or lactic acidosis. Assessment includes serum electrolytes and ketones, BG, and, if indicated, blood pH and lactate levels. Lactic acidosis is characterized by elevated blood lactate levels (greater than 5 mmol/L), decreased blood pH, and electrolyte disturbances with an increased anion gap. Because impaired hepatic function may significantly decrease the ability to clear lactate, liver function studies should be done before therapy is initiated.

● CLINICAL PEARL ●

When **metformin** is added to a **sulfonylurea**, the increased sensitivity to **insulin** caused by **metformin** results in less need for the insulin secretion generated by the **sulfonylurea**. If the BG level drops too much, the dose of the **sulfonylurea** should be reduced.

Response to metformin therapy is assessed by daily to weekly monitoring of fasting and postprandial BG and by monitoring Hb A1c every 3 months or monitoring fructosamine every 2 months. During initial therapy and with each incremental increase, FBG is used to evaluate response. After the patient is stabilized on a specific dose, monitoring with FBG and A1C levels every 6 months is sufficient.

Some patients with inadequate vitamin B$_{12}$ or calcium intake or absorption may be predisposed to developing subnormal vitamin B$_{12}$ levels. Assessment for this problem is done by red blood cell indices drawn at initiation of therapy and every 2 to 3 years thereafter.

Patient Education

Administration

Patients are taught to take the drug at the same time each day exactly as prescribed. The tablets should be swallowed whole and not cut, crushed, or chewed. Because the titrating doses will change weekly or every other week, a card or calendar is helpful to remind patients of the schedule. If a dose of metformin is missed, it is taken as soon as it is remembered unless it is about time for the next dose. Doses should not be doubled. If a dose of the ER drug is missed, patients resume taking the drug according to schedule.

Adverse Reactions

The most common adverse reactions are GI disturbances. If they occur, they may be reduced by taking the drug with food rather than before the meal. The provider should be notified of GI disturbances so that the dose may be kept at the current level until they resolve. Even with the same dose, GI disturbances will usually resolve in about 2 weeks. If the GI disturbances include vomiting or diarrhea or the patient develops a fever, the drug is stopped. Dehydration may result and presents a risk for the patient to develop lactic acidosis and decreased renal function. Patients are taught the signs and symptoms of lactic acidosis (e.g., chills, dizziness, low blood pressure, muscle pain, sleepiness, trouble breathing, slow heart rate, and weakness) and to report them immediately.

A patient who is to undergo a procedure with an iodine-based contrast medium or surgery in which fluid will be withheld should be temporarily taken off metformin; the provider should be notified if one of these procedures is anticipated.

SULFONYLUREAS

The first class of oral drugs developed to manage patients with type 2 diabetes mellitus was the sulfonylureas. They are true oral hypoglycemics and are useful only for patients with some endogenous insulin secretion. Owing to the risk for hypoglycemia and their limited action on insulin resistance, their use should be used in combination therapy.

Pharmacodynamics

Sulfonylureas cause an increase in endogenous insulin secretion by the beta cells of the pancreas related to increased cAMP generation. They may improve the binding between insulin and insulin receptors or increase the number of receptors, thereby having a limited ability to improve insulin utilization by the tissues. Hypoglycemic effects appear to be due to increased endogenous insulin production and to improved beta cell sensitivity to BG levels or suppression of glucose release by the liver. Sulfonylureas also potentiate the effect of antidiuretic hormone and may produce a mild diuresis. They appear to be similar to metformin in lowering Hb A1c levels by about 1.5% (Nathan et al, 2009). The glucose-lowering effect of these drugs is rapid compared to some other antihyperglycemic agents, but the maintenance of glycemic targets over time is not as effective as monotherapy with metformin (Nathan et al, 2009).

Pharmacokinetics

Absorption and Distribution

All sulfonylureas are well absorbed after oral administration and all except glipizide (Glucotrol) can be taken with food

(Table 21-14). Absorption of glipizide is delayed by the presence of food in the gut. Tolbutamide, glyburide, and glipizide are more effective when taken 30 minutes prior to a meal. Tolazamide (Tolinase) is absorbed more slowly than the other sulfonylureas.

Although the mechanisms of action are similar for all sulfonylureas, the first and second generations differ in absorption. Second-generation compounds are more nonpolar and lipophilic. Therapeutically effective doses and serum concentrations are lower because of their intrinsic potency and ability to cross plasma membranes. All sulfonylureas are highly bound to plasma proteins, especially albumin, but the first-generation binding is ionic, whereas the second-generation binding is not. Because they have ionic bonds, first-generation drugs are more likely to be displaced from their binding sites by drugs that competitively bind to proteins (e.g., warfarin, phenylbutazone). Displacement would result in a greater hypoglycemic effect and may account for the increased risk for hypoglycemia found with first-generation drugs.

Chlorpropamide and tolbutamide enter breast milk. Glyburide (DiaBeta) reaches high concentrations in bile and crosses the placenta.

Metabolism and Excretion

All sulfonylureas are metabolized in the liver to active or inactive metabolites. The hypoglycemic effects of these drugs may be prolonged by severe liver disease because of reduced metabolism. Differences exist among the sulfonylureas in the duration of hypoglycemic effects, in part because of their metabolism. Tolbutamide is short-acting because it is rapidly metabolized to an inactive metabolite by the liver. Tolazamide has two active metabolites that are less potent than the parent compound.

All sulfonylureas are excreted primarily in the urine; first generation are excreted 100% and second generation has both urine and feces elimination routes. Glyburide is excreted as metabolites in bile and urine, approximately 50% by each route. The renal elimination of chlorpropamide may be sensitive to changes in urine pH, with urinary alkalinization

Table 21–14 ⚙ Pharmacokinetics: Sulfonylureas

Drug	Onset (h)	Peak (h)	Duration (h)	Protein Binding	Half-Life (h)	Metabolism	Elimination
First-Generation							
Chlorpropamide	1	3–6	25–60	99%	36 (prolonged by renal disease)	80% metabolized in liver; activity unknown	Excreted 100% in urine; renal elimination may be hastened by increased urine pH
Tolazamide	4–6	1–6	12–24	99%	7	Metabolized in liver to several mildly active metabolites	Excreted 100% in urine
Tolbutamide	1	4–6	6–12	99%	4.5–6.5	Oxidized in liver to inactive metabolites	Excreted 100% in urine
Second-Generation							
Glipizide	1–1.5	1–2	10–16	99%	2–4	Metabolized in liver to inactive metabolites	Excreted 80%–85% in urine
Glyburide				99%		Metabolized in liver to weakly active metabolites	Excreted as metabolites in bile and urine, approximately 50% by each route
Nonmicronized	2–4		24		10		
Micronized	1	1.5–3	24		4		
Glimepiride	2	2–3	24	99.5%	5	Completely metabolized by liver	Excreted 60% in urine and 40% in feces

UK = unknown.

hastening its excretion. The half-life of this drug is prolonged in renal disease.

Pharmacotherapeutics

Precautions and Contraindications

All sulfonylureas are contraindicated for patients with hypersensitivity to the drugs or the compounds in which they are mixed. Cross-sensitivity may occur with other sulfonamides, including thiazide diuretics.

Sulfonylureas are listed as Pregnancy Category C (glyburide is Pregnancy Category B). Abnormal BG levels during pregnancy may be associated with a higher incidence of congenital abnormalities; thus insulin has been the drug of choice. All sulfonylureas except glyburide are teratogenic in animals. There are no adequate studies in pregnant women. Prolonged severe hypoglycemia has occurred in neonates born to mothers on a sulfonylurea at the time of delivery. If these drugs must be used during pregnancy, discontinue use 2 to 4 weeks before the expected delivery date.

Chlorpropamide and tolbutamide are known to enter breast milk; it is not known if other sulfonylureas are also excreted in breast milk. Because of the potential for hypoglycemic reactions in nursing infants, sulfonylureas are contraindicated in nursing mothers. The safety and efficacy of these drugs in children have not been established; however, with the increased incidence of type 2 diabetes in children, studies may be conducted to address the possible use of these drugs in children.

Other conditions in which sulfonylureas should not be used include type 1 diabetes; DKA or diabetic coma; and uncontrolled infection, burns, or trauma. Patients with adrenal or pituitary insufficiency are especially susceptible to hypoglycemia, and sulfonylureas should be used cautiously and patients monitored more frequently if they have these comorbid conditions. Severe hepatic impairment may cause inadequate hepatic release of glucose in response to hypoglycemia. Renal impairment may cause decreased elimination, leading to accumulation of these drugs and resulting in hypoglycemia. All sulfonylureas should be used with extreme caution for patients with hepatic or renal impairment, and liver and renal function should be monitored frequently if they must be used.

Older adults and debilitated patients are particularly susceptible to the hypoglycemic action of sulfonylureas, and the signs and symptoms of hypoglycemia may be difficult to recognize. Long-acting agents should be avoided, and short-acting agents should be used with caution in these patients.

All sulfonylureas carry a warning that states that the administration of oral hypoglycemic drugs has been reported to be associated with increased cardiovascular mortality as compared to treatment with diet alone or diet plus insulin. This warning is based on the study conducted by the University Group Diabetes Program (1970). Patients who were treated for 5 to 8 years with diet plus tolbutamide had a rate of cardiovascular mortality approximately 2.5 times that of patients treated with diet alone despite ongoing analyses of the study-identified limitations. Although only one drug in the sulfonylurea class was shown to produce this problem, this warning was extended to the entire drug class because of the close similarities in mode of action and chemical structure of drugs within the class. These concerns were not substantiated by the UK Prospective Diabetes Study (UKPDS) or Action in Diabetes and Vascular Disease: Preterax and Diamicron MR Controlled Evaluation (ADVANCE) studies (Nathan et al, 2009), but the warning remains.

Adverse Drug Reactions

All sulfonylureas may produce severe hypoglycemia. Second-generation drugs are less likely than first-generation drugs to cause this adverse reaction. Hypoglycemia may be difficult to recognize in patients who are concurrently taking beta blockers because these drugs mask the signs and symptoms of hypoglycemia, with the exception of diaphoresis. Hypoglycemia is also more likely when caloric intake is reduced, after severe or prolonged exercise, when alcohol is consumed, or when more than one glucose-lowering agent is used.

Weight gain is common following the initiation of sulfonylurea therapy. The increased insulin secretion generated by sulfonylureas has been associated with weight gain and hyperinsulinemia. Combination with metformin (Glucophage) reduces these adverse effects.

Gastrointestinal disturbances (nausea, epigastric fullness, and heartburn) are the most common adverse reactions. They tend to be dose-related and disappear when the dose is reduced. Diarrhea has been associated with glipizide use; taste alteration has been associated with tolbutamide use. Cholestatic jaundice is rare but requires discontinuation of the drug.

Dermatological reactions include rashes, pruritus, erythema, and urticaria. These tend to be transient and may disappear despite continued use of the drug. Photosensitivity can also occur, and patients should use sunblock and wear clothing when exposed to sunlight.

Syndrome of inappropriate secretion of antidiuretic hormone (SIADH) has occurred after administration of sulfonylureas, especially with patients who also have congestive heart failure or hepatic cirrhosis. These drugs stimulate ADH release, augmenting hypothalamic-pituitary release of ADH. The result is excessive water retention and dilutional hyponatremia. Glipizide, tolazamide, and glyburide are mildly diuretic.

Hemolytic anemia, agranulocytosis, leukopenia, and thrombocytopenia have occurred but are rare. Patients should have initial and annual complete blood counts done.

Drug Interactions

Sulfonylureas interact with a large number of drugs that either increase or decrease their hypoglycemic effect (Table 21-15). Alcohol interacts with these drugs to produce a disulfiram-like syndrome, characterized by facial flushing and occasional breathlessness but without the nausea, vomiting, and

Table 21–15 ⁘ Drug Interactions: Sulfonylureas

Drug	Interacting Drug	Possible Effect	Implications
All sulfonylureas	Androgens, anticoagulants,* chloramphenicol, fluconazole, gemfibrozil, histamine$_2$ blockers, magnesium salts, methyldopa, MAO inhibitors, NSAIDs (except diclofenac), phenylbutazone, probenecid, salicylates, sulfonamides, tricyclic antidepressants, urinary acidifiers	Enhance the hypoglycemic effect of the sulfonylurea	Avoid concurrent administration or monitor blood glucose levels closely if drug must be given
All sulfonylureas	Beta-adrenergic blockers, cholestyramine, diazoxide, hydantoins, rifampin, thiazide diuretics, urinary alkalinizers	Decrease the hypoglycemic effect of the sulfonylurea	Avoid concurrent administration or monitor blood glucose levels closely
Glimepiride*	In addition to drugs with all sulfonylureas: corticosteroids, phenothiazines, thyroid products, estrogens, oral contraceptives, nicotinic acid, sympathomimetics, and isoniazid	May cause loss of glucose control because these drugs can cause hyperglycemia	If concurrently administered, monitor closely for loss of glucose control; when they are withdrawn, monitor closely for hypoglycemia

The changes in prothrombin time/international normalized ratio (PT/INR) were so small that they are unlikely to be clinically significant.

*Concurrent administration of glimepiride and warfarin did not alter the pharmacokinetic properties of warfarin.

hypotension seen in a true alcohol–disulfram reaction. This reaction occurs in about 33% of patients concurrently ingesting alcohol and chlorpropamide. It is uncertain whether this reaction occurs with glyburide and glipizide.

Clinical Use and Dosing

Type 2 Diabetes Mellitus

Both first- and second-generation sulfonylureas are used to treat type 2 diabetes. They are effective as second-line therapy with patients who have previously used diet, exercise, weight control, and metformin. Equivalent therapeutic doses vary from 1 mg to 1,000 mg, depending on the drug. Micronized glyburide 3 mg tablets provide serum concentrations that are not bioequivalent to those from the conventional formulation group. When transferring patients from any sulfonylurea to micronized glyburide, the dose must be retitrated. Although all the drugs are listed as once-daily doses, many of the drugs work equally well when the daily dose is divided and given twice, especially when higher doses are required. The dose is highly individualized, based on BG readings (Table 21-16). Start with the lowest dose and increase every 4 to 7 days, based on glucose control. In general, one-half the maximum dose is usually the maximally efficient dose for glucose control. If the BG level goal is not achieved on one-half the maximum dose, consider adding a drug from a different class.

Table 21–16 ⊗ Dosage Schedule: Sulfonylureas

Drug	Initial Dose	Dosage Form	Maintenance Dose	Maximum Dose
First-Generation				
Chlorpropamide	Moderately severe, middle-aged stable adults: 250 mg	100 and 250 mg tablets	250 mg/d before morning meal	750 mg/d
	Older adults: 100–125 mg Severe disease: 250 mg		100–250 mg/d before morning meal 500 mg/d before morning meal	
Tolazamide	100 mg	100, 250, and 500 mg tablets	If FPG less than 200 mg/dL, give 100 mg/d before morning meal. If FPG more than 200 mg/dL, give 250 mg/d before morning meal. If patient malnourished, underweight, or elderly, give 100 mg/d before morning meal.	1,000 mg/d

Table 21–16 ⊗ Dosage Schedule: Sulfonylureas—cont'd

Drug	Initial Dose	Dosage Form	Maintenance Dose	Maximum Dose
			If more than 500 mg/d, divide dose and give bid before morning and evening meal.	
Tolbutamide (Orinase)	1,000 mg	500 mg	500–2,000 mg/d; divide dose and give bid before morning and evening meal	2,000 mg/d
Second-Generation				
Glipizide (Glucotrol, Glucotrol XL) (B)	5 mg Older adults, liver disease: 2.5 mg	5 and 10 mg tablets	Doses more than 15 mg/day: divide and give bid before morning and evening meal; adjust doses in 2.5–5 mg increments several days apart	40 mg/d
Glyburide				
Glyburide (DiaBeta, Micronase) (Generic available in both micronized and nonmicronized formulations)	2.5 mg	Tablets: 1.25, 2.5, 5 mg Micronized tablets: 1.5, 3, 6 mg	1.25–20 mg/d before morning meal. Dose more than 10 mg/d: divide and give bid; adjust dose in increments of 2.5 mg at weekly intervals	12 mg/d for micronized; 20 mg/d for nonmicronized
Glynase (micronized formulation)	1.5 mg		0.75–6 mg/d before morning meal. Dose more than 10 mg/d: divide and give bid before morning and evening meal; adjust dose in increments of 1.5 mg at weekly intervals	12 mg/d
Glimepiride (Amaryl) (G)	1 mg	1, 2, and 4 mg tablets	1–4 mg/d before morning meal. After reaching 2 mg dose, increase in increments of no more than 2 mg at 1–2 wk intervals.	8 mg/d

Rational Drug Selection

Age

Glyburide should be avoided in older adults because of the risk for severe hypoglycemia in this age group (Kirkman et al, 2012). Sulfonylureas in general may cause problems with hypoglycemia in older adults; they are not currently approved for use in children.

Concurrent Disease

In the presence of renal impairment, glipizide and tolbutamide are reasonable choices because they are oxidized in the liver to inactive metabolites. Glyburide is also a reasonable choice because 50% of it is excreted in bile, which gives an alternative route for excretion. Tolazamide is also safe to use with creatinine clearance (CCr) less than 30 mL/min.

Taking Multiple Medications

Second-generation sulfonylureas are best to minimize potential drug interactions and for patients who are taking multiple medications. Second-generation sulfonylureas also have the advantage of once-daily administration, thereby reducing the complexity of the drug regimen and improving adherence. Among this group of drugs, glimepiride binds to different insulin receptors than do other sulfonylureas and may be effective when others are not. It is also associated with a lower incidence of hypoglycemic reactions.

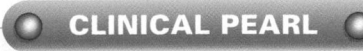

CLINICAL PEARL

Tolazamide has the added advantage that it may be crushed and put down a nasogastric tube or sprinkled on applesauce or other soft food for patients who have difficulty in swallowing tablets.

Monitoring

Hb A1c is the preferred tool for monitoring long-term glycemic control. Glycated albumin (fructosamine) is also sometimes used for monitoring, although it is not recommended as a substitute for A1C except in situations such as hemolytic anemia in which Hb A1c cannot be used. It indicates the average BG for the past 1 to 3 weeks and is used to assess short-term control. The minimum goal for fructosamine levels is 325 mmol or less, with a goal for intensive therapy of 287 mmol or less. All decreases in these monitoring parameters are beneficial, even if the goal is not met. SMBG should be performed and monitored for daily BG changes and adequacy of control.

Patient Education

Administration

Patients are taught to take the medication exactly as prescribed, at the same time each day, preferably before or with the morning meal. All sulfonylureas except glipizide may be taken with food. Glipizide must be taken 30 minutes before a meal to prevent a reduction in absorption. If a dose is missed, instruct the patient to take it as soon as remembered unless the timing of the dose will produce a risk for hypoglycemia. Doses should not be taken if the patient is unable to eat.

Adverse Reactions

The most common adverse reactions are gastrointestinal. If GI upset is a problem, notify the health-care provider. The dose may be divided and given twice daily to reduce this adverse effect. The most serious potential adverse reaction is hypoglycemia. Teach the patient the signs and symptoms of hypoglycemia and how to treat it. Caution the patient to avoid concurrent administration of other drugs without first discussing them with the health-care provider. Many drugs increase or decrease the effectiveness of sulfonylureas and can produce hypoglycemia or hyperglycemia. This is especially a problem with alcohol because it both produces hypoglycemia and masks the indications of this adverse reaction. Alcohol may also produce a disulfram-like reaction when combined with some sulfonylureas.

Because these drugs may produce alterations in red and white blood cell and platelet formation, patients should notify their provider promptly if they experience sore throat, rash, or unusual bruising or bleeding. Sulfonylureas may also produce an antidiuretic effect, and patients should promptly report unusual weight gain, swelling of the ankles, drowsiness, or shortness of breath.

ALPHA-GLUCOSIDASE INHIBITORS

The alpha-glucosidase inhibitors are oral antihyperglycemic drugs used in the treatment of type 2 diabetes mellitus. The action of this class has proved to reduce BG both as added therapy for patients who cannot achieve control on diet alone and as added therapy for patients whose BG cannot be controlled by lifestyle modifications and other oral antihyperglycemic agents. These drugs are not typically given as monotherapy; they are adjunct to other therapy for type 2 diabetes. In Asia, it is used as initial, mono therapy and is being considered as a metformin substitute if someone cannot take that drug (Yang et al, 2014).

Pharmacodynamics

Alpha-glucosidase inhibitors do not act directly on any of the defects in metabolism seen in type 2 diabetes mellitus. They competitively inhibit the absorption of complex carbohydrates (CHO) from the small bowel. Their chemical structure is a pseudo-tetrasaccharide that binds to alpha glucosidase. Because this structure is so similar to the CHO molecule, digestive enzyme activity is partially diverted from CHO digestion while it is trying to digest the alpha-glucosidase inhibitor. This effectively delays the digestion of CHO and permits CHOs that would normally have been digested in the upper

small bowel to move farther down in the bowel. The lower parts of the bowel have the necessary enzymes to digest this CHO, but, because they are not normally active in this process, enzyme induction is required. The process of induction takes weeks to months, and during this time patients may experience intestinal flatus and abdominal distention. Alpha-glucosidase inhibitors have no inhibitory activity against lactase and do not induce lactose intolerance.

Alpha-glucosidase inhibitors lower BG levels after meals. The higher that the postprandial BG level is, the larger the reduction will be that this drug can provide. As a consequence of plasma glucose reduction, they also reduce glycosylated hemoglobin levels. The mean reduction in Hb A1c is 0.77%, postprandial BG reduction is approximately 50 mg/dL, and fasting BG reduction is 20 mg/dL (*DF & C*, 2011).

Unlike other classes of antihyperglycemic agents, they do not enhance pancreatic beta cell secretion of insulin and so do not produce hypoglycemia. Like metformin, they are not associated with weight gain, and they diminish the weight-increasing effects of sulfonylureas when given in combination with them. Their activity is effective on any CHO food intake, including liquid diets taken via nasogastric tube.

Pharmacokinetics
Absorption and Distribution

Less than 2% of acarbose is systemically absorbed as an active drug. The remainder is active in the GI tract with no systemic distribution. Miglitol is completely absorbed in the GI tract at 25 mg doses, and 50% to 70% is absorbed at higher doses. Its volume of distribution of 0.18 is consistent with distribution primarily into extracellular fluids.

Metabolism and Excretion

Acarbose and miglitol are metabolized exclusively by intestinal bacteria and digestive enzymes. The minimal amount of drug absorbed is excreted by the kidneys. The plasma elimination half-life of both drugs is about 2 hours, so drug accumulation does not occur with 3-times-daily dosing. The mean steady-state AUC and maximum concentration of this drug were 1.5 times higher in older adults taking acarbose, but this was neither statistically nor clinically significant. This change was not seen with miglitol.

Pharmacotherapeutics
Precautions and Contraindications

Alpha-glucosidase inhibitors should not be used for patients with bowel diseases such as inflammatory bowel disease, bowel obstruction or risk factors for it, chronic intestinal disease associated with marked digestive disorders, or conditions that may deteriorate as a result of increased gas in the intestine.

Plasma concentrations of alpha-glucosidase inhibitors were 5 times higher in patients with severe renal impairment (CCr less than 25 mL/min); however, dosage adjustments to compensate for this are not possible because the drugs act locally (*DF & C*, 2011). Long-term studies with diabetes patients with renal impairment have not been conducted. Therefore, treatment with these drugs is not recommended for these patients.

The safety of alpha-glucosidase inhibitors in pregnant women has not been established. Although they are listed as Pregnancy Category B, they should not be used in pregnancy unless clearly needed. As previously discussed with other oral agents, insulin is the drug of choice for pregnant diabetics. In a study, a small amount of acarbose was excreted in the breast milk of rats. It is not known if it is excreted in human breast milk, and it should not be used in lactating women. Miglitol is excreted in human breast milk to a small degree. Total excretion in breast milk accounts for 0.02% of a 100 mg maternal dose. Although the levels in breast milk are exceedingly low, it also should not be used for lactating women.

Safety and efficacy in children have not been established for either drug.

Adverse Drug Reactions

GI symptoms are the most common adverse reactions seen with alpha-glucosidase inhibitors. Approximately 77% of patients taking acarbose and 41% of patients taking miglitol experience flatulence, the leading reason for discontinuance of the drug. Approximately 33% of patients taking acarbose and 29% of patients taking miglitol experience diarrhea, whereas 21% report abdominal pain while taking acarbose and 12% while taking miglitol. These adverse effects can be reduced by slow titration to maximal dose.

> ### CLINICAL PEARL
>
> Starting the **alpha glucosidase inhibitor** at 25 mg daily for 1 week and increasing the dose to 25 mg twice daily for 1 week and then to 25 mg 3 times daily for 1 week decreases the incidence of GI-adverse responses.

Because of their mechanism of action, alpha-glucosidase inhibitors alone do not cause hypoglycemia but may do so in combination with other drugs that lower BG, such as sulfonylureas and insulin. Treatment of this hypoglycemia cannot be accomplished with the usual ingestion of sucrose, fructose, or starches because alpha-glucosidase inhibitors delay the absorption of these disaccharides. Reversible increases in serum transaminases (alanine aminotransferase [ALT] and aspartate aminotransfeptidase [AST]) have occurred with doses of acarbose greater than 200 mg 3 times daily. Hepatic abnormalities improved or resolved with discontinuance of the drug. This laboratory change has not been reported with miglitol.

Drug Interactions

Acarbose may decrease serum digoxin levels. Drugs may enhance the hypoglycemic effects of acarbose and miglitol, such as neomycin, selective serotonin uptake inhibitors, salicylates, and MAO inhibitors; those that may diminish the hypoglycemic effects are somatropin, loop and thiazide diuretics, and corticosteroids (Access Pharmacy, 2013). Both acarbose and miglitol may have their therapeutic effects reduced by concurrent administration with digestive enzymes or intestinal absorbents (Table 21-17).

Clinical Use and Dosing

Management of type 2 diabetes mellitus is the only indication for these drugs. They are useful for patients with high postprandial BG levels. The initial dose of both drugs is 25 mg 3 times daily taken with the first bite of each meal. Taking the dose with the first bite is critical; a space between administration of the drug and ingestion of food decreases its effect, and no effect occurs if it is taken after a meal. The dose is increased in increments of 25 mg with each meal (75 mg/day) at 4- to 8-week intervals. The maintenance dose is usually 50 mg 3 times daily, although some patients may benefit from increasing the dose to 100 mg 3 times daily. If no further reduction in postprandial BG is achieved at the higher dose, consider reducing the dose to 50 mg 3 times daily (Table 21-18).

Because patients with low body weight are at higher risk for elevations in serum transaminase, the dose should not be higher than 50 mg 3 times daily for patients weighing less than 60 kg, and the 100 mg 3 times daily dose should be reserved for patients weighing more than 60 kg. The maximum dose is 100 mg 3 times daily.

Table 21–17 ⠿ Drug Interactions: Alpha-Glucosidase Inhibitors

Drug	Interacting Drug	Possible Effect	Implications
Acarbose, miglitol	Digoxin	Serum digoxin concentrations may be reduced with reduced therapeutic effect	Choose another antihyperglycemic drug
	Digestive enzymes and intestinal absorbents	Reduced effect of alpha-glucosidase inhibitor	Do not take concomitantly
Miglitol	Propranolol	Reduces bioavailability of propranolol by 40%	Avoid current use
	Ranitidine	Reduces bioavailability of ranitidine by 60%	Avoid current use

Table 21–18 ⊗ **Dosage Schedule: Alpha-Glucosidase Inhibitors**

Drug	Dosage Form	Initial Dose	Maintenance Dose	Maximum Dose
Acarbose (Precose) Meglitol (glyset)	25, 50, 100 mg tablets	*Wt > 60 kg* : 25 mg 3 times daily with the first bite of each meal for 4 wk *Wt < 60 kg*: 25 mg 3 times daily with the first bite of each meal for 4 wk *Poor GI tolerance*: 25 mg daily with first bite of evening meal for 2 wk	Weeks 5–8: 50 mg tid Weeks 9–12: 100 mg tid Weeks 5–8: 50 mg tid Weeks 3–4: 25 mg tid; Weeks 5–12: 25 mg tid Week 50 mg tid	100 mg tid 50 mg tid 50 mg tid

When given in combination with a sulfonylurea or insulin, hypoglycemia may occur. It is important to monitor BG levels closely when alpha-glucosidase inhibitors are added to the treatment regimen to avoid hypoglycemia. For treatment of mild–moderate hypoglycemia, oral glucose (dextrose) should be used instead of sucrose (cane sugar). For severe hypoglycemia, IV glucose or glucagon should be used.

Rational Drug Selection

Adverse Reactions

Elevated serum transaminase levels have been reported in long-term studies of acarbose, usually with doses up to 300 mg 3 times daily. These elevations appear to be dose-related and disappeared with maximum doses at 100 mg 3 times a day. There have been no reported hepatic adverse reactions and no reported changes in liver function tests with miglitol. The percentage of patients experiencing GI adverse effects in clinical trials is slightly lower with miglitol. Patients at risk for this adverse effect might be tried first on miglitol. During stress-related states, such as fever, trauma, infection, or surgery, treatment may need to be changed to insulin.

Monitoring

Before initiating therapy and at least annually thereafter, assess renal function. For patients with increased risk beyond their diabetes for developing altered renal function, the assessment timing should be related to the disease process that produces the added risk. Alpha-glucosidase inhibitors are not recommended for patients with renal impairment. Assessment of renal function includes serum electrolytes, blood urea nitrogen (BUN), and serum creatinine. A similar assessment is required related to hepatic function for patients taking acarbose. Because acarbose has been associated with reversible elevations in serum transaminase, these values should be assessed every 3 months for the first year.

Response to alpha-glucosidase inhibitor therapy is assessed by regular monitoring of fasting and postprandial BG. During initial therapy and with each incremental increase, FPG is used to evaluate response. After the patient is stabilized on a specific dose, monitoring with FPG and Hb A1c levels every 3 to 6 months is sufficient.

Patient Education

Administration

Patients are taught to take these drugs with the first bite of each meal. The need for this timing of administration must be stressed because taking it too soon reduces its effect and taking it after a meal has no effect.

Adverse Reactions

The most common adverse reactions are GI disturbances. These effects can be reduced or prevented by slow titration of the dose. Even without changing the dose, GI disturbances usually resolve in about 2 weeks.

○ **CLINICAL PEARL** ○

The delayed absorption of carbohydrates caused by **alpha-glucosidase inhibitors** results in less need for the insulin secretion generated by a **sulfonylurea**. If the BG level drops too much, the dose of the **sulfonylurea** should be reduced.

Hypoglycemia is less common than with other glucose-lowering drugs but may occur when alpha-glucosidase inhibitors are given with insulin, sulfonylureas, or repaglinide (Prandin). The usual treatment for hypoglycemia with sucrose, fructose, or starches does not resolve the problem for patients on alpha-glucosidase inhibitors because it interferes with the absorption of these carbohydrates. Treatment for mild to moderate hypoglycemia should be treated with glucose in the form of dextrose, not sucrose (table sugar, candy, cookies, etc.). Severe hypoglycemia may need to be treated with IV glucose or glucagon. Patients should wear identification that states they are taking an alpha-glucosidase inhibitor and the source of simple carbohydrate that should be used in case of hypoglycemia.

THIAZOLIDINEDIONES

The thiazolidinediones (TZDs) are oral antihyperglycemic drugs used in the treatment of type 2 diabetes. Their action lowers BG levels as monotherapy for patients who cannot achieve BG control with diet alone, and they are successful as added therapy for patients who cannot be controlled by lifestyle modifications or other antihyperglycemic agents. They are not part of initial therapy. Troglitazone (Rezulin), the first TZD, was approved in March 1997. It was removed from the market in 1999 because of the adverse reactions associated with liver damage. Pioglitazone (Actos) and rosiglitazone (Avandia) are the only TZDs on the U.S. market. TZDs are recommended in the current guidelines in two or three drug combinations if glycemic targets are not met but should be used cautiously because of the potential for cardiovascular problems, especially with rosiglitazone. In 2011, the FDA imposed restrictions on prescribing rosiglitazone-containing drugs that required health-care providers and patients be enrolled in the Avandia-Rosiglitazone Medicines Access Program (REMS) (FDA, 2011). Two FDA panels met in 2013 to relinquish many of the restrictions placed on rosiglitazone after the "Rosiglitazone Evaluated for Cardiovascular Outcomes and Regulation of Glycemia in Diabetes" (RECORD) study reanalysis (Medscape 2013). This remains controversial due to reports of severe cardiovascular (CV) compromise in some patients.

Pharmacodynamics

TZDs improve glycemic control by improving insulin sensitivity, a major pathological problem with type 2 diabetes. They are effective only in type 2 diabetes because they depend on the presence of insulin for their action. They are highly selective activators of the peroxisome proliferator-activated receptor gamma, a nuclear receptor that regulates gene transcription, resulting in expression of proteins that improve insulin action in the cell. This action leads to increased utilization of available insulin by the liver and muscle cells and also in adipose tissue. In addition, these drugs reduce hepatic glucose production. Taken together, these actions improve glucose tolerance and lower both basal and postprandial plasma glucose levels. Unlike the sulfonylureas, TZDs do not produce hypoglycemia, except in special situations, and do not cause hyperinsulinemia because they do not stimulate insulin release from the pancreatic beta cells. Like metformin, they have a modest impact on lipids because of their actions in the liver.

Pharmacokinetics

Absorption and Distribution

Pioglitazone and rosiglitazone are rapidly absorbed after oral administration. Food does not alter the extent of absorption, but it does delay the time until peak concentration is reached. Both drugs are extensively bound to plasma proteins, with a mean volume of distribution (V_d) ranging from 0.63 L/kg for pioglitazone to 17.6 L/kg for rosiglitazone. This difference in V_d might be a factor in drug choice for patients with high extracellular fluid levels.

Metabolism and Excretion

Both drugs are highly metabolized by the liver into metabolites, and pioglitazone has at least two active metabolites. Hepatic function impairment increased C_{max} for both drugs and AUC levels for rosiglitazone. The pioglitazone site of metabolism in the liver results in inhibition of the CYP450 2C8, 3A4, and 1A1 isoezymes. Drugs using these isoezymes are likely to have drug interactions. In vitro drug studies suggest that rosiglitazone does not inhibit any of the major CPY450 enzyme systems. It is predominantly metabolized by CYP450 2C8 and, to a lesser extent, 2C9.

Mean plasma elimination half-life ranges from 3 to 7 hours, with 23% of rosiglitazone and its metabolites recovered in the feces and 64% in the urine. Pioglitazone is excreted 15% to 30% in the urine.

● CLINICAL PEARL ●

When **thiazolidinediones** are added to a **sulfonylurea** in a diabetic regimen, the increased sensitivity to insulin caused by the **thiazolidinedione** results in less need for the **insulin** secretion generated by the **sulfonylurea**. If the BG level drops too much, the dose of the **sulfonylurea** should be reduced.

The mean pioglitazone C_{max} and AUC values are increased 20% and 60% in women. The mean oral clearance of rosiglitazone in women is 6% lower compared to men (*DF & C*, 2011).

Pharmacotherapeutics

Precautions and Contraindications

The metabolites of these drugs have been found in increased concentrations in patients with chronic liver disease. Serum transaminase levels must be checked at the start of therapy and frequently during therapy. These drugs should not be initiated in patients with ALT levels greater than 2.5 times the upper limit of normal. They should be discontinued if the patient develops jaundice or has laboratory measurements suggesting liver injury (e.g., ALT greater than 3 times the upper limit of normal).

An increase in plasma volume (fluid retention) with a resultant increase in body weight and decrease in hemoglobin of less than or equal to 1% with rosiglitazone and 2% to 4% with pioglitazone has been noted in some patients. In the United States, initiation of therapy is contraindicated in patients with NYHA class III or IV heart failure; in Canada, use is contraindicated in patients with any stage of heart failure (NYHA I, II, III, IV). A higher frequency of cardiovascular events has been noted in patients with NYHA class I or II heart failure treated with rosiglitazone. Use may also be associated with an increased risk of angina and myocarcial infarction (MI). Use with caution in patients at risk for cardiovascular events and monitor closely following the Black-Box Warning for cardiotoxicity (Access Pharmacy, 2013). The apparent risk for macular edema associated with pioglatizone use may more be a function of the typically higher BMI and resistant hyperglycemic status of patients on glitazone therapy rather than the medication itself (Fujimoto, 2013).

In premenopausal anovulatory patients with insulin resistance, TZD treatment may result in resumption of ovulation. This has been found to be useful in Polycystic Ovarian Syndrome patients. If pregnancy is not desired, a birth control method should be instituted prior to beginning therapy. There are no adequate and well-controlled studies of the use of pioglitazone or rosiglitazone in pregnant women. Some animal studies have shown fetal death and growth retardation. These drugs are listed as Pregnancy Category C; TZDs should not be used during pregnancy unless the potential benefit clearly outweighs the risk. Insulin is the drug of choice for treatment of diabetes during pregnancy.

It is not known whether these drugs are excreted in human breast milk. They are secreted in the milk of lactating rats. Do not administer these drugs to lactating women. The safety and efficacy in children younger than 18 years have not been established.

Adverse Drug Reactions

TZDs are generally well tolerated, with the exception of cardiovascular effects, including weight gain (5%), hypertension (4%), heart failure (2% to 3% in patients receiving insulin), and myocardial ischemia (3%). Increases in total cholesterol, HDL cholesterol, LDL cholesterol, and weight gain occur in less than 10% of patients (Access Pharmacy, 2013).

Drug Interactions

Administration of pioglitazone with an oral contraceptive that contains ethinyl estradiol and norethindrone reduces the plasma concentrations of both components by 30%. These

changes, added to the resumption of ovulation that occurs in some anovulatory women, could result in loss of contraception. A higher dose of oral contraceptive or an alternative birth control method may be needed.

Pioglitazone is metabolized by the CPY450 3A4 isoezyme system. Specific formal pharmacokinetic interaction studies have not been conducted with other drugs also metabolized by this system (e.g., erythromycin, calcium channel blockers, corticosteroids, cyclosporine, HMG-CoA reductase inhibitors). Until data are available, it is prudent to avoid these drug combinations or to carefully monitor patients concurrently taking pioglitazone and any of the drugs also metabolized by the CYP450 3A4 isoenzyme system. Table 21-19 presents drug interactions with thiazolidinediones.

Clinical Use and Dosing

The only approved indication for these drugs is as therapy for type 2 diabetes not controlled by diet alone or diet and an oral antihyperglycemic agent or insulin (Table 21-20).

Monotherapy

Clinical trials have been conducted to study the use of both pioglitazone and rosiglitazone as monotherapy for patients

Table 21–19 ▦ Drug Interactions With Thiazolidinediones

Drug	Interacting Drug	Possible Effect	Implications
Pioglitazone	Oral contraceptives	Oral contraceptives with ethinyl estradiol and norethindrone show reduced plasma contraceptive components	May result in loss of contraception; consider higher dose of contraceptive or alternative method
	Atorvastatin	Concurrent use for 7 d shows an increase in serum concentrations of both drugs	Monitor BG closely
	Ketoconazole	Coadministration shows an increase in pioglitazone AUC and C_{max}. Ketoconazole significantly inhibits pioglitazone metabolism.	Avoid concurrent use. Select different antifungal agent. If both must be given, monitor glycemic control closely.
	Nifedipine	Concurrent use shows an increase in nifedipine-ER concentrations	Unknown clinical significance
Pioglitazone and rosiglitazone	Bile-acid sequestrants	Pharmacological effects of thiazolidinedione may be decreased; bile-acid sequestrant reduces absorption	Avoid concurrent use; separate doses by 4 h, giving thiazolidinedione first

Table 21–20 ⊗ Dosage Schedule: Thiazolidinediones

Drug	Initial Dose	Dosage Form	Maximum Dose	Maintenance Dose
Pioglitazone (Actos) Pioglitazone and metformin (ActoPlus Met) ActoPlus Met XR	15–30 mg daily	15, 30, 45 mg tablets 15 mg XR: 15, 30 mg tablets	45 mg/day	45 mg/d
Rosiglitazone (Avandia) Rosiglitzaone and metformin (Avandamet)	4 mg/d in single dose or in divided doses twice daily	2 and 4 mg tablets 1, 2, and 4 mg tablets	8 mg/day	Increase to 8 mg/d in single or divided doses. With insulin: Do not exceed 4 mg/d. Decrease insulin dose by 10%–25% if hypoglycemia or FBG <100 mg/dL

previously treated only with diet. The current Standards of Medical Care in Diabetes of the American Diabetes Association (2013), however, recommend that these drugs be used as adjunctive therapy when BG targets are not achieved by lifestyle modifications and metformin. Doses of 15 to 30 mg/d of pioglitazone were associated with decreased FPG by 39 mg/dL for the 15 mg dose and 58 mg/dL for the 30 mg dose. Hb A1c was reduced by 0.9% for the 15 mg dose and 1.3% for the 30 mg dose. The initial dose of pioglitazone may be either 15 mg or 30 mg and the dose may be increased in 15 mg increments to a maximum dose of 45 mg/d (Table 21-20). Because effectiveness of therapy is best evaluated by Hb A1c, it is recommended that the adequate time period for evaluation of drug effectiveness is 3 months unless glycemic control deteriorates.

Rosiglitazone in doses of 4 mg/d reduced FPG by 25.4% and A1C by 0.27%. Rosiglitazone is usually initiated at 4 mg/d as a single dose. If single-dose therapy is not effective, the dose may be divided into twice-daily dosing or increased incrementally to a maximum dose of 8 mg/d. As with pioglitazone, evaluation of adequacy of response requires 12 weeks of therapy.

Combination Therapy With Oral Agents

When used as added therapy to management with a sulfonylurea, initiate pioglitazone with either the 15 or 30 mg dose. For rosiglitazone, initiate therapy at 4 mg/d in single or divided doses. Continue the current dose of the sulfonylurea. If the response in terms of glycemic control is inadequate, increase the dose of the TZD at 8 to 12 weeks, not to exceed the maximum mg/d.

The pharmacodynamics of TZDs is different from that of sulfonylureas so that the two drugs taken together potentiate each other's actions. Both fasting and postprandial BG levels of patients decrease. It is important to monitor BG levels closely when TZDs are added to the treatment regimen to avoid hypoglycemia.

Combination Therapy With Insulin

For patients stabilized on insulin, continue the insulin dose while initiating the TZD. For pioglitazone, initiate the dose at 15 to 30 mg once daily. For rosiglitazone, initiate the dose at 4 mg once daily and do not increase this dose. For both drugs, decrease the insulin dose by 10% to 25% if the patient reports hypoglycemia or if the FBG decreases to less than 100 mg/dL. Further adjustments are individualized based on the glucose-lowering response (see Table 21-20).

Monitoring

Serum transaminase (ALT) levels must be checked at the start of therapy. TZDs are not started if the pretreatment serum ALT level is more than 2.5 times the upper limit of normal (ULN). Once therapy is started, ALT is checked every 2 months for the first 12 months and periodically thereafter. If the ALT increases to more than 1.5 to 2 times the ULN, liver function tests are done every week until levels return to normal. The drug is discontinued if the ALT level is more than 3 times the ULN. The cost of this amount of monitoring must be considered in the total cost of therapy with these drugs.

If any patient develops symptoms suggesting hepatic dysfunction, the decision whether to continue the therapy with pioglitazone or rosiglitazone is guided by clinical judgment pending laboratory evaluation. If jaundice is observed, therapy is discontinued.

Due to contradictory evidence on the cardiotoxicity of rosiglitazone, patients taking this drug should have their cardiac function evaluated on a regular basis. This evaluation should look for indications of myocardial ischemia and heart failure. Response to TZD therapy is also assessed by regular monitoring of FPG and A1C every 3 to 6 months. During initial therapy and with each incremental increase, FPG is used to evaluate response.

Patient Education

Administration

Pioglitazone is to be taken once daily in the morning. If it is missed, it can be taken as soon as remembered. If the dose is missed for the entire day, the dose should not be doubled the next day. Explain to the patient that pioglitazone helps to control hyperglycemia, but it does not cure diabetes. The therapy is long-term.

Rosiglitazone may be taken once daily or twice daily in divided doses. The dosing schedule should not be changed without consultation with the provider. If the dose is missed for the entire day, the dose should not be doubled the next day.

Adverse Reactions

TZDs are generally well tolerated and adverse reactions are rare. The one adverse reaction of concern is hepatocellular injury. Advise the patient to report immediately any signs of hepatic dysfunction such as nausea, vomiting, abdominal pain, fatigue, anorexia, jaundice, or dark urine. Explain to the patient that hepatic function must be carefully monitored and that it is essential to keep follow-up appointments for laboratory work.

Hypoglycemia is not a risk with monotherapy but may occur when TZDs are given with another glucose-lowering drug. The usual treatment for hypoglycemia with sucrose, fructose, or starches will resolve the problem.

Cardiac risk has been discussed. Patients should report immediately any chest pain, shortness of breath, peripheral edema, or indications of impending stroke.

Female patients using oral contraceptives for birth control and premenopausal anovulatory patients should be informed about the possible need to increase the dose of oral contraceptive or choose an alternative birth control method.

MEGLITINIDES

The meglitinides are phenyalanine derivatives that are short-acting insulin secretagogues; they act by stimulation of insulin secretion to lower postprandial BG levels. They do not directly affect fasting BG levels or any of the other defects in metabolism seen in type 2 diabetes mellitus. They are most useful in patients whose primary glucose alteration is postprandial hyperglycemia and the amount of insulin released depends on existing BG levels. Current guidelines suggest these drugs be used as adjunct therapy. This section discusses the two drugs repaglinide (Prandin) and nateglinide (Starlix).

Pharmacodynamics

Meglitinides close ATP-dependent potassium channels in the beta cell membrane by binding at specific receptor sites. This potassium channel blockade depolarizes the beta cell and leads to an opening of calcium channels. The resultant influx of calcium increases the secretion of insulin. Because its time in the plasma is less than 2 hours, the effect is 4 hours with peak effect in 1 hour (Access Pharmacy, 2013). The ion channel mechanism is highly tissue selective, with low affinity for heart and skeletal muscle, which reduces the potential adverse effects on these tissues.

Pharmacokinetics

Absorption and Distribution

After oral administration, meglitinides are rapidly and completely absorbed from the GI tract. They are highly bound to albumin for distribution, primarily to beta cell membranes. Peak plasma levels occur within 1 hour. The presence of food in the gut does not affect AUC, but there is a delay in C_{max} and time to peak plasma concentration (T_{max}). Both drugs are taken 20 minutes before a meal.

Metabolism and Excretion

Both drugs are completely metabolized by oxidative biotransformation and direct conjugation with glucuronic acid. The CYP450 enzyme system, particularly 2C9 for nateglinide and 3A4 for repaglinide, is involved in their metabolism. The metabolites of nateglinide are less potent antihyperglycemic agents, but the metabolites of repaglinide do not contribute to any glucose-lowering effect.

This drug is rapidly eliminated from the plasma, with a half-life of 1 to 1.5 hours. Within 96 hours after administration of repaglinide and 6 hours of nateglinide, the drugs and their metabolites are recovered in the feces and in the urine. Table 21-11 depicts the pharmacokinetics of these drugs.

Pharmacotherapeutics

Precautions and Contraindications

These drugs should be used cautiously with patients who have hepatic impairment, and longer intervals between dosage adjustments should be used. Caution should be used in patients with severe renal impairment and adrenal/pituitary impairment because these drugs may exert more glucose-lowering effects.

Repaglinide and nateglinide are Pregnancy Category C. Nonteratogenic skeletal deformities occurred in test animals. There are no adequate and well-controlled trials in pregnant women. Meglitinides should not be used during pregnancy.

Both drugs are excreted in the breast milk of test animals. It is not known if they are excreted in human breast milk. Because the potential exists for hypoglycemia in nursing infants, the drugs should not be used with lactating women. No studies have been done to test the safety and efficacy of these drugs in children.

Adverse Drug Reactions

The risk for hypoglycemia with meglitinides is a concern, so appropriate patient selection should be used when prescribing. Patients with hepatic insufficiency, older adults, and debilitated and malnourished patients are at higher risk for hypoglycemia. The frequency of hypoglycemia is also greater for patients who have not been previously treated with oral hypoglycemic agents or whose A1C is less than 8%. Careful timing of administration with regard to meals lessens the likelihood of this adverse reaction. The risk for weight gain is similar to that of the sulfonylureas.

Drug Interactions

Because the CYP450 3A4 enzyme system is involved in the metabolism of repaglinide and both 2C9 (70%) and 3A4 (30%) in the metabolism of nateglinide, drugs that induce these isoezymes (e.g., rifampin, barbiturates, carbamazepine) may increase meglitinide metabolism (Table 21-21). These

Table 21–21 ⠿ Drug Interactions With Meglitinides and Repaglinide

Interacting Drug	Possible Effect	Implications
Drugs that induce CYP450 3A4	Increases metabolism and decreases effect of repaglinide and nateglinide	Closely monitor blood glucose levels and patient response
Drugs that induce CYP450 2C9	Increases metabolism and decreases the effect of nateglinide	Closely monitor blood glucose levels and patient response
Ketoconazole, miconazole, and potentially other "azoles"	Inhibits meglitinide metabolism and may increase risk for hypoglycemia	Closely monitor blood glucose levels and patient response Choose a different antifungal
Erythromycin and potentially other macrolides	Inhibits meglitinide metabolism and may increase risk for hypoglycemia	Closely monitor blood glucose levels and patient response Choose a different class of antimicrobial
Any drug that increases or decreases BG levels	May alter glycemic effects of meglitinide and increases risk for lack of control or hypoglycemia	Closely monitor blood glucose levels and patient response

isoezymes are among the most used widely by drugs for metabolism; other drug reactions may be found as these drugs are used.

Antifungal agents such as ketoconazole and miconazole and antimicrobial agents such as erythromycin inhibit repaglinide metabolism and may increase the risk for hypoglycemia by raising blood levels of the drug. Any drug that alters BG levels has the potential to alter the glycemic control effects of meglitinides. Meglitinides can potentiate the action of drugs that are highly protein bound by competing for their binding sites (e.g., NSAIDs, salicylates, sulfonamides, warfarin, beta-adrenergic blockers, and monoamine oxidase inhibitors). Table 21-21 shows drug interactions for the meglitinides.

Meglitinides should not be used in place of metformin monotherapy or if other insulin-stimulating drugs (sulfonylureas) have been used unsuccessfully. Using concurrently with sulfonylureas has no additional benefit and should not be prescribed (Access Pharmacy, 2013).

Clinical Use and Dosing

Monotherapy

For nateglinide, the initial and maintenance dose is 120 mg 3 times/day, 1 to 30 minutes before each meal; if the patient is near target A1C (less than 7%), dosing may be started at 60 mg 3 times daily. For repaglinide, if A1C is less than 8% or not previously treated, the dose is 0.5 mg before each meal; if the A1C is greater than 8% or the patient is being switched from another oral agent, the initial dose is 1 to 2 mg 3 times/d (Access Pharmacy, 2013).

Combination Therapy

Meglitinides may be given in conjunction with metformin or TZDs. Meglitinides are not currently on the ADA treatment algorithm for type 2 diabetes, the primary reason being more frequent dosing and less glucose-lowering effectiveness than other drugs available (Inzucchi et al, 2012). When adding meglitinides to either metformin or TZD therapy, careful monitoring and dosing is necessary to prevent hypoglycemic episodes.

For Both Uses

Dosage changes are based on FPG and Hb A1c levels. With repaglinide, the preprandial dose should be doubled, up to 4 mg, until satisfactory response is achieved. The initial dose and the maintenance dose are the same for nateglinide. Allow at least 1 week to assess patient response before adjusting a dose. The maximum daily dose is 16 mg for repaglinide and 720 mg for nateglinide. No dosage adjustments are required based on age, race, or gender. Table 21-22 shows the dosage schedules for these drugs.

Monitoring

The monitoring required with the meglitinides is periodic monitoring of FPG and Hb A1c every 3 months. These values should be determined prior to initiation of therapy to determine baseline values and contribute to the decision about initial dose. Thereafter, they are used to monitor patient response.

Patient Education

Administration

Doses are always administered 0 to 30 minutes prior to each meal and should be omitted if meals are not eaten. If extra meals are eaten, extra doses should also be taken. Timing of the drug in relation to food is critical.

Adverse Reactions

The adverse effect associated with the meglitinides is hypoglycemia. Patients should be taught how to prevent, recognize, and treat hypoglycemia, as discussed earlier in the Patient Teaching sections on insulin and oral hypoglycemics.

Table 21–22 ⚕ Dosage Schedule: Meglitinides

Drug	Initial Dose	Dosage Form	Maximum Dose	Maintenance Dose
Nateglinide (Starlix)	60–120 mg taken 20–30 min before each meal	60 mg 120 mg tablets	720 mg/day	Same as initial dose.
Repaglinide (Prandin)	0.5–2 mg taken 30 min or less before each meal If A1c less than 8%, dose is 0.5 mg If A1c is 8% or more, dose is 1–2 mg	0.5, 1, and 2 mg tablets	16 mg/d	
Repaglinide and Metformin (Prandimet)	**On metformin alone:** 1 mg repaglinide/500 metformin twice daily with meals **On repaglinide:** Start with 500 mg metformin dose and titrate as GI side effects are tolerated.	1 mg/500 mg and 2 mg/500 mg tablets		Double preprandial dose up to 4 mg. Dose increases at 1 wk intervals. 10 mg repaglinide/2,500 metformin 2–3 times daily before meals. No more than 4 mg repaglinide/1,000 metformin per meal.

DIPEPTIDYL PEPTIDASE-4 INHIBITORS

The dipeptidyl peptidasase-4 inhibitors (DPP-4) are also known as gliptins. There are currently four approved for use in the United States: sitagliptin, saxagliptin, linagliptin, and alogliptin. Vildagliptin is not yet approved in the United States but is being used in other countries. All except linagliptin require considerations for renal dysfunction.

Newer insights into the pathogenesis of type 2 diabetes have created a bigger role for the incretin hormones. The action of gliptins is different from that of other antihyperglycemic agents because gliptins act on the incretin hormone system to have an indirect effect on increasing insulin production. Although the improvement in glycemic control is moderate and no more than with metformin, gliptins are well tolerated, have a low risk for hypoglycemia, are weight neutral, and can be given orally. These effects contrast with the common adverse effects of existing antidiabetic agents. Although they have been approved for monotherapy, gliptins are best used as add-on therapy in combination with metformin as second-line therapy. Long-term impact on CV and DM outcomes is yet to be determined.

Pharmacodynamics

Glucagon-like peptide (GLP-1) is an incretin hormone derived from the gut that stimulates glucose-dependent insulin secretion, enhances insulin gene transcription and insulin biosynthesis, enhances cellular transformation from pancreatic ductal tissues to beta cell tissue, increases beta cell mass by cellular neogenesis and proliferation, inhibits beta cell apoptosis, suppresses glucagon secretion, inhibits gastric emptying, and reduces appetite and food intake (Drucker & Nauck, 2006; Pande, 2009). The actions of this peptide address several defects found in type 2 diabetes. DM GLP-1 receptors have been found in the stomach, intestine, central nervous system, kidney, heart, and lungs (Pande, 2009) and are significantly reduced in type 2 diabetes. DPP-4 is a naturally occurring enzyme that inactivates GLP-1. The DPP-4 inhibitor drug class does not directly change this reduction in GLP-1 production but extends the action of any GLP-1 still present in the system by interfering with its rate of breakdown. This effect is akin to doubling the endogenous GLP-1 available in the system.

The DPP-4 inhibitors have demonstrated efficacy in reducing pre- and postprandial glucose levels, reducing A1C levels and promoting weight loss. Although gliptins enhance the activity of any residual GLP-1, they also reduce postprandial glucose concentration by stimulating insulin secretion and suppressing glucagon secretion but have no direct effect on insulin action to increase glucose utilization and so do not address cellular insulin resistance Though not as strong in their therapeutic impact on BG and Hb A1c reduction as the GLP-1 agonist group, the fact they are oral drugs is a strong factor for patients who do not wish to use injectable medications.

Pharmacokinetics

Absorption and Distribution

After oral administration, these drugs are rapidly absorbed from the GI tract. They can be taken with or without food. The volume of distribution of sitagliptin is approximately 198 L. Older adults have a greater volume of distribution of saxagliptin than do younger patients.

Metabolism and Excretion

DPP 4s are metabolized primarily in the small intestine and they are excreted through the urine unchanged. Decreased renal function results in reduced renal clearance, and doses should be adjusted accordingly. Table 21-11 shows the pharmacokinetics of these drugs.

Pharmacotherapeutics

Precautions and Contraindications

Because of their high dependence on the renal system for elimination, these drugs should be used cautiously with those with impaired renal function. A risk for toxicity exists for patients with end-stage renal disease and for those with moderate to severe renal impairment. Dosage adjustments for renal impairment are needed but less so for linagliptin. Older adults are more likely to have renal impairment; therefore kidney function should be considered for initial dosing and periodically monitored when these drugs are used in this population. Given that, for patients without severe renal impairment, the typical progression of microalbuinuria to proteinuria in DM appears to reverse after 2 years of saxagliptin use (Udell et al, 2014). This is probably a class effect. No other DM medication has demonstrated this outcome. The same secondary analysis of the SAVOR-TIMI 53 study also indicated saxagliptin did not increase CV risk in renal patients.

Gliptins are Pregnancy Category B; however, no well-controlled trials have been performed in humans related to pregnancy. These are relatively new drugs without long-term exposure to the pregnant population with diabetes. It is unknown if gliptins pass into breast milk and infant risk has not been determined. Caution should be used when these drugs are given to nursing mothers.

The safety and efficacy in children (under 18 years of age) have not been established. These drugs are not used in type 1 diabetes.

Adverse Drug Reactions

DPP-4 medications are typically well tolerated; much better tolerated than the GLP-1 class of medications. The most common adverse effects are edema (4%), headache (7%), and urinary tract infections (7%). Hypoglycemia can occur when used in combination with insulin secretagogues (15%) (Access Pharmacy, 2013). Cases of acute pancreatitis have been reported with the DPP-4 inhibitors. Use caution if the patient has a history of pancreatitis or is at greater risk. Reports of pancreatic metaplasia are being investigated because longitudinal animal models are reporting pancreatic cellular changes even at exposures only double that for humans. Monitoring for pancreatic impact is part of the required post-marking studies currently underway. Saxagliptim has been linked to an increase in bone fractures, but there is no firm evidence that this is a drug or class effect.

Drug Interactions

Coadministration of gliptins with ACE inhibitors has been associated with increased risk of angioedema. Digoxin has an increase in concentration when coadministered with sitagliptin. Gliptins have limited hepatic metabolism with CYP 3A4 and CYP 2C8. Until there is more long-term experience with these drugs, other drugs that use these same isoenzyme systems should be monitored for potential interactions. Table 21-23 shows the drug interactions with these drugs.

Clinical Use and Dosing

Gliptins are indicated as monotherapy and in combination with or added to other antihyperglycemic drugs for the treatment of patients with type 2 diabetes who cannot achieve adequate BG control with diet, exercise, weight control, metformin, and other drugs. They are especially useful for obese patients because they are not associated with weight gain. The current guidelines typically use these drugs as adjunctive therapy. They are preferred over GLP-1 medications in those who are injection averse.

Monotherapy

All of the gliptins have been approved for monotherapy. Sitagliptin is administered in a once-daily dose of 100 mg. Saxagliptin is administered once daily with dose ranges between 2.5 and 5 mg. Linagliptin dosage is 5 mg once daily. Dosages for both sitaglipitn and saxagliptin are reduced for decreased creatinine clearance (Access Pharmacy, 2013), but reductions are not necessary for linagliptin (Table 21-24).

Combination Therapy

All of the gliptins have been approved for use in combination with other antihyperglycemic agents. The current treatment algorithm recommends using DPP-4s in two-drug combinations with metformin or three-drug combinations with sulfonylureas, TZDs, or insulin. Saxagliptin, alogliptin, and sitagliptin come in combination formulations with metformin.

TZD combinations are associated with more adverse effects, such as weight gain and potential increased cardiovascular risk. The newest gliptin, alogliptin, comes in a combination formulation with pigliozone (Osani), which was

Table 21–23 ⚏ Drug Interactions With Dipeptidyl Peptidase-4 Inhibitors (Gliptins)

Drug	Interacting Drug	Possible Outcomes	Implications
Sitagliptin	Digoxin	AUC of digoxin increased 11%	Monitor patients receiving digoxin
Alogliptin/pioglitazone	Strong CYP2C8 inhibitors (i.e., Gemfibrozil)	Significantly increases AUC and half-life of pioglitazone	Maximum recommended dose of pioglitazone is 15 mg daily if used in combination with gemfibrozil or other strong CYP2C8 inhibitors
Linagliptin	Inducers of CYP3A4 or P-gp (e.g., rifampin)	Decreases linagliptin concentrations	For patients requiring use of such drugs, an alternative is strongly recommended
Saxtagliptin	CYP3A4/5 inhibitors Diltiazem Ketoconazole	Increases saxtagliptin peak concentration by 63%; AUC increases by 2-fold	Monitor

Table 21–24 ⚘ Dosage Schedule for Dipeptidyl Peptidase-4 Inhibitors (Gliptins)

Drug	Initial Dose	Dosage Form	Maintenance Dose	Maximum Dose
Sitagliptin	100 mg once daily	Tablets: 25, 50, 100 mg	100 mg once daily	200 mg total daily dose
Sitagliptin/ metformin (Janumet) (B) (Janumet XR)	**Inadequately controlled on metformin alone:** 100 mg/day sitagliptin plus current dose of metformin **Inadequately controlled on sitagliptin alone:** 1,000 mg/day metformin PO plus 100 mg/day PO sitagliptin	Tablets: 500 mg/50 mg 1,000 mg/50 mg Tablets, extended-release: 500 mg/50 mg 1,000 mg/50 mg 1,000 mg/100 mg		Not to exceed 2,000 mg metformin and 100 mg sitagliptin

Continued

Table 21–24 ⊗ **Dosage Schedule for Dipeptidyl Peptidase-4 Inhibitors (Gliptins)—cont'd**

Drug	Initial Dose	Dosage Form	Maintenance Dose	Maximum Dose
Alogliptin (G) Nesina (B)	25 mg daily **Renal impairment:** Moderate (CrCl ≥30 to <60 mL/min): 12.5 mg daily Severe (CrCl ≥15 to <30 mL/min) or ESRD (CrCl <15 mL/min) or requiring hemodialysis: 6.25 mg daily	12.5, 25, or 6.25 mg tablets		25 mg daily
Alogliptin/ pioglitazone (Oseni) (B)	**Adjunct to diet/exercise, metformin monotherapy:** 25/15 or 25/30 mg once daily **Already on pioglitazone:** 25 mg/ 15 mg, 25 mg/30 mg, or 25 mg/ 45 mg once daily **CHF:** 25/15 mg once daily	Tablets: 12.5 mg/15 mg 12.5 mg/30 mg 12.5 mg/45 mg 25 mg/15 mg 25 mg/30 mg 25 mg/45 mg		25/45 mg once daily based on response
Alogliptin/ metformin (Kazano) (B)	Starting dose based on current regimen. Take twice daily with food and gradually titrate to decrease GI side effects.	Tablets: 12.5/500 mg, 12.5/1,000 mg		25/2,000 mg daily
Linagliptin (G) Tradjenta (B)	5 mg daily; lower dose of insulin or secretagogues may be needed when used in combination	5 mg tablets	5 mg daily	5 mg daily
Linagliptin/ metformin Jentadueto (B)	**Not currently taking metformin:** 2.5 mg/500 mg twice daily **Already taking metformin:** Base dose on current metformin dose twice daily	Tablets: 2.5/500 mg, 2.5/850 mg 2.5/1,000 mg		2.5/1,000 mg twice daily
Saxaglitpin (G) Onglyza (B)	2.5–5 mg once daily **CrCl <50 mL/min:** 2.5 mg daily	2.5, 5 mg tablets	2.5–5 mg once daily	5 mg once daily

shown in four clinical trials involving more than 1,500 patients to produce additional A1C reductions of 0.4 to 0.6 percentage points over pioglitazone monotherapy and 0.4 to 0.9 percentage points over alogliptin alone. Because of the increased risk of heart failure, it has a Black-Box Warning. The FDA is also requiring pharmacovigilance related to liver abnormalities, pancreatitis, and allergic reactions (FDA, 2013). If a gliptin is used in combination with a sulfonylurea or insulin, the dose of insulin or secretagogue should be lowered to reduce the risk of hypoglycemia. The use of basal insulin affects fasting BG; the incretin agents improve both fasting sugars and postprandial readings.

Adding a DPP-4 to insulin therapy typically requires adjustment of the insulin dose. If possible, start the DPP-4 agent and then add the insulin once glycemic impact is known. The addition of a DPP-4 can stunt the additional body weight associated with insulin.

Rational Drug Selection

Age

Gliptins have been studied in the elderly population. Despite the concerns raised above about renal function, gliptins are effective and well-tolerated treatment options in elderly patients with type 2 diabetes. They demonstrate improvement in glycemic control similar to that of metformin, for example, with similar improvements in glycemic control and better GI tolerability (Schweizer, Dejager, & Bosi, 2009). Dosage adjustments may be made as needed for renal function.

Weight/Obesity

In two separate studies comparing a gliptin with a TZD, body weight decreased for the patients on the gliptin and increased for patients on the TZD alone (Blonde et al, 2009; Bolli, Dotta, Colin, Minic, & Goodman, 2009). Both gliptins and metformin are weight neutral, but have also been associated with weight loss! These drugs are appropriate for overweight patients with diabetes.

Cost

As is usually true for new classes of drugs that have required significant research and development costs, the gliptins are expensive. To date, there is not much variability among the drugs in terms of cost. Because they are expensive, insurance coverage might be an economic barricade. A whole-picture evaluation of treatment costs over time demonstrates that early and aggressive interventions reduce onset and intensity of complications. Reduction of such events is actually cost-effective; therefore, the argument against use of incretin therapy due to cost is starting to change.

Monitoring

Before initiating therapy and at least annually thereafter, assess renal function. Assessment is by serum creatinine and CCr initially and then by serum creatinine annually. Dosage adjustments are required based on creatinine clearance. For patients with increased risk of developing altered renal function, the assessment should be made more often.

Response to gliptin therapy is assessed by daily to weekly monitoring of FPG and postprandial BG and by monitoring Hb A1c every 3 months or monitoring fructosamine every 2 months. During initial therapy and with each incremental increase, FPG is used to evaluate response. After the patient is stabilized on a specific dose, monitoring with FPG and Hb A1c levels every 6 months is sufficient.

Patient Education

Administration

All gliptins are taken once daily in the morning. If the dose is missed, it should be taken as soon as remembered. If the dose is missed for the entire day, it should not be doubled the next day. It would be prudent to SMBG in the case of missed doses.

Adverse Reactions

Gliptins are generally well tolerated and adverse reactions occur in only a small percentage of those taking the drugs. Hypoglycemia is not anticipated with monotherapy but may occur when these drugs are combined with another glucose-lowering agent. The usual treatment for hypoglycemia is recommended. In clinical trials of alogliptin, pancreatitis (2%) and hypersensitivity (6%) were reported.

SELECTIVE SODIUM GLUCOSE CO-TRANSPORTER 2 (SGLT-2) INHIBITORS

Canagliflozin (Invokana), dapglifoxin (Farxiga), and empagliflozin (Jardiance) are novel inhibitors of renal SGLT-2, block the reabsorption of glucose in the kidneys, and promote excretion of excess glucose in the urine. Canagliflozin, the first drug in this class, was approved by the FDA in 2013, with requirements to continue five post-marketing studies, which include a cardiovascular outcomes study, and a pediatric safety and efficacy study which includes inquiry into any impact on renal and bone maturation. The other drugs in the class have the same requirements. These drugs are approved for use as monotherapy or in combination with other antihyperglycemic agents for adults with type 2 diabetes. They are not recommended for treatment of type 1 diabetes or DKA (FDA, 2013).

Pharmacodynamics

Inhibition of SGLT-2 lowers reabsorption of plasma glucose concentration in the kidneys, which results in increased urinary glucose excretion and reduction of plasma glucose in type 2 diabetes (Medscape Reference, 2013). SGLT-2 works in the proximal tubule to absorb about 90% of the glucose in the ultrafiltrate. This is comparable to around 200 to 250 calories a day. If blood glucose is high, then more is excreted in the urine. There is an osmotic fluid loss which can lead to intravascular volume depletion.

In a 52 week, phase III trial of patients with type 2 diabetes who were not controlled with metformin and sulfonylurea, adding canagliflozin improved glycemic control better than adding sitagliptin. Mean Hb A1c levels dropped by 1.03% with canagliflozin versus 0.66% with sitagliptin. Canagliflozin also resulted in weight loss and reductions in FPG and BP (Schernthaner et al, 2013). Similar outcomes were demonstrated with studies for efficacy of empagliflozin and dapagliflozin across gender, age, duration of disease, and baseline BMI average. Empaglifozin also inhibits other SGLT receptors; the impact on outcomes and comparison to other drugs in the class is unknown. This new class of drugs adds another option for therapy in type 2 diabetes for selected patients, although there are significant side effects for selected populations.

Pharmacokinetics

Absorption and Distribution

Canagliflozin binds 99% primarily to albumin and has a peak plasma time of 1 to 2 hours. Dapagliflozin is 91% protein bound and empaglifozin is 86.2% bound. Both peak within 1.5–2 hours. Empagliflozin has some decrease in circulation after a fatty meal, but this is considered not clinically significant.

Metabolism and Excretion

The major metabolic elimination pathway is O-glucuronidation for these drugs. The half-life of canagliflozin for the 100 mg dose is 10.6 hours and for a 300 mg dose it is 13.1 hours. Excretion is through feces as cangliflozin (41.5%), and 33% is excreted in urine, mainly as O-glucuronide metabolites. Dapagliflozin is similarly processed with 75% renally excreted and 21% in the feces. The half-life is 12.9 hours. Empagliflozin has a half-life of 10 to 19 hours. It is excreted 41% in the urine and 55% in the feces. None of the medications require dose adjustment with mild to moderate hepatic disease. (Child-Pugh class A or B). The drug class has not been studied extensively with advanced liver issues (Child-Pugh class C). Empagliflozin has data on Child-Pugh class C which demonstrates an increasing retention of medication in the system. Appropriate precautions extend to the whole drug class. See Table 21-11 for drug class pharmacokinetic information.

Pharmacotherapeutics

Precautions and Contraindications

SGLT-2 inhibitors are contraindicated in patients with severe renal impairment (eGFR less than 30 mL/min/1.73 m²), end-stage renal disease, or who are on dialysis. Modification of the dose is suggested when eGFR is less than 45mL/min/1.73.

Severe hypersensitivity reactions were reported in clinical trials, specifically in the form of generalized urticaria. These drugs are contraindicated in the treatment of DKA or type 1 diabetes.

SGLT-2 inhibitors can cause intravascular volume depletion and symptomatic hypotension. Urine volume increases about 300 mL on day one, but stabilizes to around 135 mL extra per day after day five. There is no change in electrolyte balance in normally functioning kidneys. Precaution should be used when the eGFR is less than 60 mL/min/1.73 m^2, in older adults, in those who have low systolic BP, or in those who are on diuretics or drugs that interfere with the renin-angiotensin-aldosterone system (RAS) such as ACE inhibitors and ARBs. Volume status should be assessed and monitored prior to and during treatment with these drugs, particularly if patients have one or more of these issues (Janssen Pharmaceuticals, 2013). This drug class increases serum creatinine and decreases eGFR in longer-term DM. Patients with hypovolemia are more susceptible to renal function impairment. Their renal function should be monitored frequently. Hyperkalemia can also occur in patients with moderate renal impairment who take potassium-sparing diuretics or drugs that alter RAS are more prone to hyperkalemia. Potassium should be monitored frequently after initiating treatment (Janssen Pharmaceuticals, 2013). If renal issues do not exist, there is no suggested decrease in dosing for elders, though the risk of falls related to hypovolemia should be considered.

Interestingly, the impact of SGLT-2 medications in early diagnosis DM patients may actually induce a form of renal protection (Cherney, et al, 2014). They cause a decrease in urine protein loss, and appear to reduce the damaging hyperfiltration associated with the disease. The "renal protective" effects of the ACE and ARB class actually drops over time; about 20% of patients still progress to renal disease due to hyperfiltration damage. The SGLT2 drugs do not increase potassium like the RAS active medications. More research is needed to determine if this drug class has a true renal protective role.

There is an increased risk of hypoglycemia when SGLT-2 medications are used with insulin and secretagogues; insulin or secretagogue doses should be lowered to avoid hypoglycemia (Medscape Reference, 2013). There is no impact on natural insulin secretion. The reduction of serum glucose by renal reabsorption blockade may trigger a need to adjust other medications.

SGLT-2 medications are Pregnancy Category C. Rat studies showed these medications may affect renal development and maturation in utero. Appropriate alternative therapies should be considered for pregnant women, especially during the second and third trimesters. These medications should be used during pregnancy only if the potential benefit justifies the potential risk to the fetus. It is unknown whether the drug can be excreted through human breast milk; therefore, breastfeeding women should not take them.

Adverse Drug Reactions

Genital fungal infections, urinary tract infections, and increased urination are the most commonly reported drug reactions. This is most likely linked to the 50 to 60 g of glucose now found in the urine. The most frequently reported side effect (greater than 10%) is female genital mycotic infections or male genital mycotic infections (4%). A dose-related increase in LDL-C can also occur. Volume depletion has been reported in adults older than 75 years (4.9% to 8.7%), eGFR less than 60/mL/min/1.73 m^3 (4.7% to 8.1%), and in individuals using loop diuretics (3.2% to 8.8%) (MedScape Reference, 2013).

There are reports of bladder cancer, but too few cases for the FDA to take action. The provider must balance the small risk of cancer with the demonstrated positive impact on Hb A1c. Do not prescribe if there is a history of bladder cancer or high risk for cancer as there are other effective therapeutic choices available.

There is an increase in LDL cholesterol (2.5%) and a tendency toward intravascular volume contraction related to the osmotic diuretic impact of glucose in the urine; therefore, in patients with higher CV or DVT risk may not be the best choice of medication. There have been no studies on macrovascular risk changes in this class of drugs.

Drug Interactions

Canagliflozin should not be taken with pimizide. When digoxin was given with 300 mg of canagliflozin, there was an increase in the area AUC and C$_{max}$ of digoxin. Monitor patients who are taking digoxin and canagliflozin concomitantly. Concurrent use with canagliflozin can increase the effect of ACE and ARB medications, aliskiren, aripiprazole, dofetilide, duloxetine, eplerenone, hypoglycemic agents, lomitapide, and potassium-sparing diuretics. The impact of canagliflozin may be reduced by systemic and inhaled steroids, danazol, fosphenytoin, loop and thiazide diurectics, luteinizing hormone releasing analogs, phenobarbital, phenytoin, rifampin, ritonavir, and somatropin. It may build up to toxic levels when given with androgens, barbiturates, low-molecular weight heparin, MAO inhibitors, hypoglycemic agents, hypotensive agents of lopitapide, pimozide, and potassium-sparing diuretics. Dapagliflozin is decreased in effectiveness when mixed with both systemic and inhaled steroids, danazol, loop and thiazide diuretics somatropin, and luteinizing hormone–releasing analogs. It may build up to toxic levels when given with androgens, barbiturates, MAO inhibitors, pegvisomant, salicylates, and SSRIs. Dapagliflozin can increase the effect of duloxetine, hypotensive agents, and hypoglycemic agents. Empagliflozin package inserts put an emphasis on interactions with diuretics and hypoglycemic agents (see Table 21-25 for interactions).

Canagliflozin AUC was decreased by 51% when coadministered with rifampin, a nonselective inducer of several UGT enzymes. If coadministering canagliflozin with UGT enzyme inducers (e.g., rifampin, phenytoin, phenobarbital, ritonavir), consider increasing the dose to 300 mg/d in patients tolerating 100 mg/d, who have eGFR greater than or equal to 60 mL/

Table 21–25 ▦ **Drug Interactions With SGLT-2 Drugs**

Drug	Interacting Drug	Possible Outcomes	Implications
Canagliflozin Dapapagliflozin and empagliflozin	UGT enzyme inducers (Rifampin, phenytoin, phenobarbitol, ritonavir)	Decreased AUC Decreased efficacy	If UGT enzyme inducers and canagliflozin must be coadministered, consider increasing the dose if patients are currently tolerating and have an eGFR greater than 60 mL/min/1.73 m². Consider other antihyperglycemic therapy in patients with an eGFR of 45 to less than 60 mL/min/1.73 m² receiving concurrent therapy with a UGT inducer.
	Insulin and insulin secretogogues and any other other medication that causes hypoglycemia	Hypoglycemia increased when coadministered with SGLT-2 meds	Decrease dose of insulin or insulin secretogogue or the other medications, but maintain SGLT-2 unless at the higher dose.
	Antihypertensives	Intensified lowering of BP	Check specific interactions of larger impact: cangliflozin and ACE/ARB, aliskiren, lomitapide, and potassium-sparing diuretics, eplerenone.
Cangagliflozin and dapagliflozin	Systemic and inhaled steroids, danazol, loop and thiazide diuretics, leutinizing hormone-releasing analogues, somatropin	Effect of SGLT-2 medication is reduced	Try another medication group or consider increasing dose.
	Androgens, barbiturate, MAO Inhibitors	SGLT-2 medications are increased and may become toxic	Consider different drug classes or reduce dose of SGLT meds.
	Duloxetine	Effect of duloxetine is intensified	Reduce dose of duloxetine
Canagliflozin	Digoxin	Increased AUC 20% and mean peak drug concentration (C_{max}) of digoxin 36% when coadministered with Invokana 300 mg	Patients taking concomitant digoxin should be monitored appropriately
	Aripiprazole, dofetildide, lopitapide	Increase the effect of these meds	Coordinated possible dose reductions in these meds
	Low-molecular weight heparin, lopitapide, pimozide, and potassium-sparing diuretics	SGLT effect is increased	Consider not mixing or decreasing dose of SGLT
Dapagliflozin	Pegvisomat, salicylates, and SSRIs	SGLT effects increased to potential toxic level	Consider not mixing or decrdeasing dose of SGLT.

min/1.73 m² and require additional glycemic control. The other drugs are also UGT-mediated and have similar concerns. Decisions to increase any drug dosing should be coordinated with a specialist (Jannsen Pharmaceuticals, 2013).

Clinical Use and Dosing

Type 2 Diabetes

SGLT-2 drugs are indicated as an adjunct to diet and exercise in the treatment of adults with type 2 diabetes. Because the drugs are new on the market, they are just being included in the current standards of care. They can decrease Hb A1c by 1% and contribute to a 2–4 pound weight loss. Initial treatment with canagliflozin is initiated at 100 mg/d before the first

meal is eaten. Timing of food does not appear to clinically impact the dosing of the other SGLT-2 medications. If patients require additional glyccemic control and are tolerating the initial doses, they can be increased if eGFR levels are adequate. Volume depletion should be corrected before initiating therapy with any SGLT-2 inhibitor (Table 21-26). Dapagliflozin is started at 5 mg and adjusted up to 10 mg depending on tolerance and efficacy. Empagliflozin starting dose is 10 mg, advancing to 25 mg based on tolerability and efficacy.

Monitoring

As stated previously, select individuals may need monitoring above what is indicated for management of diabetes, including

Table 21–26 ⊗ **Dosing Schedule for SGLT2 Drugs**

Drug	Initial Dose	Dosage Form	Maintenance Dose	Maximum Dose
Cangaflozin(B)	100 mg once daily taken before the first meal of the day. Dose should be limited to 100 mg once daily in patients who have an eGFR of 45–60 mL/min/ 1.73 m². Patients with eGFR < 45 mL/min/ 1.73 m² should not take canagliflozin.	100 and 300 mg tablets		300 mg once daily (eGFR of ≥60 mL/ min/1.73 m²)
Dapagiltozin (Farixga) (B)	5 mg without regard to meals	5 and 10 mg tablets	Based on tolerability and efficacy	10 mg daily
Empagliflozin (Jardiance) (B)	Without regard to meals	10 and 25 mg tablets	See above	25 mg daily

renal function and electrolytes plus screening for genital mycotic infections. Urine dip sticks are expected to show positive for glucose, as this is an intended consequence of the medication. There an anticipated increase in hematocrit. Increases in both LDL lipids and serum inorganic phosphorus is possible.

Patient Education

Administration

Canagliflozin (Invokana) should be taken at the same time each day before the first meal; dapaglifloxin and empagliflozin can be taken without regard to meals. If a dose is missed of any drug in the class, it should be taken as soon as it is remembered, but if it is almost time for the next dose, the missed dose should be skipped and taken at the next regularly scheduled time. SMBG should be performed to assess if treatment goals are being met.

Adverse Reactions

Patients should be taught the signs and symptoms of dehydration (dizziness, hypotension, weakness) and genital yeast infections for both men and women (itching, redness/swelling of the genitals, thick white discharge). Most are minor and easily treated, but will recur.

Allergic reactions include rash, hives, and swelling of the face, lips, tongue, and throat that may cause difficulty in breathing or swallowing. The medication should be discontinued if this occurs. Emergency intervention may be required.

Hypoglycemia should be expected if other antihyperglycemics are being taken. The patient should be taught prevention, recognition of the signs and symptoms, and treatment using fast-acting CHO. Adjustment of concurrent medication dosages should be anticipated at the onset of SGLT-2 inhibitor introduction.

AMYLIN AGONISTS

Amylin agonists are a synthetic analogue of the beta cell hormone amylin for use as adjunct therapy in both types 1 and type 2 diabetes to help reduce blood glucose after eating. In type 1 diabetes, pramlintide is used for patients who use mealtime insulin therapy and have failed to achieve their glycemic target despite optimal insulin therapy. In type 2 diabetes, pramlintide is used for patients who use mealtime insulin therapy, with or without a concurrent sulfonylurea or metformin, and still have not achieved their glycemic target. Like the GLP-1 agonists, pramlintide lowers glucose by acting on glucagon secretion, slowing gastric emptying, and suppressing the appetite (Access Pharmacy, 2013). To date, there is only one drug in this class, pramlintide (Symlin). Currently, it is approved for use in the United States only as second-line therapy for those using insulin.

Pharmacodynamics

Amylin is co-located with insulin in secretory granules and co-secreted with insulin by pancreatic beta cells in response to food intake. Both amylin and insulin show similar fasting and postprandial patterns in healthy individuals. Amylin affects the rate of postprandial glucose by slowing gastric emptying; by suppressing glucagon secretion, which leads to decreased endogenous glucose output by the liver; and by centrally mediated modulation of appetite. Patients with type 1 and type 2 diabetes have dysfunctional beta cells, resulting in reduced secretion of both insulin and amylin in response to food.

Pramlintide acts as an amylin mimetic to modulate gastric emptying, prevent postprandial risk in plasma glucagons, and improve satiety, leading to decreased caloric intake and potential weight loss. In clinical studies, Hb A1c has decreased 0.5% to 0.7% and weight loss associated with this drug is about 1 to 1.5 kg over 6 months.

Pharmacokinetics

Absorption and Distribution

Pramlintide is slowly absorbed from injection sites in the abdomen or thigh. Injection into the arm results in higher exposure to the drug with greater variability compared with injection into the abdomen or thigh. The drug does not bind extensively to plasma cells or albumin, so its pharmacokinetics is relatively insensitive to changes in binding sites.

Metabolism and Excretion

Pramlintide is metabolized primarily by the kidneys, and its primary metabolite (2-37 praline) has a similar half-life and is biologically active. AUC values are relatively constant with repeat dosing, indicating lack of bioaccumulation. Table 21-11 shows the pharmacokinetics of this drug.

Pharmacotherapeutics

Precautions and Contraindications

Confirmed diagnosis of gastroparesis or the required use of drugs to stimulate GI motility is contraindicated in using this drug. It should not be used in patients with a history of nausea (Access Pharmacy, 2013).

Although pramlintide alone does not cause hypoglycemia, it is coadministered with insulin, which increases the risk for hypoglycemia. Pramlintide should not be used in patients who have recurrent episodes of severe hypoglycemia or hypoglycemic unawareness. The insulin dose should be reduced by 50% to avoid hypoglycemia (Access Pharmacy, 2013).

Do not use in patients with poor compliance with insulin regimen and/or blood glucose monitoring or with recurrent episodes of hypoglycemia. A detailed history of glucose control, including Hb A1c, incidence of hypoglycemia, glucose monitoring, medication compliance, and baseline body weight should be obtained before initiating therapy. Use caution in patients with visual or dexterity impairment. Patients should use caution when driving or operating heavy machinery until effects on blood sugar are known (Access Pharmacy, 2013).

Older adults are prone to hypoglycemic unawareness, a reason to use the drug with caution in that population. No consistent age-related differences in drug activity have been shown in clinical studies with older adults, but, given its renal metabolism, it is prudent to use caution or closely monitor older adults on this drug. Studies of patients with moderate or severe renal impairment did not show increased exposure or decreased clearance of the drug, but caution seems prudent given its renal metabolism.

Pramlintide is Pregnancy Category C. No adequate and well-controlled studies have been conducted on pregnant women. Increases in congenital anomalies were observed in fetuses of rats treated with this drug, but no such changes were noted in rabbits. The potential risks to the fetus must be balanced with the needs of the mother for the drug when deciding to prescribe it.

Whether this drug is excreted in human milk is unknown. Administer to nursing women only if it is determined that the potential benefit outweighs the potential risk to the infant.

Adverse Drug Reactions

Pramlintide has a Black-Box Warning about the increased risk for severe hypoglycemia when this drug is used in conjunction with insulin. It should also be used cautiously with certain antihypertensives (beta blockers, etc.) that may mask the signs and symptoms of hypoglycemia.

Most adverse effects are GI disturbances. The incidence of nausea was higher at the beginning of treatment and decreased with time in most patients. The incidence and severity of nausea were reduced by gradual titration to the recommended dose.

Drug Interactions

Drug interactions are based largely on other drugs that increase or decrease the actions of pramlintide. Drugs that alter GI motility and orally administered drugs that depend on gastric emptying time for absorption interact because of pramlintide's slowing of gastric emptying. Anticholinergic effects of drugs may be enhanced by pramlintide. Drugs that affect BG levels and those with an adverse effect of hypoglycemia interact because of pramlintide's BG-lowering effects. Alcohol should be avoided because of the increased risk of hypoglycemia. Herbs such as garlic, chromium, and gymnema also increase the hypoglycemic effects. Table 21-27 shows these interactions.

Table 21–27 ⠿ Drug Interactions With GLP-1 and Amylin Agonists

Drug	Interacting Drug	Possible Outcomes	Implications
Exenatide and liraglutide	Acetaminophen	Acetaminophen AUC and C_{max} decreased and T_{max} increased when coadministered	Give acetaminophen at least 1 h before or 4 h after exenatide
Exenatide and liraglutide	Digoxin	Coadministration of repeated doses of exenatide decreased digoxin C_{max} 17% and delayed T_{max} by about 2.5 h	Avoid concurrent use unless both are specifically needed. If so, monitor digoxin level and cardiac rhythm closely.
Exenatide	Lovastatin	Lovastatin AUC decreased by 40% and C_{max} by 28% and T_{max} delayed by 4 h when drugs coadministered	Give lovastatin at least 1 h before or 4 h after exenatide
Exenatide and liraglutide	Oral antibiotics and oral contraceptives	Slowed gastric emptying may reduce extent and rate of oral medications that require rapid GI absorption	Take these drugs at least 1 h before exenatide

Continued

Table 21–27 ⁜ **Drug Interactions With GLP-1 and Amylin Agonists—cont'd**

Drug	Interacting Drug	Possible Outcomes	Implications
Exenatide	Warfarin	Exenatide may lead to increased INR and increased bleeding when coadministered with warfarin	Avoid concurrent use unless both are specifically needed. If so, monitor INR closely.
Albiglutide	Simvastatin	Levels of simvastatin 80 mg increased	Unknown clinical impact as 80 mg no longer prescribed.
Pramlintide	Drugs that alter GI motility (e.g., anticholinergics)	Pramlintide may increase the effects of drugs that slow gastric emptying	Patients using these drugs have not been studied. Avoid concurrent use at this time.
Pramlintide	Orally administered drugs (e.g., analgesics, antibiotics, contraceptives)	Pramlintide has potential to delay absorption if coadministered	Administer interacting drug at least 1 h prior to or 2 h after pramlintide injection.
Pramlintide	Acetaminophen	Acetaminophen C_{max} decreased 29% and T_{max} increased 48–72 min when coadministered or given within 2 h of pramlintide injection	Separate dosing by more than 2 h. Give acetaminophen prior to pramlintide.
Pramlintide	Sulfonylureas, ACE inhibitors, fibrates, fluoxetine, pentoxifylline, propoxyphene, salicylates, and sulfonamide antibiotics	Increase the blood glucose lowering effect and susceptibility to hypoglycemia	If must be given, monitor blood glucose levels closely, which may mean frequent blood glucose testing (AC, PC, HS) and teach patient signs and symptoms of hypoglycemia.
Pramlintide	All insulin	Unknown interaction	Do not mix. Must administer each separately.

Clinical Use and Dosing

Pramlintide is used in treating type 1 and type 2 diabetes, and dosage differs depending on the type of diabetes (Table 21-28). When initiating pramlintide, reduce current insulin dose (including rapidly and mixed-acting preparations) by 50% to avoid hypoglycemia. If pramlintide is discontinued for any reason, restart therapy with same initial titration protocol (Access Pharmacy, 2013).

Type 1 Diabetes Dosing

Initiate pramlintide at a dose of 15 mcg and titrate the dosage up in 15 mcg increments as tolerated every 3 days, to a 30 or 60 mcg maintenance dose. Pre- and postprandial blood glucose and bedtime glucose levels are monitored frequently. The dose of the pramlintide is then increased to the next increment when no clinically significant nausea has occurred for at least 3 days. If significant nausea persists at the 46 or 60 mcg dosage, reduce the dose back to 30 mcg. If the 30 mcg dosage is not tolerated, consider discontinuing the drug. After a maintenance dose of pramlintide is achieved, insulin doses may be adjusted to optimize glycemic control.

Type 2 Diabetes Dosing

Initiate pramlintide at 60 mcg immediately before meals. Monitor pre- and postprandial blood glucose and bedtime glucose levels frequently. Then increase the dose of the pramlintide to 120 mcg when no clinically significant nausea has occurred for 3 to 7 days. If significant nausea continues at the 120 mcg dose, decrease the dose to 60 mcg. Adjust the insulin dose to optimize glycemic control once the target dose of pramlintide is achieved and nausea has subsided.

Monitoring

The only monitoring required for this drug is that associated with the management of diabetes.

Patient Education

Administration

Pramlintide is administered by subcutaneous injection in the thigh or abdomen but not in the upper arm because of variability of absorption. It is given immediately before each major meal containing at least 250 kcal or at least 30 g of carbohydrate. Pramlintide cannot be mixed with any form of insulin; it is administered in a separate syringe from insulin. The injection site for pramlintide should be at least 2 inches away from the injection site for the insulin. The solution should be room temperature to avoid injection site reactions (Access Pharmacy, 2013). Inform patients that if a dose is missed, they should wait until the next meal and take the usual dose of pramlintide at that meal.

Table 21–28 ✂ Dosage Schedule GLP-1 and Amylin Agonists

Drug	Initial Dose	Dosage Form	Maintenance Dose	Maximum Dose
Exenatide (Byetta) (B)	5 mcg SC every 12 h, 60 min before a.m. and p.m. meals at least 6 h apart; may increase to 10 mcg every 12 h after 1 mo	250 mcg/mL solution: 1.2 mL (5 mcg) and 2.4 mL (10 mcg) prefilled pens in 60 dose kits	5–10 mcg every 12 h	10 mcg every 12 h
Exenatide Bydureon (B) Extended release	2 mg SC once weekly May administer any time of day with or without meals	Injectable suspension 2 mg/vial; comes in a single-dose tray containing 1 vial of 2 mg exenatide, 1 vial connector, 1 prefilled diluent syringe	2 mg once weekly	2 mg once weekly
Pramlintide (Symlin) (B)	**Type 1:** 15 mcg SC before meals; increase by 15 mcg every 3 d. Reduce SA insulin dose by 50%. **Type 2:** 60 mcg SC before meals; increase to 120 mcg before meals in 3–7 d. Reduce SA insulin by 50%.	Injection solution: 0.6 mg/mL Pen injectors: 15, 30, 45, 60, 120 mcg/dose	Type 1: 30–60 mcg Type 2: 60–120 mcg	Type 1: 60 mcg Type 2: 120 mcg
Liraglutide (Victoza)	**Type 2:** 0.6 mg SC once daily without regard to meals	Prefilled pen that can deliver the 0.6, 1.2, or 1.8 mg doses	Based on glycemic response	1.8 mg daily
Albigutide (Tanzeum)	**Type 2:** 30 mg SC weekly without regard to meals	Pen that needs reconstitution. Wait 15–30 min to ensure all in solution.	Takes 4–5 wk for steady state and decision to advance dose	50 mg weekly;
Dulaglutide (Trulicity)	**Type 2:** 0.75 mg SC weekly	Single use pen that needs refrigeration; room temp no more than 14 d.	Takes 2–4 wk for steady state.	1.5 mg SQ weekly

Pramlintide is available in 5 mL vials and in a multidose prefilled pen for injection. Patients should confirm they are using the correct pen injector to deliver their prescribed dose. A package insert provides instructions for using the pen injector. Needles are not included with the pen and must be purchased separately. If drawing from a multidose vial, patients should be taught to convert to mL, not units, as the confusion could result in a 6-fold overdosage (Fig. 21-4).

Pramlintide Dose in Micrograms	Amount to Draw Up in a U-100 Insulin Syringe
15	2.5
30	5
45	7.5
60	10
120	20

Figure 21–4. Conversion of mcg to units for injecting pramlintide.

Adverse Reactions

Patients on the drug should check BG levels before and after every meal and at bedtime. Because this drug is taken with insulin, patients have an increased risk for severe hypoglycemic reactions. Hypoglycemic reactions should be reported to the provider so that dosage adjustments can be made if needed. Patients should be taught the signs and symptoms of hypoglycemia, prevention, and how to treat using 15 g of fast-acting CHO. In case of severe hypoglycemia and the inability to swallow, the patient should have glucagon available and someone who is knowledgeable in administering it.

GLUCAGON-LIKE PEPTIDE AGONISTS

Another class of drugs that acts on the incretin system is the glucagon-like peptide-1 agonists (GLP-1 or incretin mimetics). Drugs approved for use in this class include exenatide (immediate- and extended-release), liraglutide, dulaglutide, and albiglutide. Glucagon-like peptide-1 is a naturally occurring peptide produced in the small intestine that potentiates glucose-stimulated insulin secretion,Although the gliptins support endogenous GLP activity indirectly, GLP-1 agonists directly bind to the GLP-1 receptor in the pancreatic beta cell and act as an incretin mimetic. Improvement in glycemic control with a reduction in A1C of 0.5% to 1.7% has been demonstrated when GLP-1 is added to other antihyperglycemic agents. A real positive attribute is that these drugs have a low risk for hypoglycemia , but some patients are hesitant to start them because they are given by injection. That objection is less intense when weekly dosing schedules are allowed with exenatide and albigutide. GLP-1 are recommended in a two-step therapy for patients on metformin, and in a three-drug approach with metformin and a sulfonylurea, or TZD, or insulin (Inzucchi et al, 2012).

Incretin mimetics require a GLP-1 receptor in the gut to act. Part of the newly recognized pathological processes in DM is the loss of receptor numbers. When compared to the DPP-4 inhibitors, this class of drugs promotes satiety and weight loss more. It appears incretin mimetics contribute to reduction of systolic pressures and lower triglycerides. These effects are not as strong in the DPP-4 medications. The extended-release formulations have better fasting BG control than the short-acting ones.

Pharmacodynamics

The role of GLP-1 in the incretin system was discussed in a previous section. Exenatide is a homologue of the human GLP-1 sequence, but it has a longer circulating half-life. It binds avidly with the GLP-1 receptor on the pancreatic beta cell to augment glucose-mediated insulin release. It also enhances other antihyperglycemic actions of the incretins, such as moderating glucagon secretion and lowering glucagon concentrations during periods of hyperglycemia. This latter effect leads to decreased hepatic glucose output and decreased insulin demand. Each of these effects occurs only in the presence of increased glucose and subsides as BG concentrations decrease and approach euglycemia. GLP-1 agonists improve glycemic control by reducing fasting and postprandial glucose concentrations. They also slow gastric emptying and reduce appetite, making them either weight neutral or promoting weight loss, a significant factor in type 2 diabetes. Exenatide is associated with weight loss of 2 to 3 kg over 6 months (Nathan et al, 2009); the extended-release formulation produces up to a 5 kg weight loss over the same period.

Pharmacokinetics

Absorption and Distribution

Exenatide is slowly absorbed following subcutaneous injection, reaching median peak plasma concentrations in 2.1 hours. Liraglutide reaches peak concentration later, at 9 to 12 hours. Absorption is similar for both drugs, whether given in the upper arm, abdomen, or thigh. Steady state of the extended-release formulations of this drug class takes 2 to 4 weeks for dulaglutide and 4 to 5 weeks for the others. They have half-lives of 2 to 3 days for dulaglutide and 4 to 7 days for the other extended-release forms. Increasing doses, therefore, is delayed until full glycemic impact is achieved.

Metabolism and Excretion

The metabolic fate of exenatide is not clear, but it is excreted predominantly by glomerular filtration with subsequent proteolytic degradation. Liraglutide is metabolized to a number of minor metabolites, which are excreted in both urine and feces. Albigutide and dulaglutide are cleared much like natural albumin. Table 21-11 presents pharmacokinetic information on these drugs.

Pharmacotherapeutics

Precautions and Contraindications

Patients with severe GI disease (e.g., ulcerative colitis, Crohn's disease) should not use these drugs because of their effects on gastric emptying. Pancreatitis has been reported in patients treated with these drugs. Patients should report persistent, severe abdominal pain, which may be accompanied by vomiting; these are hallmark symptoms of pancreatitis. C cell thyroid tumors or hyperplasia have been associated with several of the medications when used in animals and humans; it carries a boxed warning. Patients should be assessed appropriately and counseled on this risk as well as those with a family history of medullary thyroid tumor and other endocrine neoplasia (Access Pharmacy, 2013).

GLP-1s are not recommended for use in those with moderate renal impairment or end-stage renal disease. Cases of acute renal failure and exacerbation of chronic renal failure have been reported, possibly due to the GI side effects that may cause dehydration (Access Pharmacy, 2013). Increases in LFTs have been noted on occasion, but appear to be linked to prior gallbladder and/or liver disease.

These drugs are listed as Pregnancy Category C based on studies in pregnant laboratory animals. No studies have been conducted on pregnant women. It is not known if these drugs are excreted in breast milk. The decision whether to discontinue either breastfeeding or the drug should take into account the drug's importance to the mother.

Adverse Drug Reactions

This class of medications has been associated with a relatively high frequency of GI disturbances, with 8% to 45% of treated patients experiencing one or more episodes of nausea, vomiting, or diarrhea (Access Pharmacy, 2013). These adverse reactions tend to subside over time; the extended-release formulations have a more transient nausea profile, and liraglutide has fewer reports of GI distress when compared with twice-daily exenatide. Dulaglutide at the highest doses may have 21% nausea rate. Consult with an endocrinologist if antiemetic use is considered to get over this initial-phase problem. Slower, lower-dose titration may also be helpful. Because many DM patients have a reduced satiety reflex, the slow down of gastric motility and sensation of fullness maybe reported as nausea.

Reports of pancreatic duct metaplasia are being investigated by the FDA for the entire class. Patients with new nodules or changes in thyroid function tests should be evaluated by an endocrinologist. There is the possibility of site reactions with any injectable medication. They appear to be infrequent and self-limiting.

Drug Interactions

The major interactions for these drugs relate to their action in slowing gastric emptying. Separating the administration of the interacting drug and the incretin mimetic will usually resolve the problem. The International Normalized Ratio (INR) increases and the risk of bleeding also increases when exenatide is coadministered with warfarin; these two drugs should not be used concurrently. Serum concentration of oral contraceptives is decreased by exenatide. Neither of these interactions are documented for albigutide. The effect of simvastatin is reduced when taken with albigutide. Table 21-27 lists the interactions.

Clinical Use and Dosing

This drug class is not typically used in DM type I. None of these drugs has been approved for monotherapy to treat type 2 diabetes but are being used off-label even in prediabetic patients. They typically are adjunctive therapies for patients already taking other drugs. All are administered subcutaneously. Regardless of the other antidiabetic drugs being taken, the initial dose of immediate-release exenatide is 5 mcg subcutaneously twice daily 60 minutes before morning and evening meals (or the two main meals of the day, approximately 6 or more hours apart). Based on clinical response, the dose of exenatide can be increased to 10 mcg twice daily after 1 month of therapy. Liraglutide is started as 0.6 mg/d for 1 week and 1.2 mg daily thereafter. It can be increased to 1.8 mg daily if tolerated. If more than 3 days are missed, return to a previous dose level is indicated to reduce GI distress.

Extended-release exenatide is administered 2 mg once a week. If a dose is missed or a different day dosing schedule is desired, the patient should wait no more than 3 days to administer the next dose. Liraglutide is administered once daily, initiating treatment at 0.6 mg for 1 week, then increasing to 1.2 mg daily. It may be increased to 1.8 mg if the target is not reached on 1.2 mg/d. Albigutide is started at 30 mg and advanced to 50 mg weekly depending on glycemic response. Due to its extended half-life, some patients may be stable on biweekly dosing (see Table 21-26).

Some patients do not respond to GLP-1 medications or have a reduction in effects over time. The hypothesis is that they have genetic antibody responses to the molecules or develop those antibodies over time. Antibody development against one drug may be overcome by switching to another one in the same class.

Combination Therapy

When added to metformin or TZD therapy, the current dose of metformin or TZD can be continued. Dosage adjustment is not required because the risk of hypoglycemia is low. When added to sulfonylurea therapy, a reduction in the sulfonylurea dose should be considered to reduce the risk of hypoglycemia.

Rational Drug Selection

There is no significant difference among the drugs in terms of precautions or contraindications, or serious adverse effects. Albigutide has fewer drug interactions, but extended clinical use may change that profile. Nausea is more significant with exenatide that is given twice a day; it is a much less common complaint with the extended release forms (liraglutide, albigutide, and exenatide weekly). Number of injections per day and cost are compelling factors for drug choice. Timing of glucose control is a factor when comparing short- and long-acting formulations. Short-acting medications are best for making significant reductions in postprandial glucose levels; long-acting medications are better to control FPG levels. The initial selection of formula may be guided by which glucose peak is most critical to control for the individual patient. Reduction of A1C levels is larger with the extended-release drugs; daily dosing regimens result in 0.9% reductions but extended-release drugs typically have a 1.7% reduction. Onset of action is within a few days for the shorter-acting medications; it takes up to 2 weeks for actions to be evident for the long-acting formulas.

Monitoring

Glycemic control is monitored based on diabetic guideline protocols. If the patient must also take warfarin, INR is monitored closely, and if the patient is on digoxin, the levels of this drug and cardiac response to it are monitored closely if on exenatide. Renal function studies are monitored based on diabetic guideline protocols. Thyroid and abdominal assessments for pancreatitis are critical.

Patient Education

Administration

Each dose of these medications should be administered as a subcutaneous injection in the thigh, abdomen, or upper arm. Immediate-release exenatide is given about 60 minutes before morning and evening meals and doses should be at least 6 hours apart. Do not administer after a meal. If a dose is missed, the patient should resume the treatment regimen as prescribed with the next scheduled dose. Liraglutide is a daily medication given via prefilled pen without regard to meal times. The other medications are given weekly as doses without regard to meals.

Exenatide is dispensed for injection in prefilled pens. Pens should be primed before use and a new needle used for each injection. Extended-release exenatide comes in a vial with a diluent that must be reconstituted and used immediately. The prefilled pens and vials come with a user manual that includes information on setup, storing, and disposing of the pen and needles, and cleaning the outside of the pen. Needles are not included and must be purchased separately. Albigutide comes in a single-dose pen that needs to be reconstituted by a twisting action. Waiting 15 to 30 minutes prior to injection is required to ensure full dissolving of the powder. Once reconstituted it must be given within 8 hours. Other pen formulations do not indicate a waiting period.

If using concurrently with insulin, do not mix drugs. Injections should be given separately. Sites should be rotated; the same body region may be used, but sites should not be adjacent to one another (Access Pharmacy, 2013). Dulaglutide has not be studied in combination with insulin.

Adverse Reactions

The most common adverse reactions are GI disturbances that tend to subside with time. Exenatide may reduce appetite, the amount of food eaten, and patient weight. No changes in dose are needed—the reactions are transient and actually have a positive effect on diabetes.

When taking exenatide, patient BG levels should be checked before and after every meal and at bedtime. Hypoglycemia should not occur unless the patient is also taking a sulfonylurea. Hypoglycemic reactions should be reported to the provider so that dosage may be adjusted if needed.

GLUCAGON

Glucagon is a hormone secreted by the pancreas. It has several actions, but its primary use clinically is in elevating BG levels during hypoglycemic episodes or for treating insulin overdose. It is also used to reverse the hypoglycemia induced by insulin shock therapy in psychiatric patients and to relax the GI musculature to facilitate radiographic examinations and scoping procedures. The increase in BG in patients who have been NPO for hours prior to a scheduled GI procedure can also be considered beneficial.

Pharmacodynamics

Glucagon is a polypeptide hormone produced by the alpha cells of the islets of Langerhans in the pancreas. It accelerates liver glucogenolysis by stimulating cAMP synthesis and increasing phosphorylase kinase activity. This results in increased breakdown of glycogen to glucose and inhibition of glycogen synthesis. The end result is an elevation in BG levels. Glucagon also stimulates hepatic gluconeogenesis by promoting the uptake of amino acids and converting them to glucose precursors. When administered parenterally, glucagon also produces relaxation of the smooth muscle of the GI tract, decreases gastric and pancreatic secretions, and increases myocardial contractility. These latter actions are not the primary reason for its clinical use.

Pharmacokinetics

Absorption and Distribution

Glucagon is well absorbed after parenteral administration. Its distribution is unknown.

Metabolism and Excretion

Glucagon is extensively metabolized by the liver and kidney and degraded in the plasma. Plasma half-life is about 8 to 18 minutes.

Pharmacotherapeutics

Precautions and Contraindications

The only contraindication to glucagon is hypersensitivity to it. It should be given with caution to patients with insulinoma or pheochromocytoma. It may produce an initial increase in BG in these patients, but because of its insulin-releasing effect, it may subsequently cause hypoglycemia. It also stimulates catecholamine release, causing a marked increase in blood pressure in patients with pheochromocytoma. It has positive inotropic and chronotropic effects in all patients.

Glucagon is Pregnancy Category B, but there are no adequate and well-controlled studies in pregnant women. It should be used in pregnancy only if clearly indicated. Because insulin is the drug of choice in managing gestational diabetes and other diabetic patients during their pregnancy, the potential for a hypoglycemic reaction exists. The rapid resolution of any moderate to severe hypoglycemia is clearly in the best interests of the fetus and would override any concerns about potential risk from exposure to glucagon. It is not known whether this drug is excreted in breast milk. Caution should be used in giving it to a nursing mother.

Adverse Drug Reactions

The most frequent adverse reactions to glucagon are nausea and vomiting. These may occur because of a possible reactive hypoglycemia after the initial BG rise. Rare allergic reactions resulting in urticaria, respiratory distress, and hypotension have been reported, possibly related to the phenol and glycerin in some products.

Drug Interactions

The anticoagulant effects of oral anticoagulants may be increased, with the possibility of bleeding. This interaction may occur after several days of therapy and appears to be dose-related. This interaction is not associated with single-dose therapy to resolve a hypoglycemic reaction. The hyperglycemic response is prolonged with epinephrine. The response is blunted with phenytoin.

Clinical Use and Dosing

Reversal of hypoglycemia is the main object for glucagon (Table 21-29). Because its actions depend on the presence of glycogen in the liver, glucagon is of little or no help in states of starvation, adrenal insufficiency, or chronic hypoglycemia.

Table 21–29 ⊗ **Dosage Schedule: Glucagon**

Drug	Initial Dose	Dosage Form	Maximum Dose
Glucagon	*Children, weight <20 kg:* 0.5 mg SC, IM, or IV *Adult and children, weight >20 mg:* 1 mg SC, IM, or IV *Infants:* 0.3 mg/kg (may repeat Q4 h) *Insulin shock:* 0.5–1 mg SC, IM, or IV. If no response in 10–25 min, repeat dose.	1 mg powder with 1 mL diluent for reconstitution Emergency kit with 1 mg/1 mL prefilled syringe	If response not adequate in 5–15 min, administer 1–2 additional doses; accompany with IV glucose if patient fails to respond.

Supplemental glucose is typically used to help reverse severe hypoglycemia.

Monitoring

Monitoring of BG should be done immediately prior to and after the injection.

Patient Education

Patients with diabetes who are at high risk for hypoglycemia should have this drug on hand to be mixed and injected by a family member if oral glucose supplements are contraindicated with loss of consciousness or swallowing impairment. Education of the family member would include recognition of and testing for hypoglycemia and the procedure for mixing and administering glucagon parenterally.

THYROID AGENTS

Thyroid hormones include both natural and synthetic compounds. The natural hormones are derived from pork thyroid glands. Because their content and bioavailability are not consistent from dose to dose, they have largely been replaced with the synthetic compounds. This section discusses the synthetic thyroid hormones.

Pharmacodynamics

The hypothalamus-pituitary-thyroid hormone axis begins with the secretion of thyrotropin-releasing hormone (TRH) by the hypothalamus in response to cold, stress, and decreased levels of thyroxine (T4). TRH stimulates the synthesis and release of thyroid-stimulating hormone (TSH) by the anterior pituitary. TSH, in turn, stimulates an adenylyl cyclase mechanism in the thyroid cells to (1) immediately increase the release of stored thyroid hormones; (2) increase iodine uptake and utilization; (3) increase the synthesis of the two thyroid hormones, triiodothyronine (T3) and T4; and (4) increase the synthesis and secretion of prostaglandins by the thyroid gland. When thyroid hormones are secreted, they create a negative feedback loop, inhibit TRH and TSH secretion, and decrease further thyroid hormone synthesis and secretion. Figure 21-5 depicts the hypothalamus-pituitary-thyroid hormone axis.

As shown in Figure 21-5, thyroid hormones increase all the metabolic processes of the body and are central to the growth and differentiation of body tissues. The mechanism by which thyroid hormones exert their effect is not well understood, but it is believed that most of their effects are exerted through control of DNA transcription and protein synthesis. Administration of synthetic thyroid hormones—levothyroxine (T4), liothyronine (T3), and liotrix (a 4:1 mixture of T4 and T3)—produces the same effects on body tissues as the body's own thyroid hormones and produces the negative feedback loop to reduce further secretion of TSH and thyroid hormones.

Pharmacokinetics

Absorption and Distribution

Levothyroxine (T4) is variably absorbed, with 48% to 79% of the dose absorbed after oral administration (Table 21-30). Fasting increases its absorption, and malabsorption syndromes cause excessive fecal loss of this drug. Liothyronine (T3) is 95% absorbed within 4 hours after administration. More than 99% of both circulating hormones are bound to serum proteins, including thyroid-binding globulin (TBg), thyroid-binding prealbumin (TBPA), and albumin (TBa). The higher affinity of T4 for TBg and TBPA as compared with T3 partially explains the higher serum levels and longer half-life of T4. T4 and T3 exist in the body in equilibrium between bound and free drug, but only the free drug produces the hormone's effects.

Metabolism and Excretion

Thyroid hormones are distributed to most body tissues. They do not readily cross the placenta, and minimal amounts are excreted in breast milk. Under normal body functioning, the ratio of T4 to T3 released from the thyroid gland is 20:1. Approximately 35% of T4 is converted in peripheral tissues to T3 so that 80% of T3 comes from monodeiodination of T4. This process of deiodination of T4 occurs in the liver, kidney, and other body tissues, especially the skeletal muscles. The conjugated hormones then reenter the hepatic circulation, where they are excreted in the feces via bile.

Pharmacotherapeutics

Precautions and Contraindications

Cardiovascular disease, particularly coronary artery disease, may worsen when thyroid hormones are given; however, considering the increased risk of death from CHF in African Americans with even mild hypothyroid conditions, this should not dissuade cautious use (Rhee,

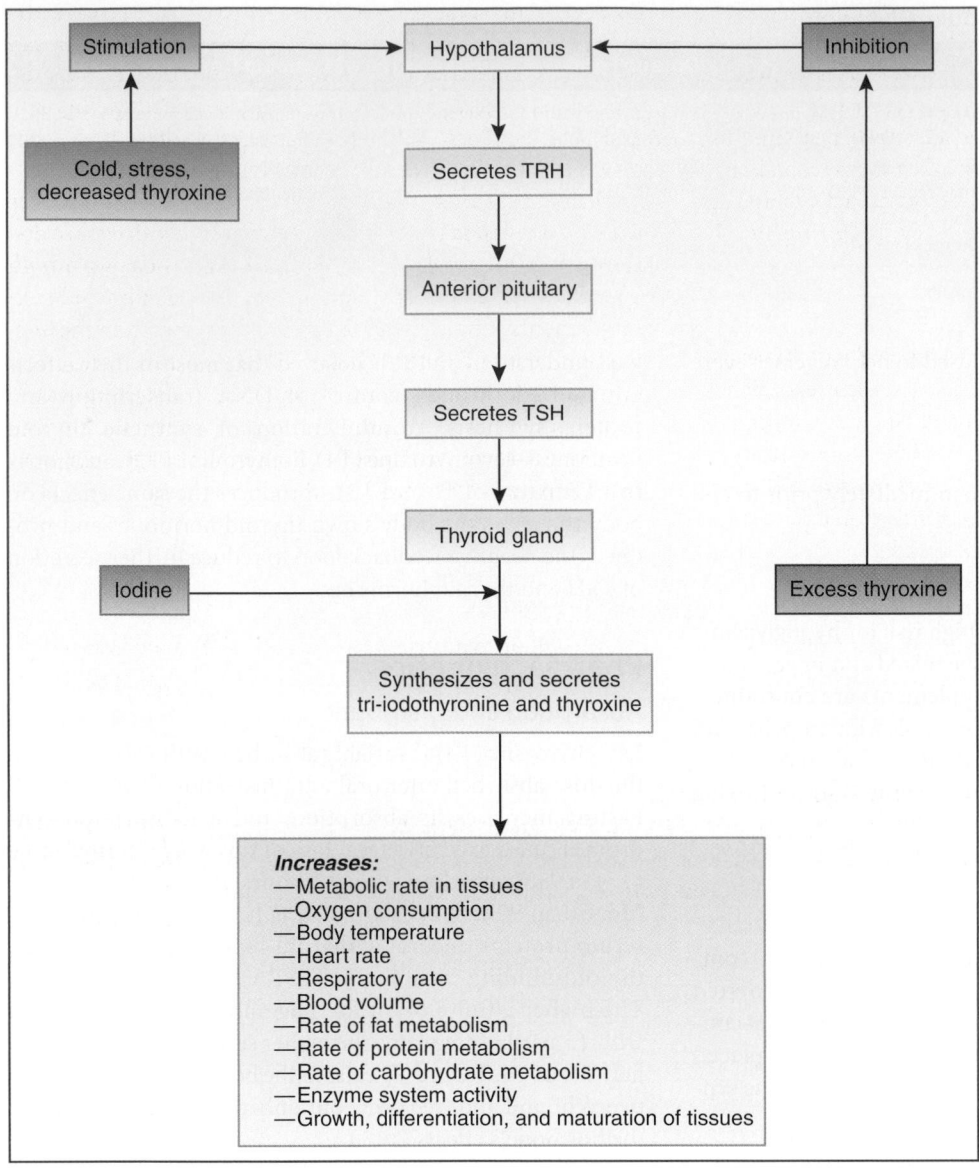

Figure 21–5. Hypothalamus-pituitary-thyroid hormone axis.

Table 21–30 ⚏ Pharmacokinetics: Oral Thyroid Hormones

Drug	Onset*	Peak*	Duration*	Biological Potency	Half-Life	Excretion
Levothyroxine (T4)	48 h	1–3 wk	1–3 wk	1	6–7 d**	In feces via bile
Liothyronine (T3)	48 h	24–72 h	72 h	4	<2.5 d	In feces via bile

*Effects on thyroid function tests.
  **3–4 d in hyperthyroidism; 9–10 d in myxedema.

Curhan, Alexander, Bhan, & Brunelli, 2013). Thyroid hormone replacement is contraindicated after recent MI. When hypothyroidism is a complicating or causative factor in MI or heart disease, judicious use of small doses may be indicated if coordinated with cardiology and endocrinology teams. The increased heart rate associated with thyroid hormone administration increases oxygen demand by the heart muscle and decreases oxygen supply by reducing diastolic filling time. A recent study has not found this CV risk as severe as traditionally considered (Hyland, Arnold, Lee, & Cappola, 2013).

Advance practice prescribers are cautioned not to change practice until major guidelines endorse this stance.

Long-term levothyroxine therapy has been associated with decreased bone density in the hip and spine in both pre- and postmenopausal women. A self-induced subclinical hyperthyroidism via insistence on unnecessary borderline-low TSH levels for "well-being" is linked to this bone loss. Use of only the lowest dose possible to achieve the desired effects, with strict periodic monitoring, is indicated for the osteoporosis patient.

Thyroid hormone therapy for patients with concomitant diabetes insipidus or adrenal insufficiency exacerbates the intensity of their symptoms. Dosage adjustments downward in thyroid hormone may be required. Severe or prolonged hypothyroidism can lead to decreased adrenocortical function. When thyroid replacement therapy is begun, the metabolism increases at a greater rate than adrenocortical activity and can precipitate adrenocortical insufficiency, requiring supplemental adrenocorticosteroids.

Adverse Drug Reactions

Adverse reactions other than those associated with hyperthyroidism due to overdose are rare. If the patient experiences indications of hyperthyroidism (increased heart rate, cardiac arrhythmias, chest pain, tremors, nervousness, insomnia, irritability, diarrhea, vomiting, weight loss, menstrual irregularities, or heat intolerance), the TSH level should be assessed and appropriate dosage adjustments made.

Drug Interactions

Bile-acid sequestrants, iron salts, and antacids decrease the absorption of orally administered thyroid preparations.

Estrogens increase TBg and may therefore decrease the response to thyroid hormone. The SSRI medications can sometimes alter thyroid dosing requirements. Thyroid hormones may decrease the effectiveness of warfarin, digoxin, and beta blockers. Table 21-31 mentions these and other drug interactions.

Many drugs affect thyroid function tests and may interfere with correct assessment of thyroid status. These drugs are discussed in Chapter 41. High-fat meals and those with high fiber may decrease absorption up to 40%. Calcium and iron supplements should be taken 2 to 4 hours apart from the hormone. Coffee and other caffeine-containing drinks are linked to less absorption, as is excess fluoride in drinking water. Some individuals are sensitive to excessive ingestion of goitrogenic foods, such as turnip greens, cabbage, soybeans, and rutabagas (Messina & Redmond, 2006).

Clinical Use and Dosing

Hypothyroidism

Treatment of hypothyroidism follows the "start low and go slow" principle to avoid excessive increase in metabolism

Table 21–31 ⠿ Drug Interactions With Thyroid Hormones

Interacting Drug	Possible Outcomes	Implications
Beta-adrenergic blockers	Actions of beta-adrenergic blocker may be impaired when patient is converted to euthyroid state	Monitor response to beta-adrenergic blockers; assess for continued need for drug or for dosage adjustment
Carbamazepine, hydantoins, phenobarbital, rifamycins	Increased hepatic degradation of T4 Increased levothyroxine requirements	Monitor thyroid function closely
Cholestyramine, colestipol	Interferes with thyroid hormone absorption with loss of efficacy	Administer at least 4 h apart
Digoxin	Serum levels of digoxin reduced when hypothyroid patient is converted to euthyroid state	Monitor response to digoxin and serum levels; assess for need for dosage adjustment
Estrogens	Increases TBg and may decrease response to thyroid hormone	Monitor therapeutic response
Glucocorticoids	Concurrent use may decrease peripheral conversion of T4 to T3	Monitor thyroid function and symptoms of hypothyroidism
Iodides (including amiodarone and iodine-based radiographic contrast agents, IV or oral)	Can trigger hypo- or hyperthyroid state that may persist for several months; IV agents have shorter impact	Monitor thyroid function and symptoms of hypo- or hyperthyroidism
Metformin, meglitinides, sulfonylureas, TZDs, and insulin	Initiating thyroid hormones may cause increases in insulin or oral hypoglycemic requirements	Monitor BG closely
Sertraline (an SSRI)	Increased levothyroxine requirements	Monitor thyroid function closely or select different SRI
Tricyclic and 3-times daily depressants	Concurrent use may increase toxic effects of both drugs. Toxic effects may include increased risk of dysrhythmias and CNS stimulation.	Avoid concurrent use
Warfarin	Increased anticoagulant action	May need to decrease dose of warfarin; monitor PT/INR carefully

INR = international normalized ratio; PT = prothrombin time.

before the body has a chance to adapt to the increase. For adults, levothyroxine is started at 50 mcg daily and is increased in increments of 25 mcg/d at 2- to 4-week intervals to 100 to 150 mcg/d. The target dose is based on TSH levels and is approximately 1.7 mcg/kg/d. Older adults may require less than 1 mcg/kg/d as their target. An initial dose for elders of 25 to 50 mcg/d is recommended, with gradual dosage increases of 12.5 to 25 mcg/d at 6- to 8-week intervals. Lower doses and longer intervals for changing doses are required for patients with cardiovascular impairment or long-standing hypothyroidism. In these cases or in severe hypothyroidism, the initial dose is 12.5 to 25 mcg/d, increased by 25 mcg/d at 4-week intervals. The target dose is also based on TSH levels. Most patients require less than than 200 mcg/d. Failure to respond adequately to doses of 300 mcg/d suggests lack of adherence or malabsorption; however, reduction in sensitivity to thyroid hormone is possible.

Liothyronine (T3) is started at 25 mcg/d. Dosage is increased by 12.5 to 25 mcg/d at 1- to 2-week intervals until a maintenance dose of 25 to 50 mcg is reached.

Liotrix is started with 50 mcg of levothyroxine/12.5 mcg of liothyronine per day. Doses are increased by 50/12.5 mcg at 4-week intervals until a maintenance dose of 50 to 100/12.5 to 25 is reached. For patients with myxedema or hypothyroidism with cardiovascular disease, the doses are reduced. This formulation is claimed to follow a more natural hormone secretion pattern; however, a meta-analysis demonstrated no benefits with combination medications, including improved mental health and quality-of-life measures (Grozinski-Glasberg, Fraser, Nashshoni, Weizman, & Leibovici, 2006). The subset of post–total thyroidectomy patients may be the exception (Garber et al, 2012).

For all of these drugs, dosages are different for infants, children, and geriatric patients. Table 21-32 presents the dosing schedules for all of these age groups.

Hashimoto's Thyroiditis

Approximately 70% or more of patients with Hashimoto's thyroiditis go on to develop permanent hypothyroidism. The treatment regimen is the same as for other causes of

Table 21–32 ⊗ Dosage Schedule: Thyroid Hormones

Drug	Indication	Dose Form	Initial Dose	Maintenance Dose
Levothyroxine T4 (G) Synthroid levoxyl	Hypothyroidism and congenital hypothyroidism	Tablets: 25, 50, 75, 88, 100, 112, 125 mcg, 137 (B only), 150, 175 mcg, 200, 300 mcg	*Adults:* 50 mcg daily (0.05 mg)	Increase dose by 25 mcg at 4 to 6 wk intervals to maintenance dose of 100–150 mcg daily
			Older adults: 12.5–25 mcg daily	Increase dose by 25 mcg daily at 6 wk intervals to maintenance dose of 100–150 mcg daily
Triosint (levothyroxine)		Liquid-filled caps 13, 25, 50, 75, 88, 100, 112, 125, 137, 150 mcg	*Children >12 yr:* 2–3 mcg/kg daily	Increase in increments of 2 mcg/kg/d at 4 to 6 wk intervals to maintenance dose of 150–200 mcg daily
			Children 6–12 yr: 4–5 mcg/kg daily	Increase in increments of 4 mcg/kg/d at 4 to 6 wk intervals to maintenance dose of 100–150 mcg daily
			Children 1–5 yr: 5–6 mcg/kg daily	Increase in increments of 3 mcg/kg/d at 2 to 4 wk intervals to maintenance dose of 75–100 mcg daily
			Children 6–12 mo: 6–8 mcg/kg daily	Increase in increments of 5 mcg/kg/d at 2 to 4 wk intervals to maintenance dose of 50–75 mcg daily
			Infants 3–6 mo: 8–10 mcg/kg daily	Increase in increments of 5 mcg/kg/d at 4 to 6 wk intervals to maintenance dose of 25–50 mcg daily
			Infants 0–3 mo: 10–15 mcg/kg	Dosage may be increased after 4–6 wk to 50 mcg daily
			Infants less than 2,000 g or at risk for cardiac failure: 25 mcg daily	For infants with congenital hypothyroidism, initiate therapy with full dose as soon as diagnosis is made
Liothyronine Synthetic T3 (G) Cytomel	Mild hypothyroidism	Tablets: 5, 25, and 50 mcg	*Adults:* 25 mcg daily	Increase in increments of 12.5–25 mcg daily at 1 to 2 wk intervals to maintenance dose of 25–75 mcg daily

Table 21–32 ⚕ Dosage Schedule: Thyroid Hormones—cont'd

Drug	Indication	Dosage Form	Maintenance Dose	Initial Dose
			Older adults or patients with cardiovascular disease: 5 mcg daily	Increase in increments of no more than 5 mcg daily at 2 wk intervals
	Congenital hypothyroidism		5 mcg daily	Increase in increments of 5 mcg every 3–4 d until desired response Maintenance dose for infants a few months old is 20 mcg daily; for children age 1 yr, dose is 50 mcg daily; above 3 yr, use adult dose
	Simple nontoxic goiter		5 mcg daily	Increase in increments of 5 mcg every 1–2 wk When dose of 25 mcg daily is reached, increase by 12.5–25 mcg daily every 1–2 wk Usual maintenance dose is 75 mcg daily
	Myxedema		5 mcg daily	Increase in increments of 5 mcg every 1–2 wk When dose of 25 mcg daily is reached, increase by 12.5–25 mcg daily every 1–2 wk Usual maintenance dose is 50–100 mcg daily
Liotrix Levothyroxine & Liothyronine (G) (Thyrolar)	Hypothyroidism	Tablets: 12.5 mcg/ 3.1 mcg; 25 mcg/ 6.25 mcg; 50 mcg/ 12.5 mcg; 100 mcg/ 25 mcg; 150 mcg/ 37.5 mcg Or the grain formulation: ¼ grain ½ grain 1 grain 2 grain 3 grain	*Adults:* 30 mg equivalent daily	Increase in increments of 15 mg (1/4 grain) every 2–3 wk to maintenance dose of 60–120 mg daily
			Children and infants with congenital hypothyroidism	Follow dosage recommendations for levothyroxine (see available dosage forms table for T4 equivalents for liotrix)

hypothyroidism. Monitoring of thyroid antibodies assumes greater significance with these autoimmune patients.

TSH Suppression in Thyroid Cancer, Nodules, and Euthyroid Goiter

The required maintenance dosage for these indications is larger than that for primary hypothyroidism. The initial dose of levothyroxine is 50 to 100 mcg/d, and the dose is increased until the TSH level declines to 0.05 to 0.3 mU/L. This therapy is relatively contraindicated in older adults and in patients with cardiovascular disease.

Thyroid Suppression Therapy

The dose is 2.5 mcg/kg daily for 7 to 10 days for this indication. These doses usually yield normal serum T4 and T3 levels without a response to TSH.

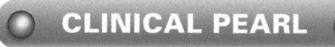

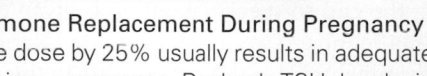

Thyroid Hormone Replacement During Pregnancy
Increasing the dose by 25% usually results in adequate coverage during pregnancy. Recheck TSH levels in 4 weeks to determine any dosage adjustment.

Pregnancy

Untreated hypothyroidism during pregnancy may increase the incidence of maternal complications, spontaneous abortion, fetal death or stillbirth, low birth weight, and abnormal fetal brain development (American Association of Clinical Endocrinologists [AACE], 2012; DeGroot et al, 2012). These outcomes can be avoided by thyroid hormone replacement.

Thyroid hormones are Pregnancy Category A, and replacement is advised for all symptomatic pregnant women. Therapy begun before pregnancy should not be stopped. The increased metabolic rate common to pregnancy often requires higher doses. Increasing a patient's maintenance dose by 25% usually provides adequate coverage but a 45% increase may be required. T4 requirements increase by the eighth week and typically plateau at 16 weeks. TSH levels should then be checked every trimester to determine the need for any further dosage adjustment. AACE, American College of Obstetricians and Gynecologists (ACOG), and The Endocrine Society recommend levothyroxine.

Hormones are excreted in breast milk but have not been associated with adverse effects in nursing infants. Infants must be monitored after birth for issues related to maternal levels. Preliminary data from studies measuring lowered thyroid levels in male infants taking formulas from BPA-containing bottles have not triggered special alerts. Concerned mothers should avoid bottles with a 7 in the recycle number, avoid placing bottles in the microwave, and use powder formula, not those shipped in plastic bottles (Chevier, 2013).

Postpartum thyroiditis (5% to 10% of deliveries and miscarriage, abortion, and ectopics) can result in either hypo- or hyperthyroid states. Current recommendations do not suggest screening before or after deliveries unless patients are symptomatic. Women with symptoms may or may not be treated within the first 8 to 12 weeks postpartum, as hormonal levels typically return to normal. Propanolol may be used for symptom control of tachycardiac symptoms. Elevated TSH is not strongly associated with postpartum depression. Those who have rebalanced levels within a few months are at risk for future thyroid imbalances within the next 5 to 10 years (DeGroot et al, 2012).

Congenital Hypothyroidism

Congenital hypothyroidism occurs in 1 in 3,000 to 4,000 newborns and requires referral to a pediatric endocrinologist. Of all the causes of mental retardation, it is the easiest to screen for and treat. Most impacted infants have no signs or symptoms. Levothyroxine is the drug of choice. Full weight-based doses are started immediately on diagnosis of the condition. Tablets may be crushed and added to infant formula. There is some evidence that soy may impair thyroxine absorption from the gut, so special attention is given to monitoring in infants requiring soy-based formula (National Institute of Environmental Health Sciences, 2010); this precaution does not pertain to adults.

Inappropriate Use of Thyroid Hormones

Obesity

In euthyroid patients, hormone replacement doses are ineffective for weight reduction. Larger doses may produce serious or even life-threatening toxicity, particularly when given with anorexiants. Use of thyroid hormones for this indication is not justified (Pierce, 2012).

Infertility

Thyroid hormone therapy is *not* justified for the treatment of infertility in male or female patients by primary care providers unless the condition is accompanied by hypothyroidism.

Depression

Undiagnosed hypothyroidism can present as a depressive state. These patients can benefit with hormone correction. However, use of thyroid supplementation for chronic depressive states without abnormal TSH is not supported by evidence. Quality of life, perceived energy levels, and complaints of hypothyroid symptoms are not altered with other than standard doses of thyroid medications; therefore, practitioners are cautioned not to up dosages "to feel better" due to the chronic bone and potential CV issues.

◉ CLINICAL PEARL ◉

Levothyroxine tablets can be crushed and suspended in a small amount of formula or water for infants who cannot swallow whole tablets. For children who cannot swallow the intact tablet, it may be crushed and sprinkled over a small amount of food such as cooked cereal or applesauce. The suspension cannot be stored for any period of time. The tablet should be crushed, mixed to form a suspension, and given immediately.

Lithium preparations are antithyroid and can cause goiter. Patients can develop overt hypothyroidism. The goiter size will eventually return TSH levels toward normal. Treated patients should be monitored using T4 levels.

Rational Drug Selection

Pharmacokinetics

Levothyroxine (T4) is the drug of choice for thyroid replacement and suppression therapy because of its longer half-life. This means that it can safely be withheld for up to 2 weeks, if necessary, without altering the patient's thyroid status. Because T4 is converted to T3 in the body, use of this drug produces both hormones. Both levothyroxine and liothyronine (T3) have content stability. Liothyronine is 3 to 4 times more active than levothyroxine, and this greater potency increases the risk for cardiotoxicity. Levothyroxine should be used with patients who have cardiovascular disease. There are no randomized controlled studies comparing T4 with "natural" thyroid extracts (Cappola, 2012).

Cost

Generic forms of levothyroxine and the brands Levoxyl and Levothroid typically have similar low costs. Cost varies between Synthroid and the other brands and the generic form of levothyroxine and also between strengths of the same drug.

Ease of Monitoring

Levothyroxine is the easiest to monitor via TSH and free T4 laboratory measurements of thyroid function. The monitoring of therapy with these laboratory tests is more difficult with liothyronine due to its rapid T3 release. It will suppress TSH, but monitoring the more expensive T3 test is also required. Liotrix offers no clear benefit on any of these parameters.

Monitoring

Thyroid function is monitored with TSH and free T4 levels. Because of the negative feedback loop between TSH and thyroid hormones, elevations in TSH indicate insufficient thyroid hormone, and TSH levels below desired levels indicate excessive thyroid hormone. TSH and free T4 levels are checked initially and at 6 weeks after the first adjustment. Recheck the levels 4 to 6 months after achieving the target dose. Remember that steady state must be present to reliable values; steady state takes 4 to 6 weeks to be achieved. Once the adult primary hypothyroid patient is stable on an appropriate dose, TSH can be checked only annually; serum T4 measurements are unreliable for monitoring levothyroxine dosing. The exception is for secondary hypothyroidism. In that case, TSH is typically suppressed and the T4 is used to regulate dosing. See Chapter 41 for additional thyroid disease care.

Infants must be checked every 1 to 2 months. Children should be monitored every 3 to 6 months, especially during growth spurts. Age-based normal values from a consistently used ordering laboratory should be used for dose adjustments.

Diagnostic TSH levels (0.5 to 5.0 mU/L) are not the same as therapeutic levels. Newest TSH levels for maintaining dosing have been revised to be 0.3 to 3.0 mU/L. Laboratory work-ups plus patient symptomology are used to find the right dosing, with most patients best maintained between 1.0 and 2.5 mU/L. Hormone overreplacement (low TSH with normal T4 and T3) results in a subclinical hyperthyroidism. Dangers include bone thinning and cardiac irregularities with a 24% increase risk of CV death and all-cause mortality (Selmer et al, 2013).

Patient Education

Administration

Thyroid hormones are taken as a single daily dose in the morning before breakfast to prevent insomnia. Taking levothyroxine on an empty stomach enhances absorption. Other types may be taken without regard to food. If a dose is missed, it may be taken that same day as soon as it is remembered. If more than three doses are missed, the health-care provider should be informed.

Caution patients not to change brands of thyroid preparation. If brands are switched to generics, titrating of doses over several months may be required. The additional costs of laboratory tests may offset any cost savings from selecting another manufacturer.

Although some health food stores may sell desiccated thyroid preparations OTC at a lower cost, these formulations do not have consistent amounts of thyroid hormone in them and should not be substituted for the FDA-approved prescribed

drug (Cappola, 2012). The serum fluctuations are more likely to cause cardiac symptoms than are the synthetic versions. Liquid formulations from compounding pharmacies are not FDA-supervised. They do not have the same shelf-life as tablets (Cappola, 2012).

Brand-name manufacturers have color-coded the tablets to assist in identification of nonstandard dosing divisions. These unusual dosing levels (i.e., 88 or 112 mcg) require careful attention. These shortened dosing intervals facilitate intermediate dosing levels that can eliminate the need for pill splitting. The potential confusion with unusual dosing formulations is compounded by most doses coming in micrograms, not milligrams. Care must be taken in writing prescriptions to avoid dosing errors, for example, 100 mcg = 0.1 mg and 75 mcg = 0.075 mg.

Adverse Drug Reactions

Teach the patient how to measure pulse rate. If the pulse rate is greater than 100 beats per minute at rest, the dose should be withheld and the health-care provider notified. This may indicate excessive amounts of hormone. Other signs or symptoms that require notification include nervousness, chest pain, hypertension and unexplained weight loss of more than 2 lb in 1 week. Extreme fatigue may indicate inadequate dosing.

Some children on thyroid hormone therapy may experience partial hair loss. This is usually temporary, but parents and children should be informed that it may happen. Elders are at higher risk of developing atrial fib; therefore, patients at higher risk for this issue might be more safely maintained at levels at the higher end of normal.

Lifestyle Management

Thyroid disorders are usually chronic illnesses managed with self-monitoring of symptoms as well as drug therapy. Emphasize the importance of keeping follow-up appointments for evaluation of thyroid function. For children, evaluation of physical and psychomotor growth and development is also central to their management. Explain to the patient that replacement therapy must be taken for life (except in transient cases). The drug will treat the disorder, but not cure it. Further patient teaching related to management of thyroid disorders is discussed in Chapter 41. Patients should be cautioned not to take "thyroid health" OTC supplements as they are potential sources of exogenous hormone, iodine, or kelp products that can counter the effectiveness of the prescription.

ANTITHYROID AGENTS

Antithyroid agents function by either inhibiting the synthesis of thyroid hormones or destroying thyroid gland tissue. They are used to treat hyperthyroidism. Hyperthyroidism, also known as *thyrotoxicosis,* occurs when there is a breakdown in the feedback loop and the body's tissues are exposed to excessive levels of thyroid hormone. The cause of this excessive secretion varies, with the most common cause an autoimmune disorder called Graves' disease. The hyperfunction of the thyroid gland leads to suppression of TSH and TRH.

Hyperfunction of the thyroid gland results in a dramatic increase in iodine uptake and thyroid gland metabolism. A disproportionate increase in T3 production is combined with a decreased concentration of TBg so that increased circulating levels of thyroid hormone are seen. Severe levels may lead to thyroid storm, a life-threatening situation not covered in this chapter.

Regardless of the etiology of hyperthyroidism, the clinical features are attributable to metabolic effects of increased circulating levels of thyroid hormone. These effects include heat intolerance and increased sensitivity to stimulation of the sympathetic division of the autonomic nervous system. Table 41-3 (Chapter 41) shows the most common systemic effects of hyperthyroidism and outlines the management of hyperthyroidism.

The two drugs used in the outpatient setting to treat hyperthyroidism are propylthiouracil and methimazole, referenced in the literature as the thionamides or thioureas. Radioactive iodine 131 (I[131]) is prescribed and administered by specialists. Nonradioactive iodine solutions can also be used to suppress thyroid levels.

Pharmacodynamics

Propylthiouracil and methimazole inhibit the synthesis of thyroid hormones. They do not inactivate existing thyroxine and tri-iodothyronine that are stored in the thyroid gland or circulating in the blood, nor do they interfere with the effectiveness of exogenous thyroid hormones. Propylthiouracil partially inhibits the peripheral conversion of T4 to T3. Both drugs are concentrated in the thyroid gland; however, neither of these drugs treats the underlying pathology in hyperthyroidism.

Iodine tablets and solutions (SSKI or Lugol's) are no longer first-line medications; however, they have a role in pre-operative thyroid cancer care, in thyroid storm, and in individuals requiring persistent thyroid suppression if first-line care does not achieve desired outcomes. A bolus increase in iodine intake can have a suppressive effect on normal hormone synthesis for up to 10 days (longer in those previously receiving I[131]). This suppression is the basis for iodine use in cases of radiation bomb or reactor accidents, a topic beyond the scope of this text. The reader is referred to http://www.fda.gov for dosing recommendations at the time of such an incident.

I[131], like other iodine substances, is preferentially taken up by the thyroid gland via the sodium/iodine symptorter. Agents that affect any iodine uptake include cigarette smoking and perchlorate, a possible water contaminant. I[131] in subtherapeutic doses can be used to help diagnose whether thyroid masses localize uptake of iodine before or after ablation therapy. Full doses are given to cancer patients postthyroidectomy to continue eradication of abnormal tissue. Because thyroid cells preferentially take up iodine molecules, the impact is mostly limited to thyroid tissue. Controversy exists whether long-term outcomes of survival or recurrence are altered for patients with low-risk masses. The endocrine team makes the decision for use.

Pharmacokinetics

Absorption and Distribution

Propylthiouracil is rapidly absorbed after oral administration, reaching a peak serum level within 1 hour (Table 21-33). This drug is highly protein bound (75% to 80%) and concentrates in the thyroid gland. Concentrations in breast milk are low. It crosses the placenta in low concentrations. Currently it is used only in adults (FDA, 2009).

Methimazole is completely absorbed after oral administration but at variable rates. This drug is not protein bound and also concentrates in the thyroid gland. Concentrations in breast milk are high. It readily crosses the placenta in high concentrations and is associated with birth defects in early pregnancy (Bahn et al, 2011; FDA, 2010).

I[131] comes in capsules and solutions that must be prepared in special nuclear isotope pharmacies. It is rapidly absorbed by the thyroid, even faster under autoimmune conditions. I[131] uptake by thyroid tissues is facilitated by following a low-iodine diet for a week prior to scanning. Research has not established optimal doses, but higher levels have been associated with phenomena wherein thyroid tissues are "stunned" and do not absorb as much isotope. This is being investigated, as is a lesser "stun" factor with different iodine isotopes (McDougall & Iaguru, 2011; Norden, Larsson, & Tedelind, 2007). The higher doses, however, have better, longer-term results.

I[131] can be the initial therapy but frequently is administered after the thionamides have returned the patient to a

Table 21–33 ✚ Pharmacokinetics: Antithyroid Drugs

Drug	Onset*	Peak*	Duration*	Bioavailability	Protein Binding	Placental Transport and Breast Milk Levels	Half-Life	Excretion
Methimazole	1 wk	4–10 wk	Weeks	80%–95%	0%	High	6–13 h	Less than 10% in urine
Propylthiouracil	10–21 d	6–10 wk	Weeks	80%–95%	75%–80%	Low	1–2 h	35% in urine

*Effect on thyroid function.

near euthyroid state. Pretreatment with methimazole may increase the success of sustained good outcomes and decreases the possible transient spike in hyperthyroid symptoms at the onset of therapy. Propylthiouracil is associated with more cases of radiation therapy failures (Ross, 2012b). Elders and those with cardiovascular disease are more vulnerable to these spike effects. Pretreatment is stopped 6 days prior to the isotope dosing. Ablation of thyroid tissue is achieved with one dose 80% of the time.

Metabolism and Excretion

Propylthiouracil is completely metabolized by the liver with a significant first-pass effect. Methimazole is mostly metabolized by the liver, but some drug (10%) is excreted unchanged in the urine. Both drugs have a short half-life, but this has little influence on the duration of antithyroid action or the dosing intervals because they are concentrated in the thyroid gland.

Pharmacotherapeutics

Precautions and Contraindications

Pregnancy creates a serious cautionary condition for the use of antithyroid drugs. I^{131} is contraindicated (Category X) due to its impact on the infant when it crosses the placenta and into breast milk (Bahn et al, 2011). Methimazole is associated with birth defects, leaving propylthiouracil as the option for early pregnancy when it is clinically necessary to administer an antithyroid drug. Propylthiouracil and methimazole cross the placenta and can induce goiter and even cretinism in the fetus. Pregnancy typically reduces Graves' disease symptoms, so dosing is lower than normal and drops as the pregnancy advances (Bahn et al, 2011). The newborn should be tested at birth.

Adverse Drug Reactions

The most common serious adverse reaction to therapy with the thionamides is agranulocytosis and possible aplastic anemia. This risk is higher for patients who already have decreased bone marrow reserve, for those older than 40 years, and for those receiving more than 40 mg/day. These drugs must be discontinued, should this adverse reaction occur. It is important to remember that about 10% of patients with untreated hyperthyroidism have leukopenia (WBC count less than 4,000/mm^3), often with related granulocytopenia.

Drug-induced hepatitis and abnormal hair loss may occur with either drug. The FDA (2010b) issued a Black-Box Warning concerning propylthiouracil and liver failure, so it should be reserved for those patients where surgery or methimazole is not appropriate. Use in pediatric patients is restricted unless there is a methimazole allergy (FDA, 2009). Less serious and less frequent adverse reactions to both thioamides include drowsiness, headache, paresthesias, vertigo, diarrhea, nausea, arthralgia, and a pruritic skin rash. The nausea and skin rash are more common with propylthiouracil, but there is an element of cross-sensitivity with metimazole.

I^{131} is considered safe for outpatient therapy. There can be localized pain and edema for 2 to 3 weeks if thionamides were not used prior to treatment. Short-dose corticosteroids help alleviate it. Precautions about household contacts are covered in Chapter 41. Dosing for thyroid cancer is higher than it is for hyperthyroidism therapy. Controversies exist over long-term (40-year) minimal increases in post-therapy malignancies. Many patients complain of dry mouth. Use of lemon candies within the first 24 hours remains contentious but is considered appropriate thereafter. Iodine-free laxatives can be used to purge residual radioactive activity from the colon if normal bowel movements do not occur within the first day. Body or blood dosimetry is not done except for those with distant metastasis.

Drug Interactions

Any drugs that produce bone marrow depression have an additive effect with antithyroid drugs (Table 21-34). Additive antithyroid effects occur with lithium, potassium iodide, or sodium iodide given with propylthiouracil. Potassium iodide and amiodarone decrease antithyroid effects when given with methimazole. The risk of agranulocytosis is increased with concurrent administration of phenothiazines with both thioamines. The anticoagulant activity of warfarin may be potentiated by the anti–vitamin K activity attributed to propylthiouracil.

Table 21–34 ▦ Drug Interactions With Antithyroid Drugs

Drug	Interacting Drug	Possible Effect	Implications
Methimazole, propylthiouracil	Any drug that produces bone marrow depression	Additive bone marrow depression	Monitor white blood cell counts with differential; dosage adjustments or discontinuance of one of the drugs may be needed.
Propylthiouracil	Lithium, potassium iodide, warfarin	Additive antithyroid effects Anticoagulant effects potentiated	Avoid concurrent administration. Monitor PT/INR closely.
Methimazole	Potassium iodide, amiodarone	Decreased antithyroid effects	Avoid concurrent administration.
Methimazole, propylthiouracil	Phenothiazines	Increased risk for agranulocytosis	Avoid concurrent administration.

INR = international normalized ratio; PT = prothrombin time.

Patients treated with I[131] and later treated with amiodarone may develop hypothyroidism, sometimes acutely. This is in contrast to the amiodarone-induced hyperthyroid effects found in most other circumstances (Ross, 2012a).

Clinical Use and Dosing

Hyperthyroidism/Graves' Disease

Any of the antithyroid drugs may be used in adults. Propylthiouracil is available in 50 mg tablets. Standard dosing varies from 150 to 300 mg daily. Because of its short half-life, the dose is divided and taken 3 times daily. Methimazole comes in 5, 10 and 20 mg tablets. Dosing is usually started at 10 to 15 mg daily. Methimazole works faster than propylthiouracil. Low doses are as efficacious as higher doses over time except when treating severe cases and enlarged goiters. For moderate disease the methimazole dose is 30 to 40 mg/d and for severe disease the dose is 60 mg/d. Patients with severe hyperthyroidism may have initial 300 to 900 mg/d doses of propothiuriacil depending on the severity of the disease. After lab values normalize, maintenance doses are 100 to 150 mg/d. Treatment is for 6 to 18 months, with most patients being treated for 1 year (Table 21-35).

Toxic Goiter

Patients with toxic goiter require higher doses of antithyroid drugs. Methimazole is initiated at a dose of 60 mg/d divided into three equal doses given 8 hours apart. Propylthiouracil is initiated with 600 to 900 mg/d in three equally divided doses given 8 hours apart. Maintenance doses are the same as for hyperthyroidism. Some treatment regimens give either medication for 1 month to "calm" the thyroid and then administer a dose of radioactive iodine.

Rational Drug Selection

Pregnancy and Lactation

Because the amount of drug that crosses the placenta is lower with propylthiouracil, the lowest effective dose of this drug is selected if one must be used. In many pregnant women, the thyroid dysfunction diminishes as the pregnancy continues, so the dose can be reduced. In some cases, the drug can be withdrawn 2 to 3 weeks prior to delivery. Postpartum patients receiving antithyroid drugs should not nurse their infants. If it is necessary, however, propylthiouracil is the preferred drug.

Cost

There is a significant difference in cost between methimazole and propylthiouracil. Unless the provider is willing to try once-daily dosing and sees this as an advantage, propylthiouracil is about 10% of the cost of methimazole. The cost of I[131] runs into thousands of dollars, with additional charges for hospital services, scanning requirements, and special handling. Costs for simple iodine (SKKI or Lugol's) are extremely low.

Monitoring

TSH and free T4 levels are evaluated prior to beginning therapy and whenever symptoms recur, whenever dosages are adjusted, and every 2 to 3 months throughout therapy. TSH levels may be misleading, especially early in therapy. T4 and T3 levels are monitored with the thionamides because the T3 may stay high even though the T4 returns to a normal baseline. Once TSH is back to normal, monitoring of T3 is no longer necessary. Overt symptoms typically resolve weeks before laboratory values stabilize. If the hyperthyroid state has been prolonged, the pituitary axis may not become rebalanced for months (Ross, 2012b). In addition to laboratory assessment, both the provider and the patient should regularly assess for signs and symptoms of hyperthyroidism (too low a dose) or hypothyroidism (too high a dose).

The majority of patients receiving antithyroid medication will develop hypothyroidism over time. Recurrent hyperthyroidism is more likely in smokers and those who do not remain euthyroid for more than 6 months. Therefore, monitoring TSH levels after therapy is completed becomes a long-term primary care responsibility (Bahn et al, 2011).

To monitor for the risk for agranulocytosis, a complete blood count, including white blood cell count and differential, is done prior to initiating therapy. This adverse reaction may develop rapidly, usually within the first 2 months of therapy. During that time, both the provider and the patient should be especially vigilant. It is more common in persons older than 40 years and those who are receiving more than 40 mg/d. Only if symptoms suggestive of this disorder occur should it be monitored after the initial period (Ross, 2012b).

Drug-induced hepatitis has become a concern. Liver function tests should be done prior to any thioamide therapy, especially if there are any indications of hepatic issues or a

Table 21–35 ⟨⟩ Dosage Schedule of Antithyroid Drugs

Drug	Indication	Dosage Form	Initial Dose	Maintenance Dose
Methimazole (G)(Tapazole)	TSH suppression	5 mg (scored) tablet 10 mg (scored) tablet 15 mg tablet 20 mg tablet	*Adults:* 10–15 mg/d *Pediatric:* per specialist	Moderate disease: 30–40 mg/d
	Severe disease			60 mg/daily
Propylthiouracil (G)	TSH suppression	50 mg tablet	*Adults:* 150 mg/d in three divided doses *Pediatric:* per specialist	150–300 mg daily in three divided doses Severe disease: 300–900 mg/d

history of liver impairment, with monitoring during and 6 months after treatment (FDA, 2009).

Patient Education

Administration

If the drug is to be taken every 8 hours, it is not necessary to awaken at night to take the drug at exactly 8-hour intervals because the drug is concentrated in thyroid tissue. If a dose is missed, the patient should take it as soon as remembered. If it is almost time for the next dose, the two doses may be taken together. The health-care provider should be notified if several doses are missed so that an assessment of thyroid function can be made.

Dietary sources of iodine should be discussed and reduced or eliminated because they interfere with the action of the antithyroid drugs. Many OTC drugs, especially those used to treat colds, have iodine in them. Teach the patient to read the labels.

Adverse Reactions

The most common potential adverse reaction related to the antithyroid medications is agranulocytosis. Patients are taught to report sore throat, fever, chills, rash, and unusual bleeding or bruising, as well as the reasons for them.

Another potential adverse reaction is drug-induced hepatitis. Patients are also taught to report headache, malaise, weakness, and yellowing of the eyes or skin and the reasons for them. The patient should be told that any abnormal hair loss is probably temporary.

I^{131} may have a slight overall mortality from cardiovascular deaths in patient cohorts followed for over 40 years. The increased risk of cerebrovascular accident is probably due to the effects of hyperthyroidism, not the radiation itself. Any suppressed testicular function returns to normal quickly. Any link to an increased risk of ophthalmopathy already associated with Graves' disease is controversial but probably unfounded.

Lifestyle Management

Hyperthyroidism and goiter are often chronic illnesses managed with self-monitoring of symptoms as well as drug therapy. Emphasize the importance of keeping follow-up appointments for evaluation of thyroid function. For children, evaluation of physical and psychomotor growth and development is also central to their management. Explain to the patient that antithyroid drug therapy will be required for 6 to 18 months and perhaps longer, because recurrence of hyperthyroidism happens when lower doses are used. Such is the case in children. Further patient teaching related to management of thyroid disorders is discussed in Chapter 41.

AROMATASE INHIBITORS

The aromatase inhibitors are typically thought of as part of the arsenal against breast cancer. Their actions within the hormone system places them within the category of endocrine medications. They can be used in both men and women.

Pharmacodynamics

Aromatase is a naturally occurring enzyme involved with estrogen synthesis; it is sometimes called estrogen synthetase or synthase in the classic literature. It is one enzyme in the complex P450 cytochrome system that plays a role in steroid hormone balance to include sexual maturity, and health of tissues of the genitals, brain, and fatty tissues; though it is found in many tissues, it has strong impact in the estrogen-sensitive tissues of the uterus, adrenal glands, placenta, gonads, and breast (McCance & Huether, 2014). Aromatase plays a critical role in estrogen generation from androgen building blocks. Testosterone is changed to estradiol and androstenedion becomes estrone through a complex series of steps. It has many other major functions to include a role in determination of gender expression in the the developing embryo and neuroprotection during brain injury.

Inhibition of the enzyme is the major role of the class of aromatase inhibitors. The drugs approved for use in post-breast cancer treatment in women are the primary focus of this section. Men can take the medications if they have estrogen sensitive breast cancer or to try to resolve gynecomastia or fertility issues associated with an imbalance of testosterone to estradiol ratio.

Pharmacokinetics

Anastrazole (Arimidex) and letrozole (Femara) are non-steroidal medications that create a reduction in circulating estrogens. Exemestane (Aromasin) is classified as a steroidal agent. All are oral medications. Anastrazole and letrozole are well absorbed with or without food; exemestane has increased circulating levels if taken after a fatty meal and shifts from a 2 hour time peak to 5 hours. Half-life of anastrazole is 24 hours, exemestane is 50 hours, and letrozole is 2 days. Fecal elimination accounts for 90% of anastrazole after metabolism. Exemestane has a 45% urine elimination with the rest in the feces. Ninety percent of letrozole is excreted in the urine.

Renal dosing is not required of any of three agents discussed. Liver impairment Child-Pugh class C requires reducing doses of letrozole; dosing may not have been tested for the other two medications in pre-release studies (Table 21-36).

Pharmacotherapeutics

Aromatase inhibitors are used as adjuvant therapy in estrogen receptor positive postmenopausal breast cancer patients. They are added to the plan after 3 to 5 years of tamoxifen therapy and continued for at least 5 years. They are also used as first-line treatment in cases of advanced or metastatic cancer. There are unlabeled uses for ovarian cancer and to stimulate ovulation in anovulatory women done within specialty care.

The aromatase inhibitors are oral agents taken once daily. Anastrazole is given as a 1 mg tablet, exemestane is a 25 mg tablet, and letrozole comes in a 2.5 mg dose. There is no increasing in dosage over time. All forms of these medications

Table 21–36 ⚙ **Pharmacokinetics of Aromatase Inhibitors**

Drug	Site of Metabolism	Peak	Protein Binding	Half-Life (in hours)	Elimination
Exemestane	Liver	1.2 h	90%	24	Urine 42%; feces 42%
Anastrozole	Liver	2 h without food; 5 h with food	40%	50	80% liver; 20% renal
Letrozole	Liver	2–6 wk for steady state	weak	48	90% renal

are considered hazardous agents that require special handling and disposal. All are contraindicated in pregnancy and breast feeding (Table 21-37).

Adverse Drug Reactions

Adverse effects for the drug class include various pain syndromes, vertigo, insomnia resulting in daytime sleepiness and confusion, increased risk of blood clots, and hair loss. A key concern is the loss of bone mass. Bone loss can be significant when considering the concurrent osteoporotic risks of postmenopause. Closer monitoring is required. All patients should be on calcium and vitamin D supplementation. A relative leukopenia can occur, but the incidence of viral and bacteria infections is not considered greater than matched groups (about 10%). Hypertension occurs in 10% of patients. A life-threatening increase in blood clotting can result in MI, stroke, or pulmonary embolus. Hot flashes can be intense.

Drug Interactions

Drug interactions vary by agent, but none should be taken with tamoxifen or an estrogen product. Anastrazole cannot be taken with pimozide. Both anastrazole and letrazole will decrease the effect of digoxin and vitamin K antagonists.

Exemestane should not be taken with axtinib or simeprevir. It will decrease the effect of aripiprazole and saxagliptin and increase the effect of methadone and vitamin K antagonists. Letrozole cannot be taken with tegafur (Table 21-38).

Education and Lifestyle Management

Patient education follows the standards for how to take the medication, when to report adverse effects, and the need for close monitoring of LFT labs. Frequent reports of weakness should be countered by encouragement for exercise and pacing of activities. Advice on how to recognize development of DVT, stroke, and MI is important. Patients should be encouraged to discuss issues of pain and fatigue with the provider prior to just stopping the medications. Switching from one drug in the class to another has sometimes proven to be an effective solution to lower the symptoms to a more tolerable level. Providers and patients need to evaluate whether the degree of fatigue and insomnia is being accelerated by the expected concurrent depressive syndrome experienced by all oncology patients or a possible alteration in thyroid function. Unlike Tamoxifen, the SSRI medications do not appear to decrease the effectiveness of the aromatase inhibitors.

Table 21–37 ⚙ **Dosing and Indications Aromatase Inhibitors**

Drug	Indication	Dosage Form	Initial Dose	Maintenance Dose
Anastrazole (Armidex)	Postmenopausal breast cancer inhibition	1mg tablet	1mg ; no change for most renal patients or elders	Usually taken for 5 yr after tamoxifen, but can be first line medication as well and extend beyond 5 yr of use.
Letrozole (Femara)	Postmenopausal breast cancer inhibition	2.5 mg tablets	2.5 mg; no renal dosing or change for elders	As above
Exemestabe (Aromasin)	Postmenopausal breast cancer inhibition	25 mg tablets	25 mg	As above
Ospemifene (Osphena)	Vaginal atrophy, dyspareunia	60 mg tablets	60 mg for moderate or severe issues	
Bazedoxifene & conjugated estrogen (Duavee)	Hot flashes and osteoporosis	20 mg–0.45 mg tablets	One tablet daily for both indications	Use for shortest duration possible to minimize estrogen-related risks

Table 21–38 ⚏ Drug interactions of Aromatase Inhibitors

Drug	Interacting Drug	Possible Effect	Implications
Anastrozole (Arimidex); Exemestane (Aromasin); Letrozole (Femara)	Estrogen products	Defeats purpose of both	Avoid coadminstration
Exemestane (Aromasin)	Rifampin	Decreases levels and effectiveness	May need to increase dose; consult oncology
	Phenytoin	Decreases levels and effectiveness	May need to increase dose; consult neurology
Letrozole (Femara)	Tamoxifen	Reduces plasma levels of letrozole	Not a combination medication
Conjugated estrogens + bazedoxifene (Duavee)	No studies conducted—see estrogen. For bazedoxifene: Rifampin, phenobarb, carbamazepine, phenytoin	No known CYP interactions with bazedoxifene UGT interactions increase metabolism of bazadoxifene	May need additional uterine protection/monitoring.

UGT = uridine diphosphate glucuronosyltransferase in the gut.

REFERENCES

Access Pharmacy. (2013). McGraw Hill Education. Retrieved from www.accesspharmacy.com

Adachi, J. (2013). Fracture patterns with the use of SSRI, Proton-Pump Inhibitors, and Glucocorticoids in a large international observational study: GLOW. Presentation American Society for Bone and Mineral Research (ASBMR) 2013 Annual Meeting, Oct 4-7, 2013, Baltimore, MD. www.asbmr.org/education/2013-abstracts accessed 20 Jan 2015.

Agency for Healthcare Research and Quality (AHRQ). (2008). Comparative effectiveness, safety and indications of pre-mixed insulin analogues for adults with type 2 diabetes. Retrieved August 28, 2009, from http://effectivehealthcare.ahrq.org

Aldasouqui, S., & Reed, A. (2014). Pitfalls of insulin pump clocks: Technical glitches that may protent[sic] affect medical care in patients with diabetes. *Journal of Diabetes Science and Technology, 8*(16), 1215–1220.

American College of Obstetricians and Gynecologists (ACOG). (2010). *Thyroid disease in pregnancy* (ACOG Practice Bulletin No. 37. Bulletin originally published 2002; reaffirmed 2010). http://www.acog.org

American Diabetes Association. (2012, January). Standards of medical care in diabetes—2012. *Diabetes Care, 32*(Suppl. 1), 13–61.

Andrews, E. B., Gilsenan, A. W., Medkiff, K., Sherrill, B., Wu, Y., Mann, B. H. et al. (2012). The US postmarketing surveillance study of adult osteoscarcoma and teriparatide: Study design and findings from the first 7 years. *Journal of Bone Mineral Research, 27*(12), 2429–2437.

Bahn, R., Burch, H., Cooper, D., Garber, J., Creenlee, M., Klein, I., et al. (2011). Hyperthyroidism and other causes of thyroid toxicosis: Management guidelines of the American Thyroid Association and American Association of Clinical Endocrinologists. *Endocrine Practice, 17*(3), 457–520.

Bianchi, M., Colombo, C., Baroukh, A., Dubini, A., Lombardo, M., Quattrucci, S., et al. (2013). Treatment of low bone density in young people with cystic fibrosis: A multicenter, prospective, open-label observational study of calcium and calcifediol followed by a randomized placebo-controlled trial of alendronate. *Lancet Respiratory Medicine, 1*(5), 377–385.

Black, D., Kelly, M., Genant, M., Palermo, L., Eastell R., Bucci-Rechtweg, C., & HORIZON Pivotal Fracture Trial Steering Committee. (2010). Bisphosphonates and fractures of the subtrochanteric or diphyseal femur. *New England Journal of Medicine, 362*(19), 1761–1771.

Blonde, N., Dagogo-Jack, S., Banerji, M., Pratley, R., Marcellari, A., Braceras, R., et al. (2009, October). Comparison of vildagliptin and thiazolidinedione as add-on therapy in patients inadequately controlled with metformin: Results of the GALIANT trial—a primary care, type 2 diabetes study. *Diabetes, Obesity and Metabolism, 11*(10), 978–986.

Bloomgarden, Z. (2003). American Association of Clinical Endocrinologists (AACE) consensus conference on insulin resistance syndrome. *Diabetes Care, 26*(4), 1297–1303.

Bolli, G., Dotta, F., Colin, L., Minic, B., & Goodman, M. (2009). Comparison of vildagliptin and pioglitazone in patients with type 2 diabetes inadequately controlled with metformin. *Diabetes, Obesity and Metabolism, 11*(6), 589–595.

Buse, J., Wolffenbuttel, B., Herman, W., Shermonsky, N., Jiang, H., Fahrbach, J., et al. (2009). Durability of basal versus lispro mix 75/25 insulin efficacy (DURABLE) trial 24 week results. *Diabetes Care, 32*(6), 1007–1013.

Cappola, A. (2012, Oct). Alternative therapies for thyroid disease examined. *Endocrine Today.* Report on abstract presented at: The American Thyroid Association 82nd Annual Meeting Sept 19–23, 2012, Quebec City, QE.

Cherney, D., Perkins, B., Soleymanlou, N., Maione, M., Laei, V., Lee, A, et al. (2014). Renal hemodynamics effect of sodium-glucose cotransporter 2 inhibition in patinets[sic] with type 1 diabetes mellitus. *Circulation, 129*(5), 587–597.

Chevier, J. Gumier, R., Bradman, A., Holland, N, Calefat, A., Eskenazi, B., et al. (2013). Maternal urinary bisphenol A during pregnancy and maternal and neonatal thyroid function in the CHAMACOS study. *Environmental Health Perspectives, 121*(1), 138–144.

Cystic Fibrosis Foundation [CFF]. (2009). CFF evidence-based guidelines for management of infants with cystic fibrosis. *Journal of Pediatrics, 155*(6), S73–S93.

Cystic Fibrosis Foundation (2014). About Cystic Fibrosis. Retrieved from http://www.cff.org/AboutCF/

DeGroot, L., Abalovich, M., Alexander, E., Amino, N., Barbour, L., Cobin, R., et al. (2012). Mangement[sic] of thyroid dysfunction during pregnancy and postpartum: An Endocrine Society clinical practice guideline. *Journal of Clinical Endocrinology and Metabolism, 97*(8), 2543–2565.

Diabetes Control and Complications Trial Research Group. (1993). The effect of intensive treatment of diabetes on the development and progression of long-term complications in insulin-dependent diabetes mellitus. *New England Journal of Medicine, 329*(14), 977–986.

Diabetes Prevention Program Research Group. J (2002). Reduction in the incidence of type 2 diabetes with lifestyle intervention or metformin. *New England Journal of Medicine, 346*(6), 393–403.

Drucker, D., & Nauck, M. (2006). The incretin system: Glucagon-like peptide-1 receptor agonists and dipeptidyl peptidase-4 inhibitors in type 2 diabetes. *The Lancet, 368*(9548), 1696–1705.

Drug facts and comparisons (DF & C). (2011). St. Louis, MO: Wolters Kluwer Health.

Duncan, A. (2012). Hyperglycemia and perioperative glucose management. *Current Pharmaceutical Design, 18*(38), 6295–6203.

Duntas, L., Orgiazzi, J., & Brabant, G. (2011). The interface between thyroid and diabetes mellitus. *Clinical Endocrinology, 75*(1), 1–9.

Feig, D. S., & Moses, R. G. (2011). Metformin therapy during pregnancy: Good for the goose and good for the gosling too? *Diabetes Care, 34*(10), 2329–2330.

Fieker, A., Philpott, J., & Armand, M. (2011). Enzyme replacement therapy for pancreatic insufficiency: Present and future. *Clincial[sic] and Experimental Gastroenterology, 4*(4), 55–73.

Fleisha, K., Jolly, A., Venkata, U., Norman, R., Saxena, D., & Glickman, R. (2013). Osteonecrosis of the jaw onset times are based on the route of bisphosphonate therapy. *Journal of Oral & Maxillofacial Surgery, 71*(3), 513–519.

Fujimoto, K. (2013). Risk for macular edema increased with pioglitazone in T2DM. Presentation at European Association for the Study of Diabetes 2013 Barcelona, Spain 27 SEP, 2013.

Garber, J., Cobin, R., Gharib, H., Hennessey, J., Klein, I., Mechanick, J., et al. (2012). Clinical practice guidelines for hypothyroidism in adults: Co-sponsored by the American Association of Clinical Endocrinologists and the American Thyroid Association. *Endocrine Practice, 18*(6), 988–1028.

Grey, A., Garg, S., Dray, M., Purvis, L., Horne, A., Callon, K., et al. (2013). Low dose fluoride in postmeopausal women: A randominzed controlled trial. *Journal of Clinical Endocrinology and Metabolism,* doi: 10.1210/jc2012-4062.

Grozinski-Glasberg, S., Fraser, A., Nashshoni, E., Weizman, A., & Leibovici, L. (2006). Thyroine-triiodothyronine combination therapy versus thyroxine monotherapy for clinical hypothyroidism: Meta-analysis of randomized controlled trails. *Journal of Clinical Endocrinology and Metabolism, 91*(7), 2592–2599.

Hellier, S., & Ross, C. (2012). Long-term bisphosphonate therapy: Possible link to rare femur fracture. *American Journal for Nurse Practitioners, 16* (9/10), 12–19.

Hyland, K., Arnold, A., Lee, J., & Cappola, A. (2013). Persistent subclinical hypothyroidism and CV risk in the elderly: The CV Health Study. *Journal of Clinical Endocrinology and Metabolism, 98*(2), 533–540.

Institute for Clinical Systems Improvement (ICSI). (2011). *Diagnosis and treatment of osteoporosis.* Bloomington, MN: Author. http://www.ICSI.org/osteoporosis

International Osteoporosis Foundation (IOF). (2012). Facts and statistics about osteoporosis and its impact. http://www.iofbonehealth.org

Inzucchi, S. (2011). Diabetes facts and guidelines. Yale Diabetes Center. Retrieved from http://endocrinology.yale.edu/patient/50135_Yale%20National%20F.pdf

Inzucchi, S., Bergenstahl, R., Buse, J., Diamant, M., Ferrannini, E., Nauck, M., et al. (2012). Medical management of hyperglycemia in type 2 diabetes: A patient centered approach. Position statement of the American Diabetes Association and the European Association for the Study of Diabetes. *Diabetes Care, 35*(6), 1364–1369.

Inzucchi, S., Lipska, K., Mayo, H., Bailey, C., & McGuire, D. (2014). Metformin in patients with type 2 diabetes and kidney disease: A systematic review. *Journal of the American Medical Association, 312*(24), 2668–2675.

Janssen Pharmaceuticals, Inc. (2013). Invokana prescribing information. Retrieved from http://www.invokanahcp.com/prescribing-information.pdf

Katznelson, l., Atkinson, J., Cook, D., Ezzat, S, Hamrahian, A., & Miller, K. (2011). American association of clinical endocrinologists (AACE) medical guidelines for clinical practice for the diagnosis and treatment of acromegaly—2001 update. *Endocrine Practice, 17*(Suppl 4), 1–44.

Kilpatrick, E., Rigby, A., & Atkin, S. (2008). A1C variability and the risk of microvascular complications in type 1 diabetes: Data from the Diabetes Control and Complications Trial. *Diabetes Care, 31*(11), 2198–2202.

Kim, S., Kim, M., Cadarette, S., & Solomon, D. (2010). Bisphonates and the risk of afib: A meta-analysis. *Arthritis Research and Therapy, 12*(1), R30. doi: 10.1186/ar2938.

Kirkman, M., Briscoe, V., Clark, N., Flores, H., Haas, L., Halter, J., et al. (2012). Diabetes in older adults. Consensus report of the American Diabetes Association and the American Geriatrics Society. *Diabetes Care, 35*(12), 2650–2664.

Kumar, P., & Khan, K. (2012). Effects of metformin use in pregnant patients with polycystic ovary syndrome. *Journal of Human Reproductive Science, 5*(2), 168–169.

Lilly USA, LLC [Eli Lilly and Company]. (2012). Forteo (teriparatide fDNA) Product Inset. Indianapolis, IN. www.forteo.com

McCance, K., & Huether, S. (2014). *Pathophysiology: The biological basis for disease in adults and children* (7th ed.). St. Louis, MO: Mosby.

McClung, M., Harris, S., Miller, P., Bauer, D., Davison, K., Dian, L., et al. (2013). Bisphosponate therapy for osteoporosis: Benefits, risks, and drug holiday. *American Journal of Medicine, 126* (1), 13–20.

McDougall, I., & Iaguru, A. (2011). Thyroid stunning: Fact or fiction? *Seminars in Nuclear Medicine, 41*(2), 105–112.

Marfella, R., Barbieri, M., Grella, R., Rizzo, M., Nicoletti, G., & Paolisso, G. (2009, March 5). Effects of vildagliptin twice daily vs. sitagliptin once daily on 24-hour acute glucose fluctuation. *Journal of Diabetes and Its Complications, 24*(2), 79–83.

Medscape Reference Drugs, Diseases, and Procedures. (2013). Canagliflozin. Retrieved from http://reference.medscape.com/drug/invokana-canagliflozin-999811

Messina, M., & Redmond, G. (2006). Effects of soy protein and soybean isoflavones on thyroid function in healthy adults and thyroid patients: A review of the relevant literature. *Thyroid, 16*(3), 249–258.

Molitch, M., Clemmons, D., Malozowski, S., Merriam, G., & Vance, M. (2011). Evaluation and treatment of adult growth hormone deficiency: An Endocrine Society clinical practice guideline. *Journal of Clinical Endocrinology and Metabolism, 96*(6), 1587–1609.

Nathan, D., Buse, J., Davidson, M., Heine, R., Holman., R., Sherwin, R., et al. (2006). Medical management of hyperglycemia in type 2 diabetes: A consensus algorithm for the initiation and adjustment of therapy. A consensus statement of the American Diabetes Association and the European Association for the Study of Diabetes. *Diabetes Care, 29*(8), 1963–1972.

Nathan, D., Buse, J., Davidson, M., Ferrannini, E., Holman, R., Sherwin, R., et al. (2009). Medical management of hyperglycemia in type 2 diabetes: A consensus algorithm for the initiation and adjustment of therapy. A consensus statement of the American Diabetes Association and the European Association for the Study of Diabetes. *Diabetes Care, 32*(1), 193–203.

National Institute for Health and Clinical Excellence (NICE). (2010). TA188 Human growth hormone (somatropin) for the treatment of growth failure in children (review). http://guidance.nice.org.uk/TA188/Guidance/pdf/English

Norden, M., Larsson, F., & Tedelind, S. (2007). Down-regulation of the sodium iodide symporter explains I[131]-induced thyroid stunning. *Cancer Research (Baltimore), 67*(15), 7512–7517.

Olansky, L. (2010, Jan 1). Do incretin-based therapies cause acute pancreatitis? *Journal of Diabetes Science and Technology, 4*(1), 228–229.

Pierce, E. N. (2012, Oct). Thyroid hormones and obesity. *Current Opinion in Endocrinology, 19*(5), 408–413.

Regulatory Focus. (2013). NICE fails to recommend dapagliflozin for type 2 diabetes. Latest Regulatory News Update, posted Feb. 1, 2013. http://www.raps.org/focus-online/news/news-article-view/article/2804/nice-fails-to-recommend-dapagliflozin-for-type-2-diabetes.aspx

Rhee, C., Curhan, G., Alexander, E., Bhan, I., & Brunelli, S. (2013). Subclinical hypothyroidism and survival: The effects of heart failure and race. *Journal of Clinical Endocrinology and Metabolism, 98*(6), 2326–2336. doi: 10.1210/jc.2013–1039.

Rizzoli, R., Akesson, K., Boouxsein, M., Kanis J., Napoli, N., Papapoulos, S., et al. (2011). Subtrochanteric fractures after long-term treatment with bisphosphonates: A European Society on clinical and economic aspects of osteoporosis and osteoarthritis, and International Osteoporosis Foundation Working Group report. *Osteoporosis International, 22*(2), 373–390.

Rogel, A. (2012, 22 Mar). Treatment of growth hormone deficiency in children. *UpToDate.* Retrieved 6 Nov 2012, from http://www.uptodate.com

Rosen, H., & Drezner, M. (2012, 10 Oct). Overview of the management of osteoporosis in postmenopausal women. *UpTo Date.* Retrieved Nov 2012, from http://www.uptodate.com

Rosenstock, J., Hollander, P., Chevalier, S., & Iranmanesh, A., for the SERENADE Group. (2009). SERENADE: The study evaluating rimonabant efficacy in drug-naïve diabetic patients. Effects of monotherapy with rimonabant, the first CB1 receptor antagonist, on glycemic control, body weight, and lipid profile in drug-naïve type 2 diabetes. *Diabetes Care, 31*(11), 2169–2176.

Ross, D. (2012a, May 23). Amiodarone and thyroid dysfunction. *UpTo Date.* Retrieved 6 Nov 2012, from http://www.uptodate.com

Ross, D. (2012b, Jun 22). Pharmacology and toxicity of thionamides. *UpToDate.* Retrieved 6 Nov, 2012, from http://www.uptodate.com

Ross, J., Quigley, C., Cao, D., Feuillian, P., Kowal, K., & Chipman, J. (2011). Growth hormone plus childhood low-dose estrogen in Turner syndrome. *New England Journal of Medicine, 364*(13), 1230–1242.

Ruggiero, S., Dodson, T., Assall, L., Landesberg, R., Mari, R., & Mehrotra, B. (2009). American Association of Oral & Maxillofacial Surgeons position paper on bisphosphonate-related osteonecrosis of the jaws. *Journal of Oral and Maxillofacial Surgery, 67*(Supp. 1), 2–12.

Schernthaner, G., Gross, J., Rosenstock, J., Guaricso, M., Min, F., Yee, J., et al. (2013). Canagliflozin compared with sitagliptin for patients with type 2 diabetes who do not have adequate glycemic control with metformin plus sulfonylurea: A 52-week randomized trial. *Diabetes Care, 36* (Supp. 2), S155–S161.

Schweizer, A., Dejager, S., & Bosi, E. (2009). Comparison of vildagliptin and metformin monotherapy in elderly patients with type 2 diabetes: A 24-week, double-blind, randomized trial. *Diabetes, Obesity and Metabolism, 11*(8), 804–812.

Selmer, C., Olesen, J., Madsen, J., Faber, J., Hansen, P., Ledersen, O., et al. (2013). Subclinical hyperthyroidism and risk of cardiovascular and all-cause mortality. *European Endocrine Conference Abstracts,* 2013-4-01, Copenhagen, DK. doi: 10.1530/endoabs.32.OC3.6

Sharma, A., Chatterjee, S., Arbab-Zadeh, A., Goyal, S., Lichstein, E., & Ghosh, J. (2013). Risk of serious atrial fibrillation and stroke with use of bisphosphonates: Evidence from a meta-analysis. *Chest, 144*(4), 1311–1322.

Udell, J., Blatt, D., Braunwald, E., Cavender, M., Mosenzen, O., & Steg, P. (2014). Saxagliptin and cardiovascular outcomes in patients with type 2 diabetes mellitus and moderate or severe renal impairment: Observations from the SAVOR-TIMI 53 Trial. *Diabetes Care,* epub ahead of print 31 Dec, 2014 doi: w-2337/dc1-4-1850.

Umpierrez, G., Jones, S., Smiley, D., Mulligan, P., Keyler, T., Temponi, A., et al. (2009). Insulin analogs versus human insulin in the treatment of patients with diabetic ketoacidosis: A randomized controlled trial. *Diabetes Care, 32*(7), 1164–1169.

U.S. Food and Drug Administration [FDA]. (2003). Approval letter (for Serostim). http://www.accessdata.fda.gov/scripts/cder/drugsatfda/index.cfm

U.S. Food and Drug Administration [FDA]. (2009). *Propylthiouracil-induced liver failure.* http://www.fda.gov/Drugs/DrugSafety/PostmarketDrugSafety InformationforPatientsandProviders/ucm162701

U.S. Food and Drug Administration [FDA]. (2010a). *Safety update for osteoporosis drugs, bisphosphonates, and atypical fracutres.* http://www.fda .gov/Drugs/DrugSafety/PostmarketDrugSafetyInformationfor Patientsand Providers/ucm 229009.htm

U.S. Food and Drug Administration [FDA]. (2010b). *FDA drug safety communication: New boxed warning on severe liver injury with propylthiouracil.* Retrieved April 21, 2010, from http://www.fda.gov/Drugs/ DrugSafety/PostmarketDrugSafetyInformationfor PatientsandProviders/ ucm209023.htm

U.S. Food and Drug Administration [FDA]. (2010c). Approval of Egrifta (tesamorelin) to treat lipodystrophy. www.fda.gov/ucm233573.htm

U.S. Food and Drug Administration [FDA]. (2011a). *New contraindication and updated warning on kidney impairment for Reclast (zoledronic acid).* http://www.fda.gov/Drugs/DrugSafety/PostmarketDrugSafetyInformationforPatientsandProviders/ucm 270199.

U.S. Food and Drug Administration [FDA]. (2011b). *Safety review update of recombinant human growth hormone (somatropin) and possible increased risk of death.* http://www.fda.gov/Drugs/DrugSafety/Postmarket DrugSafetyInformationforPatientsandProviders/ucm 26585.

U.S. Food and Drug Administration [FDA]. (2012a). *FDA approves pancreatic enzyme replacement product.* http://www.fda.gov/Drugs/DrugSafety/ PostmarketDrugSafetyInformationforPatientsandProviders/ucm 204745.htm.

U.S. Food and Drug Administration [FDA]. (2012b). *Updated Q & A for healthcare professionals and the public: Use an approved pancreatic enzyme product (PEP.)* http://www.fda.gov/Drugs/DrugSafety/PostmarketDrug SafetyInformationforPatientsandProviders/ucm209023.htm

U.S. Food and Drug Administration [FDA]. (2013). FDA Press Release January 25, 2013. *FDA approves three new drug treatments for type 2 diabetes.* http://www.fda.gov/NewsEvents/Newsroom/PressAnnouncements/ucm3 36942.htm

Walsh, J., Ward, L., Burke, V., Bhagat, C., Shiels, L., Henley, D., et al. (2006). Small changes in thyroxine dosage do not produce measurable changes in hypothyroid symptoms, well-being, or quality of life: Results of a double-blind, randomized clinical trial. *Journal of Clinical Endocrinology & Metabolism, 91*(7), 2624–2630.

Watts, N., Bilezikian, J., Camacho, P., Greenspan, S., Harris, S., Hodgson, S., et al. (2010). American Association of Clinical Endocrinologists medical guidelines for clinical practice for the diagnosis and treatment of postmenopausal osteoporosis: Executive summary. *Endocrinology Practice, 16*(6), 1016–1019.

Whelen, A., Jurgens, T., Bowles, S., & Doyle, H. (2009). Efficacy of natural health products in treating osteoporosis: What is the quality of internet patient advice? *Annals of Pharmacotherapeutics, 43*(5), 899–907.

Williams, L., Padhikasahasram, B., Ahnendeni, B., Peterson, E., Wells, K., Gonzalez-Buchard, E., et al. (2014). Differing effects of metformin on glycemic control by race-ethnicity. *Journal of Clinical Endocrinology & Metabolism, 99*(9), 3160–3168.

White, N., Chase, P., Arslanian, S., Tamborlane, W., and for the 4030 Study Group. (2009, March). Comparison of glycemic variability associated with insulin glargine and intermediate-acting insulin when used as the basal component of multiple daily injections for adolescents with type 1 diabetes. *Diabetes Care, 32,* 387–393.

Yang, W., Liu, J., Shan, Z., Tian, H., Zhou, Z., & Ji, Q. (2014). Acarbose compared with metformin as intial therapy in patients with newly diagnosed type 2 diabetes. *The Lancet, Diabetes & Endocrinology, 2*(1) 46–55.

Zhang, J., Saag, K., & Curtis, J. (2011). Long-term safety concerns of antiresorptive therapy. *Rheumatic Disease Clinics of North America, 37*(3), 387–400

CHAPTER 22

DRUGS AFFECTING THE REPRODUCTIVE SYSTEM

Diana L Dewel

There are many medications that are prescribed for reproductive problems in both men and women. This chapter discusses androgens and antiandrogens, commonly prescribed for men, as well as appropriate prescribing of these medications for women. Prescribing of estrogens and progesterone, as well as their antagonists, is reviewed, as well as drugs for lactation and erectile dysfunction. Medications discussed in this chapter are limited to medications prescribed in primary care and gynecology and do not include medications prescribed in specialty endocrine or reproductive health care.

ANDROGENS AND ANTIANDROGENS

Testosterone is the primary male androgen. In many tissues, its activity depends on reduction to dihydrotesterone, which binds to cytosol-receptor proteins. The androgen-receptor complex is then transported to the nucleus of the cell, where it initiates transcription events and cellular changes. Endogenous androgens are responsible for the following:

- Normal growth, maturation, and maintenance of the male sex organs and secondary sexual characteristics
- The skeletal growth spurt in adolescence and for the termination of linear growth by fusion of the epiphyseal growth plate
- Activation of sebaceous glands, accounting for some cases of acne during puberty
- Enhancing production of erythropoietic stimulating factor, resulting in increased red blood cell production
- Playing a role in libido

A more detailed discussion of the roles and therapeutic uses of androgens is given in the Pharmacodynamics section.

The androgens—testosterone propionate (in oil, Depo-Testerone), testosterone enanthate (in oil, Delatestryl), testosterone cypionate (in oil, Depo-Testosterone), methyltestosterone (Android, Methitest, Testred, Virilon), testosterone gel (AndroGel 1%, AndroGel 1.62%, Axiron, Testim), flu-oxymesterone, transdermal testosterone (Testoderm, Androderm), and buccal testosterone (Striant)—have been used to treat disorders in both the male and female reproductive systems. Androgens are indicated for the symptomatic treatment of (1) deficiency states in males associated with hypogonadism and (2) in both sexes for disorders such as cancer and HIV. Androgen therapy has also been used to treat libido, endometriosis, and postmenopausal symptoms in women. However, there is limited evidence supporting the correlation of testosterone levels and symptom reduction in women. Androgens have also been used illicitly to enhance athletic performance and increase muscle mass.

Antiandrogens fall into several different categories. Androgen hormone inhibitors in this section are also known as 5-alpha-reductase inhibitors. These enzyme inhibitors block the conversion of testosterone to dihydrotesterone. Key agents in this class include finasteride (Propecia, Proscar) and dutasteride (Avodart). This class of drugs is used to treat benign prostatic hyperplasia, and finasteride (Propecia) has been approved to treat male-pattern baldness. Leuprolide acetate (Lupron) is a gonadotropin-releasing hormone analogue, also known as a luteinizing hormone–releasing hormone antagonist.

These agents create a reversible chemical orchiectomy state in males and an oophorectomy state in females. Through this mechanism of action, these agents are effective in the treatment of advanced prostatic cancer and for the management of endometriosis and uterine leiomyomata (fibroids).

Flutamide (Eulexin), bicalutamide (Casodex), and nilutamide (Nilandron) are direct antiandrogens; these agents inhibit androgen uptake or nuclear binding of androgen at target tissues. These agents are used as part of a combination therapy treatment of prostatic carcinoma. Spironolactone (Aldactone) is an aldosterone antagonist and inhibitor of 5-alpha-reductase that is indicated for use as a potassium-sparing diuretic (see Chaps. 16, 36, and 40 for further discussion regarding cardiovascular use). Additionally, it has an off-labeled use in the treatment of female hirsutism and acne due to its antiandrogenic properties. Symptoms of premenstrual syndrome/premenstrual dysphoric disorder (PMS/PMDD) have also been relieved by spironolactone doses of 25 mg 4 times a day beginning on day 14 of the menstrual cycle.

Box 22-1 provides information on antiandrogens. Note that the discussion in this chapter focuses on utilization and monitoring of androgen therapy in the primary care setting rather than in specialized practice.

BOX 22–1   COMPOUNDS WITH ANTIANDROGENIC PROPERTIES

The problems of reduced potency in the oral form and the virilizing side effects of androgens led investigators to develop drugs that inhibit synthesis and block sex hormone production receptors. This approach of countering the effects of undesirable androgen excess has enabled therapy at higher dosages. Dihydrotestosterone is the essential androgen in the prostate. The effect of androgens can be reduced by inhibiting 5-alpha-reductase in its target tissues. PSA levels and digital prostate examination are required monitoring for men on these agents. Users of alpha$_1$-adrenergic antagonists may experience hypotension, syncopy, impotence, and decreased libido. Caution is advised with concurrent use of agents that potentiate the alpha$_1$-adrenergic blocking and agents that increase the risk of hypotension.

Finasteride (Propecia, Proscar)

Finasteride, a steroid-like drug, inhibits 5-alpha-reductase, an intracellular enzyme that converts testosterone to 5-alpha-dihydrotestosterone (DHT). It has a 100-fold selectivity for 5-alpha-reductase type 2, the isoenzyme found primarily in the prostate, seminal vesicles, epididymides, and hair follicles. It is well absorbed orally, and the reduction in DHT begins within 8 hours of administration and lasts for about 24 hours. Finasteride undergoes extensive hepatic metabolism, with 39% being excreted in the urine and 57% in feces.

Approximately 90% is bound to plasma proteins. The FDA approved doses of 5 mg per day to treat benign prostatic hyperplasia (BPH). Although early improvement may be seen, 6 to 12 months of therapy may be needed to determine if a beneficial response has been achieved. Most patients experience a rapid regression in prostate gland size, and about 50% experience an increase in urinary flow and improvement in BPH symptoms (*Drug Facts and Comparisons,* 2005). In 1998, the FDA approved a 1 mg dose for treating male pattern baldness. Three months of therapy are usually required to demonstrate benefits. Stopping the drugs reverses the effect within 12 months. The main undesirable adverse effects are decreased libido and impotence, which occur with both doses.

Dutasteride (Avodart)

Like finasteride, **dutasteride** inhibits 5-alpha-reductase, an intracellular enzyme that converts testosterone to 5-alpha-dihydrotestosterone (DHT). It inhibits both type 1 and type 2 forms of the isoenzyme. It does not bind to the human androgen receptor. It is absorbed well after oral administration and reaches peak serum concentration within 2 to 3 hours. However, peak clinical effect does not occur until 6 to 12 months of therapy have been completed. Heavily bound to plasma protein (99%), it is extensively metabolized by the liver, utilizing the CYP450 3A4/5 substrate. The drug and its metabolites are excreted mainly in feces (45%). Only trace amounts are found in the urine. This drug is approved for the treatment of BPH. BPH patients treated with this drug had a decrease of 94% of DHT after 1 year. Because of its long half-life, serum concentrations remain detectable for up to 6 months after discontinuance of treatment. Dutasteride is absorbed through the skin, so women who are pregnant or may become pregnant should not handle dutasteride capsules due to the potential risk of fetal anomaly to a male fetus. The main undesirable adverse effects are decreased libido and impotence.

BOX 22–1   COMPOUNDS WITH ANTIANDROGENIC PROPERTIES—cont'd

Leuprolide Acetate (Lupron)

Leuprolide is a luteinizing hormone–releasing agonist. This drug produces gonadal suppression when blood levels are continuous in the treatment of prostate cancer. It may be given in a dose of 1 mg SC daily or IM every 3 months in the depot formulation. Mean plasma levels are achieved in 4 hours and are maintained after an initial drop in concentration. It has even greater suppression when used with flutamide. In pediatric patients, its use is to treat central precocious puberty. In gynecology, its use is in reducing uterine fibroids, endometriosis, and polycystic ovary syndrome. Approximately 90% of women with unstaged endometriosis have relief of pain, and 50% regain fertility with leuprolide.

Flutamide (Eulexin, Euflex)

Flutamide behaves like a competitive antagonist at the androgen receptor site, although it is truly a nonsteroidal agent. It has been used with leuprolide for the treatment of advanced prostate cancer and with female androgen excess syndrome. The adverse effects in men are gynecomastia and reversible liver toxicity. Flutamide is rapidly absorbed orally. It is metabolized into six compounds and bound 97% to plasma proteins, reaching a steady state by the fourth dose. Flutamide is excreted in the urine but has not required changes in dose unless renal function is less than 29 mL/min. There is a Black-Box Warning regarding hepatic failure, hepatic encephalopathy, and death with this agent. Most of these events have occurred within the first 3 months of therapy. Baseline and monthly liver function testing is necessary for the first 4 months of therapy and then periodically. Medication should be discontinued if any symptoms of hepatic injury or jaundice develop.

Spironolactone (Aldactone)

Spironolactone is another competitive inhibitor of the dihydrotestosterone, aldosterone, and interferes with the androgen receptors in the prostate. It also reduces 17-alpha-hydroxylase activity, lowering plasma levels of testosterone and androstenedione. Refer to Chapter 16 for its uses as a diuretic. Spironolactone is absorbed orally, reaches peak levels in 2 hours, and is metabolized by the liver and excreted through the portal system. Spironolactone has short-term use for primary hyperaldosteronism in patients preoperatively. It is used long-term for those patients who are not good candidates for surgery or those with idiopathic hyperaldosteronism. There are also edematous conditions that require potassium conservation, such as congestive heart failure and cirrhosis of the liver associated with ascites. An off-labeled use is in females with androgen excess for the treatment of hirsutism and acne in dosages of 50 to 200 mg/day. Adverse reactions are usually dose-related and reversible when the drug is discontinued. The most common adverse reactions are GI upset, drowsiness, gynecomastia, impotence, cutaneous eruptions, and urticaria. Early animal chronic toxicity studies demonstrated tumorigenicity. Therefore, use should be balanced against risk (there is a Black-Box Warning regarding this concern). This drug is contraindicated in pregnancy, yet the American Academy of Physicians has stated that it is compatible with breastfeeding. Although this drug is classified as a diuretic, its use in premenstrual syndrome is probably effective because of its antiandrogen effect, even at low doses (25 to 50 mg daily).

Pharmacodynamics

Testosterone is the most important androgen in humans. It is highly protein bound, and only a small portion (2%) is found free in plasma and converted to dihydrotestosterone in the skin, prostate, seminal vesicles, and epididymis. In men, testosterone is produced primarily within the testes in interstitial or Leydig cells, located in the spaces between the seminiferous tubules. The testis, like the ovary, has both reproductive and endocrine functions. Women produce small amounts of testosterone in the menstruating ovary and the adrenals, and both sexes produce testosterone peripherally from androstenedione, dehydroepiandrosterone (DHEA), and dehydroepiandrosterone sulfate (DHEAS).

At puberty, the normal male produces testosterone that stimulates maturation of the male reproductive tract and causes penile and scrotal growth. Secondary sexual characteristics associated with androgens also become noticeable. Skin changes occur, resulting in pubic, axillary, and facial hair growth, along with stimulation of sebaceous glands, making the skin thicker and oilier. Even the vocal cords become thicker, resulting in a lower-pitched voice. Lean body mass increases and more growth occurs in all bones, with epiphyseal closure occurring at around 21 years of age.

Androgens continue to play a crucial role in the maintenance of sexual function across the male life span. Androgen levels remain stable until age 55 years, when a gradual decline begins. At 70 years, a more rapid decline in hormone levels occurs, and men experience decreased muscle mass, strength, and libido. Androgens have metabolic effects in protein metabolism, liver synthesis of clotting factors, and renal production of erythropoietin. Androgens affect lipoprotein metabolism, resulting in lower high-density lipoprotein (HDL). For example, men have HDLs of 20 to 40 mg/dL, and women have HDLs in the range of 40 to 60 mg/dL.

The use of synthetic androgens is intended to supplement or replace endogenous hormones. The mechanism of action and effects of synthetic androgens are similar to those described above. When men attempt to improve athletic prowess by taking large doses of exogenous testosterone, the normal feedback mechanisms in the male reproductive process are altered and spermatogenesis is reduced through suppression of follicle-stimulating hormone (FSH).

Pharmacokinetics

Absorption and Distribution

Several delivery modes for testosterone replacement are available. Oral testosterone is rapidly metabolized by the gut as methyltestosterone and fluoxymesterone and is converted in its target tissues by the enzyme 5-alpha-reductase. The further conversion of testosterone to estradiol by cytochrome P450 (CYP450) aromatase occurs in adipose tissue, the liver, and the hypothalamus. Buccal administration lengthens the half-life. IM administration (esters) in depot preparations can last 2 to 4 weeks. Depo-Testosterone is slowly absorbed into the bloodstream between dosing intervals. Varying rates of absorption from IM administration are associated with this method, and significant fluctuation in serum testosterone levels and effects are reported. For this reason, the selection of transdermal or implanted testosterone therapy may be preferred.

Transdermal application is available in either a topically applied gel or through patch delivery systems. Both gel and patch delivery methods require once-daily application to intact, nonscrotal skin. These agents (Androderm, AndroGel, Axiron, and Testim) are well absorbed through the skin and result in rises in serum testosterone levels within 2 to 4 hours of application. Testoderm is associated with a rapid return to baseline within 2 hours after removal. Other transdermal formulations have continuous absorption during a 24-hour dosing period. Specific precautions for the use of transdermal applications will be discussed later in this section. Testopel is

a subcutaneous pellet that produces sustained testosterone effects for 3 to 6 months. The use of this subcutaneous version requires specific provider training in appropriate technique for in-office administration.

Testosterone in plasma is 98% bound to a specific testosterone-estradiol-binding globulin known as sex hormone–binding globulin (SHBG). SHBG is increased in plasma by estrogen, thyroid hormone, and cirrhosis of the liver. It is decreased by androgens, growth hormone, and obesity. The final 2% remains free to enter the cell (*Drug Facts and Comparisons* [*DF & C*], 2010).

Metabolism and Excretion

Testosterone uses the CYP450 3A4 substrate for metabolism. Forty-four percent of testosterone degradation occurs in the liver, where it is inactivated to androsterone and etiocholanolone and then conjugated and excreted in the urine. The majority (90%) is excreted in the urine and 6% is excreted in the feces. There is considerable variation in the reported half-life of testosterone: from 10 to 100 minutes. The amount of bound testosterone will determine the percentage of free drug and the free drug concentration determines half-life.

Onset, Peak, and Duration

Oral administration of testosterone reaches peak levels in 2 hours, buccal in 1 hour, and IM in 8 days to 2 weeks. Onset, peak, and duration of action of transdermal forms vary. Table 22-1 depicts the pharmacokinetics of the various

Table 22–1 ❖ Pharmacokinetics: Androgens and Anti-Androgens

Drug	Onset	Peak	Duration	Protein Binding (in %)	Half-Life	Elimination
Androgens						
Testosterone cypionate (in oil) (Depo-Testerone)	UK	UK	2–4 wk	98%	8 d	90% in urine as conjugates and metabolites; 6% in feces
Testosterone enanthate (in oil) (Delatestryl)	UK	UK	2–4 wk	98%	8 d	90% in urine as conjugates and metabolites; 6% in feces
Testosterone, buccal (Striant)	UK	10–12 h	12 h	UK	10–100 min	90% in urine. Avoids first-pass effects of liver. Metabolized in liver and reproductive tissue.
Methyltestosterone (Android, Methitest, Testred)	UK	UK	1–3 d	98%	10–100 min	90% in urine as conjugates and metabolites; 6% in feces
Fluoxymesterone(Androxy)	UK	UK	UK	98%	9.2 h	90% in urine as conjugates and metabolites; 6% in feces
Testosterone (Testoderm). Must apply to scrotal skin	UK	2–4 h	*		*	90% in urine as conjugates and metabolites; 6% in feces
Testosterone (Testoderm TTS). Apply to nonscrotal skin	UK	2–4 h	*		*	90% in urine as conjugates and metabolites; 6% in feces
Testosterone (Androderm). Apply to nonscrotal skin	UK	4–6 h	24 h	24 h		90% in urine as conjugates and metabolites; 6% in feces
Testosterone gel (AndroGel 1%, Androgel 1.62%, Testim)	30 min	4 h	48 h		5 d	90% in urine as conjugates and metabolites; 6% in feces

Table 22–1 ❖ Pharmacokinetics: Androgens and Anti-Androgens—cont'd

Drug	Onset	Peak	Duration	Protein Binding (in %)	Half-Life	Elimination
Anti-Androgens						
Finasteride (Propecia)	NA	1–2 h	24 h	None	Normal renal function: 4.8–6 h Men > 70 yr: 7 h	39% urine, 57% feces
Leuprolide (Eligard, Lupron, Lupron Depot)	NA	Depot: 4 h	4 wk	45%–49%	NA	NA
Spironolactone (off-labeled use) (Aldactone)	24–28 h	48–72 h	48–72 h	90%	1.3–2 h	Total: renal Unchanged: NA

NA = not available; UK = unknown.

*Serum levels return to normal within 2 h of removal. Serum levels plateau after 3–4 wk of use.

formulations of androgens and antiandrogens, including the variable half-lives of transdermal formulations.

Pharmacotherapeutics

Precautions and Contraindications

Contraindications for the use of testosterone include male breast cancer, prostate cancer, pregnancy (Category X due to fetal harm/virilization of the female fetus), and lactation.

Transdermal systems and testosterone gel are not indicated for women and must not be used by them. Safety and efficacy of Testoderm and AndroGel products in pediatric patients have not been established. Men who use topical gels must not have skin contact with pregnant women or with children, because skin-to-skin transfer of testosterone may occur. Men should wash their hands after application and allow skin to dry before it touches clothing to decrease the risk of inadvertent transfer of medication.

Edema, with or without congestive heart failure, may be a serious complication. These drugs should be used cautiously in patients with preexisting cardiac, renal, or hepatic disease, and frequent monitoring is required (see the Monitoring section). In addition to discontinuing the drug, diuretic therapy may be needed.

Men, especially elderly men, treated with androgens are at increased risk for developing prostatic hypertrophy, prostatic hyperplasia, and prostatic carcinoma. The treatment of hypogonadal men with testosterone may potentiate sleep apnea. This risk increases in men with obesity or chronic lung disease.

The areas of clinical usage of androgens that are more controversial include stimulating growth in boys with delayed puberty and in aging men to increase strength and muscle mass. It is advisable for primary care providers to refer these populations of patients for consultation with endocrine specialists regarding initiating therapies.

Athletes try to use these drugs to illegally improve competitive performance. In this regard, there has been abuse by coaches and athletes alike. The adverse effects far outweigh the potential benefits. Because of the abuse potential of anabolic steroids, providers must supply their federal Drug Enforcement Administration [DEA] number on all prescriptions written for hormone combinations with androgens. Patients receiving steroid therapy require periodic laboratory and clinical evaluation. Prescribers may wish to limit prescription quantities and refills to match monitoring time frames to aid in adherence to follow-up evaluations and to reduce the potential for misuse.

Adverse Drug Reactions

The androgens as a class are potent agents and can have serious or even fatal reactions if used improperly. When properly used, androgens mimic the body's endogenous processes. However, prolonged use of high doses of androgens has been associated with the development of potentially life-threatening hepatitis, hepatic neoplasms, cholestatic hepatitis, jaundice, and hepatocellular carcinoma. Cholestatic hepatitis and jaundice occur at relatively low doses of fluoxymesterone and methyltestosterone. These conditions are reversible with drug discontinuance.

Gender-specific side effects have been reported with the use of androgen therapy. Men may develop gynecomastia and reduced sperm levels that threaten fertility. Acne and baldness may occur, even with short-term therapy. Men can paradoxically have decreased libido, depression, and headache with exogenous administration of androgens. Scrotal pain, groin pain, or changes in urination may be associated with stimulation and changes of the prostate gland and need further evaluation. Men may develop priapism (a sustained erection) and will require education to seek emergent evaluation if this occurs. In women, menstrual irregularities may occur with these drugs through suppression of gonadotropin secretion. Hypercalcemia and virilization are reported.

All patients on androgen therapy may experience gastrointestinal (GI) symptoms, including nausea, vomiting, change in liver function, edema, and cholestatic jaundice. Suppression of clotting factors, as well as increased red blood cell production, can contribute to hemorrhage and thrombus formation simultaneously.

Both testosterone and anabolic steroids have the potential for abuse. The anabolic steroids have a high anabolic–low androgenic ratio of activity. The U.S. Food and Drug Administration (FDA) warns that androgens may cause peliosis hepatis. Peliosis is the replacement of normal liver tissue with bloody cysts. This vascularity may cause a silent, fatal abdominal hemorrhage. Liver tumors that are benign or malignant may develop. The lipoprotein changes with these steroids may hasten coronary artery disease. Drugs classified as anabolic steroids include oxymetholone, stanozolol, oxandrolone, nandrolone phenylpropionate, and nandrolone decanoate.

Drug Interactions

Various drug interactions have been reported with androgens. The main classes of associated drug interactions with androgens include anticoagulants, diabetic agents, and corticosteroids. The interaction of anticoagulants such as warfarin (Coumadin) with the 17-alkyl testosterone derivatives poses the most significant potential problem. The 17-alkyl testosterone drugs are the methyl- and fluoxy- forms used for hypogonadism and male climacteric.

Although testosterone has been used for breast tenderness in the past, its use is discouraged because of lack of proven efficacy and the masculinizing effect that it has on women. Laboratory values of decreasing protein-bound T_4 and increased T_3 uptake need to be mentioned. But, because the free T_4 levels are not affected, no deficiency state occurs. Table 22-2 presents drug interactions.

Clinical Use and Dosing

The primary clinical use of these agents is for the replacement or augmentation of endogenous androgen for primary hypogonadal males or hypogonadotropic hypogonadism and for male climacteric. After 30 years of clinical use, the World Health Organization (WHO) selected testosterone enanthate as the prototype hormone in its contraceptive efficacy studies.

In rare situations, androgens are used in endometriosis, in refractory anemia, and with estrogen for osteoporosis and loss of libido. Androgens have anabolic effects with food and exercise for post-operative trauma patients and with some types of metastatic breast cancer. The masculinizing effect on women detracts from wider usage.

Testosterone is controversial in pediatrics as a height stimulator and in sports as a performance enhancer. Primary care providers prescribe androgens largely for replacement

Table 22–2 ▦ **Common Drug Interactions: Androgens and Anti-Androgens**

Drug	Interacting Drug	Possible Effect	Implications
Androgens			
Testosterone	Anticoagulants	Increased anticoagulant effect	More frequent monitoring of prothrombin time
	Imipramine	Paranoid response	Consider switching to another class of antidepressants
	Diabetic agents	Decrease blood sugar	Frequent blood sugar monitoring. Dose adjustment of diabetic agents.
	Cyclosporine	Impaired hepatic metabolism	Consider switching to another agent
Anti-Androgens			
Finasteride	Nevirapine	Combination induces hepatic metabolism of finasteride	Monitor for effectiveness of finasteride
Leuprolide	Pituitary, gonadotropic, and gonadal function Lab tests	Misleading results	Consider if lab test reports show unexpected values
Flutamide	Warfarin	Increased INR and risk of bleeding	Monitor INR closely. As lutamide is indicated for advanced prostate cancer, the option to select an alternative treatment may be limited.
Spironolactone	Renal impairment and agents that affect renal function	Alteration in renal function and electrolytes	Monitor potassium levels in young patients with reduced renal function and in patients >65 yr
	Digitalis	May increase or decrease digitalis half-life	Monitor closely for signs of digitalis toxicity and electrolyte and digitalis levels. Consider alternative treatments.
	Potassium	Additive effect—increases risk of hyperkalemia	Recommend alternative
	Eplerenone (aldosterone receptor antagonist used for CHF)	Severe hyperkalemia	Combination is contraindicated. Do NOT use together; select an alternative agent.

therapy, and for that reason this discussion is limited. Table 22-3 presents the dosage schedule for androgens and antiandrogens.

Rational Drug Selection

Slow-Acting Versus Long-Acting Form

As discussed previously, there are various formulations of androgen supplementation from which a provider may select. There are various advantages and concerns for each formulation that should be considered. Providers should include patient preference, adherence concerns, and lifestyle as factors in agent selection.

IM forms have longer half-lives than do oral and transdermal agents but less uniform absorption and steady serum drug levels. IM aqueous preparations need to be administered 2 to 3 times per week. The patient or a family member can be taught to administer these long-term medications to simplify daily routines. Preparations in oil can be administered at 2- to 4-week intervals. Oral preparations cause less discomfort to administer but may cause gastric irritation and require twice-daily administration. Transdermal agents have demonstrated improved steady-state hormone levels; however, transfer to partners and children is a concern. Subcutaneous pellets offer a long-acting option with infrequent administration

Table 22–3 ⨯ Dosage Schedule: Androgens and Anti-Androgens

Drug	Indication	Dosage Form	Initial Dose	Maintenance Dose
Androgens Testosterone	Replacement therapy for primary or hypogonadotropic hypogonadism			Dose adjustment based on testosterone levels
Androderm		Patch: 2 mg Patch: 4 mg	4 mg daily	Level >930 ng/dL: decrease dose to 2 mg daily Level 400–930 ng/dL: continue 4 mg daily Level <400 ng/dL: increase dose to 6 mg daily
AndroGel 1%		Gel pump: 25 mg/2.5 g 1.25 g/actuation	50 mg applied once daily to the shoulder and upper arms or abdomen	Less than normal range: increase dose 25 mg (max 100 mg) Greater than normal range: decrease dose by 25 mg. Discontinue if consistently above normal at 50 mg daily.
AndroGel 1.62%		Gel pump: 40.5 mg/2.5g 20.25 mg/actuation	40.5 mg applied once daily in the morning to the shoulder and upper arms	Level >750 ng/dL: decrease dose by 20.25 mg daily Level ≥350 ng/dL to ≤750 ng/dL: maintain current dose Level <350 ng/dL: increase dose by 20.25 mg daily to max dose 81 mg daily
Axiron		Solution pump: 30 mg/actuation	60 mg once daily applied to the axilla	Dose range 30–120 mg daily Level <300 ng/dL: increase by 30 mg daily. Level 105 ng/dL: decrease by 30 mg increments. If persistent elevation, discontinue therapy.
Fortesta		Pump 10 mg/actuation	40 mg once daily applied to the thighs	Dosing range: 10–70 mg daily Level <550 ng/dL: increase dose by 10 mg daily Level ≥500 to ≤1,250 ng/dL: maintain current dose Level ≥1250 to ≤2,500 ng/dL: decrease dose by 10 mg daily Level ≥2,500 ng/dL: decrease dose by 20 mg daily
Testim		50 mg/g	5 g applied once daily to the shoulder and upper arms	Less than normal range: increase dose from 5 g to 10 g (maximum) Greater than normal range: decrease dose. Discontinue if consistently above normal at 5 g daily.

Continued

Table 22–3 ⚕ **Dosage Schedule: Androgens and Anti-Androgens—cont'd**

Drug	Indication	Dosage Form	Initial Dose	Maintenance Dose
Testosterone cypionate (Depo-Testosterone) Testosterone enanthate (Delatestryl) Generic		Oil, generic 200 mg/mL Oil, cypionate 100 mg/mL; 200 mg/mL Generic: 100 mg/mL; 200 mg/mL Oil, enenthate 200 mg/mL Generic: 200 mg/mL	50–400 mg IM every 2–4 wk	50–400 mg IM every 2–4 wk
Anti-Androgens				
Finasteride (Proscar)	Benign prostatic hyperplasia	5 mg tablet, oral	5 mg daily, with or without meals	5 mg daily
(Propecia)	Androgenic alopecia	1 mg tablet, oral Generic: 1 mg, 5 mg tablet, oral	1 mg daily, with or without meals	1 mg daily
Flutamide	Prostatic carcinoma	Capusle, oral Generic: 125 mg	250 mg 3 times/d, alternatively, once-daily doses of 0.5–1.5 g have been used (unlabeled dosing)	250 mg 3 times/d
Leuprolide (Eligard)	Prostatic carcinoma	Kit, subcutaneous, as acetate 7.5 mg, 22.5 mg, 30 mg, 45 mg	7.5 mg monthly or 22.5 mg every 3 mo or 30 mg every 4 mo or 45 mg every 6 mo	7.5 mg monthly or 22.5 mg every 3 mo or 30 mg every 4 mo or 45 mg every 6 mo
(Lupron Depot)	Endometriosis	Kit, intramuscular, as acetate 3.75 mg, 11.25 mg, 22.5 mg, 30 mg, 45 mg Generic: 1 mg/0.2 mL	3.75 mg every mo for up to 6 mo	3.75 mg every mo for up to 6 mo
(Lupron Depot)	Uterine leiomyomata (fibroids)	Kit, intramuscular, as acetate 3.75 mg, 11.25 mg, 22.5 mg, 30 mg, 45 mg Generic: 1 mg/0.2 mL	11.25 mg every 3 months for up to 2 doses	11.25 mg every 3 months for up to 2 doses
Spironolactone (off-labeled use) (Aldactone)	Acne Hirsutism	Tablet, oral: 25 mg, 50 mg, 100 mg (scored) Generic: 25 mg, 50 mg, 100 mg	To reduce delay in onset of effect, a loading dose of 2–3 times the daily dose may be administered on the first day of therapy	25–200 mg once daily 50–200 mg daily in 1–2 divided doses

(every 3 to 6 months). However, this formulation does not afford for easy dose titration and requires specialty skill in administration.

Cost

Oral testosterone products are less expensive than those administered via other routes, in part because equipment and technical skills are not required for administration. Buccal preparations avoid the 44% metabolism in the liver, but the tablets are more costly. Transdermal patches are the most recent addition to hormone replacement therapy for men and women, and the convenience is associated with increased cost. Transdermal is the preferred route of administration for children because there are no taste issues or painful injections, and older adults with poor eyesight or swallowing problems have less difficulty with patch application.

In addition to the health-care needs and delivery preference, agent selection may also be influenced by a third-party payer source. Frequently, the patient's third-party payer (insurance) limits available formulations. Table 22-3 presents the available dosage forms.

Monitoring

Clients using supplemental and replacement androgen therapy will require monitoring for serum testosterone levels as well as therapeutic effect. In general, all patients on androgen therapy will require serum testosterone level monitoring, lipid tracking, liver function tests, and complete blood count evaluation. The goal of therapy is to maintain a normal range of serum testosterone levels. These laboratory evaluations should be performed at baseline, 3 to 6 months after initiating treatment, then annually while on therapy. Closer monitoring of serum testosterone is needed at initiation and during dose titration. Male patients will additionally require prostate-specific antigen (PSA) and digital prostate evaluation prior to initiation of therapy and throughout the duration of treatment due to the increased risk of prostate hypertrophy and cancer associated with androgens. Abnormalities of liver function and elevation of lipids can be seen with these agents, as well as polycythemia. There appears to be a trend that men with low levels of testosterone have higher death rates than those with normal levels; however, the FDA is concerned about potential CV risks for the population as a whole. This may be linked to the finding that many men on supplements actually do not have low lab values. See Chapter 49 for more information about men's health.

Calcium levels in serum and urine may become abnormal in patients with breast cancer. Methyltestosterone and fluoxymesterone are apt to cause hepatic toxicity, and liver function tests should be drawn every 6 months. Individuals with renal or cardiovascular comorbidities will also require monitoring of electrolytes and for symptoms of edema and congestive heart failure (CHF). Blood glucose levels and antidiabetic medication may be affected by androgen therapy, and closer monitoring will be required. When using testosterone in prepubertal males, perform an x-ray every 6 months for bone maturation to avoid early closure of epiphyseal centers.

PATIENT EDUCATION

Administration

Avoid coadministering with other medications that cause gastric irritation. With buccal forms, food or liquids reduce absorption. Do not swallow buccal tablets; instead, park the tablet between gums and teeth. If the skin is sensitive to the patch adhesive, a small application of aerosolized cortisone (e.g., Asthmacort or Nasacort) to the skin will reduce irritation without loss of efficacy. A specific description of how to apply transdermal systems is given in Table 22-3.

Adverse Reactions

Common adverse drug reactions and site effects of androgens have been discussed previously in this section. Some adverse effects are reversible if the drug is reduced or temporarily stopped. Significant adverse events with the use of androgens include hepatic injury, worsening of cardiovascular comorbidities, prostatic hypertrophy, and female virilization.

Hepatic injury has been associated with the use of orally administered synthetic androgen agents. Additional use of agents that are associated with risk of hepatic injury should be avoided to prevent additive hepatic risk. Patient education should include a discussion regarding the need to report abdominal pain, jaundice, anorexia, muscle pain, and weakness because these may be symptoms of hepatic injury. Patients with underlying dyslipidemia or angina may experience a worsening of symptoms and should be further evaluated. Caution women to report signs of virilization, such as hoarseness, hair thinning, and menstrual disruption. Older

men should be routinely screened with questions regarding changes in urine stream and nighttime voiding patterns; prostatic hypertrophy with secondary urinary retention may develop while they are on androgen therapy.

Lifestyle Management

Children and young adults with hypogonadism need to treat their chronic problem cautiously because long-term use of androgens can precipitate adverse reactions. If managed early and carefully, males with hypogonadism may be able to conceive a child. Adolescents requiring therapy need to know that testosterone replacement is a far different matter from anabolic steroid use by athletes looking for a competitive edge in their sport. Older patients need to reduce sodium in their diet to avoid CHF while on androgen therapy.

ESTROGENS AND ANTIESTROGENS

Estrogen, like testosterone, is an endogenous hormone with multiple actions. The primary role of estrogen is the maturation and function of the female reproductive system. However, because there are estrogen receptor sites in the bone, cardiovascular system, central nervous system, and gastrointestinal tract, estrogen exerts significant nonreproductive health effects.

The first supplemental estrogens were prescribed for replacement therapy more than 50 years ago. The first marketed estrogens were conjugated equine estrogens (Premarin). Later, estrogens were esterified (80% estrone sulfate; 15% sodium equilin sulfate), and other synthetic and bioidentical formulations have been introduced to the market. Estradiol was synthesized into oral and IM preparations, vaginal creams, transdermal patches, and vaginal rings. Ethinyl forms of estradiol became the primary forms of estrogen used in combination oral contraception (preparations containing both estrogen and progesterone). Ethinyl estradiol has approximately 10 times the potency of estradiol.

Phytoestrogens and estrogen-like herbal preparations have shown some symptomatic improvement for perimenopausal symptoms. Studies have yet to demonstrate that phytoestrogens convey the same osteoporosis prevention benefits of traditional estrogen therapy. Extensive discussion of the use of estrogens, phytoestrogens, and related herbal therapies both for hormonal replacement and for prevention of osteoporosis is found in Chapter 38.

The following section focuses the discussion on estrogen and its related pharmacodynamic/pharmacokinetic principles for prescribing. It should be noted that the use of estrogen-only products is contraindicated in women with an intact uterus. For these women, combination estrogen and progesterone products should be used. An extended discussion regarding the use of estrogen in the treatment of menopause and contraception is presented in Chapters 31 and 38. Information about a few antiestrogens is presented in Box 22-2. The aromastase inhibitors are covered in Chapter 21.

BOX 22–2 ANTIESTROGENS

Although naturally occurring hormones such as progesterone and testosterone may modify the action of **estrogen**, the following discussion focuses on the synthetic estrogen antagonists. Drugs in this class may have limited use by most practitioners in primary care. Clomiphene is used for ovulation stimulation by infertility clinics. **Danazol** is primarily used for endometriosis by gynecologists, and tamoxifen is used for female cancers by oncologists. Monitoring by primary care providers is essential.

Clomiphene (Clomid)

Clomiphene was the first chemical used to initiate ovulation in normogonadotropic, normoprolactinemic, and anovulatory patients. It has also been used as a component in the management of luteal-phase dysfunction, oligo-ovulation, artificial insemination, unexplained infertility, and in vitro fertilization. Although clomiphene has been used for 30 years, it is still a drug that remains in a specialized practice setting. The list of adverse side effects are hot flashes, multiple gestation, visual symptoms, cervical mucus abnormalities, luteal-phase defect, luteinized unruptured follicle syndrome, ovarian cancer, teratogenicity, enlargement of ovarian cysts, and liver disease.

The agonist–antagonist characteristics of clomiphene depend on the hormone climate. Clomiphene initiates ovulation in the presence of high estrogen levels in anovulatory females. It does this as long as other endogenous mechanisms trigger an LH surge and follicle rupture. Clomiphene blocks endogenous estrogen-negative feedback at the level of the hypothalamus. It also elevates estrogen and progesterone levels higher than normal. Its function may even affect the ovary and pituitary glands. Clomiphene also decreases serum insulin-like growth factors and increases SHBG, which assists those infertile women with polycystic ovary (PCO) disease. It has direct antiestrogenic effects on the endometrium and cervical mucus-producing glands. Elevated estrogen levels of women in the reproductive years can override the direct antiestrogen effects on the endometrium and cervical mucus.

This compound is active when taken orally, but little is known about its metabolism. Half of the compound is excreted in the feces within 5 days of administration. The hypothesis is that it is excreted through a slow enterohepatic pathway.

Danazol (Danocrine)

Although the major use of danazol has been to treat endometriosis, it has been employed in severe fibrocystic breast changes, hematological disorders, and idiopathic thrombocytopenic purpura. Danazol must be used with great caution in hepatic dysfunction and carries a Black-Box Warning for this and for the risk of thromboembolism. The list of adverse effects is long, which is, in part, why this drug is not indicated for most primary care settings.

Danazol suppresses the pituitary-ovarian axis, inhibiting the midcycle surge of LH and FSH to suppress ovarian function. It has weak progestational and androgenic properties, as does its major metabolite, ethisterone. Danazol binds to androgen, progesterone, and glucocorticoid receptors and alters androgen metabolism. It does not inhibit aromatase, the enzyme required for estrogen synthesis. It also increases the clearance rate of progesterone by competing with the hormone for binding proteins. Danazol is taken orally and is slowly metabolized by the liver (CYP450 3A4 inhibitor), being excreted primarily in the urine after a 24 hour half-life.

Tamoxifen (Nolvadex)

Tamoxifen is the first agent in the selective estrogen receptor modulator (SERM) class of medications used to treat conditions that respond to adding or withdrawing estrogens. As the class name implies, these agents target selective estrogen receptors, while not stimulating others. It is used primarily as part of adjuvant therapy for breast cancer in patients with estrogen receptor (ER)–positive tumors. Recent studies have demonstrated a reduction in breast cancer in those individuals at high risk for developing the disease within 5 years. In the Gail model, age, family history, medical history of premalignant biopsies, and age at first live birth calculate the patient's absolute risk.

An antiestrogen in mammary tissue, tamoxifen blunts the effect of estrogen and has direct antigrowth activity of its own in the absence of estrogen. The mechanism may be that it blocks estradiol-induced cancer cell growth by altering the local production of growth factors and/or inhibiting the development of the tumor's blood supply. Tamoxifen continues to stimulate estrogen receptors in the endometrial tissue and causes hyperplasia in the postmenopausal woman's endometrium and vagina. Several large-scale, longitudinal trials are under way to evaluate its effectiveness in preventing disease in high-risk women. The results will try to address its potential benefits on bone and lipids while reducing the risk on breast tissue.

This is a nonsteroidal agent that is given orally. Peak plasma levels are reached in a few hours with an initial half-life of 7 to 14 hours. The liver extensively metabolizes tamoxifen, and 65% of the drug is excreted through the gut within 2 weeks.

Raloxifene (Evista)

Raloxifene is also a SERM. Indications initially were for osteoporosis prevention in women who cannot or will not take hormone replacement therapy. Post-marketing studies have shown a positive lipid effect, which may improve cardiovascular disease risk. Results from the recent MORE randomized trial demonstrated a 76% reduced risk of invasive breast cancer

BOX 22–2   ANTIESTROGENS—cont'd

among the women taking raloxifene for osteoporosis. This was attributed to the effect of the drug on ER-positive tumors. This drug can be used only in women past menopause who have never had thromboembolic problems.

Raloxifene is a selective estrogen receptor modulator similar to tamoxifen with different degrees of estrogen agonist or antagonist activity in different tissues. It is an estrogen agonist on bone and an antagonist on breast and uterus. Unlike tamoxifen, it appears to be neutral on the vaginal tissues. A comparison of the beneficial effect on bone mineral density is slightly less than that of estrogen. Whether this bone effect will decrease the incidence of fractures has yet to be proved.

Raloxifene is taken orally without regard to meals, with a 60% absorption rate, but is extensively glucuronidated, and only 2% is bioavailable. It is excreted though the GI tract with a half-life of 32.5 hours.

Raloxifene is not indicated for pediatric patients or for premenopausal women. Concomitant hormone replacement therapy is not recommended.

The primary reasons sited by patients for discontinuing therapy were hot flashes and leg cramps. One reported that these symptoms may have lasted up to 6 months.

Raloxifene is highly bound (95%) to plasma proteins. Close monitoring or alternative treatments should be considered for patients using bile acid sequestrants, thyroid hormones, and warfarin.

One short-term trial indicated that it might be effective for prevention of postmenopausal bone loss without the risk for breast or uterine cancer. It may also have a beneficial effect on lipid metabolism. More studies are needed to validate that the effect on lipids actually confers a cardio-protective effect. This drug may be useful for advance practice nurses in primary care practices, but at this time, the long-term safety effects are not known. Like estrogens, there is some increase in thromboembolic disease, and it is teratogenic.

Patients on concurrent anticoagulant therapy will require frequent INR levels initially during therapy, and dose adjustments of anticoagulants may be needed. Women should also be advised to continue with supplemental calcium and vitamin D for bone health.

Raloxifene can be administered orally without regard to food. Patients need to know that hot flashes can sometimes occur at the beginning of therapy, even in postmenopausal women.

The risk of thromboembolic disease (1%) is the same as it is for estrogen users. Individuals on raloxifene should discontinue use 72 hours prior to surgery to decrease risk of thrombosis and embolism. When traveling, patients should get up and move around every hour to avoid long periods of inactivity.

Pharmacodynamics

Estrogens occur naturally in several forms. The primary sources of estrogen in the normally cycling adult woman is the ovarian follicle, which secretes 70 to 500 mcg of estradiol daily, depending on the phase of the menstrual cycle (*DF & C*, 2010). This estradiol is converted to estrone, which circulates in about equal amounts to the estradiol and to small amounts of estriol. After menopause, most endogenous estrogen is generated from conversion by peripheral tissues of androstenedione, secreted by the adrenal cortex, to estrone.

Effects of estrogen on the reproductive system include:

- Maturation of reproductive organs
- Development of secondary sexual characteristics
- Regulation of the menstrual cycle
- Endometrial regeneration postmenstruation.

Other physical effects of estrogen include:

- Closure of long bones after the pubertal growth spurt
- Maintenance of bone density by decreasing the rate of bone resorption through antagonizing the effects of parathyroid hormone (PTH)
- Maintenance of the normal structure of skin and blood vessels through its actions on the endothelial cells in the arterial walls, including the induction of nitric oxide to facilitate vasodilation and oxygen uptake by cells

- Reduction of the motility of the bowel through its modulation of sympathetic nervous system control over smooth muscle
- Altering of the production and activity of selected proteins, resulting in higher levels of thyroxine-binding globulin, sex-hormone binding globulin, transferrin, and renin substrate
- Enhancing the coagulability of blood by increasing the production of fibrinogen
- Facilitating the loss of intravascular fluid into extracellular space by its action on the renin-angiotensin-aldosterone cycle (retention of sodium and water by the kidney), resulting in edema and decreased extracellular fluid (ECF) volume
- Maintaining the stability of the thermoregulatory center in the brain

Control of estrogen secretion is by the hypothalamus through the pituitary gland. Gonadotropin-releasing hormone (GnRH) from the hypothalamus controls FSH and luteinizing hormone (LH) from the anterior pituitary. FSH and LH stimulate follicular development in the ovary. In the presence of adequate estrogen, LH surge is responsible for ovulation. Primary hormone pathways in the reproductive system are modulated by both negative and positive feedback loops.

Pharmacokinetics

Absorption and Distribution

Estrogens used as therapy are well absorbed in oral, transdermal, and parenteral administration routes. Orally administered estrogen, whether tablet or the newer chewable form, is well absorbed given its lipophilic nature. However, oral estrogens are subject to extensive hepatic first-pass metabolism and require larger doses in order to achieve significant bioavailability. Substitution of an ethinyl group along with the estrogen or estrogen stabilized with piperazine has inhibited the first-pass effect and allows for lower dosing amounts. The current dosing scheme has accounted for bioavailability, and prescribing clinicians are not required to make dosing adjustments. Conjugated estrogens are well absorbed from the GI tract. The tablet releases the drug slowly over several hours.

Compared to oral estradiol, transdermal formulations are metabolized in the skin to a small extent and are not subject to hepatic first pass. This results in a therapeutic serum level of estradiol with lower circulating levels of estrone and its metabolites so that smaller total doses are required. An additional benefit of transdermal patches is that they release a constant stream of hormone, providing a steady serum hormone level. Topical applications given vaginally for local impact can still be sufficient to cause systemic effects. Topical delivery formulations include creams, hormone-impregnated rings, and tablets. Vaginal absorption varies among women and treatment will require titration to achieve symptom control and limit unnecessary estrogen exposure. More of the hormone is absorbed if the degree of atrophy is great in the surrounding tissues.

Parenteral formulations that have an oil-based preparation have slow absorption with a prolonged duration of action. A single dose of IM estradiol valerate or estradiol cypionate is absorbed over several weeks.

The majority of estradiol estrogen (69% to 80%) binds strongly to the SHBG, and another 18% to 30% binds to albumin with less affinity. The remaining 1% to 2% of the free and unbound fraction is physiologically active and is responsible for the observed effects of estrogen. The distribution of exogenous forms of estrogen is similar to that of endogenous forms.

Metabolism and Excretion

The liver converts estradiol into less potent metabolites, estrone and estriol, which are excreted in the bile. A significant portion undergoes enterohepatic recirculation in the liver, resulting in undesirable side effects such as increased clotting factors and plasma renin substrate. The water-soluble forms that result from this recirculation are acidic, favoring renal excretion. Estrogen formulations that are administered by non-oral routes are not subject to first-pass metabolism, but they still undergo significant hepatic uptake, metabolism, and enterohepatic recycling.

Onset, Peak, and Duration

Naturally occurring estradiol levels vary during the menstrual cycle. Supplemental estrogen has a rapid onset of action ranging from less than an hour to 3 hours, depending on the route of administration. Peak concentrations occur within the first days of use, and patients generally report symptom improvement within the first few days of therapy. The duration of action depends on the route of delivery and can range from several hours to a few days. The majority of patients report symptoms of estrogen deficiency after missing several days of therapy. Table 22-4 presents the pharmacokinetics of estrogens.

Pharmacotherapeutics

Estrogens have been synthesized for several decades and are used in the primary care setting for replacement after oophorectomy and in natural menopause for treatment of hot flashes, vaginal atrophy, and irregular menstrual bleeding. The first oral contraceptive pills contained only progesterone. However, these early progesterone-only pills were associated with significant breakthrough bleeding. To combat that problem, estrogen was added to contraceptive pills in the 1960s. These early combined progesterone/estrogen pills used a much higher dose of estrogen than is currently used in combined contraceptive pills. The dose of estrogen needed for contraception is higher than the dosage needed for replacement therapy. The potency ratio of replacement estrogens to contraception estrogens is approximately 1:10.

Chapter 38 goes into greater detail about replacement estrogens, and Chapter 31 deals with estrogen use as a contraceptive. Many advance practice nurses commonly prescribe oral contraceptives for a noncontraceptive use in the treatment of dysmenorrhea, cycle control, and acne management and for other secondary benefits. Oral contraceptives may be also prescribed to treat amenorrhea and hirsutism associated with polycystic ovary disease.

Precautions and Contraindications

There are absolute and relative contraindications that clinicians must consider when initiating estrogen therapy. Absolute contraindications include current or prior history of an estrogen-dependent cancer, current pregnancy, undiagnosed dysfunctional uterine bleeding, deep vein thromboembolism, arterial thromboemboli within the prior year, clotting disorders, and severe hepatic disease. Relative contraindications require added discussion with patients regarding the risk of estrogen therapy and its perceived benefits. Relative contraindications include cardiovascular disease, uncontrolled hypertension, diabetes mellitus, gallbladder disease, obesity, endometriosis, seizure disorder, and migraine. Women who experience migraine with aura are at increased risk for stroke and should not be prescribed estrogen. Women with an intact uterus should not be prescribed unopposed estrogen because of the risk of endometrial hyperplasia and endometrial cancer.

There is not a significant risk of non-estrogen–dependent breast cancer in the short-term use of oral contraceptives.

Table 22–4 ⚙ **Pharmacokinetics: Estrogens and Antiestrogens**

Drug	Site of Metabolism	Active Metabolism	Half-Life (in hours by formulation and metabolites in individuals with normal renal function)	Elimination
Estrogens				
Ethinyl estradiol	Liver	Estradiol Estrone	1–2 4–18	Urine Feces
Conjugated estrogens	Liver	Estradiol Estrone	1–2 4–18	Urine
Estradiol transdermal system	Skin/liver	Estrone	1–4 4–18 estrone	Urine
Estradiol vaginal ring	Vagina/liver	Estrone	1–2	Unchanged: NA
Antiestrogens				
Clomiphene	NA	NA	5–7 d	42.4% feces; 7.8% in urine
Danazol	Liver	NA	24	NA
Tamoxifen	Liver	N-desmethyl-tamoxifen	5–7 d 14 d (metabolite)	Primarily in feces
Raloxifene	Liver		32.5	Primarily in feces
Ospemifene (Osphena B)	Liver	4-hydroxyospemifene	26	Feces 75% and urine 7%

NA = not available.

But, with every 10-year increment of use, there is a 14% rise in breast cancer risk (Zhu, Lei, Feng, & Wang, 2012).

Estrogens have been implicated in the risk of endometrial cancer. The rates have increased dramatically since 1969 even though the dose of estrogen for both contraception and replacement has significantly decreased. At the same time, the survival rate of woman with endometrial cancers has been higher in estrogen users than in those who do not use estrogen—perhaps in part due to early detection, as women on estrogen are required to have routine follow-up care.

"Natural" and synthetic estrogens have the same risks for users. The absolute and relative contraindications for estrogen use are looked at in more detail in Chapters 31 and 38, with special emphasis on clinical trials such as the Women's Health Initiative (WHI). The WHI findings have had a considerable impact on the prescribing patterns of clinicians and the perception of hormone therapy by the public. It is critical that prescribers understand the current literature and can adequately evaluate the risks versus the benefits of estrogen-containing therapies and partner with patients to determine the best course of treatment.

Although it was thought that estrogen replacement therapy (ERT) and estrogen plus progestin therapy (HRT) would provide some protection against coronary heart disease (CHD), the results of several trials from the PEPI trials (Writing Group of the PEPI Trial, 1996) to the WHI (Writing Group for the Women's Health Initiative Investigators, 2002) have shown that not only does HRT not provide protection, it actually causes some increase in morbidity and mortality related to CHD. The WHI study revealed a higher incidence of CHD, stroke, and thromboemboli both in women taking estrogen only or HRT therapy.

Increased risk for thromboembolic events has been a long-standing concern related to hormone replacement, whether estrogen alone or in combination with progestins. The WHI found significantly increased risk for stroke in postmenopausal women on both ERT and HRT. For HRT, the risk was apparent in each decade of age, but for ERT the risk appeared to emerge after age 60 years (Langer, 2005). The risk for venous thromboembolic disease, including pulmonary embolism, was doubled in women in the HRT arm of the study, with no difference based on age. There was a nonsignificant increase by about one-third with ERT alone (Anderson et al, 2004). There is some evidence to suggest that the timing of initiation of ERT and HRT may play a role in the CHD and atherosclerosis. The highest risk for cardiovascular events occurs within the first year of therapy until later ages.

Several design limitations have been identified in the WHI trial that deserve consideration when prescribing ERT and HRT. The majority of women in the WHI study were older (mean age of 63 years), had been menopausal for almost a decade, and were not experiencing menopausal symptoms, and many of the participants had comorbidities of obesity and cardiovascular disease. Findings from the Women's HOPE (Health, Osteoporosis, Progestin, Estrogen) study, along with age-adjusted meta-analysis, suggest that lower doses of estrogen and progesterone may not raise the risk of CVD and that women who initiate treatment at the time of menopause may not be at as great a risk for heart disease–related complications as women who started HRT at an older age (greater than age 65 years) and more distant from menopause (greater than 10 years) (Warren, 2010).

Estrogens are Pregnancy Category X. Use of estrogens during pregnancy is contraindicated because of the high rate of teratogenicity in male and female offspring. In the past, strong estrogens (DES) were used empirically to treat women who habitually spontaneously aborted in an effort to help them retain a subsequent pregnancy. Time, teratogenic outcomes, and research have shown there is no benefit in using estrogens for preventing miscarriages. The risks to the developing fetus have become understood to be mutagenic in terms of transfer of genetic abnormal tendencies toward uterine abnormalities and vaginal cancer in subsequent generations.

These precautions for any therapy that contains estrogen are the same regardless of the indication. The exception is that ethinyl estradiol is contraindicated in patients who smoke and are older than 35 years. Smoking patients may use postmenopausal hormone replacement therapy (ERT/HRT) due to the lower dosages of hormone; however, the risk of clotting and cardiovascular events remains higher than for nonsmokers. The interaction of estrogens and smoking showing dose-related morbidity and mortality has been well documented.

Adverse Drug Reactions

Most of the adverse reactions to estrogens are dose-related. As a result, the majority of adverse effects are seen in patients using oral contraceptives. Some of the most concerning adverse reactions with estrogen are cardiovascular and hematological—myocardial infarction, hypertension, alteration in clotting factors, and thromboembolism. Unopposed estrogen use in women with an intact uterus increases the risk of abnormal uterine bleeding, endometrial hyperplasia, and gynecological cancers and should not be prescribed. Women using estrogen therapy need adequate screening for risks that may predispose them to greater risk of adverse events, and should receive education on the risks and possible warning symptoms associated with these events.

Additional adverse reactions are discussed in further detail in subsequent chapters for managing migraine headaches, mood changes, eye discomfort, skin pigmentation, breast changes, weight gain, change in vaginal secretion, and leg discomforts. The adverse reactions more common with menopausal estrogens are elevation of systemic blood pressure, gallbladder disease, and irregular bleeding. Women who have estrogen-dependent tumors may have worsening of their cancer while on any form of estrogen therapy; therefore, it is not advised for women with a current cancer or a history of estrogen-dependent cancer to use estrogen therapies.

Drug Interactions

Estrogens can interfere with laboratory measurements of endocrine and liver function tests and thyroid-binding globulin; however, in most cases it does not. In addition, the prothrombin time and factors VII, VIII, IX, and X show increased levels in patients taking estrogens at the time of testing. Women may experience impaired glucose tolerance and increased triglycerides when oral estrogens are administered. The most common drug interactions are with anticoagulants, tricyclic antidepressants, barbiturates, antituberculosis drugs, corticosteroids, seizure control medication, and drugs for spasticity. Table 22-5 presents drug interactions.

Table 22–5 ⚏ Common Drug Interactions: Estrogens and Antiestrogens

Drug	Interacting Drug	Possible Effect	Implications
Estrogens	Oral anticoagulants	Estrogens increase the risk of thromboembolitic events	The use of estrogen-containing products is contraindicated in individuals at high risk for coagulopathy
	Fosamprenavir	Alter efficacy of both agents; alter hepatic metabolism	Combination is contraindicated. Use nonhormonal contraception.
	Benzodiazepines, rifampin	Barbiturates, rifampin, and other agents that induce hepatic microsomal enzymes with concomitant estrogens may produce lower estrogen levels than expected	Use a backup birth control method
	Corticosteroids	Estrogen coadministration may reduce the clearance and increase the elimination half-life of corticosteroids	It may be necessary to lower steroid dosage if there is an increase in adverse effects
	Dantrolene	Hepatotoxicity occurred more often in women >35 yr receiving dantrolene and estrogen	Check liver function tests after first 4 wk of therapy in women >35 yr
	Anticonvulsants	Breakthrough bleeding, spotting, and pregnancy have resulted when these medications were used concurrently. A loss of seizure control has also been suggested and may be due to fluid retention	Check blood levels of seizure medications after first 2 wk of therapy. Using a backup birth control method or switching to an IUD is preferred.

Table 22–5 ⚏ **Common Drug Interactions: Estrogens and Antiestrogens—cont'd**

Drug	Interacting Drug	Possible Effect	Implications
Antiestrogens			
Clomiphene	Bromsulphalein (BSP) lab studies	BSP retention of >5% reported in 10%–20% of patients; retention is usually minimal but elevated during prolonged clomiphene administration or with apparently unrelated liver disease. In some, preexisting BSP, retention decreased even though clomiphene was continued. Other liver function tests usually normal.	Use other liver function tests when patient is taking clomiphene
Danazol	Insulin and diabetic agents	Insulin requirements may increase in patients with diabetes; abnormal glucose tolerance tests may be seen	More frequent glucose monitoring; possible decreased dosing of antidiabetic agents
	Warfarin	Prolongation of PT reported with concomitant use	Measure PT more frequently
	Amiodarone, clarithromycins, erythromycins	QT prolongation, cardiac arrhythmias	Avoid combination/select alternative agents
	Statin agents	Inhibits metabolism of statin agent, increases risk of rhabdomyolysis	Avoid combination/select alternative agents
Tamoxifen	Anticoagulants	Hypoprothrombinemic effect may be increased by concurrent tamoxifen administration	Monitor PT more frequently. Consider a nonhormonal, non-SERM alternative
	Medications that utilize the CYPP450 3A4, 2C9, 2D6 pathways	Altered metabolism	Evaluate each agent individually
	Lab studies	T_4 elevations occurred in a few postmenopausal patients but not accompanied by clinical hyperthyroidism	Measure TSH instead of T_4
Raloxifene	Bile-acid sequestrants (Cholestyramine)	Raloxifene absorption and enterohepatic cycling reduced 60%	Avoid combination. Consider statins to decrease cholesterol
	Warfarin	In single-dose studies, 10% decreases in PT have been observed	Monitor PT closely, or consider alternative agent to raloxifene
	Thyroid agents	Combination may cause hypothyroidism	Separate dosing by at least 12 hours; closely monitor TSH at initiation of therapy—may require increased dose of thyroid hormones while using raloxifene
Conjugated estrogens + bazedoxifene (Duavee)	No studies conducted—see estrogen. For bazedoxifene: Rifampin, phenobarb, carbamazepine, phenytoin	No known CYP interactions with bazedoxifene UGT interactions increase metabolism of bazadoxifene	May need additional uterine protection/monitoring
Osepemifene (Osphena)	Estrogen, fluconazole, ketoconazole	May increase SE	
	Rifampin	May decrease osepemifene effect	

UGT = uridine diphosphate glucuronosyltransferase in the gut.

Clinical Use and Dosing

Relief of Perimenopausal and Postmenopausal Symptoms

Relief of menopausal vasomotor symptoms can be dramatic after the initiation of hormonal therapy. The lowest effective dose of estrogen should be used for the shortest duration possible. Estrogen is available in various formulations, including estrogens derived from animal, plant, and synthetic sources. For women who have no objections to estrogens from animal sources, conjugated equine estrogen (Premarin) is available in doses from 0.3 mg to 2.5 mg. Suppression of hot flashes has been shown to be best at 0.625 mg, followed by 0.45 mg and 0.3 mg/d (Liu, 2004). Studies reported by Liu indicate that vasomotor symptoms begin to decrease by the second week of therapy and reach maximal effect by the eighth week of therapy. Dosage increases should not occur, however, until at least a 6 to 8 week interval to give the drug time to reach maximal effect at that dose.

Micronized estradiol (Estrace, Gynodiol) is the only bioidentical estrogen-alone product that is available in pill form. It is available in 0.5 mg to 2 mg doses. Vasomotor suppression is found at 1 mg and 2 mg doses. The typical regimen is 1 mg taken daily. The lower dose (0.5 mg) has been used for osteoporosis prevention but is less useful for vasomotor symptom relief. The bisphosphonates should be considered if treatment of osteoporosis is the primary goal of therapy. They are only used together in extreme cases where both are required for full bone effect.

For women who prefer estrogens derived from plant sources, estrone-based drugs are available. In a randomized, blinded, four-arm trial conducted by Sood and associates, compounded hormones were associated with lower and inconsistent levels of serum estrogen in subjects compared to a standard estradiol patch or oral doses. They also determined that further studies were needed to find comparable doses (Sood et al, 2013). Synthetic conjugated estrogen-A (Cenestin) is available in doses from 0.3 mg to 1.25 mg. Liu (2004) found that the majority (77%) of women randomized to Cenestin required a total daily dose of 1.25 mg to relieve vasomotor symptoms, whereas the remaining 23% required 0.625 mg or less. By week 8, the vasomotor symptoms were significantly decreased. Synthetic conjugated estrogen-B (Enjuvia) is available in doses of 0.3 mg to 1.25 mg, with the lower dose producing relief in many women. Estropipate (Ogen, Ortho-EST) is also derived from plant sources and is available in 0.75 to 6 mg tablets. Following the rule to use the lowest dose to control symptoms, the dosing regimen should start at 0.75 mg.

Findings from the WHI, Women's HOPE study, and multiple meta-analyses suggest that therapy to treat the vasomotor and urogenital symptoms associated with menopause should be started early in menopause in an effort to reduce adverse cardiovascular events (Warren, 2010). When initiating therapy, begin with lowest starting dose of the selected estrogen product. Clinicians may wish to initiate an even slower taper or defer to a specialist for those women who have relative contraindications or precautions to estrogen therapy and who still elect to proceed with estrogen therapy. One proposed example is to use small doses (0.3 mg) of conjugated estrogens every other day for 2 months. Then, gradually increase the estrogens to daily use for another 2 months. If symptoms such as bleeding or breast pain do not occur, increase the estrogen up to 0.625 mg daily. Some women may need only the lower estrogen dosages to adequately control their symptoms as long as they have an adequate diet. Remember, estrogen must be partnered with progesterone to prevent endometrial hyperplasia and cancer in women with an intact uterus. ERT and HRT should be reevaluated on an annual basis, with the goal of utilizing therapy for 5 or fewer years.

Complementary and alternative therapies include phytoestrogens, botanicals, and herbs. These alternatives have varying degrees of effectiveness and research support.

Prevention and Management of Vulvovaginal Atrophy and Dryness

A decline in estrogen causes the vaginal mucosa and vulvar skin to become thin and atrophic. The result is discomfort, itching, dyspareunia, and increased cases of vaginitis. Low-dose oral ERT with estrogen from plant or animal sources has been shown to decrease vaginal pH, thus reducing vaginal infections. It also thickens and revascularizes the vaginal epithelium, increases the number of superficial cells, and reverses vaginal atrophy (Tan, Bradshaw, & Carr, 2012). Vaginal estrogen also produces these positive effects, and the changes begin in as short a time frame as 2 weeks. Topical creams and intravaginal delivery of estrogen are equally as efficacious as oral agents in the management of vulvovaginal symptoms.

An option for dryness and dyspareunia is an estrogen agonist-antagonist ospemifene (Osphena). It is technically a SERM medication, but does not have the bone health indication. The agonist action of this molecule is akin to estrogen, but at tissue level, so it increases the thickness moisture of the vaginal canal. The package insert has many similar adverse effects to estrogen such as increasing the risk of blood clots, hot flashes, and uterine cancer (though no cases have been reported). It has only weak effect on the uterus and breast, but the FDA requires listing of all the major estrogen risks without strong data to prove otherwise. Its impact on breast cancer risk is unknown, but considered weak. Therefore, this is used for the shortest possible time to overcome issues of moderate to severe painful intercourse. Because it is a newly released medication, the post-marketing data is not available to provide any reliable information on which to base a rationale drug selection. The known pharmacokinetic and drug interactions are included in the chapter tables for reference upon which to build future understanding of this medication. The starting dose is 60 mg daily. No dosage adjustments are needed in renal patients. Contraindications include prior blood clots, active thromboembolic disease or a family history of such, known estrogen-dependent hyperplasia or neoplasia, and abnormal genital bleeding.

Reduced Risk for Colon Cancer

Colorectal cancer is the third most common cancer in women in the United States and the third most common cause of cancer death in women (Thorneycroft, 2004). Because this cancer is also associated with aging, it clearly is a cancer to be considered concurrently with menopause. ERT and HRT have been shown to reduce the risk of colon cancer; however, the use of estrogen-containing products for colon cancer risk reduction alone is not approved.

Prevention and Treatment of Osteoporosis

Estrogen is associated with bone formation and has osteoprotective benefits. Until the WHI report, estrogen had been used solely for both prevention and treatment of osteoporosis. Estrogens prevent osteoporosis by reducing the bone-resorbing action of PTH. Estrogen receptors have been found in bone, which validates the hypothesis that estrogen may have direct effects on bone remodeling. Studies have shown that there is a direct correlation between the rate of bone loss in menopausal women and estradiol levels (Youngkin, Davis, Schaldewald, & Juve, 2013). Bone resorption has also been shown to be highest in the first postmenopausal year. Bone density declines between 1% and 4% in the first several years after menopause and then stabilizes to about 1% per year. Women in the immediate postmenopausal years are the ones who are most in need of protection from osteoporosis.

Chapter 38 looks at the use of estrogen alone and in combination with other drugs in the treatment of osteoporosis. ERT and HRT use can significantly slow the natural progression of bone loss in postmenopausal women. Numerous studies have shown significant improvement in bone mineral density (BMD) and the reduction of hip and vertebral fractures in women using ERT and HRT; however, current practice cautions against selecting ERT and HRT exclusively for the prevention of osteoporosis. The WHI findings that ERT and HRT raised the risk for coronary events, stroke, pulmonary emboli, and breast cancer in women who took a combination of estrogen and progesterone have led leading national women's health organizations, the FDA, and U.S. Preventative Services Task Force to encourage clinicians to consider alternative options for osteoporosis prevention and treatment when women are not experiencing moderate to severe menopausal symptoms. Balancing the risks and benefits of estrogen therapy and the availability of other drugs to prevent and treat osteoporosis should be discussed with women, who can then make an intelligent decision about whether to use estrogen. Dosing for osteoporosis may not work for menopausal symptoms. The long-term efficacy of taking estrogen in lower doses for prevention of osteoporosis remains unknown at this time. The use of SERM medications for this indication is covered in Chapter 38.

Contraception

There are currently two formulations of estrogen available in combination contraceptive preparations, ethinyl estradiol (EE) and mestranol. Mestranol is the weaker of the two preparations and must be metabolized into EE before it is able to bind with estrogen receptors. Fifty mcg of mestranol is equivalent to 35 mcg of EE. EE is the estrogen used in the vast majority of hormonal contraceptive formulations in wide use today with most preparations containing between 20 and 35 mcg of EE. The estrogen component of hormonal contraception improves efficacy by suppressing FSH release and therefore development of a dominant follicle. Estrogen also adds to cycle control, decreasing the irregular bleeding patterns commonly found with progestin-only methods.

Combined oral contraceptives come in three main formulations. The most common formulation is a monophasic combined oral contraceptive (COC) that contains the same dose of hormone in each active pill. Biphasic pills alter the hormone dose in the middle of the cycle, and triphasic pills alter the estrogen dose, the progesterone dose, or both each week during

a 28 day-dose pack. Additionally, there are progesterone-only contraceptives available; these are discussed later in this chapter. Chapter 31 summarizes the brand-name and synthetic hormone formulas commonly available.

The theoretical effectiveness of prevention of pregnancy with COCs is 99% or greater. Patients who receive education on the proper use of COCs have lower discontinuation rates and therefore fewer unwanted pregnancies. Additionally, clinicians should provide patients with information on emergency hormonal contraception and the use of a backup method such as spermicide and condoms.

Because the different COCs have similar effectiveness and are well tolerated, choosing among them may seem difficult. Although there are some advantages to selecting one type of progesterone option over another, for the majority of patients it is generally best to use a drug that has the lowest estrogen dose while still offering cycle control. Thin teens can frequently use the low-estrogen pills; women typically need a higher dose. Issues of acne breakout are dealt with by reducing the amount of androgen in the formulation selected.

Off-Label Uses

COCs have been used to treat conditions for which a formal FDA approval has not been awarded. Many of these off-label uses have considerable literature and research to support clinical use. Some pharmaceutical companies have sought FDA approval for specific indications for marketing purposes (such as acne management). Prescribers must disclose to patients when agents are being used for off-label purposes, thoroughly review the risks and benefits, and obtain informed consent. Table 22-6 presents the dosage schedule of estrogens other than those used for contraception.

Rational Drug Selection

Short-Acting Versus Long-Acting

A consistent and expected level of estrogen is maintained with same-time daily dosing. Some women may have problems remembering or difficulty in swallowing the oral form, so intravaginal, transdermal, or parenteral administration is preferable. Giving injections every 3 to 4 weeks is uncomfortable. The daily levels may vary, depending on the circulation in the muscle into which the dose is injected.

Formulation

Oral formulations of estrogen are the most commonly selected formulation by patients and prescribers, but there may be reasons for selecting another formulation. Most estrogens are available in transdermal formulation. The major advantage of transdermal formulations is their once- or twice-weekly application. A disadvantage is the incidence of skin irritation that occurs in 20% to 40% of users (Wysocki & Alexander, 2005). Vaginal instillation is possible for patients unable to tolerate oral formulations or for severe urethral and urogenital atrophy, as in vulvar dystrophies and dyspareunia. Low-dose vaginal estrogens (with the ring or cream) are not associated with as much risk of endometrial hyperplasia as are the oral forms. The estradiol-releasing

Table 22–6 ⚕ Dosage Schedule: Estrogens and Antiestrogens

Drug	Indication	Dosage Form	Initial Dose	Maintenance Dose
Estrogens				
	Moderate to severe vasomotor symptoms associated with menopause			Attempts to discontinue should be made at 3–6 mo intervals
Estrogen (Conjugated A/Synthetic) (Cenestin)		Tablet, oral: 0.3 mg, 0.45 mg, 0.625 mg, 0.9 mg, 1.25 mg	0.45 mg/d	May be titrated up to 1.25 mg/d
Esterified estrogen/ methyltestosterone (Covaryx, Covaryx HS, EEMT, EEMT HS)		Tablet, oral: Covaryx 1.25/2.5 mg Covaryx HS 0.625/1.25 mg EEMT 1.25/2.5 mg EEMT HS 0.625/1.25 mg	0.625 mg/d 3 wk on and 1 wk off	0.625–1.25 mg/d 3 wk on and 1 wk off
Estrogen (Conjugated B/Synthetic) (Enjuvia)		Tablet, oral: 0.3 mg, 0.45 mg, 0.625 mg, 0.9 mg, 1.25 mg	0.3 mg/d	May titrate up to 1.25 mg/d
Estrogen (Esterfied) (Menest)		Tablet, oral: 0.3 mg, 0.625 mg, 1.25 mg, 2.5 mg	1.25 mg/d 3 wk on and 1 wk off	1.25 mg/d 3 wk on and 1 wk off
Estrogen (Conjugated/ Equine) (Premarin)		Tablet, oral: 0.3 mg, 0.45 mg, Tablet, oral: 0.625 mg, 0.9 mg, 1.25 mg	0.3 mg/d Cyclically or daily	0.3–1.25 mg Adjust based on patient response, lowest dose to control symptoms
Estrogen (Conjugated/ Equine) and Medroxyprogesterone (Premphase, Prempro)		Premphase (pak) Conjugated estrogens 0.625 mg (14/tab) and conjugated estrogen 0.625 mg/medroxyprogesterone 5 mg (14/tab) Prempro (conjugated estrogens/medroxyprogesterone) 0.3/1.5 mg (28 tab), 0.45/1.5 mg (28 tab), 0.625/2.5 mg (28 tab), 0.625/5 mg (28 tab)	Start estrogen at 0.625 mg daily	Adjust per symptoms
	Female hypogonadism			
(Menest)		Tablet, oral: 0.3 mg, 0.625 mg, 1.25 mg, 2.5 mg	2.5 mg/d 3 wk on and 1 wk off	2.5–7.5 mg/d 3 wk on and 1 wk off
(Premarin)		Tablet, oral: 0.625 mg, 0.9 mg, 1.25 mg	0.3 mg/d cyclically	0.3–0.625mg/d
	Breast cancer Palliation therapy			
(Menest)		Tablet, oral: 0.3 mg, 0.625 mg, 1.25 mg, 2.5 mg	Males and postmenopausal females 10 mg 3 times/d for at least 3 mo	10 mg 3 times/d for at least 3 mo
(Premarin)		Tablet, oral: 0.625 mg, 0.9 mg, 1.25 mg	10 mg 3 times/d for at least 3 mo	10 mg 3 times/d for at least 3 mo
	Prostate cancer Palliation therapy			

Table 22–6 ⚕ Dosage Schedule: Estrogens and Antiestrogens—cont'd

Drug	Indication	Dosage Form	Initial Dose	Maintenance Dose
(Menest)		Tablet, oral: 0.3 mg, 0.625 mg, 1.25 mg, 2.5 mg	Advanced cancer 1.25 mg 3 times/d	1.25–2.5 mg 3 times/d
(Premarin)		Tablet, oral: 0.625 mg, 0.9 mg, 1.25 mg	1.25 mg 3 times/d	1.25–2.5 mg 3 times/d
	Vaginal dryness/ vulvar and vaginal atrophy associated with menopause			
(Enjuvia)		Tablet, oral: 0.3 mg, 0.45 mg, 0.625 mg, 0.9 mg, 1.25 mg	0.3 mg/d	0.3 mg/d
(Estrace)		Vaginal cream: 0.1 mg/g (42.5 g)	2–4 g/d for 1–2 wk; gradually reduce to ½ the initial dose for 1–2 wk	1 g 1–3 times/wk
(Estring)		Vaginal ring: 2 mg/ring	2 mg	Ring in place for 90 days
(Premarin)		Tablet, oral: 0.625 mg, 0.9 mg, 1.25 mg	0.625 mg daily	Adjust based on patient's response
(Vagifem)		Vaginal tablet: 10 mcg/tablet	1 tablet once daily for 2 weeks	1 tablet twice weekly
	Female castration; primary ovarian failure			
(Menest)		Tablet, oral: 0.3 mg, 0.625 mg, 1.25 mg, 2.5 mg	1.25 mg/d 3 weeks on and 1 week off	Adjust dosage upward or downward according to symptoms; maintenance is lowest level that will provide effective control
(Premarin)		Tablet, oral: 0.625 mg, 0.9 mg, 1.25 mg	1.25 mg/d cyclically	Adjust dosage upward or downward according to symptoms; maintenance is lowest level that will provide effective control
(Premarin)	Osteoporosis	0.625 mg, 0.9 mg, 1.25 mg	0.3 mg/d cyclically or daily	Adjust based on bone mineral density
Antiestrogens				
Clomiphene (Clomid, Serophene)	Treatment of ovulary failure in patients desiring pregnancy whose partners are potent and fertile	Clomid: 50 mg Scrophen: 50 mg Generic: 50 mg	50 mg/day for 5 days Begin 5th day of cycle	Adjust as needed; max dose 100 mg. Lower dose of 12.5–25 mg for women sensitive to med or who consistently develop large ovarian cysts
Danazol (Danazol)	Endometriosis	Tablet, oral: 50 mg, 100 mg, 200 mg Generic available	Mild disease: 200–400 mg/d in 2 divided doses Moderate to severe disease: 800 mg/d in 2 divided doses	Dosage should be individualized. Continue therapy for 3–6 mo (up to 9 mo)

Continued

Table 22–6 🕸 **Dosage Schedule: Estrogens and Antiestrogens—cont'd**

Drug	Indication	Dosage Form	Initial Dose	Maintenance Dose
	Fibrotic breast disease		100–400 mg/d in 2 divided doses	Therapy based on symptoms: Pain and tenderness to 2–3 mo Nodularity 4–6 mo
	Hereditary angioedema (males/females)		200 mg 2–3 times/d	After favorable response, decrease by 50% or less for 1–3 mo For acute attack, increase dose to 200 mg/d
Tamoxifen (Soltamox)	Breast cancer (females) Metastatic (males and females) Ductal carcinoma in situ (DCIS) (females) Breast cancer risk reduction Endometrial carcinoma, recurrent, metastatic, or high-risk (unlabeled use) Induction of ovulation (unlabeled use) Ovarian cancer, advanced or recurrent (unlabeled use) Paget's disease of the breast (risk reduction; with DCIS or without associated cancer)	Solution, oral: 10 mg/5 mL (150 mL) Generic Tablet, oral: 10 mg, 20 mg	Adjuvant therapy 20 mg/d for 5 yr ER-positive up to 10 yr 20–40 mg/d in divided dose if >20 mg 20 mg/day for 5 yr 20 mg/d for 5 yr Monotherapy: 20 mg twice daily until disease progression Combination therapy: 20 mg twice daily for 3 wk 20 mg/d for 5 days 20 mg twice daily 20 mg/d for 5 yr	20 mg/d No clinical benefit demonstrated with doses above 20 mg daily 20 mg/d 20 mg/d 20 mg/twice daily 20-80 mg/d 20 mg twice daily 20 mg/day
Raloxifene (Evista)	Prevention of osteoporosis in postmenopausal women Invasive breast cancer risk reduction (females)	Tablet, oral: 60 mg	60 mg/d 60 mg/d for 5 yr	60 mg/d 60 mg/d
Anastrazole (Armidex)	Postmenopausal breast cancer inhibition	1 mg tablet	1 mg ; no change for most renal patients or elders	Usually taken for 5 yr after tamoxifen, but can be first line medication as well and extend beyond 5 yr of use.
Letrozole (Femara	Postmenopausal breast cancer inhibition	2.5 mg tablets	2.5 mg; no renal dosing or change for elders	As above
Exemestabe (Aromasin)	Postmenopausal breast cancer inhibition	25 mg tablets	25 mg	As above
Ospemifene (Osphena)	Vaginal atrophy, dyspareunia	60 mg tablets	60 mg for moderate or severe issues	
Bazedoxifene & conjugated estrogen (Duavee)	Hot flashes and osteoporosis	20 mg–0.45 mg tablets	One tablet daily for both indications	Use for shortest duration possible to minimize estrogen related risks

vaginal ring/string also has a positive effect on urethral and vaginal atrophy symptoms. Estrace is a bioidentical vaginal cream approved for the treatment of vaginal and urinary symptoms.

The usual doses for all the creams include nightly application. Topical application with vaginal rings and vaginal tablets may be preferred by patients because they may be perceived as easier to administer and less "messy" than the creams. The differences between the oral versus topical formulations are 2-fold: (1) the oral formulations retain the positive effects of ERT that accrue because of liver metabolism and the topical formulations lose this benefit; and (2) the total amount of estrogen to which the body is exposed is less with the topical formulations, which may be a consideration for women who have risk factor concerns with ERT. A dose of 25 mcg per day of estradiol administered vaginally does not significantly raise blood levels of estrogen, especially if vaginal cornification has already taken place. Studies reported by Thorneycroft (2004) found no evidence of increased risk of CHD, breast cancer, or endometrial cancer with the use of vaginal ERT. Low-dose vaginal estrogens have not been shown to be associated with endometrial hyperplasia; however, decades of application have not been studied (Tan et al, 2012).

Cost

The pricing of oral estrogen and estrogen-combination products can vary significantly. Because oral preparations have been around the longest, several generic versions are available and are the least expensive. Several vaginal creams are also available in generic versions. The latest products and brand-name products tend to be the most expensive. Transdermal preparations, the vaginal ring, and prepackaged punch-out cards or dial packs for convenience are generally priced higher. Cost may be a determining factor in product selection for women on Medicare, those who have fixed incomes, or those who have multiple medications to purchase.

Route of Administration

As previously discussed, the route of administration affects hepatic metabolism of estrogen and can impact potential side effects and risks. Beyond these considerations, patient preference and affordability determine route selection. Oral formulations are typically preferred by patients and are easy for most patients to administer at mealtime or bedtime. A small percentage of women experience elevated triglycerides with oral estrogens; these patients can avoid liver metabolism of the medication through transdermal absorption. Transdermal patches allow patients the freedom of less frequent dosing and may be preferred by caregivers who assist patients with limited dexterity and an inability to swallow. Vaginal application reduces liver metabolism. It is systemically absorbed less after the initial vaginal atrophy is treated. Estrogen levels are not as high after the first 6 months of therapy. As some older women and the disabled lack the finger dexterity to fill an applicator and instill the cream, clinicians

should assess the ability of patients to use this route of administration. Table 22-6 presents the available dosage forms of estrogen.

Monitoring

Oral contraception, ERT, and HRT are chronic medications that are taken for months or years. All patients should have their blood pressure monitored. If the patient has a coexisting medical condition, monitoring of adverse effects is necessary (see Chaps. 31 and 38). Schedule 1-month, 3-month, 6-month, or annual evaluation appointments, depending on the degree of illness or the severity of symptoms. Patient education regarding the symptoms and reporting of potentially worrisome adverse effects are necessary at the institution of therapy. Drawing baseline blood tests, including a lipid panel, and ordering mammograms prior to prescribing ERT or HRT are recommended. Additionally, women should have annual mammograms, pelvic evaluations, and cardiovascular assessments while on ERT or HRT. Patients with diabetes need to perform daily blood glucose measurements until stable on ERT or HRT because adjustment to diabetes agents may be needed. Patients with hypertension need monthly blood pressure readings. Patients with seizure disorders will need initial increased frequency of laboratory monitoring of seizure medications and then every 6 months because estrogen therapy may alter drug metabolism, affecting therapeutic levels of antiepileptic medications.

PATIENT EDUCATION

Administration

Patients taking oral hormonal contraceptives and HRT need to take the drug daily at about the same time to avoid breakthrough bleeding. Specific patient education regarding anticipated transient and nuisance side effects at the time of initiating therapy will improve adherence to therapy. Women may experience transient adverse effects such as mild nausea and breast tenderness or midcycle spotting during the first 2 months of therapy. Sometimes taking the medication at bedtime solves the nausea problem. Advise the patient to seek follow-up to discuss alternatives to oral therapy if nausea or vomiting or other issues make oral therapy unsuccessful. Advise the patient to rotate the application sites for transdermal patches and to avoid applying patches to breast tissue.

Devices to improve adherence to a daily regimen include pill organizer boxes and ways of making the drug part of the daily routine. For example, some women find it easier to put the birth control packet by their toothbrush or alarm clock or set an alarm on their phone to avoid forgetting the medication.

Adverse Reactions

The breasts, uterus, and vagina are the more obvious organs dependent on estrogen. Although adverse drug reactions were discussed earlier in this section, clinicians need to communicate the following information to patients who are initiating or renewing estrogen-containing prescriptions. Leg pain, visual disturbances, and severe headache could herald thromboembolic phenomena that could be life-threatening. Patients who smoke and those who are diabetic are at increased risk for this type of complication. Abnormal bleeding patterns or genital pain needs to be reported in all age groups. In younger women who experience irregular bleeding, infection or pregnancy is suspected. But bleeding in a postmenopausal woman may be the first symptom of uterine or ovarian cancer. Dysfunctional uterine bleeding in any perimenopausal or postmenopausal woman should be considered to be cancer until proved otherwise, and the appropriate steps should be taken to determine the presence or absence of cancer.

Lifestyle Management

Smoking increases the risk of thrombolytic events in patients taking estrogen. The use of estrogen-containing contraception in women who smoke and are over the age of 35 is contraindicated. All patients who smoke should be counseled on the added risks associated with concurrent tobacco use and estrogen products. Patients who quit smoking for at least 1 year are considered nonsmokers.

Routine exercise and dietary changes have been associated with a reduction in vasomotor symptoms of menopause and reduced symptoms of dysmenorrhea.

The use of condoms and barrier devices to reduce the risk of sexually transmitted infections is also an important component of contraceptive management and should be assessed and encouraged at prescription initiation and refill.

PROGESTERONES AND PROGESTERONE ANTAGONISTS

The progesterones include progesterone (Prometrium, Progesterone in Oil, Crinone, Prochieve), medroxyprogesterone acetate (Provera), norethindrone (Aygestin), and megestrol acetate (Megace). Most are used in oral contraceptives and for HRT. Many formulations (sometimes referred to as "generations") of progesterone have been developed to address issues of mood change, breakthrough bleeding, and sensitivity to progesterone agents.

Currently there are several different androgen-derived progestins available in oral contraceptive preparations: norethindrone, norethindrone acetate, ethynodiol diacetate, norgestrel, desogestrel, levonorgestrel, and norgestimate. Norethindrone acetate and ethynodiol diacetate are converted to norethindrone in the body. Levonorgestrel is the levorotatory form of norgestrel and its active metabolite.

Desogestrel and norgestimate offer a decrease in androgenicity when compared to other progesterones. Desogestrel undergoes conversion to its active metabolite etonogestrel, which is the progestin used in the vaginal ring. Norelgestromin is the primary metabolite of norgestimate and is available as a contraceptive patch. Decreased androgenicity theoretically reduces adverse effects on carbohydrate and lipid metabolism found in previous formulations, as well as improves acne and hirsutism. Medroxyprogesterone acetate is available for injectable contraception.

Drospirenone is a progestin developed as a derivative of spironolactone. As a derivative of spironolactone, it has a mild diuretic effect as well as antimineralocorticoid effects. The drug has been granted FDA approval for the treatment of premenstrual syndrome and contraception when it is a component of a COC pill. Drospirenone may cause hyperkalemia and should be used cautiously with women who are using drugs that cause a potassium-sparing effect, such as ACE inhibitors, or have underlying renal disease. Box 22-3 presents information on progesterone antagonists. Drospirenone is associated with a higher risk of venous thromboembolism (VTE) than COCs containing the progestin levonorgestrel or some other progestins.

Pharmacodynamics

Effects of progestin on the reproductive organs include thickening of the endometrium and increasing its complexity in preparation for pregnancy; thickening of cervical

---

BOX 22–3 PROGESTERONE ANTAGONISTS

Mifepristone (Mifeprex)

Mifepristone was approved by the FDA on September 28, 2000, for termination of intrauterine pregnancy. It has a long half-life (18 h) and may prolong the follicular phase of the subsequent cycle. It is strongly bound to plasma proteins (98%). This binding is saturable and the drug has nonlinear pharmacokinetics with relation to plasma concentration and clearance. The antiprogestational activity results from competitive interaction with progesterone at progesterone receptor sites. The drug inhibits the activity of both endogenous and exogenous progesterone. When there is no progesterone to maintain a pregnancy, termination results. In 85% of women, mifepristone will act as an abortifacient when used in conjunction with misoprostol during the first 7 weeks of pregnancy. Women should expect to experience bleeding or spotting for an average of 9 to 16 days. Persistent heavy or moderate bleeding for more than 30 days could indicate an incomplete abortion. There are very specific requirements associated with administration of this drug, and it is best done in clinics that can meet these requirements. The drug is available only from the manufacturer and not through licensed pharmacies.

Mifepristone also exhibits antiglucocorticoid and weak antiandrogenic activity. Off-labeled uses in the treatment of endometriosis, Cushing's syndrome, and uterine leiomyomata are under study.

mucus; thinning of the vaginal mucosa; and relaxation of smooth muscles of the uterus and fallopian tube. During pregnancy, progestin maintains the thickened endometrium, relaxes myometrial muscles, thickens the myometrium for labor, is responsible for placental development, and prevents lactation until the fetus is born. In the absence of pregnancy, the reduced production of estrogen and progestin by the corpus luteum results in the shedding of endometrium to produce menstruation. Progestin is also responsible for alveolobular development of the secretory apparatus of the breast. Progestin also has actions outside the reproductive system. It stimulates lipoprotein activity and seems to favor fat deposition; increases basal insulin levels and insulin response to glucose; promotes glycogen storage in the liver; promotes ketogenesis; competes with aldosterone in the renal tubule to decrease Na^+ resorption; increases body temperature; and increases ventilatory response to CO_2, resulting in a measurable decrease in $PaCO_2$. The latter occurs only during pregnancy.

No significant differences in endometrial lining were noted with vaginal estrogen therapy alone. The North American Menopause Society states that progesterones are not indicated in low-risk, asymptomatic women on lower-dose vaginal estrogen forumlations. Endometrial monitoring is not indicated except for postmenopausal bleeding (Tan et al, 2012).

Pharmacokinetics

Absorption and Distribution

Progesterone is rapidly absorbed following any route of administration. Oral progestins are rapidly absorbed from the GI tract and quickly undergo hepatic degradation. Following IM administration, progesterone in oil is rapidly absorbed and undergoes hepatic metabolism. Long-acting forms can be maintained for 3 to 6 months. The gel formulation has sustained-release properties, so absorption can be lengthened to 50 hours. Subdermal implants of progesterone are also available. In the United States, Implanon/Nexplanon is available to providers who have completed specific training on insertion. Nexplanon is the newest subdermal implant. The difference between the two is that Nexplanon is radiopaque and the earlier Implanon is not. Subdermal implant progesterone is well absorbed through the dermis at a continuous rate and is effective for 3 years. Progesterone formulation in the form of an IUD is also available. The Mirena IUD is effective for 5 years. Progesterone binds to plasma albumin and corticosteroid-binding globulin.

Metabolism and Excretion

Oral progesterone is rapidly metabolized in the first pass through the liver. In the liver, progesterone is metabolized to pregnanediol and with the glucuronide metabolites conjugated with glucuronic acid. It is excreted in the urine. IM and implantable progesterone is extensively bound to serum proteins. Its metabolites are excreted 60% by the kidney and 10% through the bile and feces. The gel formulation is also eliminated through the renal route.

Onset, Peak, and Duration

Onset, peak, and duration vary based on the form of progesterone. After oral administration, the peak concentrations for oral progesterone occur after 1 to 2 hours. Half-life also varies by the form of progesterone and can be from 4 to 40 hours. IM preparations reach peak levels by 24 hours and have a half-life of approximately 10 weeks. The liver quickly metabolizes the gel formulation, but the long absorption half-life provides the steady serum concentrations. The absorption half-life of the vaginal gel can be from 25 to 50 hours. With the subdermal implant, maximum serum etonogestrel concentrations were reached within the first 2 weeks after insertion. Levonorgestrel in the Mirena IUD peaks at 20 mcg/d approximately 2 weeks after insertion. Table 22-7 presents the pharmacokinetics of progestins.

Table 22–7 ⚙ Pharmacokinetics: Progesterones and Progesterone Antagonists

Drug	Peak	Active Metabolite	Half-Life	Elimination
Progesterones				
Progesterone	1–2 h	5β-pregnan-3A, 20A-diol glucuronide	8–9 h	50%–60% in urine, 10% in bile and feces; small amount unchanged in bile
Progesterone gel	3.5 h (on daily dosing), 5.4 h (for bid dosing)	5β-pregnan-3A, 20A-diol glucuronide	45 h (for daily dosing), 25.9 h (for bid dosing)	50%–60% in urine, 10% in bile and feces; small amount unchanged in bile
Medroxyprogesterone acetate		5β-pregnan-3A, 20A-diol glucuronide	IM: 10 wk	15%–22% in feces; small amount unchanged in bile
Megestrol acetate	2.2 h	5β-pregnan-3A, 20A-diol glucuronide	34.2 h (mean)	50%–60% in urine, 10% in bile and feces; small amount unchanged in bile
Progesterone Antagonists				
Mifepristone (Mifeprex)	1–3 h	3 active metabolites	20–54 h	NA

NA = not available.

Pharmacotherapeutics

Precautions and Contraindications

Patients with thromboembolic disease or a history of it should not use progestins. Breast cancer may become worse under hormone influence. Patients with impaired liver function would have trouble metabolizing exogenous hormones.

Mental depression has been associated with both short-acting and long-acting progestins. The drug may need to be discontinued if depression recurs or occurs to a serious degree.

Fluid retention may occur. Patients with disorders that may be affected negatively by excess fluid (e.g., epilepsy, migraine, asthma, congestive heart failure, or renal dysfunction) require careful observation.

A decrease in glucose tolerance has been observed in a small percentage of patients on estrogen-progestin combination drugs. Diabetic patients should increase their glucose monitoring when receiving progestin therapy.

Progesterone is Pregnancy Category D and norethindrone acetate is Pregnancy Category X. Progesterone gel is used to support embryo implantation and maintain pregnancies as part of assisted reproductive technology (ART) treatments. Lactation may be enhanced by medroxyprogesterone, although the effects on the infant have not been determined.

Adverse Drug Reactions

The most common adverse reaction associated with progestins is irregular, breakthrough vaginal bleeding. Some patients may experience amenorrhea. Acne and chloasma have occurred with several of the more androgenic progestin products. Patients report increased breast tenderness and galactorrhea. Nausea, depression, and weight gain have also been reported.

Injectable and implanted progesterone for contraception use is associated with an increased incidence of weight change and irregular menstrual bleeding. Because of low estrogen levels associated with IM progestin (Depo-Provera), patients on this therapy are at increased risk for osteoporosis. In 2004, the FDA issued a Black-Box Warning for Depo-Provera. In the warning, the FDA cautioned about using this form of contraception for longer than 2 years unless other forms of contraception are not viable options. The bone density loss may extend beyond the duration of treatment. Clinicians need to perform a risk assessment and have a thorough discussion of this information with patients prior to the initiation of therapy. Delays to return to fertility may also occur with IM progestin use.

Drug Interactions

The two drugs known to have specific interactions with progestins are aminoglutethimide and rifampin. The primary result is to decrease effectiveness of progestin therapy, which can result in unplanned pregnancy. In addition to drug–drug interactions, progesterone can cause erroneous laboratory results in testing hepatic function, coagulation, thyroid, metyrapone, and other endocrine functions. Table 22-8 presents drug interactions.

Clinical Use and Dosing

Progestins are used for their effect on endometrial tissue. The major uses of progestational hormones are for perimenopausal and postmenopausal hormonal therapy and as a contraceptive alone and in combination with estrogen.

Perimenopausal and Postmenopausal Hormone Replacement

Combinations of estrogen and progestin are used when the uterus is intact. The risk for endometrial cancer secondary to endometrial hyperplasia has been consistently demonstrated in research studies of ERT and exists for all dose levels of ERT. To prevent this increased incidence, progestins, which reduce the buildup of endometrial tissue, are added to the treatment regimen. There are several combination therapies for use in menopause. These are discussed in more detail in the Rational Drug Selection section.

Table 22–8 ⊞ Common Drug Interactions: Progesterones and Progesterone Antagonists

Drug	Interacting Drug	Possible Effect	Implications
Progesterones			
Progesterone	Lab studies	Results of hepatic function, coagulation tests (increase in prothrombin; factors VII, VIII, IX, and X); thyroid, metyrapone test, and endocrine functions may be affected by progestins	Anticipate that laboratory levels of liver function and hormonal assays may not be accurate while the patient is taking these drugs
Medroxyprogesterone acetate (DMPA)	Aminoglutethimide	Aminoglutethimide may increase the hepatic metabolism of DMPA	Chemotherapy drug used for metastatic cancer. If spotting occurs, give DMPA earlier than 12 wk
Progesterone Antagonists			
Mifepristone (Mifeprex)	Agents that utilize the CYP450 3A4 pathway	Multiple interactions regarding changes in agent metabolism	Seek alternative options or close monitoring based on agents

Progestin-Only Contraception

Progestins exhibit a negative effect in the hypothalamic-pituitary-ovarian axis, essentially suppressing the LH surge necessary for ovulation. They also cause thickening of cervical mucus, making penetration by sperm difficult. Tubal motility is slowed, delaying transport of the ovum and sperm. In addition, progestins cause atrophy of the endometrium, preventing implantation.

There are several brand-name progestin-only pills available that each contain 0.35 mg of norethindrone. These pills contain no estrogen and are primarily used with special populations in which estrogen is contraindicated because of medical conditions or breastfeeding. Because progestin-only pills contain very low levels of hormone, users need to be particularly diligent to take their medications correctly.

The FDA approved the use of medroxyprogesterone acetate (Depo-Provera) for contraception in 1993. When administered IM at the recommended 150 mg dose every 3 months (12 weeks), it inhibits secretion of gonadotropins, which prevents follicular maturation and results in endometrial thinning. Most women using Depo-Provera experience disruption in menstrual bleeding patterns. These disruptions include irregular or unpredictable bleeding, spotting, or, rarely, heavy or continuous bleeding. Over half of all women on IM therapy will experience amenorrhea or some form of irregular menstrual bleeding. If abnormal bleeding persists or is severe, it should be investigated to rule out an underlying pathology. Depo-Provera has been associated with reduced bone density after chronic administration. Women using this form of contraception need to be made aware of the potential for osteoporosis, and this risk should be considered in choosing this form of contraception. Adolescents and young adults are of special concern, because growth in bone mineral density is largest during this age period and loss at this time reduces the total bone mass available later in life. As with all progestin products, there is a risk for thromboembolic events.

Off-Label Use of Progestins

Other off-label uses for progestins in the treatment of dysmenorrhea, endometriosis, hirsutism, and menstrual bleeding disorders are implemented when estrogen is contraindicated. The gel form of progesterone is used to assist in fertility programs for women with progesterone deficits. Refer to Chapter 31 for a more detailed discussion of progesterone as contraception and to Chapter 38 for its use in conjunction with estrogen for postmenopausal hormone therapy. Table 22-9 presents the dosage schedule of progestins and progesterone antagonists.

Table 22–9 ⊗ Dosage Schedule: Progesterones and Progesterone Antagonists

Drug	Indication	Dosage form	Initial Dose	Maintenance Dose
Progesterones				
Progesterone	Amenorrhea	Capsule, oral: Prometrium: 100 mg, 200 mg (contains peanut oil) (B) Generic: 100 mg, 200 mg (G)	IM: 5 10 mg/d for 6–8 consecutive days	IM: 5–10 mg/d for 6–8 consecutive days
	Amenorrhea, secondary		Intravaginal gel: 45 mg (4% gel) every other day for 6 doses	If response is inadequate, may increase to 90 mg (8% gel)
	ART in patients who require progesterone supplementation	Gel, Vaginal Crinone 4% (1.45 g); 8% (1.45 g) (B) Insert, Vaginal:	Intravaginal gel: 90 mg (8% gel) once daily	Intravaginal gel: 90 mg (8%) gel) once daily. If pregnancy occurs, may continue for 10–12 wk.
		Endometrin: 100 mg (21 each) (B) Oil, Intramuscular: Generic: 50 mg/mL (10 mL) (G)	Intravaginal tablet: 100 mg 2–3 times daily starting at oocyte retrieval and continuing for up to 10 wk	100 mg 2–3 times daily
	ART in patients with partial or complete ovarian failure	Suppository, Vaginal: First-Progesterone VGS 25: 25 mg (30 each) (B) First-Progesterone VGS 50: 50 mg (30 each)	Intravaginal gel: 90 mg (8%) gel twice daily	Intravaginal gel: 90 mg (8%) gel twice daily. If pregnancy occurs, continue treatment for 10–12 wk
	Endometrial hyperplasia prevention	First-Progesterone VGS 100: 100 mg (30 each) (B) First-Progesterone VGS 200: 200 mg (30 each) (B) First Progesterone VGS 400: 400 mg (30 each) (B)	In postmenopausal women with a uterus in conjunction with daily conjugated estrogen tablet. Oral: 200 mg every evening for 12 consecutive days in a 28-day cycle	200 mg every evening for 12 consecutive days in a 28-day cycle
	Functional uterine bleeding		IM: 5–10 mg/d for 6 doses	5–10 mg/d for 6 doses

Continued

Table 22–9 ✂ **Dosage Schedule: Progesterones and Progesterone Antagonists—cont'd**

Drug	Indication	Dosage form	Initial Dose	Maintenance Dose
Medroxyprogesterone acetate	Amenorrhea	Suspension, IM: Depo-Provera 150 mg/mL (1 mL) (B)	Oral: 5–10 mg/d for 5–10 days	5–10 mg/d for 5–10 days
	Abnormal uterine bleeding	Depo-Provera 400 mg mL (400 mg/mL (2.5 mL) (B)	Oral: 5–10 mg for 5–10 days starting on day 16 or 21 of cycle	5–10 mg for 5–10 days starting on day 16 or 21 of cycle
	Contraception	Generic: 150 mg/mL (1 mL) (G)	IM: 150 mg every 3 mo	IM: 150 mg every 3 mo
		Suspension, Subcutaneous Depo-SubQ Provera 104:	SubQ: 104 mg every 3 mo (12–14 wk)	SubQ: 104 mg every 3 mo (12–14 wk)
	Endometriosis	104 mg/0.65 mL (0.65 mL) (B)	SubQ: 104 mg every 3 mo (12–14 wk)	SubQ: 104 mg every 3 mo (12–14 wk)
	Endometrial carcinoma, recurrent or metastatic (adjunctive/palliative treatment)	Tablet, oral Provera 2.5 mg, 5 mg, 10 mg (B) Generic: 2.5 mg, 5 mg, 10 mg (G)	IM: 400–1,000 mg/wk	400–1,000 mg/wk
	Postmenopausal therapy with accompanying estrogen		Oral: 5–10 mg for 12–14 consecutive days starting on day 1 or day 16 of 28-day cycle	5–10 mg for 12–14 consecutive days starting on day 1 or day 16 of 28-day cycle
	Paraphilia/hypersexuality in males (unlabeled use)		IM: 100–600 mg weekly	100–600 mg weekly
Megestrol acetate	Breast carcinoma (females)	Suspension, oral: Megace ES: 625 mg/5 mL (150 mL) (B)	Oral, tablet: 40 mg 4 times/d	40 mg 4 times/d
	Endometrial carcinoma	Megace Oral: 40 mg/mL (240 mL) (B) Generic: 40 mg/mL (10 mL, 240 mL, 480 mL); 400 mg/10 mL (10 mL) (G)	Oral, tablet: 40–320 mg/d in divided doses	40–320 mg/d in divided doses. Maximum doses have been up to 800 mg/day
	HIV-related cachexia (males/females)	Tablet, oral: Generic: 20 mg, 40 mg (G)	Oral, suspension: 800 mg/d ES: 625 mg/d	400–800 mg found to be clinically effective
Norethindrone acetate	Contraception (females)	Tablet, oral: Camila: 0.35 mg (B) Errin: 0.35 mg (B) Heather: 0.35 mg (B) Jencycla: 0.35 mg (B)	Oral, tablet: 0.35 mg daily Start on first day of menstrual period or the day after a miscarriage or abortion	0.35 mg daily
	Amenorrhea and abnormal uterine bleeding	Jolivette 0.35 mg (B) Nor-QD 0. (B) Nora-BE 0.35 mg (B) Ortho Micronor 0.35 mg (B)	Oral, tablet: Two 5–10 mg/d for 5–10 days during the second half of the menstrual cycle	Two 5–10 mg/d for 5–10 days during the second half of the menstrual cycle
	Endometriosis	Generic: 0.35 mg (G) Tablet, oral, as acetate Aygestin 5 mg (B) Generic: 5 mg (G)	Oral, tablet: 5 mg/d for 14 days	Increase in increments of 2.5 mg/d every 2 weeks to reach 15 mg/d. Continue for 6–9 mo.
Progesterone Antagonists				
Mifepristone	Hyperglycemia in patients with Cushing's syndrome	Tablet, oral: Korlym 300 mg (B) Mifeprex 200 mg (B)	Oral, tablet: 300 mg/d	Increase in 300 mg increments every 2–4 wk. Maximum dose: 1,200 mg/d or 20/mg/dg/d

Table 22–9 ⚯ Dosage Schedule: Progesterones and Progesterone Antagonists—cont'd

Drug	Indication	Dosage form	Initial Dose	Maintenance Dose
	Termination of pregnancy (restricted use in U.S.)		Oral, tablet: Day 1: (mifepristone): 600 mg (three 200 mg tabs) Day 3: (misoprostol) 400 mcg (two 200 mcg tabs) Day 14: confirmation of complete termination by US (unlabeled use) Day 1: misepristone 200 mg Day 3: misepristone 800 mcg vaginally 24–48 h later	No maintenance dosing
	Meningioma, unresectable (unlabeled use)		Oral, tablet: mifepristone 200 mg/d	Mifepristone 200 mg/day

Rational Drug Selection

Short-Acting Versus Long-Acting

Oral contraceptive products are dosed in a convenient dial pack. These products are short-acting, and the patient chooses when to stop and become fertile again. Progesterone is available for contraception in two parenteral forms, which are long-acting, and both have greater than 99% theoretical efficacy. Patient preference is a primary concern when selecting the route for contraceptive delivery with progesterone agents. For patients who have difficulty remembering to take the medication daily, the use of a long-acting method may be preferred. Table 22-9 presents available dosage forms.

Prevention of Endometrial Cancer

Endometrial cancer is a risk associated with estrogen therapy. In an attempt to decrease this risk, combinations of estrogen and a progestin have been prescribed to perimenopausal and postmenopausal women who have an intact uterus. There are several dosing regimens and related concerns in their use. Estrogen (0.625 mg) plus medroxyprogesterone acetate (MPA) 2.5 mg daily (Prempro) is the medication combination used in the WHI study in which concern was raised about increased CHD risk. Estrogen (0.625 mg) days 1 to 25 plus MPA days 16 to 25 is an alternative regimen. It has the disadvantage of increasing hot flashes. Estrogen (0.625 mg) plus progestin Monday through Friday is less commonly used and has more vasomotor flashing reports than the continuous-use form.

When initiating therapy in older women, begin with low doses (0.3 mg) of conjugated estrogens every other day for 2 months. Next, increase the estrogens to daily doses and use for another 2 months. Add a progestin from the treatment regimens above if the patient has a uterus. If symptoms such as bleeding or breast pain do not occur, increase the estrogen to up to 0.625 mg daily. Some women may need only the lower estrogen dosages as long as they have

an adequate diet. Use of formulations other than oral may reduce the need for the addition of progestin because of reduced cancer risk. This reduced risk for different estrogen formulations is discussed in the estrogen therapy Rational Drug Selection section.

A newer alternative to using progestins for uterine protection, as well as vasomotor symptoms, is the combination of conjugated estrogen with bazedoxifene (Duavee). Because it contains conjugated estrogens, all the warnings associated with estrogen apply. The bazedoxifene, an estrogen agonist/antagonist, component is also associated with increased risk of blood clots; its impact on breast cancer is unknown. The reason for its use is that it reduces endometrial hyperplasia induced by the estrogen. Alone bazedoxifine is a SERM medication approved for osteoporosis treatment and prevention. Data comparing the impact on bone health when used together does not appear to be much greater than each medication alone. Bazedoxifine is not metabolized by the CYP450 system, but this does not mean no drug interactions. A lessor known uridine diphosphate glucuronosyltransferase (UGT) enzyme system in the gut is the site of metabolism. Therefore medications that induce UGTs like rifampin, carbazapeine, phenobarbital, and phenytoin can reduce its effectiveness in preventing vaginal lining growth.

Vaginal Bleeding

The most common reason women give for discontinuing HRT is unacceptable vaginal bleeding. Continuous regimens eliminate monthly withdrawal bleeding but are associated with a higher rate of breakthrough bleeding, especially in the first 6 months. This is most likely in women who are early into postmenopause because endogenous production of estrogen is more labile from cycle to cycle in these women. The most positive risk/benefit profiles for all indications for HRT may accrue when the therapy is started near the time of menopause onset. The use of cyclical or sequential therapy reduces the risk for breakthrough bleeding and is preferred until endogenous hormone production stabilizes, typically 2 to 3 years after menopause. Differences in potency of various progestins may result in differences in rates of bleeding. The PEPI study found micronized progestin was associated with less bleeding during the first 6 months than either continuous or cyclical MPA (Lindenfeld & Langer, 2002).

Effects on Lipids

Different types of progestin not only have differing effects on the endometrium, they also have differing effects on estrogen-associated benefits to lipids. Norethindrone acetate has been shown to reverse any estrogen impact on HDL cholesterol while still offering effective endometrial protection. MPA and micronized progestin do not attenuate the effects of estrogen on lipid levels. Norgestimate improves HDL to a level intermediate between MPA and micronized progestin, also while providing good endometrial protection (Langer, 2005). The overall impact is not favorable toward long-term CV health; hence, the caution to keep HRT therapy to a maximum of 5 years and only in younger women. Reevaluation of the WHI data implies that the worst CV outcomes occurred in women who were started on HRT years after menopause onset.

Monitoring

Pretreatment physical examination to assess health and possible contraindications to progestins is mandatory. The examination should be age specific. Patients with seizure disorders need monitoring of their symptoms because increased fluid retention may lower the seizure threshold. Women with migraines are vulnerable to any changes in physiological states, and fluid retention may give them cyclic migraines. Depression should be assessed early in therapy for those women with a history of previous affective disorders. Patients with diabetes may see changes in blood glucose levels, triggering the need for more frequent measurement. Patients with a history of or risk for thromboembolic events or who use tobacco products should not use these products. Additionally, women on injectable progesterone will require education and possible screening for osteoporosis based on age and risk factors. Women on HRT require careful monitoring for cardiovascular, thromboembolic, and cancer risks.

Patient Education

Administration

Most hormone regimens require daily dosing for efficacy, especially for the progestin-only oral contraceptive. The most common adverse effect is breakthrough bleeding, especially if doses are missed. The injectable form requires administration every 12 weeks, so a follow-up appointment should be scheduled for the time the injection is due to avoid loss of pregnancy protection. If a woman is outside the 2 week window to receive a shot, she should use alternate protection such as condoms or abstain from intercourse. She will need a repeat pregnancy test prior to restarting injections. The use of injectable progesterone for contraception requires added screening at initial administration. Patients must present for initial administration of an injectable progesterone therapy while they are actively menstruating and have a negative pregnancy test. The use of injectable progesterone is associated with significant teratogenic effects. Patient-specific education regarding the need to maintain the specific redosing schedule should also be provided.

Estrogen/progestin combinations used for HRT require daily dosing. No specific instructions are required beyond those already discussed.

Adverse Reactions

Progestins should not be used in the first 12 weeks of gestation because of masculinization of the female fetus. Depression and mood swings are common and represent a significant factor in postmenopausal HRT cessation. Irregular menstrual patterns and unpredictable spotting contribute to the proportion of women stopping progestin-only oral contraceptives. Breast tenderness and galactorrhea are the third most common reason women switch from a progesterone contraceptive and another reason that postmenopausal women stop HRT altogether.

Lifestyle Management

Progesterone therapy may be associated with hyperpigmentation and weight gain. To help reduce these complications, clinicians should encourage patients to use sunscreen to prevent skin changes, such as blotchy pigmentation. Promotion of routine physical exercise is used to combat the increase in body weight sometimes seen with Depo-Provera.

Smoking cessation is encouraged in all patients, but especially in young women using hormonal contraception. The association of both estrogen and progesterone with morbidity and mortality in patients older than 35 years who smoke may be a powerful motivator to quit smoking.

OTHER DRUGS AFFECTING THE REPRODUCTIVE SYSTEM

Other drugs affecting the reproductive system include those that are commonly used to treat infertility (GnRH, FSH, LH, and human chorionic gonadotropin [hCG]), those used as lactation inhibitors (bromocriptine), and those used in erectile dysfunction. Though the primary care advanced practice nurse may not prescribe these medications, it is important to understand all the medications that the patient is using within the role of coordination of care.

Drugs Commonly Used in Fertility Clinics

Gonadotropin-Releasing Hormone

GnRH is produced in the arcuate nucleus of the hypothalamus and controls the release of FSH and LH for both males and females. GnRH is used as a stimulant in pulsatile doses if the patient has a functional pituitary gland and an ovary to produce the LH surge initiating ovulation. GnRH agents may be used in pulsate form to stimulate ovulation and treat endometriosis and uterine fibroids and as continuous therapy to suppress prostate cancer. Leuprolide acetate (Lupron, Lupron Depot) may be administered subcutaneously (SC) or IM. Goserelin (Zoladex) is an SC implant that is used to treat prostate cancer, breast cancer, and severe endometriosis. It is administered every 28 days.

The use of GnRH is contraindicated in conjunction with medications that stimulate ovarian function. The use of GnRH for infertility treatments may result in multiple gestations. Long-term use of GnRH agents may result in bone demineralization, and DEXA (Dual Energy X-ray Absorptiometry) scans should be considered for patients who require ongoing treatment. Patients may report hot flashes, headache, and menstrual irregularities during treatment.

Follicle-Stimulating Hormone/Gonadotropins

FSH has an analogue, human menopausal gonadotropin (hMG) (follitropin [Fertinex], menotropins [Pergonal, Humegon]). The drug is used in fertility treatments for both men and women. In men, the use of gonadotropins stimulates spermatogenesis and in women stimulates the maturation of follicles and ovulation. Used in specialty practices, these agents are administered IM. Onset, peak, and duration are not established for all of them. As these agents are used to stimulate ovarian function, there is a risk of hyperstimulation syndrome that can cause ovarian enlargement, ascites, hydrothorax, hypovolemia, hemoperitoneum, fever, or arterial thromboembolism.

Luteinizing Hormone and Human Chorionic Gonadotropin

Luteinizing hormone (LH) like FSH is produced in the anterior pituitary and used in conjunction with FSH to stimulate ovulation. It also stimulates the corpus luteum to produce progesterone and androgens. No LH preparation is available for use clinically. Instead, a similar preparation, hCG, is substituted successfully (analogue hCG:A.P.L., Chorex-5, Profasi).

Lactation Inhibitors

Bromocriptine

Although not a true hormone, bromocriptine (Parlodel) has an inhibitory effect on the pituitary gland. It is widely used for shrinking pituitary prolactin-secreting tumors, reducing the prolactin levels of idiopathic prolactinemia, galactorrhea, and infertility. Bromocriptine is similar to dopamine in structure and binds to dopamine receptors within the pituitary gland to inhibit prolactin secretion. It is well absorbed from the GI tract and can begin to exert an effect within 2 hours of administration. Bromocriptine is metabolized through the CYP450 3A4 substrate and excreted primarily in bile. When used for hyperprolactinemic indications, the initial dosage is 0.5 to 2.5 mg daily with meals; 2.5 mg may be added as tolerated every 3 to 7 days or until optimal therapeutic response

is achieved. Therapeutic dosage is usually 5 to 7.5 mg, with a range of 2.5 to 15 mg/d.

For acromegaly, the initial dose is 1.25 to 2.5 mg for 3 days at time of sleep. An additional 1.25 to 2.5 mg is added as tolerated every 3 to 7 days. Therapeutic dosage is usually 5 to 7.5 mg, with a range of 20 to 30 mg/d.

Multiple drugs interact with bromocriptine. Some of the most notable interactions include acetaminophen, erythromycin, phenothiazines, sympathomimetics, isometheptene, and phenylpropanolamine.

Drugs Used for Erectile Dysfunction

Phosphodiesterase Type 5 Inhibitors

Erectile dysfunction (ED) is a common health condition that is associated with increased age and various comorbidities, such as diabetes and hypertension. The causes of erectile dysfunction are beyond the scope of this chapter. However, clinicians should complete a full history and physical to confirm proper diagnosis prior to initiating medication therapy. This section focuses on ED treatment with the use of phosphodiesterase type 5 inhibitors (PDE5 inhibitors). Additional information is found in Chapter 49.

Sildenafil citrate (Viagra), the first PDE5 inhibitor indicated for the treatment of impotence in men with ED, was originally studied as a selective vasodilator for use in angina. Although not effective in the coronary arteries, it was effective as a selective inhibitor of cyclic guanosine monophosphate (cGMP), specifically PDE5. It has found an effective role in pulmonary hypertension as well. The dosing and discussion of this indication is not included in this chapter.

The PDE5 class has a 10-fold selectivity for the enzyme that produces smooth muscle relaxation in the corpus cavernosum of the penis. As smooth muscles in the corpus cavernosum relax, blood flow into the penis is increased, resulting in an erection. There is no drug effect without sexual stimulation. They have no effect if the cause of ED is not biological in nature. The drug class also relaxes bladder smooth muscle giving a second indication of benign prostatic enlargement if used daily. They are rapidly absorbed after oral administration and eliminated by hepatic metabolism (mainly CYP450 3A4). Ingestion of food reduces its rate of absorption, especially high-fat, high-protein meals. The peak onset for sildenafil occurs 60 minutes after dosing, with a duration up to 4 hours; tadalafil is the fastest acting and lasts the longest in circulation at 17 hours with reports of up to 36 hours.

For erectile dysfunction, the dosage of sildenafil is 50 mg (25 to 100 mg, based on effectiveness) taken as needed approximately 1 hour before sexual activity for sildenafil and vardenafil, and 15 minutes for tadalafil. The intended frequency is about every 3 days. Studies in healthy elderly volunteers (over 65 years) showed a reduced clearance with free plasma concentrations 40% higher than in younger volunteers (18 to 45 years). An initial starting dose of 25 mg is recommended for men over age 65 years. Tadalafil and vardenafil starting doses are 10 mg with a maximum of 20 mg for the initial occasional use formula. The daily use dose for Tadalafil is 2.5 mg.

There is an absolute contraindication for concomitant use with any form of nitrates because of the risk of severe hypotension, cardiovascular collapse, and death. Other potential drug interactions are many, including antifungals, macrolide antibiotics (such as erythromycin), cimetidine, rifampin, alpha blockers, nonspecific beta blockers, and diuretics. These drugs should not be used concomitantly or doses of the phosphodiesterase inhibitor should be adjusted downward. Common adverse effects include headaches, flushing, dyspepsia, and blue-hue vision change (most common with sildenafil).

All PDE5 inhibitors have been shown to have equal efficacy in treating ED. The main difference between the agents is longer duration of action. Vardenafil (Levitra) shares a pharmacokinetic profile similar to that of sildenafil but is purported to have a shorter time to onset of action and lasts for up to 6 hours. Maximum plasma concentrations are reached between 30 minutes to 2 hours. Tadalafil (Cialis) has a different chemical structure than the other two PDE5 inhibitors. This allows for greater binding affinity in skeletal smooth muscle, the testes, and prostate and less affinity in the retina. This may account for the low back pain and decreased incidence of visual disturbances with tadalafil that some users report. As with sildenafil, there is reduced clearance in both of these medications in elderly patients, with plasma concentrations up to 52% higher. A lower starting dose of 5 mg is recommended with this population. No adjustments are required for renal impairment, but the same recommendations are made as related above to drug interactions.

Once-daily use of tadalfil is now approved for erectile dysfunction and benign prostatic hyperplasia at a dose lower than the initial version. Daily dosing is 2.5 to 5 mg based on efficacy and tolerability. Steady-state plasma concentration is reached after 96 hours of continuous daily use. Using the higher dose tablets in a daily pattern is not recommended due to the eventual toxicity from the prolonged duration of effects and associated acute hypotension.

All PDE5 inhibitors share the same contraindication in patients who are using nitrates because of a risk of severe hypotension. Concurrent use with alpha blockers is also not recommended because of additive hypotensive effects; they are considered contraindicated for vardenafil and tadalafil. Patients with underlying cardiovascular disease require additional pretreatment evaluation. The American College of Cardiology and the American Heart Association have suggested that patients with unstable coronary artery disease, active ischemia, heart failure, and low blood pressure, and patients on multiple antihypertensive agents or medications that inhibit the CYP 450 3A4 pathway should not take PDE5 inhibitors. They are not given after stroke, MI, or recent life-threatening dysrhythmias due to heightened sensitivity to blood pressure changes for up to 6 months. Vardenafil can cause QT prolongation and should not be used in patients with underlying arrhythmias, on dysrhythmic medications, or with hepatic insufficiency. Tadalafil is not indicated for persons with retinal pigmentosa.

Patient education regarding the anticipated effectiveness of therapy and potential side effects should be given at the initiation of therapy and at each refill. Patients who experience chest pain or dizziness with sexual activity should refrain from additional use of these agents and sexual activity until they have been reevaluated.

Priapism is a rare but emergent adverse event that can occur with PDE5 inhibitors. Patients who experience an erection that lasts for longer than 4 hours need to be evaluated in the emergency department. There have been several reports of nonarterial anterior ischemic optic neuropathy (NAION) and cyanopsia (blue vision) within hours of taking PDE5 inhibitors (Thurtell & Tomsak, 2008). NAION is a permanent loss of vision resulting from ischemia of the optic nerve head. The U.S. Federal Aviation Administration recommends that pilots do not use sildenafil or vardenafil for 6 hours prior to flying. The half-life for both is below 6 hours. Tadalafil is not approved for pilots (or workers requiring color recognition) due to its half-life of 17.5 hours. Sudden hearing loss has also been reported. While patients are on this therapy, periodic medication and health evaluation are encouraged to identify any new potential cardiovascular or health risks that may alter the ability to continue ED therapy.

The effects of PDE5 inhibitors for treating women with sexual dysfunction have been evaluated in small clinical trials. The results are mixed, with many studies unable to demonstrate efficacy. PDE5 inhibitors have been used to treat children with persistent pulmonary hypertension, although the FDA has issued a statement reiterating that sildenafil is not labeled for use in children. The FDA notes that while sildenafil is approved for use in adults with pulmonary arterial hypertension, it is not approved for this use in children, since the studies in children indicate increased mortality with long term use (FDA, 2014). The FDA notes that providers need to weigh the risk benefit when treating children with PAH. (Baquero, Soliz, Neira, Venegas, & Sola, 2006). Adults with pulmonary arterial hypertension and those with high-altitude pulmonary edema are also treated with this drug class. The identical drugs are marketed under different brand names to prevent any hesitancy to take "ED" meds for a pulmonary vascular problem (i.e., Revato, Staxyn, and Adcirca). These forms are not interchangeable for the ones marketed for ED primarily due to significant differences in dosing.

REFERENCES

Agency for Healthcare Research and Quality (2012). The 2012 hormone position statement of The North American Menopause Society. *Menopause,* 19(3), 257–271. Retrieved May 25, 2013, from http://www.menopause.org/docs/default-document-library/psht12.pdf?sfvrsn=2

Anderson, G., Judd, H., Kaunitz, A., Barad, D., Beresford, S., Pettinger, M., et al. (2003). Effects of estrogen plus progestin on gynecologic cancers and associated diagnostic procedures: The Women's Health Initiative Randomized Trial. *Journal of the American Medical Association, 290*(13), 1739–1748.

Anderson, G., Limacher, M., et al., and The Women's Health Initiative Steering Committee. (2004). Effects of conjugated equine estrogen in postmenopausal women with hysterectomy: The Women's Health Initiative randomized trial. *Journal of the American Medical Association, 291,* 1701–1712.

Archer, D. (2004). Hormonal therapy and the postmenopausal woman: Current clinical challenges. *Portraits and Passages: Women's Health Through the Prime of Life.* CE # 04-17.

Baquero, H., Soliz, A., Neira, F., Venegas, M. E., & Sola, A. (2006). Oral sildenafil in infants with persistent pulmonary hypertension of the newborn: A pilot randomized blinded study. *Pediatrics, 117*(4), 1077–1083.

Barrett-Conner, E., Grady, D., & Stefanick, M. (2005). The rise and fall of menopausal hormone therapy. *Annual Review of Public Health, 26,* 115–140.

Boyack, M., Lookinland, S., & Chasson, S. (2002). Efficacy of raloxifene for treatment of menopause: A systematic review. *Journal of the American Academy of Nurse Practitioners, 14*(4), 150–165.

Brucker, M. (2002). What's a woman to do? *Association of Women's Health, Obstetric and Neonatal Nurses Lifelines, 6*(5), 408–417.

Cummings, S., Eckert, K., Grady, D., Powles, T., Cauley, L., Norton, L., et al. (1999). The effect of raloxifene on risk of breast cancer in postmenopausal women. *Journal of the American Medical Association, 281*(23), 2189–2197.

Drug facts and comparisons. (2010). St. Louis, MO: Wolters Kluwer Health.

Garnero, P., Stevens, R., Ayres, S., & Phelps, K. (2002). Short-term effects of new synthetic conjugated estrogens on biochemical markers of bone turnover. *Journal of Clinical Pharmacology, 42,* 290–296.

Greenspan, S., Emkey, R., Bone, H., Weiss, S., Bell, N., Downs, R., et al. (2002). Significant differential effects of alendronate, estrogen or combination therapy on the rate of bone loss after discontinuation of treatment of postmenopausal osteoporosis: A randomized, double-blind, placebo-controlled trial. *Archives of Internal Medicine, 137*(11), 875–883.

Hatcher, R., Trussell, J., Stewart, F., Nelson, A., Cates, W., Guest, F., et al. (2004). *Contraceptive technology* (18th ed.). New York: Ardent Media.

Hatcher, R., Trussell, J., Nelson, A., Cates, W., & Stewart, F. (2007). *Contraceptive technology* (19th ed.). New York: Ardent Media.

Kern, L., Powe, N., Levine, M., Fitzpatrick, A., Harris, T., Robbins, J., et al. (2005). Association between screening for osteoporosis and the incidence of hip fracture. *Annals of Internal Medicine, 142*(3), 173–181.

Kong, Y., & Penninger, J. (2004). Molecular control of bone remodeling and osteoporosis. *Experimental Gerontology, 35*(8), 947.

Kovats, P. (2004). Vardenafil as an alternative to sildenafil in the treatment of erectile dysfunction. *Federal Air Surgeon's Medical Bulletin, 42*(3), 9–11. Retrieved May 25, 2013, from http://www.faa.gov/other_visit/designees_delegations/designee_types/ame/fasmb/media/f2004_3.pdf

Kritz-Silverstein, D., & Barrett-Connor, E. (1996). Long-term postmenopausal hormone use, obesity, and fat distribution in older women. *Journal of the American Medical Association, 275*(1), 46–49.

Langer, R. (2005). Postmenopausal hormone therapy. *CME Bulletin of the American Academy of Family Physicians, 4*(1), 1–10.

Lexicomp. (2013). Lexicomp pharmaceutical reference. Retrieved between January and June 2013, from http://online.lexi.com/Ico/action/home/switch?siteid=1

Lindenfeld, E., & Langer, R. (2002). Bleeding patterns of hormone replacement therapies in the postmenopausal estrogen and progestin interventions trial. *Obstetrics and Gynecology, 100,* 853–863.

Liu, J. (2004). Use of conjugated estrogens after the Women's Health Initiative. *The Female Patient, 29,* 8–13.

Liu, J., Burdette, J., Xu, H., Gu, C., van Breeman, R., Bhat, K., et al. (2001). Evaluation of estrogenic activity of plant extracts for the potential treatment of menopausal symptoms. *Journal of Agricultural and Food Chemistry, 49,* 2472–2479.

Marx, P., Schade, G., Wilbourn, S., Blank, S., Moyer, D., & Nett, R. (2004). Low dose (0.3 mg) synthetic conjugated estrogen A is effective for managing atrophic vaginitis. *Maturitas, 47*(1), 47–55.

Prentice, R. L., Manson, J. E., Langer, R. D., Anderson, G. L., Pettinger, M., Jackson, R. D., et al. (2009). Benefits and risks of postmenopausal hormone therapy when it is initiated soon after menopause. *American Journal of Epidemiology, 170,* 12–23.

Rossouw, J., Anderson, G., Prentice, R., Lacroix, A., Kooperberg, C., Stefanick, M., et al. (2002). Risks and benefits of estrogen plus progestin in healthy postmenopausal women: Principal results from the Women's Health Initiative Randomized Controlled Trial. *Journal of the American Medical Association, 288*(3), 321–333.

Sarrel, P. (2004). Vasomotor and vascular consideration. *The Female Patient* (Suppl. February), 10–18.

Siminoski, K., Leslie, W., Frame, H., Hodsman, A., Josse, R., Khan, A., et al. (2005). Recommendations for bone mineral density reporting in Canada. *Canadian Association of Radiologists Journal, 56*(3), 178–188. Retrieved October 25, 2005, from http://www.osteoporosis.ca/ english/For%20Health%20Professionals/Research

Sood, R., Warndahy, R., Schroeder, D., Singh, R., Rhodes, D., et al. (April 2013). Bioidentical compounded hormones: A pharmacokinetic evaluation in a randomized clinical trial. *Maturitas, 74*(4), 375–382. Retrieved May 19, 2013, from http://www.sciencedirect.com

Stevens, R., Roy, P., & Phelps, K. (2002). Evaluation of single- and multiple-dose pharmacokinetics of synthetic conjugated estrogens, A (Cenestin) tablets: A slow-release estrogen replacement product. *Journal of Clinical Pharmacology, 42,* 332–341.

Tan, O., Bradshaw, K., & Carr, B. (2012). Management of vulvovaginal atrophy-related sexual dysfunction in postmenopausal women: An up-to-date review. *Menopause: The Journal of the North American Menopause Society, 19*(1), 109–117. Retrieved May 19, 2013, from http://ovidsp.tx.ovid.com

Thorneycroft, I. (2004). Unopposed estrogen and cancer. *The Female Patient* (Suppl. to February), 19–26.

UpToDate. (2009a). *Overview of contraception.* Waltham, MA. Retrieved October 21, 2009, from http://www.uptodate.com/online/content/ topic.do?topicKey=gen_gyne/3029&selectedTitle=2~150&source=search_result

UpToDate. (2009b). *Treatment of menopausal symptoms with hormone therapy.* Waltham, MA. Retrieved October 21, 2009, from http://www.uptodate.com/online/content/topic.do?topicKey=r_endo_f/9609&selectedTitle=2~150&source=search_result

UpToDate. (2009c). *Treatment of male sexual dysfunction.* Waltham, MA. Retrieved October 21, 2009, from http://www.uptodate.com/online/content/topic.do?topicKey=r_endo_m/6961&selectedTitle=1~150&source=search_result

U.S. Department of Health and Human Services. (2004). *Bone health and osteoporosis: A report of the Surgeon General.* Rockville, MD: U.S. Department of Health and Human Services, Office of the Surgeon General. Retrieved from http://www.surgeongeneral.gov/library

U.S. Food and Drug Administration (FDA). (2004). *Safety Alerts: Depo-Provera (medroxyprogesterone acetate injectable suspension).* Retrieved from http://www.fda.gov/Safety/MedWatch/SafetyInformation/SafetyAlertsforHumanMedicalProducts/ucm154784.htm

Warren, M. P. (2010). Hormone therapy for menopausal symptoms: Putting benefits and risks into perspective. *The Journal of Family Practice, 59*(12), E1–E7.

Writing Group for the Women's Health Initiative Investigators. (2002). Risks and benefits of estrogen plus progestin in healthy postmenopausal women. *Journal of the American Medical Association, 288*(3), 321–323.

Writing Group of the PEPI Trial. (1996). Effects of hormonal therapy on bone mineral density: Results from the post-menopausal estrogen/progestin interventions (PEPI). *Journal of the American Medical Association, 276*(17), 1398–1396.

Wysocki, S., & Alexander, I. (2005). Bioidentical hormones for menopause therapy: An overview. *Women's Health Care: A Practical Journal for Nurse Practitioners, 4*(2), 9–17.

Youngkin, E., Davis, M., Schaldewald, D., & Juve, C. (2013). *Women's health: A primary care clinical guide* (4th ed.). New Jersey: Pearson Education, Inc.

Zhu, H., Lei X., Feng J., & Wang Y. (2012 Dec). Oral contraceptive use and risk of breast cancer: A meta-analysis of prospective cohort studies. *European Journal of Contraception & Reproductive Health Care, 17*(6), 402–414.

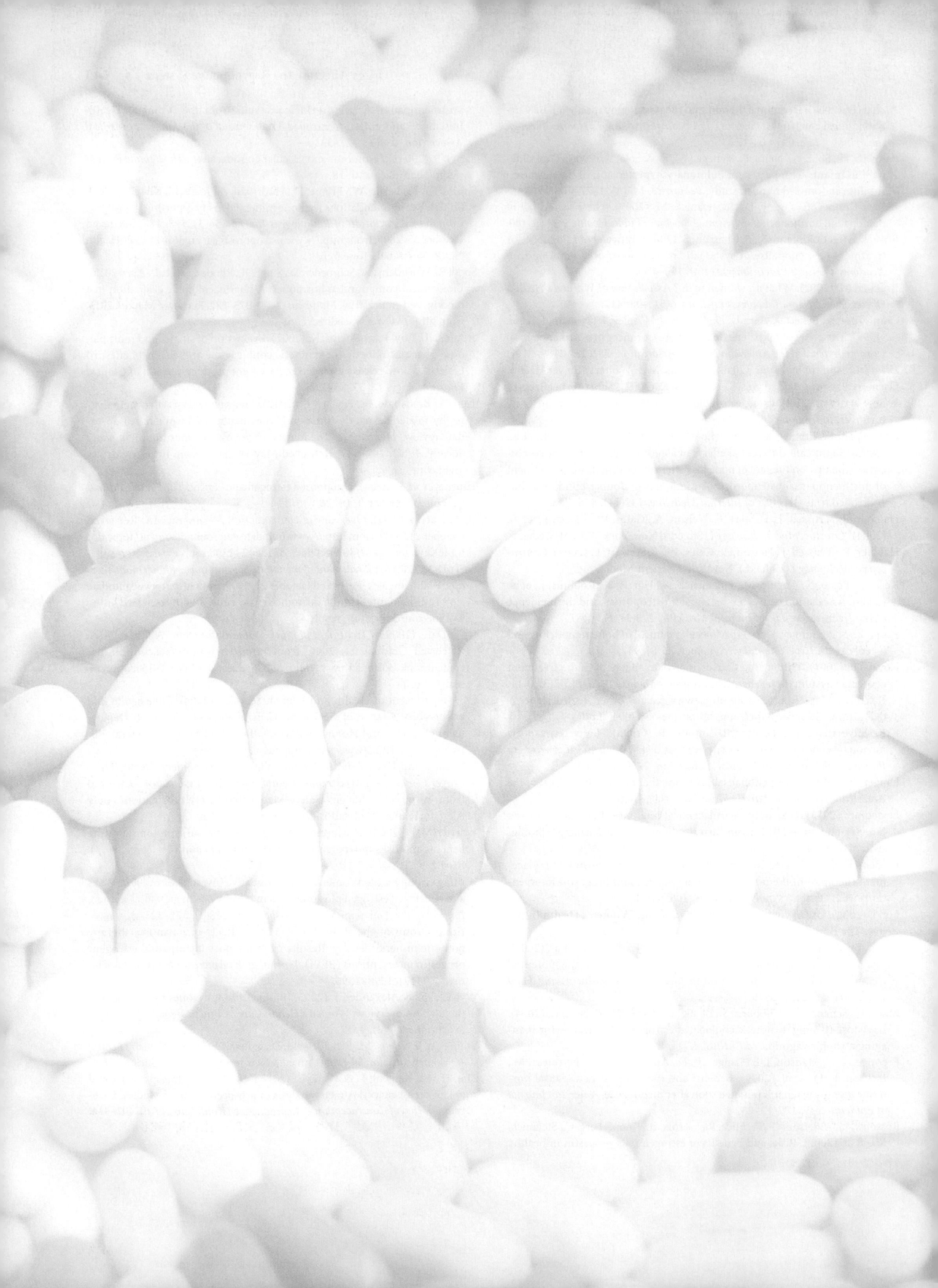

CHAPTER 23

DRUGS AFFECTING THE INTEGUMENTARY SYSTEM

Cally Bartley

This chapter discusses a wide variety of medications used to treat disorders of the skin or integumentary system, including topical anti-infective medications used to treat bacterial, fungal, and viral infections of the skin; topical corticosteroids and immunomodulators used for a variety of inflammatory diseases; and topical antipsoriasis and acne medications. Systemic medications used for skin disorders are discussed here only if not covered in another chapter. Systemic antibiotics and antifungal medications used to treat more serious skin infections, with the exception of griseofulvin and terbinafine, are discussed in Chapter 24. Systemic medications used for acne are discussed in this chapter, with the exception of systemic antibiotics, which are also covered in Chapter 24.

ANTI-INFECTIVES
TOPICAL ANTIBACTERIALS

Bacterial infections of the skin are common in patients of all ages. Antibacterial medications commonly used in primary care include topical agents and oral antibiotics. The most common pathogens seen in bacterial skin infections are *Staphylococcus aureus* and *Streptococcus pyogenes*. Skin infections with gram-negative bacilli are rare, but they may occur in patients who are immunocompromised or patients with diabetes. These patients usually require IV antibiotic therapy for their infections.

Impetigo is usually treated topically unless it is a moderate to severe case. First-line therapy for impetigo is mupirocin (Bactroban, Centany). A newer medication, retapamulin (Altabax), is also effective in treating impetigo. Over-the-counter (OTC) products like triple antibiotic ointment (neomycin, bacitracin, and polymyxin B) and double antibiotic ointment (polysporin and bacitracin) are less effective than prescribed topical agents and do not treat MRSA (*S. aureus*) (Bangert, Levy, & Herbert, 2012). Moderate to severe impetigo, a boil or abscess, perianal streptococcal infections, and cellulitis all require prompt treatment with appropriate systemic antibiotics. Methicillin-resistant *S. aureus* (MRSA) is increasing in prevalence and providers need to have a suspicion for MRSA in the differential of any skin infection. If MRSA is suspected, appropriate systemic antibiotics should be used (TMP/SMZ, doxycycline, minocycline, or vancomycin). See Table 23-1 for dosing schedules for topical antibacterials.

Table 23–1 ⊗ Dosage Schedule: Selected Anti-Infectives Used to Treat Skin Disorders

Drug	Indication	Available Dosage Forms	Dosage
Antibacterial			
Bacitracin (Baciguent)	Superficial wound infections	500 U/g ointment	Apply a small amount to the affected area 1–2×/d; do not use >1 wk
Mupirocin (Bactroban)	Impetigo	2% ointment 2% cream	Apply a small amount to the lesions 3×/d for 10 days. Reevaluate after 3–5 days if no response
	Nasal colonization with MRSA	2% nasal ointment	1/2 the ointment from a single-use tube of nasal ointment into one nostril, and the other 1/2 into the other nostril 2×/d for 5 days
Retapamulin (Altabax)	Impetigo	1% ointment	Apply thin layer 2×/d for 5 days. Reevaluate if no improvement in 3–4 days
Double antibiotic (polymyxin B, bacitracin)	Superficial wound infections	Polysporin 10,000 U/g, bacitracin 500 U/g ointment	Apply small amount to affected area 1–3×/d
Triple-antibiotic ointment (polymyxin B, neomycin, bacitracin)	Superficial wound infections	Polysporin 10,000 U/g, neomycin 3.5 mg/g, bacitracin 400 U/g	Apply a small amount to affected area 1–3×/d
Antifungals			
Butenafine (Lotrimin Ultra, Mentax)	Fungal skin infections	1% cream	Apply to affected and immediately surrounding area 1×/d for 2 wk. Pedis: 2×/d × 1 wk and then 1×/d × 2 wk
Ciclopirox olamine (Loprox) (Penlac)	Fungal skin infections and candidiasis	0.77% cream 0.77% gel 1% shampoo 8% solution 0.77% suspension 8% solution (nail lacquer)	Massage into affected skin 2×/d Nail lacquer solution: apply evenly over nail plate 1×/d to affected nails, remove with alcohol every 7 days
Clotrimazole (Mycelex Troche)	Oral candidiasis	10 mg troche	Adults and children >3 yr: 1 troche 5×/d for 2 wk; dissolve slowly in mouth

Table 23–1 ⊗ **Dosage Schedule: Selected Anti-Infectives Used to Treat Skin Disorders–cont'd**

Drug	Indication	Available Dosage Forms	Dosage
(Lotrimin, Lotrimin AF)	Fungal skin infections	1% cream 1% solution	Apply to affected area 2×/d for 4 wk
Econazole (Spectazole)	Fungal skin infections	1% cream	Apply to affected area 1×/d for 2 wk Pedis: 4 wk
Ketoconazole (Nizoral, Nizoral A-D, Xolegel)	Fungal skin infections and candidiasis	2% cream 2% foam 2% shampoo 2% gel	Candidiasis, cruris, corporis: Apply 2×/d for 2 wk Pedis: 6 wk
	Pityriasis veriscolor		Apply shampoo, leave on 5 min, rinse or apply cream 1×/d for 2 wks
Miconazole (Micatin)	Fungal skin infections	2% cream 2% powder 2% spray	Cruris: Apply to affected area 2×/d for 2 wk Corporis, pedis: 4 wk
Naftifine	Fungal skin infections	1% and 2% cream 1% gel	Apply 1% cream 1×/d for 2 wk; 2% cream for up to 4 wk; gel 2×/d for up to 4 wk
Nystatin oral suspension	Oral candidiasis	100,000 U/ML oral suspension	Adults and children: 2–3 mL in each inner cheek (total dose 4–6 mL) 4×/d; have patient hold medication in mouth as long as possible before swallowing; treat for 48 h after clinical cure to prevent relapse Infants: 1 mL each cheek 4×/d (2 mL/dose total), until 48 h after clinical cure; may apply medication to inner cheeks and tongue with cotton swab prior to administering the 1 mL dose via dropper
Nystatin	Candidiasis	100,000 U/GM cream 100,000 U/GM ointment 100,000 U/GM powder	Apply to affected areas 2–3×/d until clear
Oxiconazole (Oxistat)	Fungal skin infections	1% cream 1% lotion	Pityriasis veriscolor, corporis, cruris: Apply to affected area 1–2×/d for 2 wk Pedis: 4 wk
Sertaconazole (Ertaczo)	Tinea pedis	2% cream	Dry area Apply to affected and adjacent areas 2×/d for 4 wk
Sulconazole (Exelderm)	Fungal skin infections	1% cream 1% solution	Cruris, corporis, versicolor: Massage medication into affected area 1–2×/d for 3 wk Pedis: 4 weeks
Terbinafine (Lamisil)	Fungal skin infections	1% cream 1% spray	Pedis, cruris, corporis, versicolor: Apply to affected area 1×/d for 1–4 wk
Tolnaftate (Tinactin)	Fungal skin infections	1% cream 1% powder 1% spray	Pedis, cruris, corporis: Apply to affected area 2×/day for 2–4 wk
Antivirals			
Acyclovir (Zovirax)	Initial herpes genitalis and labialis Mucocutaneous herpes simplex virus (HSV) infections in immunocompromised patients	5% ointment 5% cream	Apply ointment to affected area every 3 h (6×/d) for 7 days Labialis: 5×/d for 4 days
Docosanol (Abreva)	Recurrent oral-facial herpes simplex episodes	10% cream	Gently rub into affected area 5×/d until healed. Begin treatment at earliest sign or symptom.
Penciclovir (Denavir)	Recurrent herpes labialis	1% cream	Apply every 2 h while awake for 4 days. Begin treatment at earliest sign or symptom.

MRSA = methicillin-resistant *staphylococcus aureus*.

Pharmacodynamics

Topical or systemic antibacterial agents may be either bacteriostatic or bactericidal. Mupirocin has a wide range of coverage against gram-positive bacteria, including MRSA, and does have limited coverage against some gram-negative organisms. Mupirocin is bactericidal at concentrations achieved by topical administration of the 2% ointment. Mupirocin acts by binding to bacterial isoleucyl-tRNA synthetase. Retapamulin is bacteriostatic against *S. aureus* and *S. pyogenes* by inhibiting bacterial protein synthesis.

Bacitracin is bacteriostatic but may also be bactericidal, depending on the antibiotic concentration and the susceptibility of the organism. Bacitracin is primarily active against gram-positive organisms; it inhibits bacterial cell wall synthesis by preventing transfer of mucopeptides into the growing cell wall. Neomycin is an aminoglycoside; it is bactericidal by binding the 30s subunit of the bacterial ribosome to inhibit protein synthesis. Polymyxin acts as a surfactant that disrupts bacterial membranes. Polymyxin has bactericidal activity against some gram-negative organisms including *P. aeruginosa*, *E. coli*, *Enterobacter* sp. and *Klebsiella* sp.

Pharmacokinetics

Absorption and Distribution

The topical agents commonly used to treat bacterial skin infections are minimally absorbed through normal skin. Mupirocin does not appear to be appreciably absorbed systemically following topical application to intact skin. If it is applied to large areas of abraded skin, it may allow for deeper penetration into the epidermal layers. Limited data is available on the absorption of mupirocin following intranasal application in adults. Distribution of mupirocin is by serum protein binding

Retapamulin ointment is minimally absorbed via intact skin; however, absorption is increased when applied to abraded skin. The distribution of retapamulin is unknown.

Bacitracin, when used topically, is minimally absorbed. However, bacitracin is readily absorbed through large areas of denuded or burned skin. Topical preparations of bacitracin that include neomycin and polymyxin B are minimally absorbed through normal skin. Distribution of bacitracin, neomycin, and polymyxin B is unknown.

Metabolism and Excretion

Metabolism and excretion of the topical antibacterial agents mupirocin, bacitracin, neomycin, and polymyxin B are unknown. Retapamulin is metabolized by liver enzymes in vitro; excretion is not known because of the low systemic absorption with topical administration.

Pharmacotherapeutics

Clinical Use and Dosing

Impetigo

Impetigo is a contagious superficial skin infection caused by *S. aureus, S. pyogenes,* or both organisms. Using an antibiotic that is effective against both organisms, either topical or oral, ensures successful treatment. Bullous impetigo is usually pure *S. aureus* and should be treated with an oral antibiotic.

The decision of how to treat impetigo depends on the number of lesions, their location (face, eyelid, or mouth), and the need to limit spread of infection to others. The first-line topical agent is mupirocin; other agents, such as bacitracin and neomycin, are considerably less effective. If the patient has up to five singular lesions, topical mupirocin ointment may be applied 2 times a day until the lesions are healed (5 days). Topical retapamulin is applied twice a day for 5 days. Mupirocin and retapamulin are available only by prescription. There are no reported drug interactions with either mupirocin or retapamulin.

Patients who have numerous lesions or who are not responding to topical agents should receive oral antimicrobials effective against both *S. aureus* and *S. pyogenes*. Antibiotics that are effective against *S. aureus* or *S. pyogenes* include cephalexin (Keflex) or dicloxacillin (Stevens et al, 2014). If MRSA is suspected, clindamycin, TMP/SMZ, or doxycycline should be prescribed depending on local resistance patterns (Stevens et al). A macrolide antibiotic such as erythromycin or azithromycin (Zithromax) or clindamycin can be used if the patient is penicillin allergic and MRSA is not suspected (Stevens et al). There is resistance of *S. aureus* to the macrolides, so the patient needs to be monitored closely. The patient treated with systemic antibiotics should be treated for 7 days (5 days with azithromycin).

Furuncle

Furuncles, commonly known as boils, are infections of the hair follicle and are usually caused by *S. aureus*. The first-line treatment for a small furuncle is use of a warm, moist compress. Larger furuncles are treated by incision and drainage. Incision and drainage alone without use of adjunctive antibiotic therapy are usually sufficient to treat a single abscess smaller than 5 cm.

Systemic antibiotics should be reserved for abscesses larger than 5 cm or if cellulitis and/or symptoms of infection are present such as temperature >38°C or 24 breaths per minute, tachycardia >90 beats per minute, or white blood cell count >12 000 /μL (Stevens et al, 2014). Other situations that warrant the use of antibiotics are occurrence on the central facial area, in pediatric or elderly patients, and in the presence of comorbidities such as immunosupression (Stevens et al). Gram's stain and culture of the drainage from the abscess can determine if the organism will be sensitive to the antibiotic of choice. Prior to Gram's stain results, an appropriate first-line antibiotic would be doxycycline or TMP-SMX (Stevens et al). Length of treatment should be 5 to 10 days.

Recurrent Skin Abcesses

Some patients may experience recurrent skin abcesses. Initial therapy is early incision and drainage, with drainage sent for culture. When culture and sensitivity results are available an antibiotic active against the identified pathogen is started (Stevens et al, 2014). Antibiotics are continued for 5 to

10 days. A 5 day decolonization regimen of twice daily nasal mupirocin, daily chlorohexadine washes, and daily washing of personal towels, sheets, and clothing may be considered (Stevens et al).

Cellulitis

Cellulitis is a skin infection involving the deep layers of the dermis and subcutaneous tissue. The patient may become septic if left untreated. Use of topical antibacterial agents is not appropriate. Patients with cellulitis need to be managed with oral or parenteral antibiotics. Use of oral antibiotics is discussed in Chapter 24.

Nasal MRSA Carrier

Eradication of nasal MRSA colonization in adult patients and health-care workers may be achieved with intranasal mupirocin. However, increased use of topical mupirocin is correlated to the development of resistance. Therefore, routine eradication therapy is not necessary unless MRSA colonization is confirmed in the nares or another site (McConeghy, Mikolich, & LaPlante, 2009). Intranasal mupirocin is supplied in 1 g, single-use tubes twice a day. The patient applies approximately half the ointment from a single-use tube of nasal ointment into one nostril and the other half into the other nostril in the morning and evening for 5 days. Children may require smaller amounts of ointment.

Rational Drug Selection

Antibacterial Activity

The choice of a topical antibiotic is based on susceptibility. Mupirocin and retapamulin are considered broad-spectrum topical antibiotics. Bacitracin and the combination of bacitracin, neomycin, and polymyxin B are OTC products that combine different antimicrobial spectrums to provide a single broad-spectrum product. Mupirocin is considered a broader-spectrum antibiotic than the double- or triple-antibiotic formula. If resistance to the topical product is suspected or if the infection is not responding to topical antibiotics, then systemic antibiotics are warranted.

Cost

The OTC topical antibiotic products are relatively inexpensive. Bacitracin is usually sold as a generic product and is quite inexpensive. The combination product of neomycin, polymyxin B, and bacitracin is available in brand names (Neosporin), which are slightly more expensive than the generic product (triple-antibiotic ointment). Likewise the double-antibiotic brand-name products (Polysporin) are more expensive than generic double-antibiotic ointment.

Combination Products

Due to the possibility of developing neomycin sensitivity, most providers are recommending that patients use double-antibiotic (Polysporin) rather than triple-antibiotic (Neomycin) products.

Monitoring

No specific monitoring is required beyond that related to the disease process for which the patient is being treated.

Patient Education

Administration

Patients should be taught how to appropriately apply the topical antibiotic ointment. They should be instructed to wash their hands before applying the ointment or to use a gloved hand or a clean cotton swab. The antibiotic ointment should be applied sparingly only to the affected infection area. Overapplication of the antibiotic ointment can increase adverse effects. Patients should not use the antibiotic ointment for longer than 1 week unless instructed to do so by their provider. To avoid contamination of the antibiotic ointment, care must be taken not to touch the tip of the antibiotic ointment container to the infected area or to any other surface.

Adverse Reactions

The patient should be instructed that adverse reactions to topical antibiotics are rare but that skin irritation is possible with any topical ointment. Any adverse reactions should be reported to the provider as soon as possible, and the antibiotic ointment should be discontinued until examined. The patient should not use the antibiotic ointment over large surface areas (more than 20% of body surface) without prior instruction from the provider.

Lifestyle Management

Patients need to be instructed on general infection control measures, especially if the patient has impetigo or if MRSA is suspected; both are highly contagious diseases. Patients should wash their hands after any contact with the infected area. Within the family, the infected patient should use care not to share towels or other utensils with other family members to prevent the spread of infection. In addition to topical or oral antibiotic therapy for impetigo, crusts should be removed by soaking with wet compresses and washing the involved areas with antibacterial soap twice a day.

ANTIFUNGALS

Fungal infections of the skin are common in all age groups. These infections, which occur in both healthy and immunocompromised persons, are caused by dermatophytes and yeasts. Dermatophyte infections are classified according to the anatomic location. Infants and immunocompromised patients may have thrush and *Candida* infections in the diaper area. Tinea corporis, also known as ringworm, can be found in patients of all ages. Tinea capitis is most common in children. Tinea pedis, also known as athlete's foot, can be found at any age but generally in postpubertal patients. Fungal overgrowth occurs in immunocompromised patients or patients on antibiotics. Antifungal medications are used to treat superficial fungal infections caused by dermatophytic fungi and yeast. Oral agents must be used in the treatment of disease that is extensive, that affects hair and nails, or does not respond to topical agents.

The topical antifungal medications can be roughly divided into four major categories: allylamine/benzylamine, imidazole, polyene, and other.

Terbinafine (Lamisil) is a topical allylamine antifungal indicated for the treatment of tinea capitis, tinea pedis, and tinea corporis. Another topical allylamine antifungal, naftifine (Naftin, Naftine-MP), is indicated in the treatment of tinea cruris, tinea corporis, and tinea pedis. Butenafine (Mentax) is a benzylamine antifungal indicated for the topical treatment of interdigital tinea pedis, tinea corporis, and tinea cruris due to *Epidermophyton floccosum, Trichophyton mentagrophytes, Trichophyton rubrum,* and *Trichophyton tonsurans.*

The category of imidazole, which includes clotrimazole (Lotrimin), ketoconazole (Nizoral, Extina), miconazole (Monistat), econazole (Spectazole), sertaconazole (Ertaczo), oxiconazole (Oxistat), and sulconazole (Exelderm), are active against common dermatophytes and yeasts. Econazole also has some antibacterial activity.

Nystatin is a polyene antifungal antibiotic that is not effective against the dermatophytes.

Ciclopirox olamine (Loprox) is a broad-spectrum *N*-hydroxypyridinone antifungal used in the treatment of tinea corporis, tinea cruris, or tinea pedis. Tolnaftate (Tinactin) is an OTC product used to treat superficial fungal infections. Systemic antifungals are used to treat tinea capitis and onychomycosis. Griseofulvin is the first-line drug choice in the treatment of tinea capitis (Goldstein & Goldstein, 2011). Onychomycosis may be treated with topical ciclopirox (Penlac) or systemic griseofulvin, itraconazole, or terbinafine.

Pharmacodynamics

Topical Antifungals

Nystatin is a topical polyene antifungal antibiotic. It is effective against most oral, mucosal, and cutaneous infections caused by *Candida* species. Nystatin binds to sterols in the cell membranes of both fungal and human cells. When the nystatin binds to the sterols in the cell membrane of the fungus, it causes a change in membrane permeability that allows leakage of intracellular components.

The topical azole antifungals all act in a similar fashion. They appear to alter the fungal cell membrane by inhibiting ergosterol synthesis through interacting with 14-alpha-demethylase, an essential component of the membrane. This causes leakage of cellular contents, such as potassium- and phosphorus-containing compounds. Clotrimazole is active against a wide variety of fungi, yeasts, and dermatophytes. Organisms that are susceptible to clotrimazole include *Aspergillus fumigatus, Candida albicans, Cephalosporium, Malassezia furfur, T. rubrum,* and some strains of *S. aureus* and *S. pyogenes.* Miconazole inhibits the growth of common dermatophytes *T. rubrum, T. mentagrophytes, C. albicans,* and the active organisms in tinea versicolor, *Pityrosporum orbiculare* and *Pityrosporum ovale.* Ketoconazole is a broad-spectrum antifungal agent that is active against the dermatophytes *T. rubrum, T. mentagrophytes, T. tonsurans, Microsporum canis, E. floccosum,* and the yeast organisms *C. albicans, C. tropicalis, P. ovale,* and *P. orbiculare.* Econazole and oxiconazole have activity

similar to that of ketoconazole. Sertaconazole is only indicated for use in the treatment of interdigit tinea pedis and is active against *T. rubrum, T. mentagrophytes,* and *E. floccosum.*

Terbinafine and naftifine are allylamine antifungals that probably exert their antifungal effectiveness by inhibiting squalene epoxidase, a key enzyme in sterol biosynthesis in fungi. This results in the accumulation of squalene within the fungal cell and causes fungal cell death. Terbinafine has fungicidal activity against dermatophytes. It is less active, however, against *Candida.*

Tolnaftate distorts hyphae and stunts mycelial growth in susceptible fungi.

Butenafine is the first of a newer class of topical antifungal agents, the benzylamines. Butenafine is effective against a wide variety of pathogenic fungi including *E. floccosum, T. mentagrophytes, T. rubrum,* and *T. tonsurans.* The inhibition of squalene monooxygenase creates a deficiency in a component of fungal membranes necessary for normal cell growth; it is less active against *Candida* species. It acts to inhibit fungal ergosterol biosynthesis by interfering with the conversion of squalene into 2,3-oxidosqualene.

Ciclopirox olamine is a broad-spectrum antifungal agent. It acts on the cell membrane to block transmembrane transport of amino acids into the fungal cell, causing intracellular depletion of essential substrates and/or ions. Ciclopirox is used to treat tinea corporis, tinea cruris, or tinea pedis. It has fungicidal activity against in vitro isolates of *T. rubrum, T. mentagrophytes, E. floccosum, M. canis,* and *C. albicans.* Ciclopirox also inhibits the growth of pathogenic dermatophytes, yeasts, and *M. furfur.* Ciclopirox nail lacquer penetrates the nail to achieve minimum inhibitory concentration (MIC) levels high enough to be fungicidal to most organisms responsible for onychomycosis.

Systemic Antifungals

The systemic antifungal agents used in the treatment of fungal infections of the skin include griseofulvin; the azoles ketoconazole, itraconazole, and fluconazole; and the oral allylamine terbinafine.

Griseofulvin is an antifungal antibiotic produced by certain species of *Penicillium.* Griseofulvin exerts its fungistatic activity by disrupting the mitotic spindle structure of the fungal cell. This arrests metaphase cell division. Griseofulvin may also produce defective DNA. Griseofulvin, which has a greater affinity for diseased tissue than for healthy tissue, has an affinity for keratin precursor cells. These are gradually exfoliated and replaced by uninfected tissue. It is tightly bound to the new keratin, which becomes highly resistant to fungal infections.

Fluconazole is a synthetic, broad-spectrum triazole antifungal agent of the imidazole class. Fluconazole has a broader spectrum than the other imidazole antifungals. It exerts its effect by altering the fungal cell membrane and is a highly selective inhibitor of fungal CYP450 and sterol 14-alpha-demethylase. This inhibition results in increased cellular permeability, causing leakage of cellular contents.

Ketoconazole alters the permeability of the cell membrane and inhibits fungal synthesis of phospholipids. Itraconazole is a synthetic triazole antifungal medication that is closely related to ketoconazole. Similar to ketoconazole, it exerts its effect by altering the fungal cell membrane. Itraconazole inhibits the CYP450-dependent synthesis of ergosterol, which increases cellular permeability and causes leakage of cellular contents.

Terbinafine is an allylamine antifungal that exerts its antifungal effect through interfering with fungal sterol biosynthesis by inhibiting the enzyme squalene monooxygenase. This causes accumulation of squalene, which weakens the cell membrane in sensitive fungi. The accumulation of squalene within the fungal cell causes fungal cell death. Terbinafine has fungicidal activity against dermatophytes; it is less active against *Candida*. Naftifine's mechanism of action is not known, but it is thought to work similarly to terbinafine.

Pharmacokinetics
Absorption and Distribution
Topical Antifungals

Topical antifungals are poorly absorbed from intact skin. Nystatin is not absorbed from intact skin or mucous membranes. The topical azoles have little or no systemic absorption following topical application. When applied topically, ciclopirox olamine is minimally absorbed (average of 1.3%). Butenafine, when applied topically, is absorbed through the skin into the systemic circulation in amounts that have not been quantified. Absorption and distribution of tolnaftate have not been described. Systemic absorption of topically administered terbinafine is significantly lower than that of orally administered terbinafine. Naftifine is minimally absorbed when applied topically, with 4.2% of the dose absorbed.

Systemic Antifungals

Griseofulvin and terbinafine are the two systemic antifungals discussed in this chapter, as they are primarily used in dermatological diseases. See Chapter 33 for further information on systemic antifungal medications.

Griseofulvin is poorly absorbed, and therefore oral formulations have been developed in an attempt to increase bioavailability. Microsize griseofulvin has a variable and unpredictable oral absorption. Ultramicrosize griseofulvin has almost complete absorption. Oral griseofulvin is absorbed mainly from the duodenum. Its absorption may be increased by the intake of high-fat food. Griseofulvin is widely distributed and concentrates in the skin, hair, nails, fat, and skeletal muscles. It does cross the placenta, and distribution in breast milk is unknown but should be assumed because of griseofulvin's affinity for fat.

Terbinafine, when administered orally, is well absorbed from the gut. Bioavailability is approximately 40%. Administration with food increases the serum area under the curve (AUC) of terbinafine by 20%. It is widely distributed, including the central nervous system (CNS), hair, and nailbeds. Following 2 weeks of therapy at recommended doses, terbinafine remains in the skin for up to 3 months. The drug may be detected in the nails for up to 90 days following treatment. It is unknown whether terbinafine crosses the placenta, but it is excreted in the breast milk of nursing mothers with a milk/plasma ratio of 7:1.

Metabolism and Excretion
Topical Antifungals

Topical antifungals are either not absorbed or absorbed minimally. Therefore, metabolism information regarding nystatin, tolnaftate, oxiconazole, sulconazole, butenafine, sertaconazole, ciclopirox olamine, and topical ketoconazole is not available. Topically administered miconazole is minimally absorbed following application to intact skin, with 1% of a dose applied 6 times daily for 14 days recovered in urine and feces. Metabolism of oral miconazole occurs mainly in the liver, and the small amount of topical medication that is absorbed is assumed to be also metabolized in this manner. Topical application of econazole results in lower systemic absorption. Less than 1% of an applied dose is recovered in urine and feces. Metabolism of econazole is unknown. There is little systemic absorption of clotrimazole following topical application. The small amounts absorbed are metabolized in the liver and excreted in the bile.

Systemic Antifungals

Griseofulvin is metabolized in the liver, mainly through oxidative demethylation and conjugation with glucuronic acid. The major metabolite is inactive. Griseofulvin is excreted through the urine, feces, and perspiration.

Terbinafine is metabolized in the liver through oxidation and hydrolysis to five inactive metabolites. Seventy percent of the oral terbinafine dose is excreted in the urine as conjugated and unconjugated metabolites. Clearance of terbinafine is decreased by approximately 50% in patients with renal impairment or hepatic cirrhosis.

Pharmacotherapeutics
Precautions and Contraindications
Topical Antifungals

There are few contraindications to the topical antifungal medications. Hypersensitivity to the antifungal agent or any of the components of the formulation is a contraindication. Patients with azole hypersensitivity are often sensitive to all azole derivatives. The antifungal agent should be discontinued if sensitization occurs. The use of antifungals around the eyes should be avoided. Ketoconazole cream contains sulfites that may cause allergic types of reactions, including anaphylactic symptoms and life-threatening or less severe asthmatic episodes in susceptible persons. Ciclopirox topical nail lacquer (Penlac) should not be used in immunocompromised or diabetic patients with onychomycosis.

The topical antifungals that are classified Pregnancy Category B are clotrimazole, oxiconazole, ciclopirox olamine, naftifine, and butenafine. The topical antifungals classified as Pregnancy Category C are nystatin, ketoconazole, sulconazole, tolnaftate, miconazole, sertaconazole, and econazole. Of these, only ketoconazole and econazole have demonstrated teratogenic effects in animal tests with doses 10 times the maximum recommended human dose. Therefore, ketoconazole and econazole should be used in pregnant women only when potential benefits to the mother outweigh the potential risk to the fetus. Although systemic absorption following topical application is extremely low, caution is advised in prescribing econazole or ketoconazole to breastfeeding women. The use of topical antifungals on the breast during lactation is not advised. If antifungal medication is needed to treat such a topical infection in a lactating woman, application of oral nystatin suspension to the affected area on the breast is suggested for safety.

The safety of topical antifungals for infants and children varies from product to product. Nystatin, oxiconazole, econazole and miconazole are all safe for use in infants and children. Tolnaftate, topical ketoconazole, and topical clotrimazole are contraindicated in children younger than 2 years. The safety of ciclopirox olamine for use in children younger than 12 years is product specific. Butenafine, sertaconazole, terbinafine, and naftifine have not had safety and effectiveness established for children younger than 12 years.

Systemic Antifungals

Griseofulvin should be used cautiously in patients with hepatic disease. It may be hepatotoxic on rare occasions. Patients with systemic lupus erythematosus (SLE) or lupus-like syndromes should use griseofulvin with caution because it has been known to exacerbate lupus. Griseofulvin is contraindicated in patients with porphyria or hypersensitivity to griseofulvin. There is a possibility of cross-sensitivity to griseofulvin in patients with penicillin hypersensitivity because griseofulvin is produced by a species of *Penicillium*. This cross-sensitivity is theoretical, and patients have been treated with griseofulvin without adverse effects.

Griseofulvin use during pregnancy is contraindicated. Men should wait at least 6 months after completion of griseofulvin therapy before fathering a child. Its use should be avoided in pregnant women because some women who received the drug during pregnancy reportedly have had spontaneous abortions or delivered infants with congenital abnormalities. Griseofulvin may be used safely in children as young as 2 years.

Terbinafine is contraindicated in patients who have known hypersensitivity to terbinafine or any of its components. Terbinafine should be used with caution in patients with hepatic disease. Terbinafine is rated Pregnancy Category B. It should be used in pregnancy only if the potential benefit to the mother outweighs the potential risk to the fetus; treatment of onychomycosis can be postponed until after pregnancy is completed. Oral terbinafine treatment is not recommended during lactation. Terbinafine may be prescribed for children 4 years of age or older to treat tinea capitis.

Adverse Drug Reactions

Topical Antifungals

Adverse reactions are minimal with topical antifungal medications. Nystatin may cause mild skin irritation when applied topically to some patients, usually related to the preservative (parabens) in the formulation. The topical azoles may all cause itching, stinging, burning, or general skin irritation. Note that cross-sensitization among the topical azoles has been reported. Adverse reactions to topical azoles occur in approximately 1% to 3% of patients treated. The only adverse reaction reported with tolnaftate is mild skin irritation. The allylamine antifungals butenafine and naftifine may cause burning, stinging, dryness, erythema, pruritus, local irritation, and rash. Ciclopirox olamine may cause skin irritation, pruritus at the application site, redness, pain, burning, and worsening of clinical symptoms. Ciclopirox nail lacquer may cause a change in shape or discoloration of the nail.

Systemic Antifungals

The most common adverse reaction with griseofulvin is hypersensitivity, such as skin rashes, urticaria, and, rarely, angioedema. Less commonly reported adverse reactions are oral thrush, nausea, vomiting, epigastric distress, and diarrhea. Several CNS effects have been reported. Headache occurs frequently in the beginning of therapy but often disappears with continued therapy. Other CNS adverse effects include fatigue, dizziness, insomnia, confusion, and impaired performance of routine activities. Hepatitis and elevated hepatic enzymes have been reported in a few patients after prolonged use or high doses of griseofulvin. A rare adverse effect of granulocytopenia or of leukopenia has been reported from prolonged use of high doses of griseofulvin. It should be discontinued if the patient exhibits these conditions. When rare serious reactions occur with griseofulvin, they are usually associated with high doses or long periods of therapy.

The most common adverse reactions with oral terbinafine are gastrointestinal (GI) symptoms such as diarrhea, dyspepsia, abdominal pain, nausea, headache, fever, rash, elevated liver enzymes, and taste disturbance. Rare but serious adverse reactions observed with oral terbinafine include serious skin reactions (Stevens–Johnson syndrome and toxic epidermal neurolysis). Rare cases of blood dyscrasia have been reported with terbinafine use. Severe neutropenia, lymphopenia, thrombocytopenia, and agranulocytosis have all been reported. In clinical trials (Novartis Pharmaceuticals, 2001) 1% to 2% of patients treated with oral terbinafine developed decreased absolute lymphocyte cells (less than 1,000/mm^3). These hematological adverse reactions are reversible with discontinuation of oral terbinafine.

Drug Interactions

Topical Antifungals

There are few drug interactions found with topical antifungal medications. The only significant interactions noted are with clotrimazole and econazole. Clotrimazole and theoretically the other azole antifungals inhibit the synthesis of the fungal sterol ergosterol; the polyene antifungals, such as amphotericin B and nystatin, act by binding to ergosterol. Therefore, the azole antifungals could interfere with the action of either amphotericin B or nystatin by depleting polyene-binding sites. This appears to be the most significant when the azole antifungal is given prior to amphotericin B. Clotrimazole intravaginal preparations should not be administered concurrently with nonoxynol-9 and octoxynol. Clotrimazole may inactivate the spermicides, leading to contraceptive failure. Corticosteroids may inhibit the antifungal activity of econazole against *C. albicans* in a concentration-dependent manner. When the concentration of corticosteroid is equal to the concentration of econazole, the antifungal activity of econazole is inhibited. When the corticosteroid concentration is 10% of that of econazole, there is no inhibition of antifungal activity.

Systemic Antifungals

Systemic antifungal medications have a number of drug interactions. Griseofulvin can increase some of the effects of ethanol, causing the patient to experience tachycardia, diaphoresis, and flushing. Griseofulvin can accelerate the hepatic metabolism of some medications. Griseofulvin may also decrease the hypoprothrombinemic activity of warfarin, which decreases its anticoagulant effect. Prothrombin time should be monitored closely if griseofulvin is either added or discontinued from warfarin therapy. Estrogens or estrogen-containing oral contraceptives can be affected by coadministration of griseofulvin. Patients may experience breakthrough bleeding, amenorrhea, or unintended pregnancy. They should use an alternative or second form of contraception while they are taking griseofulvin and for 1 month after griseofulvin is discontinued. Griseofulvin may reduce cyclosporine levels, resulting in decreased pharmacological effects. An increase in the cyclosporine dose may be necessary if griseofulvin is added. A second dosage adjustment may be necessary if griseofulvin is discontinued. Serum salicylate concentrations may be decreased with griseofulvin use. Certain medications, including barbiturates and primidone, may impair the absorption of griseofulvin, resulting in decreased serum concentrations. Food can also affect the absorption of griseofulvin. Eating a high-fat meal at the time of dosing may increase microsize griseofulvin absorption.

Terbinafine clearance is affected by a number of medications. It is decreased by cimetidine and terfenadine and increased by rifampin. Caffeine clearance is decreased by terbinafine. Cyclosporine clearance is increased by terbinafine. Theophylline clearance is decreased by terbinafine. Patients taking theophylline, aminophylline, or cyclosporine concurrently with terbinafine should be monitored closely for increased or decreased effects of these medications with a narrow therapeutic window. Terbinafine may affect the metabolism of warfarin, leading to bleeding and coagulopathy.

Clinical Use and Dosing

Candidiasis

Of the more than 150 recognized species of *Candida*, only a few cause disease in humans. The most common sites for mucocutaneous candidiasis are the mouth, where it causes stomatitis or thrush; the esophagus, where it causes esophagitis; and the vagina, where it causes yeast vaginitis. *Candida* can also be invasive or systemic, aspects that are not discussed in this chapter. In most patients, candidiasis is an opportunistic disease. *C. albicans* is the most common pathogen in humans; other

common pathogens in humans are *C. glabrata, C. parapsilosis,* and *C. tropicalis. Candida* species are normal human flora of the mucosal membranes of the gastrointestinal, genitourinary, and respiratory tracts. It normally lives in balance with other microorganisms within the body. When drugs or conditions, such as broad-spectrum antibiotics, corticosteroids, diabetes mellitus, or HIV infection, offset this balance, *Candida* may become a pathogen and cause mucocutaneous disease. *Candida* species may be transmitted from person to person, by direct contact either by hands or sexual contact, or during birth from a colonized vagina to the neonatal oropharynx. Candidiasis has emerged as the most common opportunistic fungal disease.

The first-line treatment for cutaneous *Candida* infections are the OTC azoles, miconazole and clotrimazole, which are applied twice daily to the affected skin area until clear. For thrush in patients older than 3 years, a 10 mg clotrimazole troche is slowly and completely dissolved in the mouth 5 times a day for 14 days. Longer therapy may be needed in immunosuppressed patients.

For the patient who does not tolerate the azole antifungals, nystatin can be prescribed. Nystatin in cream, ointment, or powder formulation can be applied to the affected area 2 to 3 times per day until clear (see Table 23-1). Cream is preferred to ointment in intertriginous areas. Treatment should continue for at least 2 weeks. For thrush, the dose in adults and children is 4 to 6 mL of nystatin suspension, which is swished around the mouth and swallowed 4 times per day. The dose in infants is 2 mL, with 1 mL applied on each side of the mouth 4 times per day. The dose of nystatin for neonates is 0.5 mL applied to each side of the mouth 4 times per day. Adults and older children can use nystatin troches, which are slowly dissolved in the mouth. Treatment should continue until symptoms have been resolved for 48 hours.

Second-line treatment for cutaneous *Candida* infections includes other prescription azole antifungal medications. Econazole is applied to the affected area twice daily for at least 2 weeks. Ketoconazole is applied once daily for at least 2 weeks. Oxiconazole is applied to the affected and immediately surrounding areas once or twice daily until clear. Sulconazole may be gently massaged into the affected areas and surrounding skin once daily until clear.

Other antifungals effective against *Candida* species include ciclopirox olamine, naftifine, and butenafine. Ciclopirox olamine is gently massaged into the affected skin and surrounding area twice daily until clinical improvement occurs. Naftifine is gently massaged into the affected area once a day for the cream formulation and twice a day for the gel formulation until clinical clearing is observed. Topical butenafine is used in adults and children older than 12 years, and it is applied to the affected areas once daily until clear. Safety in children younger than 12 years has not been established.

An optional second-line treatment for oropharyngeal candidiasis (thrush) is systemic fluconazole. The dosage in adults is 200 mg orally for 7 days. Dosing in children, infants, and neonates older than 14 days is 6 mg/kg PO on the first day, followed by 3 mg/kg PO once daily for 14 days. Neonates younger than 14 days have the same dose as infants, except it should be given every 72 hours instead of once daily until age 2 weeks. Clinical improvement is rapid with fluconazole, with lesions on the inner cheeks often clearing within the first 1 or 2 days of treatment, but treatment should continue for the full 14 days. This point should be stressed to patients.

Tinea Capitis

Tinea capitis is commonly called ringworm of the scalp. The causative organism is *Trichophyston tonsurans*; exposure to affected pets is associated with *M. canis*. Tinea capitis occurs mainly in children, although it may be seen at all ages. *Trichophyston* causes "black dot" tinea, which presents with tiny black dots that are the remains of broken hair shafts, flush with the scalp. Definitive diagnosis is obtained by fungal culture. As fungal cultures may take 2 to 4 weeks for results, treatment is begun while awaiting results. Microscopy by performing KOH examination of spores on the hair shaft provides the most rapid means of diagnosis.

Treatment of tinea capitis consists of oral antifungal therapy with griseofulvin and biweekly shampooing with sporicidal shampoo. Tinea capitis should always be treated with a systemic antifungal. The treatment of choice is griseofulvin, with treatment to continue for 2 to 4 months, or for at least 2 weeks after negative laboratory examinations are obtained. Griseofulvin is absorbed more easily with a high-fat meal (whole milk, cheese, or ice cream), and the patient should be instructed about this point when beginning treatment.

The patient should also be treated with a sporicidal shampoo such as selenium sulfide or ketoconazole. The patient should shampoo with either the selenium sulfide 2.5% shampoo or ketoconazole 2% shampoo twice weekly until clear. Close contacts should be empirically treated with sporicidal shampoo twice per week.

If the patient is not responding to therapy, a culture should be obtained. Cases resistant to griseofulvin may be treated with systemic terbinafine, fluconazole, or itraconazole, based on the sensitivity of the organism as determined by culture. Resistance to griseofulvin is not common. By obtaining a fungal culture from the patient at the beginning of therapy, the provider will have sensitivity studies on which to base the treatment decision if there is no response after 4 weeks of treatment. Dosing information regarding systemic terbinafine, fluconazole, and itraconazole can be found in Chapter 24.

Tinea Corporis

Tinea corporis is a superficial fungal infection of the skin, also known as ringworm. The causative organism is *T. rubrum, M. canis, T. verrucosum,* or *M. gypseum.* Tinea corporis presents as an annular lesion with raised borders and center clearing. There may be scaling and some erythema. It is spread by direct contact with an infected person or animal. Diagnosis is made by KOH scrapings, Wood's lamp, or fungal culture. Treatment is topical antifungal cream, with miconazole, tolnaftate, or clotrimazole the most common medications used. Other topical antifungals may be used, including terbinafine, butenafine, sulconazole, naftifine, ciclopirox olamine, ketoconazole, and econazole.

Tinea Cruris

Tinea cruris is also known as jock itch. It is a superficial fungal infection of the groin, upper thighs, and intertriginous folds. It is more common in males and rarely occurs before adolescence. The causative fungal organisms are *E. floccosum, T. rubrum,* and *T. mentagrophytes. C. albicans* may also be a causative organism. The lesions are pruritic, erythematous, scaly, well-demarcated patches with central clearing. The treatment for tinea cruris is the same topical antifungal medications that are used for tinea corporis, with the same dosing schedule.

Tinea Pedis

Tinea pedis is a superficial fungal infection of the skin of the feet, commonly called athlete's foot. It is caused by the dermatophytes *E. floccosum, T. rubrum,* and *T. mentagrophytes. C. albicans* may also be a causative organism. Tinea pedis is more common in males and rarely occurs before puberty. Diagnosis is made by the classic clinical presentation of scaling, maceration, fissuring, and inflammation on the feet, especially in the inner digital areas. Treatment for tinea pedis is the same topical agents used for tinea corporis. Length of treatment is extended with tinea pedis, often with 4 weeks of treatment needed.

Tinea Versicolor

Tinea versicolor is a superficial fungal infection of the skin caused by yeasts in the genus *Malassezia.* Clinically, tinea versicolor appears as hyper- or hypopigmented coalescing scaly macules on the trunk and upper arms. The treatment for tinea versicolor consists of topical application of selenium sulfide shampoo or a topical antifungal. Selenium sulfide shampoo is applied to the tinea versicolor patch and left on for 10 to 15 minutes every day for 1 week. Selenium sulfide can be used prophylactically once a month. The topical azoles miconazole, clotrimazole, and econazole may be used twice a day for 2 to 4 weeks in the treatment of tinea versicolor.

Onychomycosis

Onychomycosis, also known as tinea unguium, is a fungal infection of the nail, either fingernail or toenail. Treatment of onychomycosis usually involves months of treatment with a systemic antifungal medication. Topical treatment is usually not effective, with the exception of ciclopirox nail lacquer (Penlac). When treating onychomycosis, medications such as terbinafine and itraconazole appear to have higher rates of cure than griseofulvin. Clearing of onychomycosis takes months of treatment regardless of treatment modality.

Itraconazole may be used for first-line therapy in adult patients with onychomycosis. It may be dosed in one of two methods, either daily dosing or pulse dosing. The daily dosing regimen for adults with toenail onychomycosis is 200 mg daily for 12 weeks. The pulse regimen for adults with toenail involvement is 400 mg/d for 1 week per month for 3 to 4 consecutive months. If only the fingernail area is involved, the adult dose is 200 mg bid for 7 days, then 3 weeks without treatment, and then 200 mg bid for for 2 months. Safety in children has not been established. For onychomycosis, the pediatric pulse dose is 5 mg/kg/d for 1 week per month for

3 to 4 consecutive months. For any patient who takes itraconazole for more than 8 consecutive weeks, liver enzymes and electrolytes should be drawn prior to and every 8 weeks during treatment. Itraconazole should not be administered to pregnant women or women considering pregnancy.

Systemic terbinafine is also used as first-line treatment for onychomycosis in adults (Lipner & Scher, 2014). The dose for treating onychomycosis of the fingernail is 250 mg daily for 6 weeks. To treat an infected toenail, the dose is 250 mg daily for 12 weeks. Liver enzymes and complete blood count (CBC) should be monitored every 6 weeks if treatment lasts longer than 6 weeks.

Griseofulvin has been used extensively in the treatment of onychomycosis as second-line therapy and has a proven safety profile in adults and children. The medication should be administered for at least 4 months for onychomycosis of the fingernail. Treatment of the toenail should last at least 6 months. Renal, liver, and hematopoietic functions should be measured at least every 8 weeks during therapy. The adult dose of griseofulvin microsize for onychomycosis is 600 mg to 1 g/d; the dose for ultramicrosize is 375 mg to 750 mg/d. The dose for children is 10 to 15 mg/kg/d of microsize griseofulvin and 5 to 10 mg/kg/d of ultramicrosize griseofulvin. The medication should be taken with a high-fat meal.

Topical monotherapy with ciclopirox (Penlac) is indicated in superficial white onychomycosis, when there is distal subungual onychomycosis that affects less than 50% of the nail surface, when four or fewer nails are infected and for children with thin, fast growing nails (Gupta, Paquet, & Simpson, 2013). Topical ciclopirox nail lacquer (Penlac) is applied once daily to the infected nail, preferably at bedtime. The solution is applied to the entire nailbed and surrounding 5 mm of skin. The solution must remain on the nail 8 hours before bathing. Once a week (every 7 days) previous coats of lacquer are removed with alcohol and excess nail is trimmed and filed. This routine is repeated for 24 to 48 weeks. The patient should not use nail polish during treatment.

Combining an oral antifungal with topical ciclopirox has been found in multiple studies to be more effective than either treatment alone. The combination of terbinafine and ciclopirox has the most published studies (Avner, Nir, & Henri, 2005; Baran & Kaoukhov, 2005; Gupta, Onychomycosis Combination Therapy Study Group, 2005). Dosing ciclopirox daily for 48 weeks combined with terbinafine 250 mg/d for 12 weeks or terbinafine 250 mg/d for 4 weeks, then 4 weeks of rest and an additional 4 weeks of terbinafine produced similar cure rates (70.4% versus 66.7%) (Gupta et al, 2005). A slightly higher cure rate (88.2%) is achieved when terbinafine 250 mg/d for 16 weeks is combined with 9 months of topical ciclopirox (Avner et al, 2005). Although further studies are needed, it is reasonable to consider combining therapies in patients with onychomycosis.

Rational Drug Selection

Indication

For treating topical dermatophyte infections, generally the OTC azoles are the first-line therapy because they are easily available without prescription and are low cost. If OTC products are not effective, then a broader-spectrum antifungal can be prescribed, with little difference found in efficacy in treating common organisms that cause tinea infections.

Cost

The cost of medication varies greatly among the antifungals. Generally, OTC products are less expensive than prescriptions. In the treatment of thrush, nystatin is a low-cost, effective therapy for topical fungal infections and is usually covered by insurance plans. When treating cutaneous fungal infections, the OTC products clotrimazole and miconazole should be the first medications used because of their low cost and their safety profile. If they are ineffective, then a prescription product with a broader spectrum may be used, but it is generally more expensive. In the treatment of tinea pedis, tolnaftate is available OTC in a variety of formulations; the generic products are generally the least expensive.

> Metholated ointment (Vicks VapoRub) is a common lay treatment for onychomycosis. A small study (*n* = 18) of the use of daily topical mentholated ointment showed a positive treatment effect (83%), with mycological cure in 27.8% of study subjects and partial cure in 55.6% (Derby, Rohal, Jackson, Beutler, & Olsen, 2011).

Patient Variables

Many patients cannot tolerate systemic antifungals due to liver toxicity. Topical ciclopirox nail lacquer provides an alternative treatment for patients with onychomycosis who cannot tolerate systemic antifungals.

Monitoring

The patient being treated for oral candidiasis should be monitored for efficacy of treatment, with no laboratory monitoring necessary. The patient being treated for tinea capitis will need monitoring for adverse effects from the systemic antifungals. All of the systemic antifungal agents can possibly cause some alteration in hepatic function. If the patient is to be on continuous therapy, then baseline and ongoing monitoring of liver function is necessary. If liver enzymes become elevated, the medication should be discontinued. The patient being prescribed griseofulvin will require renal, liver, and hematopoietic function measurements every 8 weeks during therapy. Patients receiving ketoconazole require liver function tests prior to beginning therapy and monthly for the whole course of their treatment. Patients on itraconazole need liver enzyme and renal studies if the medication is prescribed for longer than 8 consecutive weeks. In that case, liver function and electrolytes should be monitored prior to beginning therapy and every 8 weeks during treatment. Liver enzymes and CBC should be monitored every 6 weeks in the patient receiving terbinafine who is treated for longer than 6 weeks.

Patient Education

Administration

Instruct patients to take the drug as prescribed for the full course of their treatment, even if they note clinical improvement. In the treatment of oral candidiasis, the patient should be instructed to continue therapy until 2 days after symptoms have disappeared. When treating infants with thrush, all pacifiers and bottle nipples should be washed in warm, soapy water and soaked in hot or boiling water for 20 minutes between each use. This step is important to prevent reinfection of the infant with candidiasis. If oral candidiasis is treated with clotrimazole troche, patients should be instructed to slowly dissolve the troche in their mouth, not chew.

Patients using topical antifungals for dermatophyte infections of the skin should be instructed to apply the medication to the infected area and the immediate surrounding area for the full length of treatment. Treatment is often continued beyond the point of clinical clearing to prevent recurrence of the infection. Generally, avoid occlusive dressings, which provide favorable conditions for yeast growth.

The treatment of tinea capitis or onychomycosis involves long-term therapy with oral antifungal medications. The patient should be encouraged to continue the medication for the full length of treatment and take the medication as prescribed. Griseofulvin must be taken with a high-fat meal to ensure adequate absorption of the medication. Itraconazole should be taken with food. Ketoconazole and terbinafine may both be taken without regard to meals.

In treating topical dermatophyte infections such as tinea corporis or ringworm, family members and pets should be checked for signs of infection and be treated also.

Adverse Reactions

The patient should be given written and oral instructions regarding the adverse drug reactions that may be expected with the medication that is being prescribed. If the patient is prescribed systemic antifungal medication, then an explanation of the possible adverse effects and the necessity for laboratory monitoring should be discussed. Patients should be instructed to immediately report to their provider any flu-like symptoms, which may be a sign of hepatic toxicity.

TOPICAL ANTIVIRALS

Topical antivirals are used to treat herpes simplex virus (HSV) and herpes zoster. The oral antiviral medications used to treat these conditions and varicella are discussed in Chapter 24. The two herpes simplex virus infections that are treated with topical medications are HSV-1 and HSV-2, with HSV-1 generally associated with nongenital infection and HSV-2 with genital infection. There are three topical antiviral medications: acyclovir (Zovirax), penciclovir (Denavir), and the OTC product docosanol (Abreva).

Pharmacodynamics

Both acyclovir and penciclovir must be phosphorylated to be active against herpes simplex virus. Intracellularly, both medications are converted to monophosphate forms by viral thymidine kinases, then further converted to diphosphate and finally to triphosphate by various cellular enzymes. Acyclovir triphosphate competes with deoxyguanosine triphosphate for a position in the DNA chain of the herpes virus. Once incorporated in the DNA chain, it terminates DNA synthesis. Penciclovir triphosphate selectively inhibits viral DNA polymerase by competing with deoxyguanosine triphosphate. This inhibits viral replication. In vitro, penciclovir triphosphate is retained inside the HSV-infected cells for 10 to 20 hours, compared with 0.7 to 1 hour for acyclovir.

Pharmacokinetics

Absorption and Distribution

After topical application of acyclovir, penciclovir, or docosanol there is minimal absorption, and no drug is detected in the blood or urine after application.

Pharmacotherapeutics

Precautions and Contraindications

The only true contraindication to acyclovir, penciclovir, or docosanol is hypersensitivity to the product or any of its components. Acyclovir should be used with caution in patients with ganciclovir hypersensitivity in that these two drugs have similar chemical structures and there may be cross-sensitivity.

Acyclovir and penciclovir are classified as Pregnancy Category B, although no complete or well-controlled pregnancy studies have been performed in humans. No adverse effects on pregnancy outcomes or fetal development are found in animal studies. However, there have been no adequate or well-controlled studies in pregnant women.

Orally administered acyclovir is excreted in breast milk. It is unknown whether topical acyclovir is excreted in breast milk. Because topical acyclovir cannot be measured in the serum, it is assumed that it is not excreted in breast milk. It is not known if penciclovir is excreted in human milk after topical administration. Both medications should be used with caution in a nursing mother until further studies clarify their safety.

Acyclovir, penciclovir, and docosanol have all been approved in the use of children older than 12 years of age.

Adverse Drug Reactions

Although systemic acyclovir has extensive adverse reactions, topical acyclovir has only transient local adverse reactions. The most common reaction to topical acyclovir use is mild pain with transient burning or stinging in 28.3% of patients. Pruritus is reported by 4.1% of patients, with rash and local edema found in less than 1%.

The only adverse reactions reported for docosanol is irritation at the site of application.

Drug Interactions

There are no known drug interactions identified with topical acyclovir, penciclovir, or docosanol.

Clinical Use and Dosing

Herpes Simplex

Acyclovir is indicated for the treatment of recurrent herpes labialis (cold sores); herpes genitalis; and in limited, non–life-threatening, mucocutaneous HSV infections in immunocompromised patients. Topical acyclovir is applied to cover all lesions every 3 hours, 6 times a day for 7 days. The dose size per application should be approximately a 0.5- to 1-inch ribbon of ointment per 4 square inches of surface area. A glove or finger cot should be used to apply the medication to prevent autoinoculation of other body sites and transmission of infection to other people.

Penciclovir is indicated in the treatment of recurrent herpes labialis (cold sores) on the lips and face. Application to mucous membrane is not recommended. In adults, penciclovir 1% cream is applied every 2 hours while awake, with treatment started as early as possible (during the prodrome or when lesions appear).

Docosanol (Abreva) is the only OTC product available for the treatment of herpes labialis. It is applied to the cold sore 5 times a day until healed. Treatment should begin at the first sign of outbreak.

Herpes Zoster

Neither topical acyclovir nor topical penciclovir is indicated in the treatment of herpes zoster.

Varicella

Although oral acyclovir is used in the treatment of varicella, topical acyclovir does not have this indication. Penciclovir is not used in the treatment of varicella.

Rational Drug Selection

Efficacy

Penciclovir is the first topical antiviral medication that has been clinically proved to be effective in the treatment of herpes labialis (cold sores). Docosanol is effective in decreasing the duration of a cold sore outbreak but must be started early in the course of the outbreak to be effective, whereas penciclovir may be started any time in the disease course. Although acyclovir may be used for herpes labialis, it has not been clinically proved to be effective in the treatment of HSV infections in immunocompetent patients. In genital herpes, acyclovir is the drug of choice for primary lesions in immunocompromised patients.

Cost

Topical acyclovir and penciclovir are both unique antiviral agents and their cost is not generally used as part of the decision of whether to prescribe the drug in treatment.

Monitoring

There is no laboratory monitoring necessary for patients treated with topical acyclovir or penciclovir. Monitoring for the adverse reactions noted previously is the only monitoring needed.

Patient Education

Administration

Patients should be instructed to start therapy with acyclovir as early as possible after the onset of the signs and symptoms of HSV infection. When applying acyclovir, patients should first wash their hands thoroughly and use a finger cot or rubber glove to apply the ointment to prevent the spread of infection. They should apply enough ointment to thoroughly cover all lesions. Patients should be instructed that acyclovir might cause transient burning, stinging, itching, and rash. They should notify their primary care provider if these symptoms become pronounced or persist.

Patients should be instructed to begin therapy with penciclovir as soon as symptoms begin, during the prodrome or when lesions appear. They should wash their hands thoroughly after applying penciclovir to prevent the spread of infection. Patients should avoid application on or near the eyes or mucous membranes. Although adverse reactions are rare, patients should be instructed to report any skin irritation to their provider.

Treatment with docosanol should begin at the earliest sign or symptom. Patients should wash hands before and after application. The medication should be rubbed in completely. Patients are to use the medication 5 times a day until cold sores are healed.

AGENTS USED TO TREAT ACNE

Acne is the most common skin condition in the United States, affecting approximately 40 to 50 million Americans (American Academy of Dermatology [AAD], 2011). Acne can occur at any age, with up to 25% of adults having some degree of acne. Acne is classified as mild, moderate, or severe, and pharmacological intervention is based on the severity of acne. The bacterium commonly found in acne is *Propionibacterium acnes (P. acnes);* thus, treatment often includes antibiotics active against *P. acnes* (Strauss, et al, 2007).

The medications used in the treatment of acne may be either topical agents or systemic. The topical agents used for acne can be divided into two categories: retinoids and antibiotics. Oral medications for systemic use are divided into three categories: oral antibiotics (discussed in Chap. 24), hormonal therapy (discussed in Chap. 31), and isotretinoin, an oral retinoid. Oral antibiotics are prescribed for moderate to severe acne, and isotretinoin is prescribed for severe nodulocystic acne.

Pharmacodynamics

Topical Retinoids

Tretinoin is a naturally occurring derivative of vitamin A that is structurally related to isotretinoin. After topical administration, tretinoin appears to reduce the cohesion between keratinized cells. They act specifically on microcomedones, causing fragmentation and expulsion of the microplug, expulsion of comedones, and conversion of closed comedones to open comedones. New comedone formation is prevented by continued use. Tretinoin thins the cell layers of the stratum corneum. Tretinoin does not affect the bacteria found in *P. acnes*. Topical tretinoin is also used in the treatment of fine wrinkling, mottled hyperpigmentation, and roughness of the skin associated with sun damage. Retinoids enhance the penetration of other topical agents such as topical antibiotics and benzoyl peroxide.

Adapalene is a topical retinoid-like drug used for the treatment of mild to moderate acne vulgaris. Adapalene binds to specific retinoic acid nuclear receptors but does not bind to the cytosolic receptor protein. Although the exact mode of action of adapalene is not known, it is suggested that topical adapalene may normalize the differentiation of follicular epithelial cells, resulting in decreased microcomedone formation. It is also a modulator of cellular differentiation, keratinization, and inflammatory processes, all of which represent important features in the pathology of acne vulgaris.

Tazarotene is a retinoid. The exact mechanism of action of tazarotene in the treatment of acne is not well defined, but it is believed that the drug works by normalizing epidermal differentiation and by reducing the influx of inflammatory cells into the skin.

Topical Antibiotics

Benzoyl peroxide has antibacterial activity against *P. acnes,* the predominant organism in sebaceous follicles and comedones of acne vulgaris. This antibacterial activity is presumably due to the release of active or free-radical oxygen capable of oxidizing bacterial proteins. Benzoyl peroxide also has a drying effect, removes excess sebum, causes mild desquamation, and has a sebostatic effect.

Erythromycin is a bacteriostatic macrolide antibiotic, which binds to the P site of the 50S ribosomal subunit, interfering with protein synthesis.

Topical clindamycin has activity against *P. acnes* in vitro. Clindamycin reversibly binds to 50S ribosomal subunits, preventing peptide bond formation and thus inhibiting bacterial protein synthesis. It can be bacteriostatic or bactericidal.

Metronidazole is classified as an antiprotozoal and antibacterial agent. The mechanism by which topical metronidazole acts in reducing the inflammatory lesions is thought to disrupt bacterial and protozoal DNA, inhibiting nucleic acid synthesis.

The mechanism of action for azelaic acid in acne vulgaris is its antimicrobial effect against *P. acnes* and *S. epidermidis*. The mechanism of action may be due to inhibition of microbial cellular protein synthesis. Azelaic acid decreases the inflammation associated with acne lesions by reducing the concentration of bacteria present in the skin. Azelaic acid may also cause normalization of keratinization, leading to an anticomedonal effect. It may also decrease microcomedone formation by reducing the number and size by of keratohyalin granules and the amount and distribution of filaggrin in epidermal layers. Azelaic acid does not effect sebum excretion.

The mechanism of action of topical dapsone in the treatment of acne is unknown.

Systemic Retinoids

Isotretinoin is an isomer of *all-trans* retinoic acid, a metabolite of retinol (vitamin A). It reduces sebum production by reducing sebaceous gland size, normalizing follicular keratinization, and indirectly reducing *P. acne* and its inflammatory sequale.

Pharmacokinetics

Absorption and Distribution

Topical Retinoids

Tretinoin and adapalene administered topically are minimally absorbed systemically. However, there are published case reports of birth defects in the literature associated with topical tretinoin use, which are consistent with retinoid embryopathy (Bozzo, Chua-Gocheco, & Einarson, 2011). Women should be encouraged to not use topical retinoids during pregnancy. Tazarotene, when administered topically to the skin, has minimal systemic absorption However, this medication is categorized as a Category X drug and women of childbearing age should be alerted and avoid usage.

Topical Antibiotic

Only about 5% of benzoyl peroxide is absorbed by the skin and then it is completely metabolized to benzoic acid within the skin and excreted unchanged in the urine. Absorption of topical erythromycin is unknown. Clindamycin, when applied topically, does exhibit some systemic absorption, depending on the surface area covered. Following multiple topical applications at a concentration equivalent to 10 mg, very low levels of clindamycin are present in the serum. Metronidazole is absorbed when applied topically but in very small amounts. Approximately 4% of topically applied azelaic acid is absorbed systemically.

Systemic Retinoids

Due to its high lipophilicity, oral absorption of isotretinoin is enhanced when given with a high-fat meal. Isotretinoin is more than 99.9% bound to plasma proteins, primarily albumin, and is not stored in adipose tissue. Although severe fetal abnormalities have been noted, it is not known whether isotretinoin crosses the placenta, due to ethical restrictions imposed on such studies.

Metabolism and Excretion

Topical Retinoids

A minimal amount of tretinoin is absorbed systemically. This trace amount is metabolized by the CYP450 hepatic enzyme system. Approximately 1% to 5% of a topically applied dose is excreted in the urine. The metabolism of topically applied adapalene is low and it is eliminated by biliary excretion. Tazarotene is rapidly metabolized in the skin to the active metabolite tazarotenic acid, which is systemically absorbed and further metabolized by the liver to sulfoxides, sulfones, and other metabolites. Elimination of the metabolites is via fecal and renal pathways.

Topical Antibiotics

Benzoyl peroxide is absorbed by the skin, where it is metabolized to benzoic acid and excreted as benzoate in the urine. Topical erythromycin absorption is minimal. Excretion of erythromycin is mainly unknown. Topical clindamycin is systemically absorbed, depending on the surface area covered. Topically applied azelaic acid is minimally absorbed and is mainly excreted unchanged in the urine.

Systemic Retinoids

Isotretinoin is metabolized in the liver primarily via oxidation. It is unknown whether its metabolite is pharmacologically active. The metabolites are eliminated renally, and unchanged drug and metabolites are excreted in the feces.

Pharmacotherapeutics

Precautions and Contraindications

Topical Retinoids and Topical Antibiotics

Topical retinoids should be avoided in patients with eczema, sunburn, or skin abrasions at the site of application. Topical retinoids are contraindicated in lactating women. Safety and efficacy in children younger than 12 years have not been established. Tretinoin and adapalene are classified as Pregnancy Category C. Tazarotene is Pregnancy Category X.

Topical antibiotics used in acne treatment have few true contraindications. Benzoyl peroxide may exhibit cross-sensitivity with benzoic acid derivatives. Erythromycin, when applied topically, is contraindicated only when the patient is hypersensitive to erythromycin or to any component of the preparation. Topical clindamycin is contraindicated in any patient who is hypersensitive to clindamycin or lincomycin. It is also contraindicated in patients with a history of regional enteritis, ulcerative colitis, or antibiotic-associated colitis. Azelaic acid products are contraindicated for use in patients with a history of hypersensitivity to any components of the preparation, and caution should be exercised in patients with dark complexion to avoid hypopigmentation. Azelaic acid is classified as Pregnancy Category B. Because small amounts of azelaic acid are absorbed systemically and may be excreted in breast milk, caution should be exercised in administering it to lactating women. Safety and efficacy of azelaic acid in children younger than 12 years have not been established. Hypersensitivity to metronidazole, nitroimidazole derivatives, or any component of the formulation is a contraindication to its use. Meteronidazole is Pregnancy Category B and use is not recommended in lactating women.

Systemic Retinoids

Isotretinoin should be avoided in patients with retinoid hypersensitivity, including vitamin A, tretinoin, and etretinate. Patients with parabens hypersensitivity should avoid isotretinoin because the drug is prepared with parabens, a preservative. Patients with a risk for osteoporosis (osteomalacia and anorexia nervosa) should avoid taking isotretinoin due to decreased bone mineral density seen during treatment. Adolescents who participate in impact sports while taking isotretinoin are at risk for bone injuries. The safety and effectiveness in children younger than 12 years have not been established for isotretinoin. Care should be exercised in administering isotretinoin to patients with hyperlipidemia, as they may have increased lipids during therapy. Isotretinoin should be prescribed cautiously to patients with psychotic disorders; it may cause major depression, psychosis, and, rarely, suicidal ideation.

Isotretinoin is classified Pregnancy Category X and is absolutely contraindicated in pregnancy. It may cause severe malformations of the craniofacial, cardiac, thymic, and CNS structures. Spontaneous abortions and premature births have been reported. The drug should not be administered to any woman of childbearing age until after pregnancy has been excluded and appropriate birth control measures are used for at least 1 month. Patients should also avoid pregnancy for at least 1 month after discontinuation of isotretinoin. Breastfeeding is not recommended during isotretinoin treatment because of the potential adverse affects to the nursing infant.

Only dermatologists prescribe isotretinoin due to its adverse effect profile. It must be stressed that, because of the safety issues, primary care providers usually do not prescribe this medication. As a requirement of the Risk Evaluation and Mitigation Strategy (REMS) program, access to this medication is restricted. All patients (male and female), prescribers, wholesalers, and dispensing pharmacists must register and be active in the iPLEDGE risk management program, designed to eliminate fetal exposures to isotretinoin (www.ipledgeprogram.com).

Adverse Drug Reactions

Topical Retinoids

Topical retinoids all cause some degree of skin irritation. Burning or pruritus immediately after applying a topical retinoid is common. All three retinoid products cause erythema, scaling, xerosis, and peeling. These symptoms occur frequently and appear to be necessary for the therapeutic effect. Because photosensitivity may occur with topical retinoid use, patients should use sunscreen to prevent severe sunburn. Both tretinoin and tazarotene may cause hyperpigmentation, or hypopigmentation, which will resolve after discontinuation of the medication.

Topical Antibiotics

Topical antibiotics used in the treatment of acne all cause some dryness, erythema, burning, peeling, and itching. Benzoyl peroxide may also cause marked peeling and desquamation, which appears to be a necessary component of the therapeutic effect. Benzoyl peroxide may also cause photosensitivity. Allergic contact sensitization may occur with any of the topical antibiotics used in the treatment of acne vulgaris. In patients with dark complexions, skin hypopigmentation may occur with the use of topical azelaic acid.

Systemic Retinoids

Isotretinoin has multiple reported significant adverse reactions. The most commonly reported adverse reactions involve mucocutaneous effects. Cheilitis (inflammation of the lips) occurs in more than 90% of patients, and dry skin, pruritus, and skin fragility occur in approximately 80% of patients. Conjunctivitis is reported by 40% of patients, with facial skin desquamation and drying of mucous membranes reported by approximately 30% of those treated with isotretinoin. Patients also report xerosis, xerostomia, and epistaxis. These mucocutaneous drying effects of isotretinoin are dose-related and are usually reversible after discontinuation of therapy.

Hypertriglyceridemia occurs in up to 45% of patients on isotretinoin therapy and elevations of total cholesterol and low-density lipoprotein are seen in approximately 30% (Zane, Leyden, Marqueling, & Manos, 2006). These elevations are transient in about 80% of subjects and are rarely severe enough to require termination of therapy. Alcohol consumption may potentiate serum triglyceride elevations. Lipid alterations occur most frequently at dosages greater than 1 mg/kg/d and are reversible upon discontinuation of isotretinoin.

Elevation of serum glucose and fasting serum blood glucose has been reported. Exacerbation of diabetes mellitus can occur. Decreases in hemoglobin and hematocrit concentrations and increased sedimentation rates have been reported. Patients may also experience anemia and thrombocytopenia.

CNS effects include headache, lethargy, and fatigue. Isotretinoin has also been associated with pseudotumor cerebri (benign increased intracranial pressure). Symptoms include headache, visual disturbances, and papilledema. In the post-marketing period, depression has been reported, as have psychosis and, rarely, suicidal ideation. If patients report depression, immediate discontinuation of therapy is indicated. Depression appears to subside with discontinuation of therapy and to recur upon reinstitution of therapy.

Adverse GI reactions include anorexia, nausea and vomiting, increased appetite, and thirst. Eighty percent of patients report dry mouth when taking isotretinoin. Inflammatory bowel disease, including regional enteritis, may occur.

Musculoskeletal adverse effects such as arthralgia and myalgia are reported in approximately 16% of patients taking isotretinoin. Skeletal abnormalities have been reported in adults and children receiving excessive doses (more than 2 mg/kg/d for prolonged periods, 6 months to 2 years). Bone mineral density (BMD) decreases have been seen in pediatric patients when administered a single course of isotretinoin at normal dosages. Adolescent or adult athletes who participate in sports with a repetitive impact may be at increased risk for bone-related injuries due to the decreased BMD seen with isotretinoin use (Bradford, 2008).

Isotretinoin has been associated with rare cases of hepatitis. Normalization of liver enzyme levels does not readily occur with dose reduction or continuation of the drug. If hepatitis is suspected during isotretinoin treatment, the drug should be discontinued.

Ophthalmic adverse effects including corneal opacification have been reported in patients receiving isotretinoin for acne. This ocular effect is reversible with complete resolution or continuing resolution at 6 to 7 weeks following discontinuation of therapy. Of patients taking isotretinoin, 25% report visual disturbances, including blurred vision, decreased visual acuity, tunnel vision, photophobia, diplopia, decreased night vision, and intolerability to contact lenses.

Drug Interactions

Topical Retinoids and Topical Antibiotics

Topical retinoids should not be used concomitantly with other topical medications that have strong drying effects, such as benzoyl peroxide, salicylic acid, or lactic acid (Table 23-2). Medicated or abrasive soaps or cleaners should also be

Table 23–2 ⚏ Drug Interactions: Selected Acne Medications

Drug	Interacting Drug	Possible Effect	Implications
Topical Acne Medications			
Retinoids			
• Adapalene	Skin irritants, like benzoyl peroxide, salicylic acid, lactic acid, medicated or abrasive cleansers	Increased skin irritation	Avoid concurrent use of topical medications that have strong drying effects
• Tazarotene			
• Tretinoin			Before beginning therapy, the effects of strong topical drying agents need to subside to prevent significant skin irritation
	Products that contain alcohol, lime, menthol, spices, or perfumes		
Topical Antibiotics			
• Azelaic acid	No known interactions		
• Benzoyl peroxide	Topical retinoids		
	PABA-containing sunscreens	May transiently discolor skin	Avoid concurrent use
• Clindamycin	Erythromycin	Antagonize each other	Avoid concurrent use
• Erythromycin	Clindamycin	Antagonize each other	Avoid concurrent use
Metronidazole	No known interactions		

Table 23–2 ⚏ Drug Interactions: Selected Acne Medications—cont'd

Drug	Interacting Drug	Possible Effect	Implications
Dapsone	TMP/SMX	Levels of dapsone and its metabolites increased in the presence of TMP/SMX	Exposure from the proposed topical dose is about 1% of that from the 100 mg oral dose, even when coadministered with TMP/SMX
	Benzoyl peroxide	Localized discoloration of skin	Avoid concurrent use
	Antimalarial agents	May enhance the adverse effect of dapsone	Avoid concurrent use
Systemic Acne Medication			
Isotretinoin	Vitamin A	Potentiate the toxic effects of isotretinoin	Do not take concurrently
	Alcohol		Avoid concurrent use
	Tetracycline	Potentiate the toxic effects of isotretinoin	Avoid concurrent use
	Skin irritants, like benzoyl peroxide, salicylic acid, lactic acid, medicated or abrasive cleansers	May increase incidents of pseudotumor cerebri	Observe for skin irritation if using concurrently
	Products that contain alcohol, lime, menthol, spices, or perfumes	Can potentiate the drying effects of isotretinoin	Postpone lipid determinations for at least 36 h following ethanol consumption, if patients are taking isotretinoin
	Ethanol	Can increase the hypertriglyceridemic effects of isotretinoin	Monitor closely if using concurrently
	Carbamazepine	Reduced carbamazepine levels with concurrent use	

PABA = para-aminobenzoic acid.
TMP/SMX = trimethoprim/sulfamethoxazole.

avoided because they can potentiate the skin irritation caused by topical retinoids. Products that contain alcohol, lime, menthol, spices, or perfumes can further dry and irritate the skin and should not be used with topical retinoids. Before topical retinoids are begun, the effects of strong topical drying agents need to subside to prevent significant skin irritation. Topical retinoids should not be used in the same areas of skin at the same time as benzoyl peroxide or topical antibiotics. A physical incompatibility between the medications or a change in pH may reduce the efficacy of topical retinoids if used simultaneously. When used together for clinical effect, these medications should be used at different times of the day, such as morning and night, to minimize possible skin irritation.

Topical antibiotics have fewer significant drug interactions than systemic antibiotics. Benzoyl peroxide can interact with topical retinoids, as noted previously. PABA sunscreens may transiently discolor the skin if used concurrently with benzoyl peroxide. All of the topical antibiotics may have possible additive irritation when used with other topical acne agents (especially abrasives or keratolytics). Azelaic acid has no known drug interactions.

Systemic Retinoids

Concomitant use of isotretinoin and other sources of vitamin A can potentiate the toxic effects of isotretinoin. Alcohol may also potentiate the toxic effects of isotretinoin. Tetracycline may increase the incidence of pseudotumor cerebri. Simultaneous use of isotretinoin and other drying agents, such as benzoyl peroxide or other medicated or abrasive soaps or alcohol-containing products, can potentiate the drying effects of isotretinoin. Ethanol can increase the hypertriglyceridemic effects of isotretinoin. Lipid determinations should be postponed for at least 36 hours after ethanol consumption.

Clinical Use and Dosing

Acne Vulgaris

Topical retinoids are applied to the skin once daily as tolerated (Table 23-3). If bothersome or excessive dryness or peeling occurs, patients should reduce the number of applications per day or week. In the evening before retiring, the patient applies a thin film of medication after washing with a gentle cleanser. Care should be taken to avoid the eyes, lips, and mucous membranes. It is recommended that the patient wait 20 to 30 minutes after cleaning before applying tretinoin. Patients should wash their hands immediately after applying topical retinoids.

Topical antibiotics are applied to affected acne areas twice daily as tolerated, in a thin film. Patients should wash their skin with a gentle cleanser and pat dry before applying. Benzoyl peroxide cream or gel is applied once or twice a day to acne-affected areas. Benzoyl peroxide cleanser may be used for cleaning once or twice daily. Patients should wet the skin areas to be treated prior to administration, rinse thoroughly after cleaning, and pat dry. If bothersome or excessive dryness or peeling occurs, patients should reduce the number of applications per day. Clindamycin should be applied to all of the affected areas twice daily. If using the pledget formulation, more than one pledget may be used. Patients should remove the pledget from the foil just before use and discard after a single use. Patients should be instructed to wash their hands thoroughly after the use of any topical antibiotic.

There are combination products available that combine a topical antibiotic with benzoyl peroxide (Benzamycin, Benzaclin, Duac). Benzamycin, a product that combines benzoyl peroxide and erythromycin gel, is unique in that

Table 23–3 ⚗ Dosage Schedule: Selected Acne Medications

Drug	Available Dosage Forms	Dosage	Notes
Retinoids			
Adapalene (Differin)	0.1% cream 0.1%, 0.3% gel 0.1% lotion	Apply to affected areas 1×/d at bedtime, as tolerated	Allow 20–30 min for skin to dry after cleansing, before applying medication
Tazarotene 0.1% (Tazorac)	0.05%, 0.1% cream 0.05%, 0.1% gel		Avoid use near eyes, lips, and mucous membranes
Tretinoin (Atralin, Retin-A)	0.025%. 0.05%, 0.1% cream 0.01%, 0.025% gel		Wash hands after application
(Retin-A micro)	0.04%, 0.1% gel		
Topical Antibiotics			
Azelaic acid (Azelex)	20% cream	Apply a thin film on affected areas 2×/d	May decrease to once a day if irritating/drying
Benzoyl peroxide (OXY Maximum Face Wash, Clean & Clear, Neutrogena On The Spot)	10% cream 2.5%, 5%, 10% gel 5%, 10% liquid 5%, 10% liquid 9% pad 4%, 5%, 6%, 8%, 10% soap 8.5% solution	Cleansers: wash affected areas 1–2×/d Other forms: apply to affected areas 1–3×/d	May decrease to once a day if irritating/drying Wash hands after application Medication can bleach fabrics
Benzoyl peroxide and erythromycin gel (Benzamycin)	Erythromycin 3% and benzoyl peroxide 5% gel	Apply to affected acne areas 2×/d	Wash hands after application Medication can bleach fabrics
Benzoyl peroxide and clindamycin gel (Benzaclin, Duac, Acanya)	Benzoyl Peroxide 5% and clindamycin phosphate 1% gel; benzoyl peroxide 2.5% and clindamycin phosphate 1.2% gel	Apply to affected areas 2×/d (Benzaclin) Apply 1×/d (Acanya, Duac)	Wash hands after application Medication can bleach fabrics
Adapalene and benzoyl peroxide (Epiduo)	Adapalene 0.1% and benzoyl peroxide 2.5% gel	Apply once a day after washing	Apply pea-sized amount for each area of the face
Clindamycin (Cleocin T, Clindagel, ClindaMax)	1% foam 1% gel 1% lotion 1% pad 1% solution	Apply to affected areas 2×/d	Wash hands after application More than 1 pledget may be used; remove from foil just before use and discard after, single-use only
Clindamycin and tretinoin (Veltin, Ziana)	Clindamycin phosphate 1.2% and tretinoin 0.025%	Apply to affected area once daily at night	Apply a pea-sized amount. Avoid the eyes, lips, and mucous membranes.
Erythromycin (Akne-Mycin, Ery, Erycette)	2% solution 2% gel 2% pad 2% solution	Apply to affected acne areas 1–2×/d	Wash hands after application
Metronidazole (Metrogel, Metrocream, Metrolotion, Noritate)	0.75%, 0.1% gel 0.75% cream 0.75% lotion 1% lotion	0.75%: Apply to affected areas 2×/d 1%: Apply to affected areas 1×/d	Wash hands after application
Dapsone (Aczone)	5% gel	Apply to affected areas 2×/d	Wash hands after application. Reevaluate if no improvement in 12 wk.
Acne Medication			
Isotretinoin (Absorica, Amnesteem, Claravis, Myorisan, Sotret)	10, 20, 30, 40 mg capsule	Initially: 0.5–1 mg/kg/d in 2 divided doses; severe acne may require 2 mg/kg/d; treatment continues for 15–20 wk	Provider registered with iPledge must prescribe medication

the medication is supplied in a package in which the two medications are separate and are then mixed immediately prior to dispensing. This combination product forms a gel and should be stirred prior to application. Benzamycin should be stored in the refrigerator and expires 3 months after reconstitution. The product should not be allowed to freeze. Benzamycin Pak is also a combination of benzoyl peroxide and erythromycin packaged in single-use foil pouch that the patient opens and then mixes the two ingredients in the palm before applying to acne-affected areas. Benzamycin Pak does not require refrigeration. Products that combine benzoyl peroxide with clindamycin (Benzaclin, Duac) are also effective in acne treatment. Patients should apply these products to clean, dry skin twice daily for Benzamycin or Benzaclin and once daily before bed for Duac. If irritation occurs, patients may decrease application to once daily. It must be pointed out that all benzoyl peroxide–containing products bleach fabrics and hair, and care should be taken when handling such products.

Dapsone gel should be applied twice a day to skin that has been washed and patted dry. A pea-size amount of dapsone gel is spread into a thin layer over all acne-affected areas. Patients should wash their hands after application.

Acne Rosacea

The topical treatment of rosacea is based on the severity of clinical presentation. The most commonly used initial therapy for the treatment of mild forms of rosacea is topical metronidazole. Metronidazole 0.75% cream or gel (Metro-Gel and MetroCream) or 1% emollient cream (Noritate) is applied in a thin film twice a day after washing with a gentle cleanser. There may be some mild skin irritation associated with topical metronidazole use. Significant therapeutic results should be noticed within 3 weeks. Patients may use cosmetics after application of topical metronidazole. If irritation occurs, patients should reduce frequency, interrupt therapy, or discontinue use. They should avoid getting metronidazole in the eyes.

Rosacea may also be treated with combination products that combine an antibacterial with a keratolytic. Formulas that combine sulfacetamide 10% and sulfur 5% (Clenia, Rosula, Sulfacet-R) are applied 1 to 3 times a day to clean skin. Sulfacetamide and sulfur washes (Clenia, Rosula Cleanser) are used once or twice a day. Another product available is azelaic acid 15% gel (Finacea), which is an antibacterial/antikeratinizing agent. It is applied to clean, dry skin twice a day. Patients should avoid getting any of these products in their eyes and wash their hands after applying.

Rational Drug Selection

Severity

The choice of acne medications is generally dependent on several factors: clinical type of acne (e.g., comedonal, inflammatory, nodular), severity of acne, skin type (dry, oily), presence of acne scarring or post-inflammatory hyperpigmentation, menstrual history, signs of hyperandrogenism in women,

history of prior successful and failed treatments, history of acne-promoting medications, and psychological impact of acne on the patient.

Noninflammatory comedonal acne is treated with topical retinoids and/or benzoyl peroxide products. Antibiotics are not considered necessary for this type of acne. Azelaic acid is also effective for noninflammatory acne.

Antibiotics (oral or topical) may be used in the treatment of inflammatory papulopustular acne. Benzoyl peroxide is an effective antimicrobial and comedolytic agent for treating inflammatory and noninflammatory acne. Resistance to topical antibiotics easily develops when used as monotherapy. Addition of a topical retinoid or benzoyl peroxide will improve outcomes. Topical dapsone and topical metronidazole may be useful for mild inflammatory acne. Adding a topical retinoid or azelaic acid to improve follicular keratinization can also be helpful.

Papulopustular or nodulocystic acne with severe inflammation is treated with a combination of a topical antibiotic, benzoyl peroxide, and an oral antibiotic. Combining antibiotic therapy with the use of benzoyl peroxide decreases the development of antibiotic resistance and improves treatment efficacy.

When acne has not responded to the above treatments, therapy with oral isotretinoin should be considered. Therapy with isotretinoin is indicated for severe nodulocystic acne or moderate noncystic inflammatory acne with the potential for scarring.

Hormonal therapy is indicated in mild to moderate acne in women (Ortho-Tri-Cyclen, Estrostep Fe, Yaz or Yasmin).

Monitoring

There is no special laboratory monitoring required with the use of topical antibiotics or topical retinoids. Monitoring of the patient who is started on isotretinoin includes baseline CBC, both baseline and monthly liver function tests throughout treatment, baseline and monthly pregnancy testing for female patients throughout treatment, and serum lipid profile. If visual difficulties occur, an ophthalmological examination is recommended, with a second examination 6 to 7 weeks after discontinuation of the medication.

Patient Education

Administration

When retinoids are applied topically, it should be explained that the increased turnover of follicular epithelial cells causes extrusion of comedones, even comedones that may not be seen on the skin surface. Clinically, this causes an initial worsening of acne, as comedones that were previously under the skin are extruded. This "worsening" of acne is not a reason for discontinuation of treatment, and the patient should be reassured that the face will likely improve after approximately 4 to 16 weeks of treatment. The patient should also be instructed to use the medication as prescribed; there is no improved response to topical retinoids if they are used more often than recommended.

Adverse Reactions

It is important to instruct patients that all topical antibiotics used in the treatment of acne may cause skin irritation to some degree. Benzoyl peroxide may cause excessive drying, photosensitivity, and allergic contact sensitization. Azelaic acid may cause skin hypopigmentation in patients with dark complexions. Patients should be instructed to notify their provider if this problem develops.

Isotretinoin has many significant adverse reactions, as previously described. Patients should be fully informed about these adverse reactions prior to beginning therapy and should have written information to refer to at home if any adverse effects occur.

Lifestyle Management

The nonpharmacological management of acne includes gentle facial cleansers such as mild soaps or facial washes. Scrubbing, picking, and squeezing of comedones should be avoided. Patients should be advised to use skin products that will not aggravate their acne. That includes avoidance of oil-based cosmetics, hair spray, mousse, and facial creams and moisturizers. Oil-free sunscreen should be used at all times because of the increased photosensitivity due to acne preparations.

TOPICAL CORTICOSTEROIDS

Topical corticosteroids are adrenocorticosteroid derivatives incorporated into a vehicle suitable for application to the skin. Topical corticosteroids are utilized for their anti-inflammatory, antimitotic, immunosuppressive, and vasoconstrictive properties. They differ widely in potency and formulation; potency ranges from super potent (group 1) to least potent (group 7). Table 23-4 contains selected forms of corticosteroids.

Pharmacodynamics

The therapeutic effects of topical corticosteroids are due to their nonspecific anti-inflammatory effects. They act against most causes of inflammation, including mechanical, chemical, microbiological, and immunological. At the cellular level, they appear to inhibit the formation, release, and activity of endogenous mediators of inflammation, such as prostaglandins, kinins, histamines, liposomal enzymes, and the complement system. When applied to inflamed skin, steroids inhibit the migration of macrophages and leukocytes into the area by reversing vascular dilatation and permeability. This results in decreasing edema, erythema, and

Table 23–4 ❊ Available Dosage Forms: Topical Corticosteroids

Drug	Potency	Dosage Form	Rx Required
Clobetasol			
• Generic	Super high	0.05% cream, foam, gel, lotion, ointment, shampoo, solution	Yes
• Temovate	Super high	0.05% cream, gel, ointment, solution	Yes
• Clobex	Super high	0.05% lotion, shampoo, solution	Yes
• Embeline	Super high	0.05% solution	Yes
Desonide			
• Generic	Mild	0.05% cream and lotion	Yes
	Low mid	0.5% ointment	Yes
• Desown	Mild	0.05% cream	Yes
• Desowen	Mild	0.05% lotion	Yes
	Low mid	0.5% ointment	Yes
• Desonate	Low mid	0.05% gel	Yes
• LoKara	Mild	0.05% lotion	Yes
• Verdeso	Mild	0.05% foam	Yes
Desoximetasone			
• Generic	Mid	0.05% cream	Yes
	High	0.25% cream, ointment	Yes
	High	0.05% gel	Yes
• Topicort LP	Mid	0.05% cream	Yes
• Topicort	Mid	0.05% cream	Yes
	High	0.25% cream, ointment	Yes
	High	0.05% gel	Yes
Fluocinonide			
• Generic	High	0.05% gel, cream, ointment	Yes
• Lidex	High	0.05% cream	Yes
• Vanos	Super high	0.1% cream	Yes

Table 23–4 ✿ Available Dosage Forms: Topical Corticosteroids—cont'd

Drug	Potency	Dosage Form	Rx Required
Fluocinolone Acetonide			
• Generic	Mild	0.01% cream, solution	Yes
	Low mid	0.025% cream	Yes
	Mid	0.025% ointment	Yes
• Synlar	Low mid	0.025% cream	Yes
	Mild	0.01% cream, solution	Yes
	Mild	0.025% ointment	Yes
Flurandrenolide			
• Cordran tape	Super high	4 mcg/cm (24 in., 80 in.) tape	Yes
Halcinonide			
• Halog	High	0.1% cream, ointment	Yes
Halobetasol Proprionate			
• Generic	Super high	0.05% cream, ointment	Yes
• Ultravate	Super high	0.05% cream, ointment	Yes
Hydrocortisone			
• Generic	Least	1% and 2.5% cream, lotion, ointment	No: 1% Yes: 2.5%
• Aveeno hydrocortisone anti-itch	Least	1% cream	No
• Cortaid	Least	0.1% ointment	No
• Cortizone	Least	0.1% ointment	No
• Locoid	Least	0.1% cream	Yes
Mometasone Furoate			
• Generic	Mid	0.1% cream	Yes
	Mid	0.1% lotion	Yes
	Upper mid	0.1% ointment	Yes
	Mid	0.1% solution	Yes
• Elocon	Mid	0.1% cream	Yes
	Mid	0.1% lotion	Yes
	Upper mid	0.1% ointment	Yes
Triamcinolone Acetonide			
• Generic	Mild	0.025% lotion	Yes
	Low mid	0.1% lotion	Yes
	Mid	0.1% cream	Yes
	Upper mid	0.5% cream, ointment	Yes
	Mid	0.025% ointment	Yes
	Upper mid	0.1% ointment	Yes
• Triamcot	Mid	0.1% cream	Yes
• Trianex	Upper mid	0.05% ointment	Yes
• Triderm	Mid	0.1% cream	Yes

pruritus by suppressing DNA synthesis. Corticosteroids applied topically have an antimitotic effect on epidermal cells. This is their primary action in proliferative disorders such as psoriasis.

At the molecular level, unbound corticosteroids readily cross the cell membrane and bind with high affinity to specific cytoplasmic receptors. Inflammation is reduced by diminishing the release of leukocytic acid hydrolyses. Corticosteroids also prevent macrophage accumulation at inflamed sites. Interference with leukocyte adhesion to the capillary wall and reduction of capillary membrane permeability and subsequent edema also reduce inflammation.

Pharmacokinetics

Absorption and Distribution

Absorption of topical corticosteroids varies, depending on the drug used, the vehicle used, the amount of skin surface area the medication is applied to, and the condition of the skin. Absorption is enhanced by increased skin temperature, hydration, and application to denuded areas, intertriginous areas, or skin surfaces with a thin stratum corneum layer (face or scrotum). Occlusive dressings enhance skin penetration and therefore increase drug absorption. Infants and children have more body surface area compared to body weight, and therefore proportionally more medication is absorbed into their system.

The penetration of topical steroid through the skin varies with the vehicle the medication is in. Ointments are more occlusive and therefore more potent. Creams are less occlusive and usually less potent. Lotions are usually the least potent. Gels, aerosols, lotions, and solutions are useful in hair-bearing areas. Occlusive dressings such as plastic wrap increase skin penetration approximately 10- to 100-fold by increasing the moisture content of the stratum corneum. This may be beneficial in resistant cases but may also lead to increased adverse effects because increased absorption of the corticosteroid may produce systemic side effects.

The relative potency of a product depends on several factors, including the characteristics and concentration of the drug, the vehicle used, and the vasoconstrictor assay. The vasoconstrictor assay is developed by applying an agent to the skin under occlusion and assessing the area of skin blanching.

Metabolism and Excretion

Following topical administration, corticosteroids enter the bloodstream and are metabolized and excreted via the same pathways as systemic steroids. Corticosteroids are metabolized in the liver, although some topical preparations are partially metabolized in the skin. Inactive metabolites, as well as a small portion of unchanged drug, are excreted in the urine.

Pharmacotherapeutics

Precautions and Contraindications

Corticosteroids are contraindicated in any patient with a history of hypersensitivity to other corticosteroids or any ingredient in the preparation.

Corticosteroids are contraindicated as monotherapy in primary bacterial infections, treatment of rosacea, or acne vulgaris. Use of high-potency or very-high-potency agents on the face, groin, or axilla is contraindicated. Ophthalmic use should be reserved for specialty practice only, because prolonged ocular exposure may cause steroid-induced glaucoma and cataracts. When applied to the eyelids or the skin near the eyes, the drug may enter the eyes.

Corticosteroids are Pregnancy Category C. They are teratogenic in animals when administered systemically at relatively low dosages. There are no adequate and well-controlled studies of topical steroid use in pregnant women. Therefore, use during pregnancy is advised only if the potential benefits outweigh the potential hazards to the fetus. In pregnant patients, they should not be used extensively.

Systemic corticosteroids are excreted into breast milk in quantities not likely to have an adverse effect on the infant. Nevertheless, exercise caution when administering topical steroids to a nursing mother.

Children may be more susceptible to the effects of topical corticosteroids because of their larger body surface area compared to weight. Therefore, in infants and young children, the lowest effective strength of topical steroid should be used to prevent systemic corticosteroid effects. Use of high-potency or very-high-potency agents should be avoided. Hypothalamic-pituitary-adrenal (HPA) axis suppression, Cushing's syndrome, and intracranial hypertension have been reported in children receiving topical corticosteroids. Many of the topical corticosteroids have been relabeled recently and are not to be used in children due to HPA suppression. Chronic high-dose corticosteroid therapy in children may interfere with growth and development.

Adverse Drug Reactions

Topical corticosteroid preparations may all cause localized skin irritation (pruritus, dryness, burning, and dermatitis). Use of topical corticosteroids also increases the risk for secondary infection due to immunosuppression. Topical corticosteroids can also worsen and alter the appearance of tinea skin infections. Other localized effects include acneiform rash, allergic contact dermatitis, folliculitis, hypertrichosis, miliaria, and maceration of the skin. Skin atrophy, hypopigmentation, striae, and xerosis may occur. Tolerance may occur with prolonged use of topical corticosteroids; it is reversible and may be prevented by interrupted or cyclic schedules of application for chronic dermatological conditions.

Systemic absorption may produce reversible HPA axis suppression, Cushing's syndrome, hyperglycemia, and glycosuria. They are more likely to occur with occlusive dressings and with more potent steroid preparations. Patients with liver failure or children may be at higher risk for systemic steroid effects.

Following prolonged application of topical corticosteroid around the eyes, cataracts and glaucoma may develop.

Changing to a less potent topical corticosteroid preparation may minimize the risk of adverse reactions.

Drug Interactions

There are no significant drug interactions noted with topical corticosteroid use.

Clinical Use and Dosing

Inflammatory Skin Diseases

Topical corticosteroids are used for numerous inflammatory or pruritic dermatoses. Some of the conditions for which topical corticosteroids have been proved effective are contact dermatitis, atopic dermatitis, nummular eczema, psoriasis, lichen planus, lichen simplex chronicus, insect bite reactions, discoid lupus erythematosus, and seborrheic dermatitis. Topical corticosteroids have a repository effect; with continuous use, one or two applications per day may be as effective as three or more (Table 23-5). One dosing schedule that may

Table 23–5 ⊗ Dosage Schedule: Selected Topical Corticosteroids

Drug	Dosage	Comments
Least Potent (group 7)		
• Hydrocortisone 1% or 2.5%	Apply a thin layer 2–4×/d	May be used in children
Mild Potency (group 6)		
• Fluocinolone acetonide 0.01% cream	Apply a thin layer 2–4×/d	May be used in children
• Triamcinolone acetonide cream, lotion 0.025%	Apply a thin layer 2–4×/d	May be used in children
• Desonide lotion, foam, cream 0.025%	Apply a thin layer 2–3×/d	May be used in children
Lower Mid-Strength Potency (group 5)		
• Fluocinolone acetonide cream 0.025%	Apply a thin layer 3–4×/d	May be used in children
• Desonide gel, ointment 0.5%	Apply a thin layer 2–3×/d	May be used in children >3 months of age
Mid-Strength Potency (group 4)		
• Desoximetasone 0.05% cream	Apply a thin layer 2×/d	If no improvement after 4 wk, reassess diagnosis
• Fluocinolone acetonide 0.025% ointment	Apply a thin layer 2–4×/d	May be used in children >3 months of age
• Triamcinolone acetonide 0.1% cream, ointment	Apply a thin layer 2–3×/d	May be used in children
Upper Mid-Strength Potency (group 3)		
• Mometasone furoate 0.1% ointment	Apply a thin layer 1×/d	Do not use longer than 3 wk in pediatrics
• Triamcinolone acetonide 0.5% cream, ointment	Apply a thin layer 2–4×/d	May be used in children
High Potency (group 2)		
• Desoximetasone 0.05%, 0.25% cream, ointment, and gel	Apply a thin layer 2×/d	If no improvement after 4 wk, reassess diagnosis
• Fluocinonide acetonide 0.05% cream, gel, ointment, solution	Apply a thin layer 2–4×/d	May be used in children
• Halcinonide 0.1% cream, ointment	Apply a thin layer 1–3×/d	If no improvement, reassess diagnosis
Super High Potency (group 1)		
• Halobetasol propionate 0.05% cream, ointment	Apply a thin layer 1–2×/d	Treatment should not exceed 2 consecutive wk and total dosage should not exceed 50 g/wk. Do not apply on face, groin, or axillae.
• Flurandrenolide tape	Apply tape to clean, dry, affected skin; replace tape every 12 to 24 h.	Use should not exceed 2 wk
• Clobetasol 0.05% cream, foam, gel, lotion, ointment, shampoo, solution	Apply a thin layer 2×/d	Treatment should not exceed 2 consecutive wk and total dosage should not exceed 50 g/wk. Do not apply on face, groin, or axillae.

be used is to apply the medication twice daily until clinical response is achieved and then only as frequently as needed to control symptoms.

Another dosing schedule that may be used to achieve therapeutic response with fewer adverse effects is short-term or intermittent therapy with high-potency agents for a short period (3 or 4 consecutive days per week or once per week). This may be more effective and cause fewer adverse effects than continuous use of lower-potency products.

It must be stressed that topical corticosteroids should not be abruptly discontinued. After long-term use or after using a high-potency agent, a rebound effect may occur. Switching to a less potent agent, alternating topical corticosteroids and emollient products, or gradually reducing the frequency of

application (similar to tapering oral corticosteroids) can prevent a rebound effect.

In children, low- to mid-potency agents should be used. Low-potency topical corticosteroids should also be used on body sites with a thinner stratum corneum layer (face, scrotum, axilla, and skinfolds). If treating large surface areas, a lower-potency agent should be used. Higher-potency agents should be used for areas such as the palms and soles, which are more resistant to treatment. Higher-potency agents are also used for crusting and thickened conditions, which are also more resistant to treatment.

Treatment with very-high-potency topical corticosteroids should not exceed 2 consecutive weeks. The total dosage should not exceed 50 g/wk because of potential HPA axis suppression.

To increase absorption of corticosteroids, occlusive dressings may be used. The technique for properly using occlusive dressings is as follows: First, the area must be soaked in water and gently washed. While the skin is still moist, the medication is gently rubbed into the affected area. The area is then covered with plastic wrap. For hands, a plastic glove may be used; for feet, a plastic bag may be used; and a shower cap may be used for the scalp. After the plastic is applied, the edges should be sealed with tape to ensure that the wrap adheres closely to the skin. Do not use for more than 12 hours in a 24-hour period.

Psoriasis

Topical corticosteroids are used to treat psoriasis because of their anti-inflammatory effects on the plaques. Moderate- to high-potency steroids are used because the psoriasis lesions are generally steroid-resistant. Occlusion with plastic may be necessary for best results. The steroid cream or ointment is applied 2 to 3 times per day. Intermittent or "pulse" therapy minimizes some of the adverse effects and has the best long-term outcome. If using topical corticosteroids in the intertriginous areas or on the face, a low-potency medication should be chosen. Longer courses of therapy may be necessary for patients with chronic diseases, and these individuals should be closely monitored for the development of adverse effects.

Rational Drug Selection

Potency

The choice of steroid based on potency is determined by the area of skin to be treated, the condition of the area, and the patient's condition (see Table 23-5). In general, low- to mid-potency topical corticosteroids are used on children. On the face or other areas with thin skin, low-potency agents should be used. High-potency agents may be used for brief periods, up to 3 weeks, in areas that are resistant to lower-potency treatment. There are many available topical steroid preparations, and it is impossible for any practitioner to be familiar with all of them. It is reasonable for the practitioner to be familiar with one or two agents in each potency category. Each provider needs to be familiar with what medications are allowed from each category in the formulary he or she is using.

Vehicle

The vehicle used may increase or decrease the potency of the corticosteroid. As previously mentioned, ointments are more occlusive and are effective for dry or scaly lesions. Creams may be used more frequently on oozing lesions on intertriginous areas, where the occlusive effects of ointments may cause increased adverse effects. Gels, aerosols, lotions, and solutions are used on hair-bearing areas. The urea that is added to some products may enhance the penetration of hydrocortisone and other steroids by hydrating the skin. Steroid-impregnated tape (Cordran) is useful for occlusive therapy in small areas.

Cost

In general, lower-potency and generic products are less expensive than higher-potency and brand-name products, although this difference may be offset by increased efficacy in short-term burst therapy with some dermatoses. Therefore, cost must be evaluated, and the practitioner must determine whether it will be a part of the drug-selection process. Cost must also come into effect when prescribing off-formulary. If possible, prescribe medications that will be covered by the patient's insurance.

Monitoring

Adrenal function should be monitored in children if a high-potency steroid or occlusion is used. Adrenal function should also be assessed in adults who are applying more than 50 g weekly of a high-potency steroid preparation. Growth should be monitored in children who are using mid- or high-potency topical corticosteroids. The patient should also be monitored for adverse effects, as noted previously.

Patient Education

Administration

The patient should be instructed to use the topical corticosteroid exactly as prescribed. Demonstration of the amount of medication that should be applied will be helpful for most patients. The provider can use a sample-size dose in the area to be treated to show the amount of medication to use. The fingertip unit (FTU) provides the means to assess how much cream to dispense and apply. A fingertip unit is the amount of ointment expressed from a tube with a 5-mm-diameter nozzle, applied from the distal skin crease to the tip of the index finger. One FTU weighs approximately 0.5 g. An estimate of the number of FTUs required to cover various areas of the body is as follows: head and neck = 4.5, trunk (front or back) = 7, one arm = 3, one hand = 1, one leg = 6, and one foot = 2 (Goldstein & Goldstein, 2012). The patient should also understand the serious adverse effects that may occur with overuse of topical corticosteroids. If mid- or high-potency topical steroids are prescribed, the patient must understand that these medications are much stronger than, for example, hydrocortisone 1% cream and that these medications therefore have more significant adverse effects associated with them if they are not used appropriately. If occlusion is to be used, clear directions regarding it need to be provided to the patient, preferably in writing.

Adverse Reactions

The patient should have written information regarding the adverse effects that may occur with overuse of corticosteroids. Patients should report any adverse effects, including worsening of their condition. When prescribing topical corticosteroids to children, the provider must clearly outline the course of treatment for the parent. If mid-potency steroids are used, the parent should understand the concern about growth in children. Patients should also be instructed not to abruptly discontinue their topical steroid medications, which also may cause adverse effects.

Lifestyle Management

Patients who are using topical corticosteroids often can benefit from nonpharmacological management. Many conditions require the use of moisturizers or emollients to provide optimal outcome in the disease process. Patients should be encouraged to use these nonpharmacological measures, in addition to the prescribed topical corticosteroid, to have the most optimal management of their skin condition. Bathing may improve the outcome with some skin conditions, but this must be individualized based on the patient and the condition.

TOPICAL IMMUNOMODULATORS

The immunomodulators are a class of topical medications used in the short-term or intermittent long-term treatment of atopic dermatitis. Pimecrolimus (Elidel) and tacrolimus (Protopic) are additional nonsteroidal options for treatment of atopic dermatitis when it's not responsive to conventional therapy or when conventional therapy is not appropriate.

Pharmacodynamics

The therapeutic effects of the topical immunomodulators are related to their ability to inhibit calcineurin. The topical immunomodulators work through inhibition of phosphorylase activity of the calcium-dependent serine/threonine phosphatase calcineurin and the dephosphorylase activity of the nuclear factor of activated T-cell protein (NF-ATp). NF-ATp is a factor necessary for the cytokines IL-2, IL-4, and IL-5. They might also inhibit the transcription and release of other T-cell proteins, which can contribute to allergic inflammation. Tacrolimus has been found to inhibit T cells, Langerhans cells, mast cells, and keratinocytes, with skin biopsy after topical tacrolimus treatment finding markedly diminished T-cell and eosinophilic activity in the epidermal cells. Pimecrolimus was specifically developed to treat inflammatory skin conditions and is active by binding to FKBP/macrophilin 12 and interfering with calcineurin action. It inhibits the release of inflammatory cytokines and mediators from mast cells.

Pharmacokinetics

Absorption and Distribution

Topical tacrolimus and pimecrolimus are minimally absorbed. It is unknown if these medications cross the placenta or are excreted into breast milk.

Metabolism and Excretion

Both tacrolimus and pimecrolimus are metabolized in the liver via the CYP3A4 system and excreted in the feces.

Pharmacotherapeutics

Precautions and Contraindications

The only contraindication to either tacrolimus or pimecrolimus is hypersensitivity to the product or any component of the cream. The products should not be applied to a site with active cutaneous viral infection. Both products have received a U.S. Food and Drug Administration (FDA, 2006) Black-Box Warning regarding the long-term safety of topical immunosuppressant calcineurin inhibitors because of rare cases of malignancy (skin and lymphoma) that have been reported in patients using the topical forms of these medications. The FDA advisory stated, "Animal studies have shown that three different species of animals developed cancer following exposure to these drugs applied topically or given by mouth, including mice, rats and a recent study of monkeys" (FDA, 2006). Both tacrolimus and pimecrolimus should be avoided in children younger than 2 years and in immunosuppressed patients. Consider discontinuing the medication if lymphadenopathy of unknown etiology or infectious mononucleosis occurs. Use of these products should be avoided in malignant or premalignant skin conditions. Any bacterial or viral skin infections should be cleared before starting either product.

Both tacrolimus and pimecrolimus are Pregnancy Category C; neither product is recommended in the breastfeeding mother, as breast milk excretion is unknown. Both products are not to be used in children younger than 2 years. If prescribing tacrolimus to children 2 to 15 years, the 0.03% ointment is recommended.

Adverse Drug Reactions

Tacrolimus and pimecrolimus both may have a local reaction at the site of application, consisting of burning, pruritus, and tingling. Other side effects include headache, fever, flu-like symptoms, acne, and folliculitis.

Drug Interactions

There are no drug interactions reported with topical application of tacrolimus or pimecrolimus. There is a theoretical interaction between CYP3A4 inhibitors (such as erythromycin, irtraconazole, ketoconazole, fluconazole, calcium channel blockers, and cidemtidine) in widespread erythrodermic diseases due to increased absorption, and patients should be observed for toxicity.

Clinical Use and Dosing

Pimecrolimus is to be used as a second-line drug in the short-term or intermittent long-term treatment of mild to moderate atopic dermatitis in immunocompetent patients older than 2 years. Pimecrolimus (Elidel) is applied to affected areas twice daily. The area where the medication is applied should not be occluded. Tacrolimus (Protopic) is used for short-term or intermittent long-term treatment of moderate to severe atopic dermatitis in children older than 2 years and in adults. Children aged 2 to 15 years should use the 0.03% strength, and patients 16 years or older can use either the 0.03% or 0.1% strength. The tacrolimus ointment is applied twice a day and should not be occluded or applied to wet skin. The patient should be reevaluated 6 weeks after therapy is started.

Rational Drug Selection

Drug selection is based on the severity of atopic dermatitis, as tacrolimus is approved for moderate to severe disease and pimecrolimus is approved for mild to moderate disease.

Monitoring

Monitor patients' skin for worsening conditions, such as pruritus, erythema, excoriation, infection, and lichenification.

Patient Education

Administration

Patients should use the medication exactly as prescribed. When applying the medication, the patient should be instructed to avoid contact with eyes, nose, mouth, and cut or scraped skin. The patient should be instructed not to occlude the area that the medication is applied to. Hands should be washed with soap and water before and after application of the medication. It may take 2 to 3 weeks for improvement and patients need to be advised of this.

Adverse Reactions

Patients should contact their provider if any signs of infection occur. Patients should also report lymphadenopathy or other adverse effects they experience.

Lifestyle Management

Patients using either tacrolimus or pimecrolimus should avoid exposure to sunlight and artificial light sources such as tanning beds. Patients should use sunscreen and lip sunscreen (SPF [sun protection factor] 30 or higher) and wear protective clothing such as wide-brimmed hats. Patients can continue to use emollients for their atopic dermatitis.

TOPICAL ANTIPSORIASIS AGENTS

The management of psoriasis consists of topical medication and phototherapy for mild to moderate psoriasis (less than 20% of the body involved), and for severe psoriasis (more than 20% of the body involved) the addition of systemic medications. Patients with severe disease are usually referred to a dermatologist, and therefore systemic treatments with immunosuppressants (Amevive, methotrexate), retinoids (Soriatane), tumor necrosis factor blocker (Enbrel), and Adalimumab (Humira) are not covered in this chapter. Providers need to be mindful of the negative emotional impact of psoriasis and refer patients for more intensive therapy and/or mental health therapy if needed (Skevington, Bradshaw, Hepplewhite, Dawkes, & Lovell, 2006.)

Topical therapy recommended by the American Academy of Dermatology evidence-based guidelines (Menter et al, 2009) for psoriasis consists of nonmedicated topical moisturizers, coal tar, topical corticosteroids, vitamin D analogues, calcineurin inhibitors, and tazarotene. Management of psoriasis is discussed in Chapter 33.

Pharmacodynamics

Calcipotriene, a vitamin D_3 derivative, regulates cell differentiation and proliferation and suppresses lymphocyte activity. In humans, the natural supply of vitamin D depends mainly on exposure to the ultraviolet rays of the sun for conversion of 7-dehydrocholesterol to vitamin D_3 in the skin. After entering the bloodstream, it is metabolized in the liver and kidneys to its active vitamin D form. Vitamin D_3 receptors occur in many parts of the body, including the skin cells known as keratinocytes. Calcipotriene has a similar affinity for the vitamin D receptor in the keratinocyte.

Coal tar affects psoriasis by enzyme inhibition and antimitotic action. It is manufactured as a by-product of the processing of coke and gas from bituminous coal and is extremely complex, rich in polycyclic hydrocarbons, and variable in composition. Little is known about its mechanism of action.

Tazarotene is a topical retinoid prodrug that is used in the treatment of psoriasis. The exact mechanism of action is unclear at this time. Following topical application, tazarotene undergoes esterase hydrolysis in skin to form its active metabolite, tazarotenic acid. Tazarotenic acid is further metabolized in skin. It is believed that the drug works by normalizing epidermal differentiation, reducing hyperproliferation, and reducing the influx of inflammatory cells into the skin.

Pharmacokinetics

Absorption and Distribution

Approximately 6% of calcipotriene is absorbed systemically when it is applied topically to psoriasis plaques. Distribution of calcipotriene is unknown. There is evidence that calcipotriene does cross the placenta. It is not known whether calcipotriene is excreted in breast milk. Absorption and distribution of anthralin are unknown, as is the absorption of coal tar.

When administered topically to the skin, tazarotene has minimal systemic absorption because of its rapid metabolism in the skin to the active metabolite, tazarotenic acid, which is systemically absorbed and further metabolized. There is no apparent accumulation of tazarotene within body tissues. Retinoids may cross the placenta, and therefore it is assumed that tazarotene is also harmful to the fetus.

It is not known if tazarotene is distributed into human breast milk; however, animal studies show detection of tazarotene in maternal milk.

Metabolism and Excretion

Calcipotriene is rapidly and extensively metabolized in the liver into inactive metabolites and excreted in the bile.

Tazarotene is rapidly metabolized in the skin to the active metabolite tazarotenic acid, which is absorbed and further metabolized. Tazarotenic acid is hydrophilic and quickly metabolized systemically. It is more than 99% plasma protein bound. Metabolism of tazarotene to tazarotenic acid occurs via esterase hydrolysis in the skin. After systemic absorption, it is hepatically metabolized to sulfoxides, sulfones, and other metabolites. Elimination is via the fecal and renal routes.

The metabolism and excretion are unknown for coal tar.

Pharmacotherapeutics

Precautions and Contraindications

Calcipotriene should not be prescribed to any patients with preexisting hypercalcemia or evidence of vitamin D toxicity. It should also not be used in any patient with hypercalciuria, as this may increase renal calculi formation. Calcipotriene should not be applied to the face, as there have been several reports of facial dermatitis following application of this drug to the face. Calcipotriene is contraindicated in any patient with known hypersensitivity to any components of the preparation.

The safety and efficacy of calcipotriene in children have not been established. Children are at a greater risk of developing systemic adverse effects. Calcipotriene should be used cautiously in the elderly because patients older than 65 years have significantly more severe skin-related reactions than do younger patients treated with topical medication.

Calcipotriene is classified as Pregnancy Category C. It should be avoided during breastfeeding because adverse effects on the nursing infant may occur.

Coal tar preparations should not be applied to abraded skin. They should also be avoided on skin that is inflamed, broken, or infected because exacerbation of the condition can occur and systemic absorption of the drug can be increased. Sunlight (UV) exposure should be avoided for at least 24 hours after application of coal tar products unless patients are otherwise directed by their health-care provider. Exposure to sunlight causes a photosensitivity reaction. Coal tar does not have an FDA pregnancy classification. It is not known what effects coal tar may have on the fetus. Whether coal tar is distributed into breast milk is unknown, although it is advised that coal tar should be used by lactating women only when clearly needed.

Tazarotene should not be used on eczematous skin because it may cause severe irritation and worsen eczema. Tazarotene should be used cautiously in patients with known retinoid hypersensitivity reactions. Exposure to sunlight should be avoided, as well as UV exposure (including sun lamps). Patients must be warned of their increased photosensitivity and their increased potential for sunburn while using tazarotene. Tazarotene is classified as Pregnancy Category X and is contraindicated in women who are pregnant or may be considering pregnancy. Adequate pregnancy prevention is essential when childbearing-age women are prescribed tazarotene. It is not known if tazarotene is distributed into human breast milk; however, it should be used cautiously for breastfeeding women. The safety and efficacy of tazarotene in children younger than 12 years have not been established.

Adverse Drug Reactions

The most common reactions reported by patients using topical calcipotriene are application site pain, dermatitis, dry skin, erythema, peeling, pruritus, and worsening of psoriasis. Rare reports of allergic contact dermatitis have also occurred. Hypercalcemia and hypercalciuria occur almost exclusively when the recommended dosage of 100 g/wk is exceeded. A significant increase in urine calcium has been seen when calcipotriene is administered at the maximum weekly dose (100 g/wk) for 4 weeks.

Coal tar may stain hair or fabrics. Excessive or long-term use may cause folliculitis, sensitization, and photosensitivity.

The most commonly reported adverse reactions from tazarotene topical use are burning, stinging, xerosis, and erythema. Worsening of psoriasis may occur. Skin irritation and skin pain may also develop. Reactions reported in less than 10% of patients include rash, desquamation, irritant contact dermatitis, and skin inflammation. Photosensitivity may occur with tazarotene.

Drug Interactions

No drug interactions with calcipotriene have been reported (Table 23-6). However, concurrent administration of high-dose calcipotriene with other agents may produce hypercalcemia. Those agents include vitamin D or vitamin D analogues or calcium supplements. Avoid prescribing large doses of calcipotriene to patients taking vitamin D analogues or calcium supplements.

No drug interactions are known for coal tar.

Concomitant use of tazarotene and other topical medications that have strong drying effects, such as benzoyl peroxide, salicylic acid, or sulfur preparations, should be avoided. The manufacturer suggests that a patient's skin "rest" until the effects of such preparations subside before using tazarotene.

Clinical Use and Dosing

Psoriasis

Calcipotriene is applied in a thin film to the affected psoriasis plaques and rubbed into the skin gently and completely (Table 23-7). In adults, the ointment is applied twice daily in the morning and evening. The patient does not exceed 100 g/wk of calcipotriene applied to the skin because of increased adverse drug reactions (ADRs) of hypercalcemia or parathyroid hormone suppression (Menter et al, 2009).

Table 23–6 ⚏ **Drug Interactions: Selected Psoriasis Medications**

Drug	Interacting Drug	Possible Effect	Implications
Calcipotriene	Agent that may cause hypercalcemia: vitamin D, vitamin D analogues, calcium supplements	Concurrent administration of *high-dose* calcipotriene may produce hypercalcemia	Avoid using large doses of calcipotriene in patients taking vitamin D analogues or calcium supplements
Coal tar products	Psoralens	Increased photosensitivity	Avoid concurrent use
Tazarotene	Topical retinoids Skin irritants, like: benzoyl peroxide, salicylic acid, lactic acid, medicated or abrasive cleansers Products that contain alcohol, lime, menthol, spices, or perfumes	Increased skin irritation	Avoid concurrent use of topical medications that have strong drying effects Before beginning therapy, the effects of strong topical drying agents need to subside to prevent significant skin irritation

Table 23–7 ⊗ **Dosage Schedule: Topical Psoriasis Medications**

Drug	Available Dosage Forms	Dosage	Notes
Calcipotriene (Calcitrene, Dovonex, Sorilux)	0.005% ointment, cream, solution	Apply to affected area 2×/d	Improvement is usually noted after 1–2 wk
Coal tar products (DHS Tar Gel) (MG217) (Balnetar) (Neutrogena T/Gel)	2.9% shampoo 10% coal tar ointment 5% coal tar lotion 2.5% oil for use in bath 2%, 4% shampoo	Cream or ointment preparations: Apply enough to cover the affected area and rub in gently, 1–2×/d Shampoo: Apply to wet hair, massage in, and rinse; repeat application and leave on for 5 min. Rinse thoroughly after application. Cleansing bar or gel formulas: Apply to the affected area, rub in gently, leave on for 5 min, and then remove excess Coal tar solution: May be used full strength or diluted in 3 parts water and applied to a cotton or gauze pad, then massaged gently into the affected area Baths: The solution may also be used as a bath by adding 4 to 6 tbsp coal tar solution to a tub of lukewarm water. The patient should be immersed into the bath to soak for 10–20 min. Bathing should be performed once daily to once every 3 d; the usual duration of therapy is 30–45 d. The patient must rinse skin thoroughly after a coal tar bath if exposure to UV or sunlight is to follow.	All products are staining
Tazarotene (Tazorac)	0.05%, 0.1% gel	The 0.05% or 0.1% gel is applied in a thin film once daily, in the evening, to psoriatic lesions	Apply to clean, dry skin. No more than 20% of body surface area should be covered

Calcipotriene is inactivated by UVA; it is important to apply calcipotriene before or after UVA exposure. Safety and efficacy in children have not been established. For the treatment of mild to moderate scalp psoriasis, the patient applies the topical solution twice daily. Improvement will be noted as soon as 1 to 2 weeks after treatment has begun. The patient should be reevaluated after 6 to 8 weeks. Calcipotriene may be used in combination with topical steroids. A combination of calcipotriene and betamethasone propionate (Taclonex) ointment is available for use.

Coal tar has been used in the treatment of psoriasis for more than 100 years. However, it is generally not used in the United States because of poor efficacy, odor, and messiness. Coal tar is still commonly used outside the United States. With newer psoriasis products available, the AAD ranks coal tar as having Level II evidence for efficacy; more effective products such as topical corticosteroids or vitamin D derivatives are available (Menter et al, 2009). Regardless, a variety of tar preparations, including creams, shampoos, ointments, lotions, gels, and oils, are available. The tar preparation is applied to the affected psoriatic lesions once or twice daily. For cream or ointment preparations, the patient should apply enough to cover the affected area and rub in gently. Shampoo should be applied to wet hair, massaged in, and then rinsed. The application is then repeated and left on for 5 minutes. The shampoo should be rinsed out thoroughly after application. The cleansing bar or gel formulas should be applied to the affected area, rubbed in gently, and left on for 5 minutes; then the excess is removed. Coal tar solution may be used full strength or diluted in 3 parts water, applied to a cotton or gauze pad, and then massaged gently into the affected area. The solution may also be used as a bath by adding 4 to 6 tablespoons of coal tar solution to a tub of lukewarm water. The patient should soak immersed in the bath for 10 to 20 minutes. Bathing should be performed once daily to once every 3 days; the usual duration of therapy is 30 to 45 days. Patients must rinse their skin thoroughly after a coal tar bath if exposure to UV or sunlight is to follow.

The AAD ranks tazarotene as having Level I evidence for efficacy in treating psoriasis, with 50% or more improvement seen in the majority of patients (Menter et al, 2009). Tazarotene should be applied to clean, dry skin. The 0.05% or 0.1% gel is applied once daily in the evening to psoriatic lesions for 12 weeks. The patient should use enough to cover only the lesions with a thin film. No more than 20% of the body surface area should be covered. Because unaffected skin may be more susceptible to irritation, avoid application of tazarotene to these areas. The AAD notes tazarotene is best used in combination with topical corticosteroids (Menter et al).

Rational Drug Selection

Potency

With multiple medications available for treatment of psoriasis, the provider must decide which medication provides the most improvement to psoriatic lesions without severe adverse effects. Response to antipsoriasis medications is highly individualized; therefore, different medications may be needed for similar presentations of psoriasis.

Vehicle

The patient's clinical presentation often determines which antipsoriasis medication should be used first. The optimal topical formulation is the oiliest one that the patient will use. Large surface areas may respond to bath emulsions of coal tar solutions, where large surface areas can be treated. For scalp psoriasis, coal tar shampoo may be used.

Monitoring

The patient who is being treated for psoriasis should be monitored for the effectiveness of therapy and for adverse effects of the medication. There is no laboratory monitoring required unless treatment levels of calcipotriene approach 100 g/wk. At that point, serum and urine calcium should be measured to determine the patient's risk for hypercalcemia or hypercalciuria.

Patient Education

Administration

Patients should be instructed to use their psoriasis medications exactly as prescribed. Vitamin D derivatives need to be applied as directed, because more than 100 g/wk may cause hypercalcemia. Coal tar may cause staining or discoloration of the skin, especially if not used correctly. Use of tazarotene on healthy skin increases adverse reaction. The patient should be advised not to increase the number of doses per day; doing so increases adverse effects.

Adverse Reactions

Proper application of topical medications will not only optimize treatment but also decrease the adverse effects of the medication. The provider should review the use of medication prior to any change in therapy. Some psoriasis medications cause photosensitivity; therefore, the patient should be instructed to apply sunscreen or avoid sun exposure during therapy.

TOPICAL ANTISEBORRHEIC MEDICATIONS

Topical antifungals are the treatment mainstay for seborrheic dermatitis (Naldi & Rebora, 2009). In addition, antiseborrheic shampoos and topical steroid preparations may be used. Selenium sulfide, pyrithione zinc, coal tar, and salicylic acid are commonly used seborrhea shampoos (Table 23-8). Sulfacetamide sodium is another option available in many formulations.

Pharmacodynamics

Seborrhea is an inflammatory dermatitis that produces greasy-looking, yellowish scales distributed on areas rich in sebaceous glands such as the scalp, the external ear, the center of the face, the upper part of the trunk, and the intertriginous areas. The mildest and most common form of scalp seborrheic dermatitis is dandruff, which occurs as fine, white scaliness on the scalp without erythema. Selenium sulfide (Selsun) appears to have a cytostatic effect on the cells of the epidermis and follicular epithelium, leading to reduced corneocyte production. Pyrithione zinc (Head & Shoulders) is a cytostatic agent that reduces the cell turnover rate; it also exhibits antifungal and antibacterial properties. The mechanism of action of pyrithione zinc is thought to be a nonspecific toxic effect on the epidermal cells. Tar derivatives treat seborrhea by correcting abnormal keratinization and by decreasing epidermal proliferation and dermal infiltration. Tar derivatives also have antiseptic, astringent, antifungal, vasoconstrictive, and photosensitizing properties. The antifungals ketoconazole (Nizoral) and ciclopirox work against dandruff and seborrheic dermatitis by altering the fungal cell membrane, particularly of *P. ovale*, a pathogen implicated in seborrhea. Sulfacetamide sodium (Sebizon) is an antibacterial

Table 23–8 ⊗ Dosage Schedule: Topical Antiseborrheic Medications

Drug	Indication	Available Dosage Forms	Dosage	Notes
Ketoconazole shampoo (Nizoral, Nizoral AD)	Dandruff, seborrheic dermatitis	1%, 2% shampoo	Apply to wet hair, massage in, leaving on scalp for 5 min, then rinse. Use 2×/wk for up to 8 wk, with at least 3 d between use	May remove curl from permanently wavy hair; can cause discoloration and changes in hair texture
Pyrithione zinc (Head & Shoulders, DermaZinc, DHS Zinc, Selsun Blue)	Dandruff, seborrheic dermatitis	1%, 2% shampoo	Shampoo is applied to wet hair, lathered, rinsed. Repeat once or twice weekly to maintain control.	
Selenium sulfide (Selsun Blue, Head & Shoulders Clinical Strength)	Dandruff, seborrheic dermatitis	1%, 2.5% shampoo	Shampoo is massaged into wet hair, left on for 2–3 min, and rinsed well. Apply 2×/wk, then 1–4×/mo, to maintain control	
Sulfacetamide sodium (Ovace Plus)	Seborrheic dermatitis	10% shampoo	Wash affected areas with 10% wash 2×/d for 8–10 d, and then decrease usage to maintain control	
Tar-derivative shampoos (Neutrogena T/Gel) (MG217 Medicated Tar Extra Strength)	Dandruff, seborrheic dermatitis	2%, 4% shampoo 15% shampoo	Apply to wet hair, lather, leave on for 5 min, then rinse. Use 2×/wk, then decrease to 1×/wk to maintain control.	

agent that exerts a bacteriostatic effect against gram-positive and gram-negative microorganisms, the common organisms isolated from secondary cutaneous infections.

Pharmacokinetics

Absorption and Distribution

Absorption and distribution of topical pyrithione zinc and sulfacetamide sodium are unknown. Topical ketoconazole does not have significant systemic absorption. Repeated topical application of ketoconazole 2% shampoo, however, will lead to absorption of the drug into hair keratin. Systemic absorption of selenium sulfide may occur if applied to open skin areas.

Metabolism and Excretion

Metabolism and excretion of topical selenium sulfide, pyrithione zinc, ketoconazole, and sulfacetamide sodium are unknown.

Pharmacotherapeutics

Precautions and Contraindications

Selenium sulfide is contraindicated in patients with acute inflammation and exudate, as absorption can be increased. It is also contraindicated in patients who are sensitive to any ingredients. There are no contraindications to the use of pyrithione zinc. Tar preparations should not be used on open or infected lesions or on areas of acute inflammation. Ketoconazole, selenium sulfide, and pyrithione zinc are contraindicated in patients who are sensitive to any ingredients.

Ketoconazole also contains sulfites, and patients who are sensitive to sulfites should be advised not to use ketoconazole shampoo. Sulfacetamide sodium should not be prescribed if sensitivity to sulfonamides is present because cross-reactions to topical sulfa preparations may occur.

Selenium sulfide and sulfacetamide sodium are Pregnancy Category C. Tar preparation (Zetar) has no FDA pregnancy classification listed. Tar preparations should not be used in children younger than 2 years. Ketoconazole shampoo is Pregnancy Category C.

Adverse Drug Reactions

Skin irritation can occur with any of the topical antiseborrheic products. They may also cause greater-than-normal hair loss, hair discoloration, and scalp and hair oiliness or dryness.

Drug Interactions

There are no identified drug interactions with any of the topical antiseborrheic products.

Clinical Use and Dosing

Seborrhea and Dandruff

Selenium sulfide shampoo is available as an OTC product, which is 1% selenium sulfide (Selsun Blue, Head & Shoulders), or by prescription, which contains 2.5% selenium sulfide (Excel, Selsun). Selenium sulfide shampoo is massaged into wet hair and left on for 3 to 5 minutes before rinsing thoroughly. It should be applied twice a week until the dandruff is under control, usually within 2 weeks, and then weekly to maintain control.

Ketoconazole shampoo is applied to wet hair, left in place for 3 to 5 minutes, lathered and rinsed. It should be used every 3 to 4 days for up to 8 weeks.

Ciclopirox shampoo (Loprox) is applied to wet hair, lathered, left in place for about 3 to 5 minutes and then rinsed, and repeated twice weekly for 4 weeks, allowing a minimum of 3 days between use.

Pyrithione zinc is the active ingredient in OTC dandruff shampoos such as Head & Shoulders. Pyrithione zinc is applied to wet skin or hair, left in place for about 3 to 5 minutes and then rinsed. The treatment is used once or twice a week to maintain control of dandruff and/or seborrheic dermatitis.

Tar shampoos are available OTC and range in strength from 0.5% (DHS Tar) to 12.5% (Extra Strength Denorex) coal tar. The different products vary in their application instructions from daily to weekly, and the patient should be advised to follow the label instructions. The variety of antiseborrheic medications and their dosage forms are found in Table 23-8.

Cradle Cap

For cradle cap in infants that is resistant to nonpharmacological treatment, selenium sulfide and zinc pyrithione have been used; however, clinical trials have not established the efficacy and safety in infants.

Rational Drug Selection

There are few clinical data to suggest that one antiseborrheic product is better than another. Selenium sulfide 2.5% shampoo is commonly prescribed or 1% shampoo purchased OTC. Ketoconazole shampoo is available OTC (Nizoral A-D) and has comparable results to selenium sulfide 2.5% in the treatment of dandruff.

Monitoring

There is no laboratory monitoring necessary for any of the topical antiseborrheic agents.

Patient Education

Administration

The patient should be instructed to use the medication exactly as directed. Overuse increases adverse effects without clinical improvement in seborrhea. Seborrheic dermatitis cannot be cured, only controlled; therefore, continued use of the medication will be necessary to maintain control. All of the medications should be rinsed well with plain water after use.

Adverse Reactions

Patients should be advised to notify their provider if they have an adverse reaction to the medication prescribed.

TOPICAL ANTIHISTAMINES AND ANTIPRURITICS

The topical antihistamine commonly used is diphenhydramine (Benadryl) to relieve itching. Doxepin (Zonalon)

cream can be used for moderate to severe pruritus associated with atopic dermatitis.

Pharmacodynamics

Topical diphenhydramine provides local relief from pruritus and edema because its local effect on the H_1-receptors suppresses the formation of edema, flare, and pruritus. It may also provide local anesthetic activity by decreasing the permeability of the nerve cell membrane to sodium ions, thus blocking the transmission of nerve impulses.

Doxepin's topical mechanism of action is unclear but probably related to its H_1- and H_2-receptor blocking action. Histamine-blocking drugs appear to compete at histamine receptor sites and inhibit the activation of histamine receptors.

Pharmacokinetics

Absorption and Distribution

Diphenhydramine can be measurable in the serum following topical administration to large areas of the body or on chicken pox or measles, in young children and infants, or when applied to large surface areas or a denuded area.

Significant amounts of doxepin for topical use can be absorbed systemically if it is used over 10% of the body surface area or for long periods. Absorption is increased by occlusion. Serum levels may be similar to those achieved with oral administration. It is unknown whether doxepin crosses the placenta.

Metabolism and Excretion

Metabolism and excretion of topical diphenhydramine are unknown.

Absorbed doxepin is metabolized in the liver into an active metabolite, N-desmethyldoxepin. Parent drug and metabolite are excreted in gastric juice. N-desmethyldoxepin is reabsorbed and further metabolized. Primary excretion is renal. Doxepin and its metabolites are known to be excreted in breast milk.

Pharmacotherapeutics

Precautions and Contraindications

Topical diphenhydramine is contraindicated if the patient is sensitive to the medication in any form. It is for external use only, and contact with the eyes should be avoided. Prolonged use of topical diphenhydramine (more than 7 days) should be avoided. Topical diphenhydramine should not be used to treat chicken pox, measles, poison ivy, or sunburn, or used on blistered or oozing skin. Applying diphenhydramine to denuded skin or to large surface areas increases the potential for toxic psychosis, especially in children. It is recommended that topical diphenhydramine be used in children 2 years and older. Diphenhydramine is Pregnancy Category B.

Drowsiness occurs in more than 20% of patients using doxepin cream, especially on more than 10% of body surface area. Patients with untreated narrow-angle glaucoma and urinary retention should not use doxepin orally or in topical form because of its anticholinergic effect, even in the topical form. Doxepin cream is contraindicated for use in children and is classified as Pregnancy Category B. Doxepin use during lactation may result in neonatal sedation; use during breastfeeding is not recommended.

Adverse Drug Reactions

Topical diphenhydramine may cause skin irritation if used for prolonged periods.

Patients have reported burning and stinging upon application of topical doxepin; 25% of those patients classify the burning as "severe." Pruritus, dry skin, and eczema exacerbation are reported in fewer than 10% of patients.

Drug Interactions

There are no known drug interactions with topical diphenhydramine (Table 23-9). Topical diphenhydramine should not be used concurrently with oral or systemic diphenhydramine; doing so increases the likelihood of toxicity.

Doxepin cream interacts adversely with alcohol, cimetidine, and monoamine oxidase inhibitors (MAOIs), and these drugs should be avoided during therapy. Doxepin may also interact with any drug that is metabolized by the CYP450 2D6 enzymes.

Clinical Use and Dosing

Local Reactions to Insect Bites, Stings, and Minor Skin Disorders (Poison Ivy, Sumac, and Oak)

Topical diphenhydramine is applied to the affected area 3 to 4 times a day for up to 7 days (Table 23-10).

Severe Pruritus

Doxepin cream (Prudoxin) is applied in a thin layer 4 times a day in 3- to 4-hour intervals for up to 8 days of treatment. Treatment for longer than 8 days may result in higher systemic levels of doxepin. Other available topical antipruritics that are safer to use than doxepin are the emollients Aveeno cream (colloidal oatmeal-based) and Sarna anti-itch lotion.

Rational Drug Selection

Selection of a topical antihistamine is based on the severity of the pruritus, with doxepin reserved for severe cases.

Table 23–9 ▦ Drug Interactions: Topical Antihistamine and Antipruritic Medications

Drug	Interacting Drug	Possible Effect	Implications
Diphenhydramine	No known drug interactions		
Doxepin	Alcohol	Increased sedative effects of doxepin	Use together with caution. Advise patients to limit alcohol use when using topical doxepin.
	Cimetidine	May affect serum doxepin levels	Avoid concurrent use
	MAOIs	Serious side effects and death reported with the use of MAOIs and drugs related to doxepin	Separate use of two medications by at least 2 wk
	Medications metabolized by CP450 2D6 enzymes	Decreased metabolism of doxepin, leading to increased plasma levels	Monitor closely. May need to adjust dosage of doxepin or other drug. Use together with caution.

MAOIs = monoamine oxidase inhibitors.

Table 23–10 ⊗ Dosage Schedule: Topical Antihistamine and Antipruritic Medications

Drug	Indication	Available Dosage Form	Dosage	Comments
Diphenhydramine (Benadryl)	Local reactions to insect bites, stings, minor skin cuts, and burns and rashes (poison ivy, oak, sumac)	2% cream, spray	Apply to affected area 3–4×/d	Avoid use >7 d
Doxepin (Zonalon, Prudoxin)	Short-term (<8 d) management of moderate to severe pruritus	5% cream	Apply a thin film 4×/d with at least 3–4 h intervals between applications	Do not occlude. If excessive drowsiness occurs, do one of the following: 1. Decrease body surface area treated 2. Reduce the number of applications/d.

Monitoring

There is no laboratory monitoring necessary with the use of topical diphenhydramine or short-term use of topical doxepin.

Patient Education

Administration

The patient should be instructed to use the medication exactly as prescribed (see Table 23-10). Overuse or incorrect use may increase the adverse effects of these topical medications.

Adverse Reactions

Parents should be cautioned against extensive use of topical diphenhydramine in infants and young children, as well as avoiding concurrent use of topical and oral products. Patients who are prescribed doxepin should be told about the potential for drowsiness and be warned against driving or operating hazardous machinery until they are reasonably certain that doxepin does not affect their ability to operate safely.

Lifestyle Management

Patients should be encouraged to use nonpharmacological measures to control their pruritus, including avoidance of sensitizing agents. OTC emollient products may be used to treat their pruritus.

MOISTURIZERS, EMOLLIENTS, AND LUBRICANTS

Moisturizers, lubricants, and emollients help to retain water in the skin. They are composed of petrolatum, lanolin, or other agents such as colloidal oatmeal in an emulsion.

Pharmacodynamics

Emollients, moisturizers, and lubricants are applied after the patient bathes. This procedure acts to trap the moisture in the skin. Ointments provide the most occlusive barrier; creams are the next best. Lotions offer the convenience of easy application over large areas of skin but are not as occlusive as ointments and creams.

Pharmacokinetics

Topical emollients interact only with the outermost layers of the skin and are not absorbed systemically.

Pharmacotherapeutics

Precautions and Contraindications

There are no true contraindications to emollients, other than to avoid getting them in the eyes. Patients who are allergic to wool should avoid lanolin-containing products.

Adverse Drug Reactions

There are minimal to no adverse drug reactions reported with the use of emollients.

Drug Interactions

There are no known drug interactions with emollients.

Clinical Use and Dosing

Dry Skin

To treat dry skin, the emollient is applied 1 to 4 times per day and after the patient bathes. Patients pat their skin dry and then liberally apply lotion, cream, or ointment to all affected areas. This procedure acts to trap the moisture in the skin. Ointments provide the most occlusive barrier; creams are the next best. Lotions offer the convenience of easy application over large areas of skin but are not as occlusive as ointments and creams. Before using a lotion, make sure it does not contain alcohol, which is drying and irritating.

There are many emollient products available, but many are eliminated from patient use by their additives of perfumes or other chemicals, to which many eczema patients are sensitive. Commonly used emollients are Aveeno cream or lotion, Eucerin cream or lotion, Aquaphor ointment, Cetaphil cream or lotion, CeraVe cream or lotion, and Vanicream cream or lotion. White petrolatum (Vaseline) or vegetable shortening (Crisco) can be used in severe cases.

Rational Drug Selection

Cost

Expense can play a role in choosing an emollient because large amounts, over a long period, are needed to be effective. White petrolatum is inexpensive and a treatment option for eczema patients who have limited resources. Discussing the cost of emollients prior to recommending them to the patient will determine if the provider needs to assist the patient in finding resources to pay for emollients, which are usually not covered by health insurance plans. The use of generic equivalents will decrease the cost of emollients.

Monitoring

No laboratory monitoring is necessary with the use of emollients. Ongoing monitoring of clinical status is necessary to determine if the emollient is effective.

Patient Education

Administration

The patient should be instructed to apply liberal amounts of the emollient to the areas of dry skin. The emollient is most effective if applied just after bathing. Daily use offers the best results.

Lifestyle Management

Nonpharmacological measures used to treat dry skin include hydrating baths and avoidance of offending agents that cause exacerbations. Patients should be told to use gloves when their hands may be exposed to harsh chemicals or detergents, which may increase dryness. They should avoid wearing irritating fabrics such as wool. Soft cotton clothing allows the skin to breathe.

Baths hydrate the skin. The patient should take a warm—not hot—brief bath. The skin is patted dry, and emollients are applied immediately (within 3 minutes) to maintain the skin's hydration. The patient should use mild soap to cleanse the groin and axillae and avoid harsh deodorant soaps. After the bath is also a good time to apply corticosteroid creams or ointments, if needed.

AGENTS USED IN THE TREATMENT OF BURNS

In primary care, the most commonly prescribed preparation for a partial-thickness burn is silver sulfadiazine (Silvadene). Alternative treatment for a partial-thickness burn includes the topical antibiotic bacitracin. Although generally not used in primary care practice, biological and synthetic dressings can also be used to treat partial-thickness burns.

Pharmacodynamics

Silver sulfadiazine is a topical anti-infective active against both bacteria and yeast. It is bactericidal; it acts on the cell membrane and cell wall to produce a toxic effect on bacteria. It is active against both gram-positive and gram-negative organisms. The organisms that are generally susceptible to silver sulfadiazine include *S. aureus, S. epidermidis,* b-hemolytic streptococci, *C. albicans, Klebsiella* sp., *Escherichia coli, Enterobacter* sp., *Proteus, Pseudomonas, Clostridium perfringens, Morganella morganii, Serratia* sp., and *Providencia* sp. Reduction of bacterial growth after a partial-thickness burn promotes spontaneous healing by preventing conversion of partial-thickness burns to full thickness by sepsis.

Pharmacokinetics

Absorption and Distribution

Silver sulfadiazine is absorbed through intact skin. On burns, up to 10% of the sulfadiazine may be absorbed from silver sulfadiazine, with only 1% of the silver absorbed. Serum concentrations of 10 to 20 mcg/mL of sulfadiazine have been reported when large surface areas have been treated. Once absorbed, sulfadiazine is distributed into most body tissues. It is not known whether it crosses the placenta or is excreted in breast milk.

Metabolism and Excretion

The portion of sulfadiazine that is absorbed is metabolized in the liver and excreted renally.

Pharmacotherapeutics

Precautions and Contraindications

Silver sulfadiazine is contraindicated in patients sensitive to any of the contents of the preparation, including sulfa-sensitive patients.

Silver sulfadiazine is Pregnancy Category B but is considered Pregnancy Category D in the near-term pregnancy. Pregnant women at or near term should not use silver sulfadiazine. It is also contraindicated in premature infants and infants 2 months or younger because the sulfonamide displaces bilirubin and causes kernicterus. Use with caution in breastfeeding women.

Silver sulfadiazine should be used cautiously in patients with G6PD deficiency because sulfonamides may cause hemolytic anemia in these patients. Silver sulfadiazine should be used with caution in patients with hepatic or renal disease, as well as patients with thrombocytopenia, leukopenia, or other hematological disorders, as they may worsen these disorders. Sulfonamides should be used with caution in patients with porphyria, as they may precipitate porphyria.

Adverse Drug Reactions

Leukopenia (white blood cell [WBC] count less than 5,000) can occur in patients who use silver sulfadiazine, especially if large surface areas are treated. This occurs within 2 to 4 days of beginning therapy and resolves spontaneously upon discontinuation of the medication. Patients may also experience discoloration of skin, pruritus, erythema multiforme, photosensitivity, or rash at the site of application. Systemic sulfonamide reactions have also been reported.

Clinical Use and Dosing

Silver sulfadiazine is applied to burns once or twice daily, in a sterile fashion. It is applied to a thickness of 1/16 inch. Silver sulfadiazine should cover the burn at all times; reapply if the medication is removed. Dressings are not necessary but are helpful to prevent the medication from getting on the patient's clothing. Silver sulfadiazine should be stopped when there is evidence of reepithelialization.

Monitoring

If the area that the silver sulfadiazine is applied to is large or if treatment is prolonged, the patient's CBC, platelet count, liver function, and renal function need to be monitored. The burn should also be monitored for signs of superinfection or delayed separation.

Patient Education

Administration

Patients can treat small partial-thickness burns themselves and apply the silver sulfadiazine at home, although the first one or two applications are best done by a trained health-care provider to teach the patient the proper technique for applying the medication in a sterile fashion.

Adverse Reactions

Patients should be informed of the possible adverse drug reactions that may occur with the use of silver sulfadiazine and report any adverse symptoms to their provider.

SCABICIDES AND PEDICULICIDES

Skin and hair infestation is a frequently seen problem in primary care, with arthropods, scabies, and lice the most common. The pharmacological management of scabies and lice consists of ectoparasiticides (Table 23-11). The specific medication used varies according to the type of infestation and the age of the patient. There is a choice of OTC products (Nix and RID) for the treatment of head lice. Prescription-strength permethrin (Elimite) and lindane are the commonly prescribed ectoparasiticides. Benzoyl alcohol (Ulesfia) was approved for use in 2009 and was the first FDA-approved non-neurotoxin for head lice. Topical ivermectin (Sklice) was approved in 2012 to treat head lice. Malathion (Ovide) is a pediculicide that is available OTC in the United Kingdom and has been reapproved as a treatment for infestations in the United States. Oral use of ivermectin will not be discussed in this chapter.

Nonpharmacological, environmental measures are a key part of the treatment of any infestation because patients can reinfect themselves or other family members and restart the infestation cycle.

Pharmacodynamics

Pyrethrins are derived from chrysanthemums and are found in combination with piperonyl butoxide in OTC pediculicide products (RID, Pronto, A-200). Pyrethrins are absorbed through the chitinous exoskeleton of arthropods. Once absorbed, pyrethrins block sodium channel repolarization of

Table 23–11 ⚗ Dosage Schedule: Ectoparasiticides

Drug	Indication	Available Dosage Forms	Dosage	Comments
Permethrin (Nix)	Head lice	1% cream rinse	Apply permethrin 1% cream rinse after shampooing. Leave in hair for 10 min, then rinse off. Remove nits with comb. Repeat treatment in 1 wk.	Treatment should be repeated in 1 wk, regardless of whether signs of infestation are present
(Elimite)	Scabies	5% cream	Apply 5% cream to entire body and leave on for 8–14 h, then shower off. Repeat application in 2 wk if living mites are present.	All family members must be treated. Dispense 30 g per adult. Usually only requires 1 treatment.
Pyrethrins (RID, Pronto, A-200)	Head, body, and pubic lice	0.33% shampoo	Pyrethrin shampoo is applied to dry hair/skin and left on for 10–20 min. Repeat in 1 wk.	It is important for the product to be applied to dry hair to enable the pediculicide to better enter the insect's body. Do not use spray on humans or animals.
Lindane	Head, body, and pubic lice	1% shampoo	Lindane is applied to dry hair, working small quantities of water in to create a good lather. Leave shampoo in hair for 4 min, then rinse with water. Remove nits with comb.	The amount of shampoo prescribed for short hair is 30 mL; for long hair, prescribe 60 mL. Sexual partners should be treated concurrently. Bedding and clothing should be washed.
	Scabies	1% lotion	Apply cream or lotion from the neck to toes, and leave on for 8 h. Then shower off.	All family members should be treated. Dispense 2 oz per adult.
Malathion (Ovide)	Head lice	0.5% lotion	Apply to dry hair, then wet hair and scalp. Let dry naturally. Shampoo after 8–12 h. Repeat second application in 7–9 d, if needed.	Flammable; do not use hair dryer
Benzyl alcohol (Ulesfia)	Head lice	5% lotion	Apply lotion to dry hair, saturating scalp; leave on 10 min, rinse with water, and then repeat in 7 d.	Hair length 0–2 in.: 4–6 oz 2–4 in.: 6–8 oz 4–8 in.: 8–12 oz 8–16 in.: 12–24 oz 16–22 in.: 24–32 oz >22 in.: 32–48 oz
Ivermectin (Sklice)	Head lice	0.5% lotion	Apply to dry scalp, working from the scalp outward, leave on 10 min, rinse well, and use a nit comb.	Single use only Children >6 months

the arthropod neuron, leading to paralysis and death. Pyrethrins are pediculicidal, not ovicidal, and have no residual activity after rinsing. Application should be repeated 7 days later to ensure resolution.

Permethrin is a synthetic compound that is related to pyrethrins. It acts on the nerve cell membrane to disrupt the sodium channel current. This disrupts the sodium channel polarization, leading to paralysis. Permethrin cream rinse has residual activity against lice for up to 10 days.

Lindane is absorbed through the exoskeleton of parasites, causing CNS excitation, which leads to convulsions and death. It has low ovicidal activity (30% to 50% of the eggs are not killed) and resistance has been documented worldwide.

Malathion is an organophosphate agent that acts as a pediculicide by inhibiting cholinesterase activity in vivo. It is very effective against head lice and is both ovicidal and pediculicidal, with 96% mortality in 30 minutes (Downs, Narayan, Stafford, & Coles, 2005). Some residual activity remains and can kill newly hatched lice for up to 7 days.

The active ingredient in benzoyl alcohol appears to stun the breathing spiracles of the lice open, enabling the vehicle to penetrate the respiratory mechanism (spiracles), leading to asphyxiation. Benzoyl alcohol does not elicit ovicidal activity.

Ivermectin interferes with the function of invertebrate nerve and muscle cells by binding to glutamate-gated chloride channels located in invertebrate nerve and muscle cells; this results in parasite paralysis and death.

Pharmacokinetics

The pharmacokinetics of pyrethrins is unknown.

Permethrin is absorbed in unknown amounts, although it is thought to be less than 2% of the dose. It is then rapidly metabolized by ester hydrolysis into inactive metabolites, which are excreted in the urine. It is unknown whether permethrin crosses the placenta or is excreted in breast milk.

Lindane is slowly and incompletely absorbed through intact skin. Absorption is increased though damaged or occluded skin. Measurable amounts of lindane are absorbed. It is stored in the body fat, metabolized by the liver, and excreted in the urine and feces. It is unknown whether lindane crosses the placenta. Lindane is excreted in breast milk.

Malathion is rapidly and effectively absorbed by practically all routes, including the gastrointestinal tract, skin, mucous membranes, and lungs. It is excreted in the urine and does not accumulate in organs or tissues. Malathion (Ovide) is Pregnancy Category B and it is unknown whether it is excreted in breast milk. The safety and effectiveness of malathion lotion have not been assessed by the FDA in children younger than 6 years of age.

Benzoyl alcohol is minimally absorbed. The metabolism and excretion of locally applied benzoyl alcohol is unknown.

The pharmacokinetics of topical ivermectin is unknown.

Pharmacotherapeutics
Precautions and Contraindications

Hypersensitivity to any component of the products is a contraindication to their use. Pyrethrins are contraindicated in people who are allergic to chrysanthemums or ragweed.

Although all of the head lice and scabies treatments are relatively safe, they are classified as neurotoxic agents and they should be used exactly as directed. To limit exposure, the medication should be washed off at a sink, rather than in a shower. Cool or lukewarm water should be used to minimize absorption caused by vasodilatation (Centers for Disease Control and Prevention [CDC], 2010c, 2011).

Permethrin should not be used near the eyes. If it gets in the eyes, they should be flushed with water immediately. Permethrin should not be used on infants younger than 2 months.

The American Academy of Pediatrics (AAP, 2012) no longer recommends the use of lindane. Lindane is a neurotoxin and has been banned in some countries and also in the state of California. It should not be used to treat premature infants, persons with HIV or a seizure disorder, women who are pregnant or breastfeeding, infants, children, the elderly, or persons who weigh less than 110 pounds. Lindane should not be used on abraded or inflamed skin, which increases the absorption of the medication. The FDA (2009) has labeled lindane with a Black-Box Warning due to association with severe neurologic toxicities.

Malathion (Ovide) is contraindicated in neonates and infants due to their scalp being more permeable and therefore leading to possibly increased absorption of the lotion. Safety has not been established in children younger than 6 years. Ovide is flammable due to its high alcohol content and care should be taken not to expose the lotion or wet hair to open flames (including cigarettes) or electric heat sources such as hair dryers or curling irons.

The safety and efficacy of benzoyl alcohol (Ulesfia Lotion) in pediatric patients below the age of 6 months has not been established. Ulesfia Lotion is Pregnancy Category B.

There are no contraindications listed in the manufacturer's labeling for topical ivermectin. It has been approved for use in children older than 6 months; it is Pregnancy Category C and has been found to be excreted in breast milk.

Adverse Drug Reactions

All of the topical ectoparasiticides can cause skin irritation, some burning, or pruritus. Contact dermatitis can occur, usually as the result of incorrect use.

CNS toxicity can occur with lindane, but this is most commonly associated with ingestion or misuse of the product.

Organophosphate poisoning and severe respiratory distress may occur with ingestion of malathion. The product should be used by adults only and care taken to avoid prolonged exposure or over large surface areas.

The common adverse effects of benzoyl alcohol (Ulesfia) during clinical trials were pruritus, erythema, and pyoderma.

The most common adverse effects of topical ivermectin (Sklice) during clinical trials were eye irritation, dandruff, dry skin, and a burning sensation of the skin.

Clinical Use and Dosing

Head Lice

Treat only those family members who are actively infested (lice or nits seen on the head). Do not treat head lice prophylactically. The CDC, Division of Parasitic Diseases, recommends that a cream rinse, combination shampoo/conditioner, or conditioner should not be used before using lice medicine. Hair should not be washed for 1 to 2 days after lice treatment (CDC, 2011). The dosing for ectoparasiticides is found in Table 23-11.

Pyrethrin shampoo is applied to dry hair and left on for 10 to 20 minutes, with the time varying by brand. It is important for the product to be applied to dry hair to enable the pediculicide to enter the insect's body more efficiently. The patient should be re-treated in 1 week, regardless of whether there is evidence of infestation.

Permethrin is a cream rinse that is applied after shampooing. It is important that the shampoo not have any conditioners in its formula, which makes the permethrin less effective. The cream rinse is left in the hair for 10 minutes and then rinsed out. Treatment should be repeated in 1 week, regardless of whether signs of infestation are present. Permethrin is not approved by the FDA for use on children younger than 2 years of age (CDC, 2011).

Lindane is applied to dry hair and left on for 4 minutes. At the end of 4 minutes, a small amount of warm water is used to lather the shampoo, then the hair is rinsed well with water. The amount of shampoo prescribed for short hair is 1 oz; for long hair, 2 oz.

Malathion (Ovide) is applied to dry hair in an amount sufficient to wet the hair and scalp. Hair should be allowed to dry naturally. Malathion lotion is flammable. The lotion and wet hair should not be exposed to open flames or electric heat sources, including hair dryers or curlers. Do not smoke while applying lotion or while hair is wet. Hands should be washed with soap after applying Ovide. Ovide is left on for 8 to 12 hours and then shampooed out. If lice are present in 7 days, Ovide may be repeated.

Benzoyl alcohol (Ulesfia Lotion) is applied to dry hair, completely saturating the hair and scalp, and left on for 10 minutes. The lotion is then rinsed off well with water. Treatment with another application of Ulesfia should be repeated in 7 days if live lice are seen.

Topical ivermectin lotion (Sklice) is applied to dry hair to coat the hair and scalp, and left on for 10 minutes. The lotion is rinsed off with water. Topical ivermectin does not have to be reapplied; one treatment is usually effective.

After use of any head lice product, a nit or fine-tooth comb should be used to remove any dead lice or eggs.

Nonpharmacological treatments for head lice are popular. With the growing problem of resistance and concern over exposing children to repeated doses of pediculicides, parents are looking for various nonmedicated therapies. Popular and safe remedies are mayonnaise (full-fat variety), olive oil, and petroleum jelly. These remedies likely asphyxiate the lice by blocking their breathing apparatus or immobilize them and affect their ability to feed. A small study of six home remedies found petroleum jelly had the highest egg mortality; only 6% of the eggs hatched (Takano-Lee, Edman, Mullens, & Clark, 2004). The authors suggested that none of the remedies they studied were as effective as pediculicides, which are insecticidal and ovicidal. If a family would like to try these treatments, they should apply a thick layer of the product and cover with a shower cap. The product is left on from 1 hour to overnight and then shampooed out. Removal of nits and lice is critical to the success of treatment.

Body Lice

Because body lice live on clothing and underwear and come to the skin only to feed, instruct patients to wash all clothing and bedding in hot water to kill lice and nits that are on it, as well as treat their bodies with a pediculicide (CDC, 2010a). A low potency corticosteroid can be prescribed for the pruritus associated with body lice.

Permethrin 5% (Elimite) is massaged into skin from the head to the soles of the feet, left on for 8 hours (overnight), and then showered off. Dispense 30 grams for an average adult.

Lindane has more ADRs than permethrin, so it is second-line therapy. It is applied to the total body as a cream or lotion and left on 8 to 12 hours (overnight). The amount needed for an adult is 2 oz.

Pubic Lice

Pubic lice are treated with the same medications used to treat pediculosis capitis (head lice), which are permethrin 1% or pyrethrin. Thoroughly saturate hair with lice medication and leave medication on for 10 minutes. Lindane is a second-line treatment that is not recommended for first-line therapy because of neurotoxicity (CDC, 2010b). If using lindane, leave on for only 4 minutes and then thoroughly rinse off the medication with water. Dry off with a clean towel. Reapply in 7 days if there is evidence of live lice. Sexual partners should be treated concurrently, and bedding and clothing should also be washed. Infestation of eyelashes by pubic lice is treated with petrolatum (Vaseline) ointment applied 3 to 4 times daily for 8 to 10 days. Nits should be removed by hand from the pubic area, axilla, and eyelashes.

Scabies

All family members should receive treatment for scabies, even those who are asymptomatic, because they may be in the incubation period and so need treatment to prevent recurrence. The CDC recommends that sexual and any close personal contacts that have had direct, prolonged, skin-to-skin contact with an infested person also be examined and treated (CDC, 2010c).

Permethrin 5% cream (Elimite, Acticin) is the drug of choice for the treatment of scabies in young children and pregnant women. The cream is massaged into the skin from the neck to the soles of the feet. It should be left on for 8 to 14 hours and then washed off in the shower. One ounce or a 30-gram tube of permethrin per family member is prescribed.

Lindane 1% lotion or cream is used for scabies in children older than 6 months and in nonpregnant adult patients. It is applied in a thin layer from the neck down to the soles of the feet, left on for 8 to 12 hours (overnight), and then washed off thoroughly. If there are crusted lesions present, a tepid bath should be taken prior to application to soften the lesions. Patients should dry the skin thoroughly before applying lindane. One ounce or a 30-gram tube of lindane per family member is recommended.

Topical corticosteroids are used after scabies treatment to treat the pruritus and inflammation associated with the scabies mite. Hydrocortisone 1% or 2.5% or a stronger corticosteroid, if indicated, is applied to affected areas twice a day until the lesions are healed.

Rational Drug Selection

Cost

The relative costs of the different OTC ectoparasiticides for head lice are similar, so cost is not usually a consideration in the treatment.

Adverse Effects

The provider may choose the drug based on the patient's age and the toxicity of the agent. Lindane and malathion should be avoided in pregnant patients. Lindane is contraindicated in children younger than 2 years, and malathion in children younger than 6 years.

Monitoring

No specific laboratory monitoring is necessary with the use of ectoparasiticides.

Patient Education

Administration

Patients should be instructed to use the prescribed medication exactly as directed. Treatment failure due to incorrect use of the medication is common. Give written instructions about how to apply the medication and the length of time that the medication should be left on the skin or hair.

Careful instruction should be given regarding the flammability of malathion (Ovide). Lotion and wet hair should not be exposed to open flames or electric heat sources, including hair dryers and electric curlers. Do not smoke while applying lotion or while hair is wet. Allow hair to dry naturally and to remain uncovered after application of Ovide Lotion.

Adverse Reactions

When used as directed, there are minimal adverse effects from the use of ectoparasiticides. Skin irritation or toxicity may occur, but the incidence increases if patients use the medication incorrectly.

Lifestyle Management

Environmental measures should be discussed and written instructions given to patients or family members to take home to refer to as they delouse the home.

CAUTERIZING AND DESTRUCTIVE AGENTS

The cauterizing agent used in primary care is silver nitrate. Podophyllum resin (Podophyllin) and podofilox (Condylox) are used for genital warts.

Pharmacodynamics

Silver nitrate is a strong caustic agent and escharotic. The silver acts as antiseptic, astringent, and germicide. The silver attaches to the protein ion and decreases the protein's solubility. The local effects of silver are self-limiting, and the spread of damage occurs only when the dose of silver overwhelms the capacity of the tissues to fix the ion at the site of application.

Podophyllum resin contains podophyllotoxin, which binds to the microtubules in the cell, causing mitotic arrest in metaphase. Podophyllum is considered cytotoxic to the wart cells.

Pharmacotherapeutics

Precautions and Contraindications

Cauterizing agents should be used with great care because they damage any skin they touch; inappropriate use may cause chemical burns

Silver nitrate used for prolonged periods discolors the skin. It also stains any clothing or linens it contacts. Only a health-care provider should apply podophyllum resin, a powerful caustic and severe irritant that must be handled carefully. Podophyllum resin should not be used in pregnancy because it has led to birth defects, fetal death, and stillbirth. It is also contraindicated in breastfeeding women. Podophyllum resin is contraindicated in diabetic patients and other patients with poor circulation. It is also contraindicated in the treatment of malignant or premalignant lesions, bleeding warts, and warts with hair growing from them. The use of podophyllum should be avoided if the wart or surrounding tissue is inflamed or irritated.

Adverse Drug Reactions

Cauterizing agents are powerful keratolytics and cauterants. Use with caution to avoid contact with healthy skin.

Irritation and ulcerative local reactions are the major side effects of podophyllum. It may also cause paresthesias. Serious neuropathy and death have occurred from the use of podophyllum in large amounts on multiple lesions.

Use and Dosing

Umbilical Granuloma

Use a silver nitrate stick and touch to the granulomatous area. One treatment is usually curative.

Aphthous Ulcer, Vesicular, or Bullous Lesion

Touch the lesion with a silver nitrate stick. One treatment is usually all that is necessary to provide styptic action.

Poorly Healing Wounds or Ulcers

Apply a cotton pad dipped in silver nitrate solution to the affected area. A silver nitrate stick may also be used.

Verruca (Warts)

Podophyllum resin is only applied by a health-care provider to genital warts; it is not to be dispensed to the patient. After the area is cleansed, podophyllum resin is applied sparingly to the lesion. Avoid contact with healthy skin. The first treatment should be left in place for 30 to 40 minutes and then washed off thoroughly with soap and water. Later treatments may require 1 to 4 hours of contact to produce the desired result. Do not treat numerous lesions or large areas in one treatment, which increases the incidence of neuropathy occurring from podophyllum use. Multiple treatments may be necessary.

Podofilox (Condylox) is used for the treatment of genital warts. The patient applies the medication twice daily to the wart for 3 days and then discontinues treatment for 4 days. Treatment may be repeated up to 4 times. It should not be used for warts on the mucous membranes.

KERATOLYTICS

Keratolytic agents are used to treat a variety of hyperkeratotic and scaling cutaneous lesions, such as corns, calluses, and warts. Salicylic acid is the only OTC product considered safe and effective by the FDA. Lactic acid is used to treat xerosis and ichthyosis vulgaris.

Pharmacodynamics

Salicylic acid produces desquamation of the horny layer of the skin without affecting the viable epidermis. It acts by dissolving the intercellular cement substance in the stratum corneum.

Lactic acid, alpha-hydroxy acid, which may act as a humectant when applied to the skin, is thought to diminish corneocyte cohesion by interfering with the formation of ionic bonds.

Pharmacotherapeutics

Precautions and Contraindications

Salicylic acid products are contraindicated if the patient is sensitive to salicylic acid. Prolonged use in infants and patients with decreased renal or hepatic function is contraindicated, because it may lead to salicylism. Topical salicylic acid use is contraindicated in patients with diabetes or impaired circulation.

Lactic acid should be used carefully on the face or in patients with fair skin because it may cause irritation. Minimize the exposure to UV light or sun when using lactic acid topically. Lac-Hydrin (12% lactic acid) lotion is Pregnancy Category C. It is not known how this medication affects normal levels of lactic acid in human milk.

Adverse Drug Reactions

Local irritation can occur from salicylic acid contact with normal skin surrounding the wart or callus.

Transient stinging or burning has been reported with the use of topical Lac-Hydrin (12% lactic acid). Erythema, peeling, dryness, hyperpigmentation, or eczema flare may also occur.

Clinical Use and Dosing

Warts, Corns, and Calluses

There are many salicylic acid products available. Products that are 5% to 17% in collodion are used for safe, effective removal of common and plantar warts. Transdermal patches are available in 40% and 15% strengths for use on warts, corns, and calluses. Patients should refer to the individual product's label for instructions for use. To ensure successful treatment, patients should soak the affected area in warm water for at least 5 minutes before applying salicylic acid. Loose tissue or dried wart tissue is removed with a washcloth or emery board.

Xerosis, Dry Skin, and Ichthyosis

Lac-Hydrin (12% lactic acid) is applied to the affected area twice a day. The lotion or cream should be rubbed in when applied. Lac-Hydrin cream is not recommended in children younger than 2 years.

Patient Education

Administration

When instructing patients to use OTC salicylic acid, the provider should tell them to soak the affected area in warm water for at least 5 minutes or to bathe just before applying the medication. This will soften the area and allow better penetration of the medication. Patients should be advised that total healing might take several weeks to months.

TOPICAL ANESTHETICS

This section discusses the use of EMLA (lidocaine-prilocaine), Synera (lidocaine-tetracaine), and LMX-4 (4% lidocaine cream) for local anesthesia. These products are unique in that they bridge the gap between topical and infiltration anesthesia. It is useful in preparing for painful procedures such as bone marrow biopsies, IV starts, and blood draws. A lidocaine 5% patch (Lidoderm) is available for the treatment of postherpetic neuralgia.

Pharmacodynamics

EMLA is a unique mixture of lidocaine 2.5% and prilocaine 2.5%. The combination has a lower melting point than does either agent alone. EMLA cream produces anesthesia to a depth of 5 mm. Local anesthetics inhibit conduction of nerve impulses from sensory nerves because of an alteration in the cell membrane permeability to ions. The onset, depth, and duration of analgesia on intact skin depend primarily on the duration of application and to the area to which it is applied. Absorption from the mucosa is more rapid and onset time is shorter. When applied to intact skin and covered with an occlusive dressing, local anesthesia is achieved in 1 hour.

Synera is a transdermal patch containing lidocaine 70 mg and tetracaine 70 mg used for local dermal analgesia for superficial venous access or superficial dermatological procedures. The patch is applied to skin 30 minutes before the procedure.

LMX-4 (previously ELA-Max) is a 4% lidocaine cream in a liposomal delivery system and is available OTC. Little information is available regarding this product although it is marketed for the treatment of minor cuts, abrasions, sunburns, and insect bites. It has been used for cosmetic procedures such as chemical peels, IV catheter placement, venipuncture, circumcision, and lumbar puncture.

Lidocaine patch 5% (Lidoderm) is composed of an adhesive material containing 5% lidocaine, which is applied to a nonwoven polyester felt backing and covered with a polyethylene terephthalate (PET) film release liner. Each adhesive patch contains 700 mg of lidocaine (50 mg per g adhesive) in an aqueous base. The penetration of lidocaine into intact skin after application of Lidoderm is sufficient to produce an analgesic effect but less than the amount necessary to produce a complete sensory block (Endo Pharmaceuticals, 2010). It is approved for pain associated with postherpetic neuralgia.

Pharmacokinetics

Absorption and Distribution

Lidocaine is absorbed systemically, with greater amounts absorbed based on the amount of medication used and where it is applied on the skin. Absorption is increased across abraded skin or mucous membranes. Once absorbed, lidocaine and prilocaine are widely distributed.

Metabolism and Excretion

It is not known if lidocaine or prilocaine are metabolized in the skin. Lidocaine is metabolized rapidly by the liver. Prilocaine is metabolized in both the liver and kidneys. Lidocaine is excreted in the urine.

Pharmacotherapeutics

Precautions and Contraindications

EMLA is contraindicated in the patient with methemoglobinemia. EMLA increases the risk of methemoglobinemia if used in patients with G6PD deficiency or in young infants. It is contraindicated in patients with known hypersensitivity to lidocaine or other local anesthetics.

If instilled into the middle ear, EMLA can be ototoxic. Therefore, use in the ear near the tympanic membrane is contraindicated.

In patients with severe hepatic disease, older adults, or debilitated and acutely ill patients, topical lidocaine should be used with caution. The minimal effective dose should be used to prevent adverse effects. Topical lidocaine is Pregnancy Category B. It should be used with caution in nursing mothers.

Adverse Drug Reactions

Adverse reactions are generally dose-related and usually result from high plasma levels of anesthetic due to excessive dosage or rapid absorption. The patient may experience local adverse effects, such as paleness of the area, erythema, and changes in temperature sensation.

Drug Interactions

Do not prescribe topical lidocaine products for use in children younger than 12 months who are concurrently taking methemoglobinemia-inducing drugs (acetaminophen, sulfonamides, nitrates, phenytoin, phenobarbital).

Class I antiarrhythmic agents (tocainide and mexiletine) may potentiate the toxicity of topical lidocaine products. See Table 23-12 for drug interactions.

Clinical Use and Dosing

Topical Anesthetic

To provide local anesthesia for minor procedures such as IV cannulation, venipuncture, or circumcision, the dose of EMLA varies by the age of the patient (Table 23-13). For adults and infants, cream is applied and occluded for 1 hour. If the patient is to self-administer the medication before a procedure, for ease of administration a 5 mg tube is dispensed and the patient instructed to apply half of the tube to the site or sites. For IV cannulation or venipuncture anesthesia, two sites may be treated. Dosing of cream for younger infants is determined by age, and the provider must refer to the dosing schedule for accurate dosing to prevent adverse effects. Higher dosing is used to harvest skin grafts, which is rarely done in primary care.

A Synera patch is applied to intact skin 20 to 30 minutes before venipuncture or 30 minutes before a dermatological procedure. Synera is approved for children age 3 years or older and adults. Patches are not to be cut. Synera patches contain iron powder and should be removed before a patient undergoes an MRI.

A Lidoderm patch is applied to intact skin at the most painful postherpetic neuralgia sites. Up to three patches may be applied at once for up to 12 hours of a 24-hour period. To adjust the dose, cut patches before release liner is removed. Do not apply to broken or inflamed skin. Avoid eyes and mucous membranes.

Monitoring

The patient being treated with topical lidocaine products should be monitored for adverse effects, such as methemoglobinemia.

Patient Education

Administration

Patients who are to self-administer topical lidocaine products should have clear instructions as to the correct use. The

Table 23–12 ⠿ Drug Interactions: Miscellaneous Topical Medications

Drug	Interacting Drug	Possible Effect	Implications
EMLA	Methemoglobinemia-inducing drugs: • Acetaminophen • Sulfonamides • Nitrates • Phenytoin • Phenobarbital	Methemoglobinemia	Methemoglobinemia can occur in very young (<12 mo) or patients with G6PD deficit, so do not use concurrently. Monitor other patients closely if using concurrently.
	Class I antiarrhythmic drugs: • Tocainide • Mexiletine	Additive toxic effects	Use concurrently with caution
Minoxidil	Topical steroids Topical retinoids Guanethidine Antihypertensives	Increased absorption of minoxidil Increased absorption of minoxidil Increased orthostatic hypertension Possible additive effect	Avoid concurrent use Avoid concurrent use Avoid concurrent use Monitor closely if using concurrently
Aluminum chloride (Drysol)	No known drug interactions		

Table 23–13 ⊗ Dosage Schedule: Miscellaneous Topical Medications

Drug	Indication	Dosage	Comments
Lidocaine 2.5% and prilocaine 2.5% (EMLA)	Topical anesthesia	Apply 2.5 g cream in a thick layer with occlusion over 20–25 cm² for 1 h	Apply to clean skin. Avoid eyes, mucous membranes, tympanic membrane, and application to large areas.
Lidocaine 70 mg and tetracaine 70 mg (Synera)	Topical analgesia	Children ≥3 yr and adults: apply patch 20 to 30 min before procedures.	Apply to intact skin. Remove before undergoing MRI (it contains iron powder). Do not cut patch.
Minoxidil (Rogaine for Women, Rogaine Extra Strength for Men)	Hair loss	Men: Use minoxidil 2% or 5%. Apply 1 mL topical 2×/d. Women: Use minoxidil 2%	Do not exceed recommended dose. Continue use or hair loss will begin again.
Aluminum chloride (Xerac 6.25% solution; Certain Dri 12% solution; Drysol 20% solution; Hypercare 20% solution)	Hyperhidrosis	Solution is applied once daily to the affected area at bedtime, then washed off in the morning. May decrease to 1–2×/wk once control is achieved.	Do not apply to recently shaven or broken skin
Eflornithine (Vaniqa)	Unwanted facial hair	Apply a thin layer to affected areas on the face and under the chin 2×/d, at least 8 h apart	For use by females only

patient should clearly understand how to apply the EMLA cream and occlude the area with the occlusive dressing or how to apply the Synera patch. If possible, the first dose should be applied by a health-care provider to demonstrate proper use.

MINOXIDIL

Topical minoxidil (Rogaine) is the first FDA-approved medication for stimulating hair growth. Alopecia androgenetica, also known as male pattern baldness, affects men and some women. It involves hair loss from the frontal, vertex, and occipital regions of the scalp in men and thinning of the hair in the frontoparietal area or diffuse hair loss in women.

Pharmacodynamics

The exact mechanism of action is unknown, but it does produce growth of epithelial cells near the base of the hair follicle. It may also induce vasodilatation of the scalp blood vessels, which also promotes hair growth. It does not appear to have an anti-androgen effect.

Pharmacokinetics

Absorption and Distribution

Topical minoxidil is poorly absorbed (2% of the dose) from an intact scalp. It is widely distributed in body tissues. It is not known whether minoxidil crosses the placenta or is distributed in breast milk.

Metabolism and Excretion

The small portion of topical minoxidil that is absorbed is extensively metabolized in the liver. Both the unchanged drug and the metabolites are excreted in the urine.

Pharmacotherapeutics

Precautions and Contraindications

Minoxidil topical solution used as directed has minimal cardiac effects, but if large amounts are applied, there is a potential for cardiac side effects, including hypotension.

Absorption of minoxidil is increased through abraded or irritated skin, leading to a slightly higher risk for cardiac side effects.

Minoxidil should not be used by pregnant patients (Pregnancy Category C) or by children younger than 18 years.

Adverse Drug Reactions

Minoxidil is generally well tolerated. The topical solution contains alcohol and therefore may be irritating upon application. Patients may be sensitive to minoxidil and develop contact dermatitis.

Drug Interactions

Topical steroids, retinoids, and other drugs that increase blood flow to the area may increase the absorption of minoxidil, leading to increased hypotension. Avoid using these topical medications concurrently on the scalp. There is a possible additive effect if minoxidil is used concurrently with antihypertensives.

Clinical Use and Dosing

Alopecia Androgenetica

Minoxidil is available OTC for the treatment of alopecia androgenetica (male pattern baldness). It is important to note that minoxidil does not treat balding of the frontoparietal areas in men; it only treats this in women. Minoxidil is effective in treating balding on the vertex of the scalp in men.

Minoxidil 2% topical solution is applied to the scalp twice daily for the entire length of treatment. Men may use the 5% solution if needed. The patient applies 1 mL directly to the affected area of the scalp (vertex area in men and frontoparietal area in women). The medication should be applied to a dry scalp. Patients should be instructed to wash their hands after using their fingers to rub medication into the scalp. Twice-daily application for at least 4 months may be needed to obtain observable hair growth. If the medication is discontinued, the hair in the treated area will shed in 3 to 4 months.

Monitoring

There is no specific laboratory monitoring needed when topical minoxidil is used.

Patient Education

Realistic expectations of therapy should be addressed. Minoxidil does not treat patients with predominantly frontal hair loss. It may take 3 to 4 months for the effects of treatment to be noticed. Treatment needs to be continued for there to be a continued effect, and the new hair will shed if the medication is discontinued. Effectiveness is variable among patients. New hair may initially be fine and almost colorless. With continued treatment, the hair should be the same color and thickness as the hair on the rest of the scalp.

Administration

Caution the patient to use the medication exactly as prescribed or, for OTC minoxidil, as the instructions indicate (see Table 23-13).

Adverse Reactions

Adverse effects of the medication should be discussed, and the patient instructed to use the medication exactly as recommended to decrease adverse effects.

MISCELLANEOUS TOPICAL MEDICATIONS

Bath Dermatologicals

Bath dermatologicals contain colloidal solids and oils that act as emollients. They are used to treat dry skin and the pruritus associated with dry skin and common dermatological conditions. Emollient baths that contain colloidal oatmeal solids (Aveeno) or oils (Alpha Keri Bath Oil, Lubriderm Bath Oil) can be used to provide relief from pruritus associated with contact dermatitis. These products are available OTC, and the patient should be instructed to use them according to the label instructions. Baths may be used as needed for comfort. Caution the patient to be careful when using bath oils to prevent slipping in the tub.

Astringents

Aluminum chloride hexahydrate (Drysol) is an astringent used for the management of hyperhidrosis (see Table 23-13). The solution is applied to the affected area at bedtime and then washed off in the morning. Excessive sweating may stop after two or more treatments. Once control of hyperhidrosis is achieved, the medication is applied once or twice weekly. Aluminum chloride hexahydrate solution should be applied to clean, completely dry skin to prevent irritation. Avoid use on broken, irritated, or recently shaved skin.

Hair-Growth Retardants

Eflornithine HCl (Vaniqa) is thought to inhibit hair growth by irreversibly inhibiting ornithine decarboxylase enzymes, which are necessary for the synthesis of polyamine. Polyamine inhibits cell division affecting the rate of hair growth. In clinical trials, 32% of women reported marked improvement in hair-growth reduction (SkinMedica, 2010). Adverse effects of eflornithine include acne, pseudofolliculitis barbae, stinging, burning, and rash. Vaniqa is Pregnancy Category C and is not recommended for use in children. It has been labeled for use in women. Vaniqa cream is applied twice a day (at least 8 hours apart) to affected areas of the face and adjacent areas under the chin. The medication is rubbed in thoroughly and the area should not be washed for at least 4 hours. Vaniqa works for most women within 8 weeks when used consistently twice a day. Women need to understand that this product only slows hair growth and they will need to continue to use other hair-removal methods (tweezing, shaving, etc.).

Sunscreens

Sunscreens provide either a chemical or physical barrier to sunlight. Chemical sunscreens are transparent and absorb portions of ultraviolet light. Some chemical sunscreens block UVA (avobenzone) and others UVB (PABA and others). Oxybenzone and dioxybenzone block both UVA and UVB light. Multiple-chemical sunscreens are usually combined in commercial products to provide broad-spectrum coverage. Physical barrier sunscreens contain large particulate ingredients (titanium dioxide, red petrolatum, or zinc oxide) that reflect and scatter UVA, UVB, and visible light.

The efficacy of sunscreens is determined by their sunscreen protective factor (SPF). Theoretically, a sunscreen with an SPF of 15 should allow the person to remain out in the sun 15 times longer before burning than if the skin is unprotected. According to the FDA (2012), sunscreen products labeled "broad-spectrum" sunscreens protect against both UVA and UVB rays. Sunscreens labeled "water resistant" sunscreens state whether the sunscreen remains effective for 40 minutes or 80 minutes when swimming or sweating. There is no longer a label of "waterproof" on sunscreen because eventually all sunscreens wash off. Sweating, reflection, and wind affect SPF.

Sunscreens must be applied liberally 15 to 30 minutes before sun exposure to allow penetration and binding to skin and must be reapplied after swimming.

Do not use sunscreens on children younger than 6 months. Sensitivity to sunscreen can occur. Contact dermatitis may occur with the use of PABA or its esters. PABA may permanently stain clothing yellow.

REFERENCES

Atanaskova, N., & Tomecki, K. (2010). Innovative management of recurrent furunculosis. *Dermatologic Clinics, 28*(30), 479–487.

American Academy of Dermatology. (2011). Acne. Retrieved from http://www.skincarephysicians.com/acnenet/index.html

American Academy of Pediatrics Committee on Infectious Diseases. (2012). Report of the Committee on Infection Diseases, Pediculosis capitis, corporis and pubis. In L. Pickering, D. Kimberlin, C. Baker, & S. Long (Eds.),. *Red book* (29th ed.) (543–552). Elk Grove Village, IL: American Academy of Pediatrics.

Avner, S., Nir, N., & Henri, T. (2005). Combination of oral terbinafine and topical ciclopirox compared to oral terbinafine for the treatment of onychomycosis. *Journal of Dermatological Treatment, 16*(5–6), 327–330.

Bangert, S., Levy, M., & Herbert, A. (2012). Bacterial resistance and impetigo treatment trends: A review. *Pediatric Dermatology, 29*(3), 243–248.

Baran, R., & Kaoukhov, A. (2005). Topical antifungal drugs for the treatment of onychomycosis: An overview of current strategies for monotherapy and combination therapy. *Journal of the European Academy of Dermatology and Venereology, 19*(1), 21–29.

Bikowski, J. (2009). Facial seborrheic dermatitis: A report on current status and therapeutic horizons. *Journal of Drugs in Dermatology, 8*(2), 125–133.

Bewley, A. (2008). Expert consensus: Time for a change in the way we advise our patients to use topical corticosteroids. *The British Journal of Dermatology, 158*(5), 917–920.

Brelsford, M. (2008). Preventing and managing the side effects of isotretinoin. *Seminars in Cutaneous Medicine and Surgery, 27*(3), 197.

Bozzo, P., Chua-Gocheco, A., & Einarson, A. (2011). Safety of skin care products during pregnancy. *Canadian Family Physician, 57*(6), 665–667.

Buys, L. (2007). Treatment options for atopic dermatitis. *American Family Physician, 75*(4), 523–528.

Centers for Disease Control and Prevention, Division of Parasitic Diseases and Malaria. (2010a). Body lice. Retrieved from http://www.cdc.gov/parasites/lice/body/index.html

Centers for Disease Control and Prevention, Division of Parasitic Diseases and Malaria. (2010b). Pubic lice infestation. Retrieved from http://www.cdc.gov/parasites/lice/pubic/index.html

Centers for Disease Control and Prevention, Division of Parasitic Diseases and Malaria. (2010c). Scabies. Retrieved from http://www.cdc.gov/parasites/scabies/

Centers for Disease Control and Prevention, Division of Parasitic Diseases and Malaria. (2011). Head lice. Retrieved from http://www.cdc.gov/parasites/lice/head/index.html

Charakida, A., Dadzie, O., Teixeira, F., Charakida, M., Evangelou, G., & Chu, A. C. (2006). Calcipotriol/betamethasone dipropionate for the treatment of psoriasis. *Expert Opinion on Pharmacotherapy, 7*(5), 597–606.

Del Roso Do, J. Q. (2006). Combination topical therapy for the treatment of psoriasis. *Journal of Drugs in Dermatology, 5*(3), 232–234.

Derby, R., Rohal, P., Jackson, C., Beutler, A., & Olsen, C. (2011). Novel treatment of onychomycosis using over-the-counter metholated ointment: A clinical case series. *Journal of the American Board of Family Medicine, 24*(1), 69–74.

Downs, A. M. R., Narayan, S., Stafford, K. A., & Coles, G. C. (2005). Effectiveness of Ovide against malathion-resistant head lice. *Archives of Dermatology, 141*, 1318.

Endo Pharmaceuticals. (2010). *Lidoderm 5% prescribing information.* Retrieved from http://www.lidoderm.com/prescrib.aspx

GlaxoSmithKline. (2005). *Bactroban ointment prescribing information.* Retrieved from http://www.gsksource.com/gskprm/en/US/adirect/gskprm?cmd=ProductDetailPage&product_id=1244166895635&featureKey=600562#section-34089-3

Goldstein, B., & Goldstein, A. (2011). Dermatophyte (tinea) infections. In B. Rose (Ed.), *UpToDate.* Available from http://www.uptodateonline.com

Goldstein, B., & Goldstein, A. (2012). General principles of dermatologic therapy and topical corticosteroid use. In B. Rose (Ed.), *UpToDate.* Available from http://www.uptodateonline.com

Graber, E. (2012). Treatment of acne vulgaris. In B. Rose (Ed.), *UpToDate.* Available from http://www.uptodateonline.com

Gupta, A. K., & Onychomycosis Combination Therapy Study Group. (2005). Ciclopirox topical solution, 8% combined with oral terbinafine to treat onychomycosis: A randomized, evaluator-blinded study. *Drugs Dermatology, 4*(4), 481–485.

Gupta, A.K., Paquet, M. & Simpson, F.C. (2013). Therapies for the treatment of onychomycosis. *Clinics in Dermatology, 31*(5), 544-54.

Habif, T. (2010). *Clinical Dermatology*, 5th ed. Retrieved from http://www.mdconsult.com/books/about.do?about=true&eid=4-u1.0-B978-0-7234-3541-9.X0001-6—TOP&isbn=978-0-7234-3541-9&uniqId=397817045-2722

iPledge. (2005). About iPledge. Retrieved from https://www.ipledgeprogram.com/Default.aspx

Lipner, S., & Scher, R. K. (2014). Onychomycosis: Current and future therapies. *Cutis, 93*(2), 60-3.

Lio, P., & Kaye, E. (2009). Topical antibacterial agents. *Infectious Disease Clinics of North America, 23*(4), 945–962.

Lorch Dauk, K. C., Conrov, E., Blumer, J. L., O'Riordan, M. A., & Furman, L. M. (2010). Tinea capitis: Predictive value of symptoms and time to cure with griseofulvin treatment. *Clinical Pediatrics, 49*(3), 280–286.

Luba, K. M., & Stulberg, D. L. (2006). Chronic plaque psoriasis. *American Family Physician, 73*(4), 636–644.

Luhman, J., Hurt, S., Shootman, M., & Kennedy, R. (2004). A comparison of buffered lidocaine versus ELA-Max before peripheral intravenous catheter insertions in children. *Pediatrics, 113*(3), e217–e220.

McConeghy, K., Mikolich, D., & LaPlante, K. (2009). Agents for the decolonization of methicillin-resistant *Staphylococcus aureus*. *Pharmacotherapy, 29*(3), 263–280.

Menter, A., Korman, N. J., Elmets, C. A., Feldman, S. R., Gelfand, J. M., Gordon, K. B., et al. (2009). Guidelines of care for the management and treatment of psoriasis with topical therapies. *Journal of the American Academy of Dermatology, 60*(4), 643–659.

Morelli, J. (2011). Cutaneous bacterial infections. In R. Kliegman (Ed.), *Nelson textbook of pediatrics* (19th ed.) (2299–2308). Philadelphia: Elsevier Saunders.

Naldi, L., & Rebora, A. (2009). Seborrheic dermatitis. *New England Journal of Medicine, 360*(4), 387–396.

Novartis Pharmaceuticals. (2001). *Lamisil prescribing information*. Retrieved from http://www.pharma.us.novartis.com/products/lamisil.shtml

Skevington, S. M., Bradshaw, J., Hepplewhite, A., Dawkes, K., & Lovell, C. R. (2006). How does psoriasis affect quality of life? Assessing an Ingram-regimen outpatient programme and validating the WHOQOL-100. *British Journal of Dermatology, 154*(4), 680–691.

SkinMedica. (2010). *Vaniqua prescribing information*. Retrieved from http://www.vaniqa.com/

Stevens, D., Bisno, A., Chambers, H., Dellinger, P., Goldstein, E. J., Gorbach, S. L., et al. (2014). Practice guidelines for the diagnosis and management of skin and soft-tissue infections: 2014 update by the Infectious Diseases Society of America.*Clinical Infectious Diseases, 59*(2), e10–e52.

Straus, A. W., Krowchuk, D. P., Leyden, J. J., Lucky, A. W., Shalita, A. R., Siegfried, E. C., et al. (2007). Guidelines for acne vulgaris management. *Journal of the American Academy of Dermatology, 56*, 651–663.

Vallerance, A., Sanoski, C., & Deglin, J. (2013). *Davis's drug guide for nurses*. Philadelphia: F.A. Davis.

Walker, G. J. A., & Johnstone, P. W. (2006). Interventions for treating scabies. *The Cochrane Database of Systematic Reviews, 2*, 1–37.

U.S. Food and Drug Administration. (2006). FDA approves updated labeling with boxed warning and medication guide for two eczema drugs, Elidel and Protopic. Retrieved from http://www.fda.gov/NewsEvents/Newsroom/PressAnnouncements/2006/ucm108580.htm

U.S. Food and Drug Adminstration (2009). Lindane shampoo and lindane lotion. Retrieved from http://www.fda.gov/Drugs/DrugSafety/PostmarketDrugSafetyInformationforPatientsandProviders/ucm110452.htm

U.S. Food and Drug Adminstartion (2012). FDA announces changes to better inform consumers about sunscreen. Retrived from http://www.fda.gov/NewsEvents/Newsroom/PressAnnouncements/ucm258940.htm

University of Massachusetts Medical School (2012). Therapeutic class overview scabicides and pediculicides. Retrieved from https://www.medicaid.nv.gov/Downloads/provider/Scabicides%20and%20Pediculicides.pdf.

Zane, L., Leyden, W., Marqueling, A., & Manos, M. (2006). A population-based analysis of laboratory abnormalities during isotretinoin therapy for acne vulgaris. *Archives of Dermatolology, 142*(8),1016.

CHAPTER 24

DRUGS USED IN TREATING INFECTIOUS DISEASES

Jennifer Jordan • R. Brigg Turner • Teri Moser Woo

In 1928, Alexander Fleming discovered the first antibiotic, penicillin. In the ensuing years, a wide variety of antibiotic, antifungal, and antiviral classes and drugs have been developed. These anti-infective agents have made a significant difference in morbidity and mortality throughout the world. Many disease processes, once incurable, are now treatable with various agents.

ANTIMICROBIAL RESISTANCE

Within 10 years of Fleming's discovery, group A streptococci and pneumococci had developed modes of resistance (Schumann & Nollette, 2000). Antibiotic resistance has continued; widespread acquisition of penicillin resistance emerged in the 1950s and 1960s, and outbreaks of resistant gram-negative organisms and beta-lactamase-producing bacteria occurred in the 1970s. In the 1980s, new pathogens began to emerge, and organisms previously susceptible to therapy developed multidrug resistance (MDR). The first known penicillin-non-susceptible pneumococcus was identified in the 1960s; by the 1980s, there was a high prevalence of antibiotic-resistant pneumococci worldwide (Linares, Ardanuy, Pallares, & Fenoll, 2010). In the 1990s, vancomycin-resistance enterococci emerged. The World Health Organization (WHO) reported an estimated 630,000 cases (3.7%) of MDR tuberculosis in 2011 (WHO, 2013b).

Factors that contribute to this phenomenon include increasing populations of immunocompromised patients, increases in the number and complexity of invasive medical procedures, and increased survival of patients with chronic diseases. Spread of resistant organisms in the community has been associated with day care for young children, overcrowding, travel, and the use of antibiotics in agriculture (American Academy of Microbiology, 2009). The leading risk factors for having a drug-resistant pathogen include recent use of antibiotics, age younger than 2 years or older than 65 years, day-care center attendance, exposure to young children, multiple medical comorbidities, recent hospitalization, and immunosuppression (Chow et al, 2012).

Excessive and inappropriate use of antibiotic agents is a major factor in the development of drug resistance (Bishai, Morris, & Scanland, 2004; Centers for Disease Control and Prevention [CDC], 2011a; Linares et al, 2010). Examples of inappropriate use include prescribing antibiotics for viral infections, inadequate dosing, excessive duration of therapy, and increased empirical use of broad-spectrum antibiotics when not required (CDC, 2009b; Schumann & Nollette, 2000). To address the public health burden caused by overuse of antimicrobials, the CDC convened a meeting in December 2011 of international experts in clinical medicine, veterinary medicine, microbiology, public health and health policy, which led to the development of a Federal Action Plan titled *A Public Health Action Plan to Combat Antimicrobial Resistance* (CDC, 2011). In 2013, the CDC published a report outlining the burden and threats posed by antibiotic-resistant organisms and their impact on health in the United States, noting that 2 million people become infected with resistant bacteria and 23,000 people in the United States die annually from resistant bacteria (CDC, 2013a). Among the strategies proposed by the *Action Plan* were increased surveillance for emergence of antimicrobial organisms and the development, implementation, and evaluation of strategies to improve appropriate antimicrobial use. In 2015 the Obama Administration released a comprehensive national plan to combat antibiotic resistance that included doubling the budget for combating antibiotic resistance.

In the 21st century, resistance has developed to *every* antibiotic class. Unless novel drug mechanisms are developed, a prospect many experts find unlikely, providers will be dependent on the current classes of drugs to treat infectious diseases. Many health systems around the world are utilizing antimicrobial stewardship programs to preserve the current antibiotic armamentarium. These programs are helpful in combatting increasingly complex problems, are multidisciplinary, and promote using the most appropriate antibiotic with the best dose, route, and duration for a specific patient.

Stewardship strategies include treatment pathways for specific infectious diseases, formulary restrictions, dose optimization, prospective audits of prescribed antimicrobials, and continued education for prescribers.

This chapter focuses on the systemic administration of drugs that are active against bacterial, fungal, viral, and parasitic organisms. Topical applications associated with dermatological conditions are presented in Chapter 23. Although many of these drugs are available in IV formulations, oral (PO) and intramuscular (IM) formulations are more commonly used in primary care and are the focus of this chapter.

ANTIBIOTICS: BETA-LACTAMS

The discovery of penicillins initiated the antibiotic era. The active moiety of penicillins is a four-member ring known as the beta-lactam ring. Other antibiotics that contain the beta-lactam ring, mainly cephalosporins, carbapenems, and monobactams, have a similar mechanism of action and share clinical effects. Beta-lactam antibiotics are bactericidal when concentrations exceed the minimum inhibitory concentration (MIC) of the pathogen for approximately 50% of the dosing interval. Efficacy is affected by the organism's susceptibility, dose, tissue concentration, and rate of organism multiplication. They are most effective against rapidly growing organisms forming cell walls. Cephalosporins are discussed in the next section. Monobactams and carbapenems are used to treat serious infections in the hospital, which is outside the scope of this textbook. Beta-lactamase inhibitors are described with the penicillins because they are usually used together as combination products.

PENICILLINS

Penicillins are characterized chemically by the 6-aminopenicillanic acid joined to the beta-lactam ring. Attachment of different substitutes to 6-aminopenicillanic acid results in different pharmacological and antibacterial characteristics, which are the basis for four penicillin subclasses: (1) penicillinase-sensitive or natural penicillins, (2) aminopenicillins, (3) penicillinase-resistant or anti-staphylococcal penicillins, and (4) anti-pseudomonal or extended-spectrum penicillins.

Pharmacodynamics

Penicillins hinder bacterial growth by inhibiting the biosynthesis of bacterial cell wall mucopeptide (also called murein or peptidoglycan). This action is dependent on the drug reaching the penicillin-binding proteins (PBPs), which include transpeptidase, carboxypeptidase, and endopeptidase enzymes involved in the terminal stages of forming the cell wall. When penicillins bind to the PBPs, the wall is weakened and lysis of the bacterial cell wall occurs. Because human cells lack a cell wall, there is virtually no action against host cells. Penicillins are bactericidal against sensitive organisms and are most effective during active cellular multiplication. Lower drug concentrations may result in bacteriostatic effects only.

Penicillin

The only natural penicillin commercially available is penicillin. Penicillin can be administered orally (Penicillin V, or oral Penicillin G which is no longer available in the United States), intramuscularly (procaine and benzathine penicillin), and intravenously (Penicillin G). This group is active against aerobic, gram-positive organisms, including *Streptococcus* species such as *S. pneumoniae* and group A beta-hemolytic *Streptococcus* (GABHS), some *Enterococcus* strains, and some non-penicillinase-producing staphylococci. Only about 5% to 15% of community-acquired *Staphylococcus aureus* remains susceptible to natural penicillins, principally because the majority of strains produce penicillinase.

The concern with penicillin-resistant *S. pneumoniae* has been somewhat decreased with less indiscriminate use of antibiotics and vaccination against pneumococcus. Resistant strains dropped from a high of 40% in 2000 to 20% by 2003 with the universal use of the PCV-7 vaccine (Thomas, 2005). Penicillin-resistant strains are also commonly resistant to cephalosporins, macrolides, and sulfonamides and, to a lesser extent, to clindamycin; they are commonly called drug-resistant *S. pneumoniae* (DRSP) (Thomas, 2005).

In addition to its bactericidal activity against most streptococcal and community-acquired enterococcal species, penicillin has reliable activity against *Pasteurella multocida*, *Actinomyces, Clostridium, Peptostreptococcus,* and *Treponema pallidum.* The American Academy of Pediatrics (AAP) *Red Book* recommends penicillin for Group A beta streptococci and for Group B beta streptococci due to low resistance (AAP, 2012a, 2012b). Penicillin G is reliable for treating *Listeria monocytogenes* but is no longer listed as active against *Neisseria gonorrhoeae* due to resistance that was first documented in 1976 (CDC, 2013b; see Chap. 44, Sexually Transmitted Infections) or against *Staphylococcus* species. Penicillinase-producing organisms have reduced the breadth of organisms that this group is used to treat.

Aminopenicillins

Like penicillin, aminopenicillins have reliable activity against gram-positive organisms, including *Streptococcus* and *Enterococcus* species. However, they have greater activity against gram-negative bacteria because of their enhanced ability to penetrate the outer membrane of these organisms. Ampicillin and amoxicillin are the only two available aminopenicillins. Because of the increasing beta-lactamase production among gram-negative pathogens and anaerobes, amoxicillin and ampicillin are often combined with beta-lactamase inhibitors, clavulanic acid, and sulbactam, respectively, for enhanced gram-negative and anaerobic activity. Beta-lactamase inhibitors prevent the destruction of beta-lactam antibiotics by serving as a competitive inhibitor of beta-lactamase. Although beta-lactamase inhibitors also contain a beta-lactam ring, they have poor antimicrobial activity alone. As combination products, ampicillin/sulbactam and amoxicillin/clavulanate have excellent activity against methicillin-susceptible *Staphylococcus aureus* (MSSA), *Streptococcus* and *Enterococcus* species, *Moraxella catarrhalis*, *Haemophilus influenzae*, *Neisseria meningitidis*, *Escherichia coli*, *Klebsiella*, *Proteus mirabilis*, *Salmonella*, some *Shigella* species, *Pasteurella multocido*, *Actinomyces*, *Clostridium*, *Peptostreptococcus*, and *Bacteroides fragilis*.

Penicillinase-Resistant Penicillins

Nafcillin, oxacillin, cloxacillin, and dicloxacillin, also called the anti-staphylococcal penicillins, have a unique spectrum of activity. Chemical modifications of penicillin produced this class of antibiotics that is stable in the presence of penicillinase produced by staphylococci; however, activity was eliminated for *Enterococcus* species, *Listeria*, gram-negative bacteria, and most anaerobes. They are active against *Streptococcus* species, MSSA, some coagulase-negative staphylococci, and *Peptostreptococcus*. Resistance by staphylococci is mediated via the mecA gene, which encodes the low-affinity PBP 2a. This will manifest as methicillin-resistant *S. aureus* (MRSA) and *Staphylococcus epidermidis* (MRSE). With the exception of ceftaroline, methicillin-resistant strains are resistant to all penicillins, cephalosporins, and carbapenems.

Anti-Pseudomonal Penicillins

The anti-pseudomonal penicillin group is comprised of piperacillin, ticarcillin, mezlocillin (discontinued in the United States), and carbenicillin (discontinued in the United States). Piperacillin and ticarcillin have enhanced activity against gram-negative bacilli, particularly *Pseudomonas aeruginosa, Enterobacter, Morganella,* and *Providencia* species. They retain activity against aminopenicillin-susceptible organisms, yet have less potency against streptococci and enterococci.

Piperacillin and ticarcillin are available as combination products with beta-lactamase inhibitors. Piperacillin/tazobactam and ticarcillin/clavulanate have a wider spectrum of activity that includes MSSA and anaerobes, including *Bacteroides* species. None of these agents is available for oral use in the United States.

Many texts and references, including the *Sanford Guide to Antimicrobial Therapy* (2012), have tables that list the organisms generally susceptible to various penicillins.

Resistance

Resistance to penicillins is due to (1) inactivation by beta-lactamases, (2) alteration in target PBPs on the bacterial cell wall, or (3) a permeability barrier preventing penetration of the antibiotic to the target cell. Beta-lactamase production is the most common mechanism. Beta-lactamases include a large group of enzymes called penicillinases, cephalosporinases, and carbapenemases. Beta-lactamases produced by *S. aureus, Haemophilus* species, and most *E. coli* have narrow specificity for penicillins. Beta-lactamase inhibitors (clavulanate, sulbactam, and tazobactam) have minimal antibacterial activity but irreversibly inactivate beta-lactamase

enzymes produced by bacteria by binding to their active site and protecting the antibiotic from inactivation. However, some *E. coli, Klebsiella* species, and *Enterobacter* species produce extended-spectrum beta-lactamases (ESBLs) that have broader specificity and will hydrolyze both penicillins and cephalosporins while sparing carbapenems. ESBLs are not inhibited by commercially available beta-lactamase inhibitors.

Alteration in PBPs is responsible for methicillin resistance in staphylococci and penicillin resistance in pneumococci. Drug penetration problems are associated with the cellular outer membrane, which is present in gram-negative but not gram-positive organisms.

Pharmacokinetics
Absorption and Distribution

The extent of oral absorption of penicillins is dependent on the specific penicillin agent, the pH of the stomach and intestine, and presence of food. Although oral penicillin formulations are generally well absorbed from the GI tract, use is limited to mild to moderate infections because higher-than-recommended doses cause GI distress and diarrhea. In addition, serum concentrations do not rise proportionately with increased doses.

Penicillin V has less individual variation in absorption than Penicillin G and is virtually the only oral natural penicillin in use. Nafcillin's oral absorption is so poor that the oral route is rarely used, whereas dicloxacillin is the best absorbed of the penicillinase-resistant group, producing blood levels twice that of orally administered oxacillin or cloxacillin. Amoxicillin is more completely absorbed than ampicillin and may be given without regard to food. Carbenicillin, the only oral anti-pseudomonal penicillin, is not adequately absorbed enough orally to attain blood levels effective for systemic infections, so it is indicated only for urinary tract and prostatic infections. It is not first-line treatment for this indication and not currently available in the United States.

All subclasses of penicillin have agents that can be given IM, but different penicillin salts have different absorption rates. The IM route is unreliable and erratic, as well as irritating to the tissue, and repeated dosing by this route should be avoided. Because the penicillin G procaine and penicillin G benzathine formulations are slowly absorbed, they are used as depot agents for deep IM use only. They are not to be injected near an artery or vein. IV injection of these depot formulations of penicillin may cause cardiac arrest and death.

Penicillins are bound to plasma proteins to varying degrees and are well distributed to most tissues and body fluids. Inflammation enhances penetration of the meninges, joints, and eye fluids, which are otherwise poorly penetrated. Penicillins cross the placenta and enter breast milk.

Metabolism and Excretion

Excluding nafcillin and oxacillin, penicillins undergo negligible metabolism and are excreted primarily as unchanged drugs in the urine, achieving high urinary concentrations.

Ninety percent of the renal excretion of penicillin is by active tubular secretion, and most other penicillins undergo extensive tubular secretion. Probenecid, which competes with penicillins for the tubular secretion carrier, will prolong the half-life and raise the peak plasma concentration of penicillins. Thus, concurrent administration of oral probenecid is used to treat some serious infections. Renal insufficiency prolongs the half-life and increases the risk for toxicity of penicillins. Table 24-1 shows the pharmacokinetic properties of each of the penicillin subclasses. Throughout this chapter, any change in dosing that is required based on renal impairment will be shown in the dosage schedule tables.

Pharmacotherapeutics

Precautions and Contraindications

Although less than 10% of patients taking these drugs have an allergic reaction, penicillins are the most likely antibiotics to cause an allergic reaction. A history of a serious hypersensitivity reaction (e.g., anaphylaxis, serum sickness, exfoliative dermatitis, hemolysis, or other blood dyscrasia) to a penicillin contraindicates the use of any penicillin on account of cross-reactivity. Severe, type I allergic reactions to cephalosporins, carbapenems, or beta-lactamase inhibitors may contraindicate use of penicillins. Although historically cross-sensitivity between penicillins and these other classes was thought to be much higher, recent data suggest that the rate is closer to 1% (Campagna, Bond, Schabelman, & Hayes, 2012; Frumin & Gallagher, 2009). Patients with a history of allergy to other substances (e.g., atopic skin conditions) should also use these drugs with caution.

Mezlocillin, carbenicillin (parenteral), and piperacillin may induce hemorrhagic manifestations, and they should be used with extreme caution by patients who have anemia, thrombocytopenia, granulocytopenia, or bone marrow depression, or who are receiving anticoagulants.

Penicillins are Pregnancy Category B, but there are not adequate and controlled studies in women. They should be used only when clearly indicated. They are excreted in low concentrations in breast milk and may cause diarrhea, candidiasis, or allergic response in the nursing infant.

The safety and efficacy of carbenicillin and the piperacillin-tazobactam combination have not been established for children younger than 12 years. Dosage adjustment of penicillins may be required for infants because of their undeveloped renal function (see the Clinical Use and Dosing section for further discussion).

Adverse Drug Reactions

Serious and occasionally fatal immediate hypersensitivity reactions (type I hypersensitivity) have occurred, with an incidence of anaphylactic shock of 0.015% to 0.04%. These reactions usually occur within 2 to 30 minutes after administration and are characterized by nausea, vomiting, urticaria, pruritus, tachycardia, severe dyspnea, diaphoresis, stridor, vertigo, and eventually loss of consciousness and circulatory collapse. Treatment is the same as for any anaphylactic reaction. Skin testing may be used to identify those at risk for penicillin allergy. A radioallergosorbent test (RAST), or a combination of RAST and minor determinant skin testing, may also be used. Patients should be referred to an allergist for skin testing. Patients with a known allergy or a positive skin test can be given desensitization therapy (Schafer, Mateo, Parlier, & Rotschafer, 2007). Other hypersensitivity reactions include skin rashes, a serum sickness–like reaction (skin rash, joint pain, fever), exfoliative dermatitis (red, scaly skin), and blood dyscrasias (hemolytic anemia, neutropenia, leukopenia).

A pruritic, maculopapular rash that does not represent a true allergy occasionally occurs with amoxicillin and ampicillin (9%). It is more common with patients who have mononucleosis (43% to 100%), chronic lymphocytic leukemia (90%), or concurrent allopurinol therapy (15% to 20%). This measles-like, pruritic, generalized rash typically appears 7 to 10 days after initiation of therapy and remains for a few days to a week after the drug is discontinued. This rash does not contraindicate subsequent use of aminopenicillins.

As with many antibiotics, common adverse reactions include GI symptoms such as nausea, vomiting, diarrhea, and epigastric distress. Amoxicillin produces these symptoms less often than ampicillin and can be taken with food, which will further decrease incidence of these adverse effects. Addition of clavulanate to amoxicillin doubles the incidence of diarrhea to 10%, but new formulations with lower concentrations of clavulanate have reduced this side effect. Although uncommon, the penicillinase-resistant penicillins are the most likely group to cause hepatotoxicity, especially when administered with other hepatotoxic drugs.

Use of broad-spectrum penicillins, or prolonged or repeat therapy with any broad-spectrum antibacterial, may result in bacterial or fungal overgrowth (i.e., superinfection) of nonsusceptible organisms. The patient should be monitored for this possibility and treated with appropriate measures. *Clostridium difficile* infection (CDI) is a superinfection that manifests as diarrhea that may occur during therapy or up to several weeks after discontinuation of the antibiotic. CDI may present with watery or bloody diarrhea, accompanied by severe abdominal cramps and pain, fever, and pseudomembranous colitis. CDI is a serious sequela that may abate with supportive therapy and discontinuance of the antibiotic, but if definitive diagnosis is made, treatment with oral metronidazole, oral vancomycin, or fidaxomicin is required.

Patients who are HIV-positive are more susceptible to hepatotoxicity resulting from cloxacillin, dicloxacillin, and oxacillin than are HIV-negative patients. Although interstitial nephritis was commonly seen with methicillin, which is no longer used, it still occurs occasionally with oxacillin, nafcillin, or any other penicillin. High doses of procaine penicillin G can cause transient mental disturbances, including combativeness, irritability, and hallucinations. Platelet dysfunction is primarily associated with parenteral carbenicillin, piperacillin, and ticarcillin. Irritability and seizures have occurred with high doses of all penicillins, especially in patients with renal insufficiency.

Table 24–1 ✛ Pharmacokinetics: Penicillins

Drug	Onset	Peak	Duration	Protein Binding	Bioavailability	Half-Life	Penicillinase Resistance	Acid Stability	Elimination
Penicillinase Sensitive									
Penicillin G sodium (IM)	Rapid	0.5–3 h	4–6 h	60%	0	0.7 h	No	NA	70% unchanged by kidney
Penicillin G potassium (IM)	Rapid	15–30 min	4–6 h	UA	0	0.5–1 h	No	NA	70% unchanged by kidney
Penicillin G benzathine (IM)	Delayed	12–24 h	7–18 d	UA	0	0.5–1 h	No	NA	70% unchanged by kidney
Penicillin G procaine (IM)	Delayed	1–4 h	12 h	UA	0	0.5–1 h	No	NA	70% unchanged by kidney
Penicillin G potassium (PO)	1 h	1 h	4–6 h	UA	UA	0.5–1 h	No	No	70% unchanged by kidney
Penicillin V (PO)	Rapid	0.5–1 h	4–6 h	65%	60%	0.5 h	No	No	70% unchanged by kidney
Penicillinase Resistant									
Cloxacillin (PO)	30 min	1–2 h	6 h	93%–95%	50%–70%	0.5 h	Yes	Yes	30%–60% by liver; 40%–70% by kidney
Dicloxacillin (PO)	30 min	1–2 h	6 h	96%–98%	50%	0.8 h	Yes	Yes	6%–10% by liver; 50% unchanged in urine
Methicillin (IM)	Rapid	0.5–1 h	4–6 h	40%	Minimal	0.4 h	Yes	NA	Unchanged by kidney
Nafcillin (IM)	Rapid	30 min	1–2 h	80%–90%	NA	0.5–1.5 h	Yes	Yes	60% by liver; rest unchanged in urine
Oxacillin (IM)	Rapid	0.5–1 h	4–6 h	90%–94%	NA	0.5–1 h	Yes	Yes Yes	49% by liver; rest unchanged in urine
Aminopenicillins									
Amoxicillin (PO)	30 min	1–2 h	8 h	20%	80%	1–1.5 h	No	Yes	30% by liver; 70% unchanged in urine
Ampicillin (PO)	Rapid	1–2 h	4–6 h	20%	50%	1–1.5 h	No	Yes	60% in urine
(IM)	Rapid	1 h	4–6 h	20%	NA	1–1.5 h	No	NA	50%–85% in urine
Anti-Pseudomonals									
Carbenicillin (PO)	Rapid	1 h	6 h	98%	30%–50%	1 h	No	Yes	85% unchanged in urine
Mezlocillin (IM)	Rapid	1–1.5 h	4–6 h	16%–42%	NA	0.7–1.3 h	No	NA	55%–60% unchanged in urine; up to 50% metabolized by liver
Piperacillin (IM)	Rapid	0.5–1 h	4–6 h	16%	NA	1h	No	NA	60%–80% unchanged in urine; 10% in bile
Combinations									
Amoxicillin/clavulanate (PO)	30 min	1–2 h	8 h	18%–25%	80%	1–1.3 h	Yes	Yes	30% by liver; 70% unchanged in urine
Ampicillin/sulbactam (IM)	Rapid	1 h	6–8 h	20%–38%	NA	1–1.3 h	Yes	NA	75% of ampicillin and sulbactam by kidney
Piperacillin/tazobactam (IM)	Rapid	0.5–1 h	4–6 h	16%–30%	NA	0.7–1.2 h	Yes	NA	Piperacillin 68% and tazobactam 80% by kidney

NA = not applicable; UA = information unavailable.

Drug Interactions

The main drug interactions with penicillins are shown in Table 24-2. Of interest is the potential for reduced efficacy of oral contraceptives (OCs), particularly with aminopenicillins. However, there are only a few case reports of such failures, which may be consistent with the normal failure rate of OCs. All antibiotics have been implicated in the failure of OCs; however, only rifampin and griseofulvin have been shown to alter serum levels of estrogen (Archer & Archer, 2002). Other proposed, but unproven, mechanisms of interaction between OCs and antibiotics include decreased absorption of OCs, decreased enterohepatic recirculation of OCs, and increased serum protein displacement by antibiotics. While potentially unnecessary, the most cautious approach is to recommend an additional form of contraception during the antibiotic course. For drug interactions specific to a particular penicillin, selecting a different penicillin may be acceptable, but selecting a different antibiotic class is preferable. Food and acidic juices decrease the oral absorption of penicillin V and the penicillinase-resistant penicillins.

Clinical Use and Dosing

A penicillin is usually the drug of choice for a susceptible organism because of limited toxicities. Amoxicillin is the top antibiotic prescribed to children and the second most prescribed antibiotic in adults (Kofke-Egger & Udow-Phillips, 2011). The most common infections treated with penicillins in ambulatory care are bacterial upper respiratory infections (URIs) (pharyngitis, otitis media, sinusitis), pneumonia, sexually transmitted infections, urinary tract infections, and wound infections. Other important indications for penicillins are endocarditis prophylaxis, eradication of *Helicobacter pylori* in gastritis and peptic ulcer disease, and Lyme disease.

Acute Bronchitis and Upper Respiratory Infection

Over the past 15 to 20 years, concern has been growing that overuse and misuse of antibiotics for URIs contribute to antibiotic resistance (AAP, 2012c; Bucher et al, 2003; Schumann & Nollette, 2000). In 1998, "Common Cold: Principles of Judicious Use of Antimicrobial Agents" was published in *Pediatrics* to begin a dialogue and recommendation for avoiding antibiotic prescriptions for the common cold (Rosenstein et al, 1998). In spite of recommendations not to prescribe antibiotics for the common cold, the CDC reported that up to 50% of patients treated for colds, bronchitis, and URIs received antibiotics inappropriately and launched a nationwide campaign called "Get Smart: Know When Antibiotics Work" (http://www.cdc.gov/getsmart) to educate providers and patients regarding the inappropriate use of antibiotics. In spite of almost 15 years of focusing on appropriate use of antibiotics, approximately 75% of antibiotic prescriptions written in pediatric practice are for otitis media, sinusitis, cough illness/bronchitis, pharyngitis, and the common cold (AAP, 2009). Because the common cold, URI, and acute bronchitis are seasonal, self-limiting illnesses usually caused by viruses, antibiotics have no role in management of uncomplicated cases (CDC, 2012c). Symptomatic treatment, rest, and proper nutrition should be mainstays of treatment; these are discussed in Chapter 46, Upper Respiratory Infections.

Table 24–2 ▦ Drug Interactions: Penicillins

Drug	Interacting Drug	Possible Effect	Implications
Penicillins	Diuretics	Potassium-wasting diuretics may have increased risk for hypokalemia; the reverse is true for potassium-sparing diuretics.	If they must be given together, monitor serum potassium levels and for indications of these electrolyte imbalances.
	Methotrexate	Increased levels of methotrexate.	Avoid concurrent administration.
	Oral contraceptives	Evidence is contradictory. The efficacy of oral contraceptives may be reduced, and increased breakthrough bleeding may occur. Although infrequently reported, contraceptive failure is possible.	It is difficult to tie contraceptive failure directly to penicillin use because no oral contraceptive is 100% efficacious. The use of an additional form of contraception during penicillin therapy should be considered.
	Probenecid	Delays renal elimination and increases blood levels.	Monitor for penicillin toxicity.
	Tetracyclines	Bacteriostatic action of tetracyclines may impair bactericidal effects of penicillins.	Rarely used therapeutically. Monitor for therapeutic efficacy.
	Warfarin	Increased effects of warfarin and risk of bleeding with penicillin, aminopenicillins, and antipseudomonal penicillins; however, decreased effects of warfarin with nafcillin, oxacillin, and dicloxacillin.	Monitor INR closely.
Ampicillin	Beta blockers	May reduce bioavailability of atenolol. Beta blockers may potentiate anaphylactic reactions of penicillin.	Select a different penicillin if patient is taking atenolol.
	Allopurinol	Higher incidence of ampicillin-induced rash.	Avoid coadministration.
Nafcillin	Cyclosporine	Concurrent administration produces subtherapeutic cyclosporine levels.	If they must be used concurrently, monitor cyclosporine levels more closely.
Penicillin G	Colestipol, cholestyramine	May decrease absorption of oral penicillin G.	Separate doses. Give penicillin G 1 h before or 4 h after colestipol or cholestyramine.

Cough of less than 3-weeks duration seldom requires treatment in adults or generally well-appearing children (CDC, 2012c). The American College of Chest Physicians produced an extensive guideline regarding the management of acute and chronic cough with clear guidelines recommending antibiotic avoidance coupled with patient education (Irwin et al, 2006). Bronchitis requires antimicrobial therapy only if there is prolonged cough with a diagnosed etiology of a specific infection, such as *Bordetella pertussis* or *Mycoplasma pneumoniae* (Irwin et al, 2006). Penicillins are generally not appropriate for the infecting organisms in these complicated cases of bronchitis. During the common cold, mucopurulent rhinitis (thick, opaque, or discolored nasal discharge) is not an indication for antimicrobials unless it persists without improvement for more than 10 days, at which point the symptoms meet the criteria for acute bacterial sinusitis, discussed in depth in Chapter 47 (Chow et al, 2012; Wald et al, 2013).

Chronic Bronchitis

It is important to distinguish acute bronchitis from an acute bacterial exacerbation of chronic bronchitis (ABECB). Chronic bronchitis, a condition largely confined to smokers, is defined as a recurrent daily cough with sputum production that persists for at least 3 months in at least 2 consecutive years (Irwin et al, 2006). Patients with underlying chronic bronchitis may periodically become infected with a wide variety of organisms. The common organisms found in the sputum of patients with chronic bronchitis are most commonly viruses, as well as *H. influenzae, S. pneumoniae, M. pneumoniae,* and *M. catarrhalis* (Rabe et al, 2007). Throat swab with Gram's stain and culture are unreliable in these patients because the respiratory tract is normally colonized below the vocal cords. The decision to use antimicrobial drugs may be based on the presence of at least two of the three cardinal symptoms: increased sputum volume, increased sputum purulence, and increased dyspnea. A radiograph of the chest may be required to rule out bronchopneumonia. Recovery usually begins 3 to 4 days after antibiotics are initiated. Amoxicillin/clavulanic acid, macrolides, and double-strength sulfamethoxazole/trimethoprim are all appropriate first-line choices (Rabe et al, 2007). Resistant organisms require selection of an antibiotic agent based on susceptibilities. Patients who don't respond to first-line therapy should be treated with a respiratory fluoroquinolone (levofloxacin, moxifloxacin, gemifloxacin). The length of treatment is 7 to 14 days.

Otitis Media

Acute otitis media (AOM) is the most common indication for antibiotic prescribing in the United States and accounts for nearly half of all pediatric diagnoses and office visits. In assessing middle-ear symptoms, it is important to distinguish between AOM and otitis media with effusion (OME). The AAP revised the AOM Clinical Practice Guideline in 2013 to define AOM as: "moderate to severe tympanic membrane (TM) bulging or new-onset otorrhea not caused by acute otitis externa; or mild bulging of the TM and recent (less than 48 hours) onset of ear pain (holding, tugging, rubbing of the ear in a nonverbal child) or intense erythema of the TM" (Lieberthal et al, 2013). The new AAP practice guidelines state that AOM should not be diagnosed in children without evidence of middle ear effusion based on pneumatic otoscopy or tympanometry (Lieberthal et al, 2013). OME is the presence of fluid in the middle ear in the absence of signs or symptoms of acute illness. OME often follows resolution of AOM and may not abate for several months after the infection. Chapter 47 discusses AOM in more depth. Observation without use of antibiotics in a child older than 24 months of age with nonsevere AOM is an option (see Chap. 47). Mixed bacterial-viral etiology may be dectected in up to 96% of AOM cases diagnosed using strict microbiologic testing (Lieberthal et al, 2013). The most common bacterial pathogens present in AOM are *S. pneumonia,* nontypeable *H. influenzae,* and *M. catarrhalis.* Because the culture of AOM requires tympanocentesis, AOM is usually treated empirically.

Amoxicillin is the first-line drug of choice for AOM with initial doses of 875 mg twice daily or 500 mg 3 times daily for adults. The pediatric dose is 80 to 90 mg/kg/d in two or three divided doses (Lieberthal et al, 2013). Recent studies indicate that 83% to 87% of *S. pneumoniae* and 58% to 82% of *H. influenzae* isolates are susceptible to high-dose amoxicillin (Lieberthal et al, 2013). Coverage for beta-lactamase is recommended for patients who have been prescribed amoxicillin in the past 30 days, have concurrent purulent conjunctivitis, or have a history of recurrent AOM unresponsive to amoxicillin. Amoxicillin/clavulanate (90 mg/kg/d of amoxicillin and 6.4 mg/kg/d of clavulanate in two divided doses) is the drug of choice (Leiberthal et al, 2013).

If symptoms worsen or there is a failure to respond to appropriate therapy within 48 to 72 hours, reassessment of the diagnosis is indicated to exclude other causes of the illness and decide if an antibiotic change is necessary. In general, if high-dose amoxicillin was the initial choice, then amoxicillin/clavulanate should be tried before moving to a different drug class. Almost 100% of *M. catarrhalis* strains produce beta-lactamase but remain susceptible to amoxicillin/clavulanate (Leiberthal et al, 2013). The AAP practice guidelines recommend the length of treatment in children under 2 years of age or with severe AOM to be 10 days (Leiberthal et al, 2013). Children 2 years to 5 years of age with mild or moderate symptoms may be treated for 7 days, and children age 6 years and older with mild to moderate disease may be treated with a 5 to 7 day course. Perforated tympanic membrane requires at least 10 days of treatment with a combination of topical and oral antibiotic therapy.

Persistent OME after therapy for AOM is expected and does not require treatment. OME should be treated with antimicrobials only if bilateral effusions, accompanied by documented hearing loss, persist for 3 or more months; however, insertion of tympanostomy tubes may be more effective.

Sinusitis

Sinus inflammation can be a response to viruses, allergy, pollution, or other irritants. Viral rhinosinusitis is 20 to 200 times more common than bacterial sinusitis, which complicates 0.5% to 2% of cases of viral URI. Clinical diagnosis of acute bacterial sinusitis requires prolonged, nonspecific upper respiratory signs such as rhinosinusitis and cough without improvement for more than 10 days, or more severe upper respiratory signs and symptoms such as substantial fever, facial swelling, or maxillary tooth or facial pain (usually unilateral) (Chow et al, 2012; Wald et al, 2013). In children, the signs and symptoms are more subtle and difficult to diagnose. The CDC and AAP guidelines recommend not treating mucopurulent nasal discharge in children as a sinus infection until it has been present for at least 10 to 14 days, if there are severe symptoms such as fever great than 39°C, facial swelling, or pain (CDC, 2009a; Wald et al, 2013). Acute bacterial sinusitis is caused by the same pathogens as otitis media (*S. pneumoniae, H. influenzae, M. catarrhalis*) (Chow et al, 2012; Wald et al, 2013). Concerns with antibacterial resistance are similar to concerns with otitis media.

Amoxicillin is first-line therapy for sinusitis in children (Wald et al, 2013). Standard-dose (45 mg/kg/d divided in two doses) is first-line therapy for children 2 years or older who do not attend day care (Wald et al, 2013). In areas with greater than 10% pencillin-resistant *S. pneumoniae,* high-dose amoxicillin (80 to 90 mg/kg/d) is recommended (Wald et al, 2013). For children treated with antibiotics in the past 4 weeks, under 2 years of age, or with moderate to severe disease, high-dose amoxicillin-clavulanate (80 to 90 mg/kg/d of the amoxicillin component with 6.4 mg/kg/d of clavulanate in two divided doses with a maximum of 2 g per dose) is recommended for 10 days or until symptom-free for 7 days (Wald et al, 2013). Failure to respond within 72 hours to first-line therapy should prompt reassessment and a change in therapy should be considered. If amoxicillin was used, high-dose amoxicillin/clavulanate should be considered (Wald et al, 2013). Treatment of sinusitis in children is more fully described in Chapter 46.

First-line treatment for sinusitis in adults at low risk for resistance is amoxicillin/clavulanate (875 mg amoxicillin/ 125 mg clavulanate) for 5 to 7 days (Chow et al, 2012). In areas with greater than 10% pencillin-resistant *S. pneumoniae,* then high-dose amoxicillin/clavulanate (2 g orally twice daily) is recommended (Chow et al, 2012). Failure to respond within 3 to 5 days should prompt reassessment and a change in therapy should be considered. Antimicrobial drugs have little efficacy in treatment of chronic sinusitis. Sinusitis treatment is discussed in depth in Chapter 46.

Pharyngitis

Pharyngitis is usually caused by a virus, and concurrent rhinorrhea, cough, hoarseness, conjunctivitis, and diarrhea strongly suggest this etiology. Most bacterial pharyngitis is self-limiting and will subside without sequelae (AAP, 2012a; Shulman et al, 2012). The exception is that caused by group A beta-hemolytic streptococci (GABHS; *Streptococcus pyogenes*), which is associated with rheumatic fever if not treated (Shulman et al, 2012). The risk of rheumatic fever is now so rare in the United States that 3,000 to 4,000 patients with GABHS would need to be treated to prevent a single case

(Thomas, 2005). An antigen detection ("rapid strep") test should be used to confirm the diagnosis, with negative results confirmed by throat culture. Antibiotics have no effect on the clinical course of patients with negative cultures. Antibiotic therapy started within 9 days of onset will prevent rheumatic fever (AAP, 2012a; Shulman et al, 2012).

Treatment for GABHS pharyngitis is best managed with narrow-spectrum agents. Due to consistent susceptibility, penidcillin remains the first choice in both adults and children (AAP, 2012a; Shulman et al, 2012). Penicillin V 250 mg 2 to 3 times a day for children weighing less than 27 kg (60 lb) and 500 mg 2 to 3 times a day for patients weighing more than 27 kg, including adolescents and adults, is recommended (AAP, 2012a; Shulman et al, 2012). To prevent acute rheumatic fever, penicillin should be given for 10 days, even if the patient is afebrile and asymptomatic (AAP, 2012a). Treatment failure is more likely with oral penicillin than IM penicillin G benzathinc (AAP, 2012a). Due to the poor taste of the oral penicillin V solution, amoxicillin 50 mg/kg/d in one dose (maximum 1,000 mg/d) for 10 days may be used in children. If nonadherence is anticipated, penicillin G benzathine as a single IM dose of 1.2 million U for patients weighing greater than 27 kg, or 600,000 U for those under 27 kg, is recommended (AAP, 2012a; Shulman et al, 2012). For patients who are allergic to penicillin, first-generation cephalosporins (cephalexin) or a macrolide (clarithromycin, azithromycin) may be substituted.

Urinary Tract Infections

Urinary tract infections (UTIs) are responsible for 8.27 million (1.41 million men; 6.86 million women) office visits per year (Litwin & Saigal, 2007). *E. coli* is responsible for 85% of community-acquired UTIs and 50% of hospital-acquired UTIs. Empirical treatment with trimethoprim/sulfamethoxazole (TMP/SMX, Septra, Bactrim) or nitrofurantoin are the first-line choice when no complicating factors are present (Gupta et al, 2011). Amoxicillin-clavulanate for 3 to 7 days can be prescribed as therapy to patients who are allergic to first-line drugs (Gupta et al, 2011). Because of its safety profile, amoxicillin/clavulanate 500 mg twice daily for 3 to 5 days is an acceptable therapy for treating asymptomatic bacteriuria or UTI during pregnancy (Hooton & Stamm, 2010). Up to 25% to 70% of *E. coli* is resistant to amoxicillin; therefore, it should not be used as first-line therapy unless patient factors warrant its use.

Sexually Transmitted Infections

Because of beta-lactamase production by many strains of *N. gonorrhoeae,* penicillins no longer have a role in the treatment of gonococcal infections. However, *T. pallidum* retains susceptibility to natural penicillins, so recommended treatment for adults with primary, secondary, or latent syphilis of less than 1-year duration is one 2.4 million U dose of penicillin G benzathine IM (CDC, 2010e). If latent syphilis is over 1-year duration or of indeterminate duration, three doses at weekly intervals are required (CDC, 2010e). Because penicillin G benzathine does not attain adequate concentrations in the brain, neurosyphilis and congenital syphilis are treated with

IV penicillin G or IM penicillin G procaine (2.4 million U daily for 10 d) plus oral probenecid (1 g daily for 10 d). Pregnant women with chlamydial infections unable to tolerate erythromycin may be treated with amoxicillin (CDC, 2010e).

Skin and Tissue Infections

Amoxicillin/clavulanate is indicated as first-line therapy for prophylaxis of infection following animal bites, including cats, dogs, and humans (AAP, 2012d). It may also be used for infected post-operative or post-traumatic wounds. Oral penicillinase-resistant penicillins (dicloxacillin) are indicated for bullous impetigo caused by *S. aureus* and erysipelas of the extremities (Stevens et al, 2014). Penicillin V and penicillin G benzathine are used in the treatment of impetigo caused by group A streptococci. Wounds accompanied by sepsis and severe tissue involvement require hospitalization and IV treatment.

Pneumonia

Although the pattern of causal organisms in pneumonia varies by age and other risk factors (e.g., smoking, HIV, alcohol abuse, IV drug abuse, airway obstruction, use of corticosteroids), the most common pathogens in community-acquired pneumonia (CAP) are *S. pneumoniae, M. pneumoniae, Chlamydia pneumoniae, H. influenzae,* and *M. catarrhalis. M. pneumoniae* lack a cell wall and are naturally resistant to penicillins. Acquired resistance is common in strains of the other organisms that cause pneumonia, so oral or IM penicillin has a minimal role in the empirical treatment of pneumonia. High-dose amoxicillin (80 to 90 mg/kg/d) is recommended for previously healthy and immunized infants as well as preschool and older children with mild to moderate CAP (Bradley et al, 2011). Amoxicillin can be combined with a macrolide as an alternative to respiratory fluoroquinolones for CAP in adults. Management of pneumonia is fully described in Chapter 42.

Helicobacter Pylori Eradication

Antral gastritis and peptic ulcer of the stomach or duodenum are associated with colonization of *H. pylori;* 95% to 100% of duodenal ulcers are colonized by this organism. Once colonized, it remains in the body for life unless eradicated by antibiotics. Eradication of the organism decreases recurrence of ulcer and promotes resolution of gastritis. Although there are many treatment regimens for *H. pylori* eradication, treatment with amoxicillin 1 g given twice daily for 10 to 14 days in combination with two other drugs is standard therapy (Lew, 2009). Because there is greater than 90% eradication with 7-day therapy with these combinations, selective pressure for resistance and adverse effects are reduced by limiting therapy to 1 week. Other antimicrobials used in *H. pylori* eradication include clarithromycin, metronidazole, tetracycline, and bismuth subsalicylate. Some experts recommend *H. pylori* eradication prior to initiation of NSAIDs to prevent NSAID-induced peptic ulcers, but further research is needed to confirm the efficacy of this strategy. Further discussion of *H. pylori* eradication is found in Chapter 34, and four treatment protocols are found in Table 34-6.

Lyme Disease

Lyme disease is caused by *Borrelia burgdorferi* and other *Borrelia* species and is transmitted by tick bite. Diagnosis is primarily clinical, although serological testing of positive findings with an enzyme-linked immunosorbent assay (ELISA) and Western blot provide confirmatory evidence. According to the Infectious Disease Society of America (IDSA) guidelines, amoxicillin 500 mg 3 times daily for 14 to 21 days may be used in early stages of the disease, characterized by erythema chronicum migrans, isolated facial nerve paralysis, or arthritis (Wormser et al, 2006). Children younger than 8 years of age are treated with amoxicillin 50 mg/kg/d (maximum 500 mg/dose) for 14 to 21 days (Wormser et al, 2006; AAP, 2012e). Alternative treatments for the early stage include doxycycline, clarithromycin, or cefuroxime axetil.

Bacterial Endocarditis Prophylaxis

Antibiotic administration has traditionally been recommended for susceptible patients prior to certain oral, GI, and pulmonary invasive procedures when bacteria may be released into the circulation. A joint task force from the American College of Cardiology and the American Heart Association recently published a document that currently recommends therapy only for those with prosthetic heart valves, previous infective endocarditis, certain patients with congenital heart disease, and cardiac transplant patients with valve regurgitation who are undergoing dental procedures that involve manipulation of either gingival tissue or the periapical region of the teeth (Nishimura et al, 2008). Patients with congenital heart disease (CHD) who require prophylaxis include those with unrepaired cyanotic CHD, completely repaired CHD repaired with prosthetic material or device during the first 6 months after repair, and repaired CHD with residual effects at the site of the prosthetic patch or device (Nishimura et al, 2008). Amoxicillin (adults 2 g and children 50 mg/kg orally 1 h before procedure) and ampicillin (adults 2 g and children 50 mg/kg IM or IV within 30 min before procedure) should be used as first-line therapy. Penicillin-allergic patients should use cephalosporins (cefazolin, ceftriaxone, cephalexin), clindamycin, or the newer macrolides (azithromycin, clarithromycin) for prophylaxis (Nishimura et al, 2008).

Group B Streptococcal Disease Prevention

Sepsis caused by group B streptococci (GBS) is the leading cause of neonatal morbidity and mortality within the United States (AAP, 2012f; CDC, 2010d). The CDC guidelines recommend all pregnant women be screened for GBS vaginal and rectal colonization at 35 to 37 weeks of gestation (CDC, 2010d). Women who have had previous GBS isolation either via urine screen or who had a previous infant with invasive GBS do not need screening; they receive intrapartum antibiotic prophylaxis. At the time of labor or rupture of membranes, intrapartum antibiotic prophylaxis is given to all women who test positive for GBS and those with unknown culture results who have one or more risk factors (less than 37 weeks' gestation, rupture of membranes greater than 18 hours, intrapartum temperature, or intrapartum testing positive for GBS) (CDC, 2010d). For women undergoing testing while in preterm labor, prophylactic antibiotics are started while awaiting results. Prophylaxis is IV aqueous crystalline penicillin G 5 million U loading dose and 2.5 to 3 million U every 4 hours until delivery or IV ampicillin 2 g loading dose and then 1 g every 4 hours until delivery (CDC, 2010d). Table 24-3 presents the dosage schedule of penicillins for their common indications.

Rational Drug Selection

Indication

The first consideration in drug selection is whether antimicrobial therapy is indicated. Antibiotic therapy is indicated only when the benefits of therapy outweigh the costs and risks of treatment. For self-limiting infections, symptomatic and

supportive treatment, rather than antibiotic therapy, is recommended. If antibiotics are deemed necessary, empirical selection or definitive, culture-derived selection are both appropriate strategies (Table 24-4).

The first step with either method is identifying a clinical diagnosis. Collection of specimens for culture or laboratory testing follows the clinical diagnosis. For some infections, such as otitis media or pelvic inflammatory disease, specimens are not available without invasive procedures, so they are not usually obtained. Additionally, specimens for culture are not helpful if the site is commonly colonized, such as in acute exacerbation of chronic bronchitis. Microbiological testing is an important tool in the rational prescribing of antibiotics, although delay in obtaining results, misinterpretation of colonization as infection, quality control (mislabeling

Text continued on page 705

Table 24–3 ⚕ Dosage Schedule: Penicillins

Drug	Indications	Dosage Forms	Initial Dose	Maximal Dose and Maintanence Dose
Amoxicillin (Amoxil, Trimox, Polymox, Wymox, generic)	Antibacterial	Tablets: 500, 875 mg Tablets (chewable): 125, 200, 250 mg Capsules: 250, 500 mg Powder for oral suspension: 50 mg/mL (drops), 125 mg/5 mL, 250 mg/5 mL, 400 mg/5 mL	*Adults:* PO: 250–500 mg q8h, 875 mg q12h *Children >3 mo:* 25–50 mg/kg/d in divided doses *Children high dose:* 80–90 mg/kg/d in two divided doses	Maximal daily dose 4.5 g Duration of therapy depends on site of infection Continue treatment 5–14 d, depending on site of infection Suspensions retain potency after reconstitution for up to 14 d at room temperature or refrigerated, depending on manufacturer
	Exacerbation of chronic bronchitis		*Adults:* 500 mg tid	Usual duration of therapy 3–10 d
	Acute otitis media		*Adults:* 500 mg tid or 875 mg bid	Usual duration of therapy 5–7 d
			Children: 80–90 mg/kg/d in 2–3 divided doses	Usual duration of therapy 10 d
	Chlamydia and non-gonococcal urethritis or cervicitis		*Adults:* 500 mg tid	Usual duration of therapy 7 d
	H. pylori eradication in peptic ulcer disease		*Adults:* 1 g bid *Children:* 90 mg/kg/d in 2 divided doses	Given as part of three-drug regimen for 10–14 d
	Sinusitis		*Adults:* 500 mg tid or 875 mg bid	
			Children: 80–90 mg/kg/d in 2–3 divided doses	4 g/d in divided doses for patients at risk for DRSP
	Suspected resistant *S. pneumoniae* (DRSP)		*Children:* PO: 80–90 mg/kg/d divided into 2–3 doses	90 mg/kg/d doses for patients at risk for DRSP
	Endocarditis prophylaxis, preprocedural		*Adults:* 2 g 1 h before procedure *Children:* 50 mg/kg 1 h before procedure	
	Lyme disease		*Adults:* 500 mg tid for 14–21 d *Children:* 50 mg/kg/d for 14–21 d	
	Urinary tract infections, uncomplicated		*Pregnant women:* 500 mg tid for 7 d	

Continued

Table 24–3 ⊗ **Dosage Schedule: Penicillins—cont'd**

Drug	Indications	Dosage Forms	Initial Dose	Maximal Dose and Maintanence Dose
Amoxicillin and potassium clavulanate (Augmentin)	*Antibacterial*	Tablets: 250 mg amoxicillin/ 125 mg clavulanate 500 mg amoxicillin/125 mg clavulanate 875 mg amoxicillin/125 mg clavulanate Tablets (chewable): 125 mg amoxicillin/31.25 mg clavulanate (chewable): 200 mg amoxicillin/28.5 mg clavulanate (chewable): 250 mg amoxicillin/62.5 mg clavulanate (chewable): 400 mg amoxicillin/57 mg clavulanate	*Children >40 kg and adults:* PO: 250 mg amoxicillin and 62.5 mg clavulanate q8h for 7–10 d *Children <40 kg:* PO: 20–40 mg/kg/d amoxicillin component q8h for 7–10 d *or* 25 to 45 mg/kg/d amoxicillin component q12h. Use 200 mg/5mL or 400 mg/5 mL amoxicillin formulation or 200 mg or 400 mg chewable	Suspensions maintain potency after reconstitution for 10 d if refrigerated Less diarrhea if daily dose in bid therapy because of lower amount of clavulanate.
	Antibacterial, pneumonia, serious or resistant infections	Tablet, extended-release: 1,000 mg amoxicillin/ 62.5 mg clavulanate (Augmentin XR) Powder for oral suspension: 125 mg amoxicillin/ 31.25 mg clavulanate per 5 mL 200 mg amoxicillin/28.5 mg clavulanate per 5 mL 250 mg amoxicillin/62.5 mg clavulanate per 5 mL 400 mg amoxicillin/57 mg clavulanate per 5 mL Powder for oral suspension: 600 mg amoxicillin and 42.9 mg clavulanate (Augmentin ES)	*Children >40 kg and adults:* PO: 500 mg amoxicillin and 125 mg clavulanate q8h *or* 875 mg amoxicillin and 125 mg clavulanate q12h *Children ≥16 yr and adults:* Extended-release tablet = 2,000 mg q12h *Children <40 kg:* PO: 80–90 mg/kg/d of amoxicillin component, 7:1 bid formulation or ES-600 suspension	Pediatric dose equivalent to 70–90 mg/kg amoxicillin/d in 2–3 divided doses. Using 600 mg amoxicillin and 42.9 mg clavulanate/5 mL formulation bid decreases clavulanate-related diarrhea. NOTE: Children <40 kg should not receive the 250 mg film-coated tablets, which contain a higher dose of clavulanic acid than the 250 mg chewable tablets.
	Acute exacerbation of chronic bronchitis		*Adults:* 875/125 mg bid	Usual duration of therapy 10 d.
	Acute otitis media and sinusitis		*Adults:* 875/125 mg bid *Children:* 80–90 mg/kg/d of amoxicillin component with 6.4 mg of clavulanate	Usual duration of therapy 5–7 d. Do not exceed 6.4 mg clavulanate.
	Animal bites (excluding spider)		*Adults:* 875/125 mg bid or 500/125 mg tid	Usual duration of therapy 5 d. For penicillin allergy, clindamycin may be substituted.
Ampicillin (Polycillin, Principen, Totacillin)	Antibacterial	Capsules: 250, 500 mg Powder for oral suspension: 125 mg/5 mL (reconstituted), 250 mg/5 mL (reconstituted) Powder for injection: 125, 250, 500 mg, 1 g, 2 g	*Children ≥20 kg and adults:* PO: 250–500 mg q6h *Children <20 kg:* PO: 12.5–25 mg/kg q6h *or* 16.7–33.3 mg/kg q8h	Maximum dose: parenteral 14 g/d; oral 4 g/d Take on empty stomach Suspensions retain their potency after reconstitution for 7 d at room temperature or 14 d in refrigerator, depending on manufacturer
Ampicillin and sulbactam (Unasyn)	Antibacterial	Powder for injection: 1.5 g (1 g ampicillin/ 0.5 g sulbactam) 3 g (2 g ampicillin/1 g sulbactam)	*Adults:* IM: 1.5–3 g q6h *Children <12 yr:* IM: 300–600 mg/kg/d divided into three–four doses	After reconstitution, the IM solution loses potency in 1 h Equivalent to 1–2 g amoxicillin and 0.5–1 g sulbactam Off-label dosage for children. Equivalent to 200–400 mg/kg/d amoxicillin and 100–200 mg/kg/d sulbactam

Table 24–3 ⚕ Dosage Schedule: Penicillins—cont'd

Drug	Indications	Dosage Forms	Initial Dose	Maximal Dose and Maintanence Dose
Carbenicillin indanyl sodium (Geocillin)	UTI and prostatitis	Tablets: 382 mg	*Adults:* PO: 500–1,000 mg q6h	Not effective in severe renal impairment (creatinine clearance [CCr] <10 mL/min)
Cloxacillin sodium (Cloxapen)	Antibacterial	Capsules: 250, 500 mg Powder for oral solution: 125 mg/5 mL	*Children ≥20 kg and adults:* PO: 250–500 mg (base) q6h *Children <20 kg:* PO: 6.25–12.5 mg/kg (base) q6h	Maximum 6 g (base)/d Suspension stable 14 d in refrigerator. Shake suspension well before measuring. Take on empty stomach, preferably 1 h before meals.
Dicloxacillin sodium (Dynapen, Dycill, Pathocil)	Antibacterial Infections in cystic fibrosis patients	Capsules: 250, 500 mg	*Children ≥40 kg and adults:* PO: 125–500 mg q6h *Children <40 kg:* PO: 3.125–6.25 mg/kg (base) q6h *Children <40 kg:* PO: 12.5–25 mg/kg (base) q6h	Maximum adult dose 6 g (base)/d Shake suspension well before measuring Take on empty stomach, preferably 1 h before meals
Oxacillin (Bactocill, Prostaphlin)	Antibacterial	Capsules: 250, 500 mg Powder for oral solution: 250 mg/5 mL (reconstituted) Powder for injection: 250, 500 mg, 1 g, 2 g, 4 g	*Children ≥40 kg and adults:* PO: 500 mg–1 g (base) q4–6h IM: 250 mg–1 g (base) q4–6h *Children <40 kg:* PO: 12.5–25 mg/kg (base) q6h IM: 12.5–25 mg/kg (base) q6h *or* 16.7 mg/kg q4h	Maximum adult daily dose 6 g Take oral forms on empty stomach, preferably 1 h before meals After reconstitution, IM solution retains potency for 4 d at room temperature or 7 d if refrigerated After reconstitution, oral solution retains potency for 7 d at room temperature or 14 d if refrigerated
Penicillin G, benzathine (Bicillin L-A)	Prophylaxis for streptococcal infections in patient with rheumatic fever history	Injection: 300,000 U per mL in 10 mL vials 600,000 U per dose in 1 mL Tubex 1,200,000 U per dose in 2 mL Tubex 2,400,000 U per dose in 4 mL syringe	*Adults:* IM: 1,200,000 U q3–4wk *Children: >27 kg:* IM: 1,200,000 U q2–3wk *Children <27 kg:* 600,000 U q2–3wk	For deep IM use only into large muscle mass.
	Pharyngitis, group A streptococci		*Adolescents and adults:* IM: 1,200,000 U as single dose *Children >27 kg:* IM: 1.2 million U as single dose *Children <27 kg:* IM: 600,000 U as single dose	IV injection causes embolic or toxic reaction. Intra-arterial injection causes necrosis of extremity or organ, especially in children. Maximum daily adult dose 2,400,000 U. Inject at slow, steady rate to avoid blockage of the needle.
	Syphilis (primary, secondary, early latent)		*Adolescents and adults:* IM: 2,400,000 U as single dose *Children:* IM: 50,000 U/kg up to 2,400,000 units as single dose	
	Syphilis (late latent or latent of unknown duration)		*Adolescents and adults:* IM: 2,400,000 U weekly for 3 wk	

Continued

Table 24–3 ✂ **Dosage Schedule: Penicillins—cont'd**

Drug	Indications	Dosage Forms	Initial Dose	Maximal Dose and Maintanence Dose
			Children: IM: 50,000 U/kg weekly up to 2,400,000 U as single dose for 3 wk	
Penicillin G, procaine	*Antibacterial*	Injection: 600,000 U per dose in 1 mL Tubex 1,200,000 U per dose in 2 mL Tubex 2,400,000 U per dose in 4 mL disposable syringe	*Adults:* IM: 600,000– *1,200,000 U/d*	For deep IM use only into large muscle mass. After large doses, some patients may experience a CNS syndrome of transient anxiety, confusion, agitation, combativeness, depression, seizures, hallucinations, expressed fear of impending death.
	Neurosyphilis		*Adults:* IM: 2,400,000 U and 500 mg probenecid qid for 10–14 d	
	Congenital syphilis		*Children:* 50,000 U/kg/d for 10–14 d	
	Diphtheria		*Adults:* IM: 300,000–600,000 U/d as adjunct to diphtheria antitoxin	
	Rat bite fever		*Adults:* IM: 600,000 U every 12 h	
Penicillin G benzathine and procaine combined (Bicillin-CR)	Antibacterial	Injectable: 300,000 U (150,000 U of each) per dose in 10 mL vials 600,000 U (300,000 U of each) per dose in 1 mL Tubex 1,200,000 U (600,000 U of each) in 2 mL Tubex 2,400,000 U (1,200,000 U of each) in 4 mL syringe 1,200,000 U (900,000 U of benzathine and 300,000 U of procaine) per dose in 2 mL Tubex	*Children >27 kg and adults:* IM: 2,400,000 U as single dose *Children 14–27 kg:* IM: 900,000–1,200,000 U as single dose *Children <14 kg:* IM: 600,000 U as *single dose*	See comments for penicillin G benzathine and penicillin G procaine May be dosed with half of dose on day 1 and half on day 3 *For deep IM use only into large muscle mass* Continue until afebrile for 48 h
	Pneumococcal infections (excluding meningitis)		*Adults:* IM: 1,200,000 U every 2–3 d *Children:* IM: 600,000 U every 2–3 d	
Penicillin V (Beepen-VK, Betapen-VK, Ledercillin-VK, Pen Vee K, Veetids, V-Cillin K, generic)	Antibacterial	Tablets: 250, 500 mg Powder for oral solution: 125 mg/5 mL (reconstituted) 250 mg/5 mL (reconstituted)	*Adults and children >12 yr:* 125–500 mg q6h *Children <12 yr:* 2.5–8.3 mg/kg q6h *or* 5–16.7 mg/kg q8h	Use higher doses for moderate-severe infections and obese patients. Maximum adult dose 7.5 g/d.
	Continuous prophylaxis of streptococcal infection in patients with history of rheumatic heart disease		*Children >12 yr and adults:* 125–250 mg q12h	Solution retains potency for 14 d if refrigerated. Shake solution well before measuring.
	Pharyngitis (GABHS)		*Adults and children >27 kg:* 500 mg PO 2 to 3 times/d for 10 d *<27 kg (60 lb):* 250 mg PO 2 to 3 times/d for 10 d	Duration dependent on response. Treatment failures have occurred and retreatment may be necessary.
Piperacillin (Pipracil)	Antibacterial Urinary tract infection, uncomplicated		*Children >12 yr and adults:* IM: 3–4 g q4–6h *Adults:* IM: 1.5–2 g q6h or 3–4 g q12h	Maximum adult daily dose 24 g. CCr <40 mL/min requires reduced dosage and/or frequency. IM injection should not exceed 2 g per site.

DRSP = drug-resistant *Streptococcus pneumoniae*; GABHS = Group A beta hemolytic streptococcus.

Table 24–4   Steps in Antimicrobial Drug Selection

Step 1	Make clinical diagnosis
Step 2	Obtain cultures and/or specimens
Step 3	Make microbial diagnosis Results of culture and/or lab test *or* most likely pathogen, references
Step 4	Select drug Results of sensitivity *or* usual susceptibility

of the specimen or using the wrong procedure), and cost are disadvantages of routine culture and sensitivity (Kolmos & Little, 1999). Procedures such as the group A streptococci antigen test, urine dipsticks, and microscopy are widely used and have the advantages of moderate cost and immediate results. However, these rapid tests are rarely definitive and require confirmatory testing for a definitive diagnosis. With the empirical method, culture results can confirm the diagnosis and allow for adjustment of therapy.

The final two steps, making the microbial diagnosis and drug selection, differ for definitive and empirical therapy. In definitive therapy, the microbial diagnosis is based on valid and reliable tests such as culture or antigen assays, and drug selection is based on laboratory and susceptibility results. The goal of susceptibility testing is to identify susceptible antibiotics.

Susceptibility tests measure the in vitro concentration of the drug required to inhibit the growth of the organism (called the minimum inhibitory concentration [MIC]) or the concentration required to kill the organism (minimum bactericidal concentration [MBC]). The MBC is rarely used clinically. The MIC can be correlated with achievable concentrations at the site of infection (e.g. middle-ear fluid, serum, cerebrospinal fluid [CSF]).

The gold standard technique for susceptibility testing is the broth dilution method. This method consists of inoculating the organism into a series of liquid media containing increasing concentrations of the antibiotic. The MIC is the lowest concentration that inhibits growth. This technique is not widely used clinically and is usually reserved for reference laboratories or in research. The most common methods used clinically include the automated and disk diffusion methods. In the disk diffusion method, fibrous disks or strips containing specific drug concentrations are placed on agar plates incubated with the organism (Kirby-Bauer or E-test). After incubation, susceptibility is determined by the diameter of the visible area of growth inhibition around the disk or strip. In the automated method, a standardized inoculum of organism is placed into a machine that performs a technique similar to that of broth dilution described above. Sensitivity and resistance represent a continuum rather than a dichotomy. For example, *S. pneumoniae* strains are defined as penicillin-susceptible if the MIC is less than 0.1 mcg/mL, intermediate if the MIC is 0.1 mcg/mL to 1 mcg/mL, and resistant if the MIC is greater than 2 mcg/mL.

In empirical testing, the microbial diagnosis and drug regimen are determined based on epidemiological studies. References that compile and update these data annually or biannually include the *Sanford Guide to Antimicrobial Therapy*, the *Handbook of Antimicrobial Therapy*, periodic updates given in the biweekly *Medical Letter on Drugs and Therapeutics*, and material available on the CDC Web site at http://www.cdc.gov. These references identify the drug with the narrowest spectrum that covers the most likely microbiological pathogens for a specific clinical diagnosis. Clinicians should also consult local sources for local trends in susceptibility.

Allergy History

Allergy history may limit antimicrobial selection. References and guidelines usually provide alternative therapies when first-line therapies cannot be used.

Age, Pregnancy, and Genetic Factors

Age is important when using penicillins because most are renally eliminated. Neonates and elderly patients often have poor renal function and are more prone to drug toxicity. Highly protein-bound drugs such as sulfonamides and the penicillinase-resistant penicillins should be avoided in late pregnancy and neonates because these agents may displace bilirubin from plasma proteins of the newborn, causing kernicterus, a central nervous system (CNS) disorder.

Pregnancy contraindicates several classes of antibiotics, such as tetracyclines and fluoroquinolones, so aminopenicillins may be used for gravid women, even though another agent is the drug of choice.

For some drugs, genetic factors predispose patients to adverse effects. Pharmacogenomics are discussed in Chapter 8.

Site of Infection

The anatomical site of the infection affects drug selection, as well as dose, route, and duration of therapy. For example, penicillins enter CSF poorly, so a CNS infection may require a different agent, higher doses, IV and/or intraventricular administration, or prolonged therapy. When the meninges are inflamed, as in meningitis, penicillin attains higher concentrations in the CSF. By contrast, penicillins enter the respiratory tract in high concentrations, permitting single-dose or short-course therapy for susceptible organisms.

Immunocompromised Status

Bactericidal drugs, such as penicillins, may be preferred to bacteriostatic drugs in immunocompromised patients.

Affordability

Affordability is another consideration in drug selection. One reason amoxicillin is the preferred drug of choice for several common infections is its low cost combined with its high efficacy and long history of safe use. Oral amoxicillin and penicillin are on most $4 or reduced-cost generic plans at pharmacies.

Taste and Convenience

Taste is a significant factor in patient acceptance of a liquid product, affecting adherence to the prescribed regimen

(Steele, Thomas, & Begue, 2001). The use of amoxicillin suspension rather than penicillin V suspension for group A streptococcal infections is an example of drug selection based on taste and convenience. Steele and colleagues (2001) provide comparative ratings on antibiotic suspensions based on overall taste and adjusts them for cost. In all categories in this study, no antibiotic scored significantly higher than amoxicillin.

Convenience is largely a matter of the number of times per day that a drug must be taken. Amoxicillin requires two or three doses daily, whereas penicillin V requires two to four doses per day. Frequent dosing decreases compliance and may be particularly problematic when the patient is away from home, such as at work or in day care, especially when the drug requires refrigeration or cannot be taken with food.

Monitoring

Both microbiological and clinical responses are used to evaluate the therapeutic outcome of antimicrobial therapy. Serial cultures of specimens from infected sites become sterile with successful treatment. Follow-up cultures may detect superinfection or development of resistance. All patients with early or congenital syphilis should have a quantitative Venereal Disease Research Laboratory (VDRL) test at 6 and 12 months after therapy.

For most infections treated in outpatient settings, it is sufficient to monitor clinical response alone. Local signs of heat, redness, swelling, tenderness, or discharge usually abate after 48 to 72 hours. Specific indicators of improvement such as the resolution of pulmonary infiltrates and normalization of pulse oximetry in pneumonia are important outcomes to monitor. Systemic signs such as fever, malaise, and leukocytosis also improve. The patient should be advised to call the prescriber if there is no improvement in 48 to 72 hours, when consideration should be given to adjusting the treatment; alternatively, the provider can initiate telephone contact to evaluate progress and improvement. Compliance is monitored throughout the course of therapy, particularly if there is therapeutic failure, as well as after symptoms resolve and the patient is less motivated to complete the therapy.

Signs of allergic reactions may occur from minutes to weeks after the antibiotic is initiated and even after the course of therapy is completed. Although immediate hypersensitivity reactions are more likely to be life-threatening, delayed reactions can also be serious. Superinfection often presents with subtle and nonspecific symptoms such as mouth or throat pain (oral candidiasis) or perineal itching or discharge (vaginal candidiasis), so it is important to attend to these minor complaints. Distinguishing between antibiotic-associated diarrhea and CDI is at times difficult, but more than three watery, unformed stools per day or blood in the stool warrant stool testing to detect *C. difficile* toxin.

Other adverse effects are almost exclusively associated with high-dose parenteral therapy, protracted oral therapy, or impaired renal function. During parenteral therapy, periodic blood urea nitrogen (BUN) and creatinine determinations should be performed, especially with agents from the penicillinase-resistant group or the anti-pseudomonal group. However, many of the penicillins, especially amoxicillin, have a wide range of tolerance for renal impairment. Amoxicillin is an especially safe drug for the elderly, who commonly have decreased renal function. When amoxicillin is combined with a beta-lactamase inhibitor, closer monitoring is appropriate. Monitor serum potassium in patients receiving piperacillin, potassium penicillin G, or other parenteral agents. Patients with low potassium, especially if they are taking cytotoxic drugs or diuretics, can develop hypokalemia. Hyperkalemia has occurred with high doses of potassium penicillin G in patients with impaired renal function. The partial thromboplastin time (PTT) and prothrombin time (PT) should be assessed at baseline and during therapy with parenteral carbenicillin, piperacillin, or ticarcillin, particularly for patients with renal impairment.

Patient Education

Administration

The most critical information to provide to patients who will self-administer antibiotics is the importance of completing the full course of therapy. They should understand that failure to complete therapy may result in resistant infections that can be passed on to family and friends or cause the patient to become more seriously ill. Doses of the medication should be spaced as evenly as possible without sleep disruption throughout the 24 hours of a day. Missed doses should be taken as soon as they are remembered, but the dose should not be doubled.

Oral penicillins that should be taken on an empty stomach, 1 hour before a meal or 2 hours after meals, include ampicillin, carbenicillin, cloxacillin, oxacillin, nafcillin, and dicloxacillin. Chewable tablets must be crushed or chewed or the drug may not absorb adequately. Oral tablets and chewable tablets of amoxicillin/clavulanate have different clavulanate content and should not be considered interchangeable.

Many penicillins are available as solutions or suspensions. Suspensions must be shaken to disperse the particles of drug immediately before measurement. Refrigerated liquid formulations maintain full activity for 14 days after reconstitution, except amoxicillin/clavulanate suspension, which lasts for 10 days in the refrigerator. Amoxicillin suspension maintains full activity for 14 days whether refrigerated or not, although some manufacturers specify refrigerated storage. Instruct patients not to use antibiotics beyond the expiration date. Liquid formulations should always be dispensed with a calibrated measuring device. Because household teaspoons vary from 2 mL to 10 mL in volume, they are unreliable for medication measurement. Clinicians should tell the patient whether there will be liquid remaining at the end of the course of therapy and urge disposal of unused medication.

Very concentrated oral forms of amoxicillin (50 mg/mL) or ampicillin (100 mg/mL) in suspension are called antibiotic drops. It is important to explain that the drops are for oral use, describe how to measure and administer the medication appropriate to the patient's developmental and physical capabilities, and specify that an appropriate measuring device be used.

Medications mixed for injection also lose potency with time, although refrigeration after reconstitution will extend the period of full potency. Consult the package insert for proper mixing and storage of reconstituted parenteral penicillins. Some of these agents (e.g., piperacillin) can be prepared with lidocaine to decrease pain on IM injection. Adhere to the manufacturer's limits on volume of injection at one site. IM injection should be slow and steady, extended over 12 to 15 seconds to minimize pain and avoid blockage of the needle, especially with procaine and benzathine preparations that are very thick. Because IV extravasation of nafcillin causes tissue necrosis, IM injection should be avoided and a Z-track injection technique used if this route is unavoidable.

Adverse Reactions

Patients should be taught to distinguish allergic reactions from other adverse effects so that they can provide an accurate drug allergy history. Many patients claim penicillin allergy because they experienced diarrhea during therapy. Patients with immediate or type 1 allergies of the anaphylactic type should wear an identification bracelet.

If severe diarrhea occurs, the patient should contact the prescriber before initiating any treatment. For mild diarrhea, they can use adsorbent antidiarrheal agents containing attapulgite (e.g., Donnagel) but should avoid antiperistaltic agents that promote the retention of toxins.

Aminopenicillins and clavulanate cause false positives on glucose urine testing by the copper sulfate technique (Clinitest). Diabetics on these penicillins should use blood glucose monitoring or urine testing based on glucose enzymatic tests (Clinstix, TesTape).

Lifestyle Management

Mild infections, especially upper-respiratory tract infections, are often self-limiting and resolve with symptomatic treatment, rest, fluids, and nutritious diet. Prevention of infection by good hand washing, shunning crowded environments, avoiding cigarette smoke including passive smoke, practicing safe sex, and maintaining a generally healthy lifestyle will limit the need for antibiotics. Other risk-reduction counseling specific to otitis media includes breastfeeding of infants, avoidance of passive smoke, enrollment in day care with a small class size if day care is unavoidable, and pneumococcal and influenza vaccine (Lieberthal et al, 2013). Because pain has been shown to inhibit the immune system, comfort measures and pain management of patients with infections will promote the antibiotic action.

CEPHALOSPORINS

Cephalosporins are beta-lactam antibiotics, structurally and chemically related to the penicillins. Cefoxitin and cefotetan are actually cephamycins, and loracarbef (no longer available in the United States) is a carbacephem, but they are usually included with the cephalosporins because of their clinical and chemical similarity. The cephalosporin class of drugs is divided into five generations, based on the order of development and spectrum of antibacterial activity.

Pharmacodynamics
Spectrum of Activity

Cephalosporins inhibit mucopeptide synthesis in the bacterial cell wall, making the bacterium osmotically unstable. As with penicillins, cephalosporins inhibit PBPs involved in the cross-linking of peptidoglycans in the cell wall. Cephalosporins are usually bactericidal, depending on organism susceptibility, dose, tissue concentration, and the rate of organism multiplication. They are most effective against rapidly growing organisms forming cell walls and when antibiotic concentrations exceed the pathogen's MIC for at least 50% of the dosing interval.

First-Generation Cephalosporins

First-generation cephalosporins are active against gram-positive cocci, including *S. aureus* and *S. epidermidis* (excluding methicillin-resistant strains), and most streptococci; however, *Enterococcus* species are intrinsically resistant to cephalosporins. First-generation cephalosporins have limited activity against aerobic gram-negative organisms, such as *E. coli, P. mirabilis,* and *Klebsiella pneumonia.* In addition, they do not readily enter the CSF.

Second-Generation Cephalosporins and Cephamycins

Examples of second-generation cephalosporins include cefaclor, cefprozil, and cefuroxime. These are active against the same organisms as the first generation but with increased activity against *H. influenzae.* The cephamycins include cefotetan and cefoxitin. These antibiotics are unique: they have a similar spectrum of activity as first-generation cephalosporins, while adding limited activity against anaerobes, including *Bacteroides fragilis.* Each of the drugs listed as a second-generation cephalosporin has a slightly different spectrum of activity, so susceptibility tests for each must be performed, rather than assuming consistency within the group.

Third-Generation Cephalosporins

Third-generation cephalosporins have activity against streptococcal species, *Streptococcus pneumoniae*, MSSA, *H. influenzae* (including beta-lactamase producing strains), *Moraxella, N. gonorrhoeae, N. meningitidis, E. coli, Klebsiella, Proteus,* and *Salmonella.* Oral and IV agents have a similar spectrum; however, cefdinir and cefpodoxime have the best gram-positive activity. Parenteral third-generation cephalosporins available in the United States include cefotaxime, ceftazidime, and ceftriaxone. With the exception of ceftazidime, their spectrum of activity is similar. Ceftazidime has reduced gram-positive potency but has increased gram-negative activity to include *Pseudomonas aeruginosa.* Historically, third-generation cephalosporins have been active against uncommon gram-negative pathogens like *Serratia, Citrobacter,* and *Enterobacter*; however, the use of third-generation cephalosporins for these pathogens is discouraged secondary to the poor ability to detect inducible beta-lactamases that are capable of inactivating these cephalosporins. None of the third-generation cephalosporins have reliable activity against anaerobes, other than *Peptostreptococcus*.

Fourth-Generation Cephalosporin

The fourth-generation cephalosporin, cefepime (Maxipime), has a broader spectrum of activity and is more resistant to beta-lactamases that inactivate many third-generation agents. Cefepime is active against both gram-positive and gram-negative organisms, including *Pseudomonas* and extended-spectrum beta-lactamase producing strains of *Enterobacter, E. coli,* and *Klebsiella.*

Resistance

The most common mechanisms of resistance that bacteria express against cephalosporins are beta-lactamase production and altered target sites. All cephalosporins are stable in the presence of penicillinases produced by *S. aureus.* Most beta-lactamases produced by *Haemophilus* and *Moraxella* only affect the first-generation cephalosporins. Third- and fourth-generation cephalosporins are generally the most stable in the presence of most beta-lactamases produced by enteric gram-negative bacteria. Emergence of cephalosporinases and carbapenemases are of great concern.

Changes of PBPs that prevent all cephalosporins from binding to receptors are accountable for the resistance of MRSA, DRSP, *E. faecalis,* and *E. faecium.* Cefepime is active against most gram-positive and gram-negative pathogens, including resistant strains, with the exception of those listed previously (see Box 24-1).

Pharmacokinetics

Absorption and Distribution

Cephalosporins that have oral formulations are well absorbed from the GI tract. Except for cefadroxil and cefprozil, absorption is delayed by food, but the amount absorbed is not affected. The absorption of the oral ester prodrugs cefpodoxime proxetil and cefuroxime axetil is increased when given with food. All IM formulations are well absorbed from muscle tissue. Differences in bioavailability exist for the suspension and tablet formulations of both cefpodoxime proxetil and cefixime, so the formulations should not be substituted.

All cephalosporins are widely distributed to most tissues and fluids. Protein binding varies, but ceftriaxone is so highly bound to albumin that it should be avoided in neonates at risk for hyperbilirubinemia, especially preterm infants. The penetration of CSF varies by generation. Except for cefuroxime, first- and second-generation drugs do not readily enter the CSF, even when the meninges are inflamed. Third- and fourth-generation drugs and cefuroxime readily enter the CSF in the presence of meningeal inflammation. Therapeutic levels are reached in bone at usual doses for most cephalosporins, and they are used prophylactically and therapeutically in orthopedic disorders.

High concentrations of ceftriaxone are found in bile. Bile levels of cefazolin can exceed serum levels by up to 5 times in patients with obstructive biliary disease.

Metabolism and Excretion

In general, hepatic metabolism is not significant for cephalosporin drug elimination. A metabolite of cefotaxime increases its spectrum of activity and extends the dosing interval because of its prolonged metabolic half-life. Cefuroxime and cefpodoxime are prodrugs metabolized to active metabolites.

Most cephalosporins are excreted via the kidney in varying degrees as unchanged drug. Increased cephalosporin plasma concentrations may occur when probenecid blocks renal tubular secretion of cephalosporins. The combination of oral probenecid and cephalosporins is used in serious infections and single-dose therapy of sexually transmitted infections. Renal impairment significantly extends the half-life of these drugs. Ceftriaxone elimination is mainly extra-renal, making its half-life stable to changes in renal function. In hepatic dysfunction, the half-life and urinary excretion of ceftriaxone are increased.

Changes Related to Pregnancy and in Children

The pharmacokinetic properties of cephalosporins change during pregnancy, tending toward shorter half-lives, lower serum levels, larger volumes of distribution, and increased clearance.

In neonates, accumulation of these drugs because of immature renal function results in prolonged half-lives. Ceftriaxone is contraindicated in neonates younger than 28 days of age with hyperbilirubinemia because of the displacement of bilirubin from plasma albumin, leading to more free bilirubin and possible bilirubin encephalopathy. In children older than 3 months, higher doses of cefoxitin have been associated with increased incidence of eosinophilia and elevated AST. In children older than 6 months, ceftizoxime has been associated with transient elevated levels of AST, ALT, and CPK.

BOX 24–1   ANTI-MRSA CEPHALOSPORINS

Ceftaroline (Teflaro) is an injectable cephalosporin approved for complicated skin and soft tissue infections and CAP. Ceftaroline inhibits cell wall synthesis by binding to the modified PBP sites expressed by MRSA and penicillin-resistant *S. pneumoniae*. Gram-negative activity is similar to third-generation cephalosporins but does not include *Pseudomonas*. Ceftobiprole is an injectable cephalosporin that has activity against MRSA and pseudomonal species. Ceftobiprole was rejected by the FDA in 2009; however, clinical investigations continue.

Table 24-5 presents the pharmacokinetics of selected cephalosporins. Half-life alterations associated with end-stage renal disease are included.

Pharmacotherapeutics

Precautions and Contraindications

Like the penicillins, cephalosporins may produce hypersensitivity reactions in a small percentage of patients. Cross-sensitivity with penicillins increases the risk and occurs in 5% to 16% of patients. Cephalosporins are generally not recommended for those who have had a type 1 (immediate, anaphylactic) reaction to any penicillin. Skin testing is not helpful for identifying individuals likely to experience anaphylactic reactions to cephalosporins.

Renal function impairment significantly affects the half-life of most cephalosporins, and they may also be nephrotoxic. Use in the presence of markedly impaired renal function (creatinine clearance [CCr] 10 to 50 mL/min) is undertaken with extreme caution. Older adults and patients with known or suspected renal impairment are monitored carefully prior to and during therapy. Dosage adjustments of 50% are recommended for oral agents only after the glomerular filtration rate (GFR) reaches less than 10 mL/minute, a condition not usually seen in primary care patients. *Drug Facts and Comparisons* (2010) recommends titrated dosage adjustments for some cephalosporins for CCr less than 30 mL/minute. Dosage adjustments are usually not required based on renal function at higher levels.

Hepatic impairment is a concern for ceftriaxone. Caution is advised if daily doses exceed 4 g.

Cephalosporins are Pregnancy Category B; however, their use during pregnancy should always be based on a risk/benefit determination because relatively few controlled studies exist. All of these drugs cross the placenta, with maternal to fetal serum ratios of 0.16 to 1. Cefotetan, however, reaches therapeutic levels in cord blood (see discussion about pharmacokinetic changes in pregnancy).

Table 24–5 ⬛ Pharmacokinetics: Cephalosporins

Drug	Onset	Peak	Duration	Protein Binding	Bioavailability	Half-Life NRF/ESRD*	Elimination (% unchanged in urine)
First Generation							
Cefadroxil (PO)	Rapid	1.5–2 h	12–24 h	20%	90%	78–96 min/20–25 h	>80%
Cefazolin (IM)	Rapid	1–2 h	6–12 h	80%–86%	NA	90–120 min/3–7 h	60%–80%
Cephalexin (PO)	15–30 min	1 h	6–12 h	10%	UA	50–80 min/19–22 h	>95%
Second Generation							
Cefaclor (PO)	15 min	0.5–1 h	6–12 h	25%	>90%	35–54 min/2–3 h	60%–85%
Cefotetan (IM)	Rapid	1–3 h	12 h	88%–90%	0NA	180–276 min/13–35 h	51%–81%
Cefoxitin (IM)	Rapid	0.5 h	4–8 h	73%	NA	40–60 min/20 h	85%
Cefprozil (PO)	Rapid	1–2 h	12–24 h	36%	95%	78 min/5.2–5.9 h	60%
Cefuroxime (PO)	2–3 h	2 h	8–12 h	50%	40%–50%	80 min/16–22 h	66%–100%
(IM)	Rapid	15–60 min	6–12 h	50%	NA	80 min/16–22 h	66%–100%
Loracarbef (PO)	Rapid	0.5–1.2 h	12 h	25%	79%	60 min/32 h	>90%
Third Generation							
Cefdinir (PO)	Slow	2–4 h	UA	60%–70%	20–25%	100 min/16 h	12%–18%
Cefixime (PO)	15–30 min	2–6 h	25 h	65%	30%–50%	180–240 min/11.5 h	85%
Cefotaxime (IM)	Rapid	0.5 h	4–12 h	30%–40%	NA	60 min/3–11 h	60%
Cefpodoxime (PO)	Rapid	1 h	12 h	21%–29%	50%	120–180 min/9.8 h	85%
Ceftazidime (IM)	Rapid	1 h	6–12 h	<10%	NA	114–120 min/14–30 h	80%–90%
Ceftibuten (PO)	Rapid	2–3 h	24 h	65%	UA	144 min/13.4–22.3 h	70%
Ceftriaxone (IM)	Rapid	1–2 h	12–24 h	85%–95%	NA	348–522 min/15.7 h	33%–67%
Fourth Generation							
Cefepime (IM)	30 min	1–2 h	12 h	20%	NA	102–138 min/17–21 h	85%

ESRD = end-stage renal disease; NRF = normal renal function; UA = information unavailable; NA = not applicable.

Most cephalosporins are excreted in breast milk in small quantities. The average breast milk plasma ratio is 0.01 to 0.5 after 500 mg to 2 g doses. Cefdinir has not been detected in breast milk and ceftibuten has not been studied.

The safety and efficacy in children vary by drug. Safety and efficacy have not been established for children younger than 1 month for cefazolin, cefotaxime, and cefaclor; younger than 2 months for cefpodoxime; younger than 3 months for cefuroxime, cephapirin, and cefoxitin; younger than 6 months for cefdinir, loracarbef, cefixime, ceftizoxime, and cefprozil; younger than 9 months for oral cephradine; and younger than 1 year for cefepime and parenteral cephradine. Cefditoren is not approved for use in children younger than 12 years.

Adverse Drug Reactions

In addition to type I allergic reactions (see the Precautions and Contraindications section), serum sickness–like reactions, consisting of erythema multiforme, other skin rashes, arthralgia, and fever, have been reported. This type III delayed reaction usually occurs following a second course of therapy and may be delayed up to 10 or more days after initiation of the drug. Between 0.1% and 1% of patients who receive cefaclor have this reaction. Antihistamines and corticosteroids may help to manage symptoms.

Several parenteral cephalosporins have been associated with induction of seizure activity, especially in the presence of renal impairment when the dose was not adjusted. Discontinuance of the drug resolved the problem in most cases.

Coagulation abnormalities have occurred in conjunction with administration of parenteral cephalosporins containing a particular chemical group and include cefotetan. Patients at risk appear to be those with renal impairment, cancer, impaired vitamin K synthesis, low vitamin K stores, or malnutrition. These cephalosporins are also associated with a disulfiram-like reaction in patients who consume or, less frequently, inhale alcohol (such as aftershave or alcohol swabs).

Immune hemolytic anemia has also been observed with cephalosporins in rare instances. Patients who develop anemia within 2 to 3 weeks of the initiation of cephalosporin therapy should be evaluated for the role the cephalosporin may play in this disorder, and the drug should be stopped until the etiology is determined.

As with almost all antibiotics, CDI is a potentially serious adverse reaction to cephalosporins. Detection and management were described earlier. Use of cephalosporins, especially prolonged or repeated therapy, may result in bacterial or fungal overgrowth of nonsusceptible organisms. The patient should be monitored for this superinfection and treated with appropriate measures.

Incidence of non–*C. difficile* diarrhea is high with some oral cephalosporins, including cefdinir (16%), cefixime (16%), and cefpodoxime (7%). There have been reports with cefpodoxime of acute liver injury, bloody diarrhea, and pulmonary infiltrates with eosinophilia. Ceftriaxone has caused accumulation of biliary sludge or pseudolithiasis, which clears on discontinuation of the drug.

Drug Interactions

Table 24-6 shows specific drugs and their interactions. Drugs that interact with all cephalosporins include probenecid,

Table 24–6 ⦙⦙⦙ Drug Interactions: Cephalosporins

Drug	Interacting Drug	Possible Effect	Implications
All cephalosporins	Probenecid	Probenecid may increase and prolong cephalosporin plasma levels by competitively inhibiting renal tubular secretion.	Avoid concurrent administration unless planned for therapeutic reasons.
	Loop diuretics	Increased risk of nephrotoxicity.	Use with caution and monitor renal function.
	Warfarin	May increase effects of warfarin and increase bleeding risk.	Monitor INR.
Cefotetan	Ethanol Anticoagulants	Alcoholic beverages consumed concurrently or within 72 h after cefotetan may produce an acute disulfiram-like reaction within 30 min of alcohol ingestion. This reaction may occur ≤3 d after last antibiotic dose. Effects of anticoagulants may be increased. Bleeding complications may occur. This interaction is also reported with some other cephalosporins.	Warn patients to avoid concurrent ingestion of alcohol. Select a different antibiotic class for patients taking anticoagulants. If they must be given together, monitor PT more closely.
Cefaclor, cefdinir, cefpodoxime	Antacids	Extended-release tablets may have reduced plasma concentration when given with antacids.	If both must be given, separate administration by at least 2 h. Cefprozil and ceftibuten do not appear to be affected by antacids and may be substituted if appropriate.
Cefpodoxime, cefuroxime	Histamine$_2$ blockers	Plasma concentrations of the cephalosporin may be reduced by coadministration.	Cefaclor does not appear to be affected and may be substituted if appropriate.
Cefdinir	Iron supplements	Iron supplements and foods fortified with iron reduce absorption of cefdinir by 80% and 30%, respectively.	If iron must be taken, separate administration by 2 h. Iron-fortified infant formula has no effect.

which increases plasma levels of cephalosporins, and loop diuretics, which increase the risk for nephrotoxicity.

Clinical Use and Dosing

Exacerbation of Chronic Bronchitis

The common organisms found in the sputum of patients with COPD with acute exacerbation of chronic bronchitis are viruses—*H. influenzae, S. pneumoniae, M. pneumoniae,* and *M. catarrhalis.* The most common organism is *S. pneumoniae* (Rabe et al, 2007). Although penicillins are among the first-line agents to treat this disorder, oral cephalosporins are also useful in mild to moderate disease based on their activity against *S. pneumoniae, H. influenzae,* and *M. catarrhalis.* For severe disease, macrolides or respiratory fluoroquinolones have a broader spectrum that includes the likely organisms and is more effective against DRSP. When cephalosporins are used, treatment is continued for 5 to 10 days at dosages shown in Table 24-7.

Acute Otitis Media

Although amoxicillin is the recognized first-line drug of choice for otitis media (see discussion in the Clinical Use and Indications section for penicillins), cephalosporins play an important role in the management of this common infection. For therapeutic failures of amoxicillin, the AAP guidelines recommend amoxicillin/clavulanate and then ceftriaxone 50 mg/kg IM or IV once daily for 3 days (Lieberthal et al, 2013). For penicillin-allergic children, cefdinir (14 mg/kg/d in one or two doses), cefuroxime axetil (30 mg/kg/d in two divided doses), or high-dose cefpodoxime (10 mg/kg/d as one or two doses) may be prescribed (Lieberthal et al, 2013). The duration of therapy is 10 days for children younger than 2 years, and 7 days for children 2 to 5 years, and 5 to 7 days in children age 6 years or older with mild to moderate symptoms (Lieberthal et al, 2013). Ceftriaxone 50 mg/kg as a daily IM dose can be given (Lieberthal et al, 2013). Ceftriaxone is approved as a single injection for first-line therapy, but three daily doses are recommended for children who have recently failed therapy with another antimicrobial.

Sinusitis

The primary organisms involved in acute sinusitis are *S. pneumoniae* (31%), *H. influenzae* (21%), viruses (15%), anaerobes (6%), *S. aureus* (4%), *M. catarrhalis* (2%), and

Text continued on page 716

Table 24–7 ⬧ Dosage Schedule Cephalosporins

Drug	Indications	Dosage Forms	Initial Dose	Maximal Dose and Comments
		First Generation		
Cefadroxil (Duricef)*	Endocarditis prophylaxis	Capsules: 500 mg Tablets: 1 g Powder for oral suspension: 125 mg/5 mL, 250 mg/5 mL, 500 mg/5 mL	*Adults:* PO: 2 g 1 h prior to surgery *Children:* PO: 50 mg/kg 1 h prior to surgery	Maximum adult daily dose 4 g. Decrease dose frequency if CCr <25 mL/min.
	Pharyngitis/tonsillitis, impetigo (children)		*Adults:* PO: 500 mg q12h *or* 1 g once daily for 10 d *Children:* PO: 15 mg/kg q12h *or* 30 mg/kg once/d for 10 d	
	Skin and soft tissue infection		*Adults:* PO: 500 mg q12h *or* 1 g once daily *Children:* PO: 15 mg/kg q12h	
	Urinary tract infection, uncomplicated		*Adults:* PO: 500 mg–1 g q12h *or* 1–2 g once daily *Children:* PO: 15 mg/kg q12h	
Cefazolin (Kefzol, Ancef)*	Endocarditis prophylaxis	Powder for injection: 250 mg, 500 mg, 1 g	*Adults:* IM: 1 g 30 min prior to surgery *Children:* IM: 25 mg/kg 30 min prior to surgery	Maximum adult daily dose 6 g, although up to 12 g/d have been used in rare instances. Reconstituted IM solution stable for 24 h at room temperature and 10 d if refrigerated.
	Urinary tract infection, uncomplicated		*Adults:* IM: 1 g q12h	
	Antibacterial, mild to moderate infections		*Adults:* IM: 250 mg–1 g q6–8h *Children:* IM: 6.25–25 mg/kg q6h *or* 8.3–33.3 mg/kg q8h	

Continued

Table 24–7 ⊗ Dosage Schedule Cephalosporins—cont'd

Drug	Indications	Dosage Forms	Initial Dose	Maximal Dose and Comments
First Generation				
Cephalexin (Keftab, Keflex)	Antibacterial, mild to moderate infection	Capsules: 250 mg, 500 mg Tablets: 250 mg, 500 mg, 1 g	*Children: >40 kg and adults:* PO: 250–500 mg q6h *Children* PO: 25–50 mg/kg/d divided q6–8h	Adult maximum daily dose 4 g. If adult dose >4 g/d is needed, substitute parenteral therapy.
	Antibacterial, severe infection	Powder for oral suspension: 125 mg/5 mL, 250 mg/5 mL	*Children >40 kg and adults:* PO: 1 g q6h *Children:* 50–100 mg/kg/d divided q6–8 h	Shake suspension well before measuring.
	Endocarditis prophylaxis (off-label use)		*Children >40 kg and adults:* PO: 2 g as single dose 1 h prior to surgery *Children ≥1 yr:* PO: 50 mg/kg as single dose 1 h prior to surgery	Potency of suspension maintained after reconstitution for 14 d if refrigerated.
	Streptococcal pharyngitis, tonsillitis		*Children > 40 kg and adults:* PO: 500 mg q12h *Children ≥1 yr:* PO: 25–50 mg/kg/d divided q12 h	Dose adjustments may be necessary if CCl <50 mL/min.
	Cystitis, uncomplicated		*Adolescents >15 yr and adults:* 50 mg q12h for 7–14 d	Dose on higher range if patient is obese.
Second Generation				
Cefaclor (Ceclor)	Bacterial infections, pharyngitis, pneumonia, skin infections due to *S. aureus* or *S. pyogenes,* tonsillitis, or urinary tract infection	Capsules: 250 mg, 500 mg Tablets, extended-release: 500 mg Powder for oral suspension: 125 mg/5 mL, 187 mg/5 mL, 250 mg/5 mL, 375 mg/5 mL	*Adults:* PO: 250–500 mg q8h *or* 375–500 mg extended-release tablet q12h *Infants >1 mo:* PO: 6.7–13.4 mg/kg q8h *or* 10–20 mg/kg q12h 500 mg q8h or 500 mg q12h for extended-release form	Adult maximum dose 2 g/d, although 4 g/d have been used in rare cases. Dose adjustments for CCl <10 mL/min. Extended-release formulation should be taken with food and not crushed or chewed. Cefaclor extended-release 500 mg bid is equivalent to capsules 250 mg tid, but not to other formulations at doses of 500 mg tid. Shake suspension well before measuring. After reconstitution, the suspension maintains potency for 14 d if refrigerated.
	Acute exacerbation of chronic bronchitis			
Cefprozil (Cefzil)	Pharyngitis, tonsillitis	Tablets: 250 mg, 500 mg Powder for oral suspension: 125 mg/5 mL, 250 mg/5 mL	*Children >12 yr and adults:* PO: 500 mg q24h for 10 d *Children 2–12 yr:* PO: 15 mg/kg/d divided q12h *Children >12 yr and adults:* PO: 250–500 mg q12h for 10 d	
	Sinusitis, acute pneumonia			

Table 24–7 ⊗ **Dosage Schedule Cephalosporins—cont'd**

Drug	Indications	Dosage Forms	Initial Dose	Maximal Dose and Comments
			Second Generation	
	Skin and soft tissue infections Otitis media		*Children 6 mo–12 yr:* PO: 7.5–15 mg/kg q12h for 10 d *Children >12 yr and adults:* PO: 500 mg q12–24h for 10 d *Children 2–12 yr:* PO: 20 mg/kg q24h for 10 d *Children 6 mo–12 yr:* PO: 30 mg/kg q12h for 10 d *Children >12 yr and adults:* PO: 500 mg q24h for 10 d	
	Urinary tract infection			
Cefotetan (Cefotan)*	Bacterial infections, mild to moderate Urinary tract infections	Powder for injection: 1 g, 2 g	*Adults:* IM: 1–2 g q12h for 5–10 d *Adults:* IM: 500 mg q12h *or* 1–2 g q12–24h for 5–10 d	Lidocaine (0.5%–1%) without epinephrine can be used as diluent for preparing IM injection. Solutions maintain potency 24 h at room temperature, 96 h if refrigerated, and 1 wk if frozen. Dosage should be decreased if CCr <30 mL/min.
Cefuroxime axetil (Ceftin, Kefurox, Zinacef)*	Pharyngitis, sinusitis, tonsillitis Otitis media or impetigo Bronchitis, skin and soft tissue infections ABECB Lyme disease, early Pneumonia Urinary tract infection, uncomplicated	Tablets: 125, 250, 500 mg Suspension: 125 mg/5 mL, 250 mg/5 mL Powder for injection: 750 mg, 1.5 g	*Children >12 yr and adults:* PO: 250 mg bid for 10 d *Children 3 mo–12 yr:* PO: 10 mg/kg q12h for 10 d *Children 3 mo–12 yr:* PO: 30 mg/kg/d divided q12h up to 1,000 mg/d for 10 d *Children >12 yr and adults:* PO: 250–500 mg bid for 10 d 250 to 500 mg q12h *Children >12 yr and adults:* PO: 500 mg bid for 20 d 500 mg bid *Adults:* 125–250 mg for 7–10 d	Studies indicate 4-to 6-day treatment effective for group A streptococcal pharyngitis. Suspension is not as well absorbed as tablets. Oral forms should be taken with food to increase absorption. Suspension does not require refrigeration and maintains potency for 10 d after reconstitution. Single-dose packets for suspension can be mixed with 10 mL or more cold water; apple, grape, or orange juice; or lemonade. Mix and consume entire volume immediately. Low rating for palatability of suspension.

Continued

Table 24–7 ⚕ **Dosage Schedule Cephalosporins—cont'd**

Drug	Indications	Dosage Forms	Initial Dose	Maximal Dose and Comments
		Second Generation		
Cefdinir (Omnicef)	Sinusitis, otitis media	Capsules: 300 mg Oral suspension: 125 mg/5 mL	*Adults:* PO: 300 mg q12h *or* 600 mg q24h for 10 d *Children:* PO: 7 mg/kg q12h *or* 14 mg/kg q24h for 5–10 d	Dose reduction if CCl <30 mL/min
	Community-acquired pneumonia, skin and soft tissue infections		*Adults:* PO: 300 mg q12h *or* 600 mg q24h for 10 d *Children:* PO: 7 mg/kg q12h for 10 d	
	Pharyngitis, tonsillitis		*Adults:* PO: 300 mg q12h for 5–10 d *or* 600 mg q24h for 10 d *Children:* PO: 7 mg/kg q12h for 5–10 d *or* 14 mg/kg q24h for 10 d	
		Third Generation		
Cefixime (Suprax)*	Bronchitis, exacerbation; pharyngitis; tonsillitis; or urinary tract infection Gonorrhea, cervical, urethral, rectum	Tablets: 200 mg, 400 mg Powder for oral suspension: 100 g/5 mL	*Children >50 kg and adults:* PO: 400 mg q24h *Children 6 mo–12 yr, <50 kg:* PO: 4 mg/kg q12h *or* 8 mg/kg q24h *Adults:* PO: 400 mg as a single dose	Palatability of suspension rated high. Oral suspension results in higher blood level than tablets, so do not substitute tablets for suspension in otitis media. Shake suspension well before measuring. Refrigeration not required. After reconstitution, it maintains potency for 14 d at room temperature. Dosage reduction required if CCr <60 mL/min.
Cefotaxime (Claforan)*	Antibacterial, uncomplicated infection	Powder for injection: 500 mg, 1 g, 2 g	*Children >50 kg and adults:* IM: 1 g q12h *Children >1 mo <50 kg:* IM: 8.3–30 mg/kg q4h *or* 12.5–45 mg/kg q6h	After preparation, the solution retains potency for 12 h at room temperature and 5 d if refrigerated in syringe and 7 d if refrigerated in original container For pneumonia, only if MIC = 2 mcg/mL

Table 24–7 ✂ Dosage Schedule Cephalosporins—cont'd

Drug	Indications	Dosage Forms	Initial Dose	Maximal Dose and Comments
Third Generation				
Cefpodoxime proxetil (Vantin)	ABECB	Tablets: 100 mg, 200 mg Granules for suspension: 50 mg/5 mL, 100 mg/5 mL	*Adolescents and adults:* 200 mg q12h *Infants >6 mo and children:* 10 mg/kg/d divided q12h max 200 mg/dose	Palatability of suspension rated low. Shake suspension well before measuring.
	Sinusitis		*Adults:* PO: 100 mg q12h for 7 d *Children >12 yr and adults:* PO: 100 mg q12h for 5–10 d *Children 2 mo–12 yr:* PO: 5 mg/kg, up to 400 mg, q12h for 10 d	Take suspension with food or alone. Tablets should be taken with food.
	Urinary tract infection Pharyngitis, tonsillitis Otitis media Pneumonia, community acquired Skin and soft tissue infection		*Children 2 mo–12 yr:* PO: 10 mg/kg, up to 400 mg, q24h for 10 d *or* 5 mg/kg, up to 200 mg, q12h for 10 d *Children >12 yr and adults:* PO: 200 mg q12h for 14 d PO: 400 mg q12h for 7–14 d	After reconstitution, maintains potency for 14 d if refrigerated.
Ceftibuten (Cedax)*	Pharyngitis, tonsillitis	Capsules: 400 mg Powder for oral suspension: 90 mg/5 mL, 180 mg/5 mL	*Children >12 yr and adults:* PO: 400 mg q24h for 10 d *Children 6 mo–12 yr:* PO: 9 mg/kg q24h for 10 d	Maximal daily adult dose 400 mg. Renal impairment (CCr <50 mL/min) requires dosage decrease. Shake suspension well before measuring. Maintains potency for up to 14 d if refrigerated.
Ceftriaxone (Rocephin)	Gonorrhea, uncomplicated; chancroid Syphilis, early Pelvic inflammatory disease Epididymo-orchitis Gonococcal conjunctivitis Otitis media Skin and soft tissue infections All other serious infections Febrile neutropenia	Powder for injection: 250 mg, 500 mg, 1 g, 2 g	*Adolescents and adults:* IM: 250 mg as a single dose 1 g daily IM or IV for 10 d to 14 d 250 mg IM as a single dose 250 mg IM as a single dose 1 g IM as a single dose *Children:* IM: 50 mg/kg, up to 1 g, daily × 3 d *Children:* IM: 50–75 mg/kg q24h or 25–37.5 mg/kg q12h, up to 2 g/d	Maximal daily dose is 4 g for adults and 2 g for children (except meningitis is 4 g). Dose should not exceed 2 g/d in patients with both hepatic and renal impairment. After reconstitution, IM solution retains potency for 24 h at room temperature and 48–96 h if refrigerated. Yellow to amber discoloration does not affect potency. Must give with doxycycline 100 mg/d for 14 d. Must give with doxycycline 100 mg/d for 10 d. Adults only. Also saline lavage of eye.

Continued

Table 24–7 🎗 **Dosage Schedule Cephalosporins—cont'd**

Drug	Indications	Dosage Forms	Initial Dose	Maximal Dose and Comments
Fourth Generation				
Cefepime (Maxipime)	Complicated intra-abdominal infections	Injectable: 500 mg/ 15 mL vial, 1 g/15 mL vial, 2 g/15 mL vial	*Adults:* IM: 1–2 g q24h or 500 mg–1 g q12h *Children:* 80–100 mg/kg/d in 1–2 divided doses (max 4 g/d) *Children:* IM: 25–37.5 mg/kg q12h up to 2 g/d	Combine with metronidazole.
	Pneumonia		*Adults:* 2 g IV q8h *Children:* 50 mg/kg/dose q8h	
	Skin and skin structure infections, uncomplicated		*Adults:* 2 g IV q8–12h for 4 to 7 d *Adults:* 1–2 g q8–12h *Children:* 50 mg/kg/dose q12h for 10 d	
	Urinary tract infections		*Children:* 50 mg/kg/dose q12h for 10 d *Adults:* Mild to moderate 0.5 to 1 g q12h for 7 to 10 d Severe 2 g q12h for 10 d	

*Required dosage adjustments for renal impairment. Frequently it means extending the time between doses. If a drug must be used in the presence of renal impairment because there is no alternative, consult the package insert for specific dosage data.

group A streptococci (2%). Second- and third-generation cephalosporins are no longer recommended for empiric sinusitis due to variable rates of resistance (Chow et al, 2012). Children with type I penicillin allergy with severe sinusitis may be treated with a combination of cefixime and clindamycin (Wald et al, 2013).

Pharyngitis

Penicillin V is the drug of choice for treatment of pharyngitis caused by group A streptococci (AAP, 2012a). A narrow-spectrum first-generation cephalosporin (cephalexin or cefadroxil) is indicated as an alternative for this infection as a 10-day course of treatment (Shulman et al, 2012). The recommended pediatric dosage of cephalexin for this indication is 40 to 50 mg/kg/d divided every 12 hours. Adult dosage for cephalexin for streptococcal pharyngitis is 500 mg every 12 hours. Cefadroxil 30 mg/kg once daily may also be prescribed (Shulman et al, 2012). A small percentage (5% to 10%) of patients allergic to penicillins may also be allergic to cephalosporins (AAP, 2012a).

Urinary Tract Infection

The cephalosporins (cephalexin, cefpodoxime, cefixime) can be prescribed as second-line therapy to patients who are allergic to sulfa drugs or fluoroquinolones or as first-line treatment for women who are pregnant. Duration of therapy for cystitis-urethritis in adults is 3 days; uncomplicated pyelonephritis requires 14 days of treatment. Children require 10 days of therapy for UTI because it is difficult to distinguish cystitis and

pyelonephritis in young children. Cefpodoxime proxetil is used in adult dosages of 100 mg twice daily for urethritis-cystitis, 200 mg twice daily for pyelonephritis, and pediatric dosages of 10 mg/kg/day divided into two doses. Cefixime is used in adult dosages of 400 mg once daily for urethritis-cystitis and pyelonephritis; pediatric dosages are 8 mg/kg/d divided into two doses. Dosages of other agents for adults and children are listed in Table 24-7.

UTI is a common cause of unexplained fever in infants and young children aged 2 months to 2 years. In this population, diagnosis requires a culture obtained by catheterization. Febrile UTI is treated aggressively in infants and children, because fever is often an indication of pyelonephritis (Gaylord & Starr, 2009). Infants and children with febrile UTI should receive parenteral antibiotics for the first 24 hours or until afebrile. Ceftriaxone 50 to 75 mg/kg/day divided every 12 to 24 hours IV/IM is often used because of the convenience of 24-hour dosing. Another appropriate parenteral antibiotic choice is cefotaxime (50 to 200 mg/kg/d in divided doses every 6 to 8 hours). The treatment of UTIs is discussed in depth in Chapter 47.

Sexually Transmitted Infections

Ceftriaxone and cefixime are the recommended antibiotics for the treatment of cervicitis, urethritis, pharyngitis, and proctitis due to *N. gonorrhoeae* (CDC, 2007). Recommended adult dosages are ceftriaxone 250 mg IM or cefixime 400 mg orally, both as single doses (CDC, 2010e). Acceptable alternative parenteral treatments include ceftizoxime 500 mg IM;

or cefoxitin 2 g IM, administered with probenecid 1 g orally; or cefotaxime 500 mg IM (CDC, 2010e). An acceptable alternative single-dose oral therapy is cefpodoxime 400 mg or cefuroxime axetil 1 g (CDC, 2010e). Ceftriaxone 1 g IM or IV every 24 hours is used for disseminated gonococcal infections with cefotaxime (1 g IV every 8 h) or ceftizoxime (1 g IV every 8 h) as alternative regimens (CDC, 2010e). Because chlamydia is commonly associated with genital gonorrhea, azithromycin 1 g as a single dose or doxycycline 100 mg twice daily for 10 days should be prescribed concurrently (CDC, 2006a). Ceftriaxone is also used in the treatment of chancroid (250 mg as a single IM dose); early primary, secondary, or latent syphilis (1 g daily IM for 8 to 10 d); pelvic inflammatory disease (250 mg IM as a single dose plus doxycycline 100 mg daily for 14 d); epididymo-orchitis (250 mg IM as a single dose plus doxycycline 100 mg daily for 10 d); and gonococcal conjunctivitis in the adult (1 g IM as single dose plus saline lavage of eye) (CDC, 2006a, 2007). Treatment of STIs is discussed in depth in Chapter 44.

Skin and Tissue Infections

First-generation cephalosporins are first-line agents in the treatment of primary and secondary skin infections, including cellulitis, erysipelas, impetigo, traumatic wound infection, and surgical incision infection. The most commonly used drug is cephalexin (Stephens et al, 2014). Other first-line drugs include dicloxacillin, amoxicillin/clavulanate, and clindamycin (Stephens et al, 2014). Dosages are listed in Table 24-7.

Coverage for MRSA is indicated in areas of high prevalence or with high clinical suspicion. Antibiotics appropriate for MRSA include TMP-SMZ, doxycycline, or clindamycin, depending on local resistance patterns (Stephens et al, 2014). Cat bites, 80% of which become infected with *Pasteurella multocida* and/or *S. aureus,* can be treated with amoxicillin/clavulanate or cefuroxime axetil 500 mg twice daily. Cephalexin and other first-generation cephalosporins should not be used for cat bite infections.

Community-Acquired Pneumonia

Macrolides are the first-line treatment for CAP in adults (Mandell et al, 2007) and high-dose amoxicillin is the first-line treatment for CAP in children under age 5 years (Bradley et al, 2011). Cephalosporins (cefpodoxime, cefuroxime, or parenteral ceftriaxone followed by oral cefpodoxime) combined with a macrolide are used as alternative therapy to respiratory fluoroquinolones in adults with CAP (Mandell et al, 2007). Ceftriaxone (50 mg/kg in one daily dose) is appropriate therapy for 1 to 2 days in toxic-appearing children who may not be able to take oral antibiotics. Treatment of pneumonia is discussed in Chapter 42.

Other Uses

Although an off-label use, oral and parenteral first-generation cephalosporins are effective in dosages listed in Table 24-7 for endocarditis prophylaxis prior to surgery for patients with a history of rheumatic heart disease. Cefuroxime axetil in adult doses of 500 mg twice a day for 21 days is used in early Lyme disease characterized by erythema migrans. Ceftriaxone in adult doses of 2 g daily for 14 to 28 days has been used for facial nerve involvement and arthritis of Lyme disease.

Rational Drug Selection

The general principles of rational antimicrobial selection, using the definitive and empirical approaches, are presented in the section on penicillins. Because there is so much variability within each generation of the cephalosporins, sensitivity testing is valuable in drug selection. Selection of cephalosporins, like selection of any antimicrobial, is based on the organism that is present (in the definitive approach) or most likely present (in the empirical approach), site of infection, resistance patterns, adverse effects, pharmacokinetics, cost, and convenience.

The oral first-generation cephalosporins are interchangeable in terms of efficacy and safety. Parenteral cefazolin has good tissue penetration and is the drug of choice for surgical prophylaxis. Oral first-generation agents are good alternatives to penicillinase-resistant penicillins in the penicillin-allergic patient, unless the allergy is a type I hypersensitivity reaction. First-generation cephalosporins have the advantage of a fairly narrow spectrum and may be used by most penicillin-allergic individuals. An off-label use is endocarditis prophylaxis prior to surgical procedures.

Second-generation oral cephalosporins are slightly less active against gram-positive cocci than first-generation oral cephalosporins, so the latter are the preferred empirical treatment for skin and tissue infections. Cefaclor is more susceptible to beta-lactamases than other oral second-generation cephalosporins and is not recommended for the treatment of otitis media in current guidelines. Cefuroxime axetil has the most consistent activity of the second-generation cephalosporins against penicillin intermediate-resistant pneumococci and *H. influenzae.* Consequently, although all second-generation oral cephalosporins are approved for URIs, the resistance pattern favors cefuroxime axetil for oral therapy for otitis media unresponsive to amoxicillin, for sinusitis, and for pneumonia if *S. pneumoniae* is suspected. For other indications including UTIs, all second-generation agents have comparable efficacy.

Generic cefuroxime axetil is among the less expensive oral second-generation cephalosporins, but the suspension formulation has been rated one of the least palatable liquid preparations (Steele et al, 2001). Cefixime suspension was

---

On The Horizon — **CEFTOBIPROLE**

Ceftobiprole is a new fifth-generation cephalosporin active against MRSA, DRSP, and *Pseudomonas aeruginosa.* It is intended for use with skin and skin structure infection and for nosocomial pneumonia. It was originally submitted to the FDA in May 2007 for the treatment of complicated skin and skin structure infections. In 2010, the FDA requested further information and studies before approving **ceftobiprole**.

also low in cost and rated as moderate to high on palatability. With the exception of cefaclor, which requires three doses daily, the oral second-generation agents are dosed twice daily. Extended-release cefaclor (Ceclor-CD) has the advantages of twice-daily dosing and daily cost comparable to other second-generation cephalosporins. Cephalexin oral formulations are on most $4 or reduced-cost generic plans at pharmacies that offer these services.

Because of the enhanced beta-lactamase resistance and extended gram-negative spectrum of third-generation cephalosporins, agents in this class are indicated for infections where resistance is a major consideration, such as gonorrhea infections and resistant otitis media. Although the incidence of GI intolerance would be expected to be lower with single-dose IM ceftriaxone, diarrhea has been observed in up to 25% of patients who receive ceftriaxone for otitis media. Additionally, IM injections may be poorly accepted by children and their parents, so the convenience and improved compliance expected with ceftriaxone may be offset by these liabilities. Cefdinir and cefpodoxime proxetil are oral agents that share similar antibacterial activity. Cefixime and ceftibuten are much less active than cefpodoxime proxetil against pneumococci, are completely inactive against penicillin-resistant pneumococcal strains, and have poor activity against *S. aureus*. Cefixime and cefpodoxime proxetil are the most active oral agents against *N. gonorrhoeae*. Parenteral ceftriaxone and cefotaxime are effective against most resistant strains of pneumococcus and are used empirically in serious infections presumed to be caused by these strains. Because they cross the blood–brain barrier, third-generation parenteral cephalosporins are used to treat meningitis. Unfortunately, this class of drugs is commonly misused for infections that could be treated by a narrower-spectrum agent. Because of long half-lives, ceftriaxone, ceftibuten, and cefixime can be dosed once daily for most infections; cefpodoxime proxetil and cefdinir require two doses daily. Third-generation cephalosporins are expensive relative to other antimicrobials. The palatability of cefixime suspension was rated moderate to high, whereas cefpodoxime proxetil suspension had one of the lowest ratings of all suspensions tested (Steele et al, 2001).

Monitoring

Monitoring for therapeutic and adverse responses to antimicrobials requires clinical, microbiological, and laboratory data (see the Monitoring section for the penicillins).

Because the cephalosporins have a broad spectrum, signs and symptoms of *C. difficile* infection (CDI), as well as other superinfections, should be noted. Diarrhea is common with some cephalosporins and must be distinguished from CDI. Perform *C. difficile* testing if there are more than three watery, unformed stools per day or if there is blood in the stool. Although hemolytic anemia is rare with the cephalosporins, signs of tiredness or weakness, yellow skin, or yellow eyes require a red blood cell (RBC) count with indices. During prolonged therapy, periodic BUN and CCr determinations should be performed to evaluate renal

function. If the CCr indicates renal impairment, dosage should be decreased according to the schedule in the package insert or drug reference. Many older patients require dosage adjustment because of age-related decrements in renal function. Patients who are receiving protracted courses of cefotetan, a parenteral cephalosporin that may affect clotting, require baseline and periodic assessment of PT. Administration of exogenous vitamin K (phytonadione; AquaMephyton) may be necessary if the PT is prolonged. Patients receiving cefotetan should also be observed for disulfiram reaction (abdominal cramping, facial flushing, headache, hypotension, palpitations, shortness of breath, sweating, tachycardia, vomiting) if exposed to alcohol.

Patient Education

Administration

Emphasize to the patient or caregiver the importance of completing the entire course of antibiotic therapy. IM cephalosporins may be irritating and painful. Inject the medication deep into a large muscle mass and avoid repeated injection by initiating IV access for therapy requiring more than a few injections. Medications mixed for injection will lose potency with time, although refrigeration after reconstitution will usually extend the period of full potency. Consult the package insert for proper mixing and storage of reconstituted parenteral cephalosporins. Adhere to the manufacturers' limits on volume of injection at one site (see also Table 24-7).

Usually, oral cephalosporins can be taken with food or milk if they cause stomach irritation. Ceftibuten is the exception because it is poorly absorbed unless taken on an empty stomach; it should be taken 1 hour before or 2 hours after meals. Cefuroxime axetil, particularly the suspension formulation, and cefpodoxime proxetil should be taken with food to enhance absorption. Tablets and suspension formulations of cefuroxime axetil and cefixime should not be used interchangeably because they have different bioavailability. Cefuroxime tablets are more completely absorbed than the suspension; however, the suspension of cefixime is better absorbed than the tablets. Cefdinir must be taken 2 hours before or 1 hour after antacids that contain magnesium or aluminum, which impairs its absorption. Patients with phenylketonuria should avoid cefprozil, which contains phenylalanine.

Suspensions and antibiotic solutions must be shaken to disperse or dissolve particles of drug immediately before measurement. Adhere to the manufacturer's specifications for storage after reconstitution and advise the patient not to use the drug after the expiration date. Describe to the patient whether there will be liquid remaining at the end of the course of therapy and urge disposal of unused medication. Ask the pharmacist to dispense a measuring device with every liquid preparation.

Adverse Reactions

If severe diarrhea occurs, the patient should contact the prescriber before initiating any treatment. For mild diarrhea, adsorbent antidiarrheal agents containing attapulgite can be used, but antiperistaltic agents that would promote the retention of *C. difficile* toxins must be avoided.

Other signs and symptoms of adverse effects that patients should be advised to report include vaginal itching or discharge, sore mouth or throat, white patches on mucous membranes of the mouth, easy bruising or bleeding, altered urine output, yellow skin or eyes, or unusual lethargy commencing after the drug is started. Development of skin rash, aching joints, hives, or respiratory problems may signal allergic response and should also be reported. Cephalosporins cause false positives on urine testing for glucose when the copper sulfate technique (Clinitest) is used. Diabetics taking cephalosporins should use blood glucose monitoring or urine testing based on the glucose enzymatic tests (e.g., Clinstix, TesTape). Anorexia, epigastric pain, nausea, and vomiting in a patient taking a course of ceftriaxone may indicate development of biliary sludge or pseudolithiasis, which abates when the drug is discontinued.

Lifestyle Management

Practicing infection control and good health hygiene, such as safe sex practices and a healthy lifestyle, helps to prevent infections. Supportive nutrition, adequate rest, appropriate fluids, and comfort measures promote recovery from an infection. Maintaining a clean, dry wound site free of excess necrotic tissue and foreign bodies is essential to resolution of a wound infection and wound healing.

FLUOROQUINOLONES

The fluoroquinolones are synthetic, broad-spectrum antibiotics chemically related to the quinolone nalidixic acid (NegGram), a narrow-spectrum antibiotic used to treat UTIs. Fluoroquinolones are a newer class of antibiotics introduced in the 1980s. The fluoroquinolones are divided into the older group (ciprofloxacin [Cipro], norfloxacin [Noroxin], ofloxacin [Floxin]) and the newer group (gemifloxacin [Factive], levofloxacin [Levaquin], and moxifloxacin [Avelox]). The newer fluoroquinolones are often referred to as the respiratory fluoroquinolones, which is a reference to their activity against *S. pneumoniae*, not to drug distribution or limited treatment indications. Two newer fluoroquinolones have been withdrawn from the market because of adverse effects: trovafloxacin (Trovan) because of liver toxicity and gatifloxacin (Tequin) because of hypoglycemia and hyperglycemia. Sparfloxacin is no longer available in the United States. An ophthalmic solution of gatifloxacin (Zymar) is still available.

Pharmacodynamics

Fluoroquinolones are bactericidal through interference with enzymes required for the synthesis and repair of bacterial DNA. The addition of two chemical moieties, including a fluorine-containing group and a piperazine group, to the structure of the quinolone nalidixic acid resulted in the greatly enhanced antimicrobial efficacy of the fluoroquinolones. The fluorine molecule added to create the fluoroquinolones provides increased potency against gram-negative organisms and broadens the spectrum to include gram-positive organisms as well. The added piperazine moiety is responsible for the anti-pseudomonal activity of fluoroquinolones. Levofloxacin, the pure L-isomer of racemic ofloxacin, has a broader gram-positive spectrum than the racemate.

Fluoroquinolones inhibit bacterial topoisomerase II (DNA gyrase) and topoisomerase IV. Inhibition of DNA gyrase prevents the relaxation of positively supercoiled DNA that is required for normal transcription and replication. Inhibition of topoisomerase IV probably interferes with separation of replicated DNA into the daughter cells during replication.

Fluoroquinolones exhibit concentration-dependent killing, with the best predictor for clinical efficacy being the ratio of exposure to the drug, expressed as AUC to MIC. Achieving an AUC:MIC of less than 125 for gram-negative bacteria and less than 30 for gram-positive bacteria has been associated with clinical failures and the development of resistance.

Spectrum of Activity

Fluoroquinolones are notable for their extensive gram-negative activity against *E. coli, Klebsiella, Enterobacter, Campylobacter, Salmonella, Shigella, Proteus, Serratia, Haemophilus, N. gonorrhoeae, N. meningitidis, M. catarrhalis,* and many others. Only ciprofloxacin and levofloxacin have full activity against *P. aeruginosa.* All fluoroquinolones have some activity against gram-positive organisms; however, only the newer fluoroquinolones (gemifloxacin, levofloxacin, and moxifloxacin) have significantly more potent activity against *Staphylococcus, Enterococcus,* and *Streptococcus,* including DRSP. The fluoroquinolones are active against atypical organisms such as *Chlamydia, Legionella,* and *Mycoplasma* species. They have varying activity against *Mycobacterium* species. Moxifloxacin is the only fluoroquinolone with significant activity against anaerobic organisms.

Resistance

Resistance is mediated by mutations in the quinolone-binding region of the target enzyme or by a change in the permeability of the organism (Piddock, 1999). Many scientists and clinicians are concerned that overuse of these agents has already eroded the utility of this group of drugs. Resistance has been documented in community-acquired isolates of *Staphylococcus, Enterococcus, E. coli,* and *Pseudomonas.* The CDC no longer recommends fluoroquinolones in the treatment of gonorrhea because of resistance (CDC, 2007). Many areas can no longer use fluoroquinolones as empiric therapy for uncomplicated cystitis since *E. coli* resistance rates exceed 20%. Fluoroquinolone-resistant tuberculosis is associated with previous exposure to fluoroquinolones (Devasia et al, 2009). To prevent increased resistance, fluoroquinolones should not be used for upper and lower respiratory infections, skin and soft tissue infections, or urinary tract infections for which other inexpensive, safe, and narrower-spectrum drugs are still effective. Rather, fluoro-quinolones should be reserved for use when alternatives are costlier and more hazardous.

Pharmacokinetics

Absorption and Distribution

All drugs in this class are well absorbed after oral adminis-tration. Recommended dosing of intravenous and oral for-mulations typically yields similar serum concentrations, making oral therapy attractive for those patients with a func-tional GI tract. Food only marginally affects absorption of fluoroquinolones; however, norfloxacin is best absorbed on an empty stomach and ciprofloxacin absorption may be decreased when administered with dairy products. Divalent (calcium, magnesium, zinc) and trivalent (aluminum, iron) cations can bind to fluoroquinolones in the GI tract and significantly decrease drug absorption.

All drugs in this class are widely distributed, with high tissue and urinary levels. For most fluoroquinolones, tissue concentrations are usually higher than plasma concentra-tions. Plasma protein binding is variable. Fluoroquinolones are also found in saliva, nasal and bronchial secretions, sputum, bile, lymph, and peritoneal fluid. They cross the blood–brain barrier poorly into uninflamed meninges, but ciprofloxacin, levofloxacin, moxifloxacin, and ofloxacin penetrate to a moderate extent in the presence of inflam-mation. All appear to cross the placenta. Although ciprofloxacin and ofloxacin are known to enter breast milk, this property has not been adequately studied for other fluoroquinolones.

Metabolism and Excretion

The predominant route of elimination varies widely be-tween fluoroquinolones. Ofloxacin and levofloxacin have predominant renal excretion with minimal (less than 10%) metabolism. In contrast, nalidixic acid and moxifloxacin undergo extensive metabolism (greater than 35%). The other drugs undergo modest metabolism but have signifi-cant renal excretion as well. A few of them are also excreted in feces. Renal impairment results in increased half-lives of those patients with substantial excretion of unchanged drug. For patients with CCr of 50 mL/min or less, dosage adjust-ments are necessary for all fluoroquinolones, except for moxifloxacin. This is especially of concern with older adults, who are likely to have some degree of reduced renal func-tion. Table 24-8 lists the pharmacokinetics of selected oral fluoroquinolones.

Pharmacotherapeutics

Precautions and Contraindications

All of the fluoroquinolones have a Black-Box Warning re-garding the risk of tendon rupture and tendonitis. The risk is increased in older patients; in patients taking cortico-steroids; and patients with a heart, kidney, or lung trans-plant. An additional Black-Box Warning has been issued for all fluoroquinolones to avoid this class in patients with myasthenia gravis.

All fluoroquinolones produce a slight prolongation of the QTc interval. The increase is not considered to be clinically significant and is rarely reported in ciprofloxacin and lev-ofloxacin. Preexisting QTc prolongation or concurrent use

Table 24–8 ⚏ Pharmacokinetics: Fluoroquinolones

Drug	Onset	Peak	Duration	Protein Binding	Bioavailability	Half-Life*	Elimination
Ciprofloxacin	1 h	1–2 h	12–24 h	20%–40%	70%	3–6 h	40%–50% unchanged in urine; remainder in feces
Gemifloxacin	Rapid	0.5–2 h	24 h	60%–70%	71%	7 h	36% unchanged in urine; 61% in feces
Levofloxacin	Rapid	1–2 h	24 h	24%–38%	99%	6–8 h	87% unchanged in urine; eliminated by tubular secretion
Lomefloxacin	Rapid	1.5 h	12–24 h	10%	95%–98%	6–8 h	60%–80% unchanged in urine; 5% metabolized; 28%–30% biliary excretion
Moxifloxacin	Rapid	1–3 h	24 h	30%–50%	90%	11–16 h	20% unchanged in urine; 52% hepatically cleared, and 25% in feces
Norfloxacin	Rapid	2–3 h	12 h	10%–15%	30%–40%	6.5 h	30% unchanged in urine; 30% in feces; 10% metabolized by liver
Ofloxacin	Rapid	1–2 h	12 h	20%–25%	89%	5–7 h	70%–80% unchanged in urine

*Half-life is increased in renal impairment and dosage adjustments may be needed.

of other drugs producing this cardiac conduction change produces additive effects with the fluoroquinolones.

Cautious use is required for patients with renal impairment. Dosage adjustments of all fluoroquinolones except moxifloxacin are needed for patients with impaired renal function. Seizures, increased intracranial pressure, and toxic psychoses have occurred with fluoroquinolones. CNS stimulation, including tremors, restlessness, sleeplessness, tiredness, dizziness, light-headedness, bad dreams, confusion, and hallucinations, may also occur. These symptoms are dose-dependent and tend to resolve with continued use. Some studies indicate fluoroquinolones inhibit bonding of gamma-aminobutyric acid (GABA) to its receptor, which may be the mechanism of CNS stimulation. Slight decreases in magnesium concentration amplify the effect (*Sanford Guide*, 2010). Patients with known or suspected CNS disorders and other factors that predispose to seizures should use these agents with caution and careful monitoring.

Older adults and dialysis patients have increased risk of tendon rupture and adverse CNS reactions. Use fluoroquinolones cautiously with these populations.

Hepatitis, hepatonecrosis, and liver failure have been observed with fluoroquinolones. Drug discontinuation should occur at the first sign of jaundice.

Fluoroquinolones are Pregnancy Category C. Use is not recommended in pregnant women because there are no adequate, well-controlled studies in this population, and teratogenesis has been demonstrated in animals. Use during pregnancy only if there is a clear benefit that justifies the risk to the fetus.

Norfloxacin is not detected in breast milk following a 20 mg dose to nursing mothers; however, this dose is much lower than recommended. Ciprofloxacin is excreted in breast milk, but the dose ingested by the infant is small. Concentration of ofloxacin in breast milk is similar to maternal plasma, and it is presumed that its L-isomer, levofloxacin, also enters breast milk. Moxifloxacin is excreted in the breast milk of rats, but the drug has not been studied in humans. Because fluoroquinolones have caused cartilage lesions on weight-bearing joints in young animals, lactating women should use fluoroquinolones only if there is no safer alternative.

Fluoroquinolones are not recommended for children younger than 18 years. Arthropathy and osteochondrosis have been demonstrated in all species of immature animals tested. Nalidixic acid, norfloxacin, and ciprofloxacin have been used in children without evidence of arthropathy or osteochondrosis, but these three agents have poorer tissue penetration than other fluoroquinolones.

The only indications for which a fluoroquinolone is licensed by the FDA for use in patients younger than 18 years are complicated urinary tract infections, pyelonephritis, and post-exposure treatment for inhalation anthrax. The AAP (2006) recommends that the systemic use of fluoroquinolones in children should be restricted to situations in which there is no safe and effective alternative to treat an infection caused by multidrug-resistant bacteria or to provide oral therapy when parenteral therapy is not feasible and no other effective oral agent is available.

Adverse Drug Reactions

CDI has been reported with nearly all antibacterial agents, including fluoroquinolones, and may be mild to life-threatening. It is important to consider this diagnosis in patients who present with diarrhea subsequent to administration of fluoroquinolones, especially if this diarrhea contains blood, pus, or mucus. Other common GI adverse reactions include abdominal pain, nausea, and altered taste, which are the most frequent adverse drug reactions.

Serious and occasionally fatal hypersensitivity reactions, including Stevens–Johnson syndrome, have occurred with fluoroquinolones. Some of the reactions occur following the first dose, presumably due to cross-allergy with other chemicals in the environment. Reactions that are anaphylactic in nature have also occurred.

Phototoxicity has been observed with all fluoroquinolones. Clinical manifestations range from mild erythema to severe bullous eruptions in the sun-exposed areas.

Use of fluoroquinolones, especially in prolonged or repeated therapy, may result in bacterial or fungal overgrowth of nonsusceptible organisms. The patient should be monitored for this superinfection and treated with appropriate measures.

Cardiovascular adverse reactions, including angina, atrial flutter, cardiopulmonary arrest, cerebral thrombosis, myocardial infarction, and ventricular ectopy, have rarely been reported. CNS symptoms such as sleep disorders, nervousness, and vertigo have also been observed uncommonly for this drug class. Fluoroquinolones have increased or decreased blood sugar in diabetics.

Rarely, fluoroquinolones are associated with acute renal failure, typically acute interstitial nephritis. Crystalluria has been reported with ciprofloxacin and other fluoroquinolones, especially in patients with alkaline urine (pH greater than 7). Ciprofloxacin has been associated with acidosis, polyuria, urinary retention, and renal calculi.

Fluoroquinolone tendinitis begins with inflammatory edema that manifests as painful and swollen tendons that are bilateral in 50% of cases. Failure to take appropriate measures to rest the tendon can result in rupture. The time from initiation of the drug to onset of tendinitis has varied from 1 week up to months after treatment (Stahlmann & Lode, 2010). The elderly are at high risk of developing tendon rupture (Stahlmann & Lode, 2010). This condition has led to a Black-Box Warning regarding the risk of tendonitis and tendon rupture with the use of fluoroquinolones.

Ophthalmological abnormalities are extremely rare but include cataracts and multiple punctate lenticular opacities. A causal relationship has not been clearly established.

Additional adverse reactions are listed in the Precautions and Contraindications section.

Drug Interactions

Table 24-9 shows the various drug interactions. Several drugs interact with this class to decrease their absorption. Some

Table 24–9 ⠿ Drug Interactions: Fluoroquinolones

Drug	Interacting Drug	Possible Effect	Implications
All fluoroquinolones	Antacids, bismuth subsalicylate, calcium, iron salts, magnesium, sucralfate, sevalamer, zinc salts	Interfere with GI absorption of the fluoroquinolone, resulting in decreased serum levels	Avoid simultaneous use; administer antacids 2–4 h before or after the fluoroquinolone
	Antidiabetic drugs	Increase or decrease blood sugar	Carefully monitor blood sugar
	Class 1 and 3 antiarrhythmics: Amiodarone, disopyramide, quinidine, bepridil, sotalol, all drugs that cause QT prolongation	Increased risk of serious adverse cardiovascular effects and fatal arrhythmias	Select different antibiotic
	Glucocorticoids	Concurrent use may increase risk for tendon rupture	Select different antibiotic
	Warfarin	Effects of anticoagulant may be increased	Monitor PT/INR
Ciprofloxacin	Caffeine	Total body clearance of caffeine reduced, with possible increased pharmacological effects	Monitor for increased blood pressure or CNS excitability
	Phenytoin	Phenytoin levels may be increased or decreased	Monitor phenytoin levels
	Probenecid	Renal clearance of ciprofloxacin reduced 50%; serum concentrations increased 50%	Avoid concurrent use
	Theophylline	Decreased clearance, increased plasma levels, and toxicity of theophylline have occurred with concurrent use of ciprofloxacin and enoxacin	Select different antibiotic or monitor theophylline levels
Levofloxacin	NSAIDs	Concurrent use increases CNS stimulation and seizures	Avoid concurrent use
Moxifloxacin	Rifampin	Rifampin may decrease moxifloxacin exposure by 31%	Use with caution
Norfloxacin	Caffeine	Total body clearance of caffeine reduced, with possible increased pharmacological effects	Ofloxacin does not appear to affect caffeine
	Cyclosporine	Nephrotoxic effects increased	Monitor renal function
	Nitrofurantoin	Antibacterial effect of norfloxacin in urinary tract may be antagonized	Avoid concurrent use

INR = international normalized ratio; PT = prothrombin time.

fluoroquinolones weakly inhibit drug metabolism by cytochrome P450 (CYP) 3A4, one of the most important enzymes in hepatic drug metabolism. Ciprofloxacin inhibits drug metabolism by CYP 1A2, which increases drug levels of caffeine, zolpidem, olanzapine, clozapine, and several other drugs. Cyclosporine's nephrotoxic effects are increased by concurrent administration with norfloxacin. Warfarin has increased effects when administered to a patient receiving a fluoroquinolone.

Food may decrease the absorption of norfloxacin. Food delays the absorption of ciprofloxacin, although total absorption is not changed. Dairy products reduce the absorption of ciprofloxacin and should not be used concurrently. Antacids, bismuth subsalicylate, iron salts, sevalamer, sucralfate, and zinc salts form an insoluble chelate with fluoroquinolones, preventing the absorption of the antimicrobial drug.

Clinical Use and Dosing

Exacerbations of Chronic Bronchitis

Because culture and sensitivity in patients with chronic bronchitis are unreliable due to bronchial colonization, empirical therapy is selected to cover the most likely pathogens. The primary organisms are viruses (20% to 50%), *C. pneumoniae* (5%), and *M. pneumoniae* (less than 1%). The treatment of

ABECB is described in the Clinical Use and Indications section for penicillins. Patients with moderate exacerbation who may require hospitalization or who do not respond to first-line therapy should be treated with a respiratory fluoroquinolone (levofloxacin, moxifloxacin, gemifloxacin), using dosages summarized in Table 24-10. Treatment of ABECB is discussed in Chapter 30.

Community-Acquired Pneumonia

In dosages listed in Table 24-10, fluoroquinolones with enhanced gram-positive activity, such as levofloxacin, moxifloxacin, and gemifloxacin, are active against strains of *S. pneumoniae*. In addition, fluoroquinolones cover *Legionella*, as well as *M. pneumoniae* and *C. pneumoniae*, which are the most common pathogens in patients with CAP without comorbidity. These atypical organisms are resistant to beta-lactam antibiotics but susceptible to macrolides. A respiratory fluoroquinolone such as moxifloxacin, gemifloxacin, or levofloxacin is used as first-line therapy when there are comorbidities, such as chronic heart, lung, liver, or renal disease; diabetes mellitus; alcoholism; malignancies; asplenia; immunosuppressing conditions or use of immunosuppressing drugs; or other risk for DRSP infection, such as use of antimicrobials within the

Table 24–10 ⊗ Dosage Schedule: Fluoroquinolones

Drug	Indications	Dosage Forms	Initial Adult Dose	Maintanence Dose
Ciprofloxacin (Cipro)	Bone and joint infections	Tablets: 100, 250, 500, 750 mg,	PO: 500–750 mg q12h for at least 4–6 wk	Maximal adult daily dose 1.5 g
	Bacterial diarrhea	Tablets: 500 mg extended-release	PO: 500 mg q12h for 1–3 days *Adults:* PO 500 mg q12h × 60 d post-exposure	Renal impairment (CCr <50 mL/min) requires dosage reduction
	Inhalation anthrax	Powder for oral suspension:	*Children:* PO 15 mg/kg/dose q12h × 60 d post-exposure	Use higher range of dosing for severely ill or obese patients
	Intra-abdominal infections	250 mg/5 mL, 500 mg/ 5 mL	PO: 500–750 mg q12h for 7–14 d in combination with oral metronidazole	Not recommended for children, but doses of 10–20 mg/kg q12h have been used where no alternative existed
	Meningococcal carrier		500 mg as a single dose	Oral suspension stable for 14 d at room temperature or in refrigerator
	Prostatitis		500 mg q12h for 28 d	
	Sinusitis		PO: 500 mg q12h 10 d	
	Typhoid fever		PO: 500 mg q12h for 10 d	Shake suspension well before measuring
	Skin and soft tissue infections		500–750 mg q12h for 7–14 d	Take with full glass of water
	Urinary tract infection: acute, uncomplicated cystitis, severe or complicated		250–500 mg q12h for 3 d *Adults:* 500 mg q12h for 7–14 d *Children:* 20–40 mg/kg/d divided q12h (max 2 g/d)	Oral and parenteral routes are bioequivalent
(Ciloxan)	Bacterial conjunctivitis		Ophthalmic solution: >1 yr: 1–2 drops every 2 h while awake for 2 d, then 1–2 drops qid while awake for 5 d	
Gemifloxacin (Factive)	Bronchitis, acute exacerbation of chronic Community-acquired pneumonia	Tablet: 320 mg	PO: 320 mg q 24 h for 5 d	Not studied in ages less than 18 yr
Gatifloxacin (Zymar)	Bacterial conjunctivitis		Ophthalmic solution: >1 yr: 1 drop every 2 h while awake for 2 d, then 1 drop qid while awake for 5 d	
Levofloxacin (Levaquin)	Bronchitis, acute exacerbation of chronic	Tablets: 250, 500, 750 mg	500 mg q24h for 7 d	Not recommended for use by children
	Community-acquired pneumonia		750 mg q24h for 5 d	Renal impairment (CCr <50 mL/min) requires dosage reduction
	Sinusitis		750 mg q24h for 5 d 500 mg q24h for 7–10 d	Take with full glass of water
	Skin and soft tissue infection		250 mg q 24 h for 3 d	Oral and parenteral routes are bioequivalent and interchangeable
	Urinary tract infection: uncomplicated cystitis, complicated or pyelonephritis prostatitis		750 mg q 24 h for 5–14 d 750 mg q24h for 4 wk	Can use oral or injectable form
(Quixin)	Bacterial conjunctivitis		Ophthalmic solution: >1 yr: 1 drop every 2 h while awake for 2 d, then 1 drop qid while awake for 5 d	
Lomefloxacin (Maxaquin)	Bronchitis, bacterial exacerbation	Tablets: 400 mg	400 mg daily for 10 d	Not recommended for use by children
	Urinary tract infection, complicated; uncomplicated due to *E. coli,* uncomplicated due to *P. mirabilis, K. pneumoniae, S. saprophyticus*		400 mg daily for 14 d 400 mg daily for 3 d 400 mg daily for 10 d	Renal impairment (CCr <40 mL/min) requires dosage reduction Take with full glass of water with or without food
Moxifloxacin (Avelox)	Acute sinusitis	Tablets: 400 mg	400 mg daily for 10 d	Not for use by children
	Acute exacerbation of chronic bronchitis		400 mg daily for 5 d	Duration dependent on organism
	Community-acquired pneumonia		400 mg daily for 10 d	

Continued

Table 24–10 🕮 **Dosage Schedule: Fluoroquinolones—cont'd**

Drug	Indications	Dosage Forms	Initial Adult Dose	Maintanence Dose
(Vigamox or Moxeza)	Bacterial conjunctivitis		Ophthalmic solution: >1 yr: 1 drop tid for 7 d	
Norfloxacin (Noroxin)	Gastroenteritis (off-label) Prostatitis Urinary tract infection, uncomplicated, due to *E. coli, K. pneumoniae, P. mirabilis* uncomplicated, due to other organisms	Tablets: 400 mg	400 mg q8–12h for 5 d 400 mg q12h for 28 d 400 mg q12h for 3 d 400 mg q12h for 7–10 d	Maximal adult daily dose 800 mg (1.2 g infectious diarrhea) Take on empty stomach with full glass of water (1 h before or 2 h after food or milk) Not recommended for use by children
Ofloxacin (Floxin)	Bronchitis, bacterial exacerbations or community-acquired pneumonia Skin and soft tissue infections *Chlamydia*, endocervical or urethral Uncomplicated; nongonococcal urethritis Pelvic inflammatory disease, acute Prostatitis Urinary tract infection, complicated Cystitis due to *E. coli, K. pneumoniae* Cystitis due to other organisms	Tablets: 200, 300, 400 mg	400 mg q12h for 10 d 400 mg q12h for 7–10 d 300 mg q12h for 7 d 300 mg q12h for 7 d 400 mg q12h for 10–14 d 200 mg q12h for 10 d 200 mg q12h for 3 d 200 mg q12h for 7 d	Maximal adult daily dose 400 mg. Not recommended for use by children Renal impairment (CCr <50 mL/min) requires dosage reduction Take with a full glass of water
(Ocuflox)	Bacterial conjunctivitis		Ophthalmic solution: >1 yr: 1–2 drops every 2–4 h while awake for 2 d, then 1 drop qid while awake for 5 d	

previous 3 months (Mandell et al, 2007). For older patients or those with underlying disease, levofloxacin may be the best choice. The usual duration of therapy for CAP is 7 to 14 days. Higher dosages of some fluoroquinolones are required for more serious infections. Pneumonia treatment is discussed in depth in Chapter 42.

Urinary Tract Infection

Although empirical first-line treatment for a UTI is trimethoprim/sulfamethoxazole (TMP/SMX, Septra, Bactrim) or nitrofurantoin, an alternative treatment in patients who are not able to take or tolerate first-line therapy is the the fluoroquinolones ofloxacin, ciprofloxacin, and levofloxacin (Gupta et al, 2011). Moxifloxacin and gemifloxacin are not approved for use with UTIs because they have poor concentration in the urine. Cross-resistance occurs with the fluoroquinolones. Fluoroquinolone resistance has been steadily increasing, with 24.2% of *E. coli* resistant to ciprofloxacin and 24% resistant to levofloxacin (Kashanian et al, 2008). Fluoroquinolones are not prescribed to children or pregnant women because of concern for adverse effects on joints and cartilage, which have been found in animal studies. The exception is ciprofloxacin, which has FDA approval as second-line therapy in complicated UTI or pyelonephritis in children.

Uncomplicated cystitis and urethritis are treated with oral fluoroquinolones for 3 days. Complicated UTI and pyelonephritis require 7 to 14 days of therapy. Dosages of some fluoroquinolones for acute cystitis are lower than dosages for more serious urinary tract and kidney infections. Treatment of UTIs is discussed in Chapter 47.

Sexually Transmitted Infections and Genital Infections

Previously, the fluoroquinolones were recommended for treatment of uncomplicated gonorrhea manifested as cervicitis, urethritis, pharyngitis, or proctitis. Unfortunately, strains of gonococci resistant to fluoroquinolones have been identified worldwide and the CDC treatment guidelines no longer recommend the use of ciprofloxacin or other fluoroquinolones (CDC, 2007).

Oflaxacin or levofloxacin are recommended by the CDC as second-line therapy for chlamydia (CDC, 2010e). The first-line therapy is azithromycin or doxycycline. If treating with a fluoroquinolone, oflaxacin 300 mg twice a day or levofloxacin 500 mg daily for 7 days is prescribed (CDC, 2010e).

The fluoroquinolones, ofloxacin and levofloxacin, are recommended for the treatment of acute epididymitis most likely caused by enteric organisms or with a negative gonococcal culture or nucleic acid amplification test (CDC, 2010e).

Dosing for the treatment of epididymitis with ofloxacin is 300 mg orally twice a day for 10 days, and with levofloxacin it is 500 mg orally once daily for 10 days.

Detailed discussion of treatment of sexually transmitted infections is found in Chapter 44.

Skin and Tissue Infections

Although approved for skin and tissue infections, use of fluoroquinolones in these infections should be avoided to decrease selection pressure for bacterial resistance. Most skin and tissue infections treated in outpatient settings respond to beta-lactam antibiotics, except wounds that have been exposed to fresh water, such as ponds, lakes, and swimming pools, which may be infected with *Pseudomonas* and *Aeromonas* species.

Infectious Diarrhea

Fluoroquinolones are first-line therapy in treatment of traveler's diarrhea and severe diarrhea not associated with antibiotic therapy. Recommended self-treatment for traveler's diarrhea is 3 days of twice-daily therapy with oral ciprofloxacin (500 mg), norfloxacin (400 mg), or ofloxacin (300 mg), combined with loperamide 4 mg initially and 2 mg after each stool (Conner, 2013). Growing resistance may limit the use of fluoroquinolones in some countries.

For mild bacterial diarrhea not associated with antibiotics, characterized by three or fewer stools per day and minimal associated symptomatology, supportive therapy is usually adequate. For moderate infectious diarrhea, evidenced by four or more stools per day or fewer stools with systemic symptoms, an antiperistaltic drug (e.g., loperamide) may be added to supportive therapy. Severe infectious diarrhea not associated with antibiotics is manifested by six or more unformed stools per day and/or a temperature of 38.8%C or more, tenesmus, blood, or fecal leukocytes. Presence of blood may be indicative of *E. coli* O157:H7 infection, which has serious sequelae and requires hospitalization. Most common pathogens in severe infectious diarrhea not associated with antibiotics are *Shigella, Salmonella, Campylobacter jejuni,* and *E. coli* (O157:H7 strains). Drugs of choice for severe bacterial diarrhea (not associated with antibiotics) are ciprofloxacin 500 mg every 12 hours or norfloxacin 400 mg every 12 hours. Therapy is continued for 3 to 5 days.

Sinusitis

The Infectious Diseases Society of America (ISDA) published updated guidelines for the treatment of sinusitis in adults and children in 2012 (Chow et al, 2012). The fluorquinolones levofloxacin (500 mg PO daily) or moxifloxacin (400 mg PO daily) may be prescribed for adult patients who are allergic to beta-lactam antibiotics, although the ISDA cautions against the use due to higher cost and increasing rsistance (Chow et al, 2012). The ISDA guidelines recommend levofloxacin (10–20 mg/kg/d PO every 12–24 h) for treatment of sinusitis in children with a type 1 allergy to beta-lactams (Chow et al, 2012), althought this is an off-label indication. The AAP issued a clinical practice guideline for sinusitis management soon after the ISDA guidelines that cautions against the use of levofloxacin due to cost, toxicity, and emerging resistance (Wald et al, 2013). The AAP guidelines state levofloxacin can be used as therapy in penicillin-allergic pediatric patients but recommends a combination of clindamycin and cefixime to be prescribed first.

Other Uses

Ciprofloxacin is approved for bone and joint infections, but many typical pathogens (*Staphylococci* and *Streptococci*) are no longer susceptible to this drug. Use should be reserved for proven susceptibility on culture and sensitivity. Ciprofloxacin may be used off-label as a single 500 mg dose as chemoprophylaxis for high-risk adult (18 years of age or older) contacts of persons with invasive meningococcal disease (MacNeil & Cohn, 2011). The CDC notes ciprofloxacin should be avoided in areas where ciprofloxacin-resistant strains of *N. meningitidis* have been detected. Ciprofloxacin should not be used as chemoprophylaxis in pregnant women or children younger than age 18, with safer options of ceftriaxone or azithromycin available (McNeil & Cohn, 2011). Ciprofloxacin is also a first-line treatment for typhoid fever in doses of 500 mg twice daily for 10 days, although resistance is increasing, especially in the Indian subcontinent (Newton & Mintz, 2013).

Rational Drug Selection

Both definitive drug selection and empirical drug selection follow the same principles described in the Rational Drug Selection section for the penicillins. Specific implications to consider in selecting fluoroquinolones are cost, resistance, pharmacodynamics parameters, and adverse effect profile. Brand-name fluoroquinolones are relatively high-cost agents. Ciprofloxacin is on multiple $4 or reduced-cost generic lists, making it a cost-effective choice if appropriate. Levofloxacin is available as a generic product. The cost of fluoroquinolones is comparable to other, newer, broad-spectrum agents, such as amoxicillin/clavulanate, clarithromycin, and cefuroxime axetil (see the available dosage forms table for these drug classes).

Another reason to use fluoroquinolones judiciously is to prevent resistance. Ciprofloxacin and levofloxacin are unique as oral agents effective for *P. aeruginosa*. In addition, the agents with enhanced gram-positive activity (levofloxacin, gemifloxacin, moxifloxacin) retain susceptibility to highly penicillin-resistant strains of *S. pneumoniae* that are also resistant to cephalosporins, tetracyclines, macrolides, and sulfonamides. Moxifloxacin and gemifloxacin achieve much higher AUC:MIC ratios than levofloxacin and ciprofloxacin, making them more desirable for the treatment of upper respiratory infections. It behooves us to guard these susceptibilities as long as possible by using definitive drug selection based on culture and sensitivity and by selecting agents with the narrowest spectrum.

Selection between agents with similar spectrums of bacterial activity may depend on the comparative adverse effects and drug interactions. Norfloxacin has much less effect on caffeine metabolism; lomefloxacin and ofloxacin appear devoid of effects on caffeine metabolism. Treated diabetics and patients with a prolonged QTc interval or taking drugs that increase the QTc interval should avoid fluoroquinolones if other equally effective antimicrobial drugs are available. Unless there are compelling reasons, fluoroquinolones should not be used by children and pregnant women. Renal impairment requires decreased dosage of all agents except moxifloxacin. Other antibacterial drugs are also preferable for patients with severe cerebral arteriosclerosis or who are otherwise seizure-prone (e.g., epilepsy, alcohol abuse, theophylline or antipsychotic drug use).

Monitoring

Monitoring for therapeutic response to antimicrobial drugs is described in the Monitoring section for penicillins. Patients on prolonged therapy with fluoroquinolones should have periodic assessment of organ function, including renal, hepatic, and hematopoietic function. Renal function should be measured or estimated with standard formulas prior to initiation of a fluoroquinolone. It is prudent to obtain a baseline electrocardiogram (ECG) prior to prescription of moxifloxacin. The drugs should be withheld and the ECG repeated if syncope occurs, which may indicate development of torsades de pointes, a potentially lethal arrhythmia. Patients taking theophylline and cyclosporine should have determinations of the plasma concentrations ("blood levels") of these agents, which are metabolized by CYP3A4, a hepatic drug-metabolizing enzyme inhibited by fluoroquinolones. Patients on warfarin who are started on fluoroquinolones should have their INR monitored closely. When either ofloxacin or levofloxacin is administered for gonorrhea, it may mask, but not cure, coexisting syphilis. Obtain serological testing for syphilis whenever a diagnosis of gonorrhea is made, with repeat testing at 3 months after treatment. Patients with epilepsy, alcohol abuse, or concurrent theophylline use should be monitored for CNS irritability (agitation, irritability) and seizure activity.

Patient Education

Administration

As with all antimicrobial drugs, the patient must understand the significance of taking all doses and completing the full course of therapy. Although the effect of food on absorption is unknown, the manufacturer suggests that the optimal time for administration of ciprofloxacin is 2 hours after meals. All fluoroquinolones should be taken with a full glass of water to help avoid dehydration, which can lead to crystalluria. Fluoroquinolones should not be taken within 2 to 6 hours of drugs that may chelate them (including antacids, sucralfate, iron preparations, sevalamer, and zinc salts) and prevent absorption. Dairy products hamper absorption of norfloxacin.

Adverse Reactions

Fluoroquinolones can cause photosensitivity or phototoxicity; therefore, all patients should be taught to avoid direct sunlight, sun lamps, and tanning beds from the first dose until several days after therapy is completed. They should withhold the drug and report any blister, rash, or itching that occurs. Recovery is prolonged and the reaction tends to recur

if the patient is exposed to sunlight again before recovery. Sunscreens, hats, and long-sleeved clothing should be suggested for even short-term exposure.

Fluoroquinolones often cause dizziness or light-headedness, so driving and hazardous activities should be avoided until a patient's reaction is known. Adequate fluid intake to maintain urine output of 1,500 mL per day will avoid crystalluria. Minimize use of urinary alkalinizers such as citrus drinks and avoid baking soda and antacids. If tenderness or inflammation occurs in any tendon, the patient should immediately discontinue the fluoroquinolone, notify the prescriber, rest, and refrain from exercise of the affected joint. Diabetics should immediately report any signs or symptoms of hypoglycemia and should perform home blood glucose testing regularly. The drug should be discontinued at any sign of an allergic reaction (hives, itching, dyspnea) because serious anaphylactic reactions have occurred during first exposure to a fluoroquinolone.

Lifestyle Management

See the Lifestyle Modification section for the penicillins.

LINCOSAMIDES

The original drug in this class was lincomycin. Although structurally different from erythromycin, lincomycin resembled it in activity. Unfortunately, it was too toxic and is rarely used; therefore, it will not be discussed in this chapter. Clindamycin (Cleocin) is a chlorine-substituted derivative of lincomycin and the only other drug in the class. Although less toxic, its indications are still limited because of its potential to cause severe diarrhea and CDI.

Pharmacodynamics

Clindamycin binds to the 50S subunit of the bacterial ribosome and suppresses protein synthesis. This is the same as the receptor for macrolides, so combined use with erythromycin and related drugs may decrease the effectiveness of both drugs. The action of clindamycin is usually bacteriostatic, but it may produce bactericidal effects if the pathogen is especially sensitive.

Spectrum of Activity

Susceptible organisms are primarily gram-positive, including *S. pneumoniae, S. pyogenes, Streptococcus viridans, S. aureus, Corynebacterium diphtheria,* and *Corynebacterium acnes.* It is also effective against selected anaerobic pathogens: *Bacteroides, Fusobacterium, Actinomyces, Peptococcus, Prevotella, C. perfringens,* and *C.tetani.* It is also effective against *Campylobacter jejuni* and *Gardnerella vaginalis,* and is used for treatment of bacterial vaginosis. In primary care, clindamycin is used for infections associated with anaerobic pathogens as well as gram-positive cocci. Clindamycin plays a significant role in treating infections secondary to staphylococcal or streptococcal species in penicillin-allergic patients. In addition, because of its inhibition of protein synthesis, clindamycin is able to decrease toxin production in the setting of septic shock caused by *Streptococcus*, susceptible *Staphylococcus*, and *Clostridium*. Clindamycin lacks clinically relevant activity against enterococci and gram-negative aerobic organisms. *C. difficile* is resistant to clindamycin, which explains the prevalence of CDI as an adverse effect of the drug.

Resistance

Mechanisms of resistance include mutation or modification of the ribosomal receptor site and enzymatic inactivation of clindamycin. Resistance to clindamycin commonly confers cross-resistance to macrolides.

Pharmacokinetics

Absorption and Distribution

Oral administration of clindamycin results in complete absorption, and it is not affected by gastric acid or food. It distributes to pleural and peritoneal fluids, with high concentrations in bile and bone but poor CSF penetration.

Plasma protein binding is high. It readily crosses the placenta and is found in breast milk at 0.7 to 3.8 mcg/mL following doses of 150 to 600 mg.

Metabolism and Excretion

Clindamycin is metabolized by the liver to active and inactive metabolites. Both the parent drug and its metabolites are excreted in the bile and in urine. Approximately 10% of the drug is eliminated in the urine. Dosage modification is not usually required for renal or hepatic impairment unless it is very severe. Table 24-11 shows the pharmacokinetics of this drug.

Pharmacotherapeutics

Precautions and Contraindications

Use with caution in patients with a history of asthma or significant allergies. Hypersensitivity may occur. Cautious use is also recommended for the patient with severe renal or hepatic impairment accompanied by severe metabolic aberrations. The routes of excretion include both hepatic and renal.

Clindamycin is Pregnancy Category B. However, it crosses the placenta in amounts approximating 50% of maternal serum levels. It also appears in breast milk. According to LactMed, the National Institutes of Health Drug and Lactation Database, if clindamycin is required by a nursing mother, breastfeeding may continue, but an alternative drug may be a better choice in breastfeeding women.

Dosages are given for infants and children. Yet clindamycin should be used only for serious infections and when other, less toxic, alternatives are not appropriate.

Adverse Drug Reactions

The main adverse reactions with this drug are GI-related, including nausea, vomiting, and a bitter or metallic taste. GI intolerance may be dose-limiting. The most serious is the risk for CDI. The provider should consider CDI in patients who present with diarrhea subsequent to administration of clindamycin, especially if the diarrhea involves three or more unformed stools per day and contains blood, pus, or mucus. Older adults are less likely to tolerate any diarrhea, and the drug should be used cautiously with that population.

Other adverse effects include dizziness, vertigo, headache, hypotension, and rare cardiac arrhythmias. Indicators of hepatic and renal dysfunction occasionally occur.

Drug Interactions

There are few drug interactions with clindamycin. Table 24-12 lists them.

Clinical Use and Dosing

Because of its anaerobic activity, clindamycin is a first-line therapy for several serious infections treated parenterally in the hospital. Clindamycin is appropriate first-line therapy for MRSA in areas of the country where resistance is low; however, these areas are very limited and may only apply to the

Table 24–11 ⚏ Pharmacokinetics: Lincosamides

Drug	Onset	Peak	Duration	Protein Binding	Bioavailability	Half-Life	Elimination
Clindamycin	Rapid	45 min	6–8 h	93%	>90%	2–3 h	>90% hepatic; 10% unchanged in urine; 3.6% in feces

Table 24–12 ⚏ Drug Interactions: Lincosamides

Drug	Interacting Drug	Possible Effect	Implications
Clindamycin	Erythromycin	Antagonistic effects have occurred for both oral and topical formulations	Avoid concurrent use
	Kaolin-pectin	GI absorption is delayed when coadministered	Give 2 h before or 3–4 h after clindamycin, or avoid concurrent use
	Neuromuscular blockers	Enhanced neuromuscular blockade that may cause severe respiratory depression	Use with caution

pediatric population. Providers will need to know their local susceptibilities to make an informed prescribing decision. Other uses of clindamycin in primary care are limited to second-line treatment of gram-positive cocci. Despite the controversy about whether clindamycin causes a higher incidence of CDI than other antimicrobials, research shows that limiting its use decreases the prevalence of CDI and decreases clindamycin resistance.

Infections in Penicillin-Allergic Patients

Clindamycin is used for bacterial endocarditis prophylaxis as an alternative to penicillins in individuals allergic to penicillin. It also can be substituted for penicillin in treatment of pneumococcal pneumonia and skin and tissue infections, although there are other effective agents.

Drug-Resistant Pneumococcal Infections

Although many strains of *S. pneumoniae* are resistant to penicillins, cephalosporins, macrolides, tetracyclines, and sulfonamides, clindamycin retains good activity. Clindamycin is recommended for second- or third-line therapy for upper and lower respiratory infections (pneumonia, sinusitis, otitis media) due to DRSP. Because it does not cover other common pathogens (*H. influenzae* and *M. catarrhalis*), clindamycin should be reserved for definitive therapy for DRSP or in otitis media nonresponders after at least 72 hours of therapy with a drug that covers *H. influenzae*.

Infections in Special Populations

Clindamycin is indicated for pregnant women and children to treat infections when first-line agents may be harmful or not tolerated. For example, clindamycin has been used for bacterial vaginosis in pregnancy in doses of 300 mg twice daily for 7 days. However, because metronidazole is now recognized as safe for use in pregnancy, the use of clindamycin is limited for this indication. Clindamycin is also used in treatment of malaria and other protozoal infections in pregnant women, children, and in patients unable to tolerate first-line therapy.

Odontogenic (Dental) Infections

Clindamycin 300 to 450 mg given every 6 hours for 3 to 5 days is first-line therapy to treat odontogenic infections because of consistent activity against oral organisms. Pediatric dosing of clindamycin for dental infections is 10 to 20 mg/kg/d in three to four divided doses. It is especially helpful in dental abscesses. Table 24-13 presents the dosage schedules of lincosamides.

Rational Drug Selection

Both definitive drug selection and empirical drug selection follow the same principles described in the Rational Drug Selection section for the penicillins. Specific implications for selection of clindamycin are spectrum of activity and adverse effects. Because clindamycin has a narrow spectrum of aerobic activity and lacks activity against *H. influenzae*, it cannot

Table 24–13 ⚔ Dosage Schedule: Lincosamides

Drug	Indication	Dosage Forms	Initial Dose	Maintenance Dose
Clindamycin (Cleocin)	Mild-moderate bacterial infections	Capsules: 75, 150, 300 mg Injection, solution: 150 mg/mL	*Adults:* PO: 150–300 mg q6h *Children:* PO: 8–20 mg/kg/d in 3–4 equal doses	Maximal daily adult dose is 1.8 g orally and 2.7 g parenterally.
	Severe bacterial infections	Topical: 1% lotion 1% gel 1% solution 1% swab	*Adults:* PO: 300–450 mg q6h *Children:* PO: 16–40 mg/kg/d in 3–4 equal doses	Take with food and a full glass of water to decrease esophageal irritation. Sit or stand for 30 min after dose.
	Endocarditis prophylaxis (off-label)		*Adults:* PO: 600 mg 1 h before procedure *Children:* PO: 20 mg/kg 1 h before procedure	Dosing for clindamycin palmitate HCl (Cleocin Pediatric) oral solution varies slightly from tablets for children.
	Malaria treatment		*Adults:* PO: 900 mg tid for 7 d with quinine *Children:* PO: 20 mg/kg divided in 3 equal doses for 7 d with quinine	Shake solution well before measuring. Shake solution well before measuring.
	Bacterial vaginosis in pregnancy (off-label)		*Adults:* PO: 300 mg bid for 7 d	Dispense with calibrated measuring device. Do not refrigerate solution because it will become thick and hard to pour.
	Pneumocystis carinii pneumonia (off-label)		*Adults:* PO: 1,200–1,800 mg/d in divided doses with 15–30 mg primaquine daily for 21 d	
	Toxoplasmosis of CNS treatment (off-label)		*Adults:* PO: 600 mg tid with pyrimethamine and leucovorin	No dosage adjustments required for renal or liver impairment.
	Odontogenic (dental) infections		*Adults:* 300–450 mg q6h for 3–5 d *Children:* 10–20 mg/kg/d divided in 3–4 doses	

be substituted for other agents typically used to treat URIs but must be used when there is reasonable certainty that the organisms are susceptible to clindamycin. Because of the high incidence of CDI associated with clindamycin, patients with a history of colitis and older patients who poorly tolerate colitis should probably not receive this agent. Severe hepatic impairment requires careful monitoring of drug response.

Monitoring

Monitoring for therapeutic response to antibiotics is described in the Monitoring section for penicillins. If significant diarrhea occurs (six or more stools daily and/or blood, mucus, or watery diarrhea), the drug should be discontinued. Cytotoxin assays or PCR testing may be used to detect the presence of *C. difficile* and its toxin. If the original infection for which clindamycin was prescribed is severe and alternative antibiotics cannot be used, therapy can continue with close observation. Hospitalization may be warranted. CDI requires treatment with metronidazole, oral vancomycin, or fidaxomicin.

Prolonged therapy with clindamycin requires assessment of liver and renal function and blood counts. Because some oral clindamycin formulations contain tartrazine, patients with asthma or aspirin allergy are at risk to develop an allergic response and should be carefully monitored.

Patient Education

Administration

The patient should be advised of the necessity of completing the full course of therapy. Because clindamycin requires multiple daily doses, the patient should be guided in planning mnemonic or other strategies to promote adherence. The drug can be taken without regard to meals, but taking the drug with food and a full glass of water will avoid esophageal irritation. Sitting or standing for a full 30 minutes after the dose will also decrease the risk of esophageal irritation.

Adverse Reactions

If severe diarrhea develops, the patient should check with the prescriber before initiating any antidiarrheal treatment. Antiperistaltic agents, which may worsen the symptoms, should not be used. For mild diarrhea, the patient may use an attapulgite-containing antidiarrheal (e.g., Kaopectate, Donnagel) at least 2 hours before or 3 to 4 hours after the clindamycin. If surgery or general anesthesia is planned during or within a day or so after therapy, the anesthetist or anesthesiologist must be advised because clindamycin can intensify neuromuscular blockade.

Lifestyle Management

See the Lifestyle Management section for the penicillins.

MACROLIDES, AZALIDES, AND KETOLIDES

The macrolides are another early antibiotic group. The prototype drug in this group, erythromycin, was discovered in 1952. The drugs in the class (erythromycin, clarithromycin [Biaxin], dirithromycin [Dynabac]) are compounds characterized by a macrocyclic lactone ring with deoxy sugars attached. A closely related drug, azithromycin (Zithromax), is chemically an azalide derived from erythromycin by the addition of a methylated nitrogen to the lactone ring. The latest addition to this group is telithromycin (Ketek), which is chemically a ketolide derived from erythromycin by the lack of alpha-L-cladinose at position 3 on the erythronolide A ring. They are generally included with the macrolide group and are discussed in the same section here. In addition to their antibiotic activity, macrolides exhibit immunomodulating properties, which increase their usefulness in infectious diseases and cystic fibrosis.

Pharmacodynamics

This group of drugs reversibly binds to the P site of the 50S ribosome subunit of susceptible organisms and may inhibit RNA-dependent protein synthesis by stimulating the dissociation of peptidyl-tRNA from ribosomes. These drugs are typically bacteriostatic but may be bactericidal depending on drug concentrations and the bacterial species tested. Macrolides are weak bases, and their activity increases in alkaline media.

Erythromycin is inactivated by acid, and erythromycin base is marketed in acid-resistant, enteric-coated form to retard gastric inactivation. Erythromycin is also formulated as acid-stable salts and esters to improve bioavailability. These salts include erythromycin ethylsuccinate, erythromycin estolate, and erythromycin stearate. Dirithromycin is a prodrug that is converted nonenzymatically during intestinal absorption into a form of erythromycin. Azithromycin, telithromycin, and clarithromycin are semisynthetic derivatives of erythromycin.

Spectrum of Activity

Macrolides are active against gram-positive organisms such as pneumococci and other *Streptococcus* species, MSSA, and *Corynebacterium*. The gram-negative spectrum of the oral macrolides includes *H. influenzae, M. catarrhalis, Neisseria* species, *B. pertussis, Bartonella quintana,* some *Rickettsia* species, *T. pallidum,* and *Campylobacter* species. Atypical and intracellular organisms commonly resistant to beta-lactam antibiotics are also susceptible, such as *Mycoplasma, Legionella, Chlamydia, Helicobacter, Listeria,* and certain strains of *Mycobacterium.*

Among the macrolides, there is some variability of spectrum. Azithromycin has the greatest activity of the macrolides against gram-negative organisms such as *H. influenzae* and *M. catarrhalis.* It is more active than erythromycin against anaerobes and has activity similar to erythromycin against gram-positive organisms. Clarithromycin has some anaerobic activity and greater activity than erythromycin or azithromycin against gram-positive organisms such as *Streptococcus* species and MSSA. Its activity against *H. influenzae* is greater than that of erythromycin but less than that of azithromycin.

Telithromycin is also effective against DRSP, including those resistant to penicillin, cephalosporins, tetracycline, trimethoprim/sulfamethoxazole, and other macrolides. Dirithromycin has the narrowest spectrum of the macrolides. The single best use for all these drugs is in treating highly intracellular organisms.

Resistance

Resistance to erythromycin is a result of (1) reduced permeability of the cell membrane or active efflux, (2) modification of the ribosomal binding site by chromosomal mutation, or (3) production of esterase by *Enterobacteriaceae* that hydrolyze macrolides. Cross-resistance is nearly complete between erythromycin and the other macrolides. Cross-resistance may also develop with other antibiotics that share the same ribosomal binding site, such as clindamycin. The prevalence of macrolide-resistant pneumococci in the United States reported in the 2011 Active Bacterial Core Surveillance was 26.2% (CDC, 2012). Telithromycin is newer but resistance has developed to *S. pyogenes* (Richter et al, 2008).

Pharmacokinetics

Absorption and Distribution

The macrolides, azalides, and ketolides are all well absorbed from the duodenum following oral administration. Food decreases the amount of absorption of azithromycin tablets by 23% and the suspension by 56%. These formulations should be taken on an empty stomach. Food does not affect the absorption of telithromycin. Absorption of enteric-coated erythromycin is delayed by food. Food also delays the absorption of clarithromycin, although bioavailability is not affected, so this drug may be taken without regard to meals. Dirithromycin is best absorbed when taken with food

or within an hour of having eaten. Erythromycin base or stearate must be taken on an empty stomach, but the absorption of the estolate and ethylsuccinate forms are not affected by food intake. Minimal absorption occurs after topical or ophthalmic use. Macrolides distribute readily to body tissues and enter pleural fluid, ascitic fluid, middle-ear exudates, and sputum. When meninges are inflamed, macrolides enter the CSF. Because of high intracellular concentrations, particularly in phagocytic cells, tissue levels are higher than serum levels and concentrations in white blood cells may remain high for many hours after the last dose of the drug.

Metabolism and Excretion

Macrolides, azalides, and ketolides are partially metabolized by the liver, and clarithromycin, dirithromycin, and telithromycin are converted to active metabolites. This class of drugs is excreted mainly unchanged in bile; the drug is also excreted unchanged in urine in varying degrees. Clarithromycin and its active metabolite are substantially eliminated by the kidneys. Because older adults often have renal impairment, dosage adjustment should be considered for this population.

Erythromycin is heavily metabolized by CYP 3A4, which explains many of its drug interactions. Telithromycin is 50% metabolized by CYP 3A4, but the remaining 50% is CYP450 independent, so dosage adjustments are not required for hepatic dysfunction. Table 24-14 presents the pharmacokinetics.

Pharmacotherapeutics

Precautions and Contraindications

Hypersensitivity to any of the macrolides and patients' use of pimozide contraindicate use of macrolides. The removal

Table 24–14 ❖ Pharmacokinetics: Macrolides, Azalides, and Ketolides

Drug	Onset	Peak	Duration	Protein Binding	Bioavailability	Half-Life	Elimination
Azithromycin	Rapid	2.5–3.2 h	24 h	7%–50%	40%	11–14 h after single dose; 68 h after multiple doses	6% unchanged in urine; remainder unchanged in bile
Clarithromycin	UA	2 h	12 h	40%–70%	55%	3–4 h for 250 mg dose; 5–7 h or 500 mg dose	20%–30% unchanged in urine
Dirithromycin	UA	2–4 h	6–8 h	15%–30%	10%	2–36 h	81%–97% fecal/hepatic
Erythromycin	1 h	1–4 h	UA	7%–90%	35%–60%	1.4–2 h	5% unchanged in urine; remainder largely in bile
Telithromycin	Rapid	0.5–4 h	24 h	60%–70%	57%	7.16 h after single dose; 9.81 h after doses	7% unchanged in feces; 13% unchanged in multiple urine; 37% metabolized by liver

UA = information unavailable.

of terfenadine and cisapride from the market was related to serious dysrhythmic reactions that frequently were triggered by inhibition of CYP 3A4 by erythromycin and other drugs. QT prolongation has been observed with erythromycin, azithromycin, clarithromycin, and telithromycin. These drugs should be avoided if possible in patients at risk for torsades de pointes or when receiving other medications that could prolong the QT interval.

The FDA issued a Drug Safety Communication in March 2013 regarding cardiac arrhythmias associated with azithromycin use. The label was changed to reflect a risk of prolonged QT interval and torsades de pointes. Groups at higher risk of cardiac rhythm disturbance with azithromycin include: patients with known prolongation of the QT interval, a history of torsades de pointes, congenital long QT syndrome, bradyarrhythmias, uncompensated heart failure, and patients on drugs known to prolong the QT interval. Patients with ongoing proarrhythmic conditions such as uncorrected hypokalemia or hypomagnesemia or clinically significant bradycardia and patients receiving Class IA (quinidine, procainamide) or Class III (dofetilide, amiodarone, sotalol) antiarrhythmic agents should be prescribed azithromycin with caution.

Telithromycin has been associated with fatal hepatotoxicity, potentially fatal exacerbations of myasthenia gravis, and visual disturbances. The FDA issued a warning in 2007 that telithromycin should not be used for minor illnesses such as upper respiratory illnesses. Erythromycin should also be avoided in patients with myasthenia gravis, because it may aggravate the condition.

Known, suspected, or potential bacteremia contraindicates use of dirithromycin because serum levels are inadequate to provide antibacterial coverage of the plasma.

Patients with Renal and Hepatic Impairment

Azithromycin is principally excreted via the liver. Patients with impaired hepatic function require cautious use of this drug. There are no data about use with renal impairment, so cautious use is also recommended in decreased renal function.

Clarithromycin is excreted via the liver and the kidney. Dosage adjustments are not required for hepatic impairment in the presence of normal renal function. Renal impairment with CCr less than 30 mL/min with or without hepatic impairment requires that dosages be halved or the dosing interval doubled.

Erythromycin is contraindicated for patients with preexisting liver disease. Erythromycin estolate has been associated with the infrequent (1 case per 1,000 patients) occurrence of cholestatis hepatitis. This has also occurred with other erythromycin salts but is rarer in children. Laboratory findings include abnormal liver function tests, peripheral eosinophilia, and leukocytosis. Symptoms include malaise, nausea, vomiting, abdominal cramps, and fever. Jaundice may or may not be present. These symptoms tend to occur after 1 to 2 weeks of continuous therapy, disappear if the drug is discontinued, and reappear within 48 hours if the drug is readministered.

Telithromycin has not shown altered AUC for patients with hepatic impairment. In severe renal impairment (CCr less than 30 mL/min), AUC was increased. To date, no dosage adjustments are recommended.

Older Adults

Although maximum plasma concentrations and AUC of clarithromycin and dirithromycin increase in older adults, no specific dosage adjustments or precautions are recommended for older adults with normal renal and hepatic function. Older adults with impaired renal function should be treated as any patient with that impairment. Younger and older adults appear to have the same pharmacokinetics for azithromycin and telithromycin.

Pregnant Women

Azithromycin and erythromycin are Pregnancy Category B and are considered safe to use during pregnancy. Clarithromycin, dirithromycin, and telithromycin are Pregnancy Category C. Animal studies with clarithromycin have shown adverse effects on pregnancy outcome and on fetal development. Animal studies with dirithromycin have shown significantly decreased fetal weight and incomplete ossification of fetal bone. These latter two drugs should not be used during pregnancy except in clinical circumstances in which no alternative therapy is appropriate. Telithromycin was not teratogenic in animals, but there are no adequate, well-controlled studies in pregnant women.

Azithromycin, clarithromycin, and erythromycin are compatible with breastfeeding. Telithromycin is excreted in the breast milk of rats and probably in human breast milk. Data are not available for the other drugs in this class, and they should be used with caution in nursing mothers.

Pediatric Patients

Erythromycin has been used extensively in infants and children and is considered safe. Azithromycin was studied and relabeled in 2008 for safety and efficacy for children as young as 6 months for otitis media, sinusitis, and CAP. Efficacy has been established for children older than 2 years for pharyngitis-tonsillitis. Clarithromycin has established safety and efficacy for children older than 6 months. The safety and efficacy of dirithromycin have not been established for children younger than 12 years. The safety and efficacy of telithromycin in children have not been established.

Adverse Drug Reactions

The most common adverse reactions to macrolides are dose-related GI symptoms, including nausea, vomiting, abdominal pain, cramping, and diarrhea. Taste disturbances have been reported with clarithromycin. In general, these reactions are transient, mild to moderate in severity, and reversible when the drug is discontinued. Erythromycin is most likely to cause GI symptoms whether given orally or parenterally because it stimulates the motilin receptor in the GI tract. An off-label use of erythromycin for the treatment of gastroparesis derives from this receptor activity. Diarrhea may also be secondary to CDI.

Azithromycin, erythromycin, and telithromycin have been associated with liver abnormalities, including hepatitis, cholestatic jaundice, and hepatic failure. Erythromycin has been associated with urticaria, bullous eruptions, eczema, and Stevens–Johnson syndrome. Allergic reactions have been reported with all available macrolides. Isolated cases of reversible hearing loss have also been reported with erythromycin, clarithromycin, and azithromycin, particularly with parenteral administration or high doses.

Hyperkinesia, dizziness, and agitation have occurred in fewer than 1% of children taking azithromycin. Stomatitis, dry mouth, and dysphagia have occurred in a small number of adults for all macrolides. Laboratory abnormalities include elevated liver function studies (azithromycin), increased platelet counts (dirithromycin and erythromycin) and elevated potassium levels (dirithromycin). In each case, less than 6% of patients were affected.

Drug Interactions

Clarithromycin, erythromycin, and telithromycin have more drug interactions than the other two drugs in this class because they are strong inhibitors of the CYP450 enzymes, particularly CYP 3A4. Object drugs in these interactions include such common drugs as cyclosporine, most statins, rivaroxaban, theophylline, carbamazepine, and select benzodiazepines. Other drug effects that will be increased with concomitant use of macrolides include colchicine, digoxin, and warfarin. The combination of most macrolides with pimozide (Orap), a drug used to treat Tourette syndrome, can result in serious dysrhythmia; the inhibited metabolism causes prolonged QT interval of the cardiac cycle, predisposing to potentially fatal cardiac dysrhythmias. Table 24-15 lists the various drug interactions by specific drug. Although azithromycin has fewer drug interactions, confirmed interactions with drugs with narrow therapeutic margins have been observed in clinical practice.

Drugs inducing CYP 3A4, such as efavirenz, rifampin, rifapentine, and rifabutin, may significantly increase the metabolism of clarithromycin and decrease effectiveness. Alternative therapy should be considered.

Caution should be used when administering any additional medications that may prolong the cardiac QT interval. These may include, but are not limited to, Class 1a and Class 3 antiarrhythmic agents, fluconazole, and promethazine.

In addition, antacids containing aluminum or magnesium slow absorption of macrolides and azalides, so they should be taken 1 hour before or 2 hours after the antimicrobial drug, particularly with azithromycin. Drug interaction testing with telithromycin indicated that no significant interactions exist with antacids, grapefruit juice, digoxin, warfarin, or the anti-ovulatory effects of oral contraceptives.

Clinical Use and Dosing

Macrolides are drugs of choice for empirical treatment of CAP due to the prevalence of intracellular organisms and the presence of other resistant strains. Relative safety in children and convenient dosing schedules have made the newer macrolides, azithromycin and clarithromycin, popular in primary care practice. In particular, azithromycin has both a 3-day dosing schedule and a 5-day dosing schedule. Clarithromycin usually requires twice-daily dosing but is available in a delayed-release formulation that can be administered once daily. Although bioavailability varies by erythromycin salt, the dosages of base, stearate, and estolate salts are the same for any indication. The dosage of erythromycin ethylsuccinate is higher because of the mass of the ethylsuccinate component. The equivalent of 250 mg base is 400 mg ethylsuccinate. Specific dosages are included in Table 24-16.

Community-Acquired Pneumonia

Pathogens in CAP that are naturally resistant to beta-lactam antibiotics are the atypical organisms *C. pneumoniae*, *M. pneumoniae*, and *Legionella pneumophila*. Other common pathogens in CAP are *S. pneumoniae*, *H. influenzae*, and *M. catarrhalis*, some of which are increasingly resistant to many antibiotics. *S. aureus* is occasionally the pathogen in postbronchitic pneumonia.

Initial empirical therapy to treat CAP in the previously healthy older child (older than age 5 years), adolescent, or

Text continued on page 737

Table 24–15 ⚏ Drug Interactions: Macrolides and Azalides

Drug	Interacting Drug	Possible Effect	Implications
All macrolides	Ergot alkaloids	Acute ergot toxicity, characterized by severe peripheral vasospasm and dysesthesia, has occurred	Use with caution, avoid concurrent use if possible
	Methadone	Additive effects on QT interval prolongation, possibly leading to torsades de pointes	Avoid concurrent use if possible
	Pimozide	Two sudden deaths occurred when clarithromycin was added to ongoing pimozide therapy	Coadministration is contraindicated
Azithromycin, dirithromycin, erythromycin	Antacids	Aluminum- and magnesium-based antacids reduce peak serum levels but not extent of absorption of azithromycin; when given immediately following antacids, dirithromycin absorption is slightly enhanced; when given immediately prior to antacids, elimination rate of erythromycin may be slightly decreased	Consider outcomes in patient education

Table 24–15 ▓ **Drug Interactions: Macrolides and Azalides—cont'd**

Drug	Interacting Drug	Possible Effect	Implications
Azithromycin, clarithromycin, erythromycin	Cyclosporine, Tacrolimus	Elevated cyclosporine or tacrolimus concentration with increased risk for toxicity	Monitor drug levels; azithromycin may be preferred
	Digoxin	Digoxin levels may be elevated based on effect of macrolide on gut flora that metabolizes digoxin in 10% of patients	Carefully monitor for signs and symptoms of digoxin toxicity
Clarithromycin, erythromycin	Rifabutin, rifampin	Antibiotic effects of macrolide reduced; increased rifabutin levels and risk of adverse effects of rifabutin	Select different macrolide; decrease dose of rifabutin when used with clarithromycin
	Alprazolam, diazepam, midazolam, triazolam	Plasma levels of benzodiazepine elevated, increasing and prolonging CNS depression effects	Azithromycin and dirithromycin not expected to react; select benzodiazepine not strongly metabolized by CYP 3A4
	Amlodipine, diltiazem, felodipine, verapamil	Calcium channel blocker levels and effects increased	Monitor closely. Azithromycin and dirithromycin not expected to react
	Buspirone	Plasma levels of buspirone elevated, increasing pharmacological and adverse effects	Azithromycin and dirithromycin not expected to react
	Carbamazepine	Increased concentration of carbamazepine	Azithromycin and dirithromycin not expected to react
	Colchicine	Increased colchicine levels	Reduce colchicine dose; concurrent use contraindicated if patient has renal or hepatic impairment
	Disopyramide	Plasma levels of disopyramide increased. Arrhythmias and prolonged QTc have occurred.	Avoid concurrent administration Carefully monitor any patient receiving both drugs
	Fluconazole, Posaconazole, Voriconazole HMG-CoA reductase inhibitors	Increased serum concentrations of macrolide Increased risk of severe myopathy or rhabdomyolysis	Use caution or select a different drug combination
	Oral anticoagulants Theophylline	Potentiates anticoagulant effects Concurrent use associated with increased serum theophylline levels	Avoid concurrent use Carefully monitor anticoagulant effects for patients receiving any macrolide Avoid concurrent use Azithromycin and dirithromycin not expected to interact
Clarithromycin	Atazanavir, Ritonavir	Increased clarithromycin levels	Decrease clarithromycin dose by 50%–75% if concurrent renal impairment
	Sildenafil, Vardenafil	Increased levels and effects of phosphodiesterase inhibitor	Coadministration not recommended
Dirithromycin	H₂ blockers	Dirithromycin absorption slightly enhanced when given immediately after H₂ blocker	Separate doses by at least 1 h or select different macrolide
Erythromycin	Alfentanil	Alfentanil clearance decreased and elimination half-life increased	Select different macrolide
	Bromocriptine	Bromocriptine levels increased; increased pharmacological and adverse effects	Select different macrolide
	Clindamycin	Potential antagonistic effects	Select a different antimicrobial regimen if possible
	Methylprednisolone	Clearance of methylprednisolone greatly reduced	Monitor for adverse effects or select a different macrolide
Telithromycin	Itraconazole, ketoconazole	Significant increase in telithromycin AUC	Select different antifungal
	Simvastatin; possibly atorvastatin and lovastatin	Significant increase in simvastatin AUC; possible increased risk for rhabdomyopathy	Avoid concurrent use
	Midazolam; BDZs metabolized by CYP3A4	Increased risk for sedation and adverse effects of midazolam and BDZs	Adjust dose of interacting drug if concurrent use cannot be avoided
	Digoxin	Peak and trough levels of digoxin increased by 73% and 21%, respectively. No increased risk for digoxin toxicity seen in research.	Monitor digoxin level closely
	Rifampin, phenytoin, carbamazepine, phenobarbital	Decreased levels of telithromycin and loss of effect	Avoid concurrent use

Note: H₂ denotes H_2 throughout.

Table 24–16 ⚄ Dosage Schedule: Macrolides, Azalides, and Ketolides

Drug	Indication	Dosage Form	Dose	Comments
Azithromycin (Zithromax)	Community-acquired pneumonia, otitis media, uncomplicated skin and soft tissue infections, acute bacterial exacerbation of chronic bronchitis	Tablets: 250, 500, 600 mg Powder for oral suspension: 100 mg/5 mL, 200 mg/5 mL Extended-release oral suspension: 2 g single-dose cup	*Adults:* 500 mg as single dose on day 1, followed by 250 mg daily on days 2–5; or 500 mg daily for 3 d *Children:* 10 mg/kg as a single dose on day 1 (not to exceed 500 mg/d), followed by 5 mg/kg as a single dose on days 2–5	Take capsules and pediatric suspension on empty stomach. Tablets and adult single-dose packets may be taken without regard to meals. Store pediatric oral suspension at room temperature after reconstitution. Stable for 10 d. Discard excess after dosing is complete.
	Pharyngitis/tonsillitis		*Adults:* Same as community-acquired pneumonia *Children:* 12 mg/kg daily for 5 d (not to exceed 500 mg daily)	Shake suspension before measurement, using calibrated dosing device. Pediatric dosing limits: 500 mg daily for pharyngitis, tonsillitis, and first day of dosing for otitis media and pneumonia; 250 mg daily for days 2–5 for otitis media and pneumonia.
	Chancroid, genital ulcer disease, nongonococcal urethritis caused by *Chlamydia trachomatis*		*Adults:* Single 2 g dose, or 1 g if combined with ceftriaxone	Do not use adult single-dose packet formulation for doses >1,000 mg.
	M. avium complex (MAC) prophylaxis Endocarditis prophylaxis		*Adults:* 1.2 g/wk *Adults:* 500 mg *Children:* 15 mg/kg	As above As above As above. Also safe for use in pregnancy. As above 30–60 min prior to procedure
Clarithromycin (Biaxin)	Pharyngitis, tonsillitis, otitis media, or skin and soft tissue infections	Tablets: 250 mg, 500 mg Granules for oral suspension: reconstituted 125 mg/5 mL, 250 mg/5 mL Extended-release: 500 mg tablet	*Adults:* 250 mg bid for 10 d *Children:* 15 mg/kg/d in 2 divided doses	May be given without regard to food. If CCr <30 mL/min, dose should be halved or dosing interval doubled.. Store suspension at room temperature after reconstitution. Stable for 14 d. Do not refrigerate. Shake suspension well before measurement with calibrated measuring device.
	Acute maxillary sinusitis		*Adults:* 500 mg bid for 14 d, 1,000 mg once daily of extended-release *Children:* Same as above for 10–14 d	As above Take extended-release formulation with food
	Acute exacerbation of chronic bronchitis caused by *S. pneumoniae*, *H. influenzae*, or *M. catarrhalis*		*Adults:* 500 mg q12h for 7 d or ER formulation 1 g daily for 7 d	As above
	Community-acquired pneumonia		*Adults:* 250 mg q12h for 7–14 d or ER formulation of 1 g daily for 7 d	As above

Table 24–16 ⊗ **Dosage Schedule: Macrolides, Azalides, and Ketolides—cont'd**

Drug	Indication	Dosage Form	Dose	Comments
	M. avium complex (MAC) treatment		*Adults:* 500 mg twice daily *Children:* 7.5 mg/kg up to 500 mg bid; give in conjunction with other antimycobacterial drugs	As above
	MAC prophylaxis		*Adults:* 500 mg bid	As above
	Active duodenal ulcer associated with *H. pylori* infection in combination with bismuth citrate		*Adults:* 500 mg bid–tid with ranitidine bismuth citrate 400 mg bid for days 1–14; followed by bismuth citrate 400 mg/d for days 15–28	As above
	Active duodenal ulcer associated with *H. pylori* infection in combination with omeprazole		*Adults:* 500 mg tid with omeprazole 40 mg bid for 4 d	As above
	Active duodenal ulcer associated with *H. pylori* infection, in combination with amoxicillin and lansoprazole		*Adults:* 500 mg clarithromycin, 1,000 mg amoxicillin, and 30 mg lansoprazole q12h for 7 d	As above
Dirithromycin (Dynabac)	Acute bacterial exacerbations of chronic bronchitis; uncomplicated skin and soft tissue infections due to methicillin-sensitive *S. aureus*	Tablets: 250 mg	*Adults:* 500 mg/d for 7 d	Take with food or within 1 h of eating. Do not crush or chew tablets.
	Community-acquired pneumonia caused by *M. catarrhalis* or *S. pneumoniae* (not for empirical therapy)		*Adults:* 500 mg/d for 14 d	As above
	Pharyngitis/tonsillitis caused by *S. pyogenes*		*Adults:* 500 mg/d for 10 d	
Erythromycin dose in mg erythromycin base	Antibacterial, mild infection, usual dose	Tablets: 250, 333, 500 mg Capsules: 250 mg		
Estolate (Ilosone)		Tablets: 500 mg Capsules: 250 mg Suspension: 125 mg/5 mL, 250 mg/5 mL	*Adults:* 250 mg base (400 mg ethylsuccinate) q6h; or 500 mg (800 mg ethylsuccinate) q12h; or 333 mg q8h	Take with 180–240 mL of water Maximum adult daily dose is 4 g
Ethylsuccinate (EryPed, E.E.S.)		Tablets: 400 mg Suspension: 200 mg/5 mL, 400 mg/5 mL		
Base (E-Mycin, E-Base, Ery-Tab, Eryc) Stearate (Erythrocin Stearate)		Tablets: 250 mg, 333 mg Tablets: 250 mg, 500 mg	*Children:* 30–50 mg/kg/d of base in divided doses (or 50–80 mg/kg/d ethylsuccinate)	Taking with food may decrease effectiveness of erythromycin stearate and certain formulations of erythromycin base. Check package insert for erythromycin base. Take erythromycin stearate and most erythromycin base at least 2 h before or after a meal.

Continued

Table 24–16 ⊗ Dosage Schedule: Macrolides, Azalides, and Ketolides—cont'd

Drug	Indication	Dosage Form	Dose	Comments
				Erythromycin estolate, erythromycin ethylsuccinate, and some enteric-coated formulations of base can be taken without regard to meals. Should be taken with meals if GI upset occurs. Do not chew or crush erythromycin base. Suspensions should be shaken before measurement, using a calibrated dispensing spoon.
	Erysipelas or nonbullous impetigo due to *S. pyogenes*		*Adults:* 250–500 mg qid for 10 d *Children:* 20–50 mg/kg/d in divided doses for 10 d	As above
	Bullous impetigo or cellulitis due to *S. aureus*		*Adults:* 250 mg q6h or 500 mg q12h to maximum of 4 g/d *Children:* 20–50 mg/kg/d in divided doses	As above
	Community-acquired pneumonia, mild to moderate		*Adults:* 250–500 mg q6h for 10–14 d; treat severe mycoplasma pneumonia with higher dose up to 21 d *Children:* 20–50 mg/kg/d in divided doses for 10–14 d	As above
	Upper respiratory tract infection, mild to moderate, due to *S. pyogenes* or *S. pneumoniae*		*Adults:* 250–500 mg qid for 10 d *Children:* 20–50 mg/kg/d in divided doses for 10 d	As above
	Pertussis (whooping cough) due to *Bordetella pertussis*		*Adults:* 500 mg qid for 10 d *Children:* 40–50 mg/kg/d in divided doses for 10 d	As above
	Newborn conjunctivitis, pneumonia of infancy due to *C. trachomatis*		*Children:* 50 mg/kg/d in 4 divided doses for 14 d (conjunctivitis) or 21 d (pneumonia)	As above
	Urethral, endocervical, or rectal infections due to *C. trachomatis*		*Adults:* 500 mg qid for 7 d or 250 mg qid for 14 d (in pregnancy)	As above
	Nongonococcal urethritis; urethral, endocervical, or rectal infections due to *N. gonorrhoeae*		*Adults:* 500 mg qid for at least 7 d	As above

Table 24–16 ✂ **Dosage Schedule: Macrolides, Azalides, and Ketolides—cont'd**

Drug	Indication	Dosage Form	Dose	Comments
	Primary syphilis		*Adults:* 20 g in divided doses over 10 d or 500 mg qid for 14 d	As above
	Endocarditis prophylaxis		*Adults:* 1 g 2 h before procedure, 500 mg 6 h after procedure *Children:* 20 mg/kg 2 h before procedure, 10 mg/kg 6 h after procedure	As above
Erythromycin ethylsuccinate and sulfisoxazole (Pediazole, Eryzole)	Acute otitis media	Granules for oral suspension. 200 mg erythromycin base activity and 600 mg ulfisoxazole/ 5 mL	*Children:* 50 mg/kg/d erythromycin and 150 mg/kg/d (to a maximum of 6 g/d) sulfisoxazole in four evenly divided doses for 10 d	May be taken without regard to mcals. Not for use in infants <2 mo.
Telithromycin (Ketek)	Community-acquired pneumonia	Tablets: 400 mg	800 mg daily for 7–10 d	Tablets should be swallowed whole and may be taken with or without food.

adult outpatient with no cardiopulmonary disease, no antibiotics in the past 3 months (no risk for DRSP), and no modifying factors is to treat with an advanced-generation macrolide (level I evidence), such as azithromycin or clarithromycin (Mandell et al, 2007). Usual dosages are azithromycin 500 mg once on day 1, followed by 250 mg daily on days 2 to 5, or 500 mg daily for 3 days (for children, 10 mg/kg on day 1, then 5 mg/kg on days 2 to 5); or clarithromycin 500 mg twice daily for 7 to 14 days (for children, clarithromycin 7.5 mg/kg twice daily). Outpatient treatment of infants and children for CAP may also be erythromycin 10 mg/kg orally 4 times daily (Bradley et al, 2011).

It is desirable to obtain sputum for culture and Gram's stain so that the treatment may be more directed, but it is impossible to identify a pathogen in up to 50% of patients with CAP. Consequently, treatment often proceeds empirically. Macrolides have high cross-resistance (50%) for highly penicillin-resistant *S. pneumoniae* strains. If the adult patient's condition deteriorates or is not improving by 48 to 72 hours, a switch to a respiratory fluoroquinolone with extended gram-positive spectrum (e.g., levofloxacin) is indicated. Detailed discussion of pneumonia and its management is found in Chapter 42.

Sexually Transmitted Infections

Nongonococcal and postgonococcal urethritis or cervicitis is most commonly caused by *C. trachomatis* (50%) or *M. hominis*. Other etiologies such as *Ureaplasma, Trichomonas, M. genitalium,* and viruses account for 10% to 15% of cases. Azithromycin 1 g as a single oral dose is a drug of choice for nongonococcal urethritis and cervicitis (CDC, 2010e). If the urethritis is recurrent or persistent, therapy includes metronidazole 2 g as a single oral dose to cover *Trichomonas,* plus azithromycin 1 g as a single dose if not used for the initial episode. If cervicitis is recurrent or persistent, the woman should be reevaluated for possible reexposure to a STI (CDC, 2010e).

Azithromycin is also first-line treatment of chancroid as a single oral dose of 1 g. An alternative is erythromycin base 500 mg orally 4 times daily for 7 days (CDC, 2010e). Azithromycin is commonly prescribed as part of the treatment of gonococcal urethritis and cervicitis as a 1 g oral dose to cover the chlamydial infections that often coexist with gonorrhea. Azithromycin is no longer indicated in the treatment of pelvic inflammatory disease due to *C. trachomatis, M. hominis,* or *N. gonorrhoeae* because of resistance (CDC, 2010e). Azithromycin 2 g as a single dose may be used as a second-line therapy for penicillin-allergic patients with early syphilis, although this has not been well studied and treatment failure has been noted (CDC, 2010e). Sexually transmitted infections are discussed in more detail in Chapter 44, Sexually Transmitted Infections.

Mycobacterium avium **Complex**

Infections with the nontuberculous mycobacterial organism *Mycobacterium avium* complex (MAC) occur in up to 40% of patients with AIDS. Advanced immunosuppression is the major risk factor for MAC. Patients with AIDS are thought to acquire this organism, usually resident in water and soil, by respiratory or GI routes. The syndrome presents with high fever, diarrhea, night sweats, weight loss, anemia, and neutropenia. Diagnosis is usually based on blood culture, although it is sometimes identified on biopsy of the liver, bone marrow, or lymph nodes. MAC prophylaxis is now strongly recommended for HIV-infected adults with a mean CD4 lymphocyte count of fewer than 50 cells/mL.

The first-line drug is clarithromycin at dosages listed in Table 24-16. An alternative treatment is azithromycin if clarithromycin is not tolerated (Benson, Kaplan, Masur, Pau, & Holms, 2004). Before prophylaxis is initiated, patients should be evaluated to assure they do not have active MAC or *Mycobacterium tuberculosis*. National guidelines indicate that treatment of MAC should include at least two antimicrobials to prevent or delay resistance, one of which should be either clarithromycin or azithromycin (Benson et al, 2004). Of these, clarithromycin, 500 mg twice daily, has the greatest evidence for efficacy (Benson et al, 2004). HIV infection and its management are discussed in Chapter 37.

Peptic Ulcer Disease

Most patients with peptic ulcers who are or are not taking NSAIDs have evidence of *H. pylori*. Eradication of *H. pylori* is recommended for all peptic ulcer patients with an active ulcer, a history of ulcer complications, or a need for maintenance therapy. Duodenal and gastric ulcers recur in up to 80% of patients treated with drugs to reduce gastric acid but not treated for eradication of *H. pylori* infection. Multiple treatment regimens for *H. pylori* eradication are available, including combining a proton pump inhibitor (PPI) and two antibiotics for 14 days (Lew, 2009). Antimicrobial agents used include clarithromycin, tetracycline, amoxicillin, levofloxacin, and metronidazole. They are given in three or four drug regimens with PPIs and bismuth subsalicylate. Approved combinations are included in Table 34-8 (Chap. 34). Two regimens include the macrolide antibiotic clarithromycin (500 mg twice daily).

Endocarditis Prophylaxis

The American Heart Association and the American College of Cardiology published joint updated guidelines for endocarditis prophylaxis in 2008, narrowing the recommendation for therapy to only those with prosthetic heart valves, previous infective endocarditis, certain patients with congenital heart disease, and cardiac transplant patients with valve regurgitation who are undergoing dental procedures that involve manipulation of either gingival tissue or the periapical region of the teeth (Nishimura et al, 2008). For patients who can take oral medications but are allergic to penicillins, a single dose of 500 mg of azithromycin or clarithromycin for adults or 15 mg/kg for children is indicated for endocarditis prophylaxis 1 hour before the procedure.

Exacerbations of Chronic Bronchitis

In patients with chronic obstructive pulmonary disease (COPD), presence of at least two of the three cardinal symptoms warrants treatment with antibiotics: increased sputum volume, increased sputum purulence, and increased dyspnea. Any of the macrolides are active against the most common pathogens (see the discussion in the penicillin section for a list of pathogens) and are appropriate first-line choices (Rabe et al, 2007). Length of treatment is 7 to 14 days. Asthma and bronchitis and their management are discussed in Chapter 30.

Upper Respiratory Infections

The common bacterial infections in the upper respiratory tract include acute otitis media (AOM), sinusitis, and pharyngitis. *S. pneumoniae, H. influenzae,* and *M. catarrhalis* are the most common pathogens found in both children and adults. Amoxicillin or amoxicillin-clavulnate is the recommended first-line treatment for both AOM and sinusitis. *S. pneumoniae* is resistant to the common macrolides erythromycin (35.3% resistance), azithromycin (35.3% resistance), and clarithromycin (35.2% resistance) (Jenkins & Farrell, 2009). A meta-analysis of 10 trials indicated greater likelihood of clinical failure if macrolides were prescribed, specifically azithromycin or clarithromycin (Courter et al, 2010). Thus the macrolides are no longer considered agents for AOM or sinusitis. The macrolides are also used for treatment of GABHS pharyngitis in penicillin-allergic patients. Dosages are shown in Table 24-16.

Skin or Soft Tissue Infections

Macrolides are primarily indicated for skin and soft tissue infections in penicillin-allergic patients, although they are not first-line treatment because of resistance. Oral and topical erythromycin has been used in the treatment of acne (see Chap. 32).

Other Uses

An accepted off-label use for erythromycin is Lyme disease in individuals who are allergic to penicillin and in children younger than age 9. However, erythromycin may be less effective than amoxicillin or doxycycline, possibly because of erratic absorption. Other accepted off-label uses for erythromycin include treatment of actinomycoses, anthrax, lymphogranuloma venereum, and relapsing fever caused by *Borrelia* species. Erythromycin and azithromycin are considered drugs of first choice for *C. jejuni*. Erythromycin is indicated in the treatment of listeriosis caused by *L. monocytogenes* and in diphtheria prophylaxis and treatment. It has been used in conjunction with oral neomycin for preoperative preparation of the bowel. Erythromycin is also approved for treatment of erythrasma caused by *Corynebacterium minutissimum*. Erythromycin is an agonist at the motilin receptor and has been effective in the treatment of gastroparesis.

Erythromycin ophthalmic ointment 0.5% is administered to all newborns to prevent ophthalmic neonatorum. During a shortage of erythromycin ointment in 2009, the CDC recommended azithromycin ophthalmic drops as an alternative, off-label treatment, but when the shortage ended the CDC issued a statement that alternatives to erythromycin ointment should no longer be used (CDC,

2010a). Erythromycin is indicated in chlamydial conjunctivitis in newborns and chlamydial pneumonia in infants caused by *C. trachomatis*. There are limited studies regarding the use of azithromycin for chlamydial pneumonia in infants, dosed at 20 mg/kg/day for 3 days (AAP, 2012f).

Rational Drug Selection

Both definitive drug selection and empirical drug selection follow the same principles described in the Rational Drug Selection section for the penicillins. Macrolides, azalides, or ketolides are often selected for susceptible organisms as alternatives in penicillin-allergic patients. Azithromycin and clarithromycin have a slightly broader spectrum than erythromycin and additional indications, such as MAC and *H. pylori*. Because of its long history, erythromycin has accumulated indications for which the newer agents have not been tested.

Increasing resistance of *H. influenzae, Staphylococcus,* and *S. pneumoniae* may increasingly limit the utility of macrolides for common bacterial infections. After consideration of antimicrobial activity and the disease state being treated, the selection of a specific macrolide may be based on cost, convenience, and adverse effect profile. Erythromycin salts are substantially less expensive than the newer drugs but have more adverse GI effects. The improved bioavailability and milder GI effects of the erythromycin estolate salt are offset by the risk of cholestatic jaundice in adults. This agent should not be prescribed for individuals with liver impairment. Patients with a history of cardiac arrhythmia or QT prolongation should avoid erythromycin or be carefully monitored. Azithromycin may be selected over erythromycin, clarithromycin, or telithromycin if the patient is taking interacting drugs whose hepatic metabolism is subject to inhibition.

Erythromycin is generally preferred over the newer agents during pregnancy and for very young infants because of greater accumulated clinical experience. A major reason for selection of azithromycin over other drugs is the enhanced compliance caused by its convenient dosing schedule. However, with its once-per-day dosing and short duration of 3 to 5 days, a single missed dose could jeopardize the successful outcome. There are no indications for dirithromycin over other drugs.

Monitoring

Monitoring for therapeutic response to antibiotics is described in the Monitoring section for penicillins. Because erythromycin, clarithromycin, and telithromycin inhibit the metabolism of many drugs, observation for altered response to concurrent medications metabolized by CYP 3A4 is essential, beginning with the first dose and continuing for several half-lives of the drugs after it is discontinued. Patients taking drugs with narrow therapeutic margins require extra scrutiny if they are taking any macrolide.

Individuals with a history of hearing loss may be at increased risk for further hearing loss, especially if they have hepatic or renal impairment and are taking high doses (more than 4 g/d) of erythromycin. These risk factors may indicate audiometric testing at baseline and whenever there is clinical evidence of hearing loss (e.g., dizziness, fullness in the ears). The hearing loss is usually reversible; it occurs from 36 hours to 8 days after treatment is initiated and begins to recover 1 to 14 days after the drug is discontinued.

ECG monitoring of QT interval is particularly recommended for patients at high risk for torsades de pointes. If the patient develops malaise, nausea, vomiting, skin rash, abdominal pain, or jaundice within 1 to 2 weeks after therapy is initiated, the drug should be discontinued and liver function tests initiated to assess for cholestatic jaundice.

Patient Education

Administration

Doses of macrolides should be evenly spaced for the best effect. Azithromycin and telithromycin are given once daily. Suspensions must be shaken thoroughly before administration, and excess medication should be discarded after the prescribed therapy is administered and never used by another individual or by the same patient for a different episode. Because it is irritating to the GI mucosa, erythromycin should be taken with a full 8 oz glass of water by adults and with at least 4 to 6 oz by children.

Food interactions are complex for these drugs. Azithromycin tablets, the adult single-dose azithromycin packet, clarithromycin, erythromycin estolate, and telithromycin can be taken without regard to meals. Erythromycin stearate, most brands of erythromycin base, erythromycin ethylsuccinate, azithromycin capsules, and azithromycin suspension must be taken on an empty stomach 1 hour before or 2 hours after eating. Dirithromycin should be taken with food or within an hour of a meal. Erythromycin ethylsuccinate has improved bioavailability if taken with food.

Because the requirements for administration with respect to food may vary by brand, the package insert is the best guide for erythromycin base. Tablets of erythromycin base, erythromycin stearate, and dirithromycin should not be chewed or crushed. If chewable tablets of erythromycin ethylsuccinate are prescribed, the necessity for chewing the dosage form should be stressed. If pediatric drops of erythromycin estolate (100 mg/mL) or erythromycin ethylsuccinate are prescribed, the prescription should specify dispensing a calibrated dropper, and the parent should be instructed on proper measurement and oral administration technique; parents have occasionally assumed drops were meant to be administered in the ear. The adult single-dose azithromycin packet should be thoroughly mixed with 2 oz (60 mL) of water and consumed immediately. An additional 2 oz of water should be added to the container, mixed, and ingested to ensure consumption of the entire dose. This form should not be used for doses greater than 1,000 mg.

Adverse Reactions

Taking erythromycin with a full glass of water decreases the GI symptoms that are the most common adverse effects. Because patients often discontinue the medication if adverse effects are intolerable, they should be urged to call the prescriber if GI distress becomes severe so that an alternative drug can be prescribed. Patients who experience signs of liver impairment (malaise, nausea, vomiting, abdominal cramps, skin rash, fever, or jaundice) should discontinue the macrolide and call the prescriber immediately. Syncope may indicate torsades de pointes related to cardiac QT interval prolongation and should also be reported. Other patient education includes information about symptoms of superinfection that is part of the education for all antibacterial drugs.

Lifestyle Management

See the Lifestyle Management section for the penicillins.

FIDAXOMICIN

Fidaxomicin (Dificid) is a macrocyclic antibiotic, currently classified as an 18-ring macrolide, which was approved by the FDA in 2011 for the treatment of *C. difficile* infection (CDI). It is not discussed in the macrolide section of this chapter because its mechanism of action, spectrum of antimicrobial activity, pharmacokinetics, and use are very different than those of the typical macrolides.

Pharmacodynamics

Fidaxomicin binds to RNA polymerase and thus inhibits RNA synthesis. Fidaxomicin is bactericidal, as is its active metabolite OP-1118.

Spectrum of Activity

Fidaxomicin has activity primarily against *Clostridium* species, *C. difficile* in particular. Minimal activity was found for staphylococci, enterococci, or *Bacteroides* spp. (Biedenbach, Ross, Putnam, & Jones, 2010; Finegold et al, 2004).

Resistance

Resistance to fidaxomicin is rare and is not related to resistance with other macrolides or other antibiotic classes.

Pharmacokinetics

Absorption and Distribution

Fidaxomicin is administered orally, but minimal amounts of drug are absorbed. Maximum plasma concentrations occur 1 to 5 hours after an oral dose. Plasma concentrations are higher in patients diagnosed with CDI than in healthy adults and range from 2 to 179 ng/mL. Fidaxomicin may be taken with or without food.

Metabolism and Excretion

Fidaxomicin is metabolized in the intestine primarily through hydrolysis. It does not undergo metabolism through CYP450 enzymes. Greater than 92% of fidaxomicin is excreted in feces, and 0.59% is excreted in the urine. Serum levels were not impacted by renal impairment.

Pharmacotherapeutics

Precautions and Contraindications

The only contraindication listed by the manufacturer is a preexisting allergy to fidaxomicin or any components of the product. Use caution if a patient has a macrolide allergy. Althought the impact of hepatic impairment on dosing has not been fully evaluated, dosage adjustments are not recommended by the manufacturer.

Fidaxomicin is Pregnancy Category B, but clinical trials in humans have not been conducted. It is unknown if fidaxomicin is excreted in human breast milk; therefore, caution is advised. Safety has not been evaluated in persons under 18 years of age.

Adverse Drug Reactions

Allergic reactions including acute dyspnea, angioedema, rash, and pruritis have been observed. In clinical trials, GI disturbances were reported in less than 6% of patients; however, these findings were consistent with CDI symptoms and had similar rates to the comparator.

Drug Interactions

Fidaxomicin may have synergistic effects with rifampin or rifaximin. No antagonistic or enhanced effects have been noted with other medications.

Clinical Use and Dosing

Fidaxomicin should only be used for CDI. In clinical trials comparing fidaxomicin to oral vancomycin, noninferiority was achieved for clinical cure. However, for non-NAP1 strains, recurrent CDI was reduced in the fidaxomicin group (Golan & Epstein, 2012). The dose of fidaxomicin for CDI is 200 mg orally twice daily for 10 days. Fidaxomicin is only available as a 200 mg tablet.

Rational Drug Selection

Fidaxomicin treatment should only be initiated for documented or highly suspected CDI. Although fidaxomicin is highly effective, safe, and has the least impact on gastrointestinal microbes, its cost has severely limited its use. Because of cost, fidaxomicin use may be limited to patients at high risk for recurrent CDI.

Monitoring

Monitoring for therapeutic response to antimicrobial drugs is described in the Monitoring section for penicillins.

Patient Education

Fidaxomicin should be taken twice daily with doses evenly spaced. It can be taken with or without food. The full course of prescribed therapy should be completed. Patients should consult their health-care provider if diarrhea does not resolve or worsens. Patients should also contact their health-care provider if a rash or other allergic symptoms develop.

OXAZOLIDINONES

Linezolid (Zyvox), approved in the United States in 2000, is the first drug in a new class of antibiotics, the oxazolidinones. Each antibiotic developed within the past 60 years has seen the emergence of resistant organisms. Recently, there has been a specific need to develop drugs effective against methicillin-resistant, penicillin-resistant, and vancomycin-resistant strains of bacteria that have produced serious illness. Unfortunately, although new variants of drugs within a class have created subclasses (e.g., azalides and ketolides), no entirely new class of antibiotics has been developed since the 1980s (Mollering, 2003). The oxazolidinones represent a unique class of totally synthetic antibiotics that make the development of naturally occurring resistance mechanism less likely.

Pharmacodynamics

The oxazolidinones are inhibitors of bacterial ribosomal protein synthesis, but unlike other antibiotics they stop the first step in synthesis in which bacteria assemble ribosomes from their dissociated subunits. Linezolid does this by binding to the 50S ribosomal subunit, thus preventing the formation of a 70S initiation complex required for protein synthesis. No other known antibiotic uses this process, so there is no cross-resistance.

Spectrum of Activity

Linezolid is bacteriostatic against most organisms, including staphylococci and enterococci, and bactericidal against others. It is most effective against aerobic gram-positive bacteria. The in vitro spectrum of activity also includes a small number of gram-negative and anaerobic bacteria. The main susceptible organisms include group A and B *Streptococcus, S. pneumoniae, E. faecalis, E. faecium, S. aureus* (both MSSA and MRSA), *S. epidermidis, C. perfringens, Peptostreptococcus* spp., *Corynebacterium jeikeium,* and *L. monocytogenes.* It is weakly effective against *H. influenzae* and *M. catarrhalis.* Linezolid also exhibits some activity against *M. tuberculosis.*

Resistance

Although linezolid resistance is not widespread and considered uncommon, reports of resistance emerged as early as 2002 (Auckland et al, 2002; Bersos, Maniati, Kontos, Petinaki, & Maniatis, 2004). Resistance has been reported in enterococci (*E. faecalis* and *E. faecium*) (Kainer et al, 2007). Linezolid resistance in *S. aureus* is associated with previous linezolid exposure, and linezolid-resistant *S. aureus* outbreaks have been reported in the hospital setting. (Sanchez Garcia et al, 2010)

Pharmacokinetics

Absorption and Distribution

Linezolid is rapidly and completely absorbed after oral administration. Food slightly delays its uptake but does not affect the total amount of drug absorbed. Linezolid may be taken without regard to meals. It is only 31% protein bound and the binding is concentration-dependent. High drug concentrations are found in the skin and other well-perfused tissues. Breast milk concentrations are similar to those in the maternal plasma.

Metabolism and Excretion

There are two inactive metabolites of linezolid created by oxidation of the morpholine ring. Because this is a nonenzymatic oxidation, this drug does not induce the CYP450 system. Nonrenal excretion accounts for 65% of the total clearance; of the remainder, 30% is excreted unchanged in urine. A small degree of nonlinearity in clearance is observed with increasing doses; however, the difference is small and not clinically significant. No dosage adjustments are required for impaired hepatic or renal function.

Clearance is altered by age; it is most rapid in the youngest age group (age 1 week to 11 years). As the age of the child increases, the clearance decreases and reaches that of the adult population during adolescence. Once again, no dosage adjustments are required, except for preterm neonates younger than 7 days because they have lower clearance values. Table 24-17 presents the pharmacokinetics of this drug.

Pharmacotherapeutics

Precautions and Contraindications

Concomitant use or use within 2 weeks of a monoamine oxidase inhibitor (MAOI) with linezolid is contraindicated. Linezolid should be used with caution with other drugs that interact with MAOIs because this may result in serotonin syndrome or increased blood pressure.

Myelosuppression (anemia, leucopenia, pancytopenia, and thrombocytopenia) has been reported in patients receiving linezolid; however, blood counts return to normal after linezolid is discontinued. Complete blood counts should be monitored weekly if a patient is on linezolid for longer than 2 weeks.

Lactic acidosis has been reported with the use of linezolid. Patients with recurrent nausea or vomiting, unexplained acidosis, or low bicarbonate level should be evaluated.

Use of linezolid for periods longer than 28 days has been associated with peripheral neuropathy and optic neuropathy.

Table 24–17 ✂ Pharmacokinetics: Oxazolidinones

Drug	Onset (h)	Peak (h)	Duration (h)	Protein Binding	Bioavailability	Half-Life (h)	Elimination
Linezolid	Rapid	1–2	12	31%	100%	4.4–5.5	30%–35% in urine; 65% nonrenal elimination

Linezolid is Pregnancy Category C. In animal studies, fetal toxicities were seen only at ranges that produced maternal toxicity. There are no adequate, well-controlled studies in pregnant women, so use during pregnancy only if the potential benefit clearly outweighs the potential risk to the fetus. Because this drug is excreted in breast milk in concentrations similar to those in maternal plasma, consider the benefit to the mother in choosing to continue the drug and/or to discontinue breastfeeding.

Linezolid is approved for use in children from birth. Preterm infants and neonates require reduced dosing per 24 hours because of reduced clearance.

Adverse Drug Reactions

The most common adverse reactions reported were diarrhea (2.8% to 11%), headache (0.5% to 11.3%), and nausea (3.4% to 9.6%). Although uncomfortable, none created serious medical consequences. CDI has been reported with nearly all antibiotics. Detection and management of CDI were described earlier. Myelosuppression has been reported, but it resolves with discontinuance of the drug. This adverse event seems to be related to duration of therapy (longer than 2 weeks). Consider discontinuing the drug if the patient develops or has worsening myelosuppression.

Drug Interactions

Linezolid was originally developed as a monoamine oxidase inhibitor (MAOI) and has properties of that inhibition. Indirect-acting sympathomimetics, vasopressors, or dopaminergic drugs may have increased effects when given concurrently, requiring decreased doses of these drugs. Because linezolid is a reversible, nonselective inhibitor of monoamine oxidase, it also has potential interactions with serotonergics such as SSRIs, tricyclic antidepressants, ondansetron, meperidine, buspirone, methadone, and tramadol. Signs and symptoms of serotonin syndrome (e.g., hyperpyrexia and cognitive dysfunction) should be watched for if concomitant therapy is required. There is also potential interaction with tyramine-rich foods and beverages. They do not need to be eliminated entirely but should not be eaten in large quantities (Table 24-18).

Clinical Use and Dosing

Pneumonia and Complicated Skin and Skin Structure Infections

The adult dose is 600 mg every 12 hours for 10 to 14 days. In pediatric patients (birth to 11 years), the dose is 10 mg/kg every 8 hours for 10 to 14 days. In each case linezolid is useful only for susceptible bacteria and only after older, less expensive agents have been tried and are found to be ineffective. The goal is to keep any new antibiotic free from resistant strains of bacteria as long as possible. It should be remembered that linezolid has poor activity against *H. influenzae* and none against *M. pneumoniae,* two common pneumonia organisms. The FDA approval for CAP is for susceptible strains of *S. pneumoniae* or *S. aureus* only.

Uncomplicated Skin and Skin-Structure Infections

The dosage is less for these uncomplicated infections and it varies with age. For adults, linezolid is approved for 400 mg every 12 hours; however, this strength is no longer available in the United States so 600 mg every 12 hours is typically prescribed. For adolescents, the recommended dose is 600 mg every 12 hours; for children aged 5 to 11 years, it is 10 mg/kg every 12 hours; and for young children (younger than 5 years), the dose is 10 mg/kg every 8 hours due to the renal clearance issues discussed above. Once again, it is not first-line therapy and is intended for resistant organisms.

Vancomycin-Resistant *Enterococcus faecium* Infections

A very useful indication for linezolid is the treatment of infections caused by vancomycin-resistant *Enterococcus.* The dose for this indication is 600 mg every 12 hours for adults and 10 mg/kg every 12 hours for children from birth to 11 years. The duration of therapy should be determined by the disease state being treated and patient response. Because these infections may include infected hardware, bone, or other deep-seated infections, long durations may be warranted. It should be noted that 28-day treatment is the outer limit of duration that has been evaluated in clinical trials and has been associated with more adverse effects, including lactic acidosis and neuropathies. Dosage schedules are found in Table 24-19.

Table 24–18 ⚏ Drug Interactions: Oxazolidinones

Drug	Interacting Drug	Possible Effect	Implications
Linezolid	Adrenergic (sympathomimetic) drugs (e.g., dopamine and epinephrine)	Increased action of the interacting drug	Reduce and titrate initial doses of interacting drug, monitor blood pressure
	Monoamine oxidase inhibitors	Increased risk of serotonin syndrome	Discontinue interacting drug 2 weeks before starting linezolid
	Serotonergics (e.g., SSRIs)	Development of serotonin syndrome	Watch for serotonin syndrome indications. Avoid concurrent use unless no appropriate alternative
	FOOD INTERACTIONS Tyramine-rich foods and drinks	Significantly increased blood pressure	No need to delete entirely from diet, but quantities of tyramine eaten should not exceed 100 mg/meal

Table 24–19 ⊗ Dosage Schedules: Oxazolidinones

Drug	Indication	Available Dosage Forms	Dose	Comments
Linezolid (Zyvox)	Community-acquired pneumonia and complicated skin and skin-structure infections	Tablets: 600 mg Powder for oral suspension: 100 mg/5 mL	*Adults:* 600 mg q12h for 10–14 d *Children birth–11 yr:* 10 mg/kg q8h for 10–14 d	May be administered without regard to food, but amount of tyramine-rich food in any meal should be kept low (<100 mg/meal)
	Uncomplicated skin and skin-structure infections		*Adults:* 600 mg q12h for 10–14 d *Adolescents:* 600 mg q12h for 10–14 d *Children 5–11 yr:* 10 mg/kg q12h	Oral suspensions should be gently inverted 3–5 times to mix; do not shake
			Children <5 yr: 10 mg/kg q8h	Store at room temperature
	Vancomycin-resistant *Enterococcus faecium* infections		*Adults:* 600 mg q12h for duration as indicated by site of infection *Children birth–11 yr:* 10 mg/kg q8h	Duration of therapy beyond 14 d is associated with more adverse effects

Note: Most preterm neonates <7 d of age (gestational age <34 wk) have lower systemic linezolid clearance values and larger AUC values than many full-term neonates and older infants. These neonates should be initiated with a dosing regimen of 10 mg/kg q12h. Consideration may be given to the use of 10 mg/kg q8h regimen in neonates with a suboptimal clinical response. All neonatal patients should receive 10 mg/kg q8h by 7 days of life (Zyvox label).

Rational Drug Selection

Although very effective for the treatment of infections caused by MRSA and VRE, linezolid's prohibitive cost, potential for drug interactions, and adverse effects associated with long-term administration have severely limited its use in the ambulatory care setting. However, with increased MRSA infections in the community, a new focus on reducing hospital admissions and length of stays, and an oral generic formulation expected in 2015, linezolid use will likely increase. Linezolid's high oral bioavailability allows for a cost-advantageous alternative to intravenous vancomycin for the treatment of complicated skin and skin-structure infections (Barron, Turner, Jaeger, Adamson, & Singer, 2012). Linezolid's use should be reserved for moderate to severe infections in which alternative antibiotics are less desirable secondary to efficacy, resistance, safety, route, or cost.

Monitoring

Because of the risk for myelosuppression, a complete blood count should be done prior to therapy at baseline and weekly if therapy exceeds 14 days.

Patient Education

Administration

Patient counseling for all antibiotics includes advice to complete the entire course of therapy, take the drug as prescribed on an evenly spaced schedule, and not double missed doses. Linezolid may be taken with or without food but should be taken with a full glass of water. Because significantly elevated blood pressure may occur if taken with tyramine-rich foods,

the amount of tyramine consumed at any one meal should be limited (less than 100 mg/meal). Oral suspensions should be gently inverted 3 to 5 times to mix; do not shake. The drug should be stored at room temperature.

Adverse Reactions

The main adverse reactions are diarrhea, headache, and nausea. Diarrhea should be reported to the health-care provider. Blood, pus, or mucus in the stool may indicate a serious problem that requires treatment. Otherwise, an antidiarrheal medication may be suggested by the provider. Patients should be instructed to consult their health-care provider if any of the following occur: visual changes; severe nausea or vomiting, or unusual bruising or bleeding.

Lifestyle Management

Lifestyle management is the same as discussed in the section on penicillins.

On The Horizon TEDIZOLID

Tedizolid is a next-generation oxazolidinone in development. It has greater potency than linezolid and a similar antimicrobial spectrum, including but not limited to MRSA, VRE, streptococci, and *M. tuberculosis*. Clinical trials with up to 21 days of therapy have not demonstrated myelosuppression. Preliminary testing suggests that tedizolid has lower potential than linezolid for MAOI drug and food interactions (Flanagan, Bartizal, Minassian, Fang, & Prokocimer, 2013). Like linezolid, tedizolid has excellent oral bioavailability and tissue penetration (Urbina et al, 2013).

SULFONAMIDES, TRIMETHOPRIM, NITROFURANTOIN, AND FOSFOMYCIN

The sulfonamides were once major antibacterials, but the development of resistant strains of bacteria and the incidence of allergic reactions to sulfa drugs resulted in their largely being relegated to treatment of UTIs, alternative therapy options for drug-resistant organisms, and treatment of specific infections in immunocompromised hosts, like nocardiosis and toxoplasmosis. Sulfasalazine (Azulfidine) is used in the treatment of ulcerative colitis and rheumatoid arthritis for its anti-inflammatory properties rather than for treatment of infection. Mafenide (Sulfamylon) and silver sulfadiazine (Silvadene) are used to prevent infection in patients with burns. Topical applications such as those for burns are not discussed in this chapter. Included in this section are drugs commonly used in combination with sulfonamides, such as trimethoprim (Proloprim, Trimpex), and agents used to treat UTIs, such as nitrofurantoin (Furadantin, Macrodantin) and fosfomycin (Monurol). The combination formulation trimethoprim-sulfamethoxazole (Bactrim, Septra, TMP-SMZ) is also considered in this section.

Pharmacodynamics

Sulfonamides and trimethoprim both have distinctive pharmacodynamic properties that are enhanced when combined.

Sulfonamides

Sulfonamides exert their bacteriostatic action by competitive inhibition of dihydrofolate synthetase, which is necessary for the conversion of para-aminobenzoic acid (PABA) to dihydrofolic acid. Inhibition of this pathway prevents folic acid synthesis, which is required by susceptible organisms for production of purines and nucleic acids. Microorganisms that use exogenous folic acid or do not synthesize folic acid are not susceptible to sulfonamides. Clinical use of sulfonamides as monotherapy is uncommon. Sulfamethoxazole is combined with trimethoprim, as described below with trimethoprim.

Spectrum of Activity

Sulfonamides inhibit both gram-positive and gram-negative bacteria. Susceptible organisms include *E. coli, Enterobacter, Klebsiella, Salmonella, S. pyogenes, S. pneumoniae, H. influenzae, Nocardia,, N. gonorrhoeae*, and some protozoa (*Pneumocystis jiroveci* and toxoplasmosis).

Resistance

The increasing frequency of resistant organisms limits the use of sulfonamides in chronic and recurrent UTI. In addition, resistance has increased in streptococci and limited their role in skin (other than MRSA infections) and upper respiratory tract infections. Mutations that result in excessive production of PABA cause organisms to develop resistance.

Dihydropteroate synthetase with a low sulfonamide affinity may be encoded on a plasmid that is transmissible and can be disseminated rapidly and widely. Cross-resistance between sulfonamides is common.

Trimethoprim

Trimethoprim inhibits bacterial dihydrofolic acid reductase. Dihydrofolic acid reductases convert dihydrofolic acid to tetrahydrofolic acid, a stage leading to the synthesis of purines and ultimately to DNA. When given with a sulfonamide, it produces a sequential blocking in the metabolic sequence, resulting in synergistic activity of both drugs. This combination is often bactericidal. The widely used formulation trimethoprim-sulfamethoxazole (TMP-SMZ) illustrates the synergy of the combination.

Spectrum of Activity

Trimethoprim is active against both gram-positive and gram-negative organisms. Gram-positive organisms include *S. pneumoniae,* and staphylococci. Its spectrum of gram-negative organisms includes *Citrobacter, Enterobacter, E. coli, K. pneumoniae, P. mirabilis, Stenotrophomonas, H. influenzae, B. pertussis, Nocardia, Salmonella,* and *Shigella.* Some *Serratia* and the protozoan *P. carinii* are also susceptible. Although enterococci may be susceptible to TMP/SMZ in vitro, these agents may not be effective because enterococci have the ability to utilize extrinsic folic acid.

Resistance

Resistance results from reduced cell permeability, overproduction of dihydrofolate reductase, or production of an altered reductase with less drug-binding ability. Mutation is possible, but the most common cause is plasmid-encoded resistant reductases. As with the sulfonamides, dissemination of resistance is rapid and widespread.

Nitrofurantoin

Nitrofurantoin is a synthetic nitrofuran that is activated by bacteria to reactive intermediates that inactivate or alter bacterial ribosomes and other macromolecules. Ultimately, protein synthesis, aerobic energy metabolism, DNA and RNA synthesis, and cell wall synthesis are inhibited. Nitrofurantoin is bacteriostatic in low concentrations and bactericidal in high concentrations in the urine.

Spectrum of Activity

Nitrofurantoin is active against most gram-positive cocci and gram-negative bacilli that cause UTIs. These include *Staphylococcus saprophyticus* and other *Staphylococcal* spp., *Enterococcus* spp., *E. coli, Klebsiella,* and *Citrobacter* spp. Most strains of *Enterobacter, Proteus,* and *Serratia* are resistant. It has no activity against *Pseudomonas* species.

Resistance

Among susceptible organisms, resistant mutants are rare. Some plasmid-mediated resistance transferable to susceptible organisms has been demonstrated. There is no cross-resistance between this drug and other antibacterial agents.

Fosfomycin

Fosfomycin is a bactericidal antibiotic available in the United States only as an oral formulation for the treatment of urinary tract infections. Fosfomycin inactivates the enzyme enolpyruvyl transferase, which ultimately leads to inhibition of cell wall synthesis. It is beneficial in the treatment of urinary tract infections because it reduces adherence of bacteria to the epithelial cells in the urinary tract.

Spectrum of Activity

Fosfomycin has clinical activity against most urinary pathogens, including *S. saprophyticus*, *Enterococcus*, *E. coli*, *Citrobacter*, *Enterobacter*, *Klebsiella*, indole-negative *Proteus*, *Serratia*, and some strains of *Pseudomonas*.

Resistance

Resistance to fosfomycin is uncommon but has been reported. The bacterial mechanisms of resistance most commonly described are enzymatic modification of fosfomycin.

Pharmacokinetics

Absorption and Distribution

Oral sulfonamides are absorbed readily from the GI tract. They are distributed widely throughout the body and found in all body tissues. They readily enter the CSF, pleura, synovial fluids, and the eye. They cross the placenta and enter breast milk. They are bound to plasma proteins in varying degrees. "Free" serum levels of 5 to 15 mg/dL are therapeutically effective for most infections.

Trimethoprim is also well absorbed following oral administration. It is widely distributed in body tissues, including prostatic tissues, and crosses the placenta. Distribution into breast milk occurs with high concentrations.

Nitrofurantoin is readily absorbed via oral administration. The macrocrystalline form is absorbed more slowly than the microcrystalline form, causing less GI distress. The monohydrate crystals are so slowly absorbed that twice-daily dosing is effective. Bioavailability is enhanced by taking nitrofurantoin with food. Because it undergoes rapid tubular secretion, therapeutic serum and tissue concentrations are achieved only in the urinary tract at usual oral doses. It is not effective in patients with severe renal impairment.

Fosfomycin has an oral bioavailability of 34% to 58%, which is not affected by food. Very little drug is protein bound. Fosfomycin distributes into the kidneys, bladder wall, prostate, and CSF fluid if the meninges are inflamed.

Metabolism and Excretion

Metabolism of sulfonamides occurs in the liver by conjugation and acetylation to inactive metabolites. Patients who are slow acetylators have increased risk for toxicity.

Renal excretion is mainly by glomerular filtration, with some acetylated metabolites being less soluble. Acetylated metabolites may produce crystalluria unless the urine is sufficiently alkaline and adequate fluid intake (more than 2,500 mL/d) is maintained. Sulfadiazine is especially prone to this problem. Small amounts are excreted in feces, bile, breast milk, and other secretions.

Liver metabolism of trimethoprim is less than 20%. Eighty percent of this drug is excreted unchanged in the urine. Because it is so dependent on the kidney for excretion, elimination is delayed and its half-life is increased in patients with renal impairment.

Approximately 50% to 70% of nitrofurantoin is rapidly metabolized by body tissues to inactive metabolites. Plasma concentrations are low and prostatic fluid concentrations are negligible. However, nitrofurantoin crosses the placenta and enters breast milk. Renal excretion is via glomerular filtration and tubular secretion. Acidic urine enhances antibacterial activity and enhances tubular reabsorption, which increases its activity in renal tissues. Serum half-life is increased in patients with severe renal impairment. Usual doses produce therapeutic urinary levels in patients with normal renal function. If CCr is less than 40 mL/minute, urinary concentrations are not therapeutic, and the increased serum levels may produce toxicity.

Fosfomycin is eliminated as unchanged drug primarily through renal excretion (up to 60% of an oral dose) and in feces (18%). Therapeutic drug levels of fosfomycin are present at 48 hours after the initial dose. The half-life of fosfomycin is increased in the setting of renal impairment; however, urinary drug concentrations may be decreased.

Table 24-20 presents the pharmacokinetics of sulfonamides, trimethoprim, nitrofurantoin, and fosfomycin.

Pharmacotherapeutics

Precautions and Contraindications

There are a number of patients in which the sulfonamides, trimethoprim, and nitrofurantoin should be used cautiously. Such patients include those with glucose-6-phosphate dehydrogenase (G6PD) deficiency, renal impairment, and folate deficiency. Neither nitrofurantoin nor fosfomycin are indicated for the treatment of pyelonephritis or perinephric abscess.

Blood Dyscrasias or Glucose-6-Phosphate Dehydrogenase Deficiency

Sulfonamides should be used with caution in patients who have blood dyscrasias or G6PD deficiency. Serious adverse reactions secondary to direct toxic effects on the bone marrow have sometimes resulted in death. They include agranulocytosis, aplastic anemia, and other blood dyscrasias. Acute hemolytic anemia resulting in increased destruction of RBCs has resulted, usually with G6PD deficiency. Sore throat, fever, pallor, purpura, or jaundice may be early indications of these serious blood disorders. These problems occur only rarely with trimethoprim and with nitrofurantoin in conjunction with G6PD deficiency.

Renal Impairment

Sulfonamides should be used cautiously for patients with renal impairment. The more soluble drugs in this class (sulfisoxazole and sulfamethoxazole) are less likely to result

Table 24–20 ⬛ **Pharmacokinetics: Sulfonamides, Trimethoprim, Nitrofurantoin, and Fosfomycin**

Drug	Onset	Peak	Duration	Protein Binding	Bioavailability	Half-Life	Elimination
Nitrofurantoin	2.5–4.5 h	0.5 h	6–12 h	90%	87%–94%	20 min*	30%–50% unchanged in urine
Sulfadiazine	Varies	3–6 h	6–12 h	32%–56%	70%–100%	13 h	Mainly in urine; small amount in feces
Sulfamethoxazole	1 h	2–4 h	12 h	65%	90%–100%	7–12 h	Mostly by liver with 80%–100% excreted in the urine as metabolites or unchanged drug (20%)
Sulfamethoxazole/trimethoprim	Rapid	2–4 h	6–12 h	65%/50%	80%/90%–100%	8–13 h	
Sulfisoxazole	1 h	2–4 h	4–6 h	90%	70%–100%	5–8 h	Mostly by liver
Trimethoprim	Rapid	1–4 h	12–24 h	50%	80%	8–11 h	80% unchanged in urine; 20% by liver
Fosfomycin	2–4 h	2 h	48 h	<10%	34%–58%	5.7 h	38% in the urine, 18% excreted in feces

UA = information not available.

*Increased in renal impairment.

in renal complications. Adequate hydration (more than 2,500 mL/d) helps to prevent crystalluria and stone formation. Cautious use of trimethoprim is recommended for patients with renal impairment. Nitrofurantoin is contraindicated in patients with CCr less than 60 mL/min. Nitrofurantoin is not effective in severe renal impairment and patients are at increased risk of toxicity.

Folate Deficiency

Because of its effect on folic acid synthesis, trimethoprim should be used with caution for patients with folate deficiency. Folate supplementation may be administered concomitantly without interfering with antibacterial action.

Pregnancy

Sulfonamides are Pregnancy Category C. These drugs cross the placenta, and fetal levels average 70% to 90% of maternal serum levels. Significant levels may persist if they are given near-term. Sulfonamides are highly bound to plasma albumin and compete for binding sites with bilirubin, resulting in increased free bilirubin concentrations. In utero, the fetus clears free bilirubin through the placental circulation. After birth, this route is no longer available and unbound bilirubin may cross the blood–brain barrier. Do not use near-term. Jaundice, hemolytic anemia, and kernicterus have occurred. Teratogenicity has occurred in animal studies.

Trimethoprim is also Pregnancy Category C. It crosses the placenta, producing similar levels in fetal and maternal plasma. Teratogenicity has occurred in animal studies. Because it may interfere with folic acid metabolism, it should be used only when its benefits clearly outweigh fetal risks. The combination product, TMP/SMZ, is Pregnancy Category D for all trimesters.

Nitrofurantoin is Pregnancy Category B. Use for women of childbearing potential only when it is clearly needed. The incidence of fetal changes in animal studies was low and the alterations minor. It should not be given, however, to pregnant patients at term, during labor and delivery, or when the onset of labor is imminent; it may induce hemolytic anemia in the newborn because of immature enzyme systems. For this reason, nitrofurantoin is contraindicated in infants younger than 1 month.

Fosfomycin is Pregnancy Category B, but limited safety information and the fact that fosfomycin crosses the placenta indicate caution in its use.

Lactation

Because sulfonamides are excreted in breast milk in low concentrations and milk to plasma ratios are as low as 0.5 to 0.6, the American Academy of Pediatrics considers breastfeeding safe during administration of sulfonamides. However, premature infants or those with hyperbilirubinemia or G6PD deficiency should not be breastfed while the mother is taking the drugs. Trimethoprim milk:plasma ratios are 1.25, indicating the drug concentrates in breast milk. Because it may interfere with folic acid metabolism, it should be used cautiously for nursing women. Nitrofurantoin is excreted in breast milk in very low concentrations. Infants with G6PD deficiency, however, should not nurse while the mother is receiving this drug. It is unknown if fosfomycin is excreted in breast milk. Its use during lactation cannot be recommended at this time due to lack of safety information.

Children

Sulfonamides are contraindicated in infants less than 2 months of age (except as adjunctive therapy with pyrimethamine for congenital toxoplasmosis). Insufficient clinical data are available on prolonged or recurrent therapy with sulfamethoxazole in children under 6 years with chronic renal disease. It is best to avoid its use in these patients.

Safety for use in infants younger than 2 months has not been established for trimethoprim. Nitrofurantoin is contraindicated in infants younger than 1 month.

Safety and effectiveness of fosfomycin in children under 12 years of age have not been well studied. In addition, the clinical studies for fosfomycin did not have sufficient numbers of patients over the age of 65 to detect a difference in therapeutic response as compared to younger patients.

Adverse Drug Reactions

As with most antibiotics, the most common adverse reactions for all these drugs are in the GI tract. Anorexia, nausea, vomiting, diarrhea, stomatitis, and abdominal pain are the main adverse reactions. CDI has been reported with all of these agents.

Rashes and generalized skin eruptions are also common adverse reactions for sulfonamides and trimethoprim. The incidence may be dose-related and is more prevalent in HIV-infected patients. Skin eruptions may include erythema multiforme, exfoliative dermatitis, toxic epidermal necrolysis, and Stevens–Johnson syndrome. Cholestatic jaundice, hepatitis, and hepatonecrosis, as a result of direct toxicity or hypersensitivity reactions, may occur with sulfonamides and nitrofurantoin. These drugs should be discontinued at the first sign of rash or jaundice. For the sulfonamides, cross-hypersensitivity occurs within the sulfonamide antimicrobial class and with dapsone. However, minimal data exist to suggest that other sulfonamide-containing compounds that lack the arylamine group or a substituted aromatic ring (sulfonylureas, thiazide and loop diuretics, carbonic anhydrase inhibitors, and sunscreens with PABA) cross-react (Brackett, Singh, & Block, 2004; Slatore & Tilles, 2004).

Photosensitivity reactions can occur with sulfonamides. Measures such as sunscreens and protective clothing may reduce these problems.

Trimethoprim is an inhibitor of the sodium channel in the renal distal tubules of the kidney, resulting in decreased urinary excretion of potassium. This has led to clinically significant hyperkalemia.

Peripheral neuropathy may develop and become severe and irreversible with nitrofurantoin. Predisposing conditions include renal impairment, anemia, diabetes, electrolyte imbalances, vitamin B deficiency, and debilitating disease. Less severe peripheral neuropathy has also occurred with sulfonamides. CNS adverse effects, including headache, dizziness, and drowsiness, have occurred with both of these drug classes. Aseptic meningitis has been associated with TMP/SMZ therapy.

Nitrofurantoin has also been associated with acute, subacute, and chronic pulmonary reactions. Pulmonary toxicity, including pulmonary fibrosis, typically occurs when nitrofurantoin treatment lasts longer than 6 months,

Other serious adverse reactions are discussed in the Precautions and Contraindications section.

Drug Interactions

Trimethoprim and nitrofurantoin have very few drug interactions. Sulfonamides interact with several commonly used drugs, including salicylates, warfarin, and hydantoins. In addition, sulfamethoxazole and trimethoprim may increase the cardiac QT interval, so they should not be used with other agents that could exacerbate this effect. Specific drug interactions are listed in Table 24-21.

Clinical Use and Dosing

Urinary Tract Infections

Lower-tract UTIs are most commonly caused by gram-negative bacteria (95%), with *E. coli* the most prevalent organism ((75% to 95%) (Gupta et al, 2011). Among community-acquired infections, *S. saprophyticus, Klebsiella,* and gram-negative enteric bacilli cause almost all UTIs not caused by *E. coli.* In children, additional organisms include *Klebsiella* in neonates and *Proteus* in boys. All of the antibiotics mentioned have a spectrum of activity that covers these organisms.

Trimethoprim-sulfamethoxazole is the most effective drug when no complicating factors are present; the recommended dose for adults is one double-strength tablet twice daily for 3 days if local *E. coli* resistance is less than 20% (Griebling, 2007; Gupta et al, 2011). If 3-day empirical therapy fails, urine should be sent for culture and subsequent therapy continued for 14 days. The recommended dosage of TMP-SMZ in children is 6 to 12 mg trimethoprim and 30 to 60 mg sulfamethoxazole per kg/d in two divided doses (1 mL suspension per kg/d). Children should be treated with a 10-day regimen. Resistance to TMP-SMZ is seen in patients who have had antibiotic therapy for any reason in the past 3 months or if they have been hospitalized recently.

Nitrofurantoin is an effective treatment for UTIs, with a low *E. coli* resistance rate of 2.1% in a recent study comparing it to TMP-SMZ, ciprofloxacin, and levofloxacin (Kashanian et al, 2008). The dose of nitrofurantoin is 50 to 100 mg twice a day. This drug can also be used prophylactically in adults and children who have recurrent UTIs more often than 3 times per year. Nitrofurantoin is useful in pregnant women because it is Pregnancy Category B. During pregnancy, the dose must be given for 7 days. Nitrofurantoin should be avoided in pregnancy near-term, in labor, and during lactation when the infant is less than 1 month of age because of the risk of the infant's developing hemolytic anemia. The pediatric dose is 5 to 7 mg/kg/d divided every 6 hours for 7 to 10 days. Shortened therapy should not be used in children.

Recurrent infections (more than three infections in 1 year) may be treated with prophylactic antibiotics. Low-dose nitrofurantoin at bedtime (50 to 100 mg) or TMP-SMZ (40 mg TMP and 200 mg SMZ or 1 single-strength tablet) at bedtime and postcoitally to prevent recurrent UTIs in women.

Pregnant women with asymptomatic bacteriuria detected during routine screening during the first trimester can be treated with TMP-SMZ, nitrofurantoin, or trimethoprim, as well as amoxicillin or oral cephalosporins. Other genitourinary indications for TMP-SMZ are treatment of acute prostatitis in men older than 35 years, chronic prostatitis, recurrent UTI (more than three in a year), and prophylaxis before and after invasive urological procedures. Although

Table 24–21 ⠿ **Drug Interactions: Sulfonamides, Trimethoprim, Nitrofurantoin, and Fosfomycin**

Drug	Interacting Drug	Possible Effect	Implications
Nitrofurantoin	Anticholinergics Magnesium salts Probenecid	Increase nitrofurantoin bioavailability by delaying gastric emptying and increasing absorption. May delay or decrease nitrofurantoin absorption. High doses decrease renal clearance and increase serum levels of nitrofurantoin.	Monitor for adverse reactions and toxicity. Avoid concurrent administration. Monitor for increased risk for toxicity.
All sulfonamides	Cyclosporine Hydantoins Methotrexate Probenecid and other uricosurics, salicylates, indomethacin Sulfonylureas Thiazide diuretics Warfarin	Increased cyclosporine concentration and risk of nephrotoxicity. Increased serum hydantoin levels. Enhanced adverse effects of methotrexate, including bone marrow suppression. Increased sulfonylureas half-life and risk of hypoglycemia. Sulfonamides may be displaced from plasma albumin resting in increased free drug. Sulfonamides may potentiate action ofuricosurics. May cause increased incidence of thrombocytopenia with purpura. Enhanced action of warfarin.	Select different antibacterial. Monitor serum levels closely. Avoid concurrent use. Unless planned for therapeutic reasons, avoid concurrent administration. Avoid concurrent use or monitor blood glucose closely. Avoid coadministration. Monitor PT/INR closely.
Trimethoprim	ACE inhibitors and Angiotensin II receptor blockers	Enhanced hyperkalemic effects.	Monitor closely.
	Phenytoin	Inhibition of hepatic metabolism may result in increased effects of phenytoin.	Avoid concurrent administration or monitor phenytoin levels closely.
Fosfomycin	Metoclopramide	Decreased fosfomycin serum and urinary concentrations.	Monitor for clinical response or select a different antibiotic.

INR = international normalized ratio; PT = prothrombin time.

infrequently used, the sulfonamides sulfadiazine, sulfamethizole, sulfamethoxazole, and sulfisoxazole are approved for treatment of cystitis and uncomplicated pyelonephritis. A more detailed discussion of UTI and its management is found in Chapter 47. For dosage schedules see Table 24-22.

Upper Respiratory Infection

TMP-SMZ is no longer recommended in patients with sinusitis or AOM due to high rates of resistance to *S. pneumoniae* and *H. influenza* (Chow et al, 2012; Lieberthal et al, 2013). Although TMP-SMZ is effective in vitro against group A beta-hemolytic *S. pyogenes,* it does not eradicate the organism or protect against rheumatic fever. Thus, it should not be used to treat streptococcal pharyngitis.

Exacerbations of Chronic Bronchitis

Although treatment of ABECB is controversial, TMP-SMZ may be a good choice for patients who have not taken antibiotics recently and therefore are less likely to be infected with a resistant strain and for those with a persistent cough (Rabe et al, 2007). Treatment is one DS tablet twice daily for 14 days. Another advantage of this formulation is low cost. However, with repeated use of TMP-SMZ, resistant organisms are likely to prevail and it is not first-line therapy.

MRSA

Methicillin-resistant *S. aureus* (MRSA) has emerged as a common pathogen in both hospital-acquired and community-acquired infections. Depending on local resistance patterns,

TMP-SMZ is an inexpensive treatment for community-acquired MRSA (CA-MRSA) (Liu et al, 2011; Stevens et al, 2014).

Other

TMP-SMZ will slightly shorten the duration of symptoms and carrier state if given for the treatment of shigellosis enteritis in adults and children (Heiman & Bowen, 2013). It also is used for the prevention and treatment of pneumonia caused by the protozoon *Pneumocystis jiroveci* (PCP) in immunocompromised patients, particularly HIV patients (Mofeson et al, 2009), although TMP-SMZ may be associated with up to 35.3% treatment failure (Rabodonirina et al, 2013). Sulfonamides are inexpensive agents used primarily outside North America to treat trachoma, inclusion conjunctivitis, toxoplasmosis, chancroid, and meningitis.

Rational Drug Selection

Both definitive drug selection and empirical drug selection follow the same principles described in the Rational Drug Selection section for the penicillins. Although no longer primary agents for upper respiratory tract infections, the sulfonamides and trimethoprim are useful, low-cost agents for proven-susceptible urinary tract infections.

Trimethoprim/sulfamethoxazole plays a key role as affordable and effective therapy to treat MRSA infections as compared to intravenous vancomycin or oral linezolid. Nitrofurantoin and fosfomycin play an important role

Table 24–22 ⊗ **Dosage Schedule: Sulfonamides, Trimethoprim, Nitrofurantoin, and Fosfomycin**

Drug	Indication	Available Dosage Forms	Dose	Comments
Nitrofurantoin (Furadantin) Nitrofurantoin macrocrystals (Macrodantin)	Urinary tract infection	Oral suspension: 25 mg/5 mL Capsules: 25, 50, 100 mg	*Adults:* 50–100 mg qid with meals and at bedtime for 3–7 d or more	Maximum daily dose 600 mg for adults or 10 mg/kg for children. Take all nitrofurantoins with food or milk to decrease GI distress.
			Children: 5–7 mg/kg/d in 4 divided doses for at least 7 d	All nitrofurantoins are contraindicated in infants under age 1 mo. Suspension should be shaken well before measurement, using a calibrated measuring device. Store at room temperature. The oral suspension can be mixed with water, milk, fruit juice, or infant formula, although it may discolor.
	Long-term suppression of urinary tract infection		*Adults:* 50–100 mg at bedtime *Children:* 1 mg/kg/24 h in 1 or 2 divided doses	As above
Monohydrate macrocrystals (Macrobid)	Urinary tract infections	Capsule: 100 mg	*Adults:* 100 mg q12h for 3–7 d	As above
Sulfadiazine	Antibacterial or antiprotozoal	Tablets: 500 mg	*Adults:* 2–4 g as initial dose, then 1 g q4–6h *Children:* 75 mg/kg as initial dose, then 37.5 mg/kg q6h or 25 mg/kg q4h	Take with a full glass of water.
Sulfamethoxazole (Gantanol)	Antibacterial or antiprotozoal, mild to moderate infections	Tablets: 500 mg	*Adults:* Initial dose of 2 g, followed by 1 g q8–10h *Children >2 mo:* 50–60 mg/kg to maximum of 2 g initially, followed by 25–30 mg/kg q12h	Maximum dose for children is 75 mg/kg. Fluid intake should be sufficient to maintain urine output of at least 1,200 mL/d. Most crystalluria-prone sulfonamide. Take with full glass of water.
Sulfisoxazole (Gantrisin)	Recurrent acute otitis media	Suspension: 500 mg/5 mL	*Children:* 50 mg/kg/d in 2 divided doses q12h	Maximum adult daily dose 8 g; maximum daily pediatric dose 6 g. Take with full glass of water. Fluid intake should be sufficient to maintain urine output of at least 1,200 mL/d. Shake suspension well before measurement, using calibrated dosing device. Store at room temperature.
	Rheumatic fever prophylaxis (secondary) Antibacterial or antiprotozoal		*Adults:* With carditis, 1 g/d for 10 yr or until age 25 Without carditis, 1 g/d for 5 yr or until age 18 *Adults:* 2–4 g initially, then 750 mg– 1.5 g q4h; 1–2 g q6h *Children >2 mo:* 75 mg/kg or 2 g/m² initially, followed by 25 mg/kg q4h or 37.5 mg/kg q6h	As above As above

Continued

Table 24–22 ⊗ Dosage Schedule: Sulfonamides, Trimethoprim, Nitrofurantoin, and Fosfomycin—cont'd

Drug	Indication	Available Dosage Forms	Dose	Comments
Trimethoprim (Polytrim, Trimpex, Triprim, Primsol)	Urinary tract infection, treatment Urinary tract infection, prophylaxis	Tablet: 100 mg, 300 mg Oral solution: 50 mg/5 mL	*Adults:* 100 mg q12h for 3–10 d or 200 mg daily *Children >2 mo:* 3 mg/kg bid for 10 d *Adults:* 100 mg/d	May be taken on an empty stomach or with food to decrease GI distress. As above
Trimethoprim (TMP)/ Sulfamethoxazole (SMZ) (Bactrim, Septra)	Urinary tract infection MRSA Chronic suppression of urinary tract infection in women Acute exacerbation of chronic bronchitis *P. carinii* pneumonia prophylaxis *P. carinii* pneumonia treatment	Tablets: 400 mg (SMZ)/ 80 mg (TMP) 800 mg (SMZ)/160 mg (TMP) Oral suspension: 200 mg (SMZ)/40 mg (TMP)/ 5 mL	*Adults:* 160 mg TMP/800 mg SMZ bid for 3 d *Children >2 mo:* 6–12 mg TMP/30–60 mg SMZ per kg/d in 2 divided doses × 10 d *Adults:* 160 mg TMP/800 mg SMZ bid for 7 to 10 d *Children >2 mo:* 4–6 mg TMP mg 1 kg/dose TMP/20–30 mg/kg/dose SMZ for 7–10 d *Adults:* 40 mg TMP/200 mg SMZ at bedtime a minimum of 3 times wk and postcoitally *Adults:* 160 mg TMP and 800 mg SMZ q12h for 14 d *Adults:* 160 TMP and 800 SMZ orally q24h or thrice weekly *Children:* 150 mg/m² TMP and 750 mg/m² SMZ/d in 2 divided doses on 3 consecutive d *Adults and Children:* 15–20 mg/kg/d of trimethoprim component, in divided daily doses for 14–21 d	If empirical 3 d treatment fails, culture urine for treatment decision. For pyelonephritis; duration of therapy is 7–14 d; in pregnancy, duration of therapy is 7 d. For prostatitis, duration of therapy is 4–6 wk. Dose is ½ of a single-strength tablet. Not first-line therapy. Only for penicillin allergy. As above As above
Fosfomycin (Monurol)	Uncomplicated urinary tract infections (acute cystitis)	3 g sachet	One sachet	Mix sachet with 3 to 4 oz water and stir to dissolve. Do not use hot water. Fosfomycin is not indicated for the treatment of pyelonephritis or perinephric abscess

in the empiric treatment of cystitis, especially in the setting of high community TMP/SMZ and fluoroquinolone resistance. Because trimethoprim and nitrofurantoin are indicated as monotherapy only for UTI, use of these agents does not contribute as much to selection pressure that promotes resistance to drugs used for other infections. A single dose of fosfomycin is an attractive option for uncomplicated cystitis, especially when medication adherence may be an issue. However, nitrofurantoin is significantly less expensive than fosfomycin and may be preferred in patients without renal dysfunction. Sulfamethoxazole/

trimethoprim oral formulations are on multiple $4 or reduced-cost generic lists, making it a cost-effective choice if appropriate.

Nitrofurantoin is available as microcrystals, macrocrystals, and monohydrate macrocrystals. Microcrystals (Furadantin) cause excessive GI irritation and should not be used. Monohydrate macrocrystals (Macrobid) form a gel that gradually releases the drug, requiring only twice-daily dosing, whereas macrocrystals (Macrodantin) require administration every 6 hours. Nitrofurantoin should be used with caution in those predisposed to its adverse effects: older patients and patients with anemia, renal impairment, electrolyte imbalance, diabetes, vitamin B deficiency, and debilitating diseases.

Monitoring

Monitoring for therapeutic response to antibiotics is described in the Monitoring section for penicillins. Culture of the urine to follow up a UTI will verify eradication of the infection. If a patient is on long-term therapy of nitrofurantoin, trimethoprim, or a sulfonamide, periodic assessment of the complete blood cell (CBC) count, hepatic function, and renal function should be conducted. For nitrofurantoin, there should also be periodic evaluation of pulmonary function for signs of fibrosis, physical examination for indications of peripheral neuropathy, and urine culture; superinfections with *Pseudomonas* or *Candida* sometimes occur with chronic therapy. Elderly patients on nitrofurantoin should be monitored closely because serious adverse effects such as acute pneumonitis and peripheral neuropathy occur more commonly in this population. Any patient on nitrofurantoin who develops cough, dyspnea, chest pain, or fever should receive a chest x-ray, sedimentation rate, and CBC to detect the signs of hypersensitivity and pulmonary fibrosis. Patients on long-term sulfonamide therapy should also have periodic urinalysis to check for crystalluria or urinary calculi formation. Patients with AIDS are prone to adverse effects of sulfonamides.

Patient Education

Administration

Patient counseling for all antimicrobials includes advice to complete the entire course of therapy, take the medications as prescribed on a regular schedule, and abstain from sharing medications with others. Sulfonamides and solid or liquid forms of trimethoprim-sulfamethoxazole should be taken with a full glass of water and sufficient daily fluid intake to maintain 1,200 mL urine output in the adult. Nitrofurantoin causes less GI distress and is better absorbed if taken with food or milk. Suspensions should be shaken before measurement and taken with a specially marked measuring spoon or comparable device. Patients receiving fosfomycin should be advised on proper preparation and administration of the sachet packet and drinking extra fluids to increase urination.

Adverse Reactions

Patients taking sulfonamides and trimethoprim or combinations containing these agents should be counseled to avoid photosensitivity or photoallergy by wearing protective clothing and sunscreens. They should not expose their skin to ultraviolet light from the sun or tanning lamps more than a few minutes until tolerance is determined. The patient who develops a rash while taking these agents should discontinue the drug and contact the health-care provider; rash may develop into Stevens–Johnson syndrome. Patients on sulfonamides should also report signs of crystalluria (blood in urine) and blood dyscrasias (sore throat, fever, chills, pale skin, unusual bleeding or bruising). Sulfonamides may cause

dizziness that can make operation of machinery and automobiles dangerous.

Counseling for patients on nitrofurantoin includes similar cautions for signs of blood dyscrasias (sore throat, fever, chills, pale skin, unusual bleeding or bruising). Patients should know that the drug may cause brownish discoloration of the urine and elicit a false positive on copper sulfate urine tests for glucose. Patients should call the health-care provider if there are signs of acute pulmonary fibrosis (sudden onset of chest pain, dyspnea, cough, fever) or subacute pulmonary fibrosis (dyspnea, nonproductive cough, malaise after 1 to 6 months of therapy). Because rechallenge with nitrofurantoin could cause rapid return of the pulmonary condition, the patient should be provided with written information to warn future health-care providers of the reaction. Other symptoms to report are signs of peripheral neuropathy (numbness, tingling, pain in extremities) and intolerable GI upset.

Lifestyle Management

See the Lifestyle Management section for the penicillins.

TETRACYCLINES

Tetracyclines are broad-spectrum antibiotics that are used extensively throughout the world. Originally introduced in 1948, they are used in the United States for a variety of bacterial, *Rickettsiae*, and spirochete infections; malaria prophylaxis for certain travel destinations; and acne vulgaris. Included in this class are oxytetracycline, tetracycline, demeclocycline, doxycycline (Doxy, Doxychel, Vibramycin), and minocycline (Minocin). Tigecycline, a glycylcycline that has an extended spectrum of activity, is only available as an intravenous formulation and is reserved for very resistant organisms due to tolerability and safety concerns. Demeclocycline is used primarily for syndrome of inappropriate antidiuretic hormone secretion (SIADH). Due to the uncommon usage of tigecycline and demeclocycline, these drugs will not be discussed further in this chapter. The second-generation drug doxycycline is the most commonly prescribed tetracycline. It has fewer problems with drug–food interactions, is dosed less frequently than tetracycline, and is generally less expensive than minocycline. Tetracycline is used both topically and orally to treat acne and is one of four drugs in the combination treatment of *H. pylori* infection. Topical application is discussed in Chapters 23 and 32.

Pharmacodynamics

Tetracyclines include a group of drugs with a common tetracycline nucleus structure and similar spectrum of activity. Tetracyclines inhibit protein synthesis by reversibly binding to the 30S subunit of the bacterial ribosome and preventing the addition of amino acids to growing peptides. The class is typically bacteriostatic but may be bactericidal against highly susceptible organisms. In addition to their antibacterial properties, tetracyclines have other anti-inflammatory mechanisms that are useful for the treatment of acne vulgaris. Tetracyclines chelate with divalent and trivalent cations, which can interfere with their absorption and activity.

Spectrum of Activity

Tetracyclines have good activity against gram-positive organisms such as *S. aureus* (including MRSA), *S. pneumoniae*, *Bacillus anthracis*, *Actinomyces* spp., *C. perfringes*, *L. monocytogenes*, *Nocardia*, and *Propionibacterium acnes*. Activity against *Enterococcus* spp. is variable.

Gram-negative organisms that tetracyclines are effective against include *Haemophilus ducreyi* (chancroid), *Yersinia pestis*, *Francisella tularensis*, *Bartonella bacilliformis*, *Vibrio cholerae*, and *Brucella*. Although not first-line therapy, they also are active against *H. influenzae*, *E. coli*, *Shigella*, and *Klebsiella* spp. Tetracyclines, particularly minocycline and tigecycline may have a role in the treatment of infections due to *Bacteroides* spp. or *Acinetobacter*. None of the tetracyclines have reliable activity against *Proteus* spp.

Tetracyclines also have activity against intracellular organisms such as *Chlamydia*, *Mycoplasma pneumoniae*, *Ureaplasma urealyticum*, and *Legionella*. This class is active against *Rickettsia* (Rocky Mountain spotted fever, typhus, Q fever, rickettsial pox, and tick fever) and spirochetes such as *Borrelia recurrentis* (relapsing fever), *Treponema pallidum*, and *Leptospira*. Tetracycline has demonstrated activity against *H. pylori*. Doxycycline is a blood schizonticidal agent and is active against the asexual erythrocytic forms of *P. falciparum*.

Resistance

The mechanisms of resistance to tetracyclines are (1) decreased intracellular accumulation due to impaired influx or increased efflux of an active transport protein pump, (2) ribosome protection by proteins that interfere with drug binding, and (3) enzymatic inactivation. Resistance to tetracycline generally predicts resistance to the entire class. For the treatment of gram-positive and gram-negative bacterial infections, susceptibilities should be verified because resistance may be an issue. For example, in the United States, up to 13% of *S. pneumoniae* and 21.6% of *N. gonorrhea* are resistant (CDC 2012).

Pharmacokinetics

Absorption and Distribution

Tetracyclines are adequately but incompletely absorbed in the fasting state. The percentage of oral dose absorbed is highest for doxycycline and minocycline (95% to 100%) and intermediate for oxytetracycline and tetracycline (60% to 70%). Achlorhydria has no effect on absorption of tetracyclines. Food and polyvalent cations (Ca^{2+}, Mg^{2+}, Zn^{2+}, Fe^{3+}, and Al^{3+}) decrease absorption of tetracyclines. Doxycycline is the least affected by food and divalent cations.

Doxycycline and minocycline are highly lipid soluble and readily penetrate body tissues and fluids, including pleural fluid, eye, and prostate, and cross placental membranes. Fetal plasma concentrations reach 60% of maternal serum levels. Minocycline displays good penetration of saliva. Tetracycline has intermediate lipid solubility, and oxytetracycline has the least. Oxytetracycline readily diffuses across the placenta into fetal circulation and into pleural fluid.

Metabolism and Excretion

Tetracyclines are eliminated by the kidney via glomerular filtration and by liver metabolism and undergo enterohepatic recirculation with excretion in the bile and feces. Dosage adjustments of tetracycline and oxytetracycline are required for renal impairment; however, doxycycline and minocycline do not significantly accumulate or require dosage reductions. Minocycline is metabolized by the liver and its half-life is prolonged in oliguria. Because it also uses nonrenal routes of excretion, dosage adjustments are not required in renal impairment. Table 24-23 describes the pharmacokinetics of selected tetracyclines.

Table 24–23 Pharmacokinetics: Tetracyclines

Drug	Onset	Peak	Duration	Protein Binding	Bioavailability	Half-Life	Elimination
Doxycycline	1–2 h	1.5–4 h	12 h	80%–95%	93%	18–22 h	30%–42% unchanged in urine; some inactivation in intestine; remainder excreted in bile and feces
Minocycline	Rapid	2–3 h	6–12 h	70%–80%	90%	11–22 h	5%–10% unchanged in urine; some metabolism by liver; remainder excreted in bile and feces
Oxytetracycline	1–2 h	2–4 h	6–12 h	20%–40%	60%	6–12 h	10%–35% unchanged in urine
Tetracycline	1–2 h	2–4 h	6–12 h	65%	60%–80%	6–12 h	20%–55% unchanged in urine

Pharmacotherapeutics

Precautions and Contraindications

There are a number of patients for whom the tetracyclines should be prescribed cautiously; such patients include those with renal impairment, those with hepatic impairment, pregnant women, lactating women, and children under 8 years of age. In addition, outdated tetracyclines should not be administered. Historically, the degradation products of these drugs were highly nephrotoxic, and reversible nephrotoxicity, including a Fanconi-like syndrome, has been reported. However, current formulations do not include citric acid as an excipient, which may have eliminated this possible adverse effect.

Renal Impairment

Extreme caution should be used in the presence of renal impairment. Usual doses of tetracyclines (except doxycycline and minocycline) may lead to excessive accumulation of the drugs and possible hepatotoxicity. The antianabolic activity of tetracyclines may be seen with renal impairment and include an increased BUN, azotemia, hyperphosphatemia, and acidosis. Therefore, lower-than-normal doses are recommended for tetracycline and oxytetracycline in renal impairment. If therapy is prolonged, an assay of drug serum concentrations may be advisable.

Hepatic Impairment

There are serious concerns related to hepatotoxicity for IV forms of tetracycline. This is not a major concern with oral administration, but liver function studies are advisable during long-term management with doxycycline or minocycline. Hepatotoxicity has been reported with minocycline, and it should be used with caution in patients with hepatic dysfunction.

Pregnancy

Doxycycline is Pregnancy Category D. Others are Pregnancy Category X and should not be used during pregnancy. They readily cross the placenta in concentrations up to 60% of maternal plasma. Tetracyclines are found in fetal tissue and can produce retardation of skeletal development in the fetus and staining of deciduous teeth.

Lactation

Tetracycline is excreted in breast milk; however, the AAP considers tetracycline to be compatible with breastfeeding because the serum concentrations of infants in the study were below detectable levels and there was no evidence of teeth staining (AAP, 2001). Doxycycline is also excreted into breast milk; however, because milk levels are low and absorption is inhibited by the calcium in breast milk, a short course is considered safe during lactation (LactMed, 2014). Minocycline may affect milk production or composition.

Children

Children younger than 8 years generally should not use any tetracycline. These drugs form a stable calcium complex in any bone-forming tissue, decreasing bone growth. They also may cause permanent yellow/gray/brown discoloration of deciduous and permanent teeth. Enamel hypoplasia has also been reported. Doxycycline is less likely to produce these problems, but the risk outweighs any potential benefit for most indications.

Adverse Drug Reactions

As with other antibiotics, the most common adverse reactions are associated with the GI tract. Anorexia, nausea, vomiting, and diarrhea are caused by direct irritation of the intestinal mucosa. Taking the drug with food (note food interactions above) or reducing the dose usually alleviates GI complaints. Esophageal ulcers have occasionally occurred but can be avoided by taking the drug with a full glass of water and remaining upright after taking the drug. As broad-spectrum antibiotics, tetracyclines can cause CDI, previously discussed in the sections on penicillins, cephalosporins, and clindamycin.

Light-headedness, dizziness, and vertigo have been reported in up to 9% of patients taking minocycline and in some patients taking doxycycline. Pseudotremor cerebri (benign intracranial hypertension) has also been associated with tetracyclines. Symptoms are headache and blurred vision. Discontinuing the drug usually resolves these problems, but the possibility for permanent sequelae exists.

Dermatological adverse reactions include photosensitivity manifested by an exaggerated sunburn reaction, as well as maculopapular and erythematous rashes. Severe skin reactions, including Stevens–Johnson syndrome and toxic epidermal necrolysis, have been reported with tetracyclines. Blue-gray pigmentation of skin and mucosa has been reported with minocycline.

Drug Interactions

The main drug–drug interactions associated with tetracyclines are with divalent and trivalent cations that are found in antacids, iron salts, sevalemer, magnesium-containing laxatives, and zinc supplements. Concurrent administration leads to the formation of poorly soluble chelated compounds, resulting in decreased antibiotic activity. Separation of these products from the administration of tetracyclines by at least 2 hours is recommended. Doxycycline and minocycline have less affinity for calcium and zinc and are not significantly affected. Tetracyclines increase the anticoagulant effects of warfarin.

Whether tetracyclines cause a decrease in efficacy of oral contraceptives is controversial, but the alleged mechanism is related to the enterohepatic recirculation of tetracycline and oral contraceptives. It seems prudent to suggest the use of a barrier contraceptive method while the patient is taking the tetracycline and until the next menses. These and other interactions of the tetracyclines are shown in Table 24-24.

Clinical Use and Dosing

The tetracyclines are prescribed for sexually transmitted infections, acne, *H. pylori*, and other less common infections.

Table 24–24 ⠿ **Drug Interactions: Tetracyclines**

Drug	Interacting Drug	Possible Effects	Implications
Tetracyclines	Antacids, dairy foods, iron salts, and sodium bicarbonate	Impair absorption because of formation of a poorly soluble chelate	Take on empty stomach or separate doses by 2 h and take tetracycline first. Doxycycline and minocycline have lower affinity for divalent cations and are not significantly affected by food or dairy products.
	Warfarin	Tetracyclines may increase warfarin effects	Choose a different antibiotic or monitor PT/INR closely.
	Barbiturates, carbamazepine, hydantoins	Increase metabolism and decrease half-life and serum levels of doxycycline	Antibacterial activity decreased. Avoid concurrent administration.
	Cimetidine	Decreased GI absorption of tetracyclines because of pH-dependent inhibition of dissolution	Antibacterial activity decreased. May be true for other H_2 blockers. Avoid concurrent administration.
	Digoxin	Serum levels of digoxin increased in 10% of patients with risk for toxicity	Effects last for months after tetracycline discontinued. Select different antibiotic class.
	Insulin	May reduce insulin requirements	Further study needed. Monitor blood glucose closely.
	Lithium	May increase or decrease lithium levels	Monitor serum levels closely.
	Oral contraceptives	May decrease effectiveness; breakthrough bleeding may occur	Controversial. Suggest barrier method for women taking tetracyclines.
	Penicillin	May interfere with bactericidal action of penicillins	Avoid concomitant administration.

INR = international normalized ratio; PT = prothrombin time.

Genitourinary Infections

One of the most important indications for doxycycline is treatment of genital *C. trachomatis* infections and nongonococcal urethritis and cervicitis. Doxycycline in doses of 100 mg twice daily for 7 days is a first-line agent because of its low cost, but it may have lower compliance than the more expensive azithromycin, which requires a single dose in these infections (CDC, 2010e). Sexual partners should be evaluated and treated. Doxycycline is contraindicated in pregnancy; the drug of choice for pregnant women is amoxicillin or azithromycin (CDC, 2010e). In penicillin-allergic patients, doxycycline (100 mg orally twice daily) or tetracycline (500 mg orally 4 times daily) for 14 days is the only recommended alternative treatment of early primary, secondary, or latent syphilis of less than 1 year's duration (CDC, 2010e). For latent syphilis of more than 1 year's duration without neurosyphilis, a longer course of treatment (28 days) is required.

Doxycycline (100 mg twice daily for 10 days) combined with ceftriaxone (250 mg IM) is indicated for empirical treatment of epididymo-orchitis in heterosexual men less than 35 years of age where the likely pathogens are *C. trachomatis* or *N. gonorrhoeae* (CDC, 2010e).

Men with acute proctitis who practice receptive anal sex should be treated with a combination of antibiotics that cover for *N. gonorrhoeae* and *C. trachomatis*. The CDC guidelines (2010e) recommend ceftriaxone 250 mg IM combined with doxycycline 100 mg twice daily for 7 days. Chronic prostatitis, the most common form, is a chronic pain syndrome of unknown etiology. Studies suggest it may have a microbial etiology, and doxycycline (100 mg twice daily for 14 days) is used empirically for treatment.

Acne

Patients with moderate, inflammatory acne who show no improvement with 6 to 8 weeks of topical therapy may be treated with oral antibiotics to treat the *P. acnes* that cause inflammatory papules and pustules. Treatment is tetracycline (Achromycin) 500 mg twice daily for 1 to 2 months; then, when acne control is achieved, the dose is lowered to 500 mg per day for 1 to 2 months, after which a maintenance dose of 125 to 500 mg daily is taken. Minocycline is an alternative, although more expensive, treatment. Dosing of minocycline is 100 mg twice daily; then the patient is weaned to 50 mg daily. Doxycycline is an oral alternative to topical metronidazole in the treatment of acne rosacea.

Peptic Ulcer Disease

Tetracycline is one component of the quadruple drug regimen used for the eradication of *H. pylori* associated with peptic ulcer disease (PUD). Tetracycline 500 mg 4 times a day is combined with metronidazole 250 mg 4 times a day, bismuth subsalicylate 525 mg 4 times a day, and a proton pump inhibitor. The quadruple drug therapy is more complex than the triple drug therapy. Full prescribing information for PUD is found in Chapter 34.

Lyme Disease

The International Lyme and Associated Diseases Society (ILADS) has released evidence-based guidelines recommending early and aggressive antibiotic treatment to prevent Lyme disease from becoming persistent or recurrent (Cameron et al, 2006). Doxycycline, 100 mg twice daily, is the first-line drug of choice for early treatment of Lyme disease, a tick-borne infection caused by *B. burgdorferi* (CDC, 2013c). Children age 8 years or older are treated with doxycycline 4 mg/kg/d divided into twice daily doses (maximum 100 mg twice daily). The duration of oral treatment varies by the presenting signs: early erythema migrans (14 to 21 days), mild cardiac involvement (21 days), arthritis (28 days), and isolated facial paralysis (21 to 28 days). Amoxicillin is the alternative for pregnant women and children younger than 8 years, for whom doxycycline is contraindicated (CDC, 2013c). The ILADS recommends early empirical treatment for patients with a likely diagnosis of Lyme disease while waiting for laboratory confirmation (Cameron et al, 2006).

Other

Doxycycline is an alternative for penicillin-allergic patients for prophylaxis of rat, bat, raccoon, and skunk bites (AAP, 2012g). The primary drug of choice for ehrlichiosis and rickettsial infections (e.g., Rocky Mountain spotted fever, typhus, Q fever, trench fever caused by *B. quintana*) is doxycycline (AAP, 2012h). Minocycline, 100 mg twice daily for 6 to 8 weeks, is the drug of first choice for infections by *Mycobacterium marinum*, an infection associated with contamination by water from aquariums. Minocycline may be used as an alternative to sulfonamides in nocardiosis. Tetracyclines are first-line therapy for a number of diseases rarely seen in North America, including trachoma, cholera, and granuloma inguinale. Doxycycline 100 mg twice daily for 6 days is an alternative therapy for post-exposure prophylaxis to anthrax (Hendricks et al, 2014). Doxycycline is also used in prophylaxis and treatment of falciparum malaria and as an adjunct in treatment of intestinal amebiasis. Table 24-25 presents the dosage schedule of tetracyclines.

Rational Drug Selection

Both definitive drug selection and empirical drug selection follow the same principles described in the Rational Drug

Table 24–25 ⚕ Dosage Schedule: Tetracyclines

Drug	Indication	Dosage Form	Dose	Comments
Doxycycline (Doxy Caps, Vibramycin)	Antibacterial	Capsules: 25, 50, 100 mg Tablets: 100 mg Syspension: 25 mg/5 mL Syrup: 50 mg/5mL	*Adults:* 50–100 mg q12h	Maximal daily adult dose 500 mg for 5 d for acute gonococcal infection; 300 mg for all other infections.
	Community-acquired MRSA		*Children >8 yr:* 2.2–4.4 mg/kg/d divided into 2 doses q12h *Adults:* 100 mg q 12h for 5 to 10 d *Children >45 kg:* 100 mg q 12 h for 5 to 10 d *Children ≤45 kg:* 2 mg/kg/dose q12 h for 5 to 10 d	Shake suspension well before measurement with calibrated device. Store at room temperature for up to 14 d. Do not take this drug within 1 h of other medicines; separation of 3 h preferable. May be administered without regard to meals.
	Anthrax (post-exposure prophylaxis)		*Children <8 yr:* 2.2 mg/kg q12h (max 100 mg/dose) *Children ≥ 8 yr and adults:* 2.2 mg/kg q12h (max 100 mg/dose)	
	Endocervical, rectal, or urethral infection caused by *C. trachomatis*		*Adults:* 100 mg q12h for 7 d	As above
	Epididymo-orchitis caused by *C. trachomatis* or *N. gonorrhoeae;* nongonococcal urethritis		*Adults:* 100 mg q12h for 10 d combined with ceftriaxone 250 mg IM	As above
	Gonococcal infections, uncomplicated		*Adults:* 100 mg q12h for 7 d combined with ceftriaxone 250 mg IM	Ceftriaxone is first-line treatment
	Lyme disease		*Adults and children >8 yr:* 100 mg q12h for 14 to 21 d	As above

Continued

Table 24–25 ⚕ **Dosage Schedule: Tetracyclines—cont'd**

Drug	Indication	Dosage Form	Dose	Comments
	Malaria prophylaxis		*Adults:* 100 mg daily beginning 1–2 days before travel, continued through visit and for 4 wk after traveler leaves the malarious area *Children >8 yr:* 2.2 mg/kg daily, up to 100 mg daily on same schedule as adult	As above
	Acne vulgaris		*Adolescents and adults:* 100 mg bid for inflammatory form	May wean
(Oracea)	Acne rosacea	Capsule: 40 mg	*Adults:* 40 mg daily in the a.m.	As above
	Acute exacerbation of chronic bronchitis		*Adults:* 100 mg q12h for 5–10 d	As above
	Bite of rat, bat, raccoon (prophylaxis)		*Adolescents and adults:* 100 mg q12h	As above
Minocycline (Dynacin, Minocin)	Antibacterial, other infections	Capsules: 50 mg, 100 mg Oral suspension: 50 mg/5 mL	*Adults:* 200 mg base initially, then 100 mg q12h; *or* 100–200 mg initially, then 50 mg q6h *Children >8 yr:* 4 mg base/kg initially, then 2 mg/kg q12h	As above
	Acne		*Adolescents ≥12 yr:* 100 mg daily for 1 to 2 mo then wean to 50 mg/d	Treat for at least 12 wk. May need to increase to 150 mg to 200 mg/day in some patients.
Oxytetracycline (Terramycin)	Brucellosis	Capsules: 250 mg	*Adults:* 500 mg q6h for 3 wk, given concurrently with 1 g streptomycin IM q12h the first wk and once/d the second wk	Maximum daily adult dose 4 g; maximum daily pediatric dose 250 mg. Take with full glass of water. Keep container tightly closed in a dry place. Store at room temperature. Parenteral dose must be given by deep IM injection; do not administer IV. Change to oral form as soon as possible.
Tetracycline (Achromycin V, Sumycin)	Acne	Oral suspension: 125 mg/5 mL Capsules: 100, 250, 500 mg Tablets: 250 mg, 500 mg	*Adults:* 1 g/d in divided doses (q 6 to 12 h) for severe cases; gradually reduce to maintenance dose of 125 mg– 500 mg/d in divided doses. Alternate-day dosing or intermittent therapy possible if in remission.	Shake suspension well before measurement with calibrated device. Not for children <8 yr. Keep container tightly closed in a dry place. Store at room temperature. Heed expiration date. Dispose of excess or leftover drug. Do not take within 1–3 h of other drugs. Take with full 8 oz glass of water, and stand for at least 90 sec after swallowing. Take drug at least 1 h before bedtime.
	Brucellosis		*Adults:* 500 mg qid for 3 wk in combination with streptomycin 1 g bid for the first wk and 1 g/d for second wk	As above
	Other bacterial infections		*Adults:* 250–500 q6h to q12h *Children >8 yr:* 25 to 50 mg/kg q6h	As above

Selection section for the penicillins. When a patient with renal impairment requires a tetracycline, doxycycline is preferred; it does not require dosage adjustment and lacks the antianabolic effects that increase azotemia when other tetracyclines are used. Another advantage of doxycycline and minocycline is decreased chelation with divalent cations, which allows them to be taken with meals if necessary. Additionally, these two agents also require fewer daily doses than other tetracyclines. Unfortunately, tetracyclines are contraindicated in children younger than 8 years and during pregnancy because of the risk of bone and teeth abnormalities in the fetus and young child, as well as increased risk of hepatotoxicity during pregnancy. Besides age and pregnancy, reasons to choose alternative agents over tetracyclines are concurrent administration of other hepatotoxic drugs and risk of noncompliance with the complex scheduling required to avoid drug–food interactions. Doxycycline is on multiple $4 or reduced-cost generic lists, making it a cost-effective choice if appropriate.

Monitoring

Monitoring for therapeutic response to antimicrobial drugs is described in the Monitoring section for penicillins. Long-term therapy with tetracyclines exceeding several weeks requires periodic hematopoietic, hepatic, and renal function tests. Because doxycycline is metabolized by the liver, other drugs can induce or inhibit its metabolism. Patients should be assessed for potential interactions of other drugs with doxycycline, particularly inducers such as rifampin, phenytoin, carbamazepine, and barbiturates that accelerate doxycycline metabolism and may result in therapeutic failure. Additionally, digoxin assays should be obtained when a patient takes broad-spectrum antibiotics concurrent with digoxin.

Patient Education

Administration

Oral solid dosing forms of tetracyclines should be stored in a tightly closed container in a dry environment to avoid accelerated decomposition that might result in toxic constituents. The patient should note the expiration date and dispose of outdated tetracycline, which can cause serious toxicity. The entire prescription should be taken, with doses evenly spaced.

Suspension products should be shaken before measurement of the dose with a calibrated dosing device. Although some tetracyclines come in liquid formulations for use by adult patients who cannot swallow solids, it should not be assumed they are indicated for children younger than 8 years. Administer tetracyclines 1 hour before or 2 hours after meals and give tetracyclines 2 hours before antacids. However, doxycycline and minocycline can be taken with meals if they cause GI upset when taken on an empty stomach. To avoid esophageal irritation, do not take tetracyclines at bedtime and administer with a full 8 oz glass of water.

Tetracyclines should not be used during pregnancy and should be avoided in children younger than 8 years.

Adverse Reactions

Tetracyclines can cause phototoxicity, so sunlight and tanning lights should be avoided. Wear sunscreen, hats, and protective clothing if it is necessary to be in the sun for more than a few minutes. Avoid hazardous activities and driving if dizziness, light-headedness, or unsteadiness develops, which is most common with minocycline. Contact the prescriber if these symptoms interfere with activities of daily living. The patient should stop taking the tetracycline and contact a health-care provider if headache and blurred vision develop; these are the symptoms of pseudotumor cerebri.

Signs of superinfection that should be reported to the prescriber include hoarseness, glossitis, sore throat, dysphagia, or vaginal itching and discharge. The patient should also report symptoms of hepatotoxicity, which include upper abdominal pain, nausea, vomiting, dark urine, clay-colored stools, or yellowing of skin or eyes. Diarrhea involving three or more unformed stools per day and blood or mucus in the stool could indicate CDI. Detection and management of CDI were described earlier.

Women of childbearing age would be prudent to use a backup barrier method of contraception during tetracycline therapy and until the next menses. Women on hormone replacement should know that broad-spectrum antibiotics can cause exacerbation of hot flashes and menopausal symptoms during therapy.

Tetracyclines can cause reversible pigmentation of skin and mucous membranes, which is more common with minocycline.

Lifestyle Management

See the Lifestyle Management section for the penicillins.

GLYCOPEPTIDES

The glycopeptide class consists of vancomycin (Vancocin) and the structurally similar lipoglycopeptides, which include telavancin (Vibativ) and a drug in phase III trials, dalbavancin (Zeven). This group of antibiotics is used for gram-positive infections that are resistant to first-line antibiotics.

Vancomycin is a narrow-spectrum antibiotic. Use of vancomycin has increased because of the development of organisms resistant to other drugs, such as MRSA. Unfortunately, its widespread use led to the development of strains of vancomycin-resistant *Enterococcus* (VRE) and *S. aureus* with reduced susceptibility, including vancomycin-intermediate *S. aureus* (VISA) and vancomycin-resistant *S. aureus* (VRSA). The decreased susceptibility of *S. aureus* and *E. faecium* has greatly reduced treatment options for some infections, especially nosocomial infections in hospitals and hemodialysis centers.

Telavancin was approved in 2009 for use in complicated skin and skin-structure infections (cSSSI) caused by susceptible gram-positive bacteria. Although telavancin does not require therapeutic drug monitoring, its use has been limited by adverse effects and lack of demonstrated superiority over vancomycin.

Pharmacodynamics

Vancomycin is a tricyclic glycopeptide antibiotic that inhibits cell wall synthesis by binding firmly to the D-A1a-D-A1a terminus of nascent peptidoglycan pentapeptide. The end result is a weakened cell wall susceptible to lysis. The cell membrane is also damaged, contributing to the antibacterial effects.

Telavancin is a lipoglycopeptide antibacterial that is a synthetic derivative of vancomycin. Telavancin inhibits cell wall synthesis by binding the bacterial membrane and disrupting the membrane barrier function.

Spectrum of Activity

Vancomycin is bactericidal for gram-positive organisms, including staphylococci, streptococci, pneumococci, *Corynebacterium, Listeria, Lactobacillus, Actinomyces,* and *Clostridium.* It kills staphylococci relatively slowly and only if cells are actively dividing.

Telavancin is active against gram-positive organisms including *S. aureus* (including MRSA), *S. pyogenes, Enterococcus* spp. (vancomycin-susceptible isolates only), *Streptococcus agalactiae,* and *Streptococcus anginosus* group (includes *S. anginosus, S. intermedius,* and *S. constellatus*). Additionally, *E. faecium* (vancomycin-susceptible isolates only), *Staphylococcus haemolyticus,* and *Staphylococcus epidermidis* are more than 90% susceptible to telavancin.

Resistance

Resistance is due to a modification of the binding site of the peptidoglycan building block. This results in loss of a critical hydrogen bond that facilitates high-affinity binding of vancomycin to the target organism. To reduce the development of resistant strains, it is recommended to limit vancomycin use to situations in which drug resistance is suspected or documented or when severe drug allergies preclude the use of beta-lactam or other preferred therapies. There is some cross-resistance between VRE strains with a high vancomycin MIC and telavancin.

Pharmacokinetics

Absorption and Distribution

Absorption of vancomycin from the GI tract is poor, although clinically significant serum concentrations have occurred. When administered intravenously, onset of action is rapid, with peak concentrations in 1 hour and a duration of effect of approximately 12 hours, depending on renal clearance. It is 52% to 56% protein bound and has less than 1% bioavailability by the oral route. Its half-life is 4 to 6 hours in adults and 2 to 3 hours in children. Distribution is wide, with 20% to 30% penetration of the CSF. The drug crosses the placenta.

Telavancin is administered IV and is 90% protein bound. Its single-dose half-life is 8 hours. Concentrations of telavancin in skin blister fluid were 40% of those in plasma.

On The Horizon **DALBAVANCIN**

A new glycopeptide antibiotic, dalbavancin (Zeven), is in phase III trials. The only other drug structurally related to dalbavancin is vancomycin. This once-weekly antibiotic is effective against MRSA and MRSE. In 2008, Pfizer withdrew its global applications to conduct further studies on dalbavancin. In 2010, Pfizer out-licensed dalbavancin to Durata Therapeutics, which will continue phase III trials.

Metabolism and Excretion

Because minimal oral absorption occurs, the majority of oral doses of vancomycin are excreted in feces. Intravenously administered vancomycin is eliminated renally, with more than 90% via glomerular filtration.

Telavancin is primarily excreted in the urine (76%). Clearance is decreased in patients with renal impairment.

Pharmacotherapeutics

Precautions and Contraindications

Because of poor oral absorption, oral forms of vancomycin should not be used to treat systemic infections. Oral formulations are unlikely to cause systemic adverse effects. However, clinically significant serum concentrations may occur in some patients who have inflammatory conditions of the intestinal mucosa. Care should be taken if this drug must be administered to these patients. Intramuscular administration should be avoided.

Vancomycin is nephrotoxic and should be used with caution in patients with impaired renal function or patients receiving other nephrotoxic agents. Vancomycin may be ototoxic, with increased risk for these problems when coadministered with other ototoxic agents or in older adults, who may have an underlying hearing loss. It should be used with caution in the elderly. Red man syndrome, including potentially severe hypotension, has been associated with rapid intravenous administration of vancomycin.

Oral vancomycin is listed as Pregnancy Category B, and IV forms are Pregnancy Category C. Telavancin is Pregnancy Category C; there are no data on the use of telavancin in pregnant women. A pregnancy test should be performed before telavancin therapy, with use avoided in pregnant females. The VIBATIV pregnancy registry at 1-888-658-4228 should be contacted to monitor outcomes of telavancin exposure during pregnancy.

Vancomycin is excreted in breast milk, although concentrations in breast milk during oral administration are low. It is unknown whether telavancin is excreted in human milk. Exercise caution when giving either drug to a nursing mother. Vancomycin has been used in serious infections in neonates and children and there are published doses for neonates, infants, and children. Vancomycin use in children is best confined to serious infections during which the child is hospitalized. Telavancin has not been studied and is not approved for children younger than age 18.

Adverse Drug Reactions

Vancomycin therapy has been associated with nephrotoxicity, presenting with increased serum creatinine and BUN. Risk factors for nephrotoxicity include the use of high-dose, prolonged therapy, preexisting renal dysfunction, and concomitant use of other nephrotoxins. Vancomycin has rarely been associated with serious ototoxicity that may be transient or permanent. It has occurred most often in patients with high IV doses, who have underlying hearing loss, or who are receiving concomitant therapy with another ototoxic drug. Serial tests of auditory function may be helpful to minimize this adverse reaction. Hematological effects include reversible neutropenia, eosinophilia, and thrombocytopenia. Skin rash is the most common adverse effect with oral therapy.

The significant adverse reaction to telavancin is nephrotoxicity, especially in patients who are at risk for decreased renal function (preexisting renal disease, diabetes mellitus, congestive heart failure) and those with CDI. Other adverse effects associated with telavancin include QT interval prolongation, GI disturbances, and hypersensitivity reactions.

If telavancin or vancomycin is infused too fast, the patient may develop red man syndrome, a flushing of the upper body, urticaria, pruritus, or rash. Stopping or slowing the infusion usually leads to resolution of the rash. Slow infusion over 60 minutes or more per gram of vancomycin may decrease the likelihood of this reaction.

Drug Interactions

The only significant interaction between vancomycin and drugs used in primary care occur with drugs that also have ototoxic or nephrotoxic effects (aminoglycosides). The concomitant administration increases the risk and should be avoided if possible.

The adverse effects of telavancin may be increased by drugs that may affect renal function, such as ACE inhibitors, loop diuretics, and NSAIDS. Renal function should be monitored and the patient observed for adverse effects.

Clinical Use and Dosing

Vancomycin (Vancocin) is used to treat CDI; however, it is recommended that metronidazole be tried first in mild to moderate cases. It is also used to treat staphylococcal enterocolitis. It is not effective in any other intestinal infections, especially when gram-negative pathogens are present. Adult dosages are 125 to 500 mg orally every 6 hours for 7 to 10 days. The maximum oral daily adult dosage is 2 g. Studies have indicated that higher dosages result in fecal concentrations far in excess of the MIC and that the 125 mg dose is as effective as higher doses. Dosage for children is 10 mg/kg, up to 125 mg, every 6 hours. Recurrences, which develop in approximately 25% of treated patients, may be treated with a second course of oral vancomycin.

Vancomycin is available for oral administration in pulvules at 125 mg and 250 mg formulations. It is also available as a powder for reconstitution as a solution of 250 mg/5 mL or 500 mg/6 mL. The more concentrated solution contains ethanol. The solution must be refrigerated after reconstitution and will maintain potency for 14 days. It should be dispensed with a calibrated measuring device.

The intravenous dose of vancomycin is 2 to 3 g per day (30 to 60 mg/kg/d) in divided doses every 8 to 12 hours, with a dosage adjustment for decreased renal function and maintainance of troughs of 10 to 20 mg/L. The usual dose for infants older than 1 month and children is 10 to 15 mg/kg every 6 hours.

The telavancin dose for complicated skin and skin structure infections is 10 mg/kg IV every 24 hours for 7 to 14 days. Infuse over 60 minutes. In patients with renal function impairment, dosing is adjusted accordingly: for CrCl 30 to 50 mL/min, give 7.5 mg/kg every 24 hours; for CrCl 30 to 10 mL/min, give 10 mg/kg every 48 hours.

Monitoring

For oral vancomycin, positive response to therapy will be manifested in cessation of diarrhea and associated symptoms. Proctosigmoidoscopy and/or colonoscopy may be useful to document the presence of pseudomembranous colitis or relapse in patients with persistent symptoms. Enzyme immunoassay of stool samples for the presence of *C. difficile* toxins may remain positive after treatment, so follow-up cultures and toxin assays are not recommended. Renal function determinations are warranted periodically during either oral or IV vancomycin therapy, especially in patients receiving high doses of vancomycin, receiving other nephrotoxins, and those with renal function impairment or severe CDI. Vancomycin troughs should be performed during intravenous therapy. The white blood cell (WBC) count or audiometry may also be monitored during extended or repeat therapy.

Renal function should be measured prior to starting telavancin and during treatment at 48 to 72 hour intervals. Pregnancy testing should be done on all women of childbearing age before the start of therapy.

Patient Education

Administration

If cholestyramine is used in conjunction with oral vancomycin, the medications should be administered several hours apart because cholestyramine binds oral vancomycin and prevents its effectiveness. The oral solution can cause a bitter or unpleasant taste and mouth irritation and should be followed by a full glass of water. Oral vancomycin can be taken without regard to meals. If the patient is too ill for oral therapy, vancomycin solution may be administered by nasogastric tube, enema, long intestinal tube, or directly into a colostomy or ileostomy.

Adverse Reactions

Skin rashes may occur and, if serious, should be reported to the health-care provider. Patients should report evidence of ototoxicity (loss of hearing; ringing, buzzing, or fullness in ears; dizziness), neutropenia (chills, coughing, difficult breathing, sore throat, fever), or nephrotoxicity (altered frequency or amount of urine, nausea or vomiting, increased thirst, difficulty breathing, weakness).

Lifestyle Management

Detection and management of CDI were described earlier. If diarrhea is present, administration of an antiperistaltic antidiarrheal (e.g., atropine and diphenoxylate, loperamide, opioids) is contraindicated because it may delay the elimination of toxins from the colon, thereby prolonging or worsening the condition. Good perianal hygiene will improve patient comfort during this illness.

Patients should be educated about how to prevent the spread of skin infections, including hand washing and covering open skin lesions.

ANTIMYCOBACTERIALS

Mycobacterial infections are among the most difficult to cure because mycobacteria (1) grow slowly and are relatively resistant to drugs that are largely dependent on how rapidly cells are dividing, (2) have a lipid-rich cell wall relatively impermeable to many drugs, (3) are usually intracellular and inaccessible to drugs that do not have good intracellular penetration, (4) have the ability to go into a dormant state, and (5) easily develop resistance to any single drug. Tuberculosis, an example of a mycobacterial infection, is a worldwide public health issue. In addition to drug–organism issues, adherence is often poor to treatment regimens that include multiple drugs and last for months.

Despite these problems, drug combinations have proved effective in the treatment of mycobacterial disease. Drugs used to treat tuberculosis include first-line drugs (isoniazid [INH], rifampin [RIF, Rifadin, Rimactane], ethambutol [EMB, Myambutol], pyrazinamide [PZA], and streptomycin) and second-line drugs used for drug-resistant or recurrent disease (para-aminosalicylic acid [PASA], ethionamide [Trecator-SC], capreomycin [Capastat], cycloserine [Seromycin], kanamycin [Kantrex], ofloxacin [Floxin], levofloxacin [Levaquin], moxifloxacin [Avelox], and bedaquiline [Sirturo]). Rifabutin (Mycobutin) is used mainly to treat or prevent *Mycobacterium avium* complex (MAC) and may be the preferred rifamycin for HIV patients when specific drug–drug interactions exist. Management of tuberculosis is further discussed in Chapter 45, and HIV infection is discussed in Chapter 37.

Pharmacodynamics

Spectrum of Activity

Isoniazid is the most active drug for the treatment of tuberculosis. It interferes with lipid and nucleic acid biosynthesis in growing organisms. It is also thought that isoniazid and ethambutol inhibit synthesis of mycolic acids. These acids are important constituents for mycobacteria cell walls and are not found in mammalian cells. Isoniazid is bactericidal

against susceptible mycobacteria, including intracellular and extracellular organisms.

Rifamycins (rifampin, rifabutin, and rifapentine) bind to the beta subunit of mycobacteria DNA-dependent RNA polymerase and inhibit RNA synthesis. Antimycobacterial action results in destruction of both multiplying and inactive bacilli. These drugs readily penetrate most tissues and can kill bacteria that are poorly accessible to many other drugs. Rifamycins are bactericidal against susceptible mycobacteria. Rifampin and rifabutin also have activity against *N. gonorrhoeae,* staphylococci, streptococci, *Mycobacterium leprae* (the cause of leprosy), MAC, and *H. influenzae* type b. Rifabutin is active against most *Mycobacterium* spp. Rifampin resistance develops rapidly when used as monotherapy; therefore, it should be combined with another active antibiotic for treatment of established infections.

Ethambutol inhibits synthesis of arabinogalactan, an essential component of mycobacteria cell walls. It also arrests cell multiplication, causing cell death. Ethambutol enhances the activity of lipophilic drugs such as rifampin and ofloxacin that cross the mycobacteria cell wall primarily in lipid portions of this wall. It is bacteriostatic against susceptible mycobacteria, including *M. tuberculosis*, *M. avium*, and *M. kansasii.*

Pyrazinamide, an analogue of nicotinamide, is bactericidal against *M. tuberculosis* in an acidic environment (pH less than 5.6). Pyrazinamide therapy is especially useful in the treatment of tuberculosis; it exhibits good activity within macrophages and plays a key role in killing intracellular organisms. This may be especially important in shortening therapy and preventing relapses. The exact mechanism of action of pyrazinamide is unknown.

Streptomycin is an aminoglycoside used now almost exclusively to treat *M. tuberculosis* infections. It is added as a fourth drug to the treatment regimen because up to 80% of patients treated with this drug harbor resistant bacilli after 4 months of treatment. Other mycobacteria except *M. avium* and *M. kansasii* are resistant to streptomycin. This drug is an irreversible inhibitor of protein synthesis. It penetrates cells poorly but is bactericidal in an alkaline extracellular environment.

Ethionamide, a thioamide with a similar binding site and mechanism of action as isoniazid, ultimately blocks the synthesis of mycolic acids. It is bacteriostatic against *M. tuberculosis,* and this drug also inhibits some other *Mycobacterium* species.

Capreomycin, a peptide antibiotic, inhibits RNA synthesis, thereby decreasing the replication of *M. tuberculosis.* Because resistance easily develops when it is given alone, it is given as part of a multidrug regimen. It is bactericidal to susceptible mycobacteria.

Bedaquiline is a unique antimycobacterial that was approved by the FDA in December 2012 specifically for the treatment of pulmonary multidrug-resistant tuberculosis. Bedaquiline inhibits mycobacterial adenosine triphosphate (ATP) synthesis and is active against replicating and dormant mycobacteria. The role of bedaquiline in the treatment of tuberculosis therapy has yet to be fully defined. The FDA issued a Black-Box Warning that bedaquiline is associated with increased mortality as compared with a placebo treatment group. Bedaquiline should therefore only be used when an effective treatment regimen cannot otherwise be provided. Bedaquiline will not be discussed further.

Para-aminosalicylic acid, structurally similar to para-aminobenzoic acid (PABA) and the sulfonamides, is a folate synthesis antagonist that is active almost exclusively against *M. tuberculosis*. It is bacteriostatic. It is not used frequently because primary resistance is common and other drugs are better tolerated and less expensive. It will not be discussed further.

Resistance

Resistance to isoniazid is mediated through the *inhA* gene or through mutation or deletion of *katG*, which encodes mycobacterium catalase. *InhA* mutants have low-level resistance and cross-resistance to ethionamide. The *katG* mutants have high-level resistance but no cross-resistance. Resistant mutants occur with a frequency of about 1 per 10^6 bacilli and are selected out if isoniazid is given alone. Globally, 3.6% of new and 20.2% of previously treated cases of tuberculosis are resistant to both isoniazid and rifampin. In the United States, only 1% of new cases and approximately 3% of retreatment cases are resistant to isoniazid and rifampin (WHO, 2013c).

Resistance to rifamycins results from point mutations that prevent binding to RNA polymerase. Cross-resistance often exists between the rifamycins. The mechanism of resistance is unknown for ethambutol, but it develops rapidly when ethambutol is used as monotherapy. Resistance to ethionamide also develops rapidly when it is used as monotherapy.

Resistance also develops rapidly to pyrazinamide, but there is no cross-resistance to other antimycobacterial drugs so that it can be given to patients exposed to a case of multidrug-resistant tuberculosis. Capreomycin is also useful for treatment of drug-resistant tuberculosis because of its lack of cross-resistance to first-line drugs. A point mutation that alters the ribosomal binding site is the mechanism of resistance for streptomycin.

Pharmacokinetics

Absorption and Distribution

All oral antimycobacterials are rapidly and well absorbed in the GI tract after oral administration.

Isoniazid is 90% bioavailable but should be taken on an empty stomach because food decreases the peak and extent of absorption. It readily diffuses into all body fluids, including CSF (90% of serum levels), pleural, and ascitic fluids; tissues; organs; and saliva, sputum, and feces. It also crosses the placenta and enters breast milk.

Meals slow the rate of absorption of rifamycins but not the extent of absorption. These drugs may be taken with or without food. Bioavailability of the oral formulations vary between 20% for rifabutin in an HIV-positive person to over 90% for rifampin. Therapeutic concentrations are achieved

for all rifamycins at recommended doses. Rifamycins and ethambutol also penetrate and concentrate in most body fluids. Adequate penetration of CSF occurs only in the presence of inflamed meninges. They both cross the placenta and enter breast milk.

Pyrazinamide is widely distributed in body tissues and fluids including the liver and lung, and it reaches high concentrations in CSF. It enters breast milk.

Streptomycin and capreomycin are widely distributed through extracellular fluid, cross the placenta, and enter breast milk in small amounts. They have poor CSF penetration except in the presence of inflamed meninges.

Ethionamide is widely distributed to body tissues and fluids. CSF concentrations are equal to those in the serum.

Metabolism and Excretion

The metabolism of isoniazid is extensive and highly variable and dependent on acetylator status. The liver, in a process that is genetically controlled, primarily acetylates it. Fast acetylators metabolize this drug 5 to 6 times faster than slow acetylators do. Approximately 50% of both blacks and whites are slow acetylators, and the rest are rapid acetylators. The majority of Alaskan natives and Asians are rapid acetylators. The rate of acetylation does not alter effectiveness but may increase the risk for toxic reactions in slow acetylators. Rapid clearance is of no consequence when the drug is given daily but may result in subtherapeutic doses when given once weekly. Isoniazid metabolites and unchanged drug are excreted in the urine. Elimination is largely independent of renal function.

Rifampin and rifapentine are also metabolized in the liver by deacetylation, with metabolites also active against *M. tuberculosis*. Rifamycins are potent inducers of liver metabolism. With repeated administration, the half-lives of rifampin and rifapentine decrease. They are excreted mainly in bile; then, through enterohepatic recirculation, the remainder is excreted in feces, with a small amount excreted in urine. Hepatic insufficiency or the age of the patient alters the pharmacokinetics of rifabutin only slightly. Somewhat reduced drug distribution and faster drug elimination are seen in renal insufficiency and may result in decreased drug concentrations.

Ethambutol is mainly excreted as unchanged drug in the urine. However, about 20% of ethambutol is metabolized by oxidation in the liver. Marked accumulation may occur in renal failure.

Approximately 70% of a pyrazinamide dose is excreted in urine by glomerular filtration. Pyrazinamide is hydrolyzed by the liver to a metabolite that also has antimycobacterial activity. Its half-life may be significantly prolonged in the presence of impaired renal or hepatic function. Streptomycin and capreomycin are excreted almost exclusively by the kidney.

Approximately 35% of ethionamide is metabolized by the liver, and the majority of the drug is excreted in urine as inactive metabolites. Less than 1% is excreted as unchanged drug.

Table 24-26 presents the pharmacokinetics of selected antimycobacterials.

Table 24–26 ▪ **Pharmacokinetics: Selected Antimycobacterials**

Drug	Onset	Peak	Duration	Protein Binding	Bioavailability	Half-Life	Elimination
Capreomycin (IM)	Rapid	1–2 h	UA	UA	UA	4–6 h	52% unchanged in urine within 12 h
Ethambutol	Rapid	2–4 h	24 h	UA	69%–85%	3–4 h*	20%–50% metabolized by liver; 50% unchanged in urine
Ethionamide	Rapid	3 h	UA	10%	100%	2–3 h	Metabolized by liver; <1% unchanged in urine
Isoniazid (PO/IM)	Rapid	1–2 h	24 h	40%–30%	90%	1–4 h	Extensively metabolized by liver; up to 66% unchanged in urine, dependent on acetylator status
Pyrazinamide	Rapid	2 h	UA	5%–10%	Nearly complete	9–10 h*	Metbolized via hydrolysis, 70% excreted in urine
Rifampin	Rapid	2–4 h	24 h	88%–90%	90%–95%	1–5 h†	40%–60% in bile and by enterohepatic circulation
Rifabutin	Rapid	2–4 h	24 h	85%	20%–53%	45 h	30% in feces; 53% as metabolites in urine
Rifapentine	Rapid	5–6 h	UA	98%	70%	13–14 h	70% in feces, 17% in urine
Streptomycin (IM)	Rapid	0.5–1.5 h	UA	0%–10%	UA	2–3 h*	>90% in urine

UA = information unavailable.

*Increased in renal or hepatic impairment.

†Varies by dose and averages 2–3 h after repeated doses.

Pharmacotherapeutics

Precautions and Contraindications

Isoniazid should be used cautiously and with careful monitoring for hepatotoxity, especially for those patients who drink alcohol daily, who have active chronic liver disease or severe renal dysfunction, who are over 35 years of age, use drugs of abuse, are pregnant or immediately postpartum. Peripheral neuropathy and other neurotoxicities may occur with isoniazid use. Special caution should be used with patients with preexisting peripheral neuropathy and those who are pregnant or are HIV-positive.

Cautious use in renal impairment is recommended for ethambutol, streptomycin, and capreomycin. Dosage adjustments may be required and are discussed in the Clinical Use and Dosing section.

Cautious use in the presence of hepatic impairment is recommended for isoniazid, rifamycins (hepatotoxic), pyrazinamide, and ethionamide (hepatotoxic). Black and Hispanic women, women postpartum, and patients older than 50 years are at special risk for development of hepatitis while taking isoniazid.

Ethionamide should be given cautiously to patients with diabetes mellitus. Management may be more difficult and hepatitis is more likely in these patients.

Hematologic alterations including various anemias and thrombocytopenia have been seen with the use of isoniazid and rifampin. Ethambutol and pyrazinamide each may precipitate gouty arthritis attacks and should be used cautiously in the presence of this disorder.

Rifamycins are potent inducers of liver metabolism. These agents may lead to subtherapeutic concentrations of other medications metabolized by CYP enzymes. Treatment failures may occur.

See Table 24-27 for specific drug–drug interactions.

Ethambutol has caused visual disturbances, including irreversible blindness. Cautious use is advised in patients with inability to appreciate or report visual changes or with preexisting optic neuritis, cataracts, or diabetic retinopathy.

Pyrazinamide should not be used during acute gout attacks.

Pregnancy categories vary by drug and country. Isoniazid is Pregnancy Category A; most other antimycobacterials are Category C. Use of antimycobacterials, particularly isoniazid and rifampin, with ethambutol added if drug resistance is a possibility, is recommended because the risk of losing the fetus is secondary to tuberculosis infection or because congenital tuberculosis poses a higher risk than the observed risks of adverse effects of the treatment. The exception is streptomycin. Streptomycin, Pregnancy Category D, may cause congenital deafness if given to pregnant women.

The infant should be observed for any evidence of adverse effects from drugs that appear in breast milk. Discontinuing the drug must take into account the importance of the drug for the mother. The drugs that enter breast milk in smaller amounts include rifampin, ethambutol, and pyrazinamide.

Table 24–27 ▦ Drug Interactions: Selected Antimycobacterials

Drug	Interacting Drug	Possible Effect	Implications
Capreomycin	Aminoglycosides and other ototoxic and nephrotoxic drugs Isoniazid, ethionamide Phenytoin	Additive ototoxicity and nephrotoxicity Additive CNS effects; increased risk for peripheral neuropathy Inhibition of phenytoin metabolism; increased toxicity risk	Avoid concurrent use If symptoms occur, discontinue one of the drugs Monitor serum levels of phenytoin
Ethambutol	Aluminum salts	Reduced absorption of ethambutol	Administer ethambutol 1–2 h before aluminum salt
Isoniazid	Alcohol	Daily ingestion increases risk for hepatitis	Avoid concurrent use
	Aluminum salts	Reduced oral absorption of isoniazid	Administer isoniazid 1–2 h before aluminum salts
	Oral anticoagulants	Enhanced anticoagulant activity	Avoid concurrent use or monitor PT/INR
	Benzodiazepines (BDZs)	Isoniazid may inhibit metabolic clearance of BDZs that undergo oxidative metabolism (e.g., diazepam, triazolam)	Avoid concurrent use
	Carbamazepine	Toxicity or hepatotoxicity may occur	Monitor carbamazepine drug levels and liver function
	Cyclosporine	Increased risk of neurotoxicity	Use with caution
	Disulfiram	Acute behavioral and coordination changes	Avoid coadministration
	Hydantoins	Increased serum hydantoin levels because of inhibition of CYP-450 enzymes. Most significant in slow acetylators	Monitor hydantoin levels and adjust doses as needed
	Itraconazole and ketoconazole	Decreased serum antifungal levels; decreased antifungal activity	Select different antifungal
	Rifampin	Increased risk for hepatotoxicity	If alterations in liver function tests, discontinue one of these drugs
	Theophylline	Increased or decreased theophylline levels	Monitor theophylline levels
	Warfarin	Increased warfarin effects and risk of bleeding	Monitor closely
	Tyramine-containing foods	Isoniazid has slight monoamine oxidase inhibition activity	Teach patient foods to avoid
	Histamine-containing foods	Diamine oxidase may be inhibited	Teach patient foods to avoid (e.g., tuna, sauerkraut, yeast extract)
Pyrazinamide	Laboratory interactions	Has been reported to interfere with Acetest and Ketostix urine tests to produce a pink/brown color	Select different method of determining ketoacidosis
Rifamycins (rifampin, rifapentine, rifabutin)	Oral anticoagulants, azole antifungals, barbiturates, BDZs, beta blockers, chloramphenicol, clofibrate, oral contraceptives, corticosteroids, cyclosporine, digitoxin, disopyramide, efavirenz, elvitegravir, etravirine, estrogens, hydantoins, methadone, mexiletine, miraviroc, nevirapine, quinidine, sildenafil, sulfonylureas, tacrolimus, tamoxifen, theophylline, tocainide, verapamil	Rifampin induces CYP-450 enzyme systems that metabolize these drugs. Therapeutic effects of these drugs may be significantly decreased. Treatment failure may occur.	Select alternative therapy

Continued

Table 24–27 ⠿ **Drug Interactions: Selected Antimycobacterials—cont'd**

Drug	Interacting Drug	Possible Effect	Implications
	Digoxin	Decreased serum levels of digoxin	Monitor serum levels or select different antimycobacterial
	Isoniazid	Increased risk for hepatotoxicity	See isoniazid above
	Protease inhibitors	Significant decrease in protease inhibitor concentrations, increased risk of HIV or hepatitis C treatment failure	Avoid concurrent use
	Laboratory interactions	Therapeutic levels of rifampin interfere with standard assays of serum folate and B_{12}	Consider alternative methods for determining concentrations
Rifabutin	Clarithromycin	Increased rifabutin levels, decreased clarithromycin levels. Increased risk of neutropenia, rash, GI disturbances.	Monitor for toxicity; select a different macrolide if possible
	Efavirenz	Decreased rifabutin levels	Increase rifabutin dose
	Fluconazole	Up to 80% increase in rifabutin levels, increased risk of rifabutin toxicity, including uveitis	Use with caution; monitor for toxicity
Streptomycin	Cephalosporins, vancomycin	Increased risk of nephrotoxicity	Monitor renal function
	Loop diuretics	Increased risk for ototoxicity. Hearing loss may be irreversible.	Avoid concurrent use

CNS = central nervous system; INR = international normalized ratio; PT = prothrombin time.

Capreomycin is excreted in such small amounts as to be undetectable in some women. Isoniazid is distributed into breast milk but is considered safe during breastfeeding.

Use in children varies by drug. Pediatric doses are listed for all of these drugs, but the age under which they should not be used varies. No age restrictions are provided for isoniazid, rifampin, and pyrazinamide. The safety and efficacy of rifabutin or rifapentine have not been established in children. Ethambutol is not FDA approved for use by children younger than 13 years. Safety and optimal dosage have not been determined for children for ethionamide and capreomycin. Ototoxicity risk precludes use of streptomycin in neonates and in older adults or patients with diminished hearing.

Adverse Drug Reactions

All of the antimycobacterial drugs have risks for hypersensitivity reactions, some of which may be severe. The usual management associated with these reactions applies here as well.

Peripheral neuropathy is the most common adverse reaction with isoniazid. It occurs in about 2% of patients taking 5 mg/kg/d. Prevalence is higher for patients taking higher doses, up to about 44% for patients taking 16 mg/kg/d. The symptoms include symmetrical numbness and tingling in the extremities. Patients predisposed to this adverse reaction include the malnourished, slow acetylators, pregnant women, older adults, diabetics, and patients with chronic liver disease, including alcoholics. Pyridoxine (B_6) prevents the development of peripheral neuropathy and is recommended for patients in these at-risk categories. Some providers use

pyridoxine for all patients on isoniazid. Recommended prophylactic doses range from 10 to 50 mg daily. Treatment of established neuropathy requires 50 to 200 mg daily.

Elevated serum transaminases (AST/ALT) are observed in 10% to 20% of patients taking isoniazid. Patients at risk were discussed previously. This condition typically occurs in the first 3 months of therapy, is asymptomatic, and will return to normal with continued isoniazid therapy. However, a small portion of patients (0.4%) may progress to hepatic failure or necrosis. The symptoms are those usually associated with the development of hepatitis, including abnormal liver function studies, jaundice, and fatigue. The frequency of progressive liver damage increases with age. Concurrent alcohol use increases the risk. When rifampin is given concurrently, the risk is increased 4-fold. Other adverse reactions associated with isoniazid include blood dyscrasias, metabolic acidosis, drug fever, and gynecomastia.

The most common adverse reactions associated with rifamycins are GI in nature: anorexia, nausea, vomiting, diarrhea, flatulence, and abdominal pain. Although hepatotoxicity is less common than it is with isoniazid, hepatotoxicity leading to hepatitis occurs with rifampin. Transient elevations of AST/ALT are seen in the first 8 weeks of therapy in 10% to 15% of patients. However, less than 1% of patients have progressive hepatotoxicity. A harmless orange-red discoloration of body fluids, including tears, saliva, urine, sweat, CSF, and feces, also occurs. Hematuria should not be confused with this discoloration because hematuria may be an indication of a hypersensitivity reaction.

Other adverse reactions associated with rifamycins include blood dyscrasias, headache, drowsiness and inability to concentrate, a pruritic rash (1% to 11% of patients), visual disturbances, lupus erythematosus, and exudative conjunctivitis. Thrombocytopenia and neutropenia have been observed with rifabutin.

Ethambutol also has the usual GI disturbances, but the most serious adverse reaction is optic neuritis, which appears to be dose-related. Signs and symptoms include decreased visual acuity, red-green color blindness, diminished visual fields, and sometimes loss of vision. These adverse reactions are generally reversible when the drug is discontinued promptly. In rare cases, recovery may take up to 1 year. Vision testing should be done before and throughout therapy. Other adverse reactions associated with ethambutol include precipitation of gouty arthritis related to elevated uric acid levels, transient impairment of liver function, and infrequent peripheral neuropathy.

The principal adverse reaction with pyrazinamide is dose-related hepatotoxicity that may appear any time during therapy. Patients at risk for this adverse reaction are the same ones mentioned in the Precautions and Contraindications section. Discontinuing the drug may be required. Because this drug inhibits the renal excretion of urates, hyperuricemia also often occurs. It is often asymptomatic but may precipitate acute gouty arthritis or arthralgias. Baseline serum uric acid levels should be drawn.

The most serious adverse effect associated with streptomycin and capreomycin is ototoxicity. Damage to the eighth cranial nerve results in vertigo, nausea, vomiting, and loss of hearing. The risk is increased with higher doses and longer duration of therapy. Nephrotoxicity is also a serious risk for patients on any aminoglycoside. Risk for this adverse reaction increases for patients with renal insufficiency and for older adults with age-related decreased renal function. Dosage adjustments are made based on renal function studies to reduce the risk for this adverse reaction. Doses taken 2 or 3 times weekly rather than daily also reduce the risk for toxicity.

Ethionamide has few adverse reactions, but it is often poorly tolerated because of its most common adverse reaction, GI distress, including nausea and diarrhea. Some patients develop a metallic taste in their mouth. Other common adverse reactions include hepatitis (rare), optic neuritis, and peripheral neuritis (common). Neurological symptoms can be alleviated by pyridoxine.

Cycloserine is associated with neurological effects, such as somnolence, psychosis, and suicidal ideation.

Drug Interactions

Drug interactions and drug–food interactions vary by drug. Many are associated with increased incidence of the common adverse reactions for the particular antimycobacterial. Some are associated with reduced effectiveness of the interacting drug. Rifamycins are potent inducers of the CYP450 enzyme system and speed the metabolism of many drugs, resulting in therapeutic failure.

Antimycobacterial agents may reduce the effectiveness of the live Bacillus Calmette Guerin (BCG) vaccine

and intravesical treatment regimens. Concomittant use should be avoided. Table 24-27 provides a list of the drug interactions.

Clinical Use and Dosing

Resistance to antimycobacterial drugs has a frequency of about 1 in 10^6 bacilli. However, with 10^8 bacilli lesions in an infected person, resistant mutants are selected out when only one drug is given. Because of the relatively high proportion of adult patients with tuberculosis caused by organisms that are resistant to isoniazid, four drugs are necessary in the initial phase of therapy for the 6-month regimen to be maximally effective (CDC, 2003). Multiple drugs with independent actions lower the prevalence of resistance. Patients with HIV infection are especially at risk for tuberculosis and resistance development. Treatment regimens include initial phase and continuation phases. Initial phases have four drugs (isoniazid [INH], rifampin [RIF], pyrazinamid [PZA], and ethambutol [EMB]) given for 2 months followed by continuation phases, usually with two drugs (INH and another drug, most often RIF) given for 4 to 7 months.

The first-line antimycobacterial drugs should be administered together; split dosing should be avoided. Fixed-dose combination preparations may be more easily administered than single-drug tablets and may decrease the risk for acquired drug resistance and drug errors. Two combination formulations have been approved for use in the United States: INH/RIF (Rifamate) and INH/RIF/PZA (Rifater). It should be noted that for patients weighing more than 90 kg, the dose of PZA in the three-drug combination is insufficient and additional PZA tablets are necessary.

Some continuation phase protocols are designed for HIV-infected individuals. These combinations are discussed in Chapter 37. Initial phase and continuation phase drug combinations and dosing for tuberculosis are discussed in Chapter 45.

Table 24-28 presents the dosage schedule for selected antimycobacterials.

Rational Drug Selection

Rifampin is also used to treat several nonmycobacterial infections. It is used as prophylaxis for close contacts of people with meningococcal infections caused by *N. meningitidis*, including household members, children and personnel in nurseries and day-care centers, and closed populations such as in college dormitories and military barracks. Health-care personnel with intimate exposure to index cases (such as mouth-to-mouth resuscitation) should receive prophylactic therapy. Prophylaxis for adults is oral rifampin 600 mg every 12 hours for four doses (two days). The dose for children is 10 mg/kg every 12 hours for four doses (two days).

Rifampin is also indicated for prophylaxis for close contacts of people with actual or suspected infections with *H. influenzae* type b. If one of the contacts in a household is an unvaccinated child 4 years or younger, it is recommended that all contacts in the household except pregnant

Text continued on page 769

Table 24–28 ✇ Dosage Schedule: Selected Antimycobacterials

Drug	Indication	Dosage Form	Initial Dose	Comments
(Capastat)	Tuberculosis, as part of combined drug therapy when first-line therapy ineffective or caused toxicity or resistance	Powder for injection: 1 g	1 g IM/IV daily for 60–120 d, then 1 g 2–3 times/wk	Maximum adult daily dose 20 mg/kg. Monitor renal function tests, audiograms, vestibular function, and sites of injection at baseline and at least weekly. Serum potassium should be measured at baseline and monthly during daily therapy. Administer deep IM into large muscle mass because superficial injections are associated with pain and sterile abscess. Administer within 24 h of reconstitution. Store in refrigerator after reconstitution. Darkening of reconstituted drug from initial nearly colorless or straw color does not affect potency. Renal impairment requires decreased dose (see package insert). Educate patients to report altered hearing, dizziness, imbalance; altered urination, nausea, vomiting, or thirst. Patients should advise prescribers they are taking capreomycin because of its potential for drug interactions.
Ethambutol (Myambutol)	Tuberculosis, as part of combined drug therapy	Tablets: 100 mg, 400 mg	*Adults:* Orally 15–25 mg/kg/d, maximum 1,500 mg/d; *or* 50 mg/kg up to 2,500 mg twice/wk; *or* 25–30 mg/kg 3 times/wk *Children <13 yr:* HIV negative: 15–20 mg/kg/d *or* 50 mg/kg twice weekly HIV exposed/infected: 15–20 mg/kg/d Not recommended for children <6 yr in whom visual acuity cannot be monitored	Maximum adult daily dose 1.5 g. Impairment of renal function may require a decreased dosage. Monitor visual fields and red and green discrimination prior to and monthly during treatment, especially for prolonged therapy or >15 mg/kg daily. Periodic uric acid and renal function tests.
	Atypical mycobacterial infections (off-label)		Orally 15–25 mg/kg/d	Educate about importance of vision monitoring. Blurred vision, eye pain, vision loss, or problems with red and green discrimination should be reported. Other reportable symptoms include evidence of peripheral neuropathy (numbness, tingling, burning pain, weakness in hands or feet), gout (chills, pain and swelling of joints, hot skin over affected joints), and hypersensitivity (rash, fever, joint aches). Take drug with food if GI irritation occurs.
Ethionamide (Trecator)	Tuberculosis, as part of combined drug therapy	Tablets: 250 mg	*Adults:* 250 mg q8–12h for 1–2 yr or more *Children:* 15–20 mg/kg/d divided into 2 or 3 doses *or* 15 mg/kg as 1 dose daily	Administer with meals to minimize GI distress. Maximal daily adult dose 1 g. In order to minimize the risk of resistance to the drug, give the highest tolerated dose (based on gastrointestinal intolerance). Monitor liver function tests periodically. Ophthalmic examinations if symptoms of visual impairment. Orthostatic blood pressure checks. Thyroid function tests if signs of hypothyroidism; serum glucose if signs of hypoglycemia. Neurological exam for peripheral neuritis.

Table 24–28 ⊗ **Dosage Schedule: Selected Antimycobacterials—cont'd**

Drug	Indication	Dosage Form	Initial Dose	Comments
				Pyridoxine decreases risk of peripheral neuropathy. Report signs of hepatitis (yellow eyes or skin, upper abdominal pain, malaise), peripheral neuritis (numbness, tingling, burning pain, weakness in hands or feet), optic neuritis (blurred vision, eye pain), hypoglycemia (poor concentration, tachycardia, hunger, shakiness), or hypothyroidism (weight gain; dry, puffy skin; coldness; irregular menses). Administer with or after meals if GI irritation occurs. Usually administered after evening meal or at bedtime as a single dose. Serum concentrations may be higher with divided doses, but GI irritation may worsen.
Isoniazid (Laniazid) (Nydrazid) Isoniazid combinations (Rifater) (Rifamate)	Inactive or latent tuberculosis	Tablets: 100 mg, 300 mg Syrup: 50 mg/5 mL Injection: 100 mg/mL Injection: 100 mg/mL Tablets: 120 mg rifampin, 50 mg isoniazid, 300 mg pyrazinamide Capsules: 150 mg isoniazid, 300 mg rifampin	*Adults:* PO or IM 5 mg/kg up to 300 mg/d *or* 15 mg/kg up to 900 mg 2 or 3 times/wk *Children:* 10–15 mg/kg, up to 300 mg, once daily *or* 20–40 mg/kg up to 900 mg/day 2 or 3 times/wk	Renal impairment does not usually require dosage adjustment if serum creatinine is <6 mcg/dL and patient is fast acetylator. For slow acetylators, adjust dose to maintain plasma concentration <1 mcg/mL at 24 h after last dose. Monitor liver function tests monthly or more often if liver impairment or clinical signs of hepatitis or prodromal symptoms. CBC and platelet count periodically or at signs of blood dyscrasia (fever, sore throat, bleeding or bruising, tiredness). Ophthalmic exam if signs of optic neuritis. Educate to report signs of clinical hepatitis (dark urine, yellow eyes or skin), hepatitis prodromal symptoms (anorexia, nausea and vomiting, unusual tiredness), optic neuritis (blurred vision or loss of vision, with or without eye pain), or peripheral neuropathy (numbness, clumsiness, burning pain of hands or feet). High risk for peripheral neuropathy (pregnant, high alcohol use, taking anticonvulsants, poor diet, malnourished, history of neuritis, chronic renal failure, diabetes, and over 65) should be prescribed 25 mg pyridoxine/d. May be taken with meals or antacids if GI irritation occurs, but do not take within 1 h of aluminum-containing antacid. Measure syrup with calibrated measuring device. Crystals may form at low temperatures, but they redissolve upon warming to room temperature.
	Tuberculosis, as part of combined drug therapy Prophylaxis or preventive TB therapy		*Adults:* PO or IM 300 mg once daily *or* 15 mg/kg, up to 900 mg, given 2–3 times/wk *Children:* 10 mg/kg, up to 300 mg, once daily, *or* 20–40 mg/kg, up to 900 mg, given 2–3 times/wk	As above. Directly observed therapy (DOT) may be administered twice weekly The following contacts with TB infection should be given prophylaxis INH therapy for 8–12 wk after exposure and until they have a negative PPD: (1) children aged <5 years; (2) contacts with HIV infection; (3) other contacts with risk factors for progression to TB disease (4); (4) contacts with documented skin test conversion; and (5) contacts of patients with positive sputum AFB smear results and cavities on chest radiography (www.CDC.gov/TB)

Continued

Table 24–28 ⊗ Dosage Schedule: Selected Antimycobacterials—cont'd

Drug	Indication	Dosage Form	Initial Dose	Comments
Pyrazinamide	Tuberculosis, as part of combined drug therapy	Tablets: 500 mg	*Adults and children:* 15–30 mg/kg once daily or 50–70 mg/kg 2–3 times/wk; patients with HIV take 20–30 mg/kg/d for first 2 mo DOT: 50 mg/kg/dose twice weekly	Maximal adult and pediatric daily dosage is 2 g when taken daily, 3 g when taken 3 times/wk, 4 g when taken twice/wk. Monitor liver function tests prior to and every 2–4 wk during treatment. Uric acid determinations may be needed. Educate that arthralgia is usually mild and self-limiting and to report signs of hepatotoxicity (dark urine, anorexia, nausea, vomiting, yellow skin or eyes) and gout (pain, swelling, heat over joints). May be taken without regard to meals.
Rifampin (Rifadin, Rimactane)	Tuberculosis, as part of combined drug therapy	Capsules: 150, 300 mg	*Adults:* 600 mg PO once daily *or* 10 mg/kg up to 600 mg 2–3 times/wk *Infants <1 mo:* 10–20 mg/kg PO once daily *or* 10–20 mg/kg 2–3 times/wk	Maximum adult or pediatric daily oral dose should not exceed 600 mg. Severe hepatic impairment requires 50% reduction in dosages. Monitor hepatic function prior to and at least monthly during treatment; CBC if signs of blood dyscrasia (sore throat, bleeding, bruising). Advise patients to report signs of hepatotoxicity (dark urine, anorexia, nausea, vomiting, yellow skin or eyes), flu-like syndrome, or blood dyscrasias. Reddish orange or reddish brown discoloration may stain clothes or soft contact lenses but is harmless. Avoid alcohol, which can increase hepatotoxicity. Advise healthcare providers of rifampin use because of high risk of drug interactions. May be taken without regard to meals. Shake suspension before measurement, using calibrated dosing device. Store suspension at controlled room temperature and discard remaining liquid 30 d after reconstitution.
	Meningococcal meningitis prophylaxis		*Adults:* 600 mg PO bid for 2 d *Children:* 10 mg/kg q12h for 2 d (max 600 mg/dose) *Infants < 1 mo:* 5 mg/kg q12h for 2 d	As above
	H. influenzae meningitis prophylaxis (off-label)		*Adults:* 600 mg PO once/d for 4 d *Children:* 20 mg/kg once daily for 4 d (10 mg/kg if infant <1 mo)	As above
	Staphylococcal infections as part of combination therapy		*Adults:* 600 mg once daily or 300 mg bid–tid	As above
Rifabutin (Mycobutin)	MAC treatment and prophylaxis, as part of combined drug therapy	Capsules: 150 mg	*Adults and adolescents:* 300 mg once daily *Infants and children:* 10–20 mg/kg once daily (maximum 300 mg/day)	May need to monitor platelet count and WBC. Rifabutin increases rate of metabolism of many drugs, including anti-HIV agents; monitor drug response and/or blood levels, if available. Also, rifabutin is affected by strong inhibitors of CYP 3A4, thus dosing of rifabutin may need to be adjusted based on specific drug interactions.

Table 24–28 ⚕ **Dosage Schedule: Selected Antimycobacterials—cont'd**

Drug	Indication	Dosage Form	Initial Dose	Comments
				Counsel patient to report allergic reaction, GI intolerance, or asthenia. May turn secretions reddish brown that can stain clothing and soft contact lenses. May be administered without regard to food. If unable to tolerate single dose, split into 2 equal doses with food. May need to adjust dose up or down for patient taking antiretrovirals.
	Tuberculosis treatment, as part of combined drug therapy		*Adults:* 300 mg daily, but may vary based on other medications	As above
Rifapentine (Priftin)	Inactive or latent tuberculosis	Tablets: 150 mg	*Adults:* 15 mg/kg once weekly with INH	Give only as directly observed therapy
	Tuberculosis treatment, as part of combined drug therapy		*Adults:* 600 mg twice weekly for the first 2 mo, then 600 mg weekly	As above
Streptomycin	Tuberculosis, as part of combined drug therapy	Injection: 400 mg/mL	*Adults:* 1 g once daily IM. Reduce to 1 g 2–3 times/wk as soon as clinically feasible. *Children:* 20 mg/kg once daily IM, not to exceed 1 g/d. *Elderly:* 500–750 mg once daily IM. Duration of therapy may be 1–2 yr	Maximum adult daily dose 4 g daily. Maximum pediatric daily dose 1 g. Renal impairment requires reduced dosage. Monitor serum concentrations: peak concentrations >50 mcg/mL are associated with nephrotoxicity and should not be >20–25 mcg/mL in patients with pre-existing renal damage. Caloric stimulation tests may be required before, during, and after prolonged therapy to detect vestibular toxicity. Do audiograms and renal function tests periodically and frequent urinalysis to detect albumin, casts, cells, and decreased specific gravity. Educate patient to report signs of hypersensitivity (skin itching, rash, swelling), vestibular ototoxicity (clumsiness, dizziness, nausea, vomiting), auditory ototoxicity (hearing loss; fullness, ringing, buzzing in ears), peripheral neuritis (burning of face or mouth, numbness, tingling), and nephrotoxicity (altered frequency or amount of urination, thirst, anorexia, nausea and vomiting). Administer deep IM, alternating injection sites. Concentration of solution should not exceed 500 mg/mL. After reconstitution, solution retains potency for 2–28 d at room temperature and 14 d in refrigerator, depending on manufacturer. See package insert. Darkening of solution does not affect potency.

women receive prophylaxis. In a day-care center attended by unvaccinated children younger than 2 years, prophylaxis with rifampin 20 mg/kg up to 600 mg once daily for 4 days for all contacts and vaccination of all unvaccinated children should be considered. If all contacts are older than 2 years, prophylaxis is not indicated. If there have been two or more cases in the center within 60 days and unvaccinated children

attend, prophylaxis is recommended for children and personnel.

Finally, rifampin has an off-label use in the treatment of leprosy and concurrently with other antistaphylococcal agents in the treatment of serious infections in hospitalized patients caused by *Staphylococcus,* including methicillin-resistant and multidrug-resistant strains.

Patient Education

Administration

Because of the long duration of therapy and complexity of the protocols in tuberculosis infections, instruction and support are essential. Multidrug therapy, essential to prevent development of resistance, presents serious challenges for adherence. Some protocols are given daily for 8 weeks (56 doses) or 5 days/week for 8 weeks (40 doses) in the initial phase and then given twice weekly for 18 weeks (36 doses) during the continuation phase. To maintain this complex two- to four-drug regimen requires commitment on the part of the patient and usually outside help. This is especially true for lower-socioeconomic populations and other high-risk groups that normally have limited contact with the health-care system. Directly observed therapy (DOT), in which each dose is observed by a health-care provider or other designated person, has proved very effective in promoting compliance and improving response to therapy. Lifestyle implications of tuberculosis include general health promotion strategies such as good nutrition, rest, and appropriate exercise.

Adverse Reactions

Adverse effects, especially GI upset, are relatively common in the first few weeks of initial phase therapy. However, first-line drugs, particularly rifampin, must not be discontinued because of minor adverse effects. Although taking the drug with food may delay or moderately decrease the absorption, the effects of food have little clinical significance. Patients who have epigastric distress or nausea with this drug should be told that they can take their whole drug protocol with meals or that the hour of dosing can be changed. Administration with food is preferable to splitting a dose or changing to a second-line drug.

Rifamycins may discolor urine, tears, saliva, and sweat. This may result in the staining of clothing, dentures, or contact lenses. Patients receiving ethambutol should be advised to contact their provider if they experience eye pain or visual changes.

Lifestyle Management

Lifestyle management related to HIV infection is discussed in Chapter 37 and in Chapter 45 related to tuberculosis. Dosages, monitoring, and patient education are summarized in Table 24-28.

ANTIVIRALS

Viral infections range from the annoying, but short-lived and self-limiting, "common cold" to the progressive and, to date, incurable HIV. Discussion in this section focuses on nucleoside analogues used to treat herpes virus infections. Chapter 37 discusses drugs to treat HIV. Drugs used to treat cytomegalovirus (CMV) retinitis and other CMV disease in HIV patients (e.g., foscarnet, ganciclovir, valganciclovir) are also discussed in Chapter 37.

Viruses are obligate intracellular agents that depend on use of the host cell's genetic material for replication. As a result, antiviral drugs must either block entry into the cells or be active inside host cells to be effective. Ideally, an antiviral medication would be selective to specific viral components or pathways; however, many antivirals are nonselective and so damage to host cells and virus may result concomitantly. To further complicate treatment, replication of the virus may peak at or before clinical symptoms appear in many viral infections, so optimal clinical efficacy depends on early recognition and treatment or prevention. Finally, many viruses depend on enzymes to reproduce and can quickly mutate in the presence of drug therapy.

Viral replication consists of several steps: (1) adsorption to and penetration into susceptible cells; (2) uncoating of viral nucleic acid; (3) synthesis of early, regulatory proteins; (4) synthesis of RNA or DNA; (5) synthesis of late, structural proteins; (6) assembly of viral particles; and (7) release from the cell. Antiviral drugs target these steps. Many of the currently available antiviral agents act on synthesis of purine and pyrimidine (step 4).

NUCLEOSIDE ANALOGUES

Pharmacodynamics

The nucleoside analogues are used mainly to treat herpes infections by interfering with DNA synthesis and inhibiting viral replication. Acyclovir (Zovirax) is an acyclic guanosine derivative that requires three phosphorylation steps for activation. It is first converted to the monophosphate derivative by the virus-specific thymidine kinase and then to the di- and triphosphate compounds by the host's cellular enzymes. Because it requires the viral kinase for the first step, it is selectively activated only in infected cells. The final step, acyclovir triphosphate, inhibits viral DNA synthesis.

Valacyclovir (Valtrex) is the L-valine ester of acyclovir. It is rapidly converted after oral administration to acyclovir and so its mechanism of action is that of acyclovir; however, serum levels are 3 to 5 times higher than those achieved with oral acyclovir.

Famciclovir (Famvir) is the diacetyl ester prodrug of 6-deoxy penciclovir, an acyclic guanosine analogue. It is rapidly metabolized to penciclovir in the intestinal mucosa and liver. Penciclovir has a mechanism of action and spectrum of activity similar to acyclovir. Activation is catalyzed by virus-specified thymidine kinase in infected cells, resulting in competitive inhibition of the viral DNA polymerase and inhibition of DNA synthesis. It has lower affinity for the viral DNA polymerase than acyclovir, but it achieves higher intracellular concentrations and has a more prolonged intracellular effect.

Another nucleoside analogue, ribavirin (Virazole), is active against a wide range of DNA and RNA viruses, including influenza A and B, parainfluenza, respiratory syncytial virus (RSV), paramyxoviruses, hepatitis C virus (HCV), and HIV-1. Oral ribavirin plays a key role when combined with interferon for the treatment of HCV; however, it has not proved beneficial for RSV or HIV-1 infections. It is given via a

SPAG-2 aerosol treatment for RSV, usually in the hospital. It is not discussed further in this chapter.

Spectrum of Activity

Acyclovir is active against herpes simplex virus (HSV) 1 and 2; varicella-zoster virus (VZV); and, to a lesser extent, Epstein-Barr virus (EBV), CMV, and herpes virus 6 (HSV-6), which is implicated as the cause of roseola and other febrile diseases in childhood. Valacyclovir is converted to acyclovir after oral administration and is active against the same viruses. Famciclovir is active against HSV-1 and HSV-2, VZV, EBV, and hepatitis B virus.

Resistance

Resistance to acyclovir can develop in HSV and VZV through alteration in either the viral thymidine kinase or viral DNA polymerase. Because most resistance is based on deficient thymidine kinase activity, cross-resistance occurs with acyclovir, valacyclovir, and famciclovir.

Pharmacokinetics

Absorption and Distribution

Absorption following oral administration varies by drug. Acyclovir is poorly absorbed orally (15% to 20%), although therapeutic levels are achieved at recommended doses. Topical formulations (acyclovir, docosanol, penciclovir) produce local concentrations that may exceed 10 mcg/mL in herpetic lesions, but systemic concentrations are undetectable. Valacyclovir is 54% bioavailable as acyclovir after oral administration. Famciclovir is absorbed in the intestine for conversion to its active form, penciclovir. Food slows absorption but does not affect the extent of absorption. Penciclovir is marketed as a topical preparation only.

Acyclovir, famciclovir, and valacyclovir are widely distributed. Areas of distribution of acyclovir include the brain, kidney, saliva, semen, herpetic lesions, and lung. CSF concentrations are 50% of plasma for acyclovir and valacyclovir. Acyclovir and penciclovir are less than 33% protein bound. Acyclovir crosses the placenta and is found in breast milk.

Metabolism and Excretion

Acyclovir is 90% eliminated in the urine as unchanged drug, primarily by glomerular filtration and tubular secretion. The liver metabolizes the remaining 10%. The kidneys also excrete the active metabolite of famciclovir (penciclovir). Because valacyclovir is rapidly converted to acyclovir, it shares the same excretion pattern. Dosage adjustments are required for each of these drugs in the presence of renal impairment because of prolonged half-lives.

Table 24-29 presents the pharmacokinetics of nucleoside analogues for herpes virus infections.

Pharmacotherapeutics

Precautions and Contraindications

Renal failure has been reported with all drugs in this group. Therefore, dose adjustment and cautious use is advised for patients with renal impairment. This caution is also important in older adults, who commonly have diminished renal function or have inadequate hydration. Other nephrotoxic agents should be avoided if possible. Thrombotic thrombocytopenic purpura/hemolytic uremic syndrome (TTP/HUS) has been reported with acyclovir therapy.

Acyclovir, valacyclovir, and famciclovir are listed as Pregnancy Category B; however, little information is available for famciclovir. Acyclovir and valacyclovir are preferred in pregnancy because there is more data supporting the safety of acyclovir. Acyclovir is excreted in breast milk; however, the concentrations are low and considered to pose minimal risk to infants. Famciclovir has not been well studied in breastfeeding; therefore, caution or alternative therapy is advised.

Among these drugs, acyclovir is the safest for children. Oral formulations are approved for children older than 2 years of age. Famciclovir does not have established safety and efficacy for children younger than 18 years. The safety and efficacy of valacyclovir have not been established for children.

Adverse Drug Reactions

Adverse drug reactions vary by drug. Acyclovir has few reactions when given orally at recommended doses. Those reactions associated with short-term administration include headache, skin rash, nausea and vomiting, and diarrhea. Oral and intravenous acyclovir therapy has been associated with renal dysfunction. This typically occurs with high doses when the maximum solubility of free drug is exceeded, leading to

Table 24–29 ⬛ Pharmacokinetics: Nucleoside Analogues for Herpes Virus Infections

Drug	Onset	Peak	Duration	Protein Binding	Bioavailability	Half-Life	Elimination
Acyclovir	UA	1.5–2.5 h	4 h	9%–33%	15%–20%	3–4 h; 20 h in anuria	>90% in urine; rest metabolized by liver
Famciclovir	Rapid	1 h	8–12 h	20%	77%	2–3 h; prolonged in renal impairment	Mostly in urine
Valacyclovir	UA	1.5–2.5 h	8–24 h	13%–18%	54%	2.5–3h; 14 h in anuria	>90% in urine; rest metabolized by liver

UA = information unavailable.

crystalluria. But acute tubular necrosis has also been reported. Patients receiving IV acyclovir, other nephrotoxic drugs, and those with preexisting renal dysfunction or who are dehydrated are at particular risk of developing renal dysfunction or failure.

Neurologic effects such as ataxia, dizziness, confusion, encephalopathy, tremor, and seizures have been reported. Elderly patients and those with renal dysfunction are more likely to experience these effects. The most frequent adverse reactions associated with famciclovir are headache, dizziness, somnolence, and paresthesias.

Because it is converted to acyclovir, the adverse reactions for valacyclovir are the same as for acyclovir. Valacyclovir does have a higher incidence of adverse reactions when compared to oral acyclovir, including serious ones (TTP/HUS) in immunocompromised patients.

Drug Interactions

Drug interactions are minimal for acyclovir, famciclovir, and valacyclovir. Table 24-30 presents the few drug interactions that exist for nucleoside analogues.

Clinical Use and Dosing

The most important variable in selecting the dosage of nucleoside analogues is renal function. The dosing interval, dosage, or both are adjusted for patients with impaired renal function, depending on the dosage and degree of impairment. For example, the usual dose of valacyclovir for herpes zoster treatment in a patient with CCr greater than 50 mL/min is 1 g every 8 hours, whereas the dosage for a CCr less than 10 mL/min is 500 mg every 24 hours; for acyclovir the usual dose is 800 mg every 4 hours (5 times per day). If CCr is less than 10 mL/min, the dose is 200 mg every 12 hours. The prescriber should consult the package insert or a comprehensive reference for specific dosing guidelines.

The nucleoside analogues are recommended for the treatment of infections by the herpes simplex virus commonly seen in primary care, specifically genital herpes, herpes zoster (shingles), varicella (chickenpox), and gingivostomatitis in children. The nucleoside analogues do not cure herpes infections but may shorten duration, decrease severity, and reduce the incidence of sequelae of the infection.

Oral forms of acyclovir, valacyclovir, and famciclovir are all indicated for primary genital herpes; they increase the rate of healing but do not prevent recurrences. Although topical acyclovir is also approved for treatment of initial herpes genitalis infections, it is less effective than the oral nucleoside analogues and is not recommended.

The oral nucleoside analogues should be initiated as soon as possible after the onset of a recurrent episode. Patients are usually provided with a prescription that can be filled at the first sign of recurrence. Topical acyclovir has no benefit in recurrent disease in immunocompetent patients, although it has some value in suppression of mucocutaneous herpes in immunocompromised individuals.

Patients with frequent recurrences can be placed on suppression therapy, which decreases subclinical shedding between active episodes and the number of symptomatic recurrences. Suppressive therapy is costly, averaging annually between $300 for acyclovir 400 mg twice a day, $3,600 for 1 g/day and $2,100 for 500 mg/day for valacyclovir, and $3,700 for famciclovir 500 mg tablets. In untreated patients, the number of recurrences tends to decrease over time during the first 5 years of the disease. By 3 to 5 years after the initial episode, the number of recurrences may have declined to the point that episodic treatment of recurrences may be preferable. Therefore, the need for suppressive therapy should be reconsidered annually.

Oral acyclovir is indicated for the treatment of varicella in immunocompetent patients when started within 24 hours of the chickenpox rash. For immunocompromised patients, parenteral acyclovir should be used. The AAP does not recommend acyclovir for the treatment of uncomplicated chickenpox in healthy children. Acyclovir is recommended for healthy, nonpregnant patients 13 years and older; children older than 12 months with a chronic cutaneous or pulmonary disorder; and children receiving short, intermittent, or aerosolized courses of corticosteroids. If possible, the steroids should be discontinued after known exposure to varicella. The CDC recommends aggressive treatment of varicella in adults 20 years and older, in that the majority of deaths from chickenpox occur in this age group. Varicella-zoster immune globulin should be given within 96 hours of known exposure of a susceptible adult. If prophylaxis fails, early initiation of

Table 24–30 ⁂ Drug Interactions: Nucleoside Analogues

Drug	Interacting Drug	Possible Effect	Implications
Acyclovir, famciclovir	Probenecid	Increased serum levels and terminal half-life of acyclovir; decreased renal clearance	Avoid concurrent use
	Nephrotoxic drugs	Potential increased risk for renal toxicity	Monitor renal function closely
Famciclovir	Cimetidine	Penciclovir AUC and urinary recovery increased 18% and 12%, respectively	No clinical significance
	Theophylline	Penciclovir AUC increased 22% Renal clearance decreased 12%	No clinical significance
	Digoxin	C_{max} of digoxin increased 19% in healthy male volunteers	Probably of no clinical significance, but to be prudent, monitor digoxin levels closely

acyclovir within 24 hours of onset of varicella rash is urged. Susceptible adults at high risk (e.g., immunosuppressed, HIV, corticosteroid users) should be vaccinated. Varicella is the leading cause of vaccine-preventable deaths in the United States, so vaccination of children is recommended (see Chapter 19 for the latest immunization schedule or go to http://www.cdc.gov).

Therapy with nucleoside analogues should be initiated within 3 days of the outbreak of the rash in herpes zoster. Therapy is most effective if initiated within 48 hours of the outbreak of the rash. Drug therapy speeds healing and reduces the duration of postherpetic neuralgia.

Other recommended uses of oral acyclovir include prophylaxis of herpes simplex and herpes zoster in immunocompromised patients, Bell's palsy, and primary gingivostomatitis in children. Parenteral acyclovir is used to treat herpes encephalitis, perinatal herpes simplex of mother and neonate, herpes pneumonia, and herpes simiae from a monkey bite.

Table 24-31 presents the dosage schedule for nucleoside analogues for herpes virus infections.

Rational Drug Selection

Three of the nucleoside analogues used to treat herpes simplex infections have shown equal efficacy in the treatment of genital herpes; hence, the selection of the specific agent is based on cost and convenience. Acyclovir is available as a generic preparation and is generally less expensive than the other nucleoside analogues. However, it must be dosed 3 to 5 times daily, which may be disruptive and promote noncompliance. Famciclovir is dosed 2 to 4 times daily, and valacyclovir requires one to two doses daily, depending on the indication. However, both of the latter drugs are more expensive.

Because of long experience and more extensive research, acyclovir is approved for the most indications, including use by children. Many experts consider valacyclovir to be the drug of choice for treatment of herpes zoster because clinical

Table 24–31 ⊗ Dosage Schedule: Nucleoside Analogues for Herpes Virus Infections

Drug	Indication	Dosage Form	Initial Dose	Comments
Acyclovir (Zovirax)	Genital herpes, initial episode (mild to moderate)	Tablets: 400, 800 mg (G); 400, 800 mg (B) Capsules: 200 mg (G), 200 mg (B) Suspension: 200 mg/5 mL (G), 200 mg/5 mL (B)	*Adults:* 200 mg q4h while awake, 5 times/d for 10 d; accepted off-label dose: 400 mg PO 3 times/d for 10 d	Severe cases and infections in immunocompromised patients require hospitalization and IV therapy. Acute or chronic renal impairment may require dosage adjustment, depending on CCr and dose. Suspension should be well shaken before measurement, using a calibrated device. Take with water. Suspension retains its potency for 24 mo from date of manufacture. Does not require reconstitution or refrigeration. May be taken without regard to meals. Cross-allergy to valacyclovir.
	Genital herpes, intermittent therapy for recurrent infections (<6 episodes/yr)		*Adults:* 200 mg q4h while awake, 5 times/d for 5 d; accepted off-label dose: 400 mg PO 3 times daily for 5 d or 500 mg bid for 5 d	As above
	Genital herpes, chronic suppressive therapy (≥6–10 episodes/yr)		*Adults:* 400 mg PO twice/d or 200 mg 3–5 times/d for up to 12 mo	As above
	Herpes zoster (shingles)		*Adults:* 800 mg PO q4h while awake, 5 times/d, for 7–10 d	As above
	Gingivostomatitis, primary, in children		*Children 2–12 yr and <40 kg:* 15 mg/kg 5 times/d for 7 d or 20 mg/kg qid for 5 d	
	Oral labial (fever blister) in normal host (off-label)		400 mg 5 times/d for 5 d	Duration of symptoms decreased by ½ d.
	Herpes simplex (Whitlow)		400 mg tid for 10 d	Risks and benefits to fetus and mother still unknown. Experts recommend treatment, especially during third trimester.

Continued

Table 24–31 ⊗ Dosage Schedule: Nucleoside Analogues for Herpes Virus Infections—cont'd

Drug	Indication	Dosage Form	Initial Dose	Comments
	Varicella during pregnancy		800 mg 5 times/d for 5 d	May add VZIG
	Varicella (chickenpox) Initiate at earliest sign of the infection (treatment of chickenpox in children 2–12 yr not recommended by American Academy of Pediatrics)		*Adolescents and adults:* 800 mg PO q4h for 5 d	As above
	Herpes simplex, mucocutaneous prophylaxis (off-label)		*Adults:* 400 mg PO q12h	As above
	Bell's palsy due to herpes simplex virus 1 or 2		*Adults:* 400 mg PO 5 times/d for 10 d	As above
Famciclovir (Famvir)	Genital herpes, initial episode (mild to moderate)	Tablets: 125, 250 mg (B), 500 mg (B)	*Adults:* (off-label) 250 mg PO 3 times/d for 7–10 d	Renal impairment may require decreased dosage. May be taken without regard to meals. Initiate as soon as possible after onset of signs or symptoms.
	Genital herpes, intermittent therapy for recurrent infections (<6 episodes/yr)		*Adults:* 125 mg twice/d for 5 d	
	Genital herpes, chronic suppressive therapy (≥6–10 episodes/yr)		*Adults:* 250 mg PO twice/d or 500 mg once/d for up to 1 yr	
	Oral labial (fever blisters) in normal host		500 mg bid for 7 d	Duration of symptoms decreased by 2 d
	Varicella (chickenpox) (off-label) Herpes zoster (shingles)		*Adolescents and young adults:* 500 mg tid for 5 d	
			750 mg daily for 7 d or 500 mg bid for 7 d or 250 mg tid for 7 d	Adjust dose for renal failure. If CCr 10–50 mL/min, change tid dose to bid and bid dose to q24h. No 750 mg dose. For CCr <10 mL/min, dose is 250 mg daily.
Valacyclovir (Valtrex)	Genital herpes, initial episode (mild to moderate)	Tablets: 500 mg (B), 1 g (B)	*Adults:* 1 g PO twice/d for 10 d	Renal impairment may require dosage adjustment. Hepatic impairment may slow rate, but not extent, of conversion to acyclovir, but dosage adjustment is not required for hepatic impairment. Not indicated for immunocompromised patients (bone marrow transplant, human immunodeficiency syndrome, renal transplantation) because of risk of thrombotic thrombocytopenic purpura/ hemolytic uremic syndrome. May be taken without regard to meals. Cross-allergy to acyclovir.

Table 24–31 🔗 **Dosage Schedule: Nucleoside Analogues for Herpes Virus Infections—cont'd**

Drug	Indication	Dosage Form	Initial Dose	Comments
	Genital herpes, intermittent therapy for recurrent infections (<6–10 episodes/yr)		*Adults:* 500 mg PO twice/d for 3 d	
	Genital herpes, chronic suppressive therapy (≥6 episodes/yr)		*Adults:* 1 g PO once/d for up to 1 yr 500 mg PO daily with 1 g given instead if breakthrough lesions	
	Herpes zoster (shingles)		1 g PO 3 times/d for 7 d	
	Oral labial (fever blisters) in normal host		2 g q12h for 1 d	Duration of symptoms decreased by 1 d
	Varicella (chickenpox) (off-label)		*Adolescents and young adults:* 1 g tid for 5 d	

Topical applications are discussed in Chapters 23 and 32.

CCr = creatinine clearance; VZIG = varicella-zoster immune globulin; CMV = cytomegalovirus.

trials have indicated that it decreased the duration of postherpetic neuralgia in patients older than 50 years better than acyclovir.

Monitoring

The characteristic herpetic lesions of genital herpes, herpes zoster, and chickenpox should be evaluated for resolution or signs of secondary bacterial infection. Temperature and general condition also reflect resolution. BUN and serum creatinine may be assessed prior to therapy in those with risk factors for renal impairment and periodically during prolonged therapy to detect changes in renal function.

Patient Education

Administration

The nucleoside analogues can all be taken without regard to meals, in that food does not alter absorption. All forms should be taken with a full glass of water. It is important that the drug be initiated at the earliest sign of recurrence of genital herpes simplex, so the patient must be taught the symptoms of recurrence and how to self-initiate the medication. Early initiation of drug therapy also increases its efficacy for treatment of varicella and herpes zoster, so public education needs to emphasize the treatability of these infections. It is particularly important for adolescents or adults with chickenpox to seek treatment at the first sign of rash or in the prodromal period if they know they are susceptible and have been exposed.

Adverse Reactions

Although acute renal failure from precipitation of acyclovir in the tubules is most common with parenteral acyclovir, patients on oral agents have developed acute renal failure and should drink sufficient fluids to remain well hydrated during therapy. Signs of declining renal function that should be reported include abdominal pain, decreased frequency or amount of urination, thirst, anorexia, and nausea or vomiting. Other reportable signs and symptoms include encephalopathic changes (coma, confusion, hallucinations, seizures, tremor), blood dyscrasias (unusual tiredness, chills, fever, sore throat, black stools, unusual bleeding, pinpoint red spots on skin, bruising), and skin reactions like Stevens–Johnson syndrome (peeling, blistering, or loosening of skin; muscle cramps, pain, or weakness; red eyes; rash, itching, or hives).

Lifestyle Management

Keeping herpetic lesions clean and dry promotes healing. Wearing loose clothing that does not rub on the lesions decreases pain and enhances healing. Herpes genitalis may be sexually transmitted even if the partner is asymptomatic. Sexual activity should be avoided whenever either partner has symptoms. Oral or topical drug therapy does not prevent transmission of the virus. A male or female condom may decrease the risk of transmission, but spermicides and diaphragms have no effect on transmission. Women with a history of genital herpes are more likely to develop cervical cancer; annual or more frequent Pap tests are required. Those who develop postherpetic neuralgia following herpes zoster should be provided with appropriate pain management for this neuropathic pain syndrome.

ANTIVIRALS FOR INFLUENZA

Amantadine (Symmetrel) and rimantadine (Flumadine) are FDA approved for prevention and treatment of respiratory infections due to influenza A virus; however, the CDC no longer recommends their use due to high levels (up to 92%) of resistance to influenza A (Fiore et al, 2011). These agents will not be discussed further in this chapter. Information on amantadine and rimantadine is discussed in Chapter 15 with Parkinson's drugs.

Zanamivir (Relenza), oseltamivir phosphate (Tamiflu), and peramivir (Rapivab) are approved for treatment of acute illness in adults. Zanamivir has been approved for children older than 7 years and oseltamivir for children older than 2 weeks. Antivirals to treat influenza are the most effective in patients who have been symptomatic less than 48 hours. Oseltamivir and zanamivir are approved for prophylaxis of influenza in patients age 1 year or older and 5 years and older, respectively. Zanamivir should not be used in patients with underlying respiratory disease. Therapy is recommended for patients who are hospitalized, have severe disease, or are at risk of developing complications. The CDC updates recommendations for antivirals annually based on prevalent influenza strains and resistance patterns. The antiviral drugs do not substitute for vaccination.

Pharmacodynamics

Mechanism of Action

Zanamivir, oseltamivir, and peramivir are neuraminidase inhibitors and are active against influenza A and B. Neuraminidase is a viral enzyme responsible for cleaving viral attachment to the host cell surface allowing for viral circulation. Inhibition of this enzyme prevents release of the virus and halts propagation of infection. Vaccination does not appear to alter the activity of zanamivir, oseltamivir, or peramivir.

Resistance

Resistance to zanamivir and oseltamivir is associated with mutations that result in amino acid changes in the viral neuraminidase. Sporadic cases of oseltamivir resistance occurred during the 2009 H1N1 pandemic. Almost all cases were associated with a H257Y mutation that retained susceptibility to zanamivir. After the 2009 pandemic, the CDC concluded that there is no evidence of continued transmission of this resistant influenza A virus (Fiore et al, 2011). Peramivir was approved in December 2014 and there is no documented resistance as this book goes to press.

Pharmacokinetics

Absorption and Distribution

Oseltamivir is available as an oral tablet and is well absorbed after administration. Oseltamivir is a prodrug of the active

---

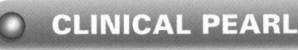

CLINICAL PEARL

CDC Influenza Antiviral Recommendations
The CDC tracks influenza worldwide to determine circulating and emerging strains. Weekly updates on flu activity and surveillance provide information on what strains are circulating in each state. The CDC also provides recommendations for the use of antivirals during influenza season, including updates as resistance patterns emerge. Providers can refer to "Information for Health Professionals," accessible at http://www.cdc.gov/flu, for the latest information.

---

compound oseltamivir carboxylate. Zanamivir is a dry powder available for oral inhalation with a provided inhalation device. Approximately 4% to 17% of the inhaled dose of zanamivir is systemically absorbed. Oseltamivir is poorly distributed into breast milk (LactMed, 2014); distribution of zanamivir into breast milk is unknown. Zanamivir is poorly absorbed orally, so it is unlikely to be absorbed by the breastfeeding infant in significant amounts. Protein binding of oseltamivir is around 42% and that of zanamivir is less than 10%. Peramivir is administered IV and is 30% bound to protein. Peramivir has not been studied in nursing mothers.

Metabolism and Excretion

Oseltamivir is almost completely converted to the active metabolite (greater than 90%). The active metabolite is excreted unchanged in the urine. Children 12 years and younger have higher clearance of oseltamivir and its metabolite, resulting in decreased drug exposure. Zanamivir is excreted as unchanged drug in the urine. Peramivir is not metabolized and is excreted unchanged via the kidneys.

Table 24-32 presents the pharmacokinetics of antivirals for influenza.

Pharmacotherapeutics

Precautions and Contraindications

Oseltamivir, peramivir, and zanamivir are listed as Pregnancy Category C. Although zanamivir crosses the placenta in animal studies, fetal blood concentrations were significantly lower than those of the mother. With no adequate, well-controlled studies in pregnant women, cautious use of all three agents is recommended. Oseltamivir is poorly excreted in breast milk and is not expected to cause adverse effects in breastfed infants. There is no information available regarding zanamivir use during breastfeeding. The inhaled medication is poorly absorbed orally, so it is assumed there would be little effect on the breastfed infant with maternal use. For zanamivir and oseltamivir, safety and efficacy have been established for children as described above. Safety and effectiveness of peramivir has not been established in children.

Adverse Drug Reactions

Bronchitis, cough, and shortness of breath are associated with use of zanamivir. These problems may be related to irritation from inhalation of the drug; however, reactions may be related to the underlying illness because the incidence of reactions was either equal or greater in the placebo-controlled groups. For oseltamivir, nausea and vomiting are the most common adverse effects and occurred more frequently than in placebo-controlled groups. Rare cases of severe skin reactions and neuropsychiatric events have been reported for all three medications.

Drug Interactions

No drug interactions are reported for oseltamivir, peramivir, and zanamivir. Although they have not been formally evaluated, these agents may impair immune response if coadministered

Table 24–32 ⁑ **Pharmacokinetics: Antivirals for Influenza**

Drug	Onset	Peak	Duration	Protein Binding	Bioavailability	Half-Life	Elimination
Oseltamivir	Rapid	2.5–6 h	UA	UA	80%	6–10 h	Prodrug; active metabolite excreted unchanged in urine
Peramivir	Rapid	30 min	UA	30%	100%	20 h	Excreted unchanged in urine
Zanamivir	Rapid	1–2 h	UA	<10%	UA	2.5–5.1 h	Excreted unchanged in urine

UA = information unavailable.

with the live attenuated influenza vaccine (LAIV). LAIV should not be administered 2 weeks before or 48 hours after administration of either drug. The inactivated virus vaccine can be administered without regard to antiviral drug administration.

Clinical Use and Dosing

Oseltamivir and zanamivir are approved for the prophylaxis and treatment of influenza types A and B. Peramivir is approved for the treatment of acute influenza in patients age 18 years or older. The CDC does not recommend routine prophylaxis with neuraminidase inhibitors. Judicious use is advised to prevent the development of resistance pathogens. The only strongly recommended indication for prophlaxis is to control outbreaks among high-risk individuals in institutional settings (Fiore et al, 2011). In times of pandemic, the neuraminidase inhibitors may be recommended for prophylaxis, particularly when an unvaccinated high-risk patient is exposed to influenza. The individual is vaccinated immediately and started on neuraminidase inhibitors to allow the antibody response to the vaccine to achieve protective concentrations.

Treatment is recommended for patients identified with influenza who are hospitalized, have severe disease, or are at risk of developing complications. No dosage adjustment is recommended for zanamivir for patients with renal impairment, but because the active metabolite of oseltamivir is excreted renally, adjustment is recommended. For patients with CCr of 10 to 30 mL/min, the treatment dose should be reduced to once daily and the prophylactic dose to once every other day. Peramivir dosage is decreased in patients with decreased renal function.

The CDC maintains an updated Web site with information regarding recommendations for antivirals based on the circulating influenza strain (http://www.cdc.gov/flu). These recommendations are updated based on emerging resistance patterns; therefore, the provider is wise to refer to the recommendations multiple times during the influenza season.

Table 24-33 presents the dosage schedule for antivirals used for influenza.

Table 24–33 ⊗ **Dosage Schedule: Antivirals for Influenza**

Drug	Indications	Dosage Form	Initial Dose	Comments
Oseltamivir (Tamiflu)	Influenza A and B treatment and prophylaxis Chemoprophylaxis	Capsules: 75 mg (B) Powder for oral suspension: 12 mg/mL (reconstituted) (B)	*Adults:* 75 mg PO twice daily for 5 d; start within 48 h of onset of symptoms *Children:* (oral suspension dosing by body weight) ≤15 kg: 30 mg bid (2.5 mL) <15–23 kg: 45 mg bid (3.8 mL) >23–40 kg: 60 mg bid (5 mL) >40 kg: 75 mg bid (6.2 mL)	For prophylaxis after exposure: Adults 75 mg daily for 7 days Children: Treat for 7 days If child is 3 months or older and younger than 1 yr old 3 mg/kg/dose once daily If 1 yr or older, dose varies by child's weight: ≤15 kg or less: 30 mg once a day >15 to 23 kg: 45 mg once a day >23 to 40 kg: 60 mg once a day >40 kg: 75 mg once a day All unimmunized patients should receive inactivated influenza vaccine. Less nausea if taken with food.
Zanamivir (Relenza)	Influenza A or B treatment	Blisters of powder for inhalation: 5 mg	*Children ≥7 yr and adults:* 2 (5 mg) inhalations twice daily for 5 d; take 2 doses on day 1 if at least 2 h apart, and start within 48 h of initial onset of symptoms	Not FDA-approved for influenza prophylaxis, although studies have indicated efficacy. For prophylaxis after exposure, immunize with inactivated flu vaccine and administer two inhalations once/d for 4 wk.
Peramivir (Rabivab)	Influenza	200 mg in 20 mL	*Adults age ≥ 18 yrs:* 600 mg IV over 15 min × 1 *CrCl 30–49 mL/min:* 200 mg IV ×1 *CrCl 10–29 mL/min:* 100 mg IV × 1	Not approved for use in children <18 yrs of age

Rational Drug Selection

The benefit of influenza drugs is tempered by the need to initiate treatment within 48 hours of the onset of the illness. Although the presence of fever, cough, myalgia, and known influenza activity in the community provide the basis for clinical diagnosis, these symptoms are not definitive. Rapid testing for influenza should be conducted if available. These tests take no more than 20 minutes, cost between $15 and $20, and have acceptable sensitivity and specificity.

The selection of an anti-influenza agent depends on the adverse effect profile, cost, and convenience. The inhaled route of administration of zanamivir has the advantage of decreased systemic effects compared with oseltamivir, but the inhalation procedure may contribute to noncompliance. Peramivir is administered IV in a single dose and may be the drug of choice in patients unable to take oral or inhaled medications.

Monitoring

Baseline evaluation of renal function should be considered for older and debilitated patients who are taking oseltamivir or peramivir. For older and debilitated patients, monitoring should include breath sounds (for evidence of heart failure or development of pneumonia), heart sounds, and weight. Vital signs will also evidence resolution of the influenza and development of adverse effects or sequelae.

Patient Education

Administration

As with all antivirals, the importance of taking the full course of therapy and following the label directions should be stressed. Patients on zanamivir require instruction on the proper use of the diskhaler. Oseltamivir can be taken without regard to food.

Adverse Reactions

If asthmatics on zanamivir experience severe bronchospasm after using the diskhaler, an alternative treatment may be needed. Nausea and vomiting are common with use of oseltamivir.

Lifestyle Management

The single most important factor in influenza prevention is annual vaccination. It is now recommended that all people 6 months and older be vaccinated. The wholesale cost of a course of therapy with a neuraminidase inhibitor is approximately $45 to $67, exclusive of diagnostic testing, whereas the cost of annual vaccination is $12 to $25. Other components of prevention include good hand washing, disposing of contaminated tissues properly, and encouraging infected individuals to convalesce at home rather than in crowded schools and workplaces.

SYSTEMIC AZOLES AND OTHER ANTIFUNGALS

Fungi are eukaryotic cells with a nucleus and a rigid cell wall. Reproduction generally occurs via asexual sporulation. Fungi occur ubiquitously in soil, water, air, and on plants. While few are capable of causing disease in humans, the incidence of infection has increased dramatically in recent years due to increased use of immunosuppressive drugs and the rising incidence of HIV. *Candida albicans,* a member of the yeast family of fungi, is now the fourth most common organism found in blood cultures in the United States (Wisplinghoff et al, 2004).

Most fungi are completely resistant to conventional antibiotics, and new classes of drugs were created to treat them. There are four main classes of antifungal drugs. The first class, macrocyclic polyenes, includes amphotericin B (Ambisome, Abelecet, Amphotec). Because this drug is available only in IV formulations, it will not be discussed further in this chapter. The second main class, the azole group, includes two subgroups, the imidazoles and the triazoles. The imidazoles are used mainly for topical treatment and will not be discussed further in this chapter. The triazoles include fluconazole (Diflucan), itraconazole (Onmel, Sporanox), posaconazole (Noxafil), and voriconazole (Vfend). The third main class, allylamines, includes terbinafine (Lamisil). The fourth main class, nuclear acid synthesis inhibitors, includes flucytosine (Ancobon), the use of which is limited to treatment of cryptococcosis.

Griseofulvin is a miscellaneous antifungal. Other antifungals used mainly as topical preparations include butoconazole (Gynazole-1), ciclopirox (Loprox), clotrimazole (Gyne-Lotrimin, Lotrimin, Mycelex), econazole (Spectazole), ketoconazole (Nizoral), miconazole (Micatin, Monistat), naftifine (Naftin), nystatin (Nystop, Nyamyc), oxiconazole (Oxistat), terconazole (Terazol), tioconazole (Vagistat), and tolnaftate (Tinactin, Absorbine, Aftate). The topical use of antifungals to treat dermatological infections is discussed in Chapters 23 and 32, and their use in treating vaginal infections is discussed in Chapter 44. This section discusses the systemic use of antifungals via the oral route of administration. The drugs most commonly used in primary care settings to be discussed here include fluconazole, itraconazole, posaconazole, voriconazole, and terbinafine.

Pharmacodynamics

Fungal cell membranes are comprised of components similar to those found in human cells with the exception of the cholesterol ergosterol. This component serves as the target for most systemic antifungal agents. Azole antifungals reduce ergosterol production by inhibition of the fungal CYP450 enzyme 14-α-demethylase. Although mainly inhibiting fungal

On The Horizon ISAVUCONAZOLE

Isavaconazole is a novel, broad-spectrum azole intended to treat most yeasts and molds, including fluconazole-resistant *Candida* strains, *Aspergillus*, and *Zygomyces*. It is currently in phase III trials.

CYP450, some inhibition of human CYP450 occurs, resulting in potential drug interactions and adverse reactions. Fluconazole appears to have the least effect on human CYP450.

In general, the azoles are fungistatic at low drug concentrations and fungicidal at higher concentrations (Hawser, 1999). Terbinafine interferes with the synthesis of ergosterol at an earlier step than the azoles through inhibition of squalene epoxide. Cell death is thought to occur by accumulation of squalene and not due to the decreased availability of ergosterol.

Spectrum of Activity

The azoles have a broad spectrum of activity that includes *Candida* species, *Cryptococcus* species, the endemic mycoses (blastomycosis, coccidioidomycosis, histoplasmosis), and the dermatophytes. In addition, itraconazole, posaconazole, and voriconazole have reliable activity against *Aspergillus* species. The azoles are approved for a variety of clinical syndromes caused by various fungi. The use of itraconazole has been mainly supplanted by voriconazole because it has superior clinical efficacy. Use of itraconazole is now limited to treatment of histoplasmosis and blastomycosis. Although possessing activity against *Aspergillus* and *Candida* species, posaconazole is used almost exclusively for prophylaxis of bone marrow transplant patients and for infection refractory to other agents.

Terbinafine (Lamisil) has in vitro activity against yeasts and a wide range of dermatophyte, filamentous, and dimorphic fungi (Garcia-Effron et al, 2004). It is fungicidal against dermatophytes, such as *Trichophyton* species, *Microsporum* species, and *Epidermophyton floccosum*. It is fungistatic against *C. albicans*. Terbinafine is only approved for treatment of onychomycosis (fungal infection of the nails) but is used off-label for tinea capitis (ringworm of the scalp), tinea corporis (ringworm of the body), tinea pedis (ringworm of the feet—athlete's foot), and tinea cruris (ringworm of the groin—jock itch). Oral terbinafine is not effective in the treatment of pityriasis versicolor; the concentrations attained by oral terbinafine in the stratum corneum are not adequate to treat this infection.

Resistance

Resistance to azoles occurs through a variety of mechanisms. Although less common, the incidence of resistance is increasing as these drugs are used for prophylaxis as well as therapy. *C. kruseii* is intrinsically resistant to fluconazole, and alternative therapy should be used. *C. glabrata* is responsible for 21% of candidemia in the United States (Pfaller et al, 2001). The Clinical and Laboratory Standards Institute developed a new classification of "susceptible dose-dependent" for fluconazole against *C. glabrata*. Isolates in this category may still be treated effectively with fluconazole if higher doses are used. The concept of dose-dependent susceptibility is restricted to *C. glabrata* that has inducible or acquired resistance (Pfaller, Diekema, & Sheehan, 2006). Cross-resistance between fluconazole and voriconazole for *C. glabrata* has been shown to be significant and caution is advised if considering voriconazole for treatment (Panackal et al, 2006). Ten to fifteen percent of *C. glabrata* is resistant to fluconazole or voriconazole. In contrast, only 1% to 2% of *C. albicans* is resistant to fluconazole or voriconazole (Rodloff, Koch, & Schaumann, 2011).

Pharmacokinetics

The pharmacokinetics of the different azoles and of terbinafine vary significantly. Table 24-34 presents these pharmacokinetic differences.

Absorption and Distribution

Fluconazole is well absorbed after oral administration, with excellent bioavailability (greater than 90%). It is widely distributed with good penetration into CSF, the eye, and the peritoneum.

Itraconazole is available for oral administration as a solution and a capsule. The bioavailability of the capsule and solution are not equivalent. The absorption of the capsule is enhanced when it is taken with food, resulting in a bioavailability of 55%. When taken on an empty stomach, absorption of the solution is about 30% greater than that of the capsule (Barone et al, 1998). Patients taking antacids (H_2 blockers and proton pump inhibitors) should not take the

Table 24–34 ⠿ Pharmacokinetics: Systemic Antifungal Agents

Drug	Onset	Peak	Duration	Protein Binding	Bioavailability	Half-Life	Elimination
Fluconazole	Slow	1–2 h	24 h	11%–12%	>90%	30 h*	>80% unchanged in urine; 11% as metabolites in urine
Itraconazole	Rapid	1.5–5 h	12–24 h	99%	55%	21 h–64 h	40% in urine as inactive metabolites; 3%–18% in feces
Ketoconazole	Rapid	1–4 h	24 h	99%	75%	8 h	85%–90% in bile and feces; 10%–15% in urine
Posaconazole	Moderate	3–5 h	UA	98%	54%	35 h	71% in feces
Terbinafine	Slow	2 h	UA	>99%	70%–80%	11–17 h	80% in urine as metabolites; 20% in feces
Voriconazole	Rapid	1–2 h	UA	58%	96%	6 h	Hepatic

*Increased in renal impairment.

capsule because absorption is markedly decreased; absorption of the solution is not affected. Due to higher bioavailability, the solution should be used preferentially in all instances (Wheat et al, 2007). Tissue concentrations are higher than plasma concentrations. Itraconazole does not enter the CSF but does enter breast milk.

Posaconazole is only available for oral administration as a suspension and delayed-release tablet. Absorption is highly variable but has been shown to be enhanced when taken with a high-fat meal. In addition, absorption is decreased with concurrent use of acid-suppressing medications (H_2 blockers and proton pump inhibitors) and avoidance is highly recommended (Krishna, Moton, Ma, Medlock, & McLeod, 2009). Despite a long half-life, absorption is saturable and administration 4 times a day is recommended. Monitoring of serum drug levels is recommended after 4 to 7 days of therapy (Andres, Pascual, & Marchetti, 2009).

Voriconazole is available in IV, oral tablet, and oral suspension formulations. The tablet and suspension are equivalent in absorption and have excellent bioavailability (greather than 90%). Voriconazole penetrates well into tissues, including the CNS (Weiler et al, 2011). Similar to posaconazole, monitoring of serum drug levels is recommended after 4 to 7 days of therapy (Andres et al, 2009).

Terbinafine is well absorbed after oral administration, with bioavailability of 70% to 85%, and is not affected by the presence of food. It is lipophilic and extensively distributed. It concentrates in the stratum corneum, attaining concentrations 25 times that in plasma. It is also distributed via the sebum to hair follicles, skin, and nails. It is not known whether terbinafine crosses the placenta, but it does enter breast milk.

Metabolism and Excretion

Fluconazole is cleared primarily by renal excretion, with 80% appearing as unchanged drug in the urine and 11% as metabolites. All azoles are inhibitors of various CYP450. Fluconazole inhibits CYP3A4 and 2C9 but has the least inhibition of the azoles discussed in this chapter. Half-life is markedly affected by renal impairment, with an inverse relationship between the elimination half-life and CCr. Dosage adjustments are required for patients with impaired renal function.

Itraconazole is extensively metabolized by the liver into several active metabolites, and fecal excretion varies from 3% to 18% of the dose. Itraconazole and its metabolites are inhibitors of CYP3A4. About 40% of the dose is excreted in urine as metabolites.

Posaconazole undergoes metabolism by CYP450, with approximately 14% of the dose excreted as an inactive metabolite in the urine. The remainder is excreted as unchanged drug in the feces. Similar to other azoles, posaconazole is a strong inhibitor of CYP3A4.

Voriconazole is extensively metabolized by CYP450, and dose reduction is required in poor metabolizers of CYP2C19 (15% to 20% of those of Asian descent) (Scholz et al, 2009). This agent is also a strong inhibitor of CYP3A4. Excretion is almost entirely nonrenal.

Terbinafine undergoes extensive first-pass metabolism. Metabolism involves only a small fraction (less than 5%) of the hepatic CYP450 capacity, so the drug interactions that are common with the azoles do not affect terbinafine. Fifteen inactive metabolites have been identified. About 80% of the dose is excreted in the urine as metabolites, and 20% is eliminated in the feces. Both liver impairment and renal impairment require dosage reduction.

Table 24-34 depicts the pharmacokinetics of these selected systemic antifungals.

Pharmacotherapeutics

Precautions and Contraindications

All of the azoles and terbinafine have been associated with hepatotoxicity. Rare cases of hepatitis that are usually reversible with discontinuance of the drug have been reported. Transaminase elevations are common with the azoles and occur in 2% to 12% of patients. Monitoring of transaminases is recommended. The azoles and terbinafine are used cautiously for patients with hepatic impairment. For those patients with renal impairment undergoing extensive renal elimination, cautious use is required. With both hepatic and renal impairment, dosage adjustments may be required. The dose of fluconazole should be reduced by 50% when the CCr is less than 50 mL/min. Because of the burden on the liver, terbinafine should be used with caution by patients with alcoholism, either active or in remission.

Voriconazole is Pregnancy Category D; the other azoles are Pregnancy Category C. Itraconazole, posaconazole, and voriconazole have teratogenic effects in animals. There are no adequate, well-controlled studies in pregnant women. These drugs should be used during pregnancy only when the potential benefits to the mother clearly outweigh the risks to the fetus and there is no reasonable alternative drug. Terbinafine is Pregnancy Category B; animal studies show no effects on fertility or fetal toxicity, but adequate studies in humans have not been conducted.

Fluconazole, itraconazole, and terbinafine are excreted in breast milk; no data exist for posaconazole and voriconazole. After a single 500 mg dose of terbinafine, 0.2 to 0.7 mg of terbinafine was detected in breast milk. In spite of these low concentrations, it is prudent to avoid administration of antifungal drugs to nursing mothers.

The safety and efficacy of these drugs in children vary. The safety and efficacy of itraconazole have not been established for children. Children aged 3 to 16 years, however, have been treated with 100 mg/d for systemic fungal infections without report of serious adverse reactions. One study with the oral solution was conducted on 26 pediatric patients receiving doses of 5 mg/kg a day for 2 weeks. Fluconazole is safe and effective for infants and children. Experience with neonates is limited, but a dosage schedule exists. Although the safety and efficacy of terbinafine have not been established in children, it has been used in a small number of children aged 3 to 16 years and was well tolerated. Although voriconazole has not been formally studied in children, its use is well established in those with hematological malignancies. Several pharmacokinetic studies of posaconazole have been conducted but use has not been standardized.

Adverse Drug Reactions

Azoles are relatively nontoxic, and the most common adverse reactions are relatively minor GI symptoms. Patients taking azoles have rarely developed exfoliative skin disorders. Patients who develop rashes should be carefully monitored and the drug discontinued if the lesion progresses. All of the azoles may cause QT prolongation. Itraconazole has been rarely associated with development of heart failure and should be used cautiously in patients with preexisting heart failure or ventricular dysfunction. Voriconazole causes visual disturbances in up to 19% of patients. These changes include photopsia (flashes of light), photophobia, and color changes. This usually occurs within 30 minutes of administration and lasts for about 30 minutes. These effects usually subside after several weeks of use. In addition to visual changes, patients may experience more serious neurological symptoms, including visual hallucinations, confusion, agitation, and myoclonus, which are usually associated with toxic drug levels.

The most common adverse reactions with terbinafine are also GI and include nausea, vomiting, and diarrhea. Reversible loss or change of taste has occurred after 5 to 8 weeks of therapy, requiring 2 to 6 months to recover after the drug was discontinued. Other adverse effects reported include hypersensitivity, hepatitis, blood dyscrasias, and Stevens–Johnson syndrome (Amichai & Grunwald, 1998).

Drug Interactions

Drug interactions are more common for the drugs with greater human CYP450 activity. All of these drugs are inhibitors of CYP3A4 and other CYP enzymes as well (see above). Additive hepatotoxicity is also possible with other hepatotoxic drugs.

Itraconazole has many drug interactions, including rifampin, histamine-2 blockers, and warfarin. Fluconazole has slightly fewer drug interactions but also interacts with rifampin and warfarin.

Additive hepatotoxicity may occur with concurrent administration of terbinafine, alcohol, or other hepatotoxins. Because terbinafine is hepatically metabolized by CYP450, drugs that induce or inhibit these enzymes may alter the clearance of terbinafine. Those interactions that have been documented for the azoles and terbinafine are listed in Table 24-35.

Table 24–35 ⠿ Drug Interactions: Selected Systemic Antifungal Agents

Drug	Interacting Drug	Possible Effect	Implications
Fluconazole	Cimetidine	Reduced fluconazole AUC.	Separate doses.
	Hydrochlorothiazide	Significant increase in fluconazole AUC, possibly because of reduced renal clearance.	Avoid concurrent use.
	Rifampin	Increased phenytoin AUC.	Monitor serum phenytoin levels.
	Phenytoin	A single dose of fluconazole after chronic rifampin resulted in a decrease in AUC and a shorter half-life for fluconazole.	If both must be taken, monitor effectiveness of fluconazole and adjust dose if needed.
	Sulfonylureas	Significant increase in AUC of tolbutamide, glyburide, and glipizide. Several patients experienced hypoglycemic episodes, some requiring oral glucose treatment.	If both must be used, monitor blood glucose levels closely while azole is taken. Monitor serum theophylline levels. Dosage adjustment may be needed.
	Theophylline	Theophylline AUC and half-life increased and clearance decreased. Increased toxicity risk.	Monitor PT/INR closely while taking azole.
	Warfarin	Fluconazole increases effects of warfarin, which results in an increase in PT/INR and risk of bleeding.	
Itraconazole	Benzodiazepines Buspirone Calcium channel blockers Phenytoin, phenobarbital, isoniazid, carbamazepine Cyclosporine, tacrolimus, oral hypoglycemic agents, and warfarin Digoxin Antacids, H₂ blockers, and other drugs that increase gastric pH	Elevated plasma concentrations of oral midazolam and triazolam. Prolonged sedative/hypnotic effects. May elevate buspirone levels, increasing the pharmacological and adverse effects. Edema with concurrent use of dihydropyridines. Increased metabolism of itraconazole. Decreased metabolism of phenytoin. Itraconazole decreases metabolism of these drugs. Increased risk for toxicity, hypoglycemia, and anticoagulant effect. Increased digoxin levels. Reduced plasma itraconazole levels.	Select different benzodiazepine. Closely monitor clinical response to buspirone. Prudent to start with conservative dose and adjust dose of buspirone as needed. Monitor cardiac status Increased dosage of azole may be needed. Monitor phenytoin levels; dosage adjustments may be needed. Monitor cyclosporine levels. Monitor for indications of hypoglycemia. Monitor PT/INR. Monitor digoxin levels closely. Much less of a problem with oral solution than with capsules.
Ketoconazole	Antacids, H₂ blockers, proton pump inhibitors, and other	Inhibit ketoconazole absorption Bioavailability and serum levels of either drug may be affected	Avoid concurrent use. Fluconazole absorption is not affected. Avoid concurrent use.

Continued

Table 24–35 ▓ Drug Interactions: Selected Systemic Antifungal Agents—cont'd

Drug	Interacting Drug	Possible Effect	Implications
	drugs that increase gastric pH Rifampin, isoniazid Hepatotoxic drug Cyclosporine, corticosteroids, warfarin Theophylline	Additive hepatotoxicity Ketoconazole decreases metabolism of these drugs. Increased risk for toxicity, anticoagulant effect. Increased serum theophylline levels	Avoid concurrent use. Monitor serum levels. Monitor PT/INR more closely. Because the effect on cyclosporine levels is consistent and predictable, this combination has been used therapeutically to reduce cyclosporine dosage. Monitor theophylline levels. Dosage adjustment may be needed.
Posaconazole	Sirolimus	Increased sirolimus levels	Contraindicated
	Drugs that prolong QT interval	Enhanced prolongation of QT interval and increased risk of torsade de pointes	Contraindicated
	HMG-CoA Reductase Inhibitors primarily metabolized by CYP 3A4	Increased levels of HMG-CoA inhibitors, increased risk of rhabdomyolisis	Contraindicated
	Ergot alkaloids Efavirenz Phenytoin Rifabutin	Increased risk of ergotism Increased posaconazole levels	Contraindicated Avoid concomitant use
	Digoxin	Increased digoxin levels	Avoid concomitant use. Monitor digoxin levels.
	Efavirenz Phenytoin Rifabutin	Decreased posaconazole levels and increased serum concentrations potentially leading to increased adverse effects or toxicity of coadministered drug	Avoid concomitant use
	Atazanavir, ritonavir	Increased exposure to protease inhibitors, which may increase adverse effects	Use with extreme caution. Do not use high-dose ritonavir with posaconazole.
	Midazolam	Inhibition of midazolam metabolism, 5-fold increase in midazolam serum concentrations	Use a different benzodiazepine
Voriconazole	Carbamazepine Rifamycins St. John's wort	Increased voriconazole metabolism and clearance leading to subtherapeutic voriconazole levels and treatment failures	Contraindicated
	Efavirenz Phenytoin	Increased voriconazole metabolism and clearance leading to subtherapeutic voriconazole levels	Increase voriconazole dose. Monitor for efficacy. Monitor phenytoin levels.
	Medications that prolong QT interval	Enhanced prolongation of QT interval and increased risk of torsade de pointes	Avoid concurrent use
	Benzodiazepines extensively metabolized by CYP 3A4 Cyclosporine Fentanyl, methadone, oxycodone NSAIDS Oral contraceptives Tacrolimus	CYP 3A4 inhibition by voriconazole increases drug levels. Enhanced effects and risk of toxicity with affected drug.	Use with caution. Monitor for toxicity and adverse events. Dose adjustments recommended for cyclosporine and tacrolimus.
	Ergot alkaloids Rifabutin Sirolimus	Significant increases in serum concentrations of affected drugs	Contraindicated
Terbinafine	Alcohol, hepatotoxins Cimetidine Phenytoin, rifampin Caffeine Cyclosporine	Additive liver damage Decreased metabolism of terbinafine Increased metabolism of terbinafine Decreased metabolism of caffeine Increased clearance of cyclosporine, possibly leading to organ rejection	Avoid concurrent use or monitor hepatic function closely. Avoid concurrent use. Avoid concurrent use or monitor response to terbinafine. Prudent use of caffeinated beverages. Avoid concurrent use or monitor cyclosporine levels.

INR = international normalized ratio; PT = prothrombin time.

Clinical Use and Dosing

Because of its long half-life, fluconazole does not achieve steady state for 5 to 10 days with standard doses but can be achieved in 2 days with a loading dose (twice the usual dose) on the first day. Hence, most dosage regimens for fluconazole include a loading dose. Because it may undergo saturation metabolism at higher plasma concentrations, the initial dose of itraconazole is often doubled, resulting in a 3-fold increase in the plasma concentration. However, patients with hepatic or renal insufficiency may need reduced maintenance doses of fluconazole and terbinafine. For serious infections, voriconazole should be administered IV as a loading dose over the first day.

Oral antifungal drugs are used to treat superficial infections by yeasts (*Candida,* pityriasis versicolor) and dermatophytes (tinea infections) and to treat invasive systemic mycoses (e.g., paracoccidioidomycosis, blastomycosis, histoplasmosis, aspergillosis, candidiasis). Indications and dosages of the oral antifungal drugs are summarized in Table 24-36.

Rational Drug Selection

Antifungal drug selection is based on susceptibility, pharmacokinetics, and adverse effects. The spectrum of terbinafine includes dermatophytes, and it is recommended for treatment of onychomycosis and tinea infections. The spectrum of the azoles includes dermatophytic and superficial fungi, as well as invasive systemic fungi. Fluconazole has more reliable bioavailability than the other azoles and is generally recommended for the treatment of mild to moderate systemic fungal infections. Fluconazole also has fewer drug interactions than other azoles and has a single-dose regimen for some indications; it is preferred by many clinicians for these reasons. It is also the drug of choice for treating vaginal yeast infections in patients with diabetes. As discussed previously, itraconazole should be reserved for blastomycosis and histoplasmosis because alternative treatments for other indications are preferred. Fluconazole is available as a generic and is the most affordable azole.

Monitoring

Prompt recognition of liver injury is essential with oral antifungal drugs. AST, ALT, alkaline phosphatase, and bilirubin should be monitored prior to initiation of therapy, monthly for 3 to 4 months, and frequently thereafter during treatment. Because of the numerous drug interactions with azoles, it is important to monitor the drug response of concurrent medications. Therapeutic response should be evaluated at 6 to 8 weeks after initiation of drug therapy for tinea infections, 4 to 6 months for fingernail onychomycosis, and 8 to 9 months for toenail mycoses. Monitoring of serum drug levels for several azoles is recommended as stated above.

Patient Education

Administration

Itraconazole capsules should be taken with food to alleviate GI symptoms and promote absorption. Antacids should not be used in conjunction with the capsule. Itraconazole solution

Text continued on page 787

Table 24–36 ⊗ Dosage Schedule: Selected Systemic Antifungal Agents

Drug	Indication	Dosage Form	Initial and Maintenance Dose	Comments
Fluconazole (Diflucan)	Vaginal candidiasis	Tablet: 50, 100, 150, 200 mg Powder for oral suspension: 10 mg/mL, 40 mg/mL	*Adults:* 150 mg as single PO dose	Maximal daily pediatric dose 600 mg. Shake suspension well before measurement, using calibrated liquid-dosing device. Store suspension in refrigerator or at room temperature. Dispose of unused suspension 2 wk after reconstitution.
	Oropharyngeal candidiasis		*Adults:* 200 mg PO on first day, followed by 100 mg once daily for 2 wk *Children:* 6 mg/kg PO on first day, followed by 3 mg/kg once daily for at least 2 wk	May be taken without regard to meals
	Esophageal candidiasis		*Adults:* 200 mg PO on first day, followed by 100 mg once daily for 2 wk; doses up to 400 mg may be used based on patient response *Children:* 6 mg/kg PO on first day, followed by 3 mg/kg once daily for at least 3 wk and 2 wk beyond resolution of symptoms; doses up to 12 mg/kg/d have been used	Doses are reduced by 50% for CCr <30 mL/min. Older adults may have impaired renal function and require lower dose.

Continued

Table 24–36 ⊗ Dosage Schedule: Selected Systemic Antifungal Agents—cont'd

Drug	Indication	Dosage Form	Initial and Maintenance Dose	Comments
	Other *Candida* infections		*Adults:* 50–400 mg/d PO *Children:* 6–12 mg/kg/d PO have been used	
Itraconazole (Sporanox)	Onychomycosis	Capsule: 100 mg, Oral solution: 10 mg/mL	*Adults:* 200 mg PO once daily with meal for 12 consecutive wk	Safety and efficacy not established for children. A small number of children aged 3–16 yr with systemic infections have taken itraconazole capsules, 100 mg daily, without serious adverse effects. In life-threatening conditions, a loading dose of 200 mg 3 times/d (600 mg/d) is given for first 3 d. Continue treatment for minimum of 3 mo until clinical parameters indicate fungal infection has subsided. Take capsules with food or cola beverage for better absorption. Oral solution should be vigorously swished in mouth, 10 mL at a time, for several seconds and swallowed. Solution should be taken on an empty stomach. Dispense solution with calibrated liquid-measuring device.
	Onychomycosis, fingernail		*Adults:* 200 mg bid for 1 wk; repeat after 3 wk period without itraconazole	Doses are reduced by 50% for CCr <30 mL/min. Older adults may have impaired renal function and require lower dose.
	Onychomycosis, toenail		200 mg once daily for 12 consecutive wk	
	Aspergillosis		*Adults:* 200–400 mg PO once daily	
	Blastomycosis or histoplasmosis		*Adults:* 200 mg PO once daily with meal; if no improvement or progression, increase in 100 mg increments to 400 mg maximum daily dose. Give doses >200 mg daily in 2 divided doses.	
	Candidiasis, esophageal		*Adults:* For solution: 100 mg PO (swish and swallow) once daily for minimum of 3 wk (2 wk after resolution of symptoms); off-label: 100–200 mg capsules PO once daily after a meal for 14 d; dose for AIDS and neutropenic patients is 200 mg for 4 wk	
	Candidiasis, oropharyngeal		*Adults:* For solution: 200 mg PO (swish and swallow) once daily for 7–14 d; if refractory to fluconazole, use 100 mg twice/d for 2–4 wk; off-label: 100–200 mg capsules PO once daily after a meal for 14 d; dose for AIDS and neutropenic patients is 200 mg for 4 wk	

Table 24–36 ⊗ **Dosage Schedule: Selected Systemic Antifungal Agents—cont'd**

Drug	Indication	Dosage Form	Initial and Maintenance Dose	Comments
	Candidiasis, vulvo-vaginal (off-label)		*Adults:* 200 mg PO once daily for 3 d	
	Coccidioidomycosis (off-label)		*Adults:* 200 mg PO twice daily	
	Histoplasmosis suppression (off-label)		*Adults:* 200 mg PO twice daily	
	Paracoccidioidomycosis (off-label)		*Adults:* 100 mg PO once daily for 6 wk	
	Tinea corporis or cruris (off-label)		*Adults:* 100 mg PO once daily for 15 d	
	Tinea manus or pedis (off-label)		*Adults:* 100 mg PO once daily for 30 d	
Ketoconazole (Nizoral)	Candidiasis, vulvovaginal	Tablets: 200 mg	*Adults:* 200–400 mg PO once daily for 5 d *Children >2 yr:* 3.3–6.6 mg/kg/d as a single dose *Children <2 yr:* Dosage not established	Maximal adult daily dosage is 1 g. Therapy should be continued 1–2 wk in candidiasis (3–5 d in vaginal candidiasis); for 1–8 wk in dermatophytic infections and mycoses of hair and scalp; for 3 mo–1 yr for paracoccidioidomycosis; and for 6 mo in other systemic mycoses. Chronic mucocutaneous candidiasis following a remission usually requires indefinite maintenance treatment to prevent relapse. Take with food to promote absorption and decrease GI irritation. In patients with hypochlorhydria or achlorhydria, take with acid drink. May be dissolved in cola or seltzer water or taken with these fluids. Shake suspension well before measurement using a calibrated liquid-measuring device. Store at room temperature.
	Paronychia		*Adults:* 400 mg PO once daily *Children >2 yr:* 5–10 mg/kg PO once daily *Children <2 yr:* Dosage not established	
	Pityriasis versicolor		*Adults:* 200 mg PO once daily for 5–10 d	
	Fungal pneumonia or septicemia		*Adults:* 400 mg–1 g PO once daily *Children >2 yr:* 5–10 mg/kg PO once daily *Children <2 yr:* Dosage not established	
	All other antifungal indications		*Adults:* 200–400 mg PO once daily *Children >2 yr:* 3.3–6.6 mg/kg PO once daily *Children <2 yr:* Dosage not established	

Continued

Table 24–36 ✂ Dosage Schedule: Selected Systemic Antifungal Agents—cont'd

Drug	Indication	Dosage Form	Initial and Maintenance Dose	Comments
	Candidiasis, esophageal		*Adults:* For solution: 100 mg PO (swish and swallow) once daily for minimum of 3 wk (2 wk after resolution of symptoms); off-label: 100–200 mg capsules PO once daily after a meal for 14 d; dose for AIDS and neutropenic patients is 200 mg for 4 wk	
Posaconazole (Noxafil)	Oropharyngeal candidiasis	Delayed-release tablet: 100 mg Oral suspension: 40 mg/mL	*Adults:* Loading dose: 100 mg bid for first day Maintenance dose: 100 mg daily for 13 d	Take during or immediately after a full meal. Other dosing regimens are recommended for prophylaxis of *Aspergillus* and *Candida* infections and for oropharyngeal candidiasis refractory to azole therapy.
Voriconazole (Vfend)	Invasive aspergillosis	Tablet: 50, 200 mg Powder for oral suspension: 40 mg/mL	*Adults:* Loading dose: 6 mg/kg IV every 12 h for first day Maintenance dose: 200 mg PO bid	If patient response is inadequate, may increase maintenance dose to 300 mg bid. Maintanence dose should be reduced by 50% in setting of hepatic impairment. When used with phenytoin or efavirenz, maintanence dose should be increased to 400 mg PO bid. Monitoring of serum voriconazole levels may be advised for severe infections or prolonged therapy.
	Candidemia or deep-tissue *Candida* infection		As above	
Terbinafine (Lamisil)	Onychomycosis, fingernail	Tablet: 250 mg	*Adults:* 250 mg PO once daily for 6 wk	May be taken without regard to meals. Patients with preexisting stable liver disease, impaired renal function (CCr <50 mL/min), or serum creatinine <3.4 mg/dL should receive 50% reduction in dosage. Safety and efficacy for children and children's dosage not established. Following dosages have been use in treatment of children age 3–16 yr: Children 12.5–18.5 kg: oral 62.5 mg once daily
	Onychomycosis, toenail		*Adults:* 250 mg PO once daily for 12 wk; extensive toenail infections may take longer	Children 18.5–25 kg: 125 mg once daily Children >25 kg: 250 mg once daily
	Tinea capitis (off-label)		*Adults:* 250 mg PO once daily for 4–6 wk	
	Tinea corporis or cruris (off-label)		*Adults:* 250 mg PO once daily for 2–4 wk	
	Tinea pedis (plantar or interdigital) (off-label)		*Adults:* 250 mg PO once daily for 2–6 wk	

CCr = creatinine clearance.

should be taken on an empty stomach; fluconazole, terbinafine, and voriconazole can be taken without regard to meals. Posaconazole should be taken with a high-fat meal. Because these drugs have many drug interactions, any time a new drug is added to the patient's treatment regimen, it should be reviewed for possible interactions.

Adverse Reactions

Because hepatotoxicity is common to all the oral antifungals, concurrent use of alcohol is discouraged. Patients should report signs of liver toxicity (unusual tiredness, anorexia, nausea and vomiting, jaundice, pale stools, dark urine), Stevens–Johnson syndrome (rash, blisters, loosening of skin, red joints), and leukopenia (sore throat or fever). Patients on terbinafine should know that loss of taste is a reversible adverse effect.

Lifestyle Management

Factors that have contributed to the rise of fungal infections are overuse of antibiotics, increased numbers of immunocompromised patients, and increased environmental exposure. Patients and providers should try to limit antibiotic use, which will decrease emergence of bacterial resistance and fungal superinfection.

ANTHELMINTICS

Infestation with parasitic worms is a major health problem throughout the world infecting billions and killing millions annually (WHO, 2010). In the United States, approximately 60 million people are estimated to harbor a helminthic parasite (VandeWaa, Henderson, White, & Nowatzke, 1998). The worms are divided into three groups: nematodes ([intestinal and tissue] roundworms), cestodes (flatworms and tapeworms), and trematodes (flukes) (McCarthy, Loukas, & Hotez, 2011). The only common helminthic infections in the United States are caused by intestinal nematodes: *Enterobius vermicularis* (pinworm), *Trichuris trichiura* (whipworm), *Ascaris lumbricoides* (roundworm), *Strongyloides stercoralis* (threadworm), and the hookworms *Ancylostoma duodenale* and *Necator americanus*. Only those drugs used to treat these infections are discussed in this chapter.

Pharmacodynamics

The benzimidazoles (mebendazole, thiabendazole [Mintezol], albendazole [Albenza]) bind to β-tubulin of the microtubule causing inhibition of polymerization and loss of function. In addition, these agents have a range of other possible inhibitory mechanisms including blocking glucose uptake.(Prichard, 1994). Thiabendazole is no longer available in the United States or Canada for human use and will not be discussed.

Pyrantel (Pinworm, Pin X, Parasitol, Pronto Plus, Vermocks) is a depolarizing neuromuscular blocking agent that creates spastic paralysis in the worm. It also inhibits cholinesterases (Robertson, Pennington, Evans, & Martin, 1994). Ivermectin (Stromectol) binds selectively to glutamate-gated chloride ion channels of the muscle and nerve resulting in hyperpolarization, paralysis, and eventual death of the parasite.

Drugs of choice for treating intestinal nematodes include mebendazole and pyrantel. Tissue nematodes are best treated with mebendazole, albendazole, or ivermectin.

Pharmacokinetics
Absorption and Distribution

Ivermectin is well absorbed with wide tissue distribution following oral administration. Albendazole, mebendazole, and pyrantel are very poorly absorbed with limited serum concentrations. The bioavailability of albendazole and ivermectin are significantly enhanced if coadministered with a fatty meal (2.5- to 5-fold increase). Absorbed albendazole is widely distributed in nearly all organs and body compartments. The distribution of mebendazole and pyrantel is not known.

Metabolism and Excretion

Albendazole is rapidly converted by the liver to the primary metabolite, albendazole sulfoxide, which is further converted to other metabolites. These metabolites undergo almost exclusive biliary elimination. Absorbed mebendazole is extensively metabolized by the liver. More than 95% is excreted in feces and the remainder by the kidney. Ivermectin is metabolized by CYP450. The parent drug and its metabolites are excreted almost exclusively in feces over an estimated 12 days. Pyrantel pamoate undergoes limited metabolism, and more than 50% is excreted as unchanged drug in the feces. Less than 7% is found in urine as parent drug and metabolites. Table 24-37 presents the pharmacokinetics of selected anthelmintics.

Pharmacotherapeutics
Precautions and Contraindications

Because the activity of these drugs is specific to the parasites, precautions and contraindications are minimal. Drugs extensively metabolized by the liver require cautious administration to patients with hepatic impairment. Drugs excreted extensively by the kidney may require careful monitoring of renal function. Albendazole and mebendazole have been linked to rare reports of bone marrow suppression.

Albendazole, mebendazole, ivermectin, and pyrantel pamoate are all designated as Pregnancy Category C. Albendazole and ivermectin have demonstrated teratogenic and embryotoxic effects in some animal studies. The WHO has determined that for albendazole, mebendazole, and pyrantel pamoate, the benefits of treatment outweigh the risks and allow administration to pregnant women in their second or third trimester (CDC, 2013d). For ivermectin, the WHO excludes pregnant patients from mass prevention campaigns (CDC, 2013c).

It is not known whether albendazole, mebendazole, or pyrantel pamoate is excreted in breast milk. Caution should

Table 24–37 ✣ **Pharmacokinetics: Selected Anthelmintics**

Drug	Onset	Peak	Protein Binding	Bioavailability	Half-Life	Elimination
Albendazole	UA	2–5 h	70%	UA	8–12 h	Mainly in urine; small amount in feces
Ivermectin	UA	4 h	UA	UA	16 h	Fecal elimination; <1% in urine
Mebendazole	UA	2–4 h	95%	2%–3%	2.5–5.5 h	>90% fecal elimination; 2% in urine
Pyrantel pamoate	UA	1–3 h	UA	UA	UA	50% unchanged drug in feces; <7% in urine
Thiabendazole	Rapid	1–2 h	UA	UA	1.2 h	5% in feces; 90% in urine

Duration of action of all of these drugs is unknown.

UA = information unavailable.

be exercised if used by a nursing mother. Ivermectin is known to be excreted in breast milk in low quantities equaling 0.98% of the weight-adjusted maternal dose (LactMed, 2014). Mebendazole and pyrantel pamoate are not recommended for children younger than age 2 years. Albendazole is not recommended for children younger than 6 years (although no adverse reactions have been found in studies of children as young as 1 year). In children weighing less than 15 kilograms, ivermectin is contraindicated.

Adverse Drug Reactions

The most common adverse reactions associated with use are nausea, vomiting, diarrhea, transient abdominal pain, fever, pruritus, and skin rash. Albendazole and mebendazole are associated with transient elevations of liver function tests and rarely hepatitis. Reversible bone marrow suppression has also occurred with both of these agents.

Some patients taking ivermectin for treatment of *Onchocerca volvulus* experience the Mazzotti reaction (fever, headache, dizziness, somnolence, weakness, rash, pruritus, diarrhea, joint pain and muscle spasms, hypotension, tachycardia, lymphadenitis, and peripheral edema). The reaction is due to the death of *Onchocerca volvulus* and is not related to ivermectin toxicity. Corticosteroids may be needed for several days to suppress the inflammatory response.

Drug Interactions

There are few drug–drug interactions with any of these drugs. Table 24-38 lists these interactions.

Clinical Use and Dosing

The five common intestinal helminthic infections in the United States are described here, with indication of the usual antimicrobial agents. Dosages of the anthelmintic drugs are summarized in Table 24-39.

Enterobius vermicularis (Pinworm)

The pinworm is named for the morphology of the posterior of the female. As many as 50 million people in the United States, primarily children, are infected with pinworm. The primary symptoms of pinworm, perianal itching and sleep disruption, are related to the fact that the female lays eggs nocturnally in the perianal area. Drugs used to treat pinworms include pyrantel pamoate, albendazole, and mebendazole.

Trichuris trichiura (Whipworm)

Some 80 million people worldwide and 2.2 million in the United States are infected with whipworm. People acquire whipworm by ingesting uncooked vegetables grown in soil contaminated by human feces. The infection is usually asymptomatic, although heavy infestations may produce anemia, bloody diarrhea, and growth retardation. Drugs used for whipworm infections include pyrantel pamoate, albendazole, and mebendazole.

Ascaris lumbricoides (Roundworm)

The roundworm is the most common helminthic parasite worldwide and affects 4 million people in the United States, primarily in the Southeast. Infection generally is derived from eating feces-contaminated raw vegetables. The parasite has a

Table 24–38 ⁘ **Drug Interactions: Selected Anthelmintics**

Drug	Interacting Drug	Possible Effect	Implications
Albendazole	Dexamethasone	Steady-state trough of main metabolite 50% higher	Avoid coadministration
Mebendazole	Carbamazepine, phenytoin	May reduce plasma levels of mebendazole; possible decrease in therapeutic effects	Avoid concomitant use
	Cimetidine	Increased plasma concentrations of mebendazole	May be used therapeutically
Pyrantel pamoate	Theophylline	May increase serum levels of theophylline	Monitor theophylline levels
Thiabendazole	Xanthines	Thiabendazole may compete with these drugs for metabolism sites; may elevate serum levels of xanthine with increased toxicity risk	Monitor serum levels of xanthine closely

Table 24–39 ⊗ **Dosage Schedule: Selected Anthelmintics**

Drug	Indication	Dosage Form	Initial Dose	Comments
Albendazole (Albenza)	Ascariasis Enterobiasis Hookworm infections Trichuriasis Strongyloidiasis Giardiasis	Tablets: 200 mg	*Children >2 yr and adults:* 400 mg PO once daily for 3 d; may repeat in 3 wk *Children <2 yr:* 200 mg PO as single dose; may repeat in 3 wk *Children >2 yr and adults:* 400 mg PO once daily for 3 d; may repeat in 3 wk *Children <2 yr:* 200 mg PO once daily for 3 d; may repeat in 3 wk *Adults:* 400 mg PO daily for 5 d	Maximal daily dose for adults and adolescents <60 kg is 800 mg. Take with food containing fat. Swallow tablets whole with small amount of liquid. Shake suspension well before measurement with calibrated liquid-measuring device. Store at room temperature.
Ivermectin (Stromectol)	Strongyloidiasis Scabies in immuno-compromised patients	Tablets: 6 mg	*Children >15 kg and adults:* 200 mcg/kg as single dose *Adults:* 200 mcg/kg as a single dose	Take with full glass of water 1 h before breakfast. Repeat in 1 to 2 wk.
Mebendazole (Vermox)	Ascariasis Trichuriasis Hookworms Roundworms Enterobiasis	Chewable tablets: 100 mg	*Children >2 yr and adults:* 100 mg PO twice daily, morning and evening, for 3 d; may repeat in 2–3 wk if required *Adults:* 100 mg PO as single dose; may repeat in 2–3 wk if required	Take with high-fat meals. Tablets may be chewed, crushed, or swallowed whole.
	Pinworms		*Children and adults:* One single 100 mg chewable tablet; repeat in 2 wk	
Pyrantel pamoate (Pin-Rid, Pin-X, Reese's Pinworm, Antiminth)	Enterobiasis Ascariasis Trichuriasis Hookworms	Capsules: 180 mg (62.5 mg of pyrantel base) Liquid: 50 mg/mL	*Children and adults:* 11 mg/kg as single dose	Maximum daily dose 1 g. May be taken with milk, food, or juice at any time of day. Shake suspension well, and measure with calibrated liquid-measuring device. Store at room temperature.
Thiabendazole (Mintezol)	Strongyloidiasis, uncomplicated Strongyloidiasis, hyperinfection	Tablets: 500 mg Oral suspension: 50 mg/mL	*Children >13.6 kg and adults:* 25 mg/kg twice daily for 2 d *Children >13.6 kg and adults:* 25 mg/kg twice daily for 5–7 d; may be repeated if required	Maximum adult daily dose 3 g. Chew or crush tablets before swallowing. Take after meals. Shake suspension well before measurement with calibrated liquid-dosing device. Take after meals.

larval stage that migrates through the lungs, causing seasonal pneumonitis, but GI symptoms are more common. Massive infections can cause intestinal obstruction. The drug used for roundworm infections is mebendazole.

Ancylostoma duodenale or *Necator americanus* (Hookworm)

Hookworms comprise pathogens from two genera, *A. duodenale* and *N. americanus*. The larvae live in the soil and must penetrate the skin to enter the circulation, where they are carried to the lungs. Here they penetrate the alveoli, crawl up the pharynx, and are swallowed. They attach to the intestinal wall and can cause anemia. A recent phenomenon is the use of hookworms to treat allergies and asthma. Although there is little evidence regarding the effectiveness of this treatment, patients can purchase hookworms via the Internet and self-medicate. Drugs used for hookworm infections include pyrantel pamoate, albendazole, and mebendazole.

Strongyloides stercoralis (Threadworm)

The larvae of the threadworm are found in warm, moist soil in the tropics and the southern United States. The larvae may penetrate the skin or be ingested. Pulmonary and

GI symptoms are common. The drug used for threadworm infections is ivermectin.

Scabies

Ivermectin may be prescribed off-label to selected patients with scabies (Currie & McCarthy, 2010). It is particularly effective in treating scabies in patients who are immunocompromised. The dose is 200 mcg/kg given as a single dose (Currie & McCarthy). Because ivermectin is not ovicidal, it should be repeated in 1 to 2 weeks.

Rational Drug Selection

The CDC Web site and guidelines should always be consulted prior to choosing and initiating drug therapy (CDC, 2013d, 2013e). Patient-specific factors such as pregnancy status and age should be carefully considered when choosing therapy. Albendazole and pyrantel pamoate are both available as a suspension. Pyrantel pamoate is also available over the counter, which may reduce inconvenience and promote adherence.

Monitoring

Evaluation of the efficacy of the anthelmintic drugs includes assessing the eradication of the helminth. For *E. vermicularis,* cellophane tape swabs of the perianal area should be obtained before starting and 1 week after drug therapy, especially in patients with persistent symptoms. The swab should be obtained every morning prior to defecation and bathing for at least 3 days to determine proof of cure.

For roundworms, hookworms, ascariasis, trichuriasis, and whipworms, stool samples are obtained before and 1 to 3 weeks after treatment to determine proof of cure. For strongyloidiasis, routine stool examinations and special examinations such as the Baermann technique may be required prior to treatment and repeated at intervals of 3 months, beginning at 6 weeks after treatment, to establish proof of cure.

Patients taking prolonged therapy with these agents should have periodic evaluation of hepatic function and CBCs. These tests should also be repeated whenever there is clinical evidence of hepatotoxicity or blood dyscrasias.

Patient Education

Administration

The available dosage forms are shown in Table 24-39. Albendazole should be swallowed whole with a small amount of water and a high-fat meal to decrease GI effects and increase absorption. Mebendazole is also taken with a high-fat meal, but it can be chewed or crushed. Ivermectin must be taken with a full glass of water on an empty stomach 1 hour before a meal. Pyrantel pamoate can be taken without regard to meals or time of the day.

Adverse Reactions

Women of childbearing capacity should take albendazole after a negative pregnancy test in the first 7 days following the onset of menses and should use a backup barrier method of contraception for 1 month after completing therapy. Albendazole should not be used in conjunction with cimetidine, which decreases clearance of albendazole. Patients who have recently taken albendazole should also report signs of neutropenia (sore throat, fever, unusual tiredness). Mebendazole should also be avoided during pregnancy.

Ivermectin can cause light-headedness, so hazardous activities should be avoided during therapy. Use may be associated with a skin rash or itching during treatment of strongyloidiasis because of the death of microfilariae in the skin. If serious, this syndrome may require short-term therapy with corticosteroids to suppress the inflammatory response.

Lifestyle Management

Patients with hookworm and whipworm infections may require iron replacement therapy. Eradication of pinworm infections usually requires simultaneous treatment of all household contacts; a vigorous hygiene program of cleaning bed linens, nightwear, and underwear; and good hand-washing habits. Contrary to popular belief, treatment of helminthic infections does not require special diets or purging with laxatives before or after the antimicrobial drug.

METRONIDAZOLE, NITAZOXANIDE, AND TINIDAZOLE

Metronidazole (Flagyl) is effective at managing bacterial as well as parasitic infections and is therefore discussed separately from the other antibiotics classes. It is available in oral, intravenous, and topical preparations. Topical applications are discussed in Chapters 23 and 32 for skin conditions and in Chapter 44 for vaginal disorders. Nitazoxanide (Alinia) is used in the treatment of diarrhea caused by *G. lamblia* and *C. parvum.* Tinidazole (Tindamax) is approved for treatment of amebiasis, bacterial vaginosis, giardiasis, and trichomoniasis. Both nitazoxanide and tinidazole are available only for oral administration.

Pharmacodynamics

Metronidazole is a nitroimidazole that disrupts DNA and protein synthesis. Upon entry into the microorganism, the nitro group of metronidazole is reduced, creating a highly reactive molecule that binds nonspecifically and deactivates DNA and other proteins. Aerobic cells lack sufficient reduction potential to produce the reactive molecule, rendering it ineffective in treatment of these organisms (Lofmark, Edlund, & Nord, 2010). Metronidazole is bactericidal against anaerobic bacteria and its efficacy is best correlated to the AUC to MIC ratio (Sprandel et al, 2006). It has reliable activity against gram-positive, and gram-negative anaerobes including *Clostridium* species, *Peptococcus* species, *Peptostreptococcus* species, *Bacteroides fragilis,* and *Fusobacterium* species. It also has activity against *H. pylori, Entamoeba histolytica, T. vaginalis, Gardnerella vaginalis,* and *G. lamblia.*

Nitazoxanide interferes with the pyruvate ferredoxin oxidoreductase (PFOR) enzyme-dependent electron transfer reaction, which is essential to anaerobic energy metabolism in the protozoa. It is active against the sporozoites and oocysts of *C. parvum* and trophozoites of *G. lamblia*.

Tinidazole is an antibacterial and antiprotozoal agent with mechanism of action similar to metronidazole. Like metronidazole, it undergoes intracellular nitro group reduction and is thought to subsequently deactivate DNA and other proteins. While the mechanism is not completely understood, tinidazole has activity against *Bacteroides* species, *Gardnerella vaginalis*, *Prevotella* species, *G. lamblia,* and *Entamoeba histolytica*.

Pharmacokinetics

Absorption and Distribution

Oral metronidazole is readily absorbed and widely distributed into most tissue and fluids, including CSF, breast milk, alveolar, bone, liver abscesses, vaginal secretions, seminal fluid, as well as crossing the placenta. Serum levels are proportional to the administered dose and are similar for oral and intravenous routes. Following administration, nitazoxanide is rapidly metabolized to two active metabolites, tizoxanide and tizoxanide glucuronide. Administration with food is recommended as the AUC and C_{max} are both decreased when taken without food. An oral suspension of nitazoxanide is available and has roughly 70% of the bioavailability of the oral tablet. The active metabolites of nitazoxanide are poorly distributed, with 99% of tizoxanide bound to plasma proteins. Tinidazole is rapidly and completely absorbed after oral administration. Administration with food does not appreciably alter absorption. It is widely distributed to virtually all tissues, crosses the blood–brain barrier and the placental barrier, and is secreted in breast milk.

Metabolism and Excretion

Metronidazole is metabolized into several degradation products with the majority (60% to 80%) being renally eliminated. Tizoxanide and tizoxanide glucuronide are mainly excreted in the feces (about two-thirds) with a small portion excreted renally (about one-third). Tinidazole undergoes extensive metabolism by CYP3A4. It is excreted by the liver and can also be recovered in the urine as unchanged drug. Table 24-40 presents the pharmacokinetics of these three drugs.

Pharmacotherapeutics

Precautions and Contraindications

Cautious use is recommended with metronidazole for patients with a history of blood dyscrasias. Seizures have occurred as an adverse reaction, and patients with a history of seizure disorder or neurological problems should use this drug with caution. Severe hepatic dysfunction may decrease plasma clearance, and metronidazole should be used cautiously with these patients. Tinidazole is also a nitroimidazole and has the same precautions and contraindications.

The pharmacokinetics of nitazoxanide in patients with compromised renal or hepatic function has not been studied. It must be administered with caution to patients with hepatic and biliary disease and to patients with renal disease or a combination of the two.

Metronidazole is listed as Pregnancy Category B. Several studies have shown the development of cleft palate when the fetus is exposed during the first trimester, but these studies have not been confirmed. Metronidazole is contraindicated for treatment of trichomoniasis during the first trimester. It has been used to treat trichomoniasis in the second and third trimesters of pregnancy, but not as a single-dose regimen. Although this drug has been used for more than 20 years with no increase in congenital abnormalities, stillbirths, or low birth weight reported, as with any drug given during pregnancy, prudence suggests that it be used only when clearly indicated.

Nitazoxanide is also listed as Pregnancy Category B. Animal studies have shown no evidence of impaired fertility or harm to the fetus. However, there are no adequate, well-controlled studies in humans. It should be used only when clearly indicated and when there is no other reasonable drug.

Tinidazole is Pregnancy Category C. It has not been studied in pregnant patients but is known to cross the placental barrier. It should not be given to pregnant patients in the first trimester. Given the long history of use of metronidazole,

Table 24–40 ⊞ Pharmacokinetics: Metronidazole, Nitazoxanide, and Tinidazole

Drug	Onset (h)	Peak (h)	Duration (h)	Protein Binding	Bioavailability	Half-Life	Elimination
Metronidazole	Rapid	1–3 h	8	<20%	100%	7.5 h	20% unchanged in urine; 6%–15% in feces
Nitazoxanide	UA	1–4; 2–8 h*	12	99%	Tablet: 100%; oral suspension: 70%	UA	As metabolites
Tinidazole	UA	1.6 h	72 h	12%		12–14 h	12% excreted in feces; 20%–25% unchanged in urine

UA = Information unavailable.

*The first number is for the tizoxanide metabolite; the second number is for the tizoxanide glucuronide metabolite.

it is a better drug choice for treatment of *G. lamblia* in pregnancy.

A nursing mother who needs metronidazole or tinidazole should interrupt nursing for 24 hours and use a single-dose regimen if clinically appropriate. Safety and efficacy in young children have not been established. It is not known if nitazoxanide is excreted in breast milk, and the choice to use it for a lactating mother should be made with extreme caution.

The safety and efficacy of metronidazole in children have been established only for treatment of amebiasis, although there are also drug dosages published for trichomoniasis and giardiasis. Elimination relates inversely to age. A single tablet of nitazoxanide contains more drug than is allowed for pediatric patients 11 years or younger; only oral suspension should be used for children aged 1 to 11 years. It should not be used for children younger than 1 year. Nitazoxanide is approved for treatment of *G. lamblia* and *C. parvum* in children. Tinidazole is approved for treatment of intestinal amebiasis and giardia in children 3 years of age or older.

Adverse Drug Reactions

Anorexia, nausea, abdominal pain, dizziness, and headache commonly occur with metronidazole. Dry mouth and a metallic taste may also develop. Although irritating, these adverse reactions are mild and transient. Infrequent adverse reactions include diarrhea, glossitis, rashes, leukopenia, seizures, aseptic meningitis, and peripheral neuropathy. Taking the drug with meals lessens the GI irritation. GI irritation with abdominal pain, nausea, and diarrhea are the main adverse reactions for nitazoxanide. Adverse effects associated with tinidazole are similar to those for metronidazole.

Drug Interactions

Drug interactions with all three drugs are few. As metronidazole undergoes metabolism by CYP450, known inhibitors (such as cimetidine) and inducers (such as phenytoin, phenobarbital) affect drug concentration. As metronidazole potentiates the anticoagulant effects of warfarin; the prothrombin time/international normalized ratio (PT/INR) should be carefully monitored. A disulfiram-like reaction may occur with alcohol ingestion, and patients are warned not to consume alcohol while taking this drug and for 48 hours after completing it.

Metronidazole may increase serum levels of lithium and close monitoring is recommended. Drug interactions are similar for tinidazole. Nitazoxanide is heavily bound to plasma proteins and may interact with other drugs that are also heavily protein bound (competition for binding sites), especially those with narrow therapeutic ranges (e.g., warfarin).

Clinical Use and Dosing

Metronidazole and tinidazole have antiparasitic and antibacterial properties. They are used against the common protozoal infections by *T. vaginalis, G. lamblia,* and *E. histolytica.* Metronidazole is also used to treat less common parasites, such as the protozoon *Balantidium coli* (with an oral dose of 750 mg 3 times daily for 5 days), as an alternative to tetracycline, and to treat the helminth *Dracunculus medinensis,* or guinea worm (with an oral dose of 250 mg 3 times daily for 10 days). Antibacterial uses of metronidazole include treatment of anaerobic bacterial infections, bacterial vaginosis, CDI, and eradication of *H. pylori* in gastritis and peptic ulcer disease. Many of the anaerobic bacterial infections treated with metronidazole are serious, even life-threatening, with treatment initiated in the hospital. Dosages of metronidazole for these diverse conditions are summarized in Table 24-41. In severe hepatic or renal disease, the dosage of metronidazole may need to be decreased; increased dosages might be required for successful therapy of patients taking inducers of hepatic CYP450, such as phenobarbital and phenytoin. Nitazoxanide is used for diarrhea casued by *G. lamblia* or *C. parvum.* Tinidazole is indicated for the treatment of trichomoniasis caused by *T. vaginalis,* giardiasis, bacterial vaginosis, intestinal amebiasis, and amebic liver abscess.

Trichomonas vaginitis

Trichomonas vaginal infection often occurs during or shortly after menses and is characterized by copious foamy discharge with a pH greater than 5, positive "whiff test," punctate hemorrhages of vaginal mucosa, and vaginal irritation. Although it is generally sexually transmitted, the organism can live for weeks on wet towels and toilet seats, so fomite transfer is theoretically possible. In the male, the infection may cause urethral discharge, but it is usually mild, if present at all. Both partners should be treated and a condom used during intercourse for a week to prevent reinfection. One-day treatment with metronidazole is 2 g as a single dose; 7-day treatment is 500 mg twice a day for 7 days (CDC, 2010e). If the infection occurs in the first trimester of pregnancy, deferral of treatment is recommended. Experts disagree over whether the long or short treatment is preferable during pregnant and nonpregnant states. Single-dose therapy promotes compliance, especially if administered under supervision.

Tinidazole is also used for this indication. The dose is 2 g as a single dose with food (CDC, 2010e). Both partners should be treated. This drug is Pregnancy Category C, so metronidazole is the preferred drug in those circumstances.

Giardiasis

The life cycle of the protozoon *G. lamblia* involves two stages: a cyst and a trophozoite. The cyst form can live in cold water for months and is ingested by the human hosts. It can also be transmitted during sexual activity. The trophozoite—or actively metabolizing, motile form—lives in the upper two-thirds of the small intestine and can be so numerous that it can mechanically interfere with digestion. *Giardia* infections may be asymptomatic or cause disease ranging from self-limiting diarrhea to a severe chronic syndrome with malnutrition.

In the United States, metronidazole, 250 mg 3 times a day for 5 days in adults and 15 mg/kg every 8 hours for 5 to 10 days in children, is used to treat giardiasis, although it is not approved for this indication. Asymptomatic cyst passers

Table 24–41 ⊗ **Dosage Schedule: Metronidazole, Nitazoxanide, and Tinidazole**

Drug	Indication	Dosage Form	Initial Dose	Comments
Metronidazole (Flagyl, Metric 21, Protostat)	Anaerobic bacterial infection	Tablets: 250 mg (G) 250 mg (F) 250 mg (P) 500 mg (G) 500 mg (F) 500 mg (P) Tablet, extended release: 750 mg (G), 750 (F) Capsules: 375 mg (F)	*Adults* 500 mg PO q8h *Children:* 7.5 mg/kg PO q6h *or* 10 mg/kg q8h	Maximum adult daily dosage is 4 g. Maximum daily dose in children is 2000 mg. Reduction in dosage may be required for patients with severe hepatic or renal impairment. May be taken with meals or a snack to decrease GI irritation. Avoid alcoholic beverages during therapy and for 48 h after completing it. Sexual partners of patients with *T. vaginalis* should be treated even if asymptomatic. Abstain from sexual contact or use condom for 7 d after therapy begins.
	C. difficile infection (CDI)		*Adults:* 500 mg PO 3 times daily *or* 250 mg PO 4 times daily for 10–14 d *Children:* 30 mg/kg/day divided qid for 7–14 days. Max 2000 mg/day	
	Bacterial vaginosis associated with *T. vaginalis* (off-label)		*Adults* 500 mg PO twice daily for 7 d	
	Giardiasis (*Giardia lamblia*) (off-label)		*Adults* 250 mg PO 3 times daily for 5–7 d *Children:* 5 mg/kg/dose PO 3 times daily for 5–7 d	
	Amebiasis (*E. histolytica*) dysentery		*Adults* 750 mg PO 3 times daily for 5–10 d *Children:* 35–50 mg/kg/24 h PO in 3 divided doses for 7–10 d *or* 11.6–16.7 mg/kg/dose PO 3 times daily for 7–10 d	
	Amebiasis (*E. histolytica*) liver abscess		*Adults:* 500–750 mg PO 3 times daily for 5–10 d *Children:* 35–50 mg/kg/24 h PO in 3 divided doses for 10 d *or* 11.6–16.7 mg/kg/dose PO 3 times daily for 10 d	
	Balantidiasis (off-label) (*Balantidium coli*)		*Adults:* 500–750 mg PO 3 times/d for 5–10 d *Children:* 11.6–16.7 mg/kg/dose 3 times daily for 10 d	
	Gastritis or peptic ulcer, *H. pylori*–associated		*Adults:* In combination with other antibiotic therapy : 500 mg PO 2–3 times daily for 7–14 d	
	Trichomoniasis (*T. vaginalis*)		*Adults:* 2 g PO as a single dose or 2 divided doses in 1 d; alternative: 250 mg PO 3 times/d for 7 d *Children:* 5 mg/kg/dose PO 3 times daily for 7 d	

Continued

Table 24–41 ⚙ **Dosage Schedule: Metronidazole, Nitazoxanide, and Tinidazole—cont'd**

Drug	Indication	Dosage Form	Initial Dose	Comments
	Anthelmintic		*Adults*: 250 mg PO 3 times daily for 10 d *Children*: 8.3 mg/kg/dose PO, up to a maximum of 250 mg, 3 times/d for 10 d	
Nitazoxanide	*G. lamblia*	Tablets: 500 mg (B) Powder for oral suspension: 100 mg/5 mL	*Children 1–3 yr*: 5 mL oral suspension* q12h *4–11 yr*: 10 mL oral suspension q12h *≥ 12 yr*: 1 tablet (500 mg) q12h or 25 mL oral suspension q12h	Take with food. Duration of therapy is 3 d.
	C. parvum		*Children 1–3 yr*: 5 mL oral suspension q12h *4–11 yr*: 10 mL oral suspension q12h	
Tinidazole	Intestinal amebiasis	Tablets: 250, 500 mg	*Adults* 2 g/d *Children ≥3 yr*: 50 mg/kg/d	Duration of therapy is 3 d.
	Giardiasis		*Adults*: 2 g *Children ≥3 yr*: 50 mg/kg	Single dose.
	Trichomoniasis		*Adults*: 2 g	Single dose.
				Partner should also be treated.

*Oral suspension is 100 mg/5 mL.

should also be treated. The nitazoxanide dose in adults is 500 mg twice daily for 3 days. Nitazoxanide is FDA approved for treatment of *G. lamblia* in children older than 1 year and will also treat intestinal parasites. Dosing of nitazaxanide for children age 1 to 3 years is 100 mg twice a day for 3 days, 200 mg twice a day in children age 4 to 11 years and children age 12 years or older prescribed the adult dose. Nitazoxanide is available in an oral suspension to make administration easier and more accurate in very young children. Tinidazole dosing to treat giardiasis in adults is a single 2 g dose with food and 50 mg/kg (up to 2 g) in children older than 3 years. Doses are provided in Table 24-41.

Amebiasis

Several species of *Entamoeba* infect humans, but *E. histolytica* is the only species known to cause disease. Like many protozoa, *Entamoeba* has two life stages: the cyst and the trophozoite. Infection of the human usually involves ingestion of cysts from fecally contaminated food, water, or hands. Transmission of cysts and trophozoites can also occur with fecal exposure during sexual contact. In the intestine, cysts undergo excystation into the trophozoite form and multiply. In many cases, the cysts remain in the intestinal lumen (noninvasive infection), resulting in asymptomatic carriers and cyst passers. In some patients, the cysts invade the intestinal lumen (invasive intestinal disease), resulting

in diarrhea or dysentery. Trophozoites also can travel through the bloodstream to form abscesses in the liver, brain, or lung (extraintestinal disease) that are manifested by local signs such as hepatomegaly or cholestasis. Drugs administered for presumptive treatment (broad-spectrum antibiotics, kaolin, bismuth, soapsuds enema, barium) can suppress shedding of amoebas into the stool and delay diagnosis. For invasive intestinal amebiasis in adults, metronidazole 750 mg orally 3 times daily for 10 days may be used (35 to 50 mg/kg/24 hours divided into three doses in children). Metronidazole can be used to treat the extraintestinal form of the disease IV or orally.

Metronidazole is so well absorbed that it is not effective against the noninvasive infection, and it may be necessary to add a luminal amoebicide like paromomycin (Humatin), 500 mg orally 3 times daily for 7 days. Paromomycin is an unabsorbable aminoglycoside similar to neomycin. If the intestinal mucosa is not intact, as in concomitant inflammatory bowel disease, paromomycin can be absorbed and cause ototoxicity and nephrotoxicity.

Tinidazole may also be prescribed for invasive intestinal amebiasis or amoebic liver abcess. The adult dose of tinidazole for invasive intestinal amebiasis or liver abcess is 2 g daily with food for 3 days. The pediatric dose of tinidazole for invasive intestinal amoebiasis or liver abcess is 50 mg/kg/day daily for 3 days. The advantage of tinidazole is the once-daily dosing.

Bacterial Vaginosis

Bacterial vaginosis develops when the bacterial flora are altered, with loss of the normally predominant lactobacilli and overgrowth of strict and facultative aerobic species such as *Bacteroides, Peptococcus, Mobiluncus, Gardnerella, Streptococcus,* and *Mycoplasma*. The infection manifests with foul-odored, clear, copious vaginal discharge with a pH greater than 4.5, positive "whiff test," and few WBCs. Untreated bacterial vaginosis has been associated with pelvic inflammatory disease, cervicitis, abnormal Pap smear cytology, preterm labor, and low birth weight. During pregnancy, symptomatic women are screened and treated if they are at high risk for preterm delivery. Treatment of low-risk and symptomatic women during pregnancy is controversial. Metronidazole, 500 mg orally twice daily for 7 days, or metronidazole intravaginal gel, 1 full applicator twice daily for 5 days, is the drug of first choice for bacterial vaginosis (CDC, 2010e). Dosing in pregnant women is 500 mg twice a day for 7 days or 250 mg 3 times a day for 7 days (CDC, 2010e).

The recommended dose of tinidazole in nonpregnant females with bacterial vaginosis is a 2 g oral dose once daily for 2 days taken with food or a 1 g oral dose once daily for 5 days taken with food. Use of tinidazole in pregnant women has not been studied. It is not necessary to treat sexual partners of women with bacterial vaginosis unless balanitis is present. Doses are provided in Table 24-41.

Cryptosporidium parvum

Nitazoxanide is the only drug in this group approved for treatment of the diarrhea caused by *C. parvum* in children 11 years old or younger. Its safety and efficacy have not been established for older children or adults, but doses are provided in the literature for these age groups. Its action appears to be caused by interference with the PFOR enzyme-dependent electron transfer reaction essential for anaerobic energy metabolism in the organism. This protein sequence is similar to the one used by *G. lamblia*. Dosing for each age group is found in Table 24-41.

Rational Drug Selection

For most of the infections for which metronidazole is used, it is the drug of choice because it is clearly more efficacious than the alternatives. Metronidazole is on many retail $4 lists, so cost is not an issue. Issues in drug selection for these conditions are the lack of effective alternatives for use in the first trimester of pregnancy, comparative efficacy of the long- and short-term oral dosing regimen, and the choice between topical and oral forms for vaginal infections.

For *G. lamblia*, nitazoxanide and tinidazole have FDA approval for this indication in children; metronidazole use is off-label. Only nitazoxanide has approval for treatment of *C. parvum* infections.

Monitoring

For most of the conditions treated with metronidazole, resolution of symptoms indicates effective treatment and further evaluation is not required. For giardiasis treated with any of these drugs, symptoms may persist for weeks or months after the organism is eradicated because of the lactose intolerance brought on by the infection (Gardner & Hill, 2001). If symptoms persist, three stool samples should be collected and cultured several days apart about 3 to 4 weeks after completion of treatment.

Patient Education

Administration

Although oral metronidazole and tinidazole can be taken without regard to meals, they should be taken with food or snacks to decrease GI irritation. Nitazoxanide should be taken with food and the oral suspension should be shaken well before administration. If vaginal or topical preparations of metronidazole are used, the patient should be provided with instruction and the opportunity to manipulate a model applicator in the office. Use of the extended-release form of metronidazole that can be administered once daily should be considered if nonadherence is an issue, although the vaginal gel and delayed-release oral form are considerably more expensive than other oral forms.

Adverse Reactions

Chewing sugarless gum or sucking on ice or candy can help to overcome the dry mouth and metallic taste that metronidazole can cause. Alcoholic beverages should be avoided during therapy with metronidazole or tinidazole and for 48 hours after the last dose because disulfiram-like reactions occur in about 40% of patients who consume alcohol. Because metronidazole can cause dizziness or light-headedness, hazardous activities should be avoided until the patient's response to the medication is established. Headache is a common adverse effect of metronidazole that can be treated with acetaminophen or an NSAID.

Metronidazole causes a harmless darkening of urine. Female patients should be counseled about the symptoms of vaginal candidiasis superinfection, which can complicate therapy and could be mistaken for recurrence of the original infection. The patient and family members should know to report CNS symptoms (ataxia, mood and mental changes, clumsiness, ataxia, seizures), peripheral neuropathy (numbness, tingling, pain, or weakness in hands or feet), and leukopenia (sore throat or fever).

Lifestyle Management

Many of the infections treated with metronidazole and tinidazole are sexually transmitted. Male or female condom usage may decrease transmittal of some, but not all, infections. Patients should be advised of the route of transmission and practices that promote transmittal of the infection. Concurrent treatment and refraining from sexual activity until the treatment is complete may be necessary to resolve the infections. Foreign travel and wilderness travel are other sources of exposure to *Giardia* and amoebas that should be considered in the history for diagnosing these conditions.

REFERENCES

American Academy of Microbiology (2009). Antibiotic eesistance: An ecological perspective on an old problem. American Academy of Microbiology. Retrieved from http://academy.asm.org/images/stories/documents/antibioticresistance.pdf

American Academy of Pedicatrics (AAP). (2001). Committee on drugs: Transfer of drugs and other chemical into human milk. *Pediatrics*,*108*(3), 776–789.

American Academy of Pediatrics (AAP). (2006). The use of systemic fluoroquinolones. *Pediatrics, 118*(3), 1287–1292. Retrieved from http://www.pediatrics.org/cgi/content/full

American Academy of Pediatrics (AAP). (2012a). Group A streptococcal infections. In L. K. Pickering (Ed.), *Red book: 2012 report of the Committee on Infectious Diseases* (29th ed., pp. 668–680). Elk Grove Village, IL: American Academy of Pediatrics. Retrieved from http://aapredbook.aappublications.org/content/1/SEC131/SEC264.body#c03-sec2-0855

American Academy of Pediatrics (AAP). (2012b). Group B streptococcal infections. In L. K. Pickering (Ed.), *Red book: 2102 report of the Committee on Infectious Diseases* (29th ed., pp. 680–685). Elk Grove Village, IL: American Academy of Pediatrics. Retrieved from http://aapredbook.aappublications.org/content/1/SEC131/SEC265.body?sid=04361975-aa77-4dde-b459-58aa30f428c3#c03-sec2-0862

American Academy of Pediatrics. (AAP). (2012c). Principles of appropriate use for upper respiratory tract infections. In L. K. Pickering (Ed.), *Red book: 2012 report of the Committee on Infectious Disease* (29th ed., pp. 802–805). Elk Grove Village, IL: American Academy of Pediatrics. Retrieved from http://aapredbook.aappublications.org/content/1/SEC295/SEC300/SEC301.body?sid=a501d0aa-1880-4888-9377-5cae8bebe82a

American Academy of Pediatrics (AAP). (2012d). Bite wounds. In L. K. Pickering (Ed.), *Red book: 2012 report of the Committee on Infectious Disease* (29th ed., pp. 203–206). Elk Grove Village, IL: American Academy of Pediatrics. Retrieved from http://aapredbook.aappublications.org/content/1/SEC70/SEC126.body?sid=09c09d7c-ade2-4cb6-9ff0-4726d6c6b38e#T38

American Academy of Pediatrics (AAP). (2012e). Lyme disease. In L. K. Pickering (Ed.), *Red book: 2012 report of the Committee on Infectious Disease* (29th ed., pp. 474–479). Elk Grove Village, IL: American Academy of Pediatrics. Retrieved from http://aapredbook.aappublications.org/content/1/SEC131/SEC212.body?sid=d7d617b2-72a2-441c-b5a7-29451020fdeb

American Academy of Pediatrics (AAP). (2012f). Chlamydial trachomatis. In L. K. Pickering (Ed.), *Red book: 2012 report of the Committee on Infectious Disease* (29th ed., pp. 276–281). Elk Grove Village, IL: American Academy of Pediatrics. Retrieved from http://aapredbook.aappublications.org/content/1/SEC131/SEC158/SEC161.body

American Academy of Pediatrics (2012g). Bite wounds. In L. K. Pickering (Ed.), *Red book: 2012 report of the Committee on Infectious Disease* (29th ed., pp 203–206). Elk Grove Village, IL: American Academy of Pediatrics. Retrieved from http://aapredbook.aappublications.org/content/1/SEC70/SEC126.body?sid=05dda433-a6ff-4dde-af72-127584257df3

American Academy of Pediatrics (AAP). (2012h). Rickettsial diseases. In L. K. Pickering (Ed.), *Red book: 2012 report of the Committee on Infectious Disease* (29th ed., pp. 620–622). Elk Grove Village, IL: American Academy of Pediatrics. Retrieved from http://aapredbook.aappublications.org/content/1/SEC131/SEC251.body?sid=350afb7c-f673-4d4a-9c6f-43fd15538837#c03-sec2-0764

Andres, D., Pascual, A., & Marchetti, O. (2009). Antifungal therapeutic drug monitoring: Established and emerging indications. *Antimicrobial Agents and Chemotherapy*, 53(1), 24–34.

Archer, J. S., & Archer, D. F. (2002). Oral contraceptive efficacy and antibiotic interaction: A myth debunked. *Journal of the American Academy of Dermatology*, 46, 917–923.

Auckland, C., Teare, L., Cooke, F., Kaufmann, M. E., Warner, M., Johnson, A. P., et al. (2002). Linezolid-resistant enterococci: Report of the first isolates in the United Kingdom. *Journal of Antimicrobial Chemotherapy*, 50, 743–746.

Barone, J. A., Moskovitz, B. L., Guarnieri, J., Hassell, A. E., Colaizzi, J. L., Bierman, R. H., et al. (1998). Enhanced bioavailability of itraconazole in hydroxypropyl β-cyclodextrin solution versus capsules in healthy volunteers. *Antimicrobial Agents and Chemotherapy*; *42*(7), 1862–1865.

Barron, J.,Turner R, Jaeger M., Adamson, W., & Singer, J. (2012) Comparing the use of intravenous antibiotic under the medical benefit with the use of oral antibiotics under the pharmacy benefit in treating skin and soft tissue infections. *Managed Care*, 21(9):44–52.

Benson, C. A., Kaplan, J. E., Masur, H., Pau, A., & Holms, K. K. (2004). Treatment of opportunistic infections among HIV-infected adults and adolescents. *Morbidity and Mortality Weekly Report*, 53(RR15), 1–112.

Bersos, Z., Maniati, M., Kontos, F., Petinaki, E., & Maniatis, A. N. (2004). First report of a linezolid-resistant vancomycin-resistant Enterococcus faecium strain in Greece. *Journal of Antimicrobial Chemotherapy*, 53, 685–686.

Biedenbach, D., Ross, J., Putnam, S., & Jones, R. N. (2010). In vitro activity of fidaxomicin (OPT-80) tested against contemporary clinical isolates of *Staphylococcus* spp. and *Enterococcus* spp. *Antimicrobial Agents and Chemotherapy*, 54, 2273–2275.

Bishai, W., Morris, C., & Scanland, S. (2004). *Treatment of community acquired pneumonia*. New York: Jobson Publishing.

Brackett, C. C., Singh, H., & Block, J. H. (2004). Likelihood and mechanisms of cross-allergenicity between sulfonamide antibiotic and other drugs containing a sulfonamide functional group. *Pharmacotherapy*, 24(7), 856.

Bradley, J. S., Byington, C. L., Shah, S. S., Alverson, B., Carter, E. R., Harrison, C., et al. (2011). The management of community-acquired pneumonia in infants and children older than 3 months of age: Clinical practice guidelines by the Pediatric Infectious Diseases Society and the Infectious Diseases Society of America. *Clinical Infectious Diseases*, 53(7), e25–e76.

Cameron, D., Gaito, A., Harris, N., Bach, G., Bellovin, S., Bock, K., et al. (2004). The International Lyme and Associated Diseases Society: Evidence-based guidelines for the management of Lyme disease. Retrieved from http://www.ilads.org/files/ILADS_Guidelines.pdf

Campagna, J, D., Bond, M. C., Schabelman, E., & Hayes, B. D. (2012). The use of cephalosporins in penicillin-allergic patients: A literature review. *The Journal of Emergency Medicine*, 42(5), 612–620.

Centers for Disease Control and Prevention (CDC). (2009a). *Careful antibiotic use: Pediatric appropriate treatment summary*. Retrieved from http://www.cdc.gov/getsmart

Centers for Disease Control and Prevention (CDC). (2009b). Get smart: Know when antibiotics work. Treatment guidelines for upper respiratory tract infections. Retrieved from http://www.cdc.gov/getsmart/campaign-materials/treatment-guidelines.html

Centers for Disease Control and Prevention (CDC). (2010a). *CDC guidance on shortage of erythromycin (0.5%) ophthalmic ointment*. Retrieved from http://www.cdc.gov/std/treatment/2006/erythromycinOintmentShortage.htm

Centers for Disease Control and Prevention (CDC). (2010b). *Drug-resistant Streptococcus pneumoniae disease*. Retrieved from http://www.cdc.gov//ncidod/dbmd/diseaseinfo/drugresisstreppneum_t.htm

Centers for Disease Control and Prevention (CDC). (2010c). Invasive pneumococcal disease in young children before licensure of 13-valent pneumococcal conjugate vaccine—United States, 2007. *Morbidity and Mortality Weekly Report, 59*(09), 253–257.

Centers for Disease Control and Prevention (CDC). (2010d). Recommendations for the prevention of perinatal group B streptococcal disease. *MMWR Recommendations and Reports, 59*(RR10), 1–32. Retrieved from http://www.cdc.gov/mmwr/preview/mmwrhtml/rr5910a1.htm

Centers for Disease Control and Prevention (CDC, 2010e). Sexually transmitted treatment guidelines, 2010. *Morbidity and Mortality Weekly Report, 59*(RR-12), 1–116. Retrieved from www.cdc.gov/std

Centers for Disease Control and Prevention. (2011). *A public health action plan to combat antimicrobial resistance*. Retrieved from http://www.cdc.gov/drugresistance/pdf/public-health-action-plan-combat-antimicrobial-resistance.pdf

Centers for Disease Control and Prevention (2012). Active Bacterial Core Surveillance (ABCs) report: Emerging Infections Program Network, *Streptococcus pneumoniae*, 2011. *Morbidity and Mortality Weekly Report.* 61(31), 590–594. Retrived from http://www.cdc.gov/abcs/reports-findings/survreports/spneu11.pdf.

Centers for Disease Control (2013a). *Antibiotic Resistance Threats in the United States, 2013.* Centers for Disease Control. Retrieved from http://www.cdc.gov/drugresistance/threat-report-2013/

Centers for Disease Control (2013b). CDC grand rounds: The growing threat of multidrug-resistant gonorrhea. *MMWR Morbity and Mortality Weekly Reports, 62*(6), 103–106.

Centers for Disease Control (2013c). *Tickbourne diseases of the United States: A reference manual for health care providers.* Retrieved from http://www.cdc.gov/lyme/resources/TickborneDiseases.pdfCenters for Disease Control (2013c).

Centers for Disease Control. (2013d). *Parasites—Strongyloides: Resources for health professionals.* Accessed on November 11, 2013, at http://www.cdc.gov/parasites/strongyloides/health_professionals/

Centers for Disease Control (2013e). *Parasites—Hookworm: Resources for health professionals.* Accessed on November 11, 2013, at http://www.cdc.gov/parasites/hookworm/health_professionals/

Cheung, O., Chopra, K., Yu, T., & Nalesnik, M. (2004). Gatifloxacin-induced hepatotoxicity and acute pancreatitis. *Annals of Internal Medicine, 140*(1), 73–74.

Chow, A. W., Benninger, M. S., Brook, I., Brozek, J. L., Goldstein, E. J. C., Hicks, L. A., et al. (2012). ISDA clinical practice guidelines for acute bacterial rhinosinusitis in children and adults. *Clinical Infectious Diseases, 54*(8), 1041–1045.

Conner, B. A. (2013). Travelers' diarrhea. *CDC health information for international travel.* Retrieved from http://wwwnc.cdc.gov/travel/yellowbook/2014/chapter-2-the-pre-travel-consultation/travelers-diarrhea

Courter, J., Baker, W., Nowak, K., Smogowicz, L., Desjardins, L., Coleman, C., et al. (2010). Increased clinical failures when treating acute otitis media with macrolides: A meta-analysis. *The Annals of Pharmacotherapy, 44*(3), 471–478.

Currie, B. J., & McCarthy, J. S. (2010). Permethrin and ivermectin for scabies. *New England Journal of Medicine, 362,* 717–725.

Devasia, R. A., Blackman, A., Gebretsadik, T., Griffin, M., Shintani, A., May, C., et al. (2009). Fluoroquinolone resistance in mycobacterium tuberculosis: The effect of duration and timing of fluoroquinolone exposure. *American Journal of Respiratory and Critical Care Medicine, 180*(4), 365–370.

Finegold, S., Molitoris, D., Vaisanen, M., et al. (2004). In vitro activities of OPT-80 and comparator drugs against intestinal bacteria. *Antimicrobial Agents and Chemotherapy; 48,* 4898–4902.

Fiore, A. E., Fry, A., Shay, D., Gubareva, L., Bresee, J. S. & Uyeki, T. M. (2011). Antiviral agents for the treatment and chemophrophylaxis of influenza. *Morbidity and Mortality Weekly Report, 60*(RR01), 1–24.

Flanagan, S., Bartizal, K., Minassian, S. L., Fang, E., & Prokocimer, P. (2013). In vitro, in vivo, and clinical studies of tedizolid to assess the potential for peripheral or central monoamine oxidase interactions. *Antimicrobial Agents and Chemotherapy, 57*(7), 3060–3066.

Frumin, J., Gallagher, J. C. (2009). Allergic cross-sensitivity between penicillin, carbapenem, and monobactam antibiotics: What are the chances? *Annals of Pharmacotherapy, 43*(2), 304–315.

Garcia-Effron, G., Gomez-Lopez, A., Mellado, E., Monzon, A., Rodriguez-Tudela, J. L., & Cuenca-Estrella, M. (2004). *In vitro* activity of terbinafine against medically important non-dermatophyte species of filamentous fungi. *Journal of Antimicrobial Chemotherapy, 53*(6), 1086–1089.

Gardner, T. B., & Hill, D. R. (2001). Treatment of giardiasis. *Clinical Microbiology Reviews, 14*(1), 114–128.

Golan, Y., & Epstein, L. (2012). Safety and efficacy of fidaxomicin in the treatment of *Clostridium difficile*-associated diarrhea. *Therapeutic Advances in Gastroenterology, 5*(6), 395–402.

Griebling, T. L. (2007). Urinary tract infection in women. In M. S. Litwin & C. S. Saigal (Eds.), *Urologic diseases in America* (NIH Publication No. 07–5512, pp. 588–617). U.S. Department of Health and Human Services, Public Health Service, National Institutes of Health, National Institute of Diabetes and Digestive and Kidney Diseases. Washington, DC: U.S. Government Printing Office.

Gupta, K., Hooton, T. M., Naber, K. G., Wullt, B., Colgan, R., Miller, L. G., et al. (2011). International clinical practice guidelines for the treatment of acute uncomplicated cystitis and pyelonephritis in women: A 2010 update by the Infectious Diseases Society of America and the European Society

for Microbiology and Infectious Diseases. *Clinical Infectious Diseases, 52*(5), e103–e120.

Heiman, K. E., & Bowen, A. (2013). Shigellosis. *CDC health information for international travel.* Retrieved from http://wwwnc.cdc.gov/travel/yellowbook/2014/chapter-3-infectious-diseases-related-to-travel/shigellosis

Hendricks, K. A., Wright, M. E., Shadomy, S. V., Bradley, J. S., Morrow, M. G., Pavia, A. T., et al. (2014). Centers for Disease Control and Prevention expert panel meetings on prevention and treatment of anthrax in adults. *Emerging Infectious Diseases, 20*(2), February 2014 online release. http://dx.doi.org/10.3201/eid2002.130687

Hooton, T. M., & Stamm, W. E. (2010). Urinary tract infections and asymptomatic bacteriuria in pregnancy. *UpToDate.* Retrieved from http://www.uptodate.com/online/content/topic.do?topicKey=uti_infe/7516&source=see_link

Hsu, K. K., Shea, K. M., Stevenson, A. E., & Pelton, S. I. (2010). Changing serotypes causing childhood invasive pneumococcal disease: Massachusetts, 2001–2007. *Pediatric Infectious Disease Journal, 29*(4), 289–293.

Irwin, R. S., Bauman, M. H., Bolser, D. S., Boulet, L. P., Braman, S. S., Brightling, C. E., et al. (2006). Diagnosis and management of cough: Executive summary. ACCP evidence-based clinical practice guidelines. *Chest, 129*(1 suppl), 1S–23S.

Jacobs, M. R., Felmingham, D., Appelbaum, P. C., Gruneberg, R. N., for the Alexander Project Group. (2003). The Alexander Project 1998–2000: Susceptibility of pathogens isolated from community-acquired respiratory tract infection to commonly used antimicrobial agents. *Journal of Antimicrobial Chemotherapy, 52,* 229–246.

Jenkins, S. G., & Farrell, D. J. (2009). Increase in pneumococcus macrolide resistance, United States. *Emerging Infectious Diseases, 15*(8), 1260–1264. Retrieved from http://www.cdc.gov/EID/content/ 15/8/1260.htm

Kainer, M. A., Devasia, R. A., Jones, T. F., Simmons, B. P., Melton, K., Chow, S., et al. (2007). Response to emerging infection leading to outbreak of linezolid-resistant enterococci. *Emerging Infectious Diseases, 13*(7), 1024–1030.

Kashanian, J., Hakimian, P., Blute, M., Wong, J., Khanna, H., Wise, G., et al. (2008). Nitrofurantoin: The return of an old friend in the wake of growing resistance. *British Journal of Urology International, 102,* 1634–1637.

Keren, R., & Chan, E. (2002). A meta-analysis of randomized, controlled trials comparing short- and long-course antibiotic therapy for urinary tract infections in children. *Pediatrics, 109*(5), e70.

Klein, J. O., & Pelton, S. (2009). Acute otitis media in children: Treatment. *UpToDate Online.* Retrieved from http://www.uptodate.com

Kofke-Egger, H., & Udow-Phillips, M. (2011) Antibiotic prescribing and use. Center for Healthcare Research & Transformation. Ann Arbor, MI. Retrieved from http://www.chrt.org/news/report-shows-high-rates-inappropriate-antibiotic-use-continue-despite-educational-efforts-improve-prescribing-patterns/

Krishna, G., Moton, A., Ma, L., Medlock, M. M., & McLeod, J. (2009). Pharmacokinetics and absorption of posaconazole oral suspension under various gastric conditions in healthy volunteers. *Antimicrobial Agents and Chemotherapy, 53*(3), 958–966.

LactMed. (2014). Toxnet Data Toxicology Network. National Library of Medicine. Retrieved from http://toxnet.nlm.nih.gov/index.html

Lew, E. (2009). Peptic ulcer disease. In N. J. Greenberger (Ed.), *Current diagnosis & treatment gastroenterology, hepatology, & endoscopy* (3rd ed.). McGraw Hill: New York.

Lieberthal, A. S., Carroll, A. E., Chonmaitree, T., Ganiats, T. G., Hoberman, A., Jackson, M. A., et al. (2013). The diagnosis and management of acute otitis media. *Pediatrics, 131,* e964–e999. Retrieved from http://pediatrics.aappublications.org/content/early/2013/02/20/peds.2012-3488

Linares, J., Ardanuy, C., Pallares, R., & Fenoll, A. (2010). Changes in antimicrobial resistance, serotypes and genotypes in *Streptococcus pneumoniae* over a 30-year period. *Clinical Microbiology and Infection, 16*(5), 402–410.

Litwin, M. S., & Saigal, C. S. (2007). Introduction. In M. S. Litwin & C. S. Saigal (Eds.), *Urologic diseases in America* (NIH Publication No. 07–5512:3–7). Washington, DC: U.S. Government Printing Office.

Liu, C., Bayer, A., Cosgrove, S. E., Daum, R. S., Fridkin, S. K., Gorwitz, R. J., et al. (2011). Clinical practice guidelines by the Infectious Diseases Society of America for the treatment of methicillin-resistant *Staphylococcus*

Aureus infections in adults and children. *Clinical Infectious Diseases, 52,* 1-38.

Lofmark, S., Edlund, C., & Nord, C. E. (2010). Metronidazole is still the drug of choice for treatment of anaerobic infections. *Clinical Infectious Diseases; 50*(Supp. 1), S16–S23.

Mandell, L. A., Wunderink, R. G., Anzueto, A., Bartlett, J. G., Campbell, G. D., Dowell, S. F., et al. (2007). Infectious Diseases Society of America/American Thoracic Society consensus guidelines on the management of community-acquired pneumonia in adults. *Clinical Infectious Disease, 44*(Suppl. 2), S27–S72.

McCarthy, J., Loukas, A., & Hotez, P. J. (2011). Chapter 51: Chemotherapy of helminth infections. In *Goodman & Gilman's The Pharmacological Basis of Therapeutics* (12th ed.). New York: McGraw Hill.

MacNeil, J., & Cohn, A. (2011). Chapter 8: Meningococcal disease. *Manual for the Surveillance of Vaccine-Preventable Diseases* (5th ed.). Retrieved from http://www.cdc.gov/vaccines/pubs/surv-manual/chpt08-mening.html

Mofeson, L. M., Brady, M. T., Danner, S. P., et al. (2009). Guidelines for the prevention and treatment of opportunistic infections among HIV-exposed and HIV-infected children: Recommendations from CDC, the National Institutes of Health, the HIV Medicine Association of the Infectious Diseases Society of America, the Pediatric Infectious Diseases Society, and the American Academy of Pediatrics. *MMWR Recommendations & Reports, 58* (RR-11), 1–166.

Mollering, R. (2003). Linezolid: The first oxazolidinone antimicrobial. *Annals of Internal Medicine, 138*(2), 135–142.

Neff, M. (2003). ATS, CDC and IDSA update recommendations of the treatment of tuberculosis. *American Family Physician, 68*(9), 1854–1862.

Newton, A. E., & Mintz, E. (2013). Typhoid and paratyphoid fever. *CDC health information for international travel.* Retrieved from http://wwwnc.cdc.gov/travel/yellowbook/2014/chapter-3-infectious-diseases-related-to-travel/typhoid-and-paratyphoid-fever

Nicolle, L., Bradley, S., Colgan, R., Rice, J., Schaffer, A., & Hootne, T. (2005). Infectious Diseases Society of America guideline for the diagnosis and treatment of asymptomatic bacteriuria in adults. *Clinical Infectious Disease, 40*(5), 643–654.

Nishimura, R. A., Carabello, B. A., Faxon, D. P., Freed, M. D., Lytle, B. W., O'Gara, P. T., et al. (2008). ACC/AHA 2008 guideline update on valvular heart disease: Focused update on infective endocarditis. *Journal of the American College of Cardiology, 52,* 676–685.

North of England Dyspepsia Guideline Development Group. (2004). *Dyspepsia: Managing dyspepsia in adults in primary care.* Center for Health Services Research. Newcastle Upon Tyne (UK): University of Newcastle. Retrieved June 15, 2005, from http://www.guideline.gov/summary/summary.aspx

Panackal, A. A., Gribskov, J. L., Staab, J. F., Kirby, K. A., Rinaldi, M., & Marr, K. A. (2006). Clinical significance of azole antifungal drug cross-resistance in *Candida glabrata. Journal of Clinical Microbiology, 44*(5), 1740–1743.

Patterson, D., Ko, W., Gottberg, A., Mohapatra, S., Casellas, J., Goossens, H., et al. (2004). International prospective study of *Klebsiella pneumoniae* bacteria: Implications of extended-spectrum β-lactamase production in nosocomial infections. *Annals of Internal Medicine, 140*(1), 26–32.

Pfaller, M. A., Diekema, D. J., Jones, R. N., et al, for the SENTRY Participant Group. (2001). International surveillance of blood-stream infections due to Candida species: Frequency of occurrence and in vitro susceptibilities to fluconazole, ravuconazole, and voriconazole of isolates collected from 1997 through 1999 in the SENTRY antimicrobial surveillance program. *Journal of Clinical Microbiology, 39,* 3254–3259.

Pfaller, M. A., Diekema, D. J., & Sheehan, D. J. (2006). Interpretive breakpoints for fluconazole and *Candida* revisited: A blueprint for the future of antifungal susceptibility testing. *Clinical Microbiology Reviews, 19*(2), 435–447.

Prais, D., Straussberg, R., Avitzur, Y., Nussinovitch, M., Harel, L., & Amir, J. (2003). Bacterial susceptibility to oral antibiotics in community acquired urinary tract infection. *Archives of Disease in Childhood, 88,* 215–218.

Prichard, R. (1994). Anthelmintic resistance. *Veterinary Parasitology, 54,* 259–268.

Rabe, K. F., Hurd, S., Anzueto, A., Barnes, P. J., Buist, S. A., Calverley, P., et al. (2007). Global strategy for the diagnosis, management, and prevention of chronic obstructive pulmonary disease. *American Journal of Respiratory Critical Care Medicine, 176,* 532–555.

Rabodonirina, M., Vaillant, L., Taffé, P., Nahimana, A., Gillibert, R.-P., Vanhems, P., et al. (2013) *Pneumocystis jirovecii* genotype associated with increased death rate of HIV-infected patients with pneumonia. *Emerging Infectious Disease, 19*(1), [Internet]. Retrieved from http://wwwnc.cdc.gov/eid/article/19/1/12-0140_intro.htm

Richter, S. S., Heilmann, K. P., Dohrn, C. L., Beekman, S. E., Riahi, F., Garcia-de-Lomas, J., et al. (2008). Increasing telithromycin resistance among *Streptococcus pyogenes* in Europe. *Journal of Antimicrobial Chemotherapy, 61*(3), 603–611.

Robertson, S. J., Pennington, A. J., Evans, A. M., & Martin, R. J. (1994). The action of pyrantel as an agonist and an open-channel blocker at acetylcholine receptors in isolated *Ascaris suum* muscle vesicles. *European Journal of Pharmacolgy, 271,*273–282.

Rodloff, A. C., Koch, D., & Schaumann, R. (2011). Epidemiology and antifungal resistance in invasive candidiasis. *European Journal of Medical Research, 16,* 187–195.

Rosenstein, N., Phillips, W. R., Gerber, M. A., March, S. M., Schwartz, B., & Dowell, S. F. (1998). The common cold—Principles of judicious use of antimicrobial agents. *Pediatrics, 101*(1 Suppl.), 181–184.

Sanchez Garcia, M. S., De la Torre, M. A., Morales, G., Pelaez, B., Tolon, M. J., Domingo, S., et al. (2010). Clinical outbreak of linezolid-resistant *Staphylococcus aureus* in an intensive care unit. *Journal of the American Medical Association, 303*(22), 2260–2264.

Schafer, J. A., Mateo, N., Parlier, G. L., & Rotschafer, J. C. (2007). Penicillin allergy skin testing: What do we do now? *Pharmacotherapy, 27*(4), 542–545.

Scholz, I., Oberwittler, H., Riedel, K. D., Burhenne, J., Weiss, J., Haefeli, W. E., et al. (2009). Pharmacokinetics, metabolism and bioavailability of the triazole antifungal agent voriconazole in relation to CYP2C19 genotype. *British Journal of Clinical Pharmacology; 68*(6), 906–915.

Shulman, S. T., Bisno, A. L., Clegg, H. W., Gerber, M. A., Kaplan, E. L., Lee, G., et al. (2012). Clinical practice guideline for the diagnosis and management of Group A Streptocolla pharyngitis: 2012 update by the Infectious Diseases Society of America. *Clinical Infectious Diseases, 55*(10), 1279–1282.

Slatore, C. G., & Tilles, S. A., (2004). Sulfonamide hypersensitivity. *Immunology Allergy Clinics of North America, 24*(3), 477.

Snow, V., Mottur-Pilson, C., & Gonzales, R. (2001). Principles of appropriate antibiotic use for treatment of acute bronchitis in adults. *Annals of Internal Medicine, 134*(6), 518–520.

Sprandel, K. A., Drusano, G. L., Hecht, D. W., Rotschafer, J. C., Danziger, L. H., & Rodvold, K. A. (2006). Population pharmacokinetics modeling and Monte Carlo simulation of varying doses of intravenous metronidazole. *Diagnostic Microbiology and Infectious Diseases; 55*(4), 303–309.

Stahlmann, R., & Lode, H. (2010). Safety considerations of fluoroquinolones in the elderly: An update. *Drugs & Aging, 27*(3), 193–209.

Steele, R. W., Thomas, M. P., Begue, R. E., & Despinasse, B. P. (1999). Selection of pediatric antibiotic suspensions: Taste and cost. *Infection Medicine, 16,* 197–200.

Steele, R. W., Thomas, M. P., & Begue, R. (2001). Compliance issues related to the selection of antibiotic suspensions for children. *Pediatric Infectious Disease Journal, 20*(1), 1–5.

Urbina, O., Ferrandez, O., Espona, M., Salas, E., et al. (2013). Potential role of tedizolid phosphate in the treatment of acute bacterail skin infections. *Drug Design, Development and Therapy, 7,* 243–265.

Wagenlehner, F., Weidner, W., & Naber, K. (2005). Emerging drugs for bacterial urinary tract infections. *Expert Opinion on Emerging Drugs, 10*(2), 275–298.

Wald, E. R., Applegate, K. E., Bordley, C., Darrrow, D. H., Glode, M. P., Marcy, S. M., et al. (2013). Clinical practice guideline for the diagnosis and management of acute bacterial sinusitis in children aged 1 to 18 years. *Pediatrics, 132*(1), e262–e280.

Weiler, S., Fiegl, D., MacFarland, R., Stienecke, E., Bellmann-Weiler, R., Dunzendorfer, S., et al. (2011). Human tissue distribution of voriconazole. *Antimicrobial Agents and Chemotherapy, 55*(2), 925.

Wheat, L. J., Freifeld, A. G., Kleiman, M. B., Baddley, J. W., McKinsey, D. S., Loyd, J. E., et al. (2007). Clinical practice guidelines for the management of patients with histoplasmosis: 2007 update by the Infectious Diseases Society of America, *45*, 807–825.

Wisplinghoff, H., Bischoff, T., Tallent, S. M., Seifert, H., Wenzel, R. P., & Edmond, M. B. (2004). Nosocomial bloodstream infections in US Hospitals: Analysis of 24,179 cases from a prospective nationwide surveillance study. *Clinical Infectious Diseases, 39*(3), 309–317.

World Health Organization (WHO. (2010). Parasitic diseases. Retrieved from http://www.who.int/vaccine_research/diseases/soa_parasitic/en/index.html

World Health Organization (WHO). (2013a). Antimicrobial resistance. World Health Organization. Retrieved from http://www.who.int/mediacentre/factsheets/fs194/en/

World Health Organization (WHO). (2013b) Global tuberculosis report 2013. www.who.int/iris/bitstream/10665/91355/1/9789241564656_eng.pdf (accessed 2013 Nov 23)

Wormser, G. P., Dattwyler, R. J., Shapiro, E. D., Halperin, J. J., Steere, A. C., Klempner, M. S., et al. (2006). The clinical assessment, treatment, and prevention of Lyme disease, human granulocytic anaplasmosis and babesiosis: Clinical practice guidelines by the Infectious Diseases Society of America. *Clinical Infectious Diseases, 43,* 1089–1134.

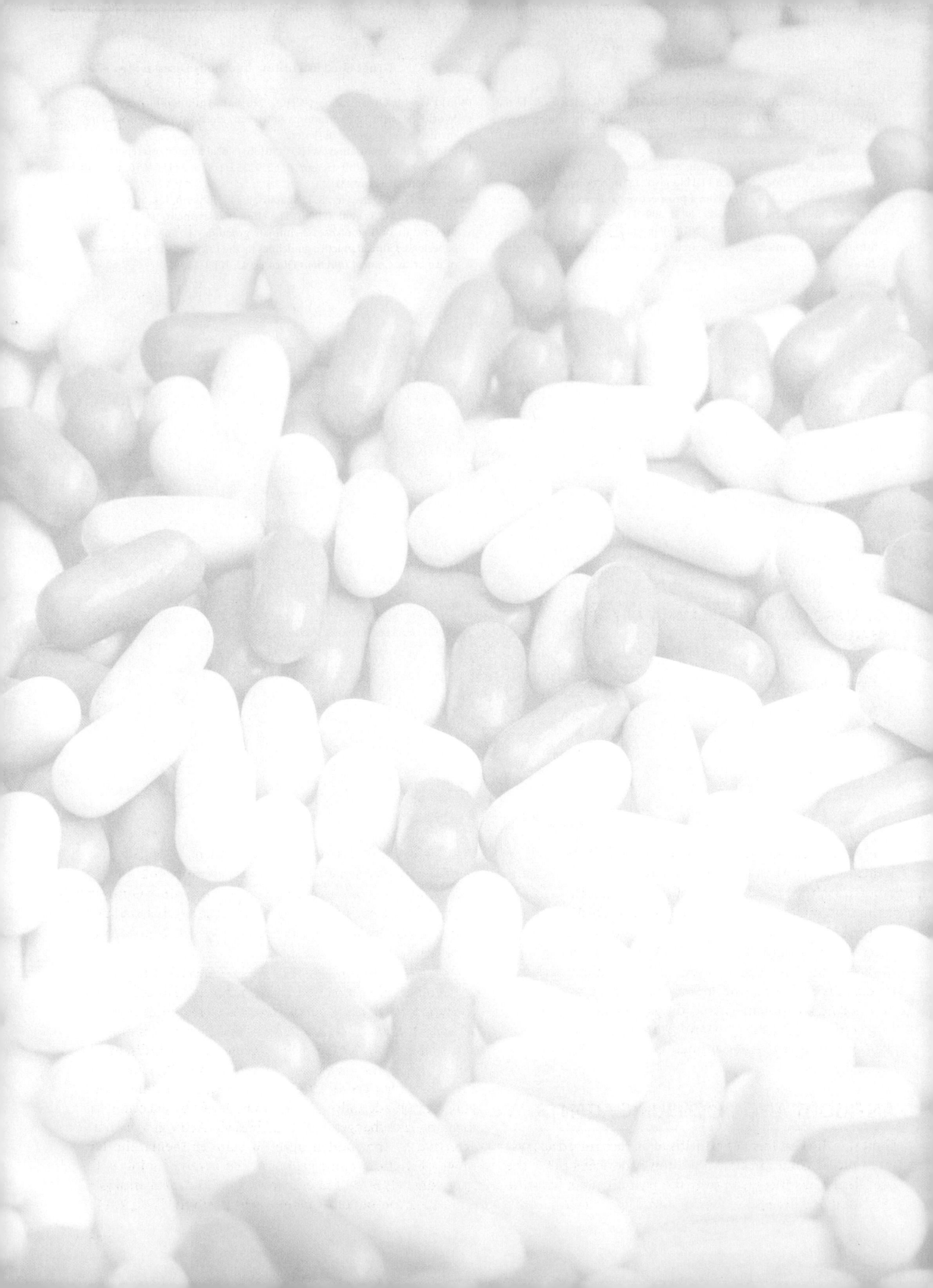

CHAPTER 25

DRUGS USED IN TREATING INFLAMMATORY PROCESSES

Teri Moser Woo

Inflammation is a common symptom of many diseases, including arthritis, with an estimated 52.5 million adults reporting they have some form of arthritis, rheumatoid arthritis, gout, lupus, or fibromyalgia according to the 2010–2012 National Health Interview Survey (Centers for Disease Control and Prevention [CDC], 2013). This chapter discusses the medication used to treat inflammation—specifically inflammation associated with gout—and the nonspecific anti-inflammatory drugs. The anti-inflammatory actions of the corticosteroids are reviewed as well as the nonsteroidal anti-inflammatory drugs (NSAIDs) and the salicylates.

ANTIGOUT AND URICOSURIC AGENTS

Gout was the first form of arthritis to be recognized as crystal induced. Gout affects 8.3 million Americans (4%); the prevalence has increased over the past 20 years with the increased incidence of obesity and hypertension (Zhu, Pandya, & Choi, 2011). The peak incidence occurs in patients 70 to 79 years old, and it is much more common in men than in women (Lawrence et al, 2008). Gout in women occurs exclusively postmenopause and is associated with hypertension, renal insufficiency, and exposure to diuretics.

The gout syndrome is caused by an alteration in purine metabolism, the end product of which is uric acid. This alteration results in hyperuricemia and in the deposition of urate crystals in various tissues. The four phases of gout are asymptomatic hyperuricemia, acute gouty arthritis, intercritical gout, and chronic tophaceous gout. Patients with asymptomatic hyperuricemia do not require treatment, but efforts are made to lower their urate levels by encouraging them to make changes in diet and lifestyle. Acute gout is characterized by the sudden onset of pain, erythema, limited range of motion, and swelling in the involved joint, with approximately 50% of cases involving the first metatarsal join of the great toe, but other joints can be involved (CDC, 2011).

The key elements in treatment of the latter three phases of this disorder are management of the acute pain and use of antigout and uricosuric agents. The drugs used to manage the pain are most often NSAIDs and corticosteroids, which are discussed later in the chapter. The three antigout drugs, allopurinol (Zyloprim), colchicine, and febuxostat (Uloric), and the two uricosuric agents, probenecid (Benemid) and sulfinpyrazone (Anturane), are the focus of this section.

Pharmacodynamics

Antigout Drugs

Antigout drugs act to reduce the inflammatory process or to prevent the synthesis of uric acid. Allopurinol and febuxostat inhibit xanthine oxidase, the enzyme responsible for the conversion of hypoxanthine and xanthine to uric acid. Allopurinol has a metabolite (alloxanthine) that is also an inhibitor of xanthine oxidase. Allopurinol acts directly on purine metabolism, reducing the production of uric acid, without disrupting the biosynthesis of vital purines. Allopurinol and febuxostat are the only drugs that act directly on the pathophysiological cause of gout.

Administration of allopurinol generally leads to a fall in both serum and urinary uric acid in 2 to 3 days. The magnitude of this decrease is dose-dependent. A week or more of treatment may be necessary before the full effects of the drug can be seen.

Febuxostat is used to treat hyperuricemia in patients with gout. The goal is to have a serum uric acid level of less than 6 mg/ dL. It may take 2 weeks or more to see the effect of febuxostat.

Unlike allopurinol, colchicine does not affect purine metabolism. It binds to microtubular proteins to interfere with the function of the mitotic spindles and inhibit the migration of granulocytes to the inflamed area. It reduces lactic acid production by granulocytes, which decreases deposition of uric acid, and it interferes with kinin formation and reduces phagocytosis. Taken together, these actions decrease the inflammatory response to the deposited urate crystals.

Although it relieves pain in acute attacks, colchicine is not an analgesic. It is also not uricosuric and does not prevent gout from progressing to chronic gouty arthritis. Its prophylactic, suppressive effect helps reduce the incidence of acute attacks and relieves the patient's occasional residual pain and mild discomfort.

Uricosuric Drugs

Uricosuric drugs, unlike antigout drugs, increase the rate of uric acid secretion. Both probenecid and sulfinpyrazone inhibit renal tubular reabsorption of urate and thus increase the renal excretion of uric acid and decrease serum uric acid levels. Effective uricosuria reduces the miscible urate pool, retards urate deposition, and promotes reabsorption of urate deposits. Sulfinpyrazone also competitively inhibits platelet prostaglandin synthesis, which prevents platelet aggregation and gives the drug an antithrombotic effect. Both drugs lack anti-inflammatory activity. They are most useful for patients with reduced urinary excretion of uric acid. They are not intended for treatment of acute attacks.

Pharmacokinetics

Absorption and Distribution

All gout drugs are well absorbed after oral administration (Table 25-1). Febuxostat absorption is decreased with a high-fat meal, but there is not a clinically significant change in serum uric acid concentration, so it may be taken without regard to food. Allopurinol is widely distributed to tissues. Colchicine concentrates mainly in white blood cells. Probenecid crosses the placenta without producing adverse effects in the fetus or infant. Sulfinpyrazone also crosses the placenta but may be hazardous to the fetus. Both probenecid and sulfinpyrazone are highly protein bound and tend to displace other drugs that have a high affinity for the same binding sites.

Metabolism and Excretion

The liver metabolizes all five drugs used in gout treatment. All have active metabolites. Both biliary and renal routes excrete allopurinol, colchicines, and febuxostat. However, colchicine is not effective in the presence of renal failure. The other two drugs are excreted primarily in urine, and the dose of probenecid may need to be reduced in the presence of renal impairment.

Pharmacotherapeutics

Precautions and Contraindications

Allopurinol (Zyloprim), colchicines, probenecid (Benemid), and sulfinpyrazone (Anturane) are associated with poor urate clearance in the presence of renal impairment. They should be used cautiously, and renal function tests should be performed regularly to determine appropriate dosage of the drug. Data are insufficient regarding the use of febuxostat in patients with renal impairment.

Allopurinol and colchicine are associated with hepatotoxicity. They are not recommended for patients with severe hepatic dysfunction. If patients taking these drugs develop anorexia, weight loss, or pruritus, evaluation of liver function should be part of the diagnostic work-up. For milder hepatic disorders, close monitoring of liver function is required.

Colchicine, probenecid, and sulfinpyrazone are all used cautiously in the presence of peptic ulcer disease or spastic colon. Gastrointestinal (GI) adverse reactions from these drugs are likely to make these disorders worse. Because probenecid and sulfinpyrazone are sulfa-based drugs, patients with known or suspected sulfa allergies should not use them.

Febuxostat, a xanthine oxidase inhibitor, is contraindicated in patients being treated with drugs requiring xanthine oxidase for metabolism (azathioprine, mercaptopurine, or theophylline) because of increased risk for toxicity.

Table 25–1 ⚙ Pharmacokinetics: Antigout and Uricosuric Agents

Drug	Onset	Peak (in plasma)	Duration	Protein Binding	Half-Life	Elimination
Allopurinol	2–3 d*	1.5 h allopurinol 4.5 h oxipurinol	1–2 wk*	NA	1–2 h allopurinol 15 h oxypurinol	20% in feces; remainder in urine
Colchicine	12 h†	0.5–2 h	UK	50%	60 min in plasma <60 h in leukocytes	10%–20% in urine; remainder in bile and feces
Febuxostat	NA	1–1.5 h	UK	99.2%	5–8 h	Urine; 49% as metabolites, feces; 45% as metabolites
Probenecid	30 min*	2–4 h	8 h	85%–95%	5–8 h dose-dependent	In urine; primarily as metabolite
Sulfinpyrazone	NA	4 h	UK	98%–99%	4 h	50% in urine: 90% of this as unchanged drug; 10% as metabolite

UK = unknown.
*Hypouricemic action.
†Anti-inflammatory action.

There is a risk of gout flare-up when febuxostat is started. Patients should be concurrently treated with an NSAID or colchicine for up to 6 months.

Pregnancy categories vary by drug. Allopurinol is Pregnancy Category C, but there are no adequate, well-controlled studies in pregnant women. Use only when benefits clearly outweigh potential risks to the fetus. Colchicine is Pregnancy Category C when given orally, D when given parenterally. This drug can cause fetal harm when administered to pregnant women and should be used only when benefits clearly outweigh risks to the fetus and other drugs are not effective. Probenecid is Pregnancy Category B. It crosses the placenta, but it has been used during pregnancy without producing harmful effects in the fetus. Sulfinpyrazone is Pregnancy Category D, but there are no adequate, well-controlled studies in pregnant women. Its use should be avoided in pregnancy unless no other drug is effective and reduction in urate levels is essential. Febuxostat is Pregnancy Category C. There are no adequate and well-controlled studies in pregnant women. Febuxostat should only be used if the benefits outweigh the risks.

Allopurinol has been found in breast milk. It is not known whether the other three drugs are excreted in breast milk. Exercise caution when prescribing these drugs for nursing women. Febuxostat is excreted in the milk of rats; it is unknown whether it is excreted in human milk.

These drugs are generally not indicated for use in children, except in hyperuricemia associated with the treatment of malignancy, and this disorder would likely be followed by a specialist. Dosage schedules are published for children only for the indication discussed and for the use of probenecid for retarding penicillin or cephalosporin excretion in selected infections.

Adverse Drug Reactions

Urates tend to crystallize out in acid urine. Fluid intake of more than 3,000 mL/d, along with sufficient sodium bicarbonate (3–7.5 g/d) or potassium citrate (7.5 g/d), maintains alkaline urine. Continue alkalization until the serum uric acid level returns to normal limits and the tophaceous deposits disappear.

Colchicine, probenecid, and sulfinpyrazone are associated with adverse reactions affecting the GI tract. Symptoms include nausea, vomiting, diarrhea, and abdominal pain. These symptoms are particularly troublesome for patients with a history of peptic ulcer disease or active peptic ulcer disease.

Probenecid and sulfinpyrazone are sulfa-based drugs. They have been associated with hypersensitivity reactions related to this base. Severe, anaphylactic reactions are rare and usually occur within several hours after administration of the first dose of a restart regimen, following prior use of the drug. The appearance of a hypersensitivity reaction requires immediate discontinuance of the drug.

Allopurinol is associated with a maculopapular skin rash that sometimes is scaly or exfoliative. The incidence of this adverse reaction is increased in the presence of renal disorders. Because skin reactions may be severe and sometimes fatal, the drug should be discontinued at the first sign of rash. The most severe reactions include fever, chills, arthralgia, cholestatic jaundice, eosinophilia, mild leukocytosis, or leukopenia.

Patients on standard therapy with colchicine who have elevated plasma levels because of renal function have developed myopathy and neuropathy that result in weakness. This problem is often unrecognized and misdiagnosed as polymyositis or uremic neuropathy. Proximal weakness and elevated serum creatinine kinase are generally present. The condition resolves 3 to 4 weeks after drug withdrawal. Colchicine also induces reversible malabsorption of vitamin B$_{12}$, perhaps because it alters the function of the ileal mucosa.

There is a risk of liver function abnormalities in patients taking febuxostat (6.6% in patients taking 40 mg/d and 4.6% taking 80 mg/d). A small number of patients (1.1%) experience nausea and arthralgia when taking 40 mg/d of febuxostat.

Drug Interactions

Colchicine has very few drug interactions. Probenecid, allopurinol, and sulfinpyrazone have many drug interactions.

Probenecid inhibits the tubular secretion of most penicillins and cephalosporins and increases plasma levels by any route these antibiotics are given. Sulfinpyrazone reduces renal tubular secretion of organic anions (e.g., antimicrobials and sulfonamides) and displaces other anions bound extensively to plasma proteins (e.g., tolbutamide, warfarin).

Salicylates have a mutually antagonistic effect with both of these drugs. Because these drugs, with the exception of colchicine, have many drug interactions, checking drug interactions before prescribing them is important. Febuxostat should not be administered with drugs that are metabolized by xanthine oxidase, including theophylline, mercaptopurine, and azathioprine, because toxicity may occur. Table 25-2 lists the drug interactions.

Table 25–2 ▦ Drug Interactions: Antigout and Uricosuric Agents

Drug	Interacting Drug	Possible Effect	Implications
Allopurinol	Angiotensin-converting enzyme inhibitors	Higher risk of hypersensitivity reaction	Avoid concurrent use
	Aluminum salts	Decreased effects of allopurinol	Separate administration
	Ampicillin	Rate of ampicillin-induced rash much higher	Warn patients
	Anticoagulants	Anticoagulant effect of some drugs enhanced; not warfarin	Use warfarin for anticoagulation; conflicting data
	Cyclophosphamide	Myelosuppressive effects enhanced; increased risk for bleeding	If must be used together, monitor for bleeding risk
	Theophylline	Theophylline clearance decreased with large doses of allopurinol; increased toxicity risk	Select different respiratory drug
	Thiazide diuretics	Increased incidence of hypersensitivity reactions	Avoid concurrent use or monitor for hypersensitivity
	Thiopurines	Clinically significant increases in pharmacological and toxic effect of thiopurines	Avoid concurrent use
	Uricosuric agents	Uricosuric agents that increase excretion of urate also likely to increase excretion of oxypurinol and lower degree of inhibition of xanthine oxidase; avoid concurrent use	Dosage adjustments may be needed if uricosuric added to treatment regimen
Colchicine	NSAIDs	Additive adverse GI effects	Avoid concurrent use; monitor for GI bleeding
Febuxostat	Drugs that are metabolized by xanthine oxidase: theophylline, mercaptopurine, azathioprine	Febuxostat may cause increased plasma levels	Concurrent use is contraindicated
Probenecid	Acyclovir	Decreased acyclovir renal clearance and increased bioavailability	Associated with IV use of drug; avoid this route
	Allopurinol	Increased blood levels for allopurinol	Beneficial effect; may be used therapeutically
	Barbiturates	Increased blood levels	Monitor central nervous system (CNS) effects
	Benzodiazepines (BDZs)	More rapid and prolonged BDZ effect	Monitor BDZ effects
	Clofibrate	Accumulation of clofibric acid; higher steady-state serum concentrations	Select different antilipidemic
	Dapsone	Possible accumulation of dapsone and its metabolites	Monitor for adverse effects or avoid concurrent use
	Dyphylline	Increased half-life, decreased clearance	May be used therapeutically to extend dyphylline dosing interval
	Methotrexate	Increased plasma level; therapeutic effects and toxicity increased	Avoid concurrent use
	NSAIDs	Increased plasma levels and toxicity	Avoid concurrent use
	Pantothenic acid	Renal transport inhibited; plasma levels increased	No specific action required
	Penicillamine	Effects of penicillamine attenuated	Avoid concurrent use
	Penicillins, cephalosporins	Inhibits tubular secretion of most	Monitor for adverse effects
	Salicylates		
	Sulfonamides		
	Sulfonylureas		
	Zidovudine		

Table 25–2 ⠿ **Drug Interactions: Antigout and Uricosuric Agents—cont'd**

Drug	Interacting Drug	Possible Effect	Implications
		penicillins and cephalosporins; usually increases plasma levels by any route these antibiotics are given	Avoid concurrent use
			Select different antimicrobial
			Monitor blood glucose closely
		Mutually antagonistic	Avoid concurrent use
		Renal transport inhibited; plasma levels increase	
		Half-life of sulfonylurea increased	
		Increased zidovudine bioavailability; cutaneous eruptions accompanied by malaise, myalgia, or fever have occurred	
Sulfinpyrazone	Acetaminophen	Risk of hepatotoxicity may be increased	Conflicting data
	Anticoagulants, oral	Anticoagulant activity of warfarin enhanced: increased bleeding risk	Use probenecid if warfarin must be used
	Niacin	Reduced uricosuric activity of sulfinpyrazone	Avoid concurrent use
	Salicylates	Mutually antagonistic	Avoid concurrent use
	Theophylline	Increased theophylline clearance and decreased plasma levels	Avoid concurrent use or adjust dosage based on serum levels
	Tolbutamide	Decreased clearance and increased half-life of tolbutamide; hypoglycemia may result	Glyburide not affected; change hypoglycemic drug
	Verapamil	Increased clearance; decreased bioavailability	Select different calcium channel blocker

Clinical Use and Dosing

Gout

Colchicine given orally is the time-honored drug for treatment of acute gouty attacks, but its efficacy is limited by the adverse reactions that commonly occur with doses adequate to manage the symptoms. In addition, dosages must be adjusted for patients with impaired renal or hepatic function, and it must be administered with caution to older adults. When colchicine is given, the usual regimen is an initial dose of 1.2 mg at the first sign of flare, followed by 0.6 mg 1 hour later (maximum 1.8 mg over 1 h).

Historically, a non-FDA approved schedule of dosing is to administer 0.6 to 1.2 mg every 1 to 2 hours until relief is obtained or until adverse reactions (usually diarrhea, nausea, and vomiting) develop, with 4 to 8 mg total administered. A randomized, double-blind, placebo-controlled, parallel-group, dose-comparison trial of a low dose (1.8 mg total over 1 h) and a high dose (4.8 mg total over 6 h) of colchicine found that low-dose colchicine had a better treatment response at 24 hours than did the high dose (37.8% versus 32.7%), with fewer adverse effects such as diarrhea (Terkeltaub, Furst, Bennett, Crockett, & Davis, 2010). The low-dose colchicine group had adverse effects similar to placebo. Therefore, the historic treatment regimen of high-dose colchicine is not recommended by this author. Articular pain and swelling usually abate within 12 hours and are usually gone in 24 to 48 hours.

Preventive therapy for patients who have fewer than one acute attack per year is 0.6 mg/d of colchicine for 3 or 4 days a week. For patients who have more than one acute attack per year, the dose is 0.6 mg every day. Serious cases may require 1.2 to 1.8 mg/d.

Allopurinol, the drug of choice for patients with a history of urinary calculi, renal insufficiency, chronic tophaceous gout, or high levels of serum urate, is given in doses of 200 to 300 mg/d for mild gout and 400 to 600 mg/d for moderately severe tophaceous gout. The minimum effective dose is 100 to 200 mg/d, and the maximum dose is 800 mg/d. Doses greater than 300 mg/d must be divided. Dosage adjustments for patients with renal insufficiency are based on creatinine clearance (CCr) values. These adjustments are listed in Table 25-3.

Febuxostat is indicated for the chronic management of hyperuricemia in patients with gout. The starting dose of febuxostat is 40 mg per day, once daily. If serum uric acid is not lowered to below 6 mg/dL after 2 weeks, then the dose is increased to 80 mg/d, once daily. Febuxostat is taken without regard to food or meals and no dosage adjustment is needed for renal or hepatic impairment. Periodic uric acid levels are drawn, the first at 2 weeks of therapy. Liver function should be tested at 2 months and 4 months after starting therapy. It is recommended that NSAIDs or colchicine be administered prophylactically for the first 6 months of febuxostat therapy to prevent acute gout flare.

Inhibitors of uric acid synthesis are more toxic, especially in older adults, and should be reserved for patients who "overproduce" urate (e.g., those who excrete more than 800 mg in 24 h). Probenecid is the uricosuric agent of choice because of its well-established safety and its relatively long duration of action. Therapy should not be initiated until the acute attack has completely resolved, because rapid decrease in serum urate levels has been shown to exacerbate a gouty attack.

Doses of probenecid are 250 mg (1/2 tablet) twice daily for 1 week and then 500 mg twice daily. Doses may be increased

Table 25-3 壿 Dosage Schedule: Antigout and Uricosuric Agents

Drug	Indication	Dosage Form	Initial Dose	Maintenance Dose
Allopurinol (Zyloprim)	Management of gout Hyperuricemia associated with treatment of malignancy Recurrent calcium oxalate stones	Tablets: 100 mg Tablets: 300 mg	*Adults:* Mild disease: 200–300 mg/d Moderately severe, topha-ceous: 400–600 mg/d *Adults:* 600–800 mg/d for 2–3 d with a high fluid intake *Children 6–10 yr:* 300 mg/d (100 mg tid) *Children <6 yr:* 150 mg/d (50 mg tid) *Adults:* 200–300 mg/d in single or divided doses	Minimum effective dose is 100–200 mg/d; maximum dose is 800 mg/d Doses >300 mg/d must be divided Dosage adjustments for renal insufficiency in adults: CCr 60 mL/min: 200 mg/d CCr 40 mL/min: 150 mg/d CCr 20 mL/min: 100 mg/d CCr 10 mL/min: 100 mg every other day CCr <10 mL/min: 100 mg 3 times/wk After 48 h titrate dose in all age groups according to serum uric acid levels Another recommended regimen for children: 1 mg/kg/d in 4 divided doses given q6h; maxi-mum dose 600 mg/d Dosage adjusted up or down based on control of hyper-uricemia according to 24 h urinary urate determinations
Colchicine	Acute gouty attacks Management of gout	Tablets: 0.5, 0.6 mg	*Adults:* 1.2 mg followed by 0.6–1.2 mg every 1–2 h up to 16 doses	Total needed during acute attack is usually 4–8 mg Wait 3 days before starting another course Adults with <1 acute attack/yr: 0.6 mg/d for 3–4 d/wk Adults with >1 acute attack/yr: 0.6 mg/d Serious cases: 1.2–1.8 mg/d
Febuxostat (Uloric)	Management of hyper-uricemia in patients with gout	Tablets: 40, 80 mg	*Adults:* Start at 40 mg once daily. If uric acid levels not <6 mg/dL after 2 wk, in-crease dose to 80 mg once a day.	40 or 80 mg/d NSAIDs or colchicine is needed in the first 6 mo of therapy to prevent acute gout attack.
Probenecid (Benemid)	Management of gout*	Tablets: 0.5 mg	*Adults:* 0.25 g bid for 1 wk	0.5 g bid; if no acute attack in >6 mo, reduce dose by 0.5 g/d every 6 mo
Sulfinpyrazone (Anturane)	Management of gout	Tablets: 100 mg Capsules: 200 mg	*Adults:* 200–400 mg/d in 2 divided doses	400 mg/d in 2 divided doses; doses as low as 200 mg/d and as high as 800 mg/d have been used

CCr = creatinine clearance.

*Probenecid is not effective for management of gout in the presence of chronic renal failure with CCr <30 mL/min.

by 500 mg/mo to a maximum of 2 to 3 g/d. Gastric intoler-ance may indicate overdose, and decreasing the dosage may ease it. The dosage that maintains normal serum uric acid levels is continued for maintenance. When the patient has had no acute attacks for 6 months, the dose is decreased by 500 mg every 6 months. Do not reduce the maintenance dose to the point at which serum uric acid levels begin to rise.

In the presence of renal impairment, a once-daily dose of 1 g probenecid may be used. The daily dose may be increased in 500 mg increments every 4 weeks (usually to less than 2 mg/d) if symptoms are not controlled or the 24-hour urate excretion is less than 700 mg. Probenecid is not effective in chronic renal failure if the glomerular filtration rate is 30 mL/min or less. Patients must maintain hydration and adequate sodium bicarbonate (2 to 7.5 g daily) or potassium citrate (7.5 mg daily) to maintain an alkaline urine while on probenecid to prevent formation of uric acid crystals. Alkalization of the urine is recommended until the uric acid level is in the normal range.

Sulfinpyrazone is a potent uricosuric agent, but it must be given several times daily, is more likely than the other drugs to cause gastric adverse reactions, and can cause platelet dysfunction. For these reasons, it is prescribed only when probenecid and allopurinol are not tolerated. Initial dosage is 200 to 400 mg daily in two divided doses. Taking the drug with meals or milk reduces its adverse GI reactions. The dose is gradually increased to a maintenance dose of 400 mg daily in two divided doses. Doses can be as low as 200 mg/d or as high as 800 mg/d to control blood urate levels. Therapy is continued even in the presence of acute exacerbations. This drug can be used concomitantly with colchicine. Patients previously controlled on probenecid may be transferred to sulfinpyrazone at the full maintenance dose.

For all of these drugs, the goal of treatment is a urate level less than 6 mg/dL. Doses are titrated upward until that goal is reached.

Hyperuricemia Associated With Malignancies

Allopurinol is approved for use in hyperuricemia associated with malignancies. Doses of 600 to 800 mg daily for 2 or 3 days, with a high fluid intake, have proved effective. Dosage is similar to the dose given for gout.

Children age 6 to 10 with hyperuricemia secondary to malignancy are given 10 mg/kg/d in two to three divided doses. Younger children are generally given 150 mg/d in three divided doses. Another suggested dosing regimen is 300 mg/d in two to three divided doses in children aged 6 to 10 years.

Recurrent Calcium Oxalate Calculi

Allopurinol 200 to 300 mg/d in single or divided doses is given to prevent recurrent calcium oxalate renal stones. Patients also benefit from dietary modifications such as increases in oral fluids and dietary fiber and reductions in animal protein, sodium, refined sugars, oxalate-rich food, and excessive calcium intake.

Off-Label Uses

Colchicine also has several off-label uses. These purposes and the recommended doses are the following:

1. Hepatic cirrhosis: 1 mg/d for 5 days each week.
2. Primary biliary cirrhosis: 0.6 mg twice daily.
3. Refractory idiopathic thrombocytopenic purpura: 1.2 to 1.8 mg/d for 2 weeks or more.
4. Skin manifestations of scleroderma: 1 mg/d.

5. Familial Mediterranean fever: 1.2 to 2.4 mg/d in one to two divided doses. Increase or decrease dose in 0.3 mg increments, to a maximum of 2.4 mg/d.

Rational Drug Selection

Specific disease processes, for which each of these drugs is most appropriate, have already been mentioned. In general, allopurinol or febuxostat is best for patients who overproduce uric acid; probenecid is best for patients who undersecrete uric acid and have adequate renal function; sulfinpyrazone is best for patients who undersecrete uric acid when on a regular diet and those who need antiplatelet activity. Additional considerations in choosing the appropriate drug are shown in Table 25-3. Table 25-3 also presents available dosage forms of gout medications.

Renal Insufficiency

Because allopurinol blocks urate production, it is especially useful for patients with a history of urinary calculi, with renal insufficiency, or with excessive basal urinary uric acid excretion (750 to 800 mg/24 h). Serious adverse reactions occur in fewer than 2% of patients, typically within the first 2 months of therapy. Patients should be kept under close surveillance during this period. Toxicity seems more likely when allopurinol is given concomitantly with thiazide diuretics.

Peptic Ulcer Disease

IV colchicine rapidly provides a therapeutic plasma level and does not cause GI adverse reactions. It is useful for patients who cannot take the drug orally, have peptic ulcer disease, or have contraindications to NSAIDs. Diluted in 20 mL of normal saline and given over 10 minutes, 2 mg usually provides relief within 6 to 8 hours. Care must be used to prevent extravasation because colchicine may cause tissue necrosis.

High Levels of Serum Urate Associated With Secondary Gout

Allopurinol is the drug of choice because it is the only drug in this group that blocks urate production.

Monitoring

All patients receiving these drugs require monitoring of the serum uric acid level. A baseline assessment is done at initiation of therapy. Uric acid levels should be normal after 1 to 3 weeks of therapy, and serum levels should be drawn again then and periodically throughout therapy or in the presence of exacerbations. The upper limit of normal for men and postmenopausal women is 7 mg/dL; for premenopausal women, it is 6 mg/dL.

For allopurinol, liver and renal function must be assessed prior to initiation of therapy and periodically during the first few months of therapy, particularly for patients with preexisting liver disease. Perform blood urea nitrogen (BUN), serum creatinine, and CCr tests, and reassess dosages based on the results.

Probenecid and sulfinpyrazone both have blood dyscrasias (anemia, hemolytic anemia) as adverse reactions. Patients taking these drugs should have periodic complete blood counts (CBCs).

Patients whose urine is being alkalinized to prevent crystallization of urates in the urine should have their acid–base balance monitored.

Patient Education

Administration

Each drug should be taken exactly as prescribed. A dose that is missed should be taken as soon as the patient remembers but without doubling doses. For allopurinol, if the dosing schedule is once daily, it should not be taken until the next day. If the dosing schedule is more than once a day, the next dose should be up to 300 mg. None of these drugs should be discontinued without first consulting the health-care provider. Uric acid levels rise when the drug is stopped.

In the event of an acute attack during maintenance therapy, allopurinol, febuxostat, probenecid, and sulfinpyrazone should be continued while colchicine is added to the regimen to treat the acute attack. Dosage adjustments of the maintenance drugs may be necessary. Allopurinol can be crushed and given with fluid or mixed with food for patients who have difficulty in swallowing.

Patients should avoid taking aspirin or salicylates while taking probenecid or sulfinpyrazone. These drugs are mutually antagonistic.

Adverse Reactions

The main adverse reaction for all these drugs is GI distress. Taking these drugs with food or milk may minimize gastric irritation.

Probenecid and sulfinpyrazone are sulfa-based drugs that have been associated with hypersensitivity reactions related to this base. Patients should be asked about sulfa allergies and taught the indications of a hypersensitivity reaction and the importance of reporting it. A hypersensitivity reaction requires immediate discontinuance of the drug. Other symptoms to report with these drugs include sore throat, fatigue, yellowing of the skin or eyes, and unusual bleeding or bruising. These drugs have been associated with blood dyscrasias and hepatotoxicity.

Allopurinol has been associated with a maculopapular rash that sometimes is scaly or exfoliative. Because this skin reaction can be severe or even fatal, patients should report the first indication of a rash to their health-care provider, who should evaluate this rash and consider discontinuance of the drug.

Drowsiness and dizziness have occasionally affected patients who are taking allopurinol. Caution patients to avoid driving or other activities requiring alertness until their response to the drug is known.

Patients taking standard doses of colchicine have developed proximal muscle weakness related to myopathy and neuropathy. Patients should be warned to report these symptoms to their health-care provider. Stopping the drug usually reverses the symptoms within 3 to 4 weeks.

Lifestyle Management

To reduce available urates, an alkaline diet may be prescribed that includes reductions in sodium, refined sugars, oxalate-rich foods (e.g., liver, kidney, anchovies, sardines, herring, mussels, bacon, codfish, scallops, trout, haddock, veal, venison, turkey), and excessive calcium intake, as well as increases in oral fluids and dietary fiber. Fluid intake in excess of 3,000 mL/day also reduces the risk for renal calculi. Because large amounts of alcohol increase uric acid concentrations and may decrease the effectiveness of medications, alcohol should be avoided or consumed in very small amounts.

CORTICOSTEROIDS

Cortisol, the endogenous glucocorticoid in the body, is produced and secreted on the basis of feedback mechanisms of the hypothalamus-pituitary-adrenal (HPA) axis. The adrenal cortex synthesizes and secretes the steroid hormones that include mineralocorticoids and glucocorticoids and, to a lesser extent, androgens. Figure 25-1 depicts this feedback system. Exogenously administered adrenal cortex hormones (corticosteroids) affect this feedback mechanism.

Corticosteroids have a major role in the management of a variety of disease processes. In primary or secondary adrenal cortex insufficiency, they are used for replacement therapy. In rheumatic disorders, they may be short-term adjunctive therapy for acute episodes or exacerbation. These drugs are also used to treat collagen disease, dermatological conditions, asthma, allergic rhinitis, neoplastic disorders, inflammatory bowel disease, and idiopathic thrombocytopenia purpura. The role of inhaled corticosteroids in the management of respiratory disorders is covered in Chapter 17. Topical corticosteroids used to manage dermatological conditions are covered in Chapter 23. This chapter focuses on the use of systemic corticosteroids to manage inflammatory conditions in primary care situations.

Pharmacodynamics

Glucocorticoids have metabolic, anti-inflammatory, and growth-suppressing effects. Cortisol is the "wake-up" hormone, and altered levels result in changes in levels of awareness and sleep patterns. Central nervous system (CNS) effects also result in labile emotional states, and high levels of cortisol are associated with decreased recent memory recall. Glucocorticoids increase blood glucose concentration by stimulating gluconeogenesis in the liver and by decreasing uptake of glucose into muscle, lymphatic, and adipose cells. In extrahepatic tissues, they stimulate protein catabolism and inhibit amino acid uptake and protein synthesis. Decreased proliferation of fibroblasts in connective tissue in concert with the poor protein synthesis leads to poor wound healing (McCance & Huether, 2010).

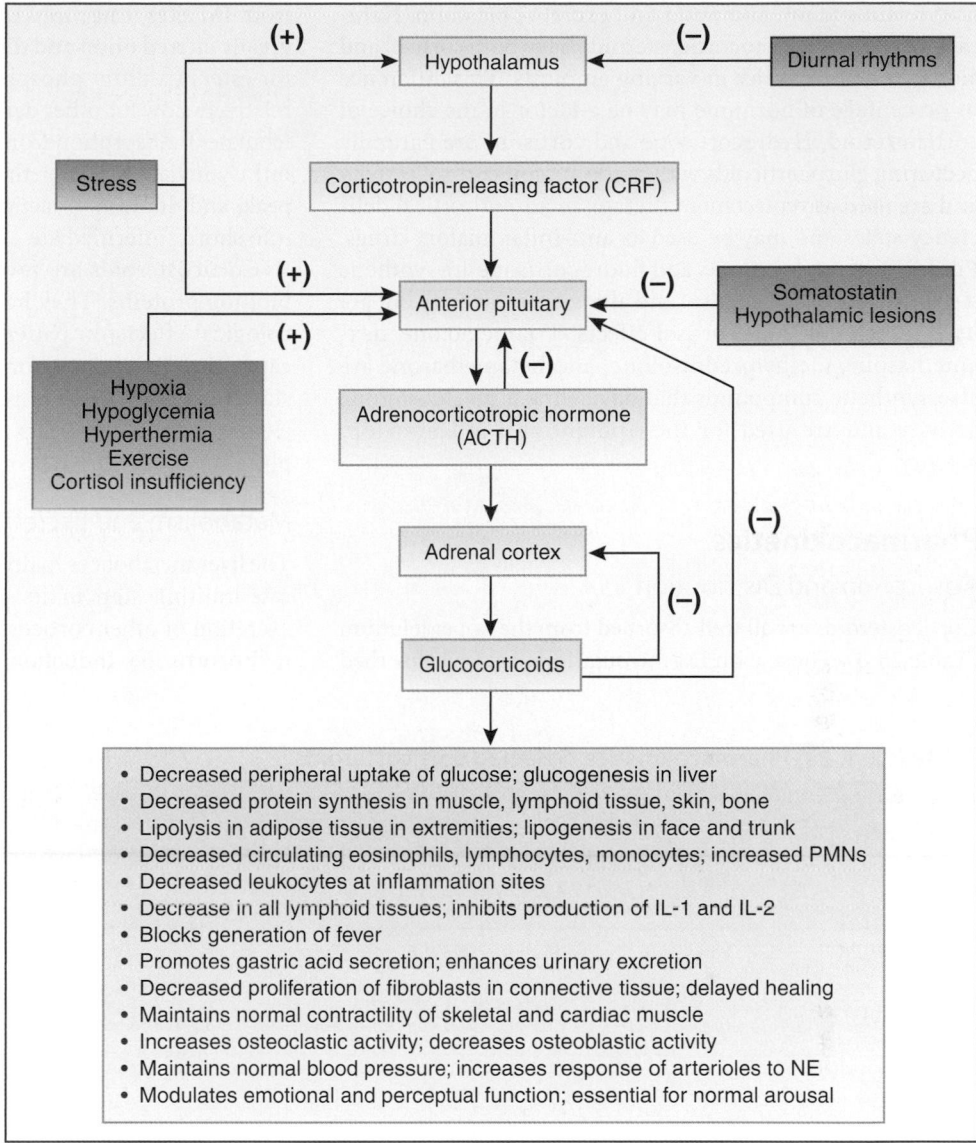

Figure 25–1. Hypothalamus-pituitary-adrenal axis and feedback control of cortisol.

Glucocorticoids inhibit the immune and inflammatory systems by their actions at several sites: depressing proliferation of T lymphocytes, including those that produce the antiviral protein interferon; decreasing natural killer cell activity; reversing macrophage activity; and suppressing the synthesis, secretion, and actions of chemical mediators involved in inflammatory and immune responses. These chemical mediators include interleukins, prostaglandins, leukotrienes, bradykinin, serotonin, and histamine.

Glucocorticoids also increase circulating erythrocytes; increase appetite; promote fat deposits in the face and cervical areas, while promoting lipolysis in the extremities; increase uric acid excretion; and decrease serum calcium levels, possibly by inhibiting GI absorption of calcium and phosphate (American College of Rheumatology, 2001 update). They also promote gastric acid secretion. In the urinary tract, glucocorticoids enhance urinary excretion. Their feedback activity on the HPA axis suppresses secretion and

synthesis of adrenocorticotropic hormone (ACTH) and suppresses prostaglandin E production of insulin-like growth hormone secretion so that somatic growth is inhibited. Skeletal wasting also occurs and is most rapid during the first 6 months of therapy. This osteoporotic process is a result of stimulation of osteoclastic activity and inhibition of osteoblastic activity. An additional factor in bone loss is the effect of glucocorticoids on sex hormones, which results in decreased circulating levels of anabolic hormones. Bone mineral density (BMD) rapidly declines beginning within the first 3 months of glucocorticoid therapy and peaks at 6 months, with continued BMD loss with ongoing therapy (Grossman et al, 2010). Finally, they potentiate the effects of catecholamines, thyroid hormone, and growth hormone on adipose tissue. Figure 25-1 depicts the control of cortisol secretion.

Mineralocorticoids (predominantly aldosterone) are also secreted by the adrenal cortex under the control of the renin-angiotensin-aldosterone system. The main role of aldosterone is to retain sodium and water and excrete potassium. Naturally occurring adrenocorticosteroids have both cortisol and aldosterone properties in varying amounts. This difference in percentage of hormone may be a factor in the choice of corticosteroid. Hydrocortisone and cortisone are naturally occurring glucocorticoids with predominant cortisol activity and are used as replacement therapy in adrenocortical deficiency states and may be used as anti-inflammatory drugs. Prednisone, prednisolone, and fludrocortisone are synthetic steroids with mixed cortisol and aldosterone activity but are used mainly for their cortisol effects. Triamcinolone, dexamethasone, methylprednisolone, and betamethasone are also synthetic compounds that have almost no aldosterone activity and are used for their potent anti-inflammatory activity.

Pharmacokinetics

Absorption and Distribution

Corticosteroids are all well absorbed from the upper jejunum (Table 25-4). Those with IM formulations are well absorbed from IM sites. Injections of suspensions and esters produce greatly altered onset and duration times. Absorption is rapid for esters (sodium phosphates and sodium succinate) and relatively slow for other derivatives (acetates, acetonides, and tebutates). Absorption from local sites (e.g., intra-articular or intrasynovial) is slower than from IM sites. Because onset, peak, and duration of action vary, these drugs are classified into short-, intermediate-, and long-acting forms.

Corticosteroids are reversibly bound to corticosteroid-binding proteins. They have significantly altered pharmacological effects on patients with altered protein-binding capacities. Pregnancy, for example, is a hyperproteinemic state in which the total plasma level of steroid would be elevated. All these drugs are widely distributed, cross the placenta, and enter breast milk.

Metabolism and Excretion

The liver metabolizes hydrocortisone (Cortef), and this is the rate-limiting step in its clearance. The metabolism and excretion of other corticosteroids generally parallel those of hydrocortisone. Induction of hepatic enzymes increases the

Table 25–4 ⬛ **Pharmacokinetics: Selected Corticosteroids**

Drug	Onset (hours)	Peak (hours)	Duration (days)	Protein Binding	Half-Life	RAP	RMP	Elimination
Cortisone* PO	Rapid	2	1.25–1.5	Very high	30 min P 8–12 h B	0.8	2	1% unchanged in urine
Cortisone* IM	Slow	20–48	1.25–1.5	Very high	—	0.8	2	1% unchanged in urine
Hydrocortisone* PO	Rapid	1	1.25–1.5	High	80–118 min P 8–12 h B	1	2	1% unchanged in urine
Hydrocortisone† IM	Slow	4–8	Varies	High	—	1	2	1% unchanged in urine
Methylprednisolone†	UK	1–2	1.25–1.5	High	78–188 min P 18–36 h B	5	0	1% unchanged in urine
Prednisolone†	1	1–2	1.25–1.5	High	115–211 min P 18–36 h B	4	1	1% unchanged in urine
Prednisone†	1	1–2	1.25–1.5	Very high	60 min P 18–36 h B	4	1	1% unchanged in urine
Triamcinolone†	UK	1–2	2.25	High	200+ min P 18–36 h B	5	0	1% unchanged in urine
Dexamethasone‡ PO	UK	1–2	2.75	High	110–210 min P 36–54 h B	20–30	0	1% unchanged in urine
Dexamethasone‡ IM	Rapid	8	6	High	—	20–30	0	1% unchanged in urine
Betamethasone‡ PO	UK	1–2	3.25	High	300+ min P 36–54 h B	20–30	0	1% unchanged in urine
Betamethasone‡ IM	1–3	UK	7	High	—	20–30	0	1% unchanged in urine

B = biological half-life; P = plasma half-life; RAP = relative anti-inflammatory potency; RMP = relative mineralocorticoid potency; UK = unknown.
*Short-acting.
†Intermediate-acting.
‡Long-acting.

metabolic clearance of all corticosteroids. The liver converts cortisone (Cortone) to hydrocortisone, and prednisone (Deltasone) is converted to prednisolone (Delta-Cortef, Prelone). These metabolites are then clinically active and metabolized by the liver for clearance. Approximately 1% of the daily dose of the drug is excreted unchanged in urine. Renal clearance is increased when plasma levels are increased.

Table 25-4 depicts the pharmacokinetics of selected corticosteroids, including their relative anti-inflammatory and mineralocorticoid activity.

Pharmacotherapeutics

Precautions and Contraindications

The wide range of contraindications and warnings about cautious use associated with corticosteroids is a factor of their numerous actions. They are contraindicated in the presence of active, untreated infections because they may mask the indications of infection, and new infections may appear during their use. A patient may also have decreased resistance, and the host defense mechanisms may be unable to prevent dissemination of the infection. Corticosteroids may exacerbate systemic fungal infections; therefore, corticosteroids are contraindicated in patients with these infections. Corticosteroids may activate latent amebiasis or tuberculosis. Although their use has been advocated for the treatment of chronic active hepatitis, they may be harmful in hepatitis positive for hepatitis B surface antigen.

For many disorders, these drugs should be used cautiously. Average and large doses of drugs with high relative mineralocorticoid potency (e.g., cortisone and hydrocortisone) can cause elevated blood pressure, salt and water retention, and increased excretion of potassium. These effects can be especially problematic for patients with hypertension and cardiovascular disorders (e.g., heart failure [HF]). Sodium restriction and potassium supplementation may be necessary. Edema can occur in the presence of renal disease with a fixed or decreased glomerular filtration rate (GFR). These drugs should be used with caution in renal insufficiency, acute glomerulonephritis, or chronic nephritis.

All corticosteroids increase calcium excretion, which creates problems for postmenopausal women and others at risk for osteoporosis (patients with a lower body mass index or parental history of hip fracture, smokers, or those who consume more than three alcoholic drinks per day) (Grossman et al, 2010).

Patients with diabetes mellitus may have difficulty maintaining glycemic control because corticosteroids alter the liver's glucose regulation. The relationship between peptic ulceration and corticosteroid therapy is unclear, with no difference seen in endoscopic peptic ulcers compared to placebo in patients treated with prednisone 60 mg daily for 3 months (Hsiang et al, 2010). Patients with ulcerative colitis or peptic ulcer disease or with concomitant use of gastric irritants (e.g., NSAIDs) and stress have an increased probability of GI bleeding and perforation.

Some of these products contain tartrazine or sodium bisulfite, both of which can cause severe allergic reactions. Patients with these allergies should notify their health-care provider, and the label of the drug should be reviewed carefully for these ingredients.

Corticosteroids cross the placenta (prednisone has the least transport), and most are Pregnancy Category C. In animal studies, large doses resulted in cleft palate, stillborn fetuses, and decreased fetal size. Chronic ingestion during the first trimester in humans has shown a 1% incidence of cleft palate. In considering use of these drugs during pregnancy or in women with childbearing potential, the benefits must be carefully weighed against the potential risks to the fetus. Infants of mothers who have taken these drugs should be observed for signs of hypoaldosteronism.

Corticosteroids appear in breast milk and could retard the nursing infant's growth, interfere with endogenous corticosteroid production, or cause other unwanted effects. Several studies suggest that the amount excreted in breast milk is negligible with prednisone or prednisolone doses of 20 mg or less per day and methylprednisolone (Medrol) doses of 8 mg or less per day. For mothers who want to nurse, waiting 3 to 4 hours after taking the drug and using one of these drugs within these doses may be tried (LactMed, 2013).

When given corticosteroids, children may experience altered growth and development, and they require monitoring of height and weight if they must be on prolonged therapy. Some of these products contain benzyl alcohol, which has been associated with a fatal "gasping syndrome" in infants.

Older adults often have chronic disorders that are worsened by corticosteroids. Consider the risk/benefit factors of steroid use. Lower doses and careful monitoring of blood pressure, blood glucose, and electrolytes at least every 6 months are appropriate.

Adverse Drug Reactions

Adverse reactions can be discussed by the body system that is affected.

Muscle and Skin

Common skin changes reported with systemic corticosteroids include atrophy and thinning of the skin, alopecia, acneiform eruptions, poor healing, purpura, striae, hirsutism, and desquamation. Myopathy is also seen, with marked muscle wasting. No relationship between dose or duration of therapy and these adverse reactions is apparent. Alteration in body fat is also noted, particularly in patients who take corticosteroids for more than 60 days, with the most common changes being truncal obesity, buffalo hump, and moon faces.

Skeletal Tissues

Osteoporosis develops in 11% to 20% of patients treated with glucocorticosteroids for more than 1 year, with decreased BMD found within the first 3 months of therapy (Grossman et al, 2010). Skeletal fractures, mainly of the spine, ribs, and pelvis, may occur secondary to the reduced bone density. Glucocorticoid therapy at doses of 7.5 mg/d or greater of prednisone for 6 or more months results in a rapid loss of trabecular bone in the spine, hip, and forearm. BMD should be measured in all individuals who are likely to be on this therapy long-term (American College of Rheumatology, 2001 update; Grossman et al, 2010). The American College of Rheumatology guidelines recommend treating patients on long-term (3 months or greater) glucocorticoid therapy with the bisphosphonates alendronate (Fosamax) or risedronate (Actonel) based on a risk-assessment algorithm (Grossman et al, 2010).

Ocular Tissues

Prolonged use of corticosterioids may produce subcapsular cataracts, glaucoma with possible damage to the optic nerve, and increased risk for secondary ocular infections due to fungi or viruses.

Gastrointestinal System

Corticosteroids have been implicated in the induction of peptic ulcer disease. Patients who appear to be at risk are those being treated for nephrotic syndrome or hepatic disease; are taking a total dose of prednisone exceeding 1 g; or have a history of ulcer disease, concomitant use of a known gastric irritant, or stress. Combining corticosteroids and NSAIDs or aspirin increases the risk of peptic ulcer disease. Prophylaxis with proton pump inhibitors (PPIs) or H_2 blockers is suggested for patients with two or more of these risk factors (Feldman & Das, 2010; Saag & Furst, 2010). Patients also taking NSAIDs may require misoprostol (Cytotec); misoprostol's use is described in Chapter 34.

Cardiovascular System

Hypertension is a common adverse reaction. This and other cardiovascular problems (e.g., fluid and electrolyte disturbances) are discussed in the Precautions and Contraindications section.

Central Nervous System

Delirium, agitation, insomnia, mood swings, and severe depression characterize steroid psychosis. The onset of symptoms is usually within 15 to 30 days. Predisposing factors include doses above 40 mg of prednisone or its equivalent dose in another drug, female gender, and a family history of psychiatric disorder. The incidence is correlated with dose. If the steroid cannot be stopped, psychotropic drugs are effective in relieving the symptoms.

Endocrine System

Prolonged therapy with corticosteroids may lead to adrenal suppression. The degree of suppression depends on dosage, relative glucocorticoid (anti-inflammatory) potency, biological half-life, and duration of therapy. As a general rule, suppression occurs with doses above the physiological range that are given for more than 1 month. It can be minimized by using intermediate-acting agents on an alternate-day dosing schedule. Abrupt withdrawal after adrenal suppression has occurred may result in a withdrawal syndrome, with symptoms similar to those seen in adrenal insufficiency. To minimize this adverse reaction, the dose

of corticosteroids used for prolonged therapy should be tapered. Recovery from HPA suppression can take up to 12 months.

The effect on glucose metabolism and regulation is discussed in the Precautions and Contraindications section. Amenorrhea, postmenopausal bleeding, and other menstrual irregularities have also been seen.

Drug Interactions

Additive hypokalemia may occur with drugs that also produce this adverse reaction. This hypokalemia increases the risk for toxicity in digoxin. Several drugs stimulate the metabolism of corticosteroids, and oral contraceptives decrease their metabolism. NSAIDs and alcohol increase the risk for GI adverse reactions. Other drug interactions are in Table 25-5.

Clinical Use and Dosing

Adrenocortical Insufficiency

In primary adrenocortical insufficiency, glucocorticoid and mineralocorticoid properties are lost; however, in secondary adrenocortical insufficiency, mineralocorticoid function is preserved. In the United States, primary adrenocortical insufficiency is an uncommon disorder. Widespread corticosteroid use has made secondary adrenocortical insufficiency due to steroid withdrawal much more common. Approximately 6 million persons are considered to have undiagnosed adrenocortical insufficiency only during times of physiological stress. The key to treatment of primary or secondary disease is replacement of the missing hormones. The drugs of choice are hydrocortisone, cortisone, and prednisone because each has both glucocorticoid and mineralocorticoid effects and requires no additional mineralocorticoid.

Initial doses for hydrocortisone are 50 mg every 8 hours for 48 hours for adults; then the dose is tapered to 30 to 50 mg/d in divided doses. In children, the dose is 2.5 to 10 mg/kg/d for children under age 12, in three to four divided doses, and then the dose is tapered to the maintenance dose over 14 days. Children over 12 years are dosed as adults. For cortisone, the initial adult dose is 25 to 300 mg/d in two divided doses, and the pediatric dose is 0.25 to 0.35 mg/kg/d IM in two divided doses. Once again, the drug is tapered over 14 days to the maintenance dose. Prednisone is started at 5 to 60 mg/d in two divided doses for adults and 1 to 2 mg/kg/d in a once- or twice-daily dose for children. This drug is tapered in the same way (Klauer, 2009).

For maintenance replacement of cortisol, under normal circumstances patients are given 15 to 20 mg of cortisol or its equivalent daily. Dosage schedules vary, but the simplest and least expensive in adults is cortisone 25 mg daily. Hydrocortisone 20 mg or prednisone 5 to 20 mg may also be used on the same schedule. To approach diurnal rhythms, the dose is given in the morning before 9 a.m. Equivalent doses of another corticosteroid may be used but have no specific advantage. In addition, other corticosteroids have less relative

Table 25–5 ▦ **Drug Interactions: Selected Corticosteroids**

Drug	Interacting Drug	Possible Effect	Implications
Betamethasone, cortisone	Insulin, oral hypoglycemics	Decreased effectiveness, resulting in altered glycemic control	Monitor blood glucose levels more closely if drugs must be given concurrently
Hydrocortisone	Cholestyramine	Hydrocortisone area under the curve (AUC) decreased	Separate dose by 4 h and give hydrocortisone first
	Insulin, oral hypoglycemics	Decreased effectiveness, resulting in altered glycemic control	Monitor blood glucose levels more closely if drugs must be given concurrently
Dexamethasone	Ephedrine	Decreased half-life and increased clearance of dexamethasone	Avoid concurrent administration
	Insulin, oral hypoglycemics	Decreased effectiveness, resulting in altered glycemic control	Monitor blood glucose levels more closely if drugs must be given concurrently
Prednisone	NSAIDs, other GI irritants	Increased risk for GI bleed	Avoid concurrent use
	Insulin, oral hypoglycemics	Decreased effectiveness, resulting in altered glycemic control	Monitor blood glucose levels more closely if drugs must be given concurrently
Methylprednisolone	Macrolide antimicrobials (e.g., erythromycin, clarithromycin)	Significant decrease in methylprednisolone clearance	Has been used therapeutically to decrease methylprednisolone dose
	Insulin, oral hypoglycemics	Decreased effectiveness, resulting in altered glycemic control	Monitor blood glucose levels more closely if drugs must be given concurrently
All corticosteroids	Barbiturates	Decrease the pharmacological effects of the corticosteroid	Avoid concurrent use
	Oral contraceptives		May require dosage adjustment
	Estrogens	Corticosteroid half-life and concentration increased; clearance decreased	May require dosage adjustment
	Hydantoins, rifampin		May require dosage adjustment
	Ketoconazole	Corticosteroid clearance decreased	Select different imidazole
	Digoxin	Corticosteroid clearance increased; reduced therapeutic effects	Avoid coadministration
	Isoniazid	Corticosteroid clearance decreased; AUC increased	If must be used together, dosage adjustments may be needed; monitor therapy closely
	Potassium-depleting agents (e.g., thiazide and loop diuretics, mezlocillin, piperacillin, ticarcillin)	May increase risk of digitalis toxicity	Avoid concurrent use; monitor serum potassium levels
	Salicylates	Isoniazid serum concentrations decreased	Avoid concurrent use
	Somatrem	Additive hypokalemia	Consult with endocrinologist for best action
		Reduced serum salicylate levels; decreased therapeutic effectiveness	
		Inhibits growth-promoting effect of somatrem	

mineralocorticoid potency, and an additional drug to provide mineralocorticoid activity might be required if they are used.

The response to any of these drugs is highly variable. Doses are highly individualized, and much higher doses given in divided doses may be needed. Specific doses and ranges for each of the corticosteroids for this indication, for both adults and children, are provided in Table 25-6.

Inflammation

Any of the corticosteroids may be used to reduce or prevent inflammation. Because the need for mineralocorticoid activity is low to absent in this indication, drugs with more anti-inflammatory activity—methylprednisolone, prednisone, and triamcinolone (Aristocort)—are appropriate. Betamethasone also has only anti-inflammatory activity, but it is 4 to 5 times more potent than the other drugs, which increases the risk for adverse reactions. Dexamethasone is used most often in

acute care to relieve the inflammation that causes intracranial pressure after closed head injury or cranial surgery. Doses are shown in Table 25-6.

Immunosuppression

Although all corticosteroids have immunosuppressive capability, the most commonly used is prednisone. It has a short half-life, low cost, negligible mineralocorticoid activity, and is available in 5 and 20 mg tablets that make dosage changes simple for the patient to manage. Post-transplant immunosuppression is often a combination of immunosuppressants and high-dose corticosteroids. Patients are often on high-dose corticosteroids for 6 to 12 months then tapered off slowly. Prednisolone, the active hepatic metabolite of prednisone, is useful in the presence of hepatic dysfunction. Other drugs in this class may also be used for this indication, and their dosing schedule is presented in Table 25-6.

Table 25–6 ✄ Dosage Schedule: Selected Corticosteroids

Drug	Indication	Dosage Form	Dose	Notes
Betamethasone (Celestone)	Inflammation, immunosuppression	Oral solution: 0.6 mg/5 mL Suspension for injection: betamethasone sodium phosphate 3 mg/mL and betamethasone acetate 3 mg/mL = 6 mg/mL Tablet: 25 mg	*Adults:* 0.6–7.2 mg/d PO as single or divided doses *Children:* 62.5–250 mcg/kg/d PO in 3 divided doses	Long-acting. Suppresses HPA at doses >0.6 mg/d.
Cortisone (generic only)	Adrenocortical insufficiency Inflammation, immunosuppression	Tablet: 25 mg	*Adults:* Initial dose 25–300 mg Maintenance dose is 10–37 mg/d in single or divided dose *Children:* Initial dose 25–300 mg orally or 0.25–0.35 mg/kg/d IM in 2 divided doses Maintenance dose is 0.56 mg/kg/d *Adults:* 25–300 mg/d PO in single or divided doses *Children:* 2.5–10 mg/kg/d PO as single or divided doses	Has mineralocorticoid activity but may need additional drug; short-acting; suppresses HPA at doses >20 mg/d. Taper initial dose to maintenance dose over 14 d. Has mineralocorticoid activity but may need additional drug; short-acting; suppresses HPA at doses >20 mg/d.
Dexamethasone (Decadron)	Adrenocortical insufficiency Inflammation, immunosuppression	Oral solution concentrate: 1 mg/mL Syrup: 0.5 mg/5 mL Tablets: 0.5 mg 0.75 mg 1 mg 1.5 mg 2 mg 4 mg 6 mg	*Children:* 23.3 mcg/kg/d PO in 3 divided doses *Adults:* 0.5–9 mg/d PO in single or divided doses *Children:* 83.3–333.3 mcg/kg/d PO in 3–4 divided doses	Not commonly used for this indication in adults; required addition of mineralocorticoid. Long-acting. Suppresses HPA at doses >0.75 mg/d.
Hydrocortisone (Cortef, Solu-Cortef)	Adrenocortical insufficiency Inflammation, immunosuppression Inflammatory bowel disease	Tablet: 5, 10, 20 mg Injection: 100, 250, 500, 1,000 mg	*Adults:* Initial dose 50 mg q8h for 48 h Maintenance dose 20–240 mg/d in single or divided doses *Adults:* 20–240 mg/d PO in 1–4 divided doses *Children:* 2–8 mg/kg/d in single or divided doses *Adults:* 100 mg nightly in retention enema for 21 d or until remission	Has mineralocorticoid activity; short-acting; suppresses HPA at doses >20 mg/d. Taper initial dose to maintenance dose over 14 d. Has mineralocorticoid activity; short-acting; suppresses HPA at doses >20 mg/d. Has mineralocorticoid activity; short-acting; suppresses HPA at doses >20 mg/d.
Methylprednisolone (Medrol) (Depo-Medrol)	Inflammation, immunosuppression Multiple sclerosis	Tablets: 2 mg 4 mg 8 mg 16 mg 32 mg Solution for injection: 20, 40, 80 mg/mL	*Adults:* 4–48 mg/d PO in single or divided doses initially; up to 240 mg/d for maintenance *Children:* 0.117–1.67 mg/kg/d PO in 3–4 divided doses *Adults:* 160 mg/d for 7 d; then 64 every other day for 1 mo	Intermediate-acting; suppresses HPA at doses of 4 mg/d Intermediate-acting; suppresses HPA at doses of 4 mg/d
Prednisolone (Prelone, Orapred, Millipred)	Adrenocortical insufficiency Inflammation, immunosuppression	Tablets: 5 mg Syrup: 5 mg/5 mL, 15 mg/5 mL	*Adults:* Initial dose and maintenance dose 5–60 mg *Children:* 1–2 mg/kg/d initial and maintenance doses	Intermediate-acting; suppresses HPA at doses >5 mg/d. Taper over 14 d.

Table 25–6 ⊗ **Dosage Schedule: Selected Corticosteroids—cont'd**

Drug	Indication	Dosage Form	Dose	Notes
	Multiple sclerosis		*Adults:* 5–60 mg/d PO in single or divided doses	Intermediate-acting; suppresses HPA at doses >5 mg/d.
			Children: 0.5–2 mg/kg/d PO in 3–4 divided doses	Intermediate-acting; suppresses HPA at doses >5 mg/d.
			Adults: 200 mg/d for 7 d; then 80 mg every other day for 1 mo	
Prednisone (Prednicolone)	Adrenocortical insufficiency	Tablets: 1, 2.5, 5 mg, 10, 20, 50 mg	*Adults:* 5–60 mg/d PO in single or divided doses	Minimal mineralocorticoid activity; intermediate-acting; suppresses HPA at doses >5 mg. Taper over 14 d.
	Inflammation, immunosuppression	Intensol syrup: 5 mg/mL Solution: 5 mg/5 mL	*Adults:* 5–60 mg/d PO in single or divided doses	Minimal mineralocorticoid activity; intermediate-acting; suppresses HPA at doses >5 mg.
	Nephrotic syndrome		*Children:* 0.14–2 mg/kg/d PO in 4 divided doses	Minimal mineralocorticoid activity; intermediate-acting; suppresses HPA at doses >5 mg.
			Children: Initial dosing 2 mg/kg/day in 1–3 divided doses (maximum 80 mg/d) until urine is protein-free. Maintenance dose 2 mg/kg/dose administered every other day. Taper and discontinue after 4–6 weeks.	
Triamcinolone (Kenalog)	Adrenocortical insufficiency	Suspension for injection: 10 mg/mL, 40 mg/mL	*Adults:* 4–12 mg/d PO in single or divided doses	No mineralocorticoid activity; requires addition of mineralocorticoid drug.
	Rheumatic disorders		*Children:* 117 mcg/kg/d in single or divided doses	Intermediate-acting; suppresses HPA at doses >4 mg/d.
	Systemic lupus erythematosus		*Adults:* 8–12 mg/d PO	No mineralocorticoid activity; requires addition of mineralocorticoid drug.
	Other inflammatory diseases or for immunosuppression		*Adults:* 20–32 mg/d PO	Intermediate-acting; suppresses HPA at doses >4 mg/d.
			Adults: 4–48 mg/d PO in single or divided doses	No mineralocorticoid activity; requires addition of mineralocorticoid drug.
			Children: 0.416–1.7 mg/kg/d PO in single or divided doses	Intermediate-acting; suppresses HPA at doses >4 mg/d.
				No mineralocorticoid activity; requires addition of mineralocorticoid drug.
				Intermediate-acting; suppresses HPA at doses >4 mg/d.

HPA = hypothalamus-pituitary-adrenal axis.

For parenteral doses, see other sources.

Rheumatoid Arthritis

Rheumatoid arthritis (RA) is a system inflammatory disorder, and treatment to reduce inflammation is appropriate. First-line therapy includes disease-modifying antirheumatic drugs (DMARDs) and biological agents, including anti-TNF (adalimumab, etanercept, infliximab, certolizumab pegol, golimumab) and non-TNF agents (abatacept, rituximab, tocilizumab) (Singh et al, 2012). Oral glucocorticoids are prescribed for moderate to severe RA to gain initial control of inflammation while awaiting response to DMARDs.

The initial dose is 5 to 2 mg per day of prednisone depending on the severity of symptoms (Schur & Cohen, 2014). Glucocorticoids should be tapered and discontinued as soon as possible.

The following principles are used when dosing corticosteroids (McCance & Huether, 2010).

1. The maximum activity of the adrenal cortex in producing cortisol is between 2 and 8 a.m. To best match this natural body rhythm, daily doses are best taken in the morning before 9 a.m.

2. The initial dose depends on the specific disease being treated. Maintain or adjust the dose until an acceptable response is achieved. Establish a time frame within which to expect this response. If such a response does not occur within that time frame, discontinue the corticosteroid and consult or refer the patient for other therapy.

3. After an acceptable response is achieved, determine the maintenance dose by decreasing the dosage in small amounts at intervals until the lowest dosage that maintains an adequate clinical response is reached. The lowest possible dose is always best, especially with long-term therapy, to avoid or reduce adverse reactions. In the presence of increased stress (e.g., trauma, surgery, or infection), a temporarily increased dosage may be needed.

4. If, after long-term therapy or because of spontaneous remission, the drug is to be stopped, withdraw it gradually to prevent an adrenal insufficiency crisis. Tapering is generally not necessary after short-term therapy (e.g., up to 3 weeks) because adrenal suppression has not occurred.

5. Most conditions that require chronic corticosteroid therapy can be well controlled on alternate-day therapy, although the therapy must usually be started with daily dosing. For alternate-day dosing, twice the daily dose is given every other morning before 9 a.m. It works best if the patient is taking an intermediate-acting drug but may be used with short-acting drugs as well. The purpose of this schedule is to provide the patient on long-term therapy the benefits of the drug while minimizing the HPA-axis suppression, withdrawal symptoms, and, for children, growth retardation. Long-acting agents may still produce HPA suppression, even with alternate-day dosing. The regimen is only for patients on long-term therapy who can be trusted to follow this schedule without needing the prompting of daily therapy. In the advent of a flare-up in the disease process, a return to daily dosing may be necessary, at least until the flare-up clears.

6. Unlike a tapering schedule, alternate-day scheduling retains the same total steroid dose. Switching is carried out by gradually increasing the dose on the first day and then decreasing it on the second day until a double dose is taken every other day with no drug on the in-between days. A rough guideline for switching is to make changes in increments of 10 mg of prednisone (or its equivalent) when the daily dose is more than 40 mg, and in 5 mg increments when the daily dosage is 20 to 40 mg. Below 20 mg, the change is made in increments of 2.5 mg. The interval between changes varies from 1 day to several weeks and is empirically based on the clinical response.

7. The schedule for tapering and withdrawing is different. The goal is to reduce the drug to physiological levels or to eliminate the drug altogether. For doses above 40 mg, the dose is reduced by 10 mg of prednisone (or its equivalent) every 1 to 3 weeks. Doses below 40 mg require reductions of 5 mg every 1 to 3 weeks. Once the physiological dose is reached (5 to 7.5 mg/d), the patient can be switched to 1 mg tablets so that dosage reductions can be continued. Weekly or biweekly reductions can then be done 1 mg at a time.

Rational Drug Selection

Length of Therapeutic Activity

Corticosteroids are classified according to their therapeutic effects into short-, intermediate-, and long-acting forms. Short-acting agents are less likely to produce HPA suppression, especially when taken only in the morning and in low doses on an alternate-day schedule. Long-acting agents are preferred if the effects of high doses must be sustained (e.g., increased intracranial pressure or organ transplant rejection).

Relative Potency

Mineralocorticoid activity is desirable in adrenocortical insufficiency but not if the primary goal of therapy is anti-inflammatory or immunosuppressive. Drugs with higher relative mineralocorticoid potency (RMP) are selected for adrenal insufficiency. Drugs high in relative anti-inflammatory potency (RAP) are selected when the goal is to reduce inflammation or suppress the immune system.

Monitoring

Monitoring is based on the common adverse reactions associated with the use of corticosteroids: weight gain, edema, hypertension, and indications of excessive potassium loss and negative nitrogen balance associated with protein catabolism. BMD testing is also appropriate for patients on long-term therapy in which osteoporosis is a significant risk. Carefully monitor the growth and development of children on prolonged therapy.

Laboratory monitoring begins with an initial assessment of serum electrolytes, glucose, and CBC. For patients on long-term therapy or high doses, annual monitoring of these parameters, as well as guaiac testing of stools and serum lipid analysis, is appropriate. For patients at risk for or with indications of GI adverse reactions, upper GI x-rays are desirable.

Systemic corticosteroids may produce subcapsular cataracts in as many as 30% of patients, and patients who have or are at risk for increased intraocular pressure (IOP) may experience increases in IOP while on these drugs. A slit-lamp examination is recommended every 6 to 12 months for patients on long-term corticosteroid therapy.

Patient Education

Administration

Instruct the patient to take the drug exactly as prescribed. Missed doses should be taken as soon as the patient remembers, unless it is almost time for the next dose. Doses should not be doubled. If the patient is being switched from daily to alternate-day therapy or is on a tapering or withdrawal protocol, make the changes as simple as possible and provide written instructions.

Corticosteroids should not be discontinued or the dosage changed without first consulting the health-care provider. Adrenal insufficiency (anorexia, nausea, weakness, fatigue, dyspnea, hypotension, and hypoglycemia) may result when the drug is stopped suddenly. If these signs appear, then the health-care provider should be notified immediately. Adrenal insufficiency can be life-threatening.

Adverse Reactions

Corticosteroids cause immunosuppression and may mask symptoms of infection. Instruct the patient to avoid people with known contagious illnesses and to report possible infections immediately. Patients should avoid vaccinations unless they first consult their health-care provider.

Review the probable adverse reactions with the patient. Patients should immediately report severe abdominal pain or tarry stools to their health-care provider. They should also report unusual swelling, weight gain, tiredness, bone pain, nonhealing sores, visual disturbances, and behavioral or mood changes.

Discuss possible changes in body image, and explore coping mechanisms for them.

Advise patients to wear medical identification that describes their disease process and drug regimen in the event of a medical emergency that prevents patients from relating their medical history. They should also inform any health-care professional who provides care that they are taking corticosteroids.

Lifestyle Management

A diet high in protein, potassium, and calcium and low in sodium and carbohydrates can counteract some of the adverse reactions associated with corticosteroids. Multivitamins with minerals, calcium, and vitamin D are appropriate. Caloric management to prevent obesity should also be implemented. Alcohol should be avoided during therapy. Osteoporosis risk can be reduced not only with calcium intake but also with regular exercise. Because stress can be a source of HPA stimulation, stress management techniques are used.

NONSTEROIDAL ANTI-INFLAMMATORY DRUGS (NSAIDS)

Inflammation, pain, and fever are common manifestations of many diseases. NSAIDs offer the advantage of having activity in all three areas, which allows a less complex and less costly regimen. They also reduce the need for opioid analgesics, which are associated with chemical dependency and addiction. These advantages have resulted in NSAIDs becoming the most widely used prescription and over-the-counter (OTC) drugs in use today.

Aspirin and other salicylates that are members of this class are discussed in the next section. Acetaminophen (Tylenol), although not an anti-inflammatory drug by chemistry, is often used to treat pain and fever and so is included in this section.

Pharmacodynamics

The inflammatory response is the same, regardless of the injury. Destruction of cell membranes results in release of chemical mediators, including histamine, prostaglandins, leukotrienes, cytokines, oxygen radicals, and enzymes. The cascade of events is depicted in Figure 25-2. Two major enzymes, lipo-oxygenase and cyclo-oxygenase, are required to produce these mediators. Although the exact mode of action of NSAIDs is not known, the major mechanism is thought to be inhibition of cyclo-oxygenase activity and prostaglandin synthesis. Inhibition of lipo-oxygenase, leukotriene synthesis, lysosomal enzyme release, neutrophil aggregation, and various cell membrane functions may also occur. These agents may also suppress rheumatoid factor.

Two cyclo-oxygenase isoenzymes have been identified: COX-1 and COX-2. COX-1 is expressed systemically and synthesized continuously so that it is present all the time in all tissues and cells, especially platelets; endothelial cells; the GI tract; and renal microvasculature, glomeruli, and collecting ducts. It has roles in homeostatic maintenance, such as platelet aggregation, the regulation of blood flow to the kidney and stomach, and the regulation of gastric acid secretion and production of protective mucus, especially in the stomach. Inhibition of these activities by NSAIDs accounts for their adverse reactions, especially on the renal and GI tracts.

COX-2 is an "inducible" enzyme that is synthesized mainly in response to pain and inflammation. However, there is some synthesis in the kidney, brain, bone, female reproductive system, and GI tract. Nonspecific NSAIDs inhibit both COX-1 and COX-2. Most NSAIDs (e.g., aspirin, ketoprofen [Actron, Orudis], flurbiprofen (Ansaid), indomethacin [Indocin], piroxicam [Feldene], sulindac [Clinoril]) are mainly selective for COX-1. Some (e.g., ibuprofen [Advil, Motrin], naproxen [Aleve, Naprosyn], diclofenac [Cambia, Cataflam, Voltaren]) are slightly selective for COX-1, and others (e.g., etodolac [Lodine], nabumetone [Relafen], meloxicam [Mobic]) are slightly selective for COX-2.

Three COX-2 selective drugs (e.g., celecoxib [Celebrex], rofecoxib [Vioxx], valdecoxib [Bextra]) have been developed that appear not to inhibit COX-1. These drugs were used for patients who had higher risks for GI bleeding. However, in 2004, research indicated that the overall risk for GI bleeding was not sufficient to compensate for the increased risk for cardiovascular events that occurred with these drugs. In September 2004, rofecoxib was voluntarily removed from the market. In April 2005, the U.S. Food and Drug Administration (FDA) requested that valdecoxib be removed from the market. At that time, a Black-Box Warning was placed on all NSAIDs and on celecoxib related to this risk. All OTC NSAIDs also had their labeling revised to

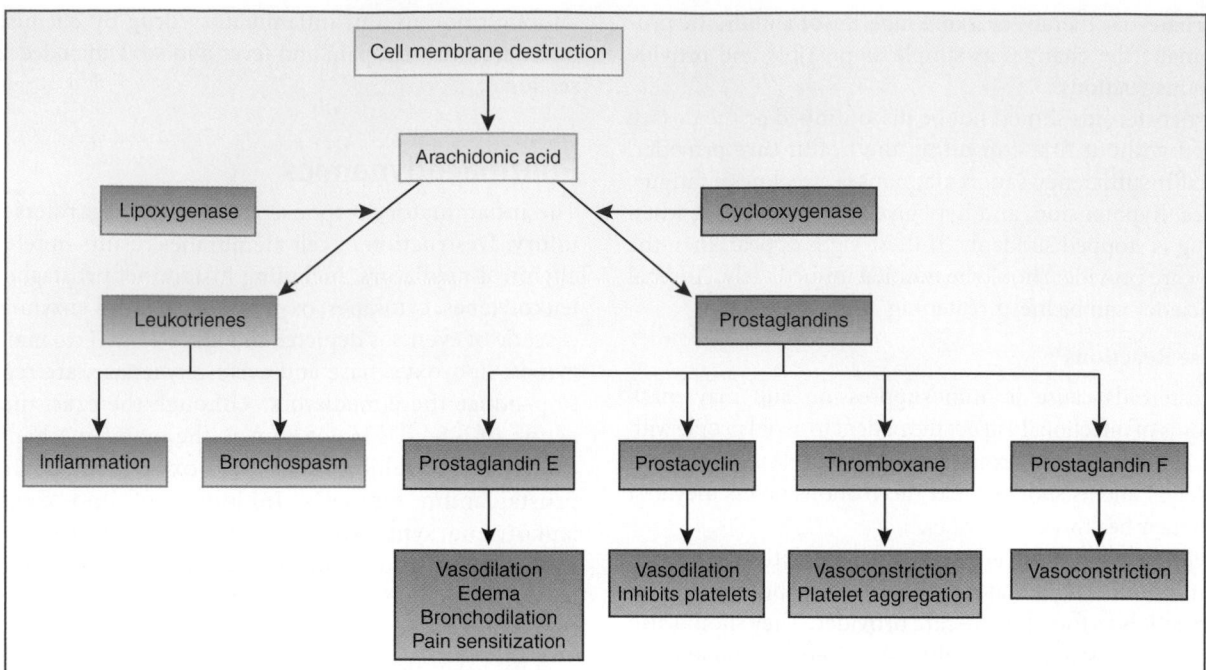

Figure 25–2. Sequence of events in inflammatory response. The sequence of events is the same, regardless of the source of injury.

include more specific information about potential GI and cardiovascular risks. In 2005, the FDA requested that sponsors of all NSAIDs and celecoxib, both prescription and OTC, add to the labeling a boxed warning about cardiovascular risk events and the well-described, serious, potentially life-threatening GI bleeding associated with their use. In addition, a Medication Guide must now be provided with each prescription.

The NSAIDs are primarily used for their anti-inflammatory activity, but they are effective analgesics useful for the relief of mild to moderate pain. They also have antipyretic properties. Because the mechanism of antiplatelet activity is reversible binding to thromboxane, antiplatelet activity exists only while the NSAID is in the blood. For this reason, NSAIDs are not used for antiplatelet therapy.

Acetaminophen is an analgesic and antipyretic with limited anti-inflammatory activity. Although its mechanism of action is not known, it is thought to act by inhibiting central and peripheral prostaglandin synthesis. The central inhibition is almost as potent as that of aspirin, but its peripheral action is minimal. It reduces fever by direct actions on the hypothalamic heat-regulating centers, which increase dissipation of body heat via vasodilation and sweating. It has the advantages of minimal GI irritation and of not affecting bleeding times, uric acid levels, or respiration.

Pharmacokinetics

Absorption and Distribution

After oral administration, NSAIDs are rapidly and almost completely absorbed (Table 25-7). Naproxen sodium (Naprosyn) is more rapidly absorbed than naproxen and is used when rapid analgesia is desired. Diclofenac potassium (Cataflam) is formulated to release the drug in the stomach, whereas the sodium formulation (Voltaren) is released in the higher pH environment of the duodenum. In general, food delays absorption of all NSAIDs but does not affect the total amount absorbed. Administration with food reduces GI adverse reactions. Ketorolac (Toradol) is the only drug in the class with an IM route of absorption.

All NSAIDs are more than 90% protein bound. They are widely distributed in tissues, cross the placenta, and enter breast milk in low concentrations.

Acetaminophen is also rapidly and almost completely absorbed after oral administration. Rectal absorption is variable. Serum protein binding is low at therapeutic concentrations but varies from 20% to 50% with toxic concentrations. It is relatively uniformly distributed in body tissues, crosses the placenta, and enters breast milk.

Metabolism and Excretion

The NSAIDs are all metabolized by the liver and excreted by the kidneys, primarily as metabolites. Sulindac and nabumetone are inactive prodrugs converted by the liver to active metabolites.

Acetaminophen is extensively metabolized by the liver and excreted by the kidneys, primarily as inactive metabolites. When it is taken regularly or in large doses, the stores of one hepatic conjugate (glutathione) become depleted, and hepatic necrosis may occur. Half-life is prolonged in neonates, and severe hepatic dysfunction is related to its dependence on a liver function for metabolism.

Table 25–7 ✖ Pharmacokinetics: Selected NSAIDs and Acetaminophen

Drug	Onset Anal/AntiR	Peak Anal/AntiR	Duration Anal/AntiR	Protein Binding	Bioavailability	Half-Life	Elimination
Propionic Acid Group							
Ibuprofen	0.5 h/7 d	1–2 h/1–2 wk	4–6 h/UK	90%–99%	>80%	1.8–2.5 h	45%–79% in urine
Ketoprofen	0.5 h/NA	0.5–2 h/NA	4–8 h/NA	99%	90%	2.1 h	80% in urine
Ketoprofen ER		ER: 6–7 h	ER: 24 h			ER: 5 h	
Naproxen	1 h/14 d	2–4 h/2–4 wk	7–12 h/UK	99%	95%	12–15 h	95% in urine
Naproxen sodium	1 h/14 d	1–2 h/2–4 wk	7–12 h/UK	99%	95%	10–20 h	95% in urine
Oxaprozin	1 h/7 d	3–5 h/UK	24–48 h/UK	>99%	95%	42–50 h	65% in urine; 35% in feces
Acetic Acid Group							
Diclofenac	1 h/1 wk	2–3 h/2 wk	4–8 h/UK	99%	50%–60%	1–2 h	65% in urine (metabolites)
Fenoprofen	UK	2 h	UK	99%	UK	3 h	Urine
Flurbiprofen	UK	1.9 h	UK	99%	UK	7.5 h	70% in urine
Indomethacin	0.5–2 h/7 d	1–2 h /1–2 wk SR: 2–4 h/NA	4–6 h/UK	99% SR: 4.5–6 h	98%	4.5 h	60% in urine; 33% in feces
Sulindac	1 h/7 d	2–4 h/2–3 wk	7–16 h/UK	93–98%	90%	7.8–16 h	50% in urine; 25% in feces
Fenamic Acid Group							
Meclofenamate	1 h/few days	0.5–1 h/ 2–3 wk	4–6 h/UK	>99%	100%	1.3 h	70% in urine; 30% in feces
Mefenamic acid	Varies/NA	2–4 h/NA	6 h/NA	90%	UK	2–4 h*	52% in urine; 20% in feces
Oxicams							
Meloxicam	UK	4–5 h/NA	24 h	99.4%	89%	15–20 h	50% in urine; 50% in feces
Piroxicam	15–30 min/ 7–12 d	3–5 h/2–3 wk	48–72 h/UK	99%	UK	50 h	Minimal amounts unchanged in urine
Naphthylalkanone Group							
Nabumetone	1–2 h/ 1–2 d	5 h/2 wk	24–48 h/UK	99%	>80	22.5–30 h*	80% in urine; 9% in feces
Pyrrolizine Carboxylic Acid Group							
	UK/NA	2–3 h	4–6 h	99%	100%	5–6 h	91% in urine; 6% in feces
Ketorolac	IM: 10 min	IM: 1–2 h	IM: ≥6 h				
Pyranocarboxylic Acid Group							
Etodolac	0.5h/d	1–2 h/UK	4–12 h/ 6–12 h	>99%	>80	7.3 h	72% in urine; 16% in feces

Continued

Table 25–7 ▪▪ **Pharmacokinetics: Selected NSAIDs and Acetaminophen—cont'd**

Drug	Onset Anal/ AntiR	Peak Anal/ AntiR	Duration Anal/ AntiR	Protein Binding	Bioavailability	Half-Life	Elimination
COX-2 Inhibitor							
Celecoxib	UK	3 h	12–24 h	97.5%	UK	11 h	27% in urine; 57% in feces
Acetaminophen	PO: 0.5–1 h	1–3 h	3–8 h	20%–50%		1–4 h	90–100% in urine (metabolites)
	Rect: 0.5–1 h	1–3 h	3–4 h				

Anal. = analgesic action; AntiR = antirheumatic action; NA = no action; not used for this indication; UK = unknown.

*Prolonged in older adults and impaired renal function.

Table 25-7 provides pharmacokinetic information on NSAIDs, including the one remaining COX-2 inhibitor, celecoxib, and acetaminophen.

Pharmacotherapeutics

Precautions and Contraindications

The only relative contraindications are for ketorolac, mefenamic acid (Ponstel), flurbiprofen, and nabumetone in the presence of preexisting renal impairment. Because NSAID metabolites are excreted primarily by the kidneys, all others should be used with caution in the presence of renal function impairment. Renal function should be assessed prior to initiation of therapy and during therapy.

The liver extensively metabolizes NSAIDs. Naproxen may exhibit an increase in unbound fraction and reduced clearance of free drug in cirrhotic patients. A reduced dose may be necessary. The area under the curve (AUC) of sulindac may be increased in patients with cirrhosis because of alterations in sulfide formation and metabolism. In patients treated with a single 15 mg dose of meloxicam, there was no marked difference in plasma concentrations in patients with mild to moderate hepatic impairment compared with healthy subjects. Protein binding was also not affected in these patients. Because the effects of hepatic disease on other NSAIDs are not known, they should be used cautiously in patients with hepatic impairment.

The liver also extensively metabolizes acetaminophen. High doses or long-term use and chronic alcoholism have been associated with hepatotoxicity. Avoid high doses or long-term use. For patients with chronic alcoholism, no safe dose has been determined. It should not be used for these patients.

GI adverse reactions are the most common reasons for cautious use. Serious GI bleeding, ulceration, and perforation can occur at any time without warning symptoms. Studies have not identified any subset of patients not at risk for these problems. A history of serious GI events, alcoholism, and smoking are the only specific factors associated with increased risk. Based on these data, active or chronic inflammation or ulceration of the GI tract relatively contraindicates use of all NSAIDs, especially indomethacin and sulindac. Other NSAIDs are sometimes used concurrently with a cytoprotective agent such as sucralfate (Carafate) or misoprostol (Cytotec). Diclofenac is produced in a combination with misoprostol under the brand name Arthrotec. Cytoprotective agents are discussed in Chapter 20. Wherever possible, however, these patients should be treated with nonulcerogenic drugs.

Indomethacin may aggravate depression or other psychiatric disturbances. A different NSAID should be chosen in this situation.

Age appears to increase the risk for adverse reactions to NSAIDs. The risk for serious ulcer disease is greater in adults over age 65. This risk appears to be dose-dependent, and reduced dosages may be necessary. Ketorolac is cleared more slowly in older adults. Nabumetone shows no difference in overall efficacy and safety between older adults and younger patients.

The NSAIDs are Pregnancy Category C (etodolac [Lodine], flurbiprofen, ibuprofen, indomethacin, ketoprofen ketorolac, mefenamic acid, nabumetone, naproxen, oxaprozin [Daypro]), piroxicam [Feldene], sulindac). Diclofenac is Pregnancy Category C before 30 weeks' gestation and Pregnancy Category D after 30 weeks' gestation. There are no adequate and well-controlled studies in pregnant women, so use during pregnancy must be carefully weighed in terms of risks and benefits. Agents that inhibit prostaglandin synthesis may cause closure of the ductus arteriosus and other untoward effects in the fetus. Use in the first trimester is less troublesome; NSAIDs should be avoided during the last trimester.

Acetaminophen is Pregnancy Category B. Although it crosses the placenta, it has been routinely used during all stages of pregnancy. At therapeutic doses, it appears safe for short-term use.

Most NSAIDs are excreted in breast milk. At doses of 400 mg bid and 400 mg every 6 hours, ibuprofen is not detected in breast milk; naproxen was detected at 1.9% of maternal concentration, and 0.18% of the maternal dose of ketorolac was detected (LactMed, 2014). Of the NSAIDS, ibuprofen is the safest during breastfeeding. Naproxen should be avoided due to its long duration of action and potential for harm to the neonate.

Acetaminophen is excreted in breast milk in low concentrations, with reported milk:plasma ratios of 0.91 to 1.42 at 1 and 12 hours, respectively. No adverse effects on nursing infants have been reported.

Mefenamic acid and meclofenamate are not recommended for children under age 14 years. Children under age 14 should not take indomethacin except in circumstances that clearly warrant the risk. Closely monitor the liver function of children between ages 2 and 14 who take it. Cases of hepatotoxicity, including fatalities, have been reported in children with juvenile rheumatoid arthritis. Indomethacin is not approved for children younger than 14, although it is used in neonates to close a patent ductus arteriosis. Flurbiprofen, diclofenac, and ketoprofen are not approved for use in children. Other NSAIDs may be used to treat children, and pediatric doses are published for these drugs. Acetaminophen is safe for infants and children.

Adverse Drug Reactions

The most common adverse reactions with NSAIDs are GI disturbances, in particular nausea, vomiting, constipation, and diarrhea. Taking the drug with food can reduce these reactions. GI bleeding and ulceration were discussed in the Precautions and Contraindications section and in the Pharmacodynamics section.

Acute renal insufficiency has occurred in patients with pre-existing renal disease or compromised renal perfusion. Patients at greatest risk are older adults, premature infants, those taking diuretics, and those with heart failure, systemic lupus erythematosus, or chronic glomerulonephritis. Stopping the drug usually brings recovery. Interstitial nephritis has occurred with increasing frequency in patients who take NSAIDs, and it may be due to altered prostaglandin metabolism.

Hematological effects are less common but can be related to the actions of the drugs. NSAIDs inhibit platelet aggregation and may increase bleeding time. Decreased hemoglobin and hematocrit levels have occurred rarely. Patients with initial values below 10 g/dL who are to receive long-term therapy should have these values regularly monitored.

Fluid retention and peripheral edema are not severe but can be problematic for patients with compromised cardiovascular function. Patients with severe heart failure may have significant deterioration in hemodynamic function, presumably related to the inhibition of prostaglandin-dependent compensatory mechanisms.

Cholestatic hepatitis, jaundice, and abnormal liver function tests have occurred rarely. Pancreatitis has developed in patients who take sulindac.

Adverse reactions associated with acetaminophen are few; however, those that do exist are significant. Acute hepatic necrosis occurs with doses of 10 to 15 g. Doses above 25 g are usually fatal. Children appear less susceptible to toxicity than adults because they have less capacity for glucuronidation, the metabolic pathway for acetaminophen. Acute poisoning is manifested by nausea, vomiting, drowsiness, confusion, liver tenderness, and renal failure, which occur within the first 24 hours and may persist for more than 1 week. Acute renal failure may also occur.

Acetaminophen Poisoning

Acetaminophen is a common cause of poisoning, either intentional or accidental, due to the lay public's underestimating the toxicity of the drug. A single dose of 150 mg/kg of acetaminophen in children or 7.5 g to 10 g in adults may be toxic. Drugs that induce CYP2E1 enzymes (carbamazepine, phenobarbitol, phenytoin, isoniazid, and rifampin) or alcohol ingestion may cause hepatotoxicity when combined with acetaminophen. The course of acetaminophen poisoning is divided into four stages:

1. 0.5 to 24 hours: Nausea, vomiting, diaphoresis, pallor, and anorexia. Some patients may be asymptomatic initially.
2. 24 to 72 hours: Clinically improved; aspartate transaminase (AST), alanine transaminase (ALT), bilirubin, and prothrombin levels begin to rise.
3. 72 to 96 hours: Peak hepatotoxicity; jaundice, confusion, AST of 10,000 not unusual.
4. 4 to 14 days: Death or recovery. Patients who survive enter a recovery phase.

Acute acetaminophen poisoning should be referred to a poison control center hospital. If this is not possible, the following treatment regimen may be followed. If the acute ingestion is more than 150 mg/kg or the dose cannot be determined, obtain a serum acetaminophen assay 4 hours after ingestion. If the level is more than 300 mg/mL, hepatic damage has occurred in 90% of patients. Minimum hepatic damage results from a level below 120 mg/mL. Treatment is by gastric lavage in all cases, preferably within 4 hours of ingestion. Oral *N*-acetylcysteine is a specific antidote for acetaminophen toxicity. Contact a poison control center for correct dosing of the antidote.

The FDA asked manufactures to reduce the amount of acetaminophen in combination products to 325 mg in each tablet or capsule. In 2014, the FDA issued a statement to prescribers recommending discontinuing prescribing and dispensing of combination acetaminophen prescription products (FDA, 2014).

Anemia, neutropenia, pancytopenia, and thrombocytopenia also occur but are not severe. The skin eruptions and urticarial skin reactions that may develop are also transient and not severe.

Drug Interactions

Both NSAIDs and acetaminophen have many drug interactions. NSAIDs decrease the effectiveness of antihypertensive drugs because of their tendency to cause fluid retention and increased extracellular fluid volume. Coadministration with anticoagulants may prolong prothrombin time because both drugs affect platelet aggregation. Drugs that have adverse reactions associated with increased risk for GI bleeding or ulceration have an even higher risk if taken with NSAIDs. Drugs that require glucuronidation for metabolism may affect the metabolism of acetaminophen by competing for metabolic sites. These and other interactions are listed in Table 25-8.

Table 25–8 ▓ Drug Interactions: Selected NSAIDs and Acetaminophen

Drug	Interacting Drug	Possible Effect	Implications
Acetaminophen	Alcohol	Increased risk for hepatotoxicity	Avoid alcohol intake
	Anticholinergics	Delayed onset of action of acetaminophen; ultimate pharmacological effects not altered	No action required
	Beta-adrenergic blockers	Propranolol inhibits the enzyme systems responsible for glucuronidation and oxidation of acetaminophen, resulting in increased pharmacological effects	Select different beta adrenergic blocker
	Contraceptives, oral	Increased glucuronidation, resulting in increased plasma clearance and decreased half-life of acetaminophen	Select NSAID for treatment if long-term therapy; not a problem with single dose
	Probenecid		
	Loop diuretics	Increases the therapeutic effectiveness of acetaminophen	Used therapeutically
	Zidovudine	Decreased effectiveness of diuretic because acetaminophen may decrease renal prostaglandin excretion and decrease plasma renin activity	Avoid concurrent use
			Avoid concurrent use; select NSAID for long-term use
		Decreased pharmacological effects of zidovudine related to enhanced nonhepatic or renal clearance of zidovudine	
All NSAIDs	Anticoagulants	May prolong prothrombin time (PT)	Avoid coadministration; monitor PT and patients closely; instruct patients to watch for indications of bleeding
	Beta adrenergic blockers	Antihypertensive effect impaired; sulindac and naproxen do not affect atenolol	Select appropriate drug match
	Hydantoins	Serum levels of phenytoin increased, resulting in increased pharmacological and toxic effects of phenytoin	If they must be used together, monitor serum levels and adjust dose accordingly
	Lithium	Serum lithium levels increased; sulindac has no effect or decreases levels	Avoid concurrent use or select sulindac; monitor serum levels
	Loop diuretics	Decreased effects of loop diuretics	Avoid concurrent use for long-term therapy or select different diuretic
	Probenecid	Probenecid may increase concentrations and toxicity risk of NSAIDs	Avoid concurrent use
	Salicylates	Decreased plasma concentrations of NSAIDs	Avoid concurrent use; offers no therapeutic advantage and significantly increases incidence of GI adverse reactions
Indomethacin	Digoxin	May decrease digoxin serum levels; ibuprofen has similar effect	Select different NSAID
	Phenylpropanolamine	Increased blood pressure	Avoid coadministration
	Dipyridamole	Additive fluid retention	Select different NSAID
Indomethacin, naproxen	Thiazide diuretics	Decreased antihypertensive and diuretic action; sulindac may enhance effects	Avoid concurrent use; select sulindac if enhanced effect is desired

Clinical Use and Dosing

Rheumatoid Arthritis

The ultimate goals in managing RA are to prevent and control joint damage, prevent loss of function, and decrease pain. NSAIDs, glucocorticoid joint injection, and/or low-dose prednisone may be used for control of symptoms (Grossman et al, 2010). The initial drug treatment involves the use of salicylates, NSAIDs, or celecoxib to reduce joint pain and swelling and to improve joint function. They have analgesic and anti-inflammatory properties but do not alter the course of the disease or prevent joint destruction, so they should not be used as the sole treatment for RA. Most patients are started on DMARDS, and NSAIDS are used as adjunct treatment.

Although most NSAIDs have been used for this indication, no one NSAID has demonstrated a clear advantage for the treatment of RA. Ketorolac and mefenamic acid do not have a labeled indication for treatment of RA. Choice is determined by adverse reactions, cost, duration of action, and patient preference. For women of childbearing age, Pregnancy Category may affect choice. Nabumetone, piroxicam, and oxaprozin have longer durations of action than the other drugs commonly used.

Ibuprofen is the least expensive and is available OTC. Diclofenac comes in a combination with a cytoprotective agent (misoprostol) to reduce the risk for GI bleeding and ulceration, but this combination is quite expensive. Doses of the drugs with this indication are presented in Table 25-9.

Osteoarthritis

OA is the most common form of arthritis in the United States. Patients have joint pain that typically worsens with weight-bearing and activity and improves with rest as well

Text continued on page 827

Table 25–9 ⚯ Dosage Schedule: Selected NSAIDs and Acetaminophen

Drug	Indication	Dosage Forms	Dosage Schedule	Comments
Acetaminophen (Tylenol)	Mild to moderate pain and/or fever Osteoarthritis	Tablets: 325 mg, 500 mg, 500 mg extra-strength Chewable tablets: 80 mg, 160 mg Caplets: 325 mg 650 mg extended-relief Gelcaps: 500 mg extra-strength Elixir: 160 mg/5 mL Liquid: 500 mg/15 mL Infant drops: 100 mg/mL Tablets: 325 mg, 500 mg, 650 mg Chewable tablets: 80, 160 mg Orally disintegrating tablets: 80, 160 mg Liquid: 160 mg/5 mL Suppository: 120, 300, 325, 650 mg	ORAL DOSES *Adults and children >14 yr:* 325–650 mg every 4–6 h *or* 1 g tid *Children* 10 to 15 mg/kg/dose every 4 h SUPPOSITORIES *Adults and children >12 yr:* 650 mg every 4–6 h *Children 3–11 mo:* 80 mg up to every 6 h *Children 1–3 yr:* 80 mg up to every 4 h *Children 3–6 yr:* 120–125 mg every 4–6 h *Children 6–12 yr:* 325 mg every 4–6 h *Adults:* Up to 1 g qid	Not to exceed 3 g/d For all ages of children, doses not to exceed 5 doses in 24 h Max dose 650 mg/dose Not to exceed 4 g/d Not to exceed 720 mg/d Not to exceed 2.6 g/d Not to exceed 4 g/d
Celecoxib (Celebrex)	Osteoarthritis, juvenile idiopathic arthritis, rheumatoid arthritis	Capsules: 100, 200, 400 mg	*Children (JIA):* ≥10 kg to <25 kg = 50 mg bid; ≥25 kg: 100 mg bid *Adults:* Acute pain: 400 mg initially followed by 200 mg bid OA: 200 mg/d RA: 100 to 200 mg bid	
Etodolac (Lodine)	Osteoarthritis, rheumatoid arthritis Analgesia	Capsules: 200 and 300 mg Tablets: 400 and 500 mg	*Adults:* 800–1,200 mg/d in divided doses, followed by dosage adjustments within the range of 600–1,200 mg/d in divided doses *Adults:* 200–400 mg every 6–8 h as needed	Not to exceed 1,200 mg/d; for patients ≤60 kg, do not exceed 20 mg/kg Not to exceed 1,200 mg/d; for patients ≤60 kg, do not exceed 20 mg/kg
Diclofenac (Voltaren) (Cataflam)	Rheumatoid arthritis Osteoarthritis Ankylosing spondylitis Analgesia, primary dysmenorrhea	Tablets: 25, 50, 75 mg Extended-release: 100 mg	*Adults:* 100–200 mg/d in divided doses (50 mg tid–qid or 75 mg bid) Chronic therapy with extended-release tablets: 100 mg/d *Adults:* 100–200 mg/d in divided doses (50 mg bid–tid or 75 mg bid) Chronic therapy with extended-release tablets: 100 mg/d *Adults:* 100–125 mg/d delayed-release tablets (25 mg qid with an extra dose at bedtime if needed) *Adults:* 50 mg tid; some patients may need 100 mg tid initially, followed by 50 mg tid	Doses above 225 mg/d not recommended Doses above 200 mg/d are not recommended Doses above 125 mg not recommended After first day, maximum dose 200 mg; doses generally should not exceed 150 mg

Continued

Table 25–9 ⨯ Dosage Schedule: Selected NSAIDs and Acetaminophen—cont'd

Drug	Indication	Dosage Forms	Dosage Schedule	Comments
Fenoprofen	Rheumatoid arthritis, osteoarthritis Mild-to-moderate pain	Capsules: 200 mg Tablets: 600 mg	*Adults:* 300–600 mg 3–4 times a day *Adults:* 200 mg q4–6 hr	Not approved for use in children <18 years. Not recommended in patients with advanced renal disease
Flurbiprofen	Rheumatoid arthritis, osteoarthritis		*Adults:* 200–300 mg/ day in two, three, or four divided doses. Maximum of 100 mg in a single dose	Not approved for use in children <18 years.
Ibuprofen (Advil, Motrin)	Rheumatoid arthritis, osteoarthritis Juvenile arthritis Acute gouty arthritis Mild to moderate pain Muscle sprain, strain (anti-inflammatory, analgesic) Primary dysmenorrhea Fever reduction OTC use for pain and/or fever	Tablets: 100, 200, 300, 500, 600, 800 mg Junior-strength tablets: 100 mg Chewable tablets: 50, 100 mg Gelcaps: 200 mg Suspension: 100 mg/5 mL Oral drops: 40 mg/mL, 50 mg/.25 mL IV solution: 10 mg/mL, 400 mg/4 mL	*Adults:* 1.2–3.2 g/d (300 mg qid or 400, 600, or 800 mg tid–qid) *Children:* 30–70 mg/kg/d in 3–4 divided doses; 20 mg/kg/d may be adequate in milder disease *Adults:* 800 mg qid; taper to eliminate as soon as pain is relieved *Adults:* 400 mg every 4–6 h as needed *Adults:* 600 mg qid or 800 mg tid for 5 d *Children:* 20–40 mg/kg/d in divided doses *Children >12 yr and adults:* 400 mg every 4 h as needed *Adults:* 200–400 mg every 4–6 h *Children 6 mo–12 yr:* 5 mg/kg for temperature <39.1°C (102.5°F) or 10 mg/kg for higher temperatures; may be repeated every 4–6 h *Adults:* 200 mg every 4–6 h while symptoms persist; if response is not adequate, may use 400 mg *Children ≥6 mo:* 5 mg–10 mg every 6–8 hr	Not to exceed 3.2 g/d; higher doses usually needed for rheumatoid arthritis Not to exceed 3.2 g/d Not to exceed 1,200 mg/d Not to exceed 3,600 mg/d Not to exceed 50 mg/kg/d Not to exceed 1,200 mg/d Not to exceed 1,200 mg/d Not to exceed 40 mg/kg/d Not to exceed 1,200 mg/d; do not take for >10 d for pain or >3 d for fever Do not administer to children <6 mo
Indomethacin (Indocin)	Moderate to severe rheumatoid arthritis, ankylosing spondylitis, and osteoarthritis Acute gouty arthritis Acute painful shoulder (bursitis or tendinitis) Acute gouty arthritis	Tablets: 200 mg, 400 mg, 600 mg, 800 mg Suspension: 100 mg/5 mL	*Children >14 yr and adults:* 25 mg bid–tid initially; increase dose by 25–50 mg at weekly intervals until satisfactory response Sustained release: 75 mg can be taken daily as alternative to 25 mg tid or bid as alternative to 50 mg tid *Adults:* 25 to 50 mg qid; taper to eliminate as soon as pain is relieved *Children >14 yr and adults:* 75–100 mg/d in 3–4 divided doses for 7–14 d *Adults:* 50 mg tid; taper to eliminate drug as soon as pain is relieved	Not to exceed 200 mg/d; for patients with persistent night pain or morning stiffness; give larger portion of dose at bedtime (up to 100 mg) Not to exceed 200 mg/d Do not use sustained-release form
Ketoprofen (Orudis)	Rheumatoid arthritis, osteoarthritis Acute gouty arthritis Mild to moderate pain, primary dysmenorrhea	Tablets: 12.5 mg Capsules: 25, 50 mg, 75 mg Extended-release: 100, 150, 200 mg	*Adults:* 75 mg tid *or* 50 mg qid initially Maintenance dose is 150–300 mg/d in 3–4 divided doses	Reduce dose by 1/2–1/3 for older adults and those with renal impairment; not to exceed 300 mg/d Not to exceed 300 mg/d

Table 25–9 ✖ Dosage Schedule: Selected NSAIDs and Acetaminophen—cont'd

Drug	Indication	Dosage Forms	Dosage Schedule	Comments
	OTC use for pain		Extended-release: 200 mg once daily *Adults:* 75 mg qid; taper to eliminate as soon as pain is relieved *Adults:* 25–50 mg every 6–8 h as needed *Children >16 yr and adults:* 12.5 mg with full glass of liquid every 4–6 h; if pain or fever persists after 1 h, follow with 12.5 mg	Doses >50 mg have not increased efficacy; not to exceed 300 mg/d Not to exceed 25 mg in a 4–6 h period or 75 mg/24 h
Ketorolac (Torodal)	Acute, moderately severe pain	Tablets: 10 mg Injection: 15 mg/mL, 30 mg/mL	*Adults <65 yr:* 60 mg IM single dose or 30 mg every 6 h (not to exceed 120 mg/d); then 20 mg PO initially, followed by 10 mg every 4–6 h as needed (not to exceed 40 mg/d) *Adults >65 yr or <50 kg or with renal impairment:* 30 mg IM single dose or 15 mg every 6 h (not to exceed 60 mg/d); then 10 mg PO every 4–6 h as needed (not to exceed 40 mg/d)	Not intended for >5 d combined IM and PO, or for minor or chronic pain; oral therapy is intended only as continuation from IM therapy
Meclofenamate	Rheumatoid arthritis, osteoarthritis Mild to moderate pain Excessive menstrual bleeding, dysmenorrhea	Capsules: 50, 100 mg	*Adults:* 200–400 mg/d in 3–4 equally divided doses *Children >14 yr and adults:* 50–100 mg every 4–6 h *Children >14 yr and adults:* 100 mg tid for up to 6 d, starting with first day of menstrual flow	Not to exceed 400 mg/d Not to exceed 400 mg/d Not to exceed 400 mg/d
Mefenamic acid (Ponstel)	Acute pain Primary dysmenorrhea	Capsules: 250 mg	*Children >14 yr and adults:* 500 mg, then 250 mg every 6 h as needed *Children >14 yr and adults:* 500 mg, then 250 mg every 6 h as needed starting at onset of bleeding or symptoms	Not to exceed 1 wk Should not be necessary for more than 2–3 d
Meloxicam (Mobic) Nabumetone (Relafen)	Rheumatoid arthritis, osteoarthritis Juvenile arthritis Rheumatoid arthritis, osteoarthritis	Tablet: 7.5, 15 mg Suspension: 7.5 mg/15 mL Tablets: 500, 750 mg	*Children >2 yr with JIA:* 0.125 mg/kg once daily; maximum 7.5 mg/daily *Adults:* 7.5 mg daily *Adults:* 1,000 mg daily; may increase to 1,500–2,000 mg/d	Not to exceed 2,000 mg/d
Naproxen (Aleve) Naproxen Sodium	Rheumatoid arthritis, osteoarthritis, ankylosing spondylitis Juvenile arthritis Acute gouty arthritis Acute gout Mild to moderate pain, dysmenorrhea, acute tendinitis or bursitis	Tablets: 250, 375, 500 mg Enteric-coated: 375, 500 mg Tablets, delayed-release: 375 mg and 500 mg Suspension: 125 mg/5 mL Tablets: 275, 550 mg	*Adults:* 250–500 mg bid; may increase to 1.5 g/d for limited periods Delayed-release: 375–500 mg bid Controlled-release: 750–1,000 mg once daily Naproxen sodium: 275–550 mg bid; may increase to 1.65 mg for limited periods	Morning and evening doses do not need to be equal; more than twice-daily dosing does not improve efficacy Not to exceed 1 g/d Not to exceed 1.25 g/d

Continued

Table 25–9 ⊗ **Dosage Schedule: Selected NSAIDs and Acetaminophen—cont'd**

Drug	Indication	Dosage Forms	Dosage Schedule	Comments
			Children: 10 mg/kg/d in 2 divided doses. Suspension: 13 kg child = 2.5 mL bid; 25 kg child = 5 mL; 38 kg child = 7.5 mL *Adults:* 500 mg bid; taper to eliminate as soon as pain is relieved Controlled-release: Same Naproxen sodium: Same *Adults:* 750 mg, then 250 mg every 8 h until attack subsides Controlled release: 1,000–1,500 mg once daily on first day, then 1,000 mg once daily until the attack subsides Naproxen sodium: 825 mg, then 275 mg every 8 h until attack subsides *Adults:* 500 mg, then 250 mg every 6–8 h as needed Controlled-release: 1,000 mg once daily; 1,500 mg/d may be used for limited period	
	OTC use for pain		Naproxen sodium: 550 mg, then 275 mg every 6–8 h as needed *Children:* Naproxen suspension, 5 mg/kg/d in 2 divided doses *Adults:* 200 mg with full glass of liquid every 8–12 h while symptoms persist; dose of 400 mg initially, then 200 mg doses, may be necessary *Adults >65 yr:* Do not take >200 mg every 12 h *Children:* Do not give to children <12 yr, except under advice/supervision of HCP	Not to exceed 1.375 g/d Not to exceed 600 mg/d
Oxaprozin (Daypro)	Rheumatoid arthritis, osteoarthritis	Caplets: 600 mg Tablet: 600 mg	*Adults:* 1,200 mg once daily; patients with low body weight or milder disease may use 600 mg once daily	Not to exceed 1,800 mg/d or 26 mg/kg, whichever is lower; doses >1,200 mg/d should be divided
Piroxicam (Feldenea)	Rheumatoid arthritis, osteoarthritis Dysmenorrhea	Capsules: 10, 20 mg	*Adults:* 20 mg once daily; may divide dose *Adults >65 yr:* 10 mg once daily initially *Adults:* 40 mg first day, then 20 mg/d	
Sulindac (Clinoril)	Rheumatoid arthritis, osteoarthritis, ankylosing spondylitis Acute gout, painful shoulder (tendinitis, bursitis)	Tablets: 150, 200 mg	*Adults:* 150 mg bid *Adults:* 200 mg bid	Therapy usually not longer than 7 d

HCP = health-care provider; OTC = over the counter.

as experience stiffness and swelling of the involved joint after periods of inactivity. Although there is no known cure for OA, treatment can help to maintain or improve joint mobility and limit functional impairment. With OA, nonpharmacological modalities are as important as drug therapy. They include weight loss; aerobic, range-of-motion, and muscle-strengthening exercises; appropriate footwear; and assistive devices for ambulation and activities of daily living when necessary. Drug therapy includes acetaminophen, NSAIDs, and COX-2 inhibitors. Topical agents such as capsaicin (hand OA only) and trolamine salicylate may also be used (Hochberg et al, 2012).

The patient's pain, disability, and comorbidities provide the guidelines for management of OA. Initially, acetaminophen in doses 650 mg 4 times a day or 1 g 3 times a day (maximum 3 g/24 h) are given to manage joint pain. If this drug fails to control pain, NSAIDs are prescribed (Hochberg et al, 2012). Patients who do not have a good response to full-dose acetaminophen should be trialed on systemic NSAIDS or intra-articular corticosteroid injections (Hochberg et al). The American College of Rheumatology recommends use of topical rather than oral NSAIDS in patients age 75 years or older (Hochberg et al, 2012). Although NSAIDs have both analgesic and anti-inflammatory actions, they do not alter the course of the disease or prevent joint destruction. All NSAIDs except ketorolac and mefenamic acid have an indication for treatment of OA. Doses are presented in Table 25-9. As in RA, the choice of NSAID to be used is determined by adverse reactions, cost, duration of action, and patient preference. For patients who experience adverse GI effects, adjunctive administration of proton pump inhibitors or cytoprotective agents (misoprostol) may be needed. Both of these drug classes are discussed in Chapter 20.

The use of both glucosamine (1,500 mg daily) and chondroitin (1,200 mg daily) for joint pain due to knee OA is a common practice among patients who are self-prescribing for OA. The evidence on the use of glucosamine and chondroitin does not consistently show improvement in pain; therefore, the American College of Rheumatology clinical guidelines do not recommend either for knee arthritis (2012). Because these two agents are available OTC and encouraged in many health food establishments, providers should ask the patient about their use and effectiveness for that patient.

Gout

Indomethacin, naproxen, and sulindac list acute gout as an indication. Ibuprofen and ketoprofen have also been used. Table 25-9 provides dosage schedules for these five drugs.

Mild to Moderate Pain

Almost every individual at some time experiences an episode of mild to moderate pain. Regardless of the source of the pain, nonopioid analgesia is the primary choice for management, especially if inflammation accompanies or is the cause of the pain. Although any NSAID may be used for this indication, several have been routinely used and proved effective.

Ibuprofen is the most commonly used because it is inexpensive, available OTC, and short-acting so that acute pain can be managed without long-term effects and adverse reactions. For women of childbearing age, it is Pregnancy Category C, and for nursing women it is not detected in breast milk. Naproxen sodium is used as an analgesic because it reaches its peak more rapidly and is longer-acting. Other drugs used for this indication include ketoprofen, ketorolac, meclofenamate, and mefenamic acid. When an injectable NSAID is needed, only ketorolac has such a formulation. Ibuprofen (Caldolor) and acetaminophen (Ofirmev) are available in IV form.

As with other indications, there is no clear difference in efficacy. Taking the drug around the clock, rather than as necessary, is most effective. Choice is based on adverse reactions, cost, duration of action, and patient preference. Health-care providers often choose one short-acting drug (ibuprofen, diclofenac, ketoprofen, ketorolac, meclofenamate), an intermediate-acting one (naproxen), and a long-acting drug (ketoprofen ER) and use the same drugs repeatedly. Because different patients seem to respond better to different NSAIDs, if one drug does not produce the desired effect, another one can be tried.

Acetaminophen is useful in treating mild to moderate pain that is not accompanied by or caused by inflammation. It is not intended for pain management for more than 5 days in children or 10 days in adults because of the increased risk for hepatic adverse reactions. For adults, a dose of 325 to 650 mg every 4 to 6 hours usually suffices. Children's doses are based on weight: 10 to 15 mg/kg per dose every 4 to 6 hours. After age 14 years, the adult dose is used. These doses are shown in Table 25-9.

Primary Dysmenorrhea

Ibuprofen, diclofenac potassium, ketoprofen, meclo-fenamate, mefenamic acid, and naproxen are the drugs used for dysmenorrhea. The best response occurs if NSAIDS are starting with the onset of menses symptoms. Doses are shown in Table 25-9.

Tendinitis and Bursitis

Indomethacin SR, naproxen, and sulindac are used for tendinitis and bursitis. Naproxen and sulindac both are intermediate-acting and provide longer duration of action than indomethacin, even in its sustained-release form. They also have fewer drug interactions. Naproxen is less likely to produce GI adverse reactions. These same three drugs are used to manage the pain in gout because it is associated with inflammation. Treatment choices are determined on the same basis.

Fever

Ibuprofen is the NSAID of choice for fever in children over age 6 months and adults. Doses are published for both adults and children. Acetaminophen may also be used for this purpose, but not for longer than 3 days. Acetaminophen is used for children younger than age 6 months and patients who do not tolerate ibuprofen (blood coagulation disorders; upper GI disease). Patients should be well hydrated if using ibuprofen for fever to decrease renal toxicity.

Rational Drug Selection

There is no clear difference in efficacy between NSAIDs, although there may be individual differences in response. The rationale for choices is provided in the Clinical Use and Dosing section. Acetaminophen is used for fever and for mild to moderate pain not associated with inflammation.

Monitoring

Monitoring is required only for long-term therapy. Because NSAIDS may produce acute renal insufficiency, assess renal function (serum creatinine) before initiation of therapy and annually throughout long-term therapy. A CBC prior to initiation of therapy and annually thereafter is appropriate because of the risk for GI bleeding. Any other monitoring is related to the disease being treated.

Patient Education

Administration

Take the drug exactly as prescribed (Table 25-12). A missed dose should be taken as soon as the patient remembers unless it is almost time for the next dose. For drugs taken more than once daily, ideally the missed dose should be taken within 1 to 2 hours of the time it was scheduled. Doses should not be doubled. Taking higher doses than those prescribed does not increase efficacy and may increase adverse reactions.

For some NSAIDs, there is a prescribed length of time beyond which the drug may not be taken. Patients should be informed of this time limitation. Taking the drug with food or a full glass of fluid and remaining in an upright position for 15 to 30 minutes may reduce GI discomfort and adverse reactions. Remind patients to avoid aspirin, alcohol, or other GI irritants while taking these drugs. Patients should be aware of products that may contain acetaminophen, including cough and cold products and combination opioid products, to avoid accidental overdose of acetaminophen.

Adverse Reactions

Advise patients about probable adverse reactions and what they should do if reactions occur. The most common adverse reaction is GI bleeding. They should contact their healthcare provider if they experience coffee-ground emesis or black, tarry stools. The provider should also be notified of skin rash, itching, visual disturbances, weight gain, edema, or persistent headache. With meclofenamate and mefenamic acid, if rash, diarrhea, or other digestive problems occur, patients should discontinue the drug and contact their healthcare provider.

These drugs may cause drowsiness. Patients should avoid activities requiring mental alertness until their response to the drug is known.

Lifestyle Management

Lifestyle modifications are only those related to the disease being treated.

ASPIRIN AND NONACETYLATED SALICYLATES

Aspirin is the prototype drug for this class, which makes it one of the most used drug classes for the treatment and prevention of a wide variety of disorders. Although salicylates are prescribed for conditions similar to those that the NSAIDs are used for, in addition to the analgesic, anti-inflammatory, and antipyretic properties common to the NSAIDs, the salicylates also possess antiplatelet properties to varying degrees. This latter property accounts for some of their adverse reactions but also for the increased breadth of their use beyond those for which NSAIDs are prescribed. The ability of aspirin to reduce platelet aggregation has given it a role in managing rheumatic fever, transient ischemic attacks (TIAs), coronary artery disease, and deep vein thrombosis. The antiplatelet role of aspirin is discussed in Chapter 18. Its nonspecific anti-inflammatory effect is invaluable in reducing cardiac workload for patients with severe carditis and heart failure. Aspirin has been shown to reduce the incidence of myocardial infarction (MI) and the incidence of death in all patients with unstable angina. These roles are discussed in Chapters 28, 33, 36, and 40. Salicylates are also used topically as keratolytic agents and counterirritants. This role is discussed in Chapters 23 and 32.

Pharmacodynamics

All salicylates have analgesic, anti-inflammatory, antipyretic, and antiplatelet actions. The pharmacological effects are qualitatively similar. Salicylates lower body temperature through their effect on the hypothalamic thermostat and vasodilation of peripheral vessels, thus enhancing dissipation of heat. The anti-inflammatory and analgesic activities are mediated through inhibition of prostaglandin synthesis in the same manner as NSAIDs. However, aspirin more potently inhibits prostaglandin synthesis and has greater anti-inflammatory activity than the NSAIDs. The acetyl group of the aspirin molecule is thought to be responsible for these differences. Aspirin acetylates the cyclo-oxygenase enzyme in the prostaglandin biosynthesis pathway; therefore, it may be theoretically classified as a COX inhibitor.

Aspirin also irreversibly inhibits platelet aggregation. Single analgesic-level doses prolong bleeding time. Acetylation of platelet cyclo-oxygenase prevents synthesis of thromboxane A, which is a potent vasoconstrictor and inducer of platelet aggregation for the life of the platelet (7 to 10 d). This drug has shown success as an antiplatelet agent for patients with thromboembolic disease. For this indication, low doses appear to be more effective than higher ones. Further discussion is found in Chapter 18.

The nonacetylated salicylates (salsalate [Disalcid], choline magnesium trisalicylate [Trilisate], and choline salicylate [Arthropan]) and diflunisal (Dolobid) are salicylic acid derivatives not metabolized to salicylic acid, are not as potent as aspirin, and do not possess the same degree of antiplatelet activity.

Pharmacokinetics

Absorption and Distribution

Salicylates are rapidly and completely absorbed after oral administration (Table 25-10). Bioavailability depends on the dosage form, gastric emptying time, gastric pH, presence of antacids or buffering agents, and particle size. The bioavailability of enteric-coated products may be erratic. The presence of food in the gut slows absorption, and absorption from rectal suppositories is also slower, resulting in lower salicylate levels.

Aspirin is partially hydrolyzed to salicylic acid during absorption and is distributed to all body tissues and fluids, including fetal tissue, breast milk, and the CNS. The highest concentrations are in plasma, the liver, the renal cortex, the heart, and lung tissues.

Protein binding of salicylates is concentration-dependent. At low concentrations (100 mcg/mL), 90% is bound; at higher concentrations (400 mg/mL), only 76% is bound.

Diflunisal is also rapidly and completely absorbed after oral administration. It crosses the placenta and enters breast milk. The first dose tends to have slower onset of pain relief than other drugs but achieves comparable peak effects. More than 99% is bound to plasma proteins.

Metabolism and Excretion

Salicylic acid is eliminated by renal excretion of salicylic acid and by oxidation and conjugation of metabolites by the liver. The amount excreted depends on urine pH. As urine pH increases from 5 to 8, renal clearance of free ionized salicylate increases from 2% to 3% to more than 80%. Alteration of urine pH is used in the treatment of salicylate poisoning to increase excretion.

Aspirin has a half-life of 15 to 20 minutes. Salicylic acid's half-life is 2 to 3 hours at low doses; at higher doses, it ranges from 6 to 12 hours. Plasma levels increase disproportionately as salicylate doses increase.

Diflunisal has a long half-life and nonlinear pharmacokinetics so that time to steady state is 3 to 4 days with 125 mg twice daily and 7 to 9 days with 500 mg twice daily. A loading dose shortens the time to steady state. Because 90% of each dose is eliminated by the kidneys, the half-life increases with renal impairment.

Pharmacotherapeutics

Precautions and Contraindications

Taking salicylates, especially aspirin, by children or adolescents with influenza or chickenpox has been associated with the development of Reye syndrome, a rare but life-threatening condition characterized by vomiting, lethargy, and eventually delirium and coma. The mortality rate is 20% to 30%, and permanent neurological deficits has been reported in survivors. Children or adolescents with influenza or chickenpox should not take salicylates.

Aspirin should be avoided for 1 week before any surgery because of the increased risk for post-operative bleeding due to its antiplatelet effects. For similar reasons, salicylates in general are contraindicated for patients with active peptic ulcer disease or other GI bleeding–related disorders or a history of such disorders. Salsalate and choline salicylate may cause less GI irritation and bleeding than aspirin. The antiplatelet effects contraindicate salicylate use for patients who are taking anticoagulants or who have anemia or a history of blood coagulation defects.

Salicylates should be used cautiously for patients with hepatic impairment. Reversible hepatic encephalopathy has occurred after even therapeutic doses for RA. Cautious use is also required for patients with renal insufficiency because salicylates may cause a transient decrease in renal function and aggravate chronic kidney diseases. Magnesium salicylates are contraindicated in the presence of renal insufficiency because the kidney cannot eliminate the magnesium, and hypermagnesemia results.

Salicylates affect uric acid accumulation. In low doses (less than 2 g/d), they decrease urate excretion and raise serum uric acid levels. At high doses (3 to 5 g/d), they have a uricosuric effect; however, they are rarely tolerated at this high a dose. They should be used with caution in the presence of gout.

Table 25–10 ⬛ Pharmacokinetics: Salicylates

Drug	Onset	Peak	Duration	Protein Binding	Half-Life	Elimination
Acetylsalicylic acid	15–20 min	1–3 h	3–6 h	90%–91%; 25%–76%*	15–20 min; 2–3 h; 15–30 h*	In urine and by liver*
Choline salicylate	5–30 min	1–3 h	3–6 h	90%–91%; 25%–76%*	15–20 min; 2–3 h; 15–30 h*	In urine and by liver*
Choline magnesium salicylate	5–30 min	1–3 h	3–6 h	90%–91%; 25%–76%*	15–20 min; 2–3 h; 15–30 h*	In urine and by liver*
Salsalate	5–30 min	1–3 h	3–6 h	90%–91%; 25%–76%*	15–20 min; 2–3 h; 15–30 h*	In urine and by liver*
Diflunisal	1 h	2–3 h	8–12 h	8–12 h		90% in urine; <5% in feces

*See discussion in text.

Aspirin is Pregnancy Category D; salsalate and magnesium salicylate are Pregnancy Category C. Ingestion during pregnancy may produce anemia in the mother and increase the risk for postpartum hemorrhage. Inhibition of prostaglandin synthesis may cause constriction of the ductus arteriosus and other possible untoward effects in the fetus. Avoid use in pregnancy, especially during the third trimester. Diflunisal is Pregnancy Category C. Although its safety during pregnancy has not been established, it should not be used, especially during the last trimester.

After aspirin ingestion salicylate is excreted in breast milk in low concentrations. Adverse effects on nursing infants have not been reported when low-dose aspirin is used (75 to 162 mg/day) as an antiplatelet (LactMed, 2014). High-dose aspirin should be avoided while breastfeeding. Diflunisal is excreted in breast milk in concentrations of 2% to 7% of the maternal plasma. Because of potential adverse effects, discontinuing either diflunisal or using a shorter-acting drug such as aspirin is recommended.

The safety and efficacy of magnesium salicylate and salsalate have not been established in children. Aspirin should not be used in children with acute febrile illness. Children with dehydration appear more at risk for salicylate toxicity.

Adverse Drug Reactions

The most common adverse reaction to salicylates is GI irritation and bleeding. Although fecal blood loss is lower with enteric-coated products, these drugs have erratic absorption and still must be used cautiously by patients with GI disorders. The amount of blood lost from GI bleeding secondary to salicylate use is usually clinically insignificant, but with prolonged use it can result in iron deficiency anemia. Patients who have developed peptic ulcers while taking salicylates have healed these ulcers with the use of proton pump inhibitors, H_2 blockers, and antacids, despite continued salicylate use. Only 20% to 25% of patients on chronic aspirin therapy for RA develop mucosal injury.

Hypersensitivity reactions have occurred with salicylates. Hypersensitivity to salicylates or NSAIDs contraindicates aspirin use and requires extremely cautious use of the other salicylates. Cross-sensitivity exists between aspirin and NSAIDs and between aspirin and tartrazine dye. This cross-sensitivity does not appear to occur with choline salicylate. Aspirin sensitivity is more prevalent in patients with asthma, nasal polyps, or chronic urticaria.

Salicylates are ototoxic at increased blood levels. They should be discontinued if dizziness, tinnitus, or impaired hearing develops. Temporary hearing loss disappears gradually when the drug is stopped.

Toxicity

The acute lethal dose of salicylates in adults is 10 to 30 g, and in children it is 3 g. Chronic salicylate toxicity can occur when more than 100 mg/kg is ingested daily for 2 or more days. Signs of salicylate poisoning appear at serum levels of 30 to 60 mg/dL. Respiratory alkalosis is seen initially. Hyperpnea and tachypnea occur as a result of increased CO_2 production and a direct stimulatory effect of the salicylate on the respiratory center in the brain. Other symptoms include nausea, vomiting, hypokalemia, tinnitus, disorientation, irritability, seizures, dehydration, hyperthermia, thrombocytopenia, and other hematological disorders.

Treatment for salicylate toxicity includes induction of emesis or gastric lavage to remove any unabsorbed drug from the stomach. Activated charcoal diminishes salicylate absorption if it is given within 2 hours of ingestion. Salicylate levels and acid–base, fluid, and electrolyte balances are carefully monitored. The rest of therapy is supportive. Forced alkaline diuresis by administering sodium bicarbonate increases salicylate excretion. Hemodialysis is reserved for those patients with severe poisoning.

Drug Interactions

Aspirin may potentiate the anticoagulant action of heparin, warfarin, or thrombolytic agents (Table 25-11). It may increase the risk for bleeding with cefamandole, cefoperazone, cefotetan, valproic acid, or plicamycin.

All salicylates may enhance the activity of penicillins, phenytoin, methotrexate, valproic acid, sulfonylureas, and sulfonamides. They may antagonize the beneficial effects of probenecid or sulfinpyrazone and blunt the therapeutic response to diuretics, antihypertensives, and some NSAIDs. Glucocorticoids decrease serum salicylate levels.

There is an increased risk for GI bleeding when aspirin is taken with any other drug with any other GI irritant, such as ethanol. The risk for ototoxicity is increased when it is taken with any other drug that causes ototoxicity (e.g., aminoglycosides, loop diuretics).

Some foods contain salicylate. Foods and spices high in salicylate include curry, paprika, licorice, Benedictine liqueur, prunes, raisins, tea, and gherkins. Foods that acidify the urine may increase serum salicylate levels, and those that alkalinize the urine may have the opposite effect.

Clinical Use and Dosing

Fever

Aspirin is the salicylate of choice for reduction of fever in adults. It is contraindicated for use with pregnant patients, however. To be used with children, the cause of the fever must first be determined. It is contraindicated in children and adolescents if the cause of the fever is influenza or chickenpox. Although not clearly stated in the literature, this warning may extend to other viral URIs. Many providers do not use it as an antipyretic for any children because there are other drugs that do not carry the concern about Reye syndrome. Acetaminophen or ibuprofen is probably better for fever management in children. Adults' and children's doses of aspirin are shown in Table 25-12.

Diflunisal is not recommended as an antipyretic. In single doses, it reduces fever in some patients but not in a clinically significant amount.

Table 25–11 ⣿ Drug Interactions: Salicylates

Drug	Interacting Drug	Possible Effect	Implications
Acetylsalicylic acid	Angiotensin-converting enzyme inhibitors, beta adrenergic blockers	Decreased antihypertensive effect because of prostaglandin inhibition	Consider discontinuing salicylate or selecting different antihypertensive
	Heparin, warfarin	Prolonged bleeding time, impaired platelet function	Avoid concurrent use
	Nitroglycerin	Unexpected hypotensive effects	Reduce nitroglycerin dose
	NSAIDs	Aspirin may decrease serum concentrations	Avoid concomitant use; no therapeutic advantage and may increase risk for GI bleed
All salicylates	Alcohol, cefamandole, cefoperazone, cefotetan, valproic acid, plicamycin	Increased risk for GI bleeding	Avoid alcohol while taking salicylates; select different antimicrobial or avoid use of salicylate
	Loop diuretics, aminoglycosides, bumetanide, ethacrynic acid	May increase risk for ototoxicity	Avoid concurrent use or monitor for tinnitus, hearing loss
	Probenecid, sulfinpyrazone	Salicylates antagonize uricosuric effects	Avoid concurrent use
	Spironolactone	Salicylates inhibit diuretic effects	Avoid concurrent use
	Sulfonylureas	Salicylates in doses >2 g/d have hypoglycemic effect; potentiate glucose-lowering effect	Select different drug combination
	Penicillins, phenytoin, methotrexate, valproic acid, sulfonamide	May enhance effects of these drugs	Monitor for potential dosage adjustments
	Foods that acidify urine*	Decreases renal excretion and increases serum levels of salicylates	May increase risk for toxicity
	Foods that alkalinize urine*	Increases renal excretion and decreases serum levels of salicylates	May be used therapeutically to treat overdose
Diflunisal	Acetaminophen	Concurrent administration may result in 50% increase in acetaminophen levels	Increased risk for hepatotoxicity; avoid concurrent use
	Heparin, warfarin	Competitively displaces warfarin from protein-binding sites; increased risk for bleeding	Avoid concurrent use; monitor PT/INR closely
	Hydrochlorothiazide (HCTZ)	Significantly decreased HCTZ plasma levels	Avoid concurrent use
	Aspirin, NSAIDs, colchicine, glucocorticoids, alcohol	Additive risk for GI bleeding	Avoid concurrent use
	Lithium	May increase serum lithium levels	Select different salicylate
	Probenecid	Increased risk of diflunisal toxicity	Avoid concurrent use or monitor closely for indications of toxicity
	Antacids	Concurrent administration decreases absorption of diflunisal	Separate administration by at least 1 h
	Indomethacin	Decreased renal clearance and significantly increased indomethacin serum levels	Avoid concurrent use
	Sulindac	Increased renal clearance and significantly decreased sulindac serum levels	Avoid concurrent use

INR = international normalized ratio; PT = prothrombin time.

*Foods that alkalinize urine: all fruits except cranberries, prunes, plums; all vegetables; milk. Foods that acidify urine: cheeses, cranberries, eggs, fish, grains, meats, plums, poultry, and prunes.

Mild to Moderate Pain

Pain associated with inflammation is especially well managed with salicylates or NSAIDs. Aspirin, choline salicylate, choline magnesium salicylate, and diflunisal are all approved for this indication. Aspirin is the gold standard against which others are judged. It is inexpensive, available OTC, the most potent analgesic in the class, and short-acting, so acute pain can be managed without long-term effects and adverse reactions. It has limitations, however. It is Pregnancy Category D, especially in the third trimester and contraindicated in children with influenza or chickenpox.

Diflunisal offers the advantage of analgesia comparable with that of aspirin, with longer-lasting responses. Like the other drugs in this group, it can be used for this indication, but all four are more often used to treat arthritic conditions.

Rheumatoid Arthritis

Salicylates or NSAIDs can be used as adjunctive treatment for RA. Serum levels can easily be measured to determine adherence and therapeutic efficacy, and it is the least expensive salicylate. Nonacetylated salicylates are less potent anti-inflammatory agents, but they have fewer adverse reactions

Table 25–12 ✂ **Dosage Schedule: Salicylates**

Drug	Indication	Dosage Forms	Dose	Comments
Acetylsalicylic acid (aspirin) (Bayer Aspirin)	Fever, pain, headache, dysmenorrhea Rheumatoid arthritis, osteoarthritis Juvenile rheumatoid arthritis Acute rheumatic fever Transient ischemic attack Myocardial infarction prophylaxis	Tablets: 325 mg Chewable tablets: 81 mg Enteric-coated tablets: 325 mg Timed-release tablets: 650 mg Caplets: 325 mg, 500 mg Tablets: 325 mg, 500 mg Enteric-coated tablets: 325 mg, 650 mg, 975 mg Suppository: 120, 200, 300, 600 mg	*Adults:* 325–650 mg every 4 h; with extra-strength may use 500 mg every 3 h *or* 1 g every 6 h; not to exceed 4 g/d *Children 2–11 yr:* 65 mg/kg/d in 4–6 divided doses* *Adults:* 3.2–6 g/d in divided doses *Children <25 kg:* 60–110 mg/kg/d in divided doses (every 6–8 h); start with 60 mg/kg/d and increase by 20 mg/kg/d after 5–7 d, then increase by 10 mg/kg/d after another 5–7 d *Children >25 kg:* 50–60 mg/kg/d with a similar dosing increase schedule *Adults:* 5–8 g/d initially in 3–4 divided doses; increase dose to reach serum salicylate level of 15–30 mg/mL; not to exceed 8 g/d *Children:* 100 mg/kg/d for 2 wk, then decrease to 75 mg/kg/d for 4–6 wk; not to exceed 130 mg/kg/d *Adults:* 50–325 mg/d *Adults:* 81–160 mg/d	*Use cautiously in children Toxicity risk increased at this dose Maintain a serum salicylate level of 15–30 mg/mL for anti-inflammatory effects Aspirin combined with extended-release dipyridamole is recommended over aspirin alone
Choline magnesium salicylate (Trilisate)	Fever, pain, rheumatoid arthritis	Tablets: 500, 750 mg, 1 g Liquid: 500 mg/5 mL	*Adults:* 2–3 g/d in divided doses or 150 mg bid *Children >37 kg:* 2.2 g/d in 2 divided doses* *Children <37 kg:* 50 mg/d in 2 divided doses*	Has fewer adverse reactions than aspirin
Salsalate (Disalsid)	Rheumatic conditions	Capsules: 500 mg Tablets: 500 mg, 750 mg	*Adults:* 1,500 mg bid *or* 750 mg qid; not to exceed 4 g/d	
Diflunisal (Dolobid)	Mild to moderate pain Osteoarthritis	Tablets: 250, 500 mg	*Adults:* 1 g initially, followed by 500 mg every 8–12 h *Adults:* 500 mg–1 g/d in two divided doses; not to exceed 1.5 g/d	Half this dose initially and following may be effective

*Dosing schedules are published for analgesia and fever reduction. Use cautiously. Not recommended for children with influenza or chickenpox because of risk for Reye syndrome.

than aspirin. The main disadvantages of aspirin are the high incidence of GI intolerance (take with food or use enteric-coated tablets), the inconvenience of taking four or five doses daily, and the relatively long interval (4 to 7 d) before a full anti-inflammatory effect is reached. A therapy trial of 3 to 4 g/d for 4 to 6 days is recommended, because 70% to 80% of patients who will respond will do so within this time frame. Older adults are predictably less tolerant to the adverse GI reactions, and their trial dose should be 2 to 3 g/d. If the response is inadequate and adherence has been good, a salicylate level should be drawn before changing drugs. If the drug level is within therapeutic parameters (20 to 25 mg/dL

in adults; 15 to 20 mg/dL in older adults) without adequate response, or if the drug is not tolerated, another drug should be tried. If the salicylate level is too low but the patient has been adherent and tolerates the aspirin, the dose should be increased by 325 to 650 mg/d until the desired anti-inflammatory level of the drug is reached.

The margin is narrow between a good therapeutic level and toxicity in treating patients with RA because the dose is higher than that used for fever or analgesia. The earliest manifestation of toxicity is tinnitus or mild deafness. Aspirin should be stopped immediately if these symptoms occur. Once they abate, it may be restarted at a lower dose, or an

NSAID may be chosen. Toxicity is discussed in the Adverse Reactions section.

For patients whose main reason for discontinuing aspirin is GI intolerance, salsalate is a good alternative. It can be given in twice-daily dosing and has a much lower incidence of GI bleeding. Choline salicylate and choline magnesium salicylate can also be used and may be given in 2 to 4 times daily dosing.

Osteoarthritis

Patients with OA may present occasionally with acute or subacute painful episodes in which the underlying problem is inflammation. No drugs have proven efficacy in altering the course of OA, but both salicylates and NSAIDs are used successfully to treat the pain associated with these exacerbations. Aspirin is an effective analgesic and anti-inflammatory that is usually well tolerated in divided doses of 1.2 to 2.4 g/d. NSAIDs tend to have more adverse reactions with no better pain relief when given at anti-inflammatory doses over the course of more than a few days. Acetaminophen is helpful for analgesia but has no anti-inflammatory effects.

The nonacetylated salicylates are also effective and have fewer GI adverse reactions than aspirin. Diflunisal has the advantage of twice-daily dosing but may take up to 2 weeks to achieve full anti-inflammatory effects. Although it is more expensive than aspirin, the cost may approach that of many of the NSAIDs. Discussion of NSAIDs is in the section preceding this one.

Juvenile Rheumatoid Arthritis

Juvenile RA is an autoimmune disease that occurs in four different forms, all of which are characterized by joint inflammation. Pediatric specialists generally follow children with the disorder and determine their treatment protocol. Salicylates and NSAIDs are commonly part of this protocol.

Aspirin is prescribed in daily doses of 60 to 110 mg/kg for children. NSAIDs are prescribed if the child does not respond to or cannot tolerate aspirin therapy.

Nonacetylated salicylates are not indicated for treatment of juvenile forms of RA.

Acute Rheumatic Fever

Acute rheumatic fever is usually a sequela of group A beta-hemolytic streptococcal infection. Rheumatic fever incidence is 0.1 to 0.2 cases per 100,000 persons in Canada, the United States, and western Europe (Madden & Kelly, 2009). There is a higher incidence (10 to 20 cases/100,000) of rheumatic fever in emerging economies, indigenous peoples, and tropical regions (Madden & Kelly). Acute rheumatic fever is treated with antimicrobials, but the inflammatory manifestations are treated with aspirin. Although this disorder is more common in children, it can also occur in adults. Dosage schedules for both are presented in Table 25-12.

Myocardial Infarction Prophylaxis

The American College of Chest Physicians (ACCP) Guidelines for Primary and Secondary Prevention of Cardiovascular Disease recommend low-dose aspirin (75 to 100 mg/d) in patients age 50 years or older for primary prevention of cardiovascular disease (Vandvick et al, 2012). The ACCP guidelines recommend low-dose aspirin (75 to 100 mg daily) or clopidogrel in patients with established coronary artery disease, patients with coronary stenosis greater than 50%, and those with evidence of cardiac ischemia. Aspirin (75 to 10 mg/d) is combined with ticagrelor or clopidogrel for the first year after coronary stent placement (Vandvick et al, 2012).

Transient Ischemic Attacks

The American Heart Association/American Stroke Association recommends the use of aspirin for the prevention of stroke in patients with stroke and transient ischemic attack (Kernan et al, 2014). Aspirin (50 to 325 mg/d) monotherapy or a combination of aspirin and extended-release dipyridamole are accepted therapy options for stroke prevention (Kernan et al, 2012). Clopidogrel and its dosing for this indication are discussed in Chapter 18. Dosing schedules for aspirin for each indication are presented in Table 25-12.

Rational Drug Selection

Rational drug selection is based largely on indication, cost, and convenience of therapy. All of these are discussed in the Clinical Use and Dosing section.

Monitoring

A random salicylate level should be drawn 7 to 10 days after initiation of chronic therapy. Periodic salicylate levels should be drawn during long-term management to check maintenance of therapeutic levels and monitor for toxic manifestations.

Because all of these drugs are eliminated by the kidneys and dosage adjustments may be required based on renal function, serum creatinine levels should be assessed before therapy is begun and annually throughout long-term therapy. Urinary pH should also be monitored regularly. Sudden acidification of urine can more than double the plasma salicylate level, resulting in toxicity.

Salicylates interfere with homeostasis. A CBC should be drawn prior to initiating therapy and at least annually throughout long-term therapy. A CBC should also be drawn and fecal occult blood studies should be done as well if there is any indication of GI bleeding.

Hepatic function should be monitored prior to antirheumatic therapy and if hepatotoxicity symptoms occur. These problems are more likely in patients with rheumatic fever, juvenile RA, or preexisting hepatic diseases, especially children.

Ophthalmic effects have been reported in patients taking diflunisal. Ophthalmic studies are appropriate for patients who develop eye complaints during therapy.

Patient Education

Administration

Instruct the patient to take salicylates exactly as prescribed. Taking with food or a full glass of water and remaining in an upright position for 15 to 30 minutes after administration can reduce GI irritation. Food slows absorption but does not alter the total amount absorbed.

Remind patients not to crush or chew enteric-coated tablets or take antacids within 1 hour of enteric-coated tablets. Chewable tablets may be chewed, dissolved in liquid, or swallowed whole. Tablets with a vinegar-like odor (acetic acid) should be discarded.

Instruct patients not to increase the dose beyond that prescribed. Increased doses increase the risk for salicylate poisoning. For patients taking aspirin for MI or TIA prophylaxis, increasing the dose has not proved to provide additional benefits but does increase the risk for adverse reactions.

Adverse Reactions

The most common adverse reactions are ototoxicity and GI irritation and bleeding. Advise patients to report tinnitus; unusual bleeding from the gums; bruising; black, tarry stools; or fever lasting longer than 3 days. Patients who are taking salicylates should not use alcohol or other substances that increase GI irritation.

Reye syndrome practically disappeared after the Centers for Disease Control and Prevention (CDC) started warning against giving aspirin to children or adolescents with influenza, influenza-like syndromes, or chickenpox (varicella) because of a possible association with Reye syndrome, a "public health triumph" (Monto, 1999). Parents should be informed of the risk of Reye syndrome and educated regarding not giving aspirin to a child with a viral illness.

Lifestyle Management

Rest, heat, exercise, and other lifestyle modifications are part of the management of arthritic conditions. The modifications are as important as the pharmacological management and should be stressed.

REFERENCES

Adams, R. J., Albers, G., Alberts, M. J., Benavente, O., Furie, K., Goldstein, L. B., et al. (2008). Update to the AHA/ASA recommendations for the prevention of stroke in patients with stroke and transient ischemic attack. *Stroke, 39,* 1647–1652.

Agency for Healthcare Research and Quality. (2009). *Three treatments for osteoarthritis of the knee: Evidence shows lack of benefit* [AHRQ Publication No. 09-EHC001-3]. Rockville, MD: AHRQ Publications Clearinghouse. Retrieved from http://www.effectivehealthcare.ahrq.gov/ehc/index.cfm/search-for-guides-reviews-and-reports/?pageAction=displayProduct&productID=134#512

American Academy of Orthopedic Surgeons. (2008). Guideline on the treatment of osteoarthritis (OA) of the knee. American Association of Orthopedic Surgeons. Retrieved from http://www.aaos.org/research/guidelines/guidelineoaknee.asp

Anderson, J., Adams, C., Antman, E., Bridges, C., Califf, R., Casey, D., et al. (2007). ACC/AHA 2007 guidelines for the management of patients with unstable angina/non-ST-elevation myocardial infarction: A report of the American College of Cardiology/American Heart Association Task Force on Practice Guidelines (Writing Committee to Revise the 2002 Guidelines for the Management of Patients With Unstable Angina/Non-ST-Elevation Myocardial Infarction) developed in collaboration with the American College of Emergency Physicians, the Society for Cardiovascular Angiography and Interventions, and the Society of Thoracic Surgeons endorsed by the American Association of Cardiovascular and Pulmonary Rehabilitation and the Society for Academic Emergency Medicine. *Journal of the American College of Cardiology, 50*(7), e1–e157. Retrieved from MEDLINE database.

Bolooki, H. M., & Askari, A. (2009). Acute myocardial infarction. *Cleveland Clinic Center for Continuing Education.* Retrieved from http://www.clevelandclinicmeded.com/medicalpubs/diseasemanagement/cardiology/acute-myocardial-infarction/#s0080

Centers for Disease Control and Prevention (CDC). (2011). Arthritis: Gout. Retrieved from http://www.cdc.gov/arthritis/basics/gout.htm

Centers for Disease Control and Prevention (CDC). (2013). Prevalence of doctor-diagnosed arthritis and arthritis-attributable activity limitation—United States, 2010–2012. *Morbidity and Mortality Weekly Report, 62*(44), 869–873.

Feldman, M., & Das, S. (2010). NSAIDs (including aspirin): Primary prevention of gastroduodenal toxicity. *UpToDate Online.* Retrieved from http://www.uptodate.com/online/content/topic.do?topicKey=acidpep/9491&selectedTitle=10~150&source=search_result#H12

Food and Drug Administration (FDA). (2014). Acetaminophen prescription combination drug products with more than 325 mg: FDA Statement—Recommendation to discontinue prescribing and dispensing. Retrieved from http://www.fda.gov/safety/medwatch/safetyinformation/safetyalertsforhumanmedicalproducts/ucm381650.htm

Grossman, J. M., Gordon, R., Ranganath, V. K., Deal, C., Caplan, L., Chen, W., et al. (2010). American College of Rheumatology 2010 recommendations for the prevention and treatment of glucocorticoid-induced osteoporosis. *Arthritis Care & Research, 62*(11), 1515–1526.

Hochberg, M. C., Altman, R. D., April, K. T., Benkhalti, M., Guyatt, G., McGowan, J., et al. (2012). American College of Rheumatology 2012 Recommendations for the use of nonpharmacologic and pharmacologic therapies in osteoarthritis of the hand, hip and knee. *Arthritis Care & Research, 64*(4), 465–474.

Hsiang, K. W., Lu, C. L., Chen, T. S., Lin, H. Y., Luo, J. C., Wu, J. M., et al. (2010). Corticosteroids therapy and peptic ulcer disease in nephrotic syndrome patients. *British Journal of Clinical Pharmacology, 70*(5), 756–761.

Kernan, W. N., Ovbiagele, B., Black, H. R., Bravata, D. M., Cimowitz, M. I., Ezekowitz, M.D., et al. (2014). Guidelines for the prevention of stroke in patients with stroke and transient ischemic attack: A guideline for healthcare professionals from the American Heart Association/American Stroke Association. *Stroke,* Published online May 1, 2014. http://stroke.ahajournals.org/content/early/2014/04/30/STR.0000000000000024

Klauer, K. M. (2009). Adrenal insufficiency and adrenal crisis: Treatment & medication. *eMedicine.* Retrieved from http://emedicine.medscape.com/article/765753-treatment

LactMed. (2013). Prednisone. Drug and Lactation Database: LactMed. Bethesda, MD. National Library of Medicine. Retrieved from http://toxnet.nlm.nih.gov/

Lawrence, R. C., Felson, D. T., Helmick, C. G., Arnold, L. M., Choi, H., Deyo, R. A., et al, for the National Arthritis Data Workgroup. (2008). Estimates of the prevalence of arthritis and other rheumatic conditions in the United States. *Arthritis & Rheumatism, 58*(1), 26–35.

McCance, K., & Huether, S. (2010). *Pathophysiology: The biological basis for disease in adults and children* (6th ed.). St. Louis, MO: Elsevier Mosby.

Monto, A. S. (1999). The disappearance of Reye's syndrome—A public health triumph. *New England Journal of Medicine, 340,* 1423–1424.

Saag, K. G., & Furst, D. E. (2010). Major side effects of systemic glucocorticoids. *UpToDate.* Retrieved from http://www.uptodate.com/online/content/topic.do?topicKey=treatme/6535&selectedTitle=1~150&source=search_result#H11

Schur, P. H., & Cohen, S. (2014). *UpToDate Online.* Retrieved from http://www.uptodate.com/contents/initial-treatment-of-moderately-to-severely-active-rheumatoid-arthritis-in-adults

Singh, J. A., Furst, D. E., Bharat, A., Curtis, J. R., Kavanaugh, F., Kremer, J. M., et al. (2012). 2012 update of the 2008 American College of

Rheumatology recommendations for the use of disease-modifying antirheumatic drugs and biologic agents in the treatment of rheumatoid arthritis. *Arthritis Care & Research, 64*(5), 625–639.

Terkeltaub, R. A., Furst, D. E., Bennett, K. A., Crockett, R. S., & Davis, M. W. (2010). High versus low dosing of oral colchicines for early acute gout flare: Twenty-four-hour outcomes of the first multicenter, randomized, double-blind, placebo-controlled, parallel-group, dose-comparison colchicines study. *Arthritis and Rheumatism, 62*(4), 1060–1068.

Vandvick, P. O., Lincoff, A. M., Gore, J. M., Gutterman, D. D., Sonnenberg, F. A., Alonso-Coello, P., et al. (2012). Primary and secondary prevention of cardiovascular disease. Antithrombotic therapy and prevention of thrombosis, 9th ed: American College of Chest Physicians Evidence-Based Clinical Practice Guidelines. *Chest, 141*(2 Suppl.), e637S–e668S.

Zhu, Y., Pandya, B. J., & Choi, H. K. (2011). Prevalence of gout and hyperuircemia in the US general population: The National Health and Nutrition Examination Survey 2007–2008. *Arthritis & Rheumatism, 63*(10), 3136–3141.

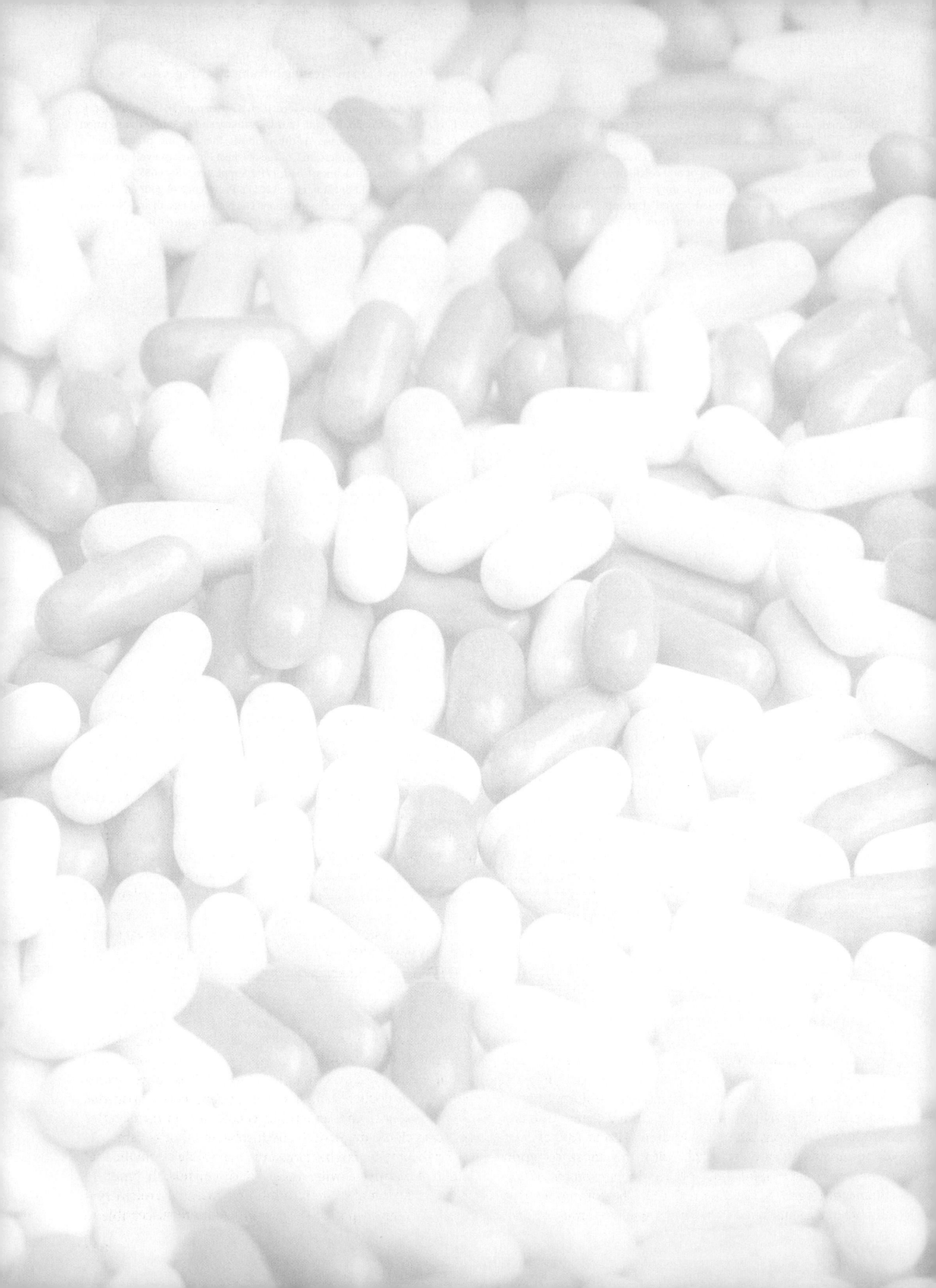

CHAPTER 26

DRUGS USED IN TREATING EYE AND EAR DISORDERS

Teri Moser Woo

This chapter discusses the medications used to treat eye and ear disorders, including the common anti-infective agents for conjunctivitis, the medications used for allergic conjunctivitis, and common anti-inflammatory agents used for ocular inflammation. Although primary care providers may not prescribe some of the glaucoma medications, many drugs interact with these ophthalmic medications and therefore a basic understanding of these agents is necessary and included. Eye lubricants and vasoconstrictors are discussed here. The use of fluorescein, a diagnostic agent commonly used in primary care, is also addressed in this chapter. The ear medications discussed here include the anti-infectives, analgesics, and ceruminolytics.

DRUGS USED IN TREATING EYE DISORDERS

OPHTHALMIC ANTI-INFECTIVES

Common eye infections that are treated by primary care providers include bacterial conjunctivitis, viral conjunctivitis, blepharitis, and hordeolum. An estimated 4 million cases of bacterial conjunctivitis occur in the United States annually (Smith & Waycaster, 2009). In children, 54% to 73% of cases of conjunctivitis are bacterial, with the most common pathogens being *H. influenzae* (29%) and *S. pneumoniae* (20%) (Buznach, Dagan, & Greenberg, 2005). The commonly used antibacterial agents for conjunctivitis are sulfacetamide sodium

(Bleph-10), bacitracin, erythromycin (Ilotycin), tobramycin (Tobrex), gentamicin (Garamycin, Genoptic), azithromycin (AzaSite) and the fluoroquinolones besifloxacin (Besivance), ciprofloxacin (Ciloxan), gatifloxacin (Zymar, Zymaxid), levofloxacin (Iquix), moxifloxacin (Moxeza, Vigamox), norfloxacin (Chibroxin, Noroxin), and ofloxacin (Ocuflox). The combination drugs Polytrim (polymyxin b/trimethoprim) and Polysporin (polymyxin b/bacitracin) Ophthalmic may also be used and are discussed here. Chloramphenicol (Chloroptic) is rarely used in primary care because of its adverse effects. More serious infectious eye disorders such as herpes simplex virus (HSV) infection, keratitis, and corneal ulcers are treated by ophthalmologists and, therefore, are not covered at great length in this chapter, although the antiviral agents that may be used to treat viral eye infections are briefly discussed.

Pharmacodynamics

Ophthalmic antibiotics may be bacteriostatic or bactericidal. Bacitracin is bacteriostatic and inhibits the incorporation of amino acids and nucleotides into the cell. It is active against many gram-positive (staphylococci, streptococci, clostridia, corynebacteria, and anaerobic cocci) and gram-negative (gonococci, meningococci, and fusobacteria) organisms.

Erythromycin is a bacteriostatic macrolide antibiotic that is active against a wide range of organisms. It binds to the 50S ribosomal subunit, inhibiting bacterial protein synthesis. The gram-positive organisms that are susceptible to erythromycin include *Staphylococcus aureus, Streptococcus pyogenes, S. pneumoniae,* the *Streptococcus viridans* group, and *Corynebacterium diphtheriae.* Erythromycin has limited gram-negative coverage. It is also active against *Chlamydia trachomatis.*

Sulfacetamide is a synthetic sulfonamide that inhibits bacterial dihydrofolate synthetase. It is active against the following susceptible organisms: streptococci, staphylococci, *Escherichia coli, Klebsiella pneumoniae, Pseudomonas pyocyanea, Neisseria gonorrhoeae,* and *C. trachomatis.*

Tobramycin is a broad-spectrum aminoglycoside. The exact mechanism by which it is bactericidal is unknown. It is active against staphylococci, streptococci, *Corynebacterium* species, *K. pneumoniae, Moraxella* species, *Proteus* species, beta-hemolytic streptococci, and *Haemophilus influenzae.* Tobramycin ophthalmic is not active against *N. gonorrhoeae* or *C. trachomatis.*

Gentamicin is a broad-spectrum antibiotic that is active against a wide range of gram-positive and gram-negative organisms. It is unclear how gentamicin causes cell death. It is active against staphylococci, *S. pneumoniae,* beta-hemolytic streptococci, *E. coli, H. influenzae, N. gonorrhoeae,* and *Enterobacter* species.

Azithromycin (AzaSite) is a macrolide antibiotic active against both gram-positive and gram-negative organisms. The manufacturer's premarketing studies indicated that azithromycin drops eradicated 88% of gram-positive bacteria and 92% of gram-negative bacteria in randomized controlled trials (RCT), including 93% of *H. influenzae,* a common pathogen in pediatric conjunctivitis (Inspire Pharmaceuticals, 2008).

The fluoroquinolones besifloxacin, ciprofloxacin, garifloxacin, levofloxacin, moxifloxacin, norfloxacin, and ofloxacin are bactericidal via inhibition of DNA gyrase. It is unclear how inhibition of DNA gyrase leads to cell death. The fluoroquinolones are active against staphylococci, *S. pneumoniae, H. influenzae, K. pneumoniae, Proteus* species, *Enterobacter* species, and *Pseudomonas aeruginosa.*

Polytrim is an ophthalmic antibacterial preparation that combines polymyxin B and trimethoprim. Polymyxin B binds to cell membranes with high affinity, specifically the phospholipids in the cell wall. This causes increased cellular permeability. Polymyxin B is generally active against gram-negative bacteria (*E. coli, P. aeruginosa, H. influenzae*). Trimethoprim inhibits bacterial dihydrofolate reductase. Trimethoprim has both gram-positive and gram-negative activity. Trimethoprim is active against *S. aureus, S. pneumoniae,* and *S. pyogenes.*

Polysporin Ophthalmic contains polymyxin B and bacitracin. This combination provides activity against gram-positive and gram-negative bacterial organisms, as discussed previously.

Antiviral ophthalmic agents that may be prescribed by an ophthalmologist are gancyclovir (Zirgan), vidarabine (Vira-A), and trifluridine (Viroptic). Gancyclovir inhibits replication by herpes simplex viruses by inhibiting the synthesis of viral DNA. Vidarabine inhibits viral DNA replication, although the exact mechanism of action is not known. Vidarabine has antiviral activity against HSV types 1 and 2, varicella-zoster virus, cytomegalovirus, vaccinia, and hepatitis B. The exact mechanism

of action of trifluridine is not known, although it is thought to interfere with DNA synthesis. Trifluridine is active against HSV-1 and HSV-2, adenovirus, and vaccinia virus.

Pharmacokinetics

Ophthalmic antibiotic and antiviral preparations generally penetrate only the ocular fluid and tissues. Systemic absorption is minimal, although there may be enough absorption for sensitization to occur, specifically with sulfacetamide. There is no information regarding the metabolism and excretion of ophthalmic anti-infectives.

Pharmacotherapeutics

Precautions and Contraindications

Hypersensitivity to any component of the preparation is a contraindication to its use. There may be cross-sensitivity between the individual aminoglycosides (tobramycin and gentamicin). The same is found with the fluoroquinolones.

The vehicles used in ophthalmic ointments may retard corneal healing after ocular trauma or ocular surgery. Improvements in ophthalmic ointment vehicles have changed this situation for the better, but manufacturers still warn that many preparations may retard corneal healing.

Purulent exudates that contain para-aminobenzoic acid may inactivate sulfacetamide antibacterial activity.

Antibacterial agents are not effective against fungal infection, viral infection, or all types of bacterial infection. If the patient is not responding to therapy, reevaluation, including appropriate cultures, is indicated.

Erythromycin, azithromycin, and tobramycin ophthalmic preparations are Pregnancy Category B. Gentamicin, ciprofloxacin, gatifloxacin, levofloxacin, moxifloxin, norfloxacin, ofloxacin, polymyxin B, and sulfacetamide are Pregnancy Category C. The antiviral ophthalmic agents gancyclovir, vidarabine, and trifluridine are all Pregnancy Category C. Safety for use during pregnancy has not been determined.

The use of the sulfacetamides and the fluoroquinolones should be avoided during lactation because they are harmful to the infant and breast milk excretion is unknown.

Erythromycin and tobramycin are safe and effective in children. The safety of the fluoroquinolones (besifloxacin, ciprofloxacin, gatifloxacin, moxifloxacin [Vigamox], levofloxacin, norfloxacin, ofloxacin, and besifloxacin) and azithromycin in children under age 1 has not been established. Moxifloxacin (Moxeza) is approved for children 4 months of age and older. Sulfacetamide and polymyxin B/bacitracin should not be prescribed to infants younger than 2 months.

Adverse Drug Reactions

All of the ophthalmic anti-infective preparations may cause local irritation, which is usually transient. Irritation may include burning, itching, and inflammation. Superinfection may occur with prolonged or repeated use of ophthalmic anti-infectives.

Bacitracin may cause blurred vision, which usually lasts only a few minutes.

Sulfacetamide ophthalmic preparations may cause a hypersensitivity reaction in patients who have previously exhibited sensitivity to sulfonamides. Stevens–Johnson syndrome is a rare adverse reaction that has been reported with sulfacetamide ophthalmic ointment use. Fever, bone marrow depression, and lupus erythematosus may rarely occur with sulfonamides, including topical preparations. There may be intense burning and stinging, especially with the 30% sulfacetamide sodium solution (Sulamyd 30%).

Aminoglycosides may cause localized ocular toxicity and hypersensitivity.

The fluoroquinolones may cause a white crystalline precipitate to form in the superficial portion of the cornea. This was observed in about 17% of the patients on ciprofloxacin. Lid margin crusting, crystals, scales, and the sensation of a foreign body in the eye are also reported with ophthalmic fluoroquinolones. Patients also report a bitter or bad taste in the mouth, specifically with ciprofloxacin solution. Fluoroquinolones may also cause photophobia, tearing, nausea, decreased vision, conjunctival hyperemia, and corneal staining.

The ophthalmic antiviral preparations may cause burning and irritation on instillation into the eye. Gancyclovir may cause blurred vision, punctate keratitis, and conjunctival hyperemia. Vidarabine may also cause photophobia, pruritus, erythema, ocular pain, and, less commonly, increased lacrimation. Patients who are using ophthalmic vidarabine may develop superficial punctate keratitis after exposure to ultraviolet (UV) light, and they should wear sunglasses to protect their eyes when exposed to bright light. Trifluridine has adverse reactions similar to those of vidarabine, with the addition of reported increases in intraocular pressure (IOP).

Drug Interactions

There are no drug interactions reported for ophthalmic preparations of bacitracin, gentamicin, tobramycin, polymyxin B, azithromycin, and erythromycin.

Sulfacetamide is incompatible with silver-containing preparations and should not be used in conjunction with ophthalmic products containing silver salts, including silver nitrate. Concomitant use of ophthalmic sulfacetamide with zinc sulfate causes a precipitate to form. Ester-type local anesthetics including benzocaine, chloroprocaine, cocaine, procaine, propoxycaine, and tetracaine should not be used concurrently with sulfacetamide because they can antagonize the therapeutic actions of the sulfonamide.

The fluoroquinolones (besifloxicin, ciprofloxacin, gatifloxacin, moxifloxacin, levofloxacin, norfloxacin, and ofloxacin) may increase theophylline levels and potentiate oral anticoagulants if significant systemic absorption occurs. These interactions are theoretical with ophthalmic use of fluoroquinolones, in that little is known regarding the amount of medication that is systemically absorbed and whether enough is absorbed to cause a drug interaction.

Table 26-1 presents drug interactions with ophthalmic anti-infectives.

Table 26–1 ⬛ Drug Interactions: Ophthalmic Anti-Infectives

Drug	Interacting Drug	Possible Effect	Implications
Sulfacetamide sodium	Silver preparations	Incompatibility	Do not use concurrently
Erythromycin	None reported		
Tobramycin	None reported		
Gentamicin	None reported		
Gatifloxacin	Theophylline, caffeine, oval anticoagulants	May raise serum levels	Monitor PT/INR levels
Levofloxacin	Theophylline, caffeine, oval anticoagulants	May raise level of these drugs	Monitor INR/PT levels
Moxifloxacin	None reported		
Norfloxacin	Warfarin, theophylline, cyclosporine	May raise levels of these systemic drugs	Monitor theophylline level and PT/PTT times
Ciprofloxacin	Warfarin, theophylline, cyclosporine	May raise levels of these systemic drugs; may increase renal toxicity from cyclosporine	Monitor theophylline level
Ofloxacin	Warfarin, theophylline, caffeine, cyclosporine	May raise levels of these systemic drugs; may increase renal toxicity from cyclosporine	Monitor PT/INR levels closely
Polymyxin B–trimethoprim	None reported		
Polymyxin B-bacitracin ophthalmic	None reported		

PT = prothrombin time; PTT = partial thromboplastin time; INR = international normalized ratio.

Clinical Use and Dosing

Conjunctivitis

The common organisms that are associated with bacterial conjunctivitis vary with the age of the patient. Newborns should be evaluated for ophthalmia neonatorum. Preschool children most commonly have bacterial conjunctivitis, with viral etiology (adenovirus) more likely in schoolchildren. *N. gonorrhoeae* conjunctivitis should be excluded in sexually active adolescents and adults. Adults may have viral or bacterial conjunctivitis. Chlamydia is seen in the neonate and sexually active teen and adult. Table 26-2 presents the clinical and laboratory features of conjunctivitis.

Ophthalmia Neonatorum

Any infant younger than 1 month who presents with conjunctivitis should have Gram's stain, antigen detection tests, and cultures of the eye discharge to rule out gonococcal, chlamydial, or HSV origin. Chlamydia is the most common cause of neonatal conjunctivitis (American Academy of Pediatrics [AAP], 2012a). Gonococcal conjunctivitis is the most serious cause of ophthalmia neonatorum owing to concerns about the bacteria causing blindness (AAP, 2012a). In the newborn, gonococcal conjunctivitis requires intramuscular (IM) ceftriaxone (50 mg/kg, maximum 125 mg) given once (AAP, 2012b). If there are extraocular manifestations, a 7-day course of IM or IV ceftriaxone is warranted. Ceftriaxone is not given to neonates with hyperbilirubinemia; cefotaxime (50 to 100 mg/kg/d divided bid for 7 d) is an alternative used in neonates with hyperbilirubinemia (AAP, 2012b). To prevent ophthalmia neonatorum, the Centers for Disease Control and Prevention (CDC) and the U.S. Preventive Services Task Force recommend prophylactic administration of antibiotic eye medication within 1 hour of delivery (CDC, 2010; US Preventive Services Task Force, 2011). The recommended antibiotic is erythromycin ointment 0.5% (0.25 to 0.5 inch ribbon in each eye).

Chlamydial conjunctivitis in the newborn requires treatment with systemic erythromycin (30–50 mg/kg/d) for 2 to 3 weeks; topical treatment is ineffective (AAP, 2012c). A short course of azithromycin 20 mg/kg per day for 3 days may also be effective (AAP, 2012c). Chlamydial conjunctivitis is not prevented by prophylactic use of erythromycin at birth; therefore, any mucopurulent eye discharge in the first few weeks of life should be evaluated for chlamydia.

Bacterial Conjunctivitis

Children between ages 3 months and 8 years are most likely to have staphylococcal, streptococcal, or *Haemophilus* conjunctivitis. Nontypable *H. influenzae* is seen more in warmer climates between May and October. *S. pneumoniae* is seen in colder climates and during the winter. *S. aureus* shows no geographic or seasonal pattern. In studies of children with acute bacterial conjunctivitis, *H. influenzae* is the most common organism isolated in children younger than 7 years (Buznach et al, 2005; Hautala, Hautala, & Koskela, 2008). *S. aureus* and *Pseudomonas aeruginosa* are the most common pathogens in the elderly (older than age 70) (Hautala et al, 2008).

Although bacterial conjunctivitis is considered a self-limited disease (unless caused by gonorrhea), patients who receive topical antibiotic therapy have faster clinical improvement. When conjunctivitis prevents the patient from going to school or work, antibiotics can speed the recovery. Most schools require treatment for the child to return to school.

Uncomplicated conjunctivitis may be treated with sulfacetamide 10% ophthalmic solution or ointment, erythromycin ointment, trimethoprim/polymyxin B (Polytrim), or bacitracin/polymyxin B (Polysporin). Sulfacetamide gives no

Table 26–2 Clinical and Laboratory Features of Conjunctivitis

Type	Common Patient Group	Common Pathogens	Clinical Features
Ophthalmia neonatorum	Infants <1 mo	*Neisseria gonorrhoeae*, *Chlamydia*	Erythema, purulent exudate, chemosis
Bacterial conjunctivitis	Most common in children between 3 mo and 8 yr; can happen at any age	*H. influenzae* *S. aureus* *S. pneumonia*	Erythema, purulent discharge, itching, burning, matted eyelashes
Conjunctivitis-otitis syndrome	Predominantly in children <6 yr	*H. influenzae* (~82% of patients)	Bacterial conjunctivitis accompanied by otitis media
Gonococcal conjunctivitis	Newborns, sexually promiscuous teens, and adults	*N. gonorrhoeae*	Eye is markedly inflamed, with copious discharge and swollen lids
Blepharitis	Any age group	May be infected with *S. aureus*	Chronic or acute inflammation of the eyelash follicles
Hordeolum	Any age group	*S. aureus*	Tender, swollen red furuncle along eyelid margin
Viral conjunctivitis	Any age group, most common in children	Adenovirus Herpes simplex virus	Redness, chemosis, photophobia

coverage against *H. influenzae* and stings with application, a consideration in choosing an antibiotic. Gram's stain or culture can further guide the choice of antibiotic. Other choices for uncomplicated bacterial conjunctivitis include tobramycin, gentamicin, azithromycin, or any of the fluoroquinolones. See Table 26–3 for dosing information.

Bacterial conjunctivitis caused by dacryostenosis is most commonly *S. pneumonia* (35%) or *H. influenzae* (20%) and may be treated with erythromycin ophthalmic ointment, tobramycin ophthalmic, or the fluoroquinolones (moxifloxacin, ciprofloxacin, ofloxacin, norfloxacin) (Paysse, Coats, & Cassidy, 2014).

Table 26–3 Dosage Schedule: Ophthalmic Anti-Infectives

Drug	Indication	Dosage Form	Dose	Comments
Sulfacetamide sodium Bleph 10 Sodium Sulamyd	Conjunctivitis Trachoma	10% solution 10% ointment	Solution: 1–2 drops q2–3h during the day, less often at night Trachoma: 2 drops q2h with systemic therapy Ointment: Small amount tid-qid and qhs	Not recommended for infants <2 mo
Erythromycin Ilotycin	Conjunctivitis and flare-ups of chronic blepharitis Prophylaxis of ophthalmia neonatorum	Ointment: 5 mg/g	Ointment: 0.25 to 0.5 in. ribbon 2–3 times/d Ointment: 0.5 in. ribbon of ointment in each conjunctival sac no later than 1 h after birth	Safe in infants Use a new tube in each infant
Azithromycin Azasite	Bacterial conjunctivitis	Solution: 1%	*Age ≥1 yr:* 1 drop in affected eye(s) bid (8–12 h apart) for 2 d and then once daily for the next 5 d	Not recommended for children <age 1 yr
Gentamicin Garamycin Genoptic	Conjunctivitis	Solution: 3 mg/mL Ointment: 3 mg/g	Severe infections: 2 drops q1h or 0.5 in. ointment q3–4h; may prolong interval as infection improves Mild/moderate infections: 0.5 drop q4h or 0.5 in. of ointment bid–tid	May be used in children
Tobramycin Tobrex	Susceptible infections of conjunctiva and cornea	Solution: 0.3% Ointment: 3 mg/g	Severe infections: 2 drops q1h or 0.5 in. ointment q3–4h; may prolong interval as infection improves Mild to moderate infections: 1–2 drops q4h or 0.5 in. of ointment bid–tid	Safe and effective in children >1 mo
Besifloxacin Besivance	Bacterial conjunctivitis	Suspension: 0.6%	One drop TID × 7 days	Not recommended for children <1 yr of age
Ciprofloxacin Ciloxan	Susceptible infections of conjunctiva and corneal ulcer	Solution: 3 mg/mL	Solution: Corneal ulcer: day 1, 2 drops q15min, then 2 drops q30min; day 2, 2 drops q1h; days 3–14, 2 drops q4h; treat for 14 d or until corneal epithelialization occurs Conjunctivitis: 1–2 drops q2h while awake × 2 d; then 1–2 drops q4h while awake for next 5 d Ointment: For conjunctivitis: 0.5 in. tid × 2 d, then bid × 5 d	Solution not recommended for children <1 yr Ointment not recommended for children <2 yr
Gatifloxacin Zymar	Bacterial conjunctivitis	0.3% solution	*Adults and children ≥1 yr:* 1 drop q2h while awake (max 8 times/day) on days 1 and 2; then 1 drop q4h while awake for next 5 d	Not recommended for children <1 yr

Continued

Table 26–3 ⊗ **Dosage Schedule: Ophthalmic Anti-Infectives—cont'd**

Drug	Indication	Dosage Form	Dose	Comments
Levofloxacin Quixin Iquix	Bacterial conjunctivitis	0.5% solution 1.5% solution	*Adults and children ≥1 yr:* 1–2 drops in affected eye q2h while awake on days 1 and 2; then 1–2 drops q4h while awake, up to 4 doses/d on days 3–7	Not recommended for children <1 yr
Moxifloxacin Vigamox Moxeza	Bacterial conjunctivitis	0.5% solution	*Adults and Children ≥1 yr:* 1 drop in affected eye tid for 7 d	Not recommended for children <1 yr
Norfloxacin Chibroxin	Susceptible infections of conjunctiva and cornea	Solution: 3 mg/mL	1–2 drops qid for up to 7 d; may administer q2h while awake on day 1	Not recommended for children <1 yr
Ofloxacin Ocuflox	Susceptible infections of conjunctiva and corneal ulcer	Solution: 3 mg/mL	Corneal ulcer: days 1 and 2, 1–2 drops q20min while awake and 4 and 6 h after retiring; days 3–9, 1–2 drops q1h while awake; thereafter, 1–2 drops qid Conjunctivitis: 1–2 drops q2–4h while awake × 2 d, then 1–2 drops qid while awake for next 5 d	Not recommended for children <1 yr
Polymyxin-trimethoprim Polytrim Ophthalmic	Susceptible infections of conjunctiva and cornea	Solution: polymyxin B 10,000 U/g, trimethoprim 1 g/mL	1 drop q3h for 7–10 d, up to 6 doses/d	Not recommended for infants <2 mo Contraindicated in ophthalmia neonatorum
Polymyxin B–bacitracinophthalmic Polysporin Ophthalmic	Susceptible infections of conjunctiva and cornea	Ointment: polymyxin B 10,000 U/g, bacitracin 500 U/g	Ointment: Apply 0.5 in. ribbon q3–4 h	May be used safely in children
Trifluridine Viroptic	Herpes simplex Type 1 and 2 keratoconjunctivitis	Solution: 1%	1 drop every 2 h while awake (max 9 drops a day). After reepithelialization, 1 drop q4h for 7 d.	Do not exceed recommended dose. Not recommended for children <6 yr

Conjunctivitis-Otitis Syndrome

The syndrome of conjunctivitis accompanied by otitis media predominantly occurs in children younger than age 6 years. *H. influenzae* is the causative organism in the majority (82%) of patients with conjunctivitis-otitis syndrome (Buznach et al, 2005). Treatment is systemic antibiotics that are effective against *H. influenzae*. Amoxicillin-clavulanate (Augmentin) with amoxicillin dosed at 80 to 90 mg/kg/d is the first-line drug of choice. If systemic antibiotics are prescribed, topical ophthalmic treatment is usually not needed. See Chapter 46 for management of otitis media.

Gonococcal Conjunctivitis

Purulent bacterial conjunctivitis usually responds to topical antibiotic therapy. An exception is hyperpurulent gonococcal conjunctivitis, which is usually found in the newborn and in sexually promiscuous teenagers and adults. The eye discharge should be gram stained and cultured to confirm the diagnosis. Treatment consists of parenteral antibiotics (ceftriaxone 1 g IM in a single dose [CDC, 2010]) and sterile saline irrigations to clear the exudate. Use of a beta-lactamase–resistant cephalosporin such as ceftriaxone is warranted due to high levels of resistance to other antibiotics. Because untreated gonococcal infection can penetrate the intact eye, treatment should begin as soon as the diagnosis is suspected.

Blepharitis

Blepharitis is an acute or chronic inflammation of the eyelash follicles and meibomian glands of the eyelids. Treatment consists of warm compresses for 5 to 10 minutes at a time 2 to 4 times a day; scrubbing the eyelashes with gentle, no-tears shampoo; and applying erythromycin ophthalmic ointment (0.25-in. ribbon to each eye twice a day) until the symptoms clear and then for an additional 7 days. Ointment is preferred in the treatment of blepharitis due to the increased contact with the ocular tissue. Azithromycin 1% ophthalmic solution for 4 weeks may also be used (Shtein, 2014). The patient should not wear contact lenses during treatment, and the contacts should be sterilized before reinserting. Eye makeup should be discarded to prevent reinfection (Shtein, 2014).

Hordeolum

Hordeolum, commonly called a *sty,* is an infection of the sebaceous gland of the eyelash or eyelid. The causative organism is *S. aureus.* Treatment consists of warm, moist compresses 4 times a day for 15 minutes each time. Antibiotic eyedrops (sulfacetamide 10% or Polytrim drops) or ointment (erythromycin 0.5%) should be applied 4 times a day until the symptoms subside and then for an additional 2 to 3 days. The hordeolum usually spontaneously ruptures; if it does not, the patient should be referred to an ophthalmologist. Multiple or recurrent hordeolum may require systemic antibiotic treatment with dicloxacillin or other antibiotic that treats staph.

Viral Conjunctivitis

Viral conjunctivitis is usually caused by an adenovirus, HSV, or herpes zoster. Simple viral conjunctivitis caused by adenovirus is treated with sulfacetamide 10% solution or ointment 4 times a day or a broad-spectrum antibiotic, such as tobramycin, to prevent secondary bacterial infection. The course of the conjunctivitis runs 12 to 15 days. Herpes keratitis is a potentially serious consequence of infection with HSV. If herpes keratitis is suspected, a referral to an ophthalmologist for diagnosis and treatment is indicated. Commonly used antiviral agents are gancyclovir, trifluridine, and vidarabine. Table 26-3 presents the dosage schedule of ophthalmic anti-infectives.

Rational Drug Selection

Efficacy

A determination of the suspected organism guides the choice of an ophthalmic antibiotic. If *H. influenzae* is high on the list of suspected organisms, then sulfacetamide should not be the first choice for treatment because it has poor coverage for *H. influenzae.* A combination product such as Polysporin or Polytrim provides good coverage for the common organisms that cause bacterial conjunctivitis. In infants, erythromycin is usually the drug of choice because of its good coverage, and ointment is more easily administered than drops.

Cost

The least expensive ophthalmic is generally generic erythromycin, bacitracin, or sulfacetamide 10%. Azithromycin and the fluoroquinolones are more expensive, up to 10 times the cost of erythromycin.

Monitoring

There is no laboratory monitoring necessary with ophthalmic anti-infectives.

Lifestyle Management

The most important nonpharmacological measure is for the patient and family members to wash their hands thoroughly whenever the infected eyes are touched and before instilling medication. Hand washing will decrease spread of the infection to other contacts.

The patient with an eye infection should not share hand towels with the rest of the family. The patient with an eye

CLINICAL PEARL

Proper Instillation of Eyedrops

- Wash hands before administering eyedrops.
- Tilt head back or lie on back.
- Gently pull down lower eyelid to form a "pocket" to place the drop of medication into.
- Squeeze the medication onto the eye without touching eye with the dropper.
- Close eye. Do not rub. Try not to blink.
- To prevent cross-contamination, do not use medication labeled for another patient.
- Wait at least 5 minutes between administrations if administering more than one eye medication.

Proper Instillation of Eye Ointment

- Wash hands prior to administering eye medications.
- Warm the ointment by holding it in the hand for 1 to 2 minutes.
- With first use of a new tube, squeeze out and discard the first 0.25 in. of medication.
- Angle head back or lie on back.
- Gently pull down lower eyelid to form a "pocket" to place the drop of medication into.
- Squeeze 0.25 to 0.5 in. of medication onto the eye without touching eye with tip of tube.
- Close eye for 1 to 2 minutes. Do not rub.
- Wipe excess medication from around the eye with a tissue.
- To prevent cross-contamination, do not use medication labeled for another patient.
- Wait at least 10 minutes between administrations if administering more than one eye medication.
- Temporary blurred vision is typical after administration of ophthalmic ointment.

infection should use a separate towel or paper towels to prevent the spread of infection to family members.

Eye makeup needs to be thrown away after an eye infection because mascara and other makeup can harbor bacteria or viruses, and the patient can become re-infected.

Crusty, purulent discharge can be irritating and may be distressing to children whose eyes become "glued shut" with the dried discharge. Purulent discharge can be removed with cotton balls moistened with warm water. The cotton ball is wiped gently from the interior canthus to the external canthus to remove discharge. A clean cotton ball should be used for each wipe and for each eye. If a washcloth is used, patients or parents should be instructed to use a clean area of the cloth for each swipe of the eye and to use a clean washcloth every time.

Patient Education

Administration

Administration of ophthalmic medications can be challenging for patients. The patient should be instructed in the importance of keeping the tip of the dropper or tube from touching the eye, fingertips, or any other surface to prevent contamination. Hands should be washed before and after instillation of eye medications. Eye medications should not be shared.

Ophthalmic ointment should be transferred from the tube onto a moistened cotton swab, then rolled into each conjunctival sac. Use one swab for each eye to prevent contamination.

Eyedrops are self-administered by holding the bottle of solution in the dominant hand and using the pointer finger of the other hand to gently pull down the lower eyelid to form a "pocket" for the solution to be dropped into. The patient can use this method for both eyes.

For children who may resist the "bull's-eye" method of instilling eyedrops, one of three methods may be used. School-age children can assist with the instillation by pulling down their own lower eyelid, while the parent or care provider instills the eyedrop into the pocket formed. If this method doesn't work, a child may lie down on his or her back and close the eyes, keeping the head still. A drop of the antibiotic or antiviral is placed on the inner canthus. After the eyedrops are placed on the internal canthus, the child should slowly open his or her eyes without moving the head. The eyedrops instill into the eyes. Younger children require immobilization to instill eyedrops or ophthalmic ointment. This can be accomplished by two people, one to hold the child and the other to administer the medication.

Adverse Reactions

The patient should be instructed that there might be transient burning or stinging with most of the ophthalmic anti-infective agents. If burning is severe or prolonged, the patient should contact the provider. Other adverse effects should be discussed with the patient, with instructions to report any unusual symptoms.

ANTIGLAUCOMA AGENTS

Glaucoma is a group of disorders in which IOP damages the optic nerve. In the United States, glaucoma affects 2.2 million people and is the leading cause of blindness in the world (Glaucoma Research Foundation, 2013). Glaucoma can affect a patient of any age; 1 in 10,000 newborns is diagnosed with congenital glaucoma and 8% of adults over age 70 years are diagnosed with glaucoma (Glaucoma Research Foundation, 2013). Blindness from glaucoma is 6 to 8 times more common among African Americans than Caucasians. The patient may have open-angle glaucoma, in which a block at the level of the trabecular meshwork impairs aqueous humor reabsorption, or the patient may have angle-closure glaucoma, which develops when the normal path of the aqueous flow is interrupted in an eye with a shallow anterior chamber. Current medical therapies are aimed at decreasing the production of aqueous humor at the ciliary body and at increasing the outflow of this fluid from the angle structures. Glaucoma or the suspicion of glaucoma requires evaluation and treatment by an ophthalmologist. Primary care providers need to be aware of the medications that are prescribed, the drug interactions that may occur, and the adverse effects of the prescribed medications.

Pharmacodynamics

The antiglaucoma agents can be roughly divided into the following categories: beta blockers, adrenergic agonists, miotics, carbonic anhydrase (CA) inhibitors, sympathomimetics, and the prostaglandin agonist latanoprost (Xalatan).

Beta Blockers

Beta-adrenergic antagonists, also known as beta blockers, reduce IOP by interference with the production of aqueous humor induced by cyclic adenosine monophosphate (cAMP) through the ciliary processes in the eye, although the exact mechanism of action is not known. IOP is reduced in patients with either elevated or normal IOP. Visual acuity, pupil size, and accommodation do not appear to be affected by ophthalmic beta blockers.

Miotics, Cholinesterase Inhibitors

Cholinesterase inhibitors are indirect-acting agents that inhibit the cholinesterase enzyme. Topical application to the eye causes intense miosis and muscle contraction. The IOP is reduced by a decreased resistance to aqueous outflow. The cholinesterase inhibitors are divided into reversible and irreversible agents. The reversible agents physostigmine and demecarium combine with cholinesterase, and as the resulting union is hydrolyzed, the cholinesterase regenerates over a number of hours. Echothiophate iodide (Phospholine) is considered an irreversible agent that binds to cholinesterase in a covalent bond that does not hydrolyze. Cholinesterase must be synthesized or drawn from other parts of the body in order for ophthalmic action to return to normal.

Miotics, Direct-Acting

The direct-acting miotics are parasympathomimetic (cholinergic) drugs with muscarinic effects. When applied topically, these drugs produce pupillary constriction, stimulate the

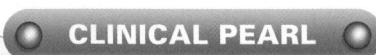
CLINICAL PEARL

Tips for Administering Eye Medications to a Child
If only one adult is available to administer eyedrops, then the adult can sit on the floor with the child between his or her legs, with the child's legs in the same direction as the adult's. The child's head can be immobilized between the adult's thighs and the arms held firmly down under the adult's thighs. This leaves the adult's hands free to instill the medication. The child may kick, but this will not affect the administration of the medication. Although this method may sound drastic, trying to administer eye medication to a squirming toddler or preschooler can be almost impossible, and with this method, the eyedrops can be effectively administered in less than 1 minute.

ciliary muscles, and increase aqueous humor outflow. They also reduce outflow resistance by contraction of the iris sphincter. IOP is decreased with the increase in outflow.

Carbonic Anhydrase Inhibitors

CA inhibitors decrease aqueous humor secretion by slowing the formation of bicarbonate ions. This reduces sodium and fluid transport, leading to decreased aqueous humor production and subsequent decreased IOP.

Sympathomimetics

Sympathomimetics applied topically cause vasoconstriction, papillary dilation, and reduction of IOP. It is believed that sympathomimetics reduce IOP by reducing the production of aqueous humor and by increasing aqueous humor outflow.

Alpha-Adrenergic Agonists

Alpha-adrenergic agonists reduce IOP by reducing the production of aqueous humor and by increasing uveoscleral outflow.

Prostaglandin Agonists

Latanoprost is a selective agonist of a prostaglandin receptor known as the FP receptor. Latanoprost increases the outflow of aqueous humor by acting on this receptor, which leads to decreased IOP. Bimatoprost (Lumigan) is a prostamide, a synthetic prostaglandin. It lowers IOP by increasing aqueous humor outflow. Unoprostone (Rescula) and Travoprost (Travatan) are synthetic prostaglandin $F_{2\alpha}$ analogues whose exact mechanism of action is unknown, although they are thought to reduce IOP by decreasing uveoscleral outflow. Bimatoprost is also marketed as Latisse for treatment of eyelash hypotrichosis. Patients should experience thicker and darker eyelashes after 2 months of treatment.

Pharmacokinetics

Little is known about the specific pharmacokinetic parameters of the beta blockers. The duration of action is noted in Table 26-4. What is known is determined by clinical observation of pharmacodynamic responses. The amount of absorption is unknown, but systemic absorption is known to occur because both cardiac and pulmonary signs of beta blocker activity can occur. Beta blockers are metabolized in the liver and excreted in the urine and feces.

The pharmacokinetics of cholinesterase inhibitors and the direct-acting miotics are not known. The duration of action is noted in Table 26–4.

Following topical administration into the eye, brinzolamide (Azopt) is absorbed systemically, although plasma concentrations remain low and generally below the level of detection. It is widely distributed, including into the breast milk in animal studies. It may cross the placenta. Brinzolamide is metabolized to *N*-desthyl brinzolamide and excreted primarily in the urine.

Dorzolamide (Trusopt), when applied topically to the eye, has some systemic absorption, although no free drug is

Table 26–4 ⸬ **Pharmacokinetics: Antiglaucoma Agents**

Drug	Duration
Beta Blockers	
Betaxolol, carteolol	12 h
Levobunolol, metipranolol, timolol	12–24 h
Miotics	
Carbachol	6–8 h
Pilocarpine	4–8 h
Echothiophate	Days/weeks
Carbonic Anhydrase Inhibitors	
Acetazolamide	8–12 h
Brinzolamide	NA
Dorzolamide	About 8 h
Methazolamide	10–18 h
Sympathomimetics	
Epinephrine, dipivefrin	12 h
Alpha-Adrenergic Agonists	
Apraclonidine	7–12 h
Brimonidine	12 h
Prostaglandin Analogues	
Latanoprost	24 h
Bimatoprost	1.5 h
Unoprostone	<1 h
Travoprost	<1 h

NA = information not available.

measured in the plasma. Dorzolamide is excreted primarily unchanged in the urine.

Methazolamide (Neptazane) is an oral CA inhibitor. It is well absorbed from the gastrointestinal (GI) tract. Methazolamide is distributed throughout the body, including the plasma, cerebrospinal fluid, aqueous humor of the eye, red blood cells, bile, and extracellular fluid. Its exact metabolism is not described. Excretion is primarily renal, with 25% of the drug excreted unchanged in the urine.

The pharmacokinetics of the sympathomimetics is not known.

Following ophthalmic administration of brimonidine (Alphagan), peak serum levels occur in 1 to 4 hours. Brimonidine is extensively metabolized in the liver and eliminated in the urine.

Latanoprost is absorbed through the cornea, where it is hydrolyzed to become biologically active. Plasma levels of latanoprost can be measured. Distribution is unknown. It is not known whether latanoprost crosses the placenta, although in animal studies adverse fetal effects were found. It is not known whether latanoprost is excreted in breast milk. Latanoprost is metabolized via fatty-acid beta oxidation in the liver. The metabolites are excreted primarily in the urine (88%).

Bimatoprost is absorbed and reaches a steady state in the plasma, with 12% remaining unbound in human plasma. It is metabolized by oxidation and is excreted in the urine (67%) and feces (25%). Travoprost is rapidly absorbed from the cornea and peaks in the plasma within 30 minutes. Travoprost is hydrolyzed by esterases in the cornea into free acid. Elimination of travoprost is rapid and within an hour of administration levels are unmeasurable. Unoprostone is rapidly absorbed from the cornea and hydrolyzed into unoprostone-free acid, which is eliminated rapidly in the urine.

Table 26-4 presents the pharmacokinetics of antiglaucoma agents.

Pharmacotherapeutics

Precautions and Contraindications

Although primary care providers do not prescribe ophthalmic antiglaucoma agents, the medications are absorbed and systemic levels reached in great enough amounts to cause complications of chronic conditions. Coordination of care with the ophthalmologist will ensure the optimal care for the patient's glaucoma and other medical problems.

The beta blocker ophthalmic medications are contraindicated in patients with asthma, a history of asthma, chronic obstructive pulmonary disease (COPD), or other pulmonary disease. There may be bronchospasm associated with the use of topical beta blockers, which may prove fatal to patients with respiratory disease.

Beta Blockers

Beta blockers suppress conduction through the atrioventricular (AV) node; therefore, topical beta blockers are contraindicated in patients with bradycardia or advanced AV block. Beta blockers should not be used in patients with compromised ventricular dysfunction, patients in cardiogenic shock, or patients with systolic congestive heart failure. Discontinue topical beta blockers at the first sign of cardiac failure. Beta blockers are contraindicated for patients with hypotension (standing blood pressure [SBP] less than 100 mm Hg).

Beta blockers should be used with caution in patients with poorly controlled diabetes mellitus because beta blockers can prolong or enhance hypoglycemia by interfering with glycogenolysis. Beta blockers may also mask the signs and symptoms of acute hypoglycemia. Because they may mask the clinical signs of hypothyroidism, beta blockers should be used with caution in patients with hyperthyroidism.

Patients using beta blockers during surgery should be monitored closely for signs of cardiac failure. Severe, protracted hypotension and difficulty in restarting the heart have been reported. Beta blockers may need to be withdrawn before surgery, with the last dose 2 days prior to surgery. Beta blockers are also contraindicated in patients with Raynaud's disease or peripheral vascular or cerebrovascular disease because decreased cardiac output can exacerbate symptoms.

Ophthalmic beta blockers are Pregnancy Category C. Fetal anomalies and fetotoxicity have been observed in animal studies. Most of the ophthalmic beta blockers are excreted in breast milk and are contraindicated in breastfeeding. Ophthalmic beta blocker agents are used in children, but they must be monitored closely.

Miotics

The miotics are contraindicated when active inflammation of the eye is present. They are also contraindicated when constriction is not wanted, for example, in iritis, uveitis, and some forms of secondary glaucoma.

The miotics are Pregnancy Category C, with demecarium (Humorsol) given the classification of Pregnancy Category X. Use with caution in lactating women. Use with extreme caution in children.

Carbonic Anhydrase Inhibitors

Dorzolamide and brinzolamide contain sulfonamide and are absorbed in amounts great enough to cause hypersensitivity reactions in patients with sulfonamide sensitivity. Dorzolamide and brinzolamide are Pregnancy Category C. They are contraindicated in lactation, and their safety for use in children is not known.

Methazolamide is contraindicated in patients with hyponatremia, hypokalemia, renal disease, liver disease, suprarenal gland failure, hyperchloremic acidosis, adrenocortical insufficiency, and severe pulmonary obstruction. It is Pregnancy Category C and not recommended for use in children.

Sympathomimetics

Apraclonidine (Iopidine) is contraindicated in patients with clonidine hypersensitivity. Dipivefrin (AKPro, Propine) is contraindicated in patients with narrow-angle glaucoma and aphakic patients. Apraclonidine is Pregnancy Category C, and dipivefrin is Pregnancy Category B. They are not recommended for use by nursing mothers or by children.

Alpha-Adrenergic Agonists

Brimonidine is contraindicated in patients taking monoamine oxidase inhibitors (MAOIs). Brimonidine should be used with caution in patients with cardiac, renal, or liver disease. It should not be instilled with contact lenses in place, and the patient should wait 15 minutes after instilling brimonidine before replacing contacts. Brimonidine is Pregnancy Category B. It should be avoided in children and lactating women.

Prostaglandin Agonists

Latanoprost should not be administered while the patient is wearing contact lenses. It should be used with caution in patients with intraocular inflammation (iritis) and aphakic patients. It is Pregnancy Category C, and it is not recommended for use during lactation or by children. Brimatoprost is Pregnancy Category C. If brimatoprost (Latisse) is being prescribed for hypotrichosis, it may lower IOP in patients with normal IOP, but the magnitude of change is not clinically significant.

Adverse Drug Reactions

All of the antiglaucoma medications may cause transient discomfort or tearing. Blurred vision, photophobia, and hyperemia may also occur. Allergic conjunctivitis may occur with any of the topical ophthalmic medications.

Headaches and dizziness may occur with the use of beta blockers. Patients may exhibit systemic beta blocker effects with the use of ophthalmic preparations. Symptoms include bradycardia, hypotension, bronchospasm, and, rarely, AV block.

Miotics may cause corneal clouding, ciliary spasm, headache, induced myopia, and retinal detachment. Patients may have systemic anticholinergic effects if excessive absorption occurs. These symptoms include headache, hypertension, salivation, sweating, nausea, and vomiting. Iris cysts may be seen with cholinesterase inhibitors.

Many patients (about 25%) report dysgeusia, or bitter taste in the mouth, after ocular administration of CA inhibitors. Superficial punctate keratitis is reported in 10% to 15% of patients using ophthalmic preparations.

Systemic CA inhibitors (methazolamide) may cause melena and GI upset, such as anorexia, nausea, and vomiting. Glycosuria and urinary frequency have been reported. Weakness, malaise, fatigue, bone marrow depression, thrombocytopenia, leukopenia, and hemolytic anemia have been reported with use of methazolamide. Renal calculi and nephrotoxicity have also been reported. Fever is a rare adverse effect of methazolamide.

The local effects of the sympathomimetics include conjunctival or corneal pigmentation. Systemic effects of topical sympathomimetic use include headache, hypertension, tachycardia, and cardiac arrhythmias (with excessive absorption).

The local effects of alpha agonists that occur in 10% to 30% of patients include the sensation of a foreign body in the eye and ocular pain. Systemic adverse effects include dry mouth, drowsiness, and headache. Corneal staining may occur.

The local adverse effects reported in 5% to 15% of patients using prostaglandin agonists include foreign body sensations, keratopathy, and iridal discoloration. The iridal discoloration may be gradual (many months) and is caused by an increase in the amount of brown pigmentation in the iris because of an increased number of melanosomes in melanocytes. The color change may be permanent. Bimatoprost (Latisse) may cause permanent brown iris pigmentation and hair growth outside the treatment area and must be applied only to the upper eyelid, using the sterile applicator supplied, and not allowed to drip down onto the cheek or other skin area.

Drug Interactions

Beta Blockers

The use of ophthalmic beta blockers with systemic beta blockers may cause additive beta blockade effects. Coadministration of ophthalmic timolol has caused bradycardia and asystole.

Miotics

Carbachol and pilocarpine solution have no reported drug interactions. Pilocarpine ocular sustained-release inserts (Ocusert Pilo) potentiate the absorption of epinephrine. Echothiophate may potentiate the effects of succinylcholine, leading to respiratory and possibly cardiovascular collapse. Echothiophate may have additive effects when used with systemic anticholinesterases used in the treatment of myasthenia gravis. There is additive toxicity (increased parasympathomimetic effects) if organic pesticides or carbamate is absorbed by someone using ophthalmic echothiophate.

Carbonic Anhydrase Inhibitors

Concurrent use of CA inhibitors (topical brinzolamide, dorzolamide, and systemic methazolamide) and high-dose salicylates may lead to metabolic acidosis and salicylate toxicity, which allow greater penetration of salicylate into the central nervous system (CNS). This interaction is theoretical with the topical CA inhibitors. CA inhibitors may inhibit excretion of basic drugs and promote excretion of acidic drugs. The concurrent use of oral and topical CA inhibitors is not recommended.

Sympathomimetics

There are no known drug interactions with ophthalmic dipivefrin. Apraclonidine may interact with cardiovascular drugs. Apraclonidine should not be used by patients who are using MAOIs because concurrent use may cause a hypertensive crisis.

Alpha-Adrenergic Agonists

The alpha-adrenergic agonists are contraindicated with the use of MAOIs. There may be additive CNS depression if topical alpha-adrenergic agonists are used concurrently with CNS depressants. Tricyclic antidepressants can affect the metabolism and uptake of circulating amines. Medications that may cause bradycardia (beta blockers, antihypertensives, and cardiac glycosides) may have additive depression of pulse and blood pressure if used concurrently with alpha-adrenergic agonists.

Prostaglandin Agonists

The only reported drug interaction noted with latanoprost is thimerosal, which can cause precipitation if administered concurrently. Advise the patient to wait at least 5 minutes between administration of two ophthalmic medications if one contains thimerosol.

Table 26-5 presents drug interactions with antiglaucoma agents.

Clinical Use and Dosing

Glaucoma

Antiglaucoma medications are prescribed by ophthalmologists. Dosage is determined by the clinical condition of the patient.

Rational Drug Selection

The ophthalmologist determines what medication should be used, based on the patient's glaucoma type and underlying medical conditions.

Table 26–5 ▦ Drug Interactions: Antiglaucoma Agents

Drug	Interacting Drug	Possible Effect	Implications
Beta Blockers			
Betaxolol, carteolol, metipranolol	Oral beta blockers	Additive effects, excessive hypotension, increased reduction of IOP	Use with caution
	Antihypertensive agents	Additive antihypertensive effects	Monitor BP
	Antiarrhythmics (diltiazem, verapamil, amiodarone, digoxin)	Additive effects; may cause significant effects on AV node conduction; may cause complete heart block	Use with caution, monitor closely
	Beta agonist bronchodilators (albuterol, metaproterenol [Alupent], salmeterol)	Beta blocker may antagonize the effects of beta agonists	Use with caution; avoid concurrent use if possible
Levobunolol	Oral beta blockers	Additive effects, excessive hypotension, increased reduction of IOP	Use with caution
	Cimetidine	Interferes with hepatic metabolism of levobunolol, potentially increasing its effects	Avoid concurrent use
	Sympathomimetics, including inhaled beta agonists	Antagonism of desired therapeutic effects	Avoid concurrent use
Timolol	Oral beta blockers	Additive effects, excessive hypotension, increased reduction of IOP	Use with caution
	Antihypertensive agents	Additive antihypertensive effects	Monitor BP
	Antiarrhythmics (diltiazem, verapamil, amiodarone, digoxin)	Additive effects; may cause significant effects on AV node conduction; may cause complete heart block	Use with caution; monitor closely
	Verapamil	Coadministration of ophthalmic timolol has caused bradycardia and asystole	Do not use concurrently
	Beta-agonist bronchodilators (albuterol, metaproterenol [Alupent], salmeterol)	Timolol may antagonize the effects of beta agonists	Use with caution; avoid concurrent use if possible
	Quinidine	Quinidine can potentiate timolol-induced bradycardia	Use with caution; monitor closely
Miotics			
Carbachol, pilocarpine	No significant interactions		
Echothiophate	Succinylcholine (anesthetic)	May potentiate succinylcholine, leading to possible respiratory and cardiovascular collapse	Do not use concurrently; consider stopping echothiophate before surgery
	Systemic anticholinesterases	Additive effects	Coadminister cautiously
	Carbamate or organophosphate insecticides and pesticides	Increased parasympathomimetic effects	Warn patients who are gardeners or workers who may be exposed to these chemicals to protect themselves with masks, frequent washing of skin, and clothing changes
Carbonic Anhydrase Inhibitors			
Acetazolamide	Barbiturates, aspirin, lithium	Excretion decreased	May lead to decreased effectiveness of interacting drugs
Brinzolamide	Amphetamines, quinidine, procainamide, tricyclic antidepressants	Excretion decreased	May result in toxicity to interacting drugs
	No known drug interactions		
Dorzolamide	Oral CA inhibitors	Potential additive effects	Concurrent use not recommended
Methazolamide	Diflunisal	Significant decrease in IOP	Avoid concurrent use
	Salicylates	Accumulation of methazolamide, resulting in CNS depression and metabolic acidosis	Avoid concurrent use
	Topiramate	Increased risk of renal stone formation	Avoid concurrent use
	Basic pH drugs	Inhibited renal excretion of basic drugs	

Table 26–5 ▓ **Drug Interactions: Antiglaucoma Agents—cont'd**

Drug	Interacting Drug	Possible Effect	Implications
	Acidic pH drugs	Promotes excretion of acidic drugs	Monitor potassium
	Corticosteroids, potassium-depleting diuretics	Hypokalemia	Monitor potassium
Sympathomimetics			
Epinephrine	Anesthetics (cyclopropane, halogenated hydrocarbons)	May cause cardiac arrhythmias	Discontinue epinephrine prior to surgery
Dipivefrin	No significant interactions		
Alpha-Adrenergic Agonists			
Apraclonidine	Cardiovascular agents: antihypertensives, cardiac glycosides, beta blockers MAOIs	Apraclonidine may reduce pulse and BP	If using concurrently, monitor pulse and BP frequently Concurrent use contraindicated
Brimonidine	CNS depressants: alcohol, barbiturates, opiates, sedatives, or anesthetics Beta blockers, antihypertensives Tricyclic antidepressants MAOIs	Additive CNS depression Brimonidine may reduce pulse pressure and BP Tricyclic antidepressants can lower circulating amines	Use with caution Use with caution; monitor cardiac status Monitor IOP closely if necessary to administer concurrently Use contraindicated
Prostaglandin Analogues			
Latanoprost	Thimerosal	Precipitation of latanoprost occurs when used concurrently	Administer at least 5 to 10 min apart
Bimatoprost	No significant interactions		Allow 5 min between application of other topical ophthalmic agents
Unoprostone	No significant interactions		Allow 5 min between application of other topical ophthalmic agents
Travoprost	No significant interactions		Allow 5 min between application of other topical ophthalmic agents

IOP = intraocular pressure; BP = blood pressure; AV = atrioventricular; CA = carbonic anhydrase; CNS = central nervous system; MAOIs = monoamine oxidase inhibitors.

Monitoring

The patient who is prescribed antiglaucoma medications may require monitoring of blood pressure and cardiovascular status. IOP is measured and monitored by the ophthalmologist. No laboratory monitoring is necessary.

Patient Education

Administration

The patient should be instructed to administer the medication exactly as the ophthalmologist has prescribed (Table 26-6). Abruptly stopping the medication can increase adverse effects.

Adverse Reactions

The patient should have been instructed by the ophthalmologist regarding the adverse effects of the medication. Reinforcement may be necessary. If the patient is experiencing adverse effects

from the medication, the primary care provider can facilitate a referral back to the ophthalmologist.

OCULAR ANTIALLERGIC AND ANTI-INFLAMMATORY AGENTS

There are several ocular antiallergic and anti-inflammatory drugs. The antiallergic medications include the mast cell stabilizers lodoxamide (Alomide), nedocromil (Alocril) and cromolyn sodium (Crolom). Levocabastine (Livostin), antazoline (Vasocon-A, Antazoline-V), azelastine (Optivar), bepotastine (Bepreve), epinastine (Elestat), emedastine (Emadine), ketotifen (Zaditor), olopatadine (Patanol, Pataday), pheniramine (Naphcon-A), and emedastine (Emadine) are antihistamines. The NSAIDs are flurbiprofen (Ocufen), suprofen (Profenal), diclofenac (Voltaren ophthalmic

Table 26–6 ❀ Available Dosage Forms: Antiglaucoma Agents

Drug	Dosage Form	How Supplied
Beta Blockers		
BETAXOLOL		
Betoptic*	Solution: 5.6 mg/mL	In 2.5, 5, 10, 15 mL
Betoptic S*	Suspension: 2.8 mg/mL	In 2.5, 5, 10, 15 mL
CARTEOLOL		
Ocupress	1% solution	In 5 or 10 mL dropper bottles
Generic	1% solution	In 5, 10, 15 mL bottles
LEVOBUNOLOL		
Betagan	0.25% solution	In 5 or 10mL bottles
AKBeta, Generic	0.5% solution	In 2, 5. 10, or 15 mL bottles
	0.25% solution	In 5 or 10 mL bottles
	0.5% solution	In 5, 10, or 15 mL bottles
METIPRANOLOL		
OptiPranolol	0.3% solution	In 5 or 10 mL dropper bottle
TIMOLOL		
Timoptic	0.25%, 0.5% solution	In 2.5,5,10, or 15 mL bottles
Timoptic-XE	0.25%, 0.5% gel	In 2.5 or 5 mL bottles
Betimol	0.25%, 0.5% solution	In 5, 10, or 15 mL bottles
Generic	0.25%, 0.5% solution	In 5, 10, or 15 mL bottles
		In 5, 10, or 15 mL bottles
COMBINATION PRODUCTS		
β blocker timolol and Carbonic anhydrase inhibitor dorzolamide Cosopt	Solution: Timolol 0.5% and dorzolamide 2%	10 mL
Miotics		
CARBACHOL		
Isopto Carbachol	0.75% solution, 1.5% solution	In 15 or 30 mL dropper bottles
Carboptic	2.25% solution	In 15 mL bottles
	3% solution	In 15 or 30 mL dropper bottles
	3% solution	In 15 mL bottle
PILOCARPINE		
Isopto Carpine	Solution: 0.25%, 0.5%, 1%, 2%, 3%, 4%, 5%, 6%, 10%	In 15 or 30 mL dropper bottles
Pilocar		In 15 or 30 mL dropper bottles
Pilopine HS	Solution: 0.5%, 1%, 2%, 3%, 4%, 6%	In 3.5 g
Generic	Gel: 4%	In 15 or 30 mL dropper bottles
	Solution: 0.5%, 1%, 2%, 4%, 6%, 8%	
ECHOTHIOPHATE		
Phospholine iodide	Powder for solution: 0.03%, 0.06%, 0.125%, 0.25%	In 5 mL diluent
Carbonic Anhydrase Inhibitors		
ACETAZOLAMIDE		
Diamox	Tablets: 125 mg, 250 mg	In 100s
BRINZOLAMIDE		
Azopt*	1% suspension	In 10, 15 mL
DORZOLAMIDE		
Trusopt*	2% solution	In 5, 10 mL
METHAZOLAMIDE		
Neptazane	Tablets: 25 mg, 50 mg	In 100s
Generic	Tablets: 25 mg, 50 mg	In 100s

Table 26–6 Available Dosage Forms: Antiglaucoma Agents—cont'd

Drug	Dosage Form	How Supplied
Sympathathomimetics		
EPINEPHRINE		
Epifrin*†	0.5% solution	In 15 mL dropper bottle
Glaucon*†	1% solution	In 10 mL dropper bottle
	2% solution	In 15 mL dropper bottle
	1% solution, 2% solution	In 10 mL dropper bottle
DIPIVEFRIN		
Propine, generic	0.1% solution	In 5, 10, or 15 mL bottle
Alpha-Adrenergic Agonists		
APRACLONIDINE		
Iopidine	1% solution	In 0.25 mL dispenser
	0.5% solution	In 5 mL drop container
BRIMONIDINE		
Prostaglandin Analogues		
LATANOPROST		
Xalatan	0.005% solution	In 2.5 mL
Latisse	0.03% solution	In 3 mL
UNOPROSTONE		
Rescula	0.15% solution	In 5 mL
TRAVOPROST		
Travatan	0.004%	In 2.5 mL, 5 mL
Travatan Z	0.004%	In 2.5 mL

*Contains benzalkonium chloride, which cannot be administered with soft contact lenses in place.
†Contains sulfites.

solution), nepafenac (Nevanac), and ketorolac (Acular). Corticosteroid ophthalmic agents are used as anti-inflammatories, although they are rarely used in primary care because of the serious adverse effects. Anti-inflammatory agents are found in single formula or in combination with antibiotics.

Pharmacodynamics

Ophthalmic Antiallergic Agents

The mast cell stabilizers limit hypersensitivity reactions by inhibiting the degranulation of sensitized mast cells that occur after exposure to specific antigens. They also inhibit the release of histamine and SRS-A (slow-reacting substance of anaphylaxis). They have no intrinsic antihistamine activity.

Ocular antihistamines are selective for the H_1 histamine receptor. They block the H_1 histamine receptors and inhibit histamine-stimulated vascular permeability in the conjunctiva. This relieves ocular pruritus associated with allergic conjunctivitis.

Ocular Anti-Inflammatory Agents

The ocular NSAIDs have analgesic, antipyretic, and anti-inflammatory activity. The ophthalmic NSAIDs reduce prostaglandin E_2 in aqueous humor by inhibition of prostaglandin biosynthesis. The mechanism is thought to be by means of the inhibition of cyclo-oxygenase enzyme, which is essential to the synthesis of prostaglandins.

Topical steroids exert an anti-inflammatory action. The exact mechanism of action for ocular corticosteroids is not known. They are thought to act by the induction of phospholipase A_2 inhibitory proteins. These proteins control the mediators of inflammation, such as prostaglandins and leukotrienes. Corticosteroids can increase IOP; the mechanism is not clear.

Pharmacokinetics

Limited systemic absorption occurs with the use of ophthalmic anti-inflammatory and antiallergic agents. The metabolism and excretion of ophthalmic antiallergic and anti-inflammatory agents are unknown.

Pharmacotherapeutics

Precautions and Contraindications

Hypersensitivity to any component of the product is a contraindication for any of the ophthalmic medications. Use caution with patients with known sensitivity to acetylsalicylic acid when prescribing NSAIDs because cross-sensitivity may occur.

Ophthalmic Antiallergic Agents

Patients should not wear soft contact lenses while inserting any ophthalmic product that contains benzalkonium chloride (cromolyn sodium, lodoxamide, ketotifen, emedastine, levocabastine). Wear can be resumed within a few hours of discontinuing cromolyn, levocabastine, lodoxamide, and nepanfenac. Patients who are using ketotifen and emedastine may wear their soft contacts if they wait at least 10 minutes after instilling the eyedrops to insert their contacts.

Emedastine, cromolyn sodium, and lodoxamide are Pregnancy Category B. Antazoline, ketotifen, levocabastine, and nepafenac are Pregnancy Category C, although no studies have been done on pregnant women. Safe use in lactation has not been established, although such minimal amounts are absorbed that use during lactation is probably safe.

Lodoxamide is safe in children as young as age 2. Cromolyn sodium ophthalmic can be prescribed to children older than age 4. The safety of emedastine and ketotifen in children younger than age 3 has not been established. Nepanfenac is not recommended for children younger than 10 years of age.

Ocular Anti-Inflammatory Agents

Referral to an ophthalmologist is warranted for patients who appear to need corticosteroid therapy. They require slit-lamp examination to rule out herpes keratitis prior to initiating therapy.

Corticosteroid eye medications should not be administered to patients with acute, untreated purulent bacterial, viral, or fungal ocular infection. Prescribing ophthalmic corticosteroids to a patient with herpes keratitis can lead to serious complications, including blindness. This may also occur with ocular NSAIDs; therefore, a referral is indicated before treatment.

The ocular NSAIDs are Pregnancy Category C, and the ocular corticosteroids are also Pregnancy Category C. Safety in children has not been established.

Adverse Drug Reactions

All ophthalmic antiallergic and anti-inflammatory medications may cause transient discomfort or tearing. Blurred vision, photophobia, and hyperemia may also develop. Allergic conjunctivitis may occur with any of the topical ophthalmic medications.

Other adverse reactions reported (1% to 5%) with the use of the mast cell stabilizer lodoxamide include dry eye, foreign body sensation, ocular itching and pruritus, and crystalline deposits. Cromolyn sodium may also cause itchy eyes, eye dryness and puffiness, and stys.

The most frequent adverse reaction reported with the use of ocular H_1 histamine blockers is headache. Conjunctival injection and rhinitis are reported in 10% to 25% of patients treated. The adverse reactions that occur in fewer than 5% of patients include asthenia, blurred vision, corneal staining, dysgeusia, hyperemia, keratitis, pruritus, rhinitis, and sinusitis.

Naphazoline may precipitate narrow-angle glaucoma. It may also cause mydriasis, increased IOP, and allergic dermatitis. Systemic adrenergic or antihistamine effects may occur with excessive use.

The ocular NSAIDs may cause minor ocular irritation on instillation (less than 40% incidence). The other reported adverse reactions noted in 1% to 10% of patients using ocular NSAIDs include superficial ocular infection, superficial keratitis, ocular inflammation, corneal edema, and iritis. Reactions reported less frequently include corneal infiltrates, corneal ulcer, keratitis, and mydriasis.

The severe adverse reactions that can occur with the use of ocular corticosteroids include glaucoma (elevated IOP) with optic nerve damage, field defects and loss of visual acuity, cataract formation, secondary infection of the eye, exacerbation of existing infections, and perforation of the globe. Systemic side effects may develop with extensive use.

Drug Interactions

There are no drug interactions noted with any of the ocular antiallergic medications. Ocular NSAIDs may potentiate oral anticoagulants; the patient should be monitored for prolonged bleeding times if the drugs are used concurrently. Ophthalmic steroids have no known drug interactions.

Clinical Use and Dosing

Allergic or Vernal Conjunctivitis

Allergic conjunctivitis can occur in response to a variety of allergens; vernal conjunctivitis refers to conjunctivitis that occurs primarily in the spring, usually because of an allergen. The mast cell stabilizers (lodoxamide, cromolyn sodium) may be used to treat vernal conjunctivitis and may be used safely for up to 3 months.

The ophthalmic H_1 blocker ketotifen can be prescribed for allergic conjunctivitis and ocular pruritus. The dose used in adults and children over age 3 is 1 drop in the affected eye every 8 to 12 hours. The dosage for levocabastine, another prescription ophthalmic H_1 blocker, is 1 drop in the affected eye 4 times a day.

The over-the-counter (OTC) products available to treat allergic conjunctivitis combine a decongestant with an antihistamine. Products that combine antazoline and naphazoline (Vasocon-A) or naphazoline and pheniramine (Opcon-A, Naphcon-A) are used for temporary relief of the minor eye symptoms of itching and redness caused by pollen and other allergens such as animal hair. Patients may self-prescribe these products; therefore, the primary care provider needs to monitor the patient for proper use and the adverse effects associated with the use of these medications.

Ocular Inflammation

Consultation with an ophthalmologist is indicated in the treatment of ocular inflammation. The patient requires a slit-lamp examination to rule out herpes keratitis or other infectious disease before beginning therapy with ocular anti-inflammatory agents. The dosing of these agents may be found in Table 26-7.

Table 26–7 ⊗ Dosage Schedule: Selected Ocular Antiallergic and Anti-Inflammatory Agents

Drug	Indication	Dosage Form	Dose	Notes
Mast Cell Stabilizers				
Cromolyn sodium Crolom* Opticrom*	Allergic or vernal conjunctivitis	4% solution	*Adults and children ≥4 yr:* 1–2 drops each eye 4–6 times daily	Safety in children <4 yr is not known Advise the patient not to wear soft contact lenses while using ophthalmic cromolyn sodium
Lodoxamide Alomide	Vernal conjunctivitis, keratoconjunctivitis, vernal keratitis	0.1% solution	*Adults and Children >2 yr:* 1–2 drops qid for up to 3 mo	Not recommended in children <2 yr
Pemirolast (Alamast)	Allergic conjunctivitis	0.1% solution	*Children ≥3 yr:* 1–2 drops each eye qid	Not recommended in children <3 yr
Nedocromil (Alocril)	Allergic conjunctivitis	2% solution	*Children ≥3 yr:* Instill 1–2 drops in each eye bid at regular intervals	Continue treatment throughout period of exposure (e.g., until pollen season is over) Not recommended in children <3 yr
Antihistamines				
Antazoline-naphazoline Vasocon-A*	Allergic conjunctivitis	Solution: antazoline 0.5%, naphazoline 0.027%	*Adults:* 1–3 drops into eyes q3–4h	OTC; use for temporary relief of allergic conjunctivitis symptoms
Azelastine (Optivar)	Allergic conjunctivitis	0.05% solution	*Adults and children ≥3 yr:* Instill 1 drop each eye bid	Not recommended in children <3 yr
Epinastine (Elestat)	Allergic conjunctivitis	0.05% solution	*Adults and children >3 yr:* Instill 1 drop each eye bid	Not recommended in children <3 yr
Emedastine Emadine*	Allergic conjunctivitis	0.025% solution	*Adults and children ≥3 yr:* 1 drop qid	Not recommended in children <3 yr Soft contact wearers may reinsert lens 10 min after administration of emedastine
Zaditor* (OTC)	Temporary prevention of ocular itching due to allergic conjunctivitis	0.05% suspension	*Adults and children ≥3 yr:* 1–2 drops q8–12h	Not recommended in children <3 yr Soft contact wearers may reinsert lens 10 min after administration of ketotifen
Levocabastine Livostin	Seasonal allergic conjunctivitis	0.05% suspension	*Adults and children ≥12 yr:* 1 drop into affected eye qid for up to 2 wk	Not recommended for use in children
Pheniramine-naphazoline Naphcon-A* (OTC) Naphazoline Plus,*	Allergic conjunctivitis	Solution: 0.3% pheniramine, 0.025% naphazoline	*Adults:* Instill 1–2 drops q3–4h	OTC; use for temporary relief of allergic conjunctivitis symptoms
Olopatadine Patanol*	Temporary prevention of ocular itching due to allergic conjunctivitis	0.1% solution	*Adults and children ≥3 yr:* 1–2 drops bid, at least 6–8 h interval	Not recommended in children <3 yr Soft contact wearers may reinsert lens 10 min after administration of olopatadine

Continued

Table 26–7 ⊗ Dosage Schedule: Selected Ocular Antiallergic and Anti-Inflammatory Agents—cont'd

Drug	Indication	Dosage Form	Dose	Notes
NSAIDs				
Diclofenac Voltaren	Post-op inflammation after cataract surgery	0.1% solution	After surgery, instill 1 drop into affected eye qid for 2 wk, beginning 24 h after surgery	Prescribed by ophthalmologists
Flurbiprofen Ocufen	Post-op inflammation after cataract surgery	0.03%	On day of surgery, instill 1 drop into eye every 30 min, beginning 2 h prior to surgery	Prescribed by ophthalmologists
Ketorolac Acular* Acular PF	Seasonal allergic conjunctivitis	0.5% solution 0.5% solution, preservative free	*Adults and children ≥12 yr:* 1 drop in affected eye(s) qid	Patients wearing hydrogel soft contact lenses may experience ocular irritation when using concurrently Advise patients not to wear contacts while using this drug
Nepafenac Nevanac	Post-op pain and inflammation following cataract surgery	0.3% solution	*Adults ≥10 yr:* 1 drop in affected eye tid beginning the day before surgery	Prescribed by ophthalmologists
Suprofen Profenal†	Post-op inflammation after cataract surgery	1% solution	On day of surgery, instill 2 drops into eye at 3, 2, and 1 h prior to surgery; after surgery, instill 2 drops into affected eye q4h for 1 d	Prescribed by ophthalmologists

*Contains benzalkonium chloride, which cannot be administered with soft contact lenses in place.
    †Contains thimerosal.

Rational Drug Selection

Safety

The ophthalmic mast cell stabilizers are quite safe to use, even in children and in pregnant patients. The ocular antihistamines are safe and can be used in children as young as 2 years (lodoxamide). The ophthalmic H₁ blockers are safe for use in adults, with ketotifen safe for use in children as young as 3 years.

The ocular NSAIDs are safe for treating a clear case of vernal conjunctivitis. If the diagnosis is unclear, an ophthalmological consult is indicated before prescribing to clarify the diagnosis and rule out herpes keratitis.

The ophthalmic corticosteroid preparations have serious adverse effects. They should be prescribed only by an ophthalmologist.

Monitoring

The primary care provider needs to monitor the patient for effectiveness of therapy. There is no specific laboratory monitoring necessary with these medications. IOP should be periodically monitored by a trained eye professional if using medications that may increase IOP, ocular corticosteroids, and naphazoline.

Patient Education

Administration

The patient should be instructed to use the medication exactly as prescribed. Overuse or underuse can adversely affect the outcome of the clinical condition. Advise the patient to avoid touching the dropper to the eye or other surface, which may contaminate the medication. To prevent cross-contamination, neither prescription nor OTC products should be shared with another person.

Adverse Reactions

Alert the patient to the adverse reaction of transient stinging and burning that may occur with the use of ocular medications. If the burning or stinging is intense or prolonged or if there is any other adverse reaction, the patient should contact the primary care provider.

OCULAR LUBRICANTS

Ocular lubricants offer tear-like lubrication for the relief of dry eyes and eye irritation. Ocular lubricants are also referred to as *artificial tears.* An artificial tear insert consisting of hydroxypropyl cellulose (Lacrisert), which may be prescribed by an ophthalmologist or optometrist, is not discussed in this chapter. The immunomodulator/anti-inflammatory cyclosporine (Restasis) is used to treat dry eye and is prescribed by an ophthalmologist.

Pharmacodynamics

Ocular lubricants contain a balanced solution of salts to maintain ocular tonicity, buffers to adjust pH, viscosity to prolong eye contact time, and preservatives.

Pharmacokinetics

Ocular lubricants are not absorbed in measurable amounts.

Pharmacotherapeutics

Precautions and Contraindications

There are no true contraindications to the use of ocular lubricants. Products that contain benzalkonium chloride (Teargen, Akwa Tears, Puralube Tears, Comfort Tears, Dry

Eyes, HypoTears, Ultra Tears, Isopto Plain, Isopto Tears, Just Tears, LubriTears, Moisture Drops, Murine, Nature's Tears, Nu-Tears, Nu-Tears II, Tearisol, OcuCoat, Tears Naturale, Tears Renewed) should not be used with soft contacts.

Adverse Drug Reactions

The ocular lubricants may cause mild stinging and temporary blurred vision.

Drug Interactions

There are no significant drug interactions with the ocular lubricants.

Clinical Use and Dosing

Dry Eye Syndrome

Ocular lubricants or artificial tears are used as needed to provide relief of dry eyes and ocular irritation. They can also be used as lubricants for artificial eyes. The patient should be instructed to instill 1 or 2 drops into the eye(s) 3 to 4 times a day or as needed. Table 26-8 presents the dosing schedule.

Table 26–8 ⊗ Dosage Schedule: Miscellaneous Ophthalmic Products

Drug	Indication	Dosage Forms	Dose	Comments
Ocular Lubricants				
Artificial tears Bion Tears Duratears Naturale Hypotears Lacri-Lube Muro 128	Ocular irritation, xerophthalmia	Preservative-free solution: dextran, hydroxypropyl methylcellulose Ointment: lanolin, mineral oil Solution: polyvinyl alcohol Preservative-free ointment: light mineral oil, white petrolatum Ointment: petrolatum, mineral oil Solution: sodium chloride	*Adults and children:* Instill 1–2 drops into affected eye(s) 3–4 times/d as needed	
Ophthalmic Vasoconstrictors				
Naphazoline Bausch & Lomb Allergy Drops Bausch & Lomb Maximum Strength Allergy Drops Clear Eyes Comfort Eye Drops	Relief of eye redness	0.012% solution 0.03% solution 0.012% solution 0.03% solution 0.012% solution 0.1% solution 0.1% solution 0.02% solution	Instill 1–2 drops qid as needed	Treatment should not continue for longer than 3 to 4 d without the supervision of an ophthalmologist
Oxymetazoline OcuClear Visine LR	Relief of eye redness	0.025% solution	*Adults and children:* 1–2 drops in affected eye(s) bid-qid but no more frequently than every 6 h	OTC
Tetrahydrozoline Visine Murine Plus	Relief of eye redness	0.05% solution	*Adults:* Instill 1–2 drops into the affected eye(s) up to 4 times/d	OTC

Continued

Table 26–8 ⊗ **Dosage Schedule: Miscellaneous Ophthalmic Products—cont'd**

Drug	Indication	Dosage Forms	Dose	Comments
Ophthalmic Diagnostic Products				
Fluorescein	Detection of corneal abrasion or defect	2% solution Strips: 0.6, 1, 9 mg	2% solution: Instill 1–2 drops into the eye; use Wood's lamp to detect staining of defect Strips: Moisten strip with sterile water and place at fornix in the lower cul-de-sac; the patient should close lid tightly and blink several times; use Wood's lamp to detect defect	After examination, excess stain can be removed with sterile saline solution Soft contact lenses can be reinserted 1 h after the eyes are flushed with saline to remove fluorescein

Monitoring

There is no laboratory monitoring needed with the use of artificial tears.

Patient Education

Administration

Advise the patient to avoid touching the dropper to the eye or another surface, which may contaminate the medication.

Adverse Reactions

Advise the patient that transient mild stinging and blurred vision may occur. The patient should contact the primary care provider if headache, eye pain, vision changes, prolonged redness, or discharge occurs.

OPHTHALMIC VASOCONSTRICTORS

Ophthalmic vasoconstrictors are used in primary care to provide temporary relief of redness of the eye due to minor eye irritants. There are ophthalmic vasoconstrictors that are used by eye-care specialists to dilate the pupil (hydroxyamphetamine Hbr, 2.5% and 10% phenylephrine); they are not covered in this chapter.

Pharmacodynamics

The ophthalmic vasoconstrictors are sympathomimetic agents that act by constricting the conjunctival blood vessels. The products used for eye redness are generally weak sympathomimetic solutions.

Pharmacokinetics

Information regarding the pharmacokinetics of the ophthalmic vasoconstrictors is not available, other than duration of action. The duration of action of naphazoline is 3 to 4 hours. Oxymetazoline's duration of action is 4 to 6 hours, and tetrahydrozoline's duration of action is 1 to 4 hours.

Pharmacotherapeutics

Precautions and Contraindications

The ophthalmic vasoconstrictors are contraindicated if the patient is sensitive to any of the components of the product. They are also contraindicated in any patient who has narrow-angle glaucoma.

The ophthalmic vasoconstrictors are Pregnancy Category C; the safety of their use in pregnancy has not been established.

Adverse Drug Reactions

The patient may experience transient stinging or burning on instillation. Blurring of vision may occur and is temporary, passing within minutes. Patients may experience mydriasis. Increased lacrimation, irritation, and discomfort may occur. The most serious adverse reaction that may occur is increased IOP.

Rebound congestion or redness can develop with frequent or extended use of ophthalmic vasoconstrictors.

Drug Interactions

There are no significant drug interactions with the use of oxymetazoline or tetrahydrozoline.

Tricyclic antidepressants and maprotiline (Ludiomil) may potentiate the pressor effects of naphazoline. If MAOIs are used with ophthalmic sympathomimetics, exaggerated adrenergic effects may result. Do not use MAOIs within 21 days of the ophthalmic sympathomimetics.

Systemic adverse effects may more easily occur if ophthalmic sympathomimetics are used with beta blockers.

Clinical Use and Dosing

Relief of Eye Redness

Ophthalmic vasoconstrictors that are used for temporary relief of eye redness due to irritation or allergic conjunctivitis include tetrahydrozoline, oxymetazoline, naphazoline, and phenylephrine. The usual adult dose is 1 or 2 drops instilled in the eyes 4 times a day. Use in children is not recommended.

Rational Drug Selection

Tetrahydrozoline, oxymetazoline, naphazoline (0.012%, 0.02%, 0.03%), and phenylephrine 0.12% are available OTC. Naphazoline 0.1% is available only by prescription. Phenylephrine 2.5% and 10% are used only for pupil dilation and are instilled by eye-care specialists.

Monitoring

There is no laboratory monitoring necessary with the use of ophthalmic vasoconstrictors.

Patient Education

Administration

Advise the patient to avoid touching the dropper to the eye or another surface, which may contaminate the medication. The patient should avoid prolonged or excessive use of ocular vasoconstrictors because rebound congestion or redness may occur.

Adverse Reactions

Advise the patient that transient mild stinging and blurred vision may occur.

OPHTHALMIC DIAGNOSTIC PRODUCTS

The ophthalmic diagnostic that is used in primary care is topical fluorescein sodium. It is used to detect corneal epithelial defects or abrasions. The injectable form of fluorescein is used by ophthalmologists as a diagnostic aid in ophthalmic angiography. Only the topical form is discussed in this chapter.

Pharmacodynamics

Fluorescein is a yellow, water-soluble dibasic acid xanthine dye. It produces an intense fluorescent green color in alkaline (pH 0.5) solution. Fluorescein detects defects in the corneal epithelium. A corneal abrasion or corneal epithelial defect will uptake the dye and appear bright green under ultraviolet light (Wood's lamp). Fluorescein does not stain the intact cornea.

Pharmacokinetics

When used for the detection of corneal abrasion, topical fluorescein is not absorbed.

Pharmacotherapeutics

Precautions and Contraindications

Hypersensitivity to fluorescein is a contraindication to its use.

Do not use fluorescein with soft contact lenses, which become stained. Lenses can be reinserted after the eyes are flushed with sterile saline and the patient waits an hour.

Fluorescein is Pregnancy Category C, although there are no reports of fetal complications or anomalies.

Adverse Drug Reactions

There are no adverse drug reactions reported with topical fluorescein use, other than staining of soft contact lenses.

Drug Interactions

There are no drug interactions with the use of topical fluorescein.

Clinical Use and Dosing

Detection of Corneal Epithelial Defects

If a corneal abrasion or foreign body is suspected, the provider instills 1 or 2 drops of fluorescein 2% solution into the eye. After a few seconds, epithelial defects will stain. The use of a Wood's lamp enhances detection of defects. Fluorescein strips may be used. The strip is moistened with sterile water and placed at the fornix in the lower cul-de-sac close to the punctum. The patient should close the lid tightly over the strip until the desired amount of staining occurs. Have the patient blink several times to distribute the stain. After examination, excess stain can be removed with sterile saline solution. An anesthetic eyedrop can be administered before instilling the fluorescein if the patient is experiencing discomfort from the initial injury.

Monitoring

There is no specific laboratory monitoring necessary with the use of topical fluorescein.

Patient Education

Administration

Advise the patient that the staining of the cornea is temporary and will resolve within a few hours. The patient should not be wearing soft contact lenses during the examination. Advise the patient to wait at least 1 hour before reinserting the contact lenses.

DRUGS USED IN TREATING EAR DISORDERS

OTIC ANTI-INFECTIVES

Otitis externa (OE) is an acute, painful inflammatory condition of the external auditory canal. Commonly known as *swimmer's ear,* OE affects people of all ages, and it is the most common cause of visits for ear pain. It can easily be treated by a primary care provider, yet it can have serious, even life-threatening, complications, especially in diabetic or immunocompromised patients.

OE occurs when there is a breakdown in several protective mechanisms. The normally acidic environment creates a hostile climate for bacterial growth. Cerumen is bacteriostatic and provides a protective layer that protects the epithelium against hyperhydration (Goguen, 2014). Factors that alter these defenses and contribute to OE include an abrasion in the ear canal, water in the ear canal, and maceration of the skin from heat and moisture. With OE, the acidic environment in the ear canal is changed to neutral or basic, usually by retained moisture. Itching and a sense of fullness develop from damage to the epithelium caused by hyperhydration. Organisms invade wet intact skin as well as damaged epithelium. Devices (hearing aids, ear phones) that occlude the ear canal can predispose one to external otitis (Goguen, 2014).

Pharmacodynamics

The medications used in the treatment of OE include combination products (Cortisporin, Pediotic, Ciprodex, Cipro HC) that contain a corticosteroid (hydrocortisone) and antibiotic(s) (neomycin, polymyxin B, ciprofloxacin); antibiotic alone (gentamycin, ofloxacin); and acid or alcohol drops (Otic Domeboro, Burow's Otic, VoSol, VoSol HC).

Hydrocortisone reduces the inflammation caused by OE. The exact mechanism of action for topical corticosteroids is not known. They are thought to act by the induction of phospholipase A_2 inhibitory proteins. These proteins control the mediators of inflammation, such as prostaglandins and leukotrienes.

Neomycin is active against *S. aureus* and *Proteus* and *Enterobacter* species. Polymyxin B is generally active against gram-negative bacteria (*P. aeruginosa, E. coli, H. influenzae*). Gentamicin is a broad-spectrum aminoglycoside that is active against *P. aeruginosa,* staphylococci, *S. pneumoniae,* beta-hemolytic streptococci, and *Enterobacter* species. The fluoroquinolones (ciprofloxacin, ofloxacin) are active against staphylococci, *S. pneumoniae, Proteus* and *Enterobacter* species, and *P. aeruginosa.*

Acid and alcohol solutions such as Otic Domeboro and Burow's Otic contain 2% acetic acid in aluminum acetate solution. Another acid solution, VoSol Otic, contains 2% acetic acid solution and 3% propylene glycol. These solutions reduce inflammation and are antibacterial and antifungal.

Pharmacokinetics

Information regarding the pharmacokinetics of otic preparations is not available.

Pharmacotherapeutics

Precautions and Contraindications

Hypersensitivity to any component of the product is a contraindication to its use.

Ciprofloxacin is contraindicated if the tympanic membrane (TM) is perforated. Cortisporin otic solution is contraindicated if the TM is perforated. Cortisporin otic suspension may be used.

Prolonged use of topical antibiotics may lead to superinfection and overgrowth of nonsusceptible organisms and fungi.

Adverse Drug Reactions

Local reactions, such as contact dermatitis, may occur with any of the otic preparations. Superinfection may develop with prolonged use. Ofloxacin otic may cause taste alteration. Dizziness, vertigo, and paresthesias have also been reported with otic ofloxacin use. Ototoxicity may occur with prolonged use of Pediotic and Cortisporin otic solution.

Drug Interactions

There are no known drug interactions for the topical otic preparations.

Clinical Use and Dosing

Acute Otitis Externa (Swimmer's Ear)

On presentation of OE, the canal is swollen and full of discharge. The organisms found in OE (swimmer's ear) are usually gram-negative rods, *P. aeruginosa, Enterobacter* species, and *Proteus mirabilis. Pseudomonas* is the most common organism found in OE. Mycotic OE is less common, usually caused by *Aspergillus, Trichophyton,* or *Candida.* Occasionally, a furunculosis (small abscess) of the external canal may be caused by *S. aureus* or *S. pyogenes,* carried there by dirty fingers.

Once it has been determined that the TM is intact, the canal can be gently cleaned with warm saline or 3% hydrogen peroxide. If the TM cannot be visualized, irrigation should not be performed.

Topical medication is the treatment of choice. A steroid/antibiotic drop that combines hydrocortisone with neomycin and polymyxin B (Cortisporin Otic, Pediotic), colistin (Coly-Mycin S Otic), a hydrocortisone/ciprofloxacin (Ciloxan HC) suspension is instilled in the affected ear 4 times a day. The usual dose is 4 drops, and treatment should continue for 7 to 10 days. Gentamicin and ofloxacin provide good coverage for the common organisms, but the combination products decrease inflammation faster. Gentamycin, acetic acid, and Cortisporin Otic cannot be used if the TM is perforated.

A topical acid or alcohol solution (Otic Domeboro, Burow's Otic, VoSol) can be instilled into the ear 4 times a day if the TM is intact. A 1:1 mixture of vinegar and rubbing alcohol is just as effective, but it can be painful to administer. If excessive inflammation is present, a combination of acid with hydrocortisone (VoSol HC) may be effective.

If the canal is too swollen to allow the drops to be instilled, a wick of 0.25 in. gauze or cotton may be inserted into the swollen external canal for 24 to 36 hours. The medication can be dropped onto the wick. To evaluate progress, the patient will need to be reexamined 48 hours after the wick has been placed.

Chronic Otitis Externa

Chronic OE can be inflammatory or infectious. Psoriasis, eczema, or seborrhea can cause inflammatory chronic OE. Chronic infectious OE may be caused by infected sinus tracts, cysts, or fungi.

The treatment for inflammatory chronic OE is determined by the severity of presentation. If the patient is complaining of chronic itching, accompanied by dry skin elsewhere on the body, the treatment consists of placing 2 or 3 drops of baby oil or mineral oil in the canal daily. If the patient has psoriasis in the external canal, it can be treated with steroid cream or lotion (see Chap. 32). Seborrhea can cause a scaly inflammation in the external auditory canal and behind the ears, usually accompanied by seborrhea of the forehead, eyelids, and face. Treatment is the use of selenium sulfide shampoo and topical corticosteroids (see Chap. 23, "Drugs Affecting the Integumentary System").

If the ear canal is greatly inflamed, treatment includes cleansing the external canal of debris and using a steroid otic solution (Decadron) 2 or 3 times a day until the swelling decreases. If needed to relieve the inflammation, a wick can be placed and Otic Domeboro or Burow's Otic dropped onto the wick for 24 to 48 hours.

Malignant Otitis Externa

Malignant OE is a rare but potentially lethal infection caused by *P. aeruginosa*. Malignant OE occurs mainly in older patients with diabetes (90%). It develops when OE extends and invades the surrounding tissues, causing osteomyelitis of the base of the skull and purulent meningitis, accompanied by multiple cranial nerve palsies. Standard treatment includes parenteral antibiotics with an aminoglycoside and carbenicillin for 4 to 6 weeks, plus surgical debridement.

Prevention of Swimmer's Ear

Most cases of acute OE (swimmer's ear) can be prevented by instilling isopropyl ear drops (Swim-Ear, EarSol) or 1 or 2 drops of rubbing alcohol into the ear canal to dry the ear after swimming. A combination of 1:1 isopropyl alcohol and white vinegar may also be used. The commercial preparations have the advantage of less stinging with application if the skin is slightly macerated.

Table 26-9 presents the dosage schedule of drugs used in treating ear disorders.

Table 26–9 ✂ Dosage Schedule: Drugs Used in Treating Ear Disorders

Drug	Indication	Dosage Forms	Dose	Comments
Otic Anti-Infectives				
Gentamicin Garamycin	Otitis externa	Solution: 3 mg/mL	Use ophthalmic drops: 4 drops in affected ear qid for 7–10 d	Broad-spectrum coverage
Ofloxacin Floxin Otic	Otitis externa Chronic suppurative otitis media with perforated tympanic membrane Otitis media in children with tympanostomy tubes	0.3% solution	*Children 6 mo–12 yr:* 5 drops in affected ear once daily for 10 d *Children ≥12 yr:* 10 drops in affected ear once daily for 10 d	To prevent dizziness, warm bottle in hand for 1–2 min prior to administering Not recommended for use in children <6 mo
Otic Anti-Infective-Steroid Combination				
Ciprofloxacin-hydrocortisone (Cipro HC Otic)	Acute otitis externa	Suspension: Ciprofloxacin 2 mg/mL hydrocortisone 10 mg/mL	*Children ≥1 yr:* 3 drops in affected ear bid for 7 d	To minimize dizziness warm suspension by holding bottle in hand for 1–2 min before use Not recommended in children <1 yr Contraindicated if tympanic membrane ruptured
Ciprofloxacin-dexamethasone (Ciprodex)	Acute otitis media in pediatric patients with tympanostomy tubes Acute otitis externa	Suspension: ciprofloxacin 0.3% dexamethasone 0.1%	*Children ≥6 mo:* 4 drops in affected ear bid for 7 d	Not recommended in children <6 mo
Hydrocortisone-neomycin-polymyxin B Cortisporin Otic Pediotic	Otitis externa Chronic suppurative otitis media with perforated tympanic membrane	Suspension: hydrocortisone 1%, neomycin 5 mg/mL, polymyxin B 10,000 U/mL Solution: hydrocortisone 1%, neomycin 5 mg/mL, polymyxin B 10,000 U/mL	*Children:* 3 drops of suspension in affected ear 3–4 times/d *Adults:* 4 drops of suspension in affected ear 3–4 times/d	Contraindicated if TM perforated
Hydrocortisone-neomycin-colistin Coly-Mycin S Otic	Otitis externa	Suspension: hydrocortisone 1%, neomycin 5 mg/mL, colistin 3 mg/mL	4 drops of suspension in affected ear 3–4 times/d	Contraindicated if TM perforated

Continued

Table 26–9 ⊗ **Dosage Schedule: Drugs Used in Treating Ear Disorders—cont'd**

Drug	Indication	Dosage Forms	Dose	Comments
Acid–Alcohol Solutions				
Acetic acid-aluminum acetate Otic Domeboro, Burow's Otic	Otitis externa	Solution	Clean ear canal; instill 4 drops 3–4 times/d for 7–10 d If canal swollen: Insert wick saturated with solution; instill 4–6 drops q2–3h; keep moist for 24 h	Contraindicated if TM perforated
Acetic acid-propylene glycol VoSol Otic	Otitis externa	Solution	Clean ear canal; instill 5 drops 3–4 times/d for 7–10 d If canal swollen: Insert wick saturated with solution; instill 4–6 drops q2–3h; after 24 h, remove wick and instill 5 drops qid	Contraindicated if TM perforated Not recommended in children ≤3 yr
Acetic acid-propylene glycol-hydrocortisone VoSol HC Otic	Otitis externa	Solution	Clean ear canal, and instill 5 drops 3–4 times daily for 7–10 d May use cotton wick for first 24 h	Contraindicated if TM perforated Not recommended in children ≤3 yr
Isopropyl alcohol-glycerine Swim-Ear	Drying solution for ear canal	Liquid: 95% isopropyl alcohol, 5% anhydrous glycerin	Instill 4–6 drops in each ear after swimming or bathing	
Isopropyl alcohol-propylene glycol EarSol	Drying solution for ear canal	Drops: 44% isopropyl alcohol, propylene glycol	Instill 6–8 drops in each ear after swimming or bathing bid	
Otic Analgesics				
Benzocaine-antipyrine-glycerin Auralgan	Analgesia in acute otitis media Adjunct in cerumen removal	Solution	Otitis media: Fill affected canal and insert cotton plug; may repeat every 1–2 h if needed Cerumen removal: Fill ear canal tid for 2–3 d	Contraindicated if TM perforated
Benzocaine-antipyrine-propylene glycol Tympagesic	Analgesia in acute otitis media	Solution	Fill ear canal and insert cotton plug; repeat q2–4h as needed	Contraindicated if TM perforated
Ceruminolytics				
Carbamide peroxide Debrox Murine Ear Auro Ear Drops	Cerumen removal	6.5% drops	Instill 5–10 drops in ear canal, keep drops in for several minutes, and repeat bid for up to 4 d	Contraindicated if TM perforated Not recommended in young children
Triethanolamine Cerumenex Drops	Cerumen removal	10% drops	Fill ear canal, insert cotton plug, allow to remain for 15–30 min, and flush ear	Contraindicated if TM perforated

TM = tympanic membrane

Monitoring

There is no laboratory monitoring necessary with these medications. The patient with a severely inflamed external canal requiring a wick should be reassessed 48 hours after treatment is begun and at the end of treatment to determine clinical cure. Patients with chronic OE need cleansing of the canal and reassessment every 2 to 3 weeks and may require alterations in topical medications, depending on clinical status.

Patient Education

Administration

Advise the patient to hold the bottle of medication in the hand for a few minutes to warm the medication before instilling. The patient should lie on her or his side with the affected ear up, instill the drops, and keep the ear up for 2 minutes or insert a soft cotton plug to prevent the medication from draining out.

Adverse Reactions

Advise patients to notify their primary care provider if adverse effects occur.

OTIC ANALGESICS

Topical anesthetics are used in the ear to treat pain associated with otitis media. The local anesthetics antipyrine and benzocaine (Americaine, Dolotic, Auralgan, Auroto) are used to provide pain relief until systemic antibiotics can take effect. Analgesic eardrops are instilled into the affected ear 3 to 4 times daily or up to once every 1 to 2 hours as needed for pain. The tympanic membrane should be examined to ensure it is intact before prescribing topical anesthetic agents.

CERUMINOLYTICS

Some patients have an excessive accumulation of cerumen, which can lead to conductive hearing loss, impaction, and an environment for OE to develop. Patients who use cotton-tipped applicators (Q-Tips) to try to remove the cerumen actually push the cerumen farther into the canal. The cerumen often forms a hard plug that is painful to remove. Treatment includes instillation of mineral oil, which softens the wax, or the use of carbamide peroxide (Debrox, Dent's Ear Wax, Murine Ear Wax Removal), which softens and emulsifies the wax. Dosage of carbamide peroxide is to instill 1 to 5 drops (depending on the size of the ear canal) twice daily for up to 4 days. Once the cerumen is softened, the ear canal can be irrigated with *warm* water or saline. If the canal is excoriated, application of antibiotic or steroid eardrops for 7 to 10 days will prevent the development of OE.

REFERENCES

American Academy of Pediatrics (2012a). Prevention of neonatal ophthalmia. In L. K. Pickering (Ed.), *Red book: 2012 report of the Committee on Infectious Diseases* (29th ed., pp. 880–881). Elk Grove Village, IL: American Academy of Pediatrics. Retrieved from http://aapredbook.aappublications.org/content/1/SEC317/SEC329.body

American Academy of Pediatrics. (2012b). Gonococcal infections. In L. K. Pickering (Ed.), *Red book: 2012 report of the Committee on Infectious Diseases* (29th ed., pp. 336–344). Elk Grove Village, IL: American Academy of Pediatrics. Retrieved http://aapredbook.aappublications.org/content/1/SEC131/SEC184.body

American Academy of Pediatrics. (2012c). *Chlamydia trachomatis.* In L. K. Pickering (Ed.), *Red book: 2012 report of the Committee on Infectious Diseases* (29th ed., pp. 276–281). Elk Grove Village, IL: American Academy of Pediatrics. Retrieved from http://aapredbook.aappublications.org/content/1/SEC131/SEC158/SEC161.body

Buznach, N., Dagan, R., & Greenberg, D. (2005). Clinical and bacterial characteristics of acute bacterial conjunctivitis in children in the antibiotic resistance cra. *Pediatric Infectious Disease Journal, 24*(9), 823–828.

Centers for Disease Control and Prevention (CDC). (2010). Sexually transmitted treatment guidelines: Gonococcal infections. Retrieved from http://www.cdc.gov/std/treatment/2010/gonococcal-infections.htm

Glaucoma Research Foundation. (2013). Glaucoma facts and stats. Retrieved from http://www.glaucoma.org/learn/glaucoma_facts.php

Goguen, L. A. (2014). External otitis: Pathogenesis, clinical features, and diagnosis. *UpToDate.* Wolters Kluwer Health. Retrieved from http://www.uptodate.com/contents/external-otitis-pathogenesis-clinical-features-and-diagnosis

Hautala, N., Hautala, T., & Koskela, M. (2008). Major age group-specific differences in conjunctival bacteria and evolution of antimicrobial resistance revealed by laboratory data surveillance. *Current Eye Research, 33,* 907–911.

Paysse, E. A., Coats, D. K., & Cassidy, M. (2014). Nasolacrimal duct obstruction (dacryostenosis) in children. *UpToDate.* Wolters Kluwer Health. Retrieved from http://www.uptodate.com/contents/nasolacrimal-duct-obstruction-dacryostenosis-in-children#H15

Shtein, R. M. (2014). Blepharitis. *UpToDate.* Wolters Kluwer Health. Retrieved from http://www.uptodate.com/contents/blepharitis

Smith, A. F., & Waycaster, C. (2009). Estimate of the direct and indirect annual cost of bacterial conjunctivitis in the United States. *BMC Ophthalmology, 9,* 13.

U.S. Preventive Services Task Force. (2011). Ocular prophylaxis for gonococcal ophthalmia neonatorium. *AHRQ Publication No. 10-05146-EF-3.* Retrieved from http://www.uspreventiveservicestaskforce.org/uspstf10/gonoculproph/gonocupsum.htm

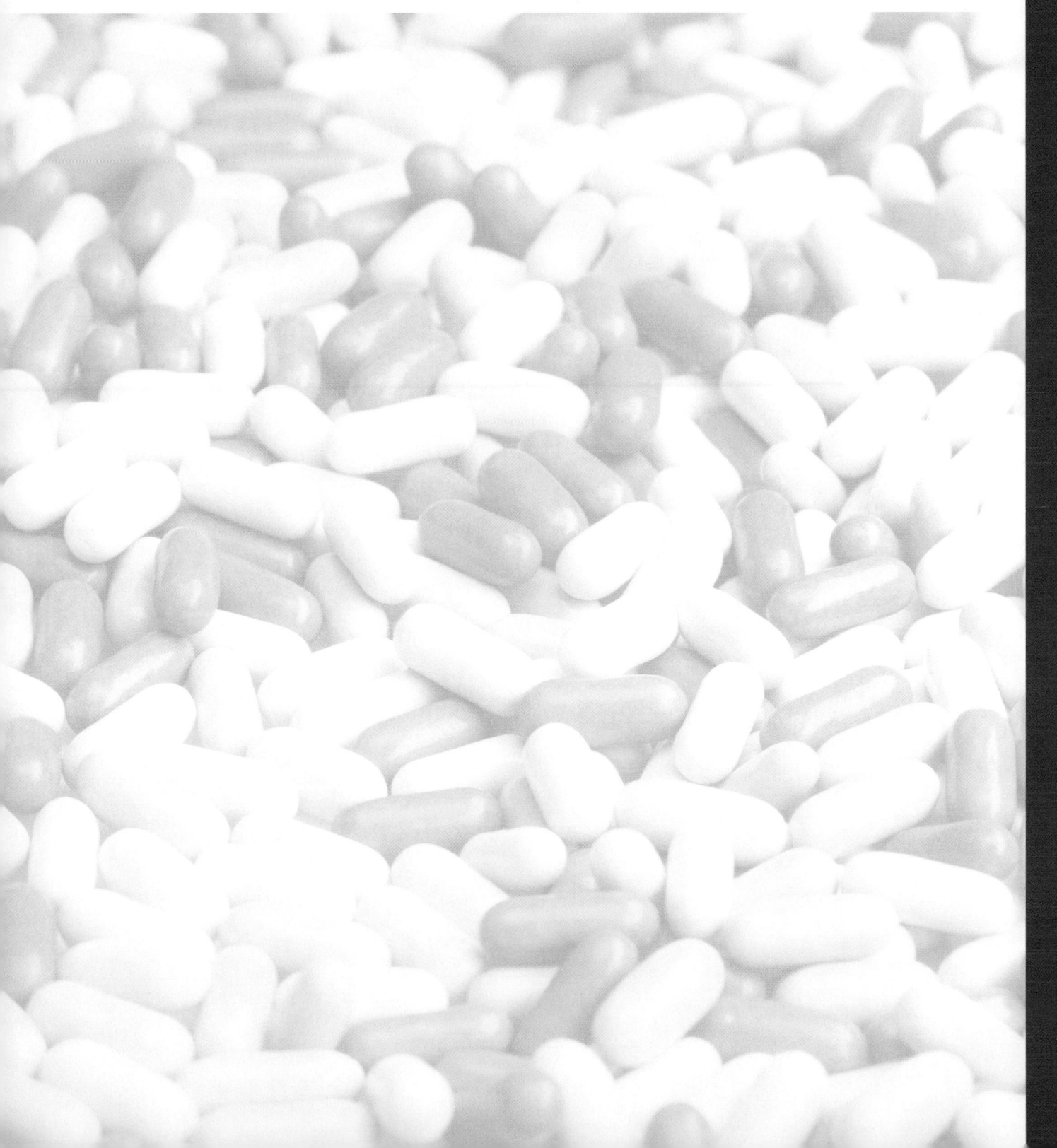

PHARMACOTHERAPEUTICS WITH MULTIPLE DRUGS

PHARMACEUTICS
WITH MULTIPLE DRUGS

ANEMIA

Teri Moser Woo • Kristen Osborn

nemias are extremely common in primary care practice; there are 5.5 million ambulatory care visits annually that list anemia as the primary diagnosis (Schappert & Rechtsteiner, 2008). The World Health Organization (WHO) estimates that 2 billion people worldwide have anemia (2013). Anemia is a sign of disease rather than a disease itself. Iron deficiency anemia (IDA) is the most common type of anemia, with a prevalence of 14% in children age 1 to 2 years and 9% in women age 12 to 49 years (Centers for Disease Control and Prevention [CDC], 2013a). Anemia of chronic disease (ACD) develops secondary to a chronic disease, cancer, or long-term infection and is the second most common form of anemia, The third major form of anemia is sickle cell disease (SCD), which affects 90,000 to 100,000 Americans, mainly of African ancestry, with SCD occurring in approximately 1 in every 500 African American births (CDC, 2011). Other forms of anemia discussed in this chapter are folic acid deficiency and pernicious anemia.

Diagnosis and treatment of the various forms of anemia entail interpretation of blood studies and peripheral smears to correctly diagnose the type of anemia. Normal blood count values are found in Table 27-1. Treatment consists of lifestyle modifications in the form of diet and energy conservation and prescription of drugs specific to each disorder. This chapter reviews the relevant pathophysiology of the common anemias seen in primary care, as well as management or comanagement of the disorder.

PATHOPHYSIOLOGY COMMON TO ALL ANEMIAS

The underlying pathophysiology in all types of anemia is a decrease in the oxygen-carrying capacity of the blood. Figure 27-1 depicts the progression and manifestations of anemia. The reasons for this decrease vary by type of anemia. Anemias are classified by erythrocyte size and hemoglobin (Hgb) content. Size is referred to by the terms *microcytic* (small), *macrocytic* (large), and *normocytic*. Hgb content is referred to by the terms *hypochromic* (low Hgb) or *normochromic*.

Regardless of the disease process, the decreased oxygen transport to tissues carries the same results. Decreased mitochondrial oxygenation at the cellular level leads to decreased ATP production and reliance on the glycolytic process, resulting in poor energy generation and the formation of lactic acid, which affects the body's acid–base balance. It also affects the functioning of the body's largest energy consumer, the sodium-potassium-ATPase pump. As this pump works less efficiently, fluid and electrolyte shifts occur. Activation of the renin-angiotensin-aldosterone system augments the fluid shifts, with resultant sodium and water retention.

A reduction in the number of circulating red blood cells (RBCs) affects the consistency and volume of blood. Less viscous blood flows faster and more turbulently and may cause ventricular dysfunction, cardiac dilation, and heart valve insufficiency. Increased venous return to the heart stimulates the heart to pump harder and faster, resulting in tachycardia

Table 27–1   Normal Blood Values by Age and Gender

Age/Gender	Hemoglobin (g/100 mL)	Hematocrit	RBC Count (million/mm³)	Mean Corpuscle Volume (mcg³) Concentration (pg/cell)	Mean Corpuscle Hemoglobin Concentration (pg/cell)	RBC Distribution Width
Infants 3 mo	9.5–14.5 Mean 12	32%–41%	2.7–4.9	78	30–33	
Infants 6 mo to children 6 yr	10.5–14	32–41%	3.7–5.3	77–81	31–34	
Children 9–12 yr	12–15	34%–43%	4.0–5.2	83–86	31–34	
Adolescents 12–14 yr Male Female	12–16 11.5–15	35%–45% 34%–44%	4.5–5.3 4.1–5.1	78–88 78–90	31–34	
Adolescents 15–17 yr Male Female	12.3–16.6 11.7–15.3	37%–48% 34%–44%	4.5–5.3 4.1–5.1	Adult levels Adult levels	31–34	
Adults 18+ yr Male Female	13.2–17.3 11.7–15.5	40%–54% 35%–47%	Both genders: 4.2–5.4 3.6–5.0	Both genders: Microcytic = <87 Normocytic = 87–103 Macrocytic = >103	Hypochromic = <32 Normochromic = 32–36 Hyperchromic = >36	Both genders: 11.5%–14.5% CU

CU = conventional units.

and the risk of heart failure. To better oxygenate the reduced number of RBCs, the respiratory rate and depth increase. If the anemia is severe enough to overcome the usual compensatory mechanisms, the patient experiences shortness of breath, a rapid pounding pulse, dizziness, and fatigue, even at rest. Laboratory values with anemias are found in Table 27-2.

Iron Deficiency Anemia (IDA)

The World Health Organization (WHO) considers iron deficiency the most common and widespread nutritional disorder in the world (2013). Iron deficiency anemia (IDA) decreases oxygen-carrying capacity because of a low hemoglobin concentration that is due to reduced RBC production (lack of adequate iron intake, poor absorption of iron by the body, or lead poisoning) or acute or chronic blood loss. This produces a microcytic-hypochromic anemia that develops slowly after the normal stores of iron have been depleted in the body and particularly the bone marrow.

IDA may be caused by increased demand for iron during pregnancy, periods of growth in children, or blood loss from menstruation. IDA affects 9% of women of childbearing age, related largely to iron loss secondary to blood loss from menstruation (CDC, 2013a). Premenopausal women who are athletes may experience iron deficiency or iron deficiency anemia at a higher rate than nonathletes (McClung, Marchitelli, Friedl, & Young, 2006; McClung, 2013). About 50% of pregnant women worldwide have IDA based in part on the use of

iron by the fetus (WHO, 2013). An estimated 14% of children 1 to 2 years of age in the United States and 40% of preschool children worldwide are anemic. IDA also affects about 4% of males (Rote & McCance, 2010). IDA associated with increased demand can be easily managed by the use of vitamins that contain additional iron or iron supplements (Office of Dietary Supplements [ODS], 2010).

Pathological iron loss occurs most often from gastrointestinal (GI) bleeding. Gastric and duodenal ulcers, diverticula, hemorrhoids, and ulcerative colitis are common sources of this bleeding. GI bleeding is such a common cause of IDA that it is recommended all men and postmenopausal women with IDA and all premenopausal women whose IDA cannot be explained by heavy menses should be evaluated for occult GI bleed (Bull-Henry & Al-Kawas, 2013). Less common causes of IDA include malabsorption syndromes, achlorhydria, steatorrhea, and unrelenting diarrhea (Montoya, Wink, & Sole, 2002). Individuals with renal failure, especially those being treated with dialysis, are at high risk for developing IDA because their kidneys do not secrete sufficient erythropoietin. Erythropoietin and iron can both be lost in dialysis. The National Kidney Foundation (2006) has a clinical practice guideline specifically addressing this issue. Lead exposure can also lead to IDA because high blood lead levels impair iron uptake and prevent Hgb formation.

Iron absorption can be affected by food intake and medications. Foods containing ascorbic acid (vitamin C) can increase iron absorption, whereas phytate found in bran, oats,

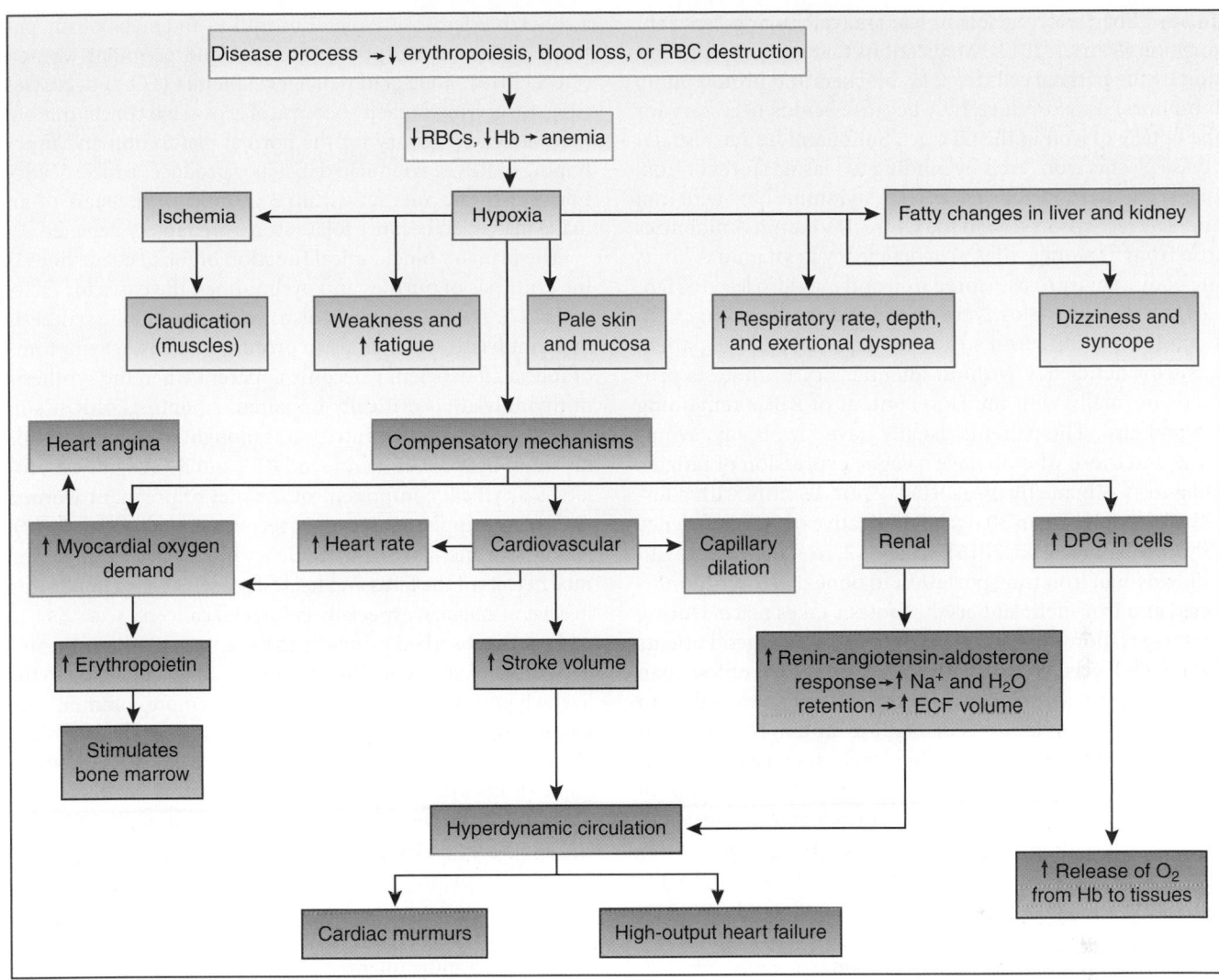

Figure 27–1. Progression and manifestations of anemia.

Table 27–2 Laboratory Findings in Selected Anemias

Test	Iron Deficiency Anemia	Folic Acid Deficiency Anemia	Pernicious Anemia	Anemia of Chronic Disease	Sickle Cell Anemia
Hemoglobin	Low	Low	Low	Low	Low (5–11 g/dL)
Hematocrit	Low	Low	Low	Low	Low (about 20%)
Reticulocyte count	Normal	Low	Low	Normal	Low (5%–20%)
Plasma iron	Low	High	High	Normal or low	Normal
Total iron-binding capacity	High	Normal	Normal	Normal or low	Normal
Ferritin	Low	High	High	Normal	Normal
Transferrin	Low	Slightly high	Slightly high	Slightly high	Normal
Mean corpuscular volume (MCV)	Low	High	High	Normal to low	Normal to low*
Serum B$_{12}$	Normal	Normal	Low	Normal	Normal
Folate	Normal	Low	Normal	Normal	Normal

*MCV will be low if a combination of sickle cell disease (SCD) and beta thalassemia are present, and normal if only SCD is present.

and rye fiber; polyphenols in tea; and calcium decrease absorption (Schrier, 2013). Medications that reduce acid secretion by the parietal cells (e.g., H$_2$ blockers and proton pump inhibitors) may produce IDA because acid is necessary for the uptake of iron in the GI tract. Sulfonamides can also decrease plasma iron levels by binding to plasma stores of iron. Bile-sequestering acids such as cholestyramine bind with iron and decrease absorption in the GI tract. Vitamin A mobilizes iron from its storage sites, so a deficiency in vitamin A limits the body's ability to use stored iron and may also lead to IDA.

IDA develops slowly in three overlapping stages. In stage 1, the body's iron stores are depleted and the patient has iron deficiency without anemia. Erythropoiesis proceeds normally with the Hgb content of RBCs remaining normal also. The patients usually have few, if any, symptoms and those who do have a vague expression of fatigue. Diagnosis is made by measuring serum ferritin, with a ferritin level of less than 30 ng/mL indicative of iron deficiency (Short & Domagalski, 2013). In stage 2, iron deficiency with mild anemia, iron transportation to bone marrow is diminished and iron-deficient erythropoiesis takes place. During this stage laboratory values begin to show changes. Patients have Hgb levels of 9 to 12 g/dL, serum ferritin of less than 20 ng/mL, and serum iron level of less than 60 mcg/dL and usually have no symptoms or vague symptoms of fatigue or headache. Those with lower Hgb levels may have more definitive symptoms, such as weakness and shortness of breath. Table 27-2 shows the laboratory values consistent with a variety of anemias. Stage 3, severe iron deficiency with severe anemia, begins when the small, hemoglobin-deficient cells enter the circulation in sufficient numbers and replace normal erythrocytes that have reached maturity and been removed from the circulation.

RBCs have a normal life expectancy of about 120 days. This stage is associated with IDA, depleted iron stores, and diminished Hgb production. Hgb levels are now 6 to 7 g/dL. Serum ferritin levels are very low at this point, less than 10 mg/mL and serum iron levels are less than 40 mcg/cL (Schrier, 2013). The earlobes, palms, and conjunctivae become pale. Nails become brittle, thin, coarsely ridged, and spoon-shaped as a result of impaired oxygen transport. The tongue becomes red, sore, and painful owing to atrophy of papillae. Dry, sore skin at the corners of the mouth and difficulty swallowing exacerbated by decreased salivation may also occur. Mental confusion, memory loss, and disorientation frequently are associated with anemia secondary to poor oxygen transport to cerebral tissue. This is especially problematic in the older adult population if they are wrongly perceived to be normal events related to aging (Rote & McCance, 2010). Severe IDA with Hgb levels below 7 g/dL may result in postural hypotension, dizziness, weakness, gastritis, irritability, numbness, and lethargy.

Folic Acid Deficiency Anemia (FOA)

Folate deficiency is rare in developed countries, but certain groups are at risk for deficiency, including alcoholics because alcohol interferes with folate absorption and metabolism, patients with malabsorptive disorders, and pregnant women (ODS, 2012). Folic acid deficiency anemia (FOA) decreases oxygen-carrying capacity because of a low Hgb concentration. Folic acid is necessary for the normal maturation and functioning of RBCs. Folic acid deficiency produces a macrocytic-normochromic anemia within 3 months of the start of an inadequate diet, because folate stores are rapidly depleted.

The primary biochemical function of folate coenzymes is the synthesis of purines and pyrimidines, the bases for DNA and RNA. These coenzymes also are involved in the synthesis of thymidylate, which is also a precursor of DNA. Symptoms of folic acid deficiency become apparent when the synthesis of thymidylate is critically impaired. Apoptosis of RBCs in the late stages of differentiation is thought to occur with this disorder. Because of its role in DNA and RNA synthesis, folate is a critical component of the diet of pregnant women and folate supplementation is recommended (ODS, 2012). Along with anemia, folate deficiency is associated with neural tube defects of the fetus and heart disease. It is also implicated in several cancers, especially colorectal cancers.

Folate is absorbed primarily in the upper small intestine independent of any facilitating factor. It is then circulated to the liver where it is stored. Folate deficiency is more common than vitamin B$_{12}$ deficiency and often associated with alcoholics, chronic malnutrition, fad diets, and diets low in vegetables. Some drugs interfere with the cobalamin-folate–dependent pathway (e.g., methotrexate and fluorouracil). Dilantin, sulfamethoxazole/trimethoprim, and oral contraceptives compete with folate metabolism and storage in the liver.

Patients with folic acid deficiency commonly complain of glossitis, stomatitis, nausea and anorexia, and diarrhea. A systolic ejection murmur may be heard. A positive Romberg's sign and increased or decreased deep tendon reflexes (DTRs) may also occur along with mild confusion, depression, apathy, and intellectual loss. Peripheral neuropathies will be present only if vitamin B$_{12}$ is also deficient.

Pernicious Anemia (PA)

Pernicious anemia (PA) also has a low Hgb concentration. Vitamin B$_{12}$ is necessary for maturation and DNA synthesis in RBCs, and when the cause of vitamin B$_{12}$ deficiency is autoimmune and linked to heredity, it is PA. PA is also associated with other autoimmune conditions, particularly those that affect the endocrine, such as Hashimoto's thyroiditis, type 1 diabetes mellitus, Addison's disease, and Graves' disease. PA produces a macrocytic-normochromic anemia that develops slowly, often over years, and it is frequently severe before it is diagnosed. In the absence of genetic mutations, vitamin B$_{12}$ deficiency is practically nonexistent because there are rich dietary sources in animal proteins. However, other patients are prone to consume too little vitamin B$_{12}$—vegetarians, particularly vegans, those with Crohn's disease, in which a section of the small intestine may be destroyed or others with resection of the bowel such as gastric bypass surgery, and pregnant women who are strict vegetarians (ODS, 2011).

Gastric parietal cells secrete intrinsic factor, which binds to dietary vitamin B_{12} during digestion and absorption of nutrients. Adequate intrinsic factor, along with hydrochloric acid, is needed to permit this vitamin to be absorbed. Patients with PA have a genetic absence of intrinsic factor. Other causes include gastrectomy and gastric atrophy of parietal cells associated with type A chronic gastritis.

Vague early symptoms of PA (e.g., infections; mood swings; and GI, cardiac, or kidney problems) are often ignored. The classic symptoms of anemia are not seen until Hgb approaches 7 to 8 g/dL. Neurological symptoms are the result of nerve demyelination, and the patient may experience loss of position and vibratory sense, ataxia, and spasticity. Concomitant symptoms include a beefy red tongue secondary to glossitis, and peripheral neuropathy; the latter is often used to clinically differentiate between FDA and PA. The liver may be enlarged, especially in older adults, indicating right-sided heart failure.

Anemia of Chronic Disease (ACD)

ACD is also associated with low Hgb, but it is caused by destruction of RBCs by a hyperactive reticuloendothelial system, decreased production of RBCs by hypoactive bone marrow, or altered iron metabolism, with defective transfer of iron from stores to the plasma. Overall, ACD appears to be produced by the activation of the cellular immune system. Specific cytokines that have been implicated in ACD include tumor necrosis factor alpha, interferon delta, interleukin-1 beta, and interleukin-6. Microvascular eruptions occur in the GI tract in response to the inflammatory mediators. This results in occult blood escaping into the intestines. Chronic use of NSAIDs, such as aspirin or ibuprofen, must also be considered as the source of occult bleeding. ACD produces a normocytic-normochromic anemia in 75% of cases but is microcytic in 25% of cases. It develops slowly and is often mild or asymptomatic.

Anemias that resemble ACD include anemias secondary to malignancy, chronic renal disease, HIV infection, and heart failure (Schrier & Camaschella, 2013). Anemia in patients with malignancy may be multifactorial in origin due to red blood cell losses, increased red cell destruction, or decreased red cell production (Drews, 2013). Patients with chronic kidney disease develop normochromic, normocytic anemia due to decreased erythropoietin production (Rosenberg, 2013). Medications used to treat HIV may cause anemia, including zidovudine (AZT) and may suppress erythropoiesis leading to anemia. Patients with heart failure may have anemia due to inflammation, dilutional anemia, iron deficiency anemia, or anemia caused by medications such as angiotension-converting enzyme inhibitors (Colucci, 2013).

Sickle Cell Anemia (SCD)

The National Heart, Lung, and Blood Institute (NHLBI, 2004) recommends universal screening for SCD. More than 98% of children born in the United States are screened for sickle cell anemia (SCA) as part of the routine newborn screening for preventable diseases (CDC, Division of Laboratory Services, 2013b).

Patients with SCA have a normal amount of Hgb (normocytic-normochromic), but their RBCs contain an abnormal type of Hgb, hemoglobin S (HbS). SCD is actually a group of autosomal recessive genetic disorders characterized by the predominance of this Hgb. These disorders include SCA, a homozygous form that is the most severe; sickle cell thalassemia syndromes and sickle cell HbC disease are heterozygous forms in which the child also inherits another type of abnormal Hgb from one parent. Sickle cell trait, in which the child inherits HbS from one parent and normal hemoglobin (HbA) from the other parent, is a heterozygous carrier state. It does not cause abnormalities in the blood count, and it does not produce vaso-occlusive symptoms under physiological conditions.

These disorders are found in people of African, Mediterranean, Indian, and Middle Eastern heritage. In the United States, SCD occurs more commonly in African Americans, with a reported incidence ranging from 1 in 400 to 1 in 500 live births. Sickle cell HbC disease is less common (1 in 800 births), and sickle cell thalassemia is the least common (1 in 1,700 births). Sickle cell trait occurs in 7% to 13% of African Americans, but the incidence among East Africans may be as high as 45%. This trait may provide some protection against lethal forms of malaria that are endemic in the areas that provide the gene pool of African Americans, but it provides no genetic advantage to persons living in the United States.

Sickle cell Hgb is produced by a recessive allele of the gene encoding the beta chain of the protein hemoglobin. A single amino acid, glutamic acid, is replaced by valine at the sixth position of the chain, producing HbS. There are two cardinal pathophysiological features of SCD: chronic hemolytic anemia and vaso-occlusion, which results in ischemic tissue injury. Low oxygen tensions in the blood from ischemia or decreased partial pressures of oxygen in the air cause HgbS to crystallize, which distorts the RBCs into a sickle shape and makes them fragile and easily destroyed. The degree of deoxygenation required to produce sickling varies with the percentage of HbS in the cells. Sickle trait cells will sickle at oxygen tensions of about 15 mm Hg, whereas those with SCD will sickle at about 40 mm Hg.

Sickling is rarely permanent, and most sickled RBCs regain a normal shape when reoxygenated and rehydrated. Some irreversible sickling occurs based on damage to the plasma membrane of the RBC. Hemolytic anemia may be related to repeated cycles of sickling and unsickling. Tissue injury is usually produced by hypoxia secondary to the obstruction of blood vessels by sickled erythrocytes. The sickled cells are unable to squeeze through the smaller blood vessels, and tissues supplied by these blood vessels undergo ischemia. The organs at greatest risk for damage are those with venous sinuses in which blood flow is low and oxygen tension and pH are low (spleen and bone marrow) and those with a limited terminal arterial blood supply (eye and head of the femur and humerus). The kidney is also at risk, especially as the patient ages.

Specific discussion of the complications associated with SCD and SCA are presented in the *Management of Sickle Cell Disease* (NHLBI, 2004). Additional information may also be found on several organizations' Web sites, including the American Sickle Cell Anemia Association (http://www.ascaa .org/); National Heart Lung and Blood Institute Sickle Cell Anemia (http:// http://www.nhlbi.nih.gov/health/health-topics/topics/sca/); and the Sickle Cell Anemia Center (scinfo .org), a program sponsored by a partnership among Emory University School of Medicine, Grady Health System, Morehouse School of Medicine, and others that offers extensive information on SCA for patients, families, and health-care providers. An expert panel is updating the NHLBI SCA guidelines, to be published in 2014.

GOALS OF TREATMENT

The ultimate goal of treatment for all types of anemia is to provide adequate oxygen transport to body tissues. For patients with IDA, FDA, and PA, this may be seen in a return to normal in the number and character of RBCs and to normal Hgb values. ACD is normocytic and normochromic, so the goal is a return to the normal number of RBCs and to normal Hgb values. Table 27-1 shows the normal blood indices for each age and sex grouping. The goal of treatment for SCA is prevention of the morbidity and mortality associated with this disease and reduction in the percentage of HgbS in the blood.

RATIONAL DRUG SELECTION

Iron Deficiency Anemia (IDA)

Risk Stratification and Screening

Growth, development, and gender factors play important roles in risk stratification. The fetus stores iron during the last trimester, providing the infant with stores that usually last about 6 months. Maternal conditions during pregnancy, including anemia, hypertension, or diabetes, can lead to low fetal iron stores (Baker, Greer, & the Committee on Nutrition, 2010). Preterm infants may have only 3 months of iron stores, and they grow at a more rapid rate, compounding the problem of poor iron stores.

The diet is the major source of iron. Human milk contains 0.35 mg/L of iron (Baker et al, 2010). The iron in breast milk is well absorbed (50% absorbed), as opposed to the iron in cow's milk, which is 10% absorbed. Breastfeeding reduces the risk for IDA in infants by providing a minimum of 0.27 mg/d of iron that term infants younger than age 6 months need (Baker et al, 2010). Due to waning iron stores between the ages of 4 and 6 months, the American Academy of Pediatrics (AAP) recommends exclusively breastfed infants be supplemented with 1 mg/kg per day of oral iron until iron-fortified foods (iron-fortified cereal) are introduced into the diet (Baker et al,

2010). Preterm infants who are breastfed should have 2 mg/kg per day of supplemental elemental iron daily until age 12 months (Baker et al, 2010). Infants, including preterm infants who are formula fed, should receive iron-fortified formula for the first 12 months of life. Partially breastfed infants (more than half their nutrition from breast milk) should receive 1 mg/kg per day of iron. The early addition of solid foods to the infant's diet may impair the ability to absorb iron, and solid foods should be introduced slowly, with conscious inclusion of foods high in iron. Cow's milk should not be introduced into the diet before age 12 months (Baker et al, 2010).

Conducting a good history of iron intake is a guide for whether screening for IDA should occur at the routine 9 or 12 month well visit. The AAP recommends all children have hemoglobin measured to screen for IDA at approximately age 12 months (Baker et al, 2010). Prematurity, low birth weight, lead exposure, or diet low in iron may indicate a need for earlier screening.

The Institute for Clinical Systems Improvement (ICSI, 2004) and the AAP (Baker et al, 2010) recommend an iron-rich diet for all children from birth to 6 years of age. Children between ages 1 and 2 are particularly prone to IDA (CDC, 2002). Toddlers require 7 mg per day of iron (Baker et al, 2010). Typically, toddlers may have somewhat picky eating habits and may consume large quantities of milk. Children age 1 to 3 years who do not have adequate dietary intake of iron should receive daily supplementation with iron in liquid, chewable, or, if in Canada, sprinkle form (Baker et al, 2010). If toddlers or preschoolers exhibit signs and symptoms consistent with anemia (tiredness, irritability, loss of appetite) or have a history of inadequate iron intake or drinking more than 32 oz of milk a day, they should be screened with Hgb and Hct tests (Baker et al, 2010). Lead poisoning can also contribute to IDA in young children; therefore, high-risk children should be screened for lead.

Iron needs increase during periods of rapid growth. Teenage girls are in a high-risk group because of their growth spurt, the onset of menstruation, and poor dietary intake of iron-containing foods (less than 15 mg of iron per day). Although IDA is more common in females, adolescent boys may be at risk during their growth spurt if they don't have adequate intake of iron (11 mg/d). Adolescents should be screened with Hgb and Hct tests at ages 12 to 14 years, based on a history of their risk factors, including dietary intake, vegan or vegetarian diet, skipping meals or disordered eating, history of heavy menstrual periods, participation in endurance sports, or intensive physical training (National Anemia Action Council, 2009).

Although anemia is common in older adults, in this population it is usually due to GI blood loss associated with ulcers, the use of aspirin or NSAIDs, or chronic disease rather than to iron deficiency. Ferritin levels increase with illness and inflammation; therefore, a ferritin of 45 ng/dL should be used to determine iron deficiency in the older adult (Bross, Soch, & Smith-Knuppel, 2010). Unexplained iron deficiency requires investigation for gastric malignancy or other source, as well as replacement of iron.

Women generally have smaller stores of iron than do men and have increased loss through menstruation, and their balance between intake and loss of iron is precarious. IDA occurs more frequently in nonpregnant women who experience menorrhagia. Pregnancy places a woman at risk of IDA because their iron requirement doubles due to the increased blood volume of the mother and iron need of the growing fetus (ODS, 2010). Women at risk should be screened for IDA at annual physical examinations, and pregnant women should have screening included as part of their regular prenatal care.

Prevention of IDA

Treatment of IDA begins with prevention, but iron deficiency cannot be overcome with increased dietary intake alone. Iron supplements are always required.

The primary goal of management for IDA is prevention. The key to prevention of IDA not due to a disease process is adequate nutrition. Prevention, for infants, starts with breastfeeding. The AAP recommends exclusive breastfeeding for the first 4 to 6 months of life (Baker et al, 2010) and that iron fortification of 1 mg/kg per day of iron be started at age 4 months and iron-rich foods be introduced at age 6 months (Baker et al, 2010). Preterm infants require iron supplementation of 2 mg/kg per day starting at age 1 month and continuing until age 12 months (Baker et al, 2010). Low-birth-weight infants or infants with hematological disorders require iron supplementation before age 6 months. The AAP recommends liquid or chewable forms of iron (Baker et al, 2010). Iron

sprinkles are available in Canada. Formula-fed infants should use an iron-fortified formula.

Children and adults need to eat sufficient amounts of iron-rich foods. Foods rich in iron that the body can readily absorb include raisins, lean meats, fish, poultry, eggs, legumes, soybeans, dark green leafy vegetables, blackstrap molasses, fortified cereals, and whole-grain rice. The iron in many vegetables is poorly absorbed, so vegetarians must pay special attention to their intake of legumes and rice. The recommended amount of iron for non-anemic pregnant women is 27 mg/d, with a recommendation that all pregnant women take a low dose (30 mg/d elemental iron) daily to prevent anemia (ODS, 2010). Table 27-3 presents iron intake recommendations for the prevention and treatment of IDA.

Learning energy conservation techniques, such as planning rest periods, pacing activities, keeping objects within reach when performing tasks, and sitting down when doing chores, are other important lifestyle modifications for the patient with IDA.

Drug Therapy

Once the decision is made to begin drug therapy, the choice of drug is based on age and gender variables. Figure 27-2 delineates the drug treatment algorithm for IDA. See Table 27-3 for the dosages of iron recommended for infants, children, adolescents, and adults and during pregnancy and lactation. Doses ranging from 60 to 185 mg of elemental iron have been used. Oral formulations of 325 mg (60 mg of elemental iron) are usually taken by mouth with each meal tid.

Table 27–3   Iron Intake Recommendations for the Prevention and Treatment of Iron Deficiency Anemia

Risk Group	Prevention	Treatment
Infants	• Breastfeeding for first yr or iron-fortified formula • Preterm infants: 2 mg/kg of iron from 1 mo to 12 mo Breastfed infants 1 mg/kg per day of iron until adequate dietary intake of iron from foods • Begin iron-rich cereals or supplement at 6 mo • Screen for IDA at approximately 12 mo	Mild to moderate deficiency: 3 mg/kg/d in 1–2 divided doses Severe anemia: 6 mg/kg/d of elemental iron in 3 divided doses
Children 1–3 yr 3–12 yr Male 12–18 yr Female 12–18 yr All adolescents	7 mg/d of iron in diet 10 mg/d of iron in diet 11 mg/d of iron in diet 15 mg/d of iron in diet Diet should include iron-rich foods	1–3 yr: 6 mg/kg/d of elemental iron in 3–4 divided doses 3–12 yr: 3 mg/kg/d of elemental iron in 3–4 divided doses 12–21 yr: 150–250 mg of elemental iron/d Ferrous sulfate is best choice for oral iron Absorption enhanced by taking it on an empty stomach or with vitamins C and E; milk, antacids, tea, and food interfere with absorption
Adults 19–50 yr Male Female	8 mg/d of iron 18 mg/d of iron Diet should be high in iron-rich foods	150–250 mg of elemental iron/d (e.g., ferrous sulfate 300–325 mg tid or qid)
Adults 51+ yr	8 mg/d	
Pregnant and lactating women	30 mg of elemental iron daily during last two trimesters and while lactating	Ferrous sulfate 300–325 mg/d

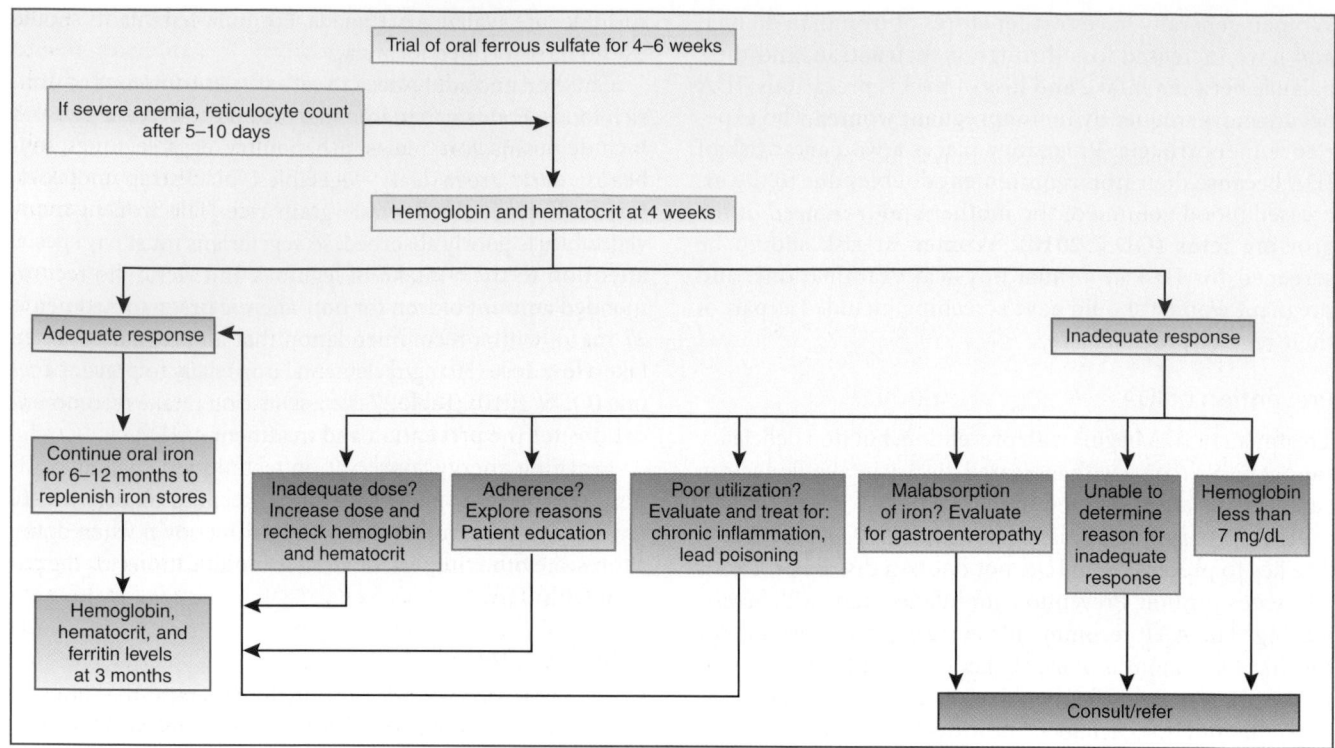

Figure 27–2. Drug treatment algorithm for iron deficiency anemia.

Chapter 18 has a more detailed discussion of iron formulations. Although Chapter 18 includes ferrous sulfate, gluconate, and fumarate formulations, ferrous sulfate is the least expensive and the most easily absorbed. Slow-release and enteric-coated compounds have been advertised to reduce GI distress, and they require only once-daily dosing. However, they dissolve slowly and can bypass the proximal small bowel, where most absorption of iron takes place. Slow-release formulas are also significantly more expensive ($24.99 for 90 tablets of Slow Fe Slow Release Iron with 50 mg of elemental iron versus $4.49 for 100 tablets of generic ferrous sulfate with 65 mg of iron). There is no evidence to suggest that these formulations are worth the extra cost. If patients experience GI upset, it can be reduced by adjusting the dosage and by taking the drug with food.

Monitoring

The response to iron therapy is apparent within 10 days of initiation. The first change noted in blood values is an increase in the reticulocyte count as soon as 4 days after treatment is started, followed by a rise in Hgb concentration of 1 to 2 g/dL per day. If the anemia is severe (Hgb less than 8 g/dL), a reticulocyte count can be obtained 5 to 10 days after initiating therapy. If the anemia is not severe, Hgb, Hct, and ferritin levels are checked at 4 weeks. If the IDA is mild (Hgb 10 to 12 g/dL and Hct 30% to 60%), follow-up every 4 to 6 months is appropriate. Referral is almost never required unless there is an inadequate response to therapy in which the Hgb remains very low (Hgb less than or equal to 7 g/dL); there is a question of possible

malabsorption that requires special GI testing; or the reason for the inadequate response is unclear.

Outcome Evaluation

Several weeks of therapy are required to bring Hgb levels back into the normal range, and replenishing iron stores may take months. Speed is not the issue, however, unless there is rapid blood loss. In that case, consultation or referral is appropriate. Hgb, Hct, and RBC indices should be evaluated at 4 weeks, 3 months, and annually. If the Hgb level does not return to normal limits within 6 weeks, the inadequate response should be evaluated. If the dose is inadequate, it may be increased. Starting with a lower dose and gradually increasing it reduces the likelihood of adverse reactions that may hamper adherence to the treatment regimen. Persistent, unrecognized blood loss should be sought with stool specimens for occult blood and ova and parasites. Referral to a gastroenterologist for x-rays and endoscopy may be necessary, and the source of the blood loss should be treated. If there is a history of poor weight gain, diarrhea and other GI symptoms, or surgery on the GI tract, malabsorption syndromes should be ruled out.

Poor iron utilization can result from chronic inflammation, lead poisoning, or sideroblastic anemia. Chronic inflammation can be demonstrated with elevated sedimentation rates, elevated iron and total iron-binding capacity levels, low percentage of iron saturation, and high ferritin levels. Lead poisoning is demonstrated with increased serum lead levels and basophilic stippling on RBC morphology. Sideroblastic anemia is usually found in infancy. Laboratory values reveal high ferritin levels, normal or high iron and total iron-binding

PATIENT EDUCATION

Patient education related to IDA should focus on:

1. Understanding the pathophysiology of IDA and its potential long-term effects.
2. Recognizing the importance of prevention and the role of diet and energy conservation.
3. Understanding the necessity of adherence to the treatment regimen.
4. Understanding the need for follow-up visits with the primary care provider because IDA can recur.

Stress to the patient that a diet with sufficient amounts of iron-rich foods may avoid the need for supplemental iron therapy but only after the IDA has been resolved. When diet alone is inadequate or when iron needs are very high, as in pregnancy, drug therapy is initiated. Patient education specific to drug therapy includes the following:

1. The reason for taking iron.
2. Doses and schedules for the drug.
3. Potential drug interactions and the need to inform other providers that they are taking iron.
4. Possible adverse reactions and ways to reduce them. The most common adverse reactions that lead to nonadherence are GI problems such as nausea and constipation. Taking iron with food reduces the total amount absorbed but can also reduce the nausea. Adequate fluids and fiber can prevent constipation. Stool softeners may be needed to treat constipation associated with iron therapy.

Additional patient education related to iron therapy is presented in Chapter 18.

capacity levels, and elevated bone marrow stores of iron. Each of these disorders must be treated before iron therapy can be successful. When the history, physical examination, and standard laboratory analyses do not lead to a determination of the cause of the inadequate response, or the initial Hgb level is less than 7 g/dL, consultation with or referral to a hematology specialist is appropriate.

Folic Acid Deficiency Anemia

Risk Groups

Several patient populations, including age-based, gender-based, and concomitant disease-based groups, are at risk for folic acid deficiency. Certain drugs are also associated with effects on dihydrofolate reductase, an enzyme critical to folate synthesis.

Infants who are fed powdered milk products or goat's milk develop this deficiency because these products are deficient in both folic acid and vitamin B_{12}. Older children who are exclusively vegetarian or who have severe nutritional deficiencies, absorption problems, or tapeworm infestations are also at risk. Prolonged cooking of vegetables destroys folates and can result in deficiency if such foods are the only source of this vitamin. Older adults whose diets lack vegetables, eggs, and meat often develop folic acid deficiency. Supplementation of cereals with folic acid has been mandatory since 1998, resulting in a prevalence of folate deficiency of less than 0.1% in the general population (Odewole et al, 2013).

Women are not especially at risk unless they become pregnant. Pregnant women have increased folate requirements (800 µg daily versus 50 to 100 µg per day) and may become deficient, especially if their diets are lacking in folic acid–containing foods such as dark green vegetables. Evidence suggests that maternal folic acid deficiency is associated with increased risk for neural tube defects in the fetus.

Disease states associated with folic acid deficiency caused by impaired absorption include sprue, Crohn's disease, giardial infections, and short bowel syndrome. Disease states that result in deficiency because of increased demand include hyperthyroidism, hemolytic anemia, malignancy, and other chronic debilitating disorders. Alcoholics and patients with liver disease develop deficiency because of poor diet and reduced hepatic storage of folates. There is also evidence that alcohol interferes with the absorption and metabolism of folates. Patients undergoing renal dialysis lose folates from the plasma during dialysis, and that results in deficiency.

Drugs that interfere with folate absorption or metabolism include the antiepileptic drugs phenytoin, carbamazepine, and valproic acid, methotrexate (Folex), oral contraceptives, isoniazid (INH), triamterene (Dyrenium), trimethoprim (Trimpex), and pyrimethamine (Daraprim). Patients who take these drugs, especially on a long-term basis, should be monitored for folate deficiency.

Lifestyle Modifications

All patients should be instructed to eat foods high in folic acid. Foods high in folic acid include dark green leafy vegetables, bran, yeast, dried beans, fortified cereals, and nuts. Females should also be educated about the increased needs for folic acid prior to and during pregnancy. The U.S. Preventive Services Taskforce recommends folic acid supplements of 400 to 800 µg daily for all females planning or capable of becoming pregnant (2009).

Drug Therapy

Oral folic acid is well absorbed, and doses of 1 to 2 mg daily result in correction of the deficiency in 4 to 5 weeks. Hgb levels begin to rise within the first week, and the anemia is completely corrected in 1 to 2 months. Because of the potential teratogenic effects of folate deficiency in pregnant women, women of childbearing age should take prophylactic doses of 0.4 to 0.8 mg daily and continue this dose throughout any pregnancy. Folic acid supplementation to prevent deficiency should also be considered in the other high-risk patients mentioned previously. Detailed discussion of clinical use and dosing of folic acid is provided in Chapters 9 and 18.

Monitoring

Response to treatment is assessed after 2 weeks and then monthly until the condition stabilizes. A rapid rise in reticulocytes follows the initial treatment, with a peak in 5 to 8 days, an improving Hgb and Hct within 1 week, and a normal Hct within 2 months. The only monitoring required is to follow Hgb and Hct levels at regular intervals. The timing of such assessment is based on the acute versus chronic nature of the cause of the deficiency.

Pernicious Anemia (PA)

Risk Groups

The underlying disorder in PA is usually defective secretion of gastric intrinsic factor, which is necessary for vitamin B_{12} absorption. It is most common in northern Europeans but can occur in any age or ethnic group. Vitamin B_{12} malabsorption occurs in 10% to 30% of adults over the age of 50 because they have reduced pepsin activity and gastric acid secretion. This reduced activity interferes with the cleavage of vitamin B_{12} from dietary protein before it is absorbed. Partial or total gastrectomy and small bowel resection are the two most common iatrogenic causes of this problem. The former surgery removes the parietal cell–containing portion of the stomach that secretes intrinsic factor, and the latter surgery removes a portion of the bowel that absorbs the vitamin B_{12}–intrinsic factor complex. Diseases of the terminal ileum, fish tapeworm, thyroid diseases, and bacterial overgrowth in the small bowel from stasis can also cause PA. Nutritional deficiency is rare but may be seen in strict vegetarians after several years without meat, eggs, or dairy products.

Screen for PA any of these risk groups and other patients who present with the neurological symptoms of peripheral neuropathy, symmetrical paresthesias in the hands and feet progressing to ataxia from loss of vibratory and position sense, memory loss, depression, agitation, personality change, or central visual scotomata. This is especially true for older adults, in which some of these changes may be confused with dementia.

Lifestyle Modifications

The underlying problem in PA is vitamin B_{12} deficiency. Patients should be taught to eat foods high in this vitamin, such as mollusks (e.g., clams), fortified breakfast cereals, liver, trout, salmon, milk, and eggs. These foods are listed in the order of highest to lowest amount of vitamin B_{12} (ODS, 2011). One serving of fortified breakfast cereal provides 100% of the daily requirement for vitamin B_{12},

Drug Therapy

Because the underlying problem in almost all cases of PA is malabsorption, therapy with vitamin B_{12} is required. Oral, IM, and intranasal replacements are available. Oral vitamin B_{12} is useful only for the rare case of nutritional deficit and for patients who cannot take the parenteral form. If the vitamin B_{12} deficiency is a nutritional deficit and not PA, 1,000 mcg of oral cobalamin is given until normal B_{12} levels are achieved, usually in 6 to 12 weeks. Intranasal cyanocobalamin (Nascobal), a synthetic vitamin B_{12}, may be used for maintenance therapy of patients with hematological remission after initial treatment. Once-weekly dosing of intranasal cyanocobalamin (one spray in one nostril) gives a 500 mcg dose. For PA, the parenteral route is often used, although oral therapy may also be effective (Oh & Brown, 2003). Vitamin B_{12} therapy is initiated with 1,000 mcg IM daily for 1 week followed by 100 to 1,000 mcg IM weekly for a month. Doses of 1,000 mcg may be used, as excess vitamin B_{12} is excreted in the urine. Because PA is not correctable, the patient must take vitamin B_{12} for life.

Parenteral, nasal, or oral therapy may be used once a patient's B_{12} levels return to normal. Parenteral therapy consists of 1,000 mcg of vitamin B_{12} monthly. Nasal therapy consists of 500 mcg of cyanocobalamin weekly. Oral therapy consists of 1,000 mcg daily for life. Oral therapy should be tried because of administration ease and cost.

The hematological response to parenteral vitamin B_{12} is rapid. The bone marrow usually returns to normal within 48 hours. Reticulocytosis begins on the second or third day and is usually maximum by the fifth to the tenth day. Patients usually show some other hematological improvements in 5 to 7 days, with deficiency resolving in 3 to 4 weeks. Hgb and Hct levels should return to normal within 1 to 2 months. It may take up to 6 months to resolve neurological symptoms. Correctable conditions require treatment of the underlying problem, and parenteral therapy continues temporarily. Sudden drops in serum potassium levels have been reported with vitamin B_{12} therapy. Serum potassium levels should be monitored and supplemental oral potassium given if needed.

Chapter 18 has a detailed discussion of rational drug selection and dosing for vitamin B_{12}. Although it is not urgent

---

PATIENT EDUCATION

Patient education for folic acid deficiency anemia focuses on prevention as well as treatment. Diet and appropriate cooking methods are central to prevention, especially for strict vegetarians. The need for folic acid supplementation should be discussed with women of childbearing age. When diet alone is inadequate or folate needs are very high, as in pregnancy, drug therapy is initiated. Patient education specific to drug therapy includes the following:

1. The reason for taking folic acid.
2. The doses and schedule for the drug.
3. The fact that some drugs may potentially interfere with folate metabolism.
4. The need to inform their providers that they are taking supplemental folic acid.

More specific discussion of patient education is found in Chapter 18.

to treat most cases of PA, the reversibility of neurological deficits is, to some extent, dependent on their duration. Patients with neurological symptoms should have this disorder promptly diagnosed and treated. When neurological symptoms are present, twice-monthly dosing is recommended for 6 months prior to beginning the usual monthly dose.

Monitoring

Reticulocyte counts, Hgb and Hct, iron, folic acid, and vitamin B_{12} serum levels are obtained prior to treatment, between the fifth and the seventh day of therapy, and then frequently until the Hgb and Hct are normal. Relapse of symptoms is not uncommon in the presence of continuing therapy. Blood counts should continue at regular intervals throughout the patient's lifetime, based on individual response to therapy.

Because of the potential for sudden drops in serum potassium levels, these should also be monitored at the same time as Hgb and Hct levels are drawn. Liver function tests (LFTs) should also be done. If LFTs (aspartate transaminase [AST] and alanine transaminase [ALT]) are elevated before the start of cobalamin therapy, they should be evaluated every 2 to 4 weeks to monitor for liver dysfunction. If LFTs elevate after the start of therapy, more frequent testing might be required to assess for hepatotoxicity. The Schilling test is used for diagnosis but not as a monitoring tool. Referral to or consultation with a hematologist and gastroenterologist should occur with the diagnosis of PA.

Anemia of Chronic Disease

Risk Stratification and Screening

Anemia of chronic disease (ACD) is the most common form of anemia in older adults and is associated with several specific chronic diseases, including osteomyelitis, tuberculosis, rheumatoid diseases, hepatitis, carcinoma, myeloma, lymphoma, and leukemia. Anemias associated with renal failure occur secondary to erythropoietin deficiency, and the National Kidney Foundation (2006) has produced a separate guideline for diagnosis and management of this subset of ACD. Anemias associated with endocrine deficiency (e.g., thyroid, adrenal, or pituitary deficiency) reduce bone marrow responsiveness by not stimulating erythropoietin secretion. These disorders also have their own management.

Older adults with any chronic illness and patients of any age with these illnesses should be evaluated for the presence of anemia. ACD may also coexist with IDA. In these patients, ACD is usually mild and asymptomatic, but some patients may present with fatigue, shortness of breath, loss of appetite, weight loss, or light-headedness after mild activity. Because these symptoms may be the same as those seen with the underlying chronic illness, it is important to include evaluation for anemia in the work-up for these disorders (Bross, Soch, & Smith-Knuppel, 2010).

Hct in patients with ACD is rarely less than 25%; other laboratory findings are shown in Table 27-2. The criterion for the coexistence of ACD and IDA is a serum ferritin level of 20 to 50 nanograms (ng)/mL. Serum ferritin, however, may elevate in the presence of an acute inflammatory reaction and may not accurately reflect total body iron stores.

Treatment of ACD

There is no effective therapy directed specifically at ACD. Treatment of the underlying chronic disease is necessary to resolve the anemia. Sometimes, patients have a concomitant IDA that is amenable to treatment with iron, but otherwise, oral iron is not necessary. The main focus of therapy for ACD, besides treatment of the underlying disease, is energy conservation.

When ACD is caused by chronic renal failure, the cause is probably associated in part with decreased production of erythropoietin by the kidney. The target for successful treatment of this form of anemia is an Hgb level of 11 to 12 g/dL and an Hct level of 33% to 36%. To achieve this level, sufficient iron should be administered to maintain greater than 20% transferrin saturation and a serum ferritin level of 100 ng/mL or higher. In this case, administration of epoetin alfa (Epogen, Procrit) may lead to an increase of 6% to 10% in the Hct within 6 weeks. During the initiation of epoetin alfa therapy and while increasing the dose in order to achieve an increase in Hgb and Hct, the percentage of transferrin saturation and the serum ferritin level should be checked every month in patients not receiving iron and every 3 months in patients receiving iron until target Hgb and Hct are reached (National Kidney Foundation, 2006).

For patients with anemia associated with chronic renal failure or zidovudine-treated HIV, epoetin alpha is started at 50 to 100 units/kg in adults and 50 units/kg in children and dosed 3 times a week. The epoetin alpha dose is titrated to keep the Hgb level between 10 and 12 g/dL. Dosage is increased by 25% if Hgb is less than 10 g/dL and has not increased by 1 g/dL after 4 weeks of therapy or if Hgb decreases

---

PATIENT EDUCATION

Patient education related to pernicious anemia (PA) should focus on:

1. Understanding the pathophysiology of PA and its potential long-term effects.
2. The importance of adherence to the treatment regimen.
3. The need for follow-up visits with the primary care provider in that PA and its symptoms can recur, even with continuing therapy.

Patient education specific to the drug therapy includes the following:

1. The reason for taking vitamin B_{12}.
2. The fact that the oral vitamin B_{12} found in multivitamin tablets is not sufficient to treat the problem.
3. The doses and schedule for the drug.
4. The fact that patients need to take the drug for the rest of their lives.

below 10 g/dL. The epoetin alpha dose is decreased by 25% if hemoglobin approaches 12 g/dL or Hgb increases more than 1 g/dL in any 2-week period. The maintenance dose for patients on dialysis is individualized for each patient. The malignant diseases causing ACD may also require the use of this drug, which is discussed in Chapter 18.

Sickle Cell Anemia

This chapter does not discuss the total management of sickle cell disease (SCD). The reader is referred to NHLBI Evidence-based Management of Sickle Cell Disease (NHLBI, 2014) for a complete discussion and guidelines for management of common problems, such as pain and infection. However, it is important to remember that treatment of pain with NSAIDs carries with it the risk for GI bleeding, which may be a source of anemia beyond that associated with sickling. Hematuria can also occur secondary to renal abnormalities in SCD and may also contribute to anemia. This chapter focuses on management of the anemia and precipitants of sickling and the resultant ischemia.

Prevention

Prevention of the morbidity and mortality associated with the hemolytic anemia of SCD is focused on avoidance of the precipitants of a sickling crisis. Serious bacterial infections, especially those due to *Streptococcus pneumoniae,* *Haemophilus influenzae,* and *Mycoplasma pneumoniae,* are a major cause of sickling. Patients and their parents need to be taught early recognition of signs and symptoms of these infections, and early aggressive treatment is critical. Dehydration is another precipitant. Adequate hydration (2 qt/d or more in children and adults) should be stressed, especially during periods of elevated environmental temperature and physical activity. Exposure to cold, with its resultant vasoconstriction, can precipitate a sickling event and should be avoided.

Children with SCD should also receive all childhood immunizations as recommended by the Advisory Committee on Immunization Practices (ACIP) as discussed in Chapter 19. Additionally children with SCD need to be immunized with pneumococcal vaccine (PCV 13 and PPSV 23). Infants with SCD are considered high risk and are vaccinated with meningococcal vaccine (HibMenCY) and persons age 9 months to 55 years are vaccinated with MenACWY (NHLBI, 2014). All children with SCD should have an annual influenza vaccine, starting at age 6 months.

Although strenuous exercise may precipitate sickling, there is no evidence that most exercise is harmful, and the beneficial effects of exercise are well known. Patients with SCD are encouraged to participate in physical activities and set their own limits. Exercise capacity is reduced by as much as 50% in adults with SCD. Participation in noncompetitive recreational activities that do not involve strenuous exercise should be encouraged. Any activity, whether recreation or employment, resulting in exhaustion should be discouraged. Exercise under adverse conditions, such as cold weather, high altitude, or cold water exposure, should also be avoided.

Dietary Counseling

Dietary counseling is an important part of patient care. Mothers should be encouraged to breastfeed their infants and give regular doses of iron supplementation per the AAP guidelines, although iron-fortified formulas are an acceptable alternative. Foods high in iron and folic acid should be encouraged in children and adults. Chapter 9 has more information on foods high in these nutrients.

Drug Therapy

Sickle cell patients should receive a daily multivitamin supplement (Tanyi, 2003). A diet rich in complex B vitamins and vitamin C and ingesting eight glasses of water daily to maintain hydration are critical.

Patients with SCA do not usually have concurrent IDA. Supplemental iron should not be prescribed unless the patient is documented to have reduced iron stores by specific assessments of the serum ferritin level or measurement of serum iron and iron-binding capacity. Children with SCA are often microcytic in the absence of iron deficiency. The incidence of the alpha thalassemia trait is also quite high in African Americans and may produce microcytosis in the absence of iron deficiency. Most patients eat poorly during painful crises, and daily supplements of 1 mg of folic acid should be prescribed during those times if not already being taken. The danger of masking a vitamin B_{12} deficiency is small, but African American patients are at risk. There is no evidence that any other form of vitamin supplementation is of value in SCD.

Infections also enhance susceptibility to vaso-occlusive events and their subsequent ischemia. Prophylactic penicillin is so effective in reducing the number of life-threatening episodes of pneumococcal sepsis in children under age 5. Most states screen newborns for SCD so they can be placed on penicillin by age 2 to 3 months. Oral penicillin VK 125 mg bid is given until age 3 years, then 250 mg bid is given until age 5 (NHLBI, 2014). Prophylaxis in older children has not been shown to be beneficial and may be unnecessary after *S. pneumoniae* and *H. influenzae* immunizations are complete and antibody titers are protective (NHLBI, 2014). Pneumococcal vaccination is also recommended for children and adults with SCD. Penicillin is discussed in more detail in Chapter 24.

A consensus statement from the National Institutes of Health published in 2008 states that evidence is strong for the use of hydroxyurea in the treatment of SCD in adults (Brawley et al, 2008). Although there is no drug to cure SCD, hydroxyurea (Droxia, Hydrea) has been shown to reduce the frequency of sickle cell pain crisis in adults, reduce the need for transfusions, and increase total hemoglobin and HgbF (NHLBI, 2014). SCD patients requiring hydroxyurea are usually managed by a specialist in hematology. The dosing schedule varies, but patients are usually started on 10 mg/kg initially, with the dose increased by

5 mg/kg every 12 weeks until the maximum dose of 25 to 35 mg/kg per day is reached, unless toxicity is observed. Toxicity is defined as absolute neutrophil counts lower than 2,000/mm³, absolute reticulocyte counts lower than 80,000/mm³, platelet counts lower than 80,000/mm³, or a fall in Hgb from greater than or equal to 7 g/dL to 4.5 to 5 g/dL if reticulocytes are lower than 320,000 or Hgb is lower than 4.5 g/dL. The BABY HUG study of hydroxyurea use in infants with sickle cell disease demonstrated significant improvement in pain, acute chest syndrome, hospitalizations, and transfusions; therefore the recommendation in the NHBLI guidelines is to start all infants with SCD on hydroxyurea at age 9 months (Lebensburger et al, 2012; McGann & Ware, 2012; NHLBI 2014).

Hydroxyurea may not be appropriate for all patients and should not be used for patients likely to become pregnant or those unwilling or unable to follow instructions regarding treatment. Hydroxyurea is a cytotoxic agent and has the potential to cause life-threatening cytopenia. The onset of leukopenia and thrombocytopenia may occur within 10 days of beginning therapy. White blood cell and platelet counts should be monitored prior to and periodically during therapy. Because hydroxyurea attacks rapidly growing cells, stomatitis, anorexia, nausea, vomiting, and diarrhea may occur. Good oral hygiene and monitoring of nutritional status are important. Patients requiring hydroxyurea are usually managed by hematology. Patients and caregivers should be instructed not to handle the hydroxyurea tablets with bare hands; gloves should be worn.

Experimental drug therapy is being tried with erythropoietin to determine its capability in augmenting the production of fetal Hgb (HgbF). HgbF interferes with the polymerization of HgbS in solution and with the sickling of HgbS RBCs. Butyrate, a simple fatty acid widely used as a food additive, is also being investigated as an agent that may increase HgbF production. Their role in therapy, alone or in combination with hydroxyurea, is still unclear. Erythropoietin is discussed in Chapter 18.

Transfusions

With the mild to moderate anemia common to SCD, body systems except the eye and the spleen adapt fairly well to the reduced oxygen-carrying capacity of the blood. Most patients with SCD are relatively asymptomatic from their anemia and do not require transfusions to improve oxygen-carrying capacity. Transfusions may be used for specific indications

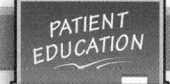

PATIENT EDUCATION

Patient and parental information related to sickle cell anemia should focus on the following:

1. Understanding the pathophysiology of SCD and the organs commonly damaged.
2. Recognizing the importance of prevention, especially the central role of prevention of infection and avoidance of precipitants of sickling.
3. Learning how to administer prophylactic antibiotics and other drugs.
4. Understanding the necessity of adherence to the treatment regimen.
5. Recognizing the need for regular follow-up visits with a primary care provider to manage this chronic disease.
6. Understanding the role of genetic counseling.

Prevention of sickling requires the parents and the patient to learn specific assessment skills. Any sign of illness in a child with SCD can be serious.

Patient education related to the administration of penicillin is discussed in Chapter 24.

Measures to minimize the risk of vaso-occlusive events beyond prevention of infection were discussed previously. The hazards of cigarette smoking and excessive alcohol intake and the benefits of a well-planned exercise program should be included.

Although IDA is not common for patients with SCD, prevention of IDA with a diet that includes sufficient amounts of iron-rich foods should be discussed. When iron is required, follow the patient education instructions for IDA.

Patient education specific to the use of hydroxyurea includes the following:

1. Take the drug exactly as prescribed, even if nausea, vomiting, or diarrhea occurs.
2. If a dose is missed, do not take it at all; do not double dose.
3. Notify the health-care provider of fever; chills; sore throat; loss of appetite; nausea; vomiting; diarrhea; bleeding gums; bruising; petechiae; or blood in the urine, stool, or emesis.
4. Avoid alcoholic beverages, aspirin, and NSAIDs, which may increase the risk of bleeding.
5. Inspect oral mucosa for erythema and ulceration. If it occurs, use a sponge brush and rinse mouth with water after eating and drinking. If mouth pain interferes with eating, contact the health-care provider for lidocaine-based mouthwash.
6. Encourage fluid intake of 2,000 to 3,000 mL of noncaffeinated fluid daily.
7. Review the need for contraception during therapy because of the teratogenic potential of this drug.

Patient education related to the other drugs used in treatment of SCD and its complications is presented in the Unit II chapters that include these drugs. Patient education related to the other complications of SCD is detailed in the NIH publications in the References section.

when the anemia is severe or to prevent chronic complications (NHLBI, 2014).

Monitoring

Hgb, Hct, reticulocyte counts, platelet counts, and white blood cell counts should be done frequently during the first year of life to establish the patient's baseline. After the first year, Hgb and Hct are relatively stable and need to be checked only once or twice a year in stable patients. Stable patients also require annual urinalysis, blood urea nitrogen (BUN), creatinine, and liver enzyme studies to monitor for evidence of organ damage. Before administration of transfusions, RBC antigens are needed. Patients with SCD are often difficult to crossmatch.

Most adults with SCD should have regular medical evaluations every 3 to 6 months. Blood counts, urinalysis, and routine chemistry tests should be done annually. With advancing age, complications such as chronic organ failure often require more frequent visits and more extensive laboratory evaluations. Attention focuses primarily on abnormalities in renal function and complications such as gallstones, aseptic necrosis, leg ulcers, and priapism.

Outcome Evaluation

The overall goal of therapy is the reduction in the number of sickling crises and prevention of organ damage. Hgb level goals are 9 g/dL or greater, but levels of at least 7 g/dL may be acceptable in asymptomatic patients. The goal for percentage of HgbS is 30% or less. Outcomes for chronic transfusion therapy were presented previously.

REFERENCES

Adams, R. J. (2000). Lessons from the Stroke Prevention Trial in Sickle Cell Anemia (STOP) study. *Journal of Child Neurology, 15*(5), 344–349.

Baker, R. D., Greer, F. R., and The Committee on Nutrition (2010). Clinical report—Diagnosis and prevention of iron deficiency and iron-deficiency anemia in infants and young children (1–3 years of age). *Pediatrics, 126*(5), 1040–1050.

Brawley, O. W., Cornelius, L. J., Edwards, L. R., Gamble, V. N., Green, B. L., Inturrisi, C., et al. (2008). National Institutes of Health Consensus Development Conference Statement: Hydroxyurea treatment for sickle cell disease. *Annals of Internal Medicine, 148*(12), 932–938.

Bull-Henry, K., & Al-Kawas, F. H. (2013). Evaluation of occult gastrointestinal bleeding. *American Family Physician, 87*(6), 430–436.

Burns, C., Dunn, A., Brady, M., Barber-Starr, N., & Blooser, K. (2009). *Pediatric primary care* (4th ed.). Philadelphia: Saunders.

Centers for Disease Control and Prevention (CDC). (2011). Sickle cell disease: Data and statistics. Retrieved from http://www.cdc.gov/ncbddd/sicklecell/data.html

Centers for Disease Control and Prevention (CDC). (2013a). Anemia or iron deficiency. CDC/National Center for Health Statistics. Retrieved from http://www.cdc.gov/nchs/fastats/anemia.htm

Centers for Disease Control and Prevention (CDC), Division of Laboratory Services. (2013b). Quality assurance and proficiency testing for newborn screening. Retrieved from http://www.cdc.gov/labstandards/nsqap.html

Colucci, W. S. (2013). Impact of anemia in patients with heart failure. *UpToDate Online*. Retrieved from http://www.uptodate.com/contents/impact-of-anemia-in-patients-with-heart-failure

Drews, R. E. (2103). Hematologic consequences of malignancy: Anemia and bleeding. *UpToDate Online*. Retrieved from http://www.uptodate.com/contents/hematologic-consequences-of-malignancy-anemia-and-bleeding

Institute for Clinical Systems Improvement (ICSI). (2004). Preventive counseling and education—*by topic*. Bloomington, MN: Institute for Clinical Systems Improvement.

Lebensburger, J. D., Miller, S. T., Howard, T. H., Casella, J. F., Brown, R. C., Lu, M., et al. (2012). Influence of severity of anemia on clinical findings in infants with sickle cell anemia: Analysis from the BABY HUG study. *Pediatric Blood & Cancer, 59*(4), 675–678.

McClung, J. P. (2013). Iron status and the female athlete. *Journal of Trace Elements in Medicine and Biology, 26*, 124–126.

McClung, J. P., Marchitelli, L. J., Friedl, K. E., & Young, A. J. (2006). Prevalence of iron deficiency and iron deficiency anemia among three populations of female military personnel in the US Army. (2006). *Journal of the American College of Nutrition, 25*(1), 64–69.

McGann, P. T., & Ware, R. E. (2012). Hydroxyurea for sickle cell anemia: What have we learned and what questions still remain? *Current Opinions in Hematology, 18*(3), 158–165.

Montoya, V., Wink, D., & Sole, M. (2002). Adult anemia: Determine clinical significance. *Nurse Practitioner, 27*(3), 38–53.

National Anemia Action Council. (2009). Anemia in adolescents—the teen scene. National Anemia Action Council. Retrieved from http://www.anemia.org/patients/feature-articles/content.php?contentid=000348

National Heart Lung and Blood Institute (2014). *Evidence-Based Management of Sickle Cell Disease: Expert Panel Report, 2014*. U.S. Department of Health and Human Services, National Institutes of Health. Retrieved from http://www.nhlbi.nih.gov/sites/www.nhlbi.nih.gov/files/sickle-cell-disease-report.pdf

National Kidney Foundation. (2006). *NKF-K/DOQI clinical practice guidelines and clinical practice recommendations for anemia of chronic kidney disease*. Retrieved November 9, 2010, from http://www.kidney.org/professionals/kdoqi/guidelines_anemia/index.htm

Office of Dietary Supplements. (2010). Dietary supplement fact sheet: Iron. National Institutes of Health. Retrieved from http://ods.od.nih.gov/factsheets/Iron-HealthProfessional/

Office of Dietary Supplements. (2011). Dietary supplement fact sheet: Vitamin B$_{12}$. National Institutes of Health. Retrieved from http://ods.od.nih.gov/factsheets/VitaminB12-HealthProfessional/

Office of Dietary Supplements. (2012). Dietary supplement fact sheet: Folate. National Institutes of Health. http://ods.od.nih.gov/factsheets/Folate-HealthProfessional/

Oh, R. C., & Brown, D. L. (2003). Vitamin B$_{12}$ deficiency. *American Family Physician, 67*(5), 979–986.

Pass, K., Lane, P., Fernhoff, P., Hinton, C. F., Panny, S. R., Parks, J. S., et al. (2000). Newborn screening system guidelines II: Follow-up of children, diagnosis, management, and evaluation. Statement of the Council of Regional Networks for Genetic Services. *Journal of Pediatrics, 137*(Suppl.), S1–S46.

Rosenberg, M. (2013) Overview of the management of chronic kidney disease in adults. *UpToDate Online*. Retrieved from http://www.uptodate.com/contents/overview-of-the-management-of-chronic-kidney-disease-in-adults

Rote, N. S., & McCance, K. L. (2010). Alterations of erythrocyte function. In K. L. McCance, S. E. Huether, V. L. Brashers, & N. S. Rote (Eds.), *Pathophysiology: The biologic basis for disease in adults and children*, 6th ed. (pp 989–1013). Maryland Heights, MO: Mosby.

Schappert, S. M., & Rechtsteiner, E. A. (2008). *Ambulatory medical care utilization estimates for 2006* (National Health Statistics Reports No. 8). Hyattsville, MD: National Center for Health Statistics.

Schrier, S. L. (2013). Causes and diagnosis of iron deficiency anemia in the adult. *UpToDate Online*. Wolters Kluwer Health. Retrieved from http://www.uptodate.com/contents/causes-and-diagnosis-of-iron-deficiency-anemia-in-the-adult

Schrier, S. L., & Camaschella, C. (2013). Anemia of chronic disease (anemia of [chronic] inflammation). *UpToDate Online*. Retrieved from http://www.uptodate.com/contents/anemia-of-chronic-disease-anemia-of-chronic-inflammation

Tanyi, R. (2003). Sickle cell disease: Health promotion and maintenance and the role of primary care nurse practitioners. *Journal of the American Academy of Nurse Practitioners, 15*(9), 389–397.

U.S. Preventive Services Task Force. (2006). *Screening for iron deficiency anemia—including iron supplementation for children and pregnant women: Recommendation statement* (Publication No. AHRQ 06-0589). Rockville, MD: Agency for Healthcare Research and Quality.

U.S. Preventive Services Task Force. (2009). Folic acid for the prevention of neural tube defects: U.S. Preventive Services Task Force recommendation statement. *Annals of Internal Medicine, 150*(9), 626–631.

World Health Organization (WHO). 2013. Micronutrient deficiencies: Iron deficiency anemia. Retrieved from http://www.who.int/nutrition/topics/ida/en/index.html

CHAPTER 28

CHRONIC STABLE ANGINA AND LOW-RISK UNSTABLE ANGINA

Laura D. Rosenthal

Angina is a clinical syndrome typically characterized by deep, poorly localized chest or arm discomfort that is reproducibly associated with physical exertion or emotional stress and promptly relieved by rest or nitroglycerin. The pathophysiology behind it is an imbalance between myocardial oxygen supply and demand (ischemia) associated with coronary artery disease (CAD). Several million Americans suffer from ischemic heart disease, and more than 600,000 die each year from this disorder or its complications. Chronic stable angina is the form most commonly seen in primary care, but even these patients have a mortality risk of 1% to 4.5% annually.

Treatment includes lifestyle modifications and pharmacological and surgical interventions. Pharmacological management includes the use of aspirin, nitrates, beta-adrenergic blockers, long-acting calcium channel blockers (CCBs), angiotensin-converting enzyme (ACE) inhibitors, ranolazine, and low-density lipoprotein (LDL) cholesterol lowering with a 3-hydroxy-3-methylglutaryl coenzyme A (HMG CoA) reductase inhibitor (statin). These drugs are discussed in detail in Chapters 14 and 16. Concomitant disorders often include diabetes mellitus, hyperlipidemia, and hypertension, so the treatment regimen can be quite complex. Chapters 33, 39, and 40, respectively, discuss management of these specific disorders. The focus of this chapter is the long-term management of chronic stable angina and low-risk unstable angina that is usually done by primary care providers.

Several guidelines have been written about this management. The central guideline to which others refer or with which others are consistent is the American College of Cardiology/American Heart Association (ACC/AHA) guideline, published in 2007. The Institute for Clinical Symptoms Improvement (ICSI) guidelines published in 2011 and American College of Physicians guidelines published in 2012 all refer to the 2007 ACC/AHA guideline as a scientifically valid, high-quality review of evidence and agree with the findings of that guideline. The recommendations in this chapter are consistent with that guideline. Other guidelines that add to or differ from this guideline are also discussed.

PATHOPHYSIOLOGY

CAD, myocardial ischemia, and myocardial infarction (MI) form a pathophysiological continuum that impairs the pumping ability of the heart by depriving it of sufficient oxygen and nutrients. Figure 28-1 depicts the physiological changes that occur when the myocardium is deprived of oxygen. The coronary arteries supply oxygen to the myocardium. Oxygen extraction from these vessels is at maximum efficiency at all times, and there is little oxygen reserve during

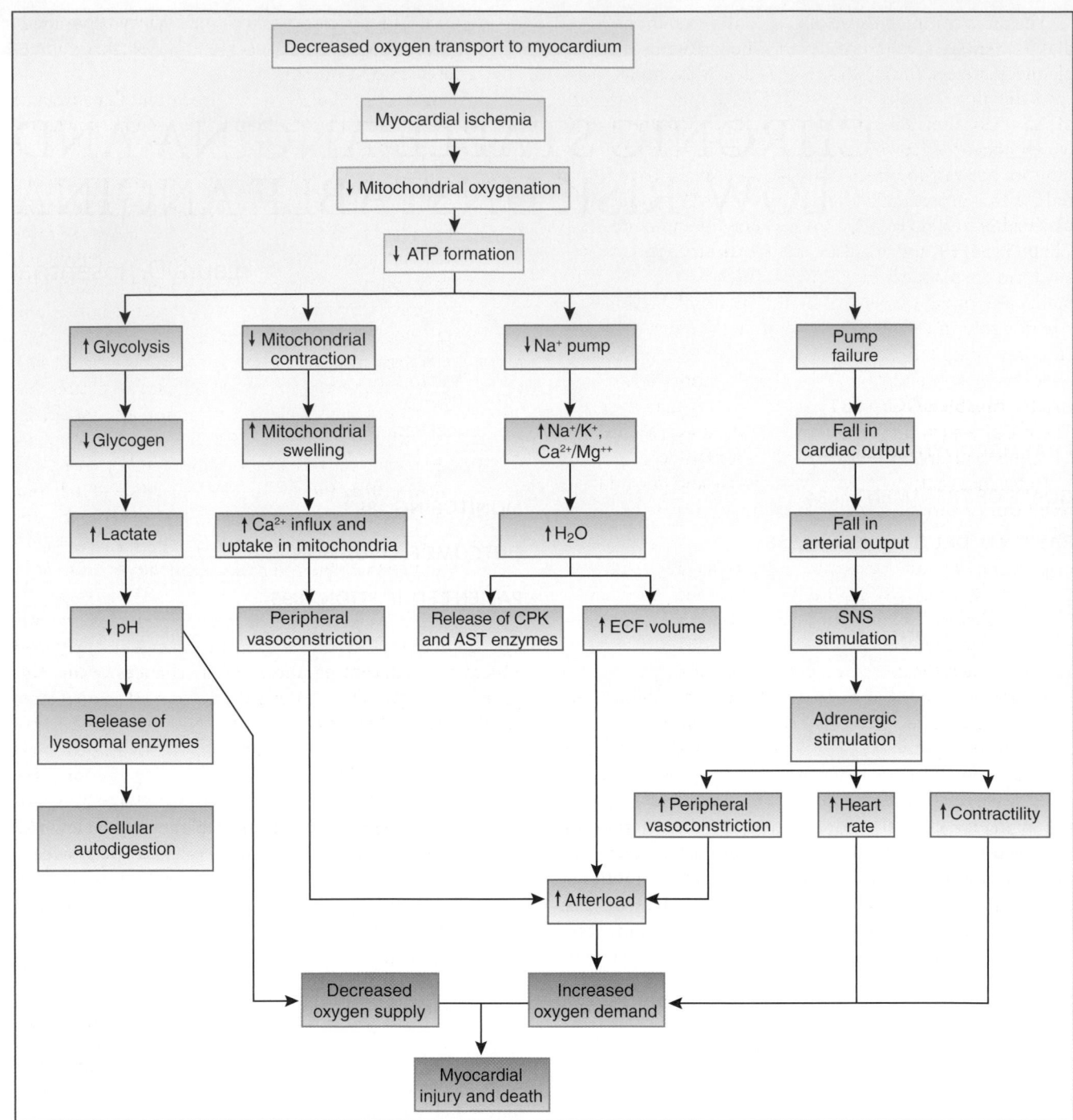

Figure 28–1. Pathophysiology of myocardial ischemia.

periods of increased oxygen demand (McCance & Huether, 2014). Ischemia occurs when demand exceeds supply. One mechanism available to increase oxygen supply is to dilate the coronary arteries and bring more blood flow to the myocardium. Nitrates can do this in patients with normal hearts. Unfortunately, in CAD, usually associated with atherosclerosis and plaque formation, the coronary arteries are often maximally dilated already or unable to dilate secondary to plaque and calcium deposits. Most of the drugs available to treat angina decrease myocardial oxygen demand by decreasing the workload of the heart. The drugs accomplish this by decreasing afterload, preload, or both. The one exception to these mechanisms is ranolazine, whose mechanism involves reducing sodium-induced calcium overload in myocytes, which leads to myocyte dysfunction and angina.

In patients with ischemia, nitrates do not increase total coronary blood flow, but redistribute the blood to the ischemic areas. Although they have some ability to dilate the coronary arteries, nitrates are also able to facilitate movement of oxygen across the arterial–myocardial membrane. Their use in CAD relates as much to this action as it does to vasodilation.

The most common cause of CAD and resultant myocardial ischemia is atherosclerosis. The growing mass of plaque, platelets, fibrin, and cellular debris eventually narrows the lumen enough to impede blood flow. The growth of this mass is related in part to the action of angiotensin II, which acts as a growth factor for vascular cells. ACE inhibitors prevent the formation of angiotensin II and thus reduce this growth. The link between CAD and elevated plasma lipoprotein concentrations is well documented (see Chapters 36, 39, and 40). The fatty streaks that will eventually form the plaque have a lipoprotein/cholesterol base, the main component of which is LDL cholesterol. Statins have a major role in reducing LDL cholesterol concentrations and preventing plaque formation. Platelet aggregations release the prostaglandin thromboxane A_2, a potent vasoconstrictor capable of causing spasms of the coronary arteries. The use of aspirin in patients with CAD is associated with its role in irreversibly blocking thromboxane A_2.

Imbalances between myocardial supply and demand can result from a variety of conditions. Supply is reduced by the following:

- Hemodynamic factors such as increased resistance in coronary vessels, hypotension, and decreased blood volume. ACE inhibitors, beta blockers, direct renin inhibitors, and the dihydropyridine CCBs decrease peripheral resistance through their vasodilatory actions.
- Cardiac factors such as decreases in diastolic filling time, increases in heart rate, and valvular incompetence. Beta blockers and non-dihydropyridine CCBs decrease heart rate. The beta blockers have the further advantage of preventing the recurrence of MIs.
- Hematological factors such as the oxygen content of the blood, the acid–base status of the blood, and anemia.
- Systemic disorders, such as shock, which reduce blood flow or the availability of oxygen.

Demand is increased by the following:

- High systolic blood pressure, which increases the work the heart has to do to move blood from the left ventricle to the systemic circulation. One focus of anginal management is control of blood pressure. ACE inhibitors, beta blockers, direct renin inhibitors, and both types of CCBs decrease blood pressure.
- Increased ventricular volume, which increases the work the heart has to do because the left ventricle must move more blood. ACE inhibitors reduce sodium and water retention.
- Increased thickness of the myocardium (ventricular hypertrophy). The same mechanism that facilitated growth of the vessel walls in atherosclerosis also increases the thickness of the myocardium. ACE inhibitors play a major role here to decrease the remodeling. Beta blockers can assist in prevention of ventricular hypertrophy but play a smaller role.
- Increased heart rate resulting from exercise, stress, hyperthyroidism, fever, anemia, hyperviscosity of the blood, or negative feedback systems' response to decreased cardiac output. Beta blockers can assist in decreasing heart rate resulting from conditions such as hyperthyroidism and from negative feedback patterns secondary to decreased cardiac output.
- Conditions that heighten the myocardium's contractile response. Beta blockers and CCBs both have negative inotropic effects.

Ischemia caused by the imbalance between myocardial oxygen supply (MOS) and myocardial oxygen demand (MOD) produces pain referred to as angina. There are three types of angina: chronic stable angina, unstable angina, and Prinzmetal's angina. Chronic stable angina (exertional angina) is caused by narrowing of the arterial lumen and hardening of the arterial walls so that the affected vessels cannot dilate in response to the increased MOD associated with physical exertion or emotional stress. Research indicates that 75% to 80% of ischemia can be asymptomatic (silent ischemia) (Conti, Berry, & Petersen, 2012; Dweck, Campbell, Miller, & Francis, 2009). Diabetes mellitus and hypertension are associated with an increased prevalence of silent ischemia (Conti et al, 2012; Dweck et al, 2009). Ischemia with or without pain has the same prognosis, because it is the presence of ischemia, not angina, that determines outcome. In both cases, the myocardium is at risk.

On the cellular level, the myocardium becomes cyanotic within the first 10 seconds of impaired oxygen supply, and ischemic electrocardiographic (ECG) changes occur. Deprived of oxygen, the myocardial cells convert to anaerobic metabolism, and lactic acid accumulates. Myocardial nerve fibers are irritated by this lactic acid and transmit a pain message to the cardiac nerves and upper thoracic posterior nerve roots. Under ischemic conditions, cardiac cells are viable for about 20 minutes. The supply–demand imbalance must be resolved during this time to prevent permanent damage.

PHARMACODYNAMICS

Nitrates affect the supply–demand equation on both sides. Low doses of nitroglycerin preferentially dilate the veins more than the arterioles. The resulting decrease in venous return to the heart decreases left ventricular end-diastolic pressure (preload), resulting in decreased wall tension and an increased transmyocardial gradient. This increased gradient improves perfusion between the coronary arteries on the outside of the heart and the subendocardium on the inside of the heart, resulting in increased oxygen supply to the myocardium. Higher doses of nitrates dilate arterial vessels, which decreases systemic vascular resistance (afterload). Additionally, the higher doses cause further dilation of venous vessels, which results in venous pooling and decreased venous return to the heart. MOD is reduced by the reduced cardiac workload. Nitrates also dilate coronary arteries to some extent, but doing so is difficult in severe atherosclerotic arteries, and this effect is now thought to be only a small part of their action in relieving ischemia.

Beta blockers affect the supply–demand equation on the demand side. Both beta$_1$-selective agents and nonselective beta blockers decrease the force of myocardial contractility and decrease heart rate and conduction velocity. Beta blockers also decrease systemic vascular resistance and blood pressure (afterload). All of these effects reduce myocardial oxygen demand and thus relieve anginal pain.

CCBs primarily affect the supply–demand equation on the demand side of the equation. By blocking calcium influx into cells, the dihydropyridines cause arterial smooth muscle relaxation, which results in peripheral vasodilation, decreased afterload, and ultimately decreased MOD. They also accomplish this at doses that do not affect cardiac smooth muscle. The dihydropyridines have the potential to cause coronary vasodilation, but again, because the coronary arteries are usually already maximally dilated in patients with angina, this will result in only a small, if any, increase in MOS. The non-dihydropyridine calcium channel blockers (Verapamil and diltiazem) depress the rate of sinoarterial (SA) node depolarization and slow atrioventricular (AV) conduction, resulting in a decreased heart rate as well as decreased contractility in cardiac smooth muscle. These two actions result in negative chronotropic and inotropic effects and ultimately decrease MOD. They accomplish this at doses that have only a small impact on vascular smooth muscle and consequently little effect on vasodilation.

ACE inhibitors also affect both the MOS and the MOD sides of the equation. Through their action on the renin-angiotensin-aldosterone system, ACE inhibitors prevent the formation of angiotensin II, a potent vasoconstrictor. This action decreases peripheral vascular resistance and thereby MOD, as the heart has decreased afterload against which it must pump. Reduced formation of angiotensin II also decreases the thickening of coronary artery walls, resulting in increased MOS (McCance & Huether, 2014) and decreases the thickening of ventricular walls, resulting in decreased MOD. They also reduce the secretion of aldosterone, which reduces the retention of sodium and water, thereby reducing extracellular fluid volume and preload.

Direct renin inhibitors (DRIs) decrease plasma renin activity, thus blocking the conversion of angiotensinogen to angiotensin I. Because of the lack of angiotension I, there is less available for conversion to angiotensin II. This decreases peripheral vascular resistance, thus decreasing MOD. As with ACE inhibitors, this also decreases the thickening of coronary artery walls, resulting in increased MOS. Aliskiren (Tekturna) is the only approved direct renin inhibitor available currently. Aliskiren causes less cough and angioedema than the ACE inhibitors but is still contraindicated in pregnancy.

Ranolazine has antianginal and anti-ischemic effects that do not depend on reduction in heart rate or blood pressure. At therapeutic levels, ranolazine inhibits the cardiac late sodium current. Through inhibition of the late sodium current, the pathophysiological cycle of myocardial ischemia and dysregulation of intracellular ion homeostasis that leads to angina is avoided.

Aspirin inhibits the synthesis of thromboxane A_2 in the production of platelets. This action reduces platelet aggregation to stop the cycle of vasoconstriction and platelet buildup. Research has demonstrated a role for low-dose aspirin for male patients older than 50 as an adjunct to risk factor management to prevent a second heart attack. Women have more adverse effects than help if aspirin is taken prior to age 65. Women get more assist for cerebral vascular events than CV events from aspirin.

Finally, statins should be included in the treatment regimen for angina. Their role is on the MOS side of the equation; reduction in LDL cholesterol levels plays a significant role in decreasing the formation of atherosclerotic plaque. This plaque is central to the narrowing of the arterial lumen.

GOALS OF TREATMENT

The immediate goals are to treat to complete, or near complete, elimination of anginal chest pain and return to normal activities; maintain the patient at a symptom level of the Canadian Cardiovascular Society (CCS) classification of angina class I with minimum adverse effects; and keep blood pressure less than 130/85 mm Hg and pulse less than 70 beats per minute (Veterans Health Administration, Department of Defense [VA/DoD], 2003). The ultimate goals of therapy are to reduce the risks of MI and death. Although the clinical course of some patients may extend for 15 or 20 years, most patients with chronic stable angina are at increased risk for cardiovascular morbidity and mortality. Patient prognosis is strongly affected by the number and locations of coronary artery stenosis, the severity of the ischemia, and the presence of other CAD risk factors, such as smoking, hypertension, hypercholesterolemia, low high-density lipoprotein (HDL) cholesterol, diabetes mellitus, and age and gender considerations. Achievement of these goals is accomplished through improving oxygen supply and decreasing oxygen demand.

RATIONAL DRUG SELECTION

Angina is associated with MI and sudden cardiac death in the mind of provider and public alike. This presents a two-edged sword in therapeutic management: recognition of the potential complications, leading to consistent adherence to the treatment regimen, versus denial of the seriousness of the disorder, leading to lack of adherence to the treatment regimen. The health-care provider can improve adherence by placing angina in a realistic perspective and tailoring treatment options to each patient's needs. For effective management, the choice of treatment should be low cost, limited in complexity, and with the fewest possible adverse reactions. To achieve these treatment outcomes, lifestyle modifications and pharmacological therapy are chosen based on risk stratification, grade of angina, and specific patient variables.

Risk Stratification

Major Risk Factors

The major risk factors for CAD are age, family history, smoking, hypertension, hypercholesterolemia, low HDL cholesterol, and diabetes mellitus. These risk factors are used in the Framingham equations for calculating the 10-year risk for the development of coronary heart disease (Anderson et al, 2007) and in the new risk equations that aim at uncovering a 7 year risk (Stone et al, 2014). In addition, conditions that decrease oxygen supply and increase oxygen demand are also major risk factors for ischemic heart disease. These include heart failure (see Chapter 36), anemia (see Chapter 27), hypertension (see Chapter 40), hyperthyroidism (see Chapter 41), valvular heart disease, and morbid obesity.

Noncardiac Factors

There are also noncardiac disorders that mimic angina because their primary symptom is chest pain. These include pulmonary embolism, pneumonia, pneumothorax, gastroesophageal spasm or reflux, cholecystitis, peptic ulcer, pancreatitis, rib fractures, herpes zoster, and panic disorder. Some of these disorders also decrease oxygen supply and can cause angina. These disorders should be ruled out before deciding a patient has angina.

Women often have symptoms of angina that are atypical and may include fatigue, shortness of breath without chest pain, nausea and vomiting, back pain, jaw pain, dizziness, and weakness (ICSI, 2011). A study of cardiovascular outcomes in women with nonobstructive CAD (Gulati et al, 2009) found that women with traditional or atypical symptoms and signs suggestive of ischemia, but without obstructive CAD, were still at elevated risk for cardiovascular events compared with asymptomatic women. In addition, a large observational study from the National Registry of Myocardial Infarction revealed that in patients hospitalized with MI, women were more likely to present without chest pain and had higher mortality than men within the same age group (Canto et al, 2012). This elevated risk for females should not be overlooked.

Classification System for Grading Angina

The New York Heart Association (NYHA) and the CCS have devised a classification system for grading the severity of angina (Table 28-1). The lower the class, the more likely the patient's angina can be controlled by lifestyle modification and intermittent nitroglycerin (Table 28-2). The higher the class, the more likely the patient will require multiple drug therapy. The ACC/AHA guidelines have a classification system that incorporates the NYHA/CCS system and additional data. Table 28-3 depicts this classification system.

Treatment Algorithms

It is not within the scope of this book to discuss the testing involved in the diagnosis and grading of angina; however, a thorough history including questions about symptoms and when they occur related to exercise, about smoking, a physical examination, laboratory testing for possible causes of the symptoms (e.g., anemia or thyroid disorders), and a resting 12-lead ECG should be obtained. For those with abnormal ECG findings, referral to or consultation with a cardiologist is recommended. The treatment protocol discussed in this chapter assumes accurate diagnosis of angina with the appropriate diagnostic tools. Once the diagnosis is made, protocols are based on the grade or class of angina and the risk profile.

All appropriate patients with angina should be on aspirin 81 to 162 mg/d (Anderson et al, 2007; ICSI, 2011; Scottish Intercollegiate Guidelines Network [SIGN], 2007). Aspirin is known to be effective for reducing mortality in patients with CAD and has been associated with a decrease in nonfatal MI, nonfatal stroke, and vascular death (Vandvik et al 2012). In multiple studies, aspirin was associated with preventing reinfarction and significantly reduced recurrent ischemic events (Antithrombotic Trialists' Collaboration, 2009).

Table 28–1   Grading of Angina by the New York Heart Association and the Canadian Cardiovascular Society

Class	New York Heart Association	Canadian Cardiovascular Society
Class I	Proven coronary artery disease without symptoms	Ordinary physical activity, such as walking or climbing stairs, does not cause angina. Angina occurs with strenuous, rapid, or prolonged exertion at work or recreation.
Class II	Angina only with unusually strenuous physical exertion	Slight limitation of ordinary activity. Angina occurs on walking or climbing stairs rapidly; walking uphill; walking or stair climbing after meals; in cold wind; under emotional stress; or only during the few hours after awakening. Walking more than two blocks on the level and climbing more than one flight of ordinary stairs at a normal pace and in normal conditions does not cause angina.
Class III	Angina during routine physical activity	Marked limitations of ordinary activity. Angina occurs on walking one to two blocks on the level and climbing one flight of stairs in normal conditions and at a normal pace.
Class IV	Angina during minimal activity or rest	Inability to carry on any physical activity without discomfort. Angina may occur at rest.

Table 28–2   Risk Profiles Associated With Angina

Risk	Lifestyle Risk	Physiological Risk
Low	• Nonsmoker • Normotensive • Low cholesterol • Negative family history	• Mild stable angina (class I–II) • Good exercise tolerance tests • Normal ventricular function on echocardiography
High	• Smoker • Hypertensive • Hypercholesterolemia • Positive family history	• Severe angina (class III–IV) • Unstable angina • Poor exercise test performance • Impaired ventricular function
Uncertain	• Obesity • Sedentary lifestyle • Type A personality • Emotional stress	• Silent ischemia

Table 28–3   American College of Cardiology/American Heart Association Risk Stratification in Patients With Chronic Stable Angina

Class	Description
Class I	• Disabling (CCS III and IV) chronic stable angina despite medical therapy • High-risk criteria on noninvasive testing regardless of anginal severity • Angina and have survived sudden cardiac death or serious ventricular dysrhythmias • Angina and symptoms of CHF • Clinical characteristics that indicate a high likelihood of severe CAD
Class IIa	• Significant LV dysfunction (ejection fraction <45%). CCS Class I or II angina and demonstrable ischemia but less than high-risk criteria on noninvasive testing • Inadequate prognostic information after noninvasive testing
Class IIb	• CCS Class I or II angina, preserved LV dysfunction (ejection fraction >45%) and less than high-risk criteria on noninvasive testing • CCS Class III or IV angina, which improves to Class I or II with medical therapy • CCS Class I or II angina, but intolerance to adequate medical therapy
Class III	• CCS Class I or II angina patients who respond to medical therapy and have no evidence of ischemia on noninvasive testing • Patients who prefer to avoid revascularization

CHF = congestive heart failure; LV = left ventricular.

If aspirin is contraindicated, clopidogrel (Plavix) 75 mg daily may be an effective substitute (Chen et al, 2011; Kaiser Permanente Care Management Institute, 2008; Vandvik et al, 2012). One large (19,000 patients) randomized controlled study of patients with a history of ischemic heart disease, MI, or atherosclerotic peripheral arterial disease found clopidogrel demonstrated a reduction in myocardial infarction when compared with aspirin 325 mg daily but failed to show a significant difference in reduction of stroke or total mortality (Vandvik et al, 2012).

There is no data to support the use of dual antiplatelet therapy (aspirin and clopidogrel) for secondary prevention of nonfatal MI or total mortality in patients with CAD who are greater than 1 year post MI with stent placement (Vandvik et al, 2012).

Patients with angina only on exertion, a normal resting ECG, and symptoms that can be controlled by rest and intermittent nitroglycerin (ACC/AHA class III) should be started on lifestyle modifications and have any concurrent aggravating factors or disease processes treated. For example, hypertension itself can cause angina, and elevated cholesterol contributes to the continued development of atherosclerosis. Severe anemia, hyperthyroidism, hypoxic lung disorders, diabetes mellitus, and critical valvular stenosis need to be treated and brought under control. Patients with known CAD, age 65 and older, with ECG changes on exertion, and with diabetes are considered high risk for unstable angina and should be started on both lifestyle modifications and drug therapy (Fraker & Fihn, 2007).

Lifestyle Modification

Fundamental to the management of all types and grades of angina is the reduction of risk factors through lifestyle modification. Lifestyle modifications may prevent the development of complications commonly associated with myocardial ischemia and have little cost. Even when they cannot control angina alone, they may reduce the number and dosage of drugs required for angina management and prevent the need for surgical intervention. All patients should be advised to stop smoking, maintain appropriate levels of blood pressure and cholesterol; follow the Dietary Approaches to Stop Hypertension (DASH) diet for control of hypertension, including the recommendation for cholesterol management and achieve, to the extent possible, their ideal body weight. Table 28-4 discusses the main lifestyle modifications appropriate for patients with angina. They are similar to those appropriate for patients with hypertension and hypercholesterolemia.

When these initial therapies have not resulted in improved exercise tolerance or decreased episodes of angina, or when the patient is ACC/AHA class I or IIa on the grading scale, initial drug therapy is begun. Figure 28-2 delineates the drug treatment protocol for chronic stable angina and low-risk unstable angina.

Drug Therapy

Initial Therapy for Symptomatic Patients

ACE inhibitors and beta-adrenergic blockers are the mainstays of initial drug therapy for patients with angina (ICSI, 2011; Kaiser Permanente Care Management Institute, 2008). The second-generation dihydropyridine CCBs (amlodipine and felodipine) and long-acting nitrates can be used for treatment of angina in patients when beta blockers and ACE inhibitors are ineffective or contraindicated (Kaiser Permanente Care Management Institute, 2008; Qaseem et al, 2012). Short-acting, sublingual nitrates can be used in patients with mild, stable CAD for immediate relief on an as needed basis (ISCI, 2011; Quaseem et al, 2012). Each drug class has a group of patients for whom they are best suited and a group for whom they are contraindicated. Detailed discussions of each of these classes of drugs are given in Chapters 14 and 16. The focus here is on their role in angina management.

ACE inhibitors are recommended by the American College of Physicians (Quaseem et al, 2012) and in other guidelines (ICSI, 2011; Kaiser Permanente Care Management Institute, 2008) for all symptomatic patients with chronic stable angina to prevent MI or death and to reduce symptoms. Anderson (2007) also recommend this drug class but limit it to patients who have diabetes, hypertension, chronic kidney disease, or left ventricular dysfunction. They recommend that ACE inhibitors be considered in CAD patients even without left ventricular dysfunction. They have been shown to improve outcomes for CAD patients through their ability to both increase MOS and decrease MOD. ACE inhibitors are discussed in more detail in Chapter 16. Table 28-5 shows concomitant diseases for which they are more useful and for which they are contraindicated.

Table 28–4 Lifestyle Modifications

Attain Ideal Body Weight.

Excess weight increases cardiac workload and increases oxygen demand. It is also associated with hypertension, and loss of as little as 10 lb can significantly reduce blood pressure.

Increase Aerobic Physical Activity Within the Limitations of Angina.

The overall goal of anginal therapy is to restore optimal exercise capacity. The presence of angina, however, indicates an imbalance in oxygen supply and demand and denotes possible damage to the myocardium. Start with a level of activity that does not produce pain, and gradually increase the activity level by 1 min each day as long as there is no angina. Even limited activity is preferred to no activity. Daily activity is preferred to intermittent activity.

Reduce Daily Sodium Intake to No More Than 1,500 mg.

Sodium helps the body retain water, which increases the amount of blood volume. This increases cardiac workload and increases oxygen demand. It is also associated with hypertension. Reduced intake of this level can often be achieved by not adding salt during cooking or on the table and by watching hidden sources of salt, such as canned foods.

Maintain Adequate Intake of Dietary Potassium (Approximately 60 mEq/d).

The heart is heavily dependent on potassium for contractility.

Reduce Intake of Dietary Saturated Fats and Cholesterol.

Cholesterol and saturated fats are implicated in the development of atherosclerosis, which narrows coronary arteries and makes angina worse. The level of reduction depends on serum cholesterol levels. Hypercholesterolemia requires lower levels than those required for patients with normal cholesterol levels. Start with the American Heart Association Step 1 diet (http://www.nhlbi.nih.gov/guidelines/obesity/e_txtbk/txgd/4321.htm).

Stop Smoking.

Nicotine is implicated in several ways in making angina worse. Absorbed nicotine increases blood pressure and heart rate, thus increasing myocardial oxygen demand. Nicotine also causes vasospasm, and the rise in carboxyhemoglobin from smoke inhalation reduces oxygen supply. Even passive smoke inhalation can reduce exercise tolerance in patients with angina. The low doses of nicotine found in nicotine replacement therapy (NRT) do not significantly elevate blood pressure or heart rate, and NRT may be used to aid in smoking cessation.

Limit Alcohol Intake.

For men and heavier patients, alcohol intake should be no more than 2 oz (30 mL) of ethanol (e.g., 24 oz beer, 10 oz wine, 2 oz 100-proof whiskey)/d. For women and lighter-weight patients, the intake should be no more than 1 oz/d.

Table 28–5   Drug Choice Based on Concomitant Disease States

Drug Choice	Effect on Concomitant Disease States	
	Favorable Effects	**Unfavorable Effects**
Nitrates	Heart failure Hypertension	Migraine headaches MI
Beta-Adrenergic Blockers	Heart failure Arrhythmias, atrial tachycardia Hypertension "Stage fright" Migraine headaches Hyperthyroidism	Advanced AV block Uncontrolled or severe reactive airway disease Claudication/Raynaud's disease (can use beta$_1$-selective drug) Diabetes mellitus (may try beta$_1$-selective drug)
	Post-MI	Depression
ACE Inhibitors	Diabetes mellitus Heart failure Hyperlipidemia Hypertension	Contraindicated in pregnancy Bilateral renal artery stenosis Angioedema history
Direct Renin Inhibitors	Hypertension	Contraindicated in pregnancy Bilateral renal artery stenosis Angioedema history
HMG-CoA Reductase Inhibitors (Statins)	Hyperlipidemia Hypertension	Contraindicated in pregnancy Myopathy history
Calcium Channel Blockers Dihydropyridines	Hypertension, isolated systolic hypertension Systolic heart failure Raynaud's disease, peripheral vascular disease	Peripheral edema
Verapamil	Atrial tachycardias Hypertension Migraine headache MI	Advanced AV block Constipation Heart failure Concurrent use with beta blockers may cause additive bradycardia
Diltiazem	Atrial tachycardia Diabetes mellitus MI	Advanced AV block Heart failure
Amlodipine	Atherosclerosis Heart failure	

ACE = angiotensin-converting enzymes; AV = atrioventricular; HMG-CoA = 3-hydroxy-3-methyl glutaryl coenzyme A; MI = myocardial infarction.

Angiotensin II receptor blocker (ARB) therapy is recommended for patients with CAD and diabetes with hypertension and for those with left ventricular systolic dysfunction when these patients are intolerant to ACE inhibitors. For other patients who are intolerant to ACE inhibitors, there is insufficient evidence to recommend for or against ARB therapy (Kaiser Permanente Care Management Institute, 2008). ARBs can be added to ACE inhibitor therapy for clinical reasons, such as uncontrolled hypertension or insufficient vasodilation, but it is not recommended as a routine combination. The combination of an ACE inhibitor and an ARB does not reduce all-cause mortality and may increase undesired side effects.

Beta blockers with no intrinsic sympathomimetic activity (ISA) properties are recommended as initial therapy by all the guidelines for all patients, with or without previous MI, unless specifically contraindicated. They especially decrease

MOD and are the drugs of choice for exertional angina (ACC/AHA all classes). Because they do not improve myocardial oxygen supply, their main role is in preventing recurrence of MIs in patients with CAD. They are especially useful for patients with exertional angina whose lifestyle involves frequent vigorous activity, patients with resting tachycardia (e.g., hyperthyroidism), and for patients who have concomitant diseases that might benefit from beta blockade. The Kaiser guidelines (2008) make a strong recommendation for giving a beta blocker to CAD patients with left ventricular systolic dysfunction (NYHA classes I through IV). Table 28-5 shows these concomitant diseases.

Beta blockers are contraindicated for patients with severe, uncontrolled reactive airway diseases and vasospastic angina. For patients with mild to moderate reversible airway disease or chronic obstructive pulmonary disease, cardioselective beta blockers may be used as long as the airway disease is stable and well controlled (Kaiser Permanente Care Management Institute, 2008). The most cost-effective and convenient beta blockers are atenolol (Tenormin) and metoprolol succinate (toprol XL), both with once-daily dosing, a low adverse reactions profile, and beta$_1$ selectivity. Beta blockers are discussed in more detail in Chapter 14

Most guidelines recommend lipid-lowering therapy with statins for all CAD patients who have LDL cholesterol levels greater than 100 mg/dL except the Veterans Health Administration (2003), which does not mention LDL levels, and Kaiser guidelines, which call for LDL less than 70 mg/dL in patients with CAD. Treatment of elevated LDL cholesterol is discussed extensively in Chapter 39 and the drugs themselves are discussed in Chapter 16.

Nitrates and CCBs are appropriate for symptom management and specific indications. Nitrates are the oldest and best studied of the antianginals, are cost-effective, and have a variety of routes of administration that allow flexibility for the patient. They are more effective than beta blockers in relieving and preventing anginal episodes in patients with vasospastic angina. Nitroglycerin 0.3 to 0.4 mg sublingual tablets or translingual spray is used for immediate symptom relief. All patients with angina should carry some form of rapid-acting nitrate with them at all times. They should be instructed to use this medication at the first sign of angina, even if they are uncertain if the symptoms are angina. If symptoms have not improved after 5 minutes of taking one dose of this drug, the patient should call 9-1-1 for medical attention. This recommendation has been updated from the previous recommendation of taking up to three doses before calling EMS. This change encourages earlier contacting of EMS by patients with symptoms suggestive of ACS. Self-medicating with prescription drugs, including nitrates, has been documented as a common cause of delay in calling EMS among patients with ACS (Anderson et al, 2011). Chapter 16 has specific information on the treatment protocol and storage of nitroglycerin in its various forms.

For patients who respond well to sublingual or translingual nitroglycerin and who experience angina episodes more than "rarely," and who are intolerant of beta blockers, long-acting oral or transdermal nitrates are generally indicated. Among the available drugs, the most cost-effective are isosorbide mononitrate (Imdur) given daily or nitroglycerin transdermal patches applied daily with a 10 to 12 hour nitrate-free interval to prevent nitrate tolerance. The timing of the nitrate-free interval should coincide with the time of fewest episodes of angina, which is typically at night. The administration schedule that seems most effective is 7 a.m. and 2 p.m. daily. Headache is the most common adverse reaction but resolves over time. Starting with low doses and slowly increasing the dose reduces the incidence of headache.

CCBs, like the nitrates, decrease MOD. They are the initial drugs of choice when coronary artery vasospasm is suspected to be a contributing mechanism to the angina. They are also effective for patients with exertional angina who have fixed atherosclerotic CAD; when optimal doses of beta blockers or nitrates are ineffective, contraindicated, or poorly tolerated; and when a concomitant disease might benefit from the use of a CCB. Table 28-5 shows these concomitant diseases. Studies have also shown one CCB, amlodipine (Norvasc), to be effective in inhibiting vascular smooth muscle cell proliferation in atherosclerosis, and it may have a protective mechanism in preventing or retarding the progression of atherosclerosis (Ikeda et al, 2009; Martin-Ventura et al, 2008). It also has the advantage of a long half-life that allows once-daily dosing without resorting to a sustained-release form.

When initial therapy with low to moderate doses of these drugs is not adequate to control angina or to reduce progression from a lower class (ACC/AHA class I or IIa) to a higher one (ACC/AHA class IIb or III), two choices are possible. One is to increase the dose of at least one of the drugs. This is always done with consideration for the potential adverse reactions associated with that drug. In some cases, the addition of another drug to minimize the adverse reactions and provide an additive effect to maximize benefits may be more appropriate than significant increases in the initial drug. The second option is to substitute a drug from a different class. Nitrates and CCBs are both effective, for example, in vasospastic angina, but not all patients respond well to nitrates. Ranolazine has been evaluated in patients with chronic symptomatic angina despite treatment with the maximum dose of other antianginal agents. Statistically significant decreases in angina attacks were observed. This drug may be used concurrently with any of the antianginal classes discussed above and with antiplatelet and lipid-lowering drugs.

Multidrug Therapy

Combinations of beta blockers and calcium channel blockers have been shown to be more effective than the individual drugs used alone. Both amlodipine and felodipine (dihydropyridine CCBs) work especially well in groups of patients who demonstrate improvement while on this combination. Their effects on reducing MOD are complementary, making it possible to use lower doses of both drugs, and many of their adverse reactions cancel out. Lower doses also reduce the risk of hypotension. Patients not adequately controlled by either drug alone tend to benefit from the addition of the second drug. They are a questionable combination for patients with left ventricular dysfunction because together they may induce heart failure or bradycardia. Verapamil and diltiazem also should be avoided in this combination.

Combinations of a long-acting nitrate and a beta blocker are also safe, effective, and low in cost. Their effects are additive, permitting lower doses of both drugs, and their adverse reactions often cancel out. The beta blocker slows any reflex tachycardia caused by the nitrate, which helps to reduce MOD.

Combinations of long-acting nitrates and CCBs are rarely used because of the high risk for hypotension and because their adverse reaction profiles are additive. This combination is usually reserved for refractory cases of vasospastic angina.

When the drug combination greatly improves angina, it is worthwhile to attempt gradual reduction of prior drug doses over time. For example, if the addition of a beta blocker to high-dose nitrate therapy greatly improves angina, gradual reduction in the nitrate doses can be tried.

Patients with severe (classes III–IV) angina frequently require at least three drugs from different classes. When this level of regimen is required, referral to a cardiologist is appropriate.

Drug Therapies That Are Not Helpful and/or Are to Be Avoided

According to ACC/AHA (2007) and Kaiser (2008), the following therapies are not helpful in treating angina based on evidence: vitamins C and E supplementation, chelation therapy, garlic, acupuncture, and coenzyme Q_{10}. Kaiser guidelines (2008) also mention folic acid, coenzyme Q_{10}, vitamin B_6, and vitamin B_{12} as being ineffective. Studies reviewed by Mente, deKoning, Shannon, and Anand (2009) showed varying degrees of evidence of causal links between dietary factors and coronary heart disease. No other guidelines specifically mention therapies that are ineffective.

Additional Patient Variables

Older Adults

The treatment protocol for angina is the same for older adults as it is for other adults, with consideration for the usual changes in pharmacokinetics in this age group. Lifestyle modifications are always first-line therapy because of their safety and cost. When drugs are chosen, consideration should be given to the risks for CAD and MI, which are higher in older adults. Older adults, however, may have chronic airway diseases, and nonselective beta blockers may be contraindicated if this concomitant disease is severe or uncontrolled. Congestive heart failure is also common and particularly lethal in older patients. ACE inhibitors and beta blockers have important roles in this disease process, whereas the negative inotropic effects of some non-dihydropyridine CCBs may make this disorder worse. The dihydropyridine CCBs amlodipine and felodipine do not have the negative inotropic effect and therefore do not seem to worsen heart failure in older adults. Hypertension and hypercholesterolemia are also more common in older adults. Table 28-5 shows the appropriate drug class selection for each of these disease processes.

Women

Initiation of hormone replacement therapy in postmenopausal women for the purpose of reducing cardiovascular risk is no longer recommended in the guidelines but is a current topic of debate in new literature. Data from the Women's Health Initiative indicated that this therapy may increase risk for some and was not helpful in others. Recent studies reveal that timing and duration of hormone replacement therapy may affect outcomes in women, but further research must be completed (Harman et al, 2011). The Heart and Estrogen/Progestin Replacement Study (HERS) (Miller & Oparil, 2003; Vittinghoff et al, 2003) concluded that women with coronary disease are at high risk for MI even in the absence of other risk factors.

Their risk increases up to 6-fold when many risk factors are present. Established drugs for secondary preventions, including aspirin, beta blockers, and lipid-lowering agents (statins), are underutilized in these women, especially those at highest risk.

Women of all ages are at higher risk for silent myocardial ischemia. Studies that have included significant percentages of female patients with CAD have found that taking aspirin produced the same lowering of all-cause mortality and lower incidence of nonfatal MI and stroke as found in men. The same findings have not proven true in women without CAD who are less than 65 years of age. Therefore, routine aspirin is not recommended in women without diagnosed CAD who are younger than 65 (Mosca et al, 2011). There is no gender-based difference in the treatment protocol for angina. There may be differences based on concomitant disease states such as hypertension and hypercholesterolemia (discussed in Chapters 39 and 40). Premenopausal women are at higher risk for anemia that may affect MOS. Treatment for anemia is discussed in Chapter 27.

Concomitant Diseases

Drugs used to treat angina may improve the management of some diseases and worsen others. Selection of an angina drug that treats a concomitant disease can simplify the overall therapeutic regimen, reduce cost, and increase the likelihood of adherence. It is not within the scope of this book to discuss all possible concomitant disease states, but those most common in patients with angina who might benefit from appropriate drug selection to treat the angina are discussed here.

Myocardial Infarction

Angina is usually associated with CAD, the major underlying mechanism behind MI. Both aspirin and beta blockers have been associated with MI prophylaxis and have the strongest evidence for their use. Aspirin is prescribed as for all patients with CAD. Diltiazem (Cardizem) in its long-acting form has been shown to decrease mortality for patients with non–Q wave MIs. Non-dihydropyridine CCBs should be avoided after MI for patients with poor ejection fractions (less than 40%) because of their negative inotropic effects. Nitrates tend to cause reflex tachycardia. The increased MOD associated with this tachycardia cannot be adjusted for with coronary arteries that are blocked and unable to be effectively dilated. They should be used with caution. ACE inhibitors are useful after MI to prevent heart failure and mortality. They are drugs of choice to treat angina in patients with diabetes or left ventricular dysfunction. Their action on angiotensin II produces antiatherogenic effects, and they diminish MOD and increase nitric oxide through their action on the bradykinin system. Post-MI patients who are given ACE inhibitors may also benefit from reduced angina. Both ACE inhibitors and beta blockers have been shown to decrease the cardiac remodeling that occurs with MI.

Heart Failure

Heart failure is commonly associated with higher grades of angina. Several drugs used to treat angina also reduce blood pressure and improve myocardial function to reduce the risk for development of heart failure. ACE inhibitors are associated with decreased morbidity and mortality from heart failure and are first-line therapy for that disorder. Clinical benefits in heart failure include less dyspnea, improved exercise tolerance, reduced need for emergency care, and improved survival. A meta-analysis of five large randomized controlled trials of ACE inhibitors for symptomatic heart failure found an overall decrease in mortality of 28% (Flather et al, 2000). The greater benefit was found in patients with lower ejection fractions, but benefit was seen in all patients treated with ACE inhibitors (Flather et al, 2000).

Their "cousins," the angiotensin II receptor blockers (ARBs), are being used for treatment of heart failure in patients who cannot tolerate an ACE inhibitor. The negative inotropic effects of beta-adrenergic blockers were thought to make heart failure worse and were avoided in the past. More recent data about their role in reducing sympathetic nervous system discharge have moved them into first-line therapy in heart failure for patients with left ventricular systolic dysfunction (Hernandez et al, 2009). The beta blockers that are indicated or approved for use in patients with reduced (less than 45%) left ventricular function are carvedilol, metoprolol succinate, and bisoprolol. The dihydropyridines amlodipine and felodipine (Plendil) are the only CCBs demonstrated to be safe in treating angina with concomitant heart failure caused by advanced left ventricular dysfunction. Non-dihydropyridine CCBs should be avoided in heart failure based on their negative inotropism. Lifestyle modifications are also central to heart failure prevention and management. Drugs and lifestyle modifications for heart failure are discussed in Chapter 36.

Hypertension

All patients with angina should have their blood pressure assessed and managed consistent with the JNC 8 guidelines to a goal of less than 150/90 mm Hg, or 140/90 mm Hg if diabetic (James et al, 2014). Lifestyle modifications are the first approach to treatment of both hypertension and angina. Emphasis is placed on control of weight; reduced intake of sodium, saturated fat, cholesterol, and alcohol; and increased physical activity for both disease processes. All drug classes used to treat angina are helpful in the treatment of hypertension. ACE inhibitors and direct renin inhibitors are useful in blood pressure control based on their vasodilating effects and their ability to reduce extracellular fluid volume. Both of these actions also assist in the treatment and prevention of angina. Beta blockers are no longer first-line therapy in hypertension. CCBs are acceptable for patients with hypertension especially African Americans. Chapter 40 discusses the use of these drugs in more detail.

Hypercholesterolemia

Because hyperlipidemia contributes to atherosclerosis and the narrowing of blood vessels that result in angina, all patients with angina should have their cholesterol checked by a lipid panel with a goal of reducing LDL from baseline levels. Though specific target values are not suggested in the ATP IV, striving for LDL levels less than 100 mg/dL for most patients and less than 70 mg/dL for those in the very-high-risk category has evidence to imply better outcomes (Boekholdt et al, 2014). Factors that favor a decision to reduce LDL-C levels to less than 70 mg/dL are those that place patients in the category of *very high risk*. Among these factors are the presence of established cardiovascular disease (CVD) plus (1) multiple major risk factors (especially diabetes); (2) severe and poorly controlled risk factors (especially continued cigarette smoking); (3) multiple risk factors of the metabolic syndrome (especially high triglycerides greater than or equal to 200 mg/dL plus non-HDL-C greater than or equal to 130 mg/dL with low HDL-C [40 mg/dL]); and (4) on the basis of PROVE IT (a research trial), patients with acute coronary syndromes (Cannon et al, 2004).

To avoid any misunderstanding about cholesterol management in general, it must be emphasized the newest guidelines do not outline specific goals for everyone, but places emphasis on treatment for those at highest risk (Stone et al, 2014). As with hypertension, lifestyle modifications are the first-line approach to treatment. The only class of antianginal drugs that negatively affects hypercholesterolemia is the beta blockers. Nonselective beta blockers can increase triglycerides and LDL cholesterol and reduce the level of HDL. New evidence has shown that cardioselective beta blockers do not have as significant an effect on serum lipids (Singh, Singh, Singh, Jain, & Singh, 2012; Wai et al, 2012). Because of the availability of cardioselective beta blockers, these should be considered for use when there are other compelling reasons for the use of a beta blocker, such as MI prophylaxis

Peripheral-Vascular Diseases

The vasoconstrictive effects of nonselective beta blockers have an adverse effect on peripheral blood flow that may limit their use for patients with concomitant peripheral-vascular disease (PVD). Although these drugs are not contraindicated, caution is advised when prescribing this drug class to patients with severe PVD. The peripheral vasodilating effects of the dihydropyridine group of CCBs have resulted in their having an off-label use in the treatment of Raynaud's disease. They are the drugs of choice for patients with concomitant PVD.

Diabetes Mellitus

Diabetic patients with angina should make every effort to optimize glycemic control with a goal of achieving a near normal A1c (Fraker & Fihn, 2007). ACE inhibitors are the drugs of choice for patients with diabetes. Not only are they recommended by all the treatment guidelines used in this chapter, but they are also recommended by JNC 8 and the American Diabetes Association (ADA) guidelines (2015). CCBs are also useful because of their lower effects on glucose metabolism. They have also been shown to have some degree of renal protection.

Beta-adrenergic blockers decrease insulin secretion and may mask the signs of hypoglycemia. The one sign of hypoglycemia that is not masked is diaphoresis, and patients with diabetes who are taking these drugs should be taught to test their blood glucose levels in the event of a diaphoretic episode. If a beta blocker must be used to treat angina for compelling reasons, blockade of these warning signs are associated with beta$_2$ blockade, and use of a beta$_1$-selective drug reduces but does not eliminate this issue. The use of beta blockers is important enough in the treatment of CAD in diabetic patients that its use in this group should not be avoided.

Elevated levels of plasma homocysteine were demonstrated to be a strong and independent risk factor for congestive heart disease events in studies of patients with type 2 diabetes or previous myocardial infarction (Agoston-Coldea, Mocan, Gatfosse, Lupu, &Dumitrascu, 2011; Soinio, Marniemi, Laasko, Lehto, & Ronnemaa, 2004). To date, research involving lowering plasma homocysteine levels through administration of vitamin B$_6$, B$_{12}$, and folic acid has not demonstrated a benefit in the prevention of cardiovascular disease.

Asthma and Chronic Airway Diseases

Beta blockers in both oral and topical ophthalmic forms may exacerbate asthma and other chronic airway diseases. Although they may exacerbate disease, they should not be avoided unless the patient has severe or uncontrolled airway disease. If they are to be used, the choice of a beta$_1$-selective oral agent and the occlusion of the nasal-lacrimal duct while administering the ophthalmic form minimize this issue. Appropriate calcium channel blockers are a good alternative for those patients with severe or uncontrolled airway disease.

Other disease processes that are affected positively or negatively by the drugs commonly used to treat angina are shown in Table 28-6.

Erectile Dysfunction

Erectile dysfunction (ED) is related to endothelial dysfunction and vascular damage, similar to hypertension and angina. Treatment of hypertension has also been associated with erectile dysfunction and may affect patient compliance with treatment of hypertension. The latest evidence, although very limited, states that beta blockers and thiazide diuretics are the drug classes most associated with erectile dysfunction (Baumhakel, Schlimmer, Kratz, Hacket, & Bohm, 2011; Manolis & Doumas, 2012). Nebivolol is the beta blocker least apt to cause ED and may even improve ED symptoms (Baumhakel et al, 2011). ACE inhibitors and ARBs have been shown to increase frequency of sexual contacts when compared with beta blockers (Baumhakel et al, 2011). No clinical trials have evaluated the effects of CCBs on erectile function.

It must be noted that phosphodiesterase-5 inhibitors (sildenafil, Viagra; vardenafil, Levitra; tadalafil, Cialis) used to treat erectile dysfunction, when taken in combination with nitrates used for chest pain, can cause severe vasodilation resulting in hypotension and syncope. In patients with CAD not taking nitrates on a regular basis, their administration in case of need should be 24 hours after the administration of sildenafil or vardenafil and 48 hours after the

administration of tadalafil. In patients taking nitrates on a daily basis, the use of phosphodiesterase-5 inhibitors is contraindicated (Chrysant & Chrysant, 2012).

Table 28–6   Drugs Commonly Used: Angina

Drug	Brand Name
ACE Inhibitors	
Captopril	Capoten
Enalapril	Vasotec
Lisinopril	Prinivil, Zestril
Ramipril	Altace
Trandolapril	Mavik
Direct Renin Inhibitors	
Aliskiren	Tekturna
Beta-Adrenergic Blockers	
Atenolol	Tenormin
Metoprolol succinate	Toprol XL
Calcium Channel Blockers	
Amlodipine	Norvasc
Diltiazem	Cardizem
Felodipine	Plendil
Nifedipine sustained release	Procardia XL
Nitrates	
Isosorbide dinitrate	Isordil
Isosorbide mononitrate	Imdur
Nitroglycerin (sublingual)	Nitrostat

ACE = angiotensin-converting enzyme; XL = extended release.

Cost

The cost of antianginal drug therapy should be considered in drug selection, especially because patients are often on multiple drugs and a significant proportion of patients who are older may be on fixed incomes. In general, generic formulations are acceptable and cheaper than brand-name drugs.

Nitrates are the cheapest of the antianginals. Among the nitrates, nitroglycerin sublingual is significantly cheaper than the translingual spray. For patients with dry mouth, however, the sublingual tablet may not dissolve completely. As a result the spray, which does not have this problem, may be more appropriate regardless of cost. The spray has a much longer shelf-life and may actually be closer in price if the patient uses the drug rarely. Isosorbide mononitrate comes in an extended-release form; isosorbide dinitrate must be taken multiple times daily. If a once-daily dosing schedule is needed, the simplified regimen using isosorbide mononitrate should be considered.

The beta blockers are in the middle in cost. An older drug, propranolol (Inderal), is relatively inexpensive, but its lipid solubility increases the adverse reactions profile, and it must be taken 2 to 4 times each day. It is a nonselective beta blocker, along with labetalol, nadolol, and timolol. Lack of selectivity results in more adverse reactions. In patients without reduced left ventricular systolic function, the drugs of choice are atenolol or metoprolol succinate. They are among the least expensive; are beta$_1$ selective; have a long half-life, enabling daily dosing; and have low lipid solubility, which results in a low adverse reaction profile.

CCBs and ACE inhibitors are the most expensive antianginals. Both classes have generic forms of some of the drugs that are less expensive. Short-acting forms are also less expensive but must be taken several times each day. Generically available, captopril is the only short-acting ACE inhibitor. Diltiazem is among the least expensive CCB; Verapamil is the least expensive, but it has limited use, and almost 100% of patients who take it develop constipation. This constipation usually requires an additional medication (stool softener) to treat the problem; therefore by the time the cost of the second drug is added in, all cost savings are lost. Amlodipine is a formulation that is also available in generic formulation. The expense needs to be weighed against its range of uses, once-daily dosing, reduced peripheral edema, decreased incidence of reflex tachycardia, and antiatherogenic properties. Aspirin brands do not appear to have significant advantages over generics. Enteric coating makes this drug more expensive, and there have been recent questions about inconsistent bioavailability with enteric coating. Therefore, use of the generic nonenteric-coated aspirin will be the most efficacious and cost-effective preparation.

MONITORING

The most important monitoring parameters are the presence, characteristics, and timing of angina episodes. Precipitating factors such as exercise, effort that involves use of the arms above the head, cold environment, walking after a meal, emotional stress, anger or anxiety, or coitus need to be reviewed. Patients should be evaluated every 4 to 6 months during the first year of therapy. After the first year, annual evaluations are recommended if the patient is stable and reliable enough to call or make an appointment when anginal symptoms become worse or other symptoms occur. The American College of Physicians (Qaseem et al, 2012) stresses the need for effective communication between providers when patients are co-managed by the primary care provider and a cardiologist.

The ACC/AHA (Anderson et al, 2007) and the American College of Physicians (Qaseem et al, 2012) recommend five questions that should be answered during the follow-up of any patient receiving treatment for chronic stable angina:

- Has the patient's level of physical activity decreased since the last visit?
- Have the patient's anginal symptoms increased in frequency or become more severe since the last visit?

If they have, has the patient decreased physical activity to avoid precipitating angina?
- How well is the patient tolerating therapy?
- How successful has the patient been in modifying risk factors and improving knowledge about ischemic heart disease?
- Has the patient developed any new comorbid illnesses or has the severity or treatment of known comorbid illnesses worsened the patient's angina?

Answers to these questions are as important as any diagnostic testing in determining whether the management plan needs alteration. Check with the patient first.

Initial laboratory studies should include an ECG and fasting lipid profile. Further tests in patients with chronic angina are based on history and physical findings and may include chest x-ray, CT angiography of the coronary arteries, or transthoracic echocardiography (Woodard et al, 2012); complete blood count (CBC); and tests for diabetes, thyroid function, and renal function (ICSI, 2011). Any further laboratory tests are largely based on the need to monitor concomitant disease states.

For ACC/AHA class III, low-risk angina patients, additional initial diagnostic tests may involve exercise treadmill testing and exercise echocardiography. After laboratory data and other monitoring parameters specific to the drugs they are taking have been taken and assessed, an annual 12-lead ECG, CBC, and blood chemistry tests are suggested. For ACC/AHA class I or II or high-risk angina patients, monitoring parameters should be determined in collaboration with a cardiology specialist. There is no clear evidence that routine, periodic testing of any sort is useful without a change in history or physical examination (Qaseem et al, 2012). The ACC/AHA (Anderson et al, 2007) consensus is that specific diagnostic tests, including chest x-ray, echocardiography, and stress testing, be done when specific changes occur in anginal symptoms, cardiac rhythms, congestive heart failure, or valvular heart disease. All of these tests require referral to a cardiologist, so it seems prudent that any significant changes in the areas mentioned trigger a consultation with a cardiologist to see if this testing is needed.

OUTCOME EVALUATION

Figure 28-2 shows the drug treatment protocol for angina management. Evaluation for angina control occurs throughout the protocol. The main indication for substitution of a drug from a different class or the addition of more drugs is inadequate control of angina or failure to reduce the grade or class to a lower grade or class of angina.

There are situations in which to worry about treating an angina patient and times when referral to a specialist is appropriate:

1. When chronic stable angina becomes unstable— Unstable angina means that it is new or accelerating or has become unpredictable in its characteristics or

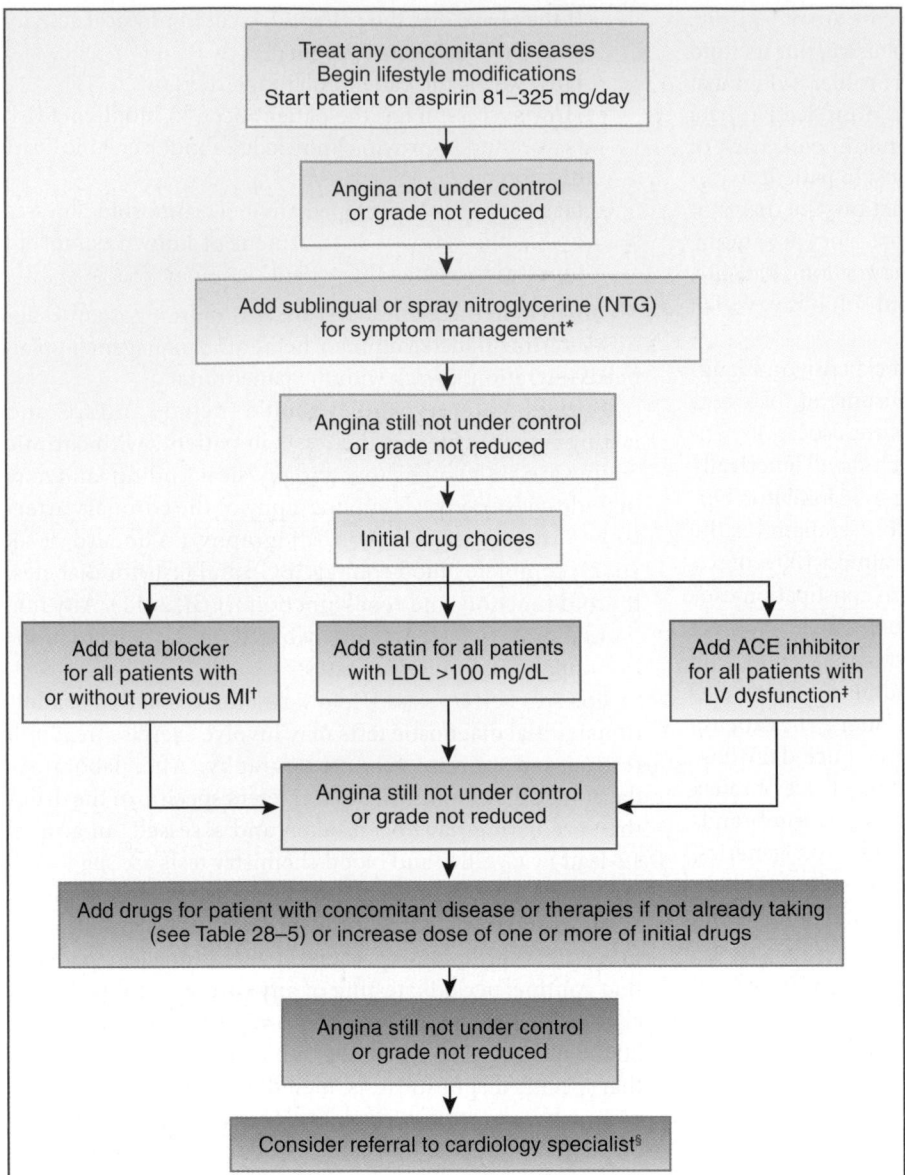

Figure 28–2. Drug treatment protocol for chronic stable angina and low-risk unstable angina.

* If patient nitrate intolerant, may use calcium channel blocker for symptom relief.

† If beta blocker contraindicated or has unacceptable side effects, may use calcium channel blocker or long-acting nitrate.

‡ ACC/AHA recommends ACE inhibitors for diabetics and patients with LV dysfunction; American College of Physicians recommends for all with no restrictions.

§ ACC/AHA class I patients may require initial referral to cardiology specialist; consultation should occur whenever needed in planning care for all classes.

precipitating factors. It is important to rule out the possibility that it is still stable angina but that changes in lifestyle or the onset of a concomitant illness is causing changes in the anginal symptoms. However, the time taken to rule this out should be very short, especially if ECG changes are noted. In general, patients with new-onset unstable angina should be referred to a specialist for urgent work-up.

2. When the patient has "ominous" findings on an exercise tolerance test—These tests are usually administered by

a specialist, who would probably be the first to notice the findings.

3. When a post-MI patient develops new-onset angina, especially with ECG changes—The more recent the MI, the higher the risk is. Urgent referral is required.

4. When an MI is suspected, based on anginal and other symptoms—Obtain an ECG, draw appropriate laboratory studies, and obtain a consultation with a physician.

5. When standard therapy is not successful in improving exercise tolerance and reducing the incidence of

PATIENT EDUCATION: ANGINA

PATIENT EDUCATION

Related to the Overall Treatment Plan/Disease Process

☐ Pathophysiology of angina and its prognosis

☐ Role of lifestyle modifications in improving prognosis and keeping down the number and cost of required drugs

☐ Importance of adherence to the treatment regimen

☐ Indications of complications that need to be reported and the need for regular follow-up visits with the primary care provider

Specific to the Drug Therapy

☐ Reason for taking the drug(s) and the anticipated action of the drug(s) on the disease process

☐ Doses and schedules for taking the drugs

☐ Possible adverse reactions and what to do when they occur

☐ Interactions between lifestyle modification and these drugs

Reasons for Taking the Drug(s)

Specific information related to angina includes reasons for the drugs being given. Antianginal drugs are given to reduce cardiovascular morbidity (especially MI) and mortality. Some drugs do both of these things; most do either one or the other. The expectation should be clear about what these drugs can and cannot do. Stable angina is a chronic condition that requires lifelong treatment, and so the regimen should be incorporated into the daily life of the patient. Even well-managed angina can become unstable and may require urgent management. Knowledge of when and how to use sublingual or translingual nitroglycerin is important.

Drugs as Part of the Total Treatment Regimen

Angina therapy is based on lifestyle modification. These modifications are not always easy to maintain, but they are equally as important as drugs in successful control of symptoms and prevention of complications. Among the lifestyle modifications is sodium restriction to reduce extracellular fluid volume, decrease afterload, and reduce MOD. Care should be taken not to reduce salt and fluid too quickly, which may result in fluid volume deficit, leading to hypotension and a reduction in MOS. Patients should be taught signs and symptoms of fluid volume deficit to report. None of the antianginal drugs directly reduces fluid volume, but all except aspirin have vasodilating actions that may make fluid volume deficit worse. Sodium reduction may also lead some patients to seek salt substitutes that have potassium as part of their contents. Changes in potassium levels can significantly affect myocardial functioning, so these substitutes should be used sparingly. Use of nonsalt herbal seasoning is encouraged.

Another central lifestyle modification is regular aerobic exercise, such as walking or cycling. The amount and type of exercise must be carefully monitored and targeted to anginal symptoms. Patients can be referred to a cardiac rehabilitation program at the start of their exercise program so that their response can be monitored. Later, they can monitor their own response and determine the pace and amount of exercise that works for them. The key is gradually increasing regular aerobic exercise. Several of the antianginal drugs, especially the nitrates, have the potential to cause orthostatic hypotension. Exercise should be timed to avoid this adverse reaction, and adequate fluids should be taken while exercising.

angina symptoms, when a secondary cause of the angina that may require surgical intervention is suspected, or when the patient has complex concomitant disease processes—Consultation is appropriate. This may result in a referral, but it is generally not urgent.

PATIENT EDUCATION

Patient education should include a discussion of information related to the overall treatment plan as well as that specific to the drug therapy, reasons for taking the drug, drugs as part of the total treatment regimen, and adherence issues.

REFERENCES

Agoston-Coldea, L., Mocan, T., Gatfosse, M., Lupu, S., & Dumitrascu, D. (2011). Plasma homocysteine and the severity of heart failure in patients with previous myocardial infarction. *Cardiology Journal, 18*(1), 55–62.

American Diabetes Association (ADA). (2015). Standards of medical care in diabetes-2015: Summary of revisions. *Diabetes Care, 38 (Suppl: 1),* S4.

Anderson, J., Adams, C. Antman, E., Bridges, C., Califf, R., Casey, D., Jr., et al, the American College of Cardiology/American Heart Association Task Force on Practice Guidelines (ACC/AHA). (2007). ACC/AHA 2007 guidelines for the management of patient with unstable angina/non-ST-elevation myocardial infarction. *Journal of the American College of Cardiology, 50*(7), e1–e157.

Antithrombotic Trialists' Collaboration. (2009). Aspirin in the primary and secondary prevention of vascular disease: Collaborative meta-analysis of individual participant data from randomized trials. *The Lancet, 373,* 1849–1860.

Baumhakel, M., Schlimmer, N., Kratz, M., Hacket, G., & Bohm, M. (2011). Cardiovascular risk, drugs and erectile function—A systematic analysis. *International Journal of Clinical Practice, 65*(3), 289–298.

Boekholdt, S., Hovingh, G., Mora, S., Arsenault, B., Amerenco, P., Pedersen, T., et al. (2014). Very low levels of atherogenic lipoproteins and the risk for cardiovascular events: A meta-analysis of statin trials. *Journal of the American College of Cardiology, 64*(5), 485–494.

Cannon, C., Brunwald, E., McCabe, C., Rader, D., Rouleau, J., Belder, R., et al. (2004). Intensive versus moderate lipid lowering with statins after acute coronary syndromes. *New England Journal of Medicine, 350*(15), 1495–1504.

Canto, J., Rogers, W., Goldberg, R., Peterson, E., Wenger, N., Vaccarino, V., et al. (2012). Association of age and sex with myocardial infarction symptom presentation and in-hospital mortality. *Journal of the American Medical Association, 307*(8), 813–822.

Chen, J., Shi, C., Mahoney, E., Dunn, E., Rinfret, S., Caro, J., et al. (2011). Economic evaluation of clopidogrel plus aspirin for secondary prevention of cardiovascular events in Canada for patients with established cardiovascular disease: Results from the CHARISMA trial. *Canadian Journal of Cardiology, 27*, 222–231.

Chrysant, S., & Chrysant, G. (2012). The pleiotropic effects of phosphodiesterase 5 inhibitors on function and safety in patients with cardiovascular disease and hypertension. *The Journal of Clinical Hypertension, 14*(9), 644–649.

Conti, C., Berry, A., & Petersen, J. (2012). Silent ischemia: Clinical relevance. *Journal of the American College of Cardiology, 59*(5), 435–441.

Dweck, M., Campbell, I., Miller, D., & Francis, C. (2009). Clinical aspects of silent myocardial ischaemia: With particular reference to diabetes mellitus. *British Journal of Diabetes & Vascular Disease, 9*(3), 110–116.

Flather, M., Yusef, S., Kober, L., Pfeffer, M., Hall, A., Murray, G., et al. (2000). Long-term ACE-inhibitor therapy in patients with heart failure or left-ventricular dysfunction: A systematic overview of data from individual patients. *The Lancet, 355*(9215), 1575–1581.

Fraker, T., & Fihn, S. (2007). 2007 chronic angina focused update of the ACC/AHA 2002 guidelines for the management of patients with chronic stable angina: A report of the American College of Cardiology/American Heart Association task force on practice guidelines writing group to develop the focused update of the 2002 guidelines for the management of patients with chronic stable angina. *Circulation, 116*, 2762–2772.

Gulati, M., Cooper-DeHoff, R., McClure, C., Johnson, D., Shaw, L., Handberg, E., et al. (2009). Adverse cardiovascular outcomes in women with nonobstructive coronary artery disease: A report from the Women's Ischemia Syndrome Evaluation Study and the St. James Women Take Heart Project. *Archives of Internal Medicine, 169*(9), 843–850.

Harman, S., Vittinghoff, E., Brinton, E., Budoff, M., Cedars, M., Lobo, R., et al. (2011). Timing and duration of menopausal hormone treatment may affect cardiovascular outcomes. *The American Journal of Medicine, 124*(3), 199–205.

Hernandez, A., Hammill, B., O'Connor, C., Schulman, K., Curtis, L., & Fonarow, G. (2009). Clinical effectiveness of beta-blockers in heart failure: Findings from the OPTIMIZE-HF (organized program to initiate life-saving treatment in hospitalized patients with heart failure) registry. *Journal of the American College of Cardiology, 53*(2), 184–192.

Ikeda, H., Minamikawa, J., Nakamura, Y., Hamamoto, Y., Wada, Y., et al. (2009). Comparison of effects of amlodipine and angiotensin receptor blockers on the intima-media thickness of carotid arterial wall (AAA study: amblodipine vs ARB in atherosclerosis study). *Diabetes Research and Clinical Practice, 83*(1), 50–53.

Institute for Clinical Symptoms Improvement (ICSI). (2011, April). *Stable coronary artery disease* (14th ed., 58 pp.). Bloomington, MN: Institute for Clinical Symptoms Improvement (ICSI). Retrieved November 16, 2012, from http://www.icsi.org/coronary_artery_disease/coronary_artery_disease__stable_.html

James, P., Oparil, S., Carver, B., Cushman, W., Dennison-Himmelfarb, C., Handler, J., et al. (2014). Evidence-based guideline for the management of high blood pressure in adults: Report from the panel members appointed to the Eight Joint National Committee (JNC 8). *Journal of the American Medical Association, 311*(5), 507–520.

Kaiser Permanente Care Management Institute. (2008). *Coronary artery disease (CAD) clinical practice guidelines* (9 pp.). Oakland, CA: Kaiser Permanente Care Management Institute. Retrieved November 16, 2012, from http://f.i-md.com/medinfo/material/52b/4eb0fa3887f2a38683db452b/4eb0fa5287f2a38683db452e.pdf

Manolis, A., & Doumas, M. (2012). Antihypertensive treatment and sexual dysfunction. *Current Hypertensive Reports , 14*, 285–292.

Martin-Ventura, J., Munoz-Garcia, B., Blanco-Colio, L., Martin-Conejero, A., Madrigal-Matute, J., Vega, M., et al. (2008). Treatment with amlodipine and atorvastatin has additive effect on blood and plaque inflammation in hypertensive patients with carotid atherosclerosis. *Kidney International, 111*, S71–S74.

McCance, K., & Huether, S. (2014) *Pathophysiology: The biological basis for disease in adults and children* (7th ed.). St. Louis, MO: Mosby.

Mente, A., deKoning, L., Shannon, H., & Anand, S. (2009). A systematic review of the evidence supporting a causal link between dietary factors and coronary heart disease. *Archives of Internal Medicine, 169*(7), 659–669.

Miller, A., & Oparil, S. (2003). Secondary prevention of coronary heart disease in women: A call to action. *Annals of Internal Medicine, 138*(2), 150–151.

Mosca, L., Benjamin, E., Berra, K., Bezanson, J., Dolor, R., Lloyd-Jones, D., et al. (2011). Effectiveness-based guidelines for the prevention of cardiovascular disease in women—2011 update. A guideline from the American Heart Association. *Circulation, 123*, 1243–1262.

Qaseem, A., Fihn, S., Dallas, P., Williams, S., Owens, D., & Shekelle, P. (2012). Management of stable ischemic heart disease: Summary of a clinical practice guideline from the American College of Physicians/American College of Cardiology Foundation/American Heart Association/American Association for Thoracic Surgery/Preventive Cardiovascular Nurses Association/Society of Throacic Surgeons. *Annals of Internal Medicine, 157*(10), 735–743.

Scottish Intercollegiate Guidelines Network (SIGN). (2007). *Management of stable angina: A national clinical guideline*. Scottish Intercollegiate Guidelines Network (SIGN) Pub. No. 96.

Singh, R., Singh, S., Singh, S., Jain, I., & Singh, S. (2012). Study of alteration in serum lipids by cardiooselective beta blockers in albino rabbits. *Asian Journal of Pharmacy and Life Science, 2*(2), 166–173.

Soinio, M., Marniemi, J., Laasko, M., Lehto, S., & Ronnemaa, T. (2004). Elevated plasma homocysteine level is an independent predictor of coronary heart disease events in patients with type 2 diabetes mellitus. *Annals of Internal Medicine, 140*(2), 94–100.

Stone, N., Robinson, J., Lichtenstein, A, Merz, C., Blum, C., Eckel, R., et al. (2014). ACC/AHA guideline on the treatment of blood cholesterol to reduce atherosclerotic cardiovascular risk in adults. A report of the American College of Cardiology/American Heart Association Task Force on Practice Guidelines. *Journal of the American College of Cardiology. 63*(25 PA), 2889–2934.

Vandvik, P., Lincoff, A., Gore, J., Gutterman, D., Sonnenberg, F., Alonso-Coello, P., et al. (2012). Primary and secondary prevention of cardiovascular disease. *Chest, 141*(2 Suppl.).

Veterans Health Administration, Department of Defense (VA/DoD). (2003). *VA/DoD clinical practice guidelines for the management of ischemic heart disease*. Washington, DC: Veterans Health Administration, Department of Defense.

Vittinghoff, E., Shiplak, M., Varosy, P., Furberg, C., Ireland, C., Khan, S., et al. (2003). Risk factors and secondary prevention in women with heart disease: The Heart and Estrogen/Progestin Replacement Study. *Annals of Internal Medicine, 138*(2), 81–89.

Wai, B., Kearney, L., Hare, D., Ord, M., Burrell, L., & Srivastava, P. (2012). Beta blocker use in subjects with type 2 diabetes mellitus and systolic heart failure does not worsen glycaemic control. *Cardiovascular Diabetology, 11*(14) doi: 10.1186/1475-2840-11-14

Woodard, P., White, R., Abbara, S., Araoz, P., Cury, R., Dorbala., S., et al. (2012). *ACR Appropriateness Criteria chronic chest pain—low to intermediate probability of coronary artery disease* (5 pp.). Reston, VA: American College of Radiology (ACR). Retrieved November 29, 2012, from http://www.acr.org/~/media/ACR/Documents/AppCriteria/Diagnostic/ChronicChestPainLowIntermediateProbabilityCoronaryArteryDisease.pdf

CHAPTER 29

ANXIETY AND DEPRESSION

Mary Weber • Krista Estes

According to the World Health Organization (WHO), major depressive disorder (MDD) is considered one of the top reasons for disability in the United States (WHO, 2012). Worldwide, it affects 350 million people across the life span, more women than men (Bromet et al, 2011; WHO, 2012). Depression, like many other chronic illnesses, can go undetected for many years, often leading to increased morbidity from other physical illnesses, substance use, and increased suicide rates (Rihmer & Angst, 2009). The most serious complication of MDD, a completed suicide, is often preventable. Suicide is a growing problem in the United States over the last few years, becoming more frequent than homicides, and in 2009 it was the 10th leading cause of death in those over age 10 (Centers for Disease Control and Prevention [CDC], 2009; Rihmer & Angst, 2009; U.S. Surgeon General, 2012).

Anxiety is a much more common and yet a misunderstood symptom. Approximately 18% of the U.S. population of adults in a given year will have an anxiety disorder (Kessler, Chiu, Demler, Merikangas, & Walters, 2005), and more women than men report having any type of anxiety disorder (McLean, Asnaani, Litz, & Hofmann, 2011). Disorders related to anxiety symptoms have changed over the years in the *Diagnostic and Statistical Manual (DSM)* and continue to evolve and change as more is learned about the neurobiology behind fear, panic, and worry. In 2013, the *DSM-V* (American Psychiatric Association [APA], 2013), differentiates between panic disorder (PD), generalized anxiety disorder (GAD) or "worry" disorder, obsessive and compulsive disorder (OCD), and post-traumatic stress disorder (PTSD). Each has a distinct set of symptoms, neurobiology, and some important differences in treatment. Anxiety disorders share similar comorbidities with multiple chronic physical illnesses as well as depression, substance use, and increased suicide (Sadock & Sadock, 2010; Stahl, 2013).

Primary care providers (PCPs) are often the health-care providers to identify both depression and anxiety disorders and are instrumental in screening, early identification, assessment, treatment, and referral. This chapter will discuss the screening and identification of these disorders, current medications used to treat anxiety disorders and depression, the neurobiology that continues to evolve, evidence-based treatment strategies, and reasons for referral. For the purpose of this chapter, any clinician who provides individual, group, or family therapy will be referred to as a "mental health provider" and a psychiatric mental health nurse practitioner (PMHNP) or psychiatrist who prescribes psychiatric medication will be referred to as a "psychiatric provider."

ASSESSMENT AND SCREENING

According to the latest *DSM-V* (APA, 2013), definitions, the symptoms of what is called a major depressive episode must include at least a 2 week period of either a depressed mood or anhedonia (loss of pleasure in previously enjoyed people, places, and things). In addition to one or both of those symptoms, at least four of the following symptoms must be present: significant changes in weight not due to physical causes or self-restricting; sleep patterns that are different from baseline; fatigue or loss of energy that is new and not due to a medical condition; feelings of worthlessness or excessive or inappropriate guilt that occur nearly every day; as well as recurrent thoughts of death, wishing for death, up to and including plans to kill oneself (APA, 2013). As with all psychiatric disorders, medical disorders must always be ruled out first.

Assessment and screening for depressive disorders must include a work-up that excludes disorders such as hypothyroidism, anemia, kidney or renal impairment, cancers, or cardiac illnesses such as congestive heart failure. Additionally, other chronic illnesses such as HIV and hepatitis must also be ruled out because they can also cause some of the neurovegetative symptoms such as fatigue and weight loss (Sadock & Sadock, 2010). Careful assessment and screening will assist providers in early identification of a depressive disorder.

One of the most important screening tools is the Mood Disorder Questionnaire (MDQ), which can help the PCP rule in or out a depressive disorder or a bipolar disorder (APA, 2013; Hirschfield et al, 2000; Sadock & Sadock, 2010). The MDQ helps the provider differentiate whether an individual has had prior hypomania or mania episodes, which may be indicative of a bipolar disorder and would lead to a very different treatment strategy. For the individual with a positive bipolar screen, a referral to a psychiatric provider would be indicated. The Patient Health Questionnaire (PHQ-9) and the Center for Epidemiological Studies Depression Scale (CESDS) have also been used in primary care for depression screening (Kerr & Kerr, 2001). Both screening tools are not diagnostic of depression but can help as a waiting-room tool

prior to a visit to help screen for mood disorders. An evaluation, in addition to screening tools, has the best evidence to support the detection of depressive disorders given cultural and somatic issues that can make a screening tool difficult to interpret (Kerr & Kerr, 2001).

There are a number of diagnostic tools that have both reliability and validity in the diagnosis of depression as well as a way to measure outcomes of care. Some of these tools are available on the Web, and others are copyrighted and require permission to use in clinical practice. There is the Beck Depression Inventory (Beck, Ward, Mendelson, Mock, & Erbaugh, 1961) that has been translated into several languages, the self-administered Montgomery-Asberg Depression Rating Scale (MDRS-S) (Montgomery & Asberg, 1979), and The Inventory of Depressive Symptomatology (IDS): Clinician (IDS-C) and Self-Report (IDS-SR) ratings of depressive symptoms (Rush, Carmody, & Reimitz, 2006). Each of these can be used as tools by the patient and the clinician to help diagnose and then monitor progress of treatment. It is recommended that some type of consistent tool be used to evaluate the outcomes of care (Kurian, Grannemann, & Trivedi, 2012; Trivedi, et al., 2006; Zimmerman, Martinez, Friedman, Boerescu, Attiullah, & Toba, 2012).

Assessment of anxiety symptoms starts with differentiation of fear, worry, and panic. All of these feelings are "hardwired" in humans as part of the fight-flight response to danger (Stahl, 2013). However, when these symptoms cause distress leading to impairment at work, school, relationships, and general functioning, the provider must consider whether there is one or more anxiety disorders present, as they are comorbid with each other.

The first and most difficult differential diagnosis is panic disorder. A panic attack is described as a sudden, recurrent, and unexpected set of feelings and intense discomfort, both physical and psychological, that include palpitations, sweating, tremors, chest pain, shortness of breath, numbness and tingling, dizziness, light-headedness, and a fear of losing control or dying (APA, 2013). There are a number of physical causes of each of these symptoms that must be ruled out before a diagnosis of panic disorder is made. Common differential diagnoses for panic include hyperthyroidism, heart failure, cardiac arrhythmias, kidney or liver damage, anemia, a myocardial infarct, cerebral vascular accident or injury, disc disease, pulmonary embolism, and substance use disorders including alcohol withdrawal, amphetamine use, and other recreational drug use. There is a Hamilton Rating scale for Anxiety (Hamilton, 1959) that can help with identifying symptoms, as well as improvement, but it does not help differentiate whether the symptoms are physically based.

Another very common anxiety disorder is generalized anxiety disorder (GAD). This disorder is seen commonly in primary care and often overlooked and undertreated (Kessler et al, 2005; Parmentier, Garcia-Campayo, & Prieto, 2013). Symptoms of GAD include excessive worry that occurs more days than not, that is difficult to control, and that is associated with restlessness, difficulty concentrating, fatigue, irritability, and sleep disturbances (APA, 2013). As in panic, differentiating physical causes of these symptoms, including hypoglycemia, hyperglycemia, asthma, COPD, and sleep apnea, is important before a GAD diagnosis is given.

Obsessive-compulsive disorder (OCD) is often not identified in primary care because of the shame and secrecy around some of the compulsive behaviors. The Yale-Brown Obsessive-Compulsive Scale (YBOCS) has been a good screening, assessment, and measurement tool (Goodman et al, 1989) that can be used in primary care. Because of the complexity of treatment of OCD, it is recommended that the PCP refer these patients to a psychiatric provider for treatment.

Because of the variety of responses to distress following exposure to different levels of catastrophic events, the concept of PTSD has been reclassified as a number of disorders under Trauma and Stressor-related disorders (APA, 2013). As of 2013, the criterion for PTSD has now been expanded to include children and adolescents. There are criteria for children under 6 to include direct experience or witnessing or learning about traumatic events (APA, 2013). Other criteria continue to include recurrent, involuntary, and intrusive memories and nightmares, intense distress, and physiological reactions to triggers or cues of the stressor to make the diagnosis of PTSD (APA, 2013). Like many anxiety disorders, PTSD is often unrecognized in primary care. The post-traumatic stress disorder checklist (PCL) and the civilian version are used in both veteran populations and other adult populations to screen for the residual effects of a traumatic event but must be followed up with a full evaluation to determine if the disorder is present (McDonald & Calhoun, 2010).

There is a screening tool that has a child and parent report version to assess for potential traumatic events called the Traumatic Events Screening Inventory (TESI) (Ippen et al, 2002; Ribbe, 1996). The TESI and a revised parent version have been made more developmentally sensitive to young children (Ippen et al, 2002). This TESI tools allow the PCP to screen for events such as domestic violence, physical abuse, physical injuries, and hospitalizations. With the new *DSM-V* criteria, there will most likely be revised screening tools developed in the next few years.

One of the key screening and assessments necessary for those with either a mood and/or anxiety disorder is to assess for the presence of suicidality and level or severity of risk. According to the CDC (2010), suicide is the third leading cause of death among those aged 15 to 24 years, the second among those between 25 and 34, and the fourth leading cause of death for those aged 35 to 54. Assessment for the presence and risk of suicide is imperative in the early diagnosis of an anxiety or mood disorder as well as during treatment. The Substance Abuse and Mental Health Services Administration (SAMSA, 2009) has developed a five-step suicide assessment, evaluation, and triage method (see Table 29-1). The assessment includes identifying both risk and protective factors. Risk factors include prior suicide attempts, the presence of past psychiatric disorders including substance use disorders, family history of suicide attempts, significant stressors, and

Table 29–1 SAFE-T Assessment of Suicide Risk

Suicide Assessment Five-Step Evaluation and Triage	
Identify Risk Factors	What can be modified to reduce risk?
Identify Protective Factors	What factors can be enhanced?
Conduct Suicide Inquiry	Ask about suicidal thoughts, plans, behavior, and intent
Determine Risk/Level of Intervention	Determine risk. Choose appropriate intervention to address and reduce risk
Document	Assessment of risk, rationale, intervention, and follow-up

U.S. DEPARTMENT OF HEALTH AND HUMAN SERVICES Substance Abuse and Mental (IHHS SAMSA); HHS publication number 09-4432, 2009.

access to firearms (SAMSA, 2009). Protective factors against suicide include having strong and positive relationships, feeling responsible for children or pets, strong social supports, religious beliefs, and a good ability to cope with stress (SAMSA, 2009). Assessment of risk also includes whether the individual has thoughts of death with no plan or intent, has thoughts of suicide with a plan but no intent, or has current suicidal thinking with a strong plan to die (SAMSA, 2009). All of these risk levels are important and need referral to a psychiatric provider immediately because even low-risk poses a significant risk for a completed suicide. Finally, it is essential to establish the appropriate level of care needed now, whether immediate hospitalization or referral with careful monitoring and a suicide-prevention plan in place. Specifics of a suicide prevention plan are discussed later in this chapter.

Assessment and screening for mood and anxiety disorders as well as risk factors for suicidal intent and behavior is just the beginning of treatment decisions. Anxiety disorders and depressive disorders have some distinct and overlapping neurobiology and often drive decisions about treatment. The next section will discuss the neurobiology of these disorders and how understanding these concepts will help the practitioner make good pharmacological decisions.

NEUROBIOLOGY

The neurobiology of depression has been evolving and changing over the last decade. In the classic monoamine theory of depression, the emphasis was on a deficiency of norepinephrine (NE), serotonin (5HT), and dopamine (DA). Although this theory corresponds to the use of the current antidepressants, there is little data to support it and some research results give conflicting evidence (Stahl, 2013). This theory has been supplemented with a more complicated view that involves how the neurotransmitter system regulates information processing in key areas of the brain that correspond to the symptoms of depression (Stahl, 2013).

Another theory about the cause of core symptoms of depression involves complex dysregulation of brain circuits in different parts of the brain. For example, the symptom of depressed mood is linked to problems in processing in the areas of the amygdala and the prefrontal cortex. Sleep and appetite are linked to dysfunction in the hypothalamus; fatigue is linked to NE and DA dysregulation in the prefrontal cortex and nucleus accumbens. Guilt, suicidality, and worthlessness theoretically are linked to dysregulation in the prefrontal cortex and the amygdala (Stahl, 2013).

There continues to be a significant amount of genetic research effort aimed at discovering why certain individuals develop depression and others never develop the illness. Although there is no specific gene or mutation identified, the information gathered suggests there are candidate genes that confer risk for depression that coupled with environmental stressors may contribute to the development of MDD (Stahl, 2013). There is also interest in both brain-derived neurotropic factors (BDNF) and vascular endothelial growth factor (VEGF) in the development of depression. Kotan, Sarandöl, Kırhan, Özkaya, and Kırlı (2012) described limited findings suggesting that BDNF levels might be associated with the recurrence of depression and that VEGF levels might be a determinant of the severity of depression. Although there are no medications to date that target these levels, research is pursuing leads in this area for newer medications.

The neurobiology of each of the anxiety disorders is more complex than traditionally described. Worry is a core symptom across most of the anxiety disorders. Worry and obsession have been linked to dysfunction of the cortico-striatal-thalamo-cortical (CSTC) loops in the brain. Specific dysfunction of these loops may be what differentiates worry from panic and then from obsession (Stahl, 2013). In GAD, dysfunction of the circuits and the amygdala that are persistent may be the cause of persistent worry, whereas a repetitive loop may be involved in OCD (Stahl).

The neurobiology of PTSD is more complicated in that the dysfunction of the amygdala in interpretation of traumatic events and the hippocampus in the memory and re-experiencing of these events is also involved. Finally, malfunctioning of neurotransmitters that include the monoamines as well as gamma-aminobutyric acid (GABA), glutamate, and other complex circuits are involved in panic and phobias (Stahl, 2013). Neurotransmitters such as GABA, glutamate, NE, and 5HT have all been associated with the CSTC loops as well as information processing in the amygdala in all of the anxiety disorders. In this way, the neurobiology leads to more understanding of why certain medications that involve increasing GABA and 5HT have been helpful in the treatment of anxiety disorders.

EVIDENCE-BASED TREATMENTS OF MAJOR DEPRESSIVE DISORDER AND ANXIETY DISORDERS

Effectiveness trials of the use of antidepressants were conducted over several years, using individuals from primary care, university settings, and public mental health settings with MDD, including subjects with multiple comorbidities, to better reflect actual practice. The National Institute of Mental Health (NIMH) study was called the Sequenced Treatment Alternatives to Relieve Depression (STAR*D) study (Fava et al, 2006; Neirenberg et al, 2006; Trivedi et al, 2006). This was the first effectiveness research study to test the efficacy of one antidepressant and to answer the question of "What next?" This was also one of the first large randomized controlled studies in the treatment of MDD that looked at remission and not just response.

In the STAR*D trial, it was noted that it took up to 14 weeks of citalopram to reach a remission rate between 25% to 35% (Trivedi et al, 2006). The subject not remitted was then given the option of augmenting with a medication such as bupropion or switching to the same class of selective serotonin reuptake inhibitors (SSRI) or another class of antidepressant. After this second trial of the nonremitters, remission rates varied from 29% to 39% with no statistically significant difference between whether the approach was augmentation or switching within or between classes (Trivedi et al, 2006). There were a number of important findings from this large NIMH study: the goal of treatment of MDD is remission; titrate to optimal doses to reach remission; achieving remission may take up to 14 weeks; and the fact that the patients' treatment was augmented or switched on the first failure of an antidepressant doesn't matter—there is still a chance to remit with another trial of medication (Trivedi et al, 2006).

There are also a number of algorithms, such as the Texas Implementation of Medication Algorithms (2008), for the treatment of MDD and clinical guidelines from the American Psychiatric Association (2010) that support the results of the STAR*D study. Figure 29-1 is a general algorithm on the treatment of depression using the latest evidence-based research. The major emphasis from this large effectiveness study as well as guidelines and algorithms is to treat to remission and use other options as available. Patients who experienced symptom remission have an improved long-term prognosis over patients with a partial response (Rush,Trivedi et al, 2006; Sadock & Sadock, 2010; Suehs et al, 2008).

Unfortunately, there are no large effectiveness studies looking at anxiety in general. However, there are many randomized controlled trials and review articles that support the use of antidepressants as the first-line treatment of GAD (Reinhold, Mandos, Rickels, & Lohoff, 2011). In a large systematic review (SR) studying the effectiveness of antidepressants in panic disorder (PD), it was found that the following antidepressants were significantly effective in the treatment of PD: citalopram, sertraline, paroxetine, fluoxetine, and venlafaxine (Andrisano, Chiesa, & Serretti, 2013). There are also practice guidelines from the APA on the treatment of specific anxiety disorders (http://www.psych.org/practice/clinical-practice-guidelines). Figure 29-2 is an evidenced-based algorithm on the general approach to the treatment of anxiety disorders.

In a meta-analysis and SR, Stein, Ipser, and Seedat (2006) reported that SSRIs are often the first-line treatment for

General Algorithim for the Treatment of Depression Based on STAR*D Effectiveness Research

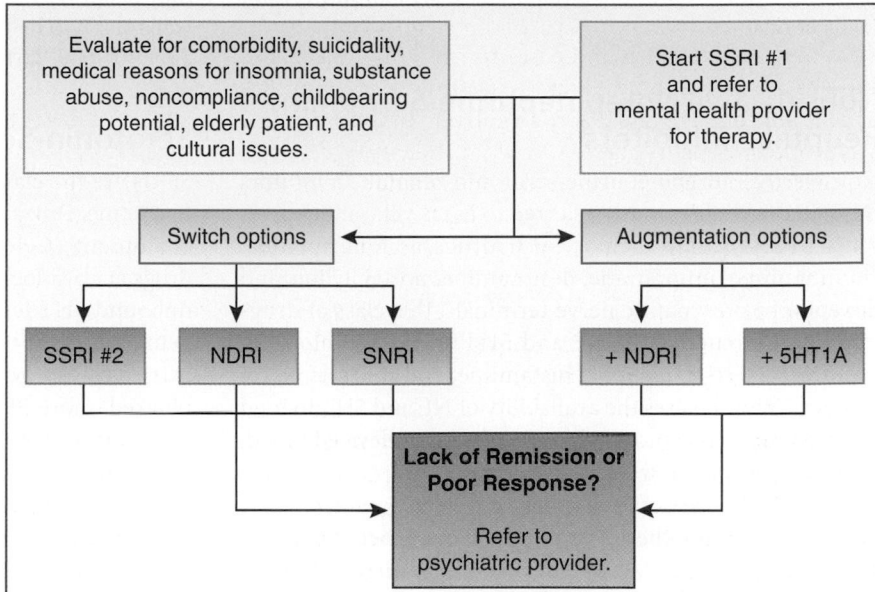

Figure 29–1. General algorithm for the treatment of depression based on the STAR*D effectiveness research.

General Algorithim for the Treatment of Adults With Anxiety Disorders

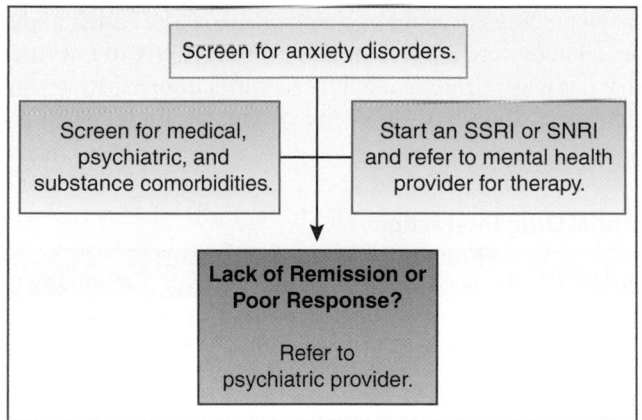

Figure 29–2. General algorithm for the treatment of anxiety disorders.

PTSD, but there are significant gaps in evidence about this disorder. The Department of Defense (2010) reviewed the literature on SSRIs and alternative medications such as atypical antipsychotics in the management of this complicated illness. There are mixed results for all classes of medications with more of a symptom-based treatment approach for PTSD (http://www.healthquality.va.gov/Post_Traumatic_Stress_Disorder_PTSD.asp). For primary care, screening for these individuals and referral to a psychiatric provider is the most prudent given the significant comorbidities associated with PTSD (Sadock & Sadock, 2010).

There has been significant evidence mounting over the years for the role of exercise in many mental illnesses

(Weber, 2010). In a Cochrane SR of exercise and depression, exercise was found to be helpful in the reduction of depressive symptoms (Rimer et al, 2012). Although no SR of exercise in anxiety disorders has been published, there are a growing number of studies supporting the use of exercise as adjunctive treatment in anxiety disorders (Asmundson et al, 2013). In smaller studies, exercise has shown reduction in symptoms in GAD and panic disorder (Herring, Jacob, Suveg, Dishman, & O'Connor, 2012; Merom et al, 2008), OCD (Abrantes et al, 2012), and PTSD (Newman & Motta, 2007).

Cognitive behavior therapy as well as other types of therapies specific to disorders, such as exposure therapy, eye movement desensitization, and reprocessing (EMDR), and short-term psychodynamic psychotherapy have been found to be efficacious alone and as adjunct treatment in depression (Driessen et al, 2009), and anxiety disorders (Fjorback, Arendt, Ørnbølel, Fink, & Walach, 2011; Sadock & Sadock, 2010). Discussion of these techniques is beyond the scope of this chapter, but it is important for the primary care provider to refer individuals with anxiety and depressive disorders to mental health providers who can augment the pharmacological therapy with these interventions.

CLASSES OF MEDICATIONS

Classes of drugs used for anxiety and depression treatment include: nonselective norepinephrine-serotonin reuptake inhibitors (tricyclic and heterocyclic), serotonin-selective reuptake inhibitors (SSRIs), serotonin-norepinephrine reuptake inhibitors (SNRIs), norepinephrine-dopamine reuptake inhibitors (NDRIs), serotonin-agonist reuptake inhibitors (SARIs), norepinephrine-serotonin specific agonists (NaSSAs),

MAO inhibitors (MAOIs), and benzodiazepines (BZDs). Each class acts on neurotransmitters in a different way. The following is a review of the different classes of antidepressant medications.

Nonselective Norepinephrine-Serotonin Reuptake Inhibitors

Nonselective norepinephrine-serotonin reuptake inhibitors (NNSRIs) were previously referred to as tricyclic antidepressants (TCAs); they include such drugs as amitriptyline, clomipramine, imipramine, desipramine, nortriptyline, and doxepin. In presynaptic nerve terminals, this class of drugs inhibits the reuptake of NE and 5HT while also blocking serotonergic, α–adrenergic, histaminic, and muscarinic receptors. This increases the availability of NE and 5HT to bind to postsynaptic receptors, which results in an elevated mood, improved sleep, and weight gain (Stahl, 2011).

The NNSRI class of drugs is equally efficacious in treating depression as the other classes and is less expensive. However, these drugs are no longer considered first-line treatment due to their greater side-effect profile and risk of overdose and death. Sedation is a common side effect; therefore, it is recommended that these drugs be taken at bedtime (Stahl, 2011). Weight gain and autonomic side effects are also common (Stahl, 2011). Often less than a week's worth of these medications can produce life-threatening cardiac arrhythmia, hypotension, seizures, and extreme sedation, and death can occur (Stahl, 2011). Due to a narrow therapeutic index and risk for overdose, these medications should not be prescribed to anyone at moderate or high risk of suicide. In patients with other medical conditions, such as benign prostatic hyperplasia, epilepsy, preexisting cardiac arrhythmias, and unstable angina, exacerbation of their condition may occur (Khouzam, 2012). These drugs are generally not well tolerated by the elderly due to their anticholinergic side effects (Stahl, 2011).

Serotonin-Selective Reuptake Inhibitors

SSRIs are the class of drugs that include paroxetine (Paxil), fluoxetine (Prozac), sertraline (Zoloft), fluvoxamine (Luvox), citalopram (Celexa), and escitalopram (Lexapro). These drugs act by blocking the transport mechanism that returns unbound 5HT left in the synaptic cleft into the presynaptic neuron, thereby terminating the transmission of the message carried by that receptor. When the transport mechanism is blocked, more 5HT is available to bind to the postsynaptic serotonin receptor (Stahl, 2013).

Vilazodone (Viibryd) is a newer antidepressant to treat major depressive disorder in adults (Stahl, 2011). It is considered to be a serotonin partial agonist reuptake inhibitor (SPARI) with $5HT_1$ a partial agonist activity. Its activity is hypothesized to increase serotonin from several mechanisms (Stahl, 2011).

There is little evidence for superior effectiveness of one SSRI over another (Riley, McEntee, Gerson, & Dennison, 2009). To a significant degree, the SSRIs interact with many other drugs. They are highly protein bound and inhibit the CYP450 isoenzyme system to varying extents, leading to many potential drug interactions (Stahl, 2011). Patients who are taking several other drugs may benefit from a drug choice that has fewer drug interactions. For a chart of substrate and inhibitory drugs in the CYP450 system, see Table 29-2.

Table 29–2 ▦ Four Cytochrome P-450 Isoenzymes and Potential Drug Interactions

Isoenzyme	Substrates	Inhibitors
1A2	Acetaminophen, caffeine, theophylline, trimipramine, doxepin, clomipramine, amitriptyline, tacrine, propranolol, clozapine, trazodone, mirtazapine, alprazolam	Citalopram, fluoxetine, fluvoxamine, nefazodone, fluoroquinolones, grapefruit juice
2D6	Fluoxetine, sertraline, amitriptyline, clomipramine, desipramine, imipramine, nortriptyline, trimipramine, maprotiline, venlafaxine, nefazodone, trazodone, paroxetine, bupropion, flurazepam, Type I antiarrhythmics, dextromethorphan, oxycodone, codeine, haloperidol, perphenazine, risperidone, propranolol, alprenolol, timolol, metoprolol, indoramin, vilazodone (Viibryd)	Citalopram, fluoxetine, fluvoxamine, paroxetine, sertraline, nefazodone, trazodone, venlafaxine, amitriptyline, clomipramine, quinidine, fluphenazine, haloperidol, perphenazine, methadone
2C19	Citalopram, clomipramine, nortriptyline, desipramine, trimipramine, diazepam, omeprazole, phenytoin, fluoxetine, venlafaxine, phenelzine, vilazodone (Viibryd)	Citalopram, fluvoxamine, fluoxetine, paroxetine, sertraline, venlafaxine, mirtazapine, imipramine, tranylcypromine, diazepam, cimetidine, omeprazole
3A4	Loratadine, alprazolam, clonazepam, diazepam, midazolam, triazolam, estazolam, flurazepam, carbamazepine, amitriptyline, imipramine, clomipramine, bupropion, nefazodone, sertraline, trazodone, venlafaxine, citalopram, calcium channel blockers, amiodarone, disopyramide, lidocaine, propafenone, quinidine, erythromycin, acetaminophen, codeine, androgens, dexamethasone, estrogens	Fluvoxamine, fluoxetine, paroxetine, sertraline, nefazodone, venlafaxine, mirtazapine, diltiazem, verapamil, clarithromycin, itraconazole, ketoconazole, cimetidine, dexamethasone, grapefruit juice

SSRIs are commonly the initial drug of choice for patients with depression and many of the anxiety disorders. These drugs demonstrate equal efficacy to the nonspecific SNRIs with a safer and more tolerable side-effect profile. The more common adverse side effects include dizziness, sexual dysfunction, nervousness, nausea, sleep disturbance, and weight changes (Stahl, 2011). Serotonin syndrome is a potentially life-threatening condition resulting from excess serotonin agonist activity. This can result from too rapid titration of medication, overdose, a drug interaction, or an adverse drug reaction. This syndrome is more common than once thought. Medications such as tramadol, meperidine, St. John's Wort, and the over-the-counter medications dextromethorphan and decongestants often can interact with the SSRIs and cause serotonin syndrome (Stahl, 2013). The symptoms start out as diarrhea and diaphoresis and can progress to mental status changes, autonomic dysfunction, and neuromuscular abnormalities, up to death (Sadock & Sadock, 2010; Stahl, 2013). Treatment consists of discontinuation of the offending drug, supportive care, control of agitation, and possible hospitalization (Stahl, 2011; Wu, 2012).

In 2011, the U.S. Food and Drug Administration (FDA) issued a *Drug Safety Communication* stating that citalopram should no longer be used at doses greater than 40 mg per day because it could cause potentially dangerous abnormalities in the electrical activity of the heart. Its use at any dose is discouraged in patients at risk for QT prolongation. The revised labeling in 2012 describes what precaution needs to be taken when citalopram is used in these patients and those over the age of 60. Recommendations include the periodic use of ECG monitoring and/or electrolyte monitoring in patients with risk conditions, the discontinuation of citalopram in patients found to have persistent QTc measurements greater than 500 ms, and the limitation of the maximum recommended dose of citalopram to 20 mg per day for patients older than 60 years of age. The labeling recommendation for patients with congenital long QT syndrome who are at particular risk of torsade de pointes, ventricular tachycardia, and sudden death when given drugs that prolong the QT interval has been changed from contraindicated to not recommended (U.S. FDA, 2012).

Discontinuation syndrome may occur when a patient takes an NNSRI or an SSRI for more than 5 weeks and the dose is sharply reduced or stopped suddenly. Symptoms include agitation, anxiety, balance problems, bad dreams, concentration issues, dizziness, diarrhea, nausea, vomiting, electric shock-like sensations and flu-like symptoms (Stahl, 2011). This can occur in up to 30% of patients anywhere from days to weeks after stopping or reducing the medication and is more common in medications with a shorter half-life. Gradual tapering may prevent discontinuation syndrome symptoms (Wu, 2012). Fluoxetine has the lowest risk of causing these symptoms (Stahl, 2011). A few controlled studies as well as clinical experience has shown that among the SSRIs, discontinuation symptoms are more likely with paroxetine than with sertraline, citalopram, or escitalopram and all of the NNSRIs (Stahl, 2011).

Serotonin-Norepinephrine Reuptake Inhibitors

SNRIs block the reuptake mechanism of NE and 5HT, thus permitting greater availability of these neurotransmitters to bind with the respective receptors in the brain. Several SNRIs are available in the United States for the treatment of depression, including venlafaxine (Effexor and Effexor XR), duloxetine (Cymbalta), and desvenlafaxine (Pristiq) (Stahl, 2011). Levomilnacipran (Fetzima) is the newest medication approved in this class, but it should only be used in major depressive disorder (MDD) in adults and is not indicated for the treatment of fibromyalgia (FDA, 2013). Duloxetine was approved by the FDA to treat diabetic neuropathy in addition to depression (Riley et al, 2009). Prescribers are cautioned that there are other medications in this class that should not be considered interchangeable with these drugs. For example, Milnacipran (Savella) is pharmaceutically categorized as an SNRI but does not have FDA indication for depression; it is used for fibromyalgia treatment.

SNRIs elicit adverse reactions similar to those of SSRIs. In addition, common side effects include insomnia and elevated blood pressure. These drugs would not be the first choice for those with uncontrolled hypertension, preexisting sleep disturbance, and autonomic instability. As with the SSRIs, abrupt cessation should be avoided because discontinuation symptoms may occur (Stahl, 2011). Because of the addition of the norepinephrine neurotransmitters, these SNRIs are also found to be lethal in overdose, and limiting the quantity prescribed is warranted (Stahl, 2011).

Norepinephrine-Dopamine Reuptake Inhibitors

Only one NDRI is available in the United States: bupropion (Wellbutrin, Wellbutrin SR, Wellbutrin XL). Its mechanism of action is not fully understood, but it has been found to increase NE and DA by weakly inhibiting their neuronal reuptake. Bupropion is indicated in the treatment of major depressive disorder, including seasonal affective disorder, and it can also be used as an adjunct in smoking cessation (Stahl, 2011).

Due to the short half-life of bupropion, more than once-a-day dosing for major depressive disorder may be required, which may have an impact on sleep. The use of the slow-release (SR) preparation (bupropion SR) or extended-release (XL) preparation once a day (bupropion XL) facilitates once-a-day dosing. The XL formulation, with a half-life of approximately 24 hours, is only intended for once-a-day dosing in the morning. The XL formulation, although now generic, is often more costly than the SR. The SR formulation has a half-life of 10 to 14 hours and can be dosed twice a day. If a second dose of the SR is required, it is usually recommended to give the second dose no later than 5 hours before bedtime because of the stimulating effect of the drug and the possible effect on sleep. There is an increased risk of seizures at high doses so it is recommended that prescribers stay within the recommended maximum total daily dose of 450 mg and use should be avoided in patients at risk for seizures (Stahl, 2011). Bupropion has a dose-dependent increased risk for seizures in patients with eating disorders or those with chronic medical conditions that require the use of diuretics (Sadock & Sadock, 2010). Side effects may include dry mouth, sweating, tremor, and nervousness (Stahl, 2011). Due to a lack of direct effects on serotonergic neurotransmission, there is a lower incidence of sexual side effects (Sadock & Sadock, 2010; Thase et al, 2005). NDRIs are not effective in treating symptoms of anxiety because they may actually exacerbate anxiety and agitation (Riley et al, 2009; Sadock & Sadock, 2010).

Serotonin Agonist Reuptake Inhibitors

There are two SARIs: nefazadone and trazadone. They not only inhibit the reuptake of 5HT but also block the postsynaptic $5HT_2$ receptor subtype (Sadock & Sadock, 2010). With long term use, these drugs have the ability to increase serotonin release through the desensitization of $5HT_{1A}$ receptors. Both of these drugs also have a mild to moderate α_1-receptor antagonism (Stahl, 2011).

Nefazadone has an FDA Black-Box Warning related to hepatotoxicity; the drug is available only in generic form at this time. This drug has beneficial effects on sleep and is associated with minimal sexual side effects (Sadock & Sadock, 2010). On rare occasions, trazodone has been associated with priapism and anticholinergic side effects (Stahl, 2011). Both of these drugs are usually not recommended as a first-line antidepressant due to the potential side effects of sedation and orthostatic hypotension (Sadock & Sadock, 2010).

Norepinephrine- and Serotonin-Specific Agonist

Mirtazapine (Remeron) is a unique addition to antidepressants used to treat anxiety and depression. It is a 5HT agonist and reuptake inhibitor that blocks the reuptake of NE and the somato-dendritic reuptake of 5HT, resulting in an increase in 5HT available for release from the presynaptic neuron and more NE available in the synaptic cleft (Stahl, 2011). Mirtazapine specifically blocks the $5HT_2$ and $5HT_3$ receptors. This results in less sexual, gastrointestinal, and anxiogenic side effects (Sadock & Sadock, 2010). Unfortunately, it also blocks histamine, which contributes to the commonly observed side effects of drowsiness and weight gain at some doses (Sadock & Sadock, 2010). This may be an advantage for treatment in patients who are depressed with difficulty sleeping or patients with weight loss. Mirtazapine does not have the anti-muscarinic side effects of NNSRIs (Stahl, 2011).

Monoamine Oxidase Inhibitors (MAOI)

Monoamine oxidase is an enzyme found in nerve and other tissues, such as the liver and gut, that contributes to degradation

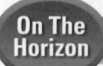

On The Horizon **PSYCHOPHARMACOLOGY RESEARCH**

What to look for during the next 5 years in psychopharmacology:

- New mechanisms of action, especially targeting glutamate/GABA interaction
- Targeting antagonism of the glutamate receptor to treat depression
- Development of drugs targeting the second messenger system for faster response rates and possibly neuroprotective qualities in preventing further depression
- Corticotropin-releasing factor antagonists to mediate effects of stress on the pathophysiology of depression

of the monoamines (DA, 5HT, and NE). In doing so, more of these neurotransmitters are available for postsynaptic binding (Stahl, 2011). The MAOIs block monoamine oxidase by binding to the enzyme and permanently inactivating it. Synthesis of replacement MAO requires about 2 weeks. This allows for levels of the catecholamines (DA and NE) and 5HT to rise, but it also decreases MAO availability for two other amines found in human diets, tyramine and phenylethylamine. MAO is a natural rate-limiting substance needed to detoxify tyramine in the human body before it causes such severe events as a sudden rise in pulse and blood pressure. Therefore, use of the MAOIs requires dietary restrictions of tyramine-containing foods, such as any aged meats and cheeses and fermented products (e.g., wine, beer, sauerkraut, soy sauce) (Stahl, 2011).

The MAOIs phenelzine, tranylcypromine, isocarboxazid, and selegiline inhibit MAO. Because there are significant dietary restrictions that, if neglected, can contribute to lethal side effects, these drugs are used less often than are other antidepressants and should only be prescribed by psychiatric providers (Sadock & Sadock, 2010). Hypertensive crisis is another potential major side effect of MAOIs. Patients may complain of occipital headache radiating frontally, sweating, photophobia, palpitations, stiffness in the neck, and nausea or vomiting. MAOIs can have dangerous interactions with many medications, including over-the-counter medications and herbal remedies. After discontinuing an SSRI or other serotoninergic, MAOIs must not be administered for 2 to 5 weeks (Stahl, 2011). This is considered a "wash-out" period.

Selegiline is available as a transdermal patch (Ensam), which avoids first-pass metabolism and produces less inhibition of the liver and gut MAO. This drug is associated with fewer food restrictions, but higher doses may cause an interaction with tyramine-containing foods and is a risk factor in elevated doses (Stahl, 2011). Transdermal selegiline is not FDA approved for use in children less than 12 years of age (Stahl, 2011). Given the risks, in depression treatment this drug should be given only by a psychiatric provider.

Benzodiazepines/GABA-ergics (BZDs)

The BZD medications are controlled substances occasionally used to treat acute anxiety. The legal implications of prescribing controlled substances are found in Chapter 4. BZDs are no longer considered first-line agents for the treatment of anxiety disorders and have been replaced by the SSRIs and SNRIs. The BZDs are divided into short-acting agents: oxazepam (Serax) and triazolam (Halcion); intermediate-acting agents: alprazolam (Xanax), lorazepam (Ativan), estazolam (Prosom), and temazepam (Restoril); and long-acting agents: diazepam (Valium), quazepam (Doral), clorazepate (Tranxene), chlordiazepoxide (Librium), and flurazepam (Dalmane) (Stahl, 2011). BZDs act on the chloride ion channel of GABA-A receptors when they are bound to their adjacent BZD receptor. In doing so, they enhance GABA neurotransmission, which then lengthens hyperpolarization of the impulse, thus slowing down responses to successive impulses. The net effect is to decrease reactivity of the brain (Stahl, 2013). BZDs have five main effects: anxiolytic, anterograde amnesia, anticonvulsant, muscle relaxation, and sedation (Stahl, 2011).

The advantages of BZDs are rapid onset of action, tolerability, inexpensive in generic form, and little effect on the cardiovascular system. The disadvantages of the BZDs far outweigh the benefits for the treatment of anxiety disorders and will make depressive symptoms worsen. The use of BZDs is associated with dependence and withdrawal, risk of overdose, respiratory depression and death, sedation, interaction with alcohol, impaired motor coordination, and impaired cognition. A sign of dependence is the need for larger dosing to achieve therapeutic effect and inability to function without the medication (Stahl, 2011).

When used for a prolonged period of time, withdrawal symptoms may occur when benzodiazepines are stopped. If addiction or withdrawal is suspected, a referral to a psychiatric provider with experience in addiction is required to help the dependent individual withdraw safely (Sadock & Sadock, 2010). Abrupt discontinuation of long-term use of any benzodiazepine has been associated with seizures, and withdrawal may involve hospitalization (Sadock & Sadock, 2010). The two most common side effects of BZDs are drowsiness and confusion. Precaution should be used when prescribing these drugs to patients with liver disease and acute narrow-angle glaucoma. Sedative effects can be enhanced in patients who drink alcohol and take other CNS depressants (Stahl, 2011).

Buspirone (Buspar) is a nonbenzodiazepine GABA agonist that is FDA approved to treat anxiety disorders (Stahl, 2011). It does not act directly on the GABA receptor but as a partial agonist to the 5HT1A receptor. It also has some affinity for the DA2 receptors and 5HT2A receptors. Buspirone has minimal side effects and low risk of dependence, but the 3 to 4 week therapeutic lag time, multiple daily dosing, and subtle effects make it less popular among patients than are other anxiolytic agents (Stahl, 2011). It does not produce cognitive or memory impairment or disinhibition euphoria as the BZDs do but does interact with alcohol (Stahl, 2011).

ADVERSE DRUG REACTIONS

The adverse drug reactions seen with antidepressants can often be explained by understanding their action on the receptors in the CNS. The SSRIs are not specific for the receptor subtype to which 5HT binds. Instead, all the available SSRIs can bind with any 5HT receptor subtype. The binding of 5HT to the $5HT_2$ receptor may be implicated in the adverse sexual reactions of the SSRIs. With $5HT_2$ antagonists (e.g., nefazodone and trazodone) and the $5HT_{1A}$ agonist buspirone (BuSpar), however, the sexual dysfunction effects are minimal (Kennedy & Rizvi, 2009). Because the SSRIs have minimum to no effect on norepinephrine, dopamine, histamine, or acetylcholine, there are few adverse reactions associated with blockade of these receptors (e.g., anxiety, restlessness, drowsiness, constipation, and orthostasis) (Stahl, 2011). Serotonin syndrome, another adverse reaction, was discussed earlier.

Reduced sexual desire, delayed or absent orgasm, premature ejaculation, and erectile disturbance can occur when taking any antidepressant, but they are most common with SSRIs (Stahl, 2011). These adverse reactions usually do not become evident for about a month, which may be more noticeable as the depressive symptoms are reduced. The patient may also have a primary reason for sexual dysfunction that needs to be evaluated. Educating patients about this possible side effect and informing them of other treatment options early can reduce the risk of patients decreasing their dosage or stopping treatment due to sexual dysfunction (Stahl, 2011). As the advanced practice nurse treating the patient, it is important to ascertain that the patient is experiencing sexual side effects due to the medication and not a co-occurring medical disorder or other reason. If the antidepressant is the cause of the sexual side effects, consider lowering the dose or changing to another antidepressant with less sexual side effects, such as bupropion. If the patient does not want to try a different medication and the lowered dose does not help, other strategies for male patients might include adding sildenafil or tadalafil (Stahl, 2011).

RATIONAL DRUG SELECTION

General Principles in Selecting an Initial Antidepressant

Clinical guidelines recommend that symptoms of depression and anxiety are best treated with a combination of medications and psychotherapy (Black, 2006; Eddy, Dutra, Bradley, & Westen, 2004; Mitte, 2005; Pampallona, Ballini, Tibaldi, Kupalnick, & Munizza, 2004; Rush, Trivedi et al, 2006; Thase et al, 2007). Many of the medications commonly used to treat anxiety are also used to treat depression (Posmontier & Breiter, 2012). For example, paroxetine is FDA approved to treat MDD, OCD, panic, GAD, and PTSD. Escitalopram is approved for the treatment of MDD and GAD. Sertraline is indicated for use in MDD, panic disorder, PTSD, and OCD. Fluoxetine is approved to treat MDD for ages 8 and older, OCD for ages 7 and older, bulimia, and panic disorder. Fluvoxamine has the approval to treat OCD and social anxiety disorder. Venlafaxine XR is indicated for MDD, GAD, and panic disorder (Stahl, 2011).

Research suggests that all antidepressants are equally effective; therefore the most important considerations are differences in onset of action and adverse events (Gartlehner et al, 2008). In one meta-analysis, the clinical effectiveness (a 50% reduction in symptoms after 8 weeks) of 12 new-generation antidepressants and patient acceptability (low dropout rates) in adults being treated for major depression were assessed. Escitalopram and sertraline were found to be the most effective (Cipriani et al, 2009). The Agency for Healthcare Research and Quality (AHRQ, 2012) did a comparative analysis and did not find differences in outcomes between antidepressants. Continued research and systematic reviews are needed to give providers more assistance in better rationales for antidepressant choice.

According to the APA practice guidelines (2010) for depression, the effectiveness of antidepressant medications is generally comparable between and within classes of medications. Therefore, it is suggested that a comprehensive psychiatric assessment be performed and initial selection of an antidepressant be largely based on the preference and prior response of the patient, clinical features, safety and anticipated side effects, coexisting medical conditions (both physical and mental), the pharmacological properties of the medications, and cost. For example, in an overweight individual, mirtazapine may not be the first choice because of the higher risks of weight gain. In addition, because mental disorders are often familial, it is helpful to know if anyone else in the family has similar symptoms and what medications have worked for them. When several choices are reasonable, select the medication that other blood relatives have had success with because they are likely to affect the patient in the same manner (Stahl, 2011). All of the antidepressants discussed in this chapter usually take 2 to 4 weeks to produce the full therapeutic effect, with gradual improvement beginning with the vegetative symptoms, then arousal symptoms, before the relief of mood symptoms. Refer to the general treatment algorithm for depression (Fig. 29-1).

Anxiety

As discussed above, anxiety is a normal emotion in response to threat or anticipation of harm. The total body responds through the autonomic system by preparing the body to flee the situation, remain and fight, or remain and freeze (Cash & Glass, 2011). Clearly, anxiety serves an adaptive purpose, and to automatically medicate anxiety may be countertherapeutic. When a patient maladaptively responds to stress and meets criteria for one of the anxiety disorders, the provider should consider medication and therapy (Cash & Glass, 2011; Sadock & Sadock, 2010).

The primary neural pathways involved in anxiety include 5HT, NE, and GABA. Therefore, pharmacological intervention can use nonselective norepinephrine-serotonin reuptake inhibitors, SSRIs, and/or SNRIs, or serotonin agonists. (Sadock & Sadock, 2010; Stahl, 2011). SSRIs and SNRIs can be used for GAD, PTSD, obsessive-compulsive disorders, and panic attacks. They usually take 2 to 4 weeks to provide the full therapeutic effect. Anxiety symptoms often resolve earlier than depressive symptoms, and they usually require a much lower dosage. For all anxiety disorders, starting low and going slow is the best way to avoid excessive serotonin adverse effects (Stahl, 2011). Refer to Figure 29-2 for a general algorithm for the treatment of anxiety disorders.

Buspirone does not produce tolerance or dependency. It requires about 2 weeks to reach the full therapeutic level, which may be intolerable to those with severe anxiety. Behavioral strategies can complement the medication effect, especially while waiting for the full therapeutic medication effect. It cannot be taken as needed and must be taken on a regular basis, usually more than once a day. Buspirone seems to be especially effective with patients who have generalized anxiety disorder.

Post-Traumatic Stress Disorder

There is evidence that cognitive behavioral therapy (CBT) (Mueser et al, 2007) and eye movement desensitization and reprocessing (EMDR) (van den Berg & van der Gaag, 2012) have been effective for the treatment of PTSD. Some patients may further benefit from medication in addition to psychotherapy (Sadock & Sadock, 2010). Medications prescribed to treat PTSD symptoms act primarily upon 5HT, NE, GABA, and DA neurotransmitters associated with the fear and anxiety circuitry of the brain. The FDA has approved two SSRIs, sertraline and paroxetine, for PTSD treatment. All other medication uses are off-label, although there is growing evidence supporting the use of the SSRI fluoxetine (Prozac) and for the SNRI venlafaxine (Effexor). Caution is needed in treatment of individuals with PTSD because comorbidity with traumatic brain injury or other mood and substance disorders is common (Department of Defense, 2010). More studies are needed at this time (National Center for PTSD, 2012).

Obsessive-Compulsive Disorder

Treatment of OCD is most effective when medication is combined with cognitive-behavioral therapy (Sadock & Sadock, 2010). OCD is typically treated with serotonin reuptake inhibitors. The mechanism by which these drugs work in the brain of an OCD patient is not fully understood despite numerous studies (Stein & Steckler, 2010). Clomipramine, a tricyclic antidepressant, and SSRIs (fluvoxamine, fluoxetine, sertraline, and paroxetine) have all been shown to be effective medications for OCD treatment. FDA-approved treatment for children with OCD includes fluoxetine and sertraline (Stahl, 2011).

MONITORING AND PATIENT EDUCATION

It is important to build a trusting relationship and be optimistic when discussing treatment options with patients. Make sure that the patient knows that recovery is possible and that confidentiality will be respected. Information about treatment and support groups should be provided (National Institute for Health and Clinical Excellence, 2012). Once treatment is initiated, the patient's status needs to be frequently monitored for response to treatment, possible side effects, safety, increased suicidal thinking, and adherence to treatment at least every 1 to 2 weeks. This should begin 1 or 2 weeks after the initiation of therapy (Qaseem, Snow, Denberg, Forciea, & Owens, 2008). When considering frequency of follow-up appointments, consider the severity of the illness, co-occurring medical conditions, available support systems, progression of symptom change, and the patients' cooperation with treatment (Stahl, 2011). If a patient needs closer monitoring, refer to a psychiatric provider. (See Table 29-3 for recommendations about when to refer to a psychiatric provider.)

Currently, all antidepressants have a Black-Box Warning regarding an increased risk of suicidal thinking and behavior in children, adolescents, and young adults to age 24 (FDA Consumer Health Information, 2009). Because depression itself is associated with an increase in suicidal ideation, the chances of such ideation must be considered when making a choice about appropriate treatment (Sadock & Sadock, 2010). All patients who are prescribed an antidepressant and the parents of children or adolescents should be educated to monitor for an increase in suicidal ideation or behavior. It is especially important to assess for suicidality at the time of diagnosis, after initiating treatment, and as treatment progresses. The antidepressants begin to work on sleep, appetite, and energy, with mood as one of the last symptoms to remit. This puts all individuals being treated for depression and anxiety at risk for suicidal thinking.

The assessment, evaluation, and triage system discussed above and in Table 29-1 must be used every 1 to 2 weeks early in treatment and when increasing dosage (FDA Consumer Health Information, 2009; Sadock & Sadock, 2010). Immediate referral and possible hospitalization need to be considered if the patient persists in suicidal thinking (U.S. FDA, 2007). Some antidepressants, such as the NNSRIs and the SNRIs, can be lethal in overdose. When using these medications early on in treatment, consider dispensing weekly quantities and be aware of the possibility of hoarding. For patients who are having suicidal ideation, consider a safer medication in overdose, such as an SSRI (APA, 2010).

Planning ahead for the potential for suicidal ideation must always be considered as the treatment plan for each

Table 29–3　When to Refer

When to refer to a psychiatric provider
- Bipolar disorder
- Suicidality
- Psychosis
- Significant substance disorder comorbidities
- Comorbid PTSD or OCD
- Comorbid eating disorder
- Failure of two antidepressants
- Possibility of a personality disorder

individual is established. According to the U.S. Surgeon General's 2012 report on a Comprehensive National Strategy on Suicide Prevention, there needs to be support and treatment available at multiple points of entry. At the primary care provider and emergency department level:

- Screening improves the likelihood that the person will receive appropriate evaluation and treatment;
- Training on recognition of risk and quality of care increases the likelihood of a good outcome;
- The care provider accurately diagnoses and records the problems and ensures that the appropriate public health surveillance systems are notified or made aware of the diagnoses;
- The implementation of trauma-informed policies and practices ensures that the person is treated with respect and in a way that promotes healing and recovery;
- Easy access to mental health care referrals for individuals with suicide risk increases the likelihood of a better outcome;
- Education efforts by health-care providers increase knowledge of the warning signs of suicide risk among the individual and his or her family and/or support network; and
- Continuous care and improved aftercare lead to better monitoring and follow-up of the at-risk individual over time (U.S. Surgeon General, 2012, p 12).

During the acute treatment phase, it is important to monitor the patient's response to ensure the treatment has been given for a sufficient duration, frequency, or dose. A patient needs about 4 to 8 weeks of optimal dosing of medication treatment to appropriately evaluate whether or not there is a partial response or no response at all. Treatment should be modified if remission has not been obtained in at least a 14 week period of optimal dosing or there has been little symptomatic improvement (Qaseem et al, 2008; Rush, Trivedi et al, 2006). If there is a mild-moderate response, increasing the dose or switching antidepressants or using of augmenting agents discussed earlier from the STAR*D results should be considered (Rush, Trivedi et al, 2006 Trivedi et al, 2006).

It is important to know when to refer someone who is not responding to treatment. Table 29-3 gives a list of possible reasons for referral to a psychiatric provider. Consider referring any individual with a poor response to two adequate trials of antidepressants, a chronic suicide history, comorbid PTSD, comorbid eating disorders, or if this person shows indications of a more complicated mood disorder. Refer to psychiatric providers immediately those with any psychotic disorder and those who are dependent on substances (Sadock & Sadock, 2010).

When reassessing and modifying a treatment plan, it is important to consider the patient's diagnosis, side effects, treatment adherence, psychotherapy, pharmacology, co-occurring conditions, and psychosocial factors (Stahl, 2011). Once the patient shows relief and response from the original symptoms and adverse reactions are tolerable, both the medication and psychotherapy should be continued for at least

4 to 9 months to reduce the risk of relapse (Qaseem et al, 2008). It is important to monitor for signs of relapse during this time. A patient's family can be helpful in the identification of relapse (Stahl, 2011).

Maintenance therapy may be necessary for some patients, especially those with a history of three or more major depressive disorders, a recurrent illness, or another medical and/or psychiatric disorder (Sadock & Sadock, 2010). If maintenance therapy is needed, the same treatment that was effective in the acute and continuation phases should be used. The patient should continue to be regularly monitored for signs of reoccurrence (Stahl, 2011).

When planning with the patient to discontinue antidepressant medication, it is important to select a target time when ordinary stresses are low; holidays, major family events, or return to school are not good times to discontinue medication. The medication should be tapered over at least several weeks. Relapse risk is high in the first 2 months after discontinuation. It is important to follow up with the patient during this time period. Educate the patient about the signs, symptoms, and potential for relapse as well as the need to restart treatment should this occur (Stahl, 2011).

COMORBIDITY OF MEDICAL AND PSYCHIATRIC DISORDERS

The diagnoses of anxiety and depressive disorders complicate the diagnosis and management of chronic medical diseases and contribute to poor outcomes. The choice of medication in treating depression and anxiety depends on the prominent symptoms the patient presents, comorbid conditions, other medications the patient is taking, and tolerance to adverse reactions (Stahl, 2011). Chronic illness and chronic disease progression can exacerbate concomitant depression and anxiety disorders. It remains important to treat these comorbid anxiety and depressive disorders, but slower titration and lower doses may be necessary if liver or kidney functions are compromised (Stahl, 2011).

Various studies indicate that migraines (Lake, Rains, Penzien, & Lipchik, 2005); pulmonary diseases such as asthma (Cooper et al, 2007); pulmonary hypertension, chronic obstructive pulmonary disease (COPD), and chronic bronchitis (Goodwin, Kroenke, Hoven, & Spitzer, 2003); fibromyalgia (Thieme, Turk, & Flor, 2004); cardiovascular diseases (Frasure-Smith & Lesperance, 2005) such as carotid atherosclerosis (Jones, Bromberger, Sutton-Tyrrel, & Matthews, 2003); irritable bowel disease (Mussell et al, 2008); and diabetes (Anderson, Freedland, Clouse, & Lustman, 2001) all have remarkable association with depression and/or anxiety (Howard, El-Mallakh, Rayens, & Clark, 2007).

Furthermore, frequent users of primary care and emergency services are twice as likely to have anxiety and depression than are mid- and low-range users (Ford, Trestman, Steinberg, Tennen, & Allen, 2004; Roy-Byrne & Wagner, 2004). Current research clearly demonstrates that treatment

of depression and anxiety symptoms are an essential element of patients' general health state, their ability to cope with physical illnesses, and their quality of life with chronic illness. Primary care providers are the gatekeepers for these patients and recognition of the comorbidity can influence the outcomes for these patients if the PCP recognizes and treats the mental health features along with the physical health features.

SPECIAL POPULATIONS

There is growing evidence to support early detection of depressive and anxiety symptoms in children and adolescents and the use of developmentally appropriate assessment tools (Birmaher et al, 1999; Connolly, Bernstein, & Work Group on Quality Issues, 2007). The Screen for Child Anxiety-Related Disorders (SCARED) screening tool has both a child and parent version. (Birmaher et al, 1999). This is a short screening tool for children ages 8 to 11 that can help the PCP to look for generalized anxiety disorder and social or significant school phobias. It is recommended that questions be clarified with the child and that the tool be used with the adult caregiver (Birmaher et al, 1999). There is a recent systematic review that supports the use of cognitive behavioral therapy in children with anxiety disorders (James, James, Cowdrey, Soler, & Choke, 2013). Positive results from the screen should prompt the PCP to refer the child and parent to mental health providers for further evaluation.

According to the United States Preventive Services Taskforce (USPS, 2009), there is not enough evidence to support the use of routine screening for depression in children ages 7 to 11. Screening for adolescents ages 12 to 18 for MDD is recommended only when there is a system in place for accurate diagnosis, psychotherapy, and follow-up (USPS, 2009). The Guidelines for Adolescent Depression-Primary Care (GLAD-PC) was developed from 2005 to 2007. Its purpose is to provide a clinical guideline, information, recommendations, education resources, and tools for depression management of adolescents aged 10 to 21 in primary care. The guideline can be viewed at http://www.gladpc.org/ (GLAD-PC, 2010).

There is growing evidence for the use of antidepressants in children and adolescents for anxiety and depressive disorders. An SR of antidepressants for depressive disorders in children and adolescents provided some data to support the use of SSRIs in depressive disorders but also noted risks for increased suicidality (Hetrick, McKenzie, Cox, Simmons, & Merry, 2012). The evidence to support the use of SSRIs in children with OCD is not sufficient to support the use of medications in children with other anxiety disorders (Ipser, Stein, Hawkridge, & Hoppe, 2009). Fluoxetine is FDA approved for MDD and OCD in children 7 and older. Escitalopram is approved for MDD for children ages 12 and older (Stahl, 2011). Caution should be used when SSRIs are used in children and teenagers. One out of 50 report suicidal ideation as a result of treatment (Sadock & Sadock, 2010). As suicidal depressed patients begin to improve with treatment, they begin to have the physical energy to carry out the act, whereas before they did not have the will to do so (Sadock & Sadock, 2010). These child and adolescent patients should be closely monitored for worsening depression and suicidal thoughts whenever treatment is initiated or the dose is adjusted (U.S. FDA, 2007).

Symptoms of depression and anxiety are not different in older adults. The evidence described above, including the STAR*D trial and other systematic reviews of anxiety disorders, support the use of antidepressants in elders with depression and anxiety disorders with remission the outcome of treatment. The major differences in treating older adults with anxiety and depression include starting low and going slow on dosages and being more aware of medical comorbidities and drug-drug interactions that occur more frequently with older adults (Sadock & Sadock, 2010). The American Geriatrics Society (2012) Beers Criteria for Potentially Inappropriate Medication Use in Older Adults cautions against BZD use because studies have found an increased sensitivity, which may result in an increased risk of falls, delirium, cognitive impairment, motor vehicle accidents, and fractures.

The one population that deserves special attention is the childbearing woman. There is some evidence of mild congenital abnormalities, an increase in low-birth-weight babies, and premature deliveries in those pregnant women taking antidepressants (Udechuku, Nguyen, Hill, & Szego, 2010). There has also been increased incidence of primary pulmonary hypertension in neonates in women treated with SSRIs (Udechuku et al, 2010). However, there is also evidence of poor neonatal outcome and poorer cognitive scores in children born to women with untreated depression (Guedeney, 2007; Tronick & Reck, 2009). This is a significant risk/benefit discussion that must take place prior to pregnancy. Once pregnant, the primary care provider needs to refer this woman to a psychiatric provider and an obstetrical provider so that a therapeutic plan can be created and used by all providers from pregnancy through the postpartum period (Sadock & Sadock, 2010).

Postpartum depression (PPD) is a significant illness with an impact on the mother as well as the infant (Deave, Heron, Evans, & Emond, 2008). In primary care, PPD is often undetected and untreated (Boyd, 2012). A recent review of the literature shows that PPD screening improves clinical outcomes (Gjerdingen & Yawn, 2007). Use of the Edinburgh Postnatal Depression Scale (EPDS) increases the diagnosis of PPD by approximately 20% (Georgiopoulos, Bryan, Wollan, & Yawn, 2001).

Finally, an ongoing debate is whether the breastfeeding woman who has significant anxiety and depression should take antidepressants. There are levels of risk that have been determined by the FDA, but these ratings can change with more evidence. The best plan is for the health-care provider and pregnant woman to review the U.S. National Library of Medicine, Drugs, and Lactation Database (LactMed) (http://toxnet.nlm.nih.gov/newtoxnet/lactmed.htm) for the latest information on risks to the infant from any drug while breastfeeding to make a decision based on the latest evidence.

OUTCOME EVALUATION

Outcome evaluation and appropriate referral points have been discussed in this chapter. Remission is the desired outcome of all treatment of anxiety and depressive disorders. Advanced practice primary care nurses are likely to see patients with depressive and anxiety symptoms in their practice, whether or not the patients directly identify their concerns as depression or anxiety. Therefore, it is important to assess possible physical reasons for the depressive and anxiety symptoms first. A thorough examination, including laboratory studies such as a complete blood count, liver and kidney function, and thyroid function, can help the practitioner rule out medical causes of symptoms that can mimic depression and anxiety symptoms, narrow the clinical options, and treat appropriately (Richardson & Puskar, 2012).

Medications target symptoms and the neural pathways in different parts of the brain. Some of the psychological and social symptoms, such as low self-esteem, social withdrawal, and poor communication, can be better treated with psychotherapy. Because the physiological, psychological, and social symptoms occur together in depression and anxiety, it would serve the patient best by not only prescribing medications but also discussing psychotherapy and referring the patient to a therapist to learn some new ways of coping with stress (Sadock & Sadock, 2010). When making a referral, it is equally important to inquire about the attendance and effectiveness of the referral at later appointments. If the patient has not followed up on the referral, the clinician should ask about this and offer additional referrals if necessary.

Working with the patient who is depressed and/or anxious can be challenging. Frequently, the primary care provider takes on the prescribing and medication management role while the patient is in therapy and after therapy is concluded. The primary care advanced practice nurse is in a pivotal position to assist the patient to find a therapist that best fits his or her own needs. It is important, therefore, to have readily available a list of therapists of both genders who are culturally diverse. When recommending therapy, the patient should ideally be provided with two or three names of therapists. Discussing with the patient the therapists' features that would make the patient feel the most comfortable (e.g., gender, discipline, geographical area, ethnicity) invites the patient to follow up on the referral. It is also helpful to tell the patient a little about each referral specific to therapeutic style (e.g., interactive, a good listener), theoretical orientation (e.g., cognitive-behavioral, interpersonal), and special interests (e.g., family conflicts, developmental transitions, sexual orientation). Of course, this requires that the advanced practice nurse know something about the therapists. That information is acquired through networking and collaboration.

Maintaining an open line of communication between the therapist and the PCP, with a patient's signed authorization for the release of information, reduces confusion in treatment direction. Respectful and collaborative consulting with mental health professionals yields rewarding outcomes for both patient and provider. Probably the greatest reward for the

PCP is seeing and hearing about the improvement the patient is making. It is tempting for both patient and primary care provider to attribute success to the medications, but to do so invalidates the power and capacity of patients. Medications can only help the brain return to its normal functioning. It is the whole person who makes the changes necessary for recovery to mental health.

● CLINICAL PEARLS ●

Treatment and Monitoring of Patients with Anxiety and Depression

1. Always evaluate a patient for hypomania or mania before starting an antidepressant because these conditions can worsen bipolar symptoms.
2. When there is any anxiety disorder, consider starting all antidepressants low and going slow.
3. Start low and go slow when treating older adults with depression and/or anxiety.
4. Always monitor for suicidal thoughts throughout the entire treatment.
5. Always discuss the risks of fetal damage with a woman of childbearing potential who is taking an antidepressant BEFORE she gets pregnant so that she knows the risks and benefits of treatment.
6. Always monitor for signs and symptoms of serotonin syndrome, especially asking about new medications prescribed or any over-the-counter medications taken.
7. Taper off antidepressants slowly; most have discontinuation side effects.
8. Withdrawal or discontinuation symptoms include dizziness, nausea, diarrhea, sweating, irritability, and increased anxiety. If these occur, raise the dose to stop symptoms and taper even more slowly.
9. Do not start monoamine oxidase inhibitors (MAOIs) within 14 days of stopping other antidepressants; do not start another antidepressant until 14 days after stopping an MAOI.
10. It is tempting for both the patient and primary care provider to attribute success to the medications, but to do so invalidates the power and capacity of patients.
11. Medications can only help the brain return to its normal functioning. It is the whole person who makes the changes necessary for recovery to mental health.

CONCLUSIONS

Primary care providers carry a major responsibility for screening, assessing, and providing overall health care for the majority of patients within the health-care system. This is complicated by the need to control costs, time efficiency, and range of services. Because many patients first seek help for any health problem from their primary care provider, the primary care provider also has an essential role in identifying mental health issues that influence health care and quality of life. By collaborating with mental health-care and psychiatric providers, including advanced practice psychiatric mental health nurse practitioners, the primary care providers can increase success rates in the treatment of both mental health and physical disorders. Some primary care settings include mental health-care providers as consultants and providers within the same clinic. This enhances collaboration and coordination of care and provides more satisfaction for providers and patients.

REFERENCES

Abrantes, A. M., McLaughlin, N., Greenberg, B. D., Strong, D. R., Riebe, D., Mancebo, M., et al. (2012). Design and rationale for a randomized controlled trial testing the efficacy of aerobic exercise for patients with obsessive-compulsive disorder. *Mental Health and Physical Activity, 5*(2), 155–165.

Agency for Healthcare Research and Quality (AHRQ). (2012). *Second-generation antidepressants for treating adult depression: An update.* Retrieved March 7, 2013, from http://www.ncbi.nlm.nih.gov/books/NBK99902/pdf/clindep2.pdf

American Geriatrics Society (2012). *AGS Beers criteria for potentially inappropriate medication use in older adults.* Retrieved March 7, 2013, from http://www.americangeriatrics.org/files/documents/beers/2012AGSBeersCriteriaCitations.pdf

American Psychiatric Association (APA). (2010). *American Psychiatric Association practice guidelines.* Retrieved March 7, 2013, from http://psychiatryonline.org/guidelines.aspx

American Psychiatric Association (APA). (2013). *Diagnostic and statistical manual of mental disorders (DSM)* (5th ed.). Washington, DC: Author.

Anderson, R. J., Freedland, K. E., Clouse, R. E., & Lustman, P. J. (2001). The prevalence of comorbid depression in adults with diabetes: A meta-analysis. *Diabetes Care, 24,* 1069–1078.

Andrisano, C., Chiesa, A., & Serretti, A. (2013). Newer antidepressants and panic disorder: A meta-analysis. *International Clinical Psychopharmacology, 28*(1), 33-45.

Asmundson, G. J., Fetzner, M. G., Deboer, L. B., Powers, M. B., Otto, M. W., & Smits, J. A. (2013). Let's get physical: A contemporary review of the anxiolytic effects of exercise for anxiety and its disorders. *Depression and Anxiety, 8,* doi: 10.1002.

Beck, A. T., Ward, C. H., Mendelson, M., Mock, J., & Erbaugh, J. (1961). An inventory for measuring depression. *Archives of General Psychiatry, 4,* 561–571.

Birmaher, B., Brent, D. A., Chiappetta, L., Bridge, J., Monga, S., & Baugher, M. (1999). Psychometric properties of the Screen for Child Anxiety Related Emotional Disorders (SCARED): A replication study. *Journal of the American Academy of Child and Adolescent Psychiatry, 38*(10), 1230–1236.

Black, D. (2006). Efficacy of combined pharmacotherapy and psychotherapy versus monotherapy in the treatment of anxiety disorders [Review]. *CNS Spectrums, 11*(12 Suppl.), 29–33.

Boyd, R. (2012). Primary care-based screening, diagnosis and management of postpartum depression effective for improving symptoms, *Evidence-Based Medicine,* doi: 10.1136/eb-2012-100972. Retrieved March 7, 2013, from http://ebm.bmj.com/content/early/2012/10/11/eb-2012-100972.full.pdf+html

Bromet, E., Andrade, E. H., Hwang, I., Sampson, N. A., Alonso, J., Girolamo, G., et al. (2011). Cross-national epidemiology of DSM-IV major depressive episode. *BMC Medicine, 9*(90), doi: 10.1186/1741-7015-9-90. Retrieved from http://www.biomedcentral.com/1741-7015/9/90

Cash, J. C., & Glass, C. A. (2011). *Family practice guidelines* (2nd ed.). New York: Springer.

Centers for Disease Control and Prevention (2009). *National suicide statistics at a glance.* Retrieved March 7, 2013, from http://www.cdc.gov/ViolencePrevention/suicide/statistics/leading_causes.html

Centers for Disease Control and Prevention (2010). *Injury prevention and control: Data and statistics (WISQARS).* Retrieved March 7, 2013, from www.cdc.gov/injury/wisqars/index.html

Cipriani, A., Furukawa, T. A., Salanti, G., Geddes, J. R., Higgins, J., Churchill, R., et al. (2009). Comparative efficacy and acceptability of 12 new-generation antidepressants: A multiple-treatments meta-analysis. *The Lancet, 373*, 746–758.

Connolly, S., Bernstein, G., & Work Group on Quality Issues (2007). Practice parameter for the assessment and treatment of children and adolescents with anxiety disorders. *Journal of the American Academy of Child and Adolescent Psychiatry, 46*, 267–283.

Cooper, C., Parry, G., Morice, S., Hutchcrof, B., Moore, J., & Esmonde, L. (2007). Anxiety and panic fear for adults with asthma: Prevalence in primary care. *Bio Medical Central (BMC) Family Practice, 8*, 162.

Deave, T., Heron, J., Evans, J., & Emond, A. (2008). The impact of maternal depression in pregnancy on early child development. *British Journal of Obstetrics and Gynecology, 115*, 1043–1051.

Department of Defense (2010). *The management of post traumatic stress disorder.* Retrieved March 7, 2013, from http://www.healthquality.va.gov/Post_Traumatic_Stress_Disorder_PTSD.asp

Driessen, E., Cuijpers, P., de Maat, S. C., Abbass, A. A., de Jonghe, F., & Dekker, J. J. (2009). The efficacy of short-term psychodynamic psychotherapy for depression: A meta-analysis. *Clinical Psychology Review, 30*(1), 25–36.

Eddy, K. T., Dutra, L., Bradley, R., & Westen, D. (2004). A multidimensional meta-analysis of psychotherapy and pharmacotherapy for obsessive-compulsive disorder. *Clinical Psychology Review, 24*(8), 1011–1030.

Fava, M., Rush, A., Wisniewski, S., Nierenberg, A., Alpert, J., McGrath, P., et al. (2006). A comparison of mirtazapine and nortriptyline following two consecutive failed medication treatments for depressed outpatients: A STAR*D report. *American Journal of Psychiatry, 163*, 1161–1172.

Fjorback, L. O., Arendt, M., Ornbol, E., Fink, P., & Walach, H. (2011). Mindfulness-based stress reduction and mindfulness-based cognitive therapy—A systematic review of randomized controlled trials. *Acta Psychiatrica Scandinavica, 124*(2), 102–119.

Food and Drug Administration Consumer Health Information. (2009). *Understanding antidepressant medications.* Retrieved March 7, 2013, from http://www.fda.gov/downloads/ForConsumers/ConsumerUpdates/ucm095990.pdf

Food and Drug Administration (FDA). (25 July 2013). *New drug approvals.* www. fda.gov.

Ford, J. D., Trestman, R. L., Steinberg, K., Tennen, H., & Allen, S. (2004). Prospective association of anxiety, depressive, and addictive disorders with high utilization of primary, specialty and emergency medical care. *Social Science & Medicine, 58*(11), 2145–2148.

Frasure-Smith, N., & Lesperance, F. (2005). Reflections on depression as a cardiac risk factor. *Psychosomatic Medicine, 67*(1 Suppl.), 19–25.

Gartlehner, G., Gaynes, B., Hansen, R., Thieda, P., DeVeaugh-Geiss, A., Krebs, E.E., et al. (2008). Comparative benefits and harms of second generation antidepressants: Background paper for the American College of Physicians. *Annals of Internal Medicine, 149*(10), 734–746.

Georgiopoulos, A., Bryan, T., Wollan P., & Yawn, B. (2001) Routine screening for postpartum depression. *Journal of Family Practice, 50*, 117–122.

Gjerdingen, D., & Yawn, B. (2007). Postpartum depression screening: Importance, methods, barriers, and recommendations for practice. *Journal of the American Board of Family Medicine, 20*, 280–288.

GLAD-PC. (2010). *Guidelines for adolescent depression in primary care: GLAD-PC toolkit.* Retrieved from http://www.gladpc.org/

Goodman, W. K., Price, L. H., Rasmussen, S. A., Mazure, C., Fleischmann, R. L., Hill, C. L., et al. (1989). The Yale-Brown Obsessive Compulsive Scale. I. Development, use, and reliability. *Archives of General Psychiatry, 46*(11), 1006–1011.

Goodwin, R. D., Kroenke, K., Hoven, C. W., & Spitzer, R. L. (2003). Major depression, physical illness, and suicidal ideation in primary care. *Psychosomatic Medicine, 65*(4), 501–505.

Guedeney, A. (2007). Withdrawal behavior and depression in infancy. *Infant Mental Health Journal, 28*(4), 393–408.

Hamilton, M. (1959). The assessment of anxiety states by rating. *British Journal of Medical Psychology, 32*(1), 50–55.

Herring, M. P., Jacob, M. L., Suveg, C., Dishman, R. K., & O'Connor, P. J. (2012). Feasibility of exercise training for the short-term treatment of generalized anxiety disorder: A randomized controlled trial. *Psychotherapy and Psychosomatics, 81*(1), 21–28.

Hetrick, S., McKenzie, J., Cox, G., Simmons, M., & Merry, S. (2012). Newer generation antidepressants for depressive disorders in children and adolescents. *Cochrane Database Systematic Review.*

Hirschfeld, R., Williams, J., Spitzer, R. L., Calabrese, J. R., Flynn, L., Keck, P. E., et al. (2000). Development and validation of a screening instrument for bipolar spectrum disorder: The Mood Disorder Questionnaire. *The American Journal of Psychiatry, 157*, 1873–1875.

Howard, P., El-Mallakh, P., Rayens, M., & Clark, J. (2007). Comorbid medical illnesses and perceived general health among recipients of Medicaid mental health services. *Issues in Mental Health, 28*, 255–274.

Ippen, C. G., Ford, J., Racusin, R., Acker, M., Bosquet, M., Rogers, K., et al. (2002). *Traumatic Events Screening Inventory—Parent report revised.* Retrieved July 24, 2013, from http://www.ptsd.va.gov/professional/pages/assessments/tesi.asp

Ipser, J., Stein, D., Hawkridge, S., & Hoppe, L. (2009). Pharmacotherapy for anxiety disorders in children and adolescents. *Cochrane Database Systematic Review,(3)*: CD005170. doi: 10.1002/14651858.CD005170.pub2

James, A., James, G., Cowdrey, F., Soler, A., & Choke, A. (2013). Cognitive behavioral therapy for anxiety disorders in children and adolescents. *Cochrane Database Systematic Review, Jun 3*;6:CD004690. doi: 10.1002/14651858.CD004690.pub3

Jones, D. J., Bromberger, J. T., Sutton-Tyrrel, K., & Matthews, K. A. (2003). Lifetime history of depression and carotid atherosclerosis in middle-aged women. *Archives of General Psychiatry, 60*(2), 153–160.

Kennedy, S. H., & Rizvi, S. (2009). Sexual dysfunction, depression, and the impact of antidepressants. *Journal of Clinical Psychopharmacology, 29*(2), 157–164.

Kerr, L. K., & Kerr, Jr., L. D. (2001). Screening tools for depression in primary care: The effects of culture, gender, and somatic symptoms on the detection of depression. *Western Journal of Medicine, 175*(5), 349–352.

Kessler, R., Berglund, F., Demler, O., Jin, R., Merikangas, K. R., & Walters, E. E. (2005). Lifetime prevalence and age-of-onset distributions of DSM-IV disorders in the National Comorbidity Survey Replication. *Archives of General Psychiatry, 62*(6), 593–602.

Kessler, R., Chiu, W. T., Demler, O., Merikangas, K. R., & Walters, E. E. (2005). Prevalence, severity, and comorbidity of 12-month DSM-IV disorders in the National Comorbidity Survey Replication. *Archives of General Psychiatry, 62*(6), 617–627.

Khouzam, H. R. (2012). Depression in the elderly: How to treat. *Consultant,* 267–278.

Kotan, Z., Sarandöl, M., Kırhan, E., Özkaya, G., & Kırlı, S. (2012). Serum brain-derived neurotropic factor, vascular endothelial growth factor and leptin levels in patients with a diagnosis of severe major depressive disorder with melancholic features. *Therapeutic Advances in Psychopharmacology, 2*, 65–74.

Kurian, B., Grannemann, B., & Trivedi, M. (2012). Feasible evidence-based strategies to manage depression in primary care. *Current Psychiatry Reports, 14*, 370–375

Lake, A. E., III, Rains, J. C., Penzien, D. B., & Lipchik, G. L. (2005). Headache and psychiatric comorbidity: Historical context, clinical implications, and research relevance. *Headache, 45*(5), 493–506.

Lowe, B., Willand, L., Eich, W., Zipfel, S., Ho, A. D., Herzog, W., et al. (2004). Psychiatric comorbidity and work disability in patients with inflammatory rheumatic diseases. *Psychosomatic Medicine, 66*(3), 395–402.

Merom, D., Phongsavan, P., Wagner, R., Chey, T., Marnane, C., Steel, Z., et al. (2008). Promoting walking as an adjunct intervention to group cognitive behavioral therapy for anxiety disorders—A pilot group randomized trial. *Journal of Anxiety Disorders, 22*(6), 959–968.

McDonald, S. D., & Calhoun, P. S. (2010). The diagnostic accuracy of the PTSD checklist: A critical review. *Clinical Psychology Review, 30*(8), 976–987.

McLean, C. P., Asnaani, A., Litz, B. T., & Hofmann, S. G. (2011). Gender differences in anxiety disorders: Prevalence, course of illness, comorbidity and burden of illness. *Journal of Psychiatric Research, 45*(8), 1027–1035.

Mitte, K. (2005). A meta-analysis of the efficacy of psycho- and pharmacotherapy in panic disorder with and without agoraphobia. *Journal of Affective Disorders, 88*, 27–45.

Montgomery, S. A., & Asberg, M. (1979). A new depression scale designed to be sensitive to change. *The British Journal of Psychiatry, 134*, 382–389.

Mueser, K. T., Bolton, E., Carty, P., Bradley, M. J., Ahlgren, K. F., DiStaso, D., et al. (2007). The Trauma Recovery Group: A cognitive-behavioral program for post-traumatic stress disorder in persons with severe mental illness. *Community Mental Health Journal, 43*(3), 281–304.

Mussell, M., Kroenke, K., Spitzer, R., Williams, J., Herzog, W., & Lowe, B. (2008). Gastrointestinal symptoms in primary care: Prevalence and association with depression and anxiety. *Journal of Psychosomatic Research, 64*(6), 605–612.

National Center for PTSD. (2012). *Clinician's guide to medications for PTSD*. Retrieved March 7, 2013, from http://www.ptsd.va.gov/professional/pages/clinicians-guide-to-medications-for-ptsd.asp

National Institute for Health and Clinical Excellence. (2012). *NICE pathways: Depression overview*. Retrieved March 7, 2013, from http://pathways.nice.org.uk/pathways/depression#content=view-node%3Anodes-service-organisation-and-training

Newman, C. L., & Motta, R. W. (2007). The effects of aerobic exercise on childhood PTSD, anxiety, and depression. *International Journal of Emergency Mental Health, 9*(2), 133–158.

Nierenberg, A, Fava, J, Trivedi, M., Wisniewski, S., Thase, M., McGrath, P., et al. (2006). A comparison of lithium and T3 augmentation following two failed medication treatments for depression: A STAR*D report. *American Journal of Psychiatry, 163*, 1519–1530.

Pampallona, S., Ballini, P., Tibaldi, G., Kupalnick, B., & Munizza, C. (2004). Combined pharmacotherapy and psychological treatment for depression: A systematic review. *Archives of General Psychiatry, 61*(7), 714–719.

Parmentier, H., García-Campayo, J., & Prieto, R. (2013). Comprehensive review of generalized anxiety disorder in primary care in Europe. *Current Medical Opinion and Research, 29*, 1–14.

Posmontier, B., & Breiter, D. (2012). Managing generalized anxiety disorder in primary care. *The Journal for Nurse Practitioners, 8*(4), 268–274.

Qaseem, A., Snow, V., Denberg, T. D., Forciea, M. A., & Owens, D. K. (2008). Using second-generation antidepressants to treat depressive disorders: A clinical practice guideline from the American College of Physicians. *Annals of Internal Medicine, 149*(10), 725–733.

Reinhold, J., Mandos, L., Rickels, K., & Lohoff, F. (2011). Pharmacological treatment of generalized anxiety disorder. *Expert Opinion in Pharmacotherapy, 12*(16), 2457–2467.

Ribbe, D. (1996). Psychometric review of Traumatic Event Screening Instrument for Children (TESI-C). In B. H. Stamm (Ed.), *Measurement of stress, trauma, and adaptation* (pp 386–387). Lutherville, MD: Sidran Press.

Richardson, L., & Puskar, K. (2012). Screening assessment for anxiety and depression in primary care. *The Journal for Nurse Practitioners, 8*(6), 475–480.

Rihmer, Z., & Angst, J. (2009). Mood disorders: Epidemiology. In Sadock, Sadock, and Ruiz (Eds.), *Kaplan & Sadock's comprehensive textbook of psychiatry* (9th ed.). Philadelphia: Lippincott, Williams and Wilkins.

Riley, A., McEntee, M., Gerson, L., & Dennison, C. (2009). Depression as a comorbidity to diabetes: Implications for management. *The Journal for Nurse Practitioners, 5*(7), 523–534.

Rimer, J., Dwan, K., Lawlor, D. A., Greig, C. A., McMurdo, M., Morley, W., et al. (2012). Exercise for depression. *Cochrane Database of Systemic Reviews, 11*(7), CD004366.

Roy-Byrne, P. P., & Wagner, A. (2004). Primary care perspectives on generalized anxiety disorder. *Journal of Clinical Psychiatry, 65*(12 Suppl.), 20–26.

Rush, J. A., Carmody, T., & Reimitz, P. E. (2006). The Inventory of Depressive Symptomatology (IDS): Clinician (IDS-C) and Self-Report (IDS-SR) ratings of depressive symptoms. *International Journal of Methods in Psychiatric Research, 9*(2), 45–59.

Rush, A., Trivedi, M., Wisniewski, S., Nierenberg, A. A., Stewart, J. W., Warden, D., et al. (2006). Acute and longer-term outcomes in depressed outpatients requiring one or several treatment steps: A STAR*D report. *American Journal of Psychiatry, 163*, 1905–1917.

Sadock, B., & Sadock, V. (2010). *Pocket handbook of clinical psychiatry* (5th ed.). Philadelphia: Lippincott Williams & Wilkins.

Stahl, S. (2011). *The prescriber's guide (Essential Psychopharmacology Series)*. New York: Cambridge University Press.

Stahl, S. (2013). *Stahl's essential psychopharmacology: Neuroscientific basis and practical applications*. New York: Cambridge University Press.

Stein, D., Ipser, J., & Seedat, S. (2006). Pharmacotherapy for post-traumatic stress disorder. *Cochrane Database Systematic Review*

Stein, M., & Steckler, T. (Eds.). (2010). *Behavioral neurobiology of anxiety and its treatment*. New York: Springer.

Substance Abuse and Mental Health Services Administration (SAMSA). (2009). *Suicide Assessment Five-Step Evaluation and Triage (SAFE-T)*. Retrieved March 7, 2013, from http://store.samhsa.gov/shin/content//SMA09-4432/SMA09-4432.pdf

Suehs, B., Argo, T., Bendele, S., Crismon, M., Trivedi, M., & Kurian, B. (2008). *Texan Medication Algorithm Project procedural manual: Major depressive disorder algorithms*. Retrieved March 7, 2013, from http://www.pbhsolutions.org/pubdocs/upload/documents/TMAP%20Depression%202010.pdf

Thase, M. E., Haight, B. R., Richard, N., Rockett, C. B., Mitton, M., Modell, J. G., et al. (2005). Remission rates following antidepressant therapy with bupropion or selective serotonin reuptake inhibitors: A meta-analysis of original data from 7 randomized controlled trials. *Journal of Clinical Psychiatry, 66*, 974–981.

Thase, M., Friedman, E., Biggs, M., Wisniewski, S. F., Trivedi, M. H., Luther, J. F., et al. (2007). Cognitive therapy versus medication in augmentation and switch strategies as second-step treatments: A STAR*D report. *American Journal of Psychiatry, 164*(5), 739–752.

Thieme, K., Turk, D. C., & Flor, H. (2004). Comorbid depression and anxiety in fibromyalgia syndrome: Relationship to somatic and psychosocial variables. *Psychosomatic Medicine, 66*(6), 837–844.

Trivedi, M., Rush, A., Wisniewski, S., Nierenberg, A., Warden, D., Ritz, L., et al. (2006). Evaluation of outcomes with citalopram for depression using measurement-based care in STAR*D: Implications for clinical practice. *The American Journal of Psychiatry, 163*(1), 28–40.

Tronick, E., & Reck, C. (2009). Infants of depressed mothers. *Harvard Review of Psychiatry, 17*(2), 147–156.

Udechuku, A., Nguyen, T., Hill, R., & Szego, K. (2010). Antidepressants in pregnancy: A systematic review. *The Australian and New Zealand Journal of Psychiatry, 44*(11), 978–996.

U.S. Food and Drug Administration (FDA). (2007). *FDA proposes new warnings about suicidal thinking, behavior in young adults who take antidepressant medications*. Retrieved March 7, 2013, from http://www.fda.gov/NewsEvents/Newsroom/PressAnnouncements/2007/ucm108905.htm

U.S. Food and Drug Administration (FDA). (2012). *FDA Drug Safety Communication: Revised recommendations for Celexa (citalopram hydrobromide) related to a potential risk of abnormal heart rhythms with high doses*. Retrieved March 7, 2013, from http://www.fda.gov/Drugs/DrugSafety/ucm297391.htm

U.S. National Library of Medicine. (n.d.). Drugs and Lactation Database (LactMed). Retrieved March 7, 2013, from http://toxnet.nlm.nih.gov/cgi-bin/sis/htmlgen?LACT

U.S. Preventive Services Taskforce. (2009). *Screening and treatment for major depressive disorder in children and adolescents*. Retrieved from http://www.uspreventiveservicestaskforce.org/uspstf09/depression/chdeprrs.htm

U.S. Surgeon General. (2012). *2012 National strategy for suicide prevention: GOALS AND OBJECTIVES FOR ACTION*. Retrieved March 7, 2013, from http://www.surgeongeneral.gov/library/reports/national-strategy-suicide-prevention/full-report.pdf

Weber, M. (2010). The importance of exercise for individuals with chronic mental illness. *Journal of Psychosocial Nursing and Mental Health Services, 48*(10), 35–40.

Williams, J. W., Katon, W., Lin, E., et al. (2004). The effectiveness of depression care management on diabetes-related outcomes in older patients. *Annals of Internal Medicine, 140*, 1015–1024.

World Health Organization (WHO). (2012). *Depression*. Retrieved March 7, 2013, from http://www.who.int/mediacentre/factsheets/fs369/en/index.html

Wu, B. (2012). Major depression: Treatment in primary care. *Consultant*, 17–22.

van den Berg, D. P., & van der Gaag, M. (2012). Treating trauma in psychosis with EMDR: A pilot study. *Journal of Behavioral Therapy and Experimental Psychiatry, 43*(1):664–671.

Zimmerman, M., Martinez, J. H., Friedman, M., Boerescu, D. A., & Attiullah, N. (2012). How can we use depression severity to guide treatment selection when measures of depression categorize patients differently? *The Journal of Clinical Psychiatry, 73*(10), 1287–1291.

CHAPTER 30

ASTHMA AND CHRONIC OBSTRUCTIVE PULMONARY DISEASE

Benjamin J. Miller

Asthma and chronic obstructive pulmonary disease (COPD) are two of the most common chronic respiratory illnesses worldwide. According to the National Heart, Lung, and Blood Institute (NHLBI) and the World Health Organization (WHO), asthma affects more than 300 million people worldwide (Global Initiative for Asthma, 2013). COPD affects 6% of the adult U.S. population, is the third-leading cause of death, and is the 12th-leading cause of morbidity (Global Initiative for Chronic Obstructive Lung Disease [GOLD], 2014; Qaseem et al, 2011). This chapter discusses the pharmacological management of these two diseases.

ASTHMA

More than 22 million Americans, including 6 million children, have asthma (National Asthma Education and Prevention Program [NAEPP], 2007). Canada has similar statistics, with 2.3 million Canadians diagnosed with asthma in 2009 (Statistics Canada, 2010). This chapter focuses on the pharmacological management of asthma according to the current guidelines established by the NAEPP *Expert Panel Report 3: Guidelines* (2007). It includes a brief discussion of the pathophysiology of asthma to help explain the rationale for selecting appropriate medications. Monitoring and outcome evaluations are essential in asthma therapy because adjustments can have a significant impact on a patient's activity level, and patient education is the key to having patients with asthma feel that they have control over a chronic illness. The overall goal of the asthma portion of the chapter is to enable the health-care provider to render optimal care for patients with asthma.

Pathophysiology

In the past, asthma was seen as episodic bronchospasm occurring in response to specific and nonspecific stimuli. It is now known that asthma is a chronic inflammatory disorder of the airways. The airway inflammation is present even between flare-ups and can significantly alter lung function. Based on this information, the NAEPP offers the following definition:

> Asthma is a chronic inflammatory disorder of the airways in which many cells and cellular elements play a role: in particular, mast cells, eosinophils, neutrophils (especially in sudden onset, fatal exacerbations, occupational asthma, and patients who smoke), T lymphocytes, macrophages, and epithelial cells. In susceptible individuals, this inflammation causes recurrent episodes of coughing (particularly at night or early in the morning), wheezing, breathlessness, and chest tightness. These episodes are usually associated with widespread but variable airflow obstruction that is often reversible either spontaneously or with treatment (NAEPP, 2007, p 9).

When asthma therapy is adequate, inflammation can be decreased over the long term, thereby preventing most asthma-related problems.

Chronic Inflammation

The lungs of patients who have died from asthma are visually noted to be overinflated. Both large and small airways are plugged with mucus and a mixture of cell debris, inflammatory cells, and serum proteins. Microscopic examination reveals extensive infiltration of the airway lumen and wall with eosinophils, mononuclear cells accompanied by vasodilation, evidence of microvascular leakage, and epithelial disruption (NAEPP, 2007). The airway smooth muscle is often hypertrophied, with new vessel formation, increased numbers of epithelial goblet cells, mucous gland hyperplasia, and deposition of interstitial collagen beneath the epithelium. These changes further support the theory of chronic inflammation in asthma.

A series of interrelated cellular mechanisms—mast cells, eosinophils, epithelial cells, macrophages, and activated T cells—have been shown to cause inflammation and affect lung function (Fig. 30-1). These cells can influence airway function by a number of routes. The release of histamine and leukotrienes can lead directly to bronchoconstriction. The release of proinflammatory cytokines from the mast cells, macrophages, and T cells activates the neutrophils, eosinophils, and macrophages, and this activation leads to the chronic inflammation associated with asthma. Cytokines can also cause the changes found on autopsy in patients with asthma: smooth muscle hypertrophy, increased vascular permeability, and mucus secretion.

Airway Hyperresponsiveness

Airway hyperresponsiveness is a hallmark of asthma, leading to the clinical symptoms of wheezing, chest tightness, and dyspnea after exposure to stimuli such as allergens, environmental irritants, viral infections, exercise, and cold air. The inclination of airways to narrow too easily and too much is a major aspect of asthma, along with the chronic inflammation noted previously. In the past, treatment of asthma focused on treating acute attacks with bronchodilator therapy. It is now known that the underlying inflammation influences the airway in such a way as to cause airway hyperresponsiveness. An allergen may trigger the release of a multitude of cellular mediators, cytokines, and chemokines, which results in increased smooth muscle responsiveness. Therefore, treating only the bronchoconstriction without treating the underlying inflammation leads to treatment failure if inflammation is present. Treatment of asthma and decreasing airway inflammation

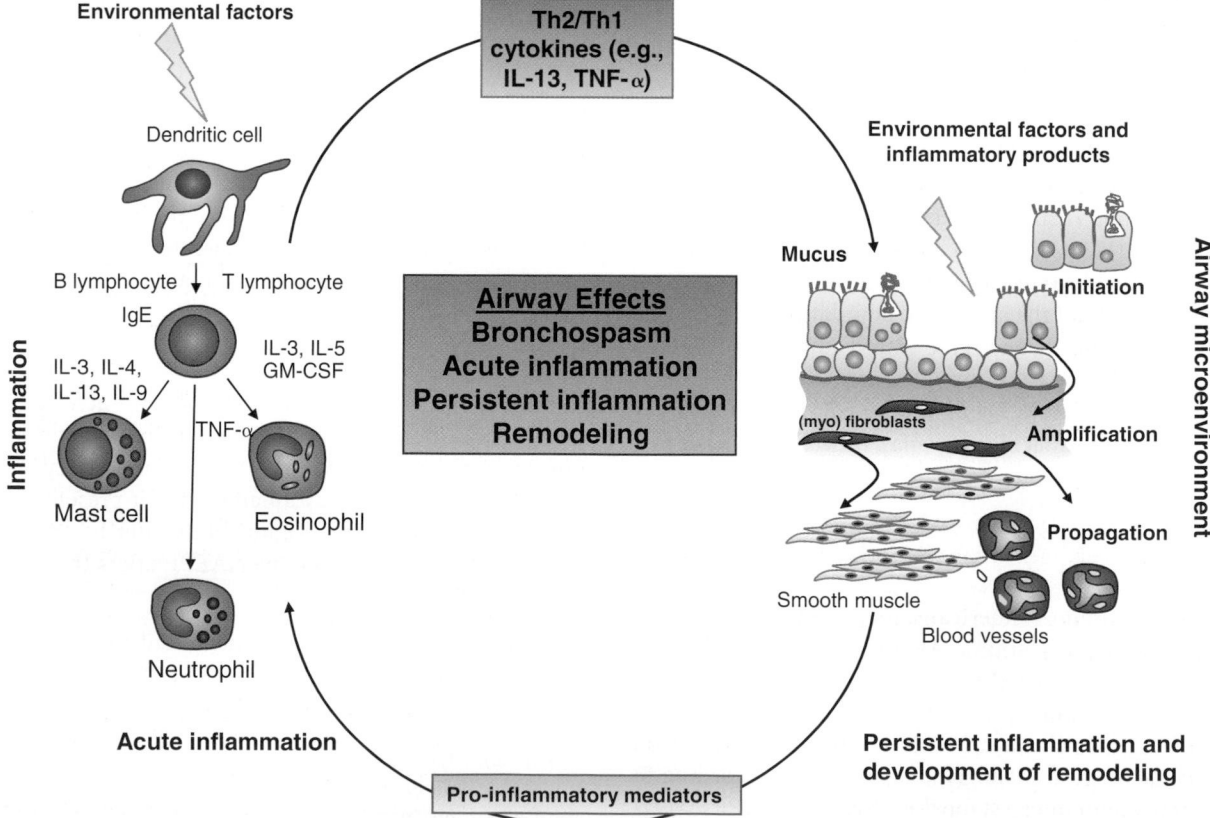

Figure 30–1. Factors limiting airflow in acute and persistent asthma. Key: GM-CSF, granulocyte-macrophage colony-stimulating factor; IgE, immunoglobulin E; IL-3, interleukin 3 (and similar); TNF-α, tumor necrosis factor-alpha. (*Source:* Holgate, S. T., & Polosa, R. [2006]. The mechanisms, diagnosis, and management of severe asthma in adults. *The Lancet, 368,* 780–793.)

not only reduces symptoms but also decreases airway hyperresponsiveness.

Airflow Obstruction

Airflow obstruction is caused by a variety of changes in the airway. Acute bronchoconstriction and airway edema are two causes already discussed. Chronic mucous plug formation caused by increased mucus secretion can also influence airflow. It is now known that in some patients, airway changes are only partially reversible. Chronic inflammation leads to airway remodeling. Histological evidence indicates that there is an alteration in the amount and composition of the extracellular matrix in the airway wall. This change is not fully understood but suggests a rationale for early, aggressive treatment with anti-inflammatory therapy.

Understanding the role of inflammation and the cellular mechanisms involved has led to new treatment strategies. Understanding the multiple mechanisms involved in airway inflammation has led to treatment aimed at either multiple components (inhaled corticosteroids) or specific mediators of inflammation. For example, leukotriene modifiers are a treatment aimed at specific mediators. Leukotrienes are responsible, in part, for increased mucus production, bronchoconstriction, and eosinophil infiltration. Leukotriene modifiers, as described in Chapter 17, are either leukotriene receptor agonists (LTRAs) (zafirlukast and montelukast) or 5-lipoxygenase pathway (zileuton). Research continues to develop a better understanding of the pathology of asthma and treatment targeted at controlling the cellular changes that occur in acute and chronic asthma.

Classification of Asthma

According to *Expert Panel Report 3: Guidelines* (NAEPP, 2007), asthma severity in children 12 years or older and adults is determined by clinical features before treatment. There are four classifications of severity, based on need for medication to relieve symptoms, nighttime symptoms, and lung function:

1. Mild intermittent asthma: Symptoms occur less often than twice a week and the patient is asymptomatic between exacerbations; nighttime symptoms occur less than twice a month; and peak expiratory flow (PEF) is greater than 80% predicted. The use of short-acting beta$_2$ agonists (SABA) should be less than twice a week, unless used for exercise-induced bronchospasm (EIB).
2. Mild persistent asthma: Symptoms occur more often than twice a week but less often than once a day and exacerbations may affect activity; nighttime symptoms occur 3 to 4 times a month; and PEF is greater than 80% predicted. Patients with mild persistent asthma may use their short-acting beta$_2$ agonists more than twice a week but not daily, and not more than once daily.
3. Moderate persistent asthma: The patient is having daily symptoms; requires daily use of a beta$_2$ agonist; exacerbations affect normal activity; nighttime symptoms

occur more often than once a week; and PEF is greater than 60% to less than 80%.
4. Severe persistent asthma: The patient has some degree of symptoms all the time; extremely limited physical activity and frequent exacerbations; frequent nighttime symptoms, often 7 days a week; and decreased lung function (PEF less than 60% predicted). Table 30-1 outlines the classifications of asthma severity in patients aged 12 years or older.

In children, classification of asthma is based on severity and frequency of symptoms (NAEPP, 2007). Table 30-2 discusses classification of asthma severity and initiating therapy in children.

1. Mild intermittent asthma: Symptoms occur less often than twice a week and the patient is asymptomatic between exacerbations. Children aged 0 to 4 years have no nighttime symptoms, and children aged 5 to 11 years have nighttime symptoms less than twice a month and PEF is greater than 80% predicted. The use of short-acting beta$_2$ agonists should be less than twice a week, unless using for EIB. Exacerbations requiring oral systemic corticosteroids occur no more than once a year.
2. Mild persistent asthma: Symptoms occur more often than twice a week but less often than once a day and exacerbations may affect activity. In children aged 0 to 4 years, nighttime symptoms occur 1 to 2 times a month, and in children aged 5 to 11 years, nighttime symptoms occur 3 to 4 times a month; PEF is greater than 80% predicted. Patients with mild persistent asthma may use their short-acting beta$_2$ agonists more than twice a week but not daily, and not more than once daily. Children younger than age 4 years with mild persistent asthma have more than two exacerbations in 6 months requiring systemic steroids or four episodes of wheezing in a year lasting more than a day and risk factors for persistent asthma. Children aged 5 to 11 with mild persistent asthma have exacerbations 2 or more times a year.
3. Moderate persistent asthma: The child is having daily symptoms; requires daily use of a beta$_2$ agonist; and exacerbations affect normal activity. In children aged 4 years or younger, nighttime symptoms occur 3 or 4 times a month, and in children aged 5 to 11 years nighttime symptoms occur more than once a week but not nightly; PEF is greater than 60% to less than 80%. Children with moderate persistent asthma have exacerbations 2 or more times a year.
4. Severe persistent asthma: The patient has some degree of symptoms all the time; extremely limited physical activity; frequent nighttime symptoms (more than once a week in children younger than age 4 years and in older children often occurring 7 days a week); and decreased lung function (PEF less than 60% predicted). Children aged 5 to 11 with severe persistent asthma have exacerbations 2 or more times a year.

Table 30–1 Classification of Asthma Severity ≥12 Years of Age

Assessing severity and initiating treatment for patients who are not currently taking long-term-control medications

Components of Severity		Classification of Asthma Severity ≥12 years of age			
	Symptoms	Intermittent	Persistent		
			Mild	Moderate	Severe
		≤2 days/week	>2 days/week but not daily	Daily	Throughout the day
Impairment	Nighttime awakenings	≤2×/month	3–4×/month	>1×/week but not nightly	Often 7×/week
	Short-acting beta₂-agonist use for symptom control (not prevention of EIB)	≤2 days/week	>2 days/week but not daily, and not more than 1× on any day	Daily	Several times per day
Normal FEV₁/FVC:	Interference with normal activity	None	Minor limitation	Some limitation	Extremely limited
8–19 yr 85% 20–39 yr 80% 40–59 yr 75% 60–80 yr 70%	Lung function	• Normal FEV₁ between exacerbations • FEV₁ >80% of predicted • FEV₁/FVC normal	• FEV₁ >80% of predicted • FEV₁/FVC normal	• FEV₁ >60% but <80% of predicted • FEV₁/FVC reduced 5%	• FEV₁ <60% of predicted • FEV₁/FVC reduced >5%
Risk	Exacerbations requiring oral systemic corticosteroids	0–1/year (see note)	≥2/year (see note)		
		Consider severity and interval since last exacerbation. Frequency and severity may fluctuate over time for patients in any severity category. Relative annual risk of exacerbations may be related to FEV₁.			
Recommended Step for Initiating Treatment. (See "Stepwise Approach for Managing Asthma" for treatment steps.)		Step 1	Step 2	Step 3	Step 4 or 5 and consider short course of oral systemic corticosteroids
		In 2–6 weeks, evaluate level of asthma control that is achieved and adjust therapy accordingly.			

Key: EIB, exercise-induced bronchospasm; FEV₁, forced expiratory volume in 1 second; FVC, forced vital capacity; ICU, intensive care unit

Notes:
- The stepwise approach is meant to assist, not replace, the clinical decision making required to meet individual patient needs.
- Level of severity is determined by assessment of both impairment and risk. Assess impairment domain by patient's/caregiver's recall of previous 2–4 weeks and spirometry. Assign severity to the most severe category in which any feature occurs.
- At present, there are inadequate data to correspond frequencies of exacerbations with different levels of asthma severity. In general, more frequent and intense exacerbations (e.g., requiring urgent, unscheduled care, hospitalization, or ICU admission) indicate greater underlying disease severity. For treatment purposes, patients who had ≥2 exacerbations requiring oral systemic corticosteroids in the past year may be considered the same as patients who have persistent asthma, even in the absence of impairment levels consistent with persistent asthma.

Source: From National Asthma Education and Prevention Program (NAEPP). (2007). The Expert Panel Report 3: Guidelines for the diagnosis and management of asthma. Bethesda, MD: National Heart, Lung, and Blood Institute, National Institutes of Health.

Goals of Therapy

The Expert Panel Report 3: Guidelines (NAEPP, 2007) clearly define the goals of asthma therapy:

Reduce Impairment

1. Prevent chronic and troublesome symptoms (e.g., coughing or breathlessness in the night, in the early morning, or after exertion).
2. Require infrequent use (less than twice a week) of inhaled short-acting beta₂ agonists for relief of symptoms (not including use for EIB).

3. Maintain (near) "normal" pulmonary function.
4. Maintain (near) normal activity levels.
5. Meet patients' and families' expectations of and satisfaction with asthma care.

Reduce Risk

1. Prevent recurrent exacerbations of asthma and minimize the need for emergency department visits or hospitalizations.
2. Prevent loss of lung function; for children, prevent reduced lung growth.

Table 30–2 Classification of Asthma Severity and Initial Therapy in Children

Classifying Asthma Severity and Initiating Therapy in Children

| Components of Severity | Intermittent | | Persistent | | | | | |
| | | | Mild | | Moderate | | Severe | |
	Ages 0–4	Ages 5–11	Ages 0–4	Ages 5–11	Ages 0–4	Ages 5–11	Ages 0–4	Ages 5–11
Impairment								
Symptoms	≤2 days/week		>2 days/week but not daily		Daily	Daily		Throughout the day
Nighttime awakenings	0	<2×/month	1–2×/month	3–4×/month	3–4×/month	>1×/week but not nightly	>1×/week	Often 2×/week
Short-acting beta₂-agonist use for symptom control	≤2 days/week		>2 days/week but not daily		Daily			Several times per day
Interference with normal activity	None		Minor limitation		Some limitation		Extremely limited	
Lung function • FEV₁ (predicted) or peak flow (personal best) • FEV₁/FVC	N/A	Normal FEV₁ between exacerbations >80% >80%	N/A	>80% >85%	N/A	60%–80% 75%–80%	N/A	<60% <75%
Risk								
Exacerbations requiring oral systemic corticosteroids (consider severity and interval since last exacerbation)	0–1/yr (see notes)		≥2 exacerbations in 6 months requiring oral systemic corticosteroids, or ≥4 wheezing episodes/1 year lasting >1 day AND risk factors for persistent asthma	≥2×/year (see notes) Relative annual risk may be related to FEV₁				
Recommended Step for Initiating Therapy. (See "Stepwise Approach for Managing Asthma" for treatment steps.) The stepwise approach is meant to assist, not replace, the clinical decision making required to meet individual patient needs.	Step 1 (for both age groups)		Step 2 (for both age groups)		Step 3 and consider short course of oral systemic corticosteroids	Step 3: medium-dose ICS option and consider short course of oral systemic corticosteroids	Step 3 and consider short course of oral systemic corticosteroids	Step 3: medium-dose ICS option OR step 4 and consider short course of oral systemic corticosteroids

In 2–6 weeks, depending on severity, evaluate level of asthma control that is achieved.
• Children 0–4 years old: If no clear benefit is observed in 4–6 weeks, stop treatment and consider alternative diagnoses or adjusting therapy.
• Children 5–11 years old: Adjust therapy accordingly.

Key: FEV₁, forced expiratory volume in 1 second; FVC, forced vital capacity; ICS, inhaled corticosteroids; ICU, intensive care unit; N/A, not applicable

Notes:
• Level of severity is determined by both impairment and risk. Assess impairment domain by caregiver's recall of previous 2–4 weeks. Assign severity to the most severe category in which any feature occurs.
• Frequency and severity of exacerbations may fluctuate over time for patients in any severity category. At present, there are inadequate data to correspond frequencies of exacerbations with different levels of asthma severity. In general, more frequent and severe exacerbations (e.g., requiring urgent, unscheduled care, hospitalization, or ICU admission) indicate greater underlying disease severity. For treatment purposes, patients with ≥2 exacerbations described above may be considered the same as patients who have persistent asthma, even in the absence of impairment levels consistent with persistent asthma.

Source: From National Asthma Education and Prevention Program (NAEPP). (2007). The Expert Panel Report 3: Guidelines for the diagnosis and management of asthma. Bethesda, MD: National Heart, Lung, and Blood Institute, National Institutes of Health.

3. Provide optimal pharmacotherapy with minimal or no adverse effects.

Rational Drug Selection

Asthma Step Therapy

The Expert Panel Report 3: Guidelines (NAEPP, 2007) recommends a stepwise approach to the pharmacological management of asthma. Management can begin at a higher level and gradually step down or start low and move up, depending on the patient's status when beginning treatment. The panel recommends that medications be categorized into two general classes: long-term-control medications to achieve and maintain control of persistent asthma and quick-relief medications to treat acute symptoms and exacerbations. Asthma severity determines the amount and frequency of medication, with suppression of airway inflammation the goal. One essential component of asthma treatment is the patient's cooperation in keeping a log of asthma symptoms. This patient self-assessment enables the provider to track the effectiveness of therapy and make treatment decisions based on medication use, nighttime symptoms, and PEF. Although step therapy is a helpful framework, the clinician must individualize therapy based on a patient's individual circumstances and response to therapy.

Initiating Control of Asthma

The *Expert Panel Report 3: Guidelines* (NAEPP, 2007) prefers an aggressive approach of gaining quick control with a higher level of therapy and then stepping down the care. A stepwise approach for managing asthma incorporates assessment of severity to initiate therapy or assessment of control to monitor or adjust therapy. New to the 2007 *Expert Panel Report 3: Guidelines* is the recommendation to assess asthma control and adjust therapy accordingly at regular intervals (NAEPP, 2007). Asthma control is "the degree to which the manifestations of asthma are minimized by therapeutic intervention and the goals of therapy are met" (NAEPP, 2007).

Once patients have received initial treatment for their asthma, they need ongoing monitoring to assess the degree of control. Control is based on level of impairment (symptoms, nighttime awakenings, interference with normal activity, SABA use, and spirometry or peak flows. Validated questionnaires can be used to measure level of impairment found in the *Expert Panel 3 Report: Guidelines* (Asthma Therapy Assessment Questionnaire, Asthma Control Questionnaire and Asthma Control Test) (NAEPP, 2007). Patients should be assessed regarding risk in relation to exacerbations. Table 30-3 outlines assessment of control in youths 12 years of age or older and adults; Table 30-4 is the assessment of control for children. The stepwise approach to treating asthma in adults is found in Table 30-5 and in children in Table 30-6. Drugs commonly used to treat asthma are shown in Table 30-7. Additional components of care include patient education and environmental control measures. See also Tables 30-7 and 30-8.

Mild Intermittent Asthma

Treatment for mild intermittent asthma symptoms consists of using short-acting inhaled beta$_2$ agonists as needed for symptoms, including patients who have asthma symptoms only when exposed to their asthma triggers (e.g., allergens, viral respiratory illness, chemical inhalants), people who have only exercise-induced asthma, and infants and children who wheeze with viral upper respiratory infections (NAEPP, 2007). Using short-acting beta$_2$ agonists more than twice a week may indicate a need to step up to step 2 therapy or to initiate long-term-control therapy. Education at this step is introducing the patient and family to the use of medication and teaching them about asthma, proper inhaler technique if appropriate, care during exacerbation of symptoms, and environmental controls to known allergens.

The *Expert Panel Report 3: Guidelines* (NAEPP, 2007) recommends that patients with mild asthma use their albuterol inhaler on an as-needed basis, which enables patients to feel that they have some control over their asthma. More frequent use (more than twice a week) indicates a need to step up therapy. Mild intermittent asthma is not inconsequential, as attacks can be severe, and it varies from patient to patient.

Mild Persistent Asthma

The recommended treatment for patients with mild persistent asthma is one long-term-control medication daily. The primary treatment is inhaled anti-inflammatory medication. Treatment is started with inhaled low-dose corticosteroids (ICS) for all age groups.

The suggested beginning dose of inhaled steroids is 80 to 240 mcg/d of beclomethasone HFA (QVAR) or 180 to 600 mcg/d of budesonide (Pulmicort Turbuhaler) or the equivalent. Sustained-release theophylline to serum concentrations of 5 to 15 mcg/mL is an alternative therapy, but it should be used with caution and with close monitoring of serum theophylline levels. Inhaled short-acting beta$_2$ agonists are used as needed to relieve symptoms. If symptoms persist, inhaled corticosteroids should be increased to 240 to 480 mcg/d of beclomethasone HFA (QVAR), which is three to six puffs per day of an 80 mcg/puff or the equivalent. If a patient is requiring daily use of inhaled beta$_2$ agonists and is using the medications correctly, then step 3 therapy is indicated. Patient education at this step is teaching self-monitoring and developing and reviewing the self-management plan.

An alternative to ICS is the use of mast cell stabilizers such as cromolyn (Intal) and nedocromil (Tilade). Mast cells are associated with asthma and other inflammatory processes. Specifically with asthma, there is hyperplasia of mast cells within the bronchial linings. With mast cell degranulation, histamines are released, resulting in bronchial constriction and acute asthma exacerbations. This class of medication prevents the breakdown of mast cells, thus stabilizing the bronchial epithelial cells, and has been found especially useful in exercise-induced bronchospasm or mild persistent asthma (Netzer, Küpper, Voss, & Eliasson, 2012; Schofield, 2014). A

(Text continued on page 928)

Table 30–3   Assessing Asthma Control and Adjusting Therapy in Youths >12 Years and Adults

Components of Control		Classification of Asthma Control (≥12 years of age)		
		Well Controlled	*Not Well Controlled*	*Very Poorly Controlled*
Impairment	Sᴍᴘᴛᴏᴍs	≤2 days/week	>2 days/week	Throughout the day
	Nighttime awakenings	≤2×/month	1–3×/week	>4×/week
	Interference with normal activity	None	Some limitation	Extremely limited
	Short-acting beta₂-agonist use for symptom control (not prevention of EIB)	≤2 days/week	>2 days/week	Several times per day
	FEV₁ or peak flow	>80% of predicted/ personal best	60%–80% of predicted/ personal best	<60% of predicted/ personal best
	Validated questionnaires			
	ATAQ	0	1–2	3–4
	ACQ	<0.75*	≥1.5	N/A
	ACT	≥20	16–19	≤15
Risk	**Exacerbations requiring oral systemic corticosteroids**	0–1/year	≥2/year (see note)	
		Consider severity and interval since last exacerbation		
	Progressive loss of lung function	Evaluation requires long-term follow-up care.		
	Treatment-related adverse effects			
		Medication side effects can vary in intensity from none to very troublesome and worrisome. The level of intensity does not correlate to specific levels of control but should be considered in the overall assessment of risk.		
Recommended Action for Treatment (See "Stepwise Approach for Managing Asthma" for treatment steps.)		• Maintain current step. • Regular follow-up at every 1–6 months to maintain control. • Consider step down if well controlled for at least 3 months.	• Step up 1 step. • Reevaluate in 2–6 weeks. • For side effects, consider alternative treatment options.	• Consider short course of oral systemic corticosteroids. • Step up 1–2 steps. • Reevaluate in 2 weeks. • For side effects, consider alternative treatment options.

*ACQ values of 0.76–1.4 are indeterminate regarding well-controlled asthma.

Key: EIB, exercise-induced bronchospasm; ICU, intensive care unit

Notes:

- The stepwise approach is meant to assist, not replace, the clinical decision making required to meet individual patient needs.

- The level of control is based on the most severe impairment or risk category. Assess impairment domain by patient's recall of previous 2–4 weeks and by spirometry or peak flow measures. Symptom assessment for longer periods should reflect a global assessment, such as inquiring whether the patient's asthma is better or worse since the last visit.

- At present, there are inadequate data to correspond frequencies of exacerbations with different levels of asthma control. In general, more frequent and intense exacerbations (e.g., requiring urgent, unscheduled care, hospitalization, or ICU admission) indicate poorer disease control. For treatment purposes, patients who had ≥2 exacerbations requiring oral systemic corticosteroids in the past year may be considered the same as patients who have not-well-controlled asthma, even in the absence of impairment levels consistent with not-well-controlled asthma.

ATAQ = Asthma Therapy Assessment Questionnaire

ACQ = Asthma Control Questionnaire

ACT = Asthma Control Test

Minimal Important

Difference: 1.0 for the ATAQ; 0.5 for the ACQ; not determined for the ACT.

Before step up in therapy:

—Review adherence to medication, inhaler technique, environmental control, and comorbid conditions.

—If an alternative treatment option was used in a step, discontinue and use the preferred treatment for that step.

Source: From National Asthma Education and Prevention Program (NAEPP). (2007). *The Expert Panel Report 3: Guidelines for the diagnosis and management of asthma.* Bethesda, MD: National Heart, Lung, and Blood Institute, National Institutes of Health.

Table 30–4 Assessing Asthma Control and Adjusting Therapy in Children

Components of Control		Well Controlled		Not Well Controlled		Very Poorly Controlled	
		Ages 0–4	*Ages 5–11*	*Ages 0–4*	*Ages 5–11*	*Ages 0–4*	*Ages 5–11*
	Sᴍᴘᴛᴏᴍs	≤2 days/week but not more than once on each day		>2 days/week or multiple times on ≤2 days/week		Throughout the day	
	Nighttime awakenings	≤1×/month		>1×/month	**≥2×/month**	>1×/week	**≥2×/week**
	Interference with normal activity	None		Some limitation		Extremely limited	
Impairment	Short-acting beta₂-agonist use for symptom control (not prevention of EIB)	≤2 days/week		>2 days/week		Several times per day	
	Lung function • FEV₁ (predicted) or peak • FEV₁/FVC flow personal best	N/A	>80% >80%	N/A	60%–80% 75%–80%	N/A	<60% <75%
	Exacerbations requiring oral systemic corticosteroids	0–1×/year		2–3×/year	≥2×/year	>3×/year	≥2×/year
Risk	Reduction in lung growth	N/A	**Requires long-term follow-up**	N/A		N/A	
	Treatment-related adverse effects	Medication side effects can vary in intensity from none to very troublesome and worrisome. The level of intensity does not correlate to specific levels of control but should be considered in the overall assessment of risk.					
Recommended Action for Treatment (See "Stepwise Approach for Managing Asthma" for treatment steps.) The stepwise approach is meant to assist, not replace, the clinical decision making required to meet individual patient needs.		• Maintain current step. • Regular follow up every 1–6 months. • Consider step down if well controlled for at least 3 months.		Step up 1 step.	Step up at least 1 step.	• Consider short course of oral systemic corticosteroids. • Step up 1–2 steps.	

• Before step up:
  Review adherence to medication, inhaler technique, and environmental control.
  If alternative treatment was used, discontinue it and use preferred treatment for that step.
• Reevaluate the level of asthma control in 2–6 weeks to achieve control; every 1–6 months to maintain control.
  Children 0–4 years old: If no clear benefit is observed in 4–6 weeks, consider alternative diagnoses or adjusting therapy.
  Children 5–11 years old: Adjust therapy accordingly.
• For side effects, consider alternative treatment options.

Key: EIB, exercise-induced bronchospasm; FEV₁, forced expiratory volume in 1 second; FVC, forced vital capacity; ICU, intensive care unit; N/A, not applicable

Notes:
• The level of control is based on the most severe impairment or risk category. Assess impairment domain by patient's or caregiver's recall of previous 2–4 weeks. Symptom assessment for longer periods should reflect a global assessment, such as whether the patient's asthma is better or worse since the last visit.
• At present, there are inadequate data to correspond frequencies of exacerbations with different levels of asthma control. In general, more frequent and intense exacerbations (e.g., requiring urgent, unscheduled care, hospitalization, or ICU admission) indicate poorer disease control.

Source: From National Asthma Education and Prevention Program (NAEPP). (2007). *The Expert Panel Report 3: Guidelines for the diagnosis and management of asthma.* Bethesda, MD: National Heart, Lung, and Blood Institute, National Institutes of Health.

Table 30–5 Stepwise Approach for Managing Asthma in Youths >12 Years and Adults

Stepwide Approach for Managing Asthma in Youths 12 Years of Age and Adults

Intermittent Asthma

Persistent Asthma: Daily Medication
Consult with asthma specialist if step 4 or higher is required.
Consider consultation at step 3.

Step 1
Preferred:
SABA PRN

Step 2
Preferred:
Low-dose ICS
Alternative:
Cromolyn, LTRA, Nedocromil, or Theophylline

Step 3
Preferred:
Low-dose ICS + LABA
or
Medium-dose ICS
Alternative:
Low-dose ICS + either LTRA, Theophylline, or Zileuton

Step 4
Preferred:
Medium-dose ICS + LABA
Alternative:
Medium-dose ICS + either LTRA, Theophylline, or Zileuton

Step 5
Preferred:
High-dose ICS + LABA
and
Consider Omalizumab for patients who have allergies

Step 6
Preferred:
High-dose ICS + LABA + oral corticosteroid
and
Consider Omalizumab for patients who have allergies

Step up if needed
(first, check adherence, environmental control, and comorbid conditions)

Assess control

Step down if possible
(and asthma is well controlled at least 3 months)

Each step: Patient education, environmental control, and management of comorbidities
Steps 2–4: Consider subcutaneous allergen immunotherapy for patients who have allergic asthma (see notes).

Quick-Relief Medication for All Patients
- SABA as needed for symptoms. Intensity of treatment depends on severity of symptoms: up to 3 treatments at 20-minute intervals as needed. Short course of oral systemic corticosteroids may be needed.
- Use of SABA >2 days a week for symptom relief (not prevention of EIB) generally indicates inadequate control and the need to step up treatment.

Key: **Alphabetical order is usually more than one treatment option listed within either preferred or alternative therapy.** ICS, inhaled corticosteroid; LABA, inhaled long-acting beta₂-agonist, LTRA, leukotriene receptor antagonist; SABA, inhaled short-acting beta₂-agonist.

Notes:

- The stepwise approach is meant to assist, not replace, the clinical decision making required to meet individual patient needs.

- If alternative treatment is used and response is inadequate, discontinue it and use the preferred treatment before stepping up.

- Zileuton is a less desirable alternative due to limited studies as adjunctive therapy and the need to monitor liver function. Theophylline requires monitoring of serum concentration levels.

- In step 6, before oral corticosteroids are introduced, a trial of high-dose ICS + LABA + either LTRA, theophylline, or zileuton may be considered, although this approach has not been studied in clinical trials.

- Step 1, 2, and 3 preferred therapies are based on Evidence A; step 3 alternative therapy is based on Evidence A for LTRA, Evidence B for theophylline, and Evidence D for zileuton. Step 4 preferred therapy is based on Evidence B, and alternative therapy is based on Evidence B for LTRA and theophylline and Evidence D zileuton. Step 5 preferred therapy is based on Evidence B. Step 6 preferred therapy is based on (EPR—2 1997) and Evidence B for omalizumab.

- Immunotherapy for steps 2–4 is based on Evidence B for house-dust mites, animal danders, and pollens; evidence is weak or lacking for molds and cockroaches. Evidence is strongest for immunotherapy with single allergens. The role of allergy in asthma is greater in children than in adults.

- Clinicians who administer immunotherapy or omalizumab should be prepared and equipped to identify and treat anaphylaxis that may occur.

Source: From National Asthma Education and Prevention Program (NAEPP). (2007). *The Expert Panel Report 3: Guidelines for the diagnosis and management of asthma*. Bethesda, MD: National Heart, Lung, and Blood Institute, National Institutes of Health.

Table 30–6 Stepwise Approach for Managing Asthma Long Term in Children

Stepwide Approach for Managing Asthma Long Term in Children 0–4 Years and 5–11 Years of Age

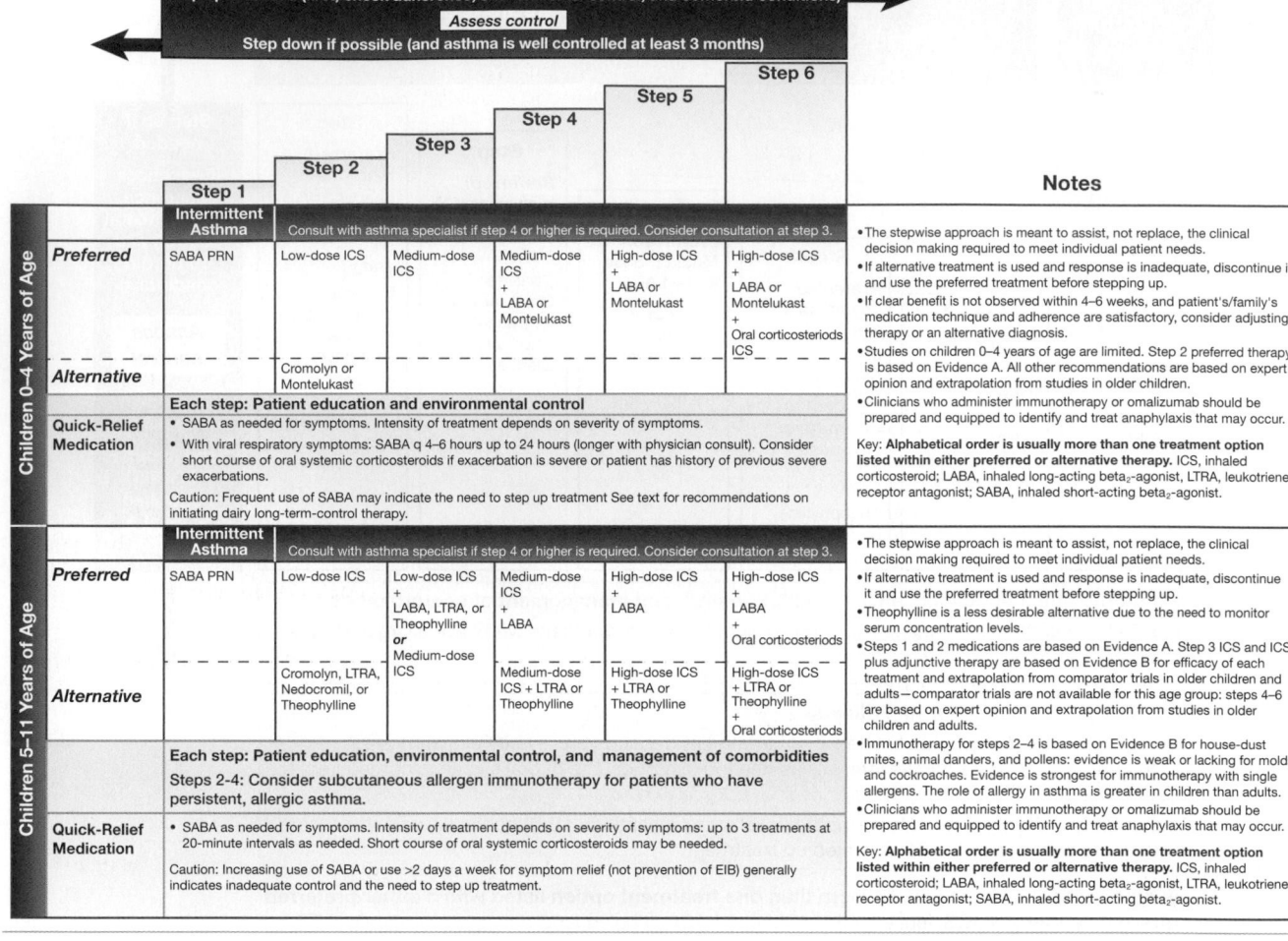

Step up if needed (first, check adherence, environmental control, and comorbid conditions)

Assess control

Step down if possible (and asthma is well controlled at least 3 months)

Children 0–4 Years of Age

		Step 1	Step 2	Step 3	Step 4	Step 5	Step 6	Notes
		Intermittent Asthma	Consult with asthma specialist if step 4 or higher is required. Consider consultation at step 3.					• The stepwise approach is meant to assist, not replace, the clinical decision making required to meet individual patient needs.
Preferred		SABA PRN	Low-dose ICS	Medium-dose ICS	Medium-dose ICS + LABA or Montelukast	High-dose ICS + LABA or Montelukast	High-dose ICS + LABA or Montelukast + Oral corticosteriods ICS	• If alternative treatment is used and response is inadequate, discontinue it and use the preferred treatment before stepping up. • If clear benefit is not observed within 4–6 weeks, and patient's/family's medication technique and adherence are satisfactory, consider adjusting therapy or an alternative diagnosis.
Alternative			Cromolyn or Montelukast					• Studies on children 0–4 years of age are limited. Step 2 preferred therapy is based on Evidence A. All other recommendations are based on expert opinion and extrapolation from studies in older children.
		**Each step: Patient education and environmental control**						• Clinicians who administer immunotherapy or omalizumab should be prepared and equipped to identify and treat anaphylaxis that may occur.
Quick-Relief Medication		• SABA as needed for symptoms. Intensity of treatment depends on severity of symptoms. • With viral respiratory symptoms: SABA q 4–6 hours up to 24 hours (longer with physician consult). Consider short course of oral systemic corticosteroids if exacerbation is severe or patient has history of previous severe exacerbations. Caution: Frequent use of SABA may indicate the need to step up treatment See text for recommendations on initiating dairy long-term-control therapy.						Key: **Alphabetical order is usually more than one treatment option listed within either preferred or alternative therapy.** ICS, inhaled corticosteroid; LABA, inhaled long-acting beta₂-agonist, LTRA, leukotriene receptor antagonist; SABA, inhaled short-acting beta₂-agonist.

Children 5–11 Years of Age

		Step 1	Step 2	Step 3	Step 4	Step 5	Step 6	Notes
		Intermittent Asthma	Consult with asthma specialist if step 4 or higher is required. Consider consultation at step 3.					• The stepwise approach is meant to assist, not replace, the clinical decision making required to meet individual patient needs.
Preferred		SABA PRN	Low-dose ICS	Low-dose ICS + LABA, LTRA, or Theophylline **or** Medium-dose ICS	Medium-dose ICS + LABA	High-dose ICS + LABA	High-dose ICS + LABA + Oral corticosteriods	• If alternative treatment is used and response is inadequate, discontinue it and use the preferred treatment before stepping up. • Theophylline is a less desirable alternative due to the need to monitor serum concentration levels.
Alternative			Cromolyn, LTRA, Nedocromil, or Theophylline		Medium-dose ICS + LTRA or Theophylline	High-dose ICS + LTRA or Theophylline	High-dose ICS + LTRA or Theophylline + Oral corticosteriods	• Steps 1 and 2 medications are based on Evidence A. Step 3 ICS and ICS plus adjunctive therapy are based on Evidence B for efficacy of each treatment and extrapolation from comparator trials in older children and adults—comparator trials are not available for this age group: steps 4–6 are based on expert opinion and extrapolation from studies in older children and adults.
		Each step: Patient education, environmental control, and management of comorbidities Steps 2-4: Consider subcutaneous allergen immunotherapy for patients who have persistent, allergic asthma.						• Immunotherapy for steps 2–4 is based on Evidence B for house-dust mites, animal danders, and pollens: evidence is weak or lacking for molds and cockroaches. Evidence is strongest for immunotherapy with single allergens. The role of allergy in asthma is greater in children than adults.
Quick-Relief Medication		• SABA as needed for symptoms. Intensity of treatment depends on severity of symptoms: up to 3 treatments at 20-minute intervals as needed. Short course of oral systemic corticosteroids may be needed. Caution: Increasing use of SABA or use >2 days a week for symptom relief (not prevention of EIB) generally indicates inadequate control and the need to step up treatment.						• Clinicians who administer immunotherapy or omalizumab should be prepared and equipped to identify and treat anaphylaxis that may occur. Key: **Alphabetical order is usually more than one treatment option listed within either preferred or alternative therapy.** ICS, inhaled corticosteroid; LABA, inhaled long-acting beta₂-agonist, LTRA, leukotriene receptor antagonist; SABA, inhaled short-acting beta₂-agonist.

Source: From National Asthma Education and Prevention Program (NAEPP). (2007). *The Expert Panel Report 3: Guidelines for the diagnosis and management of asthma.* Bethesda, MD: National Heart, Lung, and Blood Institute, National Institutes of Health.

Table 30–7 Drugs Commonly Used: Asthma and COPD

Drug	Dosage	How Supplied	Comments
Short-Acting Bronchodilators			
Albuterol HFA (Ventolin HFA, Proventil HFA, ProAir HFA)	*Inhaler* 2 puffs q4–6h 2 puffs 15 min prior to exercise	*Metered-Dose Inhaler* 90 mcg/puff	• May repeat dose in 5–10 min during exacerbations
Albuterol	*Nebulizer* (run over 10–15 min) *Adults:* Dilute 0.5 mL of 0.5% solution in 3 mL normal saline *or* give 1 unit dose Tablets: 2 mg, 4 mg *Children:* 0.01–0.03 mL/kg of 0.5% solution diluted in 2 mL normal saline *Oral* *Adults:* 2–4 mg tid or qid up to a max of 32 mg/d *Children 6–12 yr:* 2 mg tid or qid *Children <6 yr:* 0.1 mg/kg divided tid	*Solution for Nebulizer* 0.5% (5 mg/mL) 0.083 in unit-dose vial *Oral* Extended-release tabs: 4 mg, 8 mg Syrup: 2 mg/5 mL	• Check proper inhaler technique with every clinic visit

Table 30–7   Drugs Commonly Used: Asthma and COPD—cont'd

Drug	Dosage	How Supplied	Comments
Levalbuterol (R-albuterol, Xopenex)	*Nebulizer* 0.31 mg/3 mL 0.63 mg/3 mL 1.25 mg/3 mL *Adults:* 0.63 mg–2.5 mg q4–8 h *Children:* 0.025 mg/kg (min 0.63 mg, max 1.25 mg) q4–8h *Inhaler* *Children ≥5 yr and adults:* 2 puffs every 4–6 h *Children <5 yr:* not FDA approved	*Nebulizer Solution* 0.63 mg of levalbuterol is equivalent in efficacy and side effects to 1.25 mg of racemic albuterol. The product is a sterile-filled preservative-free unit dose vial. *Inhaler* 45 mcg/puff	Levalbuterol has not been evaluated for continuous nebulization therapy
Terbutaline (Brethine)	*Oral* *Children >15 yr and adults:* 5 mg tid; maximum 15 mg/24 h *Children 12–15 yr:* 2.5 mg tid; maximum 7.5 mg/24 h *Parenteral* *Adults:* 0.5 mg SC in the lateral deltoid; may repeat in 15–30 min; maximum dose 0.5 mg in 4 h	*Oral* Tablets: 2.5 mg, 5 mg *Parenteral* 1 mg/mL	• Not recommended for children <12 yr • Terbutaline is used to control premature contractions in pregnant women; use with care in the patient in the third trimester nearing her expected date of confinement (EDC), because it may affect labor
Bitolterol (Tornalate)	*Inhaler* *Children >12 yr and adults:* For bronchospasm: 2 puffs 1–3 min apart, followed by a third puff if needed For prevention of bronchospasm: 2 puffs every 8 h	*Inhaler* 0.37 mg/puff	• Not recommended for children <12 yr
Pirbuterol (Maxair inhaler)	*Inhaler* *Children >12 yr and adults:* 1–2 puffs q 4–6 h; maximum 12 puffs/day	*Inhaler* 0.2 mg/puff	Not recommended for children <12 yr
Long-Acting Bronchodilator			
Salmeterol (Serevent Diskus)	*Diskus Inhaler* *Children >4 yr and adults:* For asthma and control of bronchospasm: 1 inhalation bid For exercise-induced asthma: 1 inhalation 30–60 min prior to exercise	*Discus Inhaler* 50 mcg/inhalation	**Not to be prescribed as monotherapy for persistent asthma.** Not to be used for short-term relief. Patients need to have a short-acting bronchodilator also prescribed for short-term relief and told not to use drug for acute exacerbations. If using salmeterol twice a day, do not use another dose for exercise-induced asthma; a short-acting bronchodilator or cromolyn should be used.
Formoterol (Foradil)	DPI 12 mcg/single-use capsule *Children ≥5 yr and adults:* Inhale 1 capsule q12h Note: Capsule is not to be swallowed	12 mcg capsule	Each capsule is for single use only; additional doses should not be administered for at least 12 h. Capsules should be used only with the Aerolizer inhaler and should not be taken orally. Efficacy and safety have not been studied in children <5 yr.

Continued

Table 30–7 Drugs Commonly Used: Asthma and COPD—cont'd

Drug	Dosage	How Supplied	Comments
Anticholinergic Agents			
Ipratropium bromide (Atrovent, Atrovent HFA)	*Inhaler* *Children >12 yr and adults:* 2–3 puffs qid; maximum 12 puffs/24 h 500 mcg per unit-dose vial *or* 0.25 mg/mL *Children:* 1–2 puffs q6h *Nebulizer* 1-unit dose *Adults:* 0.5 mg q30min for 3 doses, then 0.25 mg q6h *Children:* 0.25 mg q20min for 3 doses, then 0.25 mg q6h 0.5 mg/3 mL ipratropium bromide and 2.5 mg/ 3 mL albuterol *Adults:* 2–3 puffs q6h *Adults:* 3 mL q4–6h *Children:* 1.5–3 mL q8h	*Inhaler* 17 mcg/puff *Solution for Nebulizer* • Contraindicated in patients with soybean or peanut allergy.	• Can be mixed with albuterol 0.5% solution for nebulizer use if used within 1 h.
Tiotropium (Spiriva)	*HandiHaler* *Adults with COPD:* 2 inhalations of the powder contents of a single capsule once daily	DPI capsule: 18 mcg/capsule	Not approved for use in children. Approved for use in COPD.
Combination Inhaled Medications			
Albuterol/ipratropium bromide (Combivent)	*Inhaler* *Children:* 1–2 puffs q8h *Adults:* 2 puffs qid	*Inhaler* Ipratropium 18 mcg/puff combined with albuterol 90 mcg/puff	• Primarily used for COPD patients
	Nebulizer *Adults:* 3 mL every 30 min for 3 doses, then q2–4h prn *Children:* 1.5 mL q20min for 3 doses then every 2–4 h	*Solution for Nebulizer* Each 3 mL vial contains 0.5 mg ipratropium bromide and 2.5 mg albuterol.	• Simplifies medication regimen by combining two commonly prescribed medications • Not recommended for children
Fluticasone/Salmeterol (Advair Diskus)	DPI 100 mcg, 250 mcg, or 500 mcg/50 mcg *Adults:* 1 inhalation bid; dose depends on severity of asthma *Children:* 1 inhalation bid; dose depends on severity of asthma	Not FDA approved in children <12 yr. 100/50 for patient not controlled on low-to-medium dose inhaled corticosteroids. 250/50 for patients not controlled on medium- to-high dose inhaled corticosteroids.	
Budesonide and formoterol (Symbicort)	*Inhaler* *Children 5 to 11 yr:* Symbicort 80/4.5, 2 inhalation bid *Children ≥12 yr and adults:* Symbicort 80/4.5, 2 inhalations bid *or* Symbicort 160/4.5, 2 inhalations bid (medium dose steroid)	*Inhaler* Symbicort 80/4.5 containing 80 and 4.5 mcg of formoterol fumarate dihydrate per inhalation Symbicort 160/4.5 containing 160 mcg of budesonide and 4.5 mcg of formoterol fumarate dihydrate per inhalation.	

Table 30–7   Drugs Commonly Used: Asthma and COPD—cont'd

Drug	Dosage	How Supplied	Comments
Systemic Corticosteroids			
Prednisone	*Adults:* "Burst" therapy 40–60 mg/d in 1 or 2 doses *Children:* "Burst" 1–2 mg/kg/d in 1–2 doses; maximum of 60 mg/d	*Tablets* 5, 10, 20 mg	If given in short "bursts" of 3–10 days, dose does not have to be tapered
Prednisolone (Prelone, Pediapred syrup)	*Children:* "Burst" 1–2 mg/kg/d in 1–2 doses; maximum of 40–50 mg/d	*Syrup* Pediapred 5 mg/5 mL Prelone 15 mg/5 mL	Same as for prednisone
Inhaled Anti-Inflammatory Agents			
Cromolyn (Intal)	*Nebulizer* *Children >2 yr and adults:* 1-unit dose qid, weaning down to bid	*Solution for Nebulizer* 20 mg/2 mL ampule	• Must be used continuously for 3–4 wk before maximum effect is achieved • Very safe to use in children, with fewer adverse reactions than inhaled steroids
Nedocromil (Tilade)	*Nebulizer* *Adults and children >2 yr:* 1 ampule via nebulizer qid	*Solution for Nebulizer* 11 mg/2.2 mL ampule	
Inhaled Corticosteroids			
Beclomethasone dipropionate Beclomethasone HFA (QVAR)	*Adults:* *Low dose:* 80–240 mcg *Medium dose:* 240–480 mcg *High dose:* >480 mcg *Children:* *Low dose:* 80–160 mcg *Medium dose:* 160–320 mcg *High dose:* >320 mcg	QVAR MDI 40 mcg/puff 80 mcg/puff	
Budesonide (Pulmicort Flexihaler)	*Adults:* *Low dose:* 180–600 mcg daily (1 or 2 inhalations daily) *Medium dose:* 600–1,200 mcg daily (2–3 inhalations daily) *High dose:* >1,200 mcg daily (>3 inhalations daily) *Children:* *Low dose:* 200 mcg daily (1 inhalation daily) *Medium dose:* 200–400 mcg daily (2–3 inhalations daily) *High dose:* >400 mcg/d (>2 inhalations daily)	*Turbohaler DPI* 90 mcg/puff 180 mcg/puff 200 mcg/puff	
Budesonide Inhalation suspension (Pulmicort Respules) for nebulization (child dose)	*Children 4 yr:* *Low dose:* 0.25 to 0.5 mg/d *Medium dose:* 0.5 mg to 1.0 mg/d *High dose:* 2.0 mg *Children 5–11 yr:* *Low dose:* 0.5 mg/d *Medium dose:* 1.0 mg/d *High dose:* 2.0 mg/d	*Suspension for Nebulizer* 0.25 mg/mL 0.5 mg/mL	
Flunisolide (Aerobid)	*Children ≥12 yr and adults:* *Low dose:* 500–1,000 mcg daily (2–4 puffs daily divided in bid dose) *Medium dose:* 1,000–2,000 mcg daily (4–8 puffs divided bid)	*Inhaler* 250 mcg/puff	Rinse mouth after use.

Continued

Table 30–7 Drugs Commonly Used: Asthma and COPD—cont'd

Drug	Dosage	How Supplied	Comments
	High dose: >2,000 mcg daily (>8 puffs divided bid) *Children 5–11 yr:* *Low dose:* 500–750 mcg (2–3 puffs daily) *Medium dose:* 1,000–1,250 mcg daily (4–5 puffs daily divided bid) *High dose:* >1,250 mcg daily (>5 puffs divided bid)		
Fluticasone (Flovent)	*Adults:* *Low dose:* 88–264 mcg daily (2–6 puffs of 44 mcg divided bid) *Medium dose:* 264–660 mcg daily (2–6 puffs of 110 mcg daily divided bid) *High dose:* >660 mcg (>6 puffs 110 mcg *or* >3 puffs 220 mcg) *Children 5–11 yr:* *Low dose:* 88–176 mcg daily (2–4 puffs of 44 mcg divided bid) *Medium dose:* 176–440 mcg daily (2–4 puffs 110 mcg divided bid) *High dose:* >440 mcg (>4 puffs 110 mcg *or* >2 puffs 220 mcg)	***Inhaler*** 44 mcg/puff 110 mcg/puff 220 mcg/puff	Not recommended for children <6 mo Exhibits a flat dose–response curve. Doses >10 mg do not produce a greater response in adults. Chewable tablets contain phenylalanine.
Fluticasone dry powder inhaler (Advair Diskus)	*Adults:* *Low dose:* 100–300 mcg *Medium dose:* 300–600 mcg *High dose:* >600 mcg *Children:* *Low dose:* 100–200 mcg *Medium dose:* 200–400 mcg *High dose:* >400 mcg	DPI: 50, 100, or 250 mcg/ inhalation 50 mcg/puff 100 mcg/puff 250 mcg/puff	
Leukotriene Modifiers			
Montelukast (Singulair)	*Adults:* 10 mg once daily in the p.m. *Children 6–14 yr:* 5 mg once daily in the p.m. *Children 6 mo–5 yr:* 4 mg qhs	***Oral*** 10 mg tablets 5 mg chewable tablets 4 mg chewable tablets Granules: 4 mg/packet	• Not recommended for children <5 yr • Must be taken on an empty stomach
Zafirlukast (Accolate)	*Children ≥12 yr and adults:* 20 mg bid *Children 5–11 yr:* 10 mg bid	***Oral*** 20 mg tablets 10 mg tablets For zafirlukast, administration with meals decreases bioavailability; take at least 1 h before or 2 h after meals	
Zileutin (Zyflo)	*Adults:* 600 mg qid	***Oral*** 600 mg tablets 300 mg tablets	• Not recommended for children • Evaluate liver function prior to initiating therapy and routinely during therapy; contraindicated in acute liver disease

Table 30–8 Comparative Daily Dosages for Inhaled Corticosteroids

Drug	Low Daily Dose			Medium Daily Dose			High Daily Dose		
	Child 0–4 Years of Age	Child 5–11 Years of Age	≥12 Years of Age and Adults	Child 0–4 Years of Age	Child 5–11 Years of Age	≥12 Years of Age and Adults	Child 0–4 Years of Age	Child 5–11 Years of Age	≥12 Years of Age and Adults
Beclomethasone HFA 40 or 80 mcg/puff	NA	80–160 mcg	80–240 mcg	NA	>240–480 mcg	>160–320 mcg	NA	>320 mcg	>480 mcg
Budesonide DPI 90, 180, or 200 mcg/ inhalation	NA	180–400 mcg	180–600 mcg	NA	>400–800 mcg	>600–1,200 mcg	NA	>800 mcg	>1,200 mcg
Budesonide Inhaled Inhalation suspension for nebulization	0.25–0.5 mg	0.5 mg	NA	>0.5–1.0 mg	NA	1.0 mg	>1.0 mg	2.0 mg	NA
Flunisolide 250 mcg/puff	NA	500–750 mcg	500–1,000 mcg	NA	1,000–2,000 mcg	1,000–1,250 mcg	NA	>1,250 mcg	>2,000 mcg
Flunisolide HFA 80 mcg/puff	NA	160 mcg	320 mcg	NA	320–640 mcg	320 mcg	NA	≥640 mcg	>640 mcg
Fluticasone HFA/MDI: 44, 110, or 220 mcg/puff	176 mcg	88–176 mcg	88–264 mcg	>176–352 mcg	>264–440 mcg	>176–352 mcg	>352 mcg	>352 mcg	>440 mcg
DPI: 50, 100, or 250 mcg/ inhalation	NA	100–200 mcg	100–300 mcg	NA	>300–500 mcg	>200–400 mcg	NA	>400 mcg	>500 mcg
Mometasone DPI 200 mcg/inhalation	NA	NA	200 mcg	NA	400 mcg	NA	NA	NA	>400 mcg
Triamcinolone acetonide 75 mcg/puff	NA	300–600 mcg	300–750 mcg	NA	>750–1,500 mcg	>600–900 mcg	NA	>900 mcg	>1,500 mcg

Key: DPI, dry powder inhaler; HFA, hydrofluoroalkane; MDI, metered-dose inhaler; NA, not available (either not approved, no data available, or safety and efficacy not established for this age group)
Source: From National Asthma Education and Prevention Program (NAEPP). (2007). *The Expert Panel Report 3: Guidelines for the diagnosis and management of asthma.* Bethesda, MD: National Heart, Lung, and Blood Institute, National Institutes of Health.

disadvantage to the mast cell stabilizers are that they take weeks to reach full effectiveness for asthma.

Leukotrienes are biologically active products of the arachidonic acid metabolism and result in inflammatory disorders including asthma. Antagonism of specific pulmonary receptors has provided a target for asthma therapy (Henderson, 1994). Medications in this class of therapeutics include montelukast (Singulair), zafirlukast (Accolate), and zileuton (Zyflo). Any of these medications may be used as alternatives to ICS in step 2 management of asthma.

Moderate Persistent Asthma

Patients with moderate persistent asthma require long-term preventive medication to maintain control of their asthma. The dose of inhaled corticosteroids should be 240 to 480 mcg of beclomethasone HFA (3 to 6 puffs per day of 80 mcg/puff) or low-dose inhaled corticosteroids combined with a long-acting beta-agonist bronchodilator (Advair). The long-acting beta-agonist salmeterol (Serevent) should not be prescribed without the concurrent use of inhaled corticosteroids because of increased risks of catastrophic events (asthma-related intubations and death), as discussed in Chapter 17. Quick relief of symptoms is obtained with short-acting inhaled beta$_2$ agonists. A more severe exacerbation may require oral corticosteroids. If control of symptoms is not achieved and the patient is adhering to the asthma plan, including correct inhaler technique, then increasing the treatment to step 4 is indicated. Having patients record their medication use and symptoms is essential at all steps but critical at step 3 because documentation is helpful in determining whether referral to an asthma specialist is indicated if the patient needs step 4 therapy.

Severe Persistent Asthma

Treatment for patients with severe persistent asthma symptoms requires step 4, 5, or 6 therapy. Step 4 therapy is daily medium-dose inhaled corticosteroids (240 to 480 mcg/d of beclomethasone HFA or the equivalent) and a long-acting beta agonist (arformoterol, formoterol, indacaterol, and salmeterol). An alternative approach is a medium dose of inhaled corticosteroid and a leukotriene modifier or theophylline. Step 5 therapy is daily inhaled high-dose corticosteroids combined with daily long-acting bronchodilators. The inhaled corticosteroid dose should be in the high range, which is greater than 480 mcg of beclomethasone HFA (more than 6 puffs/d at 80 mcg/puff) or the equivalent. Step 6 therapy for severe persistent asthma consists of high-dose corticosteroids combined with daily long-acting bronchodilators and oral corticosteroids.

If long-term oral corticosteroids are required, the lowest dose possible to achieve results should be used and on an alternate-day schedule if possible. Oral steroids are dosed at 2 mg/kg/d, not to exceed 60 mg/d. Inhaled corticosteroids are preferable to systemic corticosteroids, and the maximum dose should be used before long-term systemic therapy is initiated. Exacerbations require short bursts of high-dose systemic corticosteroids.

Severe persistent asthma requiring step 5 or step 6 therapy and associated with allergies may benefit from omalizumab (Xolair) therapy, which is a recombinant humanized mouse monoclonal antibody that binds to free immunoglobulin E (IgE) in the circulation and prevents them from responding to relevant allergens (dust mite, cockroach, cat, or dog) (NAEPP, 2007). It is administered every 2 to 4 weeks via subcutaneous route and has been demonstrated to reduce exacerbations and total emergency visits (Abramowicz, 2005; Bousquet, et al, 2005; Chiang, Clark, & Casale, 2005). All patients who require step 4 treatment need referral to an asthma specialist.

Emerging Therapies

Vitamin D

Recent reports indicate that persons with low vitamin D have a higher mortality from asthma (Zittermann, Gummert, & Borgermann, 2009), most likely due to the immunomodulator role that vitamin D plays (Rance, 2013). Low vitamin D levels may be responsible for the increase in childhood asthma, with 35% of children with mild-to-moderate persistent asthma presenting with low vitamin D levels (Brehm et al, 2010). Vitamin D decreases the allergic response by shifting the ratio of T1-helper cells to T2-helper cells to predominately T2-helper cells (Rance, 2013). There are no official recommendations for supplementing asthma patients with vitamin D, but measuring vitamin D levels in patients with asthma is warranted to determine if they are deficient. All asthma patients should consume at least the minimum daily intake for their age, which is 400 IU/d in infants 1 to 12 months and 600 IU/d in children age 1 year or older and adults through age 70 years. Adults over age 70 years are recommended to take 800 IU/d.

CFC Free Inhalers

Changes in the delivery of meter-dose inhalers from chlorofluorocarbons (CFC) to hydrofluoroalkanes (HFA) have resulted in a smaller particle size of delivery, which has enhanced the lung deposits from 20% to 50%, resulting in greater efficacy (Schofield, 2014).

Monitoring Control

Once control is achieved, patients need to be monitored every 1 to 6 months to determine if a step up or step down in therapy is indicated. Step therapy is meant to be a dynamic program of therapy in which changes in a patient's symptoms require movement up or down. To make appropriate treatment decisions, it is essential that patients be monitored frequently and that they maintain a self-assessment record. The *Expert Panel Report 3: Guidelines* (NAEPP, 2007) says that the dose of inhaled corticosteroids may be reduced about 25% to 50% every 2 to 3 months to the lowest dose possible to maintain asthma control. Most patients with persistent asthma require daily medication to suppress underlying airway inflammation, and they may relapse if inhaled corticosteroids are withdrawn completely.

If at any time control of asthma symptoms is not achieved and sustained, the health-care provider has a number of actions to take. First and most important, the provider must review and observe the patient's medication administration. Improper inhaler technique can create havoc in the management of asthma because the patient is not getting relief at increasing "doses" of medication. This problem can lead to unnecessary changes in therapy. The patient's inhaler technique should be reviewed at every visit because research has shown that technique deteriorates between visits (Self, George, Wallace, Patterson & Finch, 2014).

The provider needs to be aware that the prescribed regimen may not be followed at home. In a study of Medicaid patients age 2 to 17 years (N = 4262), 63% had discontinued their preventive asthma medications within 90 days of the prescription being written (Campo-Ramos Duran, Simon, Akinbami, & Schoendorf, 2014). Educating the patient on the necessity of taking preventive medication is critical to successful treatment.

Managing Exacerbations

A temporary increase in anti-inflammatory therapy may be needed to reestablish control or treat exacerbations. The need for oral steroids is characterized by increased need for short-acting bronchodilators or decreased PEF (20% or greater), reduced tolerance to activity, and increased nocturnal symptoms. A short "burst" of oral prednisone is often effective. The appropriate dose is 40 to 60 mg/d as a single or divided (twice a day) dose (1 to 2 mg/kg in children to a maximum of 60 g/d) for 5 to 10 days in adults and 3 to 10 days in children. If the steroid burst is successful (the PEF returns to normal and symptoms improve), then no other treatment is necessary. If the prednisone burst does not control symptoms, then a step up to a higher level is indicated. If frequent bursts of steroids are required, then higher-level care is needed. Doubling the dose of inhaled corticosteroids is not effective in treating asthma exacerbations (NAEPP, 2007).

Maintaining Control of Asthma

Factors that influence maintaining control of asthma include exposure to allergens, barriers to care (e.g., financial), and self-management issues. Allergy testing and referral to an allergy specialist may be necessary to maintain effective control of asthma symptoms. Families in crisis have difficulty in maintaining a complex medication regimen, and every effort should be made to simplify the treatment for all patients regardless of their resources.

Home Management of Exacerbations of Asthma

Home management of asthma exacerbations is an integral part of asthma management. Patients need to be educated to recognize early symptoms of decreasing lung function and to adjust their medications accordingly. The *Expert Panel Report 3: Guidelines* (NAEPP, 2007) recommends the following home pharmacological therapy, which is described in detail in Figure 30-2.

First, assess severity. Patients at high risk for a fatal asthma attack require immediate attention after initial treatment. Patients at risk include those having previous severe exacerbations requiring intubation or intensive care unit (ICU)

admission for asthma, two or more hospitalizations or more than three emergency department visits in the past year, use of more than two short-acting beta-agonist canisters per month, difficulty perceiving airway obstruction or worsening asthma, or low socioeconomic status or inner-city residence.

Initial home treatment consists of increased frequency of inhaled beta$_2$ agonists, up to two treatments (2 to 6 puffs of MDI) 20 minutes apart or nebulizer treatment. If the response is good, the patient should continue the inhaled short-acting beta agonists and contact the provider to discuss whether a short course of oral corticosteroids is required. If the response is incomplete to initial therapy and persistent wheezing or tachypnea is present, the patient should be started on systemic oral corticosteroids, continue the short-acting beta agonists, and contact the provider urgently (the same day). If the response is poor to initial therapy, determined by marked wheezing and dyspnea, the patient should repeat the short-acting beta agonist immediately and start oral corticosteroids. If the distress is severe, the patient should be transported to the emergency department (consider calling 911).

Patients with good response to therapy need to continue more intensive therapy (step up in care) for several days until the PEF returns to normal. Patients should contact their health-care provider any time they begin oral steroids if the attack is severe or if emergent treatment is necessary.

Patient Variables

Pregnancy

Asthma affects between 3.5% and 13.9% of pregnant women in the United States (Kwon, Belanger, & Bracken, 2003; Louik, Schatz, Hernandez-Diaz, Werler, & Mitchell, 2010). Pregnant women with asthma need to be monitored closely for changes in lung function because the effects of pregnancy on the course of asthma are unpredictable and the asthma may worsen, improve, or remain unchanged (Hanania & Belfort, 2005; Louik et al., 2010). Adequate oxygenation is essential for the fetus to develop normally. Poorly controlled asthma can lead to low birth weight, increased perinatal morbidity, and prematurity.

In general, asthma therapy is the same for pregnant women as for other patients with asthma. They need to be educated and monitor their PEF throughout the pregnancy, with the *Expert Panel Report 3: Guidelines* (NAEPP, 2007) recommending monitoring of asthma status at prenatal visits. Any changes in PEF require prompt treatment and modification in pharmacological therapy. Most medications used to treat asthma are Pregnancy Class C, as noted in Chapter 17. Oral forms of beta$_2$ agonists should be used minimally in patients who are in labor, as terbutaline is a tocolytic (off-label use). Inhaled forms of beta$_2$ agonists are less likely to affect uterine contractions, and albuterol is the beta agonist of choice for pregnant women because of its safety profile (NAEPP, 2007).

Inhaled corticosteroids (ICS) are the long-term-control medications of choice, with budesonide the ICS with the most data available in pregnant women (NAEPP, 2007). Minimal data are available regarding the safety of

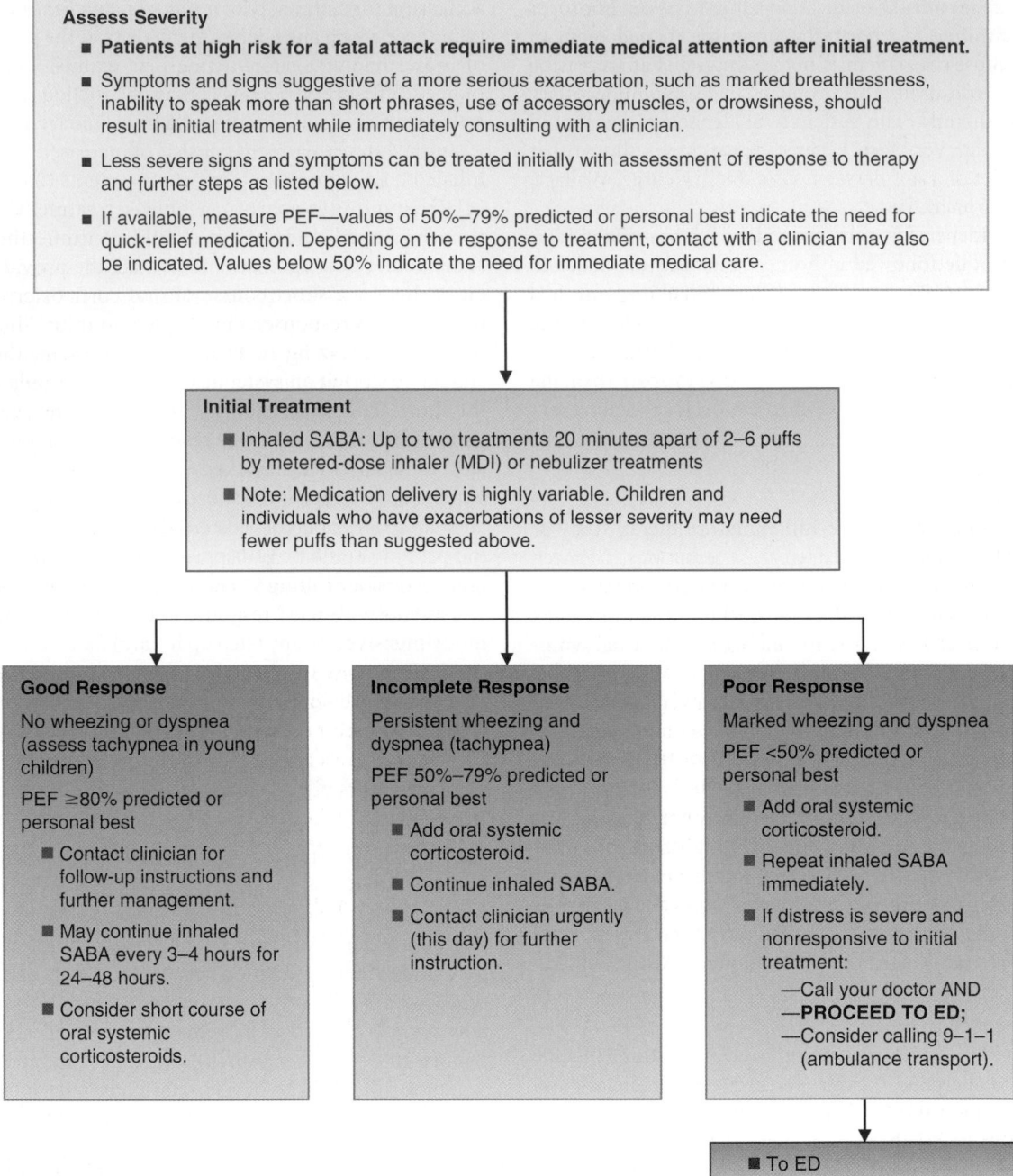

Figure 30–2. Management of asthma exacerbations: Home treatment. Key: ED, emergency department; MDI, metered-dose inhaler; PEF, peak expiratory flow; SABA, short-acting beta$_2$ agonist (quick-relief inhaler). (*Source:* From National Asthma Education and Prevention Program [NAEPP]. [2007]. *The Expert Panel Report 3: Guidelines for the diagnosis and management of asthma.* Bethesda, MD: National Heart, Lung, and Blood Institute, National Institutes of Health.)

leukotrienes in pregnant women, but animal data do not indicate a concern for use during pregnancy (NAEPP, 2007).

Pediatric Patients

Approximately 6.8 million children (9.3%) in the United States have asthma (Centers for Disease Control, 2015). The Global Initiative for Asthma (2009) describes three categories of wheezing in children younger than age 5 years: transient early wheezing, persistent early-onset wheezing, and late-onset wheezing/asthma. Transient early wheezing is associated with

prematurity and parental smoking and is often outgrown by age 3 years. Persistent early-onset wheezing occurs before age 3 years and is characterized by recurrent episodes of wheezing associated with viral upper respiratory infections. The symptoms usually persist through school age and early adolescence. Children with early-onset wheezing have no evidence of atopy. Late-onset wheezing/asthma is often associated with atopy, often eczema.

Pediatric patients under age 5 years require special management strategies. The *Expert Panel Report 3: Guidelines* (NAEPP, 2007) breaks out the treatment of children younger than age 5 years to address the needs of the population. First, diagnosing asthma in infants and young children is difficult. Asthma is often underdiagnosed and undertreated in this age group because objective measures of lung function are difficult to obtain and treatment decisions are made on clinical assessment. Some health-care providers are reluctant to label children as having asthma, and often the child is given a label of chronic bronchitis, wheezy bronchitis, "happy wheezer," or the like and therefore does not receive adequate treatment. Note that not all wheezing and coughing are asthma, and the patient may have less common conditions such as cystic fibrosis, vascular ring, tracheomalacia, congenital heart disease, foreign body aspiration, and primary immunodeficiency.

As noted, among children younger than 5 years, the most common cause of asthma symptoms is viral respiratory infection. As most infants and toddlers contract repeated viral respiratory infections, susceptible children may have repeated episodes of asthma symptoms. Parents are often frightened and frustrated with these repeated exacerbations. Parental stress associated with frequent health-care visits, uncertain diagnosis, missed work because of the child's illness, or parental guilt about needing to work instead of being at home with the child can make working with these families a challenge for the provider. Open communication between health-care provider and parents should be used to clearly define roles and expectations of care." The *Expert Panel Report 3: Guidelines* (NAEPP, 2007) stresses collaborating with parents and meeting their expectations regarding the care of their child with asthma.

Lieu and colleagues (1997) found that having a written asthma management plan and starting medications at the onset of a cold or flu lowered the odds of an emergency department visit in a case-control study of children up to age 14 with asthma in a large regional health management organization. The *Expert Panel Report 3: Guidelines* (NAEPP, 2007) concurs with this older study and recommends parents can be taught how to identify and anticipate asthma symptoms, such as the beginning of a child's upper respiratory infection symptoms. Parents can learn to identify objective parameters of concern, such as respiratory rate or use of accessory muscles for breathing. Asthma education must be written and frequently repeated to stressed and often fatigued parents. It is best to provide in-depth teaching when the child is well so the parents can be at their optimal and not distracted by the child's condition.

The *Expert Panel Report 3: Guidelines* (NAEPP, 2007) recommends that all children with asthma symptoms be given a therapeutic trial of bronchodilators, specifically inhaled short-acting beta$_2$ agonists. The *Expert Panel Report 3: Guidelines* (NAEPP, 2007) includes a stepwise approach for managing infants and young children 0 to 4 years with asthma symptoms. Use of bronchodilators more than twice a week is an indication of the need for step 2 therapy: daily anti-inflammatory medication. Daily long-term therapy should begin with low-dose inhaled corticosteroids delivered via nebulizer or metered-dose inhaler (MDI) with holding chamber with or without mask. Alternative medications include cromolyn (nebulizer is preferred) or montelukast.

Step 3 therapy is indicated for moderate persistent asthma (symptoms daily or more than 3 to 4 nights/mo) and requires therapy with medium-dose inhaled corticosteroids. Poor response to the step 3 regimen indicates a need to step up to step 4 therapy, a combination of low-dose inhaled corticosteroids and a montelukast. If step 3 therapy is required, the *Expert Panel Report 3: Guidelines* (NAEPP, 2007) says that control should be established quickly with higher doses of inhaled corticosteroids and that therapy should be stepped down after 2 to 3 months to the lowest dose required to maintain control. Referral to an asthma specialist is essential for all children who require step 3 or higher care. Poor control at step 2 may also be a reason to consider referral.

Exacerbations caused by viral upper respiratory infections can be quite severe, and systemic corticosteroids may be needed often in this age group because of the number of viral upper respiratory infections that children get in infancy. A short burst of oral corticosteroids may be needed to establish control of asthma in children with moderate or severe asthma (NAEPP, 2007). A "burst" dose is 1 to 2 mg/kg/d (maximum 30 mg/d) of prednisone in two divided doses for 3 to 10 days. Table 30-6 discusses the stepwise approach to managing children with asthma.

Delivery of medication to infants and young children can be a challenge. There are several delivery devices available, but the dose of medication received can vary considerably among devices and age groups. Nebulizer therapy is preferred for children younger than 2 years. Nebulizers may be used in older children who are unable to use MDIs well enough to get therapeutic effects. MDIs with either a spacer or a face mask can be used. An MDI and spacer with face mask is an alternative strategy in infants if there is a need for portable treatment, such as for traveling or day care. It is also a good choice if the family is financially stressed and the cost of a nebulizer and medication is prohibitive. Prior to changing or stepping up therapy, patients and parents must be assessed for proper use of delivery devices. It should be noted that Pulmicort Respules (budesonide inhalation suspension) should be administered with a compressed-air-driven jet nebulizer, *not* an ultrasonic nebulizer.

The *Expert Panel Report 3: Guidelines* (NAEPP, 2007) added a separate diagnosis and management category for children aged 5 to 11 years. The management of school-age children is similar to that of younger children, with the addition of theophylline as alternative long-term control medication in step 2 therapy and the use of long-acting beta-agonists combined with inhaled corticosteroids in step 3 or higher therapy (see Table 30-6). The U.S. Food and Drug Administration (U.S. FDA, 2010) recommends long-acting beta agonists not be prescribed without inhaled corticosteroids to children, and preferably a combination product (Advair) is to be prescribed.

Older children and adolescents often have to manage symptoms at school or otherwise away from parents, and the *Expert Panel Report 3: Guidelines* (NAEPP, 2007) recommends a written asthma action plan be shared with the school or day care. School-age children are developmentally interested in learning and mastering new skills, and should be involved with their treatment plan. School-age and adolescent children need to be able to effectively administer inhaled medications. Therefore, as children with asthma get older and gain independence, the provider needs to observe the child's inhaler technique and make adjustments as necessary. Many schools do not allow students to carry and self-administer medications. The NAEPP (2007) has endorsed a resolution allowing students to carry and self-administer medications if the provider and parent consider it appropriate. The plan has to be worked out among the parent, the school, and the health-care provider.

Sports and physical activities are essential to a healthy lifestyle for children. Every attempt should be made to control asthma symptoms so that children can participate in physical activities. Treatment just prior to activity may prevent the cough and wheeze some children experience with exercise. Poor exercise tolerance is an indication of poorly controlled asthma and the need to modify the asthma management plan. Adding a long-term-control medication usually improves exercise tolerance. Guidance from the health-care provider can assist parents and children in choosing appropriate sports. Often, children allergic to pollens cannot play outdoor sports such as baseball or soccer yet can participate in swimming, basketball, and gymnastics without problems. Restricting physical activity should be a last resort.

Older Adults

Older adults with asthma symptoms often present with a variety of other disease processes. The provider must first determine how much of the airflow obstruction is reversible and how much is due to other obstructive lung disease (chronic bronchitis, emphysema). Often a trial of 2 to 3 weeks of systemic corticosteroids is necessary to determine the extent of reversibility of airway disease. Inhaled long-term-control medications can then be introduced if indicated.

The medications used to treat asthma have increased adverse effects in the older patient. Those with preexisting ischemic heart disease may also be more sensitive to beta$_2$-agonist adverse effects, including tremor and tachycardia. Concomitant use of anticholinergics, muscurinics, and beta$_2$ agonists may be beneficial in the older patient. Theophylline clearance is reduced, causing increased serum theophylline levels. Frequent monitoring of blood levels is necessary if theophylline is used for the older patient. Systemic corticosteroids can cause confusion, agitation, and changes in glucose metabolism. There is also a dose-dependent reduction in bone mineral content that may be associated with inhaled corticosteroid use. Low-to-medium doses appear to have no major effect on bone density. Older patients may be at more risk because of preexisting osteoporosis, lower estrogen levels (in women), and a sedentary lifestyle. Consider treatment with calcium and vitamin D supplements and, as appropriate, estrogen replacement for older patients on high-dose inhaled corticosteroid therapy.

Another concern in older patients is that the medications used to treat other chronic diseases may cause asthma exacerbations or require medication adjustments. Patients who are taking theophylline need to be assessed for medications that affect theophylline clearance. The nonselective beta blockers, including some beta blockers in eyedrops used to treat glaucoma, can result in mutual inhibition of therapeutic effects if used with beta$_2$ agonists. NSAIDs used to treat arthritis may cause asthma exacerbation. At each visit for asthma-related symptoms, it is essential to assess the patient's complete history, including all medications the patient takes.

Special Situations

Seasonal Asthma

Seasonal asthma is identified when patients appear to have asthma symptoms only in relationship to certain pollens and molds. Seasonal asthma is managed by the same stepwise approach to long-term management of asthma previously discussed. If the patient has predictable seasonal asthma—each spring, for example—long-term anti-inflammatory treatment should be initiated approximately 1 month before the anticipated onset of symptoms and continued through the season.

Cough Variant Asthma

Cough variant asthma is seen especially in young children. It is diagnosed when cough, usually at night, is the principal symptom. Daytime examination may be normal, thereby often delaying or confusing the diagnosis. A therapeutic trial of bronchodilator medication is often diagnostic of cough variant asthma. Monitoring PEF changes between morning and evening readings may also assist in the diagnosis. Management is according to the stepwise approach to long-term management of asthma.

Montelukast demonstrated in a small double-blind randomized controlled study to reduce cough 75.7% from baseline by week 4 in the treatment group, whereas the placebo group had a 20.7% reduction in cough (Spector & Tan, 2004). A more recent study of the use of montelukast for the treatment of cough variant asthma found a clinical significant improvement in health status, but no additional benefit over inhaled corticosteroids (Boom, Vaessen, Uil, Kerstjens & van den Berg, 2011).

Exercise-Induced Bronchospasm

EIB should be anticipated in all patients with asthma, with 50% to 90% of asthmatics having airways that are hyperreactive to exercise (Parsons & Mastronarde, 2005). Some patients (less than 10%) exhibit asthma symptoms only when exercising. Bronchospasm is due to hyperventilation of air that is cooler and dryer than that of the respiratory system, which causes loss of heat and water from the lungs. The diagnosis of EIB is made first by history of cough, shortness of breath, chest pain or tightness, or wheezing during or right after exercise. Formal diagnosis can be made in a laboratory or by having patients exercise strenuously enough to increase their heart rate to 80% of maximum for 4 to 6 minutes. Otherwise healthy patients can run in the hallway or stairway of the clinic if appropriate. The PEF measurements are taken before and at 5-minute intervals for 20 to 30 minutes. A 15% decrease in PEF is compatible with EIB.

The goal of EIB therapy is for patients to be able to participate in any activity they choose without asthma symptoms. Teachers and coaches need to be notified that a child or an athlete has EIB. The *Expert Panel Report 3: Guidelines* (NAEPP, 2007) recommends the following treatment strategies:

1. Short-acting beta$_2$ agonists used just prior to exercise prevent EIB in 80% of patients for 2 to 3 hours. Salmeterol has been shown to prevent EIB for 10 to 12 hours. Long-acting beta agonists used daily will have decreased effectiveness; therefore, if daily pretreatment for exercise is needed, an alternative should be used.
2. Cromolyn and nedocromil inhaled shortly before exercise are also effective in preventing EIB but are not as effective as short-acting beta$_2$ agonists.
3. A lengthy warm-up before exercise may decrease the need for repeated medications if the patient can tolerate continuous exercise without symptoms.
4. Long-term-control therapy with inhaled anti-inflammatory medication may be indicated and helpful in reducing airway responsiveness and therefore decreasing EIB. Inhaled corticosteroids are recommended as first-line therapy for athletes who have persistent asthma to prevent worsening of symptoms during exercise.
5. A mask or scarf over the mouth may attenuate cold-induced EIB.
6. Leukotriene modifiers may attenuate EIB in up to 50% of patients.

Surgery

Surgery places patients with asthma at risk for complications both during and after a procedure. These complications include acute bronchoconstriction triggered by intubation, hypoxemia, and possible hypercapnia; impaired cough effectiveness; atelectasis; and respiratory infections. The more severe the patient's asthma before surgery, the higher the likelihood of complications will be. Prior to surgery, the asthmatic patient should have an evaluation that includes symptoms, review of medications, and pulmonary function testing. If possible, patients ought to be at their personal best PEF. A short burst of systemic corticosteroids may be necessary to reach ideal lung function. Patients who have received systemic corticosteroids in the past 6 months require IV hydrocortisone during the surgical period.

Monitoring

Monitoring patients with asthma is a continuous process, beginning with the initial diagnosis. The *Expert Panel Report 3: Guidelines* (NAEPP, 2007) recommends ongoing monitoring of the following six areas: signs and symptoms, pulmonary function, quality of life and functional status, history of asthma exacerbations, pharmacotherapy, and patient–provider communication and patient satisfaction.

Monitoring Signs and Symptoms of Asthma

All patients should be taught to monitor and recognize their asthma symptoms. Recording symptoms and PEF on a self-assessment diary enables the patient and the provider to track asthma symptoms and determine if there is adequate control. Clinical signs of asthma should be assessed at each visit through physical examination and appropriate questioning of the patient. Questions should be asked about the recent past (e.g., In the past 2 weeks, how many times have you had nighttime symptoms?). Questions about longer periods give a more generalized response (e.g., Have your symptoms been better or worse since your last visit?). Assessment of symptoms should differentiate between daytime symptoms, nighttime symptoms, and symptoms that occur in the early morning and that do not improve after inhaling a short-acting beta$_2$ agonist.

Monitoring Pulmonary Function

Monitoring lung function is essential to diagnosis and management of asthma. Lung function can be monitored by spirometry and peak flow monitoring. The *Expert Panel Report 3: Guidelines* (NAEPP, 2007) recommends that spirometry tests be done at the time of initial assessment, after treatment is initiated and PEF has stabilized to determine "normal" airway function for the individual patient, and then every 1 to 2 years to assess the maintenance of airway function. Spirometry may also be needed to check the accuracy of PEF readings before making major treatment decisions if there is a question about the reliability of the PEF. Peak flow meters are used for ongoing monitoring, not diagnosis, of asthma. Patients who have frequent exacerbations or require long-term therapy need to have a peak flow meter at home and be comfortable with its use. Monitoring PEF is essential to management of moderate to severe asthma in order to determine the severity of exacerbations and to guide treatment decisions. Daily PEF readings help to detect early changes in asthma status, help to evaluate response to changes in medication therapy, and provide a quantitative measure of airflow obstruction.

The *Expert Panel Report 3: Guidelines* (NAEPP, 2007) does not recommend long-term daily peak flow monitoring of patients with mild intermittent or mild persistent asthma, although PEF may be helpful during exacerbations. Patients should be given in-depth teaching regarding peak flow meter use, which may require more than one visit or referral to a nurse clinician who can teach proper peak flow meter use. Patients need to establish their personal best PEF and use that reading as the basis of their action plan. The patient should use the same brand of peak flow meter or reestablish personal best PEF if changing brands because there is no universal normative value for peak flow meters and the PEF may vary between brands. Peak flow meters are usually covered by insurance if the provider writes a prescription for the item.

Monitoring Quality of Life and Functional Status

Monitoring quality of life and functional status is essential to determine if the goals of asthma therapy are being met. The *Expert Panel Report 3: Guidelines* (NAEPP, 2007) recommends that the following areas of quality of life be periodically assessed:

1. Missed work or school because of asthma.
2. Reduction in usual activities.
3. Any disturbances in sleep due to asthma.
4. Any change in caregiver activities due to child's asthma (for caregivers of children with asthma).

Monitoring History of Asthma Exacerbations

Monitoring the history of asthma exacerbation is essential at every visit. The provider must question the patient and evaluate self-monitoring records to determine exacerbation, both self-treated and those treated by other health-care providers (e.g., emergency department visit, hospitalization). Changes in drug treatment are based on the exacerbation history.

Monitoring Pharmacotherapy

Monitoring the effectiveness of pharmacological therapy is key to successful asthma treatment. The following should be monitored: patient adherence to the regimen, inhaler technique, level of usage of as-needed inhaled short-acting beta$_2$ agonist, frequency of oral corticosteroid "burst" therapy, and changes in dosages of inhaled anti-inflammatory or other long-term-control medication. The provider must also determine if the patient is at the appropriate level of step therapy and if changes need to be made. At each visit, an up-to-date asthma action plan has to be reviewed and revised as appropriate.

Monitoring Patient–Provider Communication and Patient Satisfaction

Patient satisfaction and patient–provider communication should be assessed routinely. Two aspects of patient satisfaction should be assessed and addressed as appropriate: satisfaction with asthma control and satisfaction with quality of care (NAEPP, 2007).

Outcome Evaluation

Evaluating the effectiveness of asthma therapy is an ongoing process, as described in the Monitoring section. The best outcome for asthma patients is being able to accomplish their activities of daily living, whatever their lifestyle, with minimum asthma symptoms.

The *Expert Panel Report 3: Guidelines* (NAEPP, 2007) recommends that referral to an asthma specialist be made if there are difficulties in achieving or maintaining control, if immunosuppressive therapy is being considered, or if a patient requires step 4 care (step 3 if patient is an infant or young child).

Patient Education

Patient education should include a written asthma action plan, which includes a discussion of information related to the overall treatment plan as well as that specific to the drug therapy, reasons for taking the drug, drugs as part of the total treatment regimen, and adherence issues. The *Expert Panel Report 3: Guidelines* (NAEPP, 2007) provides a systematic review of the evidence related to written asthma action plans compared with medical management alone and clearly recommends the use of a written plan based on the evidence to date in decreasing emergency department visits and hospitalizations.

The key to asthma patient education is to establish and maintain a partnership among the patient, the family, and the health-care team. Patients and families are being asked to manage complex medical regimens, detect and self-treat most

---

PATIENT EDUCATION

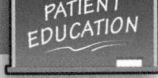

Asthma

RELATED TO THE OVERALL TREATMENT PLAN AND DISEASE PROCESS

BASIC FACTS ABOUT ASTHMA

Use a variety of teaching methods such as illustrations, videos, written pamphlets or books, and models. Repeat key facts at every visit until the patient and/or family demonstrates an understanding of asthma. An example would to be to show the patient a drawing of a normal airway and an airway affected by asthma. The provider can then demonstrate how different medications act on different components of asthma (bronchodilator relaxes smooth muscle, anti-inflammatory decreases inflammation, etc.). This information can be repeated when reviewing medications at each visit until a clear understanding is demonstrated.

MEDICATION SKILLS

This includes proper inhaler use, spacer use if appropriate, when to take quick-relief medications, and nebulizer use if appropriate.

SELF-MONITORING SKILLS

This includes self-assessment of symptoms, peak flow monitoring, and how to record symptoms and peak expiratory flow (PEF) on a self-assessment diary. Recognizing early signs of declining lung function is essential knowledge for the patient and family.

Environmental control and avoidance strategies will enable the patient and family to avoid possible asthma triggers. Discussion of how environmental exposure to allergens and irritants can worsen asthma symptoms and how to avoid triggers at home, work, and school will assist patients in learning self-management.

PATIENT EDUCATION—cont'd

SPECIFIC TO THE DRUG THERAPY

Reason for the drug being given and its anticipated action in the disease process.
Doses and schedules for taking the drug.
Coping mechanisms for complex and costly drug regimens.
Interactions between other treatment modalities and these drugs.

REASONS FOR THE DRUG(S) BEING TAKEN

Patient education about specific drugs is provided in Chapter 17.

DRUGS AS PART OF THE TOTAL TREATMENT REGIMEN

Information should be provided concerning drugs as part of the total treatment regimen and individualized to the patient's age and asthma severity.

Many educational resources are available, the best of which are from the National Institutes of Health (NIH) and the Global Initiative for Asthma. These documents include the following:

National Asthma Education Prevention Program (2007). *The Expert Panel Report 3: Guidelines for Management of Asthma.* Includes copy-ready patient handouts on use of peak flow meter, inhalers, and asthma action plans.
Global Initiative for Asthma (2009). Global strategy for asthma management and prevention. http://www.ginasthma.org. Includes a patient guide to asthma and interactive learning modules on asthma in adults and children.

INTERNET-BASED PATIENT EDUCATION RESOURCES ON ASTHMA

The *Expert Panel Report 3: Guidelines* can be found at http://www.nhlbi.nih.gov/guidelines/asthma/index.htm and the NIH/WHO Global Initiative for Asthma documents can be found at http:/www.ginasthma.com
Other resources include the following:

Allergy and Asthma Network, Mothers of Asthmatics. http://www.aanma.org/
American Academy of Allergy, Asthma, and Immunology. http://www.aaaai.org
Asthma and Allergy Foundation of America. http://www.aafa.org
Canadian Network for Respiratory Care. http://www.cnrchome.net/
National Asthma Education and Prevention Program. NHLBI http://www.nhlbi.nih.gov/health/public/lung/index .htm#asthma
National Institutes of Health National Heart Lung and Blood Institute. Asthma. http://www.nhlbi.nih.gov/health/dci/ Diseases/Asthma/Asthma_WhatIs.html

exacerbations (unless severe), and communicate appropriately with the team. Asthma education is cost-effective and can reduce morbidity for both adults and children.

CHRONIC OBSTRUCTIVE PULMONARY DISEASE

Chronic obstructive pulmonary disease (COPD) is the term commonly used to refer to conditions of chronic airflow limitation that is not fully reversible. The airflow restriction is usually progressive and involves both the airways and lung parenchyma. Other terms used include *chronic obstructive airway disease* and *chronic obstructive lung disease.* The primary risk factor is cigarette smoking, although occupational exposure (grain, coal, asbestos) and air pollution are also known factors. Not all cigarette smokers develop COPD, so genetic factors may influence who will develop the disease. Four professional organizations have published guidelines regarding COPD: the American Thoracic Society (ATS), the European Respiratory Society (ERS), the Global Initiative for Chronic Obstructive Lung Disease (GOLD), and the American College of Physicians (ACP).

COPD is a heterogeneous disorder that includes primarily chronic bronchitis and emphysema but also comprises peripheral airway disease and asthmatic bronchitis. The diagnosis of obstructive lung disease is determined by spirometry tests of lung function. A positive diagnosis of COPD is made when the FEV in 1 second (FEV_1) and the ratio to the forced vital capacity (FVC) is less than 70%. COPD can be classified as mild, moderate, severe, or very severe by the ATS and the ACP (Table 30-9).

The differences between the clinical presentations of emphysema and of chronic bronchitis are clear, although patients can have components of both diseases. Patients with emphysema are older at diagnosis and often thinner than patients with chronic bronchitis (Table 30-10). The pathological changes in emphysema consist of permanent enlargement of the airspaces distal to the terminal bronchioles and destruction of the bronchiole wall. The primary symptom seen in emphysema is dyspnea. Chronic bronchitis is defined by chronic cough with copious sputum production for 3 months in 2 successive years (American Thoracic Society [ATS]/European Respiratory Society Task Force, 2004). Physical presentation differs in that patients with emphysema are typically barrel chested and breathe through pursed lips ("pink-puffers"), whereas patients with

Table 30–9 Stages of COPD

Classification	Definition by Spirometry
At Risk Patients who: smoke or have exposure to pollutants have cough, sputum or dyspnea have family history of respiratory disease	$FEV_1/FVC > 0.70$ $FEV_1 \geq 80\%$ of predicted
Mild	$FEV_1/FVC < 0.70$ $FEV_1 \geq 80\%$ of predicted
Moderate	$FEV_1/FVC < 0.70$ $50\% \leq FEV_1 < 80\%$ of predicted
Severe	$FEV_1/FVC < 0.70$ $30\% \leq FEV_1 < 50\%$ of predicted
Very Severe	$FEV_1/FVC < 0.70$ $FEV_1 < 30\%$ of predicted, or $FEV_1 < 50\%$ of predicted plus chronic respiratory failure

Source: Derived from American Thoracic Society, 2004; Qaseem et al, 2007.

Table 30–10 Clinical Features of Chronic Bronchitis and Emphysema

Characteristic	Chronic Bronchitis	Emphysema
Age at onset of symptoms	40–50 yr	50–60 yr
Primary symptoms	Cough	Dyspnea
Sputum	Copious, usually purulent	Scant, usually mucoid
Chest x-ray	Peribronchial thickening, often evidence of old inflammatory disease diaphragm	Hyperlucent, overinflated lung, flattened
Weight	Frequently obese	Thin, often marked weight loss
Total lung capacity	Normal or slightly decreased	Increased
Chest examination	Noisy chest, slight hyperinflation	Clear, may have slight end-expiration wheeze, marked hyperinflation
Cor pulmonale with heart failure	Common	Infrequent until end stages of disease

chronic bronchitis are typically obese and suffer from significant hypoxemia, cyanosis, and carbon dioxide retention ("blue-bloaters").

Pathophysiology

The pathophysiology of COPD is characterized by both acute and chronic inflammation. There are also changes in cellular proliferation, leading to tissue destruction, loss of structural ciliated columnar cells, squamous and goblet cell metaplasia, glandular and smooth muscle hypertrophy, and scarring. Clinically, these changes lead to worsened obstruction, hyperinflation of the lungs, increased sputum production, recurrent respiratory infections, and altered gas exchange. As the disease progresses, the patient experiences respiratory muscle fatigue, ventilatory disorders, cardiovascular compromise, and poor quality of life.

The immune response is implicated in the pathophysiology of COPD, with macrophages having a pivotal role in COPD exacerbations. Environmental triggers, including cigarette smoke, are suggested in stimulating Toll-like receptors (TLR), which initiate the innate immune response contributing to bronchial construction and mucous production. These receptors offer promising targets for pharmaceutical interventions (Bezemer et al, 2012; Rovina, Koutsoukou, & Koulouris, 2013).

Emphysema

Emphysema is closely linked to cigarette smoking and the damage to the respiratory tract from the chronic cellular changes smoking produces. The chronic, progressive destruction of the alveolar structures found in emphysema is thought to be caused by an imbalance between proteases and antiproteases in the lower respiratory tract. Proteases, specifically polymorphonuclear neutrophil (PMN) elastase and pulmonary alveolar macrophage (PAM) elastase, work unchecked to destroy alveolar structures and their elastin network. Cigarette smokers have increased numbers of PMNs and PAMs in their lungs, which result in the loss of elastic recoil and structural support found in the lungs of smokers with emphysema. These findings are also found in patients with genetic alpha$_1$ antitrypsin deficiency, which accounts for 2% of patients with emphysema. Alpha$_1$ antitrypsin functions as an antiprotease in the lung to inhibit neutrophil elastase. Therefore, the same structural changes occur in these patients as occur in smokers with emphysema.

Chronic Bronchitis

Cigarette smoking is also the major contributor to the development of chronic bronchitis. Other inhaled irritants are also known to cause chronic bronchitis, among them dust, grain dust, fumes, and asbestos. Three direct effects of inhaling bronchial irritants contribute to the development of chronic bronchitis: (1) stimulation of mucus secretion in the airways, (2) impaired mucus clearance due in part to interference with ciliary activity, and (3) decreased resistance to bronchopulmonary infection because of altered alveolar macrophage function. Clinically, the patient presents with a chronic cough that is due to accumulation of the secretions. Airflow obstruction is due to inflammation of the airways and the thick secretions. The increased mucus is an excellent medium for recurrent bronchial infections, which cause further damage to the airways.

Goals of Therapy

The major goals of treatment for patients with COPD are to slow the disease process and maintain quality of life. Although medications such as antibiotics, bronchodilators, and corticosteroids are part of the treatment, other nonpharmacological measures have just as much impact. Most important, the patient must quit smoking. Nutrition and infection protection are key in maintaining optimal health. Exercise and pulmonary rehabilitation improve function and quality of life. A wellmanaged regimen of medication and nonpharmacological therapies enhances the outcome for patients with COPD.

Rational Drug Selection

The medication regimen for the COPD patient often includes different medications, each treating a different aspect of the disease. The ACP conducted an evidence-based review of therapies and made recommendations for treatment: maintenance monotherapy (long-acting beta agonists, long-acting inhaled muscarinics, or inhaled corticosteroids) for symptomatic patients with COPD and FEV_1 less than 60% of predicted; consideration of combination inhaled therapies for symptomatic patients with COPD and FEV_1 less than 60% of predicted (Qaseem et al, 2011). Drugs commonly used to treat COPD are shown in Table 30-7.

Bronchodilators

Beta Agonists

Bronchodilators are the mainstay of pharmacological therapy for COPD patients. They treat the reversible component of COPD and maximize airflow by relaxing the airway smooth muscle and improving lung emptying during tidal breathing (ATS/European Respiratory Society Task Force, 2004). Three types of bronchodilators are used in COPD management: $beta_2$ agonists, anticholinergic drugs, and methylxanthines (theophylline).

Inhaled $beta_2$ agonists have been the mainstay for COPD therapy, and short-acting $beta_2$ agonists should be prescribed for acute symptomatic relief of all persons with airflow obstruction. The ACP recommends long-acting beta agonists as monotherapy or in combination with an inhaled anticholinergic or inhaled corticosteroid (Qaseem et al, 2011). The long-acting beta agonists are effective in reducing COPD exacerbations and as of this writing may still be used for monotherapy in COPD patients, whereas they have received a Black-Box Warning not to be used as monotherapy in asthma (U.S. FDA, 2010). The long-acting beta agonists, salmeterol (Serevent) or formoterol (Perforomist), can be prescribed singly or in combination with an inhaled corticosteroid (Advair or Symbicort) or long-acting muscarinic antagonist (Tiotropium). In two large studies, the use of combination therapy was slightly better than single therapy in reducing the frequency of COPD exacerbations and hospitalizations. The combination of a short-acting beta agonist (albuterol) and ipratropium (an inhaled anticholinergic) reduces the duration of COPD exacerbations compared to albuterol alone (Qaseem et al, 2011).

Ultralong-acting beta agonists (Ultra LABA) activate the $beta_2$ receptors on the smooth muscle cells, resulting in activation of the cAMP pathway and muscle relaxation similar to short- and long-acting beta agonists. In 2011, the FDA approved the first Ultra LABA, indacaterol (Arcapta). Indacaterol is a once-daily long-acting bronchodilator that has an onset of 5 minutes and a duration of 24 hours (Reid & Pham, 2013). When combined with a long-acting muscarinic antagonist, the benefit is additive, resulting in an improvement of respiratory symptoms (Cope, Kraemer, Zhang, Capkun-Niggli, & Jansen, 2012).

Methalyxanthine

Theophylline is not included in the ACP 2011 recommendations, but is in the GOLD 2014 guidelines as a second-line drug, noting low-dose theophylline reduces exacerbations of COPD. Theophylline was historically a first-line agent used to treat asthma and COPD; however, the margin between therapeutic levels and toxic levels was small. Many patients developed toxicity and the use of theophylline decreased with the development of $beta_2$ agonists and anticholinergics. There has been a recent interest in theophylline, not only for the bronchodilator properties but also as a selective phosphodiesterase (PDE) inhibitor. Specifically, with blocking the PDE-3 resulting in bronchodilation and PDE-4 decreasing macrophage activation and inflammation, low-dose theophylline is showing promising results, especially in severe COPD patients who are resistant to steroids (Barnes, 2013; Hakim, Adcock, & Usmani, 2012).

Muscarinic Agents

Muscarininc agents that have anticholinergic properties, such as ipratropium bromide (Atrovent) and tiotropium (Spiriva), reduce the volume of sputum without changing the viscosity, which in addition to their bronchodilation effects may make them the drugs of choice in COPD. Tiotropium (Spiriva HandiHaler), a long-acting muscarinic antagonist (LAMA), is delivered as a dry inhalation powder once daily. Titropium has been found to reduce exacerbations and hospitalizations of COPD patients compared with placebo and ipratropium (ATS/ European Respiratory Society Task Force, 2004; Qaseem et al, 2011). One caution is that the inhaled LAMA are not effective for immediate relief of bronchospasm because of their slow onset of action; therefore, regular dosing is necessary. Combining agents such as albuterol and ipratropium (Combivent) or formoterol and tiotropium (Symbicort) produces a greater change in spirometry over 3 months than either agent alone. The ACP recommendations note clinicians may consider combination inhaled medications for COPD if FEV_1 is less than 60% of predicted (Qaseem et al, 2011). Combination medications may be more convenient and economical for patients with COPD who require both medications. The combination of albuterol and ipratropium is also available in solution for nebulizer use (DuoNeb).

Recently, acridinium bromide (Tudorza Pressair) has been approved as a long-acting muscarinic antagonist (LAMA) for the treatment of COPD; it is delivered as a dry powder inhaler twice a day.

Corticosteroids

Corticosteroids have nonspecific anti-inflammatory activity at multiple points in the inflammatory process. Because of the cellular-level airway changes that define COPD, corticosteroids' effects are less dramatic in COPD than those seen in asthma. Yet corticosteroids are key components in the management of stable COPD and COPD exacerbations.

The use of daily inhaled corticosteroids (ICS) in the COPD patient has mixed results in clinical studies (ATS/European Respiratory Society Task Force, 2004; GOLD, 2014; Man & Sin, 2005; Qaseem, et al, 2011). The consensus of the expert panel groups based on the evidence to date is that inhaled corticosteroids do not modify the long-term decline in FEV_1 seen in COPD, but as both monotherapy and in combination with inhaled bronchodilators they decrease exacerbations and improve health status in patients with symptomatic COPD (GOLD, 2014; Qaseem et al, 2011). Therefore, the current ACP and GOLD guidelines recommend starting a patient on moderate- to high-dose inhaled corticosteroids (see Table 30-1). Combination therapy of ICS and a long-acting beta agonist, such as Advair (salmeterol/fluticasone), is more effective in decreasing exacerbations than either agent alone (level A evidence in the GOLD report); therefore, combination therapy should be considered in any patient with moderate to severe COPD defined by FEV_1 less than 60% of predicted (GOLD, 2014; Qaseem et al, 2011).

Education about the slow onset of ICS is necessary so that patients do not become frustrated as the inhaled steroids are introduced. Patients need to be cautioned to rinse their mouths after inhaled steroid use to prevent oral candidiasis. There have been conflicting reports suggesting a higher incidence of pneumonia in patients receiving ICS; however, there is evidence to suggest causality (Hanania 2013).

Oral corticosteroids are useful in the short-term treatment of acute COPD exacerbation (ATS/European Respiratory Society Task Force, 2004; GOLD, 2014). There is level A evidence for the use of oral corticosteroids because they shorten recovery time, improve lung function, and decrease hypoxemia

during the exacerbation (GOLD, 2009). If, in spite of maximum therapy with bronchodilators, the patient continues to have significant airway obstruction, a course of systemic corticosteroids is indicated. Prednisone is given as a dose of 30 to 40 mg daily for 10 days (ATS/European Respiratory Society Task Force, 2004; GOLD, 2009). At that time, the patient should have a 20% to 30% increase in pulmonary function (FEV_1). Some patients respond to a 10-day burst of corticosteroids, and the medications can be discontinued. Other patients require a taper of medication to the lowest prednisone level required to prevent recurrent attacks and relieve bronchospasm. The prednisone dose is tapered over 1 to 2 weeks and then to 5 mg over 5 days. Tapering may lead to recurrence of symptoms, and patients should be educated regarding monitoring their symptoms and PEF during tapering. Long-term treatment with oral corticosteroids is not recommended in COPD (level A evidence), and patients should be transitioned to inhaled corticosteroids either as monotherapy or in combination with inhaled long-acting beta agonists (GOLD, 2014).

Phosphodiesterase-4 Inhibitors

An emerging therapy in the treatment of severe COPD associated with chronic bronchitis is phosphodiesterase-4 (PDE-4) inhibitors. This class of medications inhibits activation of the PDE-4 receptor sites located in the smooth muscles of the airways, resulting in bronchial relaxation and a decrease in the activation of the immune response (Lipari, Benipal, & Kale-Pradhan, 2013). Theophylline is a bronchodilator with nonspecific PDE-inhibition properties, but in 2011, roflumilast (Daliresp) was the first PDE-4 inhibitor approved by the FDA to prevent COPD exacerbation. Roflumilast is not intended as a rescue medication and should be taken daily as a 500 mcg tablet (Lipari et al, 2013; Reid & Pham, 2013).

Oxygen

For some patients, home oxygen therapy is necessary. Oxygen therapy can be used short-term during acute exacerbations or long-term in chronically hypoxemic patients. The goals of supplemental oxygen therapy are to correct arterial hypoxemia and prevent secondary organ damage; ideally, oxygen saturation should be greater than 90%. In patients experiencing an acute exacerbation of COPD, a drop in partial pressure of oxygen in arterial blood (Pa_{O_2}) to below 55 mmHg is an indication for short-term supplemental oxygen. Oxygen saturation of hemoglobin (Sa_{O_2}) has replaced arterial blood gas values in the outpatient setting. An Sa_{O_2} of 88% corresponds with a PaO_2 of 55 mm Hg (McDonald & Khor, 2013).

Patients should be started on continuous oxygen therapy if they demonstrate persistent hypoxemia at rest (Pa_{O_2} less than 55 mmHg or less than 88% oxygen saturation). These patients should be monitored to determine when oxygen therapy can be discontinued. For the chronically hypoxemic COPD patient, continuous home oxygen therapy for 15 hours or more per day is associated with increased survival rate in patients with severe airway obstruction (Qaseem et al, 2014). Patients with cor pulmonale or polycythemia with PaO_2 less than 59 mm Hg and less than 89% oxygen saturation require supplemental oxygen.

Patients on continuous oxygen therapy require arterial blood gas studies after 1, 3, and 6 months of therapy. Supplemental oxygen improves exercise tolerance, neuropsychological function, and quality of life—all key factors in the patient's emotional health in learning to live with this chronic disease.

Antibiotics

Patients with COPD have an excess of thick pulmonary mucus and decreased ciliary clearance of secretions; therefore, they are susceptible to repeated bronchial infections. Infection is considered present when the patient is producing a purulent sputum. The common organisms found in the sputum of patients with COPD patients are *Haemophilus influenzae, Streptococcus pneumoniae, Mycoplasma pneumoniae,* and *Moraxella catarrhalis.* The most common organism is *S. pneumoniae* (Rabe et al, 2007). Antibiotic choices have to cover these organisms until sputum cultures are available to determine sensitivity. Amoxicillin/clavulanic acid, macrolides, and double-strength sulfamethoxazole/trimethoprim are all appropriate first-line choices (Rabe et al, 2007). Resistant organisms require a change in antibiotic therapy after drug susceptibility studies are completed. Patients with moderate exacerbation who may require hospitalization or who don't respond to first-line therapy should be treated with a respiratory fluoroquinolone (levofloxacin, moxifloxacin, gemifloxacin). Length of treatment is 7 to 14 days.

Macrolide antibiotics have an immunomodulatory effect that has been effective for patients with moderate to severe COPD to prevent severe exacerbations (Kanoh & Rubin, 2010). Several small studies (Albert et al, 2011; Milstone, 2008; Spagnolo, Fabbri, & Bush, 2013) and one meta-analysis (Yao, Ma, Zhang, & Gao, 2013) have demonstrated a reduction in exacerbations and improvement of quality of life. The chronic use of macrolide antibiotics in patients with COPD has not been widely accepted because of FDA warnings regarding potential cardiac dysrhythmias, ototoxicity and antibiotic resistance. This therapy is under evaluation and may have a consensus for routine use in the future.

Leukotrienes

There are no data to support the use of leukotriene receptor antagonists in the treatment of COPD.

CLINICAL PEARL

Oxygen Therapy
One note of caution in providing oxygen therapy to some patients with COPD who have poor ventilatory capacity: These patients, known as "carbon dioxide retainers," no longer rely on rises in $PaCO_2$ as the primary drive to breathe. If these patients receive too much oxygen, raising their PaO_2 above their normal baseline, hypoventilation may occur. This results in CO_2 retention and the somnolence, lethargy, and coma that occur with carbon dioxide narcosis. Monitoring arterial blood gases is essential in all patients receiving oxygen therapy.

Alpha-Trypsin Augmentation Therapy

Patients who have emphysema related to genetic alpha$_1$ antitrypsin deficiency may benefit from augmentation therapy with an alpha$_1$-proteinase inhibitor (Prolastin, Aralast, Zemaira). These medications are administered weekly via IV. Patients with alpha$_1$ antitrypsin deficiency should be referred to a specialist for therapy.

Immunizations

Infection prevention is essential in management of patients with COPD, and vaccination against respiratory infections is an integral component in preventing illness in these patients. Protection against influenza virus is recommended annually. Optimally, the influenza vaccine should be administered between October and January, the earlier in the influenza season the better, to allow adequate antibody response. Patients with COPD also require a pneumococcal vaccine every 6 years regardless of age. Patients should be taught the importance of these vaccines so that they remember to get them.

Smoking Cessation

Smoking is a major contributor to COPD. Cigarette smoking results in severe destruction of lung tissue, and the damage is largely irreversible. To halt the progression of COPD, the patient must stop smoking. The benefits of smoking cessation include an eventual return to a nearly normal age-related rate of ventilatory function.

There are many new medications that can help the patient stop smoking. Smoking cessation is discussed in depth in Chapter 43.

Monitoring

Monitoring patients with COPD has four aspects related to pulmonary function and quality of life: signs and symptoms of COPD, pulmonary function, pharmacotherapy, and quality of life.

All patients should be taught how to monitor their symptoms for worsening pulmonary function. Patients with chronic bronchitis need to monitor their sputum for changes in color from their baseline to more purulent. Any symptoms of respiratory infection must be reported to their health-care provider so that appropriate antibiotic therapy can be started. During times of poor outdoor air quality, these patients need to remain indoors and report any signs of respiratory distress to their health-care provider. Patients with COPD may require increased use of bronchodilators or oxygen during these times.

Monitoring pulmonary function is done by spirometry, peak flow meter, oxygen saturation (pulse oximetry), and arterial blood gases. Patients can be taught to use a peak flow meter to monitor lung function at home and determine their need for changes in their medication regimen in times of illness or poor air quality. All patients with COPD need objective monitoring of lung function on a regular basis to identify worsening of function and, therefore, need for a change in their treatment regimen.

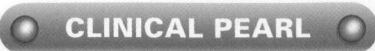

CLINICAL PEARL

Influenza Vaccine Reminders
The health-care provider should keep an electronic "tickler file" of chronic respiratory patients (those with asthma and COPD) so they can remind patients each fall to get their influenza vaccine.

Patients should bring their medications on every visit to the health-care provider. MDI use should be reviewed and technique monitored with each visit. Patients who use more than the recommended amounts of beta$_2$ agonists need to be assessed closely to determine the reason for the increased use. Is the patient using the inhaler incorrectly or is the disease progressing? Increased use of inhaled bronchodilators is an indication for reevaluation of the medication regimen and a possible need for systemic steroids. Patients on supplemental oxygen therapy require arterial blood gases, as previously mentioned, at 1, 3, and 6 months after beginning therapy. Any change in respiratory status is an indication for repeat arterial blood gas determination. All patients require a written medication management plan that is reviewed at every visit.

Monitoring quality of life at every visit can determine if the treatment regimen is successful. Is the patient able to tolerate activities of daily living without assistance? Exercise tolerance, activity level, and nutrition all need to be evaluated.

The financial burden of a chronic illness such as COPD is significant, and referral to a social worker may be necessary to help the patient pay for prescribed treatment.

Outcome Evaluation

Successful management of patients with COPD includes their self-assessment of quality of life, as well as physical parameters of optimal treatment. As COPD is chronic and for the most part irreversible, outcome evaluation is based on the patient's having the best quality of life for the disease state. The successfully managed patient with COPD has optimal activity tolerance, which varies for each patient. Pharmacological management is aimed at decreasing bronchospasm and secondary infections. Therefore, the amount of bronchospasm and the number of infections determine if treatment is successful.

Patient Education

Patient education should include a discussion of information related to the overall treatment plan as well as that specific to the drug therapy, reasons for taking the drug, drugs as part of the total treatment regimen, and adherence issues. Patient education for the COPD patient centers on maintaining optimal pulmonary function and quality of life. Teaching self-management is the basis of successful treatment.

PATIENT EDUCATION

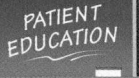

Chronic Obstructive Pulmonary Disease

RELATED TO THE OVERALL TREATMENT PLAN AND DISEASE PROCESS

The patient needs to be taught the following areas of self-management:

SMOKING CESSATION

This is a difficult area of education because of the physical and psychological addiction to cigarettes. Many patients have attempted to quit smoking previously and need to be encouraged to try again, using some of the pharmacological interventions available to aid in tobacco cessation.

PATHOPHYSIOLOGY OF CHRONIC OBSTRUCTIVE PULMONARY DISEASE

A basic understanding of the changes in the pulmonary system that occur with COPD will assist the patient in understanding the role that the different medications play in the treatment regimen.

MEDICATION SKILLS

Patients with COPD often have other chronic illnesses that require routine medications. Administering a complex regimen of multiple medications can be overwhelming, especially to older patients. Written schedules (in large print) and divided pill boxes are two strategies for medication management. Providing the patient with the generic and trade names of medications will decrease medication confusion. Having the patient bring all medications in for review will prevent medication errors. Often, the patient may be seeing other providers, including specialists who may also be prescribing medications. It is the role of the primary care provider to coordinate between specialty providers and monitor medications the patient is taking. Encourage patients to use a magnifying glass to read the generic names on the meter dose inhaler (MDI) canisters, as the canister color may change with different brands of the same medication.

SPECIFIC TO THE DRUG THERAPY

Reason for the drug being given and its anticipated action in the disease process.
Doses and schedules for taking the drug.
Coping mechanisms for complex and costly drug regimens.
Interactions between other treatment modalities and these drugs.

PATIENT EDUCATION—cont'd

REASONS FOR THE DRUG(S) BEING TAKEN

Patient education about specific drugs should be provided, including how to use inhalers appropriately.

DRUGS AS PART OF THE TOTAL TREATMENT REGIMEN

The total treatment regimen also includes teaching self-monitoring skills, including, if indicated, proper use of a peak flow meter.

Infection control measures are also taught. Patients with COPD are at high risk for respiratory infections. They need to be taught the importance of annual influenza vaccine and the need for a pneumococcal pneumonia vaccine every 6 years. They need to avoid crowds and people, especially children, with respiratory infections.

ADHERENCE ISSUES

Health-care providers should be aware of the potential problem of nonadherence with the treatment regimen and should discuss the importance of adherence with the patient and family members.

REFERENCES

Abramowicz, M. (Ed.). (2005). Drugs for asthma. Treatment guidelines from the medical letter, 3(33), 33–38.

Albert, R. K., Connett, J., Bailey, W. C., Casaburi, R., Cooper, J. A. D., Criner, G. J., et al. (2011). Azithromycin for prevention of exacerbations of COPD. New England Journal of Medicine, 365(8), 689–698. doi: 10.1056/NEJMoa1104623

American Medical Association. (1997). Managing asthma today: Integrating new concepts. Chicago: American Medical Association.

American Thoracic Society (ATS)/European Respiratory Society Task Force. (2004). Standards for the diagnosis and management of patients with COPD (Version 1.2). New York: American Thoracic Society. Retrieved from http://www.thoracic.org/clinical/copd-guidelines/resources/copddoc.pdf

Barnes, P. J. (2013). Theophylline. American Journal of Respiratory and Critical Care Medicine, 188(8), 901–906. doi: 10.1164/rccm.201302-0388PP

Bezemer, G. F. P., Sagar, S., van Bergenhenegouwen, J., Georgiou, N., Garssen, J., Kraneveld, A., et al. (2012). Dual role of toll-like receptors in asthma and chronic obstructive pulmonary disease. Pharmacologic Reviews, 64(2), 337–358.

Boehringer Ingelheim Pharmaceuticals. (2009). SPIRIVA Handihaler prescribing information. Retrieved from http://bidocs.boehringer-ingelheim.com/BIWebAccess/ViewServlet.ser?docBase=renetnt&folderPath=/Prescribing+Information/PIs/Spiriva/Spiriva.pdf

Boom, L., Vaessen, D., Uil, S., Kerstjens, H. & van den Berg, J. (2011). The effects of montelukast in patients with chronic cough and bronchial hyperreactivity. Chest, 140(4 Meeting Abstracts), 918A.

Bousquet, J., Cabrera, P., Berkman, N., Buhl, R., Holgate, S., Wenzel, S., et al. (2005). The effect of treatment with omalizumab, an anti-IgE antibody, on asthma exacerbations and emergency medical visits in patients with severe persistent asthma. Allergy, 60(3), 302–308.

Brehm, J., Schuemann, B., Fuhlbrigge, A., Hollis, B., Strucnk, R., Zeiger, R., et al. (2010). Serum vitamin D levels and severe asthma exacerbations in the childhood asthma management program study. Journal of Allergy and Clinical Immunology, 126(1), 53–58.

Centers for Disease Control (2015). FastStats: Asthma. Retrieved from http://www.cdc.gov/nchs/fastats/asthma.htm

Chiang, D. T., Clark, J., & Casale, T. B. (2005). Omalizumab in asthma: Approval and postapproval experience. Clinical Reviews in Allergy and Immunology, 29(1), 3–16.

Cope, S., Kraemer, M., Zhang, J., Capkun-Niggli, G., & Jansen, J. P. (2012). Efficacy of indacaterol 75 µg versus fixed-dose combinations of formoterol-budesonide or salmeterol-fluticasone for COPD: A network meta-analysis. International Journal of Chronic Obstructive Pulmonary Disease, 2012(7), 415–420. doi: 10.2147/COPD.S31526

Covar, R. A., & Spahn, J. D. (2003). Treating the wheezing infant. Pediatric Clinics of North America, 50(3), 631–654.

Drazen, J. M., Israel, E., Boushey, H. A., Chinchilli, V. M., Fahy, J. V., Fish, J. E., et al. (1996). Comparison of regularly scheduled with as-needed use of albuterol in mild asthma. New England Journal of Medicine, 335(12), 841–847.

Global Initiative for Asthma. (2013). Global strategy for asthma management and prevention. Retrieved from http://www.ginasthma.org

Global Initiative for Chronic Obstructive Lung Disease [GOLD]. (2014). Global strategy for the diagnosis, management, and prevention of chronic obstructive pulmonary disease: Medical communications resources. Retrieved from www.goldcopd.org

Hakim, A., Adcock, I., & Usmani, O. (2012). Corticosteroid resistance and novel anti-inflammatory therapies in chronic obstructive pulmonary disease. Drugs, 72(10), 1299–1312. doi: 10.2165/11634350-000

Halbert, R. J., Isonaka, S., George, D., & Iqbal, A. (2003). Interpreting COPD estimates: What is the true burden of disease? Chest, 123(5), 1684–1692.

Hanania, N. A., & Belfort, M. A. (2005). Acute asthma in pregnancy. Critical Care Medicine, 33(10 Suppl.), S319–S324.

Henderson, W. R. (1994). The role of leukotrienes in inflammation. Annals of Internal Medicine, 121(9), 684–697. doi: 10.7326/0003-4819-121-9-199411010-00010

Kanoh, S., & Rubin, B. K. (2010). Mechanisms of action and clinical application of macrolides as immunomodulatory medications. Clinical Microbiology Reviews, 23(3), 590–615. doi: 10.1128/cmr.00078-09

Kwon, H. L., Belanger, K., & Bracken, M. B. (2003). Asthma prevalence among pregnant and childbearing-aged women in the United States: Estimates from national health surveys. Annals of Epidemiology, 13, 317–324.

Lieu, T. A., Quesenberry, C. P., Capra, A. M., Sorel, M. E., Martin, K. E., & Mendoza, G. R. (1997). Outpatient management practices associated with reduced risk of pediatric asthma hospitalization and emergency department visits. Pediatrics, 100(3), 334–341.

Lipari, M., Benipal, H., & Kale-Pradhan, P. (2013). Roflumilast in the management of chronic obstructive pulmonary disease. American Journal of Health-System Pharmacy, 70(23), 2087–2095. doi: 10.2146/ajhp130114

Louik, C., Schatz, M., Hernandez-Diaz, S., Werler, M. M. & Mitchell, A. A. (2010). Asthma in pregnancy and its pharmacologic treatment. Annals in Allergy and Immunology, 105(2), 110–117.

Man, S. F. P., & Sin, D. D. (2005). Inhaled corticosteroids in chronic obstructive pulmonary disease: Is there a clinical benefit? Drugs, 65(5), 579–591.

Milstone, A. P. (2008). Use of azithromycin in the treatment of acute exacerbations of COPD. International Journal of Chronic Obstructive Pulmonary Disease, 3(4), 515–520.

National Asthma Education and Prevention Program (NAEPP). (2007). The Expert Panel Report 3: Guidelines for the diagnosis and management of asthma. Bethesda, MD: National Heart, Lung, and Blood Institute, National Institutes of Health. Retrieved from http://www.nhlbi.nih.gov/guidelines/asthma/

Netzer, N., Küpper, T., Voss, H., & Eliasson, A. (2012). The actual role of sodium cromoglycate in the treatment of asthma—A critical review. Sleep and Breathing, 16(4), 1027–1032. doi: 10.1007/s11325-011-0639-1

Parsons, J. P., & Mastronarde, J. G. (2005). Exercise-induced bronchoconstriction in athletes. Chest, 128(6), 3966–3974.

Qaseem, A., Wilt, T., Weinberger, S. E., Hananua, N. A., Criner, G., & Shekelle, P. (2011). Diagnosis and management of stable chronic obstructive pulmonary disease: A clinical practice guideline from the American College of Physicians. *Annals of Internal Medicine, 155,* 179–191.

Rabe, K. F., Hurd, S., Anzueto, A., Barnes, P. J., Buist, S. A., Calverley, P., et al. (2007). Global strategy for the diagnosis, management, and prevention of chronic obstructive pulmonary disease. *American Journal of Respiratory Critical Care Medicine, 176*(6), 532–555.

Rance, K. (2013). The emerging role of vitamin D in asthma management. *Journal of the American Association of Nurse Practitioners.*

Reid, D. J., & Pham, N. T. (2013). Emerging therapeutic options for the management of COPD. *Clinical Medicine Insights: Circulatory, Respiratory and Pulmonary Medicine, 2013*(7), 7–15. doi: 10.4137/CCRPM.S8140

Rovina, N., Koutsoukou, A., & Koulouris, N. (2013). Inflammation and immune response in COPD: Where do we stand? *Mediators of Inflammation, 2013,* Article ID 413735, 9 pp. doi: 10.1155/2013/413735

Schofield, M. L. (2014). Asthma pharmacotherapy. *Otolaryngologic Clinics of North America, 47*(1), 55–64. doi: http://dx.doi.org/10.1016/j.otc.2013.09.011

Self, T. H., George, C. M., Wallace, J. L., Patterson S. J., & Finch, C. F. (2014). Incorrect use of peak flow meters: Are you observing your patients? *Journal of Asthma, 51*(6), 566–572.

Spagnolo, P., Fabbri, L. M., & Bush, A. (2013). Long-term macrolide treatment for chronic respiratory disease. *European Respiratory Journal, 42*(1), 239–251. doi: 10.1183/09031936.00136712

Spector, S. L., & Tan, R. A. (2004). Effectiveness of montelukast in the treatment of cough variant asthma. *Annals of Allergy, Asthma, and Immunology, 9*(3), 232–236.

Statistics Canada (2010). Asthma, by sex, provinces and territories. Retrieved from http://www40.statcan.ca/l01/cst01/health50a-eng.htm

U.S. Food and Drug Administration. (2010). FDA drug safety communication: New safety requirements for long-acting inhaled asthma medications called long-acting beta-agonists (LABAs). Retrieved from http://www.fda.gov/Drugs/DrugSafety/PostmarketDrugSafety InformationforPatientsand Providers/ucm200776.htm

Yao, G., Ma, Y., Zhang, M., & Gao, Z. (2013). Macrolide therapy decreases chronic obstructive pulmonary disease exacerbation: A meta-analysis. *Respiration, 86*(3), 254–260. doi: 10.1159/000350828

Zittermann, A., Gummert, J., & Borgermann, J. (2009). Vitamin D deficiency and mortality. *Current Opinion in Clinical Nutrition and Metabolic Care, 12*(6), 634–639.

CONTRACEPTION

Teral Gerlt

Choosing a method of contraception (birth control) is an intimate process and one in which patients, male and female, often seek advice from their health-care provider. Unintended pregnancy rates remain high in the United States. Mosher, Jones, and Abma (2012) report that in the years from 2006 to 2010, just over 37% of all pregnancies in women age 15 to 44 were unplanned. Considerations that must be addressed include the safety of the method chosen, age of the patient, the health and medical conditions of the patient, ability to comply with method use, frequency of sexual relations, risk of sexually transmitted infections, and cost. The most important of these considerations after safety is compliance; any method that offers safety to the patient offers very little protection from pregnancy if use of the method does not fit the patient's lifestyle.

Many contraceptive options are available with varying efficacy rates (Hatcher et al, 2011). These options and their efficacy rates for first year of use are presented in Table 31-1. This chapter focuses on the pharmacological methods of contraception that offer the highest rates of effectiveness. Over the past several years, novel modes of delivery for contraceptive hormones have been introduced. The new delivery modes offer potentially lower rates of failure due to user error because they involve less frequent administration intervals, therefore increasing the user's ability to comply with proper use. Pharmacological methods include oral contraceptives (OCs), topical patches, vaginal rings, subdermal implants, injections, and intrauterine devices (IUDs). These methods include progestin-only preparations and preparations that include various combinations of estrogen and progestin.

PHYSIOLOGY OF THE NORMAL MENSTRUAL CYCLE

The menstrual cycle is regulated by positive and negative feedback in the hypothalamic-pituitary-ovarian axis. The pituitary gland releases stimulating and inhibiting hormones. Release of these hormones is regulated by pulses of gonadotropin-releasing hormone (GnRH) from the hypothalamus. GnRH pulses regulate follicle-stimulating hormone (FSH) and luteinizing hormone (LH) that in turn regulate the secretion of estrogen and progesterone from the ovary. The most obvious manifestation of this complex system is cyclic menstrual bleeding.

Table 31–1　Contraceptive Options

Method	Advantages	Disadvantages	Perfect Use Efficacy	Typical Use Efficacy
Estrogen/Progestin Combination Contraception				
Pills	Menstrual cycle control	Daily administration may be difficult for some users	>99%	91%
Patch	Menstrual cycle control Weekly administration	Patch may cause some local irritation Patch may fall off partially or completely	>99%	91%
Ring	Menstrual cycle control Once per cycle administration	User must be comfortable with vaginal administration	>99%	91%
Progestin Only				
Oral contraception	No estrogen; may be useful for users in whom estrogen is contraindicated	Daily administration may be difficult for some users Unpredictable bleeding pattern	>99%	92%
Progestin injectable contraception	Administration once every 12 wk Use of method discreet from others	Administration requires office visit Unpredictable bleeding pattern	>99%	94%
Progestin implant	Offers contraception for 3 yr	Insertion and removal requires office procedure Unpredictable bleeding pattern	>99%	>99%
Intrauterine Device (IUD)				
Copper	Hormone free Offers contraception for 10 yr	Insertion and removal requires office visit Dysmenorrhea and menstrual flow may be increased in first few months after insertion	>99%	>99%
Progestin-releasing	Decreased menstrual flow Offers contraception for 3 or 5 yr	Requires office visit for insertion and removal	>99%	>99%
Barrier Methods				
Male condom	Protection from most STIs Available without prescription	Use linked to coitus and partner-dependent	98%	82%
Female condom	Protection from most STIs Available without prescription	Use linked to coitus	95%	79%
Spermicide	Available without prescription	Use linked to coitus	82%	71%
Diaphragm	May be inserted several hours before intercourse	Available only with provider fitting and prescription Must be used with spermicide User must be comfortable with vaginal insertion technique	94%	88%
Cervical cap	May be inserted several hours before intercourse	Available only with provider fitting and prescription Must be used with spermicide User must be comfortable with vaginal insertion technique Lower efficacy for parous women	74%–91%	68%–84%
Vaginal sponge	Available without prescription Contains spermicide May be inserted several hours before intercourse	Lower efficacy for parous women	80%–91%	68%–84%

STIs = sexually transmitted infections.

The menstrual cycle is divided into four phases: follicular, ovulatory, luteal, and menstrual. During the follicular phase, FSH stimulates several follicles to develop, with one ultimately becoming dominant. The dominant follicle synthesizes enough estradiol to create negative feedback and decrease FSH levels. During the ovulatory phase, estradiol levels peak and exert positive feedback to induce an LH surge, which in turn facilitates release of the mature ovum. Estrogen also promotes proliferation of the endometrium, and development of progesterone receptors in the endometrium.

During the luteal phase, progesterone dominates; it is produced predominantly by the corpus luteum and prevents new follicle development as well as differentiation of the endometrium. If pregnancy does not occur, the corpus luteum degenerates. Once the corpus luteum degenerates, estrogen and progesterone levels decline, resulting in endometrial shedding or menstrual bleeding. Other gynecological organs are also influenced by estrogen and progesterone. The fallopian tubes exhibit increased proliferation, differentiation, and tubular contractility under the influence of estrogen; these processes are inhibited under the influence of progesterone. Cervical mucus water content is increased and penetration of sperm is facilitated by estrogen, whereas it is decreased by progesterone.

Estrogen exerts effects on other body systems, including positive effects on bone mass, increasing serum triglycerides, improving high-density lipoprotein (HDL) to low-density lipoprotein (LDL) ratios, and stimulating coagulation and fibrinolytic pathways. Progesterone increases body temperature, increases insulin levels, and may slightly depress the central nervous system (Chrousos, 2012).

PHARMACODYNAMICS

The major difference between endogenous estrogen and progestins and pharmacological preparations is their oral bioavailability. All orally available estrogen and progestins undergo first-pass metabolism in the liver. Currently, the vast majority of contraceptive preparations use ethinyl estradiol (EE) as the estrogen component. Mestranol is used in only three brands of OCs and must be metabolized into EE before it is able to bind with estrogen receptors. The last estrogen is estradiol valerate, a synthetic prodrug of 17ß-estradiol, used only in the quadriphasic Natizna.

Most progestins used in hormonal contraception are derivatives of testosterone. The alteration of testosterone not only makes them bioavailable but also changes their activity from androgenic to much more selective progestational activity. Currently, several different androgen-derived progestins are available in oral contraceptive preparations. Norethindrone, norethindrone acetate, and ethynodiol diacetate are first-generation progestins. Both norethindrone acetate and ethynodiol diacetate are converted to norethindrone in the body. As the amount of these progestins used in the formulations decreased, women experienced more spotting and breakthrough bleeding. In response, the second-generation progestins, norgestrel and levonorgestrel,

were developed. Levonorgestrel is the levorotatory form of norgestrel and its active metabolite. These progestins increased androgenic activity, thereby decreasing breakthrough bleeding; however, increasing the androgenic activity may lead to problems with acne, hirsutism, and dyslipidemia (Hatcher et al, 2011).

Desogestrel and norgestimate are third-generation progestins, which offer a decrease in androgenicity. Desogestrel undergoes conversion to its active metabolite etonogestrel, which is the progestin used in the vaginal ring and the subdermal implant. Norelgestromin is the primary metabolite of norgestimate and is available in the contraceptive patch. Decreased androgenicity theoretically reduced adverse effects on carbohydrate and lipid metabolism found in previous formulations, as well as lessening acne and hirsutism. Medroxyprogesterone acetate is available for injectable contraception.

Two fourth-generation progestins are now in use in the United States. Drospirenone is a derivative of spironolactone; as such, it has a mild diuretic effect as well as antimineralocorticoid effects. Drospirenone may cause hyperkalemia and should be used cautiously in women who are using drugs that cause a potassium-sparing effect, such as angiotensin-converting enzyme (ACE) inhibitors. Drospirenone should not be used in women with abnormal adrenal, renal, or hepatic function (*Drug Facts and Comparisons*, 2013; Speroff & Darney, 2011). The last progestin is dienogest, which displays properties of 19-nortestosterone derivatives as well as properties associated with progesterone derivatives, producing an anti-androgenic action (Speroff & Darney, 2011).

Mechanism of Pregnancy Prevention

Progestins are primarily responsible for the contraceptive effect in hormonal preparations. Progestins exhibit a negative effect in the hypothalamic-pituitary-ovarian axis, essentially suppressing the LH surge necessary for ovulation. They also cause thickening of cervical mucus, making penetration by sperm difficult. Tubal motility is slowed, delaying transport of the ovum and sperm. Finally, progestins cause atrophy of the endometrium, preventing implantation.

The estrogen component of hormonal contraception improves efficacy by suppressing FSH release, and therefore development of a dominant follicle. Estrogen also adds to cycle control, decreasing irregular bleeding patterns commonly found with progestin-only methods (Chrousos, 2012; Speroff & Darney, 2011).

GOALS OF TREATMENT

Treatment goals of pharmacological contraception are to use the safest, best-tolerated, and most effective method that the patient desires. In order to help the patient determine which contraception method may be best for her, the provider needs to be aware of any cultural or religious determinants, as well as partner acceptance.

NEW OCS

In the last few years most of the research on new OCs has involved changing the type of estrogen and/or progestin in the formulations and the dosing pattern to decrease side effects and enhance ease of use (Sitruk-Ware, Nath, & Mishell, 2013). Natazia was released in 2010 and is the only four-phasic oral contraceptive on the market. It is the first OC to contain estradiol valerate, a synthetic prodrug of 17ß-estradiol and a new progestin, dienogest, which displays properties of 19-nortestosterone derivatives as well as properties associated with progesterone derivatives.

The only chewable OC on the market, Generess, combines 0.8 mg norethindrone and 0.025 mg ethinyl estradiol with four 75 mg ferrous fumarate placebo tablets. The 24/4 regimen is intended to decrease breakthrough bleeding and provide short, light, predictable periods (Shrader & Dickerson, 2008).

A combination OC, Zoely, utilizing natural estrogen (17β estradiol), and a new progestin (nomegesterol acetate), manufactured by Merck have been approved in the United Kingdom and several European and Latin American countries (Bahamondes & Bahamondes, 2014). The estrogen component, 17β estradiol, is structurally identical to endogenous 17β estradiol (Merck, 2014). Nomegesterol acetate has a 46-hour half-life, which increases efficacy (Merck, 2014). It has not received U.S. approval yet.

Safety

The fear over increased risk of breast cancer with oral contraceptive use is largely media induced. A meta-analysis of breast cancer data (Kahlenborn, Modugno, Potter, & Severs, 2006) suggests a small overall increase in breast cancer risk (OR = 1.19) across different use patterns. In studies that controlled for parity, the data indicated that the risk of breast cancer in nulliparous women was OR equal to 1.24, and length of hormonal contraceptive use did not increase risk. The most interesting finding was the increased risk of breast cancer in parous women who used OCs for more than 4 years prior to their first full-term pregnancy (OR = 1.52). However, Speroff and Darney (2011) put this in perspective by pointing out that because most of the women using OCs are in an age bracket during which breast cancer is very rare, the overall increase in breast cancer cases is relatively small.

A recently reported prospective study of over 116,000 women did find a RR = 1.33 of breast cancer with current use and no significant risk with past use (Hunter et al, 2010). One interesting finding was an increased risk (RR = 3.05) only in current use of a triphasic formulation containing levonorgestrel. When the use of this formulation was controlled for, it was found to account for the majority of breast cancer cases.

Current studies find no increase in the frequency of liver cancer in women who use OCs. Studies do show a negligible increase in the incidence of gallstones in current users, but the data point to this in women who have underlying asymptomatic disease and its acceleration, rather than an actual increase in the population.

Cardiovascular disease risk related to lipid metabolism is difficult to quantify because so many other risk factors are involved. Formulations with less than 50 mcg of estrogen seem to have no detrimental effects. In general, the cardiovascular risk factors other than OC use play the predominant role in the occurrence of ischemic stroke and myocardial infarction. Patients who smoke share an increased risk for heart attack, stroke, and thromboembolic phenomena (deep venous thrombosis [DVT] and pulmonary embolism) as they approach 35 years of age (Speroff & Darney, 2011). Findings from the Women's Health Initiative are discussed in Chapter 38 in relation to hormone replacement therapy. These findings should be considered in prescribing OCs, but the risk for these low doses of estrogen and progesterone were not part of this study.

Tolerance

More than 40 years of experience in prescribing OCs have provided much data with which to knowledgeably help patients decide when choosing an OC. Current OCs have less estrogen; therefore, they cause fewer of the pregnancy-like symptoms that had earlier been so distressing. The third- and fourth-generation progestins show fewer weight changes, improved complexion, and reduced mood swings. Improvements in packaging have also improved compliance by providing cues in the packaging for the day of the week each pill should be taken.

Effectiveness

The theoretical effectiveness is 99% or greater with most hormonal therapies. Patients have lower discontinuation rates and therefore fewer unwanted pregnancies if they are well educated about emergency hormonal contraception and use a backup method such as spermicide and condoms. Vomiting and diarrhea that accompany gastrointestinal illnesses can decrease oral contraceptive effectiveness by decreasing absorption; women should be advised to use a backup method for at least 7 days after a gastrointestinal illness (Speroff & Darney, 2011).

RATIONAL DRUG SELECTION

Guidelines

A good place to start in helping a patient choose a new hormonal contraceptive is to exclude those methods that are absolutely or relatively contraindicated because of existing health concerns and patient age. Deciding whether the patient has any contraindications to the use of estrogen narrows the choices considerably. Then review which delivery mode appeals to the patient based on her perceived ability to comply with the dosing regimen. Choices can then be fine-tuned based on acceptability of likely changes in bleeding pattern and side-effect profile. The provider should also discuss the theoretical and typical failure rates with the patient to ascertain if these are congruent with the patient's desire to avoid pregnancy. Other factors to consider are a patient's need for discreetness in the use of her method: a patient may wish to conceal her contraceptive method from partners or other family members and taking a daily pill or wearing a patch may preclude these choices. Timing of a subsequent pregnancy should also be considered; for some methods a return to fertility is delayed after cessation of use. For patients who are satisfied with their current hormonal contraceptive choice, and for whom no new contraindications because of health issues are present, changing from a product or method to one that is newer to the market is unnecessary.

More than four dozen formulations of monophasic combined oral contraceptives (COCs), about two dozen multiphasic COCs, and several formulations of progestin-only pills (POPs), as well as several nonoral contraceptive hormone delivery methods, are available. Table 31-2 summarizes the name brand and generic hormone formulas currently available (Chrousos, 2012; *Drug Facts and Comparisons,* 2013; Hatcher et al, 2011; Shrader & Dickerson, 2008).

Table 31–2 Oral Contraceptives

Brand Name	Estrogen Dose (mcg)	Progestin Dose (mg)
Progestin-Only Tablets		
Camilla, Errin, Heather, Jencycla, Jolivette, Micronor, Nor-QD, Nora-BE		Norethindrone 0.35
Monophasic Combination Tablets		
Viorele	Ethinyl estradiol 20	Desogestrel 0.15
Gianvi, Loryna, Yaz	Ethinyl estradiol 20 (24 d)	Drospirenone 3 (24 d)
Amethyst	Ethinyl estradiol 20	Levonorgestrel 0.09
Aviane, Falmina, Lessina, Lutera, Orsythia, Sronyx	Ethinyl estradiol 20	Levonorgestrel 0.1
Junel 21 1/20, Junel Fe 1/20 Loestrin 21 1/20, Loestrin 24 Fe, Loestrin Fe 1/20, Microgestin 1/20, Microgestin Fe 1/20, Minastrin 24 Fe	Ethinyl estradiol 20	Norethindrone acetate 1
Generess Fe 24/4 (Chewable)	Ethinyl estradiol 25	Norethindrone 0.8
Apri, Desogen, Emoquette, Enskyce, Ortho-Cept, Reclipsen	Ethinyl estradiol 30	Desogestrel 0.15
Ocella , Syeda, Vestura, Yasmin, Zarah	Ethinyl estradiol 30	Drospirenone 3
Altavera, Jolessa, Kurvelo, Levora, Marlissa, Nordette, Portia, Quasense	Ethinyl estradiol 30	Levonorgestrel 0.15
Junel 21 1/30 w/Fe	Ethinyl estradiol 30	Norethindrone acetate 1
Junel 21 1.5/30, Junel Fe 1.5/30 Loestrin 21 1.5/30, Loestrin Fe 1.5/30, Microgestin 1.5/30, Microgestin Fe 1.5/30	Ethinyl estradiol 30	Norethindrone acetate 1.5
Cryselle, Elinest, Lo/Ovral, Low-Ogestrel	Ethinyl estradiol 30	Norgestrel 0.3
Kelnor, Zovia 1/35	Ethinyl estradiol 35	Ethynodiol diacetate 1
Balziva, Femcon Fe, Gidagia, Ovcon 35, Zenchent, Zenchent Fe, Zeosa	Ethinyl estradiol 35	Norethindrone 0.4
Brevicon, Modicon, Necon 0.5/35, Nortrel 0.5/35, Wera	Ethinyl estradiol 35	Norethindrone 0.5
Alyacen 1/35, Cyclafem 1/35, Dasetta 1/35, Necon 1/35, Norinyl 1/35, Nortrel 1/35, Ortho-Novum 1/35, Pirmella 1/35	Ethinyl estradiol 35	Norethindrone 1
Estarylla, Mono-Linyah, MonoNessa, Ortho-Cyclen, Previfem, Sprintec	Ethinyl estradiol 35	Norgestimate 0.25
Necon 1/50, Norinyl 1/50, Ortho-Novum 1/50	Mestranol 50 (equivalent to 35 ethinyl estradiol)	Norethindrone 1
Zovia 1/50	Ethinyl estradiol 50	Ethynodiol diacetate 1
Ovcon 50	Ethinyl estradiol 50	Norethindrone 1
Ogestrel 28	Ethinyl estradiol 50	Norgestrel 0.5
Extended Cycle Packs		
Introvale, Jolessa, Seasonale	Ethinyl estradiol 30 (84 d)	Levonorgestrel 0.15 (84 d)
Amethia, Camrese, Daysee, Seasonique	Ethinyl estradiol 30 (84 d)	Levonorgestrel 0.15 (84 d)
	Ethinyl estradiol 10 (7 d)	

Continued

Table 31–2   Oral Contraceptives—cont'd

Brand Name	Estrogen Dose (mcg)	Progestin Dose (mg)
Amethia Lo, CamreseLo, LoSeasonique	Ethinyl estradiol 20 (84 d)	Levonorgestrel 0.1 (84 d)
	Ethinyl estradiol 10 (7 d)	
Lybrel (Continuous dosing)	Ethinyl estradiol 20	Levonorgestrel 0.09
Biphasic Combination Tablets		
Lo Loestrin Fe	Ethinyl estradiol 10 (24d)	Norethindrone 1 (24 d)
	Ethinyl estradiol 10 (2)	Norethindrone 0 (2 d)
Necon 10/11	Ethinyl estradiol 35	Norethindrone 0.5 (10 d)
	Ethinyl estradiol 35	Norethindrone 1 (11 d)
Triphasic Combination Tablets		
Mircette, Kariva	Ethinyl estradiol 20	Desogestrel 0.15 (21 d)
	Placebo (2 d)	
	Ethinyl estradiol 10 mcg (5 d)	
Caziant , Cyclessa, Velivet	Ethinyl estradiol 25	Desogestrel 0.1 (7 d)
	Ethinyl estradiol 25	Desogestrel 0.125 (7 d)
	Ethinyl estradiol 25	Desogestrel 0.15 (7 d)
Ortho Tri-Cyclen Lo, Tri-Lo-Sprintec	Ethinyl estradiol 25	Norgestimate 0.18 (7 d)
	Ethinyl estradiol 25	Norgestimate 0.215 (7 d)
	Ethinyl estradiol 25	Norgestimate 0.25 (7 d)
Ortho Tri-Cyclen, Tri-Estarylla, Tri-Linyah, Tri-Previfem, Tri-Sprintec, TriNessa	Ethinyl estradiol 35	Norgestimate 0.18 (7 d)
	Ethinyl estradiol 35	Norgestimate 0.215 (7 d)
	Ethinyl estradiol 35	Norgestimate 0.25 (7 d)
Estrostep Fe	Ethinyl estradiol 20	Norethindrone acetate 1 (7 d)
	Ethinyl estradiol 30	Norethindrone acetate 1 (7 d)
	Ethinyl estradiol 35	Norethindrone acetate 1 (7 d)
Enpresse, Myzilra, Trivora	Ethinyl estradiol 30	Levonorgestrel 0.05 (6 d)
	Ethinyl estradiol 40	Levonorgestrel 0.075 (5 d)
	Ethinyl estradiol 30	Levonorgestrel 0.125 (10 d)
Alyacen 7/7/7, Cyclafem 7/7/7, Dasetta 7/7/7, Necon 7/7/7, Nortrel 7/7/7, Ortho-Novum 7/7/7, Pirmella 7/7/7	Ethinyl estradiol 35	Norethindrone 0.5 (7 d)
	Ethinyl estradiol 35	Norethindrone 0.75 (7 d)
	Ethinyl estradiol 35	Norethindrone 1 (7 d)
Aranelle, Leena, Tri-Norinyl	Ethinyl estradiol 35	Norethindrone 0.5 (7 d)
	Ethinyl estradiol 35	Norethindrone 1 (9 d)
	Ethinyl estradiol 35	Norethindrone 0.5 (5 d)
Tilia Fe, TriLegest Fe	Ethinyl estradiol 20	Norethindrone acetate 1 (5 d)
	Ethinyl estradiol 30	Norethindrone acetate 1 (7 d)
	Ethinyl estradiol 35	Norethindrone acetate 1 (9 d)

Table 31–2   Oral Contraceptives—cont'd

Brand Name	Estrogen Dose (mcg)	Progestin Dose (mg)
Quadriphasic Combination Tablets		
Natazia 28 d	Estradiol valerate 3mg (2 d)	Dienogest 0mg (2 d)
	Estradiol valerate 2mg (5 d)	Dienogest 2mg (5 d)
	Estradiol valerate 2mg (17 d)	Dienogest 3mg (17 d)
	Estradiol valerate 1mg (2 d)	Dienogest 0mg (2 d)

If all OCs are similar in effectiveness and well tolerated, then choosing among them may seem difficult. In general, using a hormonal contraceptive with the lowest dose that still offers cycle control is best. Many experienced practitioners have a few favorite formulations that they use in clinical practice; they only venture from these choices if a patient has a particular side effect that may be improved by switching to another formulation based on increasing or decreasing the dose of its component drugs. This is also a good place for new practitioners to start when becoming comfortable with contraceptive counseling and prescribing. A short list should include one preparation that does not contain estrogen, an ultra-low dose, or 20 mcg EE pill (e.g., to use for women older than 35 years of age or those who smoke more than 15 cigarettes per day), a monophasic COC, a multiphasic COC, and a nondaily administration method for women who have difficulty with daily regimens. One factor that may influence what is on the short list is the availability of samples or products for purchase at the clinical site. Another influence may be patients' request for a particular brand-name product because of direct-consumer advertising practices of the drug companies. Additionally, the provider should be aware of what OCs are covered by the patient's insurance and what OCs are available on the $4 retail plans locally.

Cost

Cost can be a major barrier to contraceptive use for patients who do not have health insurance or prescription drug coverage. Most communities have county or private not-for-profit contraceptive centers with a sliding-scale fee schedule based on income to assist women without health insurance. The average cost for most forms of cyclical hormonal contraception is $30 to over $100 per cycle. Generic substitutions at lower prices are now available for many formulations, including formulations on the $4 retail plans. The cost of injectable contraception could be higher because of the office visit required for administration.

The initial cost of an IUD insertion may rule this out as an easy choice, but the cost spread over the life of the device may be less than that of other forms. Even for women who have prescription drug coverage, cost can be an issue.

Many insurance companies have implemented two- or three-tier co-payment schedules, resulting in higher costs for the client if a drug is not on the first-line formulary. The insurance companies are to provide formulary information to patients and providers to assist in decision making.

The Affordable Care Act (ACA) covers all prescription birth control methods as of 2014. The ACA spells out that barrier methods, hormonal methods, implanted devices (IUDs), emergency contraception, and sterilization procedures are all covered.

Patient Variables

Differences in a woman's physiological and psychological responses to estrogens and progestins make choosing OCs more art than science. However, taking a thorough personal and family history, performing a complete physical examination, and performing screening laboratory tests appropriate for patient age will identify those for whom OCs should not be prescribed. Patient variables that require withholding OCs or monitoring more closely are listed in Table 31-3.

The primary indication for using hormonal contraceptive preparations is to prevent pregnancy. These methods offer effectiveness and reversibility. In addition, users may experience the following noncontraceptive benefits (Hatcher et al, 2011; Speroff & Darney, 2011).

- Decreased dysmenorrhea, menstrual irregularities, and menstrual blood loss
- Lessening of acne and hirsutism
- Fewer ovarian cysts
- Significantly reduced endometrial and ovarian cancer risk
- Lower incidence of benign breast conditions such as fibrocystic changes and fibroadenoma
- Increased bone density
- Suppression of endometriosis for women who do not currently desire pregnancy

Drug Variables

Drug Interactions

Hormonal contraception that is administered orally undergoes first-pass metabolism in the liver; therefore, drugs that induce liver enzymes will decrease their contraceptive efficacy. Agents that treat tuberculosis, barbiturates, anticonvulsants,

Table 31–3   WHO Contraindications to Initiation of Combined Contraception with 35 mcg EE or Less

Risk	Contraindication
WHO Category 2 Contraceptive benefits usually outweigh risks; may require more frequent monitoring	Age >40 yr Smoker <35 yr BMI >30 due to increased VTE risk Hx HTN during pregnancy, BP now normal Known hyperlipidemia First-degree relative with DVT/PE Major surgery without prolonged immobilization Superficial thrombophlebitis SLE on immunosuppressive therapy or with severe thrombocytopenia Rheumatoid arthritis Sickle cell disease Valvular heart disease, uncomplicated Migraine without neurological aura, age <35 yr Unexplained vaginal bleeding, suspicious for serious underlying condition Cervical intraepithelial neoplasia Cervical cancer, awaiting treatment Undiagnosed breast mass Diabetes, insulin dependent or non-insulin-dependent, without vascular disease Asymptomatic gallbladder disease or postcholecystectomy Benign focal nodular hyperplasia of the liver Hx of cholestasis in pregnancy Ulcerative colitis or Crohn's disease Postpartum & breastfeeding, 4–6 wks PP with normal risk of DVT and >6 wks PP Postpartum & not breastfeeding, 3–6 wks PP with normal risk of DVT
WHO Category 3 Risks usually outweigh contraceptive benefits	Postpartum & breastfeeding, 3–4 wks and 4–6 wks with increased risk of DVT Postpartum & not breastfeeding, 3–4 wks with increased risk of DVT Age >35 yr and smoker <15 cigarettes/d Several drug interactions: protease inhibitors; anticonvulsants; lamotrigine; rifampin Multiple risk factors for coronary artery disease (based on age, smoking, diabetes, hypertension) Hypertension, adequately controlled and monitored • Systolic 140–159 or diastolic 90–99 Migraine without neurological aura, age >35 yr Hx of breast cancer, no disease >5 yr Diabetic with nephropathy, neuropathy, retinopathy Diabetic with vascular disease Diabetic >20 yr Symptomatic gallbladder disease Past COC-related cholestasis
WHO Category 4 Unacceptable risk	Postpartum <3wk Age >35 yr and smoker >15 cigarettes/d HTN, not controlled or with vascular disease • Systolic ≥160 or diastolic ≥100 Current or hx of DVT/PE Major surgery with prolonged immobilization Known thrombogenic mutations Current or hx of ischemic heart disease Current or hx of stroke Valvular heart disease, complicated Migraine with neurological aura SLE with positive or unknown antiphospholipid antibodies Current breast cancer Active viral hepatitis Cirrhosis, severe/decompensated Benign hepatocellular adenoma or malignant liver tumor

BMI = body mass index; BP = blood pressure; COC= combined oral contraceptives; DVT/PE = deep venous thrombosis/pulmonary embolism; EE = ethinyl estradiol; Hx = history; HTN = hypertension; SLE = systemic lupus erythematosus; WHO = World Health Organization.

and the herbal preparation St. John's wort have all been shown to increase liver metabolism of OCs; irregular bleeding and a decrease in contraceptive effectiveness may occur (*Drug Facts and Comparisons*, 2013). Common broad-spectrum antibiotics have not been shown to decrease serum concentrations of OCs. Penicillin and tetracycline are known to alter steroid metabolism in the gut because of changes in intestinal flora; this may potentially reduce their absorption and effectiveness. Therefore, product labeling and *Drug Facts and Comparisons* (2013) still advise caution and the use of a backup method of contraception during and for 7 days after their use. However, both Hatcher and colleagues (2011) and Speroff and Darney (2011) agree that a backup method is not necessary unless accompanied by vomiting and diarrhea.

Another area of concern has been the effect of OCs on laboratory values. Previous thyroid test methods were affected by protein binding, but the new TSH is not. Lipid levels (cholesterol, triglycerides, and high-density lipoprotein cholesterol) may be affected by OCs. (Chrousos, 2012). A baseline lipid profile should be performed in women who have a significant family history or other risk factors for cardiovascular disease.

Adverse Effects/Contraindications

Many studies have investigated the incidence of venous thromboembolism (VTE) in COC users. The incidence of VTE is low in young women, one to three cases per 10,000 per year. VTE risk is increased by 2 to 5 times in COC users without other significant risk factors. The increase in risk is attributable to the estrogen component of COCs, which influences clotting factors and is dose-dependent. The incidence of VTE is extremely low; therefore, for any individual user this increase in risk still represents a very low chance of an adverse event. Risk factors such as inherited clotting disorders, strong family history of inherited clotting disorders, being older than 35 years, smoking more than 10 cigarettes per day, or obesity (body mass index [BMI] greater than 30) increase the risk 3 to 10 times. Such factors illustrate the need for screening patients diligently by taking a detailed family history before prescribing hormonal contraception.

In a MEGA (multiple environmental and genetic assessment of risk factors for venous thrombosis) case-controlled study, van Hylckama Vlieg, Helmerhorst, Vandenbroucke, Doggen, and Rosendaal (2009) found that overall, the use of COCs increases the risk of DVTs 5-fold over that of nonusers. The data also showed a significant difference in odds ratios in formulations using different progestins, but all using low-dose estrogens. Norethindrone and levonorgestrel had the lowest odds ratios of 3.9 and 3.6, respectively, whereas the odds ratio for norgestimate was 5.9, drospirenone 6.3, and desogestrel 7.3. These are third- and fourth-generation progestins that allow greater estrogenic activity, thereby increasing the risk. The authors' conclusion is "the safest option with regard to the risk of venous thrombosis is an oral contraceptive containing levonorgestrel combined with a low dose of estrogen" (van Hylckama Vlieg et al, 2009, p 7).

In a recently published comparison study of new users of low-dose COCs using levonorgestrel, norethindrone, or norgestimate versus a COC containing drospirenone, a transdermal patch containing norelgestromin, or a vaginal ring containing etonogestrel, Sidney and colleagues (2013) again found an increased risk of cardiovascular events with the use of drospirenone. The hazard ratio for drospirenone in relation to low-dose COCs was 1.77 for DVTs and 2.01 for arterial thrombotic events. Interestingly, the venous events were

in women under 35 years and the arterial events were in women over 35 years.

Other major, but rare, adverse effects can occur with hormonal contraception: cholestatic jaundice, benign hepatic neoplasms, myocardial infarction, stroke, and neurological migraines. Patients should be counseled about the symptoms associated with these events and instructed to call their provider immediately if they experience them. Table 31-3 lists absolute and relative contraindications to hormonal contraceptives with 35 mcg of EE or less, as recommended by the World Health Organization (WHO) (2009).

Dosing Regimens
Combined Contraceptives

Oral contraceptive pills are traditionally dispensed in packages containing 28 pills, with the first 21 pills containing active synthetic hormone and the last 7 pills containing inert ingredients (or iron), during which withdrawal bleeding occurs. Several brands are available containing only the 21 active pills; the user then takes no pill for 7 days, during which withdrawal bleeding occurs. COCs come in many different formulations. The primary difference between brand names is the type and dose of progestin used. Monophasic preparations use the same dose of estrogen and progestin for each of the active pills. Biphasic preparations vary the dose of progestin, with an increase in the amount of progestin in the latter half of the active pills; these are rarely used today. More popular today are triphasic preparations, which vary the dose of estrogen, progestin, or both.

Several products now offer extended menstrual cycling. Seasonale, which contains active pills for 84 days, with 7 days off, produces withdrawal bleeding once every 3 months. Two newer products, Seasonique and LoSeasonique, are classified as monophasic but contain 10 mcg of EE in the last week of one cycle of dosing. Lybrel uses a continuous cycle without any hormone-free weeks for 1 year. Although these are the only pills using an extended-cycle dosing schedule approved by the U.S. Food and Drug Administration (FDA), other monophasic pills may be used similarly to space or manipulate the timing of menstrual periods, using the active pills continuously with less frequent intervals of inert pills (*Drug Facts and Comparisons,* 2013). The newest dosing regimen is monophasic COCs, having 24 active and 4 nonactive pills per cycle.

● CLINICAL PEARL ●

Multiphasic Pills
Triphasic pill packs with pills of various colors may be confusing to some patients. If confusion is a concern, start with a monophasic OC for simple instructions.

Dosing Options

Numerous studies are under way experimenting with various dosing schedules, not only for COCs but also the patch and vaginal ring. The traditional monophasic 21/7 dosing schedule may soon be a thing of the past.

Starting Methods

COCs may be started in several different ways, each offering different advantages in the timing of starting the first and subsequent packs.

First-Day Start

The first pill is taken on the first day of the menstrual cycle. No backup method is needed using this initiation method because ovulation will be suppressed with the first cycle. Many pill packages allow the user to mark the start day to help keep track of pill taking, although many pill packages mark Sunday as the default start day.

Sunday Start

The first pill is taken on the Sunday following the start of menses; a backup method is recommended for the first 7 days. Starting on Sunday may offer the user the convenience of having menses occur only during the week.

Quick Start

The first pill is taken on the day of the office visit; a backup method is recommended for the first 7 days. This method can be used if the clinician is reasonably sure that the user is not currently pregnant (Hatcher et al, 2011).

Side-effect tolerance and compliance with daily pill taking are important factors in a woman's success with oral contraception. Missed pills occur much more frequently than either the user or prescriber realize. One study showed that 23% of women missed a pill the previous cycle; most were missed in the first week of the pack (Aubeny et al, 2004). Another study showed that 48% of women missed two or more pills in a 3-month period; the most common reasons were being away from home, forgetting, or not having a new pill available (Smith & Oakley, 2005). Helping the patient choose a time to take the pill when she is most likely going to be near the pill pack and helping her to associate pill taking with another daily activity may help increase compliance. The patient should also be instructed on what to do if pills are missed. Table 31-4 gives instructions for what to do about missed pills. Instructions are also found in the patient information included in each pill package (*Drug Facts and Comparisons,* 2013).

Side effects women experience may lead to discontinuation of OCs. Studies have found that discontinuation rates because of side effects are in the range of 17% to 34% and access issues are the most common reasons for discontinuation (Frost, Singh, & Finer, 2007; Westhoff et al, 2007). The majority of the side effects resolve with continued use (Hatcher et al, 2011).

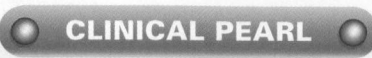

CLINICAL PEARL

LMP Notation

Last menstrual period (LMP) should be considered a vital notation to be displayed at the top of each chart note in a female patient's medical record.

Speroff and Darney (2011) state there are three major influences on continuation: the amount of side effects, concerns over medical risks (i.e., cancer, blood clots), and lastly nonmedical factors such as not understanding directions and complicated packaging. Good patient education in all aspects is essential for successful contraception.

Topical Patch

Ortho Evra is a topical patch that releases 20 mcg of EE and 150 mcg of norelgestromin, which is the primary active metabolite of norgestimate. Norelgestromin still undergoes liver metabolism; however, the resulting metabolite, levonorgestrel, is highly bound to sex hormone-binding globulin, limiting its biological impact (Speroff & Darney, 2011). The patch is applied once a week for 3 weeks, with 1 week being patch-free, during which withdrawal bleeding occurs. Patch use should be initiated on the first day of menses; if it is started on any other day, a backup method should be used for 7 days. Patch location should be rotated with each patch change, and it should be placed on skin that is clean and dry. It may be placed on the abdomen, upper torso, outer arm, or buttock. Side-effect profiles for the patch are similar to those for COCs, with the exception of skin irritation, which may occur at the application site (*Drug Facts and Comparisons,* 2013). There has been concern of decreased efficacy in women with high BMI; however, this is still uncertain. Speroff and Darney (2011) do recommend using continuous or extended schedules in this group of women for increased efficacy.

Vaginal Rings

NuvaRing is a soft, flexible plastic ring that releases 15 mcg of EE and 120 mcg of etonogestrel daily. The ring is placed in the vagina, left in place for 3 weeks, and then removed for a week when withdrawal bleeding occurs. It does not require fitting by a provider and is easily placed by the user. In addition, it releases steady, low doses of hormones, which offer better cycle control in the form of decreased breakthrough bleeding when compared to OCs (Oddsson et al, 2005). The primary advantage is the convenience of once-monthly self-administration, which may be particularly useful for the patient who has difficulty remembering to take a pill daily.

Table 31–4 Instructions for Missed Oral Contraceptives

Missed 1 active pill	Take pill as soon as you remember, taking two pills in 1 d if missed pill was d prior	Use backup contraception for 7 d
Missed 2–4 active pills	Take two pills for 2–3 d	Use backup contraception for 7 d
Missed 5 or more active pills	Start new pack on next start day (e.g., Sunday for Sunday starters)	Use backup contraception until 7 d of active pills taken

Other features of this method are the lower systemic exposure to EE, which is approximately 50% of what is typically seen in COCs with 30 mcg of EE (Timmer & Mulders, 2000) and 30% of those levels measured with patch use (van den Heuvel, van Bragt, Alnabawy, & Kaptein, 2005). Despite lower systemic levels of EE, ovulation is completely suppressed (Mulders & Dieben, 2001). As with COCs, evidence indicates that serum concentrations of EE are not affected by concomitant use of amoxicillin or doxycycline (Dogterom, van den Heuvel, & Thomsen, 2005).

As with all hormonal contraceptives, neither estrogens nor progestins should be used by women who have medical conditions that preclude their use. Other possible contraindications to use of NuvaRing are in women who have significant pelvic prolapse (Hatcher et al, 2011).

On the horizon are progestin-only vaginal rings that may be used for 3 months. These are currently on the market in several South American countries and used primarily for breastfeeding women. There is also research on a vaginal ring with the dual purpose of contraception and protection from STIs (Brache, Payán, & Faundes, 2013).

Progesterone-Only Contraceptives

Progestin-Only Pills

Two brand-name progestin-only pills are currently available: Micronor and Nor-QD. Three generics also contain 0.35 mg norethindrone. These pills contain no estrogen and are primarily used with special populations in which estrogen is contraindicated because of medical conditions or breastfeeding. Because these pills contain very low levels of hormone, users need to be particularly diligent with accurate pill taking. The primary contraceptive effect is through thickening of cervical mucus and prevention of sperm penetration, which occurs 2 to 4 hours after administration and diminishes after 22 hours of administration. If a pill is taken even a few hours late, a backup method is recommended for the following 48 hours. As with other progestin-only methods, common side effects are changes in bleeding patterns and breast tenderness (Speroff & Darney, 2011).

Injectable Progestins

Depot medroxyprogesterone acetate (DMPA), Depo-Provera, is a long-acting, injectable, progestin-only contraceptive. One injection of 150 mg IM is effective at suppressing ovulation for 12 to 13 weeks. DMPA also thickens cervical mucus and atrophies the endometrium (Hatcher et al, 2011). In 2005, Pfizer released a 104 mg SQ dose of DMPA that offers a lower overall hormone dose with no change in efficacy, even in patients with a high BMI. SQ administration can be done by the user without an office visit (Jain et al, 2004).

Injection offers the advantage of dosing once every 12 weeks, with very reliable efficacy. User errors can occur if the patient does not return for doses within the prescribed time, although it is acceptable to give a repeat dose up to 1 week late without clinical assessment to exclude pregnancy. DMPA will change a woman's bleeding pattern, causing an increased number of days of spotting or amenorrhea. This side effect may be unacceptable for some users and is the primary reason women discontinue use. Women in our society are socialized to believe that they need to have a monthly period. Patient education regarding expected bleeding pattern changes can increase the acceptance of these changes and contribute to the patient's success with this method. Weight gain may also be of concern for some patients; average weight gain is several pounds per year of use. Users of DMPA may also have a delay of return to fertility, on average 9 to 10 months (Hatcher et al, 2011).

Before initiating Depo-Provera the provider should exclude the possibility that the patient is currently pregnant. If a client discovers that she is pregnant after the drug's administration, the intramuscular injection cannot be reversed. The drug can be started while the client is menstruating, or if the client has had two negative urine pregnancy tests spaced 2 weeks apart, only if the client has not had unprotected intercourse during that time.

In 2004, the FDA issued a Black-Box Warning for Depo-Provera users in response to data showing a decrease in bone density with longer-term use. The warning states that it should not be used for more than 2 years consecutively if other alternatives are acceptable. Of particular concern is use in adolescents when bone accretion is still under way. Recommendations were made to assess bone density if women were to continue use for longer than 2 years (Omar, 2005). The Black-Box Warning applied to the lower SQ dose prior to published data. However, in a randomized 2-year study comparing IM DMPA with sub-Q DMPA, the authors found similar to slightly less bone loss in the first 2 years of use (Kauntiz, Darney, Ross, Wolter, & Speroff, 2009). Increasingly, however, data suggest that most if not all of the bone mineral density changes are reversed after discontinuation of the drug (Kauntiz, Arias, & McClung, 2008) and that increasing calcium intake and stopping smoking can significantly modify bone loss (Rahman & Berenson, 2010).

Intrauterine Progestin

Mirena is an intrauterine device that releases 20 mcg of levonorgestrel daily and can be left in place for 5 years. The local release of progestin creates only small levels of systemic circulating hormone, and the incidence of systemic side effects is small. Mirena causes thickening of cervical mucus and endometrial atrophy but has only a minimal effect on ovulation suppression. Changes in menstrual bleeding are common; many women experience a notable difference in menstrual flow or amenorrhea that may be more pronounced over time. Normal endometrial function typically returns within 1 to 3 months after discontinuation (Jensen, 2005).

In 2013, a second levonorgesterel intrauterine device, Skyla, was approved by the FDA. Skyla releases 14 mcg/d of levonorgesterel initially and declines to 5 mcg/d after 3 years. Skyla is smaller in length and width than Mirena, has a smaller insertion tube, and has a silver ring at the top for visualization on ultrasound (Bahamondes & Bahamondes, 2014). The smaller size may make it easier to insert in nulligravida women. The efficacy is the same as the Mirena.

Many studies have found various noncontraceptive therapeutic uses for the Mirena. In a recent review article, Fraser (2013) found evidence for its use with menorrhagia of various etiologies. These include leiomyomas, adenomyosis, endometrial hyperplasia, and ovulation disorders. It is also effective for iron deficiency and pelvic pain with or without endometriosis.

Progestin Implants

Implanon provides contraception for up to 3 years and is the only implant currently available in the United States. It consists of one rod that contains 68 mg of etonogestrel, an active metabolite of desogestrel (Hatcher et al, 2011). Implanon has an overall serum progestin concentration that is lower than Norplant, which is no longer available in the United States, and has less variation (Speroff & Darney, 2011). Because it is only one rod, insertion and removal are simpler than with Norplant.

Emergency Contraception

Emergency contraception (EC) is a term used to describe methods of pregnancy prevention after an episode of improperly protected intercourse. EC should be taken as soon as possible, within 72 hours, but may be initiated within 120 hours (5 days). Improperly protected intercourse may occur if no method of pregnancy prevention was used, if the method used failed (condom broke or slipped off; diaphragm/cap/sponge became dislodged), or if the method was used improperly (missed pills).

Plan B One-Step (one tablet of 1.5 mg levonorgestrel) and Next Choice (two pills of 0.75 mg levonorgestrel) are progestin-only products packaged specifically for use as EC. These products are available over-the-counter for women over 17 years of age. The traditional dosing is to take one tablet 12 hours apart, but taking both doses at the same time does not decrease efficacy and is easier (Speroff & Darney, 2011). The newest EC is ella, a single 30 mg tablet containing ulipristal that requires a prescription. Existing pregnancy is the only contraindication to EC use; therefore, a urine pregnancy test should be performed before EC use.

CLINICAL PEARL

Depo-Provera and Osteoporosis
Counsel patients using Depo-Provera to increase dietary calcium intake and weight-bearing exercise. These interventions along with stopping smoking will mitigate bone mineral density changes.

MONITORING

Traditionally, hormonal contraception is provided during an annual examination, consisting of detailed personal and family histories, blood pressure measurement, general physical examination, breast and pelvic examinations, Pap smear, and sexually transmitted infection (STI) screening. These are important for evaluation of a woman's health; however, blood pressure measurement and personal and family histories provide the clinically relevant information necessary to initiate hormonal contraception safely. In fact, the latest American College of Obstetricians and Gynecologists (ACOG, 2012) and U.S. Preventive Services Task Force (USPSTF, 2012) guidelines concur that Pap smears should not start until age 21 and then, with negative results, every 3 years until age 29 is appropriate. Clinical breast exams may also only be every 3 years for women 20 to 39 years.

Monitoring for the adverse effects of OCs should be done initially at 3 months and then annually. Serious effects that could be caused by OCs include abnormal vaginal bleeding; hypertension; amenorrhea; unilateral numbness, weakness, or tingling, indicating possible cerebral spasm or occlusion; breast pain or mass; leg pain; chest pain; sudden loss of vision from possible thromboembolic phenomena; and jaundice (Hatcher et al, 2011).

In addition to screening for adverse drug effects, the provider should use these well-patient visits to screen for asymptomatic STIs, review breast self-awareness, and reinforce barrier protection for patients at risk for disease. Use of tobacco and alcohol are the two most common lifestyle habits that contribute to morbidity and mortality at all ages. Both have interaction effects on the organ systems of patients who use an OC. Patients with a chronic disease such as diabetes, seizure disorder, or migraine headache require more frequent monitoring visits based on their conditions.

CLINICAL PEARL

Emergency Contraception
During each office visit, provide patients under 17 with an emergency contraception prescription and instructions for use in case their primary contraception method fails.

OUTCOME EVALUATION

Symptoms of serious adverse effects require immediate evaluation and discontinuation of OCs until the cause of the adverse symptom rules out OC etiology. Symptoms that can be handled less urgently are irregular vaginal bleeding, amenorrhea, and mild-to-moderate blood pressure elevation. Breakthrough bleeding frequently occurs in the initial cycles of use of any OC formulation, is most common in the first three cycles, and usually resolves with continued use. If the patient has not missed any doses, reassure her that breakthrough bleeding has not been associated with reduced efficacy. Some women may experience breakthrough bleeding after longer use; this is due to the decidualization and fragility of the endometrium, which is a progestational effect. Stopping the dosing regimen is unnecessary while resolving the problem. Use 1.25 mg conjugated estrogens or 2 mg estradiol for 7 days no matter where in the cycle spotting occurs. If this treatment is not effective, schedule an examination to rule out infection or other pathological causes. Amenorrhea is a common concern that may result after several months or years of OC use. Progestins atrophy the endometrium, and some women welcome scanty or no menses. Amenorrhea caused by DMPA may be a result of low estrogen levels (less than 30 mcg) (Speroff & Darney, 2011). For many women, no monthly cycle produces anxiety, which is usually relieved by a negative pregnancy test.

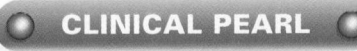

CLINICAL PEARL

Report of Bleeding

Patient reports of irregular or abnormal bleeding should be quantified with a menstrual calendar; have the patient differentiate between days on which spotting occurs and days on which bleeding is as heavy as her menses. Keeping a count of sanitary napkins or tampons used per day of bleeding may help further quantify bleeding. Bleeding may be excessive if a patient is using tampons and pads together and experiencing bleeding accidents. Serial hematocrit measurement several days or a week apart may assist in evaluating excessive bleeding. Excessive bleeding should be evaluated for underlying etiology, such as uterine cancer or polyps, thyroid disorders, or bleeding dyscrasias (Hatcher et al, 2011).

PATIENT EDUCATION

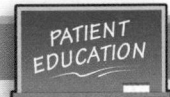

Overall Treatment Plan/Physiological Process

☐ Physiology of normal menstrual cycle.

☐ Need for follow-up visits: BP monitoring 3 months after initiation of methods containing estrogen, then annually. Breast and pelvic examinations, per national standards of care with client's age, history, and risk factors taken into consideration.

☐ Breast self-awareness education.

☐ Safe-sex practices, including male or female condom use in conjunction with hormonal contraception for STI prevention.

☐ Emergency contraception access and use, which can be used with failures of all methods.

SPECIFIC TO THE DRUG THERAPY

☐ How contraceptives prevent pregnancy through suppression of ovulation in the hypothalamic-pituitary-ovarian axis or endometrial and cervical changes.

☐ Doses and schedules for taking the drug. Specifically start method, active versus inactive pills, when to expect menses, what to do if pills are missed, suggestions for optimizing compliance with dosing schedule.

☐ Anticipated menstrual changes because of method use, such as lighter or shorter menses, amenorrhea, or irregular bleeding patterns.

☐ Common side effects with method use, such as breakthrough bleeding in first few cycles of OC use, breast tenderness, nausea, possible weight changes.

☐ Serious side effects, their symptoms, and how to access care in an emergency.

☐ Interactions between hormonal contraception and other treatment modalities or lifestyle habits. Emphasize the dangers of smoking with combined hormonal contraception at any age and the increased risk in women over age 35. Also advise patients to stop combined hormonal contraception 4 weeks before and 2 weeks after major surgery to prevent thrombus formation.

☐ Review time frame for return to fertility after discontinuation for specific method.

REASONS FOR TAKING THE DRUG(S)

Hormonal contraception offers very high efficacy; this may be particularly important for women between 15 and 35 years of age when fertility is highest. Methods can be used for long- or short-term deferment of childbearing, allowing control over timing and spacing of pregnancies.

DRUGS AS PART OF THE TOTAL TREATMENT REGIMEN

☐ Women who use hormonal contraception may also enjoy noncontraceptive benefits, such as less menstrual discomfort or lighter flow and the ability to predict or manipulate timing of menses for vacation or other social events.

☐ Use of hormonal contraception also confers protection against uterine and ovarian cancer (Speroff & Darney, 2011).

Continued

PATIENT EDUCATION—cont'd

PATIENT
EDUCATION

ADHERENCE ISSUES

☐ Access to clinic appointments and prescription refills is one of the reasons for gaps in OC use. If medically indicated, give the patient a full year of refills.

☐ Counseling, education, and use of written materials can increase a patient's success with any method. Thorough patient education is the cornerstone of contraceptive success.

☐ The following are most important for patients taking OCs—they should take a pill every day in the correct order, and they should never just stop. If there are questions or concerns, they should always call the clinic first.

REFERENCES

American College of Obstetricians and Gynecologists (ACOG) committee opinion no. 534 (2012). Well-woman visit. *Obstetrics & Gynecology, 120*(2), 421–424.

Aubeny, E., Buhler, M., Colau, J. C., Vicaut, E., Zadikian, M., & Childs, M. (2002). Oral contraception: Patterns of non-compliance. The Coraliance study. *European Journal of Contraception & Reproductive Health Care, 7*(3), 155–161.

Aubeny, E., Buhler, M., Colau, J. C., Vicaut, E., Zadikian, M., & Childs, M. (2004). The Coraliance study: Non-compliant behavior. Results after a 6-month follow-up of patients on oral contraceptives. *European Journal of Contraception & Reproductive Health Care, 9*, 267–277. doi: 10.1080/13625180400017776

Brache, V., Payán, A. J., & Faundes, A. (2013). Current status of contraceptive vaginal rings. *Contraception, 87*(3), 264–272.

Bahamondes, L., & Bahamondes, M. V. (2014). New and emerging contraceptives: A state-of-the-art review. *International Journal of Women's Health, 6*, 221–234. Retrieved from http://www.ncbi.nlm.nih.gov/pmc/articles/PMC3933723/

Chrousos, G. P. (2012). Chapter 40. The gonadal hormones & inhibitors. In B. G. Katzung, S. B. Masters, & A. J. Trevor (Eds.), *Basic & clinical pharmacology* (12th ed.). New York: McGraw-Hill. Retrieved from http://www.accesspharmacy.com/content.aspx?aID=55828264

Dogterom, P., van den Heuvel, M. W., & Thomsen, T. (2005). Absence of pharmacokinetic interactions of the combined contraceptive vaginal ring NuvaRing with oral amoxicillin or doxycycline in two randomized trials. *Clinical Pharmacokinetics, 44*(4), 429–438.

Drug facts and comparisons. (2013). St. Louis, MO: Wolters Kluwer Health. Retrieved from https://online-factsandcomparisons-com.liboff.ohsu.edu/References.aspx?book=DFC

Fraser, I. S. (2013). Added health benefits of the levonorgestrel contraceptive uterine system and other hormonal contraceptive delivery systems. *Contraception 87*(3), 273–279.

Frost, J. J., Singh, S., & Finer, L. B. (2007). U.S. women's one-year contraceptive use patterns, 2004. *Perspectives on Sexual and Reproductive Health, 39*(1), 48–55. doi: 10.1363/3904807

Hatcher, R. A., Trussell, J., Nelson, A. L., Cates, W., Jr., Kowal, D., & Policar, M. S. (2011). *Contraceptive technology* (20th ed.). New York: Ardent Media.

Hunter, D. J., Colditz, G. A., Hankinson, S. E., Malspeis, S., Spiegelman, D., Chen, W., et al. (2010). Oral contraceptive use and breast cancer: A prospective study of young women. *Cancer, Epidemiology, Biomarkers, and Prevention, 19*(10), 2496–2502. doi:10.1158/1055-9965.EPI-10-0747

Jain, J., Dutton, C., Nicosia, A., Wajszczuk, C., Bode, F. R., & Mishell, D. R. (2004). Pharmacokinetics, ovulation suppression and return to ovulation following a lower dose subcutaneous formulation of Depo-Provera. *Contraception, 70*(1), 11–18.

Jensen, J. T. (2005). Contraceptive and therapeutic effects of the levonorgestrel intrauterine system: An overview. *Obstetrical Gynecological Survey, 60*(9), 604–612.

Kahlenborn, C., Modugno, F., Potter, D. M., & Severs, W. P. (2006). Oral contraceptive use as a risk factor for premenopausal breast cancer: A meta-analysis. *Mayo Clinic Proceedings, 81*(10), 1290–1302.

Kaunitz, A. M., Arias, R., & McClung, M. (2008). Bone density recovery after depot medroxyprogesterone acetate injectable contraception use. *Contraception, 77*, 67–76. doi: 10.1016/j.contraception.2007.10.005

Kaunitz, A. M., Darney, P. D., Ross, D., Wolter, K. D., & Speroff, L. (2009). Subcutaneous DMPA vs. intramuscular DMPA: A 2-year randomized study of contraceptive efficacy and bone mineral density. *Contraception, 80*, 7–17. doi: 10.1016/j.contraception.2009.02.005

Merck. (2014). Zoely. Retrieved from http://www.zoely.co.uk/hcp/index.php

Mosher, W. D., Jones, J., & Abma, J. C. (2012). Intended and unintended births in the United States: 1982–2010. *National Health Statistics Reports, 55*, 1–28.

Oddsson, K., Leifels-Fischer, B., de Melo, N. R., Wiel-Masson, D., Benedetto, C., Verhoeven, C. H., et al. (2005). Efficacy and safety of a contraceptive vaginal ring (NuvaRing) compared with a combined oral contraceptive: A 1-year randomized trial. *Contraception, 71*(3), 176–182.

Omar, H. (2005). Depot medroxyprogesterone acetate (DMPA, Depo-Provera) in adolescents: What is next after the FDA black box warning. *Journal of Pediatric and Adolescent Gynecology, 18*(3), 183–188.

Rahman, M., & Berenson, A. B. (2010). Predictors of higher bone mineral density loss and use of depot medroxyprogesterone acetate. *Obstetrics & Gynecology, 115*(1), 35–40. doi: 10.1097/AOG.0b013e3181c4e864

Shrader, S. P., & Dickerson, L. M. (2008). Extended- and continuous-cycle oral contraceptives. *Pharmacotherapy, 28*(8), 1033–1040. doi: 10.1592/phco.28.8.1033

Sidney, S., Cheetham, T. C., Connell, F. A., Ouellet-Hellstrom, R., Graham, D. J., Davis, D., et al. (2013). Recent combined hormonal contraceptives (CHCs) and the risk of thromboembolism and over cardiovascular events in new users. *Contraception 87*(1), 93–100.

Sitruk-Ware, R., Nath, A., & Mishell, Jr., D. R. (2013). Contraception technology: Past, present and future. *Contraception 87*(3), 319–330.

Smith, J. D., & Oakley, D. (2005). Why do women miss oral contraceptive pills? An analysis of women's self-described reasons for missed pills. *Journal of Midwifery & Women's Health, 50*(5), 380–385.

Speroff, L., & Darney, P. D. (2011). *A clinical guide for contraception* (5th ed.). Philadelphia: Lippincott Williams & Wilkins.

Timmer, C. J., & Mulders, T. M. (2000). Pharmacokinetics of etonogestrel and ethinylestradiol released from a combined contraceptive vaginal ring. *Clinical Pharmacokinetics, 39*(3), 233–242.

U.S. Preventive Services Task Force (USPSTF). (2012). Screening for cervical cancer: U.S. preventive services task force recommendation statement. AHRQ Publication No. 11-05156-EF-2. Retrieved from http://www.uspreventiveservicestaskforce.org/uspstf11/cervcancer/cervcancerrs.htm

van den Heuvel, M. W., van Bragt, A. J., Alnabawy, A. K., & Kaptein, M. C. (2005). Comparison of ethinylestradiol pharmacokinetics in three hormonal contraceptive formulations: The vaginal ring, the transdermal patch and an oral contraceptive. *Contraception, 72*(3), 168–174.

van Hylckama Vlieg, A., Helmerhorst, F. M., Vandenbroucke, J. P., Doggen, C. J. M., & Rosendaal, F. R. (2009). The venous thrombotic risk of oral contraceptives, effects of estrogen dose and progestogen type: Results of the MEGA case-control study. *British Medical Journal, 339*, b2921. doi: 10.1136/bmj.b2921

Westhoff, C. L., Heartwell, S., Edwards, S., Zieman, M., Stuart, G., Cwiak, C., et al. (2007). Oral contraceptive discontinuation: Do side effects matter? *American Journal of Obstetrics & Gynecology, 196*, 412.e1–412.e7. doi: 10.1016/j.ajog.2006.12.015

World Health Organization (WHO). (2009). *Medical eligibility criteria for contraceptive use* (4th ed.). Geneva, Switzerland: Author.

DERMATOLOGICAL CONDITIONS

Teri Moser Woo

The skin is the body's largest organ, and it is uniquely accessible for diagnosis and treatment. Primary care providers see patients with dermatological problems on a daily basis, with skin-related problems accounting for 5% of clinic visits and 74 million prescriptions for dermatologic agents (Centers for Disease Control, 2010).

The most common dermatological diagnosis reported in the National Ambulatory Medical Care Survey, 1993–2005, is dermatitis (13 million office visits per year), with skin and soft tissue infections diagnosed at 6.3 million visits per year (Pallin, Espinola, Leung, Hooper, & Camargo, 2009). This chapter addresses the pharmacological management of common dermatological conditions seen in primary care. Accurate diagnosis of the condition is assumed.

DERMATITIS

Eczema (atopic dermatitis), contact dermatitis, diaper dermatitis, and seborrheic dermatitis are four common forms of dermatitis seen in primary care.

Eczema is a chronic skin disorder that affects all ages. It often begins in infancy and affects 10% to 15% of children. It may resolve during puberty, only to recur in adolescence or adulthood. The pattern of rash with eczema varies with age. Infants have the rash on the face, scalp, trunk, and the extensor surface of the extremities. In infants, the rash is usually acute or subacute, red, and vesicular. Eczema in adolescents and adults is usually chronic, with scaling, dryness, and lichenification on the flexure surfaces of the extremities, face, neck, hands, and upper chest. Eczema tends to worsen during the winter months.

Contact dermatitis is an acute inflammatory reaction of the skin to an irritant or allergen. It can be differentiated from eczema because it is generally not chronic or recurring and is usually distributed on exposed skin.

Diaper dermatitis (diaper rash) can occur in any patient who is incontinent and uses an occlusive barrier type of garment or diaper; however, it is most commonly seen in infants and toddlers.

Seborrheic dermatitis is a common inflammatory dermatitis characterized by erythematous, eczematous patches with yellow, greasy scale. It is usually localized to hairy areas and to areas with high concentrations of sebaceous glands. It can be found on the forehead, eyebrows, nasolabial folds, ear canals, neck, chest, intertriginous areas, the diaper or groin area, and intergluteal fold. In infants younger than 6 months, the scaling on the scalp without inflammation is commonly called cradle cap, and in adolescents and adults it is called dandruff.

Pathophysiology

Eczema

The exact etiology of eczema is unknown. Patients with eczema have high immunoglobulin E (IgE) antibody levels, but an exact immune cause has not been proved. A predisposition to pruritus and a reduced threshold of irritant responsiveness are believed to be key elements. Pruritus leads to increased scratching, which increases skin trauma, leading to increased itching (itch-scratch-itch cycle). Stroking the skin causes an abnormal reaction of dermatographism, a white line.

A high correlation exists between eczema and other atopic diseases, with 50% to 80% of children with eczema later developing asthma, allergic rhinitis, or hay fever. Often a positive family history for allergic disorders or asthma exists as well. The prevalence of eczema and skin allergies in children increased from 7.4% in 1997–1999 to 12.5% in 2009–2011 (Jackson, Howie, & Akinbami, 2013).

Contact Dermatitis

Contact dermatitis has two types: irritant and allergic. Both are usually confined to the point of contact with the irritant or allergen. This contact usually produces erythema, papules, and/or vesicles.

Irritant contact dermatitis is caused by contact of the skin with an irritating substance. The effect may be mild to severe. Irritating substances can be acid or alkali, solvents, or detergents. There is no immunological response as part of the inflammatory response in irritant contact dermatitis.

Allergic contact dermatitis is a delayed hypersensitivity response to an allergen. The allergen can be a variety of items in the environment, usually a small-molecular-weight substance that binds to the proteinaceous components of the skin to form a sensitizing antigen. Sensitization to the substance or allergen takes 10 to 14 days to develop after the first exposure. Dermatitis occurs within 1 to 7 days of subsequent exposure to the allergen. The most common allergens causing allergic contact dermatitis are certain plants (poison oak, ivy, and sumac), metals (especially in snaps, zippers, and jewelry), clothing (wool), cosmetics (fragrance or preservatives), topical medications (neomycin, anesthetics such as benzocaine, topical antihistamine), hair dyes, and soaps. Avoidance usually prevents the allergic response.

Diaper Dermatitis

Diaper dermatitis is an inflammatory disorder of the skin caused by a breakdown of the skin's natural barrier in the perineal or "diaper" area. The rash is often striking for its clear borders that coincide with the borders of the diaper or protective undergarment.

Forms of diaper dermatitis include irritant dermatitis, caused by chemical or mechanical irritation. Chemical irritation is caused by contact with urine and feces. Mechanical irritation is due to chafing of the diaper or undergarment on the skin folds. If the irritant dermatitis becomes chronic, the skin may appear dry. The rash may become more generalized and inflammatory, involving the creases and all the area that the diaper covers. The skin can become ulcerated or eroded with chronic irritation.

Infectious dermatitis may be caused by *Candida albicans* (candidiasis) and is usually a superinfection that can occur after a patient has had irritant dermatitis in the diaper area for 3 to 5 days. Candidiasis is suspected when there is a beefy red confluent rash with satellite lesions that are either red papules or pustules.

Other forms of diaper dermatitis include seborrheic dermatitis, psoriasiform napkin dermatitis, and atopic dermatitis. These disorders in the diaper area are treated the same as dermatitis on other parts of the body.

Seborrheic Dermatitis

The exact cause of seborrheic dermatitis is unknown. It is possibly related to increased production of sebum or an abnormal lipid composition of sebum. Seborrheic dermatitis is rare in children older than 6 to 12 months and in those who are prepubertal because the sebaceous glands are involuted and dormant during this time and become active again with puberty. Saprophytic *Malassezia* colonizes the skin of many patients with seborrhea, with the inflammation of seborrhea thought to be a host response to the fungal infection (Weston & Howe, 2010).

Goals of Treatment

With all forms of dermatitis, the primary goals are to decrease the inflammation and discomfort caused by the dermatitis.

Rational Drug Selection

With all forms of dermatitis, rational drug selection is based first on decreasing the symptoms of an acute exacerbation and then on preventing, decreasing, and/or controlling the frequency and severity of further exacerbations.

Eczema

Acute Exacerbations

Topical Corticosteroids

Topical corticosteroids are adrenocorticosteroid derivatives incorporated into a vehicle suitable for application to the skin. The anti-inflammatory effect of topical steroids is related to their action on immune cells and by suppressing the release of proinflammatory cytokines. At the cellular level, they appear to inhibit the formation, release, and activity of the endogenous mediators of inflammation. When applied to inflamed skin, steroids inhibit the migration of macrophages and leukocytes into the area by reversing vascular dilation and permeability. This decreases edema, erythema, and pruritus.

Variable amounts of the drug are absorbed through the skin, depending on the drug used, the vehicle used, the amount of skin surface area the medication is applied to, and the condition of the skin. Absorption is enhanced by increased skin temperature, hydration, and application to denuded areas, intertriginous areas, or skin surfaces with a thin stratum corneum layer (face or scrotum). Occlusive dressings enhance skin penetration and therefore increase drug absorption. Infants and children have a higher proportion of body surface area to body weight, and therefore they absorb proportionally more medication. Following topical administration, corticosteroids enter the bloodstream and are metabolized and excreted the same as systemic steroids. Therefore, in infants and young children, the lowest effective strength of topical steroid is used to prevent systemic corticosteroid effects.

Topical corticosteroids are Pregnancy Category C. In pregnant patients, do not use corticosteroids extensively, for long periods, or in large amounts. Many topical steroids have been relabeled due to studies indicating many formulations cause hypothalamic-pituitary-adrenal (HPA) axis suppression in children; providers need to stay current with labeling changes, which may be found at the U.S. Food and Drug Administration (FDA) Web site, http://www.fda.gov.

The penetration of the topical steroid varies with the medication's vehicle. Ointments are more occlusive and usually more potent and are good for scaly areas. Creams are less occlusive and usually less potent. Lotions are usually the least potent and contain the most water. Table 32-1 presents the common topical steroids used for eczema. The potency of any steroid can be increased approximately 10-fold by occlusion with plastic wrap. Therefore, to increase the effects of a steroid, apply an occlusive dressing over the area. Do not use occlusive dressings more than 12 hours per day, or systemic steroid effects may occur. In young children, occlusive dressings are rarely used. A diaper is considered occlusive, and steroid use should be avoided in the diaper area unless a low-potency steroid is needed for short periods (e.g., 2 d).

Table 32–1 Drugs Commonly Used: Dermatitis and Psoriasis

Drug	Indication	Strengths Available	Dose	Comments
Topical Corticosteroids				
Low Potency				
Hydrocortisone (Hytone, Cortisporin, Cortaid)	Dermatitis	Cream, lotion, ointment: 1%, 2.5%, 0.5%	Apply a thin layer 2–4 times/d until healed.	Available OTC
Triamcinolone acetonide (Aristocort, Aristocort A, Kenalog)	Dermatitis	Cream, lotion, ointment: 0.025%	Apply a thin layer 3–4 times/d until healed.	Prescription required
Intermediate Potency				
Hydrocortisone valerate (Westcort)	Dermatitis	Cream, ointment: 0.2%	Apply a thin layer 2–3 times/d until healed.	Should be used with caution on the face; choose lower potency on face.
Hydrocortisone butyrate 0.1% (Locoid)	Dermatitis	Cream, ointment solution: 0.1%	Apply thin layer 2–3 times/d until clear.	Should be used with caution on the face; choose lower potency on face.
Mometasone furoate 0.1% (Elocon)	Dermatitis	Cream, ointment, lotion: 0.1%	Apply thin layer once daily. Maximum 3 wk therapy in children.	Cream & ointment for children ≥2 yr. Lotion not to be used in children <12 yr.

Continued

Table 32–1   Drugs Commonly Used: Dermatitis and Psoriasis—cont'd

Drug	Indication	Strengths Available	Dose	Comments
Triamcinolone acetonide (Aristocort, Kenalog)	Dermatitis	Cream, lotion, ointment: 0.1%	Apply a thin layer 3–4 times/d until healed.	Should be used with caution on the face; choose lower potency on face.
High Potency				
Betamethasone dipropionate, augmented (Diprolene)	Dermatitis	Emollient cream, lotion: 0.05%	Apply a thin film 1–2 times/d until healed; maximum of 45 g of cream or 50 mL of lotion/wk.	Avoid abrupt cessation if used for chronic conditions; not recommended in children ≤12 yr due to documented HPA suppression.
Triamcinolone acetonide (Aristocort A, Kenalog)	Dermatitis	Cream: 0.5%	Apply sparingly to affected area 2–3 times daily until healed.	Avoid abrupt cessation if used for chronic conditions; use with caution and sparingly in children.
Super-High Potency				
Betamethasone dipropionate augmented 0.05% (Diprolene AF)	Dermatitis	Ointment, cream: 0.05%	Apply thin film 1–2 times daily. Maximum: ointment 45g/wk, gel 50 g/wk.	Not recommended in children ≤12 yr. HPA axis suppression documented in children using this product (32%).
Topical Immunomodulators				
Pimecrolimus (Elidel)	Short-term or intermittent long-term treatment of mild to moderate atopic dermatitis	Cream: 1%	Apply to affected area twice daily.	Not recommended in children <2 yr. Pregnancy Category C. Not recommended in nursing mothers. Long-term safety has not been established.
Tacrolimus (Protopic)	Short-term or intermittent long-term treatment of moderate to severe atopic dermatitis	Ointment: 0.03%, 0.1%	Apply to affected area twice daily. Apply to dry skin. Do not occlude. *Children 2–15 yr:* use 0.03% strength.	Not a first-line therapy. Not recommended in children <2 yr. Pregnancy Category C. Not recommended in nursing mothers. Long-term safety has not been established. Do not use as first-line therapy.
Oral Corticosteroids				
Prednisone	Contact dermatitis (severe or if large skin surface area is involved)		*Adults:* 0.5–1 mg/kg/d (40–60 mg/d; maximum 60 mg/d). *Children:* 1 mg/kg/d; maximum 40 mg/d.	Dose is usually tapered after the first 10–14 d, with tapering taking 1–2 wk. Severe cases may need a 2 to 3 wk course; 2 wk is the minimum length of treatment for severe poison oak or ivy dermatitis.
Methylprednisolone (Medrol Dosepak)	Contact dermatitis (severe or if large skin surface area is involved)		Premeasured dose pack; dose is preset at 24 mg on day 1, tapering 4 mg/d to a dose of 4 mg on day 6.	Allows for easy tapering over 6 d. 6 d course may not be long enough for some patients.

Table 32–1   Drugs Commonly Used: Dermatitis and Psoriasis—cont'd

Drug	Indication	Strengths Available	Dose	Comments
Antipruritic Agents				
Diphenhydramine (Benadryl)	Pruritus associated with dermatitis	Elixir: 12.5 mg/5 mL Chewable tablets: 12.5 mg Tablets: 25 mg	*Adults:* 25–50 mg every 4–6 h *Children 2–6 yr:* 6.25 mg; maximum 37.5 mg/24 h *Children 6–12 yr:* 12.5–25 mg q4–6h; maximum 150 mg/24 h	May cause drowsiness.
Hydroxyzine (Atarax)	Pruritus associated with dermatitis	Syrup: 10 mg/5 mL Tablets: 10, 25, 50, 100 mg	*Adults:* 25 mg 3–4 times/d *Children <6 yr:* 12.5 mg 3–4 times/d; maximum 50 mg/24 h *Children ≥6 yr:* 12.5–25 mg 3–4 times/d; maximum 50–100 mg/24 h	May cause drowsiness.
Cetirizine (Zyrtec)	Pruritus associated with dermatitis	Syrup: 1 mg/mL Tablets: 5, 10 mg	*Adults:* 5–10 mg once daily *Children 6–24 mo:* 2.5 mg once daily *Children 2–5 yr:* 2.5 mg initially; can increase dose to 5 mg/d either as one 5 mg dose or 2.5 mg q12h *Children ≥6 yr:* 5–10 mg once daily	Less sedation than other antihistamines. Should not be used concurrently with alcohol or other CNS depressants as it may potentiate the depressant effect.
Doxepin (systemic: Sinequan)	Pruritus associated with dermatitis	Capsules: 10, 25, 50, 75, 100, 150 mg	Dose range in 25–150 mg/d in single or divided doses; suggested starting dose is 75 mg/d, then titrate up or down as indicated. Use dose that achieves effect with fewest adverse effects.	Not recommended in children. Do not use within 14 d of monoamine oxidase inhibitors (MAOIs). May potentiate drugs metabolized by CYP2D6 (cimetidine, tricyclic antidepressants, SSRIs, phenothiazines, carbamazepine, quinidine, etc.); avoid these drugs during therapy. Contraindicated in patients with acute myocardial infarction (MI), urinary retention, or glaucoma. Pregnancy Category C; not recommend during pregnancy.
Doxepin (topical: Zonalon)	Moderate to severe pruritus associated with atopic dermatitis (eczema)	Cream: 5%	Apply a thin film to affected areas 4 times/d in 3 to 4 h intervals.	Interacts adversely with alcohol and MAOIs. Contraindicated in children. Pregnancy Category B. Patients with untreated narrow angle glaucoma and urinary retention should not use PO or topical form.
Shampoos for Seborrheic Dermatitis				
Ketoconazole shampoo (OTC: Nizoral)	Seborrheic dermatitis	2% shampoo	Apply to wet scalp, massage for 1 min, rinse, and repeat; leave on scalp for 3 min, then rinse well.	See package. Pregnancy Category C. Not recommended in children.

Continued

Table 32–1   Drugs Commonly Used: Dermatitis and Psoriasis—cont'd

Drug	Indication	Strengths Available	Dose	Comments
Selenium sulfide shampoo (Selsun Blue, Head & Shoulders Intensive Treatment, Excel)	Seborrheic dermatitis	OTC: 1% shampoo Rx: 2.5% shampoo	Apply to wet hair and massage in for 2–3 min before rinsing completely; apply twice/wk until control is achieved, then weekly thereafter. For cradle cap: Apply 1% shampoo to scalp, avoiding eyes; rinse thoroughly.	See package. Advise patient that the shampoo will loosen crusted scales and that these scales may appear loose in the hair after the first few shampoos; brush to remove the scales from the hair; this will resolve after a few treatments.
Coal tar shampoo (OTC: Zetar, Neutrogena T/Gel, Tegrin Medicated, Denorex, Theraplex T)	Seborrheic dermatitis	1% Zetar, Theraplex T 2% Ionil T Plus, Ionil-T Therapeutic 1% coal tar shampoo, Neutrogena T/Gel 5%: Tegrin Medicated 7% Tegrin Medicated Extra conditioning 9% Denorex 12.5%: Extra Strength Denorex	Rub into wet hair and scalp and then rinse: repeat and leave shampoo in for 5 min, rinse well; may be used daily–weekly; follow package directions.	See package. Do not use if there are open infected lesions. May cause sun sensitivity for 24 h after application.
Pyrithione zinc (OTC: Head & Shoulders shampoo, Zincon, Danex, DHS, Sebulon, ZNP Bar)	Seborrheic dermatitis	1% shampoo: Head & Shoulders, Zincon, Danex 2% shampoo: DHS Zinc, Sebulon 2% soap: ZNP Bar	Shampoo: apply, lather, rinse, and repeat; use once or twice weekly. Soap: wet skin, lather, rinse, and repeat; use once or twice/wk.	See package.
Sulfur and salicylic acid shampoo (Fostex, Sabex, Sebulex)	Seborrheic dermatitis	5% sulfur and 3% salicylic acid: Maximum Strength Meted 3% salicylic acid and 5% colloidal sulfur: MG400 2% sulfur and 2% salicylic acid: Fostex Medicated Cleansing, Sebex, Sebulex	Follow package directions.	See package.
Coal tar (OTC: Zetar, Medotar, Pentrax MG217 Medicated, MG217 Dual Treatment, Fototar, Tegrin for Psoriasis, Oxipor VHC)	Psoriasis	Emulsion: 30% (Zetar)	Follow package directions.	May cause staining.
		Ointment: 1% (Medotar, Taraphilic), 2% (MG217 Medicated) Cream: 2% (Fototar) Lotion: 5% (MG217 Dual Treatment, Tegrin for Psoriasis); 48.5% (Oxipor VHC) Various generics: 20%	Rinse well after use.	Contraindicated if patient is taking tetracycline, psoralens, and topical retinoids. May cause contact irritant dermatitis. Pregnancy Category C.
Anthralin (Dithrocreme, Anthra-Derm, Dithro-Scalp)	Psoriasis	Cream: 0.1%, 0.25%, 0.5%, 1% Scalp cream: 0.25%, 0.5%	Begin with a low concentration (0.1%); apply a small amount to affected areas; rub in gently, avoiding healthy surrounding skin; leave on for 10 min, then wash off; after 1 wk, may increase to 15–20 min. Increase strength in incremental steps until lesions are healed and skin looks and feels normal.	May stain skin and clothes. Pregnancy Category C; safety in young children unknown. May alternate with other therapies (retinoids, topical steroids, UV light).

Table 32–1   Drugs Commonly Used: Dermatitis and Psoriasis—cont'd

Drug	Indication	Strengths Available	Dose	Comments
			Scalp cream: begin with low concentration (0.25%); apply to scalp after combing hair to remove scales; leave on for 10–20 min; use daily for at least 1 wk; increase strength if needed.	
Calcipotriene (Dovonex)	Psoriasis	Ointment, solution, cream: 0.0005%	Apply twice daily to affected area; rub in gently and completely. Treat for 6–8 wk; improvement usually noted after 1–2 wk.	Pregnancy Category C; should not be used during pregnancy or in children. Older patients have a higher incidence of adverse skin reactions. Rare reports of rapid onset of hypercalcemia.
Calcitriol (Vectical Ointment)	Psoriasis	3 mcg/g ointment	Apply twice a day a.m. & p.m. to affected areas. Maximum dose is 200 g/wk.	Pregnancy Category C; should not be used during pregnancy or in children. Hypercalcemia may occur.

OTC = over the counter; UV = ultraviolet; CNS = central nervous system; HPA = hypothalamic-pituitary-adrenal axis; SSRI = selective serotonic reuptake inhibitor.

There are many topical steroid preparations available, and it is impossible for any practitioner to be familiar with all of them. Familiarity with one or two agents in each category is reasonable. The most commonly used low-potency topical steroid is 1% hydrocortisone. Intermediate-potency topical steroids include hydrocortisone butyrate 0.1% (Locoid) and triamcinolone acetonide 0.1% (Kenalog). High-potency steroids include betamethasone dipropionate, augmented 0.05% (Diprolene lotion, Diprolene AF), and triamcinolone acetonide 0.5% (Kenalog). Super-high-potency topical steroids include betamethasone dipropionate, augmented 0.05% (Diprolene ointment or gel), and halobetasol propionate 0.05% (Ultravate). Providers need to know what medications are allowed from each category in the formulary or formularies they are using.

Oral Corticosteroids

Oral corticosteroids are occasionally used to treat severe eczema. Patients with eczema who receive oral corticosteroids for another disease, such as asthma, see a striking improvement in their skin. Improvement in acute exacerbations is often dramatic, a mixed blessing in the treatment of this chronic illness. Patients often feel so good that they may have the false impression that the steroids "cured" their eczema. Given the major adverse effects observed with prolonged or frequently repeated corticosteroid therapy, routine use of oral steroids for eczema is contraindicated. If oral steroid therapy for severe eczema is considered, consultation with a dermatology specialist is indicated. A patient who is using oral steroids must understand that the effects are short-term and that oral steroid preparations cannot be used frequently. When the oral preparation is started, patients must be started on a comprehensive prevention routine to prevent severe exacerbations. They need to be warned that their eczema will return after the steroid effect wears off.

Immunomodulators

The immunomodulators are a class of topical medications used in the short-term or intermittent long-term treatment of atopic dermatitis. Pimecrolimus (Elidel) and tacrolimus (Protopic) are a second-line therapy after topical corticosteroid treatment failure for atopic dermatitis. They act by interrupting the inflammatory process (Eichenfield et al, 2014). Tacrolimus has been found to inhibit T cells, Langerhans cells, mast cells, and keratinocytes in the epidermal cells. Pimecrolimus was specifically developed to treat inflammatory skin conditions; it inhibits the release of inflammatory cytokines and mediators from mast cells. The immunomodulator cream is chosen based on the severity of the eczema; tacrolimus (Protopic) is prescribed for moderate to severe eczema and pimecrolimus (Elidel) is prescribed for mild to moderate eczema. Neither product is to be used in children younger than 2 years, in immunocompromised patients, or in pregnant or lactating women (Pregnancy Category C). The immunomodulators have no steroid effects. Immunomodulators may be preferable to topical steroids on the face, skin folds, and anogenital area, or if the patient's eczema is recalcitrant to topical steroids or the patient has developed steroid-induced atrophy (Eichenfield et al, 2014).

The immunomodulator creams are applied twice a day to the affected area(s). Patients are to be instructed not to occlude the area. It may take 2 to 3 weeks for patients to notice improvement. Providers need to reexamine patients every 6 weeks. If using tacrolimus (Protopic) in children aged 2 to 15 years the

0.03% strength should be prescribed. See Table 32-1 for full prescribing information.

Both pimecrolimus and tacrolimus have received an FDA Black-Box Warning regarding the long-term safety of topical immunosuppressant calcineurin inhibitors due to rare cases of malignancy (skin and lymphoma) reported in patients using the topical forms of these medications. The FDA advisory states the following: "Animal studies have shown that three different species of animals developed cancer following exposure to these drugs applied topically or given by mouth, including mice, rats, and a recent study of monkeys" (U.S. FDA, 2006). Long-term studies are ongoing to determine risk, with interim results indicating no increase in malignancy rates (Eichenfield et al, 2014).

Antipruritics

Antipruritics are used to control the itching associated with eczema and to break the itch-scratch-itch cycle. Commonly used oral agents are the antihistamines diphenhydramine (Benadryl) and hydroxyzine (Atarax). These drugs have antipruritic and sedative actions. Pruritus can disrupt sleep; therefore, mild sedation can be helpful to prevent nocturnal itching, especially in children. Cetirizine (Zyrtec), a metabolite of hydroxyzine without its sedative effects, can be used during the day to achieve an antipruritic effect without sedation. Another antipruritic is the tricyclic compound doxepin (Sinequan), which has potent histamine$_1$- and histamine$_2$-blocking action.

Topical antipruritics can be used and should be considered if severe pruritus is present. Doxepin cream (Zonalon) can be used for moderate to severe pruritus associated with eczema. Care should be taken when prescribing doxepin for topical use because significant amounts can be absorbed systemically if it is used over 10% of the body surface area or if used for a long time. Drowsiness occurs in more than 20% of patients using doxepin cream, especially if it is used on more than 10% of the body surface area.

Available topical antipruritics that are safer to use than doxepin are Aveeno cream (colloidal oatmeal-based) and Moisturel emollient cream or lotion (petrolatum, glycerine-based). These over-the-counter (OTC) agents can be used liberally on large surface areas with no harmful effects.

Emollients

Emollients play a key role in both acute exacerbations of eczema and in long-term therapy. Wet dressings and emollients can be used to soothe the skin, reduce redness, and treat pruritus caused by eczema (Weston & Howe, 2010; Eichenfield et al, 2014). Emollients are applied to the skin and a wet cotton dressing is applied; then the dressing is covered with dry cloths or clothing. This can be done nightly to decrease pruritus and redness. The use of emollients is further discussed in the Long-Term Therapy section.

Antibiotics

Antibiotics may be necessary to treat secondary infections of *Staphylococcus aureus,* beta-hemolytic streptococci, a virus, or a fungus. If a bacterial infection is suspected, a culture should be obtained prior to beginning treatment. The likelihood of community-acquired methicillin-resistant *S. aureus* (MRSA) needs to be considered. For a patient with a localized infection, mupirocin (Bactroban) or retapamulin (Altabax) ointment can be used. Most infected eczema will require treatment with an oral antibiotic that is effective against *S. aureus* and streptococci. Cephalexin (Keflex), amoxicillin/clavulanate (Augmentin), and cefprozil (Cefzil) are all effective; treatment should be for 7 days. If there is recurrent bacterial infection, a 3-week course of treatment is necessary.

Long-Term Therapy

Eczema is a chronic disorder, and the patient often cycles between mild to moderate dry skin and exacerbations that can be mild to severe. Once an exacerbation quiets, patients must continue to care for their skin to prevent further exacerbations. The keys to long-term therapy are adequate hydration of the skin and avoidance of agents that cause exacerbations.

Emollients

Moisturizers, lubricants, and emollients help retain water in the skin. They are composed of petrolatum, lanolin, or other agents such as colloidal oatmeal in an emulsion. The emollient is applied 1 to 4 times per day after patients bathe. They pat their skin dry and then apply the lotion or cream liberally to all affected areas within 3 minutes after bathing. This procedure traps the moisture in the skin. Ointments provide the most occlusive barrier; creams are the next-best option. Lotions offer the convenience of easy application over large areas of skin but are not as occlusive as ointments and creams. Patients often decrease their use of emollients between exacerbations, and a review and reinforcement of their use during each clinic visit will increase compliance.

Of all the emollient products available, many are eliminated because they have additives such as perfumes or other chemicals, to which many patients with eczema are sensitive. Commonly used emollients are Aveeno cream or lotion, Eucerin cream or lotion, Lubriderm lotion, and Moisturel lotion. If the patient uses a lotion, make sure it does not contain alcohol, which is drying and irritating. Occasionally, patients are sensitive to the lanolin in Eucerin, which is a natural product derived from sheep's wool. Because large amounts are needed to be effective, expense can play a role in choosing an emollient. White petrolatum is inexpensive and a treatment option for patients with limited resources.

Nonpharmacological Measures

Nonpharmacological measures include hydrating baths and avoiding skin irritation and offending agents that cause exacerbations. Patients should be told to wear plastic or nitrile gloves when their hands may be exposed to harsh chemicals or detergents. They should avoid irritating fabrics such as wool. Soft cotton clothing allows the skin to breathe. Careful avoidance of perfumed lotions and soaps prevents flare-ups related to the additives in these products. Some patients have food sensitivities that exacerbate their eczema.

Baths are used to hydrate the skin. The patient should take a warm—not hot—bath for 20 minutes. The skin is patted dry, and emollients are applied immediately to maintain the skin's hydration. The patient should use a mild soap for cleansing the groin and axillae, not harsh deodorant soaps. After a bath is also a good time to apply corticosteroid creams or ointments, if needed.

Contact Dermatitis

The treatment for both types of contact dermatitis is the same. If a small area of skin is affected, a topical corticosteroid cream is usually effective. If more than 10% of the skin surface must be treated or if the allergic contact dermatitis is severe, oral corticosteroids are used. Wet dressings or baths are soothing to the inflamed skin. Oral antihistamines may help control pruritus.

Topical Corticosteroids

Topical corticosteroid creams or ointments are effective in treating mild to moderate contact dermatitis. A low-potency (hydrocortisone 1% or 2.5% cream) or intermediate-potency (hydrocortisone valerate 0.2% or triamcinolone acetonide 0.1%) cream can be used. Intermediate- or high-potency corticosteroids should be used for plant dermatitis from poison ivy or oak (Prok & McGovern, 2014). See Table 32-1 for prescribing information. The patient should begin to experience relief in 2 to 3 days, with complete healing in 2 to 3 weeks.

Oral Corticosteroids

Oral corticosteroids (prednisone or methylprednisolone) are used if the contact dermatitis is severe or if a large skin surface area is involved. A 2 to 3 week course of therapy may be needed for severe cases, with 2 weeks usually the minimum length of therapy required for severe poison oak or ivy dermatitis. Oral prednisone is started at 1 mg/kg/d (maximum 60 mg/d) and tapered over 2 to 3 weeks, 40 mg/d during week 2 and 20 mg/d during week 3 (Prok & McGovern, 2014). A too short course may lead to rebound dermatitis when treating poison oak or ivy dermatitis (Prok & McGovern, 2014). See Table 32-1 for prescribing information.

Wet Dressings or Baths

Wet dressings or baths provide comfort. Aluminum acetate solution (Burow's, Domeboro) is an astringent wet dressing applied for 30 minutes 4 times a day for relief of inflammation associated with contact dermatitis. Emollient baths that contain colloidal oatmeal solids (Aveeno) or oils (Alpha Keri Bath Oil, Lubriderm Bath Oil) can be used to provide relief from pruritus associated with contact dermatitis. Baths may be used as needed for comfort.

Diaper Dermatitis

Drug therapy in the treatment of diaper dermatitis is aimed at protecting the skin, decreasing inflammation, and treating *Candida* infection. Nonpharmacological interventions are also used to prevent irritant diaper dermatitis.

Barrier Medications

Barrier medications are used to protect the skin from the irritant effects of contact with urine and feces. Plain white petrolatum is an effective and inexpensive barrier agent. Vitamins A and D are added to petrolatum to create a barrier OTC medication, A&D Ointment. Zinc oxide is a commonly used barrier that has a drying effect as well. It is combined with a variety of other agents such as petrolatum (Diprotex, Diaparene, Bottom Better), cod liver oil and talc (Desitin), and balsam of Peru (Balmex), which is thought to promote wound healing. Plain zinc oxide is an effective barrier that is less expensive than the many diaper rash products. Barrier medications should be used at the first sign of irritation.

Anti-Inflammatory Medications

Anti-inflammatory medications are used to decrease the inflammation associated with diaper dermatitis. Because of the occlusive nature of diapers and undergarments, a low-dose hydrocortisone (0.5% or 1%) should be used for a brief period. Low-dose hydrocortisone can be used for 2 to 3 days in the diaper area safely if it is applied sparingly (pea-sized amount) and used 2 to 3 times a day. Stronger corticosteroid preparations or combination medications containing mid-potency steroids with an antifungal (Lotrisone) should not be used in the diaper area.

Antifungal Medications

Candidiasis is treated with a topical antifungal agent that is effective against *C. albicans*. Commonly used medications are nystatin (Mycostatin), miconazole (Monistat-Derm), and clotrimazole (Lotrimin). All of these medications are applied twice daily until the *Candida* infection is clear. Miconazole and clotrimazole are available OTC and are usually not covered by insurance plans. Nystatin is available by prescription only and is usually covered by insurance. If a patient does not respond to the OTC products, a trial of nystatin is warranted.

Wet Soaks

Wet soaks or sitz baths are used to decrease inflammation and provide comfort from diaper dermatitis. Burow's solution soaks or compresses can be used if the rash is weepy. Commercial diaper wipes often contain alcohol, which stings, and they should be avoided during diaper dermatitis. A spray bottle of clean water allows adequate cleansing without further irritating the area.

CLINICAL PEARL

Dermatitis

- Occluding the surface with plastic wrap will increase penetration of the topical corticosteroid. Do not do this in children, as it will increase the systemic absorption of the steroid.
- For contact dermatitis, caution the patient using bath oils against slipping in the tub. Children should be supervised at all times when using bath dermatologicals, which can all cause the tub to be slippery. Older adults should also be monitored.
- For the patient with hand dermatitis, wearing cotton gloves overnight after applying a thick layer of **emollient** will increase absorption, and the patient will often see a significant improvement overnight.

Nonpharmacological Management

Nonpharmacological management includes exposure to air, frequent diaper changes, and changing the brand of diaper or protective garment. Expose the affected area to air by leaving the diaper off, or blow-dry the area with a hair dryer on low/cool setting held several inches away from the skin 2 to 3 times a day.

Seborrheic Dermatitis

The mainstay of treatment for seborrheic dermatitis is topical antiseborrheic shampoos. Topical corticosteroids may also be used for nonhairy areas such as the face.

Antiseborrheic Shampoos

Antiseborrheic shampoos should be used as prescribed to control dandruff. A variety of preparations are available to treat scalp seborrhea or dandruff. Selenium sulfide 1% shampoos (Selsun Blue, Head & Shoulders Intensive) and ketoconazole (Nizoral) are the most commonly prescribed shampoos for seborrhea and are available OTC. Selenium sulfide prescription formulas (Exsel, Selun) contain 2.5% selenium sulfide. Coal tar shampoos are available OTC and range in strength from 0.5% (DHS Tar) to 12% (Extra Strength Denorex) coal tar. Pyrithione zinc, the active ingredient in OTC shampoos such as Head & Shoulders, may also be used to treat seborrheic dermatitis. Bar soap containing pyrithione zinc is available for use on body areas with scalp seborrhea (ZNP Bar). Shampoos that combine sulfur and salicylic acid can also be used (Sebulex, Fostex). For treating cradle cap, low-strength selenium sulfide (1%) is generally recommended, and care should be taken to keep the shampoo out of the infant's eyes and to rinse the hair well. Table 32-1 presents prescribing information.

Topical Corticosteroids

Topical corticosteroids are used for inflammatory seborrhea that does not respond to medicated shampoo. Low-potency steroid lotion or gel is applied 2 to 3 times daily to affected areas. Ongoing use of topical steroids may be needed when seborrheic dermatitis recurs. Table 32-1 presents prescribing information.

Monitoring

Monitoring for all forms of dermatitis includes assessing the patient for effectiveness of therapy and determining if the patient has experienced any adverse effects or developed a secondary infection.

Outcome Evaluation

For all forms of dermatitis, effective management controls exacerbations and provides comfort measures to decrease pruritus or other symptoms. If the initial therapy has not controlled the exacerbation, increasing the potency of the initial medication or switching to another medication may be indicated. However, before switching to another medication, the provider should observe the patient's medication administration technique, which may be the problem.

Secondary skin infections, if they occur, should be treated promptly. Referral to a dermatologist may be necessary if therapy is not managing the dermatitis, if high-potency topical corticosteroids are indicated, or if the patient has an unusual presentation.

Patient Education

Patient education should include a discussion of information related to the overall treatment plan as well as that specific to the drug therapy, reasons for taking the drug, drugs as part of the total treatment regimen, and adherence issues.

PSORIASIS

Psoriasis is a chronic skin condition that affects 2% of the population worldwide (Menter et al, 2009). It is characterized by sharply defined, symmetrical, erythematous patches with a distinctive silver scale. There are two peak age ranges of onset: from 16 to 22 years and from 57 to 60 years. However, it may occur at any age. Men and women are equally affected, but it is more common in whites than in darker-skinned people. There is a positive family history for the disease in 30% of patients. The disease may remain localized to a few areas, or it may become generalized. The condition is lifelong and may occur in an intermittent or a continuous pattern.

Pathophysiology

The exact pathogenesis of psoriasis is unclear, although it is thought to be an immune-mediated disease (Feldman & Pearce, 2010a). There is a significant decrease in the amount of time that it takes for a psoriatic epidermal cell to travel to the skin surface and be cast off. A normal skin cell travels to the surface in 26 to 28 days; with psoriasis, the cells take only 3 to 4 days. This decreased time does not allow normal cell maturation to take place.

Lesions of active psoriasis can develop in areas of epidermal trauma. Surgical incisions, a sunburn, or scratch marks can all heal, leaving psoriatic lesions in their place (Koebner phenomenon). Exacerbations may be triggered by beta-hemolytic streptococcal infections, as well as by some medications (e.g., lithium, beta-adrenergic antagonists, angiotensin-converting enzyme inhibitors, antimalarial drugs, and indomethacin).

Extensor surfaces are affected more commonly, with other common sites being the intergluteal fold, the eyebrows, and around the ears. Nails may develop pits and ridges, may be thick and discolored, and have splinter hemorrhages.

Goals of Treatment

Although psoriasis is a chronic, lifelong, recurrent disease, the goal of therapy should be control of symptoms and clearing of psoriatic lesions. It should be emphasized to the patient that psoriasis is a treatable disease and that control is possible with continued, conscientious use of medication.

PATIENT EDUCATION

PATIENT
EDUCATION

Dermatitis

RELATED TO THE OVERALL TREATMENT PLAN/DISEASE PROCESS

☐ Pathophysiology

☐ Role of preventive and nonpharmacological measures if appropriate

☐ Importance of adherence to the treatment regimen

☐ Self-monitoring of symptoms

☐ What to do when symptoms worsen

☐ Need for follow-up visits with the primary care provider

SPECIFIC TO THE DRUG THERAPY

☐ Reason for taking the drug and its anticipated action on the disease process

☐ Doses and schedules for taking the drug

☐ Possible adverse effects and what to do if they occur

☐ Interactions between other treatment modalities and these drugs

REASONS FOR TAKING THE DRUG(S)

☐ Patient education about specific drugs is provided in the appropriate chapter

SPECIFICALLY FOR ECZEMA

☐ Pathophysiology of eczema, that it is a chronic disorder requiring ongoing care, and that there is an itch-scratch-itch cycle that needs to be addressed, but that it is a recurring disease that can be controlled

☐ Avoidance of offending agents that cause exacerbations

☐ Appropriate use of **topical corticosteroids** should be demonstrated. With a sample, the provider can demonstrate how far a pea-sized amount of topical medication can be spread. The patient or caregiver applying the medication should be aware of the adverse effects of overuse of **topical corticosteroids**.

☐ Avoidance of irritants or agents that cause exacerbation of the eczema should be taught, with a written list of common Irritants provided to the patient

☐ Long-term therapy (skin hydration and **emollient** use) versus acute therapy

SPECIFICALLY FOR CONTACT DERMATITIS

☐ Pathophysiology

☐ Appropriate application of **topical corticosteroids** should be demonstrated

☐ Appropriate use of **antipruritic medication**

SPECIFICALLY FOR DIAPER DERMATITIS

☐ The parent or patient should be educated about the underlying pathophysiology of diaper dermatitis, in that it is usually an irritant dermatitis caused by chemical irritation from urine or feces, complicated by mechanical irritation of the diaper or undergarment rubbing and chafing the skin.

☐ Describing the characteristics of a secondary infection with *Candida* will assist with early identification and treatment of this common complication in diaper dermatitis.

☐ Nonpharmacological management such as sitz baths, air drying, and frequent diaper changes should be discussed.

☐ If properly treated, the skin should return to normal in the area in 3 to 4 days. If the patient is not responding to treatment in 48 hours, then a reevaluation is necessary.

SPECIFICALLY FOR SEBORRHEIC DERMATITIS

☐ The patient should know that seborrheic dermatitis cannot be cured and can only be controlled and that treatment will probably need to be continued long-term in adolescents and adults. In infants with cradle cap, it will usually resolve around age 6 months.

☐ The patient should contact the health-care provider if signs and symptoms of a secondary infection occur.

DRUGS AS PART OF THE TOTAL TREATMENT REGIMEN

☐ The total treatment regimen includes pharmacological and nonpharmacological measures. Be sure the patient and/or family members are aware of the specific measures to be taken.

ADHERENCE ISSUES

☐ Health-care providers should be aware of the potential problem of nonadherence and should discuss the importance of completing the entire treatment regimen with the patient and/or family members.

Rational Drug Selection

The management of psoriasis consists of topical medication and phototherapy for mild to moderate psoriasis (less than 5% of the body involved) and the addition of systemic medications for severe psoriasis (more than 5% to 10% of the body involved) (Feldman & Pearce, 2010b; Menter et al, 2009). Not covered in this chapter because they are prescribed only by dermatology specialists are systemic treatments with immunosuppressants (alefacept [Amevive], efalizumab [Raptiva], cyclosporine [Neoral], ustekinumab [Stelara]), retinoids (acitretin [Soriatane]), methotrexate, and tumor necrosis factor blockers (etanercept [Enbrel], adalimumab [Humira], infliximab [Remicade]).

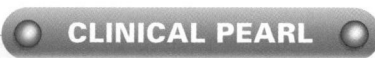

CLINICAL PEARL

Psoriasis
Psoriasis may affect a patient's self-esteem and may exacerbate depression. The patient's mood should be monitored. Referral to a support group or an organization such as the National Psoriasis Foundation (http://www.psoriasis.org) may be helpful.

Topical Therapy

Topical therapy for psoriasis consists of topical steroids, coal tar, or keratolytic shampoos for scalp involvement, keratolytic agents for thick plaques, anthralin, and calcipotriene. Topical immunomodulators may also be used.

Topical Steroids

Topical steroids are used to treat psoriasis because of their anti-inflammatory effects on the plaques. Moderate- to high-potency steroids are used because the lesions are generally steroid-resistant (Menter et al, 2009). The steroid cream or ointment is applied 2 to 3 times per day (see Table 32-1). Chronic topical corticosteroid use can cause tachyphylaxis and may have adverse effects such as atrophy and telangiectasia. Intermittent or "pulse" therapy minimizes some of these effects. If topical corticosteroids are used in the intertriginous areas or on the face, a low-potency medication should be chosen. Regardless of the topical steroid used, 2 to 4 weeks of continuous use is the limit, with gradual reduction in frequency of application to prevent rebound (Feldman & Pearce, 2010b). Patients should be discouraged from using steroids for longer periods. Topical corticosteroids should be reserved for psoriasis flare, and another medication used for ongoing therapy.

Coal Tar

Coal tar (Zetar, Medotar, Tegrin for Psoriasis) affects psoriasis by enzyme inhibition and antimitotic action. Tar preparations include creams, shampoos, ointments, lotions, gels, and oils. They range in strength from 1% to 20%. Tar has few adverse effects and is safer to use than topical steroids and anthralin, although tar has decreased in use in the United States (Menter et al, 2009). The major problem is that tar products are messy and can stain the skin and clothes. The tar preparation is applied to the affected areas once or twice daily. If using coal tar shampoo or bath emulsion, the patient should be instructed to rinse well after use. Tar preparations make the patient photosensitive; therefore, the patient should be instructed to avoid sunlight and ultraviolet light (see Table 32-1).

Anthralin

Anthralin (Dithrocreme, Dithro-Scalp) is an antimitotic agent that is used for chronic psoriasis. It has an antiproliferative effect. Although it is effective, anthralin has the disadvantages of being irritating and of staining skin and clothing. Anthralin's use has decreased over the past few years with the availability of preparations that are more cosmetically acceptable (Menter et al, 2009). Careful instructions for use increase the likelihood of a successful outcome with this difficult-to-administer medication.

When prescribing anthralin to a patient who has never used it, choose a low-concentration product (0.1%). The medication is applied to the psoriatic lesions and rubbed gently until the medication is absorbed. Take care not to get the anthralin on the healthy surrounding skin. It is important not to apply excessive medication, which increases the staining of skin and clothes. After the medication is rubbed in, it is left on 10 to 20 minutes; then it is washed off in the shower. After 1 week, the length of time the medication is in contact with the skin can be increased to 15 to 20 minutes. The strength of anthralin can be increased in increments (0.25%, 0.5%, 1%) as tolerated. Some patients require the medication to be applied and left on for 60 minutes to have improvement in their psoriatic lesions. Treatment should be continued until the lesions are completely healed (when nothing is felt with the fingers and the texture of the skin is completely normal). Table 32-1 presents prescribing information for anthralin.

Vitamin D$_3$ Derivatives

Calcipotriene (Dovonex) is a vitamin D$_3$ derivative that regulates cell differentiation and proliferation and suppresses lymphocyte activity. Calcipotriene is available in a cream, ointment, or solution preparation. It is effective and safe for short- or long-term treatment. Calcipotriene is applied in a thin film to the affected psoriasis plaques and rubbed into the skin gently and completely. In adults, the ointment is applied twice daily in the morning and evening. It is important that the patient does not exceed 100 g/wk of calcipotriene applied to the skin. Safety and efficacy in children have not been established. For the treatment of mild to moderate scalp psoriasis, the patient applies the topical solution twice daily. Improvement will be noted as soon as 1 to 2 weeks after treatment has begun. The patient should be reevaluated after 6 to 8 weeks. Calcipotriene may be used in combination with topical steroids, which is more effective than either treatment alone. Table 32-1 presents prescribing information for calcipotriene.

Topical calcitriol (Vectical Ointment) is a vitamin D$_3$ derivative similar to calcipotriene. Calcitriol inhibits keratinocyte proliferation and inhibits T-cell proliferation and other inflammatory mediators (Feldman & Pearce, 2010b). Calcitriol is applied to affected psoriatic plaques twice a day.

The maximum weekly dose should not exceed 200 g. Hypercalcemia may occur and calcitriol should be discontinued until normocalcemia returns.

Phototherapy

Patients with psoriasis respond very well to phototherapy. Phototherapy with ultraviolet-B (UVB) light is effective in managing psoriasis by reducing DNA synthesis of epidermal cells. UVB light treatment is easy for the patient to use and can produce long-lasting remissions of 2 to 4 months. UVB therapy is usually prescribed by a dermatologist. The use of commercial tanning beds is not recommended.

Systemic Medications

Systemic medications used for psoriasis are methotrexate, oral retinoids, immunosuppressants (alefacept [Amevive], efalizumab [Raptiva], cyclosporine [Neoral], ustekinumab [Stelara]), retinoids (acitretin [Soriatane]), and tumor necrosis factor blockers (etanercept [Enbrel], adalimumab [Humira], infliximab [Remicade]). They have serious adverse effects and therefore should be prescribed only by a dermatologist and only if the patient meets criteria determined by the American Academy of Dermatology. To try to decrease the adverse effects, the medications may be prescribed intermittently or on a rotational basis. Patients should be advised to avoid pregnancy before, during, and for a period of time after taking these drugs. The primary care provider will need to consult with the dermatologist and observe the patient for adverse effects if any of these medications are prescribed.

Monitoring

The patient who is being treated for psoriasis should be monitored for effectiveness of therapy and for adverse effects of the medication.

Outcome Evaluation

Psoriasis lesions should eventually clear, with the skin returning to the patient's normal look and feel. If the patient is using the medication correctly and there is unsatisfactory clinical response, or if skin irritation occurs, then either the medication needs to be changed or the strength increased. Skin irritation is a common adverse effect of psoriasis medications, especially if the patient gets the medication on the surrounding skin. Review proper administration technique prior to changing the therapy.

Patient Education

Successful treatment of psoriasis requires educating the patient on the following key points:

1. The patient should understand the pathophysiology of psoriasis: that it is a chronic disease but that remission is possible if adequately treated.
2. Proper application of topical medications will not only optimize treatment but also decrease adverse effects of the medications.
3. Many of the medications stain the skin and clothing. The patient should be aware of this problem and instructed on how to minimize the staining.
4. Some medications cause photosensitivity; therefore, the patient needs to understand the hazards of sun exposure and use protective clothing and sunscreen.

ACNE AND ACNE ROSACEA

Acne affects an estimated 17 to 28 million Americans, accounting for 4.4% of internist visits. It is the number-one condition seen by dermatologists, accounting for 18% of visits (Fleischer, Herbert, Feldman, & O'Brien, 2000). Acne can occur in girls as young as 9 or 10 years of age, with 70% to 87% prevalence in adolescents (Eichenfield et al, 2013), although acne can also occur in patients in their twenties to forties. Adolescent acne is more common in boys than in girls; however, adult acne is more common in women than in men. Males have a higher incidence of severe acne at all ages. Although acne may be a minor problem from a medical standpoint, studies have determined that acne has a significant impact on the patient's quality of life (Dalgard, Gieler, Holm, Bjertness, & Hauser, 2008). The practitioner needs to address the patient's concerns about acne with this in mind.

Pathophysiology

The underlying cause of acne is multifactorial. A genetic susceptibility appears to predispose some people to acne. Acne begins below the skin surface in the pilosebaceous unit of the sebaceous glands. In acne, the sebaceous glands are enlarged and sebum production is increased, probably because of adrenogenic hormones. In patients with acne, there is an alteration in the keratinization process in the follicular infrainfundibulum. This causes the extra sebum to occlude the hair follicle and produce microcomedones. These may enlarge with time and form closed comedones (whiteheads) or open comedones (blackheads). *Propionibacterium acnes (P. acnes)* organisms colonize the follicles and convert the triglycerides in the sebum into free fatty acids. Free fatty acids are a factor in the synthesis of chemoattractants that draw inflammatory elements, leading to the inflammation associated with acne. The patient may have superficial papules and/or pustules or deeper nodules, depending on the intensity of the inflammatory process.

Goals of Treatment

At this time, acne has no cure. The goal is to control the acne and keep visible lesions and medication adverse effects to a minimum. Management goals that will control acne are (1) controlling the inflammatory process associated with acne by altering the bacterial flora, and (2) decreasing the obstruction of the sebaceous ducts.

Rational Drug Selection

Acne treatment should be approached in a stepwise manner. If the acne is mild or moderate, a beginning therapy might include topical retinoids and/or topical antibiotics. If after 6 to 8 weeks this is not completely effective, an oral antibiotic might be added or a change in topical therapy initiated. For moderate to somewhat severe acne, the patient is usually started on an oral antibiotic and topical preparations combined. For severe, recalcitrant, nodular acne, the patient is prescribed isotretinoin (Accutane). Figure 32-1 presents an algorithm of the pharmacological management of acne.

Topical Agents

The topical agents used for acne can be divided into two categories: topical retinoids and topical antibiotics.

Topical Retinoids

Topical retinoids (tretinoin [Retin-A]), retinoid-like compounds (adapalene [Differin]), or retinoid prodrugs (Tazarotene [Tazorac]) are used to treat inflammatory and noninflammatory acne. They act to alter the abnormal keratinization process of acne that leads to microcomedome formation. Additionally, they stimulate mitotic activity and increase the turnover of follicular epithelial cells, causing extrusion of the comedones. Clinically, this causes an initial worsening of acne, as comedones that were previously under the skin are extruded. This worsening is not a reason for discontinuation of treatment. Patients should be reassured that their faces will clear after approximately 6 to 8 weeks of treatment.

All retinoid preparations can cause some skin irritation, especially in fair-skinned patients or patients with sensitive skin. Irritation may be decreased in patients with sensitive skin by initiating 3-times-a-week or every-other-day therapy and increasing to daily use as tolerated (Eichenfield et al, 2013). Atopic people can be quite sensitive to these products. The patient should not use any harsh toners, astringents, scrubs, or cleansers while on topical retinoid therapy because these increase irritation. The patient's skin is more photosensitive when topical retinoids are used, and the patient should be advised to use noncomedogenic sunscreen for any sun exposure.

The patient should avoid the eyes and mucous membranes when applying these products. There may be transient stinging, burning, or pruritus immediately after applying topical

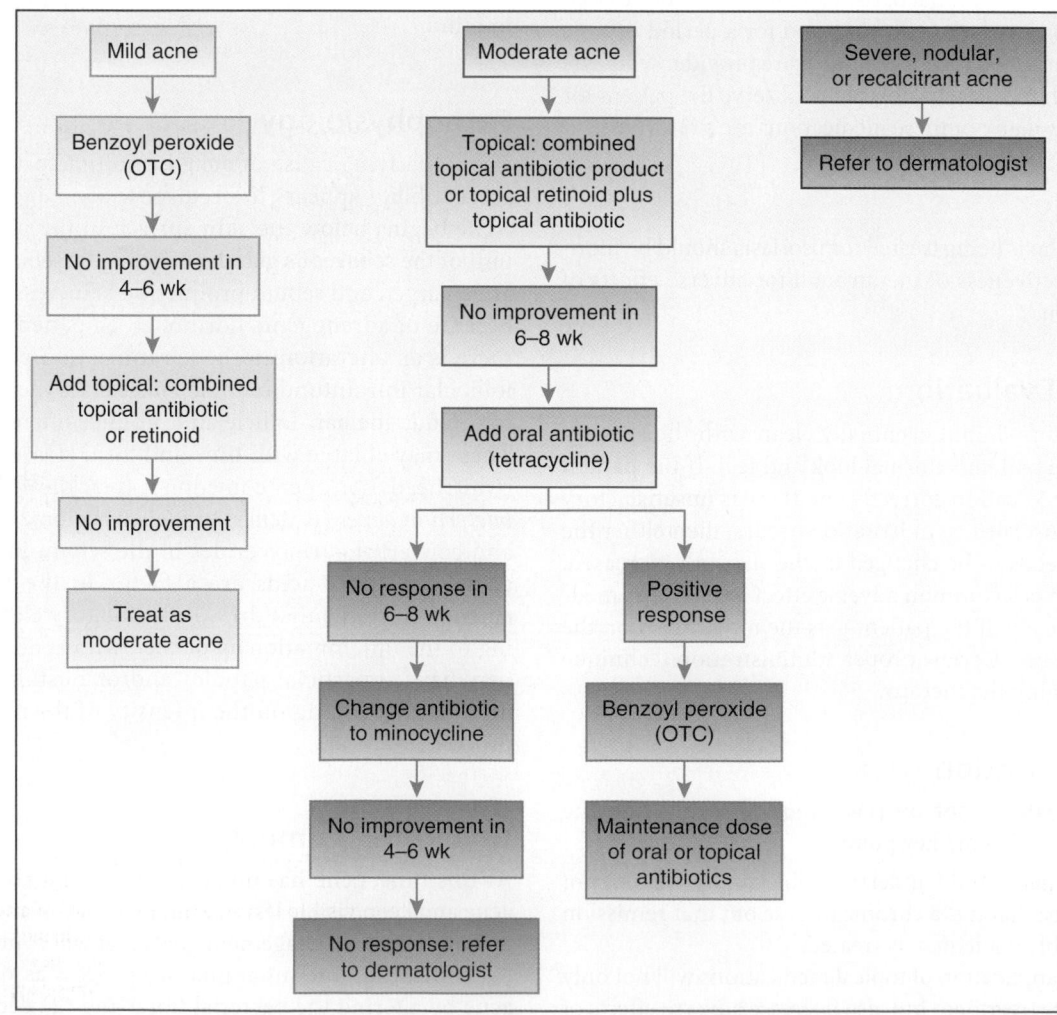

Figure 32–1. Algorithm: Pharmacological management of acne.

retinoids. Redness and peeling may occur with excessive application. If topical retinoids are used more than recommended, a dramatic increase in skin irritation occurs, but no improved response.

Table 32-2 presents the drugs commonly used to treat acne.

Topical Antibiotics

Topical antibiotics are thought to act to control acne by their bacteriostatic or bactericidal activity against *P. acnes.* They control the inflammatory process, probably by decreasing the free fatty acids that *P. acnes* produces. Applied topically,

Table 32–2   Drugs Commonly Used: Acne

Drug	Indication	Strengths Available	Dose	Comments
Topical Retinoids				
Tretinoin (Retin-A)	Acne	Cream: 0.025%, 0.05%, 0.1% Gel: 0.025%, 0.01% Liquid: 0.05%	Apply to affected areas once daily after washing face with a mild cleanser; begin with 0.025% cream and increase strength or to bid if needed. Sensitive-skin patients may need to dose every other night.	Wash hands after application. Normal use of cosmetics is permissible, but instruct patient to use noncomedogenic products. Pregnancy Category C; pregnant women should be switched to another product.
Adapalene (Differin)	Acne	Gel: 0.1% (alcohol-free) Lotion: 0.1% (30% alcohol)	Apply to affected areas once daily (HS) after washing with a gentle cleanser; avoid eyes, lips, and mucous membranes.	Avoid harsh soaps, cleansers, or alcohol-containing products, which increase skin irritation while using adapalene. Pregnancy Category C. May be used in children >12 yr.
Adapalene and benzoyl peroxide (Epiduo)	Acne	Adapalene 0.1% and benzoyl peroxide 2.5% gel	*Adults and children >12 yr:* Apply thin film once daily after washing. Reduce frequency if irritation occurs.	Avoid harsh soaps, cleansers, or alcohol-containing products, which increase skin irritation while using adapalene. Pregnancy Category C. May be used in children >12 yr.
Topical Antibiotics				
Benzoyl peroxide (Rx: Benzac, Desquam-X, Desquam-E) (OTC: Dryox, Fostex, Neutrogena AcneMask, Clearasil)	Acne	Liquid wash: 2.5%, 5%, 10% Bar: 5%, 10% Mask: 5% Lotion: 5%, 5.5%, 10% Cream: 5%, 10%	For cleansers, wash once or twice daily; rinse well and pat dry. For other forms, apply once daily; gradually increase to 2–3 times daily if needed; apply after cleansing skin.	Has a drying action that causes comedolysis and has a mild desquamation effect (irritating to the skin). Pregnancy Category C; topical application during pregnancy is generally considered safe.
		Gel: 2.5%, 4%, 5%, 10%, 20%		May be used in children >12 yr. Bleaches fabrics. Inactivates tretinoin and cannot be applied simultaneously.
Benzoyl peroxide/ clindamycin (Benzaclin, Duac)	Acne	5% Benzoyl peroxide 1% Clindamycin gel	Benzaclin: Apply to affected areas bid. Duac: Apply to affected areas once daily.	Has a drying action, causes comedolysis, and has a mild desquamation effect (irritating to the skin). Pregnancy Category C; topical application during pregnancy is generally considered safe.

Continued

Table 32–2   Drugs Commonly Used: Acne—cont'd

Drug	Indication	Strengths Available	Dose	Comments
				May be used in children >12 yr. Bleaches fabrics. Inactivates tretinoin and cannot be applied simultaneously. Rare reaction: colitis.
Erythromycin (Staticin, Akne-Mycin, A/T/S, Eryderm, Erymax, Ery-Sol, T-Stat, Erygel)	Acne	Solution: 1%, 2% Gel: 2% Ointment: 2%	Apply to affected areas bid after washing face with a mild cleanser.	Pregnancy Category B. Do not use concurrently with clindamycin.
Benzoyl peroxide/ erythromycin (Benzamycin)	Acne	Gel	Apply to affected areas once or twice/d (gel dries to a crusty white appearance; therefore, patient may prefer evening application; patient may use plain benzoyl peroxide in the morning if this is concern).	Pregnancy Category C. Bleaches fabrics. Must be kept refrigerated; stable for only 3 mo after mixed. Adverse effects include skin irritation and sun sensitivity.
Clindamycin (Cleocin, Clinda-Derm, C/T/S)	Acne	Gel, lotion, topical solution	Apply thin layer to affected areas bid.	Use with caution in patients with eczema. Although rare, there are reports of colitis with topical administration. If patient develops diarrhea, stop medication and investigate cause. Pregnancy Category B. Do not use in children <12 yr. Adverse effects include skin dryness and irritation, burning, and peeling.
Tetracycline (Topicycline)	Acne	Topical solution: 2.2 g/mL	Apply to affected areas bid; apply until skin is thoroughly wet (stinging and burning may occur but subside after a few minutes).	Pregnancy Category B. May be staining to clothes; yellowing of skin may be removed by washing. Assess patient for sulfite sensitivity. Topicycline contains sodium bisulfite.
Metronidazole (Metro-Gel, Noritate)	Acne rosacea	Gel: 0.75% Emollient cream: 1%	Apply a thin film bid to entire affected area after washing.	Improvement should be noted within 3 wk, but there may be continued improvement through 9 wk of treatment. Pregnancy Category B. Some mild skin irritation may be noted.
Oral Antibiotics				
Tetracycline (Achromycin)	Acne (long-term treatment)	Capsules: 250, 500 mg Tablets: 250, 500 mg	Initially, 500 mg bid for 1–2 mo. After control is achieved, dose may be lowered to 500 mg daily for 1–2 mo; then determine maintenance dose of 125–500 mg daily.	Must be taken on an empty stomach; poorly absorbed if taken with calcium-containing foods, milk, or antacids. Pregnancy Category D; do not prescribe to lactating women or children under age 8 (may cause staining of teeth).

Table 32–2   Drugs Commonly Used: Acne—cont'd

Drug	Indication	Strengths Available	Dose	Comments
Minocycline (Minocin)	Acne	Capsules: 50, 100 mg Tablets: 50, 100 mg	Initially, 100 mg bid, then wean to 50 mg daily after control is achieved.	Expensive. Must be taken on an empty stomach. Pregnancy Category D; do not prescribe to lactating women or children <8 yr.
Doxycycline (Monodox, Vibramycin)	Acne	Capsules: 50, 75, 100 mg	50–100 mg qd or bid	Take with a full glass of water and remain upright for 1 hour. May be taken with meals. Sunscreen must be worn.

antibiotics have an uneven, erratic penetration into the follicles. Therefore, they are usually used in mild acne, for maintenance after a course of oral antibiotics, or in conjunction with topical retinoids. There is a concern that resistant *P. acnes* may develop if topical antibiotics are overused.

The topical antibiotics that are approved for use include benzoyl peroxide, available by prescription (Benzac, Desquam-X, Desquam-E) or OTC (Dryox, Fostex, Neutrogena Acne Mask, Clearasil); erythromycin (Staticin, Akne-Mycin, A/T/S, Eryderm, Erymax, Ery-Sol, T-Stat, Erygel), clindamycin (Cleocin, Clinda-Derm, C/T/S); and tetracycline (Topicycline). A combination of benzoyl peroxide and adapalene (Epiduo Gel) is available. Ziana is a combination of clindamycin and tretinoin. The combination of benzoyl peroxide and an antibiotic erythromycin (Benzamycin) or clindamycin (Acanya, Benzaclin, Duac) is superior to either agent alone. Prescribing information is given in Table 32-2.

Oral Agents

Oral agents used for acne are divided into three categories: oral antibiotics, hormonal therapy, and isotretinoin (an oral retinoid). Oral antibiotics are prescribed for moderate to severe acne and are within the scope of practice of primary care providers. Isotretinoin is prescribed for severe nodulocystic acne but only by dermatologists because of its adverse effects.

Oral Antibiotics

Oral antibiotics are active against *P. acnes,* which helps transform comedones into inflammatory pustules and papules. Oral antibiotics do not affect existing lesions, but they prevent future lesions by decreasing sebaceous fatty acids by decreasing *P. acnes* colonization. They may also have an anti-inflammatory effect independent of their action against *P. acnes.* There is level I evidence for the use of tetracycline, doxycycline, minocycline, erythromycin, trimethoprim-sulfamethoxazole, trimethoprim, and azithromycin in the treatment of acne (Strauss et al, 2007). Azithromycin is effective against acne, but its routine use may lead to increased resistance (Graber, 2014). Increasing resistance to erythromycin has led to decreased use (Eichenfield et al, 2013). Doxycycline and minocycline are recommended due

to efficacy and once daily dosing (Eichenfield et al, 2013; Graber, 2014) Table 32-2 presents prescribing information for tetracycline (Achromycin V), doxycycline (Vibramycin) and minocycline (Minocin).

Hormonal Therapy

Hormonal therapy can be prescribed to women who require birth control who also have mild to moderate acne. Multiple oral contraceptives currently have FDA approval for use in acne: Ortho Tri-Cyclen, Ortho-Cyclen, Estrostep Fe, and Tri-Sprintec. The oral contraceptives appear to control the inflammatory component of acne. The patient is prescribed a premeasured-dose pack and takes one pill daily. Effects on acne are seen in 3 to 6 months of continued use. For full prescribing information, see Chapter 31.

> **CLINICAL PEARL**
>
> **Acne**
> Tell patients using **benzoyl peroxide** products that benzoyl peroxide can bleach clothes and towels. Advise them to use an old or white pillowcase on their bed and an old or white towel to dry their hands after using these agents.

Isotretinoin

Isotretinoin (Accutane) is the most potent agent for treating acne. It is reserved for severe, recalcitrant cystic acne. Its exact mechanism of action is unknown but thought to be related to decreased sebum production (by 90%) and isotretinoin's ability to decrease abnormal keratinization. Isotretinoin is prescribed for a period of 15 to 20 weeks and may need to be repeated. The toxicity profile and its ability to cause fetal malformations require that the prescriber provide extensive education and close monitoring throughout therapy. The adverse effects of dry skin, cheilitis, and pruritus are seen in almost all patients taking the drug. Patients may experience elevated serum triglycerides and clinical hepatitis, including elevated liver enzymes. Therefore, liver enzyme and lipid levels should be obtained before beginning therapy and monitored throughout therapy. Patients may develop depression or suicide ideation; all patients taking isotretinoin should have their mood monitored.

The major concern is the use of the drug in women who may become pregnant; therefore, there are very stringent requirements and consent that must be met before the drug is prescribed. For female patients, a pregnancy test needs to be performed before beginning therapy and then monthly throughout therapy. Isotretinoin is Pregnancy Category X. It should not be prescribed to teenagers who have not completed their linear growth. Because of the toxic effects of isotretinoin, it is rarely prescribed by a primary care provider and is usually prescribed only by a dermatologist. All providers and female patients need to be registered with iPledge, a pregnancy-prevention program committed to preventing pregnancy while patients are taking isotretinoin. To register, go to http://www.iPledgeprogram.com.

Acne Rosacea

Acne rosacea, commonly referred to as rosacea, is a skin condition that usually affects middle-aged patients. It is a chronic inflammatory disorder that affects the blood vessels and pilosebaceous glands of the face. The patient often has a characteristic red-colored nose. An important hallmark characteristic is easy facial flushing and blushing associated with the ingestion of alcohol, spicy foods, or caffeine-containing beverages.

Patients with acne rosacea have papules and pustules superimposed on diffuse erythema and telangiectasia over the central portion of the face. Hyperplasia of the sebaceous glands, connective tissue, and vascular bed can lead to a large, bulbous red nose, called rhinophyma. The patient may also have ocular involvement that may require the care of an ophthalmologist.

Skin care includes use of a gentle facial cleanser and daily use of a sunscreen with a 30 sun protection factor (SPF) or greater to protect the skin (Del Roso et al, 2013a). Topical metronidazole (Metro-Gel, Noritate) and azeliac acid (Finacea) are FDA-approved to treat acne rosacea. The mechanism by which metronidazole works to improve the inflammation of rosacea is unknown but is probably related to its antibacterial effect. Likewise, the mechanism of action of azelaic acid to treat rosacea is unknown. Rosacea usually responds well to metronidazole or azeliac acid, but the antibiotic must be continued, because the rosacea will recur if the medication is discontinued (Del Roso et al, 2013b). Table 32-2 presents prescribing information.

PATIENT EDUCATION

Acne

RELATED TO THE OVERALL TREATMENT PLAN/DISEASE PROCESS

☐ Pathophysiology

☐ Role of preventive and nonpharmacological measures if appropriate

☐ Importance of adherence to the treatment regimen

☐ Self-monitoring of symptoms

☐ What to do when symptoms worsen

☐ Need for follow-up visits with the primary care provider

SPECIFIC TO THE DRUG THERAPY

☐ Reason for the drug's being given and its anticipated action on the disease process

☐ Doses and schedules for taking the drug

☐ Possible adverse effects and what to do if they occur

☐ Interactions between other treatment modalities and these drugs

REASONS FOR TAKING THE DRUG(S)

☐ Patient education about specific drugs is provided in the appropriate chapter.

SPECIFICALLY FOR ACNE

☐ The patient should understand that it will take at least 6 weeks to determine if treatment is effective. Tying this into the explanation of normal skin growth will help the patient understand why it takes so long for the medication to work.

☐ Whatever level of treatment the patient is started on, the patient needs to understand what alternatives there are if the chosen treatment is not effective.

DRUGS AS PART OF THE TOTAL TREATMENT REGIMEN

☐ The total treatment regimen includes pharmacological and nonpharmacological measures. Be sure the patient and/or family members are aware of the specific measures to be taken.

ADHERENCE ISSUES

☐ Health-care providers should be aware of the potential problem of nonadherence and should discuss the importance of completing the entire treatment regimen with the patient and/or family members.

Monitoring

The patient needs to be monitored for effectiveness and adverse effects of the acne medication.

Laboratory testing before and during therapy may be indicated for some patients. The primary care provider may be involved in obtaining and monitoring these tests. For female patients, especially those taking tetracycline, doxycycline, minocycline, and isotretinoin, pregnancy testing is recommended prior to beginning treatment and as indicated throughout therapy.

Outcome Evaluation

The patient needs to use an acne medication for at least 6 to 8 weeks before effectiveness can be determined. If there is no response after that time, then a change in therapy can be considered—either adding another medication or changing the regimen completely. Before determining the medication is not effective, review administration of the medication with the patient. The adverse effects associated with topical acne treatments include skin irritation and some redness and peeling. Mild symptoms usually improve if the frequency of administration is decreased slightly. If possible, the strength of the topical medication can be decreased if there is mild to moderate irritation. Severe skin irritation warrants discontinuing the medication and switching to another.

Patient Education

Patient education should include a discussion of information related to the overall treatment plan as well as that specific to the drug therapy, reasons for taking the drug, drugs as part of the total treatment regimen, and adherence issues.

SKIN INFECTIONS

Skin infections commonly seen in primary care include bacterial, viral, and fungal skin infections.

Bacterial skin infections are common and seen in patients of any age. The skin infections seen in primary care include impetigo, a furuncle (boil or abscess), perianal streptococcal infection, and cellulitis. All require prompt treatment with the appropriate antibiotic.

Many viral skin infections can affect the skin, often causing rashes. Herpes simplex virus infection, herpes zoster (shingles), and varicella (chickenpox) are the common viral infections seen in primary care.

Fungal skin infections can be divided into two types: *Candida* infections and dermatophyte infections. Dermatophyte or tinea infections include tinea of the scalp (tinea capitis or ringworm of the scalp), tinea of the skin (tinea corporis or ringworm), tinea cruris ("jock itch"), tinea of the feet (tinea pedis or athlete's feet), and tinea versicolor. Onychomycosis, a fungal infection of the nails, is another type of fungal skin infection.

Pathophysiology

Bacterial Skin Infections

The most common bacterial organisms found in skin infections are *S. aureus* and *Streptococcus pyogenes*. The organism usually enters through a break in the skin. The bacteria cause an inflammatory infectious process to begin.

Viral Skin Infections

Viral skin infections include herpes viral infections, varicella, and herpes zoster.

Herpes viral infections are spread by intimate contact between a person shedding the virus and a susceptible host. With inoculation into the skin or mucous membrane, herpes simplex virus (HSV) begins to replicate. The incubation period is 4 to 6 days. As replication continues, local inflammation and cell lysis lead to the distinctive vesicle with an erythematous region. The virus generally ascends the peripheral sensory nerves to the dorsal root ganglia. HSV replicates in the dorsal root ganglia and then enters an inactive or latent stage. The herpes virus is unique in that it establishes latency for varying periods of time. HSV can be reactivated and enter a replication cycle at any time. There are two HSV infections, HSV-1 and HSV-2, with HSV-1 generally associated with nongenital infection and HSV-2 associated with genital infection.

Varicella (chickenpox) is a highly contagious disease caused by the varicella zoster virus, a herpes virus. It is spread by direct contact, in droplets, and by airborne transmission. The virus infects individuals by the conjunctivae or respiratory tract, replicating in the nasopharynx and upper respiratory tract. It spreads systemically to cause a viremia, resulting in a disseminated vesicular rash after an incubation period of 10 to 14 days. The patient is contagious for 1 to 2 days prior to the rash eruption and until all the lesions are dry. After the rash clears, the virus enters a latent phase and remains inactive in the dorsal root ganglia.

Herpes zoster (shingles) is caused by reactivation of latent varicella zoster virus. The reason for the reactivation is unknown, although stress seems to have some impact. The incidence of the disease increases with age and immunosuppression. The patient usually experiences burning and pain along the dermatome prior to the vesicles erupting. The lesions are generally unilateral and appear along a dermatome, although there may occasionally be scattered lesions. The diagnosis is confirmed with Tzanck smear or viral culture.

Fungal Skin Infections

Candida infections are caused by *C. albicans*, which is commonly found on the skin and mucosal tissues in the oral, intestinal, and vaginal areas. Considered a normal flora in these areas, an overgrowth can lead to infection and erythema, ulceration, and characteristic white plaques. In the mouth, oral candidiasis is known as thrush. In women, a vaginal *Candida* infection is often referred to as a "yeast infection." *Candida* is diagnosed by examination of scrapings from the area, using potassium hydroxide (KOH) preparation.

Dermatophytes are a group of fungi that live on the keratin of the stratum corneum, nails, and hair. Symptoms of dermatophyte infection include pruritus, scaling, occasional vesicles, and, in tinea corporis, characteristic annular lesions with raised edges and clearing in the center. Tinea versicolor can have clinical findings of multiple scaling, discrete macules that can be hypopigmented or hyperpigmented.

Onychomycosis is a fungal infection of the fingernails or toenails.

Goals of Treatment

The goals of treatment for skin infections are to decrease the severity of the infection or eradicate it (as appropriate), alleviate symptoms, and heal the skin area and return it to normal (as appropriate).

Rational Drug Selection

Bacterial Skin Infections

Impetigo

Impetigo is a bacterial infection (*S. aureus* or *S. pyogenes*) of the superficial layers of the skin, which begins as vesicles rupture, leaving a hallmark golden or honey-colored crust. Topical mupirocin ointment (Bactroban) or retapamulin (Altabax) for 5 days is used if the impetigo is mild (up to five singular lesions) (Stevens et al, 2014). The OTC ointments bacitracin and combinations of bacitracin, polymyxin B sulfate, and neomycin (Polysporin, Neosporin, Double Antibiotic Ointment, and Triple Antibiotic Ointment) are not recommended in the 2014 Infectious Disease Society guidelines for the treatment of skin infections (Stevens et al, 2014). Topical antibiotic ointments that contain neomycin (Neosporin) should not be used, as neomycin sensitivity is a concern. Oral antibiotics, such as cephalexin (Keflex) or dicloxacillin, are indicated if the patient has more than five lesions or ecthyma or if the lesions continue to worsen after 2 to 3 days of topical therapy (Stevens et al, 2014). Gram's stain and culture of exudate or pus is recommended to determine if MRSA is present. If MRSA is confirmed, treat with doxycycline, clindamycin, or sulfamethoxazole-trimethoprim (SMX-TMP) based on local resistance patterns (Stevens et al, 2014).

Furuncle

Treatment of a small furuncle, which is usually caused by *S. aureus,* may respond to warm packs and not need systemic antibiotics. A larger boil or abscess may require incision and drainage, as well as systemic antibiotics. Gram's stain and culture of the drainage will determine if the organism will be sensitive to the antibiotic of choice. Prior to Gram's stain results, an appropriate first-line antibiotic would be cephalexin or dicloxacillin (Stevens et al, 2014). Empiric therapy should include coverage for MRSA in areas of high prevalence. Antibiotics appropriate for MRSA include TMP/SMZ or

doxycycline, depending on local resistance patterns. Length of treatment should be 5 to 10 days, unless longer treatment is indicated by clinical progress.

Perianal Streptococcal Infection

Perianal streptococcal infection, a localized infection of the perianal area, usually occurs in children. The rash is caused by group A beta-hemolytic streptococci. The diagnosis is confirmed by a perianal swab and culture. The treatment of choice is penicillin, with erythromycin or cephalexin prescribed to penicillin-allergic patients.

Cellulitis

Cellulitis is a painful, erythematous, spreading bacterial infection involving the soft tissue. The patient can become quite ill if untreated, including developing sepsis. The causative organisms are most commonly *Streptococcus pneumoniae, S. aureus,* or, in children, *Haemophilus influenzae.* Treatment is with systemic antibiotics that are effective against these organisms. If the clinical assessment warrants it, an initial dose of an intramuscular or intravenous antibiotic (ceftriaxone, cefazolin, clindamycin) can be given, followed by oral antibiotic treatment. Oral antibiotic treatment with a broad-spectrum antibiotic such as dicloxacillin or a cephalosporin is indicated. Blood and tissue aspirate cultures will guide the practitioner in determining if the organism is sensitive to the antibiotic of choice. Close follow-up, usually within 24 hours, is indicated to determine if the clinical status is improving or worsening. The provider should consider MRSA if patients are not responding to initial therapy or have risk factors for MRSA. If MRSA is suspected, oral TMP/SMZ, clindamycin, or doxycycline (child older than age 8 years) are the drugs of choice. Parenteral antibiotics (vancomycin) may be needed if cellulitis is severe or the patient does not respond to oral antibiotics within 24 to 48 hours.

Viral Skin Infections

HSV Infections, Varicella, and Herpes Zoster

The treatment of HSV infections, varicella, and herpes zoster includes the use of acyclovir (Zovirax), which can be used topically or systemically. Acyclovir has inhibitory action against HSV-1, HSV-2, and varicella-zoster virus. It decreases the duration of acute infections in HSV-2 infections and, when used to treat herpes zoster, shortens the time to lesion scabbing and decreases the length of viral shedding. When prescribed for patients with varicella, acyclovir decreases the number of vesicular lesions, shortens the time to healing, and decreases fever by the second day.

Other antiviral agents that may be prescribed include famciclovir (Famvir) and valacyclovir (Valtrex), which are the drugs of choice for recurrent outbreaks of HSV infection. Famciclovir can also be used for treatment of herpes zoster. It decreases the healing time by shortening the time to crusting and healing and decreases the length of viral shedding. Valacyclovir is a hydrochloride salt of L-valyl ester of acyclovir; is rapidly converted to acyclovir; and is active against HSV infections, varicella, and herpes zoster. See Table 32-3 for prescribing information.

(Text continued on page 982)

Table 32–3 Drugs Commonly Used: Skin Infections

Drug	Indication	Strengths Available	Dose	Comments
Topical Antibiotics				
Mupirocin (Bactroban)	Bacterial skin infections	2% ointment (15, 30 g; available Rx only)	Apply to affected area tid until healed.	Pregnancy Category B Safe in children
Polymyxin B/neomycin/ bacitracin (Neosporin, Triple Antibiotics Ointment)	Bacterial skin infections	Triple antibiotic combination (available OTC)	Apply a small amount to affected area 1–3 times/d until healed.	Do not use if the patient has a neomycin sensitivity. Topical use is safe in pregnancy and in young children.
Polymyxin B/bacitracin (Polysporin, Double Antibiotic Ointment)	Bacterial skin infections	Double antibiotic combination (available OTC)	Apply a small amount to affected area 1–3 times/d until healed.	Topical use is safe in pregnancy and in young children.
Bacitracin (Baciguent)	Bacterial skin infections	Bacitracin only ointment (available OTC)	Apply to affected area 1–3 times/d until healed.	May use in patients with neomycin sensitivity. Safe during pregnancy and in young children.
Retapamulin (Altabax)	Bacterial skin infections	1% ointment	*Children age >9 mo and adults*: Apply to skin lesion twice a day for 5 days. May cover with gauze or bandage.	Safe during pregnancy and in infants age 9 mo and older. Not for intranasal use. Reevaluate if no improvement in 3–4 weeks after starting therapy.
Systemic Oral Antibiotics				
Cephalexin (Keflex)	Bacterial skin infections	Capsules: 250, 500 mg Suspension: 125 mg/5 mL, 250 mg/5 mL	*Adults:* 500 mg every 12 h for 7–10 d *Children:* 25–50 mg/kg/d divided qid or tid; treat for 7–10 d.	Inexpensive Pregnancy Category B Safe in children Well tolerated
Amoxicillin/clavulanate (Augmentin)	Bacterial skin infections	Tablets: 250 mg amoxicillin with 125 mg clavulanate; 500 mg with 125 mg	*Adults:* 500 mg of amoxicillin every 12 h *or* 250 mg every 8 h for 7–10 d	Broad-spectrum coverage Moderately expensive Pregnancy Category B
		Chewable tablets: 125 mg amoxicillin with 31.25 mg clavulanate; 200 mg with 28.5 mg; 250 mg with 62.5 mg; 400 mg with 57 mg; 125 mg with 31.25 mg/5 mL; 200 mg with 28.5/5mL; 250 mg with 62.5 mg/5 mL; 400 mg with 57 mg/5 mL	*Children >3 mo:* 25–45 mg/kg/d of amoxicillin divided every 12 h (use 200 mg/5 mL or 400 mg/5 mL strength suspension) or 20–40 mg/kg/d of amoxicillin if using 125 mg/5 mL or 250 mg/ 5 mL strength suspension; treat for 7–10 d; use higher amounts with more severe infections.	May cause gastrointestinal (GI) upset, especially at higher doses. Children's dose is based on amoxicillin content. Due to clavulanate content, two 250 mg tablets are not the same as one 500 mg tablet; suspension doses are also not equivalent. Children should not be given the 250 mg tablet until they weigh >40 kg.
Cefadroxil (Duricef)	Bacterial skin infections	Tablets: 1 g Capsules: 500 mg Suspension: 125 mg/5 mL, 250 mg/5 mL, 500 mg/5 mL	*Adults:* 1 g once/d for 10 d *Children:* 30 mg/kg/d divided into 2 doses every 12 h	Pregnancy Category B First-generation cephalosporin Convenient dosing
Cefprozil (Cefzil)	Bacterial skin infections	Tablets: 250, 500 mg Suspension: 125 mg/5 mL, 250 mg/5 mL	*Children ≥12 yr and adults:* 250–500 mg every 12 h for 7–10 d	Broad-spectrum coverage Expensive Pregnancy Category B *Children 2–12 yr:* 20 mg/kg/d divided into 2 doses 12 h apart for 7–10 d

Continued

Table 32–3   Drugs Commonly Used: Skin Infections—cont'd

Drug	Indication	Strengths Available	Dose	Comments
		Erythromycin estolate: 250, 500 mg tablets; 125 mg/ 5 mL, 250 mg/5 mL suspension Erythromycin ethylsuccinate: 200 mg chewable tablets; 400 mg tablets; 200 mg/5 mL, 400 mg/ 5 mL suspension	*Children:* 20–50 mg/kg/d qid for 10 d	May cause GI upset: take with food or milk.
Clindamycin (Cleocin)	Bacterial skin infections (MRSA)	Capsules: 75, 150, 300 mg	*Adults:* 150–300 mg qid	Pregnancy Category B
		Pediatric granules for oral solution: 75 mg/5 mL	*Children:* 8 mg/kg/d divided in 3–4 doses	May cause severe and possibly fatal colitis. Discontinue drug if significant diarrhea occurs.
Doxycycline (Doryx, Monodox) (Vibramycin)	Bacterial skin infections (MRSA)	Capsules: 50, 75, 100 mg	*Adults:* 100–200 mg/d in 1–2 divided doses	Contraindicated in children <8 yr
		Suspension: 25 mg/5 mL	*Children >8 yr:* 2–4 mg/kg/d in 1–2 divided doses maximum 200 mg/d	Pregnancy Category D Photosensitivity may occur.
Antivirals				
Acyclovir (Zovirax), topical	HSV infection, herpes zoster, varicella	3% ointment (3, 15 g)	Apply to lesion every 3 h 6 times/d for 7 d	Pregnancy Category C Use a finger cot or glove when applying ointment to prevent spread of virus.
Acyclovir (Zovirax), oral	HSV infection, herpes zoster, varicella	Tablets: 400, 800 mg	*Adults:*	Pregnancy Category C
		Suspension: 200 mg/5 mL	Genital herpes: Initial: 200 mg every 4 h 5 times/d for 10 d Chronic: 400 mg bid or 200 mg 3–5 times/d for up to 12 mo Intermittent: 200 mg q4h 5 times/d for 5 d; begin at first sign of occurrence Herpes zoster: 800 mg q4h 5 times/d for7–10 d Varicella: 20 mg/kg 4 times/d for 5 d; maximum 800 mg/dose; begin within 24 h of first lesion *Children ≥2 yr:* Varicella: 20 mg/kg 4 times/d for 5 d; maximum 800 mg/dose; begin within 24 h of first lesion	Decrease dose in renal patients.
Famciclovir (Famvir B)	HSV infection, herpes zoster	Tablet: 135, 250, 500 mg	Genital herpes: Initial episode: 125 mg q12h for 5 d; begin as soon as symptoms appear Recurrent episodes: 125 mg q12h for 5 d Suppression therapy: 250 mg q12h for up to 12 mo Herpes zoster; 500 mg q8h for 7 d; begin within 72 h of lesions appearing	Not recommended in patients <18 yr. Decrease dose in renal patients. Pregnancy Category B. Register pregnant patients exposed by famciclovir by calling 800-366-8900 ext 5231.

Table 32–3   Drugs Commonly Used: Skin Infections—cont'd

Drug	Indication	Strengths Available	Dose	Comments
Valacyclovir (Valtrex)	HSV infection, herpes zoster	Caplet: 500 mg, 1 g	Genital herpes: Initial episode: 1 g daily for 10 d Recurrent episodes: 500 mg q12h for 5 d started within 24 h of first symptom of outbreak Herpes zoster: 1g q8h for 7 d; begin within 48–72 h of first lesions appearing	Not recommended in children. Decrease dose in renal patients. Pregnancy Category B. Register pregnant patients exposed by valacyclovir by calling 800-722-9292, ext 39437.
Antifungals				
Nystatin (Mycostatin, Nilstat)	Oral *Candida* infection	Suspension: 100,000 U/mL Pastilles: 200,000 U each	*Children and adults*: 2–3 mg in each inner cheek qid (total dose 4–6 mL); have patient hold medication in mouth as long as possible before swallowing; treat for 48 h after clinical cure to prevent relapse. *Infants*: 1 mL each cheek qid (2 mL/dose total) until 48 h after clinical cure; may apply medication to inner cheeks and tongue with cotton swab prior to administering the 1 mL dose via dropper.	Safe in pregnancy and in young children and even in debilitated infants Well tolerated, even with prolonged administration
Nystatin (Mycostatin, Nilstat, Nystex)	Cutaneous *Candida* infection	Cream, ointment, powder	Apply to affected areas 2–3 times/d until healed.	Safe in pregnancy and in children
Clotrimazole (Mycelex)	Oral *Candida* infection	Troches: 10 mg	*Adults and children >3 yr and adults*: 1 troche 5 times/d for 14 d; dissolve slowly in mouth	Not recommended in children Pregnancy Category C; not recommended for use in pregnancy May cause elevated liver function tests
Clotrimazole (Lotrimin, Mycelex)	Dermatophyte infections of the skin	1% cream (Rx and OTC); 1% solution (Rx and OTC); 1% lotion (Rx)	Apply to affected area bid for 2 wk. Tinea pedis: treat for 4 wk.	Pregnancy Category B Safe in children
Gentian violet	Oral *Candida* infection	Solution: 1%, 2% (available OTC)	Apply with cotton swab to entire inner surface of the mouth 2 times/d until healed	Stains everything it touches purple; warn patient/parents about staining of mouth; stain resolves within a couple of days of discontinuing therapy.
Fluconazole (Diflucan)	Oral *Candida* infection	Tablets: 50, 100, 150, 200 mg Suspension: 10 mg/mL 40 mg/mL	*Adults*: 200 mg first day, then 100 mg daily for 2 wk minimum *Infants and children*: 6 mg/kg on the first day, then 3 mg/kg daily for 2 wk minimum	Pregnancy Category C Interacts with cimetidine, hydrochlorothiazide, rifampin cyclosporine, phenytoin, and theophylline; monitor closely if patient is taking one of these medications with fluconazole.
Miconazole (Micatin, Monistat-Derm, Micatin)	Dermatophyte infections of the skin	2% cream (Micatin, Monistat-Derm); 2% powder (Micatin); 2% spray (Micatin Liquid) (available OTC)	Apply to affected area 2–3 times/d for 2 wk. Tinea pedis: treat for 4 wk.	Topical use safe in pregnancy and in children

Continued

Table 32–3 Drugs Commonly Used: Skin Infections—cont'd

Drug	Indication	Strengths Available	Dose	Comments
Tolnaftate (Tinactin, Ting, Aftate, Absorbine)	Dermatophyte infections of the skin, tinea pedis	1% cream, solution, gel, powder, spray powder, spray liquid (available OTC)	Apply to affected area bid for 2–3 wk; if skin is thickened, treatment may take 4–6 wk.	Safe for topical use in pregnancy Not recommended for use in children <2 yr
Terbinafine (Lamisil)	Dermatophyte infections of the skin	Cream	Apply to affected and immediate surrounding areas 1–2 times/d until symptoms are significantly improved (usually 1–4 wk). Tinea pedis: apply to affected and immediate surrounding areas until symptoms are significantly improved.	Pregnancy Category B; safety in children <12 yr has not been established. Clinical improvement may continue for 2–4 wk after therapy is stopped.
Sulconazole (Exelderm)	Dermatophyte infections of the skin	1% cream; 1% solution (Rx required)	Massage medication into affected area 2 times/d for 2 wk. For tinea pedis, apply for 4 wk.	Pregnancy Category C; use only if clearly needed.
Ciclopirox (Loprox)	Dermatophyte infections of the skin	1% cream; 1% lotion (Rx required)	Massage medication into affected area 1–2 times/d for 3 wk. For tinea pedis, apply bid for 4 wk.	Pregnancy Category C; safety in children <10 yr has not been established.
Ciclopirox (Penlac)	Onychomycosis of fingernails or toenails	8% topical solution (nail lacquer)	*Adults:* Apply thin layer to entire nail and surrounding 5 mm. Leave on 8 h before washing; once a week remove with alcohol. Trim and file nails while free of drug. Repeat for 4–8 wk.	Not recommended in children. Pregnancy Category B. Product is flammable.
Ketoconazole (Nizoral)	Dermatophyte infections of the skin	2% cream	Massage medication into affected area once/d for 2 wk. For tinea pedis, apply for 6 wk.	Pregnancy Category C May be used to treat cutaneous *Candida* infections
Econazole (Spectazole)	Dermatophyte infections of the skin	1% cream (Rx required)	Massage medication into affected area once/d for 2 wk minimum. For tinea pedis, apply for 4 wk minimum.	Pregnancy Category C; do not use in first trimester; use in second and third trimesters only if clearly needed.
Oxiconazole (Oxistat)	Dermatophyte infections of the skin	1% cream; 1% lotion (Rx required)	Massage medication into affected area 1–2 times/d for 2 wk. For tinea pedis, apply for 4 wk.	Pregnancy Category B; use only if clearly needed.
Griseofulvin Microsize (Fulvicin, U/F, Grifulvin V, Grisactin)	Tinea capitis, onychomycosis	Tablets: 250, 500 mg	Tinea capitis:	Pregnancy Category C; safe in children >2 yr
		Capsules: 125, 250 mg	*Adults:* 500 mg daily for 4–6 wk	
		Suspension: 125 mg/5 mL	*Children:* 11 mg/kg/d for 4–6 wk Onychomycosis: *Adults:* 750–1,000 mg daily in divided doses; treat fingernail infection for 4 mo; toenail infection for 6 mo. *Children:* 11 mg/kg/d; treat fingernail infection for 4 mo; toenail infection for 6 mo.	Renal, liver, and hematopoietic function tests need to be drawn and monitored every 8 wk if on prolonged therapy. Best absorbed if taken with a high-fat meal.

Table 32–3   Drugs Commonly Used: Skin Infections—cont'd

Drug	Indication	Strengths Available	Dose	Comments
Griseofulvin Ultramicro-size (Fulvicin P/G, Grisactin Ultra, Gris-PEG)	Tinea capitis, onychomycosis	Tablets: 125, 165, 250, 330 mg	Tinea capitis: *Adults:* 330–375 mg daily for 4–6 wk	Pregnancy Category C; safe in children >2 yr
			Children: 7.3 mg/kg/d for 4–6 wk Onychomycosis: *Adults:* 660–750 mg daily in divided doses; treat fingernail infection for 4 mo; toenail infection for 6 mo.	Renal, liver, and hematopoietic function tests need to be drawn and monitored every 8 wk if on prolonged therapy.
			Children: 7.3 mg/kg/d; treat fingernail infection for 4 mo; toenail infection for 6 mo	Best absorbed if taken with a high-fat meal.
Ketoconazole (Nizoral)	Tinea capitis, onychomycosis	Tablets: 200 mg	*Adults:* 200 mg daily; may increase to 400 mg daily if inadequate clinical response; minimum length of treatment is 4 wk.	Monitor hepatic function prior to initiating therapy and monthly during therapy.
			Children ≥2 yr: 3.3–6.6 mg/kg/d	Pregnancy Category C; may be prescribed to children >2 yr. Not first-line treatment for onychomycosis because of possible hepatotoxicity. Use with caution if patient is taking medications that are primarily metabolized by the liver.
Itraconazole (Sporanox)	Onychomycosis	Capsules: 100 mg	*Adults:* Daily dosing schedule: toenails: 200 mg daily for 12 wk Pulse schedule: toenails: 400 mg daily for 1 wk/mo for 3–4 mo; for fingernails: 200 mg bid for 7 d, then 3 wk without medication, then 200 mg bid for 7 more days *Children:* Pulse schedule: 5 mg/kg/d for 1 wk/mo for 3–4 consecutive mo	Coadministration with astemizole is absolutely contraindicated because of secondary cardiotoxic effects. If used for more than 8 consecutive weeks, liver enzymes and electrolytes should be drawn prior to and every 8 wk during treatment. Pregnancy Category C; do not administer to pregnant women or women considering pregnancy. In children use griseofulvin as first-line therapy. Coadministration with astemizole is absolutely contraindicated because of secondary cardiotoxic effects. Coadministration with cisapride, midazolam, triazolam, simvastatin, and lovastatin is also contraindicated.

Continued

Table 32–3   Drugs Commonly Used: Skin Infections—cont'd

Drug	Indication	Strengths Available	Dose	Comments
Terbinafine (Lamisil)	Onychomycosis	Tablets: 250 mg	Fingernail infection: 250 mg daily for 6 wk Toenail infection: 250 mg daily for 12 wk	Not recommended for use in children; safety not established. Liver enzymes and complete blood count (CBC) should be monitored every 6 wk. Pregnancy Category B; delay treatment until after pregnancy.

HSV = herpes simplex virus; MRSA = methicillin-resistant *Staphylococcus aureus;* OTC = over the counter.

Three topical antiviral medications are available: acyclovir (Zovirax), penciclovir (Denavir), and the OTC product docosanol (Abreva). Acyclovir is indicated in the management of initial episodes of herpes genitalis and in limited, non–life-threatening, mucocutaneous HSV infections in immunocompromised patients. There is no clinical evidence for the benefit of using acyclovir in the immunocompetent patient, although decreased viral shedding may be noted. Topical acyclovir is applied to cover all lesions every 3 hours 6 times a day for 7 days. Penciclovir is indicated in the treatment of recurrent herpes labialis (cold sores) on the lips and face. Application to the mucous membrane is not recommended. In adults, penciclovir 1% cream is applied every 2 hours while awake, with treatment started as early as possible (during the prodrome or when lesions appear). Docosanol (Abreva) is the only OTC product available for the treatment of herpes labialis. It is applied to the cold sore 5 times a day until healed. Treatment should begin at first sign of outbreak. All of the topical products are most effective if started as early as possible, in the prodrome phase, and need to be applied with a glove or finger cot to prevent spread to other areas.

Comfort measures with antipruritics, such as antihistamines, and wet soaks are also part of the treatment plan for viral skin infections. Table 32-3 presents prescribing information.

Fungal Skin Infections

Oral Candidiasis

Oral candidiasis (thrush) is commonly found in infants and immunocompromised patients. Prompt treatment is essential to maintain adequate nutrition and for patient comfort. The treatment of choice is a topical application of an antifungal agent, such as nystatin (Mycostatin), clotrimazole (Mycelex), or gentian violet, or oral administration of the systemic antifungal fluconazole (Diflucan). Table 32-3 presents prescribing information.

Tinea Capitis

With tinea capitis (ringworm of the scalp), the patient presents with a characteristic bald patch, with crusting or scaling. *Microsporum* species usually present with broken hairs and a fine gray scale. *Trichophyton tonsurans* (black dot tinea) presents with tiny black dots that are the remains of broken hair shafts.

Treatment of tinea capitis consists of oral antifungal therapy with griseofulvin (Grifulvin V, Grisactin) and biweekly shampooing with a sporicidal shampoo (selenium sulfide or ketoconazole). Tinea capitis should always be treated with a systemic antifungal, never a topical agent. Treatment should continue for 6 to 8 weeks or until 2 weeks after the KOH or culture is negative. Close contacts should be empirically treated with sporicidal shampoo twice a week. Resistant cases can be treated with terbinafine, fluconazole, or itraconazole, based on the sensitivity as determined by culture. Table 32-3 presents prescribing information.

Tinea Corporis and Tinea Cruris

Tinea corporis (ringworm) is commonly caused by *Microsporum canis, T. tonsurans,* or *Epidermophyton floccosum.* The classic presentation is an annular lesion with raised borders and a clear center. There may be scaling and usually some erythema. The infection spreads by direct contact with an infected person or animal, with household pets being a common source of infection.

CLINICAL PEARL

Thrush
Infants (and some older or very ill patients) are unable to hold nystatin suspension in their mouth. To achieve better results with nystatin administration, instruct the parents or caregivers to dip a clean cotton-tipped applicator into the nystatin solution, then rub the medication into the areas of thrush on the inner cheeks. Use a clean swab for each side and do not redip the applicator into the nystatin. After swabbing on the nystatin, the parent or caregiver can then administer 1 to 2 mL to each cheek.

Tinea cruris ("jock itch") affects the skin of the groin, upper thighs, and intertriginous folds. It is more common in males and rarely occurs before adolescence. It is caused by the dermatophytes *E. floccosum, Trichophyton rubrum, Trichophyton mentagrophytes,* and *C. albicans.* Tinea cruris is worse in hot, humid weather. The lesions are scaly with a raised border, erythematous, and slightly brown in color. Treatment for both tinea corporis and tinea cruris is topical antifungal cream, with miconazole (Micatin, Monistat-Derm), tolnaftate (Tinactin), and clotrimazole (Lotrimin, Mycelex) the least expensive and most commonly prescribed. Other topical antifungals that may be used include terbinafine (Lamisil), sulconazole (Exelderm), ciclopirox (Loprox), ketoconazole (Nizoral), econazole (Spectazole), and oxiconazole (Oxistat). Table 32-3 presents prescribing information.

Tinea Pedis

Tinea pedis (athlete's foot) is caused by the dermatophytes *E. floccosum, T. rubrum, T. mentagrophytes,* and *C. albicans.* It is more common in males and rarely occurs before puberty. It can present in three forms: interdigital maceration, scaling, and fissuring; a "moccasin" distribution of persistent dry scale with minimal inflammation; or scattered pustules and vesicles on the sole and lateral aspects of the feet. The nonpharmacological management includes measures to keep the feet dry and well aired, such as wearing sandals whenever possible, wearing clean cotton socks, and drying the feet carefully after bathing. Pharmacological management is with topical antifungals, similar to those used for tinea corporis: miconazole, clotrimazole, tolnaftate, terbinafine, sulconazole, ciclopirox, ketoconazole, econazole, and oxiconazole. However, the length of treatment is usually longer than for tinea cruris. Table 32-3 presents prescribing information.

Tinea Versicolor

Tinea versicolor (pityriasis versicolor) is caused by *Pityrosporum orbiculare* (formerly called *Malassezia furfur*). Clinically, the infection appears as multiple scaling, discrete, oval-shaped macules that may be hypopigmented or hyperpigmented. The color of the macules ranges from salmon to brown, and they are usually seen on the trunk, neck, and shoulders. The infection is associated with warm, humid weather. Treatment consists of topical application of selenium sulfide shampoo (Selsun) or a topical antifungal, commonly one of the imidazoles (miconazole, clotrimazole, econazole). The patient should be educated to observe for recurrence, which up to 50% of patients experience. The shampoo is applied to the affected area and left on for 10 to 15 minutes every day for 1 week. It may also be used prophylactically once a month. The topical antifungal is used for 2 to 4 weeks and is rubbed into the affected area twice a day.

Onychomycosis

Onychomycosis is a fungal infection of the nail, either fingernail or toenail. The common dermatophyte that is found in onychomycosis is tinea unguium, with *Candida* infections also a cause. Effective treatment usually involves months of a systemic antifungal medication, commonly griseofulvin, ketoconazole, itraconazole, or terbinafine. Topical treatment is usually not effective, with the exception of ciclopirox nail lacquer (Penlac). Recent studies have demonstrated added effectiveness when topical ciclopirox and systemic antifungals are combined. Regardless of treatment modality, clearing of onychomycosis takes months of treatment. Table 32-3 presents prescribing information.

Monitoring

For all skin infections, the patient should be monitored to determine the effectiveness of the medication in treating the infection, compliance with the prescribed therapy, adverse effects, and the development of secondary infection.

Outcome Evaluation

For skin infections, improvement should be noted, usually within 24 to 48 hours. If not, a change in therapy may be indicated, with resistance suspected. Secondary skin infections, if they occur, should be treated promptly. Referral to a dermatologist may be necessary if therapy is not managing the infection.

Patient Education

Patient education should include a discussion of information related to the overall treatment plan as well as that specific to the drug therapy, reasons for taking the drug, drugs as part of the total treatment regimen, and adherence issues.

SKIN INFESTATIONS

Skin and hair infestation with arthropods, most commonly lice and scabies, is a frequently seen problem in primary care. Head lice infestation is at epidemic levels in school-age children, with 6 to 12 million people in the United States affected each year. Scabies can occur at any age and is more common when poor hygiene or crowded living conditions are present.

Pathophysiology

Lice

Pediculosis is infestation of the body with lice. The affected body area helps to determine what arthropod is present. The skin signs seen with pediculosis are pruritus, excoriation from scratching, adenopathy (occasionally) in the affected region, and the presence of lice or nits.

The common name for infestation with *Pediculus humanus capitis* is head lice (pediculosis capitis). The mite of head lice is usually visible, and the nits or eggs are visualized attached to the hair shaft. The female louse lays approximately four eggs per day and has a life span of 2 to 4 weeks. Head lice are spread by direct contact with another infected person or by indirect contact with a hairbrush, hat, or article of clothing that the lice or nits have been transferred to. Outbreaks in schools are seen when children share hats or hairbrushes. When outer garments are hung in a close group, which is often the case in school, the lice can travel from coat to coat and spread to an unsuspecting new household. Diagnosis is made by observing mites or nits.

Body lice (pediculosis corporis), the common name for infestation with *P. humanus corporis,* are uncommon. They usually are not seen on the body but on the seams of clothing and undergarments. They come onto the body to feed and

PATIENT EDUCATION

PATIENT
EDUCATION

Skin Infections

RELATED TO THE OVERALL TREATMENT PLAN/DISEASE PROCESS

☐ Pathophysiology

☐ Role of preventive and nonpharmacological measures if appropriate

☐ Importance of adherence to the treatment regimen

☐ Self-monitoring of symptoms

☐ What to do when symptoms worsen

☐ Need for follow-up visits with the primary care provider

SPECIFIC TO THE DRUG THERAPY

☐ Reason for taking the drug and its anticipated action on the disease process

☐ Doses and schedules for taking the drug

☐ Possible adverse effects and what to do if they occur

☐ Interactions between other treatment modalities and these drugs

REASONS FOR TAKING THE DRUG(S)

☐ Patient education about specific drugs is provided in the appropriate chapter.

SPECIFICALLY FOR BACTERIAL SKIN INFECTIONS

☐ Explanation regarding the suspected cause of the infection and the rationale for the **antibiotic** treatment chosen

☐ Hand washing should be stressed to prevent spread of the skin infection to the patient or others.

☐ Give clear guidelines regarding notifying the practitioner if the infection is getting worse.

☐ Improvement should be noted in 24 to 48 hours; if not, a change in therapy may be indicated.

SPECIFICALLY FOR VIRAL INFECTIONS

Expectations of the medication. The healthy patient will have resolution of the vesicular lesions even without pharmacological intervention. Effective antiviral therapy decreases the time to scabbing and healing of lesions and decreases viral shedding time. In immunocompromised patients, the medication will help decrease the severity of the outbreak.

☐ Explain how the virus can become dormant and recur at a later time, even many years later.

☐ Patients using topical antivirals need to be instructed to use a glove or finger cot to apply the ointment to prevent getting the virus on their hands and spreading it; also, the patient may experience a transient burning when the medication is applied.

☐ It should be stressed to the patient and/or family members that the patient is contagious until the lesions are healed or scabbed over, even if antiviral agents are being taken; the patient should avoid contact with immunocompromised individuals and avoid sexual intercourse if the patient has genital herpes lesions.

SPECIFICALLY FOR FUNGAL INFECTIONS

☐ The patient and/or family members should understand how the fungal infection is spread and how contagious the infection is.

☐ Family members and pets should be checked for signs of infection and treated if indicated.

☐ The provider should stress the possibility of relapse if the medication regimen is not followed correctly and for the full treatment time.

DRUGS AS PART OF THE TOTAL TREATMENT REGIMEN

☐ The total treatment regimen includes pharmacological and nonpharmacological measures. Be sure the patient and/or family members are aware of the specific measures to be taken.

ADHERENCE ISSUES

☐ Health-care providers should be aware of the potential problem of nonadherence and should discuss the importance of completing the entire treatment regimen with the patient and/or family members.

---

leave hemorrhagic pinpoint macules where they extract blood. There is often excoriation from scratching. The common sites for body lice are the belt line, collar, and underwear areas. Diagnosis is made by examining the clothing and underwear for the presence of mites and nits.

Infestation with *Phthirus pubis* is commonly called pubic lice (pediculosis pubis). Patients often refer to it as crabs. The mites are quite small and may need to be examined under a handheld magnifying glass because they may be mistaken for a freckle. The mites and nits are found on the pubic hair and the hair of the perianal region. They may extend up to the hair on the abdomen and to the hair on the upper thighs. The eyelashes and axillary hair may also be involved. Pubic lice are never seen before pubertal hair development. They are often sexually transmitted. Diagnosis is made by observing the mite or nits in the pubic hair.

Scabies

Scabies is a highly contagious infestation with *Sarcoptes scabiei.* The female scabies mite burrows under the skin and lays eggs as she tunnels. The eggs hatch in about 2 weeks. The surface of the skin has characteristic curving burrows and excoriated papules. The burrows are in the horny layer of the skin and are seen most frequently on the sides of the fingers; the interdigital webs; and flexor surfaces of the wrists, elbows, axillae, and genitalia. In infants, the scabies mite can often be found on the entire body, including the trunk and face. There may be a secondary infection present.

The incubation period is 1 to 2 months after contact with another infested person or with unwashed clothing recently worn by an infected person. Bed partners can be infected even if there is no body contact. Often the first sign of infestation with scabies is intense pruritus, which occurs 2 to 6 weeks after the first exposure to the mite. The itching is caused by sensitization to the mite feces. Definitive diagnosis is made by scraping a burrow that reveals mites or eggs.

Goals of Treatment

The goals of treatment are to completely eradicate the arthropods and to educate the patient and family about the disease and how to prevent further infestations.

Rational Drug Selection

Pharmacological management of lice and scabies consists of the use of ectoparacides. The specific medication used varies by the type of infestation and the age of the patient. For head lice, there is a choice of OTC products and, in the case of resistance to OTC products, prescription lindane or malathion. Benzoyl alcohol (Ulesfia), ivermectin lotion (Sklice), and spinosad (Natroba) are prescription products that are FDA approved for head lice. There is also variety of nonpharmacological remedies. For body lice, the treatment of choice is lindane or permethrin 5% (Elimite) and washing infested clothing and bedding. Pubic lice are treated with lindane shampoo. Scabies is treated with permethrin or lindane. Nonpharmacological, environmental measures are a key part of the treatment of any infestation because patients can reinfect themselves or other family members and restart the infestation cycle.

Head Lice

Head lice can cause great distress to the family. It is necessary to treat head lice aggressively and completely to prevent recurrence. Unfortunately, resistance to some pediculicides has made treating head lice at times a clinical challenge. The OTC products available include pyrethrins and permethrin. Benzoyl alcohol (Ulesfia), ivermectin lotion (Sklice), or spinosad (Natroba) may be prescribed for head lice. Malathion (Ovide) is a prescription drug used as a second-line agent for resistant head lice (Centers for Disease Control and Prevention, Division of Parasitic Diseases [CDC], 2013a).

Although all of the head lice treatments are relatively safe, they are classified as neurotoxic agents (except benzoyl alcohol), and they should be used exactly as directed on the package or prescription. To limit exposure, the medication should be washed off at a sink, rather than in a shower. Cool or lukewarm water should be used to minimize absorption caused by vasodilation. After treatment, the hair should be combed to remove all the nits. There are special combs available for this, or slow, patient combing can be effective. Advise parents to comb hair a minimum of 20 minutes, dividing hair in sections. Treat only family members who are actively infested. Do not treat head lice prophylactically.

With the use of malathion (Ovide) careful instruction should be given regarding the flammability of the product. Lotion and wet hair should not be exposed to open flames or electric heat sources, including hair dryers and electric curlers. Do not smoke while applying lotion or while hair is wet. Allow hair to dry naturally and to remain uncovered after application of Ovide lotion.

Pyrethrins

Pyrethrins are combined with piperonyl butoxide (RID, Pronto, A-200) and are available OTC. Pyrethrins are 100% insecticidal and 70% to 80% ovicidal. The shampoo is applied to dry hair and left on for 10 to 20 minutes, with the time varying by brand. It is important for the product to be applied to dry hair to enable the pediculicide to enter the insect's body better. The patient should be retreated in 1 week regardless of whether there is evidence of infestation. Pyrethrins have no residual activity and can be used in young children and pregnant women if used as directed.

Permethrin

Permethrin is a synthetic compound related to pyrethrins. It is available OTC in 1% cream (Nix) or prescription strength 5% cream (Elimite). Only Nix has FDA approval for use on head lice. It is 97% percent insecticidal and 70% to 80% ovicidal. Permethrin is a cream rinse that is applied after shampooing. It is important that the shampoo not have any conditioner in the formula, which makes the permethrin less effective. The cream rinse is left in the hair for 10 minutes before rinsing off. Treatment should be repeated in 1 week, regardless of whether signs of infestation are present. Permethrin cream rinse has residual activity against lice for up to 10 days.

Lindane

Lindane is a prescription product used as a second-line agent for head lice. The popular brand of lindane, Kwell, is no longer on the market, but multiple generic brands of the product are available. Lindane is 67% insecticidal and 45% to 70% ovicidal. Lindane is neurotoxic and should not be used in pregnant women or in infants. It is applied to dry hair, working in small quantities of water to create a good lather. The shampoo is left on for 4 minutes. The amount of shampoo prescribed for short hair is 1 oz, and for long hair, 2 oz. The shampoo should be rinsed well. Lindane has no residual activity against head lice.

Malathion

Malathion (Ovide) is a pediculicide that is available OTC in the United Kingdom and has been recently reapproved as a treatment for head lice in the United States. Malathion is an organophosphate agent that acts as a pediculicide by inhibiting cholinesterase activity in vivo. It is very effective against head lice, with 96% mortality in 30 minutes (Downs, Narayan, Stafford, & Coles, 2005). Some residual remains and can kill newly hatched lice for up to 7 days.

Ovide is applied to dry hair in an amount sufficient to wet the hair and scalp. Hair should be allowed to dry naturally. Hands should be washed with soap after applying Ovide. Ovide is left on for 8 to 12 hours and then shampooed. After rinsing, use a nit (or fine-tooth) comb to remove dead lice and eggs. If lice are present in 7 days, Ovide may be repeated.

With the use of Ovide, careful instruction should be given regarding the flammability of the product. Lotion and wet hair should not be exposed to open flames or electric heat sources, including hair dryers and electric curlers. Do not smoke while applying lotion or while hair is wet. Allow hair to dry naturally and to remain uncovered after application of Ovide lotion.

Benzoyl Alcohol

Benzoyl alcohol (Ulesfia) was the first non-neurotoxin treatment for head lice. The active ingredient in benzoyl alcohol appears to stun the breathing spiracles of the lice open, enabling the vehicle to penetrate the respiratory mechanism (spiracles) and leading to asphyxiation.

Benzoyl alcohol (Ulesfia lotion) is applied to dry hair, completely saturating the hair and scalp and left on for 10 minutes. The lotion is rinsed off well with water. Treatment with another application of Ulesfia should be repeated in 7 days.

Ivermectin

Ivermectin lotion 0.5% (Sklice) causes the death of parasites by binding with the chloride channels, causing increased permeability of the cell membrane to chloride ions and resulting in paralysis and death of the parasite. It is not ovicidal. Ivermectin lotion can be used in patients 6 months or older and is applied to dry hair and left on for 10 minutes. After 10 minutes, the lotion is rinsed off with water. Retreatment is usually not necessary.

Spinosad

Spinosad suspension 0.9% (Natroba) is derived from soil bacteria and is approved to treat head lice in patients age 4 years or older. Spinosad causes neuronal excitation, causing the lice to become paralyzed and die. It kills live lice and unhatched eggs. The suspension is applied to dry hair and left on for 10 minutes, then rinsed with warm water. Retreatment is usually not needed.

Nonpharmacological Treatments

With the growing problem of resistance and concern over exposing children to repeated doses of pediculicides, there are anecdotal reports about the success of various nonmedicated therapies. Popular and safe remedies are hair conditioner, mayonnaise (full-fat variety), olive oil, and petroleum jelly. It is thought that they asphyxiate the lice by blocking their breathing apparatus or immobilize them and affect their ability to feed. A patient who would like to try these treatments should apply a thick layer of the product and cover with a shower cap. The product is left on from 1 hour to overnight, then shampooed out.

The provider may be asked by a frustrated parent about other nonpharmacological remedies. It is important to give the parent clear guidelines regarding the use of unproven and possibly dangerous interventions, such as using lamp oil or other flammable liquid. Products developed for animals, such as dog lice shampoo, are also not advised.

Using a nit comb will assist in removing nits, which will decrease the number of lice hatching. Parents will need support as they treat the head lice, which can be frustrating.

Body Lice

The treatment for body lice is topical pediculicides: lindane and permethrin (CDC, 2013b). Body lice live on clothing and underwear and come to the skin only to feed, so it is important to instruct the patient to wash all clothing and bedding in hot water to kill lice and nits that are on the clothing.

Lindane

Lindane is applied to the total body as a cream or lotion and left on for 8 to 12 hours (overnight). The amount needed for an adult is 2 oz. Lindane should not be used in infants. It is Pregnancy Category B but should not be used as a first-line medication in pregnant patients because there have been no adequate studies in pregnant patients. If it is prescribed during pregnancy, then it should not be used more than twice during a pregnancy.

Permethrin

Permethrin 5% (Elimite) may be used for body lice. It is slightly safer in pregnant patients and can be used in children as young as 2 months. Permethrin is applied from head to toe and left on for 8 hours (overnight), then showered off.

Pubic Lice

Lindane

Pubic lice are treated with an application of lindane 1% cream, lotion, or shampoo. A thin layer of cream or lotion is applied to the hair and skin surrounding the pubic area and left on for 12 hours. If lindane shampoo is used, the shampoo is massaged into dry pubic hair and left on for 5 to 10 minutes. If axillary or thigh hair is also infested, then use the cream or lotion. Reapply in 7 days if there is evidence of live lice. Sexual partners should also be treated concurrently. Bedding and clothes should be washed.

Pyrethrins

Pubic lice may also be treated with pyrethrins, which are permethrin 1%, pyrethrin lotion, or shampoo. Advise the patient to thoroughly saturate hair with lice medication. Leave medication on for 10 minutes then thoroughly rinse off with water. Dry off with a clean towel (CDC, 2013c). Reapply in 7 days if there is evidence of live lice.

Sexual partners should be treated concurrently, and bedding and clothes should also be washed. Infestation of eyelashes by pubic lice is treated with petrolatum (Vaseline) ointment applied 3 to 4 times daily for 8 to 10 days. Nits should be removed by hand from the pubic area, axillae, and eyelashes.

Scabies

When treating scabies, the provider may choose among permethrin, lindane, or crotamiton (Eurax, Crotan). Crotamiton lotion or cream is only approved for use in adults. The provider may choose the drug based on patient age and the toxicity of the agent. All family members should receive treatment, even if asymptomatic, because they may be in the incubation period (4 wk), and so all members of the household need treatment to prevent recurrence. Although one treatment is curative, the inflamed burrows and pruritus may last for up to 3 weeks after treatment with a scabicide. Families need to be educated regarding this prolonged healing phase. Patients should not be re-treated unless living mites are observed.

Permethrin

Permethrin 5% cream (Elimite, Acticin) is the drug of choice for the treatment of scabies in young children and pregnant women. It is 90% effective against the scabies mite and can be used in infants as young as 2 months old and in pregnant women. The cream is massaged into the skin from the neck to the soles of feet. It should be left on for 8 to 14 hours and then washed off in the shower. Infants require special application of permethrin to the scalp, temple, forehead, hands, and feet. One to 2 oz of permethrin per family member are prescribed.

Lindane

Lindane 1% lotion or cream is used for scabies in children older than 6 months and in nonpregnant adult patients. It is applied in a thin layer from the neck down to the soles of the feet and left on for 8 to 12 hours (overnight) and then washed off thoroughly. If there are crusted lesions present, a tepid bath should be taken prior to application to soften the lesions. The patient should dry the skin thoroughly before applying lindane. Two oz of lindane per family member are prescribed.

Crotamiton

Crotamiton (Eurax) has scabicidal and antipruritic actions. The exact mechanism of action is not known. Crotamiton lotion or cream is massaged into clean skin of the whole body from the chin down. Medication should be applied under fingernails because scabies may remain under nails. A second application is advised 24 hours later. The medication is washed off in a bath 48 hours after the last application.

Topical Corticosteroids

Topical corticosteroids are used after scabies treatment to treat pruritus and inflammation associated with the scabies mite. Hydrocortisone 1% or 2.5% or a stronger corticosteroid, if indicated, is applied to affected areas twice a day until lesions are healed.

Monitoring

Patients and families need to be monitored for appropriate use of the medication and for effectiveness of treatment. The patient should be monitored for sensitivity to the medication prescribed. If medications are used appropriately, there is rarely an adverse reaction from them, although skin irritation or sensitivity may occur.

Outcome Evaluation

If effective treatment has been implemented, then the lice or scabies should be eradicated. Before resistance is assumed, the provider should review how the patient or family used the medication and if environmental measures were adequate.

Patient Education

Patient and family education is the key to effective eradication of lice and scabies. In prescribing treatment for lice or scabies, the following are key areas of education that need to be covered:

1. Explanation of how the patient was most likely infected with the lice or scabies and how they can be passed on to other family members or, in the case of pubic lice, sexual partners. The incubation period and early symptoms should be discussed to identify other contacts that may be infected, such as school contacts.
2. Proper use of the prescribed medication and environmental measures that may be taken should be explained. Written instructions should also be provided.
3. Environmental measures that should be taken for lice and scabies include washing sheets, towels, clothing, and headgear worn recently in hot water and laundry soap. They need to be tumbled in a hot dryer for at least 20 minutes to kill any remaining nits or scabies that may be on the clothing. Clothing that cannot be put in a hot water wash must be dry-cleaned or pressed with a hot iron. Remind parents to wash coats and car seat covers if indicated. Items that cannot be washed or dry-cleaned, such as stuffed animals, should be placed in a plastic bag for 3 to 4 weeks; for scabies, only 4 days is needed. Brushes and combs should be washed in hot water and soaked for 1 hour in disinfectant such as Lysol or rubbing alcohol and then rinsed with hot water. Vacuuming play areas, floors, rugs, and furniture will pick up any nits or lice that may have been transferred to these areas. Parents/patients should be told that insecticidal sprays or bombs are not necessary.

ALOPECIA ANDROGENETICA (MALE PATTERN BALDNESS)

Alopecia androgenetica (male pattern baldness) affects men and some women. It involves hair loss from the frontal, vertex, and occipital regions of the scalp in men and thinning of the hair in the frontoparietal area or diffuse hair loss in women.

Pathophysiology

Common male pattern baldness is genetically determined. The process can begin at any time after puberty. There is not actual hair loss, but a conversion of thick hair to fine, unpigmented vellus hairs, which are poorly seen.

The process is androgen-dependent. A male who has a disorder that lowers testosterone production will never go bald, regardless of genetics; a woman who has a masculinizing disorder that raises androgen levels will develop classic male pattern baldness.

Goals of Treatment

A realistic goal is to achieve moderate to dense hair growth with continued use of topical minoxidil (Rogaine) for at least 4 months. If treating with finasteride (Propecia), a realistic goal would be increased hair growth after 3 months of continued treatment.

Rational Drug Selection

Alopecia androgenetica can be treated topically with minoxidil or systemically with finasteride. Choosing between the two medications can often be a simple task based on the patient profile. If the patient is also being treated for benign prostatic hypertrophy (BPH), then finasteride is the drug of choice. For a female patient, minoxidil is the only choice available.

Minoxidil

Minoxidil, the first drug approved by the FDA to treat male pattern baldness, is available OTC. The patient may be seeking a recommendation from the prescriber or self-prescribing and seeking information regarding its use. It is important to note that minoxidil does not treat balding of the frontoparietal areas in men, only in women. Minoxidil is effective in treating balding on the vertex of the scalp in men.

Minoxidil 2% topical solution is applied to the scalp twice daily for the entire length of treatment. The patient applies 1 mL directly to the affected area of the scalp (vertex area in men and frontoparietal area in women). The medication should be applied to a dry scalp. Patients should be instructed to wash their hands after using their fingers to rub the medication into the scalp. Twice-daily application for at least 4 months may be needed to obtain observable hair growth. If the medication is discontinued, the hair in the treated area will shed in 3 to 4 months.

Minoxidil should not be used by pregnant patients (Pregnancy Category C) or by children under age 18 years. Minoxidil is generally well tolerated. The topical solution contains alcohol and therefore may be irritating upon application. Patients may be sensitive to minoxidil and develop contact dermatitis. Minoxidil topical solution used as directed has minimal cardiac effects, but if large amounts are applied there is a potential for cardiac adverse effects.

Finasteride

Finasteride is a type II 5-alpha reductase–specific inhibitor that inhibits the conversion of testosterone into 5-alpha dihydrotestosterone (DHT). Development of alopecia androgenetica is dependent on DHT, as is the prostate gland. Finasteride is also used in treatment of BPH. Finasteride is effective in treating vertex and anterior midscalp baldness in men. Hair regrowth is noted after 3 months of daily treatment, with full treatment effect achieved after 6 to 12 months of use.

The dose of finasteride is 1 mg once daily with or without food. Continued use is necessary to have continued benefit. If treatment is stopped, hair will return to untreated levels within 12 months.

Finasteride should be prescribed with caution in patients with hepatic dysfunction because the drug is metabolized extensively in the liver. It causes a decrease in serum prostate specific antigen (PSA) levels, even in the presence of prostate cancer. It is Pregnancy Category X. Finasteride exposure during pregnancy, even in small quantities, may produce abnormalities of the external genitalia in male offspring. Pregnant women or a woman planning a pregnancy should not handle crushed tablets. Finasteride may be potentially absorbed from the semen. When a male patient's sexual partner is pregnant or may become pregnant, the patient should either avoid exposing his partner to his semen or discontinue finasteride. There is a small possibility (3% or less) of developing decreased libido, erectile dysfunction, or ejaculation disorder while taking finasteride.

Monitoring

The patient being treated for male pattern baldness needs to be monitored for effectiveness of treatment and adverse effects of the medication. The major adverse effect seen with minoxidil is dermatitis or sensitivity to the topical solution, which is treated by discontinuing the medication. Topical steroids should not be used concurrently with minoxidil. The patient should also be observed for possible cardiac adverse effects.

Finasteride is generally well tolerated, and adverse effects are usually mild. If the patient experiences sexual dysfunction, then the drug should be discontinued. The patient should be monitored for prostate cancer with a digital rectal examination and PSA levels because finasteride causes a low PSA level, even in the presence of prostate cancer. If the patient's sexual partner is of childbearing age, he should be warned about the severe effects that finasteride can have on the developing fetus.

Monitoring for use of birth control, with condoms used to prevent semen exposure, is necessary if there is a possibility of the patient's partner becoming pregnant.

Outcome Evaluation

It may take 3 to 4 months to determine if minoxidil or finasteride is effective. The provider should schedule a follow-up appointment with the patient for 3 to 4 months after beginning therapy to determine effectiveness.

Patient Education

In treating a patient with alopecia androgenetica, the following key points should be covered in patient education:

1. The pathophysiology and cause of male pattern baldness.
2. Realistic expectations of therapy, including what type of hair loss the drug treats; how long therapy takes until effects are noticed; that if treatment is stopped, hair shedding will occur; and that the new hair initially may be fine and almost colorless, but with continued treatment the hair should develop the same color and texture as the rest of the hair on the scalp.
3. Caution that the patient should take the medication exactly as prescribed or as indicated by the instructions if taking OTC minoxidil.
4. Adverse effects of the medications, especially the hazards to women from finasteride exposure.

REFERENCES

Centers for Disease Control and Prevention, Division of Parasitic Diseases (CDC). (2010). Parasites—Scabies. Retrieved from http://www.cdc.gov/parasites/scabies/

Centers for Disease Control and Prevention. (2010). National Ambulatory Medical Care Survey: 2010 Summary Tables. Retrieved from http://www.cdc.gov/nchs/data/ahcd/namcs_summary/2010_namcs_web_tables.pdf

Centers for Disease Control and Prevention, Division of Parasitic Diseases (CDC). (2013a). Parasites—Head lice. Retrieved from http://www.cdc.gov/parasites/lice/head/index.html

Centers for Disease Control and Prevention, Division of Parasitic Diseases (CDC). (2013b). Parasites—Body lice. Retrieved from http://www.cdc.gov/parasites/lice/body/index.html

Centers for Disease Control and Prevention, Division of Parasitic Diseases (CDC). (2013c). Parasites—Pubic lice. Retrieved from http://www.cdc.gov/parasites/lice/pubic/index.html

Charakida, A., Dadzie, O., Teixeira, F., Charakida, M., Evangelou, G., & Chu, A. C. (2006). Calcipotriol/betamethasone dipropionate for the treatment of psoriasis. *Expert Opinion on Pharmacotherapy, 7*(5), 597–606.

Dalgard, F., Gieler, U., Holm, J. O., Bjertness, E., & Hauser, S. (2008). Self-esteem and body satisfaction among late adolescents with acne: Results from a population survey. *Journal of the American Academy of Dermatology, 59*(5), 746–751.

Del Roso, J. Q. (2006). Combination topical therapy for the treatment of psoriasis. *Journal of Drugs in Dermatology, 5*(3), 232–234.

Del Roso, J. Q., Thiboutot, D., Gallo, R., Webster, G., Tanghetti, E., Eichenfield, L. F., et al. (2013a). Consensus recommendations from the American Acne & Rosacea Society on the management of rosacea, Part 1: A status report on the disease state, general measures and adjunctive skin care. *Cutis, 92*, 234–240.

Del Roso, J. Q., Thiboutot, D., Gallo, R., Webster, G., Tanghetti, E., Eichenfield, L. F., et al. (2013b). Consensus recommendations from the American Acne & Rosacea Society on the management of rosacea, Part 2: A status report on topical agents. *Cutis, 92*, 277–284.

Downs, A. M. R., Narayan, S., Stafford, K. A., & Coles, G. C. (2005). Effectiveness of Ovide against malathion-resistant head lice. *Archives in Dermatology, 141*, 1318.

Eichenfield, L. F., Krakowski, A. C., Piggott, C., Del Rosso, J., Baldwin, H., Friedlander, S. F., et al. (2013). Evidence-based recommendations for the diagnosis and treatment of pediatric acne. *Pediatrics, 131*(3 Suppl.), S163–S186.

Eichenfield, L. F., Tom, W. L., Berger, T. G., Krol, A., Paller, A. S., Schwarzenberger, K., et al. (2014). Guidelines of care for the management of atopic dermatitis. Section 2. Management and treatment of atopic dermatitis. *Journal of the American Academy of Dermatology, 71*(1), 116–132.

Graber, E. (2014). Treatment of acne vulgaris. *UpToDate*. Wolter Kluwer. Retrieved from http://www.uptodate.com/contents/treatment-of-acne-vulgaris

Jackson, K. D., Howie, L. D., & Akinbami, L. J. (2013). Trends in allergic conditions among children: United States, 1997–2011. *NCHS Data Brief, 121*. Retrieved from http://www.cdc.gov/nchs/data/databriefs/db121.pdf

Menter, A., Korman, N. J., Feldman, S. R., Gelfand, J. M., Gordon, K. B., Gottlieb, A., et al. (2009). Section 3. Guidelines of care for the management and treatment of psoriasis with topical therapies. *Journal of the American Academy of Dermatology, 60*(4), 643–659.

Pallin, D. J., Espinola, J. A., Leung, D. Y., Hooper, D. C., & Camargo, C. A. (2009). Epidemiology of dermatitis and skin infections in United States physicians' offices, 1993–2005. *Clinical Infectious Diseases, 49*(6), 901–907.

Prok, L., & McGovern, T. (2014). Poison ivy *(Toxicodendron)* dermatitis. *UpToDate*. Retrieved from http://www.uptodate.com/contents/poison-ivy-toxicodendron-dermatitis

Stevens, D. L., Bisno, A. L., Chambers, H. F., Dellinger, P., Goldstein, E. J. C., Gorbach, S. L., et al. (2014). Practice guidelines for the diagnosis and management of skin and soft tissue infections: 2014 update by the Infectious Diseases Society of America. *Clinical Infectious Diseases*, Advance Access published June 18, 2014.

Strauss, J. S., Krowchuk, D. P., Leyden, J. J., Lucky, A. W., Shalita, A. R., Siegfried, E. C., et al. (2007). Guidelines for acne vulgaris management. *Journal of the American Academy of Dermatology, 56*(4), 651–663.

U.S. Food and Drug Administration (2006). *FDA Approves updated labeling with boxed warning and medication guide for two eczema drugs, Elidel and Protopic*. Retrieved from http://www.fda.gov/ NewsEvents/Newsroom/PressAnnouncements/2006/ucm108580.htm

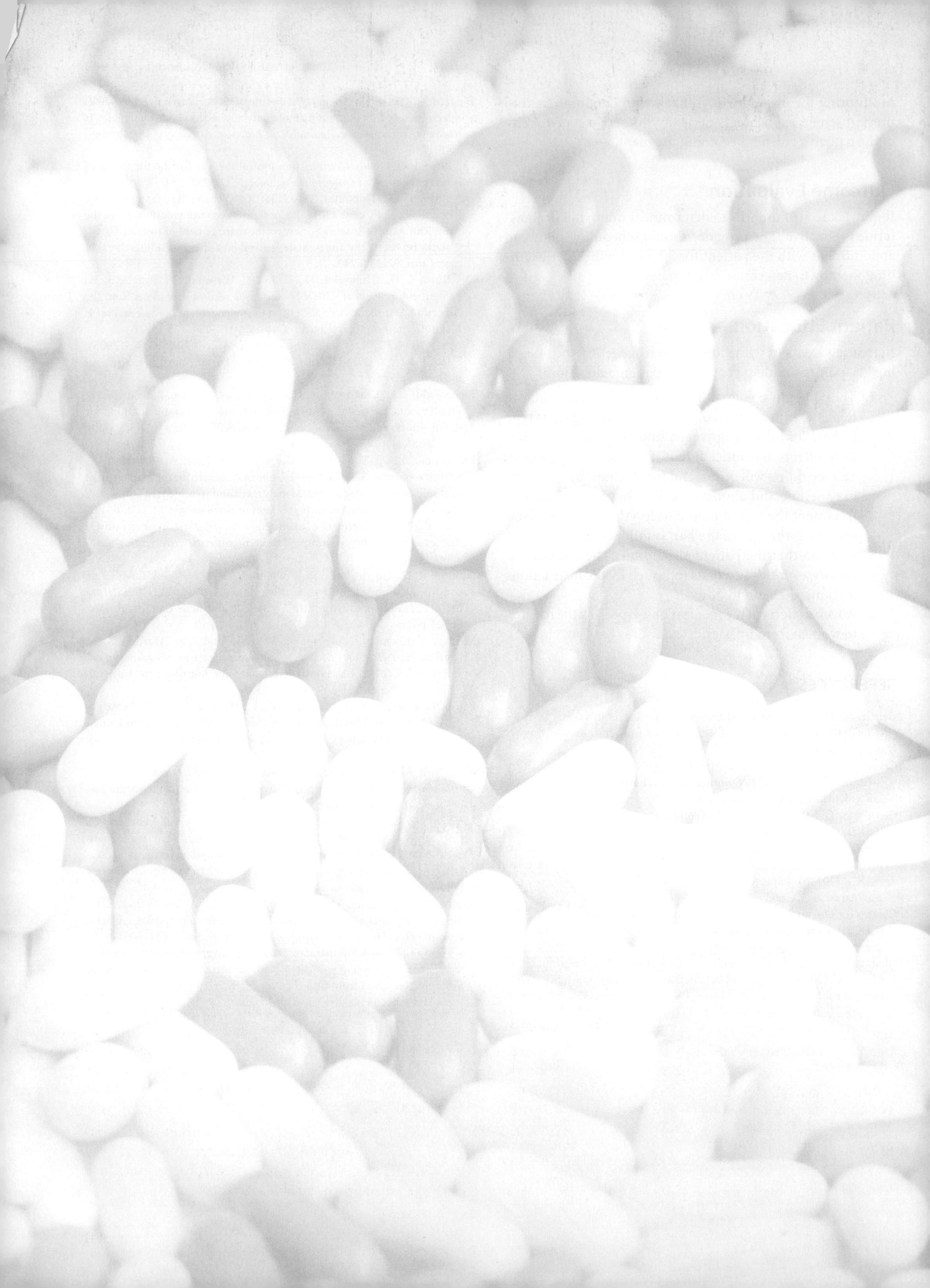

CHAPTER 33

DIABETES MELLITUS

Kathy Shaw • Marylou Robinson

Diabetes and the ensuing complications remain a major cause of morbidity and mortality in the United States and around the world. According to the National Diabetes Fact Sheet, 29.1 million adults and children have diabetes (Centers for Disease Control [CDC], 2014). This number represents 9.3% of the U.S. population; 21 million people are diagnosed while 8.1 million remain undiagnosed. The prevalence of diabetes mellitus (DM) in the United States is growing year by year with many more young people impacted than ever before. Approximately 37% of U.S. adults have pre-diabetes and that number is growing (CDC, 2014).

The annual cost of DM care in 2012 was estimated to be more than $245 billion, with $176 billion attributed to direct medical care and $69 billion attributed to indirect care, which includes work loss, disability, and premature mortality (CDC, 2014). DM is the leading cause of blindness, lower extremity amputations, and end-stage renal disease, and a major cause of heart disease and stroke. Diabetes is the seventh leading cause of death in the United States, but that number may be underreported.

Diabetes mellitus is a chronic, progressive metabolic disorder from abnormalities in glucose, protein, and fat metabolism, which results in hyperglycemia. Diabetes is categorized into four clinical classes:

- Type 1 diabetes, which results from beta-cell destruction, leading to absolute insulin deficiency
- Type 2 diabetes, which results from a progressive insulin secretory defect or insulin resistance

- Diabetes due to other causes, e.g., genetic defects in beta-cell function, genetic defects in insulin action, diseases of the exocrine pancreas (such as cystic fibrosis), and drug- or chemical-induced causes (such as in the treatment of HIV/AIDS or after organ transplantation)
- Gestational diabetes mellitus (GDM), which is diagnosed during pregnancy but is not overt after delivery (American Diabetes Association [ADA], 2015).

Some patients cannot be clearly classified as having type 1 or type 2. Clinical presentation and disease progression may vary considerably in both types and diagnosis may be difficult for some individuals. Presentation and progression differ in age of onset, genetic predisposition, treatment options, and complications. Table 33-1 provides a brief comparison of the differences between type 1 and type 2, the two major types. This chapter focuses on the pharmacological management of type 1 and type 2 DM. Gestational diabetes, which requires consultation with an obstetrical provider, is briefly mentioned.

Diabetes mellitus is clearly interrelated with hyperlipidemia, hypertension, and coronary heart disease. Because these disorders go hand in hand with DM, treatment protocols now include management of all these disorders as part of diabetes management. This chapter discusses these disorders as they relate to diabetes mellitus.

PATHOPHYSIOLOGY

Type 1 Diabetes Mellitus

Several pathogenic processes are involved in the development of type 1 diabetes mellitus. Type 1, which accounts for 5% to 10% of all persons with diabetes, results from an autoimmune destruction of the beta cells of the islet of Langerhans of the pancreas and leads to absolute insulin deficiency (Bardsley & Magee, 2011). Type 1 was previously known as juvenile diabetes and insulin-dependent diabetes. Risk factors can be genetic, autoimmune, and environmental. Seventy percent of type 1 cases are diagnosed before the age of 30, although type 1 can occur at any age (Bardsley & Magee, 2011).

Type 1 diabetes has two subtypes: immune mediated (autoimmune disease) and nonimmune (idiopathic). Active autoimmunity directed at the pancreatic beta cells and their products are the first identification of type 1. Autoantibodies to

Table 33–1 Comparison of Type 1 and Type 2 Diabetes Mellitus

Characteristic	Type 1	Type 2
Age at onset	Usually during childhood or adolescence, but can occur at any age, even in eighth and ninth decades	Usually after age 40 and risk for it increases with age, obesity, and lack of physical activity
Type of onset	Signs and symptoms abrupt, but disease process may be present for years	Insidious and gradual
Genetic susceptibility	HLA-DR3 and DR4 and others; 50% concordance in monozygotic twins	Frequent genetic background, but no relation to HLA; almost 100% concordance in monozygotic twins
Environmental factors	Viruses, toxins	Obesity, nutrition; more common in women with prior gestational diabetes and in patients with hypertension or hyperlipidemia
Etiology	Unknown; postulated causes include heredity, autoimmune disease, and viral infections	Unknown; heredity is highly associated
Islet cell antibody and pancreatic cell-mediated immunity	Present at onset	Absent
Endogenous insulin	Secretion is markedly diminished early in disease; may be totally absent later	Levels may be low (insulin deficiency), normal, or high (insulin resistance)
Nutritional status	Thin, catabolic state	Obesity is common
Symptoms	Polydipsia, polyphagia, polyuria, fatigue, and weight loss	May be asymptomatic; polydipsia or polyuria may be present
Ketosis	At onset or during insulin deficiency	Resistant except during infection or stress
Control of blood sugars	Often difficult with wide glucose fluctuations	Variable
Dietary management	Essential	Essential; sometimes controlled with diet and exercise
Insulin	Insulin therapy required	Usually required as disease progresses
Metformin, sulfonylureas, and other oral agents	Not efficacious	Efficacious
Complications	Occur in a majority of patients after >5 yr, but reduced incidence for those with good control	Frequent, but reduced incidence for those with good control

tyrosine phosphatases IA-2 and IA-2 beta to islet cells, to insulin, and to glutamic acid decarboxylase (GAD65) are seen in 85% to 90% of patients with the immune-related subtype of type 1 diabetes. A small percentage (10% to 15%) of patients with type 1 DM have no known etiology (idiopathic). Most patients with idiopathic type 1 DM are African American or Asian American. This chapter focuses on the immune-related form.

Abnormalities at six genetic loci associated with type 1 DM have been identified to date. The most common is associated with mutation of the hepatic transcription factor (hepatocyte nuclear factor [HNF]-1 alpha) on chromosome 12. A second form involves the glucokinase gene on chromosome 7p. The latter form results in a defective glucokinase molecule. Because glucokinase converts glucose to glucose-6-phosphate, which then stimulates insulin secretion, defects in this gene result in increased levels of glucose needed to elicit normal levels of insulin secretion. Less common forms result from mutations in other transcription factors: HNF-4 alpha, insulin promoter factor (IPF)-1, and NeuroD-1. Genetic mutations that result in the inability to convert pro-insulin to insulin and some that affect insulin action rather than production have also been identified.

Susceptibility to type has been linked to these genetic mutations. Current theories maintain that islet-cell destruction occurs predominantly in persons who are genetically susceptible. When a person with the appropriate genetic characteristics is exposed to a trigger, the beta cells are destroyed directly or when an autoimmune process is triggered, which in turn destroys the beta cells. Environmental factors such as toxins, food antigens, and viral infections are suspected to be responsible for the induction of type 1 (Bardsley & Magee, 2011).

Type 1 has a long preclinical period. Signs and symptoms and clinical presentation of type 1 are abrupt, although a decline in insulin secretion begins long before the symptoms develop, possibly as long as 9 years before clinical presentation (Bardsley & Magee, 2011). Research has demonstrated the presence of islet-cell autoantibodies (ICA) for years before the occurrence of symptoms. ICAs precede beta cell deficiency and have been found in 85% to 90% of type 1 diabetes at the time of onset of clinical symptoms. Autoantibodies against insulin (IAA) have also been found. ICAs and IAA are probably the result of the beta cell

---

On The Horizon   CURE FOR TYPE I DM?

Two recent research endeavors are exploring the use of older non-diabetic medications to intervene in early cases of DM I. Mice given verapamil essentially eradicated a protein that causes the death of beta cells. Trials funded by the Juvenile Diabetes Foundation with humans are planned to test this "cure" of type 1 DM (Shalev, 2014). Other researchers at Massachusetts General are exploring an interesting positive effect on pancreas recovery after administration of the old BCG vaccine originally developed to assist with TB care (Faustman et al, 2012).

---

destruction rather than its cause, and they tend to disappear with time.

The clinical difference between type 1 and type 2 is not always clear; there can be similarities between both types. Latent autoimmune diabetes in adults (LADA) is a slow, progressive form of type 1 that may be confused with type 2 and accounts for approximately 10% of older persons who require insulin. In LADA, there is a presence of autoantibodies that suggest it is an autoimmune disorder like type 1. However, there are differences such as T-cell reactivity, autoantibody clustering, and genetic susceptibility, which suggest different disease processes. In LADA, significant insulin resistance is present, which causes earlier beta cell destruction. Persons with LADA are usually over 35 years of age, are not obese, and require oral agents and progression to insulin within a relatively short period of time. Clinical presentation includes weight loss, unstable blood glucose, propensity for ketosis, and low C-peptide reserves (Bardsley & Magee, 2011).

Before hyperglycemia occurs, 80% to 90% of the function of insulin-secreting beta cells must be lost. DM may be precipitated by acute illness or stress at any time during the progressive decline in beta cell function, thus increasing the insulin demand of the damaged islet cells. Beta cell abnormalities are present long before the acute clinical onset of type 1 diabetes, and the event that precipitates the acute onset of symptoms may be far removed from the event that initiates the pathology.

Regardless of the cause, considerable evidence suggests that the pathology is probably disequilibrium between the relative excess production of glucagon by the pancreatic A cells and the lack of insulin produced by the beta cells. This ratio of insulin to glucagon in the portal vein, not the concentration of each hormone, controls hepatic glucose and fat metabolism, two major problems in type 1 diabetes. The recognition that the totality of the metabolic pathology is a factor of both of these hormones is leading to a different approach to diabetes management. Figure 33-1 depicts the pathological cause of the various symptoms of type 1 diabetes.

Due to lack of insulin production by the beta cells of the islet of Langerhans, treatment requires insulin replacement. If the disease progresses without treatment, diabetic ketoacidosis (DKA), weight loss, muscle wasting, and death may occur. Once treatment is initiated, the patient may enter temporary partial remission, despite the continued destruction of beta cells ("honeymoon phase"). Beta cell destruction eventually reaches a point at which hyperglycemia occurs again, and insulin therapy is required throughout the rest of the disease process. The assumption that C-peptides, an indication of native insulin production, would not be found in type 1 patients is being undermined by a report that up to one-third of type 1 patients have a small, clinically unimportant production of insulin (Wang, Lovejoy & Faustman, 2012).

Type 2 Diabetes Mellitus

Type 2 diabetes is much more common than type 1, affecting approximately 90% to 95% of persons with diabetes. Prevalence

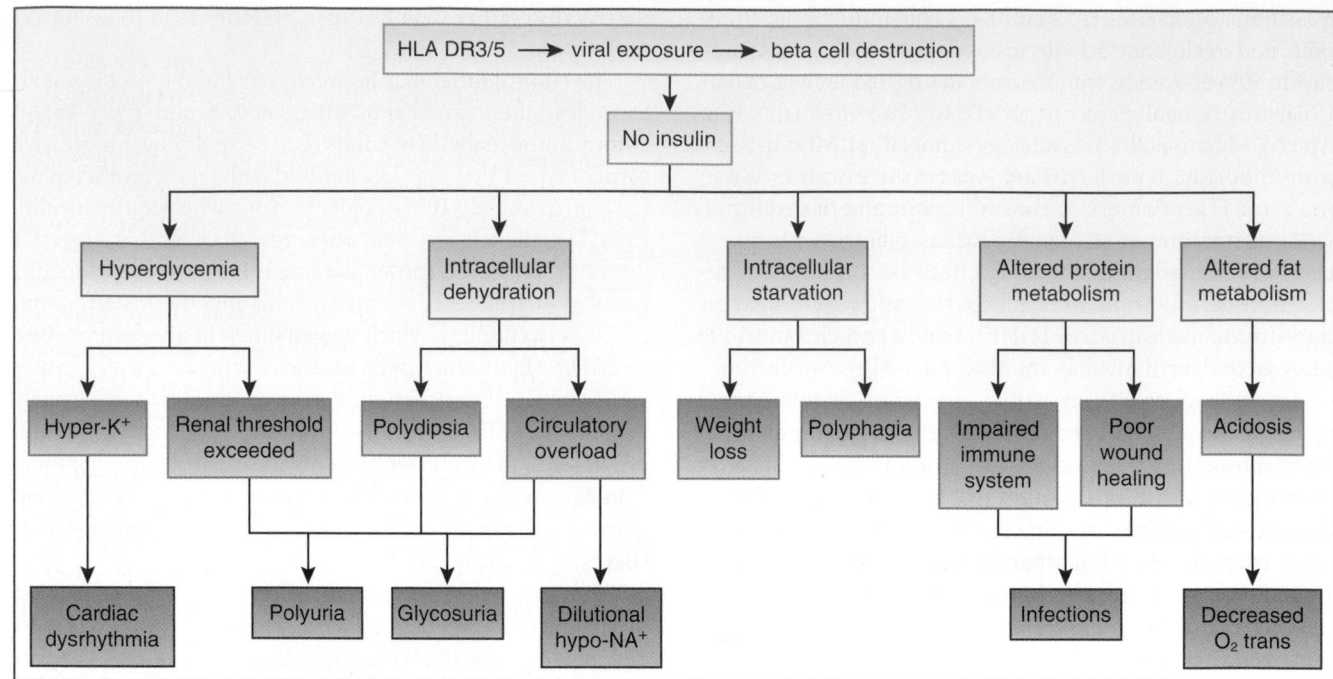

Figure 33–1. Pathophysiology of type 1 diabetes.

of type 2 varies in the United States by ethnic group, with a higher frequency in Native Americans, Asian Americans, Latinos, Pacific Islanders, and African Americans (ADA, 2015). Other risk factors include obesity, sedentary lifestyle, hypertension, dyslipidemias, family history, gestational history, and age. Genetics have a strong influence, and a locus has been found on chromosome arm 7q that may be related to insulin resistance, one underlying alteration in type 2 diabetes (Bloomgarden, 2003). The offspring of parents who both have type 2 DM have a 15% chance of developing DM. Although there is disparity in incidence between ethnic groups for having DM, there is no racial disparity in rates of pre-diabetes that progresses to DM (Dagogo-Jack, Edeoga, Ebenibo, Nyenwe, & Wan, 2014). This means that without regard to genetic background, the risk of developing full DM is an equal to 11% per year for anyone diagnosed with pre-diabetes.

The pathogenesis of type 2 diabetes is complex and multifactorial, with symptoms that can vary greatly across patients. Plasma insulin levels in type 2 diabetes may be low, normal, or high. Although the specific etiology of type 2 is unknown, autoimmune destruction of beta cells does not occur. The main physiological alteration in type 2 DM is insulin resistance and/or decreased insulin secretion. Insulin resistance is a suboptimal response of sensitivity to insulin, especially in the liver, muscle, and adipose tissue. The result is an increased rate of endogenous glucose production secondary to increased glucagon levels. The gastrointestinal system also plays a role in regulating the secretion of insulin. Incretin peptides secreted from endocrine cells in the intestinal tract are released in response to the ingestion of food. Glucagon-like peptide-1 (GLP-1) and alterations in levels of the regulatory enzyme dipeptidyl peptidase-4 (DPP-4), which impacts the presence and duration of GLP-action, are recognized as factors in type

2 DM. GLP-1 is deficient in people with DM and pre-DM and contributes to the excessive hepatic glucose production, lack of postprandial glucagon suppression, and uncontrolled eating (Bardsley & Magee, 2011). Type 2 DM causes few and nonspecific pancreatic changes.

Many years of compensatory hyperinsulinemia may occur before the onset of clinical symptoms of diabetes. Eventually, the beta cell responsiveness to glucose stimulus diminishes and hyperglycemia prevails. Adipose tissue does not use glucose in response to insulin, resulting in obesity and a large amount of fat in the bloodstream, which results in increased plasma FFA levels. Increased visceral fat shows an inverse relationship with insulin sensitivity. Many people with type 2 DM are obese; obesity triples the risk for insulin resistance. Patients who are not obese by traditional weight standards may have an increased percentage of body fat distributed predominantly in the abdominal region. The gradual onset and progression of type 2 diabetes allows patients to adapt to the symptoms without realizing that the disease process is producing them.

Insulin resistance has also been linked to three other important disorders: hyperlipidemia, hypertension, and coronary artery disease. The Framingham Offspring Study (Bloomgarden, 2003) was among the first to suggest a central metabolic syndrome with high triglyceride levels, low high-density lipoprotein (HDL) levels, obesity, and hyperglycemia, which was also associated with hypertension. Because both dyslipidemia and hypertension are linked with atherogenesis, DM is an independent risk factor for coronary heart disease. Individuals with any one of these disorders should be screened for the others. Screening is discussed below.

Insulin resistance and the metabolic syndrome are also associated with a prothrombotic state that contributes to the vascular complications seen in this disorder. Insulin has a direct antiplatelet effect, and loss of insulin results in increased adhesiveness and exaggerated aggregation and thrombus generation (Randriamboavonjy & Fleming, 2009).

Because an endogenous insulin supply exists early in the disease state, insulin may not be required initially. In older protocols, insulin was used later in the disease process or during acute illness or stress. However, current guidelines suggest that insulin may have a role earlier in the disease process, especially in light of the prevention of the three complications: dyslipidemia, hypertension, and atherogenesis. Oral hypoglycemic agents are also effective in addressing one or more of the metabolic defects in type 2 DM.

Maturity onset diabetes of the young (MODY) has a monogenetic defect in beta cell function that is inherited in an autosomal dominant pattern, resulting in impaired insulin secretion but no defects in insulin action. It usually occurs in adolescence or early adulthood and accounts for approximately 1% to 5% percent of all diabetes. Persons with MODY are not usually overweight and do not have the features of metabolic syndrome that commonly occur in type 2 DM. MODY can often be treated with oral agents (Bardsley & Magee, 2011).

Complications

Long-term complications of all types of DM are based on target organ damage from micro- and macrovascular involvement. Microvascular involvement affects the eyes, heart, kidneys, and nervous system. Complications such as retinopathy with potential loss of vision, nephropathy leading to renal failure, peripheral neuropathy with risk of foot ulcers, amputation, and Charcot's joint and autonomic neuropathy with gastrointestinal, genitourinary, and cardiovascular symptoms and sexual dysfunction may occur. Macrovascular complications from DM occur in the form of atherosclerotic cardiovascular, peripheral vascular, and cerebrovascular diseases and increase the risk for hypertension, abnormalities of lipid metabolism, abnormalities of platelet function, and periodontal disease. The management of each of these complications is discussed below.

Pre-Diabetes

Individuals whose glucose levels do not meet the criteria for diabetes but are too high to be considered normal are classified as having pre-diabetes. These patients have impaired glucose tolerance (IGT) or impaired fasting glucose (IFG). Patients with these two disorders are at risk for diabetes and cardiovascular disease and may have insulin-resistance syndrome. The United States Diabetes Prevention Program (USDPP) showed that lifestyle modification and the administration of metformin (in adults) may prevent or delay the development of type 2 diabetes in patients with pre-diabetes (U.S. Diabetes Prevention Program Research Group, 2002; 2003).

Although discussion and research continue concerning the management of pre-diabetes, the current recommendations specify lifestyle change, which includes modest weight loss by increasing physical activity and making dietary changes and effectively managing known risk factors for DM and the complications. This therapy is more effective in the pre-diabetic state than after the disease state is reached. The biggest impact comes from diet and exercise even without weight loss (Senechal, Slaght, Bharti, & Bouchard, 2014). The current Standards of Medical Care in Diabetes also recommends that metformin be considered for those at high risk for developing diabetes, who are obese (BMI > 35) and under 60 years of age (ADA, 2015).

Diagnosis and Screening

Diagnostic Criteria for Diabetes and Pre-Diabetes

The diagnostic criteria for diabetes mellitus and pre-diabetes are shown in Table 33-2. There are four tests used for diagnosis, and the tests should be confirmed on a subsequent day, unless there are overt clinical symptoms. It is preferable to confirm with the same test or one that is considered more predictive; fasting plasma glucose (FPG) levels are the most reliable. If a repeated test is below the diagnostic criteria, the test should be repeated in 3 to 6 months (ADA, 2015). The criteria for such testing are listed in Table 33-3.

Table 33–2   Diagnostic Criteria for Diabetes Mellitus and Pre-Diabetes

Diagnostic Category	Diagnostic Criteria
Diabetes mellitus	Acute symptoms of diabetes plus casual plasma glucose concentration ≥200 mg/dL. *Casual is defined as any time of day without regard to time since last meal. The classic symptoms of diabetes are polyuria, polydipsia, and unexplained weight loss.
	Fasting plasma glucose ≥126 mg/dL. *Fasting is defined as no caloric intake for at least 8 h.
	2-h postload plasma glucose in an oral glucose tolerance test ≥200 mg/dL. The test uses a glucose load containing the equivalent of 75 g anhydrous glucose dissolved in water.
	Hb A1c ≥6.5%
Pre-diabetes	Fasting plasma glucose 100–125 mg/dL (IFG) *or*
	plasma glucose 140–199 mg/dL (IGT) 2 hr post-ingestion of standard glucose load (75 g) *or*
	Hb A1c 5.7%–6.4%

IFG = impaired fasting glucose; IGT = impaired glucose tolerance.

Table 33–3   Criteria for Testing Asymptomatic Adults for Diabetes

Individuals ≥45 yr and who have a BMI ≥25 kg/m² should be tested. If normal, the test should be repeated at 3 yr intervals.
Individuals <45 yr and who have a BMI ≥25 kg/m² and have additional risk factors should have more frequent testing.
Additional risk factors are the following: <ul><li>Physically inactive</li><li>First-degree relative with diabetes</li><li>Members of high-risk ethnic group (African American, Hispanic, Native American, Asian American, Pacific Islander)</li><li>Delivered a baby weighing >9 lb or previously diagnosed with GDM</li><li>Hypertensive (B/P ≥140/90 mm Hg)</li><li>HDL cholesterol ≤35 mg/dL and/or triglyceride level ≥250 mg/dL</li><li>Have polycystic ovary syndrome (PCOS)</li><li>IGT or IFG on previous testing</li><li>Have other clinical conditions associated with insulin resistance (PCOS or acanthosis nigricans)</li><li>History of CVD</li></ul>

Source: Adapted from American Diabetes Association. (2015). Standards of medical care for patients with diabetes mellitus.

Screening Recommendations for Diabetes and Pre-Diabetes

Screening recommendations vary by specialty groups, but the most respected and used recommendations in the United States come from the ADA and therefore will be used here. The ADA (2015) recommends testing to detect pre-diabetes and type 2 diabetes in asymptomatic adults of any age who are overweight or obese (body mass index [BMI] greater than 25 kg/m²) and who have one or more additional risk factors for diabetes. In those without these risk factors, testing should begin at age 45 years. The Hb A1c, FPG, or 2 h 75 g OGTT (oral glucose tolerance test) are appropriate to test for diabetes or pre-diabetes (ADA, 2015).

Evidence from type 1 prevention studies suggests that measurement of islet autoantibodies identifies individuals who are at risk for developing type 1 DM. High-risk individuals, such as those with transient hyperglycemia or those who have relatives with type 1 diabetes, may be appropriate for this type of testing (ADA, 2015). Widespread screening of symptomatic low-risk individuals is not recommended.

In 2010, the ADA adopted the use of the Hb A1c with a threshold of ≥6.5% for diagnosis, provided the test is performed using a method that is certified by the National Glycohemoglobin Standardization Program (NGSP) and standardized or traceable to the Diabetes Control and Complications Trial (DCCT) reference assay. Point-of-care Hb A1c assays, for which proficiency testing is not mandated, are not sufficiently accurate at this time to use for diagnostic purposes (ADA, 2015). FPG or Hb A1c can be used for screening all age groups. The OGTT is impractical and expensive for general screening purposes; however, it is used to diagnose GDM.

Diagnostic Criteria for Pregnant Women

The ADA (2015) provides diagnostic screening criteria for pregnant women:

- Screen for undiagnosed type 2 diabetes at the first prenatal visit in those with risk factors, using standard diagnostic criteria.
- In pregnant women not previously known to have diabetes, screen for GDM at 24–28 weeks' gestation, using

a 75 g 2 h OGTT and the diagnostic cut points as outlined below:

- At 24–28 weeks' gestation in women not previously diagnosed with overt diabetes, perform a 75 g OGTT, with plasma glucose measurement fasting and at 1 and 2 hr.
- The OGTT should be performed in the morning after an overnight fast of at least 8 hr.
- Screen women with GDM for persistent diabetes at 6–12 weeks' postpartum, using the OGTT and nonpregnant criteria (ADA, 2015).
- Women with a history of GDM should have lifelong screening for the development of diabetes or pre-diabetes at least every 3 years.
- Women with a history of GDM found to have pre-diabetes should receive lifestyle interventions and/or metformin to prevent DM.
- GDM diagnosis is made when any of the following plasma glucose values are exceeded: fasting ≥92 mg/dL, 1 h ≥180 mg/dL, or 2 h ≥153 mg/dL.

Screening Criteria for Children

The incidence of type 2 diabetes in adolescents has increased dramatically in the past 10 years, especially in minority populations. The ADA (2015) recommends testing asymptomatic children who meet the following criteria:

- Overweight (BMI >85th percentile for age and sex, weight for height >85th percentile, or weight >120% of ideal for height), plus any two of the following risk factors:
- Family history of type 2 diabetes in first- or second-degree relative
- Race/ethnicity (Native American, African American, Latino, Asian American, Pacific Islander)
- Signs of insulin resistance or conditions associated with insulin resistance (acanthosis nigricans, hypertension, dyslipidemia, polycystic ovary syndrome, small-for-gestational- age birth weight)
- Maternal history of diabetes or GDM during the child's gestation

Such testing should begin at age 10 years and occur every 3 years thereafter.

PHARMACODYNAMICS

General Diabetes Management and Glycemic Control

The treatment goals for both type 1 and type 2 DM are near-normal glucose levels. Recent studies show that tighter glycemic control can lead to higher mortality rates in some populations, especially older adults, those with comorbidities, and those who have preexisting complications. The current guidelines recommend an individualized approach that is both acceptable to the patient and provider while preventing both acute complications, such as hypoglycemia, and the development and progression of chronic complications from DM.

Insulin

Insulin is a hormone produced in the beta cells of the isles of Langerhans in the pancreas that is released by stimulation from an elevated blood glucose level (BGL). Administration of the exogenous insulin produces the same effect as the naturally occurring hormone. Currently, all insulin is manufactured to be chemically identical to human insulin through DNA technology.

Insulin lowers blood glucose levels by the following mechanisms (Sisson & Cornell, 2011):

- Promotes protein synthesis by increasing amino acid transport into cells
- Stimulates glucose entry into cells as energy source
- Increases storage of glucose as glycogen (glycogenesis) in muscle and liver cells
- Inhibits glucose production in liver and muscle cells (glycogenolysis)
- Enhances fat storage (lipogenosis) and prevents mobilization of fat for energy (lipolysis and ketogenesis)
- Inhibits glucose formation from noncarbohydrate sources, such as amino acids (gluconeogenesis)

The action of insulin is discussed in greater detail in Chapter 21. In summary, insulin receptors "open the gate" to allow utilization of glucose by the cells. The total number of insulin receptors can be mitigated by such factors as obesity and long-standing hyperglycemia, which may explain why weight loss can be a significant factor in diabetes management.

Current treatment recommendations for insulin indicate a regimen that most closely mimics endogenous insulin production; this regimen includes basal insulin, once or twice daily, and bolus insulin before meals or to correct hyperglycemia. Insulin regimens should be designed with basal, nutritional, correction elements, and work and activity schedules to achieve and maintain glucose control. Insulin preparations are categorized by onset, duration, and peak of action following subcutaneous injection: rapid, fast, intermediate, and long-acting. There are also various pre-mixed combinations of intermediate-acting preparations with short- or rapid-acting preparations. See Table 33-4 and Chapter 21.

The two long-acting insulin analogs, glargine and detemir, are important breakthroughs in DM management and treatment. They can be used in conjunction with oral medications in type 2 or with rapid- or fast-acting insulin in both type 1 and type 2. Both provide peakless basal coverage but vary greatly in terms of how they work. Though marketed as 24 hour insulins, they do not fully meet that expectation. Until wider dissemination of a new class of ultra-long insulins, there are no better alternatives.

Glargine can be given at bedtime or at any time of day but should be given consistently at the same time each day. It cannot be mixed in the same syringe with other insulin nor can the syringe contain any other medication residue. Insulin detemir has a prolonged absorption and provides a more consistent 24-hour basal effect due to its albumin binding effect in the plasma and near the injection site. Insulin detemir cannot be diluted or mixed with any other insulin preparations.

Although insulin has been the drug of choice in managing diabetes in pregnancy, approaches to therapy vary greatly to include the use of metformin and glyburide. Women who have preexisting DM will have increased insulin requirements and should be treated aggressively. Women who have GDM and are obese will usually need higher insulin doses due to insulin resistance. The Endocrine Society now calls for all women who have had GDM to be tested for pre-diabetes

Table 33–4 Common Insulin Types, Onset, Peak, and Duration

Type	Insulin	Onset	Peak	Duration
Rapid-Acting	Humalog (Lispro) Novalog (Aspart) Apidra (Glulisine)	5–30 min	0.5 h–3 h	3–4 h
Short-Acting	Regular (Humulin R, Novalin R)	30–60 min	2–4 h	3–7 h
Intermediate-Acting	Isophane(NPH, Humulin N)	1–2 h	4–10 h	10–16 h
Long-Acting	Lantus (Glargine) Levimir (Detemir)	1–2 h 1–2 h	None	20–24 h 20–24 h
Fixed Combination	70/30 (NPH/regular ratio) 50/50 (NPH/regular ratio) 75/25 (NPH/lispro) 70/30 (NPH/aspart)	30–60 min 30–60 min 5–15 min 5–15 min	Dual	10–16 h

On The Horizon

ULTRA-LONG-ACTING INSULIN

An ultra-long-acting basal insulin analogue, insulin degludec, has just been approved. Duration of action nears 42 hours, so it might have an irregular dosing schedule. It is thought to have lower rates of nocturnal hypoglycemia compared to glargine. Its higher cost will be an issue. There are concerns about adverse CV effects.

or continued diabetes with an OGTT 6 to 12 weeks after delivery (Blumer et al, 2013).

Various insulin regimens can be used for type 1, including short-acting (SAI) or rapid-acting insulin (RAI) boluses combined with intermediate-acting (IAI) or long-acting insulin (LAI) for basal. This can also be achieved with the premixed preparations.

Because of progressive beta cell dysfunction, insulin will usually be required in type 2 after a period of time. It is theorized that earlier use may "rest" the pancreas and reduce the intensity of the progression of DM, but this is not yet established as fact. Administration of basal insulin once or twice daily is preferred initially, either with IAI or LAI, to achieve desired normal glycemic patterns throughout the day and night. Glargine and detemir may have less nocturnal hypoglyemica than NPH; detemir may have slightly less weight gain. Both of the LAI are more expensive than NPH, which may be an important consideration (Inzucchi et al, 2012).

Providers should be aware of issues related to insulin use that can affect initiation, use, and adherence. Insulin is a necessary treatment for glucose toxicity and is the necessary replacement for insulin deficiency when oral agents alone become ineffective. One of the greatest obstacles to insulin use is patient and provider resistance. This inertia, or lack of intensification of treatment when warranted, is widely documented and must be overcome in order to provide optimal treatment for patients. In a systematic review of barriers to insulin progression in insulin-naïve and insulin-experienced users, Polinski and colleagues (2013) found that patient knowledge and experience with insulin were important attributes that impacted attitudes and willingness to intensify treatment with insulin. Only two articles on physician barriers were included in this review, but the consistent themes were the lack of knowledge, experience, and resources needed to provide insulin progression. Interestingly, providers overestimate patient resistance to injectable medication use (Peyrot et al, 2005).

Oral Agents

There are many pharmacological treatment options for type 2 DM. Oral agents are only effective for type 2 and most act on different aspects of the metabolic defects. Monotherapy with any of the agents will result in the reduction of Hb A1c by 0.5% to 2.0%. Combination therapy, either with two or more oral agents or an oral agent and insulin, results in a further decrease in the Hb A1c level (Sisson & Cornell, 2011).

CLINICAL PEARL

Rules for Fine-Tuning Insulin Doses

- The correction factor (CF) and insulin: carbohydrate ratio (I:C) for patients with either type 1 or 2 taking insulin.
- The rule of 1,500 enables the provider to find the CF or how much 1 unit of insulin will drop blood sugar for high blood glucose levels (usually greater than 140 to 150). First, calculate the total daily dose (TDD) of insulin as basal + bolus—about 50% of each. Then divide 1,500 by the TDD. For example, 1,500 divided by 30 units per day of insulin equals 50. One unit of short-acting insulin will drop glucose 50 points. For rapid-acting insulin use 1,800 as the basis for calculation.
- The rule of 500 enables the provider to find the I:C ratio. Divide 500 by TDD. For example, 500 divided by 30 units per day of insulin equals 16.7. One unit will cover 16 to 17 g of carbohydrate (CHO). For ease of use, round down to 1 unit:15 g.

Insulin is the preferred treatment for pregnant women, but metformin or glyburide may also be used. Primary care providers should coordinate start of medications with an OB or endocrine specialist. Metformin is the only U.S. Food and Drug Administration [FDA] oral agent approved for use in children. There are multiple classes of orally administered drugs used for type 2, which have been discussed in Chapter 21, but are summarized here.

Biguanides

Biguanides are not considered hypoglycemic drugs; their pharmacological action does not increase insulin release from the pancreas or increase hypoglycemic effects. They are indicated as the initial drug of choice or as an adjunct in combination therapy. Metformin is the only drug in this class used clinically in the United States and is the only FDA-approved oral drug for use in children 10 years or older.

Metformin works primarily by decreasing hepatic glucose production by decreasing gluconeogenesis. It also increases peripheral glucose uptake and utilization, improves hepatic response to blood glucose levels so that the liver produces appropriate amounts of glucose, and decreases intestinal absorption of glucose. Insulin production is necessary for metformin to be effective. In contrast to some of the other drugs, patients taking metformin do not gain weight. In fact, they often lose weight. Because obesity is a major factor in the pathogenesis of type 2 diabetes, weight loss is an important action of this drug. Initial metformin therapy is indicated for type 2 DM with dyslipidemia, obesity, insulin resistance, and an elevated FPG. It can reduce Hb A1c by 1.5% to 2%.

Therapy is initiated at a low dose with slow titration to achieve desired glycemic control. The lowest dose is 500 mg once or twice daily, and the maximum dose is 2,550 mg. To reduce the gastrointestinal (GI) adverse reactions that are common with metformin, the dose is titrated up from 500 mg taken once or twice daily to the maximum effective dose. Beneficial side effects include weight loss, reduction in LDL-C, total cholesterol, and triglycerides, and an increase in HDL-C. Gastrointestinal disturbances subside over time.

The Diabetes Prevention Program Research Group (2002) tested metformin and lifestyle modifications as methods for preventing the conversion of pre-diabetes to type 2 diabetes. Lifestyle interventions reduced the incidence of conversion by 58% and metformin by 31%. The cost effectiveness of the intervention was also investigated, and both metformin and lifestyle interventions were cost-effective across subjects, regardless of age, ethnicity, or gender and affordable in routine clinical practice. Therefore, the use of metformin is recommended for the prevention of the development of diabetes in patients with diagnosed pre-diabetes.

Sulfonylureas

Sulfonylureas increase endogenous insulin secretion by the beta cells and may improve the binding between insulin and insulin receptors or increase the number of receptors. Hypoglycemic effects appear to be due to increased endogenous insulin production and to improved beta cell sensitivity to blood glucose levels or suppression of glucose release by the liver. Sulfonylureas were the first class used to treat type 2 DM, but they are now considered secondary agents partially due to their hypoglycemic risks.

Sulfonylureas are absorbed quickly and completely and are not affected by food. They can reduce Hb A1c by 1.5% to 2%. Dosing should be started at the lowest dose and titrated as needed. Sulfonylureas are Pregnancy Category C with the exception of glyburide. A person who is not overweight and who does not have dyslipidemia is a good candidate for a sulfonylurea. Common side effects include hypoglycemia and weight gain. Less common side effects include skin rashes and mild GI disturbances. A newer concern is the link with additional risk for hypoglycemia with concurrent use of antibiotics (clarithromycin, levofloxacin, sulfamethoxazole-trimethoprim, metronidazole, and ciprofloxacin) (Parekh et al, 2014).

Alpha-Glucosidase Inhibitors

Alpha-glucosidase inhibitors do not act directly on any of the defects in metabolism seen in type 2 diabetes mellitus. They competitively inhibit and delay the absorption of complex CHO from the small bowel and lower BG levels after meals. Alpha-glucosidase inhibitors have no inhibitory activity against lactase and do not induce lactose intolerance. They are not associated with weight gain and diminish the weight-increasing effects of sulfonylureas when given in combination with them. Alpha-glucosidase inhibitor activity is effective on any CHO food intake, including liquid diets taken via a nasogastric tube. They have a limited role as adjunct therapy except in individuals who cannot take metformin. They can reduce Hb A1C by 0.5% to 1%.

Thiazolidinediones

Thiazolidinediones (TZD) are oral antihyperglycemic drugs that are best classified as insulin sensitizers. Pioglitazone (Actos) and rosiglitazone (Avandia) are the only FDA-approved agents. Thiazolidinediones activate a nuclear receptor that regulates gene transcription, resulting in increased utilization of available insulin by the liver and muscle cells and adipose tissue. In addition, these drugs reduce hepatic glucose production so that the liver produces appropriate amounts of glucagon. TZDs are recommended in the guidelines for the two- or three-drug combinations. These drugs, especially rosiglitazone, should be used cautiously because of the potential for cardiovascular problems. The 2011 FDA imposed restriction on prescribing rosiglitazone-containing drugs has been lifted, but the requirement for close monitoring of heart failure signs and symptoms associated with a class effect of fluid retention remains (FDA, 2011). The fear of bladder cancer associated with these medications has not demonstrated a causal effect (Levin et al, 2015). There is a higher risk of bladder cancer in North American and European diabetic patients. There is not a dose response to cancer incidence. These agents can reduce Hb A1C by 1.5% to 2%.

Meglitinides

The meglitinides have a different mechanism of action from any of the other drugs used to treat type 2 DM. The meglitinides are short-acting insulin secretagogues. Two drugs, repaglinide (Prandin) and nateglinide (Starlix) are in this class. They work by closing the adenosine triphosphate (ATP)–dependent potassium channels in the beta cell membrane by binding at specific receptor sites. This potassium channel blockade depolarizes the beta cell and leads to an opening of calcium channels. The resultant influx of calcium increases the secretion of insulin. Because their time in the plasma is less than 2 hours, the effect is very short. Plasma insulin levels fall to baseline by 4 hours after dosing. The end result of their stimulation of insulin secretion is a lowering in postprandial blood glucose levels. To achieve this effect, they are dosed 3 times daily no more than 20 minutes before meals. They do not directly affect fasting blood glucose levels or any of the other defects in metabolism seen in type 2 diabetes. They are most useful in patients whose primary glucose alteration is postprandial hyperglycemia. These drugs are not commonly used because adherence is difficult, GI side effects can be distressing, and they are expensive. They can reduce Hb A1c by 0.5% to 1%.

Selective Sodium Glucose Co-transporter 2 (SGLT-2)

Canagliflozin (Invokana), dapglifoxin (Farxiga), and empagliflozin (Jardiance) inhibit renal SGLT-2 action, thereby blocking about 90% of the reabsorption of glucose in the kidneys and promoting excretion of excess glucose in the urine. This translates to nearly 250 calories a day. If blood glucose is high, then more is excreted in the urine. There is an osmotic fluid loss which can lead to intravascular volume depletion. Because the drug class also decreases renal hyperfiltration akin to ACE inhibitors, they are being evaluated for an indication to be nephroprotective (Cherney et al, 2014).

Major side effects are genital yeast infections in both genders related to the continuous presence of glucose in the urine. They can be used with some renal insufficiency which helps cover patients previously on medications that must be stopped when GFR begins to decline. They are combined with many other agents to help reduce glycemic levels.

Incretin Therapy

Recent research and attention has been focused on new treatment options for type 2 DM: incretin hormones and their impact on glycemic control. Glucagon-like peptide-1 (GLP-1), a normally occurring hormone released from the gut after ingesting a meal, promotes satiety, decreases gastric emptying, increases glucose-dependent insulin release from pancreatic beta cells, and decreases glucagon release from pancreatic alpha cells (Sisson & Cornell, 2011). GLP-1 is rapidly inactivated by the enzyme dipeptidyl peptidase-4 (DPP-4).

Two therapies that block DPP-4 activity include the GLP-1 agonists and DPP-4 inhibitors. Both are effective therapies in the treatment of type 2 DM that do not cause hypoglycemia and can be used as monotherapy or in combination with metformin. When choosing between GLP-1 agonists and the DPP-4 inhibitors, the patient's age, the time from initial diabetes diagnosis, body weight, compliance, and finances should be considered (Dicker, 2011).

In recent studies, both drug groups have shown promise in lowering Hb A1c levels, contributing to weight stability, and providing protective cardiovascular function. Longitudinal studies have addressed the fear of negative cardiovascular impact; there appears to be no negative impact even in patients with renal insufficiency (Udell et al, 2014). A difference between these two classes is their mode of administration: GLP-1 agonists are injectable peptides, whereas the DPP-4 inhibitors are oral agents.

In the older population, DPP-4 inhibitors may be the best choice due to their glucose-lowering effect, the neutral effect on caloric intake, and therefore less negative effect on muscle and total body protein mass. In younger patients recently diagnosed with type 2 diabetes, abdominal obesity, and abnormal metabolic profile, treatment with GLP-1 agonists have a beneficial effect on weight loss and improve the metabolic profile. An additional factor to take into consideration when using these drugs is that DPP-4 inhibitors (in reduced doses) are safe for treating patients with moderate and severe renal failure, whereas GLP-1 is contraindicated in most of these patients (Dicker, 2011).

Dipeptidyl Peptidase-4 Inhibitors

The dipeptidyl peptidase-4 inhibitors (DPP-4) include sitagliptin (Januvia), saxagliptin (Onglyza), linagliptin (Tradjenta), and alogliptin (Nesina). All except linagliptin require considerations for renal dysfunction. The action of DPP-4 inhibitors is different from all other oral agents because they act on the incretin hormone system to have an indirect effect to increase insulin production. They improve glycemic control by increasing insulin synthesis and secretion, reducing glucagon, slowing gastric emptying by prolonging the action of the remaining GLP-1 hormones, and suppressing the appetite. One main advantage is the oral preparation. (See Chapter 21 for more detail.)

Glucagon-Like Peptide-1 Receptor Agonists (GLP-1s)

The first GLP-1 agonist receiving FDA approval was Exenatide (Byetta), a synthetic form of protein found in the saliva of the Gila monster. Exenatide and the other GLP-1 medications liraglutide (Victoza), albiglutide (Tanzeum), and dulaglutide (Trulicity) activate GLP-1 receptors, which decreases fasting and postprandial glucose levels. They increase insulin synthesis and secretion in the presence of elevated glucose levels and improve first-phase insulin release, lowering glucagon, slowing gastric emptying, and reducing food intake. These drugs are given by subcutaneous injection for type 2 DM but are not a substitute for insulin. They have been noted to produce lower Hb A1c levels of 0.5% to 1.5% and weight loss. Liraglutide has been given formal FDA indication for obesity therapy; the others in the class may soon follow suit. They come in many combinations with other medications. The advent of long-acting, once weekly formulations has helped overcome much resistance to these being injectable medications. There are some concerns with medullary thyroid cancer (see Chapter 21).

Other Injectable Drugs

Amylin is a pancreatic hormone that is stimulated to release by the presence of a meal. Its role is to slow down gastric emptying rates, allowing a more gradual release of glucose into the system. The "satiety effect" suppresses appetite. The slower glucose absorption prevents a sudden postprandial spike. Pramlintide (Symlin) is an injectable amylin hormone derivative that mimics these natural effects. It is not popular due to a high rate of severe nausea and the need to inject prior to most meals (see Chapter 21).

GOALS OF TREATMENT

The overall goals for the treatment of diabetes are (1) near normalization of blood glucose, (2) prevention of acute complications such as hypoglycemia, (3) prevention of progression of the disease to target organ damage, and (4) appropriate patient-oriented self-management. Table 33-5 highlights the targets for glycemic control and prevention of complications (ADA, 2015). Although the American Diabetes Association/European Association for the Study of Diabetes [ADA/EASD] guidelines have targeted an Hb A1c of less than 7 (Inzucchi et al, 2012), the recommendation by the American Association of Clinical Endocrinologists/American College of Endocrinology [AACE/ACE] (2009) is a primary glycemic goal of an A1c of 6.5%, which must be individualized for the patient. The DCCT (1993), the Stockholm Diabetes Study of type 1 diabetes (Reichard, Nilsson, & Rosenqvist, 1993), the UK Prospective Diabetes Study [UKPDS] (1998), as well as the Kumamoto study (Ohkubo et al, 1995) conclusively demonstrated that in patients with type 1 diabetes, the risk for development or progression of retinopathy, nephropathy, and neuropathy is reduced by intensive treatment regimens when compared with conventional regimens. New data support complete normalization of glycemic levels may prevent microvascular complications even in type 2 DM. This is especially important

Table 33–5 American Diabetes Association Treatment Targets for Persons With Diabetes

Hb A1c	<7%
Preprandial Plasma Glucose	80–130 mg/dL
2-hour Postprandial Plasma Glucose	<180 mg/dL
Blood Pressure	<140–150 systolic patients with DM and HTN <90 diastolic mm Hg all patients with DM <130 systolic may be appropriate for some patients
LDL	<100 mg/dL (not a target; level per highest risk)
Triglycerides	<150 mg/dL
HDL	>50 mg/dL
Excess Urinary Albumin Excretion	<30

Key Concepts in Setting Goals:

- Individualize goals
- Special considerations for children, pregnant women, and older adults
- Less intensive glycemic goals for patients with severe or frequent hypoglycemia
- More intensive glycemic goals may further reduce microvascular complications at the risk of increasing hypoglycemia
- Postprandial glucose may be targeted if Hb A1c goals are not met despite reaching preprandial glucose goals
- Lipid goals should follow ATP IV guideline based on risks; initial evaluation at age 40.

Source: Adapted from American Diabetes Association. (2015). Standards of medical care in diabetes

considering many patients are not diagnosed for years. The microvascular system is thereby exposed to the destructive influence of heightened glucose levels for a long time. Earlier, more aggressive therapy at the time of diagnosis has long-term impacts with an unanticipated decrease in microvascular complications when compared to the traditional "easing into" more complex therapeutic approach used in the past.

However, there is less compelling evidence to support macrovascular risk reduction and glycemic control in type 2 diabetes. Several recent studies on macrovascular complications (ACCORD, ADVANCE, VADT) have actually shown increased cardiovascular disease (CVD) mortality in patients who were on the intensive control arm of the study in which the Hb A1c target was 6% (ADVANCE Collaborative Group, 2008; Duckworth, Abraira, & Moritz, 2009; Riddle et al, 2010). Because patients in all three trials had long-standing diabetes and either CVD or risk factors suggesting the presence of atherosclerosis, glycemic targets in the 6.4% to 6.9% range may play a greater role before macrovascular disease is well developed and a minimal or no role when it is advanced.

The ACCORD, ADVANCE, and the VADT studies were all large randomized controlled trials that did not conclude

tight glycemic control resulted in a reduction in cardiovascular events. The current theory is that early intervention may be the key; the UKPDS and the DCCT interventions were conducted early in the diabetes disease process, whereas the latter studies were conducted in patients who had longer durations of diabetes and preexisting illnesses. It should be noted that the ADVANCE trial did show evidence of benefits on microvascular and neuropathic complications. The ACCORD was stopped prematurely due to an increase in mortality in the control group.

APPROPRIATE TREATMENT

Initial Assessment

The initial assessment for patients with diabetes is complex and includes an extensive history about symptoms of the disease and the chronic complications associated with diabetes, current drugs being taken including over-the-counter (OTC) drugs, and alternative therapies that might affect glucose levels, family history of diabetes, CVD, cerebrovascular disease, or dyslipidemia, gestational history, and alcohol or drug use. Especially critical is assessment of risk factors for CVD, including smoking, hypertension, or dyslipidemia. After a thorough physical examination, which includes an inspection of the feet, laboratory data are collected. The results of this assessment will determine whether intensive or conventional therapy for glycemic control is better and whether treatment or referral for complications should be started early.

Setting a Glycemic Target

Many studies have shown that treatment regimens that reduce average Hb A1c <7% are associated with fewer long-term microvascular and neuropathic complications (ADA, 2015). For selected patients, a lower goal of 6.5% can be suggested if it can be achieved without significant hypoglycemia or other adverse effects of treatment. Such patients might include those with short-term duration of diabetes, long life expectancy, and no significant CVD (ADA, 2015). Glycemic targets recommended by the ADA and key concepts in setting these goals are shown in Table 33-5. Less stringent glycemic targets are recommended for patients with long-standing diabetes and/or advanced macrovascular and microvascular complications; older adults (65 years or older) in whom hypoglycemic awareness may be suppressed; children under 13 years; those with extensive comorbid conditions; those with severe or frequent hypoglycemia; and those with limited life expectancies of 5 to 15 years (ADA, 2015; ADA/EASD, 2012). Correlation between A1c levels and mean plasma glucose levels are shown in Table 33-6. Goals for children were tightened in 2014. The old goals of 8.5% for kids under 6, <8% for those 6–12 years of age and <7.5% for teens 13–19 have been supplanted with the target of <7.5% (ADA). Of course, individualization may be required based on the risks of hypoglycemia and comorbidities.

Table 33–6   Correlation Between Hb A1c Level and Mean Plasma Glucose Level

Hemoglobin A1c Levels	Mean Plasma Glucose (mg/dL)
6	126
7	154
8	183
9	212
10	240
11	269
12	290

Source: ADA. (2015). Standards of medical care for patients with diabetes mellitus.

Lifestyle Modifications

The incidence of DM and the incidence of obesity in the United States are increasing at approximately the same rate. This increased incidence of obesity is a primary culprit in the DM epidemic. Evidence from the USDPP (2002; 2003) found that even modest lifestyle changes, including eating less fat, modest weight loss of ~7% of body weight, and exercising 150 minutes weekly, cut the incidence of diabetes dramatically. Two studies of lifestyle modification have shown persistent reduction in the rate of conversion of pre-diabetes to type 2 diabetes in follow-up at 3 and 14 years' post-intervention (Li et al, 2008; Lindstrom et al, 2006). The recent questioning of dietary fat guidelines deals with a quality of evidence argument (Harcombe et al, 2014). There is a much evidence that reduction in fat has led to better outcomes in diabetes; therefore, it is suggested not to alter current therapeutic guidance until the national guideline authors make that suggestion.

Current ADA guidelines (2015) continue to support lifestyle changes that include a modest weight loss of 7% and increasing physical activity to 150 minutes of moderate-level cardiovascular exercise per week. Patients with pre-diabetes should receive an individualized consultation with a CDE or dietitian to provide guidance in healthy food choices, increasing physical activity, and moderate weight loss. Metformin therapy to prevent type 2 DM should be considered in those with IGT, IFG, or an Hb A1c of 5.7% to 6.4%, especially for those individuals with BMI greater than 35, less than 60 years of age, and women with prior GDM (ADA, 2015). Individuals with pre-diabetes should be reassessed at least annually for the presence of DM (ADA, 2015).

Lifestyle modifications should always be addressed with patients upon diagnosis of diabetes or pre-diabetes. To make these modifications more acceptable to many persons, it is suggested to place an emphasis on altered eating patterns, not "dieting." The traditional mantra of "diet and exercise" should be replaced with "exercise first" intervention. Severe dieting can create a loss of muscle (see below). Approximately 10% of patients with type 2 achieve glycemic targets with lifestyle modifications alone. All patients with DM should have an individualized consultation with a CDE for diabetes self-management education (DSME) to address lifestyle and behavior changes, which include:

- physical activity, healthy eating, tobacco cessation, weight management, effective coping
- disease self-management, which includes medication-taking management and self-monitoring of glucose and blood pressure when appropriate
- prevention of complications, including foot inspection; screening for eye, foot, and renal complications; and immunizations

Patients with pre-diabetes or diabetes should have individualized Medical Nutrition Therapy (MNT) through consultation with a registered dietitian familiar with the components of diabetes. Goals of MNT include the following:

- Attain and maintain recommended metabolic outcomes, including glucose and Hb A1c level; low-density lipoprotein (LDL) cholesterol, HDL cholesterol, and triglyceride levels; BP; and body weight.
- Modify nutrient intake as appropriate for the prevention and treatment of obesity, dyslipidemia, CVD, HTN, and nephropathy.
- Address individual nutritional needs, taking into consideration personal and cultural preferences and lifestyle while respecting the individual's wishes and willingness to change.
- For youth with type 1 diabetes, provide adequate energy to ensure normal growth and development and integrate insulin regimens into usual eating and physical activity patterns.
- For youth with type 2 diabetes, facilitate dietary changes that reduce insulin resistance.
- For pregnant and lactating women, provide adequate energy and nutrients needed for optimal outcomes.
- For older adults, provide for the nutritional and psychosocial needs appropriate to their age.

Regular exercise has been shown to improve glucose control, reduce cardiovascular risk factors, contribute to weight loss, and improve overall well-being. Exercise may also prevent type 2 diabetes in high-risk individuals (ADA, 2015). A regular physical activity program is recommended for all patients with diabetes who are capable of participating. Adaptations should be made if complications are present. Recommendations for patients with diabetes are moderate to intensive aerobic activity (50% to 70% of maximum heart rate) at least 150 minutes a week and resistance training at least 2 times a week unless it is contraindicated (ADA, 2015). Resistance exercise improves insulin sensitivity almost as much as aerobic exercise. Interval training of alternating 3 minute bursts of fast and slow walking may be more beneficial than walking at a steady rate (Karstoft et al, 2013). Before beginning an exercise program, patients should be evaluated for macro- and microvascular changes that may be worsened by exercise. A graded exercise test is appropriate only for symptomatic patients and those with cardiovascular disease who are older than 35 years, or older than 25 years with type 2 diabetes of more than 10 years' duration, or type 1 diabetes of more than 15 years' duration; those with any additional risk factor for coronary heart disease; or those with microvascular disease, peripheral vascular disease, or autonomic neuropathy. Exercise is not recommended if the patient is in poor glycemic control.

Use of tobacco products is a concern in individuals with diabetes who are at higher risk for morbidity and premature death associated with the development of macrovascular complications. Smoking is also related to the premature development of microvascular complications in diabetes. Smoking cessation is a necessary lifestyle modification that should be addressed with all patients with diabetes. Table 33-7 lists the appropriate lifestyle modifications.

All members of the diabetes health-care team should be knowledgeable and supportive of the patient making lifestyle changes. Web sites that provide low- or no-cost diabetes meal planning and self-management educational materials include the American Diabetes Association (www.diabetes.org), National Institute of Diabetes and Digestive and Kidney Diseases (www.niddk.nih.gov), and the Academy of Nutrition and Dietetics (www.eatright.org/catalogue). Many of these resources are available in Spanish. Table 33-7 provides a summary of these recommendations.

Immunizations

Immunizations are safe and effective in preventing communicable diseases. People with diabetes and other chronic illnesses are at higher risk of mortality and morbidity from common communicable diseases than the general population. Therefore, it is recommended that all people with

Table 33–7   Lifestyle Modifications for Patients With Diabetes

Nutrition	
Type 1	• Eat at consistent times synchronized with the action of the insulin preparation and the consumption of carbohydrate.
	• Eat a bedtime snack consisting of 1–2 carbohydrate servings (15–30 g).
Type 1 and type 2	• Moderate caloric restriction if needed.
	• Space meals, spreading nutrient intake, especially carbohydrates, throughout the day.
	• Eat on a regular schedule.
	• Patients using insulin are encouraged to eat at consistent times synchronized with the action of the insulin preparation.
	• In the presence of reduced kidney function, total protein intake of 0.7–0.8 g/kg/d with 10%–20% of caloric intake from protein.
	• 7% of calories from saturated fats and minimum trans fat intake; the lessened attention to cholesterol intake for the general population may not apply to those with glucose metabolism issues.
	• Total carbohydrate content is more important than type of carbohydrate. The goal for most patients is 3–4 carbohydrate servings (45–60 g) per meal. 1–2 snacks per day may also be indicated and should include 1–2 carbohydrate servings (15–30 g).
	• Healthy eating to include carbohydrate intake from vegetables, fruits, whole grains, legumes, and dairy products should be advised over intake from other carbohydrate sources, especially those that contain added fats, sugars, or sodium.
	• Low-glycemic-load foods should not be emphasized over a well-balanced diet (Sacks et al, 2014). Fiber recommendations are the same as for persons without diabetes. High-fiber content in meals may slow the rate for glucose rise postprandially.
	• Sodium restriction, if any, is related to any concomitant hypertension.
	• Abstention from alcohol is advised. If consumed, it is best done with meals. No more than 2 drinks of alcohol/d for men and no more than 1/d for women (1 alcoholic beverage = 12 oz beer, 5 oz wine, or 1.5 oz distilled spirits).
Exercise	
Both types	• Exercise affects uptake of glucose by muscle and fat tissue and can affect plasma glucose levels. Time the exercise to coincide with caloric intake. May need to decrease basal and bolus insulin for extended exercise (e.g., all-day hike, ski, etc.). Persons with type 1 should exercise at the same time daily.
	• Carbohydrate-based food should be readily available during and after exercise.
	• Increase aerobic activity to 50%–70% of maximum heart rate for 30 min 5 days/wk; goal is 150 min/week. Obese or low-activity patients may need to start with as little as 3 min of activity/d and increase the activity by 1 min/d until the desired 20–30 min is achieved.
	• Resistance training at least 2×/wk is recommended.
	• Do not exercise if ketones are present. Monitor blood glucose before and after exercise. If BG ≤100 mg/dL, eat snack containing 10–30 g carbohydrate.
	• Patients should learn their own glycemic response to different exercise conditions. They should keep records to understand their glycemic response.
	• Reduction of sedentary time to less than 90 minutes at a time (ADA, 2015).
Weight Loss	
Type 1 and type 2	• Weight loss is recommended for all overweight or obese individuals who have or are at risk for diabetes.
	• Low-carbohydrate, low-fat, calorie-restricted, or Mediterranean diets may be effective for short-term weight loss (up to 2 yr).
	• Monitor lipid profiles, renal function, protein intake (in those with nephropathy), and adjust hypoglycemic therapy as needed for patients on low CHO diets.
	• Physical activity and behavior modification are important components of weight-loss programs and are most helpful in maintenance of weight loss.
	• Moderate weight loss (7% of body weight), regardless of starting weight, has been shown to affect insulin sensitivity.

diabetes be immunized according to the following (ADA, 2015):

- Annual influenza vaccinations for all persons greater than 6 months of age.
- Pneumococcal polysaccharide vaccine should be given to all patients greater than 2 years of age. This should be administered as a one-time vaccination for those greater than 64 years if previously immunized if they were less than 65 and the vaccine was administered greater than 5 years ago.
- Hepatitis B vaccine should be given to all unvaccinated adults 19 to 59 years of age; consider vaccinating adults greater than 60.

Considerations in Special Populations

Children

Since the majority of all newly diagnosed cases of type 1 diabetes occur in patients younger than age 18 years, care of these patients requires integration of diabetes management with the growth and development needs of children, adolescents, and their families. Young patients with diabetes are best cared for by a team that can deal with these special needs. Glycemic targets may need to be modified because children younger than 7 years lack the cognitive capacity to recognize and respond to hypoglycemic signals. Considerations for level of control also should be undertaken with caution in children 2 to 7 years because hypoglycemia may impair normal brain development, but hyperglycemia is also neurotoxic. Overly aggressive dietary manipulation can contribute to lack of adherence, especially in adolescents. Schools and day-care settings must be involved in the treatment of diabetes, often participating in the administration of drugs. Treatment regimens must take all of these needs into account.

Children with type 1 diabetes also have a high risk for CVD and other complications from DM. The number of children with type 2 diabetes is currently too small to make a statement about their risk, but CVD is a strong risk factor in adults and likely exists for children as well. Management of complications is discussed in the Hyperlipidemia section.

Children may also develop type 2 diabetes. Prevention of the development of diabetes from pre-diabetes must take highest priority in children and should focus on decreasing the risk, incidence, and consequences of type 2 diabetes, especially in high-risk ethnic groups. Modifiable risks for type 2 diabetes in children that can be addressed with primary prevention include the prevention of obesity and the promotion of breastfeeding. The use of alcohol, tobacco, and drugs should be evaluated in all children and adolescents on diagnosis and reevaluated at every visit. Alcohol may increase hypoglycemic episodes caused by sulfonylureas or insulin and increase the risk of lactic acidosis in patients who use metformin. Family support is essential to the child or adolescent with type 2 diabetes. The whole family should be involved in dietary and activity changes, prevention of complications, as well as drug therapy management and self-monitoring of blood glucose.

For children, the goal weight should be the expected BMI for their age. Weight stabilization rather than weight loss is recommended for prepubertal children. Children who are morbidly obese may be referred to a specialist in weight reduction or a multidisciplinary child obesity clinic.

The BP goal is less than the 90th percentile on the basis of height and weight standards. Fasting lipid levels are best obtained after the initial metabolic stabilization (1 to 3 months after diagnosis). The lipid goals are LDL less than 100 mg/dL and total cholesterol less than 170 mg/dL. Treatment of children with dyslipidemia is discussed in Chapter 39 and hypertension is discussed in Chapter 40.

The Hb A1c goal for children depends on age and type of DM. Currently the only drugs approved for diabetes in children are metformin and insulin. Liver function tests should be performed before initiation of oral therapy. If multiple drugs are required, referral to a pediatric endocrinologist may be necessary.

Older Adults

Older adults (older than 65 years) are more likely to have type 2 diabetes and use oral agents to treat their disease. They may suffer severe consequences from a hypoglycemic episode, especially patients with significant atherosclerosis who may be vulnerable to permanent injury. Weight loss in overweight older adults should be carefully evaluated. In this population, low body weight has been associated with greater morbidity and mortality. Exercise training can significantly reduce the decline in maximal aerobic capacity that occurs with age, improve risk factors for atherosclerosis, slow the decline in age-related lean body mass, decrease central adiposity, and improve insulin sensitivity; all are beneficial in the older adult with diabetes.

Glycemia, glucose homeostasis, and the prevalence of diabetes all increase with age; therefore, this should be taken into consideration as glycemic targets for older adults are identified. Pani and colleagues (2008) examined a large cohort of patients without diabetes and found a positive correlation between increased Hb A1c levels and age. Current guidelines state that glycemic targets for older adults are generally more relaxed than younger adults. An Hb A1c of 7.5% is appropriate for the patient if cognitively intact, functional, and with a good life expectancy. The glycemic target can be less than 8.0% for those with complex needs such as multiple co-morbidities, ADL impacts, and mild cognitive impairment. They are further relaxed to less than 8.5% with moderate to severe cognitive impact, two or more ADL deficiencies, in skilled nursing facilities, and with end-stage chronic illness (ADA, 2015). There needs to be awareness of the risk for hypoglycemic and hyperglycemic complications (ADA). The presence of CVD risk factors should also be evaluated. Current research shows that more benefit may be received from the treatment of CVD and hypertension in older adults with DM than strict glycemic control. Although it is important and necessary to prevent complications from poor glycemic control, it is prudent to find the balance between adequate glycemic control and minimizing episodes of hypoglycemia.

The risk for hypoglycemic episodes in the older adult and the lack of hypoglycemic awareness due to physical, cognitive, or pharmacological effects should be assessed regularly. Recent studies have noted that ED visits for hypoglycemia outnumber those for hyperglycemia. Additionally, the median time from first hypoglycemic episode to a CV event was 1.5 years without consideration of prior CV health (Khunti et al, 2015). Sulfonylureas may produce severe hypoglycemia. Second-generation drugs are less likely than first-generation drugs to have this adverse reaction. Glimepiride (Amaryl), a third-generation sulfonylurea, is least likely to cause this adverse reaction. Glyburide is the most likely to cause hypoglycemia and is not recommended for the elderly. TZDs should not be used in patients with heart failure because of the fluid-retention side effect. Metformin is often contraindicated in older adults because they may have renal insufficiency or heart failure. Alpha-glucosidase inhibitors, which are not part of the usual algorithm, have a good safety profile in this population, but are not well tolerated. The use of insulin requires that the patient or caregiver have good vision and motor skills and be cognitively intact. Regardless of the treatment regimen, all medications should be started at the lowest possible dose and titrated according to patient response and tolerance (ADA, 2015).

Race and Ethnic Groups

While minority populations are more likely to be diagnosed with DM, the rates of complications vary by ethnicity and race. According to the CDC, the age-adjusted percentage for Hispanics with diagnosed diabetes in the United States was 6.3% in 1997 and 12.8% in 2012. For that same time period, the age-adjusted percentage of diagnosed diabetes was 7.6% for whites, 13.2% for non-Hispanic blacks, and 9% among Asians. American Indians/Alaska Natives was 15.9% (CDC, 2014). These percentages are further broken down by regions and specific subsets of these populations. Interested providers are directed to the CDC report.

There are currently no specific guidelines addressing treatment for ethnicity or racial groups. The AACE evaluated the differences in diabetes presentation and complications across ethnic groups (Bloomgarden, 2003). Asian populations, who have low rates of obesity, have high rates of diabetes and cardiovascular disease. This runs contrary to the typical picture of the type 2 patient being obese; therefore, providers are cautioned not to dismiss the differential when screening for risks. This is especially so, because normal-weight diabetics actually have higher all-cause mortality (Carnethon et al, 2012). The prevalence of diabetes appears to be higher in the migrant population. Despite low obesity rates, increased intra-abdominal fat showed stronger correlation with hypertension and dyslipidemia than did insulin sensitivity per se and was a marker for diabetes risk. The prevalence of cardiovascular disease may be associated with the higher total and LDL cholesterol, higher triglycerides, lower HDL, and higher concentrations of homocysteine and lipoprotein(a) found in persons of South Asian ethnicity. These data suggest that treatment of hypertension and dyslipidemia and lifestyle modification are also necessary in this population.

The SEARCH for Diabetes in Youth Study Group (Liu et al, 2009) looked at Asian and Pacific Islanders younger than 20 years of age. This study found that most participants in the study who had type 2 diabetes were obese (Asian 71% and Pacific Islanders 100%), with a mean BMI greater than 33 kg/m^2. Of those with type 1 diabetes, Pacific Islanders were more likely to be obese, with a mean BMI of 26. The incidence of type 2 diabetes in these populations was almost double that of type 1 diabetes. The study group's recommendation is that a stronger public health effort needs to be focused on these youths in the area of type 2 DM and obesity.

Hispanics in the United States have a high incidence of obesity, high triglycerides, low HDL-C, hypertension, and high FPG. Predictors of conversion from pre-diabetes to diabetes in this population are high LDL and triglycerides and low HDL, high BP, and high BMI. Treatment of hypertension and dyslipidemia, and lifestyle modifications related to nutrition and weight loss are critical in this group. Metformin is indicated as an early intervention in this population to prevent conversion from pre-diabetes to diabetes.

African Americans have a greater prevalence of diabetes and hypertension than other ethnic groups. Treatment of both issues is essential in this population. Compared to others, African American adolescents have had a huge increase in development of type 2 diabetes. African American children have higher insulin secretion both before and during puberty and lower insulin sensitivity during adolescence. If the extrapolation is made that African American adults may continue this lower insulin sensitivity, then selecting drugs that improve insulin sensitivity to treat type 2 diabetes in African Americans of all ages is appropriate. Drugs with this characteristic include metformin and pioglitazone. Metformin is also a drug of choice related to the increasing prevalence of obesity among African Americans, particularly women.

The SEARCH study with African American youth (Mayer-Davis et al, 2009) looked at children from infancy to 19 years. This study found that the incidence of type 1 diabetes was high in this group, especially for those older than age 10. The study also found that both types of diabetes substantially affect adolescents in this ethnic group. Among adolescents with either type of diabetes, more than 90% were overweight or obese and 60% of those with type 2 diabetes came from households with an annual income of less than $25,000. Although lifestyle modifications are a major emphasis in this group, cost variables should especially be taken into account when choosing any drug for this population.

According to the CDC (2014), 24.1% of American Indians in the southwestern United States and 6% of Alaska Natives age 20 years or older who received care from Indian Health Services had diagnosed diabetes. The vast majority of youth had type 2 diabetes. These young people are likely to have poor glycemic control, a high prevalence of unhealthy behaviors, and evidence of a severely depressed mood. They have more metabolic factors associated with obesity and insulin resistance (abdominal fat, dyslipidemia, and a higher albumin-to-creatinine ratio). Intervention efforts should be targeted at primary prevention and efforts to prevent or delay the development of chronic complications associated with metabolic factors. Failure to treat the depression will undermine any effort to increase self-management.

In non-Hispanic white youth, there are more cases of type 1 than type 2 diabetes; they have the highest rate of new cases of type 1 diabetes than any other group (CDC, 2014). In the SEARCH study, it was reported that 40% of the subjects in this study had elevated LDL echolesterol and less than 3% met traditional recommendations for the intake of saturated fat (Bell et al, 2009). Of those with type 1 diabetes, 18% were smokers, and 26% of those with type 2 smoked. Lifestyle and cardiometabolic risk factors require attention in this population.

Pharmacological Management

Diabetes is a lifelong disease that may have few symptoms until organ damage occurs. For this reason, health-care providers often find themselves prescribing lifestyle modifications or drugs to treat a problem that patients have no clear evidence that they have and at a point when they may not feel acutely ill. The choice of treatment should be low cost, limited in complexity, have the fewest possible adverse reactions and should be chosen based on the type of diabetes, the desired glycemic target, the severity of hyperglycemia, and specific patient variables.

Type 1 Diabetes

Patients with type 1 diabetes require insulin. The pattern of administration of insulin is based on the patient's blood glucose, dietary, lifestyle and exercise patterns. Regardless of the type of insulin used, appropriate therapy should mimic endogenous insulin secretion delivered before meals or to correct hyperglycemia. This can be achieved by intensive insulin therapy, split-mixed insulin therapy, or continuous subcutaneous insulin injections (CSII) (ADA, 2015). An insulin analog is recommended, especially if hypoglycemia is a problem for the patient.

The total daily insulin requirement is 0.3 to 0.5 units/kg body weight/d with titration to glycemic targets. Higher doses may be indicated during an acute illness. Adjustments should be made after reviewing patterns of control over at least 3 days, taking food intake and activity into consideration. Hypoglycemia is addressed first and then hyperglycemia. Make adjustments up or down in increments of 1 unit until sensitivity to insulin is well understood (Texas Diabetes Council, 2010; Sisson & Cornell, 2011).

In the split-mixed regimen, insulin is given 2 to 3 times daily by splitting the dose—two-thirds given in the morning and one-third given in the evening. Two-thirds of the total daily dose (TDD) is administered before breakfast using a ratio of 1:2 rapid-acting (RAI) or short-acting insulin (SAI) to intermediate-acting insulin (IAI); one-third of the TDD is given at bedtime using a 1:1 or 1:2 ratio of RAI or SAI to IAI (Texas Diabetes Council, 2010; Sisson & Cornell, 2011). Another possibility is to use premixed 70/30 insulin with two-thirds of the dose in the morning and one-third of the dose in the evening.

When using the intensive insulin therapy approach, three to four injections are administered per day. This regimen involves 1:1 basal bolus dosing with LAI basal administered either at breakfast or bedtime with either RAI or SAI bolus doses before each meal. Prandial insulin should be matched to carbohydrate intake, preprandial blood glucose levels, and anticipated activity. Patients who are intelligent, motivated, and reliable can be taught to regulate their blood sugar with intensive control. Less capable patients risk hypoglycemic reactions on this regimen and might not be appropriate candidates or might need higher fasting blood sugar targets than more capable patients (Table 33-8).

Bolus premeal insulin doses should include the following:

- Insulin to cover carbohydrate ingested: 1 unit RAI covers 500/TDD g carbohydrate from meals.
- Additional insulin to correct high SMBG: 1 unit RAI lowers PG by approximately 1,800/TDD mg/dL (regular lowers PG by ~1,500/TDD).
- Adjustments should be made for exercise. Decrease 1 unit for every 30 minutes of moderate-intensity exercise (Texas Diabetes Council, 2010).

Initial and annual assessments of blood pressure (BP) and lipids are also done. If hypertension or hyperlipidemia are found, drugs to treat these conditions are also started early in diabetes management. Screening for other autoimmune disorders, such as thyroid dysfunction, celiac disease, and vitamin B_{12} deficiency should be done based on signs and symptoms.

Figure 33-2 shows the algorithm for management of type 1 diabetes. See Table 33-9 for commonly used insulin regimens.

Table 33–8 Basal Bolus Insulin

Rapid-Acting (RAI)	Short-Acting (SAI)	Intermediate-Acting (IAI)	Long-Acting (LAI)	Mix
Bolus	Bolus	Basal	Basal	Basal
• Correction • Preprandial	• Correction • Preprandial	• a.m./p.m. breakfast and dinner	• HS or breakfast	• a.m./p.m. breakfast and dinner
3–4×/d	3–4×/d	2×/d	1×d	2×d
Novolog Humalog	Regular	NPH	Lantus Levimir	70/30 (IAI/SAI) 50/50 (IAI/SAI) 75/25 (IAK/RAI)

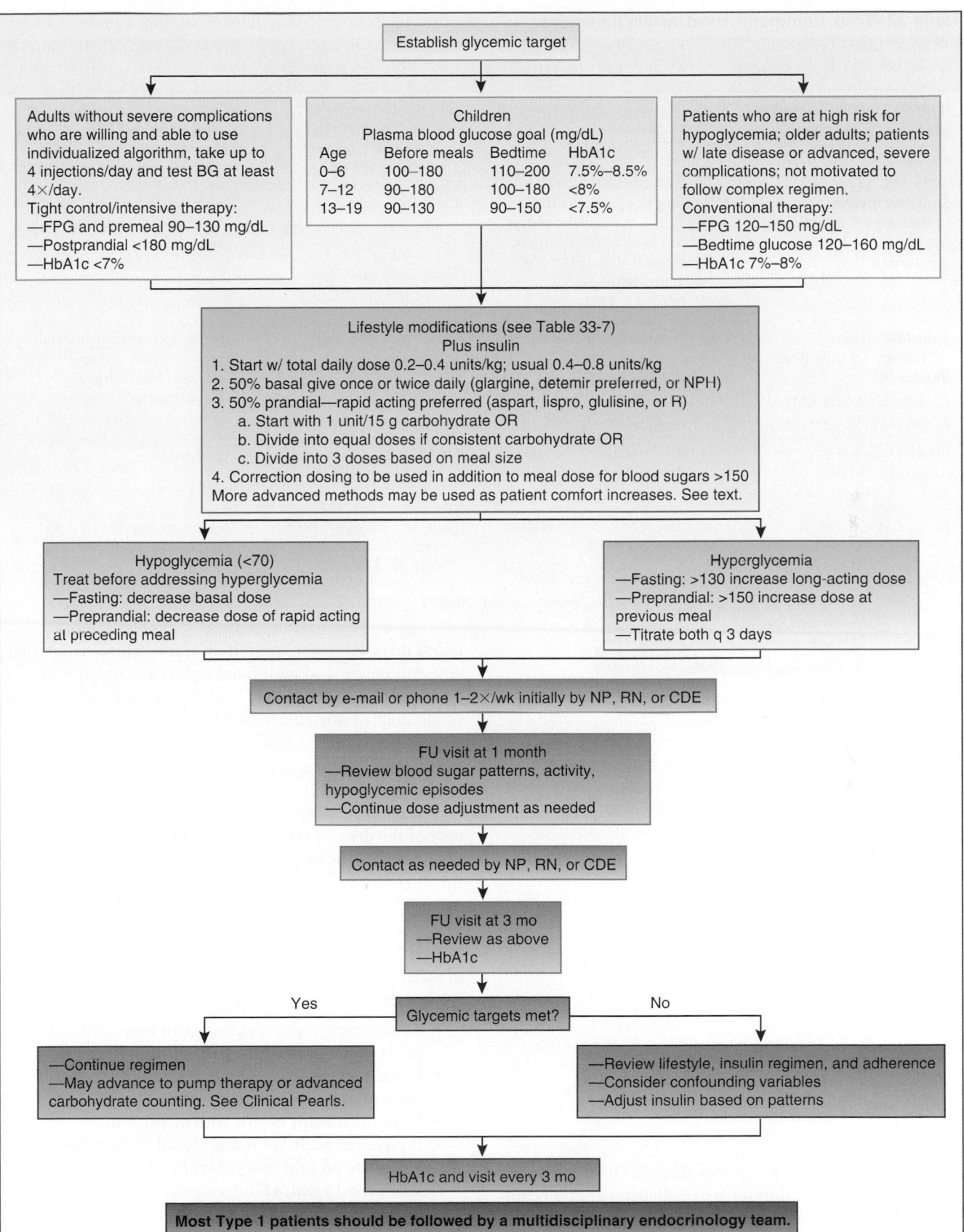

Figure 33–2. Treatment algorithm for type 1 diabetes.

Table 33–9 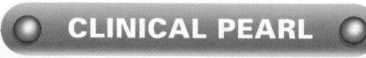 **Commonly Used Insulin Regimens**

Insulin Therapy Type Insulin	Schedule	Advantages	Disadvantages
Intensive Insulin Therapy Basal = LAI Bolus = RAI	Basal at breakfast or bedtime, or basal at evening meal Start 0.3–0/5 units/kg/d	Consistent insulin dose throughout the day with basal; bolus insulin only when food present	Requires 4 injections and pre-meal + bedtime SMBG. LAI not compatible with other insulin; requires separate syringe.
Split-Mix Insulin Therapy—3 injections Basal= LAI (or IAI) Bolus = RAI	Long-acting to = 50% TDD HS; 50% TDD RAI remainder of dose of mixed insulin at breakfast and evening meal. If using IAI, give before breakfast and HS. Start 0.3–0.5 units/kg/d	Consistent insulin dose throughout day with basal	Glargine not compatible with other insulin; needs separate syringe. Premeal SMBG
Split-Mix Insulin Therapy—2 injections Basal = IAI Basal/Bolus = SAI or RAI mix 2:1 ratio a.m., 1:1 ratio p.m.	Basal at breakfast and dinner or HS; bolus before each meal. 2/3 NPH, 1/3 SAI or RAI *or* Premix 70/30, 75/25, or 50/50	Consistent insulin dose throughout day	Multiple injections required and premeal SMBG. IAI may reduce risk of nocturnal hypoglycemia.
Basal = IAI or LAI 3	Start with 6–10 units or 0.1–0.2 unit/kg body weight/d at breakfast or HS to initiate therapy.	Start with low dose to reduce hypoglycemic risk.	**Type 2 only**
Basal = LAI + oral agent	Long-acting at bedtime or breakfast; oral agent 1–2 × daily	Once-daily dosing of insulin. Consistent insulin dose throughout day.	Requires injection as well as oral agent. **Type 2 only**

In any of the regimens using fast-acting insulin, rapid-acting insulin may be substituted.

● CLINICAL PEARL ●

Type I Diabetes Treatment
- Most patients should see an endocrinologist and diabetes treatment team; treatment can be challenging and a team approach works best. Consultation with a Certified Diabetes Educator is a must.
- Make small changes gradually with close follow-up (every 1 to 2 wk) until adequate control is achieved.
- Ongoing follow-up has been shown to be very beneficial; this can be done by phone or electronically.
- It is normal to have wide variability in BGL even with adherence to the treatment plan. Variability does not necessarily mean nonadherence.
- Consistency in mealtimes, injection sites, and timing and frequency of exercise is vital.
- The treatment plan must be individualized with adjustments preplanned for anticipated sudden increases in physical activity such as summer sports camps or ski vacations.

Type 2 Diabetes

Type 2 diabetes can be a complex disease. Once a glycemic target is set, the algorithm for type 2 diabetes always begins with lifestyle modification and DSME. Intensive glycemic targets are often difficult to reach with lifestyle modifications alone, so monotherapy should be initiated after 3 months if there is no reduction in Hb A1c.

Using a stepped approach with the recommendations published by the ADA/EASD (2012), metformin is used initially unless there are major contraindications. Combination therapy with one or two additional agents are added if there is no reduction in the Hb A1c level in 3 months, with the goal of minimizing side effects (ADA, 2015). See Figure 33-3 for current treatment recommendations. Metformin should be continuously used regardless of the addition of other agents (Iznucchi et al, 2012).

The guidelines base the choice of a drug on the effectiveness of the drug in efficacy, reducing long-term complications, weight gain, major side effects, and expense. The ADA/EASD consensus document lists the various classes of antihyperglycemic drugs and provides information about these variables. Figure 33-3 shows the algorithm for management of type 2 diabetes. Please note Inzucchi published this prior to SGLT-2 medication inclusion into guidelines. The algorithm emphasizes the following:

- Achievement and maintenance of near normal glucose levels (Hb A1c less than 7%).
- Initial therapy with lifestyle interventions, which include diet, exercise, and education.
- First-line therapy begins with metformin.
- If glycemic goals are not achieved or sustained within 3 months on oral monotherapy at maximum dose, a second oral agent, a GLP-1 agonist, DPP-4 inhibitor, or insulin should be added (ADA, 2015).
- Early addition of insulin therapy in patients who do not meet target goals.

At some point in their disease, many patients with type 2 diabetes will require the addition of insulin and can use a variety of insulin regimens; many patients can be successfully

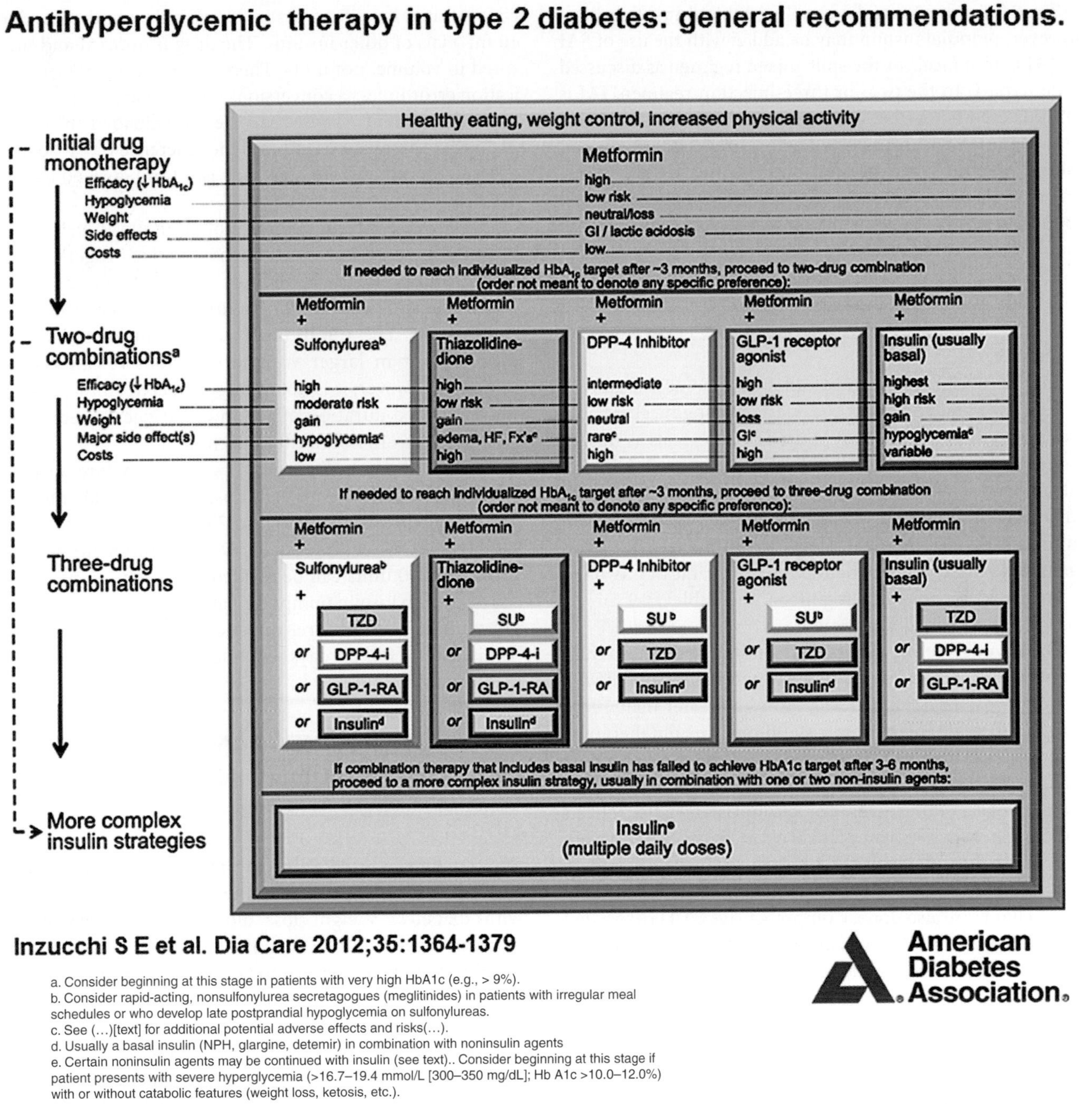

Antihyperglycemic therapy in type 2 diabetes: general recommendations.

Healthy eating, weight control, increased physical activity

Initial drug monotherapy

Metformin

Efficacy (↓ HbA₁c)	high	
Hypoglycemia	low risk	
Weight	neutral/loss	
Side effects	GI / lactic acidosis	
Costs	low	

If needed to reach individualized HbA₁c target after ~3 months, proceed to two-drug combination (order not meant to denote any specific preference):

Two-drug combinations[a]

	Metformin + Sulfonylurea[b]	Metformin + Thiazolidine-dione	Metformin + DPP-4 Inhibitor	Metformin + GLP-1 receptor agonist	Metformin + Insulin (usually basal)
Efficacy (↓ HbA₁c)	high	high	intermediate	high	highest
Hypoglycemia	moderate risk	low risk	low risk	low risk	high risk
Weight	gain	gain	neutral	loss	gain
Major side effect(s)	hypoglycemia[c]	edema, HF, Fx's[e]	rare[e]	GI[e]	hypoglycemia[c]
Costs	low	high	high	high	variable

If needed to reach individualized HbA₁c target after ~3 months, proceed to three-drug combination (order not meant to denote any specific preference):

Three-drug combinations

Metformin + Sulfonylurea[b] +	Metformin + Thiazolidine-dione +	Metformin + DPP-4 Inhibitor +	Metformin + GLP-1 receptor agonist +	Metformin + Insulin (usually basal) +
TZD	SU[b]	SU[b]	SU[b]	TZD
or DPP-4-i	or DPP-4-i	or TZD	or TZD	or DPP-4-i
or GLP-1-RA	or GLP-1-RA	or Insulin[d]	or Insulin[d]	or GLP-1-RA
or Insulin[d]	or Insulin[d]			

If combination therapy that includes basal insulin has failed to achieve HbA1c target after 3-6 months, proceed to a more complex insulin strategy, usually in combination with one or two non-insulin agents:

More complex insulin strategies

Insulin[e] (multiple daily doses)

Inzucchi S E et al. Dia Care 2012;35:1364-1379

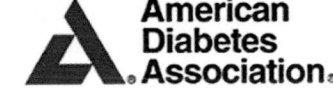

a. Consider beginning at this stage in patients with very high HbA1c (e.g., > 9%).
b. Consider rapid-acting, nonsulfonylurea secretagogues (meglitinides) in patients with irregular meal schedules or who develop late postprandial hypoglycemia on sulfonylureas.
c. See (…)[text] for additional potential adverse effects and risks(…).
d. Usually a basal insulin (NPH, glargine, detemir) in combination with noninsulin agents
e. Certain noninsulin agents may be continued with insulin (see text).. Consider beginning at this stage if patient presents with severe hyperglycemia (>16.7–19.4 mmol/L [300–350 mg/dL]; Hb A1c >10.0–12.0%) with or without catabolic features (weight loss, ketosis, etc.).

Figure 33–3. General recommendations for antihyperglycemic therapy in type 2 diabetes. *Inzucchi et al (2012). Management of hyperglycemia in type 2 diabetes: A patient centered approach. Position Statement of the American Diabetes Association (ADA) and the European Association for the Study of Diabetes (EASD). Diabetes Care, 35(6), 1364–1379.*

managed on one injection of basal insulin alone, but because of the progressive nature of the disease, the addition of prandial insulin may be needed (Inzucchi et al, 2012). The likelihood of insulin requirements over time needs to be discussed early in the disease process with all type 2 patients. Once-daily injections, split mix, or intensive insulin therapy may be used. See Table 33-9 for common insulin regimens.

When initiating insulin in type 2, LAI or IAI is administered in a single dose at bedtime or in the morning; the typical starting dose is 6 to 10 units or 0.1 to 0.2 units/kg body weight/d. Larger doses, as high as 0.7 to 2.5 units/kg body weight/d, may be needed due to the presence of insulin resistance. The single dose is usually given in conjunction with one or more oral agents. The dose is increased by 2 units every 2 to 3 days until daily FPG levels are consistently within the glycemic goal range. If the FPG is greater than 180, the dose can be increased by 6 units every 3 days. If hypoglycemia occurs, the dose can be reduced by 4 units or 10%, whichever is greater. Once the FPG is in target range, testing of blood glucose before each meal will help determine the dose of additional injections of insulin to be added.

Type 2 can be controlled well with basal insulin alone; however, prandial insulin may be added with the use of SAI or RAI before meals or the split-mixed regimen as discussed under type 1. In the two- or three-injection regimen, IAI is administered before breakfast and before the evening meal or at bedtime with an SAI given before breakfast and dinner, using a 2:1 ratio in the morning and 1:1 ratio in the evening. LAI may also be used daily or twice daily at breakfast and bedtime. Premixed agents may also be used. Starting dose should be 0.3 to 0.5 units/kg body weight/d; if the current dose is greater than 0.5 units/kg body weight/d, use 80% of once-daily insulin and divide as two-thirds IAI and one-third RAI or one-half LAI with one-half RAI (Texas Diabetes Council, 2010).

In intensive insulin therapy, a 1:1 basal bolus is used with an LAI once daily or IAI at breakfast, evening meal, or bedtime with either an SAI or RAI used before meals as in type 1. The same guidelines should be used for premeal dosage calculations. The starting dose should be 0.3 to 0.5 units/kg body weight daily. The advent of glucometers that have an automatic insulin dose calculator might make this option available to many more patients who are unable or unwilling to undertake any of these regimens. See Table 33-9 for the commonly used insulin regimens.

Oral hypoglycemic agents have limited ability to reduce hyperglycemia; therefore, patients who initially present with blood glucose levels above 300, Hb A1c greater than 10, or with significant hyperglycemic symptoms, insulin therapy is strongly recommended to lower PG to less than 180 before oral agents are begun. This treatment is mandatory in the presence of catabolic features or ketonuria; the latter reflects profound insulin deficiency (Inzucchi et al, 2012). Treatment options are once-daily insulin or intensive insulin therapy.

As with type 1 diabetes, initial and annual assessments of BP and lipids are also done. Comprehensive CVD risk reduction should be a major focus of treatment, and drugs to treat these conditions are also started early in diabetes management. The guidelines for both BP and lipid control are discussed in the Complications section. A long time "Rule of 15" can be taught to reliable patients for milder hypoglycemia episodes. They should take 15 gm of carbohydrate and recheck their sugars in 15 minutes.

Severe Insulin Resistance Therapy: U-500 Insulin

In cases of long-term DM, the volume of insulin required in each injection can become larger and larger. The obesity epidemic has accelerated the number of patients who require larger doses for adequate control. In the rare cases when individual injections are over 200 units, the prescriber should consider a consultation with endocrinology to initiate use of a concentrated insulin. Typical insulin concentrations are 100 units per mL. A specialized insulin of 500 units per mL must be specially ordered from the manufacturer Eli Lilly.

Of key importance is understanding that the dosages are not simple arithmetic division of the U-100 doses by five. Presently, there are no insulin syringes for this concentration of insulin; therefore, a standard 1 cc (TB) syringe is used. The

concentrated insulin comes in 20 mL vials, not the standard 10 mL vials of other insulins. The drug is ordered and measured in volume, not units. There is significant risk of medication error unless a conversion chart is referenced for every dose adjustment. These can be downloaded from the Eli Lilly Web site. An example of the difference is that 50 units of U-500 is only 0.1 mL, 55 units is 0.11mL and 60 units is 0.12mL.

U-500 is a concentrated form of Humulin R insulin, but it cannot be used in IV titrations nor mixed together with other insulins like the U-100 formulation. Its onset is 30 to 45 minutes and peaks in 2 to 4 hours like its less concentrated counterpart. The duration of action can be the typical 8 hours, but in larger volume injections it can last for 24 hours; however, it is not to be considered a basal insulin. This extended duration of action can trigger severe hypoglycemia 15 to 18 hours after injection.

Concentrated insulin is given twice daily before breakfast and dinner if the standard daily dose is around 200 units/day. For patients who require 300 to 750 units daily, the U-500 can be dosed three times daily. Dose requirement between 750 and 2,000 units can be divided into 4 injections. U-500 can be used in insulin pumps for patients requiring 2,000 plus units a day. Manufacturer directions indicate the vial must be discarded after 31 days without regard to the amount of medication remaining.

PREVENTION AND MANAGEMENT OF COMPLICATIONS IN DIABETES

Obesity

Obesity contributes to diabetes by affecting insulin receptors, and it contributes to many of the complications associated with diabetes. Weight loss alone improves short-term glycemic levels and has the potential to improve long-term metabolic control. Metformin is the oral agent most associated with fostering weight loss and is the drug of choice in the treatment algorithm for patients with central obesity. The lack of weight gain associated with alpha-glucosidase inhibitors suggests that these drugs might also be helpful as adjunct therapy for patients with diabetes who are obese, but they are not currently included on the treatment algorithm. GLP-1 agonists, DPP-4 medications, and SGLT-2 medications have also been shown to promote weight loss or at least

On The Horizon | **U-300 INSULIN**

The FDA has just approved a U-300 insulin (Toujeo), which is a long-acting basal insulin with a lower glucose lowering effect per unit than glargine, but lower risks of hypoglycemia. Lower-volume injections will be beneficial. The precautions about mixing solutions in a syringe also pertain. This insulin uses units per dose like glargine; this is unlike the U-500 insulins, which are volume based.

not to contribute to weight gain. Sulfonylureas, TZDs, and insulin are associated with weight gain.

Post-bariatric surgical insulin and drug therapy requires specialty consultation. There can be wild swings in glucose levels. The six mini-meal dietary plan needs specific attention for insulin coverage that should be modified by the specialist. Many patients have a nausea and emesis pattern and dumping syndrome associated with initial overeating. It takes time to find a new rhythm. As the expected weight loss accelerates over time, the amount and degree of dose adjustments requires close coordination to avoid hypoglycemic episodes.

Concomitant disease processes also affect drug choice. Often these disease processes reflect target organ damage from diabetes. The pathophysiological changes associated with the disease process and/or the drugs commonly used to treat it contribute to determining the best drug therapy, especially for patients with type 2 diabetes. The ADA (2015) has specific recommendations for screening and management of chronic complications of diabetes based on concomitant disorders. They are discussed in the sections that follow.

Coronary Artery Disease and Heart Failure

CVD is the leading cause of morbidity and mortality in people with DM; 65% of deaths in persons with diabetes are due to CAD or cerebrovascular events. Stroke, MI, and sudden death are higher in people with diabetes.

Large epidemiological studies have shown that in patients with diabetes, hyperglycemia increases the incidence of CVD (UKPDS, 1998; Khaw et al, 2004). The UKPDS found that for every percentage point reduction in Hb A1c levels, there was a reduction in microvascular complications by 35%; and for every 1% reduction in Hb A1c, there was a 25% reduction in diabetes-related deaths, a 7% reduction in all-cause mortality, and an 18% reduction in combined fatal and nonfatal MI (ADA, 2002). In the EPIC-Norfolk study, it was found that an increase in 1% Hb A1c level was associated with a 20% to 30% increase in CVD events in both men and women (Khaw et al, 2004). It is also recommended that patients with IGF, IGT, and borderline Hb A1c levels be screened for CVD risks (ADA, 2015).

Despite earlier studies suggesting better glycemic control would reduce CVD, three recent studies, the ACCORD, VADT, and ADVANCE studies, did not show a reduction in macrovascular events with stricter glycemic control (6.4% to 6.9%) compared with the standard control of 7%. Decline in macrovascular events is more likely related to control of BP, lipid reduction, and smoking cessation.

All patients with known CVD should be treated with an angiotension-converting enzyme (ACE) inhibitor and statins (if not contraindicated); in patients with acute MI, beta blockers should be used for up to 2 years after infarction in individuals at lower risk of hypoglycemia (ADA, 2015). Atherosclerosis occurs earlier in patients with diabetes than in those without elevated glucose levels. A major mechanism is increased production of thromboxane, a potent vasoconstrictor and platelet aggregant. Aspirin blocks the formation of thromboxane by acetylating cyclo-oxygenase and has been used as both primary and secondary prevention for cardiovascular events.

According to the current ADA recommendations (2015), aspirin therapy (75 to 162 mg/d) should be used as a primary prevention strategy in patients with type 1 or type 2 diabetes at increased cardiovascular risk, including men older than 50 years and women older than 60 years who have additional risk factors such as family history, smoking, dyslipidemia, or albuminuria. The same dose should be used as secondary prevention for those patients with a history of CVD. If aspirin is contraindicated (e.g., known aspirin allergy), clopidogrel (Plavix) 75 mg/d should be used as antiplatelet therapy. Combination antiplatelet therapy is reasonable for up to 1 year after an acute coronary syndrome (ADA, 2015). Aspirin therapy is not recommended for patients at low risk, which includes men younger than 50 years and women younger than 60 years with no CVD risk factors. With the diagnosis of DM now considered a CV event equivalent, few diabetic patients should go without a basic consideration of aspirin therapy.

Metformin has been associated with improving cardiovascular risk through its action in improving lipid levels. However, patients with congestive heart failure who take metformin have an increased frequency of lactic acidosis. This drug is not recommended for HF patients with lower ejection fractions. Insulin may be required for these patients.

Among the oral agents, sulfonylureas are the most associated with risk of hypoglycemia, which may be difficult to recognize in patients concurrently taking beta blockers because beta blockers mask the signs and symptoms of hypoglycemia, with the exception of diaphoresis. Patients with coronary artery disease, heart failure, or hypertension are commonly treated with beta blockers. If sulfonylureas must be given concurrently with beta blockers, glimepiride is less likely to cause hypoglycemia than other drugs in the class.

In a recent RCT in China, in patients diagnosed with type 2 DM for more than 5 years with coronary artery disease for 3 years, treatment with metformin for 3 years reduced death from cardiovascular causes, death from any cause, nonfatal MI, nonfatal stroke, and arterial revascularization by 46% compared with use of glipizide (Hong et al, 2013).

ACE inhibitors are central to the management of heart failure and hypertension. ACE inhibitors and angiotensin II receptor blockers (ARBs) promote ventricular remodeling. These drugs also have been shown to significantly reduce the trajectory of diabetic nephropathy. All patients with diabetes and hypertension should be treated with either an ACE or ARB (ADA, 2015). When renal insufficiency progresses to moderate levels of GFR reduction, they must be discontinued.

Coronary artery disease is further discussed in Chapter 28, "Chronic Stable Angina and Low-Risk Unstable Angina," and heart failure is discussed in Chapter 36, "Heart Failure."

Hyperlipidemia

Having diabetes is now considered equivalent in cardiovascular risk to having established cardiovascular disease and is listed by the National Cholesterol Education Program (NCEP) as an independent risk factor for coronary heart disease (CHD). The NCEP and ADA both recommend aggressive lipid management aimed at lowering LDL cholesterol, raising HDL cholesterol, and lowering triglycerides to reduce macrovascular disease and mortality in patients with DM. Patients diagnosed with type 1 in childhood have a high risk of developing early subclinical and clinical CVD. Adult patients with type 2 diabetes have an increased prevalence of lipid abnormalities. Although evidence is lacking on type 2 diabetes in children, the assumption is that they will also demonstrate these abnormalities.

Diabetes, particularly type 2, can cause a lipid abnormality with a high level of very-low-density lipoprotein (VLDL) and a low level of HDL (ADA, 2015). This is seen clinically as high triglyceride levels (200 to 400 mg/dL) and low HDL levels (less than 35 mg/dL). The target lipid levels recommended by the ADA are shown in Table 33-5. All patients with diabetes should have a fasting lipid profile at least annually. Children older than 2 years should have a lipid profile after the diagnosis of diabetes and when glucose control has been established. If values are normal, the test should be repeated every 5 years.

Lifestyle intervention, which includes MNT, increased physical activity, weight loss, and smoking cessation, may allow some patients to reach lipid goals. Each patient's age, type of diabetes, pharmacological treatment, lipid levels, and other medical conditions should determine the type of nutritional interventions used, with a focus on the reduction of saturated fat, cholesterol, and trans-fatty acids. Glycemic control can also positively impact plasma lipid levels, particularly in patients with very high triglycerides TG (ADA, 2015).

For those patients who have CVD or are over 40 years old with other CVD risk factors, pharmacological therapy is warranted. Statin therapy should be considered in addition to lifestyle therapy if LDL cholesterol remains greater than 100 mg/dL or in those with multiple CVD risk factors (ADA, 2015).

HMG-Co-A reductase inhibitors (statins) have consistently demonstrated the ability to reduce cardiovascular risk for adults and for children over the age of 10 years when the main goal is reduction of LDL cholesterol. These drugs have also been shown to improve endothelial function and cause regression of carotid intimal thickening (McCrindle et al, 2007; Wiegman et al, 2004). Their action is less prominent in reduction of VLDL and triglycerides, but they also have this action. Although other drugs will be discussed here, the current ADA recommendations (2015) stress treating all patients with DM with statins unless contraindicated.

Fibrates act more directly on VLDL and triglycerides (TGs), while also increasing HDL-C. They are most commonly used for lowering TGs but can be used concomitantly with statins to address multiple dyslipidemias. If used in combination, risks of serious side effects are increased, so close monitoring is necessary.

Ezetimibe is a cholesterol absorption inhibitor whose primary effect is reduction of LDL-C. It has been shown to be safe in combination with a statin to enhance the effects. Vytorin is a combination of simvastatin of varying doses and ezetimibe 10 mg. The initial systematic review of this combination, however, found that the drug was no more effective than either drug taken alone (Sharma et al, 2009). This finding provided additional support for the findings from the 2008 ENHANCE trial, which did not show a clinical outcome demonstrating efficacy for combined therapy of ezetimibe and simvastatin, although there was a decrease in LDL (Kastelein et al, 2008). The recent release of reviewed MPROVE-IT data has cast a more favorable light on the drug combination (Blazing et al, 2014). It has yet to be determined if use of ezetimibe will increase again. Because large changes in cholesterol fractions are rarely achieved by monotherapy with one drug class, providers should use individual patient response to select drugs to be used to treat hyperlipidemia.

Bile acid sequestrants affect LDL-C with a modest increase in HDL-C. They are not commonly prescribed to treat dyslipidemias in patients with diabetes. Not only do they increase TGs but they may pose problems for patients with diabetic gastroparesis. The increase in TG is especially of concern in diabetics because the pancreas is already under stress.

Nicotinic acid (niacin) has been used to increase HDL-C; it has a modest lowering effect on TGs and LDL-C. However, it is associated with increased BGL particularly in pre-diabetes or newly diagnosed patients. Although niacin is relatively inexpensive, it has unpleasant side effects for the patient and can also increase hyperglycemia (Cornell & Sisson, 2011). The recently appreciated increase in CV event risk has led to niacin falling out of favor for use.

Omega-3 fatty acids can be useful in lowering TGs with a secondary effect of increasing HDL-C. They can also increase LDL. Because these drugs cause increased bleeding, they should be used cautiously in patients on anticoagulant therapy or aspirin.

Interventions to improve glycemic control usually lower triglyceride levels but have little effect on HDL levels. Metformin has a modestly favorable impact on lipids because of its actions in the liver. In clinical studies, metformin alone or in combination with a sulfonylurea lowered mean fasting serum triglycerides, total cholesterol, and LDL and had no adverse effect on HDL. Therefore, it is an appropriate oral agent for patients with diabetes who also have lipid abnormalities. The combination of gemfibrozil with metformin and an NCEP lipid-lowering diet is the most efficacious in both controlling lipid and lowering blood glucose levels. TZDs may increase HDL and LDL, but the long-term effect of such changes is unknown. Acarbose (Precose), an alpha-glucosidase inhibitor, has also shown beneficial effects for patients with hypertriglyceridemias. Acarbose acts on the pathogenesis of these disorders, lowering production of endogenous triglycerides. Chapter 39 presents more information on treatment of hyperlipidemia.

Hypertension

Hypertension (HTN) is a common comorbidity in patients with diabetes, affecting 20% to 60% depending on age, obesity, and ethnicity (ADA, 2015). HTN is also a risk factor for CHD and microvascular complications such as retinopathy and nephropathy. In type 1 diabetes, HTN is often a manifestation of diabetic nephropathy. In type 2 diabetes, HTN is often part of a syndrome that includes glucose intolerance, insulin resistance, obesity, hyperlipidemia, and coronary artery disease. In both types of diabetes, the presence of HTN is associated with increased cardiovascular risk, especially for stroke and ischemic heart disease. Control of HTN has been demonstrated to reduce the rate of progression of diabetic nephropathy and hypertensive cerebrovascular disease.

Blood pressure should be measured at every routine visit with a health-care provider. According to ADA standards, which have changed from previous recommendations, the target for people with HTN and diabetes is <150 systolic; the target systolic BP <130 is appropriate for younger patients and for those for whom the goal can be achieved without difficulty. Diastolic BP should be treated to <90 mg Hg, per JNC-8 standards, but opinion in diabetic communities believes this might be too lenient in diabetic patients. Standard treatment for HTN should include pharmacotherapy and lifestyle modifications. These include MNT, increased physical activity, moderate alcohol consumption, and modest weight reduction.

Pharmacological treatment should be initiated with either an angiotensin converting enzyme (ACE) inhibitor or angiotensin II receptor blocker (ARB); if one drug is not tolerated, another should be initiated. Multiple drugs are usually needed to achieve BP targets in many patients (ADA, 2015). Some drugs used to treat HTN also address other complications of diabetes. ACE inhibitors have been shown to improve cardiovascular outcomes in high-risk cardiovascular patients even without HTN. In patients with congestive heart failure, ACE inhibitors are associated with better outcome than are ARBs. ARBs improve cardiovascular outcomes in patients with HTN, diabetes, and end-organ damage. ACE inhibitors reduce the risk for diabetic nephropathy through their reduction of intraglomerular pressure and a reduction in glomerulosclerosis. They have a unique, specific, and beneficial effect on the kidneys of both normotensive and hypertensive patients with diabetes. ARBs (lorastan [Cozaar] and irbesartan [Avapro]) have been approved for use in treating diabetic nephropathy.

Alpha adrenergic blockers are not usually prescribed for treatment of HTN in persons with diabetes. The alpha-blocker arm of the Antihypertensive and Lipid-Lowering Treatment to Prevent Heart Attack Trial (ALLHAT) was terminated after interim analysis showed that alpha blockers were substantially less effective in reducing congestive heart failure than diuretic therapy (Wright et al, 2009). Alpha blockers are beneficial for treatment of benign prostatic hypertrophy (BPH) and can be used as an option for men with BPH and diabetes (Cornell & Sisson, 2011).

Diuretics can also be used to treat HTN but are not typically the first-line treatment for HTN in diabetes. In low doses, diuretics may safely be used for patients with diabetes (AACE, 2006; ADA, 2015), but at moderate to high doses they adversely affect glucose metabolism. They may also potentiate orthostatic hypotensive changes in patients with diabetic autonomic neuropathy. Thiazide diuretics have been shown to increase peripheral insulin resistance and hepatic glucose release. Other side effects are changes in electrolytes, such as hypokalemia, hyperglycemia, hyperlipidemia, and hyper/hypocalcemia. Therefore, serum electrolytes should be monitored throughout therapy; baseline renal function and potassium levels are necessary when choosing therapy (Cornell & Sisson, 2011).

Beta blockers are not typically used to treat HTN in patients with DM as an addition or as first-line therapy but may be used for patients with existing cardiac problems (prevention of second MI). Beta blockers may inhibit release of insulin as well as mask hypoglycemic symptoms, such as tachycardia. Nonselective beta blockers can also reduce the B2-mediated hepatic glucose output, which could have negative impacts during a hypoglycemic episdoe. Beta blockers can also increase total cholesterol, LDL, and triglycerides, while decreasing HDL.

Nondihydropyridine calcium channel blockers (CCBs) can be considered for patients who are unable to tolerate ACE inhibitors or ARBs. CCBs are now used as first-line therapy for HTN in African Americans. HTN is discussed in more detail in Chapter 40.

On The Horizon **RENAL INSUFFICIENCY**

Metformin and other medications are curtailed when creatinine values rise. Several recent calls to continue with drug use if monitoring for lactic acidosis is not yet FDA-approved.

Nephropathy

Diabetic nephropathy (DN) occurs in 20% to 40% of patients with diabetes and is the single cause of end-stage renal disease. Elevated urinary albumin excretion (30 to 300 mg/24 h) has been shown to be the earliest stage of diabetic nephropathy in type 1 diabetes and a marker for development of nephropathy in type 2. It is also a well-established marker for increased cardiovascular disease risk (ADA, 2015). Patients with elevated urinary albumin excretion are likely to progress to clinical albuminuria and a decreased glomerular filtration rate over a period of years (Remuzzi, Schieppati, & Ruggenenti, 2003). HTN may accelerate the decline in glomerular filtration rate and the progression to end-stage renal disease.

Screening for excessive urinary albumin excretion should be done with a random spot urine sample for albumin excretion in type 1 diabetes once a child is 10 years of age and has had diabetes for 5 years and in adults once they have had diabetes for 5 or more years. All patients with type 2 should have such screening at time of diagnosis.

Elevated or high levels of urinary albumin excretion (30 to 299 mg/24 h) in nonpregnant adults should be treated with an ACE inhibitor or ARB, but not both concurrently. Reduction in dietary protein is not recommended for patients with

DM and diabetic kidney disease (albuminuria >30 mg/24 h) because it will not alter glycemic response, cardiovascular risk, or rate of glomerular filtration rate (GFR) decline (ADA, 2015). Serum creatinine and potassium levels should be monitored when ACE, ARB, or diuretics are used. Continued monitoring of urine albumin excretion to assess response to therapy and progression of disease is indicated. Serum creatinine should also be measured at least annually in all adults with diabetes regardless of urine albumin excretion (ADA, 2015).

ACE inhibitors, ARBs, and non-dihydropyridine CCBs reduce the rate of urinary albumin excretion and may give false-negative tests. To diagnose DN, excessive albumin excretion should be confirmed by at least two tests over a period of 3 to 6 months. An estimate of GFR using the CKD-EPI is becoming standard in hospitals because it also has values specific for gender, ethnicity, and age. This tool to calculate GFR can be found at the National Kidney Foundation (www.kidney.org) and the National Kidney Disease Education Program (www.nkdep.nih.gov). A more expensive test of Cystatin-C may be more useful if determination of renal insufficiency stage is unclear with standard methods. A referral to a specialist experienced in the care of DN should be considered in advanced kidney disease or when difficulties in management issues develop.

To reduce the risk or slow the progression of nephropathy, the recommendations are to optimize glucose and BP control. Intensive management and maintenance of BP to target goals have been effective in reducing the rate of progression to end stage. In patients with type 1 diabetes, with or without HTN, ACE inhibitors have been demonstrated to significantly delay the progression of DN. In patients with type 2 diabetes, HTN, and albuminuria 30 to 299 mg/24 h, ACE inhibitors and ARBs have been shown to delay the progression to albuminuria greater than 300 mg/h. In patients with type 2 diabetes, HTN, macroalbuminuria, and renal insufficiency, ARBs have been shown to delay the progression to nephropathy (AACE, 2006; ADA, 2015). The non-dihydropyridine CCBs (diltiazem and verapamil) may reduce albuminuria 30 to 299 mg/24 hours to an extent comparable with ACE, but the dihydropyridine CCBs may increase it (AACE, 2006).

Neuropathy

There are two kinds of diabetic neuropathy: autonomic and peripheral. Diabetic autonomic neuropathy (DAN) is often insidious and screening for it may require several tests. A detailed history and physical should include screening for signs and symptoms, including resting tachycardia, exercise intolerance, orthostatic hypotension, constipation, gastroparesis, erectile dysfunction, sweat gland dysfunction, impaired neurovascular function, and the potential for autonomic failure in response to hypoglycemia. Cardiovascular autonomic dysfunction (CAN) is a CVD risk factor and is the most clinically important form of DAN.

Hypotheses of etiologies of DAN include metabolic insult to nerve fibers, neurovascular insufficiency, autoimmune damage, and neurohormonal growth factor deficiency (Vinik,

Maser, Mitchell, & Freeman, 2003). Hyperglycemic activation of the polyol pathway leading to accumulation of sorbitol and potential changes in the nicotinamide adenine dinucleotide (NAD) to nicotinamide adenine dinucleotide hydride (NADH) ratio may cause direct neuronal damage. Activations of protein kinase C induces vasoconstriction and reduces neuronal blood flow. Increased oxidative stress, with increased free radical production, causes vascular endothelium damage and reduces nitric oxide bioavailability. Immune mechanisms may also be involved. Reduced neurotrophic growth factors, deficiency of free fatty acids, and formation of advanced glycosylation end products also result in reduced neuronal blood flow. In summary, a multifactorial process is probably involved in DAN; multiple body systems are affected. Major clinical manifestations are shown in Table 33-10.

Screening for signs and symptoms of CAN should be performed upon diagnosis of type 2 and 5 years after the diagnosis of type 1. Special testing is not usually needed (ADA, 2015).

CAN is a serious component of DAN because it is associated with increased morbidity and possibly mortality. CAN is the most clinically significant type of DAN. Indications can include resting tachycardia (>100 bpm) and orthostasis (fall in systolic BP 20 mm Hg upon standing without an appropriate heart rate response). Recommendations include management of HTN, lipids, and glucose control because currently there are no treatment options for treating the underlying nerve damage (ADA). Glucose control can slow progression but does not reverse existing nerve loss or damage.

Autonomic involvement can affect GI dysfunction, manifested by gastroparesis, constipation, and diarrhea. Metoclopramide (Reglan), a prokinetic agent, is the most commonly used drug to treat gastroparesis; however, it has a relatively high incidence of adverse reactions, especially in children and older adults. This increased risk for adverse reactions is significant because gastric emptying problems are more common in older adults. Diet modification (liquids or softer diet) and referral to a dietitian can be helpful.

Table 33–10   Major Clinical Manifestations of Diabetic Autonomic Neuropathy

Body System	Manifestations
Cardiovascular	Resting tachycardia, exercise intolerance, orthostatic hypotension, silent myocardial ischemia
Gastrointestinal	Esophageal dysmotility, gastroparesis, constipation, diarrhea, fecal incontinence
Genitourinary	Neurogenic bladder, erectile dysfunction, retrograde ejaculation, loss of vaginal lubrication
Metabolic	Hypoglycemia unawareness, hypoglycemic-associated autonomic failure
Skin	Anhidrosis, heat intolerance, dry skin
Pupillary	Pupillomotor function impairment, Argyll Robertson pupil

Source: Adapted from Vinik, A., Maser, R., Mitchell, B., & Freeman, R. (2003). Diabetic autonomic neuropathy. *Diabetes Care, 26*(5), 1554–1555.

Genitourinary dysfunction includes reduced bladder contraction force, resulting in urinary stasis, increased risk for bladder infections, and impotence. Bladder contraction force can be enhanced by the use of a cholinergic agonist such as bethanechol (Urecholine). Erectile dysfunction has been successfully treated with alpha blockers that increase vascular blood flow. The phosphodiesterase type 5 inhibitors sildenafil (Viagra), tadalafil (Cialis), and vardenafil (Levitra) are used for treatment of this problem. Other interventions, such as intracorporeal or intraurethral prostaglandins, vacuum devices, or penile prostheses, can also improve the quality of life for the patient suffering from erectile dysfunction.

Peripheral diabetic neuropathy, also known as distal symmetric polyneuropathy (DPN), may result in pain, loss of sensation, and muscle weakness and is a major risk factor for development of ulceration and lower extremity amputations. All patients with DM should be screened for DPN at diagnosis and at least annually thereafter, with a thorough examination that includes inspection and assessment of peripheral pulses and testing for loss of protective sensation using simple tests, such as two-point sensation, vibration perceptions using a 128 Hz tuning fork, 10 g monofilament pressure sensation, and assessment of ankle reflexes (ADA, 2015).

In addition to maintaining glycemic control, therapies are also directed at management of other symptoms in DPN and prevention of complications. Neuropathic pain is often severe and intractable. Treatment is based on individual patient response. Tricyclic antidepressants have been used for their effect on the intrinsic pain-suppressing pathways. Nortriptyline (Aven, Pamelor) and desipramine (Norpramin) are more useful when the patient also experiences orthostatic hypotension. Gabapentin (Neurontin), an anticonvulsant, acts by stabilizing neuronal membranes. The impact is very subtle in most cases. Therapy is begun at low doses, followed by gradual titration. Cymbalta (duloxetine) and Lyrica (pregabalin) are both approved for DPN. These drugs are discussed in more detail in Chapter 29. Capsaicin cream (0.025% to 0.075%), a substance P inhibitor, is also helpful in reducing DPN pain. It is applied 3 or 4 times daily. Treatment should also include smoking cessation. Patients should also be educated on the importance of foot care, proper footwear and daily foot inspection.

Retinopathy

Diabetic retinopathy (DR) is a highly specific vascular complication of both type 1 and type 2 diabetes. DR is the most frequent cause of blindness among adults ages 20 to 74 years. After 20 years of diabetes, nearly all patients with type 1 and more than 60% of patients with type 2 have some degree of retinopathy. One study found that an earlier age of onset of type 2 diabetes significantly affected the development of DR, even more than disease duration and degree of hyperglycemia (Wong, Molyneaux, Constantino, Twigg, & Yue, 2008). This finding supports the importance of delaying or preventing the development of diabetes from pre-diabetes and the need for the more stringent metabolic targets for younger patients. Additionally, other factors associated with increased risk of DR are hypertension and nephropathy, thus lowering BP has been shown to decrease risk for DR. Use of pioglitazone has been linked with macular edema, but it is unclear whether this is a drug effect or the fact that most patients on these medications have less controlled sugars, greater BP, and more obesity (Fugimoto, 2013).

Adults and children ages 10 years or older with type 1 diabetes should have an initial dilated and comprehensive examination by an ophthalmologist or optometrist within 5 years after the onset of diabetes. Patients with type 2 should have the examination shortly after the diagnosis of diabetes. These examinations should be repeated annually for both types, but if there is no evidence of retinopathy for 1 or more years, then exams may be extended to every 2 years (ADA, 2015). Women with diabetes who are planning pregnancy should have an eye examination in the first trimester with close follow-up throughout the pregnancy and 1 year postpartum (ADA, 2015). One of the main reasons for screening is the established efficacy of laser photocoagulation surgery in preventing vision loss.

The DCCT study clearly demonstrated that near-normal glycemic control reduced or prevented the development of retinopathy by 76% as compared with conventional therapy and reduced the progression by 54% (Kilpatrick, Rigby, & Atkin, 2008). Other large studies have also confirmed the protective effect of glycemic control in patients with type 2 diabetes (UKPDS, 1998; ACCORD Study Group and ACCORD Eye Study Group, 2010). It was also found that patients assigned to intensive BP control had a 34% reduction in progression of retinopathy and a 47% reduced risk of deterioration in visual acuity with a reduction of as little as 10/5 mm Hg in BP (UKPDS, 1998), although a more recent study found that tight targets (systolic <120 mm Hg) had little effect on DR (ACCORD Study Group, ACCORD Eye Study Group, 2010). The FDA has approved two vascular endothelial growth factor (VEGF) inhibitors, ranibizumbab (Lucentis) and aflibercept (Eyelea), for use by specialists to help treat diabetic macular edema.

◉ CLINICAL PEARL ◉

Pumps and Daylight Savings Time
Some pumps may not automatically adjust for changes in daylight savings time. This will not impact basal insulin rates, but bolus doses can be impacted. Time-zone travel can also impact timing of doses if the pump is not GPS-enabled.

Thyroid Function

The presence of thyroid disorders may cloud the diagnosis and complicate the treatment of diabetes. Patients with type 1 diabetes should be screened for thyroid peroxidase and thyroglobin antibodies at diagnosis. Thyroid-stimulating hormone (TSH) concentrations should be measured after metabolic control has been established. If normal, recheck them every 1 or 2 years. Metformin may alter TSH levels in the first 3 to 6 months of use. The pituitary feedback loop may be impaired in patients with prior hypothyroid issues without overt signs of hyperthyroidism. The clinical significance is undetermined (Duntas, Orgiazzi, & Brabant, 2011).

Autoimmune Disorders

Individuals diagnosed with type 1 diabetes should be assessed for the presence of other autoimmune diseases such as thyroid dysfunction, celiac disease, and B_{12} deficiency (ADA, 2015).

ASSESSMENT OF GLYCEMIC CONTROL

The ADA (2015) recommends evaluation of glycemic control at the initial visit and as part of continuing care for patients with DM. There are two mechanisms for assessing glycemic control: Hb A1c and patient self-monitoring of blood glucose (SMBG).

Hb A1c

Hb A1c provides baseline data and should be used for ongoing evaluation of glycemic control. Because Hb A1c reflects mean glycemia over the preceding 2 to 3 months, it should be measured at least twice a year if patients are meeting treatment goals or have stable glycemic control; it should be measured every 3 months if therapy has changed or if patients are not meeting treatment goals (ADA, 2015). Although the Hb A1c goal for most patients is generally less than 7% per ADA guidelines, a more stringent goal of 6.5% (AACE, 2009) may be established for some patients if there is no significant hypoglycemia or other adverse effects. Such patients include those who are young, have a long life expectancy, and no risk of CVD. Less stringent goals below 8% are appropriate for those individuals who have a history of hypoglycemia, advanced complications or comorbidities, or who have DM of a long duration with poor control. A level of 8.5% is considered acceptable for those in long-term care facilities with advanced dementia, limited life expectancy, and significant issues with ADLs.

Multiple long-term studies support glycemic control through the current recommendations for Hb A1c testing and goal setting to reduce the risk of both micro- and macrovascular complications (DCCT, UKPDS, VADT, ADVANCE, ACCORD). The availability of point of care (POC) Hb A1c testing may increase Hb A1c monitoring and providers' adherence to current guidelines. Egbunike and Gerard (2013) found that in a small sample size ($n = 41$) of chart reviews in a practice, the documentation of POC Hb A1c testing increased from 65.9% pre-implementation to 82.9% 3 months' post-implementation of POC testing in a practice.

There are a few instances when Hb A1c may be unreliable. See Table 33-11 for a list of factors that create some doubt of the values obtained. Of major import when considering the care for diverse patients, having hemoglobin composed of other than the standard hemoglobin A can make the value too high or too

low based on the average RBC life span and altered glucose binding sites (Xavier & Carmichael, 2013). There are over 700 types of altered hemoglobin, including thalassemia variants and differing sickle cell presentations; persons with Afro-Caribbean heritage are especially of concern. Also, individuals who have had multiple transfusions have unreliably high values for several months because the donor cells are preserved with a dextrose medium. This is compounded by the possibility the transfusions were required due to acute blood loss, which triggers a falsely low reading. Spherocytosis, altered splenic function, chronic liver or kidney disease, HIV patients on antiretrovirals, and individuals who take mega doses of vitamin supplements (especially A and C) also have unreliable numbers. Having high triglycerides can give falsely elevated readings. In these circumstances, it is recommended that using the same laboratory, avoiding POC testing, and concurrent monitoring of other glucose markers, including postprandial and fasting values, become a required part of the treatment plan.

Self-Monitoring of Blood Glucose (SMBG)

Regular testing provides the patient and provider with more detailed information about daily glucose fluctuations and response to medication, meals, activity, and stress. It can be useful in guiding both in successful initial management. An important factor in this equation is whether the patient and/or caregiver has adequate instruction and ongoing evaluation of SMBG technique and knows how to use the results to problem solve. All patients on inhaled or insulin pump therapy should perform SMBG 3 to 6 times daily and at least preprandial, at bedtime, prior to exercise, when hypoglycemia is suspected, after treatment of hypoglycemia, and prior to driving. SMBG may be helpful for patients on oral therapy or on less frequent insulin regimens. Those who are stable can avoid daily measurements and check with symptoms or on a less vigorous schedule.

Table 33–11 Situations Where Hb A1c May Be Unreliable

Disease or Situation	Impact on Hb A1c Value
Acute blood loss within 3 months	Too low
Multiple transfusions within 3 months	Too high
Sickle cell Hg F; thalassemia Hg S	Too low
Hemoglobin S, G, D, C, & E	Too high
Vitamin A and C supplements	Too low
Liver disease	Too low
Hyperbilirubinemia	Too high
HIV on antiretroviral medications	Too low
High triglycerides	Too high
African Caribbean heritage	Too high

Based on National Glycohemoglobin Standardization Program information (www.ngsp.org) and Xavier & Carmichael (2013).

DIABETES MELLITUS

Related to the Overall Treatment Plan/Disease Process

☐ Pathophysiology of diabetes and the long-term effects of inadequate management on target organs

☐ Role of lifestyle modification, especially dietary therapy, in improving outcomes and keeping the number and cost of required drugs down

☐ Importance of adherence to the treatment regimen

☐ Need for regular follow-up visits with the primary care provider and other specialists

SPECIFIC TO THE DRUG THERAPY

☐ Reason for taking the drug(s) and the anticipated action of the drug(s) on the disease process

☐ Doses and schedules for taking the drugs

☐ Possible adverse reactions (especially hypoglycemia, DKA, and hyperosmolar hyperglycemic non-ketotic coma), how to prevent them, and what to do if they occur

☐ Interactions between lifestyle modifications and these drugs

REASONS FOR TAKING THE DRUG(S)

Patient education about specific drugs is provided in Chapter 21. Specific information related to diabetes includes the following: glycemic control and management of hypertension and hyperlipidemia are central to reducing morbidity and mortality from cardiovascular disease and preventing retinopathy and end-stage renal disease. The risks of these complications while maintaining the potential for a good quality of life with appropriate treatment must be discussed.

DRUGS AS PART OF THE TOTAL TREATMENT REGIMEN

Expectations should be clear about what the drugs can and cannot do. Dietary and other lifestyle modifications complement drug therapy and are equally important. Diabetes is a chronic, progressive disease. Self-management requires incorporating a combination of medications, healthy eating, exercise, stress management, and SMBG into the everyday life of the patient with diabetes.

ADHERENCE ISSUES

Nonadherence to the treatment regimen may result in increased risk for complications and reduced life expectancy. Healthcare providers should be aware of potential problems with nonadherence, discuss the importance of adherence at each follow-up visit, and assist patients in removing barriers to adherence such as lack of social support and cost of the treatment regimen. A team approach with the patient as an active partner should be maximized. Ways to deal with nonadherence are discussed in Chapter 6. Patient education booklets are available from the ADA, which can be accessed on the Internet at www.diabetes.org.

OUTCOME EVALUATION

Outcome evaluation is measured by glycemic targets and prevention or development of the complications of diabetes. Current recommendations stress the importance of establishing treatment goals and glycemic targets using a patient-centered team approach. Collaboration with specialists, CDEs, dietitians, and the primary care provider is critical throughout treatment.

Because diabetes is a self-managed disease, goals and glycemic targets should take into account patient characteristics, such as the patient's capacity to understand and carry out the treatment regimen, the risk for severe hypoglycemia, and other factors that may increase risk or decrease benefit (e.g., very young or very old, end-stage renal disease, advanced cardiovascular or cerebrovascular disease, or other concomitant diseases that will materially shorten life expectancy). In addition, children with diabetes require integration of factors associated with growth and development into their treatment regimen.

PATIENT EDUCATION

Patient education includes a comprehensive overview of all aspects of management of the disease, including medications, meal planning, monitoring as appropriate, exercise, problem solving, coping, and prevention of complications. All patients should be referred to a DSME program initially and on an ongoing basis as life events occur, living situation changes, and as the disease progresses.

Patient education should focus on understanding the pathophysiology of diabetes and prevention of complications, the role of lifestyle modification, improving outcomes and keeping the number and cost of required drugs manageable, the importance of adherence to the treatment regimen, the need for regular follow-up visits with the primary care provider, and regular screenings and preventive care. Special attention must be given to planning what to do in event of illness that impacts the ability to eat. A small cache of diabetic testing supplies and a rotating emergency stock of medications should be set aside for blizzard and other weather emergencies and placed in a durable container in regions with tornados and earthquakes. Plans for extended vacations such as cruises and international travel need to include consideration of crossing time zones and erratic meal schedules for those on insulin regimens.

Many patients want information on the use of dietary supplements such as chromium and cinnamon. Though chromium is an essential nutrient, issues of deficiency are very uncommon and the evidence is not there to support its use. Cinnamon use requires much better quality studies before the conflicting results of smaller studies can be verified. The use of artificial sweeteners has also become of concern; these sugar substitutes may actually increase weight gain, metabolic syndrome, and CV disease, but they are credited with helping individuals overcome high consumption of full sugar foods. The evidence is not clear.

REFERENCES

Action to Control Cardiovascular Risk in Diabetes (ACCORD) Study Group. (2008). Effects of intensive glucose lowering in type 2 diabetes. *New England Journal of Medicine, 358*, 2545–2559.

ACCORD Study Group and the ACCORD Eye Study Group. (2010). Effects of medical therapies on retinopathy progression in type 2 diabetes. *New England Journal of Medicine, 363*, 233–244.

ADVANCE Collaborative Group. (2008). Intensive blood glucose control and vascular outcomes in patients with type 2 diabetes. *New England Journal of Medicine, 358*, 2560–2572.

American Association of Clinical Endocrinologists and the American College of Endocrinology Glycemic Control Consensus Panel [AACE/ACE]. (2009). AACE/ACE consensus statement. AACE/ACE consensus panel on type 2 diabetes mellitus: An algorithm for glycemic control. *Endocrine Practice, 15*(6), 541–559.

American Association of Clinical Endocrinologists (AACE) Hypertension Task Force. (2006). American Association of Clinical Endocrinologists medical guidelines for clinical practice for the diagnosis and treatment of hypertension. *Endocrine Practice, 12*(2), 193–222.

American Diabetes Association (ADA). (2002). Implications of the United Kingdom prospective diabetes study. Position Statement. *Diabetes Care, 25*(1 Suppl.), S28–S32.

American Diabetes Association (ADA). (2015). Standards of medical care in diabetes 2015. *Diabetes Care, 38* (1 Suppl.), S1–S94.

Bardsley, J., & Magee, M. (2011). Pathophysiology of the metabolic disorder. In Mensing, McLaughlin, & Halstenson (Eds.), *The art and science of diabetes self management education desk reference* (pp 285–308). Chicago: American Association of Diabetes Educators.

Bell, R., Mayer-Davis, E., Beyer, J., D'Agostino, R., Lawrence, J., Linder, B., et al, & The SEARCH for Diabetes in Youth Study Group. (2009). Diabetes in non-Hispanic white youth: Prevalence, incidence and clinical characteristics: The SEARCH for diabetes in youth study. *Diabetes Care, 32*(3), S102–S111.

Blazing, M., Giugliano, R., Cannon, C., Musliner, T., Tershakovec, A., White, J., et al. (2014). Evaluating cardiovascular event reduction with ezetimibe as an adjunct to simvastatin in 18,144 patients after acute coronary syndromes: Final baseline characteristics of the IMPROVE-IT study population. *American Heart Journal 168*(2), 205–212.

Bloomgarden, Z. (2003). American Association of Clinical Endocrinologists (AACE). Consensus conference on insulin resistance syndrome. *Diabetes Care, 26*(4), 1297–1303.

Blumer, I., Hader, E., Hadden, D., Jovanovic, L., Mestman, J., Murad, M., et al. (2013). Diabetes and pregnancy: An endocrine society clinical practice guideline. *Journal of Clinical Endocrinology and Metabolism. 98*(11), 4227–4249.

Carnethon, M., DeChavez, P., Biggs, M., Lewis, C., Pankow, J. Bertoni, A., et al. (2012). *Journal of the American Medical Association, 308*(6), 581-590.

Centers for Disease Control and Prevention (CDC). (2014). National diabetes statistics report. Estimates of diabetes and its burden in the United States. Atlanta, GA: U.S. Department of Health and Human Services, Centers for Disease Control, 2014.

Cherney, D., Perkins, B., Soleymanlou, N., Maione, M., Laei, V., Lee, A, et al. (2014). Renal hemodynamics effect of sodium-glucose cotransporter 2 inhibition in patients with type 1 diabetes mellitus. *Circulation, 129*(5), 587–597.

Cornell, S., & Sisson, E. (2011). Pharmacotherapy: Dyslipidemia and hypertension in persons with diabetes. In Mensing, McLaughlin, & Halstenson (Eds.), *The art and science of diabetes self management education desk reference* (pp 459–493). Chicago: American Association of Diabetes Educators.

Dabelea, D., DeGroat, J., Sorrelman, C., Glass, M., Percy, C., Avery, C., et al, & The SEARCH for Diabetes in Youth Study Group. (2009). Diabetes in Navaho youth: Prevalence, incidence, and clinical characteristics: The SEARCH for diabetes in youth study. *Diabetes Care, 32*(3), S141–S147.

Dagogo-Jack, S., Edeoga, C., Ebenibo, S., Nyenwe, E., & Wan, J. (2014). Lack of racial disparity in incident prediabetes and glycemic progression among black and white offspring of parents with type 2 diabetes: The pathobiology of prediabetes in a biracial cohort (POP-ABC) study. *Journal of Clinical and Endocrinology & Metabolism, 99*(6), E1078–E1087. doi: 10.1210/jc.2014-1077

Dicker, D. (2011). DPP 4 inhibitors. *Diabetes Care, 34*(2 Suppl.), S276–S278.

Duntas, L., Orgiazzi, J., & Brabant, G. (2011). The interface between thyroid and diabetes mellitus. *Clinical Endocrinology, 75*(1), 1–9.

Duckworth, W., Abraira, C., & Moritz, T. (2009). Glucose control and vascular complications in veterans with type 2 diabetes. *New England Journal of Medicine, 360*(2), 129–139.

Faustman, D., Wang, L., Okubo, Y., Burger, D., Ban, L., Man, G., et al. (2012). Proof-of-concept, randomized, controlled clinical trial of Bacillis-Calmette-Guerin for treatment of long-term type 1 diabetes. *PLoS ONE 7*(8), e41756.

Fujimoto, K. (2013). Risk for macular edema increased with pioglitazone in T2DM. Presentation at European Association for the Study of Diabetes 2013 Barcelona, Spain 27 SEP, 2013.

Harcombe, A., Baker, J., Cooper, S., Davies, B., Sculthorpe, N., DiNicolantonio, J., et al. (2014). Evidence from randomized controlled trials did not support the introduction of dietary fat guidelines in 1977 and 1983; a systematic review and meta-analysis. *Open Heart, 2*(1) e000196. doi: 10.1136/openhrt-2014-000196.

Hong, J., Zhang, Y., Lai S., Lv, A., Su, Q., Dong, Y., et al, on behalf of the SPREAD NIMCAD Investigators. (2013). Effects of metformin versus glipizide on cardiovascular outcomes in patients with type 2 diabetes and coronary artery disease. *Diabetes Care, 35* (6), 1304–1311.

Inzucchi, S., Bergenstall, R., Buse, J., Diamont, M., Ferrannini, E., Nauck, M., et al. (2012). Management of hyperglycemia in type 2 diabetes: A patient centered approach. Position Statement of the American Diabetes Association (ADA) and the European Association for the Study of Diabetes (EASD). *Diabetes Care, 35*(6), 1364–1379.

Jose, T., & Inzucchi, S. (2012*).*Cardiovascular effects and the DPP 4 inhibitors. *Diabetes and Vascular Disease Research, 9*(2), 109–116.

Karstoft, K., Winding, K., Knudsen, S., Nielsen, J., Thomsen, C. Pedersen, B., et al. (2013). The effects of free-living interval-walking training on glycemic control, body composition, and physical fitness in type 2 diabetic patients: A randomized controlled trial. *Diabetes Care, 36*(2) 228–236.

Kastelein, J., Akdim, F., Stroes, E., Zwinderman, A., Bots, M., Stalenhoef, A., et al, for the ENHANCE Investigators. (2008). Simvastatin with or without ezetimibe in familial hypercholesterolemia. *The New England Journal of Medicine, 358*, 1431–1443.

Khaw, K., Wareham, N., Bingham, S., Luben, R., Welch, A., & Day, N. (2004). Association of hemoglobin A1c with cardiovascular disease and mortality in adults: The European prospective investigation into cancer in Norfolk (EPIC-Norfolk). *Annals of Internal Medicine, 141*(6), 413–420.

Kilpatrick, E., Rigby, A., & Atkin, S. (2008). A1c variability and the risk of microvascular complications in type 1 diabetes: Data from the DCCT. *Diabetes Care, 31*(11), 2198–2202.

Kunti, K., Davies, M., Majeed, A., Thorsted, B., Wolden, M., & Paul, S. (2014). Hypoglycemia and risk of cardiovascular disease and all-cause mortality in insulin-treated people with type 1 and type 2 diabetes: a cohort study. *Diabetes Care 38*(2), 316–322.

Lawrence, J., Mayer-Davis, E., Reynolds, K., Beyer, J., Pettit, D., D'Agostino, R., et al, and The SEARCH for Diabetes in Youth Study Group. (2009). Diabetes in Hispanic American youth. *Diabetes Care, 32*(3), S123–S132.

Levin, D., Bell, S., Sund, R.,Hartikainen, S., Tuomilehto, J., Pukkala, E., et al. (2015). Pioglitazones and bladder cancer risk: A multipopulation polled, cumulative exposure analysis. *Diabetologia 58*(3), 493–504.

Li, G., Zhang, P., Wang, J., Gregg, E., Yang, W., Gong, Q., et al. (2008). The long-term effect of lifestyle interventions to prevent diabetes in China DaQing Diabetes Prevention Study: A 20-years follow-up study. *The Lancet, 368,* 1783–1789.

Lindstrom, J., Ilanne-Parikka, P., Peltonen, M., Aunola, S., Eriksson, J., Hemio, K., et al. (2006). Sustained reduction in the incidence of type 2 diabetes by lifestyle intervention: Follow-up of the Finnish Diabetes Prevention Study. *The Lancet, 368,* 1673–1679.

Liu, L., Yi, J., Beyer, J., Mayer-Davis, E., Dolan, L., Dabelea, D., et al, and The SEARCH for Diabetes in Youth Study Group. (2009). Type 1 and type 2 diabetes in Asian and Pacific Islander U.S. youth. *Diabetes Care, 32*(3), S133–S140.

Mayer-Davis, E., Beyer, J., Bell, R., Dabelea, D., D'Agostino, R., Imperatore, G., et al, and the SEARCH for Diabetes in Youth Study Group. (2009). Diabetes in African American youth: Prevalence, incidence and clinical characteristics. *Diabetes Care, 32*(3), S112–S122.

McCrindle, B., Urbina, E., Dennison, B., Jacobson, M., Steinberger, J., Rocchini, A., et al. (2007). A scientific statement from the American Heart Association Atherosclerosis, Hypertension and Obesity in Diabetes, American Heart Association Council of Cardiovascular Disease in the Young, American Heart Association Council on Cardiovascular Nursing. Drug therapy of high-risk lipid abnormalities in children and adolescents. *Circulation, 115*(14), 1948–1967.

Nathan, D., Buse, J., Davidson, M., Ferrannini, E., Holman, R., Sherwin, R., & Zinman, B. (2009). Medical management of hyperglycemia in type 2 diabetes: A consensus algorithm for the initiation and adjustment of therapy. A consensus statement of the American Diabetes Association and the European Association for the Study of Diabetes. *Diabetes Care, 32*(1), 193–203.

Ohkubo, Y., Kishikawa, H., Araki, E., Miyata, T., Isami, S., Motoyoshi, S., et al. (1995). Intensive insulin therapy prevents the progression of diabetes microvascular complications in Japanese patients with non-insulin-dependent diabetes mellitus: A randomized prospective 6-years study. *Diabetes Research and Clinical Practice, 28,* 103–117.

Pani, L., Korenda, L., Meigs, J., Driver, C., Chamany, S., Fox, C., et al. (2008). Effect of aging on A1c levels in individuals without diabetes: Evidence from the Framingham Offspring Study and the National Health and Nutrition Examination Survey 2001–2004. *Diabetes Care, 31*(10), 1991–1996.

Parekh, T,, Raji, M., Lin, Y-L, Tan, A, Kuo, Y-F, & Goodwin, J. (2014). Hypoglycemia after antimicrobial drug prescription for older patients using sulfonylureas. *Journal of the American Medical Association Internal Medicine. 174*(10), 1605–1612.

Peyrot, M., Rubin, R. Lauritzen, T., Skovlund, S., Snoek, F., Matthews, D., et al, and the International DAWN advisory panel. (2005). Resistance to insulin therapy among patients and providers. *Diabetes Care, 28*(11), 2673–2679.

Polinski, J., Smith, B., Curtis, B., Seeger, J., Choudhry, N., Connolly, J., et al. (2013). Barriers to insulin progression among patients with type 2 diabetes: A systematic review. *The Diabetes Educator, 39*(1), 53–65.

Randriamboavonjy, V., & Fleming, I. (2009). Insulin, insulin resistance, and platelet signaling in diabetes. *Diabetes Care, 32*(4), 528–530.

Reichard, P., Nilsson, B., & Rosenqvist, U. (1993). The effect of long-term intensified insulin treatment on the development of microvascular complications of diabetes mellitus. *New England Journal of Medicine, 329,* 304–309.

Riddle, M., Ambrosius, W., Brillon, D., Buse, J., Byington, R., Cohen, R., et al. (2010). Epidemiologic relationships between A1c and all-cause mortality during a median 3.4-year follow-up of glycemic treatment in the ACCORD trial. *Diabetes Care, 33,* 983–990.

Sacks, F., Carey, V., Anderson. C., Miller, E., Copeland, T., Charleston, J., et al. (2014). Effects of high vs low glycemic index of dietary carbohydrates on cardiovascular disease risk factors and insulin sensitivity: The omnicarb randomized clinical trial. *Journal of the American Medical Association, 312*(23), 2531–2541.

Senechal, M., Slaght, J., Bharti, N. & Bouchard, D. (2014). Independent and combined effect of diet and exercise in adults with prediabetes. *Diabetes Metabolic Syndrome & Obesity., 2014*(7), 521–529.

Shalev, A. (2014). Minireview: Thioredoxin-interacting protein regulation and function in the pancreatic beta cell. *Molecular Endocrinology, 28*(8), 1211–1220.

Sharma, M., Ansari, M., Abou-Setta, A., Soares-Weiser, K., Ooi, T., Sears, M., et al. (2009). Systematic review: Comparative effectiveness and harms of combinations of lipid-modifying agents and high-dose statin monotherapy. *Annals of Internal Medicine, 151*(9), 622–630.

Sisson, E., & Cornell, S. (2011). Pharmacotherapy for glucose management. In Mensing, McLaughlin, & Halstenson (Eds.), *The art and science of diabetes self management education desk reference* (pp 417–457). Chicago: American Association of Diabetes Educators.

Texas Diabetes Council. (2010). Insulin algorithm for type 1 diabetes mellitus in children and adults. Publication Number: E45-11649. Retrieved from http://www.tdctoolkit.org/algorithms_and_guidelines.asp

Udell, J., Blatt, D., Braunwald, E., Cavender, M., Mosenzen, O., & Steg, P. (2014). Saxagliptin and cardiovascular outcomes in patients with type 2 diabetes mellitis and moderate or severe renal impairment: Observations from the SAVOR-TIMI 53 Trial. *Diabetes Care,* epub ahead of print 31 Dec, 2014 doi: w-2337/dc1-4-1850.

UK Prospective Diabetes Study Group (UKPDS). (1998). Effect of intensive blood-glucose control with metformin on complications in overweight patients with type 2 diabetes. *The Lancet, 352,* 854–865.

U.S. Department of Food and Drug Administration (FDA). (2011). FDA drug safety communication: Updated risk evaluation and mitigation strategy (REMS) to restrict access to rosiglitazone-containing medicines including avandia, avandamet, and avandaryl. Safety announcement. Retrieved from http://www.fda.gov/Drugs/DrugSafety/ucm255005.htm

U.S. Diabetes Prevention Program Research Group (USDPP). (2002). Reduction in the incidence of type 2 diabetes with lifestyle intervention or metformin. *New England Journal of Medicine, 346*(6), 393–403.

U.S. Diabetes Prevention Program Research Group (USDPP). (2003). Within-trial cost-effectiveness of lifestyle intervention or metformin for the primary prevention of type 2 diabetes. *Diabetes Care, 26*(9), 2518–2523.

Vinik, A., Maser, R., Mitchell, B., & Freeman, R. (2003). Diabetic autonomic neuropathy. *Diabetes Care, 26*(5), 1554–1555.

Wang, L., Lovejoy, N., & Faustman, D. (2012). Persistence of prolonged C-peptide production in type 1 diabetes as measured with an ultrasensitive C-peptide assay. *Diabetes Care, 35*(3), 465–470.

Wiegman, A., Hutten, B., deGroot, E., Rodenburg, J., Bakker, H., Buller, H., et al. (2004). Efficacy and safety of statin therapy in children with familial hyperlipidemia: A randomized controlled trial. *Journal of the American Medical Association, 292,* 331–337.

Wong, J., Molyneaux, L., Constantino, M., Twigg, S., & Yue, D. (2008). Timing is everything: Age of onset influences long-term retinopathy risk in type 2 diabetes, independent of traditional risk factors. *Diabetes Care, 31*(10), 1985–1990.

Wright, J., Jr., Probstfield, J., Cushman, W., Pressel, S., Cutler, J., Davis, B., et al, for the ALLHAT Collaborative Research Group. (2009). ALLHAT findings revisited in the context of subsequent analyses, other trials, and meta-analyses. *Archives of Internal Medicine, 169*(9), 832–842.

Xavier, N., & Carmichael, K. (2013). When the A1c is unreliable. *Consultant, 53*(10), 728.

CHAPTER 34

GASTROESOPHAGEAL REFLUX AND PEPTIC ULCER DISEASE

Teri Moser Woo

Primary care providers see a variety of gastrointestinal disorders, including gastroesophageal reflux disease (GERD) and peptic ulcer disease (PUD). Over the past few years, many of the medications used to treat these two disorders have become available over-the-counter (OTC), leading to patients' attempting to self-manage a disorder before they decide to seek care from their provider. This chapter discusses the continuum of care for GERD and PUD from simple OTC antacids to chronic acid suppression therapy.

GASTROESOPHAGEAL REFLUX DISEASE

GERD is a common problem in primary care and is listed as the primary diagnosis for 6,859,000 ambulatory care visits annually, a rate of 2,332 per 100,000 (National Institutes of Health, 2009a). The prevalence of GERD is 10% to 20% (Katz, Gerson, & Vela, 2013). The severity of the disease varies from occasional postprandial discomfort to severe esophageal inflammation, stricture, bleeding, and even esophageal carcinoma. Gastroesophageal reflux is common and is often called acid reflux because of the acid taste in the back of the mouth or "heartburn" for the burning sensation patients feel in their chest. A presumptive diagnosis is made based on these symptoms of heartburn and regurgitation (Katz et al, 2013). GERD

may also present as chest pain, epigastric pain, laryngitis, asthma, or chronic cough (Katz et al, 2013). Persistent acid reflux can cause damage to the esophagus due to chronic irritation of the esophageal mucosa (National Digestive Diseases Information Clearing House [NDDICH], 2007).

Evaluation and management of GERD is based on the American College of Gastroenterology clinical practice guidelines. In most cases, the primary care provider can manage diagnosis and treatment. Ten to 15 percent of patients with GERD require referral to a gastroenterologist. Although the focus of this chapter is drug therapy, lifestyle modification is central to successful management of GERD and is also discussed.

Pathophysiology

GERD results from the reflux of chyme from the stomach into the esophagus. The physiological action of the lower esophageal sphincter (LES) is critical to maintaining a pressure barrier between the stomach and the esophagus. In patients with GERD, the resting tone of the LES tends to be less than normal, permitting transient relaxation of the LES 1 to 2 hours after eating. This relaxation allows gastric contents to regurgitate into the esophagus. Greenberger (2003) reports on a study that found that gastric juice can separate and form layers over ingested gastric contents in a pocket. After a meal, this highly acidic, unbuffered gastric juice can reflux into the distal esophagus for a distance of 1.8 cm. The median pH of this refluxed gastric juice was 1.6, compared to the pH of 4.7 in the stomach. This acidic layer may be a key factor in the high prevalence of disease in the distal esophagus and explain why the acid that is usually neutralized and cleared from the esophagus by peristaltic action within 1 to 3 minutes cannot be overcome. About 1 to 2 hours after eating, a mean LES tone is restored, but the LES is a complicated region of smooth muscle and many factors can contribute to poor functioning of the LES.

The function of the LES is regulated by the interaction of hormonal, neural, and dietary factors. The hormone gastrin increases resting tone, whereas estrogen, progesterone, glucagon, secretin, and cholecystokinin all decrease sphincter tone. The vagus nerve and alpha-adrenergic stimulation help to maintain resting tone. Tobacco, alcohol, peppermint, chocolate, and foods with high concentrations of fat or carbohydrate all decrease LES tone.

Medications can increase or decrease LES tone. Drugs that increase LES tone include bethanechol (Urecholine), metoclopramide (Reglan), pentobarbital (Nembutal), histamine, and antacids. Some of these (metoclopramide, antacids) are used to treat GERD. Anticholinergics, theophylline, caffeine, meperidine (Demerol), and calcium channel blockers are among the drugs that decrease LES tone. Drugs also contribute to LES tone (Table 34-1).

Factors that increase intra-abdominal pressure can also contribute to GERD by affecting the pressure gradient. Vomiting, coughing, and bending all increase intra-abdominal pressure. Obesity increases intra-abdominal pressure and GERD increases as BMI increases (Katz et al,

2013). Increased abdominal pressure during pregnancy may contribute to GERD, but the underlying reflux cause is the increased circulating estrogen and progesterone, which affect LES tone.

Transient relaxation of LES tone is not the only factor in GERD. Decreased secondary peristalsis and defective mucosal resistance to caustic liquids have also been implicated. Disorders that delay gastric emptying increase exposure time to the acid. Such disorders include gastric or duodenal ulcers, which can cause pyloric edema; strictures that narrow the pylorus; and hiatal hernia, which can weaken the LES. These factors are also targets of treatments for GERD.

The severity of the esophagitis that results from GERD depends on the composition of the gastric contents, the length of time they are in contact with the esophageal mucosa, and the epithelial resistance to acid. If the chyme is highly acidic (see above) or contains bile salts and pancreatic enzymes, reflux esophagitis can be severe. Patients with decreased esophageal peristalsis have longer exposure times between the chyme and the esophageal mucosa. Delayed gastric emptying contributes to reflux esophagitis by lengthening the period during which reflux is possible and by increasing the acid content of chyme.

Reflux esophagitis causes an inflammatory response in the esophageal wall, which results in hyperemia, increased capillary permeability, edema, tissue fragility, erosion, and ulcerations. Fibrosis and basal cell hyperplasia are common and precancerous lesions (Barrett's esophagus) can be a long-term consequence (McCance & Huether, 2010).

Signs and Symptoms

Most patients complain of burning substernal pain that radiates upward, often aggravated by meals and by lying down and relieved by sitting up. The burning substernal pain can be confused with the chest pain associated with angina or myocardial infarction and cause considerable patient distress. Nocturnal aspiration of reflux contents can cause recurrent pneumonia, bronchospasm, and cough.

Sore throat, hoarseness, and halitosis are associated with reflux into the back of the throat. A reflex salivary hypersecretion is sometimes described, especially in children.

Dysphagia usually suggests long-standing GERD with acute inflammation, stricture, or both. Solid food may stick in the distal esophagus; repeated swallows and significant amounts of liquid may be required to ensure passage into the stomach.

Table 34-2 shows the signs and symptoms of GERD and potential complications. A predominance of heartburn, regurgitation, or both, occurring after meals (particularly large or fatty meals) are highly specific to GERD. Older adults, who may have decreased gastric acidity or decreased pain perception, may not report these symptoms despite significant disease. They are also more likely to self-treat. Infants and children also have slightly different signs and symptoms and they are discussed in the sections about these specific patient populations.

Table 34–1 Foods and Drugs That Influence GERD

Foods and Drugs	Action on LES Tone
Foods	
Chocolate, spearmint, peppermint, decaffeinated coffee, high-fat or high-carbohydrate meals, alcohol	Decrease LES tone
Acidic foods, citrus fruit and juices, caffeine	Increase gastric acid secretion
Fatty foods	Delay gastric emptying
Drugs	
Tobacco	Decreases LES tone and increases gastric acid secretion
Anticholinergics, theophylline, meperidine, calcium channel blockers	Decrease LES tone
Bethanechol, metoclopramide, pentobarbital, histamine, antacids	Increase LES tone

LES = lower esophageal sphincter.

Table 34–2 Signs and Symptoms of GERD and Potential Complications

Signs and Symptoms	Common	Unusual	Extra-esophageal	Potential Complication	Suggestive of Cancer (Alarm)
Heartburn	X				
Regurgitation	X				
Dysphagia	X				X
Hypersalivation		X			
Nausea		X			
Painful swallowing		X			X
Asthma			X		
Noncardiac chest pain			X		X
Chronic cough			X		
Dental disease			X		
Hoarseness			X		
Laryngitis			X		
Respiratory symptoms			X		
Abdominal mass				X	
Hematemesis/melena				X	X
Anemia				X	
Weight loss				X	X
Choking					X

Source: Adapted from VHA/Department of Defense. (2003). *Clinical practice guideline for management of adults with gastroesophageal reflux disease in primary care practice.* Washington, DC: Author.

Diagnosis

Signs and symptoms alone are rarely sufficient to diagnose GERD; however, guidelines differ on their recommendations for diagnostic testing. The American College of Gastroenterology (ACG) guidelines recommends no routine testing for straightforward GERD (Katz et al, 2013). The ACG recommends diagnostic testing if patients do not respond to twice-daily proton pump inhibitors (PPIs), or gastric malignancy or misdiagnosis is a concern. The ACG (2013) recommends endoscopy for elderly patients, those with noncardiac chest pain, those at risk for Barrett's esophagitis, and those nonresponsive to PPIs (Katz et al). The ACG guidelines indicate "alarm symptoms" of melena, persistent vomiting, dysphagia, hematemesis, anemia, or involuntary weight loss greater than 5% that warrant endoscopy. Diagnostic testing is done by a gastroenterology specialist. The treatment protocol presented here assumes appropriate diagnosis of GERD.

Pharmacodynamics

Each of the contributing factors to the development of GERD is a target for pharmacological management. Drugs can be used to increase LES tone, to reduce the amount of acid in the chyme, to improve peristalsis and thereby decrease the time chyme is available to produce reflux, and to decrease the exposure of the mucosa to highly acid material. The classes of drugs with these actions include antacids, histamine₂ blockers, cytoprotective agents, prokinetics, and PPIs. Figure 34-1 depicts the site of action of each of these classes of drugs.

Drugs to Improve Lower Esophageal Sphincter Tone

Metoclopramide and bethanechol improve LES tone and have a prokinetic function but are not considered for monotherapy in the treatment of GERD. They are most useful in combination with acid suppression for patients with gastroparesis. Metoclopramide and bethanechol have not demonstrated significant healing of esophageal lesions.

Antacids also serve a dual purpose: they improve LES tone and increase gastric pH. They are usually patient-initiated drug therapy, along with lifestyle modifications.

Drugs to Reduce the Amount of Acid

Two main classes of drugs are used to reduce acid secretion: histamine₂ receptor antagonists (H₂RAs) and PPIs. H₂RAs act on the parietal cells to decrease the amount of acid

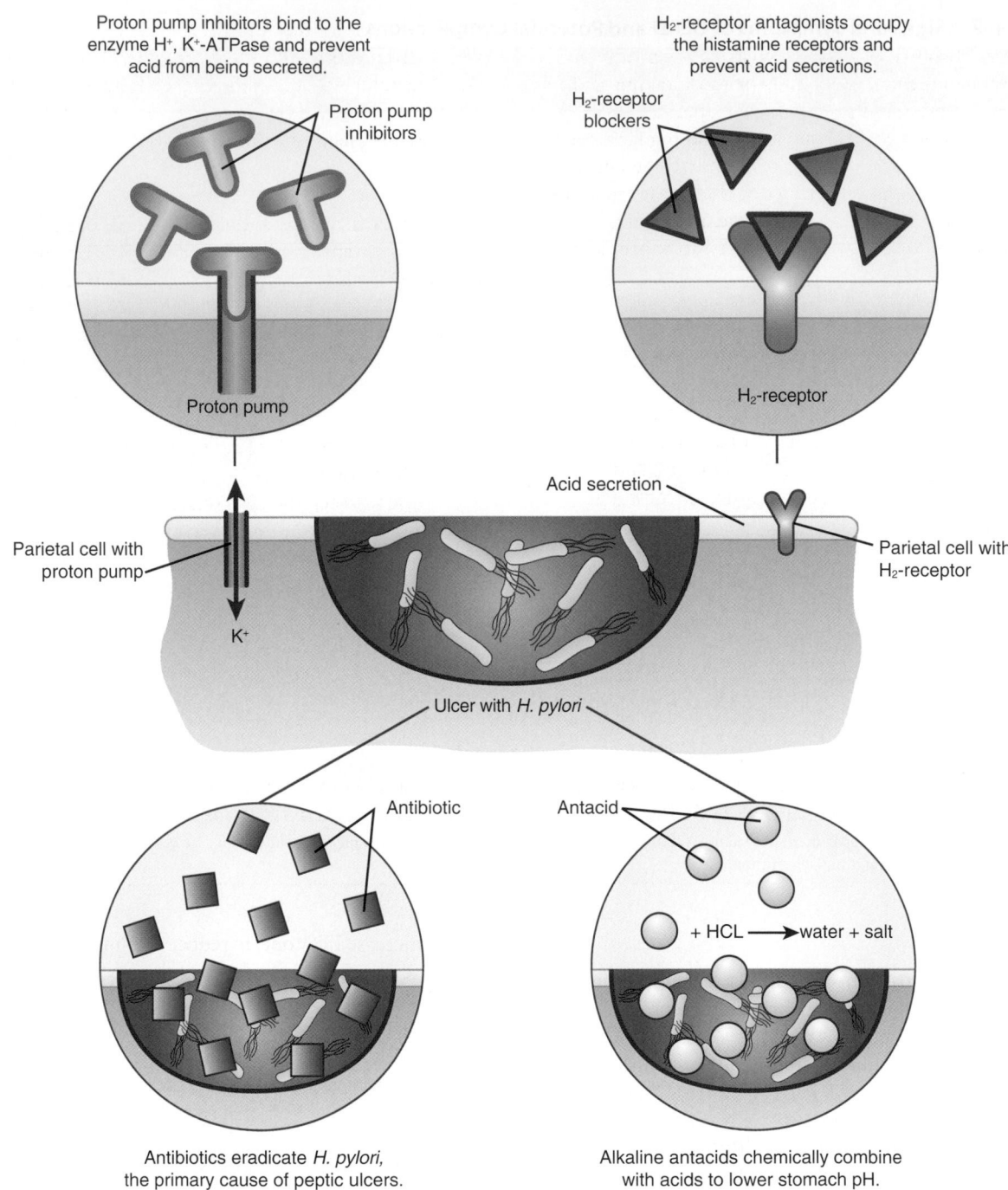

Proton pump inhibitors bind to the enzyme H⁺, K⁺-ATPase and prevent acid from being secreted.

Proton pump inhibitors

Proton pump

Parietal cell with proton pump

K⁺

H₂-receptor antagonists occupy the histamine receptors and prevent acid secretions.

H₂-receptor blockers

H₂-receptor

Acid secretion

Parietal cell with H₂-receptor

Ulcer with *H. pylori*

Antibiotic

Antacid

+ HCL → water + salt

Antibiotics eradicate *H. pylori*, the primary cause of peptic ulcers.

Alkaline antacids chemically combine with acids to lower stomach pH.

Figure 34–1. Sites of action of drugs used to treat GERD and PUD.

produced. Because most of these drugs are available OTC, many patients may have used these drugs as self-initiated therapy before seeking care. Providers need to determine self-medication for GERD in the initial history. H₂RAs may be used as maintenance acid suppression or heartburn therapy in patients who do not have erosive GERD (Katz et al, 2013). The ACG guidelines recommend a trial of nighttime H₂RAs for patients taking daytime PPIs to treat nighttime reflux (Katz et al, 2013).

PPIs are standard first-line therapy for GERD and decrease acid secretion by almost 100%. PPIs improve esophageal healing to about 80%.

Drugs to Improve Peristalsis

A few patients continue to report symptoms despite reduced acid secretion. These patients may benefit from prokinetics, which improve both LES tone and peristalsis. Metoclopramide may provide some benefit but has limited usefulness because of adverse drug reactions.

Drugs to Decrease Mucosal Exposure

Two cytoprotective agents are available to decrease the exposure of the gastric mucosa to acid: sucralfate (Carafate) and misoprostol (Cytotec). Sucralfate acts largely as a Band-Aid to cover sites having erosive damage but is more often used with ulcers. Misoprostol acts by increasing the production of cytoprotective mucus. Older adults or those taking multiple drugs may benefit from sucralfate. Misoprostol is reserved largely for use when NSAIDs are a contributing factor to the increased acid load. These drugs are not mentioned in GERD guidelines, although discontinuance of NSAIDs is mentioned.

The pharmacokinetics and pharmacodynamics of each of the categories of drugs are discussed in more detail in Chapter 20.

Goals of Treatment

Therapy for patients with GERD has four goals: (1) reduce or eliminate the symptoms; (2) heal any esophageal lesions; (3) manage or prevent complications such as stricture, Barrett's esophagus, or esophageal carcinoma; and (4) prevent relapse. Meeting these goals requires a combination of lifestyle modification and drug therapy.

Rational Drug Selection

Algorithm

For most patients, GERD is treated with PPI therapy. Figure 34-2 presents an algorithm for GERD treatment.

Lifestyle Modifications

Antireflux maneuvers, dietary changes, and cessation of smoking are central to the management of GERD regardless of the step. Antireflux maneuvers reduce back pressure on the LES from intra-abdominal contents. Dietary changes reduce the total volume and acid content of the stomach. Smoking reduces LES tone and increases gastric acid secretion. Box 34-1 lists appropriate lifestyle modifications.

Drug Therapy

Lifestyle modifications and OTC antacids are a logical first step for treatment of heartburn, dyspepsia, or mild nonerosive GERD. Most patients have tried an OTC antacid before they seek health care. This step alone may be sufficient. H_2RAs may be sufficient if symptoms are mild and no erosive disease is evident. Tachyphylaxis may occur with H_2RAs.

PPIs are first-line therapy for patients with moderate or severe GERD or erosive disease. PPI therapy continues for 8 weeks and 70% to 80% of patients should have complete relief with PPIs (Katz et al, 2013). There are no major differences in response between the PPIs (Katz et al, 2013). Maintenance PPI therapy should be prescribed for patients who have symptoms that recur after PPI therapy is discontinued or patients with complications such as erosive esophagitis or Barrett's esophagitis (Katz, et al). The patient should be reassessed in 6 to 12 months to determine if he or she can be weaned off therapy. Patients who do not respond to PPIs need to be referred to a gastroenterology specialist.

Patient Variables

Patient variables are also considered in treatment choices. Primary among them is the age of the patient.

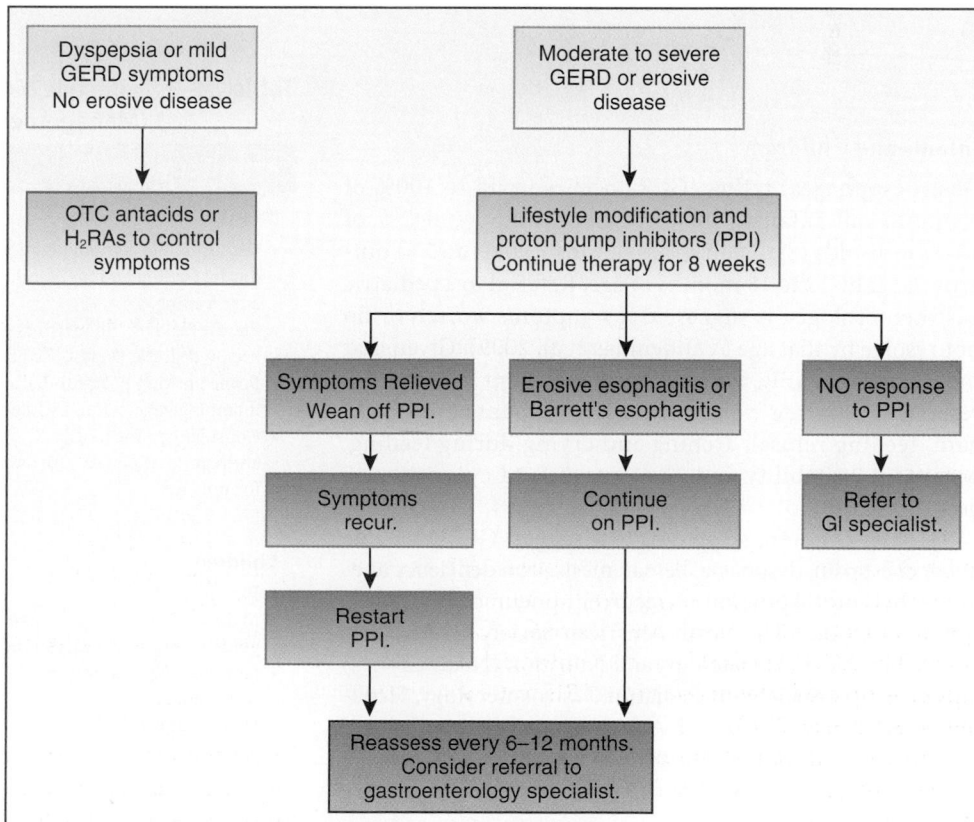

Figure 34–2. Algorithm for gastroesophageal reflux disease (GERD).

Antireflux Maneuvers

- Sleep with the head of the bed elevated 6 to 8 inches with bed blocks or wedges or by using a hospital bed.
- Avoid the recumbent position within 3 hours after eating.
- Avoid bending over within 3 hours after eating.
- Avoid exercise, especially strenuous exercise, within 3 hours after eating.
- Attain and maintain appropriate body weight.

Dietary Considerations

- Avoid spicy, acidic, tomato-based, or fatty foods.
- Avoid chocolate, peppermint, onions, and citrus fruits and juices.
- Limit your intake of coffee, tea, alcohol, and colas.
- Eat moderate amounts of food at each meal. Do not gorge yourself.
- Avoid eating meals or bedtime snacks within 3 hours of going to bed.
- Reserve fluid intake for after or between meals.

Smoking Cessation

- Stop smoking. Smoking both lowers LES tone and increases the secretion of gastric acid.
- Smoking cessation is a high priority.

Weight Loss

- Weight loss may improve symptoms

Infants and Children

Gastroesophageal reflux (GER) occurs in up to 100% of 3-month-old infants, 4% of 6-month-olds, and 2% of 12-month-olds (Stansbury, 2004). Most (90% to 95%) outgrow GER by 12 to 18 months of age. Referral to a pediatric gastroenterologist is suggested if symptoms worsen or do not resolve by that age (Vandenplas et al, 2009). Given that most outgrow GER, aggressive management in infants is reserved for the few experiencing concomitant poor weight gain, feeding refusal, arching and crying during feeding, persistent irritability and pain, apnea, and cyanosis suggesting GERD.

In older children, symptoms that suggest GERD include lower chest pain, dysphagia, hematemesis, iron deficiency anemia, wheezing, aspiration or recurrent pneumonia, chronic cough, or stridor. The North American Society for Pediatric Gastroenterology, Hepatology, and Nutrition (NASPGHAN) and European Society for Pediatric Gastroenterology, Hepatology, and Nutrition (ESPGHAN) developed an international consensus on the diagnosis and management of GER and GERD and the consensus is used as the guideline for care (Vandenplas et al, 2009).

Diagnosis of GERD in both infants and children is usually done through a thorough history and physical exam with the symptoms being reported (Stansbury, 2004; Vandenplas et al, 2009). Any infant with poor weight gain and vomiting should first have a thorough physical exam and be assessed for adequate caloric intake. If caloric intake is adequate, the patient should have the following studies: a complete blood count (CBC), electrolytes, and blood urea nitrogen (BUN). The NASPGHAN/ESPGHAN do not recommend an upper GI series because of low sensitivity and specificity in infants and children (Vandenplas et al, 2013). Esophageal pH monitoring or combined multiple intraluminal impedance (MII) and pH monitoring are the most sensitive and accurate way to diagnose GERD in infants and young children (Vandenplas et al, 2013). Older children or adolescents may be empirically treated with an empirical trial of PPIs for 4 weeks (Vandenplas et al, 2013). No evidence supports empirical treatment of GERD in infants (Vandenplas et al, 2013). Children who present with atypical or extra-esophageal symptoms, do not respond to initial therapy, or have recurrent progressive symptoms should be referred to a gastroenterologist. In children with recurrent vomiting or regurgitation, or difficult or painful swallowing, endoscopy and other invasive tests may be required and referral is appropriate.

Lifestyle modifications are similar to those for adults. Table 34-3 lists the modifications for infants and children.

Infants With GERD

Consultation with a pediatric gastroenterology specialist is needed for infants with suspected GERD because of the

Table 34–3 Lifestyle Modifications in GERD Management for Infants and Children

Antireflux Maneuvers	Dietary Considerations
Infants	
• Keep infant in upright position during feeding and for 30 min after feeding.	• Do not thicken formulas with rice cereal.
• Elevate head of crib mattress or bed 30 degrees. Do not use pillow.	• Try 2 wk on hypoallergenic formula.
• Prone position postprandially when infant is awake, but not while asleep.	• In breastfed infants, consider cow's milk protein intolerance. A
• Consider commercial antiregurgitation (AR) formula if formula fed.	trial of withdrawal of cow's milk and eggs from maternal diet for 2 wk is warranted.
Children	
• Elevate head of bed.	• Avoid substances that can cause LES relaxation, including caffeine, chocolate, peppermint, garlic, citrus fruits, tomatoes, and alcohol.
• Maintain weight according to guidelines or lose weight if indicated.	
• Stop smoking (parents or adolescents who smoke).	
• Do not eat within 1–3 h of going to bed.	

LES = lower esophageal sphincter.
Source: Vandenplas et al, 2009.

difficulty in accurately diagnosing GERD. Empirical medication treatment without studies is not appropriate in infants (Vandenplas et al, 2009). A number of randomized controlled trials in infants have not found consistent improvement in symptoms (back arching, irritability, crying, fussing, vomiting) with either PPIs or H$_2$RAs (Davidson et al, 2013; Vandenplas et al, 2013). Neonates and infants with acid reflux confirmed by esophageal pH monitoring may be treated with esomeprazole, which is FDA-approved for infants down to 1 month of age (Davidson et al; Food and Drug Administration [FDA], 2011).

Children With GERD

Older children and adolescents need a history and physical examination to confirm the suspicion of GERD. Education regarding disease pathology and lifestyle changes should be implemented. No randomized placebo-controlled trials evaluating lifestyle changes or medications in treating heartburn or GERD in children have been done (Vandenplas et al, 2009). Therefore an approach similar to that used in adults with GERD should be used.

H$_2$RAs may be prescribed in infants and children with GERD, although this is not recommended by guidelines. Ranitidine (Zantac), cimetidine (Tagamet), and famotidine (Pepcid) have liquid formulations that make pediatric dosing easier and have been used successfully in children ages 3 months to 16 years.

Alternatively, a trial of 2 to 4 weeks of PPIs may be started in older children or adolescents. If the patient does not improve, treatment continues for 8 to 12 weeks. After 12 weeks of therapy, the PPI should be discontinued. If symptoms recur, the PPI should be restarted. If there is no response to the initial 2 to 4 week trial of PPIs, the patient should be referred to a gastroenterology specialist (Vandenplas et al, 2009).

The FDA has approved four PPIs for use in children: omeprazole (Prilosec), esomeprazole (Nexium), lansoprazole (Prevacid), and rabeprazole (Aciphex Sprinkle Delayed-Release Capsules). Because the long-term effects of their use in children are not known, there is some concern regarding chronic acid suppression. Long-term PPI treatment has been associated with increased rates of community-acquired pneumonia, gastroenteritis, and entercolitis (Vandenplas et al, 2009). Long-term therapy with PPIs in children warrants consultation with a specialist.

Metoclopramide has adverse reactions in children, including restlessness, insomnia, somnolence, dystonia, and extrapyramidal symptoms. Some of the drug's antidopaminergic adverse reactions do not resolve with drug withdrawal. The NASPGHAN/ESPGHAN GERD guidelines do not recommend the use of prokinetics in most children (Vandenplas et al, 2009). Consultation with or referral to a pediatric gastroenterologist is suggested before these drugs are prescribed.

Older Adults

Gastroesophageal reflux is more common in the elderly than younger adults (Fock & Poh, 2010; Poh, Navarro-Rodriguez,

& Fass, 2010). Older patients have an age-related decrease in upper esophageal sphincter pressure and delayed gastric emptying (Fock & Poh, 2010). More elderly patients have grade III–IV esophagitis yet are less likely to report classic symptoms of heartburn, regurgitation, or epigastric pain (Poh et al, 2010). Elderly patients are more likely to present with atypical symptoms of anorexia, vomiting, respiratory symptoms, and dysphagia (Poh et al, 2010; Scholl, Dellon, & Shaheen, 2011).

Antacids are generally safe in older adults, but antacids with constipation as an adverse reaction may be more problematic for them. In addition, many antacids have high sodium content, and some older adults are on low- to moderate-sodium diets. Among the H$_2$RAs, famotidine (Pepcid) is generally safe in the older population but should be used with caution in cases of renal insufficiency. Nizatidine (Axid) may cause asymptomatic ventricular tachycardia and carries a risk of hepatocellular injury. Ranitidine (Zantac) and cimetidine (Tagamet) carry risks for mental status changes in older adults (Poh et al, 2010). Because older adults are often taking several prescription and OTC drugs, the increased number of drug interactions associated with cimetidine also makes it a less attractive choice.

PPIs are generally safe in the elderly and provide rapid relief of symptoms and healing of erosive esophagitis (Poh et al, 2010; Scholl, Dellon, & Shaheen, 2010). Patients with hepatic impairment will have decreased clearance of PPIs and may need a dosage adjustment. Of concern are drug interactions associated with PPIs that are metabolized by CYP2C19 and CYP3A4, including interactions with warfarin, phenytoin, diazepam, and clopidrogrel (Poh et al, 2010). Patients taking PPIs and drugs with a narrow therapeutic range, such as warfarin or phenytoin, should be monitored closely during therapy. Elderly patients taking PPIs are at increased risk of community-acquired pneumonia, *Clostridium difficile* infections, and possible bone fractures in immobile patients (Scholl, Dellon, & Shaheen, 2011).

Among the prokinetics, metoclopramide has a risk for central nervous system (CNS) toxicity. In addition, it is contraindicated in congestive heart failure, renal failure, and hypokalemia, all of which are more common in older adults. Metoclopramide requires careful thought and monitoring in older adults.

Monitoring

Esophagitis is the cause of 5% to 10% of all cases of upper GI bleeding. Monitoring by complete blood count at annual exams is appropriate. The remainder of monitoring is clinical evaluation of symptoms.

Endoscopy to demonstrate the presence of lesions and their healing is the gold standard. It is shown in each algorithm at various steps of therapy. For patients requiring ongoing step 3 or 4 therapy, some specialists recommend endoscopy. Given its cost, others suggest endoscopy every 2 to 3 years because Barrett's esophagus is not reversible.

Long-term use of PPIs presents concerns. One concern is the development of precancerous cells due to hypochlorhydria, with enterochromaffin cell–like hyperplasia changes found in chronic PPI use (Lodato et al, 2010; Vandenplas et al, 2009). Another concern is an increase in hip fractures in at-risk patients who are on PPIs longer than 2 years and on higher doses of PPIs (Corley, Kubo, Zhao, & Quesenberry, 2010). Vitamin B_{12} deficiency is also a concern with chronic acid suppression.

Outcome Evaluation

Figure 34-2 shows the treatment algorithm for GERD. Outcome evaluation targets relief of symptoms. Evaluation also includes the other goals for therapy: healing of lesions, prevention of complications, and prevention of relapse.

Relapse rates are high for patients with GERD. Lifestyle modifications and some drug therapies are commonly required for life. H$_2$RAs or PPIs may be required chronically but at reduced doses. Return of symptoms for a patient who has been pain-free and is adherent to the treatment regimen suggests that the provider should increase the dosage of the current drug or move the patient to the next step in the algorithm and arrange for endoscopy evaluation.

Referral to a pediatric specialist is warranted for any infant younger than 2 months who presents with vomiting or other symptoms of GERD. Children and infants older than 2 months who are unresponsive to short-term (2 to 4 wk at each step) empirical treatment or have suspected or demonstrated complications also require referral.

Patients who have mild or typical symptoms and who respond to conservative treatment can be managed by the primary care provider. Patients who do not respond to 4 to 8 weeks of step 2 therapy should have a referral to a gastroenterologist, which means at least consultation with a gastroenterologist. Patients with erosive disease or who do not respond to step 3 therapy require referral to a specialist. These patients are at high risk for Barrett's esophagus, which carries with it a 30-fold greater risk for developing esophageal cancer than the general population.

Patient Education

Patient education should include a discussion of information related to the overall treatment plan as well as that specific to the drug therapy, reasons for the drug being taken, drugs as part of the total treatment regimen, and adherence issues.

PEPTIC ULCER DISEASE

Peptic ulcer disease (PUD) is a common clinical problem estimated to have a lifetime incidence of 12% in men and 10% in women (Lew, 2009). PUD is listed as the primary diagnosis in 712,000 ambulatory care visits annually, and 1,473,000 visits annually have PUD listed as one of the diagnoses (National Institutes of Health, 2009b). The rate of hospital admission for uncomplicated ulcer has decreased significantly, but the incidence has not decreased, making this largely a disease that is treated in the primary care setting. Risk factors for PUD include smoking and habitual use of NSAIDs or alcohol, but the main culprit is *H. pylori* infection, which has been firmly established as a major cause of PUD. Reduction of stress and other factors that increase gastric acid secretion are still included in disease management.

Peptic ulcers fall into two categories: duodenal ulcers and gastric ulcers. Each has a slightly different pathology and treatment, although they share many aspects of both. They are addressed separately here.

Pathophysiology

PUD is a chronic inflammatory condition of the stomach and duodenum. It is the result of increased acid and pepsin secretion; impaired mucosal cytoprotection; use of NSAIDs; *H. pylori;* personal factors such as genetics, smoking, and stress; or a combination of these causes. Definitive diagnosis is via esophagogastroduodenoscopy.

The incidence of gastric ulcers differs from that of duodenal ulcers. Gastric ulcer disease is about one-fourth as common as duodenal ulcer disease. The pathophysiology of the disorders also varies. Table 34-4 compares the incidence, pathophysiology, and signs and symptoms of the two disorders.

Gastric Ulcer Disease

Gastric ulcers tend to develop in the antral region, adjacent to the acid-secreting mucosa of the body. Although the pathogenesis of gastric ulcer disease is unclear, it is generally thought that the underlying defect is a disruption that increases the gastric mucosal barrier's permeability to hydrogen ions. *H. pylori* is seen in 75% to 85% of patients with gastric ulcers. Gastric acid secretion may be normal or less than normal. A variety of substances can disrupt this barrier. They are summarized in Box 34-2.

Another suggested contributing factor is increased duodenal gastric reflux of bile across an incompetent pyloric sphincter. An increased concentration of bile salts disrupts the gastric mucosa and decreases the electrical potential across the gastric mucosal membrane. This altered electrical potential permits the diffusion of hydrogen ions into the mucosa, where they disrupt permeability and cellular structure. Once the barrier is broken, the damaged submucosal areas exposed to hydrogen ions release histamine, which stimulates an increase in acid and pepsinogen production, causes local vasodilation, and increases capillary permeability. The pepsinogen produces mucosal erosion, resulting in the formation of ulcers. The disrupted mucosa becomes edematous and loses plasma proteins. Destruction of small blood vessels results in bleeding.

Pyloric stenosis has also been given as a possible cause of gastric ulcer formation. With pyloric deformity, gastric emptying is poor, resulting in stasis and antral distention. This distention leads to increased gastrin release and gastric acid production.

Chronic gastritis has also been associated with the development of gastric ulcers. It may precipitate ulcer

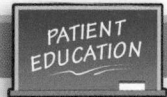

PATIENT EDUCATION

Gastroesophageal Reflux Disease

RELATED TO THE OVERALL TREATMENT PLAN/DISEASE PROCESS

☐ Pathophysiology of gastroesophageal reflux and its long-term risks for permanent esophageal damage and cancer of the esophagus

☐ Central role of lifestyle modifications in improving prognosis and keeping the number and cost of required drugs down

☐ Importance of adherence to the treatment regimen

☐ Need for follow-up visits with the primary care provider if the symptoms do not resolve or if they recur

SPECIFIC TO THE DRUG THERAPY

☐ Reason for the drug(s) being given and the anticipated action of the drug(s) on the disease process

☐ Doses and schedules for taking the drug(s)

☐ Possible adverse reactions and what to do when they occur

☐ Coping mechanisms for complex and costly drug regimens

☐ Interaction between lifestyle modifications and these drugs

REASONS FOR TAKING THE DRUG(S)

Patient education about specific drugs is provided in Chapter 20. Specific information related to GERD: drugs used to treat GERD are given to reduce symptoms, heal any esophageal ulcers, reduce the risk for permanent esophageal damage or cancer, and prevent relapse of symptoms. Different drugs have different roles with each of these. The expectations should be clear about what the drugs can and cannot do. Drugs alone will not correct the disorder.

DRUGS AS PART OF THE TOTAL TREATMENT REGIMEN

Lifestyle modification is equally important in disease management. GERD is a chronic condition. Patients with GERD must understand the lifelong nature of the disorder and the need to incorporate the treatment regimen into their everyday lives.

ADHERENCE ISSUES

Any disease process where lifestyle modifications are central to management is prone to problems with adherence. Health-care providers should be aware of the potential problem of nonadherence, discuss the importance of adherence at each follow-up visit, and assist patients in removing barriers to adherence, such as the complexity and cost of the treatment regimen and the presence of adverse reactions.

Table 34–4 Comparison of Gastric and Duodenal Ulcer Disease

Characteristic	Gastric Ulcer	Duodenal Ulcer
Age at onset	50–70 yr	20–50 yr
Gender	Equal in men and women	More common in men
Cancer risk	Increased	Not increased
Pathophysiology		
Parietal cell mass	Normal or decreased	Increased
Acid production	Normal or decreased	Increased
Serum gastrin	Increased	Normal
Serum pepsinogen	Normal	Increased
Associated gastritis	More common	Usually not present
Helicobacter pylori	Present in 60%–80% of cases	Present in 95%–100% of cases
Clinical manifestations: pain	Located in upper abdomen intermittent	Located in upper abdomen intermittent
	Pain > antacid > relief pattern	Pain > antacid or food > relief pattern
	Food > pain pattern	Nocturnal pain common
Clinical course	Chronic ulcer without pattern of exacerbation and remission	Pattern of exacerbation and remission for years*

*This pattern is significantly affected by eradication of *H. pylori.*

BOX 34–2 SUBSTANCES THAT CAN DISRUPT THE GASTRIC MUCOSAL BARRIER

Drugs

Alcohol
Aspirin
Caffeine
Corticosteroids
NSAIDs
Tobacco

Other Causes

H. pylori infection
Bile and pancreatic secretions
Physiological and psychological stress
Salmonella
Spicy, irritating foods*
Staphylococcus organisms
Uremia associated with renal failure

---

formation by limiting the ability of the mucosa to secrete a protective layer of mucus. Decreased mucosal synthesis of prostaglandin (e.g., NSAIDs) may also create an ulcerogenic environment.

Duodenal Ulcer Disease

Infection with *H. pylori* is the major cause of duodenal ulcers. With the exception of patients taking NSAIDs, 95% to 100% of patients with duodenal ulcer are infected with this organism. It is a spiral-shaped bacterium that lives attached to or just above the gastric mucosa. Once *H. pylori* is acquired, colonization continues for life unless the organism is eliminated by antimicrobial treatment or the usually late-in-life development of atrophic gastritis. Essentially everyone who carries the organism in the gastric mucosal layer has evidence of some tissue reaction (e.g., an inflammatory response and chronic active gastritis), yet most colonized patients remain asymptomatic for life. The strain of *H. pylori* with which an individual is colonized (spiral shape, flagella, and specific ability to attach to Lewis B antigens in persons with type O blood) affects risk for disease.

Once attached to the mucosal layer, *H. pylori* releases toxins, proteases, and phospholipase enzymes that promote inflammation and impair the integrity of the mucosal layer. The inflammatory process includes the release of histamine, which acts the same on the duodenal mucosa and on the gastric mucosa. The end result is ulceration. Eradication of *H. pylori* reduces ulcer recurrence (Lew, 2009).

Diagnosis

Diagnosis of ulcerative disease involves radiographic and endoscopic evaluation of the upper GI tract and testing for *H. pylori* colonization. The American College of Gastroenterology guidelines recommend all patients with peptic ulcers should be tested for *H. pylori* (Chey, Wong, & the Practice Parameters Committee of the American College of Gastroenterology, 2006). A number of tests can be used, including endoscopic testing for cytology and noninvasive tests, including serological testing, urea breath test, stool antigen test, and rapid stool antigen test (Crowe, 2013a).

Invasive diagnostic procedures are determined in consultation with or by referral to a gastroenterologist. Endoscopy is the gold standard for confirming peptic ulcer disease and to rule out gastric cancer (Lew, 2009). For further discussion of the diagnostic process associated with PUD, the reader is referred to management texts. The treatment protocol presented here assumes appropriate diagnosis of PUD.

Pharmacodynamics

Eradication of *H. pylori* is critical to PUD treatment; therefore, all recommended treatment regimens include a combination of a PPI and antimicrobial therapy. Antimicrobial agents used include clarithromycin, tetracycline, amoxicillin, levofloxacin, and metronidazole. They are given in a triple drug regimen or a quadruple drug regimen that includes bismuth subsalicylate. Acid suppression by the PPI in conjunction with the antimicrobial helps alleviate the ulcer-related symptoms, heals gastric mucosal inflammation, and may enhance the efficacy of the antimicrobial agent against *H. pylori* at the mucosal surface. Antimicrobials are discussed in more detail in Chapter 24.

Goals of Treatment

Goals of treatment for PUD are (1) to eradicate *H. pylori*, (2) heal any ulcers, (3) manage or prevent complications such as GI bleeding or the development of gastric carcinoma, (4) prevent relapse, and (5) reduce or eliminate symptoms. Meeting these goals requires both lifestyle modification and drug therapy, but lifestyle modification is less important in PUD than it is in GERD.

Rational Drug Selection

Algorithm

The treatment algorithm outlines the steps in treating peptic ulcers that consist of healing the ulcer and preventing ulcer recurrence through eradication of *H. pylori*. Ulcers that are associated with NSAID use are discussed in Chapter 25.

As with GERD, step 1 involves lifestyle modifications and OTC antacids or histamine₂ blockers. Most patients have tried some step 1 interventions before they seek health care. This step alone may be sufficient for patients with mild disease and only occasional symptoms, but this step alone is not likely to heal any ulcers. Progression to step 2 is usually required, especially for duodenal ulcers and for those that are a result of *H. pylori* infection. Figure 34-3 shows the stepped algorithm for peptic ulcer disease. See Table 34-5 for diagnostic tests.

Step 2 for patients with uncomplicated gastric ulcers includes testing and treating for *H. pylori* and acid suppressive therapy with PPIs. Multiple treatment regimens for *H. pylori*

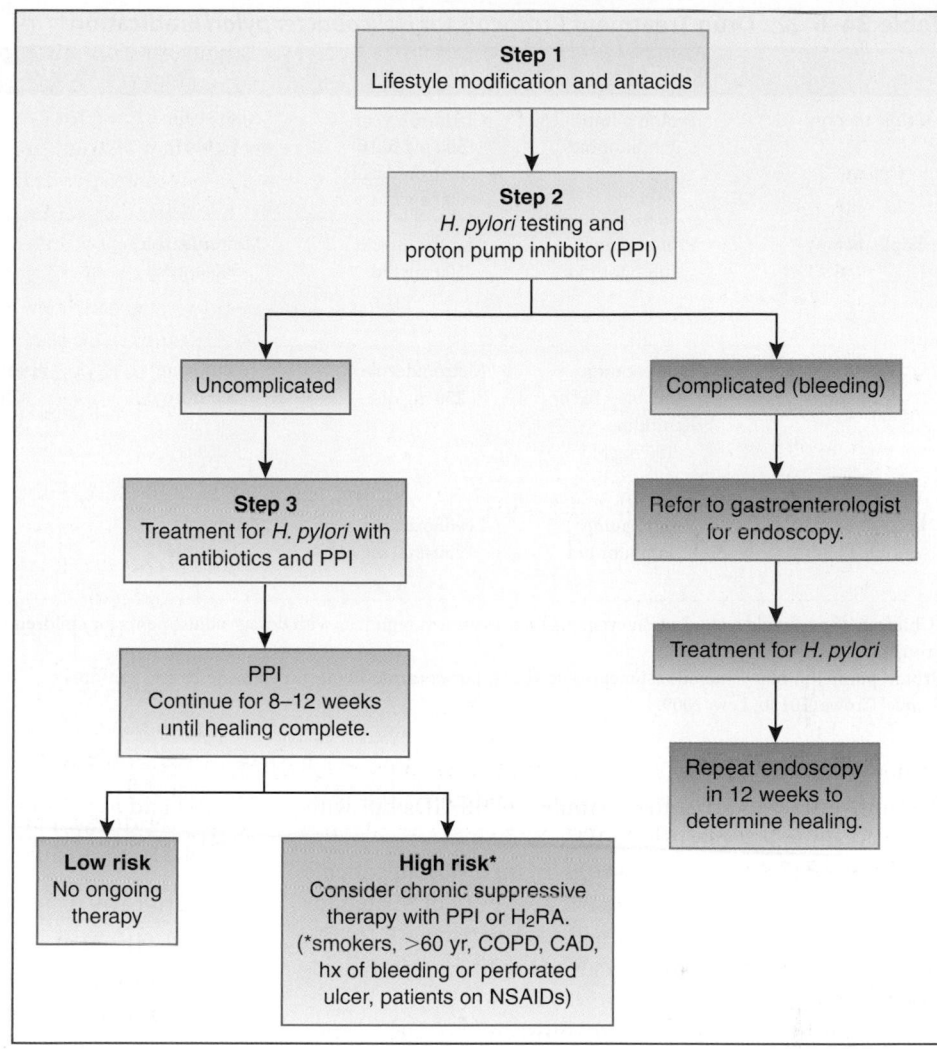

Figure 34–3. Stepped-approach algorithm for peptic ulcer disease.

Table 34–5 Invasive and Noninvasive Diagnostic Tests for *Helicobacter pylori*

Test	Sensitivity	Specificity	Comments
Noninvasive			
Serological ELISA	85%	79%	Detects *H. pylori*; cannot be used to confirm successful cure
Urea breath test	95%–100%	91%–98%	Can be used for screening and confirming cure. PPIs and recent antibiotics can cause false negative.
H. pylori stool antigen test	91%–98%	94%–99%	Can be used for initial diagnosis and test of cure
Invasive			
Rapid urease test	93%–97%%	95%–100%	
Culture of biopsy specimen	70%–80%	100%	
Histological evaluation	>95%	95%–98%	

PPI = protein pump inhibitor.

eradication are available, including combining a PPI and two antibiotics for 14 days (Lew, 2009; Soll, 2011). Maintenance therapy with an antisecretory agent, usually a PPI, at the full healing dose is necessary. Table 34-6 presents the multiple evidence-based treatment regimens.

Ulcers complicated by bleeding require endoscopy for diagnosis of the lesion. Healing should also be documented by endoscopy after 12 weeks of antisecretory therapy (usually PPIs) to document healing. Patients who are taking NSAIDs should be switched to a COX-2 inhibitor to achieve analgesic

Table 34–6 ⊗ **Drug Treatment Protocols for *Helicobacter pylori* Eradication**

	Drug 1	Drug 2	Drug 3	Drug 4	Comments
Triple therapy	Proton pump inhibitor bid	Clarithromycin 500 mg bid or metronidazole 500 mg bid	Amoxicillin 1 g bid	—	Treat for 10–14 d Usual first-line therapy
Triple therapy	Proton pump inhibitor bid	Clarithromycin 500 mg bid	Metronidazole 500 mg bid	—	Treat for 7–14 d Use as first-line therapy in penicillin-allergic patients
Quadruple therapy	Proton pump inhibitor bid *or* Ranitidine 150 mg bid	Metronidazole 250 mg qid	Tetracycline* 500 mg qid	Bismuth sub-salicylate 525 mg qid	Treat for 10–14 d Usually used as second-line therapy in patients who fail first-line therapy
Levofloxacin-based triple therapy	Proton pump inhibitor bid	Levofloxacin 250–500 mg bid	Amoxicillin 1 gm bid		Treat for 10–14 d Second-line or rescue therapy

*Children <8 yr should not take tetracycline. Other treatment regimens with dosage adjustments for children are acceptable. Some come with drugs grouped in packets.

Proton pump inhibitors include esomeprazole 40 mg, lansoprazole 30 mg, omeprazole 20 mg, pantoprazole 40 mg, rabeprazole 20 mg.

Source: Crowe, 2013b; Lew, 2009.

and anti-inflammatory effects similar to NSAIDs but with fewer GI complications (Soll, 2011).

Duodenal and gastric ulcers recur in up to 80% of patients treated with drugs to reduce gastric acid but not treated for eradication of *H. pylori* infection. By comparison, 6% to 15% of patients have recurrent ulcers when their *H. pylori* infection is cured.

Maintenance therapy with an antisecretory agent is not generally required after eradication of *H. pylori*. However, it is prudent to prescribe maintenance therapy for certain high-risk groups: smokers; patients older than 60 years; patients with chronic obstructive pulmonary disease, coronary artery disease, or renal failure; patients with a history of bleeding or perforated ulcer; patients with persistent symptoms; and those who must take NSAIDs or other ulcerogenic drugs.

Patients with gastric or duodenal ulcers who fail to become symptom-free or who develop complications such as GI bleeding while on antisecretory therapy require a referral to a gastroenterologist. Surgery is contemplated for gastric ulcer patients.

Lifestyle Modifications

Evidence is lacking that dietary modifications affect the course of PUD. Frequent small meals and decreased consumption of spices, alcohol, caffeine, and fruit juices have never been demonstrated to affect healing. Dietary changes should be directed at those substances that cause symptoms in each particular patient. An important lifestyle modification is smoking cessation. Smoking both increases the risk for gastric and duodenal ulcers and delays their healing (Soll & Vakil, 2012).

Aspirin and NSAIDs are known to be ulcerogenic. Their use should be discouraged and a high index of suspicion for

NSAID and aspirin use is required because patients do not always report OTC use (Soll & Vakil, 2012).

Drug Therapy

Currently, the FDA approves eight treatment regimens; however, several other combinations have been used successfully. Regimens include triple or quadruple drug therapy with a variety of drugs. The treatment regimens that have the highest rate of success in eradication, the best likelihood of adherence related to number of drugs taken, and adverse effects are presented in Table 34-6. All include a twice-daily dose of a PPI. The most popular antibiotics are clarithromycin (Biaxin) and amoxicillin. Because all these drugs can be taken twice daily, the regimen is simple and has a limited number of drugs.

Selection among the protocols is based on cost, convenience, ability to tolerate the adverse drug reactions of the total regimen, antimicrobial resistance, patient variables, and eradication rates. For each patient, assess the likelihood of adherence and use the most cost-effective but simplest drug regimen that will get the job done.

Adverse Drug Reactions for the Total Regimen

Adverse drug reactions have been reported in up to 70% of patients taking bismuth-based four-drug regimens. Metronidazole-based regimens have increased adverse reactions. Overall, the best regimen for tolerability appears to be a PPI-based three-drug regimen. Happily, these regimens also are highly efficacious.

Antimicrobial Resistance

Concern about antimicrobial resistance has increased, regardless of the disease process for which these drugs are being used. Chapter 24 discusses resistance to the various antimicrobials. Resistance associated with *H. pylori* eradication has been linked to the length and complexity of the treatment regimen and the tolerability of adverse reactions. Resistance to metronidazole is most common and higher in women (Crowe, 2013b). Resistance to clarithromycin is low (10%), as is resistance to amoxicillin and tetracycline. Acquired resistance occurs in up to two-thirds of treatment failures. Changing drugs and trying a different treatment regimen may be useful in these instances. First- and second-line therapy options are presented in Table 34-6.

Patient Variables

Several patient variables need to be considered. Patients with allergies to any of the drugs in a treatment regimen require a different regimen. Women of childbearing age should use a regimen that does not include tetracycline because of the risk for fetal harm. The same is true for children younger than 8 years because of problems related to discoloration of teeth. Each of the drugs in these regimens has potential drug interactions. Other drugs the patient may be taking must be taken into account.

Given all these parameters, the treatment regimen with good to excellent eradication rates, a low to medium adverse reactions profile, likelihood of adherence based on complexity of the regimen and moderate cost, and limited antimicrobial resistance appears to be clarithromycin plus amoxicillin plus a PPI, all taken twice a day for 10 to 14 days.

Monitoring

Monitoring parameters for each of the drugs in these treatment regimens are presented in Chapters 20 and 24. Documentation of ulcer healing by endoscopy 12 weeks after the end of therapy is the gold standard. Cost considerations suggest reserving it for patients who are at high risk for complications, patients with recurrence, and those who will be on long-term therapy. The urea breath test or stool antigen testing can be used to screen symptomatic patients who are suspected of having recurrent ulcers associated with *H. pylori* infection. Note that serological testing for *H. pylori* may be falsely negative if the patient is on PPIs or recently on antibiotics. Documentation by endoscopy is optional for low-risk patients.

Outcome Evaluation

Figure 34-3 shows the treatment algorithm for PUD. Outcome evaluation targets eradication of *H. pylori* and relief of symptoms. Evaluation also includes the other goals for therapy: healing of lesions, prevention of complications, and prevention of relapse. Relapse rates are high for patients with PUD but can be significantly reduced with appropriate maintenance therapy or eradication of *H. pylori* infection.

Patients with PUD who remain symptom-free without drugs or on maintenance therapy require no more frequent follow-up than their annual physical examination.

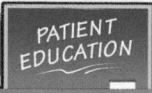

PATIENT EDUCATION

Peptic Ulcer Disease

RELATED TO THE OVERALL TREATMENT PLAN/DISEASE PROCESS

☐ Understanding the pathophysiology of ulcer formation and its long-term risks for bleeding and cancer of the stomach

☐ Role of lifestyle modifications in total treatment regimen

☐ Importance of adherence to the treatment regimen, especially in light of antimicrobial resistance

☐ Need for follow-up visits with the primary care provider if the symptoms recur or do not resolve

SPECIFIC TO THE DRUG THERAPY

☐ Reason for the drug(s) being given and the anticipated action of the drug(s) on the disease process

☐ Doses and schedules for taking the drug(s)

☐ Possible adverse reactions and what to do when they occur

☐ Coping mechanisms for complex and costly drug regimens

☐ Interactions between lifestyle modifications and these drugs

REASONS FOR TAKING THE DRUG(S)

Patient education about specific drugs is provided in Chapters 20 and 24. Specific information related to PUD includes the following: drugs used to treat PUD are given to treat *H. pylori,* reduce symptoms, heal any ulcers, reduce the risk for complications, and prevent relapse of symptoms. Different drugs have different roles with each of these.

DRUGS AS PART OF THE TOTAL TREATMENT REGIMEN

Lifestyle modification is important in disease management. PUD is often a chronic condition, requiring lifelong maintenance therapy.

ADHERENCE ISSUES

Any disease process in which lifestyle modifications are required or in which a complex regimen of three or four drugs over a period of weeks is required is likely to have problems with adherence. Health-care providers should be aware of the potential problem of nonadherence, discuss the importance of adherence, and assist patients in removing barriers to adherence, such as the complexity and cost of the treatment regimen and the presence of adverse reactions.

Patients with *H. pylori* infection–associated ulcers that do not respond to the first course of antimicrobial therapy should be evaluated for noncompliance. Ask about missed doses, adverse effects of medications, and completion of the therapy prescribed (Crowe, 2013b; Lew, 2009). Antibiotic resistance may occur. Culture and sensitivity are not routinely used in PUD treatment. A second course of therapy with a different drug combination for 14 days is recommended (Crowe, 2013b; Lew, 2009). If the patient still has symptoms and eradication fails, referral to a gastroenterologist is appropriate. Other causes, such as Zollinger-Ellison syndrome, may be present.

Patient Education

Patient education should include a discussion of information related to the overall treatment plan as well as that specific to the drug therapy, reasons for the drug being taken, drugs as part of the total treatment regimen, and adherence issues.

REFERENCES

American Gastroenterological Association (AGA) Institute Medical Position Panel. (2008). American Gastroenterological Association medical position statement on the management of gastroesophageal reflux disease. *Gastroenterology, 135*, 1383–1391.

Chey, W. D., Wong, B. C. Y., & the Practice Parameters Committee of the American College of Gastroenterology. (2007). Management of *Helicobacter pylori* infection. *American Journal of Gastroenterology, 102*, 1808–1825.

Corley, D. A., Kubo, A., Zhao, W., & Quesenberry, C. (2010). Proton pump inhibitors and histamine-2 receptor antagonists are associated with hip fractures among at-risk patients. *Gastroenterology, 139*(1), 93–101.

Crowe, S. E. (2013a). Indications and diagnostic tests for *Helicobacter pylori* infection. *UpToDate Online.* Retrieved from http://www.uptodate.com/contents/indications-and-diagnostic-tests-for-helicobacter-pylori-infection?source=see_link#H12

Crowe, S. E. (2013b). Treatment regimens for *Helicobacter pylori. UpToDate Online.* Retrieved from http://www.uptodate.com/contents/treatment-regimens-for-helicobacter-pylori?source=see_link#H7

Davidson, G., Wenzl, T. G., Thomson, M., Omari, T., Barker, P., Lundborg, P., et al. (2013). Efficacy and safety of once-daily esomeprazole for the treatment of gastroesophageal reflux disease in neonatal patients. *Journal of Pediatrics, 163*, 692–698.

Fock, K. M., & Poh, C. H. (2010). Gastroesophageal reflux disease. *Journal of Gastroenterology, 45*, 808–815.

Food and Drug Administration. (2011). Pediatric drug labeling database: Esomeprazole. Retrieved from http://www.accessdata.fda.gov/scripts/sda/sdDetailNavigation.cfm?sd=labelingdatabase&id=BE1FD14F9DDF6997E040A8C0744D54EE&rownum=1

Gold, B., Colletti, R., Abbot, M., Czinn, S., Elitsur, Y., Hassall, E., et al. (2000). *Helicobacter pylori* infection in children: Recommendations for diagnosis and treatment. *Journal of Pediatric Gastroenterology, 31*(5), 490–497.

Greenberger, N. (2003). Update in gastroenterology. *Annals of Internal Medicine, 138*(1), 45–53.

Haruma, K., Mihara, M., Okamoto, E., et al. (1999). Eradication of *Helicobacter pylori* increases gastric acidity in patients with atrophic gastritis of the corpus—Evaluation of 24-h pH monitoring. *Alimentary Pharmacology & Therapeutics, 13*, 155–162.

Institute for Clinical Systems Improvement (ICSI). (2006). *Initial management of dyspepsia and GERD.* Bloomington, MN: Institute for Clinical Systems Improvement. Retrieved from http://www.icsi.org

Katz, P. O., Gerson, L. B., & Vela, M. F. (2013). Guidelines for the diagnosis and management of gastroesophageal reflux disease. *American Journal of Gastroenterology, 108*(3), 308-28.

Lew, E. (2009). Peptic ulcer disease. In N. J. Greenberger (Ed.), *Current diagnosis & treatment gastroenterology, hepatology, & endoscopy* (3rd ed.). New York: McGraw-Hill.

Lodato, F., Azzaroli, F., Turco, L., Mazzella, N., Buonfiglioli, F., Zoli, M., et al. (2010). Adverse effects of proton pump inhibitors. *Best Practices in Research and Clinical Gastroenterology, 24*(2), 193–201.

McCance, K., & Huether, S. (2010). *Pathophysiology: The biological basis for disease in adults and children* (10th ed.). St. Louis, MO: Elsevier Mosby.

National Digestive Diseases Information Clearing House (NDDICH). (2007). *Heartburn, gastroesophageal reflux (GER), and gastroesophageal reflux disease (GERD).* (NIH Publication No. 07–0882). Bethesda, MD: National Institutes of Health. Retrieved from http://digestive.niddk.nih.gov/ddiseases/pubs/gerd/

National Institutes of Health. (2009a). Gastroesophageal reflux disease. In *Burden of digestive diseases in the United States, 2008* (NIH Publication No. 09-6443). Bethesda, MD: National Institutes of Health. Retrieved from http://www2.niddk.nih.gov/AboutNIDDK/ReportsAndStrategicPlanning/

National Institutes of Health. (2009b). Peptic ulcer disease. In *Burden of digestive diseases in the United States, 2008* (NIH Publication No. 09-6443). Bethesda, MD: National Institutes of Health. Retrieved from http://www2.niddk.nih.gov/AboutNIDDK/ReportsAndStrategic Planning/

Opekun, A., Abdalla, N., Sutton, F., Hammoud, F., Kuo, G., Torres, E., et al. (2002). Urea breath testing and analysis in the primary care office. *Journal of Family Practice, 51*(12), 1030–1032.

Poh, C. H., Navarro-Rodriguez, T., & Fass, R. (2010). Review: Treatment of gastroesophageal reflux disease in the elderly. *The American Journal of Medicine, 123*(6), 496–501.

Soll, A. H. (2011). Overview of the natural history and treatment of peptic ulcer disease. *UpToDate Online.* Retrieved from http://www.uptodate.com/contents/overview-of-the-natural-history-and-treatment-of-peptic-ulcer-disease

Soll, A. H., & Vakil, N.B. (2012). Peptic ulcer disease: Genetic, environmental, and psychological risk factors and pathogenesis. *UpToDate Online.* Retrieved from http://www.uptodate.com/contents/peptic-ulcer-disease-genetic-environmental-and-psychological-risk-factors-and-pathogenesis

Stansbury, A. (2004). GER and GERD in children. *American Journal for Nurse Practitioners, 8*(3), 37–44.

Thjodleifsson, B. (2002). Treatment of acid-related disease in the elderly with emphasis on the use of proton pump inhibitors. *Drugs and Aging, 19*(12), 911–927.

Vandenplas, Y., Rudolph, C. D., DiLorenzo, C., Hassall, E., Liptak, G., Mazur, L., et al. (2009). Pediatric gastroesophageal reflux clinical practice guidelines: Joint recommendations of the North American Society for Pediatric Gastroenterology, Hepatology, and Nutrition (NASPGHAN) and the European Society for Pediatric Gastroenterology, Hepatology, and Nutrition (ESPGHAN). *Journal of Pediatric Gastroenterology and Nutrition, 49*, 498–547.

HEADACHES

Theresa Mallick-Searle

Headaches are a common presenting complaint in primary care, accounting for 18 million outpatient visits per year in the United States. This makes headaches the seventh-leading chief complaint in ambulatory clinics. More than 80 percent of adult Americans report that they experience recurrent headache, with 35% to 50% labeling their headache severe enough to disrupt their activities of daily living (Marin, 1998; Smith, 1998). Globally, the percentages of the adult population with an active headache disorder are 47% for headache in general, 10% for migraine, up to 70% for tension-type headache in some populations, and 5% for medication-overuse headache (World Health Organization, 2012). These numbers indicate that the disability attributable to tension-type headache is larger worldwide than that due to migraine.

In the United States, 12% of the general population affected, with women affected more frequently than men (Cutrer, Bajwa, & Sabahat, 2014), the cost of direct medical care for migraine is $1.25 to $11 billion, and the cost to American employers is $13 billion annually because of an estimated 113 million missed workdays and impaired work function (Migraine Research Foundation, 2014). Successful pharmacological management of headache can improve the quality of life for millions of Americans. The Institute for Clinical Systems Improvement (ICSI, 2009) provides guidelines for treatment of multiple types of headaches, while the U.S. Headache Consortium provides evidence-based guidelines for the treatment of migraine (Matcher et al, 2000). These two evidence-based guidelines are used for treatment recommendations in this chapter.

Headaches affect all age groups, from preverbal children to the older patient. When asked, 20% to 40% of school-age children report having had headaches. The onset of migraine usually occurs between the ages of 15 and 25, although younger children may experience migraine. The peak incidence of headache is in young adulthood (25 to 34 years), with the incidence waning as a patient gets older. Onset of headache after age 50 or headaches increasing in frequency or severity should lead to the investigation of underlying neurological disease.

The most common types of headaches can be classified as migraine, tension-type, and chronic daily headache, which may present as a mixed form of tension type and migraine, or chronic migraine. Medication-overuse is also identified as a cause of chronic daily headache. Cluster headaches are uncommon, but severely debilitating. Where still little is known regarding the specific pathophysiology in post-concussive headaches, much research and focus has recently been placed on this underrecognized type of headache. The pharmacological management of common types of headaches is discussed in this chapter. Pathological headaches, caused by space-occupying lesions, alterations in intracranial pressure, or other pathology, are not discussed here, other than to note when the differential should lead to pathology rather than to common headaches. To assist the provider in diagnosing the correct type of headache, it is helpful to use a headache screening questionnaire that addresses four questions adopted by the American Academy of Neurology:

1. How often do you get severe headaches (i.e., without treatment it is difficult to function)?
2. How often do you get other (milder) headaches?
3. How often do you take headache relievers or pain pills?
4. Has there been any recent change in your headaches? (Bajwa & Wootton, 2013).

MIGRAINE

Migraine headaches are a complex multifactorial condition, which may be classified in three categories: migraine with aura (classic migraine), migraine without aura (common migraine), and complicated migraine. Classification of migraine, although important for accurate diagnosis, does not affect the pharmacological management. This chapter discusses acute or abortive therapy and preventive therapy, as well as nonpharmacological therapy for treating migraine.

Pathophysiology

There are several theories regarding the pathogenesis of migraine headache. The vascular theory proposes that the aura preceding migraine is caused by vasoconstriction of intracranial vessels, and vasodilation of the affected vessels results in the typical vascular headache pain that throbs in unison with the pulse. The vascular theory has been disputed because not all migraine sufferers have a pulsatile quality to their headache pain.

Considerable evidence associates migraine with changes in serotonin activity that result in release of vasoactive neurotransmitters (substance P, bradykinin, neurokinin A, and calcitonin gene-related peptides). This produces an inflammatory response around the blood vessels of the dura mater and pia mater and is accompanied by dilation of cerebral blood vessels. Specific excitatory serotonin receptors ($5-HT_2$), when activated, can lead to migraine. Many of the abortive agents used for migraine appear to stimulate inhibitory serotonin receptors ($5-HT_1$ and $5-HT_{1D}$) or block $5-HT_2$ receptors.

There is a strong familial component to migraine, with 20% to 60% of patients reporting a family history of migraine. Migraine is 2 to 3 times more prevalent in women than in men. Women with migraines may have increased headaches around the time of their menstrual periods and if they are taking estrogen-containing medications, such as oral contraceptives. Other known triggers of migraine include alcohol, strong light, noxious odors, extreme fatigue, and certain foods. Table 35-1 lists common triggers that may precipitate a migraine headache in patients prone to migraine.

Goals of Treatment

The overall goal of therapy is to minimize the impact of migraine headaches on patients' quality of life, social functioning, and ability to work. A second goal is prevention of migraine by avoiding each patient's identified triggers and prophylaxis for frequent migraine sufferers. Minimizing adverse effects of pharmacotherapy and avoidance of medication overuse/abuse that can lead to medication-overuse headaches should also be goals of both the provider and the patient.

Rational Drug Selection

Pharmacological management of migraine is divided into two major components: acute or abortive therapy and preventive or prophylactic therapy. Most patients with migraine need only abortive therapy for their headaches. If migraine frequency is greater than twice a month and/or severely debilitating or if abortive agents are ineffective, the health-care provider should consider prescribing daily preventive therapy.

Acute Therapy

Acute or abortive therapy is aimed at reversing, aborting, or reducing pain and accompanying symptoms of an attack that is in progress or is anticipated. Acute therapy for migraines can range from simple over-the-counter (OTC) analgesics to intramuscular (IM) dihydroergotamine, which needs to be

Table 35–1   Common Migraine Triggers

Factor	Triggers
Environmental factors	Noxious smells and fumes Bright light or glare Tobacco smoke
Foods	Caffeine (coffee, tea, caffeine-containing medications or beverages) Nuts, peanut butter, pea pods, lima or navy beans Alcohol (red wine, beer, liquor) Aged cheese Monosodium glutamate (MSG) (in Chinese food, seasoning salt, processed foods, soups) Chocolate (sweets, foods, drinks) Nitrites and nitrates (processed meats, hot dogs) Onions Avocados Dairy products (ice cream, yogurt, cheese, sour cream, milk, cream) Pickled or smoked foods (pickled herring, smoked fish) Citrus fruits, bananas, figs, raisins Aspartame (in many foods and drinks labeled "sugar free") Sulfites Yeast products (in bread, donuts)
Lifestyle	Hunger/fasting Oversleeping Inadequate sleep Stress Lack of exercise Prolonged sitting in an uncomfortable position Extended computer usage
Hormonal	Menses Menopause Oral contraceptives Hormonal replacement therapy
Medications	Nitroglycerin Oral contraceptives Antihypertensives Theophylline Antibiotics (TMP/SMZ, griseofulvin) Histamine$_2$ blockers (cimetidine, ranitidine) Analgesic or ergotamine overuse Indomethacin

TMP/SMZ = trimethoprim/sulfamethoxazole.

administered in a clinic or emergency room setting. Oral (PO) therapy may not be effective in patients with associated nausea or vomiting. The stepwise approach to selecting migraine medications for acute treatment is helpful, based on the severity of the pain and associated symptoms. Figure 35-1 is an algorithm that addresses the steps in acute migraine therapy.

The US Headache Consortium, consisting of the American Academy of Family Physicians (AAFP), American Academy of Neurology (AAN), American Headache Society (AHS), American College of Emergency Physicians (ACEP), American College of Physicians (ACP), American Osteopathic Association (AOA), and the National Headache Foundation (NHF), has evaluated the evidence regarding the clinical effectiveness of pharmacological treatment of acute attacks and their guidelines

are used in this chapter (Matcher et al, 2000). Although this section discusses pharmacological treatment, nonpharmacological therapy—specifically applying ice to the head and/or lying down in a darkened room—must accompany the medication. The patient must be advised not to try to "work through" a migraine by just taking medication.

Simple Analgesics

Simple analgesics such as aspirin (ASA) and acetaminophen (APAP) or NSAIDs are the first step in the acute treatment of mild to moderate migraine that is not associated with severe nausea or vomiting. Patients often self-medicate with OTC analgesics, relying on advertising messages to choose a medication. The health-care provider needs to be aware that most patients have already self-medicated to treat their migraines and that they are often seeking care because their treatment is no longer effective. If the provider decides to begin treatment with an OTC product, educating the patient about the rationale for starting with an OTC product will increase compliance.

Clinical experience and population-based studies have demonstrated the effectiveness of OTC analgesics in treating migraine, especially if taken early. The mechanism of action for the various OTC preparations is not completely understood. ASA is thought to have antiprostaglandin and antiplatelet activity that might deliver relief from migraine attack. There is evidence that ASA may also act centrally and has serotoninergic activity. APAP is thought to act centrally and inhibit prostaglandin synthesis. NSAIDs also inhibit prostaglandin synthesis and have a central analgesic mechanism of action. Their anti-inflammatory and antipyretic activity may also contribute to migraine relief. Caffeine is an ingredient in many OTC "headache" preparations (Table 35-2) and plays a role as an analgesic adjuvant when added to ASA or in combination with APAP. The U.S. Food and Drug Administration (FDA) has approved two OTC medications to be labeled specifically for migraine pain: one is a combination of ASA, APAP, and caffeine (Excedrin Migraine), and the other is ibuprofen in a liquid-filled capsule (Advil Migraine).

The dosing of ASA or APAP should be limited to a 1,000 mg dose (10 to 15 mg/kg for children) at the beginning of migraine symptoms or aura, with a maximum of 4,000 mg per day. The U.S. Headache Consortium recommends the combination of acetaminophen plus aspirin plus caffeine (Excedrin Migraine) as a "Group 1 drug with proven pronounced statistical and clinical benefit" (Matcher et al, 2000). APAP has varied results for acute migraine treatment and may not be any better than placebo (Matcher et al, 2000). Medication-overuse headaches are possible if ASA or APAP is used more than 3 days per week.

The NSAIDs have been found to diminish the severity and duration of migraine attacks. Although no NSAID has been found to be better than another in clinical trials, there is a variable response to the different agents that differs from patient to patient. Ibuprofen and naproxen are both group 1 drugs with proven clinical efficacy (Matcher et al, 2000). The use of NSAIDs can involve trying multiple medications

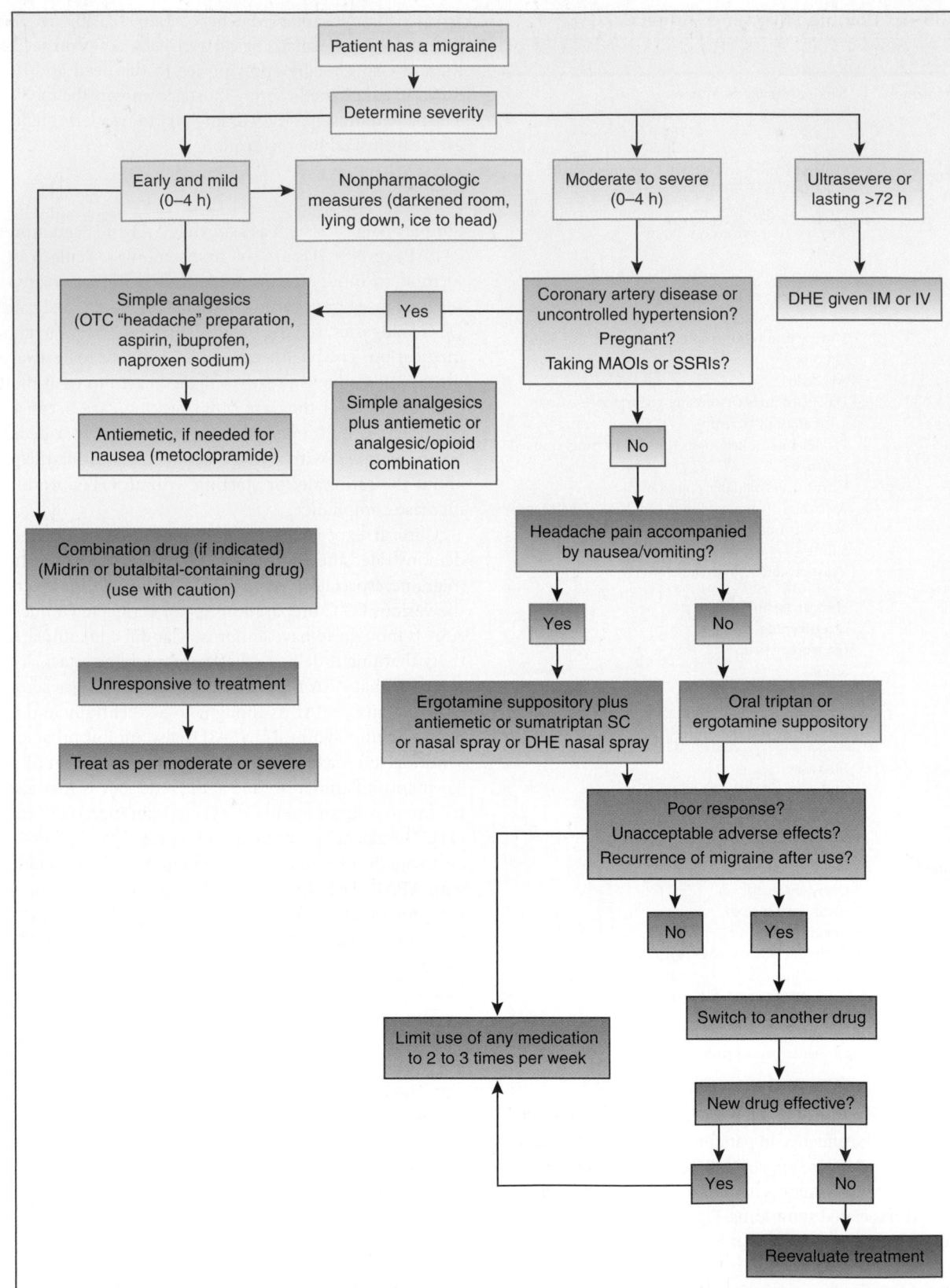

Figure 35–1. Treatment algorithm for acute migraine headache.

before an effective agent is found. Naproxen sodium (Anaprox, Aleve) is often a first choice for migraine, as it is quickly absorbed and well tolerated. The initial starting dose of naproxen sodium is 550 mg, followed by 550 mg twice a day

or 275 mg every 6 to 8 hours. The dose of naproxen sodium for children is 10 to 20 mg/kg/d divided in twice-daily dosing. Although the majority of NSAIDs are given PO, indomethacin (Indocin) is also available in suppository form,

(Text continued on page 1047)

Table 35–2 Drugs Commonly Used: Headaches

Drug	Initial Dose	Maximum Dose	Strengths Available	Rebound Potential	Comments
			Acute Therapy		
Nonnarcotic Analgesics					
Acetaminophen (OTC: Tylenol)	*Adults:* 650–1,000 mg at onset and every 4–6 h *Children:* 10–15 mg/kg/dose	*Adults:* 4,000 mg/day 2–3 d/wk 30 dosages/mo *Children:* 5 doses in 24 h	*Tablets:* 160, 325, 500, 650 mg *Liquid:* 80 mg/0.8 mL; 160 mg/5 mL *Chewable:* 80, 160 mg *Suppositories:* 80, 120, 325, 650 mg	Yes	Safe in pregnancy, lactation, and in most patients Not recommended for first-line therapy except in pregnant patients Risk for drug medication-overuse HA
Aspirin (OTC: Bayer, Bufferin, Ecotrin)	*Adults:* 650–1,000 mg at onset and every 4–6 h *Children:* Not recommended	*Adults:* 4,000 mg/d 2–3 d/wk 30 dosages/mo	*Tablets:* 325, 500, 650, 975 mg *Suppositories:* 300, 600 mg	Yes	Contraindicated in pregnancy (Category D) Avoid use within 1 wk of surgery Risk for medication-overuse HA
Ibuprofen (OTC: Motrin IB, Advil, Nuprin; Rx: Motrin)	*Adults:* 200–800 mg at onset, then every 6 h *Children:* 5–10 mg/kg initially; may repeat every 6–8 h	*Adults:* 2,400 mg/d *Children:* 40 mg/kg/d	*OTC tablets:* 100, 200 mg *Rx tablets:* 400, 600, 800 mg *Suspension:* 100 mg/5 mL *Chewable:* 50, 100 mg	Unlikely	Contraindicated in third trimester of pregnancy; safe during lactation Use with caution in kidney disease, ulcer disease, gastritis
Naproxen (Rx: Naprosyn)	*Adults:* 500 mg at onset, then 250 mg every 6–8 h *Children:* 2.5–5 mg/kg initially and may repeat every 12 h	*Adults:* 1,000 mg/d *Children:* 15 mg/kg/d	*Tablets:* 250, 375, 500 mg *Suspension:* 125 mg/mL	Unlikely	Contraindicated in third trimester of pregnancy; safe during lactation Absorbed more slowly than naproxen sodium Use with caution in kidney disease, ulcer disease, gastritis
Naproxen sodium (OTC: Aleve; Rx: Anaprox)	*Adults:* 825 mg at onset, then 200–550 mg in 3–4 h *Children:* Use suspension form of naproxen	*Adults:* 1,375 mg/d	*OTC tablets:* 200 mg *Rx tablets:* 275, 550 mg	Unlikely	Contraindicated in third trimester of pregnancy; safe during lactation Naproxen sodium absorbed more quickly than naproxen; reaches peak levels in half the time Use with caution in kidney disease, ulcer disease, gastritis
Ketorolac (Rx: Toradol, Sprix nasal spray)	*Adults:* 30–60 mg initially, may repeat 30–60 mg every 6 h *Children:* Not recommended in children <16 yr	*Adults:* 120 mg/d	*Injection:* 15 mg/mL, 30 mg/mL for IM injection *Oral:* 10 mg every 4–6 h; maximum 40 mg daily *Intranasal:* 15.75 mg/spray 1 spray in 1 nostril every 6–8 h.; maximum 4 sprays daily	Unlikely, but frequent use should be avoided	Contraindicated in pregnancy, lactation, kidney disease, ulcer disease, gastritis Use for emergency treatment of severe migraine in patients who cannot use other medications. Do not exceed 5 consecutive days of use.

Continued

Table 35–2 Drugs Commonly Used: Headaches—cont'd

Drug	Initial Dose	Maximum Dose	Strengths Available	Rebound Potential	Comments
Diclofenac (diclofenac potassium, Cambia)	*Adults:* 50 mg tid *Children:* Not recommended in children <16 yr.	*Adults:* 150 mg/day	50 mg pwdr pkt to be given on an empty stomach ×1 (Cambia)		Renal and hepatic dosing. Pregnancy (C); lactation is probably safe.
Aspirin/ acetaminophen/ caffeine combination (OTC: Excedrin, Vanquish)	*Adults:* 2 tablets every 6 h	*Adults:* 8 tablets/d, 2 d/wk	Excedrin: APAP 250 mg, ASA 250 mg, caffeine 65 mg Vanquish: APAP 165 mg, ASA 227 mg, caffeine 33 mg	Yes	Same precautions as for ASA and APAP
Tramadol (Rx: Ultram, Ultram ER, Rybix ODT)	Adults: 50–100 mg every 4–6 h 100–300 mg daily for extended dosing Children: Not recommended in children <16 yr	*Adults:* Maximum 400 mg daily			Renal and hepatic dosing. Increased risk of serotonin syndrome when combined with triptans, SSRI, SNRI Pregnancy (C); possibly unsafe in lactation.
Tramadol/ Acetaminophen (Ultracet)	37.5/325 mg every 4–6 h.	Maximum 8 tab/day			
Combination Analgesics					
Butalbital compounds (Rx: Fiorinal, Fioricet, Esgic Plus)	*Adults:* 2 tablets at onset, then 1 tablet every 4–6 h *Children:* Not recommended	*Adults:* 6 tablets per attack 2 d/wk 30 tablets per month Fioricet: One or 2 tablets every 4 hours PRN	Fiorinal: Butalbital 50 mg, ASA 325 mg, caffeine 40 mg Butalbital 50 mg, APAP 325 mg, caffeine 40 mg Esgic Plus: Butalbital 50 mg, APAP 500 mg, caffeine 40 mg	Yes	Same as for ASA and APAP Not for first-line therapy Risk for medication-overuse headache, if taken in greater than recommended dosage or more than 2 d/wk
Isometheptene compound (Rx: Midrin, Isocom)	*Adults:* Migraine: 2 capsules at onset, then 1 capsule every h if needed for relief Tension headache: 1 or 2 capsules at onset, followed by 1 capsule every 4 h *Children:* Not recommended	Migraine: 5 per 12 h, 2 d/wk, 20 per mo Tension headache: 8 per 24 h, 2 d/wk, 20 per mo	Midrin, Isocom: Isometheptene 65 mg, dichloralphenazone 100 mg, APAP 325 mg	Yes	Adverse interaction with MAOIs Contraindicated in uncontrolled hypertension, CAD, PVD Not considered first-line therapy
Narcotic Analgesics					
Codeine-containing compounds (Rx: Tylenol #3, Empirin #3)	*Adults:* 1 or 2 tablets at onset of attack, then 1 every 4–6 h *Children:* Aspirin-containing	*Adults:* 6 tablets per attack, 2 d/wk, 10–15 doses/mo	Tylenol #3: APAP 300 mg with codeine 30 mg APAP with codeine liquid: Codeine 12 mg	Yes and habit-forming Monitor use carefully; if patient is needing more than 15 tablets/mo,	Relatively safe during pregnancy Should not be considered first-line therapy Contraindicated in substance-abuse patients

Table 35–2   Drugs Commonly Used: Headaches—cont'd

Drug	Initial Dose	Maximum Dose	Strengths Available	Rebound Potential	Comments
	preparations contraindicated		and APAP 120 mg/5 mL Empirin #3: ASA 325 mg with codeine 30 mg	reevaluate treatment	Should not be prescribed for chronic daily headache
Meperidine (Rx: Demerol)	*Adults:* Maximum initial dose 150 mg, can repeat 50–100 mg every 3–4 h if needed		*IM injection:* 25 mg/mL, 50 mg/mL, 75 mg/mL, 100 mg/mL	Yes Patients must have someone to drive them home after receiving medication	May be used in pregnancy Use only as "rescue" medication Use sparingly and infrequently when other treatments have been ineffective
Butorphanol (Rx: Stadol NS)	*Adults:* 1 spray to one nostril; may be repeated in 1 h *Children:* Not recommended	*Adults:* 2 sprays (2 mg) per attack, 2 d/wk	Stadol NS: Nasal spray 1 mg/spray	Probably Side effects of orthostasis and sedation	Can be used as a "rescue" medication Effective for nocturnal headaches May be used with caution in pregnancy
Ergot Derivatives					
Ergotamine tablets (Rx: Ergostat, Ergomar)	*Adults:* 1 tablet sublingual at onset of attack; may repeat every 30 min; max 3 tablets per attack *Children:* Not safe in children	*Adults:* 3 tablets/d, 2 d/wk and 10 mg/wk	Sublingual 2 mg tablets	Yes	Contraindicated in pregnancy (Category X) and lactation Contraindicated in CAD and PVD May cause severe nausea and vomiting
Ergotamine and caffeine combination (Rx: Cafergot, Wigraine)	*Adults:* Tablets: 2 tablets at onset, then 1 tablet every 30 min if needed, up to 6 tablets per attack Suppositories: 1/3–1 suppository at onset; may repeat 1 suppository in 1 h, if needed *Children:* Not recommended	*Adults:* 6 tablets or 2 suppositories per attack, 2 d/wk, 10 mg/wk	Cafergot & Wigraine tablets: Ergotamine 1 mg, caffeine 100 mg Cafergot & Wigraine suppositories: Ergotamine 2 mg, caffeine 100 mg	Yes Suppository form better absorbed	Pregnancy Category X; contraindicated in lactation, CAD, PVD May cause nausea and vomiting May premedicate with an antiemetic
Dihydroergotamine (Rx: DHE 45, Migranal)	*Adults:* Injection: 1 mg IV/IM at onset; may repeat 1 mg dose hourly for total maximum of 3 mg IM or 2 mg IV Intranasal: 1 spray each nostril at onset; may repeat in 15 min *Children:* Not recommended	*Adults:* IM: 3 mg/attack IV: 2 mg/attack IM/IV: 6 mg/wk IM home use: 18 doses/mo Intranasal: 6 sprays/ 24 h, 8 sprays/wk	DHE 45 injection; 1 mg/mL Migranal 0.5 mg/spray	Unlikely	Contraindicated in pregnancy, lactation, CAD, PVD, hypertension, and severe renal or hepatic dysfunction. Premedicate with antiemetic: Zofran or metoclopramide for greater effectiveness

Continued

Table 35–2 Drugs Commonly Used: Headaches—cont'd

Drug	Initial Dose	Maximum Dose	Strengths Available	Rebound Potential	Comments
Serotonin Receptor Agonists					
Alomotriptan (Axert)	*Adults ≥18 yr:* 6.25 mg or 12.5 mg once. May repeat ×1 after 2 h *Adolescents age 12–17 yr:* 6.25 mg or 12.5 mg in a single dose. May repeat after 2 h *Children:* Not recommended	2 doses/24 h	6.25 mg tablets 12.5 mg tablets	Likely	Contraindicated in pregnancy, ischemic heart disease, CAD, and uncontrolled hypertension None of the triptans can be used within 24 h of ergotamine-containing medications or other triptans. Concurrent use of a triptan or use within 2 wk of MAOIs is contraindicated. All the triptans interact with SSRIs, causing serotonin syndrome. Serious adverse effects rarely reported in adults (stroke, visual loss, and death); have been reported in children after use of SC, oral, and/or nasal sumatriptan. Don't use >4× per mo
Eletriptan (Relpax)	*Adults ≥18 yr:* 20 mg or 40 mg ×1. Reevaluate if no response. May repeat ×1 in 2 h *Children:* Not recommended	Max: 80 mg/d	20 mg tablets 40 mg tablets	Likely	Contraindicated in pregnancy, ischemic heart disease, CAD, and uncontrolled hypertension. None of the triptans can be used within 24 h of ergotamine-containing medications or other triptans. Concurrent use of a triptan or use within 2 wk of MAOIs is contraindicated. All the triptans interact with SSRIs, causing serotonin syndrome. Serious adverse effects rarely reported in adults (stroke, visual loss, and death); have been reported in children after use of SC, oral, and/or nasal sumatriptan. Same as sumatriptan. Don't use >3× per mo
Frovatriptan (Frova)	*Adults ≥18 yr:* 2.5 mg with fluids. May repeat ×1 after 2 h *Children:* Not recommended	Max: 7.5 mg/24 h	2.5 mg tablets	Likely	Longer half-life. Slower onset of action, lower rate of migraine recurrence. Don't use >4× per mo

Table 35–2   Drugs Commonly Used: Headaches—cont'd

Drug	Initial Dose	Maximum Dose	Strengths Available	Rebound Potential	Comments
Sumatriptan (Rx: Imitrex, Sumavel, DosePro (Sumatriptan Injection))	*Adults ≥18 yr:* Oral: 25–100 mg initially; may be repeated every 2 h for up to 24 h SC injection 6 mg; may repeat ×1 in 1 h Intranasal: 5, 10, or 20 mg; may repeat once after 2 h if needed	*Adults:* Oral: 300 mg/d, 4 headaches per mo SC injection: 2 injections/ day, 4 headaches per mo Intranasal: 40 mg/day, 4 headaches per mo 2 tab/24 h	*Tablets:* 25, 50 mg *SC injection:* 6 mg/mL single-dose vial *Nasal spray:* 5 mg/spray, 20 mg/spray	Likely	Contraindicated in pregnancy, ischemic heart disease, CAD, and uncontrolled hypertension. None of the triptans can be used within 24 h of ergotamine-containing medications or other triptans. Concurrent use of a triptan or use within 2 wk of MAOIs is contraindicated. All the triptans interact with SSRIs, causing serotonin syndrome. Serious adverse effects rarely reported in adults (stroke, visual loss, and death); have been reported in children after use of SC, oral, and/or nasal sumatriptan.
Zecuity (sumatriptan iontophoretic transdermal system)	Transdermal: single dose 6.5 mg *Children <18 yr:*		*Transdermal:* Single-use battery-powered patch 6.5mg/4 h application		
Treximet (sumatriptan and naproxen)	Not recommended 85/500 mg oral, may repeat dosing after 2 h				
Naratriptan (Rx: Amerge)	*Adults:* One 1 mg or 2.5 mg tablet at onset of migraine; may repeat dose in 4 h, if needed *Children 12–17 yr:* Adult doses are used *Children <12 yr:* Safety has not been established	*Adults:* 5 mg/24 h, 4 headaches per mo	*Tablets:* 1 mg, 2.5 mg	Likely	Same contraindications as for sumatriptan Longer half-life than other triptans, less likely to cause medication-overuse headache Interacts with oral contraceptives
Rizatriptan (Rx: Maxalt, Maxalt-MLT)	*Adults (either form):* Take 5–10 mg at onset of migraine; may repeat in 2 h, if needed *Children:* Not recommended in patients <18 yr	*Adults:* 30 mg/24 h, 4 headaches per mo Propranolol patients: use 5 mg dose, up to 3 doses in 24 h	*Maxalt tablets:* 5, 10 mg Maxalt-MLT orally disintegrating tablets: 5, 10 mg	Likely	Same contraindications as for sumatriptan Use with caution in patient concurrently taking propranolol
Zolmitriptan (Rx: Zomig)	*Adults:* 2.5 mg or less initially (may break 2.5 mg tablet in half); repeat if headache returns after 2 h *Children:* Safety not established	*Adults:* 10 mg/24 h, 4 headaches per mo	*Tablets:* 2.5 mg, 5 mg	Likely	Same contraindications as for sumatriptan Use with caution in patients with hepatic dysfunction (<2.5 mg dose) Interacts with oral contraceptives and cimetidine

Continued

Table 35–2   Drugs Commonly Used: Headaches—cont'd

Drug	Initial Dose	Maximum Dose	Strengths Available	Rebound Potential	Comments
Alpha Agonist, Central					
Guanfacine (Rx: Tenex)	*Adults:* 1 mg daily ×12 weeks *Children:* No recommended dosing for migraines		*Tablets:* 1 mg & 2 mg		Centrally acting antihypertensive.
Antiemetics					
Metoclopramide (Rx: Reglan)	*Adults:* 10 mg either orally or IV either before ergotamine derivative or concurrently with analgesic *Children:* Not recommended	*Adults:* 40 mg/d	*Tablets:* 5 mg, 10 mg *Injection:* 5 mg/mL	N/A	Interacts with cimetidine, digoxin, MAOIs, and cyclosporine Safe in pregnancy, Category B
Ondansetron (Zofran, Zofran ODT)	*Adult:* 4–8 mg every 6–8 h *Children ages 4–11:* 4 mg every 4 h *Ages >11 =* adult dosing	*Adult:* 24–36 mg daily *Children:* <24 mg daily	*Tablets:* 4 mg & 8 mg *Parenteral:* 4mg/5mL	N/A	Safe in pregnancy (B), lactation is unknown. Prolong cardiac QTc
Promethazine (Phenergan	*Adult:* 12.5–25 mg every 4–6 h *Children:* *>2 yr:* 0.25–1 mg/kg every 4–6 h	*Adult:* 100 mg daily Maximum: 25 mg/dose.	*Tablets/suppository:* 12.5, 25, 50 mg *Parenteral:* (same as oral)	N/A	Use with caution in hepatic impairment.
		Preventive Therapy			
Beta Blockers					
Propranolol (Rx: Inderal, Inderal LA)	*Adults:* Start with 60–80 mg/d, and increase every 3–7 d *Children:* 0.5–1 mg/kg/d divided bid and increased every 3–4 d	*Adults:* 240–320 mg/d (monitor blood pressure [BP] and heart rate [HR]: systolic [BP] should be >100 mm Hg and HR >50 bpm) *Children:* 2–4 mg/kg/d	*Tablets:* 10, 20, 40, 60, 80, 120 mg, 160 mg ER	N/A Pregnancy Category C but safer than some other preventive agents	Contraindicated in CHF, asthma, COPD, PVD, diabetes mellitus, depression, Wolff-Parkinson-White syndrome. Start with a trial of 3 mo; as response improves over time, it needs to be tapered slowly (over a week) if discontinued. Interacts with many drugs, including cimetidine, oral contraceptives, calcium channel blockers.
Timolol (Rx: Blocadren)	*Adults:* Start at 20 mg/d; increase slowly *Children:* Not recommended	*Adults:* 60 mg/d	*Tablets:* 5, 10, 20 mg	N/A	Pregnancy Category C. Contraindications and drug interactions similar to propranolol.

Table 35–2 Drugs Commonly Used: Headaches—cont'd

Drug	Initial Dose	Maximum Dose	Strengths Available	Rebound Potential	Comments
Metoprolol (Rx: Lopressor, Toprol-XL)	*Adults:* Start at 100 mg/d; increase slowly *Children:* Not recommended	*Adults:* 250 mg/d	*Tablets:* 25, 50, 100 mg 200 mg ER	N/A	Pregnancy Category C. Contraindications include bradycardia, second- or third-degree heart block, overt heart failure. Interacts with many drugs, including calcium channel blockers, digoxin, clonidine, and oral contraceptives.
Atenolol (Rx: Tenormin)	*Adults:* 100 mg/d *Children:* Not recommended	*Adults:* 200 mg/d	*Tablets:* 25, 50, 100 mg	N/A	Pregnancy Category D. Contraindications include bradycardia, second- or third-degree heart block, overt heart failure. Interacts with many drugs, including calcium channel blockers, digoxin, clonidine, and oral contraceptives.
Tricyclic Antidepressants					
Amitriptyline (Rx: Elavil)	*Adults:* Start with 10 mg qhs and increase every 2 wk to a total daily dose of 20–50 mg *Children:* Not recommended for children <12 yr	*Adults:* 150 mg/d	*Tablets:* 10, 25, 50, 75, 100 mg	N/A	Contraindicated in patients with narrow-angle glaucoma, urinary retention, pregnancy, breastfeeding, concurrent use of MAOIs (within 14 d of each other), and in suicidal patients.
Nortriptyline (Pamelor)	*Adults:* Start 25–50 mg qhs; increase every 2–3 days. *Children:* Not recommended for headache.	*Adults:* 150 mg/d	*Tablets:* 10, 25, 50, 75 mg	N/A	Do not abruptly stop; wean dosing when discontinuing
Anticonvulsants					
Divalproex (Rx: Depakote, Depakote ER, Depakote Sprinkles)	*Adults:* Initial dose is 125–250 mg bid; may increase 125 mg weekly *Children:* Safety and effectiveness for migraine prevention has not been studied in children <16 yr	*Adults:* 1,000 mg/d	*Tablets:* 125, 250, 500 mg, 500 mg ER, 125 mg DR	N/A	Requires baseline assessment of liver function, platelet count, and bleeding time, as hepatic failure and thrombocytopenia are rare adverse effects Monitor LFTs and CBC every 2 wk ×3 Pregnancy Category D
Topiramate (Topamax)	*Adults:* Start on 25 mg qhs; increase to 25 mg bid in week 2.	*Adults:* 400 mg/d	*Tablets:* 25, 50, 100, 200 mg *Capsules:* 15, 25 mg		Renal dosing adjustment Pregnancy Category D

Continued

Table 35–2 Drugs Commonly Used: Headaches—cont'd

Drug	Initial Dose	Maximum Dose	Strengths Available	Rebound Potential	Comments
	During week 3 the dose is increased to 25 mg in the morning and 50 mg at night. In week 4 a dose of 50 mg twice a day. 25 mg bid may be effective in some *Children:* Not recommended for headache				
Oxcarbazepine (Trileptal)	*Adults:* Start 300 mg bid and increase 600 mg/d every week *Children:* Not recommended for headache	*Adults:* 1,200 mg bid	*Tablets:* 150, 300, 600 mg *Solution:* 300 mg/5 mL	N/A	Pregnancy Category C Monitor for hyponatremia, thrombocytopenia, Stevens–Johnson syndrome. Do not abruptly stop; wean off.
Gabapentin (Neurontin, Gralise)	*Adults:* 300 mg bid-tid, increase by 300–600 mg every week. *Children:* Not recommended for headache	*Adults:* 3,600 mg/d	*Tablets:* 100, 300, 400, 600, 800 mg, 600 mg ER *Solution:* 50 mg/mL	N/A	Pregnancy Category C Do not abruptly stop; wean off.
NSAIDs					
Naproxen sodium (OTC: Aleve; Rx: Anaprox)	*Adults:* 550 mg bid	*Adults:* 1,375 mg/d	TC tablets: 200 mg Rx tablets: 275, 550 mg	Unlikely	Contraindicated in third trimester of pregnancy; safe during lactation Use with caution in kidney disease, ulcer disease, gastritis
Calcium Channel Blockers					
Verapamil (Rx: Calan, Isoptin)	*Adults:* Start with 40 mg bid and slowly increase *Children:* Not recommended	*Adults:* 480 mg/d	*Tablets:* 40, 80, 120, mg	N/A	Contraindicated in pregnancy (Category C), Parkinson's disease, and depression. May be first-line choice in patients with hypertension who cannot take beta blockers.
Serotonin Antagonist					
Methysergide (Rx: Sansert)	*Adults:* Start with 2 mg bid; increase slowly *Children:* Not recommended	*Adults:* 8–14 mg/d	*Tablets:* 2 mg	N/A	Most serious side effect is retroperitoneal fibrosis or related conditions with prolonged therapy. Patient should have a drug-free period of 3–4 wk after every 6 mo of treatment. Contraindicated in pregnancy, CAD, PVD, impaired renal or liver function, and hypertension.

Table 35–2 Drugs Commonly Used: Headaches—cont'd

Drug	Initial Dose	Maximum Dose	Strengths Available	Rebound Potential	Comments
Antispasmodic/Neurotoxin (inhibits acetylcholin release from nerve endings)					
Onabotulinum-toxinA (Rx: Botox)	*Adults:* 155 U injected IM divided in 31 sites every 12 wk. *Children:* Not indicated for headaches		*Injectable units:* 100-unit single dose vial	N/A	Contraindicated in hypersensitivity to the drug. Caution if neuromuscular or facial nerve disorder.
Nutraceuticals	*Adults:*				
Riboflavin	400 mg/d				
Coenzyme Q10	150 mg/d				
Magnesium	600 mg/d				
Feverfew	100 mg of 0.2% parthenolide/d				
Butterbur	50–100 mg bid				

APAP = acetaminophen; ASA = acetylsalicylic acid; CAD = coronary artery disease; CBC = complete blood count; CHF = chronic heart failure; COPD = chronic obstructive pulmonary disease; HA = headache; LFTs = liver function tests; MAOIs = monoamine oxidase inhibitors; N/A = information not available; OTC = over the counter; PVD = peripheral vascular disease; SSRIs = selective serotonin reuptake inhibitors.

which may be helpful if the patient is nauseated or vomiting. Ketorolac (Toradol) is the only NSAID available in an injectable form, which can also be used if the patient is vomiting. Table 35-2 shows the dosing for commonly used NSAIDs.

Midrange Analgesics

Midrange analgesics are commonly prescribed to treat both migraine and tension-type headaches. Combination products that combine either butalbital with ASA or APAP (Fiorinal or Fioricet) or isometheptene with acetaminophen and dichloralphenazone (Midrin) are effective in treating mild to moderate migraine, although the U.S. Headache Consortium guidelines rate these drugs as group 3 drugs, with inconsistent or conflicting clinical efficacy data (Matcher et al, 2000). These products should be used cautiously because medication-overuse headaches can occur if they are taken in greater-than-recommended dosages or more than 2 days per week. Medication-overuse headaches are discussed later in this chapter.

High-Range Analgesics

High-range analgesics include the commonly used opioids, which act centrally to treat the pain of migraine. Although opioids are controversial in the treatment of migraine, there are patients for whom an opioid is the drug of choice. An opioid can be prescribed if the patient is pregnant, if vasoconstrictor medications are contraindicated, or if the migraine is not responsive to ergotamine or serotonin agonists (discussed later). The opioids are group 2 drugs with moderate clinical and statistical benefit (Matcher et al, 2000).

Codeine either alone or in combination with ASA (Aspirin with codeine #3) or APAP (Tylenol with codeine #3) is the opioid most commonly used to treat migraine. The dose of codeine should be 30 to 60 mg, with the lowest effective dose used. Meperidine (Demerol) can be given IM if the patient is unable to take oral medications because of nausea and/or vomiting. The maximum initial dose is 150 mg in an adult, and a dose of 50 to 100 mg can be repeated every 3 to 4 hours. Intranasal butorphanol (Stadol) can be tried in patients who fail nonopioid therapy or who have contraindications to other migraine medications. The dose of one spray in one nostril has a rapid onset (less than 15 minutes) and can be repeated in 1 hour if needed. Adverse effects include orthostasis and sedation. The patient should limit its use to no more than twice a week. Other opioids that are prescribed for migraine include oxycodone and hydrocodone, even though there is little clinical information to support their effectiveness over newer nonnarcotic agents and their use is not supported by the U.S. Headache Consortium. Opioids must be prescribed carefully because of their potential for physical dependence, tolerance, and addiction. Therefore, they should be limited to patients with severe but infrequent headaches or the occasional headache that is unresponsive to nonnarcotic agents.

Ergot Derivatives

Ergot derivatives have been used for many years to treat migraine. Ergotamine and dihydroergotamine (DHE) act as vasoconstrictors that lead to a decline in the amplitude of pulsation in the extracranial arteries and decreased hyperperfusion of the basilar artery area, without decreasing cerebral hemispheric blood flow. Ergotamine controls up to 70% of acute migraine attacks, but its adverse effects of nausea and vomiting and its unpredictable oral absorption limit routine use. Pretreatment with an antiemetic decreases the nausea and vomiting associated with ergotamine use. Ergotamine suppositories (Wigraine, Cafergot) are better absorbed than PO preparations and can be quite effective if administered at the beginning of migraine symptoms. Misuse of ergotamine may lead to medication-overuse headaches, and use should be limited to two doses, twice a week or less (total weekly dose of 10 mg maximum), up to 12 doses per month. Another caution with ergotamine is that the vasoconstriction can have serious effects on patients with peripheral vascular disease, coronary heart disease, hypertension, and impaired hepatic or renal function. Exceeding recommended amounts of ergotamine can lead to vasospastic adverse effects. Ergotamine derivatives are contraindicated in pregnancy because they can produce prolonged uterine contractions that can result in abortion. Thus, all forms of ergotamine are Pregnancy Category X. Ergotamine is not recommended for children. Most ergotamine preparations are group 3 drugs in the U.S. Headache Consortium guidelines, demonstrating conflicting or inconsistent evidence for their use in acute migraine (Matcher et al, 2000).

CLINICAL PEARL

Ergotamine Suppositories
Ergotamine suppositories can provide relief if taken at the beginning of a migraine attack. If a patient has not used ergotamine before, instruct the patient to use one-third of a 2 mg suppository initially and repeat in 30 to 60 minutes. Refrigeration makes the suppository easier to slice.

DHE, although chemically similar to ergotamine, does not cause the same peripheral vasoconstrictor effects, making it safer to use and listed as a group 1 drug by the U.S. Headache Consortium (Matcher et al, 2000). It also causes less nausea than ergotamine and does not require pretreatment with an antiemetic. DHE is effective even well into the course of a headache, unlike ergotamine, which must be taken at the beginning of migraine symptoms. DHE can be administered IM (DHE 45) or intranasally (Migranal). DHE has a longer duration of action than does sumatriptan, and so headache recurrence rates are lower. The dosage of DHE 45 is 1 mg (or 1 mL) IM or IV initially and can be repeated at 1-hour intervals to a maximum of 3 mg IM or 2 mg IV. IM DHE can be prescribed for home use if the patient has proper instructions regarding administration. A monthly limit for IM DHE is 18 ampules or 12 headache events. The dose of intranasal DHE is 1 spray (0.5 mg) in each nostril, repeated after 15 minutes, for a dose of 2 mg. Maximum dose is 6 sprays in a 24-hour period and 8 sprays per week. Although intranasal DHE is easier to administer, the patient should be warned that it has a slow onset of action. Precautions for DHE are the same as for ergotamine; it is contraindicated in pregnancy, coronary artery disease, peripheral vascular disease, and hypertension. DHE is not recommended for children.

Serotonin Receptor Agonists

Serotonin receptor agonists act selectively as 5-HT$_1$ receptor agonists, causing vasoconstriction and apparently blocking release of vasoactive substances that lead to migraine.

Sumatriptan (Imitrex, Alsuma, Sumavel Dosepro, Treximet) was the first selective serotonin receptor agonist developed specifically to treat migraine; other agents include almotriptan (Axert), frovatriptan (Frova), naratriptan (Amerge), rizatriptan (Maxalt), and zolmitriptan (Zomig). As they differ slightly in pharmacokinetics and individual response, trial of a different serotonin receptor agonist is warranted if one is not effective.

CLINICAL PEARL

Triptans
It is advisable to administer the first dose of any of the triptans under direct supervision to monitor for unrecognized coronary disease. The patient should receive the first dose in the clinic (or urgent care center) and be monitored for any adverse cardiovascular effects. Sumatriptan is effective in decreasing the severity of headache in 54% to 80% of patients.

It is also effective in relieving the nausea, photophobia, and phonophobia that can accompany migraine. Sumatriptan should be taken after the aura of migraine passes because it has been found to be effective only after the headache symptoms appear. Sumatriptan is available in PO, subcutaneous (SC), and intranasal forms. The dose for PO sumatriptan is 25 to 100 mg initially and may be repeated every 2 hours for up to 24 hours (maximum 300 mg in 24 hours). Although an initial dose of 25 mg should be tried with a patient who has never had sumatriptan, research has shown that an initial dose of 50 to 100 mg is superior in relieving migraine symptoms (Carpay, Schoenen, Ahmad, Kinrade, & Boswell, 2004). Carpay and colleagues studied the efficacy and tolerability of fast-disintegrating, rapid-release sumatriptan and found that 51.1% of patients who received 50 mg of sumatriptan were pain-free after 2 hours, whereas 66.2% of those who received 100 mg were pain-free at 2 hours after dosing. The initial SC dose of sumatriptan is 6 mg, and 82% of patients report relief in 20 minutes. The dose may be repeated in 1 hour if there is no relief, for a maximum of two 6 mg doses in 24 hours. Intranasal sumatriptan has a slower onset than does SC (2 h versus 20 min) and is less effective in relieving headache (62% at 2 h), yet intranasal dosing may be more appealing for children and for patients who fear self-administering injectable medication. After a dose of sumatriptan, up to 40% of headaches recur within 10 to 14 hours, and a second dose may be necessary. Do not repeat the dose of sumatriptan if the patient does not respond to the first dose.

Almotriptan binds with high affinity with 5-HT receptors 1D, 1B, and 1F. Almotriptan is rapidly absorbed from the gastrointentinal (GI) tract with a peak of 1 to 3 hours after administration. Two hours after administration of 6.25 mg of almotriptan, 55% of study subjects reported pain relief from their migraine. When 12.5 mg is administered, 58.5% to 64.9% of subjects reported relief (Ortho-McNeil Neurologics, 2009). Almotriptan has a mean half-life of 3 to 4 hours and is primarily excreted renally. Axert is FDA approved for use in adolescents aged 12 to 17 years.

Frovatriptan is a 5-HT 1B/1D receptor agonist that binds with high affinity to 5-HT$_{1B}$ and 5-HT$_{1D}$ receptors. Frovatriptan peaks in 2 to 4 hours after administration, with food delaying peak by an hour. Bioavailability of frovatriptan is 20% in women and 30% in men. In clinical trials, when 2.5 mg of frovatriptan was administered orally, 37% to 46% of patients had mild or no headache after 2 hours (Endo Pharmaceuticals, 2013). If headache recurs after initial relief, dosing recommendations are that the dose be repeated if it has been at least 2 hours since the last dose. The total daily dose of frovatriptan should not exceed three 2.5 mg tablets per 24 hours.

Naratriptan is similar to sumatriptan in its mechanism of action but differs in its pharmacokinetics. Naratriptan has a higher PO bioavailability (about 70%) and a longer half-life (6 hours) than does sumatriptan. This might lead to a lower rate of headache recurrence, with only 17% to 28% of patients reporting recurrence (Mathew, 1997). These differences may lead the practitioner to choose naratriptan as the first-line triptan. Naratriptan has been studied in adolescents (12 to 17 years), and the reported adverse events do not differ from the adult studies. One factor that may prevent the use of naratriptan is that its half-life and plasma levels are increased with concurrent use of oral contraceptives, and the dose should be lowered.

Rizatriptan, also a 5-HT$_1$ serotonin receptor agonist, has oral bioavailability that is better than sumatriptan (about 45% versus 15%) but not as good as that of naratriptan. Because its half-life is similar to sumatriptan (both 2 to 3 hours), cost and PO absorption may be factors when choosing between rizatriptan and sumatriptan. Rizatriptan is available in PO tablet or PO disintegrating tablet, which may be preferred for some patients with nausea as a major symptom of migraine. One caution with rizatriptan is that plasma levels of rizatriptan are increased significantly when taken with propranolol, and concurrent use should be avoided.

Zolmitriptan has a higher PO bioavailability than do sumatriptan and rizatriptan (60% in females, 38% in males) and a similar half-life. Zolmitriptan is the only triptan that interacts with cimetidine (doubles the half-life and plasma levels of zolmitriptan), and this may be a factor in prescribing. Zolmitriptan's half-life and clearance are also affected by oral contraceptives.

All triptans are contraindicated in patients with coronary artery disease or uncontrolled hypertension because of their potential to constrict coronary artery vessels. The triptans are contraindicated in pregnancy. None of the triptans can be used if ergotamine derivatives have been used in the prior 24 hours because of increased vasospastic reactions; their effects may be additive. The triptans sumatriptan, zolmitriptan, and rizatriptan interact with monoamine oxidase inhibitors (MAOIs) and should not be used concurrently or within 2 weeks of discontinuing the MAOI. All of the triptans interact with selective serotonin reuptake inhibitors (SSRIs), causing serotonin syndrome. Sumatriptan can be used in children, but consultation with a pediatric neurologist is advisable.

Antiemetics

Antiemetics are an integral part of migraine management. Gastric emptying and oral absorption of medications are decreased in migraine patients, especially those patients with nausea and vomiting as a component of their migraine. A dose of metoclopramide (Reglan) is often recommended as part of migraine therapy (ICSI, 2009). Other commonly used antiemetics recommended as adjunct therapy by ICSI (2009) are the phenothiazine antiemetics, perphenazine (Trilafon), prochlorperazine (Compazine), and chlorpromazine (Thorazine).

Preventive Therapy

Preventive therapy should be considered for any patient who experiences severely incapacitating or frequent severe migraines (more than two per month) and patients who cannot tolerate abortive medications because of either chronic illness (coronary artery disease or hypertension) or the adverse effects of abortive medications. Preventive medication is also recommended if the patient is taking abortive medication more than twice a week. The primary goal of preventive therapy is to use the least amount of medication with the fewest side effects to decrease migraine symptoms. If medication overuse is suspected, it must be treated first before starting the patient on preventive therapy; this topic is covered later in this chapter.

Patients must understand that preventive therapy will not completely eliminate migraine and that a 50% reduction in migraine attacks is considered a success. Fewer than 10% of patients become headache-free with preventive therapy. The patient must also be aware that it may take 4 weeks before preventive therapy begins to be effective and that there is an increase in effectiveness for 3 months. It is common for patients to discontinue preventive therapy after only a couple of weeks and label it as ineffective. Education is the key to success for preventive therapy. Another component to preventive therapy is a headache diary that is initiated prior to preventive therapy and then maintained to determine the frequency, severity, and duration of migraine. This tool enables the provider to assess the effectiveness of preventive therapy. Examples of daily, weekly, and monthly headache diaries can be found at the American Headache Society's Web site (http://www.americanheadachesociety.org).

Because preventive therapy cannot completely eliminate migraines, the patient should also have acute or abortive medications to take for migraine. The provider should recognize interactions between preventive and acute therapies and prescribe accordingly (see Table 35-2). The significance of avoiding migraine triggers, which cannot be overlooked in migraine prevention, is discussed later in the chapter.

Beta Blockers

Beta blockers are one of the first-line choices for migraine preventive therapy (ICSI, 2009), with up to a 44% reduction in migraine reported. The mechanism of action in migraine prevention is not clear, but it is thought that beta blockers may affect the central catecholaminergic system and brain serotonin (5-HT$_2$) receptors. They also block beta receptors in vascular smooth muscle to prevent arterial dilatation. Propranolol (Inderal) and timolol (Blocadren) are the only beta blockers that have been FDA approved for migraine preventive therapy, although nadolol (Corgard), metoprolol (Lopressor), and atenolol (Tenormin) have also been shown to be effective.

Propranolol is typically started at a dose of 60 to 80 mg a day and slowly increased every third or fourth day to a maximum of 240 mg per day in adults. Twice-daily dosing has the highest compliance rate. Individual response varies, and the patient should be monitored closely. A pulse below 50 or a systolic blood pressure below 100 mm Hg in the adult suggests that the maximum dosage has been reached. The dose in children is 0.5 to 1 mg/kg/d, divided into two doses and titrated every 3 to 4 days, to a maximum of 2 to 4 mg/kg/d. Pediatric patients should be monitored closely, and consultation with a pediatric neurologist before initiating and during therapy is advisable. A trial of 3 months in both adult and pediatric patients is necessary because the response improves over time. Treatment should be reassessed every 6 months, and it may be discontinued. Propranolol needs to be tapered slowly (over a week) to prevent drug withdrawal headache. Adverse effects of propranolol include fatigue, lethargy, and depression, and it should not be the first-line drug in depressed patients. It is also not well tolerated by athletes. Propranolol is contraindicated in patients with congestive heart failure, asthma, chronic obstructive pulmonary disease, peripheral vascular disease, diabetes mellitus, or Wolff-Parkinson-White syndrome. Propranolol is Pregnancy Category C, but it is safer than some of the other preventive agents.

If propranolol is not effective or not well tolerated, one of the other beta blockers can be tried; failure to respond to one beta blocker does not predict response to another. If a patient has asthma or other respiratory disorders, metoprolol and atenolol may be used because they are cardioselective (see Table 35-2 for dosing of these agents).

Tricyclic Antidepressants

Tricyclic antidepressants, specifically amitriptyline (Elavil), are effective in reducing the frequency, severity, and duration of migraine attacks. Amitriptyline modulates neurotransmitters and appears to affect the central serotonin receptor function. Its antimigraine effect is unrelated to its antidepressant effect, and the antimigraine effect can often be achieved at lower doses than are required to treat depression. The patient should be started on 10 mg a day taken before bed and increased every 2 weeks to a total daily dose of 20 to 50 mg. Adverse effects that should be monitored include drowsiness (most common), dry mouth, weight gain, constipation, and orthostatic hypotension. Amitriptyline is contraindicated in patients with narrow-angle glaucoma, urinary retention, pregnancy, breastfeeding, and concurrent use of MAOIs. Other tricyclic antidepressants that may be used include nortriptyline (Pamelor, Aventyl), which causes less drowsiness and anticholinergic effect than does amitriptyline.

Antiepileptic Drugs

Antiepileptic drugs (AEDs) are thought to work on migraines in a fashion similar to their effect on seizures. The AEDs are thought to decrease brain excitability by increasing the threshold for activation of the brainstem areas that are thought to be important for initiating migraine (Carmona & Bruera, 2009). The AEDs that are used in migraine include divalproex (valproate), gabapentin, and topiramate (ICSI, 2009).

Divalproex (Depakote) has FDA labeling as a preventive treatment for migraine. Divalproex reduces the number of migraine attacks and also reduces the duration and intensity. It is notably appropriate to use in a patient with coexisting seizure disorder. The initial dose for migraine preventive therapy is 125 to 250 mg twice daily. The dosage can be increased by 125 or 250 mg weekly, to a maximum dose of 1,000 to 1,250 mg per day. Patients who are started on divalproex require baseline assessment of liver function, platelet count, and bleeding time, as hepatic failure and thrombocytopenia are rare adverse effects. Clinical monitoring of symptoms for liver failure or bleeding disorders is more indicative of potential problems than routine laboratory monitoring. Divalproex serum concentrations should be monitored during therapy if poor compliance, toxicity, or drug reactions are suspected. Divalproex is Pregnancy Category D.

Gabapentin has proven efficacy as migraine prophylaxis for some patients and is one of the recommended ICSI migraine prophylaxis drugs (2009). In a controlled clinical trial of gabapentin for migraine prophylaxis, 46.4% of the gabapentin group (2,400 mg/d) had a significant reduction in migraine after 4 weeks of treatment (Neal et al, 2001). Patients should be started on gabapentin 300 mg daily and titrated up to 2,400 mg per day. A suggested titration is 300 mg daily, titrated up to 900 mg daily at the end of week 1, then titrated up to 1,500 mg per day at the end of week 2. During week 3, the dose is increased to 2,100 mg per day and in week 4 the dose increases to 2,400 mg/d (ICSI, 2009; Mathew et al, 2001). Gabapentin is generally well tolerated, although fatigue, somnolence, and weight gain are known adverse effects.

Topiramate (Topamax) has an FDA indication for migraine prophylaxis. It is rapidly absorbed from the GI tract and has a long duration of action. Migraine patients are started on a dose of 25 mg per day and titrated up in 1 week intervals. During week 1, patients take 25 mg before bed, then 25 mg twice a day in week 2. In week 3, patients take 25 mg in the morning and 50 mg in the evening, then 50 mg twice a day. Dosages of 25 mg of topiramate twice daily may be effective (Carmona & Bruera, 2009). Topiramate adverse effects include weight loss, somnolence, fatigue, and kidney stones. The AEDs are described in detail in Chapter 15.

NSAIDS

NSAIDs may also be used for migraine preventive therapy. The most commonly used NSAID is naproxen sodium, dosed at 550 mg twice a day. NSAIDs are particularly effective in treating menstrual migraines if daily dosing is started the week before menses and continued for a week after. In older patients, NSAIDs may pose a higher risk of causing nephrotoxicity or gastrointestinal problems.

Calcium Channel Blockers

Calcium channel blockers are also commonly used for migraine preventive therapy, although their effectiveness has had mixed results and they should not be a first-line choice. Calcium channel blockers are thought to prevent migraine by inhibiting vasospasm of the cerebral arteries and by preventing cerebral hypoxia during migraine attacks. Verapamil (Calan, Isoptin) is the most commonly used for migraine prevention. Nifedipine and diltiazem are not as effective in controlling migraines and probably should not be prescribed for this use. Calcium channel blockers may be the first-line choice for patients with hypertension who cannot take beta blockers. Dosing of verapamil is shown in Table 35-2. Adverse effects include sedation, weight gain, depression, and extrapyramidal symptoms. Calcium channel blockers are contraindicated in pregnancy, Parkinson's disease, and depression.

Methysergide

Methysergide (Sansert) is an ergot derivative that is a 5-HT$_2$ receptor agonist that inhibits or blocks the effects of serotonin. Methysergide is not commonly used because of its potential for adverse effects (reported in 30% to 50% of patients). The most serious adverse effect is retroperitoneal fibrosis or related conditions with prolonged therapy. If methysergide is prescribed, the patient should have a drug-free period of 3 to 4 weeks after every 6 months of treatment. Methysergide is contraindicated in pregnancy. Ergot derivatives should be avoided in patients with coronary artery disease, peripheral vascular disease, impaired renal or liver function, or hypertension.

Botulinum Toxin

In 2010, onabotulinumtoxinA (Botox) was FDA approved for preventive treatment of chronic migraines. Botox is injected in 31 sites divided across seven head and neck muscle areas and may be repeated every 12 weeks.

Nonpharmacological Management of Migraine

Nonpharmacological management of migraine includes a variety of interventions and alternative therapies. The first and most important is migraine trigger identification and avoidance. Alternative therapies, including herbs (feverfew and butterbur), vitamins (riboflavin), and coenzyme Q10, are all commonly used in migraine therapy (Taylor, 2009). Nontraditional health care should be addressed; up to 70% of patients who seek alternative therapy never discuss it with their health-care provider. Lifestyle issues such as stress and work environment can be modified to decrease migraine attacks or make them more manageable.

Identifying Triggers

Identifying and avoiding triggers can significantly decrease migraines. Many patients identify certain foods, odors, or medications that may cause headache. Table 35-1 lists common migraine triggers. Patients need to be encouraged to use their headache diary to determine if something is a trigger. Common foods like chocolate, yogurt, or the food additive aspartame can trigger a migraine, and patients are often not aware that something is provoking their headaches. Smoking

cessation and sleep regulation may also prove helpful in headache prevention.

Alternative Therapies

Alternative therapies that may assist in the treatment of migraine vary considerably. MigraLief, a commonly used herbal supplement containing feverfew, riboflavin, magnesium, and other vitamins, is available OTC. A naturopath may prescribe additional herbal medicine to treat migraines. Other alternative therapies that may be beneficial include acupuncture, aromatherapy, chiropractic manipulation, hypnosis, and reflexology. Patients can try massage therapy, relaxation therapy, and yoga, which all appear to reduce the tension and stress that may lead to migraine. The health-care provider should have access to local health education classes that teach yoga and relaxation classes or a local massage therapist for referral. A simple technique of applying ice to the head can often decrease the severity of pain associated with migraine; patients can be encouraged to try this simple technique as an adjunct to or a substitute for their medication.

Biofeedback

Biofeedback techniques are helpful for many patients. Biofeedback is thought to change vascular dilatation. Although the exact mechanism is unclear, some patients do report improvement in their migraine symptoms. Biofeedback is often combined with other relaxation therapies and may give the patient a feeling of control and mastery over the migraine symptoms.

 MIGRAINES

A number of medications are in the pipeline for treatment of migraines. An inhaled form of dihydroergotamine (Semprana) will be reviewed by the FDA in 2015. Two monoclonal antibody preparations that target calcitonin gene-related peptide (CGRP) are in experimental trials. CGRP is a protein that is thought to trigger migraines. ALD403 (Alder Biopharmaceuticals) and LY2951742 (Lilly) have both demonstrated reduction in migraines compared to placebo. Boehringer Ingelheim Pharmaceuticals' olcegepant, a CGRP antagonist, is undergoing phase II trials in Europe.

Monitoring

Patients with migraine headaches should keep a headache diary, especially when a new treatment is begun or if modifications are made in the therapy. The health-care provider can use the diary to determine if the treatment is decreasing the frequency, duration, or severity of the migraine. The diary can also track adverse side effects of the medication prescribed. Overuse of medication can be determined and an alternative plan developed. Patients should also have their blood pressure monitored for hypertension if they are on a triptan, ergotamine derivative, beta blocker, or calcium channel blocker. Patients on divalproex should have their liver function and complete blood count (CBC) tested every 2 weeks for a total of 6 weeks.

Outcome Evaluation

The goal of migraine treatment is to minimize the impact of migraine headaches on patients' quality of life, social functioning, and ability to work. It is evaluated by discussing with patients how their migraine is affecting their quality of life and by having them record in their headache diary when their headaches adversely affect their quality of life and ability to work. Modification of the treatment plan multiple times until the optimal treatment is found is important in achieving the goal of minimal impact from migraine on quality of life.

Avoidance of patients' identified migraine triggers often decreases the frequency of headache. It is evaluated by having patients record in their headache diaries any headache associated with a specific trigger. If patients are unable to determine if a specific item is a trigger, an elimination diet may be tried. Patients eliminate one item from the common triggers list for 2 weeks and then reintroduce it into their diet. This process may take weeks or months, but the reward of identifying a trigger is worth the perceived inconvenience.

Before beginning preventive therapy for frequent migraine sufferers, patients must be clear that the final goal is to reduce the frequency of migraine by 50% and that total elimination of migraine is not a realistic goal. Evaluating the success of preventive therapy by use of the headache diary and by demonstrating a decrease in frequency to patients will assist in clarifying the true success of treatment. It is essential to treat patients for an adequate amount of time (2 to 3 months) before a change in treatment.

Patient Education

Patient education should include a discussion of information related to the overall treatment plan as well as that specific to the drug therapy, reasons for taking the drug, drugs as part of the total treatment regimen, and adherence issues (see the Patient Education box).

Patient education is the key to successful migraine treatment. Patient education related to migraine should focus on the following:

1. An understanding of the diagnosis and nature of migraines.
2. The nonpharmacological measures to prevent and treat migraines, such as trigger identification and avoidance and the use of relaxation, massage, or ice to counter pain.
3. Education about the medication that is prescribed. Specifically, expected side effects, adverse side effects, interactions with other medications, and maximum dosages should be explained. Medication overuse should be addressed at the beginning of treatment.
4. The patient as an integral part of the treatment plan. Therapy is less effective if the patient does not keep a headache diary or uses the medication in a way different from how it was prescribed.
5. Realistic expectations of treatment. The patient will probably not be migraine-free, but the goal is to decrease the severity and frequency of migraines. Acute treatment should provide relief within an hour or two, or a change in therapy may be indicated.
6. Caution the patient about using OTC medications to treat the headache unless they are part of the treatment plan.

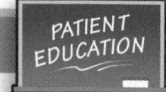

PATIENT EDUCATION

Headaches

RELATED TO THE OVERALL TREATMENT PLAN/DISEASE PROCESS

☐ Pathophysiology of headache

☐ Role of lifestyle modifications

☐ Importance of adherence to the treatment regimen

☐ Self-monitoring of symptoms and associated symptoms

☐ What to do when symptoms and associated symptoms worsen

☐ Need for regular follow-up visits with the primary care provider

SPECIFIC TO THE DRUG THERAPY

☐ Reason for taking the drug and its anticipated action in the disease process

☐ Doses (including maximum dosage) and schedules for taking the drug

☐ Possible adverse effects and what to do if they occur

☐ Interactions between other treatment modalities and these drugs

☐ Potential for medication-overuse headache

REASONS FOR TAKING THE DRUG(S)

Patient education about specific drugs is provided in the appropriate chapters. Specific reasons for taking the drug(s) should be discussed on an individual basis, depending on the diagnosis and nature of the headache. Medication overuse should also be discussed at the beginning of treatment.

DRUGS AS PART OF THE TOTAL TREATMENT REGIMEN

The total treatment regimen includes pharmacological and nonpharmacological measures, as well as the headache diary. A realistic expectation and goals of the individualized treatment plan should be presented.

ADHERENCE ISSUES

Nonadherence with the treatment regimen may affect functional status. Health-care providers should be aware of the potential problem of nonadherence and discuss the importance of adherence with the patient and family.

Education resources available for both the patient and the provider on the Internet and in print enable better understanding of the pathology and treatment of migraine and other headaches. The patient needs to be directed to reliable information. There are numerous patient-health organizations, pharmaceutical manufacturers, online support groups, and even Web sites that are maintained by private individuals. Box 35-1 provides a short list of the patient-health sites and provider information sites that are considered reliable, comprehensive, and trustworthy and that may be helpful for the health-care provider who cares for patients with headaches.

TENSION-TYPE HEADACHES

Up to 90% of all headaches could be classified as tension-type headaches. At least 15% of patients have experienced their first tension headache by age 10. Tension-type headaches can

---

BOX 35–1 HEADACHE RESOURCES FOR PATIENTS AND HEALTH-CARE PROVIDERS

American Headache Society

http://www.americanheadachesociety.org

The American Headache Society (AHS) is a professional society of health-care providers dedicated to the study and treatment of headache and face pain. Founded in 1959, AHS brings together physicians and other health-care providers from various fields and specialties to share concepts and developments about headache and related conditions.

American Council for Headache Education

http://www.achenet.org

This site is geared for patients and is connected with the American Headache Society. There is patient information on headaches in general, migraines, and prevention and treatment of headaches, as well as a discussion forum for patients. There are specific sections for children and women.

National Headache Foundation

www.headaches.org

Nonprofit organization dedicated to educating headache sufferers and health-care professionals about headache causes and treatments.

International Headache Society

www.ihs-headache.org

The International Headache Society (IHS) is an international professional organization working with others for the benefit of people affected by headache disorders. The purpose of IHS is to advance headache science, education, and management, and to promote headache awareness worldwide. *Note*: The Web site asks about membership but nonmembers can access all guidelines.

---

occur daily and may become persistent and intractable. As with migraine patients, 75% of patients with chronic tension-type headaches are women. Patients may suffer from both tension-type and migraine headaches.

The patient usually describes a bandlike pressure that is a persistent, dull pain. The pain is usually bilateral in location and nonpulsating. The headache may change in intensity and last from 30 minutes to 7 days. Unlike migraine, tension-type headaches are not worsened by physical activity. The patient may have mild nausea or photophobia, but severe nausea, vomiting, and aura are absent. Tension headaches may increase in frequency and severity in times of stress or emotional upheaval. Chronic tension-type headache is diagnosed when the headache is present for more than 15 days per month.

Pathophysiology

The pathology of tension-type headaches is poorly understood. It was thought that muscle contraction was the primary cause of tension headache, and it was previously called muscle contraction headache. The patient may exhibit tenderness of the extracranial soft tissue and of the cervical or masseter muscles. The muscle pain and tenderness in tension headaches may resemble fibromyalgia. Prolonged stress, eyestrain, and sitting for long periods, such as when using a computer, may lead to increased tension headaches. There is little agreement currently about the cause of tension headaches.

Goals of Therapy

The primary goal of tension-type headache treatment is to decrease the frequency and severity of headache and to provide acute relief of headache once it begins. Although total eradication of headaches may not be possible, a combination of relaxation therapy and preventive medication, when necessary, usually decreases the frequency of headache.

Rational Drug Selection

The pharmacological management of tension-type headaches, as with migraine, focuses on acute or abortive treatment and preventive therapy. A key distinction between tension headache and migraine treatment is that tension headaches do not respond to ergotamine derivatives or triptans.

Acute Therapy

Acute therapy in the treatment of tension-type headaches includes a combination of pharmacological and nonpharmacological therapy.

Mild Analgesics

For mild to moderate tension headaches, OTC analgesics are quite effective. ASA, acetaminophen, or one of the NSAIDs (ibuprofen or naproxen), taken at the beginning of a tension headache, can be effective in relieving headache pain. The dosing is the same as for migraine. Patients should be cautioned not to use OTC analgesics for headache more than 2 to 3 times per week because they can cause medication-overuse headache.

Patients often self-medicate with OTC products prior to seeking care for their headaches, and therefore a history of what the patient has taken for headache relief and in what amounts is necessary. This history assists the health-care provider in determining if the headache has received adequate amounts of analgesic or if the tension headache is complicated by medication-overuse headache.

Combination Medications

Combination medications are commonly prescribed to treat both migraine and tension-type headaches. Products that combine either butalbital with ASA or APAP or isometheptene with APAP and dichloralphenazone are effective in treating tension headache. These products should be used cautiously because medication-overuse headaches can occur if dosages are higher than recommended or if they are taken more than 2 days per week. The provider should distribute a maximum of 30 tablets of either of these medications per month to make sure the patient is not overusing them.

Preventive Therapy

Preventive therapy should be considered if the patient is having more than one to two headaches per week. Used more than twice a week, the medications used for acute tension headache therapy all have the potential for causing medication-overuse headaches. A trial of preventive medication is likely to be helpful and should be considered early in treatment.

Beta Blockers

Beta blockers can be used for prophylactic treatment of tension headache. The dosing and contraindications are the same as for migraine preventive therapy.

Tricyclic Antidepressants

Tricyclic antidepressants are successful in reducing tension headaches both in patients who are depressed and in those who are not. They appear to enhance the endogenous pain-suppressing systems in the brain. Amitriptyline and nortriptyline are used in the same dosages as for migraine (see Table 35-2). Patients with tension-type headaches may also have depression, and dosing for depression may be successful if a lower dose is not effective.

Nonpharmacological Therapy

Nonpharmacological therapy is central in the preventive treatment of tension-type headaches. Stress management, biofeedback, and regular exercise can help to reduce medication use for tension headaches (ICSI, 2009). Topical heat or cold packs should be applied. Massage therapy and relaxation therapy help to relax the muscle tension that can aggravate tension headaches. Alternative therapies such as acupuncture and herbal medicine prescribed by a naturopath may improve headache symptoms. Referral to a psychologist or psychiatrist may assist in identifying and treating underlying anxiety that may be contributing to the tension headaches.

Monitoring

Monitoring for effectiveness of acute or preventive medication prescribed for tension headache should be done frequently (every 1 to 2 months) at the beginning of treatment. The patient must keep a headache diary to assist in determining if treatment is successful. Once a patient is stable on an acute or preventive medication, the patient can be seen less frequently. The provider should continue to monitor the use of combination drugs (butalbital and isometheptene compounds) to safeguard against potential medication-overuse headaches developing from overuse.

Outcome Evaluation

Evaluating the success of tension-type headache therapy is achieved by monitoring the patient's headache diary to determine if there is a decrease in the frequency or severity of headaches. If the patient develops new skills, such as stress reduction or relaxation, or begins exercising regularly, these efforts ought to be acknowledged by the health-care provider. As tension-type headaches often last off and on for many years, reevaluation and reworking the treatment regimen may happen multiple times.

Patient Education

Patient education should include a discussion of information related to the overall treatment plan as well as that specific to the drug therapy, reasons for taking the drug, drugs as part of the total treatment plan, and adherence issues. For general patient education information, see the previous Patient Education section.

Patient education information specific to treating tension-type headaches should focus on the following principles:

1. Patients need to know what tension-type headaches are and how they differ from migraines or pathological headaches.
2. Medication education ensures that the acute or preventive medications are taken appropriately. Prevention of medication overuse should be addressed early in the treatment.
3. Nonpharmacological therapies should be encouraged and the patient given local resources available, such as yoga classes, relaxation tapes, and massage therapists.
4. The importance of the patient's participation by keeping a headache diary needs to be stressed. Because most treatment decisions are based on response to therapy, the headache diary is invaluable to the successful management of headaches.

CHRONIC DAILY HEADACHES

Chronic daily headache is defined as headaches 15 or more days a month for longer than 3 months (Garza & Schwedt, 2014a). Chronic daily headaches (CDH) can be divided into five subtypes: chronic tension-type headache, chronic migraine, hemicrania continua, medication-overuse headache, or new daily persistent headache. Chronic tension-type headaches have already been addressed. Use of drugs for acute headache treatment more than 9 days a month is associated with increased risk of chronic daily headaches (ICSI, 2009). Medication-overuse is addressed later in this chapter. New persistent daily headache (NPDH) is uncommon, the onset is usually abrupt (patients can often pinpoint the date), and it is usually self-limiting. The cause is thought to be Epstein-Barr virus–induced immune changes. Treatment of NPDH is not discussed in this chapter because little information is available; these patients should be referred to a neurologist for care.

Pathophysiology

The pathology of CDH is often unclear and of mixed origin. There is a clear difference between chronic migraine and hemicrania continua. The boundary between chronic tension-type headache and chronic migraine is less clear and may require a neurology referral for treatment.

The term *chronic migraine* refers to CDH that starts as episodic migraine (less than 15 days a month) that transforms into a chronic pattern of greater than 15 days a month of migraine headache (Garza & Schwedt, 2014b). It was formerly called "transformed migraine." The initial migraines have the pathogenesis of migraine discussed earlier. Chronic migraine is not well understood, but is thought to be related to a combination of atypical pain processing, cortical hyperexcitability, neurologic inflammation, and central sensitization (Garza & Schwedt, 2014b). Risk factors for chronic migraine include female gender, history of head or neck injury, life stress, psychiatric disorders, and comorbid pain disorders (Garza & Schwedt, 2014b).

Hemicrania continua, also known as *chronic paroxysmal hemicrania*, is a rare headache syndrome where the patient, most often a woman, suffers from multiple (10 to 20) and short-lived (less than 20 minutes) episodes of severe unilateral, excruciating pain in the area of the eye, forehead, and temple. Exact pathology is not known but positive emission tomography (PET) scans demonstrate activation of the contralateral posterior hypothalamus and ipsilateral rostral pons during pain episodes (Garza & Schwedt, 2014c). Patients often have autonomic symptoms, including tearing, congestion, eyelid edema, flushing, sweating, or conjunctival injection.

Goals of Treatment

The first goal of treatment for CDH is to break the pattern of daily headache. The patient is then stabilized on prophylactic or preventive therapy.

Rational Drug Selection

Chronic Migraine

In most patients with chronic migraine, the daily headache cycle can be broken by using repeated doses of IV DHE. Approximately 70% to 80% of patients respond to DHE. The patient is given a test dose of 0.33 mL of DHE (1 mg/mL

solution) with 5 mg of metoclopramide or 10 mg of prochlorperazine (Compazine), followed by 0.5 mL of DHE and one of the antinausea medications every 6 hours for 48 to 72 hours. This usually requires inpatient treatment. DHE is contraindicated in coronary and peripheral vascular disease.

Alternatives to DHE include chlorpromazine (Thorazine) and prochlorperazine. If the patient has medication-overuse headache due to misuse of analgesics, ergots, or combination medications, the patient has to be detoxified, which is discussed later in this chapter. Treatment of chronic migraine may require consultation with a neurologist.

Preventive pharmacotherapy can be started after the headache cycle is broken. The patient usually responds to migraine-preventive medications such as propranolol, divalproex, or a tricyclic antidepressant. Amitriptyline is a good choice if the patient is also depressed. The seizure medications topiramate or valproic acid may be used. The patient is on preventive medication until the headache days are reduced by 50%, and then an additional 3 to 4 weeks, for a total of 6 to 12 weeks.

The patient should also receive alternative therapy to treat CDH. Behavioral counseling, biofeedback therapy, relaxation therapy, physical exercise, and acupuncture are all valid alternative therapies for treatment of CDH.

Hemicrania Continua

Hemicrania continua or chronic paroxysmal hemicrania is a rare disorder that responds completely to indomethacin and to nothing else. Indomethacin (Indocin) 75 to 150 mg is given daily; doses up to 200 mg daily may be needed. Referral to a neurologist is recommended.

Monitoring

Monitoring of patients with CDH who are on preventive therapy requires the patient to keep a diary of headache and medication use. Patients' blood pressure should be monitored if they are on a beta blocker, and liver function monitored if on divalproex, as per migraine therapy monitoring. Ongoing monitoring of headache is necessary because 31% may have recurrence of headache in spite of preventive medication.

Outcome Evaluation

Patients with CDH are difficult to treat. Treatment success is determined by how effective it has been in breaking the cycle of daily headaches and how effective the preventive treatment is. The patient's headache diary is key in the evaluation of the success of treatment.

Patient Education

Patient education should include a discussion of information related to the overall treatment plan as well as that specific to the drug therapy, reasons for taking the drug, drugs as part of the total treatment plan, and adherence issues.

Patient education information specific to treating CDH should focus on the following principles:

1. Education about the nature of the disorder, particularly that it is biological in origin, with neurochemical changes producing the headache.
2. Overuse of analgesics, leading to medication-overuse headache, must be emphasized.
3. The influence of stress, anxiety, depression, and inability to relax should be discussed, and the patient encouraged to use nonpharmacological therapies to decrease headache.

CLUSTER HEADACHES

Cluster headaches are characterized by intense pain lasting for 15 minutes to 2 hours; they occur in "clusters" of several weeks or months, with the headache subsiding for months at a time, often to recur. The patient can experience one to three attacks a day, usually at the same time of day. They occur most frequently at night, awakening the patient from sleep. Men are affected more than women, with onset in their late twenties. The pain of a cluster headache is unique in that it occurs behind or around one eye, with tearing, conjunctival injection, and drooping of the eyelid common symptoms. There may be nasal congestion, facial flushing, and sweating. The pain is so severe that the patient is unable to lie down or sit still, often pacing the floor in pain.

Pathophysiology

There is no clear etiology for cluster headaches. They are most likely a neuronal disorder originating in the hypothalamus. The clockwork-like timing of cluster headaches suggests that the circadian pacemaker or biological "clock" is dysfunctional.

Goals of Treatment

Relieving the pain of an acute cluster headache and decreasing the length of time of the cluster are the goals of cluster headache management.

Rational Drug Therapy

Most patients with cluster headaches require acute and preventive therapy. The acute attacks are severe and last only a short time; therefore, the intervention must be fast-acting. The patient usually requires both acute and preventive medications to manage the headache.

Acute Therapy

Oxygen therapy administered via a 100% nonrebreather mask for 15 to 30 minutes often provides immediate relief of cluster headache (ICSI, 2009; May, 2014b). Sumatriptan, administered SC, or intranasal sumatriptan or zolmitriptan may provide relief of acute cluster headaches (May, 2014b).

Intranasal lidocaine is thought to be effective in treating cluster headache. The patient lies supine, hyperextends the head at 45 degrees, and rotates it 30 degrees to the side of the headache. The lidocaine nasal solution is then dripped into the nostril on the affected side over 30 seconds. The onset is approximately 5 minutes.

Ergotamine derivatives are also effective for acute cluster headaches. Sublingual 2 mg tablets are administered at the beginning of the cluster headache. Ergotamine suppositories or DHE intranasally or IM may also be used (see Table 35-2 for dosing). Ergotamine may also be administered in a 2 mg dose given before bed if nocturnal attacks occur frequently.

Preventive Therapy

Verapamil can prevent cluster headaches in some patients. Calcium channel blockers are thought to prevent cluster headache by inhibiting vasospasm of the cerebral arteries. Dosing of verapamil is given in Table 35-2. Cluster headaches appear to need dosing in the high range to achieve headache reduction.

Divalproex can be effective in preventing cluster headaches. The dosing is the same as for migraine prophylaxis (see Table 35-2).

Lithium appears to have some effect on cluster headaches in some patients, and a trial of lithium is warranted if the patient does not respond to other preventive medications. The dose for cluster headache prevention is 300 mg daily to a maximum of 300 mg 3 times a day. The patient needs careful monitoring for adverse effects, including electrocardiogram (ECG), electrolytes, thyroid function, creatinine, and CBC studies.

Nonpharmacological therapies include avoidance of all alcohol during the clustering of headaches because alcohol often precipitates a headache. Patients often are able to drink alcohol between headache clusters without adverse effects. Tobacco, stress, anger, and vigorous physical activity should be avoided. The patient needs to maintain a normal sleep pattern, if possible. Cluster headaches do not appear to respond to self-care measures such as massage and relaxation.

Monitoring

Cluster headaches can be severely disabling, and the intense pain and loss of sleep can significantly affect the patient's quality of life. The health-care provider needs to monitor the patient for suicidal thoughts during the headache. The headache diary helps to monitor the effectiveness of acute and preventive medications. A patient treated with lithium requires careful monitoring of ECG and chemistries throughout treatment.

Outcome Evaluation

Cluster headaches by definition are self-limiting and will eventually stop, regardless of treatment. The focus of care is to provide measures that shorten or prevent cluster headaches during the cluster. Evaluation of the effectiveness of acute and preventive therapy is accomplished by self-report with a headache diary. Modifications in pharmacological management of cluster headaches should be based on the headache diary.

Patient Education

Patient education should include a discussion of information related to the overall treatment plan as well as that specific to the drug therapy, reasons for taking the drug, drugs as part of the total treatment plan, and adherence issues.

Patient education information specific to treating cluster headaches should focus on the following principles:

1. Educating the family about cluster headache, particularly the fact that it is a benign condition, in spite of the severe pain experienced during attacks.
2. Self-management of acute medications. The headache is usually brief, and therefore the patient must be able to self-medicate to provide relief. The pain may be gone by the time the patient can get transportation to a medical clinic.
3. Avoidance of alcohol is crucial during clusters of headaches.

MEDICATION-OVERUSE HEADACHES

Drug-rebound or drug-induced headache was reclassified by the International Headache Society as medication-overuse headache in 2008 (Ferrari, Coccia, & Sternieri, 2008). Medication-overuse headache should be considered in any patient who reports daily use of analgesics or combination medications such as butalbital or ergotamine derivatives or one of the triptans, with medication overuse reported in one-third of patients with chronic daily headaches (Maizels, 2004). Caffeine can also cause withdrawal headache when abruptly discontinued. The headache recurs as the medication wears off, compelling the patient to take another dose of medication, which causes a cycle of medication overuse and rebound. The patient may never have complete relief of pain, leading to a patient concern about serious pathology. A careful history of all the medications, including OTC analgesics that the patient takes on a daily basis, can help to determine if drug rebound is the issue or if a patient has CDH. A thorough history and physical examination with negative findings other than medication use is reassuring to the provider, but not always initially to the patient.

The health-care provider needs to be aware of the clinical features of medication-overuse headaches. According to the International Headache Society diagnostic criteria, the following clinical characteristics are found in medication-overuse headache (Silberstein et al, 2005):

1. Headache presents on more than 15 days/month, fulfilling criteria 3 and 4 below.
2. Regular overuse for more than 3 months of one or more drugs that can be taken for acute and/or symptomatic treatment of headache.
3. The headache has developed or markedly worsened during medication overuse.

4. Headache resolves or reverts to its previous pattern within 2 months after discontinuation of overused medication.

Other symptoms reported may be worsening of headache as analgesia wears off and the slightest physical or mental exertion brings on the headache. An accurate diagnosis is essential because chronic daily headaches and medication-overuse headache have similar presentation (Silberstein et al, 2005).

Pathophysiology

Dependence on either ergotamine or the OTC analgesics is thought to have physical and psychological elements. The overuse of simple analgesics (ASA or APAP), either alone or in combination with butalbital or caffeine, has a high potential for causing medication-overuse headache. Although the exact process is unclear, it is thought to suppress or alter the central pain-control mechanism. Ergotamine causes a clear pharmacological dependence and subsequent withdrawal. When a patient has analgesic-rebound headache, other headache therapies used for acute or preventive therapy may be resistant to treatment. The patient must be detoxified before preventive therapy can be started.

Goals of Therapy

The goal of treating medication-overuse headache is that the patient will no longer be taking daily doses of analgesics or ergotamine and will be stabilized on preventive medication. The goal during the withdrawal period should be minimizing the intensity of the withdrawal headache.

Rational Drug Therapy

Treatment of medication-overuse headache involves (1) withdrawal from offending agents, including caffeine; (2) transition therapy to support the patient during detoxification; and (3) initiation or adjustment of prophylaxis medication (Garza & Schwedt, 2014b; Maizels, 2004;). Anticipating withdrawal from daily or near-daily use of analgesics, butalbital-containing drugs, triptans, or ergotamine can make the patient anxious. The provider needs to adequately prepare the patient prior to the detoxification process, as discussed in the Patient Education section. Preventive therapy can be started when the withdrawal process is started or 2 to 3 weeks before or after the withdrawal process. Preventive therapy for migraine and tension-type headache has already been discussed. The practitioner should consult with a neurologist prior to embarking on detoxification of a patient with medication-overuse headache.

Withdrawal from the simple analgesics, ASA and APAP, or caffeine-containing medications is usually done on an outpatient basis. Naproxen may be used to provide pain relief while the overused medication is withdrawn. Naproxen is dosed at 550 mg twice daily for 2 to 4 weeks or 550 mg twice daily for 1 week then 550 mg daily for a week.

Butalbital-containing drugs (Fiorinal, Fioricet) may need to be tapered slowly because severe problems can develop with abrupt cessation. Serious withdrawal symptoms, such as delirium and seizures, can appear without warning. Butalbital use of less than 8 pills (400 mg) per day can be treated on an outpatient basis. Suggested regimens include Midrin *plus* clonazepam (Klonopin) for 1 week and then taper *or* phenobarbital for 1 week *plus* promethazine (Phenergan) for 1 to 2 weeks. If the patient is using more than eight pills per day, then inpatient drug detoxification is necessary, using IV DHE, metoclopramide, and IV fluids.

Some patients may require inpatient management to get their headache under control. Prevention and astute diagnosis are the roles of the primary care provider in the care of medication-overuse headache. Consultation with a headache specialist is warranted to provide optimal evidence-based care for medication-overuse headache.

Monitoring

Monitoring begins with the provider's regulating the number of doses of acute relief medication the patient is allowed to have each month. If OTC analgesic overuse is suspected, then the provider needs to determine the number of doses the patient is taking in a day or a week. During the withdrawal period, the patient's symptoms need to be monitored. If the patient requires IV medication or fluid intervention, the patient may need to be hospitalized. After the patient has been successfully detoxified from the medication, the provider needs to monitor the effectiveness of the preventive medication in preventing headaches. Effective preventive medication decreases the need for acute therapy. Ongoing assessment of analgesic, triptan, and ergotamine use will determine if the patient is overusing again.

Outcome Evaluation

The successful outcome in medication-overuse headache is a patient who is detoxified from the offending medication and is somewhat headache-free. The patient may still have an occasional headache and need acute or preventive therapy. Monitor for overuse of headache medications and relapse.

Patient Education

Patient education should include a discussion of information related to the overall treatment plan as well as that specific to the drug therapy, reasons for taking the drug, drugs as part of the total treatment plan, and adherence issues. Patients may have an exacerbation of headache in the first 2 weeks after withdrawal, and it may take 4 to 12 weeks after withdrawal for the patient to show improvement (Maizels, 2004). Educating the patient about what to expect during the withdrawal process will reduce anxiety during the process.

When discussing medication-overuse headache with the patient, the provider must be careful to avoid terms such as *drug abuse*. Patients with medication-overuse headache began with a primary headache disorder and fell into a pattern of overuse, and to label them as "abusers" can be devastating. Before and during the detoxification period, the provider should explain the plan of care and establish a patient's trust. The patient is about to embark on a process that will surely cause moderate to severe headache, a state that the patient has been trying to avoid.

The following principles regarding medication-overuse headache and the withdrawal process need to be discussed with the patient:

1. A clear description of medication-overuse headache and how it develops should be given to the patient.
2. After stopping the medication, the headache will get worse within 24 hours (72 hours for ergotamine) and may last from days to weeks.
3. Patients must be assured that interventions will be taken to make them comfortable and to decrease the severity of headache, including hospitalization, if needed.
4. It may take 1 to 3 months for the patient to have a normal response to acute therapy.

POST-TRAUMATIC (POST-CONCUSSIVE) HEADACHES

The post-traumatic headache syndrome is a common sequelae following injuries to the head or neck. In many patients, particularly those with more severe trauma, headaches may be a problem for months, years, or a lifetime. If the headaches develop within 2 weeks of the event, and persist for more than several months, we would consider this to be the chronic phase of the post-traumatic headache syndrome (Robbins, 2000).

Post-traumatic headache (PTH) is divided into acute and chronic groups whose management and prognosis are clearly different. Although IHS criteria stipulate that PTH should have an onset within 2 weeks of the trauma, it has been observed that a headache linked to the trauma can start later. PTH can be clinically divided into the following groups: migraine-like headache, tension-type-like headache, cluster-like headache, cervicogenic-like headache, and others. Based on these clinical distinctions, therapy can be administered accordingly. However, the distinction is relative and numerous clinical features may be common to all. There seems to be a weak inverse relationship between the severity of the head trauma and the occurrence of a PTH, especially chronic. A holistic approach is not only useful but is necessary for a therapeutic success (Lenaerts & Couch, 2004).

Pathophysiology

The mechanism of post-traumatic headache is poorly understood. Current research is investigating the interplay of biochemical, molecular, and physiological contributors that follow brain injury. Trauma-induced headaches are usually heterogeneous in nature, often including both tension-type pain and intermittent migraine-like attacks. Rebound headaches may develop from overuse of analgesic medications, and the occurrence of such may complicate significantly the diagnosis of post-traumatic headache. Adequate treatment typically requires both "peripheral" and "central" measures (Lane & Arciniegas, 2002). Other complicating contributing factors to the diagnosis and management of PTH is the presence of post-dural puncture resulting in a chronic "low-flow" dural leak, or the presence of a traumatic brain injury (TBI).

The key pathological sequelae of concussion are glutamate excitotoxicity, inflammation, priming and activation of microglia, blood–brain barrier disruption, axonal damage from mechanical injury and secondary events, calcium dysregulation, and alteration in cerebral blood flow and autoregulation (Neal, Wilson, Hsu, & Powers, 2012).

There are many other symptoms that often accompany the post-traumatic headache syndrome. These tend to be similar in most patients. They include some or all of the following: poor concentration, becoming easily angered, sensitivity to noise or bright lights, depression, dizziness or vertigo, tinnitus, memory problems, fatigue, insomnia, lack of motivation, decreased libido, nervousness or anxiety, irritability, becoming easily frustrated, and decreased ability to comprehend complex issues (Jeter et al, 2012).

Goals of Therapy

Early and aggressive treatment and empathy are essential to the patient's improvement. Prompt recognition and treatment of laceration, peripheral nociceptive sources such as cervical joint displacement, and vascular factors may diminish chronicity. Neuromodulation of pain with prophylactic agents is recommended early. Although it is less necessary for the acute PTH, it will be crucial for the chronic form and should be initiated no later than the 2 months' cut-off time between acute and chronic PTH. Recognition and treatment of psychiatric factors such as depression and anxiety will lessen the risk of chronicity (Lenaerts & Couch, 2004).

Rational Drug Therapy

Medication is the cornerstone of treatment because it is consistently the most effective therapeutic modality to assist with the management of symptoms associated with post-concussive headaches, although no medication has been identified to expedite recovery for TBI. We have available both abortive and/or preventive medication. In the first 3 weeks of the headaches, we usually only utilize abortive medication. If the headaches persist beyond this point, and remain moderate or severe, preventive medicine should be instituted.

Amitriptyline has been widely used for post-traumatic tension-type headaches as well as for the nonspecific symptoms, such as irritability, dizziness, depression, fatigue, and insomnia.

An inpatient program of repetitive intravenous dihydroergotamine and metoclopramide may provide relief of refractory chronic post-traumatic headaches. Greater occipital neuralgia frequently responds to greater occipital nerve block with a local anesthetic, which can also be combined with an injectable corticosteroid. A trial of propranolol or amitriptyline alone or in combination produced a 70% response rate in 21 of 30 adequately treated patients with post-traumatic migraine. Analgesia overuse was a common contributor to post-traumatic headache in 19% to 42% of patients. These patients responded to analgesic withdrawal as favorably as patients whose headaches were not post-traumatic. Patients with post-traumatic paroxysmal hemicrania and hemicrania continua have responded to treatment with indomethacin. (Evans, 2012).

Sleep aids such as melatonin have been used to treat sleep disturbances after concussion. Antidepressants, beta blockers, calcium channel blockers, valproic acid, topiramate, triptans, dihydroergotamine, and gabapentin have all been discussed as potential medical therapies for persistent headaches after concussion (Neal et al, 2012).

In the absence of controlled studies specific to post-concussive syndrome, these data suggest that post-traumatic headaches will likely respond to those treatments used for migraine and tension headache that are used in other settings. Clinicians caring for these patients note that delayed recovery from post-traumatic headaches may be due to inadequately aggressive treatment, analgesia overuse, or comorbidity (Evans, 2012).

Acute or abortive therapy is aimed at reversing, aborting, or reducing pain and accompanying symptoms of an attack that is in progress or is anticipated. The choice of abortive therapy depends upon the type of headache that is being treated. The principle medications for treating post-traumatic migraine, cluster, or tension-type headaches are the same as those outlined in earlier respective sections of this chapter.

Anti-inflammatories are often utilized in the post-traumatic situation where bleeding is not suspected, so as to aid the accompanying cervical or back pain. Muscle relaxants are more helpful than in routine tension headaches, because of cervical muscle spasm. If patients require excessive amounts of abortive medication, we need to consider the use of preventive medication. We do not want to create the rebound headache situation.

Most patients with migraine, and the majority of patients with post-traumatic migraine, simply require abortive medications for their headaches. However, if the migraines are frequent and/or severe, we need to progress to daily preventive therapy. The decision as to when to progress to daily preventive therapy is a difficult one, but most patients with severe post-traumatic migraines also suffer from daily headaches, and they usually benefit from preventive medication (Neal et al, 2012).

Preventive therapy should be considered for any patient who experiences severely incapacitating or frequent severe migraines (more than two per month) and patients who cannot tolerate abortive medications because of either chronic illness (coronary artery disease or hypertension) or the adverse effects of abortive medications. Preventive medication is also recommended if the patient is taking abortive medication more than twice a week. The primary goal of preventive therapy is to use the least amount of medication with the fewest side effects to decrease migraine symptoms. If medication overuse is suspected, it must be treated first before starting the patient on preventive therapy; this topic is covered earlier in this chapter.

The most commonly employed preventives for the post-traumatic headaches are the antidepressants, particularly amitriptyline (Elavil) or nortriptyline (Pamelor), and the beta blockers. The anti-inflammatories often serve a dual purpose, functioning as both abortives and preventives. The antidepressants that are sedating, particularly amitriptyline, often decrease the daily headaches, migraines, and the associated insomnia. In severe cases, we need to use both a beta blocker and an antidepressant. The selection of preventive medication differs depending upon which headache type is predominant (Neal et al, 2012).

Although the first choices for prevention medication in the post-traumatic situation are usually antidepressants and/or beta blockers, alternative medications may be utilized. Calcium blockers (verapamil) are used for migraines as a first-line therapy. Valproate (Depakote), methysergide (Sansert), and MAO inhibitors (phenelzine) are employed if initial approaches have not been successful. IV DHE, used repetitively in the office or in the hospital, is very useful with severe post-traumatic headaches. Use IV DHE relatively early in the patient's course, often after 1 or 2 months, if the headaches are very severe. Concurrently, daily preventive medication is employed in these patients (Neal et al, 2012).

Monitoring

Clinicians who specialize in the assessment and management of this diagnosis encounter patients with prolonged recovery courses, persistent symptoms, and significant deficits in cognitive functioning. These patients require more involved therapy, which may include additional education, academic accommodations, physical therapy, cognitive rehabilitation, and medication (Meehan, 2011). Monitoring is based on medication choice (see monitoring for migraine, chronic daily headache, medication overuse headache). If OTC supplements are used for "neuroprotection," the prescriber needs to keep abreast of drug-to-supplement interactions.

Patient Education

Patient education should include a discussion of information related to the overall treatment plan as well as that specific to the drug therapy, reasons for taking the drug, drugs as part of the total treatment plan, and adherence issues. Patients may have an exacerbation of headache in the first 2 weeks after withdrawal, and it may take 4 to 12 weeks after withdrawal for the patient to show improvement (Maizels, 2004). Educating the patient about what to expect during the withdrawal process will reduce anxiety during the process. The following information may be useful in communications with patients (Evans, 2012):

What is post-concussion syndrome?—Post-concussion syndrome is a condition that happens after a mild brain

---

On The Horizon

DRUGS THAT MAY PROVIDE NEUROPROTECTION FOR TBI

Magnesium has demonstrated neuroprotective properties in numerous TBI models. Magnesium has been shown to have many beneficial effects, including noncompetitive NMDA receptor blockade, inhibition of presynaptic excitatory neurotransmitter release, blockade of voltage-gated calcium channels, and reduction in inflammatory cascades (Burd, Breen, Friedman, Cha, & Elovitz, 2010). Unfortunately, the data are lacking in specific and safe recommendations for the use of magnesium in this population. Additional studies should help clarify the clinical utility of magnesium supplementation following TBI (Maas & Murray, 2007).

Progesterone is an agent that appears to provide neuroprotection by multiple mechanisms. After TBI, progesterone has been shown to decrease oxidative stress by reducing membrane lipid peroxidation, reduce BBB disruption, and ameliorate the brain's inflammatory response. A phase III clinical trial, the Progesterone for the Treatment of Traumatic Brain Injury (ProTECT III), is currently underway to further assess the clinical efficacy of progesterone (Vink & Nimmo, 2009).

Erythropoietin has been identified as a neuroprotective agent that appears to ameliorate TBI by multiple avenues. The Erythropoietin in Traumatic Brain Injury (EPO-TBI) trial is currently underway to assess whether erythropoietin can improve neurological outcome in severe TBI patients (Vink & Nimmo, 2009).

Minocycline has been extensively studied in mice and has been shown to be an effective antioxidant and attenuator of the inflammatory sequelae of TBI. The study, A Safety and Feasibility of Minocycline in the Treatment of Traumatic Brain Injury, is currently underway, which will likely lead to additional clinical investigation of this drug (Schouten, 2007).

Cyclosporin is another multifactorial compound that has neuroprotective effects, including improving mitochondrial functioning, blocking free radical production, and inhibiting calcium accumulation. The animal data have been compelling that cyclosporin A (CsA) has therapeutic benefits in TBI models. However, the variability of study designs from the clinical studies has made the outcome data difficult to interpret. The safety of CsA use in TBI has been demonstrated, but additional investigation is needed to clarify the efficacy of the drug (Lulic, Burn, Bae, van Loveren, & Borlongan, 2011).

Numerous other vitamins, minerals, and antioxidant agents are being investigated as potential therapeutic modalities. These include **nicotinamide**, a soluble B-group vitamin. Animal TBI models have demonstrated beneficial effects, including reduced cortical damage, inflammation, and behavioral disruption in animals receiving infusions (Goffus, Anderson, & Hoane, 2010).

Omega-3 essential fatty acids (EFAs) have been shown in experimental TBI models to improve the blood flow, reduce the toxic effects of glutamate, and stabilize membranes. Animal models have shown that specific fatty acids can be supplemented in the diet and provide a protective function for the brain, especially in regard to seizures (Pages et al, 2011).

An antioxidant, *α-lipoic acid*, has also shown neuroprotective effects in an animal model by reducing inflammatory markers, preserving BBB permeability, and reducing brain edema (Toklu et al, 2009). Another agent called *Resveratrol*, which is a polyphenol, also has antioxidant properties and has been shown to improve behavioral outcome in a rat TBI model (Maroon & Bost, 2011). **Zinc protoporphyrin** has also been shown to attenuate brain edema and BBB permeability in an animal model (Vannemreddy et al, 2006).

injury. A "concussion" is another word for a mild brain injury. Common causes of mild brain injuries include:

- Car accidents
- Falling down and other accidents that can happen from daily activities
- Injuries from playing sports such as football, ice hockey, soccer, and boxing
- Injuries that can happen to soldiers during combat. These include injuries from blasts and bullet wounds.

What are the symptoms of post-concussion syndrome?—The symptoms include:

- Headache
- Dizziness
- Feeling very tired
- Feeling irritable or anxious
- Memory problems or problems paying attention
- Problems with sleep
- Being easily bothered by noise

How is post-concussion syndrome treated?—The treatments are different depending on which symptoms a person has. There are medicines that can help with headaches, dizziness, and other problems.

How is headache treated?—There are lots of prescription and nonprescription medicines that can ease the pain of headaches. There are also prescription medicines that can help prevent headaches from happening in the first place. The right medicine for you will depend on what type of headaches you get, how often you get them, and how bad they are.

If you get headaches often, work with your doctor to find a treatment that helps. Do not try to manage frequent headaches on your own with nonprescription pain medicines. Taking nonprescription pain medicines too often can actually cause more headaches later.

REFERENCES

American Headache Society. (2011). *Information for patients: Types of headaches.* Retrieved January 27, 2013, from http://www.achenet.org/resources/types_of_headaches/

Bajwa, Z. H., & Wootton, R. J. (2013). Evaluation of headache in adults. *UpToDate.* Wolters Kluwer. Retrieved on January 27, 2013, from http://www.uptodate.com./contents/evaluation-of-headache-in-adults

Burd, I., Breen, K., Friedma, N. A., Cha, I J., & Elovitz, M. A. (2010). Magnesium sulfate reduces inflammation-associated brain injury in fetal mice. *American Journal of Obstetrics and Gynecology, 202*(292), e1–e9.

Carmona, S., & Bruera, O. (2009). Prophylactic treatment of migraine and migraine clinical variants with topiramate: An update. *Therapeutic and Clinical Risk Management, 5,* 661–669.

Carpay, J., Schoenen, J., Ahmad, F., Kinrade, F., & Boswell, D. (2004). Efficacy and tolerability of sumatriptan tablets in a fast-disintegrating, rapid-release formulation for the acute treatment of migraine: Results of a multicenter, randomized, placebo-controlled study. *Clinical Therapeutics, 26*(2), 214–223.

Chawla, J. (2013). *Migraine headache.* Medscape. Retrieved on February 10, 2013, from http://emedicine.medscape.com/article/1142556-overview

Endo Pharmaceuticals. (2013). *Frova.* Retrieved from http://www.endo.com/File%20Library/Products/Prescribing%20Information/FROVA_Prescribing_Information.html

Evans, R. W. (2012). Postconcussion syndrome. *UpToDate.* Wolters Kluwer. Retrieved on January 27, 2013, from http://www.uptodate.com./contents/postconcussion-syndrome

Ferrari, A., Coccia, C., & Sternieri, E. (2008). Past, present and future prospects of medication-overuse headache classification. *Headache, 48,* 1096–1102.

Gagne, J. J., Leas, B., Lofland, J. H., Goldfarb, N., Freitag, F., & Silberstein, S. (2007). Quality of care measures for migraine: A comprehensive review. *Disease Management, 10*(3), 138–146.

Garza, I., & Schwedt, T. J. (2014a). Overview of chronic daily headache. *UpToDate.* Wolters Kluwer. Retrieved from http://www.uptodate.com/contents/overview-of-chronic-daily-headache

Garza, I., & Schwedt, T. J. (2014b). Chronic migraine. *UpToDate.* Wolters Kluwer. Retrieved from http://www.uptodate.com/contents/chronic-migraine

Garza, I., & Schwedt, T. J. (2014c). Hemicrania continua. *UpToDate.* Wolters Kluwer. Retrieved from http://www.uptodate.com/contents/hemicrania-continua

Goffus, A. M., Anderson, G. D., & Hoane, M. (2010). Sustained delivery of nicotinamide limits cortical injury and improves functional recovery following traumatic brain injury. *Oxidative Medicine and Cellular Longevity, 3,*145–152.

Institute for Clinical Systems Improvement (ICSI). (2009). *Health care guide line: Diagnosis and treatment of headache* (9th ed.). Bloomington, MN: ICSI. Retrieved from http://www.icsi.org/headache/headache__diagnosis_and_treatment_of_2609.html

Jeter, C. B., Hergenroeder, G. W., Hylin, M. J., Redell, J. B., Moore, A. N., & Dash, P. K. (2012, October 12). Biomarkers for the diagnosis and prognosis of mild traumatic brain injury/concussion. *Journal of Neurotrauma, 30*(8): 657–670.

Lane, J. C, & Arciniegas, D. B. (2002, January). Post-traumatic headache. *Current Treatment Options in Neurology, 4*(1), 89–104.

Law, S., Derry, S., & Moore, R. A.(2010, April 14). Triptans for acute cluster headache. *Cochrane Database Systemic Review,* (4), CD008042.

Lenaerts, M. E., & Couch, J. R. (2004). Posttraumatic headache. *Current Treatment Options in Neurology, 6*(6), 507–517.

Lulic, D., Burn, S. J., Bac, E. C., van Loveren, H., & Borlongan, C. V. (2011). A review of laboratory and clinical data supporting the safety and efficacy of cyclosporin A in traumatic brain injury. *Neurosurgery, 68*(5), 1172–1185.

Maas, A. I., & Murray G. D. (2007). Magnesium for neuroprotection after traumatic brain injury. *Lancet Neurology , 6,* 20–21.

Maizels, M. (2004). The patient with daily headaches. *American Family Physician, 70*(12), 2299–2306.

Maizels, M., & Burchette, R. (2003). Rapid and sensitive paradigm for screening patients with headache in primary care settings. *Headache: The Journal of Head & Face Pain, 43*(5), 441–450.

Mannix, L. K., Frame, J. R., & Solomon, G. D. (1997). Alcohol, smoking and caffeine use among headache patients. *Headache, 37,* 572–576.

Marcus, D. A., Cope, D. K., Deodhar, A., & Payne, R. (2009). Headache. In *An atlas of investigation and management of chronic pain* (pp 39–57). Oxford, UK: Clinical Publishing.

Marin, P. A. (1998). Pharmacology update: Pharmacologic management of migraine. *Journal of the American Academy of Nurse Practitioners, 10*(9), 407–412.

Maroon, J. C., & Bost, J. (2011). Concussion management at the NFL, college, high school, and youth sports levels. *Clinical Neurosurgery, 58,* 51–56.

Matcher, D. B., Young, W. B., Rosenberg, J. H., Pietrzak, M. P., Silberstein, S. D., Lipton, R. B., et al, & US Headache Consortium. (2000). *Evidence-based guidelines for migraine headache in the primary care setting: Pharmacological management of acute attacks.* Retrieved from http://tools.aan.com/professionals/practice/pdfs/gl0087.pdf

Mathew, N. T. (1997). Transformed migraine, analgesic rebound and other chronic daily headaches. *Neurologic Clinics, 15*(1), 167–186.

Matthew, N.T., Rapoport, A., Saper, R.A., Magnus, L., Klapper, J., Ramadan, N., et al. (2001). Efficacy of gapapentin in migraine prophylaxis. *Headache, 4*192), 119–128.

May, A. (2014a). Cluster headache: Epidemiology, clinical features, and diagnosis. *UpToDate.* Retrieved February 10, 2013, from http://www.uptodate.com/contents/cluster-headache-epidemiology-clinical-features-and-diagnosis

May, A. (2014b). Cluster headache: Treatment and prognosis. *UpToDate.* Retrieved from http://www.uptodate.com/contents/cluster-headache-treatment-and-prognosis

Meehan, W. P., 3rd. (2011, January). Medical therapies for concussion. *Clinical Sports Medicine, 30*(1), 115–124.

Mendizabal, J. E. (1998). The clinical challenge of chronic daily headaches. *Patient Care Nurse Practitioner, 1*(5), 41–46.

Migraine Research Foundation (2014). *Migraine fact sheet.* Retrieved from http://www.migraineresearchfoundation.org/fact-sheet.html

Moore, K. L., & Noble, S. L. (1997). Drug treatment of migraine: Part I. Acute therapy and drug-rebound headache. *American Family Physician, 56*(8), 2039–2048.

Neal, M. T., Rapoport, A., Saper, J., Magnus, L., Klapper, J., Ramadan, N., et al. (2001). Efficacy of gabapentin in migraine prophylaxis. *Headache, 41*, 119–128.

Neal, M. T., Wilson, J. L., Hsu, W., & Powers, A. K. (2012). Concussions: What a neurosurgeon should know about current scientific evidence and management strategies. *Surgical Neurology International, 3*, 16.

Noble, S. L., & Moore, K. L. (1997). Drug treatment of migraine: Part II. Preventive therapy. *American Family Physician, 56*(9), 2279–2286.

Ortho-McNeil Neurologics. (2009). *Axert.* Retrieved from http://www.axert.com

Pages, N., Maurois P., Delplanque, B., Bac, P., Martin, J. C., Du, Q., et al. (2011). Brain protection by rapeseed oil in magnesium-deficient mice. *Prostaglandins, Leukotrienes, and Essential Fatty Acids, 85*, 53–60.

Ramadan, N. M., Silberstein, S. D., Freitag, F. G., Gilbert, T. T., & Frishberg, B. M. *Evidence-based guidelines for migraine headache in the primary care setting: Pharmacological management for prevention of migraine.* Retrieved February 10, 2013, from http://www.aan.com/professionals/practice/pdfs/gl0090.pdf

Rapoport, A., Stang P., Gutterman, D. L., Cady, R., Markley, H., Weeks, R., Saiers, J., & Fox, A. W. (1996, January). Analgesic rebound headache in clinical practice: Data from a physician survey. *Headache, 36*(1), 14–19.

Robbins, L. (2000). *Management of headache and headache medications: Post traumatic headache.* Retrieved January 26, 2013, from http://www.headachedrugs.com/archives/post_traumatic.html

Schouten, J.W. (2007). Neuroprotection in traumatic brain injury: A complex struggle against the biology of nature. *Current Opinions in Critical Care, 13*, 134–142.

Silberstein, S. D., Olesen, J., Bousser, M.-G., Diener, H.-C., Dodick, D., First, M., et al, on behalf of the International Headache Society. (2005). The International Classification of Headache Disorders (2nd ed.) (ICHD-II)—Revision of criteria for 8.2 Medication-overuse headache. *Cephalalgia, 25*, 460–465.

Stovner, L. J., Hagen, K., Jensen, R., Katsarava, Z., Lipton, RB, Scher, AI, Steiner, TJ & Zwart, J-A. (2007). The global burden of headache: A documentation of headache prevalence and disability worldwide. *Cephalalgia, 27*, 193–210.

Taylor, F. R. (2009). Headache prevention with complementary and alternative medicine. *Headache, 49*(6), 966–968.

Thompson, J. (2013). *Postconcussion headache.* Retrieved on February 12, 2013, from http://now.aapmr.org/pain-neuro/pain-medicine/Pages/Postconcussion-Headache.aspx

Toklu, H. Z., Hakan, T., Biber, N., Solakoglu, S., Ogunc, A. V., & Sener, G. (2009). The protective effect of alpha lipoic acid against traumatic brain injury in rats. *Free Radical Research, 43*, 658–667.

Vannemreddy, P., Ray A. K., Patnaik, R., Patnaik, S., Mohanty, S., & Sharma, H. S. (2006). Zinc protoporphyrin IX attenuates closed head injury-induced edema formation, blood-brain barrier disruption, and serotonin levels in the rat. *Acta Neurochirurgica, 96*, 151–156.

Vink, R., & Nimmo, A. J. (2009). Multifunctional drugs for head injury. *Neurotherapeutics, 6*, 28–42.

Warner, J. S. (2001). The outcome of treating patients with suspected rebound headache. *Headache, 41*, 685–692.

Weiner, R. S. (2002). Primary headache disorders. In *Pain management: A practical guide for clinicians* (6th ed., pp 195–205). Boca Raton, FL: CRC Press LLC.

HEART FAILURE

Laura Rosenthal

Heart failure (HF) is a major health problem that the American College of Cardiology Foundation (ACCF) and the American Heart Association (AHA) estimate affects more than 5.1 million Americans annually (Yancy et al, 2013). The underlying HF incidence increases with age; the prevalence has increased over the past decade as the U.S. population ages. With the aging population growth, it is expected to increase significantly, especially in the black male population. Despite aggressive investigation into treatment options, the 5-year mortality rate remains 50% within 5 years of diagnosis. Of particular importance in HF management is the design of a treatment program targeted at the patient's underlying pathophysiology. Such a carefully designed program maximizes outcomes and prevents such treatment complications as prerenal azotemia and dehydration. Because multidrug regimens are often necessary, patient education is essential to limit complications, hospitalizations, and hospital readmissions that result from poor adherence to the treatment regimen.

PATHOPHYSIOLOGY

Heart failure is a complex clinical syndrome that can result from any structural or functional cardiac disorder that results in a cardiac output that is inadequate to satisfy the oxygen demands of the body. In HF, several abnormalities occur. Coronary artery disease (CAD) causing myocardial ischemia is the underlying cause in about two-thirds of patients with left ventricular dysfunction. Left ventricular dysfunction (systolic heart failure) begins with injury to the myocardium and is usually a progressive process, even in the absence of additional myocardial insults. The principal mechanism relates to remodeling, which occurs as a homeostatic mechanism to decrease wall stress through increases in wall thickness. The cells generated during remodeling are often abnormal and include a proliferation of connective tissue cells. These cells use energy inefficiently and have little contractile ability. The ultimate result is a change in the structure of the left ventricle in which the chamber dilates, hypertrophies, and becomes more spherical. This process generally precedes the development of symptoms but continues after their appearance and may contribute to the worsening of symptoms despite treatment. One of the advantages of the use of angiotensin-converting enzyme (ACE) inhibitors is their action in reducing remodeling.

As the left ventricle hypertrophies, the sarcomeres of the muscle cells lengthen so that limited numbers of cross-bridges can form and function appropriately and contractile force degenerates. Contractility of heart muscle is a function of the interaction of calcium with the actin-troponin-tropomyosin system. Activator calcium released from the sarcoplasmic reticulum facilitates the interaction of actin with myosin to create the cross-bridging that produces contraction. The amount of calcium released depends on the amount in stores and the amount that enters the cell during the plateau phase of the action potential. The reduced force at systole causes the ventricles to supply inadequate blood volume to the body and blood pressure (BP) drops, even though the ventricle is very full and overstretched. This triggers counterregulatory mechanisms in the rest of the body, activating the sympathetic nervous system (SNS) and the renin-angiotensin-aldosterone (R-A-A) system (Fig. 36-1). The SNS increases heart rate, tries to increase contractile force, and increases venous tone. A major role of beta blockers in HF treatment relates to reducing the SNS activation. The R-A-A system triggers the retention of sodium and water to increase blood volume and venous return (increased preload). Initially, this brings more venous return to the heart and increases the amount of blood available to the body.

In the long-term, these adaptive mechanisms actually create more failure. The ventricle that is already full and stretched is required to deal with more volume. Diuretics, another cornerstone of pharmacological therapy, assist by reducing increased extracellular fluid volume. The pathology of HF is further compounded by the denial of adequate oxygen as the increased heart rate shortens the diastolic filling time and the coronary arteries have less time to fill. The heart demands more oxygen supply and has less.

Risk factors for HF include hypertension, diabetes mellitus (DM) and metabolic syndrome. (Yancy et al, 2013). Increased systolic and diastolic pressures especially long term, increase the risk and treatment can reduce the risk of developing HF by 50%. Metabolic syndrome, with or without overt DM, now impacts 40% to 50% of the U.S. population over age 40. The coordinated treatment of dyslipidemia, insulin resistance, and hypertension can significantly reduce HF risk.

Types of Heart Failure

Three main forms of HF can occur. Systolic dysfunction typically occurs acutely and often follows a myocardial infarction (MI). Other potential causes include nonischemic cardiomyopathy, generally from use of alcohol, cocaine, chemotherapy and other drugs that depress the myocardium, and conditions that lead to volume overload. The problem is inadequate force generated to eject blood from the ventricles, resulting in decreased cardiac output and ejection fractions of less than 40%. Forty to 60% of patients with HF have this form.

Diastolic dysfunction, also known as heart failure with preserved ejection fraction (HF-pEF), results from inadequate relaxation and loss of muscle fiber elasticity, resulting in a slower filling rate and elevated diastolic pressures. Although cardiac output is reduced, ejection fractions remain within normal limits. Potential causes include valvular dysfunction, hypertrophic and ischemic cardiomyopathy, uncontrolled

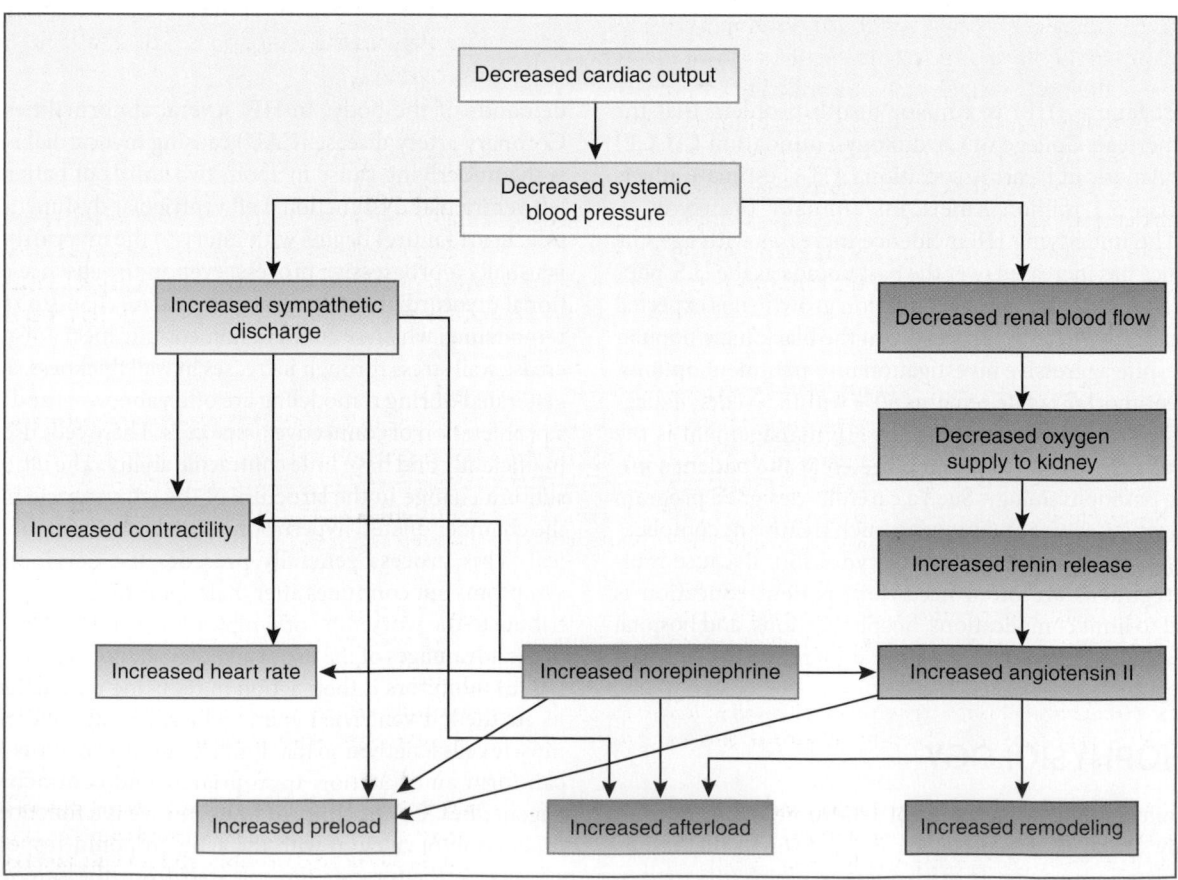

Figure 36–1. Compensatory responses in heart failure.

hypertension (HTN), and hypothyroidism. Many of the changes that occur in the cardiovascular system as a result of aging have a greater impact on diastolic function than systolic function. Heart failure with preserved systolic function is primarily a disease of elderly women (greater than 75 years), most of whom have hypertension. Up to 60% of patients with HF have this form; however, the percentage increases with age.

Coronary artery disease (CAD) and atherosclerosis are significant contributing factors for combined systolic-diastolic dysfunction. Framingham data suggest that 76% of patients with HF have hypertension or CAD alone or in combination as the cause. Treatment of these underlying disorders often improves the performance of the heart muscle.

"High-output" failure is a fairly rare form that takes place when the demands of the body are so great that even increased cardiac output is insufficient. Causative factors include hyperthyroidism, anemia, and arteriovenous shunts. Treatment for this form is directed at the underlying pathology and is not discussed here.

Classifications of Heart Failure

The New York Heart Association (NYHA) has classified HF based on the severity of symptoms. This functional classification reflects the amount of activity needed to produce symptoms. It is fairly subjective in nature and treatments used do not differ significantly across the classes. In addition, this system does not deal with patients who are asymptomatic or at high risk for the development of HF. The ACCF/AHA committee (Yancy et al, 2013) sought to develop a staging system that would objectively identify patients throughout the course of their disease and would be linked to treatments that were uniquely appropriate for each stage of their illness. In addition, this classification scheme recognizes that HF, like HTN and CAD, has established risk factors; that evolution of the disorder has asymptomatic as well as symptomatic phases; and that treatment prescribed at each stage can reduce the morbidity and mortality of HF. Table 36-1 compares these two classifications.

Symptoms of Heart Failure

Symptoms have been described as depending on whether the left or the right ventricle is affected. Lung-focused symptoms (often referred to as "congestion") are associated with left-sided failure, and body-focused symptoms, such as edema, are associated with right-sided failure. With the exception of cor pulmonale, which is clearly right-sided in nature, progression of the disease usually involves both ventricles, and the terminology of left-sided versus right-sided failure is less useful clinically. In older adults, the peripheral edema thought to be associated with right-sided HF is actually more often related to venous insufficiency. It should be noted that over 21% of community adults have asymptomatic LV dysfunction. If untreated it results in more than 8% risk of death annually (Redfield et al, 2003).

Peripheral venous disease should be considered as a causative or contributing factor to symptoms in older adults. Regardless of which ventricle is more involved, patients with HF may have a number of symptoms, the most common being breathlessness, fatigue, exercise intolerance, and weight gain secondary to fluid retention. None of these symptoms is specific to HF and several other disorders may present with similar symptoms. Therefore, symptoms alone cannot be relied upon to make the diagnosis, which depends upon good history taking and physical examination, supplemented by diagnostic tests. Diagnostic evaluation will be presented later. The clinical course of the disease depends in large part on the point at which the patient is diagnosed and treatment is started, the appropriate targeting of that treatment, and the underlying pathology.

PHARMACODYNAMICS

Only a small number of HF cases are attributable to specific disorders that can be treated with or improved by surgery. The mainstay of HF therapy is lifestyle management and drug treatment targeted to altering the physiological mechanisms

Table 36–1 Comparison of Classification Systems for Heart Failure (HF)

New York Heart Association	American College of Cardiology/ American Heart Association
Class I. No limitations. Ordinary physical activity does not cause fatigue, breathlessness, or palpitation. (Asymptomatic left-ventricular dysfunction is included in this category.)	**Stage A.** Patient at high risk for developing HF but without structural heart disease
Class II. Slight limitations of physical activity. Comfortable at rest, but ordinary physical activity results in fatigue, palpitation, breathlessness, or angina pectoris (symptomatically "mild" HF).	**Stage B.** Patient with a structural disorder of the heart but who has never developed symptoms of HF
Class III. Marked limitations of physical activity. Although patient is comfortable at rest, less than ordinary physical activity will lead to symptoms (symptomatically "moderate" HF).	**Stage C.** Patient with past or current symptoms of HF associated with underlying structural disease
Class IV. Inability to carry on any physical activity without discomfort. Symptoms of congestive HF are present even at rest. With any physical activity, increased discomfort is experienced (symptomatically "severe" HF).	**Stage D.** Patient with end-stage disease who requires specialized treatment strategies such as mechanical circulatory support, continuous inotropic infusions, cardiac transplantation, or hospice care

that create or arise from HF. Four main categories of drugs are used to treat HF, whether it is systolic or diastolic in nature. The four categories of drugs: diuretics, angiotensin-converting enzyme (ACE) inhibitors, cardiac glycosides, and the beta blockers, are listed in Table 36-2.

Diuretics reduce preload by decreasing extracellular fluid volume and can be used to decrease hypertension that increases afterload. ACE inhibitors act on the R-A-A system to decrease preload and afterload. They also affect heart tissue remodeling so that fewer abnormal myocardial cells are

Table 36–2   Drugs Commonly Used: Heart Failure

Drug	Indication	Dosage Form	Initial Dose	Target Dose
Thiazide Diuretics				
Hydrochlorothiazide (Microzide)	Initial therapy for volume overload.	Tablets: 12.5, 25, 50, 100 mg Liquid: 50 mg/5 mL	25 mg daily	50 mg daily
Loop Diuretics				
	Added therapy when resistant to standard therapy or for decompensation			
Furosemide (Lasix) Bumetanide (Bumex) Torsemide (Demadex)	Furosemide is first choice. Torsemide is best when high doses of furosemide are required.	Tablets: 20, 40, 80 mg Injection: 40 mg/5 mL Injection: 0.5, 1, 2 mg Injection: 5, 10, 20, 100 mg	20–40 mg daily or twice daily 0.5–1 mg daily or twice daily 10–20 mg daily	As needed As needed As needed
Angiotensin-Converting Enzyme (ACE) Inhibitors				
Captopril (Capoten) Enalapril (Vasotec) Lisinopril (Zestril) Quinapril (Accupril)	All subsets of patients. Initial therapy or if symptoms not relieved by diuretic. Drug of choice for patients with diabetes.	Tablets: 12.5, 25, 50, 100 mg Tablets: 2.5, 5, 10, 20 mg Tablets: 2.5, 5, 10, 20, 30, 40 mg Tablets: 5, 10, 20, 40 mg	6.25 mg three times a day 2.5 mg twice a day 2.5–5 mg daily 5 mg twice a day	50 mg tid 10 mg bid 20 mg daily 20 mg daily
Angiotensin II Receptor Antagonist				
Losartan (Cozaar) Valsartan (Diovan) Candesartan (Atacand)	Patients intolerant to ACE inhibitors	Tablets: 25, 50, 100 mg Tablets: 40, 80, 160, 320 mg Tablets: 4, 8 mg, 16, 32 mg	12.5–25 mg daily 20–40 mg daily 4–8 mg daily	100 mg daily 160 mg daily 32 mg daily
Digoxin (Lanoxin)	If symptoms unrelieved by ACE inhibitor and diuretic	Tablets: 0.125, 0.25 mg Injection: 0.05 mg/1 mL	0.125 mg daily	As needed
Hydralazine (Apresoline)	With isosorbide dinitrate for intolerance to ACE inhibitor	Tablets: 10, 25, 50, 100 mg Injection: 20mg/mL	37.5 mg 4 times daily	75 mg 4 times daily
Isosorbide dinitrate (Isordil)	With hydralazine for intolerance to ACE inhibitor	Tablets: 5, 10, 20, 30, 40 mg ER Sublingual: 2.5, 5 mg	20 mg 4 times daily	40 mg 4 times daily
Beta Blockers				
Carvedilol (Coreg, Coreg CR) Metoprolol Succinate (Toprol-XL) Bisoprolol (Zebeta)	Patients with diastolic dysfunction or cardiomyopathy in whom reduced heart rate can improve cardiac output	Tablets: 3.125, 6.25, 12.5, 25 mg Extended-release tablets: 10, 20, 40, 80 mg Tablets: 25, 50, 100, 200 mg Tablets: 5, 10 mg	3.125 mg twice a day 12.5-25 mg daily 1.25 mg daily	6.25–25 mg twice daily 200 mg daily 10 mg daily
Aldosterone Antagonists				
Eplerenone (Inspra)	Diastolic HF	Tablets: 25, 50 mg	25 mg daily	50 mg daily
Spironolactone (Aldactone)	Diastolic HF	Tablets: 25, 50, 100 mg	25 mg daily	25 mg daily

generated. Digoxin, a cardiac glycoside, improves myocardial contractility and cardiac output. Beta-adrenergic blockers affect the SNS counterregulatory mechanism of HF. Aldosterone antagonists augment the actions of ACE inhibitors on the R-A-A system.

Three other classes of drugs are used in special circumstances. Nitrates improve systolic and diastolic ventricular function by improving oxygen transport to the myocardium for patients with HF who also have angina. Anticoagulants are used for patients with HF who also have chronic atrial fibrillation. Antiplatelets are used to prevent MI and death in patients with HF who have underlying CAD.

GOALS OF TREATMENT

There are three goals of therapy used to determine treatment options: improvement of symptoms, reduction in morbidity, and reduction in mortality. Specific drug therapies are supported by research documenting their efficacy in attaining one or more of these goals. Physiological goals are to decrease overload (preload and/or afterload), improve contractility, and decrease heart rate. Rational drug selection can be based on these goals, on the mechanism behind the dysfunction, and on the symptom severity of the disease process.

RATIONAL DRUG SELECTION

Guidelines

Although the ACCF/AHA classification system is intended to complement, not replace, the NYHA classification, the ACCF/AHA guidelines will be the main source of recommendations throughout this chapter. It should be noted that these guidelines are not inconsistent with those produced by the National Institute for Health and Clinical Excellence (NICE, 2010), the Veterans Health Administration, Department of Veterans Affairs (2007), the European Society of Cardiology (McMurray et al, 2012), or the Institute for Clinical Systems Improvement (ICSI, 2013). These latter guidelines are used where noted. These clinical practice guidelines describe the management of patients with both left-ventricular (systolic) dysfunction and diastolic dysfunction and include steps in accurate diagnosis, pharmacological and nonpharmacological therapies, counseling, and patient education. Figure 36-2 depicts the stages in the evolution of HF and the recommended therapy at each stage. All recommendations also follow the same evidence-based format of the previous ACCF/AHA guidelines (Yancy et al, 2013), which are:

- Class I. Conditions for which there is evidence for and/or general agreement that the procedure or treatment is useful and effective.
- Class II. Conditions for which there is conflicting evidence and/or a divergence of opinion about the usefulness/efficacy of a procedure or treatment.
- Class IIa. The weight of evidence or opinion is in favor of the procedure or treatment.
- Class IIb. Usefulness/efficacy is less well established by evidence or opinion.

- Class III. Conditions for which there is evidence and/or general agreement that the procedure or treatment is not useful/effective and in some cases can be harmful. Class III interventions will be mentioned in this chapter only when they may be harmful and are to be avoided.

Diagnosis of Heart Failure

A complete history and physical examination are always important in the diagnosis of any disorder. This includes history of current or past alcohol use, chemotherapy exposure, illicit drug use, or use of alternative medical therapies. Specific diagnostic tests useful in evaluation of HF include the following:

1. Two-dimensional echocardiograms coupled with Doppler flow studies. This is probably the single most useful diagnostic tool because it facilitates identification of any structural abnormalities. Confirmation by echocardiography of HF diagnosis and/or cardiac dysfunction is mandatory and should be performed shortly after the diagnostic suspicion of HF. Echocardiography is the most practical measurement of ventricular dysfunction and can be used to distinguish between systolic dysfunction and preserved systolic function where the ejection fraction is normal (left-ventricular ejection fraction [LVEF] greater than 45% to 50%) (Heart Failure Society of America [HFSA], 2010; Yancy et al, 2013; Krum, Jelinek, Stewart, Sindone, & Atherton, 2011; McMurray et al, 2012; Scottish Intercollegiate Guidelines Network [SIGN], 2007). These patients generally have HF related to diastolic dysfunction.

2. Chest x-rays may show cephalization of the vascular supply and 12-lead ECGs may show left-ventricular hypertrophy and axis deviation (HFSA, 2010; Krum et al, 2011; SIGN, 2007). Although both provide baseline information, neither alone should form the primary basis for determining the specific cause of HF because they are insensitive and nonspecific.

3. Complete blood count, urinalysis, serum electrolytes (including calcium and magnesium), blood urea nitrogen (BUN), serum creatinine, Hb A1c, liver function studies, fasting lipid profiles, and thyroid-stimulating hormone are useful in determining possible treatable underlying causes of HF and in determining end-organ damage (HFSA, 2010; Krum et al, 2011; SIGN, 2007).

4. The measurement of circulating levels of brain natriuretic peptide (BNP) has been used to identify patients with elevated left-ventricular filling pressures who are likely to exhibit signs and symptoms of HF. The peptide measurement has also been used as an aid in differentiating dyspnea due to HF from dyspnea due to other causes in the emergency setting. Although the assessment of this peptide cannot reliably distinguish patients with systolic from those with diastolic dysfunction, evidence exists supporting its use in both diagnosis and management.

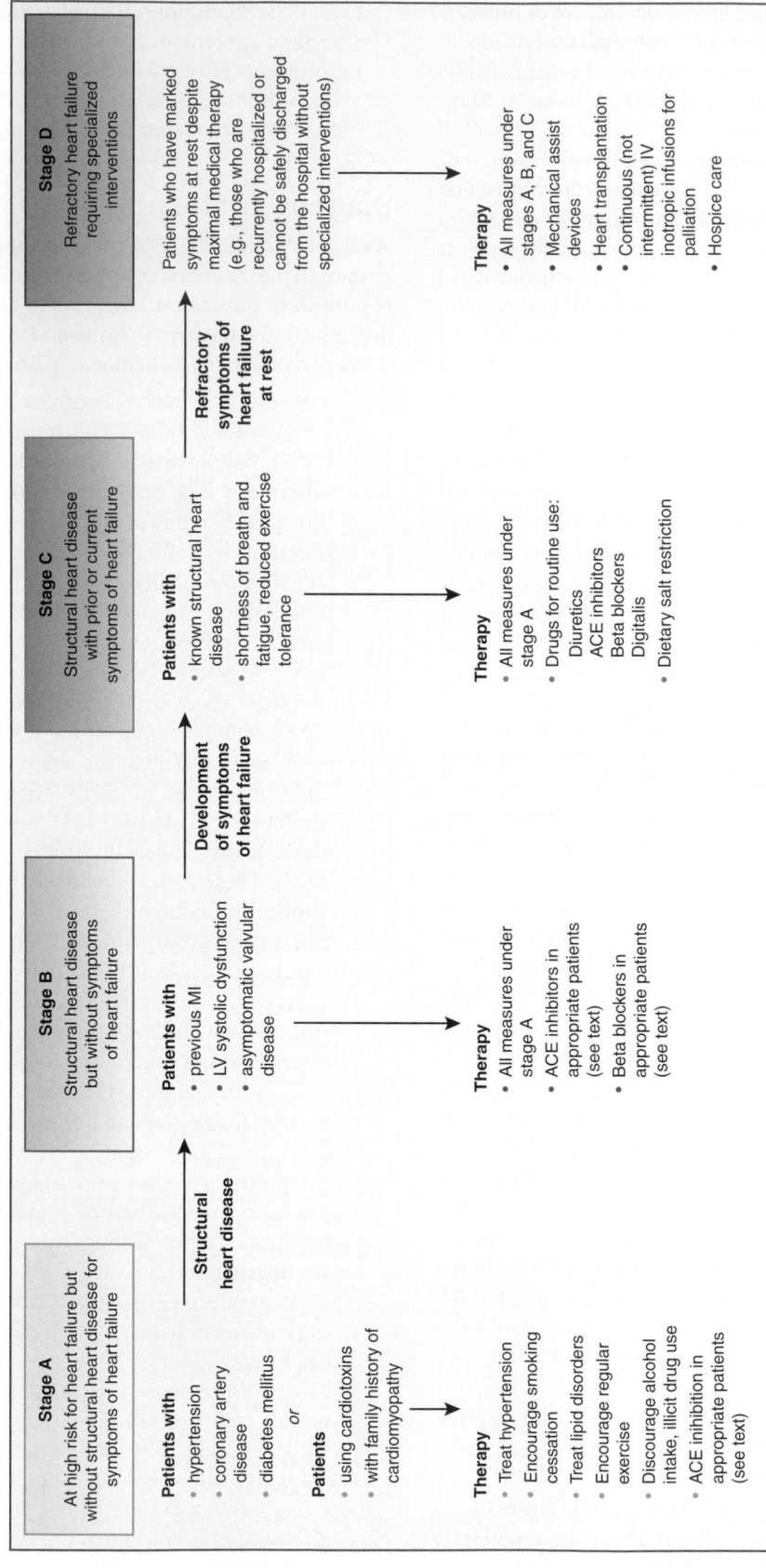

Figure 36–2. Stages in the evolution of HF and recommended therapy by stage.

Levels of the peptide have been shown to identify patients at risk for clinical events; therefore NICE (2010) recommends urgent referral to a specialist in all patients with a BNP level above 400 pg/mL. Although recent studies reveal that serum BNP levels have been shown to parallel the clinical severity of HF as assessed by NYHA functional class, their role in monitoring and adjusting drug therapy is less clearly established (Yancy et al, 2013). HFSA (2010) and Krum and colleagues (2011) do not recommend BNP determination for screening in patients without symptoms. They do recommend determination in all symptomatic patients suspected of having HF when the diagnosis is not certain. SIGN (2007) suggests BNP evaluation for widespread use as a screening tool in patients with suspected HF. Because BNP levels tend to fall after commencing therapy for HF, the sensitivity is lower in patients already on treatment, and SIGN does not recommend it for management.

5. Troponin I or T may be tested when the clinical picture suggests an acute coronary syndrome. Elevated troponin levels can also identify a cohort of patients with heart failure who are at higher risk. An initial determination of troponin is suggested by ICSI (2013) for patients presenting to the hospital with acute heart failure to assess for ACS as well as provide guidance regarding risk stratification. An increase in cardiac troponins indicates myocyte necrosis and may identify the patient for whom revascularization should be considered (McMurray et al, 2012).

The ACCF/AHA guidelines list specific recommendations for the evaluation of patients with HF using the class system discussed above. For class I, in addition to the history and physical examination, they recommend assessment of the patient's ability to perform activities of daily living (ADLs), assessment of volume status, and the tests mentioned in the first three sections above. Referral for cardiac catheterization with coronary angiography is recommended for patients with angina who may be candidates for revascularization.

For class IIa, noninvasive imaging, exercise testing, and measurement of ejection fraction are included. Screening for hemochromatosis is also listed, as is measurement of antinuclear antibody, rheumatoid factor, HIV antibodies, urinary vanillylmandelic acid (VMA), and evaluation for obstructive sleep apnea in selected patients.

Treatment Recommendations Based on Stage of Heart Failure

Stage A

Patients with stage A HF are at high risk for developing HF but do not have structural heart disease or symptoms of HF. Initial treatment for HF is focused on reversing underlying pathologies if possible and treating precipitating factors. Lifestyle modification is the first step and includes avoidance of behaviors that may increase the risk for HF, such as smoking, poor diet choices, obesity, sedentary lifestyle, and consuming alcohol or illicit drugs.

Equally important at this stage is control of systolic and diastolic HTN and treatment of lipid disorders in accordance with recommended guidelines found in Chapters 39 and 40. Controlling blood pressure and lipids can reduce the demands on the heart, decrease the risk for or facilitate the treatment of hypertension and CAD, and remove a drug that directly depresses the myocardium. Large, controlled studies have demonstrated that optimal blood pressure control decreases the risk of new HF by approximately 50% (Yancy et al, 2013). For patients with diabetes mellitus, blood glucose levels should be controlled in accordance with current guidelines. Chapter 33 discusses the guidelines for this disorder.

Lifestyle modification (e.g., stopping smoking, not consuming excessive alcohol, cessation of illicit drug use) is appropriate in all stages of HF and is an adjunct to successful drug therapy. The Web site http://www.heartfailurematters.org is an Internet tool provided by the Heart Failure Association of the European Society of Cardiology (ESC) that permits patients, their relatives, and caregivers to obtain useful, practical information in a user-friendly format.

Drug therapy is also instituted in stage A. ACE inhibitors, the cornerstone of therapy for HF in all the guidelines, are recommended for patients with a history of atherosclerotic vascular disease, diabetes mellitus, or HTN and associated cardiovascular risk factors to prevent HF in these high-risk patients. Beta blockers are also recommended for stage A in the ACC/AHA guidelines to control HTN and prevent HF (Yancy et al, 2013).

Angiotensin-Converting Enzyme Inhibitors

ACE inhibitors have been shown to improve symptoms, decrease morbidity, and increase life expectancy in all populations (Flather et al, 2000; Garg & Yusef, 1995; Jong, Yusef, Rousseau, & Bangdiwala, 2003; Keyhan, Chen, & Pilote, 2007; Neal, MacMahon, Chapman, & Blood, 2000; Rochon et al, 2004). They affect both preload and afterload through their vasodilating effects, decrease the incidence of remodeling by reducing the local generation and action of angiotensin II in heart muscle (Mancini, 2000), and prevent neurohormonal counterregulatory mechanisms that worsen HF through their action on the R-A-A system.

Patients taking ACE inhibitors show moderate increases in ejection fraction, decreased left-ventricular end-diastolic filling pressures, and improved myocardial energy metabolism. Because they are the only drugs that address all of the pathological mechanisms that produce HF, the ACE inhibitors are appropriate for all subsets of patients unless these patients are pregnant, have bilateral renal artery stenosis, serum potassium levels above 5.5 mEq, or a history of angioedema. They are also useful for preventing the development of HF in patients with ventricular dysfunction but no overt symptoms (stage B). A significant reduction in the development of symptomatic HF and death from any cause has been demonstrated in these patients.

As monotherapy or in combination with beta blockers, ACE inhibitors are superior to all other drugs and drug combinations used to treat heart failure. The NICE (2010) recommends that "all patients with HF due to left ventricular systolic dysfunction should be considered for treatment with an ACE inhibitor" (p. 15) and that such therapy should be started in addition to a beta blocker as first line treatment.

Although ACE inhibitors are most effective with systolic dysfunction, it is often difficult to ascertain if the patient has systolic or diastolic dysfunction at the time of the initial examination. However, 90% of patients with HF have some left-ventricular dysfunction (LVD). ACE inhibitors are the drugs of choice for LVD and create few adverse effects for patients with diastolic dysfunction, even though they are less efficacious with diastolic dysfunction. These drugs are safe to start before it is clear which of the two types of dysfunction exists.

Therapy should be started immediately. There is no need to wait until the disease has progressed. ACE inhibitors are commonly used as primary therapy, with other drugs added if symptoms persist or if volume overload develops at a later time. This is consistent with all of the above guidelines. Start with a low dose to prevent risks of hypotension and hypoperfusion, especially of the kidneys. Beginning with 6.25 mg captopril (Capoten), the only short-acting ACE inhibitor, permits discontinuance with rapid clearance of the drug should a renal problem occur. Gradually increase ACE inhibitor therapy to improve exercise tolerance and relieve symptoms, while monitoring BP and renal function. BP monitoring is critical not only to assure renal perfusion but also to prevent dizziness and falls. Many patients with heart failure are older adults at high risk for falls with even a limited decrease in cerebral perfusion. Renal function must also be closely watched with BUN, creatinine, and urinalysis. Any deterioration in renal function may require dosage reductions. Because ACE inhibitors alter aldosterone function, potassium levels may rise. Regular monitoring of serum electrolytes is important. Use of potassium-wasting diuretics as concurrent therapy may be helpful. Potassium-sparing diuretics are not used with ACE inhibitors.

Debate continues on the choice of the best ACE inhibitor for long-term therapy, although enalapril is the most studied drug in this class. In randomized, controlled studies, both short-acting and long-acting formulations were equally effective. The long-acting formulations demonstrate some greater risk of prolonged hypotension and impairment of renal function, but only at high doses. However, long-acting forms provide a higher affinity for the ACE receptors and more stable drug levels. They also provide a less complex treatment regimen that is more likely to result in adherence because all ACE inhibitors except captopril have once-daily dosing. The dosing schedule for different ACE inhibitors and the process for changing to a long-acting form is discussed in Chapter 16.

A dry, "tickle" cough occurs in up to 15% of patients and is the leading reason patients give for choosing to discontinue therapy. This adverse effect appears to be related to the action of ACE inhibitors on the bradykinin system. Because they do not affect this system, angiotensin II receptor blockers (ARBs) have actions similar to ACE inhibitors but do not produce the cough. ARBs can be considered an effective substitute for patients who are intolerant of an ACE inhibitor. Valsartan (Diovan) and candesartan (Atacand) are the two ARBs approved for treatment of HF. Although losartan (Cozaar) is not FDA approved for treatment of HF, there seems to be a beneficial class effect (ICSI, 2013). ARBs at higher doses have been shown to reduce mortality risk in HF, and in patients with acute myocardial infarction, valsartan was found to be equally as effective as captopril (Dickstein & Kjekshus, 2002; Konstam et al, 2009; Packer et al, 2001; Pfeffer et al, 2003). Although these are promising findings, current recommendations state that ARBs should be reserved for patients for whom ACE inhibitors are indicated but who are unable to tolerate them; this approach is supported by NICE (2010), as well as the ACCF/AHA (Yancy et al, 2013) and the ESC (McMurray et al, 2012).

Beta Blockers

Unless contraindicated or not tolerated, a beta blocker should be given to all patients with a recent or remote history of MI regardless of ejection fraction or presence of HF (Yancy et al, 2013). These drugs improve ventricular function through their action on the HF counterregulatory mechanisms and have cardioprotective properties.

Other class I recommendations for stage A patients include control of ventricular rate in patients with supraventricular tachyarrhythmias, restoration of normal sinus rhythm, treatment of thyroid disorders, and periodic evaluation for signs and symptoms of HF. Two interesting class III statements are made. Exercise to prevent the development of HF is thought to be ineffective, as is reduction in dietary salt beyond that which is prudent (generally considered to be 2,500 mg/d) for healthy individuals without HTN or fluid retention.

Stage B

Patients with structural heart disease who have not developed symptoms, also known as patients with asymptomatic LV dysfunction (ALVD), are classified as stage B. They include patients without symptoms who have had an MI and those with evidence of left-ventricular dysfunction. These individuals are at high risk for developing HF, but the likelihood of developing it can be diminished by the use of therapies that reduce the risk of additional injury, the process of remodeling, and the progression of left-ventricular dysfunction.

As with stage A, the first drugs of choice are ACE inhibitors for these patients as well. ACE inhibitors are recommended for all patients with cardiac structural abnormalities and low LVEF who have not yet developed HF (Yancy et al, 2013). If the patient has entered the algorithm at stage A, ACE inhibitors should be continued. If they enter the algorithm at stage B, ACE inhibitors should be started. This is the stage, however, where beta blockade is added regardless of the previous HTN medication regimen. Beta blockers are recommended for all patients without a history of MI who have a reduced ejection fraction (less than or equal to 40%) with no HF symptoms (Yancy et al, 2013; McMurray et al, 2012) and for patients with recent or remote MI regardless of ejection fraction. Beta blockers should be started in conjunction with an ACE inhibitor as soon as possible after diagnosis (McMurray et al, 2012).

Beta blockers are also important for MI prophylaxis for patients who develop HF secondary to an acute MI. Care must be taken in prescribing these drugs because they may precipitate acute decompensation. Patients should be clinically stable (e.g., optimal volume status achieved, lack of dependence on intravenous ionotropic support, no symptomatic bradycardia) prior to starting a beta blocker. Initially, low doses are used, and several months are required to show improvement.

Many large clinical trials (Bonet et al, 2000; Bouzamondo, Hulot, Sanchez, Cucherat, & Lechat, 2001; Brophy, Joseph, & Rouleau, 2001; Hernandez et al, 2009; McMurray et al, 2012; Ong, Ong, & Kow, 2012; Packer et al, 2001; Shibata, Flather, & Wang, 2001; Whorlow & Krum, 2000) have shown that some beta blockers increase life expectancy in patients with HF due to left-ventricular systolic dysfunction compared with placebo. This effect has been seen in patients in all NYHA functional classes of HF (NICE, 2010). The three beta blockers that have the strongest evidence to reduce mortality are bisoprolol, carvedilol, and metoprolol succinate (sustained release formulation) (Yancy et al, 2013). The evidence is strongest for carvedilol (which is actually an alpha$_1$ beta blocker) and modified-release metoprolol. There is little evidence of benefits from other beta blockers.

There is also little evidence to show a clinically significant difference based on selectivity of the beta blocker or on those with or without vasodilating properties. There are no randomized clinical trials of atenolol in patients with HF. The suggestion by the NICE (2010) is that patients who have systolic HF who are not already on a beta blocker should be started on one as first-line treatment along with an ACE inhibitor. Although not specifically mentioned in the guidelines, labetalol (Normodyne) has the same action as carvedilol. Labetalol is not recommended, however, for patients with LVEF less than 45%. Both can also be used safely with digoxin because they do not abolish this drug's inotropic action and in combination with ACE inhibitors to improve left-ventricular function. If patients developed HF while already on a different beta blocker for a concomitant condition such as angina or HTN, the health-care provider has the option to leave them on that drug or change to one of the drugs above. In any case, the "start low and go slow" paradigm should be used with these drugs.

The guidelines also recommend beta blockers for all NYHA classes of HF and mention the same ones named above. The guideline recommends that carvedilol be started at 3.125 mg twice daily and titrated as tolerated up to 25 mg twice daily maximum with 50 mg twice daily maximum for patients weighing more than 85 kg. Metoprolol succinate can be started at 12.5 mg once daily for 2 weeks and doubled upward every 2 weeks as tolerated to a target dose of 200 mg/d. The Veterans Affairs guideline (Veterans Health Administration, Department of Veterans Affairs, 2007) specifies the use of beta blockers related to recent MI and also specifically mentions the drugs above. Beta blockers are also used for a subset of patients with diastolic dysfunction or cardiomyopathies for whom decreased heart rate could improve cardiac output.

All guidelines suggest that treatment with digoxin is not effective in stage B patients who are in sinus rhythm. In addition, the risk for harm is not balanced with any known benefit (Yancy et al, 2013). In the Veterans Affairs guideline (2007), digoxin may be used in stage B when the patient has a rapid ventricular response to atrial fibrillation and there is a need to control the rate. The other guidelines would also support its use under these circumstances. Calcium channel blockers with negative inotropic effects may be harmful in asymptomatic patients with low LVEF. Other interventions that are useful in selected patients are discussed below.

Stage C

Patients with left-ventricular dysfunction with current or prior symptoms of HF are classified as stage C. They are the first stage to have active HF symptoms. The bulk of patients with HF are at this stage. All the class I recommendations for stages A and B are also appropriate here. In addition, moderate sodium restriction (1,500 mg/day) along with daily weight monitoring are indicated to facilitate the most effective use of drugs. Physical activity at this stage should be encouraged, except during periods of acute exacerbations, because restriction of activity promotes physical deconditioning and may contribute to the exercise intolerance common with this stage.

Most patients in this stage will require a combination of three to four types of drugs: ACE inhibitors, beta blockers, cardiac glycosides (digoxin), and a diuretic. The value of these drugs has been established in numerous large-scale clinical trials and the evidence supporting their use is strong. ACE inhibitors and beta blockers have already been discussed. Diuretics and digoxin will be discussed here.

Diuretics

Diuretics are the key of any successful approach to the treatment of heart failure with volume excess (McMurray et al, 2012; Yancy et al, 2013). They should be given until a euvolemic state is achieved and continued to prevent the recurrence of fluid retention. Because of their central role in control of HTN, diuretics may be drugs of choice for earlier stages of HF where the goal is control of HTN. This will be discussed later in the section "Concomitant Diseases." Even if the patient responds favorably to the diuretic, ACE inhibitors and beta blockers should be initiated or continued after euvolemia has been achieved because diuretics cause activation of the R-A-A system and ACE inhibitors and beta blockers have been shown to improve the long-term prognosis of HF.

Diuretics improve symptoms of dyspnea. There is no evidence that they affect morbidity or mortality. Their main function is to reduce preload associated with volume overload. Thiazide diuretics have long been and remain the drugs of choice for patients with HTN. However, for patients with heart failure, loop diuretics are more effective and have become the preferred diuretic agents for use in most patients with HF. Potassium-sparing diuretics (aldosterone antagonists) are too weak to be of benefit as monotherapy. They can be useful as concurrent therapy with thiazide or loop diuretics to counterbalance the potassium loss common to these latter two groups of drugs.

Two drugs in the aldosterone antagonist class (spironalactone and eplerenone) have shown increased life expectancy and reduced hospitalizations when added to a treatment regimen that included a loop diuretic and an ACE inhibitor (Pitt et al, 2003; Zannad et al, 2011). The ACCF/AHA guideline recommends spironalactone for patients with recurrent class IV symptoms, preserved renal function, and a normal potassium level. The NICE guideline (2010) and Krum and colleagues (2011) also recommend aldosterone antagonists for patients who remain symptomatic despite optimal therapy with beta blockers and ACE inhibitors. The guideline suggests a starting dose of 12.5 mg once daily and seeking advice from a specialist. For eplerenone, the recommended starting dose is 25 mg once daily (Jessup et al, 2009). The doses then may be increased to 50 mg for each of these drugs if needed.

For diastolic HF, spironalactone has a questionable role. The hormone aldosterone contributes to diastolic stiffness by promoting fibrosis. Preliminary studies have shown aldosterone antagonists such as spironalactone reduce systolic and diastolic blood pressures, as well as decrease ventricular remodeling (Pieske, 2012), but there remains conflicting data on whether these agents can improve quality of life and median NYHA class in diastolic HF (Daniel, Wells, Stewart, Moore, & Kitzman, 2009; Pieske, 2012). Two trials are currently underway that further examine the role of the aldosterone antagonist in diastolic heart failure.

For mild to moderate disease, start therapy with furosemide 40 mg twice daily. Loop diuretics can cause marked diuresis. Before starting them, discontinue any thiazide diuretic currently being used. For loop diuretics, divide the daily dose to prevent great diuresis at one time. If the patient does not respond adequately to the divided dose, try giving the entire daily dose in the morning before increasing the dose. The goal with diuretics is to give the lowest possible dose that achieves the desired effect. Doses should be titrated to increased urine output and promote weight loss of 0.5 to 1 kg daily. Single daily doses are effective, but during times of increased pathology, oral absorption may be compromised, and the IV route or high doses of oral formulations may be needed. Dosing schedules are given in Chapter 16. Monitor weight gain, changes in exercise tolerance, and electrolytes. Diuretic resistance may occur in the presence of decreased renal perfusion or renal stenotic or obstructive pathologies, or with the concurrent administration of NSAIDs. If symptoms seem resistant to the standard doses of the diuretic, check creatinine clearance. Thiazide diuretics cannot be used with creatinine clearances that are lower than 25 mL/min. Loop diuretics can be used with these low creatinine clearances. Patients may also benefit from the addition of metolazone (Zaroxolyn) for its synergistic action on diuresis, but

it is not recommended for chronic daily use because of potential for severe electrolyte shifts.

Although initiation of diuretic therapy is important for patients who have HF with volume overload, it is also important to avoid excessive diuresis, especially for patients who are also on sodium restrictions. Volume depletion can lead to hypotension and prerenal azotemia. For patients concurrently taking ACE inhibitors, renal insufficiency can be induced. Diuretics may be stopped, if necessary, to allow rehydration before restarting an ACE inhibitor. They can be reintroduced after the dose of the ACE inhibitor has been stabilized. ACE inhibitors augment the effectiveness of thiazide and loop diuretics because they decrease glomerular filtration fractions and increase the delivery of solute and water to the distal nephron segments that are responsive to the action of these diuretics.

Long-term use of diuretics can stimulate increased R-A-A activity and sodium retention, which are both counterproductive in treating heart failure. This result is less likely with low doses. In addition to the potential for fluid volume changes, thiazide and loop diuretics present risks for acid–base and electrolyte disturbances that can be proarrhythmic. Monitoring for these problems is discussed in Chapter 16.

The most common electrolyte problem is hypokalemia. Any potassium supplementation must be based on serum levels because not all patients become hypokalemic or require supplementation beyond dietary changes. Potassium supplements must be used cautiously, if at all, for patients concurrently taking ACE inhibitors, which cause elevated potassium. Oral potassium supplements should provide chloride as well to prevent diuretic-induced hypokalemic alkalosis. Hypomagnesemia is also common and may impair potassium repletion. Diuretics also contribute to abnormal glucose and lipid metabolism. Care must be taken and diagnostic tests frequently monitored when diuretics must be used for patients with diabetes or lipid abnormalities.

Cardiac Glycosides

Digitalis was once the only effective drug to treat HF. Its ability to increase contractility by increasing intracellular calcium and inhibiting the sodium-potassium-ATPase pump deals directly with one primary deficit in HF. In addition to its ionotropic effects, digitalis may act as a neurohormonal attenuator. Recent evidence suggests that by inhibiting the sodium-potassium-ATPase in the kidney, digitalis reduces the renal tubular reabsorption of sodium, leading to the suppression of renin secretion from the kidneys. Although digoxin increases the force of contraction and modulates the RAAS, thereby improving functioning and symptoms and reducing hospitalizations, it has little if any effect on mortality. Published data suggest that digoxin does not improve quality of life, symptoms, or mortality rates (Amhed, 2006; Digitalis Investigation Group, 1997; Lader et al, 2003).

The development of ACE inhibitors, combined with the risks of toxicity and multiple drug interactions associated with the cardiac glycosides (CGs), has moved digoxin to a third-line drug except for selected cases. It is recommended for worsening HF due to left-ventricular dysfunction despite ACE inhibitor, beta blocker, and diuretic therapy. Although beta blockers are first-line therapy for heart failure because they also control HTN and have a role in tachycardia-medicated cardiomyopathy associated with atrial fibrillation, digoxin remains a useful adjunctive drug for HF secondary to atrial fibrillation with a rapid ventricular response because it slows heart rate (McMurray et al, 2012).

Digoxin also remains a consideration for treatment for HF in patients with reduced systolic dysfunction (ejection fraction <40%) while receiving standard therapy with a beta blocker and ACE inhibitor. Digoxin is less beneficial with ejection fractions of more than 40% or in HF secondary to hypertrophic cardiomyopathies. Digoxin is also not useful in HF associated with idiopathic hypertrophic subaortic stenosis, also known as hypertrophic obstructive cardiomyopathy (which it actually worsens), recurrent transient ischemia, or mitral stenosis (unless the patient also has atrial fibrillation). Digoxin can also be problematic when treating older adults and patients with renal insufficiency. Renal function may decrease during heart failure treatment and the drug may not be adequately excreted, allowing it to increase to toxic levels. Digoxin levels should be closely monitored in these patients.

For stable patients, therapy can be started with an oral maintenance dose without resorting to a loading dose. Using a daily dose of 0.25 mg, a therapeutic blood level can be achieved in 5 to 7 days. Check the serum level in 1 week and make any needed adjustments on the basis of clinical response and serum level. Less stable patients require hospitalization for loading doses. Monitor patients on digoxin by following heart rate and rhythm, potassium levels, and renal function. Routine monitoring of serum digoxin levels is generally overdone. Monitoring should occur in addition to clinical judgment rather than as a substitute for it. Chapter 16 has detailed discussion of the reasons for and the process of monitoring associated with the use of digoxin, as well as the process of initiating and maintaining digoxin therapy.

The decision to begin digoxin therapy should not be made lightly. It should be used only when there is clear evidence of chronic systolic dysfunction or one of the disease processes just mentioned. Digitalis toxicity occurs in as many as 25% of patients but is declining in recent years secondary to reduction in overall use as well as dose reductions (Haynes, Heitjan, Kanetsky, & Hennessy, 2008). The mortality rate from this toxicity is usually 4% to 10%, rising as high as 50% with digitalis levels greater than 6 ng/mL.

Patients with mild to moderate heart failure often become asymptomatic on optimal doses of ACE inhibitors and diuretics and do not require digoxin. Digoxin should be added for those patients whose symptoms persist despite optimal doses of these two drugs. For patients already on digoxin, research evidence supports symptom deterioration when it is suddenly withdrawn. For these patients, digoxin should not be withdrawn unless a reversible cause of heart failure has been fully corrected or there is no basis for using the drug in the first place.

Angiotensin II Receptor Blockers

Angiotensin II receptor blockers (ARBs) are recommended as substitutes for ACE inhibitors in patients who are being treated with diuretics, beta blockers, and digoxin and who cannot be given an ACE inhibitor (Jessup et al, 2009; McMurray et al, 2012). The use of these drugs was discussed in earlier guidelines. It should be noted that using an ARB before a beta blocker in patients who are taking an ACE inhibitor is a class III recommendation, meaning it is not effective, and a triple combination of ACE inhibitor, ARB, and beta blocker should be avoided because it may lead to additional undesired side effects.

Calcium Channel Blockers

While the pathology of HF is associated with altered contractility in part associated with calcium movement within the cell, calcium channel blockers (CCBs) are used with considerable caution (Yancy et al, 2013). The NICE (2010) guidelines state that patients should not be routinely treated with calcium channel blockers for HF. These same guidelines do acknowledge that amlodipine, a long-acting dihydropyridine, is not harmful in terms of adverse events and may be considered for treatment of comorbid HTN and/or angina in patients with HF. All other CCBs should be avoided.

Nitrates

Nitrates are effective for a subset of patients whose primary pathology is increased preload. Their use is discussed related to concomitant conditions. They are also accepted therapy in combination with hydralazine when the patient has an intolerance to both an ACE inhibitor and an ARB. Its use in these patients may reduce the risk of death (McMurray et al, 2012). Randomized controlled trials show that isosorbide dinitrate in combination with hydralazine is of significant benefit, reducing both morbidity and mortality, in treatment of heart failure in African American patients on standard therapy with an ACE inhibitor and beta blocker (ICSI, 2013; McMurray et al, 2012; Yancy et al, 2013).

Stage D

Stage D includes patients with refractory end-stage HF. These patients have marked symptoms at rest despite maximal medical therapy. ACE inhibitors and beta blockers are still suggested for treatment of HF in this population, but these patients may only tolerate small doses of medications. Initiation of a beta blocker or ACE inhibitor is contraindicated in patients with a systolic blood pressure less than 80 mm Hg, or who show signs of peripheral hypoperfusion (Yancy et al, 2013). Management of fluid status is also crucial in stage D heart failure. Addition of a second, complementary diuretic to a loop diuretic, as well as strict monitoring of fluid and sodium intake, can assist in the control of fluid retention.

Patients with stage D heart failure may be referred for cardiac transplantation and should be referred to a heart failure program with expertise in the management of refractory HF (Yancy et al, 2013). Routine intermittent infusions of vasoactive and positive inotropic agents are not recommended for patients with stage D heart failure, although they may be used in the inpatient setting during acute decompensation (Yancy et al, 2013).

Patients With Heart Failure With Preserved Ejection Fraction (HF-pEF)

As many as half of the patient population have heart failure with preserved left ventricular ejection fraction. Unfortunately, there is limited evidence to show the benefit of ACE inhibitors and beta blockers in this population. Three trials using ACE inhibitors and ARBs showed no reduction in morbidity and mortality in patients with HF-pEF. The main underlying causes of HF-pEF include hypertension and CAD. Therefore, treatment in HF-pEF should target these causes. As with all heart failure patients, diuretics should be used in the presence of volume overload to improve symptoms. ACE inhibitors should be considered in patients with diabetes and one additional risk factor or those with symptomatic atherosclerotic cardiovascular disease. Beta blockers should be used in all patients with prior myocardial infarction or atrial fibrillation requiring control of ventricular rate (Yancy et al, 2013).

Cost

The drugs used to treat HF vary in cost from minimal to quite expensive. Diuretics are among the least expensive, but they vary from indapamide (Lozol) ($25 per month) to generic HCTZ ($1.04 per month). HCTZ is the drug of choice for a variety of reasons, and cost certainly also makes it desirable. The ACE inhibitors have become less expensive because several of them are now available as a generic formulation. Because digitalis has been used for so long, it is among the least expensive.

Additional Patient Variables

Concomitant Diseases

Coronary Artery Disease and the Use of Nitrates

The underlying pathology of HF in the presence of CAD relates to poor oxygenation of the myocardium, which results in angina pectoris. Chapter 28 discusses angina and ischemic heart disease. When these disorders occur with or result in HF, nitrates are often added to the treatment regimen for relief of angina symptoms. Nitrates are relatively selective to epicardial vasculature and improve systolic and diastolic ventricular function by increasing coronary blood flow. The mechanism includes both coronary artery vasodilation and improvement of the uptake of oxygen by the myocardial muscle itself. This mechanism is discussed in Chapter 16.

Nitrates are also effective after MI and for those with CAD as the primary cause of their HF. They reduce symptoms and have some effect on mortality when used in the acute setting. Improvement in mortality in primary care has been demonstrated only when isosorbide dinitrate is combined with hydralazine, a peripheral vasodilator. This combination is usually reserved for patients who are intolerant of ACE inhibitors or for African Americans who remain symptomatic on standard treatment with a beta blocker, ACE inhibitor, and diuretic. Problems with nitrate tolerance require special timing of doses, with nitrate-free intervals daily. Chapter 16 includes discussion of this problem. The dosage of isosorbide dinitrate that produces the most sustained hemodynamic effects and minimizes the development of tolerance appears to be 40 mg every 8 hours. The dosage of hydralazine is up to 800 mg every 8 hours to reduce afterload. NICE (2010) guidelines suggest consultation with a specialist prior to initiation.

Antiplatelet drugs such as aspirin have evidence to support their use in patients with atherosclerotic arterial disease, including CAD. Evidence (Eikelboom, Hirsh, Spencer, Baglin, & Weitz, 2012) supports aspirin's role in reducing the risk of vascular events in these patients. It is recommended by the ACCF/AHA for patients with CAD, although specific evidence for its benefits in patients with HF is lacking (Yancy et al, 2013). The NICE (2010) recommends aspirin 75 to 150 mg once daily for patients with a combination of HF and CAD. Some questions have been raised about the possibility that aspirin may reduce some of the benefits of ACE inhibitors when taken together (Kindsvater, Leclerc, & Ward, 2003; Takkouche, Etminan, Caamano, & Rochon, 2002), but the evidence is not robust. It is worth considering this possibility when prescribing both. If there is true concern for lack of efficacy, alternative antiplatelet drugs, such as clopidogrel (Plavix), may not be affected by concomitant administration of aspirin (CAPRIE, 1996).

Chronic Atrial Fibrillation and the Use of Anticoagulants

Beta blockers have already been discussed as the drug of choice for HF patients who have concomitant atrial fibrillation. Anticoagulants are also helpful in this situation. Randomized control trials have demonstrated that warfarin reduces the risk of stroke in patients with HF and atrial fibrillation (Yancy et al, 2013; McMurray et al, 2012). No such benefit is shown for patients with HF who are in sinus rhythm (Lip & Chung, 2010). It should be noted that in patients with atrial fibrillation, aspirin reduced mortality when compared to lack of treatment. The addition of clopidogrel to aspirin further decreased mortality. Yet, when this combination was compared to warfarin, results showed that clopidogrel used in conjunction with aspirin carried an increased risk of bleeding and there was no evidence of decreased mortality from thrombosis (Hansen et al, 2010).

Diabetes and the Use of ACE Inhibitors

Based on data from the Diabetes Complications Control Trial and more recent trials, the American Diabetes Association recommends the use of ACE inhibitors as the drugs of choice for the treatment of HTN for persons with diabetes, because of their demonstrated effect in reducing diabetic nephropathy. The role of ACE inhibitors in diabetes is discussed in Chapter 33. The same rationale for their use in diabetic patients with HTN holds for patients with HF. The ACCF/AHA guidelines (Yancy et al, 2013) mention this preference. ARBs may also reduce diabetic nephropathy, but this effect has yet to be demonstrated by longitudinal studies.

Patients with diabetes may experience increased glucose levels with diuretics. Recent evidence shows there may be a relationship between glucose metabolism and hypokalemia caused by thiazide diuretics (Elliott, 2012; Stears et al, 2012). Elevated serum glucose may be prevented with the initiation of potassium supplementation, combination treatment with an ACE inhibitor, or use of potassium-sparing agents (Grossman, Vedecchia, Shamiss, Angeli, & Reboldi, 2011). Thiazide diuretics in low doses are the least likely to cause this adverse response, followed by loop diuretics. ARBs are also acceptable drugs for patients with diabetes because of their limited effects on glucose metabolism, lipid profiles, and renal function.

Providers sometimes avoid the use of beta-adrenergic blockers in patients with diabetes because they have an adverse effect on peripheral blood flow, prolong hypoglycemia, and mask most hypoglycemic symptoms. Recent evidence suggests that these effects may not be as problematic as once thought and therefore beta blockers should not be avoided (Erdmann, 2009). The majority of diabetic patients eventually develop coronary disease, with or without heart failure, and beta blockers are a first-line drug for cardioprotection. Patients with diabetes who need MI prophylaxis and have concurrent heart failure may be placed on low doses of beta blockers and taught to monitor their blood glucose more closely and to recognize diaphoresis as their main indicator of hypoglycemia.

Hypertension and the Early Use of Diuretics

HTN is a common concurrent disorder with heart failure and may contribute to its etiology. Initial therapy for HTN is with diuretics, especially for sodium-sensitive patients such as African Americans, older adults, those who are obese, and those with renal insufficiency. Target blood pressure levels should be <130/<80 if tolerated. The most effective diuretics for both HTN and HF are the thiazides. Loop diuretics are less effective for HTN but have some use, and they are helpful for subsets of patients with stage C HF. ACE inhibitors are drugs of choice for treating HTN in young and Caucasian patients. The dose for treating HTN, however, is double the dose used to treat HF; the lower dose is required for patients who have both disorders.

In patients with low ejection fractions (less than 40%), the vasodilating effects of ACE inhibitors provide adequate perfusion, even with systolic blood pressure (SBP) at or below 90 mm Hg. Because a primary goal for all HF patients, including those in stages A and B, is the control of HTN, drugs that assist with both disorders should have preference in rational drug selection. Chapter 40 discusses in more detail the drugs helpful in treating HTN.

Hyperlipidemia and the Use of Statins

Hyperlipidemia leading to atherosclerotic changes is also a common concurrent disorder that may contribute to the etiology of HF. Treatment of lipid disorders based on the most

current guidelines is a class I recommendation for all HF patients, starting with stage A (Yancy et al, 2013). The newest ACCF/AHA lipid guidelines (2013) recommend the use of HMG-Co-A reductase inhibitors (statins) as first-line therapy when LDL cholesterol-lowering drugs are indicated to achieve treatment goals (Stone et al, 2014). Statins reduce the frequency of ischemic events (Dickstein et al, 2002) and prolong life expectancy in patients with known CAD (Gutierrez, Ramirez, Rundek, & Sacco, 2012). The risk of developing HF is also reduced. The benefits of statins appear to be universal and not restricted by age, although the ESC guideline (McMurray et al, 2012) limits their recommendation to patients with CAD, as two trials revealed lack of evidence that adding a statin to the medication regimen of a patient with normal lipid levels improves HF itself (Kjekshus et al, 2007; Tavazzi et al, 2008). Chapter 39 discusses these recommendations in detail and Chapters 16 and 39 discuss the various statins and rational drug selection among them.

Thiazide diuretics have been associated with elevation in total cholesterol and LDL cholesterol by 5% to 7% (Grossman et al, 2011). This rise is dose-dependent and greater in African Americans. The majority of studies are limited to a span of 3 to 5 years, so long-term effects are unknown, but this problem does not rule them out. ACE inhibitors, ARBs, CCBs, and digoxin do not affect lipid levels and may be used for patients with hyperlipidemia. Beta-adrenergic blockers increase triglycerides transiently and reduce levels of high-density lipids (Bell, Bakris, & McGill, 2009).

Other Comorbidities

Hyperuricemia can be a problem for patients with gout. Diuretics can produce this adverse effect. The least likely to do so are the thiazides, followed by the loop diuretics. This effect may be dose-related. It is recommended that lower doses of thiazides be used if there is concern for hyperuricemia. ACE inhibitors do not affect uric acid levels directly but can influence renal function, which may indirectly affect uric acid metabolism. Digoxin does not affect uric acid metabolism.

Asthma or chronic airway disease may occur with heart failure, especially in older adults. Chronic airway obstruction is the underlying cause of cor pulmonale, right-sided heart failure. Bronchial activity is unchanged by ACE inhibitors. In the 10% to 15% of patients taking these drugs who experience a cough, angiotensin II receptor blockers are an alternative. Alpha-beta-adrenergic blockers and beta-adrenergic blockers should not be avoided in asthma unless the underlying disease is poorly controlled. The use of these drugs is not contraindicated in patients with COPD.

Impaired renal function and electrolyte disturbances also influence drug selection. Because digoxin is excreted essentially unchanged by the kidney, renal impairment suggests cautious use and close monitoring of serum drug levels. Renal impairment is also associated with increased potassium levels, and the administration of potassium-wasting diuretics often results in decreased potassium levels. Both of these situations increase the risk for digitalis toxicity. Patients with a glomerular filtration rate (GFR) of less than 60 have significantly higher digoxin levels at one month (Shlipak, Smith, Rathore, Massie, & Krumholz, 2004). Dosage adjustments of digoxin are required for patients with decreased renal function, especially older adults. Renal clearance is a factor in the choice of diuretic, as previously discussed. Thiazide and loop diuretics may cause hypokalemia. ACE inhibitors are contraindicated in bilateral renal artery stenosis and should be adjusted for patients with a creatinine clearance less than 30. Careful monitoring of renal function is required with their use.

Age and Gender

Digoxin has a long history of use in infants and children. Thiazides, loop diuretics, ACE inhibitors, and beta blockers are also approved for use with pediatric patients. These drug groups have specific pediatric formulations and dosing schedules.

An initial post hoc analysis of women taking digoxin revealed that digoxin use increased mortality, but a large study cohort of over 20,000 patients with heart failure on digoxin failed to show a gender difference in mortality (The Digitalis Investigation Group, 1997; Flory et al, 2012). Older adults have a higher risk for digitalis toxicity. The indications of toxicity are different in children and older adults than they are in most adults. Digitalis toxicity is discussed in Chapter 16.

HF is the leading cause of death and hospitalization for adults older than 65 years (Hall, Levant, & DeFrances, 2012; Kochanek, Xu, Murphy, Minini, & Kung, 2011) and remains one of the most common Medicare diagnoses-related groups. A large portion of HF risk in this population is attributable to modifiable risk factors. The Health, Aging and Body Composition study (Kalogeropoulos et al, 2009) researched these factors and suggests that racial differences in risk factors and in hospitalization rate need to be considered in prevention and treatment efforts. ACE inhibitors and beta blockers are still the drugs of choice for older adults.

Research that includes older adults often excludes patients with serum creatinine levels above 2.0 because older adults often have elevated serum creatinine levels related to the changes associated with aging, as well as polypharmacy and the presence of multiple comorbidities. Consideration of serum creatinine alone presents some problems. Creatinine clearance may be more accurate in assessing renal function than serum creatinine due to decreased muscle mass in the older adult. The primary reason given in the literature for not reaching goal doses of ACE inhibitors in older adults with HF is renal dysfunction, symptomatic hypotension, cough, and hyperkalemia. There are few clinical trials including older adults with HF on goal doses, but several studies indicate that ACE inhibitors at target doses would benefit the older adult (Chen, Wang, Radford, & Krumholz, 2001; Cleland et al, 2006; Levine, Levine, Bolenbaugh, & Green, 2002; McDonald, 2001).

Pregnancy

ACE inhibitors are contraindicated in pregnancy. Digoxin has been used, but blood levels must be monitored closely to avoid toxicity. Diuretics decrease plasma volume and may decrease plasma placental perfusion. They are used during pregnancy only when benefits clearly outweigh risks. Jaundice and thrombocytopenia have been seen in neonates after diuretic use in the mother. Beta blockers are considered safe in the latter part of pregnancy. A general rule of thumb sometimes proposed is that drugs safe to be used in infants are safe for use in pregnancy, but it is important to remember that consideration must be given to the maternal–fetal drug concentration ratio. Some drugs develop much higher levels of concentration in the fetus than they do in the maternal circulation, and the dose that is therapeutic for the mother may be too high for the neonate. It is best to avoid any drug during pregnancy unless the benefits clearly outweigh the risk to the fetus. Pregnant women with HF are best treated in consultation with a specialist (NICE, 2010).

Drug Combinations

Adherence to any treatment regimen is less likely as the regimen becomes more complex. Drug combinations can increase that complexity. In order to avoid confusion, prevent unintentional medication overdose, and improve adherence, attempts should be made to decrease the number of pills and medications that compose a patient's treatment regimen.

Common combinations include diuretics and ACE inhibitors. When using this combination, withholding or decreasing the dose of the diuretic to permit rehydration prior to initiating the ACE inhibitor reduces the chances of renal dysfunction and hypotension. The diuretic may be reintroduced later. With this combination, monitor BP, potassium, BUN, and creatinine levels, and decrease the diuretic dose if BP falls or prerenal azotemia develops.

Diuretics are also commonly used with digoxin for patients with systolic dysfunction. The diuretics reduce afterload, and digoxin improves contractility. Care must be taken with this combination concerning serum potassium levels, as was previously discussed.

For patients who remain symptomatic on a combination of an ACE inhibitor, beta blocker, and a diuretic, digoxin may be added. With this combination, fluid status and serum potassium levels must be carefully monitored. For patients with persistent dyspnea after optimal doses of diuretics, ACE inhibitors, beta blockers, and digoxin, referral to a specialist is appropriate. The addition of a vasodilator to an ACE inhibitor may relieve symptoms, particularly for patients with hypertension or evidence of severe mitral regurgitation.

For those who cannot tolerate or do not respond to beta blockers, have a heart rate above 70 and an EF below 35%, Ivabradine (Corlanor), a new antianginal medication, was approved to help stablize heart rates and reduce hospitalizations (FDA, 2015).

MONITORING

Monitoring to assess effectiveness in treating the pathology includes a variety of tools. NICE (2010) recommends the following assessments:

1. Functional capacity, chiefly using the NYHA class, specific quality-of-life questionnaires, or a maximal exercise test.

2. Assessment of fluid status, chiefly by physical assessment (e.g., daily weights, jugular venous distention, lung crackles, hepatomegaly, peripheral edema, and orthostatic BP).

3. Assessment of cardiac rhythm, chiefly by clinical examination, but a 12-lead ECG may be used if an arrhythmia is suspected. The ACCF/AHA guidelines specifically state that Holter monitoring is class IIb and could be considered in patients who have a history of MI and are being considered for electrophysiological study to document ventricular tachycardia inducibility (Yancy et al, 2013).

4. Laboratory assessment, including electrolytes and serum creatinine and urea, with special attention to potassium and sodium. Other tests such as thyroid function, hematology, liver function, and level of anticoagulation may be required depending on the medication prescribed and the comorbidity.

Monitoring specific to each drug class is presented in Chapter 16. Serum drug level monitoring is important for digoxin, although it is only recommended routinely in the settings of dose adjustment and suspicion of toxicity. Hypokalemia, which may result from diuretic therapy, enhances sensitivity to the toxic effects of digoxin and is proarrhythmic in all patients with HF. Hypomagnesemia may impair the effectiveness of potassium replacement therapy and should be assessed for patients with refractory hypokalemia. Repeated testing may be useful for patients with a new heart murmur or sudden deterioration even though they are adherent to the treatment regimen.

OUTCOME EVALUATION

A careful history and physical examination should be the mainstay in determining outcomes and directing therapy. The history includes questions about physical functioning, appetite, mental health, sleep disturbances, sexual functioning, cognitive functioning, and ability to perform the usual ADLs, including occupational and social activities. Specific questions are asked about the presence of weight gain, orthopnea, paroxysmal nocturnal dyspnea, edema, and dyspnea on exertion. The patient should report weight increases greater than 2 lb in any single day, increased pulmonary symptoms, and ankle edema. A worsening of any of these parameters requires evaluation of the treatment regimen and may indicate the need to adjust the therapy, especially diuretic dosage.

HF is generally a chronic condition that can be adequately managed in primary care. Consultation or referral to a cardiologist is appropriate when any of the following occurs:

1. Symptoms markedly worsen or the patient becomes excessively hypotensive or experiences syncope.

2. The patient is refractory to standard therapy.

3. There is evidence of renal failure or digitalis toxicity.

4. Adequate support is not present in the home to permit the patient to be treated in that situation.

5. Patients who remain symptomatic on a combination of an ACE inhibitor, a beta blocker, a diuretic, and digoxin should be seen by a cardiologist at least once. Persistent volume overload despite standard pharmacological management may require more aggressive administration of the current diuretic, more potent diuretics via the IV route, or a combination of diuretics. The ICSI (2013) recommends developing a plan for early specialty referral for patients with ischemia or those who are refractory despite optimal medical therapy. Additional testing beyond the usual monitoring may demonstrate evidence of concurrent disorders that may be the source of the resistance to therapy. These disorders may be amenable to other therapies. Surgical intervention may be needed, and hospitalization may be appropriate. Appropriate cardiac consultation should occur during the initial evaluation and at any time that it is felt appropriate (ICSI, 2013).

As with all chronic conditions, lack of adherence to a therapeutic regimen is unfortunately common. Nonadherence with diet and drugs can rapidly and profoundly affect the clinical status of HF patients, and increases in body weight and minor changes in symptoms commonly precede the major clinical episodes that require emergency care or hospitalization. Several factors in the management of heart failure foster this nonadherence. Lifestyle management is central to the treatment regimen for all stages and types of HF, and difficulty in achieving and maintaining lifestyle changes is well documented. Adverse drug reactions and drug costs are also factors. Table 40-9 (Chapter 40) on hypertension details some activities that can improve adherence, and Chapter 6 has additional material to improve positive outcomes.

PATIENT EDUCATION

Patient education should include a discussion of information related to the overall treatment plan as well as lifestyle management and exercise instruction (Davies et al, 2010; Levitan, Wolk, & Mittleman, 2009), information specific to the drug therapy, reasons for the drug being taken, drugs as part of the total treatment regimen, and adherence issues. Unless contraindicated, all patients should also be encouraged to obtain an annual influenza vaccination. Pneumococcal immunization should be provided at diagnosis of HF, if not previously vaccinated. For older adults, if initial vaccination was at 65 years or less, revaccination at 65 years or 5 years after initial immunization, whichever is later, should be done.

Preemptive education for adults based on the Cardiovascular Pooled Risk research projects (Ahmed, 2015) may add up to 13 years of life for patients if they prevent the chronic disease precursors of HF including HTN, DM, and obesity before age 45. Prevention of all of these HF risk factors yields up to an 85% relative risk reduction for women. Men reduce their risk of HF by 73%.

HEART FAILURE

PATIENT EDUCATION

Related to the Overall Treatment Plan and Disease Process

☐ Pathophysiology of heart failure, its prognosis, and its long-term effects on other organs of the body besides the heart

☐ Role of lifestyle modifications, including dietary and activity modifications, in improving prognosis and keeping the number and cost of required drugs down

☐ Importance of adherence to the treatment regimen

☐ Self-monitoring of symptoms of worsening failure, including daily weights

☐ What to do when symptoms worsen

☐ Need for regular follow-up visits with the primary care provider

Specific to the Drug Therapy

☐ Reason for the drug being given and its anticipated action in the disease process

☐ Doses and schedules for taking the drug

☐ Possible adverse effects and what to do if they occur

☐ Coping mechanisms for complex and costly drug regimens

☐ Interactions between other treatment modalities and these drugs

Reasons for Taking the Drug(s)

Patient education about specific drugs is provided in Chapter 16. Specifically for HF, additional information includes the following: These drugs are given to reduce mortality, reduce symptoms, and improve functional status. Some drugs do all of these (**ACE inhibitors**); most do only one. The expectations should be clear about what the drugs can and cannot do. HF is a chronic condition that rarely occurs in a short period of time, and it is not likely to be corrected in a short period of time, if at all. Patients with HF must understand the seriousness of this diagnosis, including the 5-year mortality rate of 50% and the potential need for surgeries such as heart transplantation. All of this must be done while maintaining hope and emphasizing that a good quality of life is possible.

Drugs as Part of the Total Treatment Regimen

The total treatment regimen includes sodium restriction and avoidance of excessive fluid intake. **Diuretics** reduce fluid volume and may interact with dietary restrictions, resulting in orthostatic hypotension. Care should be taken not to reduce fluid volume too quickly, which exacerbates the problem of decreased cardiac output and may lead to hypotension or renal insufficiency. Patients should report symptoms of fluid volume deficit. They should be told to rise slowly from a supine to a standing position to permit the body to redistribute body fluids. Sodium restriction may lead some patients to seek salt substitutes that have a potassium salt as part of their contents. For patients taking **ACE inhibitors**, this can result in excessively high potassium levels. Such salt substitutes should be avoided. Nonsalt herbal seasoning is more appropriate.

Regular aerobic exercise such as walking or cycling may improve functional status and decrease symptoms. Regular, gradually increased exercise may lead to enough improvement, in some cases, to reduce the drugs needed. Timing of exercise with the peak action of drugs is important. Patients are often able to predict the timing of voiding after taking a diuretic or times when other drugs are more likely to produce dizziness. Exercise timing should take these into consideration.

Adherence Issues

Nonadherence with the treatment regimen in HF may reduce life expectancy and certainly affects functional status. Health-care providers should be aware of the potential problem of nonadherence, discuss the importance of adherence at each follow-up visit, and assist patients in removing barriers to adherence (e.g., cost, adverse effects, or complexity of the regimen).

REFERENCES

Amhed, A. (2006). Effects of digoxin on morbidity and mortality in diastolic heart failure: The Ancillary Digitalis Investigation Group Trial. *Circulation, 114*(5), 397–403.

Ahmad, F. (2015, Mar). XXXXXX, Abstract 1126M-05. 64th Annual Scientific Sessions American College of Cardiology, San Diego, CA.

Bell, D., Bakris, G., & McGill, J. (2009). Comparison of carvedilol and metoprolol on serum lipid concentration in diabetic hypertensive patients. *Diabetes, Obesity and Metabolism, 11*, 234–238.

Bonet, S., Agusit, A., Arnau, J., Vidal, X., Diogene, E., Galve, E., et al. (2000). Beta-adrenergic blocking agents in heart failure: Benefits of vasodilating and non-vasodilating agents according to patients' characteristics: A meta-analysis of clinical trials. *Archives of Internal Medicine, 160*, 621–627.

Bouzamondo, A., Hulot, J., Sanchez, P., Cucherat, M., & Lechat, P. (2001). Beta-blocker treatment in heart failure. *Fundamental and Clinical Pharmacology, 15*, 95–109.

Brophy, J., Joseph, L., & Rouleau, J. (2001). Beta-blockers in congestive heart failure: A Bayesian meta-analysis. *Annals of Internal Medicine, 134*, 550–560.

CAPRIE Steering Committee. (1996). A randomized, blinded, trial of clopidogrel versus aspirin in patients at risk of ischaemic events (CAPRIE). *The Lancet, 348*, 1329–1339.

Chen, Y., Wang, Y., Radford, M., & Krumholz, H. (2001). Angiotensin-converting enzyme inhibitor dosages in elderly patients with heart failure. *American Heart Journal, 141*(3), 410.

Cleland, J., Tendera, M., Adamus, J., Freemantle, N., Polonski, L., & Taylor, J. (2006). The perindopril in elderly people with chronic heart failure (PEF-CHF) study. *European Heart Journal, 27*(19), 2338–2345.

Daniel, K., Wells, G., Stewart, K., Moore, B., & Kitzman, D. (2009). Effect of aldosterone antagonism on exercise tolerance, Doppler diastolic function, and quality of life in older women with diastolic heart failure. *Congestive Heart Failure, 15*, 68–74.

Davies, E., Moxham, T., Rees, K., Singh, S., Coats, A., Ebrahim, S., et al. (2010). Exercise based rehabilitation for heart failure (review). *Cochrane Database Systematic Review*, CD003331.

Dickstein, K., & Kjekshus, J. (2002). Effects of losartan and captopril on mortality and morbidity in high-risk patients after acute myocardial infarction: The OPTIMAL randomized trial. Optimal Trial in Myocardial Infarction with Angiotensin II Antagonist Losartan. *The Lancet, 360*, (9348), 1893–1906.

Digitalis Investigation Group. (1997). The effect of digoxin on mortality and morbidity in patients with heart failure. *The New England Journal of Medicine, 336*, 525–533.

Eikelboom, J., Hirsh, J., Spencer, F., Baglin, T., & Weitz, J. (2012). Antithrombotic therapy and prevention of thrombosis, 9th ed: American College of Chest Physician evidence-based clinical practice guidelines. *Chest, 141* (2 Suppl.), 89s–113s.

Elliot, W. (2012). Effects of potassium-sparing versus thiazide diuretics on glucose tolerance: New data on an old topic. *Hypertension, 59*, 911.

Erdmann, E. (2009). Safety and tolerability of beta-blockers: Prejudices and reality. *European Heart Journal Supplements, 11*, A21–A25.

FDA (2015, April 15). FDA approves corlanor to treat heart failure. Accessed May 8, 2015, at http://www.fda.gov/NewsEvents/Newsroom/Press Announcements/ucm442978.htm.

Flather, M., Yusuf, S., Kober, L., Pfeffer, M., Hall, A., Murray, G., et al. (2000). Long-term ACE-inhibitor therapy in patients with heart failure or left-ventricular dysfunction: A systematic overview of data from individual patients. ACE-Inhibitor Myocardial Infarction Collaborative Group. *The Lancet, 355*, 1575–1581.

Flory, J., Ky, B., Haynes, K., Brunelli, S., Munsun, J., Rowan, C., et al. (2012). Observational cohort study of the safety of digoxin use in women with heart failure. *British Medical Journal Open, 2*, e000888.

Garg, R., & Yusef, S. (1995). Overview of randomized trials of angiotensin-converting enzyme inhibitors on mortality and morbidity in patients with heart failure. *Journal of the American Medical Association, 273*, 1450–1456.

Grossman, E., Vedecchia, P., Shamiss, A., Angeli, F., & Reboldi, G. (2011). Diuretic treatment of hypertension. *Diabetes Care, 34*(2 Suppl.), S313–S319.

Gutierrez, J., Ramirez, G., Rundek, T., & Sacco, R. (2012). Statin therapy in the prevention of recurrent cardiovascular events: A sex-based meta-analysis. *Archives of Internal Medicine, 172*(12), 909–919.

Hall, M., Levant, S., & DeFrances, C. (2012). *Hospitalization for congestive heart failure: United States, 2000–2010*. National Center for Health Statistics Data Brief, no. 108, October 2012. Accessed October 31, 2012, at http://www.cdc.gov/nchs/data/databriefs/db108.pdf

Hansen, M., Sorensen, R., Clausen, M., Fog-Petersen, M., Raunso, J., Gadsboll, N., et al. (2010). Risk of bleeding with single, dual, or triple therapy with warfarin, aspirin, and clopidogrel in patients with atrial fibrillation. *Archives of Internal Medicine, 170*(16), 1433–1441.

Haynes, K., Heitjan D., Kanetsky, P., & Hennessy, S. (2008). Declining public health burden of digoxin toxicity from 1991 to 2004. *Nature Publishing Group, 84*(1), 90–94.

Heart Failure Society of America (HFSA). (2010). Executive summary: HFSA 2010 comprehensive heart failure practice guideline. *Journal of Cardiac Failure, 16*(6), 475–539.

Hernandez, A., Hammil, B., O'Connor, C., Schulman, K., Curtis, L., & Fonarow, G. (2009). Clinical effectiveness of beta-blockers in heart failure: Findings from the OPTIMIZE-HF (Organized Program to Initiate Life-saving Treatment in Hospitalized Patients with Heart Failure) registry. *Journal of the American College of Cardiology, 53*(2), 184–192.

Institute for Clinical Systems Improvement (ICSI) (2013). Heart failure in adults. *Institute for Clinical Systems Improvement*. Retrieved February 15, 2015, from www.icsi.org/guidelines

Jong, P., Yusef, S., Rousseau, M., & Bangdiwala, S. (2003). Effect of enalapril on 12-year survival and life expectancy in patients with left ventricular systolic dysfunction: A follow-up study. *The Lancet, 361*(9372), 1843.

Kalogeropoulos, A., Georgiopoulous, V., Kritchevsky, S., Psaty, B., Smith, N., Newman, A., et al. (2009). Epidemiology of incident heart failure in a contemporary elderly cohort. *Archives of Internal Medicine, 169*(7), 708–715.

Keyhan, G., Chen, S., & Pilote, L. (2007). Angiotensin-converting enzyme inhibitors and survival in women and men with heart failure. *European Journal of Heart Failure, 9*(6–7), 594.

Kindsvater, S., Leclerc, K., & Ward, J. (2003). Effects of coadministration of aspirin or clopidogrel on exercise testing in patients with heart failure receiving angiotensin-converting enzyme inhibitors. *American Journal of Cardiology, 91*, 1350–1352.

Kjekshus, J., Apetrei, E., Barrios, V., Bohm, M., Cleland, J., Cornel, J., et al. (2007). Rosuvastatin in older patients with systolic heart failure. *The New England Journal of Medicine, 357*, 2248–2261.

Kochanek, K., Xu, J., Murphy, S., Minini, A., & Kung, H. (2011). Deaths: Final data for 2009. *National Vital Statistics Reports, 60*(3).

Konstam, M., Neaton, J., Dickstein, K., Drexler, H., Komajda, M., Martinez, F., et al. (2009). Effects of high-dose versus low-dose olosartan on clinical outcomes in patients with heart failure (HEAAL study): A randomized, double-blind trial. *The Lancet, 374*, 1840–1848.

Krum, H., Jelinek, M., Stewart, S., Sindone, A., & Atherton, J. (2011). 2011 Update to National Heart Foundation of Australia and Cardiac Society of Australia and New Zealand guidelines for the prevention, detection and management of chronic heart failure in Australia, 2006. *Medical Journal of Australia, 194*(8), 405–409.

Lader, E., Egan, D., Hunsberger, S., Garg, R., Czajkowski, S., & McSherry, F. (2003). The effect of digoxin on the quality of life in patients with heart failure. *Journal of Cardiac Failure, 9*(1), 4–12.

Levine, T., Levine, A., Bolenbaugh, J., & Green, P. (2002). Reversal of heart failure remodeling with age. *American Journal of Geriatric Cardiology, 11*(5), 299–304.

Levitan, E., Wolk, A., & Mittleman, M. (2009). Consistency with the DASH diet and incidence of heart failure. *Archives of Internal Medicine, 169*(9), 851–857.

Lip, G., & Chung, I. (2010). Anticoagulation for heart failure in sinus rhythm. *Cochrane Database Systematic Review*, CD003336.

Mancini, G. (2000). Long-term use of angiotensin-converting enzyme inhibitors to modify endothelial dysfunction: A review of clinical investigations. *Clinical and Investigative Medicine, 23*, 144–161.

McDonald, K., Ledwidge, M., Cahil, J., Kelly, J., Quigley, P., Maurer, B., et al. (2001). Elimination of early rehospitalization in a randomized, controlled trial of multidisciplinary care in a high-risk, elderly heart failure population: The potential contributions of specialist care, clinical stability and optimal angiotensin-converting enzyme inhibitor dose at discharge. *European Journal of Heart Failure, 3*(2), 209–215.

McMurray, J., Adamopoulos, S., Anker, S., Auricchio, A., Bohm, M., Dickstein, K., et al. (2012). ESC guidelines for the diagnosis and treatment of acute and chronic heart failure 2012: The Task Force[trunc]. *European Heart Journal, 33*, 1787–1847.

National Institute for Health and Clinical Excellence (NICE). (2010). Chronic heart failure: Management of chronic heart failure in adults in primary and secondary care. NICE clinical guideline 108. Retrieved October 22, 2012, from www.nice.org/uk/guidance/CG108

Neal, B., MacMahon, S., Chapman, N., & Blood, P. (2000). Effects of ACE inhibitors, calcium antagonists, and other blood-pressure-lowering drugs: Results of prospectively designed overviews of randomized trials. Blood Pressure Lowering Treatment Trials Collaboration. *The Lancet, 356*, 1955–1964.

Ong, H., Ong, L. & Kow, F. (2012). Beta-blockers for heart failure: An evidence based review answering practical therapeutic questions. *Medical Journal of Malaysia, 67*(1), 7–11.

Packer, M., Coats, A., Fowler, M., Jatus, H., Krum, H., Mohacsi, P., et al. (2001). Effect of carvedilol on survival in severe chronic heart failure. *The New England Journal of Medicine, 344*, 1651–1658.

Pfeffer, M., McMurray, J., Velazquez, E., Rouleau, J., Kober, L., Maggioni, A., et al. (2003). Valsartan, captopril, or both in myocardial infarction complicated by heart failure, left ventricular dysfunction, or both. *The New England Journal of Medicine, 349,* 1893–1906.

Pieske, B. (2012). Aldo-HF: Aldosterone receptor blockade in diastolic heart failure. European Society of Cardiology 2012 Congress; August 26, Munich, Germany.

Pitt, B., Remmer, A., Zannad, F., Neaton, J., Martinez, F., Roniker, B., et al. (2003). Eplerenone, a selective aldosterone blocker, in patients with left ventricular dysfunction after myocardial infarction. *The New England Journal of Medicine, 348,* 1309–1321.

Redfield, M., Jacobsen, S., Burnett, J., Mahoney, D., Bailey, R., & Rodefeffer, R. (2003). Burden of systolic and diastolic ventricular dysfunction in the community: Appreciating the scope of the heart failure epidemic. *Journal of the American Medical Association, 289,* 194–202.

Rochon, P., Sykora, K., Bronskill, S., Mamdani, M., Anderson G., Gurwitz, J., et al. (2004). Use of angiotensin-converting enzyme inhibitor therapy and dose-related outcomes in older adults with new heart failure in the community. *Journal of General Internal Medicine, 19*(6), 676.

Scottish Intercollegiate Guidelines Network (SIGN). (2007). *Management of chronic heart failure: A national clinical guideline.* Edinburgh, Scotland: Scottish Intercollegiate Guidelines Network (SIGN). 53 pp. Retrieved on June 5, 2009, from http://guideline.gov/Compare/comparison.aspx

Shibata, M., Flather, M., & Wang, D. (2001). Systematic review of the impact of beta blockers on mortality and hospital admissions in heart failure. *European Journal of Heart Failure, 3,* 351–357.

Shlipak, M., Smith, G., Rathore, S., Massie, B., & Krumholz, H. (2004). Renal function, digoxin therapy, and heart failure outcomes: Evidence from the digoxin intervention group trial. *Journal of the American Society of Nephrology, 15*(8), 2195–2203.

SOLVD investigators. (1991). Effect of enalapril on survival in patients with reduced left ventricular ejection fractions and congestive heart failure. *The New England Journal of Medicine, 325,* 293–302.

Stears, A., Woods, S., Watts, M., Burton, T., Graggaber, J., Mir, F., et al. (2012). A double-blind, placebo-controlled, crossover trial comparing the effects of amiloride and hydrocholorthiazide on glucose tolerance in patients with essential hypertension. *Hypertension, 59,* 934.

Stone, N., Robinson, J., Lichtenstein, A., Merz, C., Blum, C., Echel, R., et al. (2013). 2013 ACC/AHA guideline on the treatment of blood cholesterol to reduce atherosclerotic cardiovascular risk in adults: A report of the American College of Cardiology/American Heart Association task force on practice guidelines. *Circulation.* Accessed at http://circ.ahajournals.org/content/early/2013/11/01.cir.0000437738.63853.7a.citation.

Takkouche, B., Etminan, M., Caamano, F., & Rochon, P. (2002). Interaction between aspirin and ACE inhibitors: Resolving discrepancies using meta-analysis. *Drug Safety, 25,* 373–378.

Tavazzi, L., Maggioni, A., Marchioli, R., Barlera, S., Franzosi, M., Latini, R., et al. (2008). Effect of rosuvastatin in patients with chronic heart failure (the GISSI-HF trial): A randomized, double-blind, placebo-controlled trial. *The Lancet, 372,* 1231–1239.

Veterans Health Administration, Department of Veterans Affairs. (2007). *PBM-MAP clinical practice guideline for the pharmacologic management of chronic heart failure in primary care practice.* Washington, DC: Veterans Health Administration, Department of Veterans Affairs. Retrieved October 25, 2012, from www.pbm.va.gov

Whorlow, S., & Krum, H. (2000). Meta-analysis of effect of beta-blocker therapy on mortality in patients with New York Heart Association class IV chronic congestive heart failure. *American Journal of Cardiology, 86,* 886–889.

Yancy, C., Jessup, M., Bozkurt, B., Butler, J., Casey, D., Drazner, M., et al. (2013). 2013 ACCF/AHA guideline for the management of heart failure. *Circulation.128*: e240-e327.

Zannad, F., McMurray, J., Krum, H., van Veldhuisen, D., Swedberg, K., Shi, H., et al. (2011). Eplerenone in patients with systolic heart failure and mild symptoms. *The New England Journal of Medicine, 364*(1), 11.

CHAPTER 37

HUMAN IMMUNODEFICIENCY VIRUS DISEASE AND ACQUIRED IMMUNODEFICIENCY SYNDROME

James Raper • Gina Dobbs

Now in the third decade of treating patients with HIV infection, we can celebrate our many successes. In a short time, we have transitioned a terminal illness into a manageable chronic disease. Since the discovery of human immunodeficiency virus (HIV) in 1981, we have learned a great deal about HIV-associated epidemiology, natural history, pathogenesis, therapy, and immunological host response. However, HIV disease and its sequel, acquired immunodeficiency syndrome (AIDS), remain a global health problem of unprecedented dimensions. Since the beginning of the epidemic, more than 60 million people have been infected with the HIV virus, and approximately 30 million people have died of AIDS. In 2010, there were an estimated 34 million people living with HIV, 2.7 million new infections, and 1.8 million

AIDS-related deaths (World Health Organization, 2012). On a global scale, the HIV epidemic has stabilized, although with unacceptably high levels of new HIV infections and AIDS deaths. Globally, an estimated 34 million people were living with HIV in 2011. The annual number of new HIV infections declined from an estimated 3.0 million in 2001 to 2.5 million in 2011. Overall, 1.7 million people died due to AIDS in 2011, compared with an estimated 1.7 million in 2001.

While the percentage of people living with HIV has stabilized since 2000, the overall number of people living with HIV has steadily increased as new infections occur each year, HIV treatments extend life, and new infections still outnumber AIDS deaths. Women account for more than half of the cases of HIV worldwide, and nearly 60% of HIV infections in sub-Saharan

Africa. Over the past 15 years, the proportion of women with HIV has remained stable globally but has increased in many regions. Young people aged 15 to 24 years account for an estimated 45% of new HIV infections worldwide. An estimated 330,000 children younger than 15 years became infected with HIV in 2011. Globally, the number of children younger than 15 years living with HIV increased from 1.6 million in 2001 to 3.3 million in 2011. More than two-thirds (60%), 23.5 million, live in sub-Saharan Africa (AMFAR, 2012). In the United States and dependent areas, the cumulative estimated number of diagnoses of AIDS through 2010 was 1,163,575 (Centers for Disease Control and Prevention [CDC], 2010). The cumulative estimated number of deaths of persons with AIDS in the United States and dependent areas in 2009 was 641,976, including 614,394 adults and adolescents and 4,986 children under age 13 years (CDC, 2010).

Thanks to increasingly effective antiretroviral therapy (ART), the natural history of HIV disease has been favorably altered. A developing list of potent medications, used in combination therapy, has slowed the progression of HIV disease and has dramatically reduced the death rates for people living with HIV. In 2009, the most recent estimates, there were 1,291,739 persons (1,257,942 adults and adolescents and 3,491 children under age 13 years) living with HIV/AIDS in the United States and six dependent U.S. areas (CDC, 2010).

PATHOPHYSIOLOGY

HIV induces defects in host cell–mediated and humoral responses, making the person susceptible to opportunistic infections and certain neoplasms. It is essential to understand the complex pathogenesis of HIV in order to appreciate the impact of HIV on the immune system and the development of interventions to prevent viral replication and advance immunological recovery.

AIDS is a clinical syndrome characterized by progressive immune system suppression, resulting in the development of opportunistic diseases. It is caused by chronic HIV infection. The first reported cases were described in 1981, the causative agent of AIDS was identified as HIV in late 1983, a serological test for HIV infection was available in 1985, and the first therapy was licensed in 1987 (Bennett, 2003). HIV is a member of a family of viruses known as retroviruses, so named because they are able to create DNA copies of their RNA genome, thus reversing (retro) the usual flow of genetic information. HIV is a lentivirus, a type of virus that characteristically produces diseases with a long incubation period leading to cancer, severe immune suppression, or both. The basic pathology in AIDS is a loss of CD4-positive T lymphocytes, cells critical to maintaining cell-mediated immune function. This damage results in progressively severe immune dysfunction.

HIV-1

The retrovirus HIV can be divided into two serotypes, HIV-1 and HIV-2; HIV-1 is predominantly responsible for HIV infection worldwide. Retroviruses are RNA-containing viruses

that require the formation of proviral DNA within the host to complete their life cycle and infect other cells (Colagreco, 2003). The HIV-1 virus, like other retroviruses, is covered by a lipid bilayer derived from host-cell membranes. Viral glycoproteins are incorporated into the bilayer, as well as host adhesion molecules that may be involved in attachment to target cells (Kilby & Eron, 2003). The early characterization of HIV-1 centered on the CD4 T lymphocytes as the primary target of the HIV virus, the helper cells that are responsible for cell-mediated immune reaction (Ansari & Etzel, 2000; Kilby & Eron, 2003). The infectivity of HIV requires the surface glycoprotein (gp120) and the transmembrane glycoprotein subunit (gp41) of gp160, a viral precursor protein that binds to the CD4 receptor. The presence of a chemokine coreceptor, CCR5, also is required for cell entry (Colagreco, 2003).

Following uncoating, the viral RNA is transcribed by the reverse transcriptase enzyme into proviral DNA. The integrase enzyme then integrates the proviral DNA into the host nucleus. The integrated viral genes may remain inactive or become transcribed back into genomic RNA and messenger RNA, which are then translated into viral proteins. Late stages of viral processing involve cleavage of viral proteins by the protease enzyme into new HIV particles, followed by assembly and the release of new infectious virions to infect other cells (Colagreco, 2003).

Viral replication is a dynamic process, involving continuous rounds of de novo virus infection and replication in infected host cells with rapid turnover of both free virus and virus-producing cells (Kilby & Eron, 2003). One billion to 10 billion virions are produced daily. One of the difficulties in eradicating the virus is the existence of an HIV reservoir of latently infected memory CD4 T cells carrying integrated provirus. Those reservoirs of replication-competent virus can persist in resting CD4 T cells of patients that are receiving ART. Low-level, ongoing replication of HIV may occur despite suppression of the HIV virus with potent combination ART (Kilby & Eron, 2003). To date, complete restoration of immune function has not been possible with ART, although partial restoration of pathogen-specific immunity to recall antigens is possible. ART can increase the number of circulating CD4 T cells, which is associated with prolonged survival and a diminished rate of common opportunistic infections.

Following initial HIV infection, immediate widespread dissemination of the virus to other lymphatic systems and organs occurs (Ansari & Etzel, 2000). Infectivity is high during primary infection, with high plasma viremia detected in blood and the presence of virus in sexual organs and secretions. During acute infection, the immunological host response involves potent, cytotoxic CD8 T lymphocytes, which limits viral replication and reduces symptomology as plasma viremia declines. In adults, a new steady-state plasma HIV RNA "viral set point" is established approximately 6 months or longer after the initial infection that can remain stable for months or years before progression to AIDS. The time course of progression to AIDS varies in adults, with average durations of 10 to 11 years reported in the absence of antiretroviral therapy (Ansari & Etzel, 2000).

HIV-2

Although HIV-1 is found around the world, the prevalence of HIV-2 is highest in West Africa. HIV-2 is a zoonosis disease believed to have first infected humans as early as the 1940s by jumping from sooty mangabeys to humans as a result of bush meat hunting and slaughtering. HIV-2 has a lower transmission rate and a less pathogenic course. HIV-2 is common in the following countries: Angola, Benin, Burkina Faso, Cape Verde, Cote d'Ivoire (Ivory Coast), Gambia, Ghana, Guinea, Guinea-Bissau, Liberia, Mali, Mauritania, Mozambique, Niger, Nigeria, Sao Tome, Senegal, Sierra Leone, and Togo.

Transmission

Three principal means of HIV transmission have been identified: blood, sexual contact, and mother-to-child (vertical) transmission (Kirton, 2003). The frequency of transmission is influenced by the amount of infectious virus present in the body fluid and the extent of contact an individual has with body fluids.

HPTN 052 was a clinical trial of 1,763 HIV serodiscordant couples that examined the extent to which antiretroviral therapy (ART) can, when taken by HIV-infected people, decrease their infectivity and thereby reduce the chance that they will pass HIV on to their heterosexual partners. The results of the study were so compelling that the study's Data and Safety Monitoring Board (DSMB) asked the research team to share the results with all study participants and offer ART to the control group before the study ended (Matassa, 2011).

Stages—Natural History of HIV

The natural history of HIV disease progresses through several stages. After viral transmission, a symptomatic primary HIV infection, often called acute retroviral syndrome, occurs in 50% to 90% of the people infected. The onset of symptoms is usually 2 to 4 weeks following infection, but the incubation may be as long as several months in rare cases. Typically, a flulike viral syndrome develops, with fever, lymphadenopathy, pharyngitis, rash, and myalgias or arthralgias (Freeman & Winland-Brown, 2001). Diarrhea, headaches, and nausea and vomiting are also common. Early detection of acute HIV infection provides an opportunity to follow patients prospectively soon after infection and thereby reduce disease progression and incidence of opportunistic infections. Because patients with a recent diagnosis of HIV are more likely to reduce risk behaviors if they are linked to primary HIV care than if they are not receiving care, early detection may also be a critical component of preventing further transmission, a significant public health initiative.

At this stage, serological tests are not helpful because seroconversion to a positive HIV antibody test usually occurs at 4 to 12 weeks after exposure and infection. When acute HIV infection is suspected, an HIV serological screening test should be performed in conjunction with a plasma HIV RNA test (viral load). The plasma RNA test should be performed even if the serologic screening test is negative; a fourth-generation HIV antigen/antibody combination test is the preferred serologic screening test if available. The detection of HIV RNA or antigen in the absence of HIV antibody should be considered a preliminary positive result. HIV RNA testing from a new specimen should be repeated immediately to confirm the presence of HIV RNA. In order to exclude a false-positive result, both serological and RNA testing should be repeated when low-level quantitative results (<5,000 copies/mL) from an HIV RNA assay are reported in the absence of serological evidence of HIV infection.

Generally, 95% or more of patients seroconvert within 6 months after HIV transmission. The period from infection to 6 months following HIV transmission is known as early HIV disease. At around 6 months after infection, HIV establishes a "set point," representing a stable balance between immune suppression of the virus and ongoing viral replication. In any individual patient, this steady-state set point seems to be relatively stable over a period of years in the absence of ART. One possible effect of early therapy is to alter this set point to a level associated with longer survival.

The next stage is asymptomatic infection. During this period, the patient is clinically asymptomatic and generally has no abnormal findings on physical examination except enlarged lymph nodes (Freeman & Winland-Brown, 2001). Symptomatic HIV infection is marked by the development of common infections and other conditions that are more severe and persistent in the presence of HIV infections but by themselves do not define AIDS. Examples of the conditions include thrush, oral hairy leukoplakia, peripheral neuropathy, cervical dysplasia, constitutional symptoms, and recurrent herpes zoster. Advanced HIV disease is the development of AIDS as defined by the 1993 CDC case definition (CDC, 1992). This definition includes a list of conditions indicative of severe immunosuppression, as well as the inclusion of all patients with a CD4 count below 200 cells/mm^3.

Viral Structure and Genetic Material

HIV particles appear spherical and their genetic material is enclosed in a special protein shell known as a capsis. HIV also has an outer layer known as an envelope, which is picked up from the host cell membrane as HIV buds out of the cell. Projecting out from the envelope are numerous spikes or knobs that originate from the virus. Each spike consists of three or four molecules of a protein called gp120, which is linked to another protein called gp41; together, the proteins are called gp41. The knobs bind to receptors on cells of the immune system that carry a marker known as the CD4 molecule.

HIV Life Cycle

There are seven steps in the HIV replication cycle (Fig. 37-1) (NIAID, 2013).

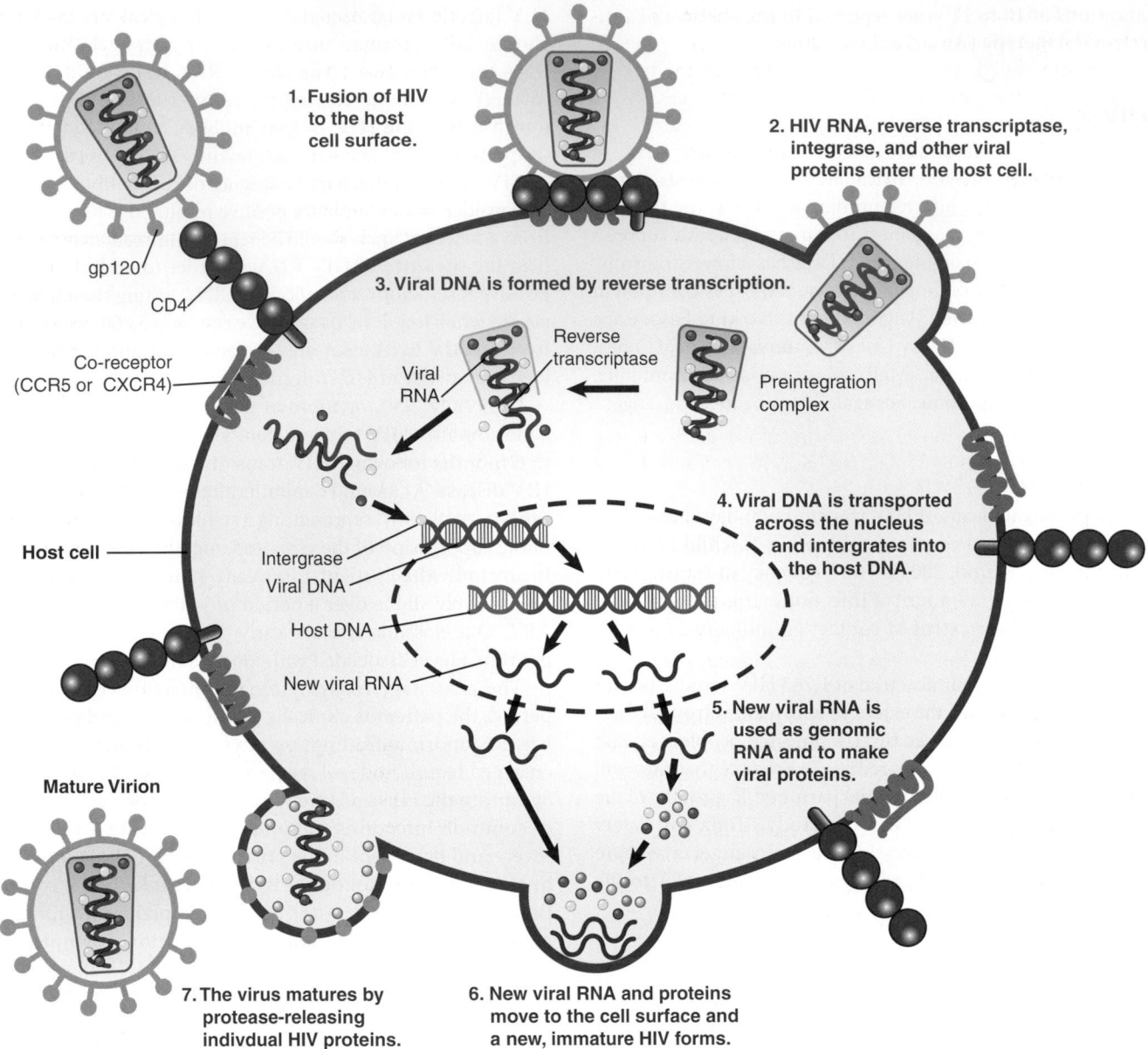

Figure 37–1. HIV replication cycle. Courtesy: National Institute of Allergy and Infectious Diseases (NIAID, 2013).

Fusion and Entry

HIV can replicate only inside human cells. The process typically begins when a virus particle bumps into a cell that carries on its surface a special protein called CD4. The spikes on the surface of the virus particle stick to the CD4 and allow the viral envelope to fuse with the cell membrane (Step 1). The contents of the HIV particle (reverse transcriptase, integrase, and other viral proteins) are then released into the cell, leaving the envelope behind (Step 2).

Reverse Transcription and Integration

Once inside the cell, the HIV enzyme reverse transcriptase converts the viral RNA into DNA (Step 3), which is compatible with human genetic material. This DNA is transported to the cell's nucleus, where it is spliced into the human DNA by the HIV enzyme integrase (Step 4). Once integrated, the HIV DNA is known as provirus.

Transcription and Translation

HIV provirus may lie dormant within a cell for a long time. But when the cell becomes activated, it treats HIV genes in much the same way as human genes. First, using human enzymes, it converts them into messenger RNA. Then the messenger RNA is transported outside the nucleus, and is used as a blueprint for producing new HIV proteins and enzymes (Step 5).

Assembly, Budding, and Maturation

Among the strands of messenger RNA produced by the cell are complete copies of HIV genetic material. These gather together with newly made HIV proteins and enzymes to form new viral particles, which are then released from the cell (Step 6). The enzyme protease plays a vital role at this stage of the HIV life cycle by chopping up long strands of protein into smaller pieces, which are used to construct mature viral cores.

The newly matured HIV particles are ready to infect another cell and begin the replication process all over again (Step 7). In this way the virus quickly spreads through the human body. And once a person is infected, that person can pass HIV on to others in bodily fluids.

GOALS OF TREATMENT

The goals of treatment with ART medication are listed in Box 37-1. The most important goals are to (1) reduce HIV-associated morbidity and prolong the duration and quality of survival, (2) restore and preserve immunological function, (3) achieve maximal and durable suppression of plasma HIV viral load, (4) and prevent HIV transmission.

These goals are achieved by reducing HIV-related morbidity and mortality, improving quality of life, and restoring and preserving immunological function in persons infected with HIV (Moyle et al, 2008).

Unfortunately, complete eradication of HIV infection is not possible with the available antiretroviral medications because latently infected CD4 T cells that are established during the earliest stages of acute HIV infection (Chun et al, 1998) persist with a long half-life in spite of prolonged suppression of HIV plasma viremia (Chun et al, 1997; Finzi et al, 1997, 1999; Wong et al, 1997).

Providers who follow approved treatment guidelines and strategies recognize substantial reductions in HIV-related morbidity and mortality (Mocroft et al, 1998; Mofenson et al, 1999; Palella et al, 1998; Delaney et al, 1998; Vittinghoff et al, 1999) and reduced vertical transmission from infected mother to infant (Garcia et al, 1999). Higher HIV plasma viral loads are associated with more rapid disease progression (Mellors et al, 1996), whereas other factors, such as heightened T-cell activation with cellular turnover and expression of immune activation markers, probably contribute as well to clinical disease progression and the rate of CD4 T-cell decline (Rodriguez et al, 2006).

The goal of maximal viral suppression with initial ART may be difficult in some patients who have preexisting medication resistance. Unfortunately, about one of every six new HIV cases diagnosed in 2007 involved virus with ARV drug-resistance mutations (CDC, 2010). To be successful, ART regimens need to contain at least two, and preferably three, active medicines from multiple medication classes. If maximal initial suppression below the level

of HIV detection (less than 50 copies/mL) is not achieved or is lost, it is important to change medication regimens to include at least two active medicines to achieve the maximal suppression goal. If it is not possible to achieve the HIV RNA less than 50 copies/mL goal in a clinically and immunologically stable patient, a time period of persistent detectable viremia may be acceptable while waiting for the availability of new medicine.

In general, viral load reduction to less than 50 copies/mL in most treatment-naïve patients occurs within the first 12 to 24 weeks of therapy. Predictors of virological success are presented in Box 37-2. Virological suppression is always observed. Viral suppression rates in clinical practice may be lower than the 80% to 90% seen in clinical trials. However, the use of current, easier-to-take, coformulated, and potent ART regimens probably decreases the differences in outcomes between clinical trials and clinical practice (Moore, Keruly, Gebo, & Lucas, 2005). To achieve treatment goals, clinicians and patients must work together to define priorities, investigate options, and mutually determine the best treatment plan.

BOX 37–2 PREDICTORS OF ART VIROLOGICAL SUCCESS

- High-level patient adherence to ART regimen
- High potency of antiretroviral medication regimen
- Higher baseline CD4 T-cell count
- Low baseline HIV plasma viral RNA level
- Rapid (i.e., equal to or greater than 1 $\log_{10}$ in 1 to 4 mo) reduction of viral RNA level in response to ART

Rationale for ART Medication Selection

The clinical management of HIV is complex. Practical strategies must be identified so that virological suppression can be attained with therapy plans that patients can adhere to consistently. The treatment of HIV disease is a dynamic, rapidly changing arena, as newer drugs are developed and different combinations evaluated. Selecting the initial combination ART regimen is extremely important. Today, there are more than 22 U.S. Food and Drug Administration (FDA) approved antiretroviral medicines from six mechanistic classes from which to design combination ART regimens. HIV medications are always used in combination to reduce the amount of HIV in the blood (plasma viral load) by helping to block or "inhibit" certain steps during the HIV replication process.

Principles of Therapy

The U.S. Public Health Service has identified certain principles of therapy of HIV infection (CDC, 1998; Panel on Antiretroviral Guidelines for Adults and Adolescent, 2012). First, ongoing HIV replication leads to immune system damage

---

BOX 37–1 HIV TREATMENT GOALS

- Improve quality of life
- Obtain maximal and durable suppression of HIV
- Prevent vertical HIV transmission
- Prolong survival
- Reduce HIV-related morbidity
- Reduce transmissibility of HIV
- Restore and preserve immunological function

and progression to AIDS. HIV infection is always harmful, and long-term survival free of clinically significant immune dysfunction is unusual. The extent of HIV replication and its rate of CD4 T-cell destruction are indicated by plasma HIV RNA levels. The extent of HIV-induced immune damage that has already occurred is indicated by the CD4 T-cell counts. Therefore, plasma HIV RNA and CD4 T-cell levels must be regularly measured (every 3 to 6 months) to determine the risk for disease progression in an HIV-infected person and to identify when to initiate or modify antiretroviral treatment regimens (Panel on Antiretroviral Guidelines for Adults and Adolescents, 2012). Treatment decisions should be individualized based on the risk of disease progression as indicated by plasma HIV RNA levels and CD4 measurements. The goal of therapy should be the maximum achievable suppression of HIV replication. The use of potent combination ART to suppress HIV replication to below the levels of detection of sensitive viral-load assays limits the potential for selection of ART-resistant HIV variants.

The most effective way to achieve sustained suppression of HIV replication is the concomitant initiation of combinations of effective anti-HIV medications that are not cross-resistant with ART agents. Because there is a finite number of available and effective ART drugs and cross resistance between specific drugs has been shown, it is critical that every ART drug used in combination therapy be used according to optimal schedules and dosages.

These dosing principles should be applied to HIV-infected children, adolescents, and adults. However, the treatment of HIV-infected children involves unique pharmacological, virological, and immunological considerations (Panel on Antiretroviral Guidelines for Adults and Adolescents, 2012). Women should receive optimal ART even if they are pregnant. In fact, ART of the pregnant woman with zidovudine alone or with standard three-drug combinations has dramatically reduced the rates of vertical transmission from mother to child (Perinatal HIV Guidelines Working Group, 2009). Treatment of acute HIV infection should be considered optional at this time (Panel on Antiretroviral Guidelines for Adults and Adolescents, 2012).

INITIATING ART MEDICATIONS

The most current recommendations (Panel on Antiretroviral Guidelines for Adults and Adolescents, 2012) suggest ART for all HIV-infected individuals. The strength of the recommendations depends on stage of the disease. Randomized controlled trials provide definitive evidence supporting the benefit of ART in patients with CD4 counts <350 cells/mm³. Since results from multiple observational cohort studies demonstrate benefits of ART in reducing AIDS- and non-AIDS–associated morbidity and mortality in patients with CD4 counts ranging from 350 to 500 cells/mm³, the recommendation is for ART for patients with CD4 (CD4 count <350 cells/mm³).

The recommendation to initiate therapy at CD4 count >500 cells/mm³ is based on growing awareness that untreated HIV infection or uncontrolled viremia may be associated with development of many non-AIDS–defining diseases, including cardiovascular disease (CVD), kidney disease, liver disease, neurological complications, and malignancy; availability of ART regimens that are more effective, more convenient, and better tolerated than earlier ART combinations no longer widely used; and evidence from one observational cohort study that showed survival benefit in patients who started ART when their CD4 counts were >500 cells/mm³.

Regardless of CD4 count, initiation of ART is strongly recommended for individuals with the following conditions:

- History of an AIDS-defining illness
- HIV/hepatitis B virus (HBV) co-infection
- HIV-associated nephropathy (HIVAN)
- Pregnancy
- Effective ART also has been shown to prevent transmission of HIV from an infected individual to a sexual partner; therefore, ART should be offered to patients who are at risk of transmitting HIV to sexual partners

However, the potential benefits of early intervention must be weighed against the risks of early therapy. One major factor is nonadherence for patients who are not yet ready to commit to a complex drug regimen and potential adverse effects that may decrease their quality of life. Therefore, the clinician and the patient need to have an in-depth discussion of the potential toxicities and the complexities of the ART regimen. Box 37-3 presents these risks and benefits.

Patients initiating antiretroviral therapy should be willing and able to commit to lifelong treatment and should understand the benefits and risks of therapy and the importance of adherence. Patients may choose to postpone therapy, and providers may elect to defer therapy, based on clinical and/or psychosocial factors on a case-by-case basis.

The recommended treatment for HIV infection is a combination of three or more medications from two different classes (Table 37-1). The six different mechanistic classes or "families" of HIV antiretroviral medications include nucleoside reverse transcriptase inhibitors (NRTIs), also called "nukes"; nonnucleoside reverse transcriptase inhibitors (NNRTIs), also called "nonnukes"; protease inhibitors (PIs); fusion inhibitors (FIs), also called "entry inhibitors"; integrase strand transfer inhibitors (INSTIs); and CCR5 antagonists. Each class of HIV medications inhibits HIV replication in a different way. The primary difference among the classes is the stage of the HIV life cycle that the medications target.

The main mechanism of action of NRTIs is the inhibition of replication of retroviruses, including HIV, by interfering with viral RNA-directed DNA polymerase (reverse transcriptase). NNRTIs also inhibit replication of HIV by acting as a specific, noncompetitive, reverse transcriptase inhibitor and by disrupting the catalytic site of the enzyme. PIs are selective and competitive inhibitors of HIV protease. PIs play an essential role in preventing cleavage of protein precursors essential for HIV maturation, infection of new cells, and replication. FIs work by blocking an important step in the process of HIV entry into CD4 cells known as fusion. By blocking fusion, FIs may prevent HIV from entering and infecting CD4 cells. Integrase inhibitors (IIs) work by blocking

---

BOX 37–3 POTENTIAL BENEFITS AND RISKS OF ART

Potential Benefits of Early Therapy

- Maintenance of a higher CD4 T-cell count and prevention of potentially irreversible damage to the immune system
- Decreased risk for HIV-associated complications that can sometimes occur at CD4 counts more than 350 cells/µL, including tuberculosis, non-Hodgkin lymphoma, Kaposi's sarcoma, peripheral neuropathy, HPV-associated malignancies, and HIV-associated cognitive impairment
- Decreased risk of nonopportunistic medical conditions, including cardiovascular disease, renal disease, liver disease, and non–AIDS associated malignancies and infections
- Decreased risk of HIV transmission to others, which will have positive public health implications

Potential Risks of Early Therapy

- Treatment-related side effects and toxicities
- Viral resistance to medications because of incomplete viral suppression, resulting in loss of future treatment options
- Less time for the patient to learn about HIV and its treatment and less time to prepare for the need for adherence to ART
- Increased total time exposed to medication, with greater chance of treatment fatigue
- Premature use of ART before the development of more effective, less toxic, and/or better studied combinations of antiretroviral medications
- Transmission of medication-resistant virus in patients who do not maintain full viral suppression

---

Table 37–1 ART Medications and Treatment Strategies, Naïve Patients

- 2 NRTIs + 1 drug from one of the following classes; NNRTI, PI (preferably boosted with ritonavir), INSTI, or a CCR5 antagonist.

Preferred regimens are those with optimal and durable efficacy, favorable tolerability and toxicity profile, and ease of use.
The preferred regimens for nonpregnant patients are arranged by order of FDA approval of components other than nucleosides, thus, by duration of clinical experience.

	Comments
NNRTI-Based Regimen	Efavirenz should not be used during the first trimester of pregnancy or in women trying to conceive or not using effective and consistent contraception.
• Efavirenz/emtricitabine/tenofovir	
PI-Based Regimens (in alphabetical order)	
• Atazanavir/r + emtricitabine/tenofovir	Tenofovir should be used with caution in patients with renal insufficiency.
• Darunavir/r (once daily) + emtricitabine/tenofovir	Atazanavir/r should not be used in patients who require >20 mg omeprazole equivalent/day.
INSTI-Based Regimen	
• Raltegravir + tenofovir/emtricitabine	
Preferred Regimen† for Pregnant Women	
• Lopinavir/r (twice daily) + zidovudine/lamivudine	

Alternative regimens are those that are effective and tolerable but have potential disadvantages compared with preferred regimens. An alternative regimen may be the preferred regimen for some patients.

	Comments
NNRTI-Based Regimens (in alphabetical order)	• Rilpivirine should be used with caution in patients with pretreament HIV RNA >100,000 copies/mL.
• Efavirenz + (abacavir or zidovudine)/lamivudine	• Use of PPIs with rilpivirine is contraindicated.
• Rilpivirine + emtricitabine + tenofovir	Abacavir:
• Rilpivirine + abacavir + lamivudine	• Should not be used in patients who test positive for HLA B*5701.
PI-Based Regimens (in alphabetical order)	• Use with caution in patients with high risk of cardiovascular disease or with pretreatment HIV-RNA >100,000 copies/mL.
• Atazanavir/r + abacavir /lamivudine	Once-daily lopinavir/r is not recommended in pregnant women.
• Daranavir/r + abacavir /lamivudine	
• Fosamprenavir/r (once or twice daily) + either abacavir/lamivudine or tenofovir/emtricitabine	
• Lopinavir/r (once or twice daily) + either abacavir/lamivudine or tenofovir/emtricitabine	
INSTI-Based Regimen	
• Raltegravir + abacavir /lamivudine	

Acceptable regimens are those that may be selected for some patients but are less satisfactory than preferred or alternative regimens.

	Comments
NNRTI-Based Regimen	Nevirapine should not be used in patients with moderate to severe hepatic impairment (Child-Pugh B or C).
• Efavirenz + zidovudine/lamivudine	
• Nevirapine + (emtricitabine/tenofovir or zidovudine/ lamivudine)	Nevirapine should not be used in women with pre-ART CD4 count >250 cells/mm³ or in men with pre-ART CD4 count >400 cells/mm³.
• Nevirapine + abacavir/lamivudine	Use nevirapine and abacavir together with caution. Both can cause hypersensitivity syndrome reactions within the first few weeks after initiation.
• Rilpivirine + zidovudine/lamivudine	

Continued

Table 37–1 ART Medications and Treatment Strategies, Naïve Patients—cont'd

PI-Based Regimen

- Atazanavir + (abacavir or zidovudine)/+ lamivudine
- Atazanavir/r + zidovudine/lamivudine
- Daranavir/r + zidovudine/lamivudine
- Fosamprenavir/r + zidovudine/lamivudine
- Lopinavir/r + zidovudine/lamivudine

INSTI-Based Regimen

- Raltegravir + zidovudine/lamivudine

CCR5 Antagonist-Based Regimens

- Maraviroc + zidovudine/lamivudine
- Maraviroc + (emtricitabine/tenofovir or zidovudine/lamivudine)

Zidovudine can cause bone marrow suppression, lipoatrophy, and rarely lactic acidosis with hepatic steatosis.

Lopinavir/r (twice daily) + zidovudine/lamivudine is the preferred regimen for use during pregnancy.

Atazanavir/r is generally referred over unboosted atazanavir. Unboosted atazanavir may be used when ritonavir boosting is not possible.

Perform tropism testing **before** initiation of maraviroc. Maraviroc may be considered in patients who have only CCR5-tropic virus.

*Lamivudine may substitute for emtricitabine or vice versa.

†For more detailed recommendations on antiretroviral use in an HIV-infected pregnant woman, refer to "Recommendations for Use of Antiretroviral Drugs in Pregnant HIV-Infected Women for Maternal Health and Interventions to Reduce Perinatal HIV Transmission in the United States," at http://aidsinfo.nih.gov/guidelines

FIs = fusion inhibitors; INSTIs = integrase strand transfer inhibitor; NNRTIs = nonnucleoside reverse transcriptase inhibitors; NRTIs = nucleoside reverse transcriptase inhibitors; PI = protease inhibitors.

the integrase enzyme that HIV needs to make more virus. CCR5 antagonists work by blocking a molecule called CCR5 that is found on the surface of CD4 cells so HIV cannot enter.

The most extensively studied combination ART regimens for treatment-naïve patients include either (1) one NNRTI with two NRTIs or (2) one PI (with or without ritonavir boosting) with two NRTIs. The potent inhibitory effect of ritonavir on metabolism of the cytochrome P450 (CYP450) 3A4 isoenzyme allows the addition of low-dose ritonavir to other PIs (except nelfinavir) as a pharmacokinetic booster to increase medication levels and prolong plasma half-lives of the active PIs. This "boosting" allows for reduced dosing frequency and/or pill burden, which may improve overall adherence to the ART regimen. The increased trough concentration (C_{min}) may improve the antiretroviral activity of the active PIs, which can be beneficial when the patient harbors HIV-resistant strains to PIs (Dragsted et al, 2003, 2005; Shulman et al, 2002). The potential for increased risk of hyperlipidemia and drug–drug interactions is the major drawback associated with ritonavir boosting.

Both NNRTI- and PI-based regimens result in suppression of HIV RNA levels and CD4 T-cell increases in a large majority of patients (Gallant et al, 2004; Gulick et al, 2006; Riddler et al, 2006; Squires et al, 2004; Staszewski et al, 1999). A list of several preferred and alternative ART regimens is available from which to choose (see Table 37-1). ART regimens vary in efficacy, pill burden, and potential side effects. A patient-specific individualized regimen that maximizes adherence may be more successful in achieving full viral suppression. Many patient-specific characteristics are considered in the selection of an ART regimen. These characteristics include the following:

- Comorbid conditions (e.g., cardiovascular disease, chemical dependency, liver disease, psychiatric disease, pregnancy, renal diseases, or tuberculosis)
- Convenience (e.g., pill burden, dosing frequency, and food and fluid considerations)
- Gender and pretreatment CD4 T-cell count if considering nevirapine

- Genotypic drug resistance testing
- HLA B*5701 testing if considering abacavir
- Patient adherence potential
- Potential adverse drug effects
- Potential drug interactions with other medications
- Pregnancy potential

Medications Used to Treat HIV

There are currently six different mechanistic classes or "families" of HIV antiretroviral medications that include nucleoside reverse transcriptase inhibitors (NRTIs), nonnucleoside reverse transcriptase inhibitors (NNRTIs), protease inhibitors (PIs), fusion inhibitors (FIs), integrase strand transfer inhibitor (INSTIs), and CCR5 antagonists. The characteristics of FDA-approved ART medications are presented in Table 37-2 and the mechanistic classes are discussed in the following section.

Reverse Transcriptase Inhibitors

Reverse transcriptase inhibitors come in several forms. We will discuss nucleoside and nucleotide inhibitors in this section and nonnucleoside reverse transcriptase inhibitors in the following section. Nucleoside and nucleotide analogue reverse transcriptase inhibitors (NRTIs and NtRTIs) are a class of antiretroviral medicines that inhibit the activity of reverse transcriptase, a viral DNA polymerase enzyme that retroviruses need to reproduce. This class of antiviral medicine was the first to be used to treat HIV and remains a backbone for most ART regimens. Available HIV NRTIs include abacavir, didanosine, emtricitabine, lamivudine, stavudine, and zidovudine. The only HIV NtRTI is tenofovir.

Nucleoside Reverse Transcriptase Inhibitors

In order for NRTIs to work, they must undergo chemical changes (phosphorylation) to become active in the body. Nucleotide analogues bypass this step. Thus, NtRTIs are already chemically activated. When HIV infects a cell, reverse

Table 37–2 Antiretroviral Agent Characteristics

Drug Name	Form	Usual Adult Dose	Food Effects	Renal Failure Dosing			Liver Failure Dosing	Toxicity
				CrCl 30–59 mL/min	CrCl 10–29mL/min	CrCl <10 or Dialysis		
Nucleoside Reverse Transcriptase Inhibitors (NRTIs)								
Abacavir (Ziagen)	300 mg tab; (see also: Trizivir); 20 mg/mL po soln	300 mg bid	No effect	Standard			Usual	Hypersensitivity: fever, rash, GI sx, dyspnea[3,6]
Combivir	Zidovudine 300 mg + lamivudine 150 mg (tab)	1 bid	No effect	Fixed formulation not recommended			Usual	Zidovudine side effects[3]
Didanosine (Videx EC)[1]	125, 200, 250, and 400 mg EC caps[2]	— EC caps with Tenofovir; >60 kg 400 mg qd; 250 mg qd; <60 kg 250 mg/d; 200 mg/d	½ hr before or 2 hr after meal Separate dosing of ATV, TPV/r	>60 kg 200 mg/d; <60 kg 125 mg/d	>60 kg 125 mg/d; <60 kg 100 mg/d	>60 kg 125 mg/d; <60 kg 75 mg/d[5]	Usual	Pancreatitis, peripheral neuropathy, GI intolerance[3]
Emtricitabine (Emtriva)	200 mg cap	200 mg qd	No effect	200 mg q72h		200 mg q96h	Usual	Minimal[3] HBV flare[10]
Lamivudine (Epivir)	150, 300 mg tab (see also: combivir & trizivir); 10 mg/mL po soln	150 mg bid or 300 mg qd	No effect	150 mg ×1 then 100 mg/d		150 mg ×1then 25–50 mg/kg/d	Usual	Minimal[3] HBV flare[10]
Epzicom	Lamivudine 300 mg + abacavir 600 mg	1 qd	No effect	Fixed formulation not recommended in renal failure			Usual	Abacavir hypersensitivity HBV flare[10]
Stavudine (Zerit)[1]	15, 20, 30, 40 mg cap; 1 mg/mL po soln	Wt >60 kg; 40 mg bid Wt <60 kg; 30 mg bid	No effect	>60 kg 20 mg q12h; <60 kg 15mg q12h	>60 kg 20 mg q24h <60 kg 15 mg q24h	>60 kg 20 mg q24h <60 kg 20 mg q24h[5]	Usual	Peripheral neuropathy, pancreatitis, lipoatrophy, ascending paresis (rare)[3]
Tenofovir (Viread)	300 mg tab (see also: truvada)	300 mg qd	Take with meal	300 mg q48h	300 mg 2 d/wk	300 mg q7d[5]	Usual	Minimal. Renal toxicity (rare)[3] HBV flare[10]

Continued

Table 37–2 Antiretroviral Agent Characteristics—cont'd

Drug Name	Form	Usual Adult Dose	Food Effects	Renal Failure Dosing			Liver Failure Dosing	Toxicity
				CrCl 30–59 mL/min	CrCl 10–29mL/min	CrCl <10 or Dialysis		
Trizivir (TZV)	Zidovudine 300 mg + lamivudine 150 mg + abacavir 300 mg (tab)	1 bid	No effect	Fixed formulation not recommended in renal failure			Usual	Hypersensitivity-reaction (abacavir), bone marrow suppression (z), GI Intolerance (zidovudine)[3] HBV flare[10]
Truvada	Tenofovir 300 mg + emtricitabine 200 mg	1 qd	No effect	Fixed formulation not recommended in renal failure			Usual	Minimal. Renal toxicity, HBV flare[10]
Zidovudine (Retrovir)	100 cap, 300 mg tab; (see also: combivir & trizivir) 10 mg/mL IV soln 10 mg/mL po soln	300 mg bid 200 mg tid	No effect	300 mg bid	300 mg qd	100 mg tid	Usual	Peripheral neuropathy, stomatitis[3]
Protease Inhibitors (PIs)								
Atazanavir (Reyataz)	100, 150, and 200 mg capsules	400 mg qd; ATV 300 mg/retonavir 100 mg qd. Boosting is often preferred and is required if ATV is combined with tenofovir or EFV	Take with food. Avoid concurrent buffered ddI, antacids.	Standard			CPS 7–9: 300 mg qd CPS >9: Avoid	Benign increase in indirect bilirubin, GI intolerance, transaminitis, prolongation of QTc (caution with conduction defects or drugs that do this)[9]
Fosamprenavir[2] (Lexiva)	700 mg tabs	1,400 mg bid or 700 mg/retonavir 100 mg bid or 1,400 mg/retonavir 200 mg qd	No effect	Standard			CPS 5–8: 700 mg bid CPS >9: Avoid	Rash, GI intolerance, transaminitis, headache, hepatitis[9]

Drug (Brand)	Formulation	Dose	Food	Hepatic	Renal	Adverse Effects
Indinavir (Crixivan)	200, 333, 400 mg caps	800 mg q8h; separate buffered didanosine ≥1 hr IDV 400 mg/retonavir 400 mg bid or IDV 800 mg/retonavir 100–200 mg bid[4]	1 hr before or 2 hr after meal unless with retonavir	Standard	600 mg q8h	GI intolerance nephrolithiasis, transaminitis, benign increase in indirect bilirubin[9]
Lopinavir/ Ritonavir (Kaletra)	200/50 mg tabs; LPV 80 mg + retonavir 20 mg/mL po soln[2]	400 mg LPV + 100 mg retonavir (2 tabs) bid soln: 5 mL bid	No effect	Standard	7	Transaminitis, GI intolerance (esp. diarrhea), asthenia[9]
Nelfinavir (Viracept)	250, 625 mg tabs; 50 mg/g powder	1,250 mg bid or 750 mg tid	Take with high-fat meal	Standard	7	GI intolerance, diarrhea, transaminitis[9]
Ritonavir (Norvir)	100 mg caps, 600 mg/ 7.5 mL po soln	600 mg q12h[4]; separate didanosine ≥2 h	Food improves GI tolerance	Standard	7	GI intolerance, paresthesia, transaminitis, taste perversion[9]
Saquinavir[2] (Invirase)	200 mg caps, 500 mg tabs	SQV 1,000 mg bid + retonavir 100 bid[2] SQV 2,000 mg qd + retonavir 100 mg qd[2]	Take within 2 hr of meal	Standard	7	GI intolerance, transaminitis[9]
Tipranavir (Aptivus)	250 mg caps	500 mg bid with retonavir 200 mg bid	Take TPV and retonavir with food	Standard	CPS B or C: Avoid	Hepatotoxicity - monitor ALT, skin rash, GI intolerance, multiple drug interactions

Nonnucleoside Reverse Transcriptase Inhibitors (NNRTIs)

Drug (Brand)	Formulation	Dose	Food	Hepatic	Renal	Adverse Effects
Delavirdine (Rescriptor)	100, 200 mg tabs	400 mg tid	No effect	Standard	7	Rash
Efavirenz[8] (Sustiva)	50, 100, 200 mg caps, 600 mg tabs	600 mg hs	Avoid high-fat meal	Standard	7	CNS ×2–3 wk, rash, hepatitis, false + cannibinoid test
Nevirapine (Viramune)	200 mg tabs 50 mg/5 mL po susp	200 mg qd ×14 d, then 200 mg bid	No effect	Standard	Avoid	Standard; give post-dialysis; Rash, hepatitis; hepatic necrosis esp women with CD4 >250 in first 6 wk

Continued

Table 37–2 Antiretroviral Agent Characteristics—cont'd

Drug Name	Form	Usual Adult Dose	Food Effects	Renal Failure Dosing			Liver Failure Dosing	Toxicity
				CrCl 30–59 mL/min	CrCl 10–29mL/min	CrCl <10 or Dialysis		
Rilpivirine (Edurant)	50 mg tabs	50 mg/d	Take with a meal of ~400 kcal (13 g of fat. Avoid PPIs.)					Rash and psychiatric disorders
Fusion Inhibitors								
Enfuvirtide (Fuzeon, T-20)	90 mg single-use vials to be reconstituted with 1.1 mL H₂0	90 mg (1 mL) SQ q12h into upper arm, anterior or abdomen (rotate sites)	N/A	Standard			Usual dose	Site reactions
CCR5 Antagonists								
Maraviroc (Selzentry)	150 & 300 mg tabs	300 mg bid with all NRTIs; nevirapine, tipranavir; enfuvirtide 150 mg bid CYP3A inhibitors (with or without a strong CYP3A inducer); protease inhibitors (other than tipranavir); delavirdine 600 mg bid CYP3A inducer (if used without a strong CYP3A inhibitor [see above]): CYP3A inducer (if used without a strong CYP3A inhibitor [see above]): efavirenz; etravirine	N/A	Standard	Not recommended	Not recommended	Monitored closely for adverse events	Rash and hepatotoxicity
Integrase Strand Transfer Inhibitors								
Raltegravir (Isentress)	400 mg tabs	400 mg bid	N/A	Standard			Monitor for toxicity	Rash & insomnia

1 The combination of didanosine and stavudine "should be used in pregnant women only when the potential benefit clearly outweighs the potential risk." Efavirenz should be avoided in first trimester of pregnancy and used with caution in women with reproductive potential. Avoid APV liquid in pregnancy.

2 The following are no longer available: buffered didanosine, lopinovir/r 133/33 mg cap, amprenavir, or fortovase.

3 Class adverse reaction: lactic acidosis with steatosis. Most common with stavudine, ddl, and zidovudine.

4 Various dosing recommendations when using dual PI, PI plus NRTI, or dual PI plus NNRTI.

5 Give post-dialysis

CPS = Child Pugh Score

6 Registry for hypersensitivity: 1-800-270-0425.

7 More frequent monitoring required. Drug change or dose change could be considered on a case-by-case basis noting the risk of resistance with underdosing.

8 Efavirenz should be avoided in first trimester of pregnancy and used with caution in women with reproductive potential. Avoid APV liquid in pregnancy.

9 Class adverse effects include lipodystrophy with hyperglycemia, fat redistribution, hyperlipidemia, and possible increased bleeding with hemophilia. ATV does not cause hyperlipidemia. All PIs may cause elevated transaminases.

10 Lamivudine, emtricitabine, and tenofovir; risk of flare of chronic HBV if discontinued.

Adapted from "Tools for Grantees: A Pocket Guide to Adult HIV/AIDS Treatment February 2006 edition" (HRSA, 2006).

transcriptase copies the HIV single-stranded RNA genome into a double-stranded HIV DNA. The HIV DNA is then integrated into the host chromosomal DNA, which allows host cellular processes such as transcription and translation (supra) to reproduce HIV. NRTIs/NtRTIs block the function of reverse transcriptase and prevent completion of synthesis of the double-stranded HIV DNA, thereby preventing HIV from reproducing. Whereas NRTIs/NtRTIs are analogues of the naturally occurring deoxynucleotides needed to synthesize the viral DNA, their mode of action is to compete with the natural deoxynucleotides for incorporation into the growing viral DNA chain. However, unlike the natural deoxynucleotides substrates, NRTIs/NtRTIs lack a 3'-hydroxyl group on the deoxyribose moiety. Thus, following incorporation of an NRTI/NtRTI, the next incoming deoxynucleotide cannot form the next 5'-3' phosphodiester bond needed to extend the DNA chain. So, when an NRTI/NtRTI is incorporated, viral DNA synthesis is prevented, a process known as chain termination. All NRTIs/NtRTIs are competitive substrate inhibitors.

Most NRITs/NtRTIs are eliminated via the kidneys so as to require renal adjustment when creatinine clearance is less than 50 mL/minute. Abacavir is eliminated by a complex mechanism in the liver. Therefore, it does not require renal function adjustment. However, the half-life of abacavir is increased in mild hepatic impairment and must be dose-adjusted for Child-Pugh class A and it is contraindicated for classes B and C. Common side effects of the NRTI/NtRTI class include anemia, bone marrow suppression, flatulence, headache, myopathy, nausea, rash, renal issues, and vomiting.

Symptomatic and life-threatening lactic acidosis may occur with NRTIs. Lactic acidosis occurs more commonly in patients with hepatomegaly and hepatic steatosis. Abacavir is contraindicated in HLA B*5701 positive patients. Genetic screening for B*5701 effectively predicts the high probability of abacavir-associated hypersensitivity reaction, a multisystem syndrome that produces a constellation of symptoms that may include rash, fever, respiratory symptoms, or gastrointestinal symptoms. Abacavir-associated hypersensitive reaction can be fatal if abacavir is continued or is rechallenged. Didanosine and stavudine are associated with peripheral neuropathy and pancreatitis. Tenofovir is associated with a variety of side effects, including decreased bone mineral density; increased biochemical markers of bone metabolism; acute renal failure; acute tubular necrosis; decreased urine volume; Fanconi syndrome; renal impairment; increased creatinine; interstitial nephritis (including acute cases); nephritis; nephrogenic diabetes insipidus; new onset or worsening renal, proximal renal tubulopathy, renal failure, and renal insufficiency.

NRTI/NtRTIs are sometimes prescribed in fixed-dose (fd) combination formulations with other NRTI/NtRTIs and other antiretrovirals agents to decrease pill burden and simplify ART regimens. Emtricitabine, lamivudine, and tenofovir are also active against hepatitis B virus.

Nonnucleoside Reverse Transcriptase Inhibitors

Nonnucleoside reverse transcriptase inhibitors (NNRTIs), also known as nonnucleosides or nonnukes, attach themselves to reverse transcriptase and prevent the enzyme from converting RNA to DNA. As a result, HIV's genetic material cannot be incorporated into the healthy genetic material of the cell, which prevents the cell from producing new virus. The pharmacokinetics of NNRTIs are complex. Although possessing a common mechanism of action, the approved NNRTIs—delavirdine, efavirenz, etravirine, nevirapine, and rilpivirine—differ in structural and pharmacokinetic characteristics. Each undergoes biotransformation by the CYPP450 enzyme system. This makes them prone to clinically significant drug interactions when combined with other ARTs. NNRTIs interact with other concurrent medications and complementary/alternative medicines, acting as either inducers or inhibitors of drug-metabolizing CYP450 enzymes. These drug interactions become an important consideration in clinical use when designing combination regimens, as recommended by current guidelines. Common side effects of the NNRTI class include: difficulty sleeping, dizziness, drowsiness, fatigue, headache, liver problems (which can be severe and life-threatening), nausea, vomiting, diarrhea, rash (which can be severe), and vivid dreams.

Protease Inhibitors

Protease inhibitors (PIs) are a class of medications used to treat or prevent viral infection such as HIV and hepatitis C. HIV-PIs prevent viral replication by inhibiting the enzyme activity of HIV-1 protease in the CD4 cell that cleaves nascent proteins for final assembly of new virions. All PIs have a similar mechanism of action and do not depend on intracellular conversion to be active in the host cell. Available PIs include atazanavir, fosamprenavir, indinavir, lopinavir/ritonavir, nelfinavir, ritonavir, saquinavir, and tipranavir. Like NNRTIs, PIs are metabolized by CYP450 enzymes. This makes PIs subject to drug interactions with other medicines that use the CYP450 pathway. Ritonavir is a very potent CYP450 inhibitor of other PIs (except nelfinavir) and therefore is commonly paired in low doses to pharmacokinetically intensify the half-life of other PIs in a prescribing practice known as ritonavir boosting. Drug interactions with boosted and nonboosted PIs must be considered when devising an effective, well-tolerated ART regimen. PIs are eliminated in the feces and do not require renal dosing adjustment. Common side effects of the PI class include: bleeding problems, diarrhea, gastrointestinal disturbance, hyperglycemia, hyperlipidemia, lipodystrophy, and liver problems that can be severe.

Integrase Strand Transfer Inhibitors

Integrase strand transfer inhibitors (INSTIs) prevent insertion of HIV DNA into the human DNA genome, thereby blocking the ability of HIV to replicate. Integrase is an enzyme that allows HIV genetic material to integrate into the DNA of human CD4 cells, making it possible for the infected cell to make new copies of HIV. By interfering with integrase, INSTIs prevent HIV genetic material from integrating into the CD4 cell, thus stopping viral replication. The stage in which HIV genetic material is integrated into human DNA is not fully understood. For that reason, developing an effective integrase inhibitor was not easy and many INSTIs failed very early in clinical trials.

However, raltegravir (2007) and cobicistat-boosted elvitegravir (2012) were approved by the FDA. They act at the final phase of integration when the viral strand is transferred into the host cell. Integrase inhibitors should be used with caution when administered with strong inducers of uridine diphosphate glucuronosyltransferase (UGT1A1), including rifampin. These inducers of UGT1A1 may reduce plasma concentrations of raltegravir. Similar to rifampin, ritonavir-boosted tipranavir reduces plasma concentrations of raltegravir. The most common side effects related to raltegravir are creatinine kinase elevations, diarrhea, headache, myopathy, nausea, pyrexia, and rhabdomyolysis. The most common side effects of elvitegravier include nausea and diarrhea, upper respiratory tract infections and bronchitis, back and joint pain, and urinary tract infections; cobicistat is associated with gastrointestinal side effects, including nausea, vomiting, and diarrhea. Cobicistat may also exacerbate kidney impairment in some people.

CCR5 Antagonists

CCR5 antagonists selectively bind to the human chemokine receptor CCR5 present on the cell membrane, preventing the interaction of HIV-1 gp120 and CCR5, which is necessary for CCR5-tropic HIV-1 to enter cells. Maraviroc is only one CCR5 antagonist licensed by the FDA. CXCR4-tropic and dual-tropic HIV-1 entry are not inhibited by maraviroc. Maraviroc is a selective, slowly reversible, small molecule. It is a substrate of CYP3A and Pgp; therefore, its pharmacokinetics are modulated by inhibitors and inducers of these enzymes/transporters. The CYP3A/Pgp inhibitors ketoconazole, lopinavir/ritonavir, ritonavir, darunavir/ritonavir, saquinavir/ritonavir, and atazanavir ± ritonavir all increase the C_{max} and the area under the curve (AUC) of maraviroc. The CYP3A inducers rifampin, etravirine, and efavirenz decreased the C_{max} and AUC of maraviroc. The most common adverse events reported with maraviroc are cough, dizziness, pyrexia, rash, and upper respiratory tract infections. Additional adverse events include diarrhea, edema, esophageal candidiasis, influenza, parasomnias, rhinitis, sleep disorders, and urinary abnormalities.

Fusion Inhibitors

Fusion inhibitors work by attaching themselves to proteins on the surface of CD4 cells or proteins on the surface of HIV and thereby prevent fusion of HIV-1 with CD4 cells. Enfuvirtide, the only FDA-approved entry inhibitor that targets the gp120 or gp41 proteins on HIV's surface, was licensed in 2003. By binding to the first heptad-repeat (HR1) in the gp41 subunit of the viral envelope glycoprotein and preventing the conformational changes required for the fusion of viral and cellular membranes, enfuvirtide interferes with the entry of HIV-1 into cells by inhibiting fusion of viral and cellular membranes. Enfuvirtide is not an inhibitor of CYP450 enzymes. Coadministration of enfuvirtide and other drugs that are inducers or inhibitors of CYP450 is not expected to alter the pharmacokinetics of enfuvirtide. Common side effects of enfuvirtide include skin itchiness, swelling, and pain at the site of the injection (injection site reactions). Other side effects may include dizziness, fatigue, insomnia, and numbness in feet or legs.

COST CONSIDERATIONS

HIV medicines are very expensive. Medication costs vary widely, depending on the choice of medications; the complexity of the ART regimen; where medications are purchased, neighborhood pharmacy versus mail order; and who is doing the purchasing, government versus individual. For most patients, private insurance providers, Medicare, state Medicaid, drug assistance programs, state AIDS Drug Assistance Programs (ADAPs), or community resources pay most of the cost. Patient co-payments also vary widely by individual prescription insurance plan. Many pharmaceutical manufacturers of HIV drugs have implemented co-pay programs to provide financial assistance to patients who qualify financially and medically. Although HIV medications are very costly, not taking them can be even more costly (Chen et al, 2006). Table 37-3 provides some indication of the expense involved in the treatment of HIV.

AIDS Drug Assistance Program

The national AIDS Drug Assistance Program (ADAP) is a major source of medications for the treatment of HIV disease. The program is funded through Part B of the Ryan White HIV/AIDS Treatment Modernization Act (formerly known as the Ryan White Comprehensive AIDS Resources Emergency [CARE] Act), which provides grants to states and territories. Program funds may also be used to purchase health insurance for eligible clients and for services that enhance access to, adherence to, and monitoring of drug treatments. Grants are awarded to all 50 states, the District of Columbia, Puerto Rico, Guam, the U.S. Virgin Islands, and the Pacific jurisdictions. Congress mandates funds that must be used for the ADAP, an important distinction because other part B spending decisions are made locally.

Patient Assistance Programs

Over 250 pharmaceutical companies operate Patient Assistance Programs to assist the uninsured who cannot afford their medicine, including HIV medications. However, very few people know about these important programs and those that do often find that applying for them is a confusing and prohibitive process. It is very easy to learn how to advocate for financially challenged patients. There is a common HIV Patient Assistance Program application available at the federal Health Resources and Services Administration HIV/AIDS Programs Web site (http://hab.hrsa.gov/patientassistance).

Table 37–3 Brand-Name Antiretroviral Medications, Usual Adult Dosing, and Monthly Average Wholesale (AWP) Price by Mechanistic Class

Generic Name	Brand Name	Usual Adult Dose	AWP	RTV AWP Price*	Total
Nucleoside and Nucleotide Reverse Transcriptase Inhibitors (N/NTRTIs)					
Abacavir (ABC)	Generic	300 mg bid or 600 mg daily	$603		$615
Abacavir/lamivudine (ABC/3TC)	Epzicom	600/300 mg daily	$1,170		$1,073
Abacavir/lamivudine/ zidovudine (ABA/AZT/3TC)	Trizivir	300/150/300 mg bid	$1,840		$1,608
Didanosine (ddI)	Generic	400 mg EC daily if >60 kg or 250 mg EC daily if <60 kg	$236 $236		$425 $272
Emtricitabine (FTC)	Emtriva	200 mg daily	$544		$437
Emtricitabine/ tenofovir (FTC/TDF)	Truvada	200/300 mg daily	$1,467		$1,118
Lamivudine (3TC)	Generic	150 mg bid or 300 mg daily	$430		$458
Lamivudine/zidovudine (ZDV/3TC)	Generic	300/150 mg bid	$931		$993
Stavudine (d4T)	Generic	40 mg bid if >60 kg or 30 mg bid if <60 kg	$411 $403		$456 $448
Tenofovir (TDF)	Viread	300 mg daily	$942		$772
Zidovudine (ZDV)	Retrovir	300 mg bid	$360		$535
Nonnucleoside Reverse Transcriptase Inhibitors (NNRTIs)					
Efavirenz (EFV)	Sustiva	600 mg daily at bedtime	$785		$785
Etravirine (ETV)	Intelence	200 mg bid with a meal	$978		$978
Nevirapine (NVP)	Viramune	200 mg bid; dose if initiated at 200 mg daily for 14 d to reduce rash risk	$650		$650
	Viramune XR	400 mg daily	$708		$708
Rilpivirin (RPV)	Edurant	50 mg daily	$804		$804
Protease Inhibitors (PIs)					
Atazanavir (ATV)	Reyataz	400 mg daily (2 caps daily) or 300 mg daily + 100 mg RTV daily	$1,222 $1,165	$308	$1,222 $1,473
Darunavir (DRV)	Prezista	600 mg bid + 100 mg RTV bid	$1,230	$616	$1,846
		800 mg daily + ritonavir 100 mg daily	$1,102	$616	$1,846
Fosamprenavir (FPV)	Lexiva	1,400 mg daily + 100 mg ritonavir daily or 1,400 mg bid	$994 $1,988	$308	$1,302 $1,988
Indinavir (IDV)	Crixivan	800 mg q8h or 800 mg bid + 100–200 mg ritonavir bid	$548 $548	$616	$548 $1,164
Lopinavir/ritonavir (LPVr)	Kaletra	400/100 mg bid (2 tabs bid)	$871		$871
Nelfinavir (NFV)	Viracept	1,250 mg bid (2 bid)	$965		$965
Ritonavir (RTV)§	Norvir	100 mg daily 200 mg daily	$308 $616		$308 $616
Saquinavir mesylate (SQV)	Invirase	1,000 mg bid + RTV 100 mg	$1,121	$616	$1,737
Tipranavir (TPV)	Aptivus	500 mg bid with RTV 200 mg bid	$1,415	$1,242	$2,657

Continued

Table 37–3   **Brand-Name Antiretroviral Medications, Usual Adult Dosing, and Monthly Average Wholesale (AWP) Price by Mechanistic Class—cont'd**

Generic Name	Brand Name	Usual Adult Dose	AWP	RTV AWP Price*	Total
Fusion Inhibitors (FIs)					
Enfuviritide (T-20)	Fuzeon	90 mg by subcutaneous injection bid	$3,248		$3,248
CCR5 Antagonists					
Maraviroc (MVC)	Selzentry	300 mg bid	$1,260		$1,260
Integrase Strand Transfer Inhibitors (INSTIs)					
Raltegravir (RAL)	Isentress	400 mg bid	$1,228		$1,228
Fixed-Dose Tablets From More Than One Class					
Emtricitabine‡/ rilpivirine/tenofovir	Complera	200/50/300 mg once daily	$2,323		$2,323
Efavirenz/emtricitabine/ tenofovir	Atripla	600/200/300 mg once at hs	$2,253		$2,253
Elvitegravir/Cobicistat†/ Emtricitabine/Tenofovir	Stribild	150/150/200/ 300 mg once daily	$2,810		$2,810

§RTV (Norvir) coadministration as a "boosting-agent" that is required to achieve therapeutic drug levels and thereby adds to the ART cost.

‡ Elvitegravir is only available in the fixed-dose preparation, Stribild.

†Cobicistat is not active against HIV. It works by inhibiting an enzyme called CYP3A4 that is responsible for breaking down (or metabolism) of certain medications, including several HIV drugs. This helps boost the effectiveness of these drugs, while allowing fewer pills or doses on a daily basis.

Source: (AmerisouceBergen, 2013).

MEDICATION RESISTANCE

Antiretroviral medication resistance occurs when HIV replicates while the patient is taking ART. The replication may be the result of poor patient adherence to the ART regimen or possible drug–drug or drug–food interactions, abnormal absorption, distribution, metabolism, or excretion of the medicine, resulting in HIV replication and genetic mutational changes. The first sign of HIV resistance to ART is the presence of detectible plasma viral RNA on two separate viral load measurements. Various assays are used to determine the nature of HIV medication resistance. The most commonly used resistance assays are phenotypic and genotypic assays.

Phenotype assays are used to measure sensitivity to various antiretroviral agents. The assay reports HIV sensitivity in terms of a ratio above the normal or wild-type IC_{50}. In other words, it is the half-maximal (50%) inhibitory concentration (IC) of a medicine (50% IC, or IC_{50}). This information allows a provider to determine the relative extent of resistance. Genotype assays are used to identify the presence of specific resistance mutations of the HIV genes known to be associated with resistance to specific antiretroviral agents (Table 37-4).

Genotype testing identifies viral mutations on the reverse transcriptase (RT), protease (PR), envelope, and integrase genes. Notation of the specific mutations is standardized by identifying the first letter of the usual amino acid, the location on the gene (number), followed by the first letter of the amino acid change related to the mutation. For example, the M184V mutation conveys that on the 184 position of the RT enzyme, the methionine amino acid residue was replaced with a valine amino acid residue. This is one of the most commonly associated cytosine analogue-resistant mutations to confer high-level resistance to medications such as emtricitabine and lamivudine. Other RT gene mutations, such as M41L, D67N, K70R, L210W, T215Y/F, and K219O/E, are more commonly known as thymidine analogue mutations, or TAMs. The presence of these mutations affects all NRTIs. K65R reduces viral sensitivity to abacavir, didanosine, emtricitabine, lamivudine, and tenofovir while increasing sensitivity to zidovudine (Grant et al, 2010). K103N, a major RT mutation, renders cross-resistance to efavirenz and nevirapine.

PR gene mutations are classified as critical and secondary. When present, PR mutations render HIV resistant to various PI agents. As the number of mutations emerges, HIV develops increasingly high-grade resistance whereby mutation can prevent the PI from binding to the catalytic site of action, allowing the normal gag-pol protein to be cleaved and form new virus. Like some RT mutations, some PR mutations confer broad, PI class cross-resistance to multiple medicines. L90M and I50L are two examples of very significant critical PR cross-resistance mutations.

Medication resistance to most PIs requires multiple mutations in the HIV protease and seldom develops following early virological failure, especially when ritonavir boosting is used. However, medication resistance to efavirenz or nevirapine is conferred by a single mutation in reverse transcriptase and develops rapidly following virological failure (Hirsch et al, 2003).

Table 37–4 Resistance Mutations to Antiretroviral Medicine

Antiretroviral Medicine	Codon Mutation	
Mutation in reverse transcriptase gene associated with resistance to NRTIs (nucleoside reverse transcriptase inhibitors)		
Multi-NRTI Resistance: 69 Insertion Complex (affects all NRTIs)		
	M41L, A62V, 69, K70R, L210W, T215Y/F, K219O/E	
Multi-NRTI Resistance: 151 Insertion Complex (affects all NRTIs)		
	A62V, V75I, F77L, F116Y, Q151M	
Multi-NRTI Resistance: Thymidine Analogue-Associated Mutations (TAMS; affects all NRTIs)		
	M41L, D67N, K70R, L210W, T215Y/F, K219O/E	
Abacavir (ABC)	K65R, L74V, Y115F, M184V	
Didanosine (ddI)	K65R, L74V	
Emtricitabine (FTC)	K65R, M184V	
Lamivudine (3TC)	K65R, M184V	
Stavudine (d4T)	M41L, K65R, D67N, K70R, L210W, T215Y/F, K219Q/E	
Tenofovir (TDF)	K65R, K70E	
Zidovudine (ZDV)	M41L, D67N, K60R, L210W, T215Y/F, K219Q/E	
Nonnucleoside Reverse Transcriptase Inhibitors (NNRTIs)		
Efavirenz (EFV)	L100I, K101P, K103N/S, V106M, V108I, Y181C/I, Y188L, G190S/A, P225H	
Etravirine (ETV)	V90I, A98G, L100I, K101E/H/P,V106I, E138A/G/K/Q,V179D/F/T, Y181C/I/V, G190S/A, M230L	
Nevirapine (NVP)	L100I, K101P, K103N/S, V106A/M, V108I, Y181C/I, Y188C/LH, G190S/A	
Rilpivirine (RPV)	L100I, K101P, K103N/S, V106A/M, V108I, Y181C/I, Y188C/L/II, G190S/A	

Mutation in the Protease Gene Associated With Resistance to Protease Inhibitors (PIs)		
PIs	*Critical*	*Secondary*
Atazanavir (ATV)	I50L, I84V, N88S	L10I/F/V/C, G16E, K20R/M/I/T/V, L24I, V32I, L33I/F/V, E34Q, M36I/L/V, M46I/L, G48V, F53L/Y, I54L/V/M/T/A, D60E, I62V, I64L/M/V, A71V/I/T/L, G73C/S/T/A, V82A/T/F/I, I85V, L90M, I93L/M
Darunavir/ritonavir (DRV/r)	I47V, I50V, I54M/L,	V11I, V32I, L33F, I47V, I50V, I54M/L, T74P, L76V, I84V, L89V
Fosamprenavir (FPV)	I50V, I84V	L10F/I/R/V, V32I,M46I/L, I47V, I50V, I54L/V/M, G73S, L76V, V82A/F/S/T, I84V, L90M
Indinavir/Ritonavir (IDVr)	M46I/L, V82A/F/T, I84V,	L10I/R/V, K20M/R, L24I, V32I, M36I, M46I/L, I54V, A71V/T, G73S/A, L76V, V77I, V82A/F/T, I84V, L90M
Lopinavir/Ritonavir (LPVr)	V32I, I47V/A, L76V, V82A/F/T/S	L10F/I/R/V, K20M/R, L24I, V32I, L33F, M46I/L, I47V/A, I50V, F53L, I54V/L/A/M/T/S, L63P, A71V/T, G73S, L76V, V82A/F/T/S, I84V, L90M
Nelfinavir (NFV)	D30N, L90M	L10F/I, D30N, M36I, M46I/L, A71V/T, V77I, V82A/F/T/S, I84V, N88D/S L90M
Saquinavir (SQV)	G48V, L90M	L10I/R/V, L24I, G48V, I54V/L, I62V, A71V/T, G73S, V77I, V82A/F/T/S, I84V, L90M,
Tipranavir (TPV)	I47V, Q58E, T74P, V82L/T, I84V	L10V, L33F, M36I/L/V, K43T, M46L, I47V, I54A/M/V, Q58E, H69K/R, T74P, V82L/T, N83D, I84V, L89I/M/V

Mutations in the Envelope Gene Associated With Resistance to Fusion Inhibitors (FIs) and CCR5 Antagonists		
Enfuviritide (T-20)	G36D/S, I37V, V38A/M/E, Q39R, Q40H, N42T, N43D	
Maraviroc (MVC)	Activity limited to CCR5 virus only. CXCR4-CCR5 mixed and CXCR4 viruses do not respond.	

Mutations in the Integrase Gene Associated With Resistance to Integrase Inhibitors (IIs)		
Raltegravir (RAL)	E92Q, Y143R/H/C, Q148H/K/R, N155H	

Adapted from Johnson et al, 2011.

Pretreatment

About one of every six new HIV cases diagnosed in 2007 involved virus with ARV drug-resistance mutations (CDC, 2010). The presence of transmitted medication-resistant viruses, particularly those with nonnucleoside reverse transcriptase inhibitor (NNRTI) mutations, may be responsible for not achieving the treatment goal of HIV suppression of less than 50 copies/mL (Wheeler, Mahle, & Bodnar, 2007). Therefore, pretreatment HIV genotypic resistance testing should be considered in selecting the best ART regimen.

Although covered by most insurance providers, resistance assays are expensive. Clinicians should be familiar with the important considerations and limitations associated with HIV resistance testing (Box 37-4) and be able to explain these to the patient. It is critical that, whenever possible, collection of blood for resistance testing should be performed when the patient is taking ART or within 4 weeks of stopping antiretroviral medicine. Resistance testing is not recommended when viral load (VL) is less than 1,000 copies/mL.

Virological Failure

Virological failure, defined as the failure to achieve or maintain suppression of viral replication to less than 50 copies/mL, may be categorized as either (1) incomplete virological response (as when two consecutive HIV RNAs are greater than 400 copies/mL after 24 wk or when HIV RNA is greater than 50 copies/mL by 48 wk in a treatment-naïve patient who is initiating ART), or (2) virological rebound (when HIV RNA is repeatedly detected at greater than 50 copies/mL after virological suppression). Baseline HIV RNA affects the time course of suppression. Some patients take longer than others to suppress HIV RNA levels. The timing, pattern, and/or slope of HIV RNA decrease may predict ultimate virological response (Weverling et al, 1998).

Unfortunately, there is no consensus on the optimal time to change ART when virological failure occurs. The more aggressive approach is to change the medication regimen for any repeated detectable viremia after suppression to less than 50 copies/mL in a patient taking ART. Again, an assessment of adherence is essential. Other approaches for when to change ART allow for detectable viremia up to an arbitrary level (e.g., 1,000 to 5,000 copies/mL when resistance testing can more easily be performed). However, ongoing viral replication in the presence of ART promotes the selection of drug-resistance mutations (Barbour et al, 2002) and may limit future ART options. Isolated episodes of viremia ("blips," e.g., single levels of 51 to 1,000 copies/mL) may simply represent laboratory variation (Nettles et al, 2005) and are not usually associated with subsequent virological failure. Rebound to higher viral load levels or more frequent episodes of viremia increase the risk of failure (Greub et al, 2002).

Causes of ART Failure

Although ART is highly successful, it is not without failure. Many factors are associated with an increased risk of ART treatment failure (Box 37-5). Suboptimal adherence and toxicity

---

BOX 37–4 HIV DRUG RESISTANCE TESTING: EIGHT IMPORTANT CONSIDERATIONS AND LIMITATIONS

1. Biological cutoffs are based on normal distribution of susceptibility to drug for wild-type strain from treatment-naïve patients.
2. Clinical cutoffs are based on data from clinical trials or cohort studies to determine change in susceptibility that results in reduced virological response.
3. Clinical phenotypic cutoff values include diminished versus no response; partial activity may be useful when treatment options are limited. Analysis complicated by prior drug exposure and activity of other drugs in salvage regimen.
4. Consider phenotyping over genotyping when treatment history is complex and/or significant resistance is expected.
5. May detect resistance only in species that make up more than 10% to 20% of viral population.
6. Measures susceptibility to individual medicines, not medication combinations.
7. Phenotypic resistance reported as fold change in IC_{50} for the test strain versus reference wild-type strain.
8. Testing should be performed on therapy whenever possible or within 4 weeks of stopping antiretroviral medicines and is not recommended when VL is less than 1,000 copies/mL.

BOX 37–5 FACTORS ASSOCIATED WITH ART FAILURE

Patient factors at baseline:
- AIDS diagnosis
- Comorbid conditions (e.g., affective mental health disorders and active substance use)
- Earlier calendar year of starting ART when less-potent regimens or more poorly tolerated antiretroviral medicines were used
- Higher pretreatment HIV RNA level (regimen-specific)
- Lower pretreatment or nadir CD4 T-cell count
- Pretreatment drug-resistant virus
- Prior ART failure, with development of drug resistance or cross-resistance
- ART adverse effects and toxicity
- Nonadherence to ART and medical appointments
- Suboptimal pharmacokinetics caused by variable absorption, metabolism, and/or penetration into HIV reservoirs, food or fasting requirements, adverse drug–drug interactions with concomitant medications and foods
- Suboptimal potency of the ART regimen
- Unknown causes

may account for 28% to 40% of treatment failures and regimen discontinuations (D'Arminio Monforte et al, 2000). Multiple risk factors for treatment failure can occur simultaneously. Factors not associated with treatment failure include gender, pregnancy, and history of past substance use.

When ART failure occurs, determining the cause(s) is essential. Candid conversation with the patient and his or her family member(s) coupled with investigation of pharmacy records allows the clinician to explore the various risk factors for ART failure. In assessing ART failure, it is important to identify as many contributing factors as possible. Careful identification of the reasons for failure allows the clinician to address patient needs more effectively and reduces the potential for subsequent ART failure.

Other circumstances should be considered when assessing for virological failure and planning for optimal patient outcomes. In some patients with extensive prior treatment and drug resistance (e.g., when new ART that contains at least two fully active agents cannot be identified), viral suppression below 50 copies/mL is difficult to achieve. When maximal virological suppression cannot be achieved, the goals are to preserve immunological function and to prevent clinical progression. Even partial virological suppression of HIV RNA greater than $0.5 \log_{10}$ copies/mL from baseline is associated with clinical benefits (Murray, Elashoff, Iacono-Connors, Cvetkovich, & Struble, 1999). However, these marginal benefits must be balanced with the ongoing risk for accumulating additional resistance mutations. It is reasonable to maintain a patient on the same regimen, rather than changing the regimen, depending on the stage of HIV disease.

DISCONTINUATION OR INTERRUPTION OF ANTIRETROVIRAL MEDICATIONS

Discontinuation or interruption of ART is associated with HIV viral rebound, immune decompensation, and clinical progression. Similarly, discontinuation of ART regimens containing emtricitabine, lamivudine, or tenofovir in patients with hepatitis B co-infection may experience an exacerbation of hepatitis on ART discontinuation (Bessesen, Ives, Condreay, Lawrence, & Sherman, 1999). Nonetheless, unplanned interruption of ART may become necessary for a number of reasons. Concurrent illness, severe drug toxicity, surgery that precludes oral therapy, and antiretroviral medication nonavailability are some of the common reasons patients discontinue ART. Potential risks and benefits of interruption vary according to a number of factors, including the clinical and immunological status of the patient, the reason for the interruption, the type and duration of the interruption, and the presence or absence of resistant HIV at the time of interruption.

Monitoring

Although ART prolongs life and improves quality of life by suppressing HIV replication and decreasing symptoms of uncontrolled HIV, ART is potentially harmful if not periodically monitored. Monitoring is multidimensional in the care of an HIV-infected patient. In addition to monitoring the effectiveness of ART, it is a standard of care to monitor the following:

- Adherence to medications and medical visits
- Affective mental health problems
- Alterations in metabolism of lipids and glucose
- Cardiovascular risk
- Hepatitis B and C co-infection
- High-risk behaviors
- Immunization status
- Renal and hepatic function
- Sexually transmitted infections
- Somatic signs and symptoms
- Tobacco, alcohol, and substance use

Plasma HIV RNA by PCR or "viral load" measures the effectiveness of ART to control viral replication. Sequential measurement of the CD4 count is performed to determine the degree of immune system reconstitution. When available, a viral load test is performed shortly after ART is started. If the treatment is working effectively, the viral load will drop to below the level of detection—less than 50 copies/mL. Ideally, this occurs within 24 weeks of initiating ART, but for some patients it can take 6 months. Viral load tests are performed every few months. As there can be some variability in viral load test results, they are monitored over a period of time. An increase in viral load may be followed by a fall in CD4 count and a greater risk of developing opportunistic infections. If viral load is increasing, it is important to determine the cause. Causes for loss of virological control are usually related to impaired medication adherence, drug interactions, altered medication absorption, and development of drug resistance.

OUTCOME EVALUATION

The patient-lived experience of HIV disease and the medications used to treat it are uniquely individual. Patients present to care at various stages of the disease, frequently challenged by multiple life circumstances that complicate the treatment plan. These challenges include, among others, active substance abuse, chronic pain, comorbid medical conditions, domestic violence, lack of child care, lack of health insurance, lack of transportation, mental illness, nonadherence to ART and provider visits, opportunistic infection(s), pregnancy, sexual abuse, stigma, unstable living conditions, and victimization. These challenges require a multidisciplinary team to optimize patient outcomes. Owing to complex social and medical problems, optimal patient outcomes are difficult to achieve. Thus, it is critical to formulate attainable treatment plans that are appropriately adapted to the individual patient and his or her living situation. A variety of personal and system barriers can potentially diminish patient resolve and confidence in lifelong treatment with ART. Positive predictors of success entail adherence to ART and routine surveillance for effectiveness of therapy and its potentially harmful events.

Although the path to treatment success is arduous without access to specialty HIV health care and modern ART, and drug toxicities and resistance continue to be formidable challengers, effective, well-tolerated therapies coupled with a pipeline of

On The Horizon: FIVE DRUGS FOR THE FUTURE

New HIV-drug development continues.

- **GS-7340** (tenofovir alafenamide, TAF), a new oral pro-drug, was well tolerated and had better antiviral activity at lower doses than tenofovir disoproxil fumarate (Viread, TDF) in early studies. Reportedly, in 38 people over 10 days, 25 mg of GS-7340 outperformed 300 mg of the currently approved tenofovir formulation. Along with fewer side effects, GS-7340 showed higher potency, which could mean longer and better viral suppression over time.

- **Dolutegravir** (GSK-572) is an investigational integrase inhibitor, but it has distinguished itself from the two approved integrase inhibitors, raltegravir (Isentress) and elvitegravir. Dolutegravir has a long half-life of 15 hours, indicating it can be taken once a day. It does not require pharmacokinetic boosting. Although resistance can occur, dolutegravir shows activity against raltegravir- and elvitegraivr-resistant viral strains. The drug may be coformulated in a once-daily pill with abacavir and lamivudine.

- **S/GSK-1265744 (744)**, an integrase inhibitor similar to dolutegravir, shows high potency and an exceedingly long half-life. Orally at once-daily doses of 30 mg, patients showed a median 2.6 log reduction in viral load. Interestingly, when using nanotechnology to formulate 744 to be injected subcutaneously or intramuscularly, a single dose showed a half-life between 21 and 50 days. After a single dose, patients had detectable levels of 744 up to 48 weeks after injection. Like dolutegravir, 744 seems to have a high barrier to drug resistance. 744 showed activity against raltegravir- and elvitegraivr-resistant viral strains. In terms of safety, there were some injection-site reactions and nodules associated with subcutaneous dosing. But conceivably, 744 could be taken as infrequently as every 3 months for treatment, or even as PrEP (pre-exposure prophylaxis).

- **Cenicriviroc (CVC),** an investigational CCR5 antagonist, not only antagonize CCR5 binding, it also antagonizes CCR2 binding. CCR2 is a receptor that sits on the surface of macrophages and may be involved in inflammation. CVC showed potent antiretroviral activity. Cenicriviroc has been found to be well absorbed and within the expected therapeutic range of potency. Further studies will assess the safety, efficacy, and effect of CCR2 inhibition on inflammatory biomarkers.

- **Albuvirtide** is a fusion inhibitor like enfuvirtide that offers a lot of activity against HIV but requires twice-daily injections. Albuvirtide, on the other hand, is an investigational fusion inhibitor that when given intravenously has a long average half-life of 11 days, warranting weekly dosing. Albuvirtide has a similar design to enfuvirtide. It is a peptide that is an analogue of gp41, one of the envelope proteins on HIV's surface, and thereby blocks HIV through CD4 membrane fusion. In very early studies, Albuvirtide was generally well tolerated, with no injection-site reactions and no serious adverse events.

evolving new medications herald a bright future for those chronically infected with HIV. HIV clinicians have immediate Internet access to current comprehensive treatment guidelines from the U.S. Department of Health and Human Services (DHHS) and the International AIDS Society—USA (IAS-USA).

CONCLUSION

Medical care for HIV-infected persons has grown increasingly complex and is beyond the scope of this chapter. However, a multiplicity of available resources exists to assist clinicians in providing high-quality care to their HIV-infected patients. The U.S. Department of Health and Human Services AIDSinfo Web site (http://www.aidsinfo.nih.gov/) is a dependable source of up-to-date information for the following:

- Fact sheets on HIV/AIDS-related drug interactions
- HIV treatment guidelines
- Locating resources on HIV/AIDS-related topics
- Preventive and therapeutic HIV vaccine research
- Research studies on investigational drugs, vaccines, and other new or existing treatments for HIV/AIDS

The Health Resources and Services Administration (HRSA) also provides multiple HIV medical care performance measures at ftp://ftp.hrsa.gov/hab/habGrp1PMs08.pdf. These performance measures can be used to help establish and measure the quality of HIV care being rendered. The performance measures include the following:

- ART adherence assessment and counseling
- ART for pregnant women
- Cervical cancer screening
- Frequency of CD4 measurement
- Hepatitis B vaccination
- Hepatitis C screening
- HIV risk counseling
- Lipid screening
- Medical evaluation visits
- Oral examination
- PCP prophylaxis
- Prescription of ART
- Syphilis screening
- TB screening

The following recommendations and treatment guidelines from the Centers for Disease Control and Prevention are also available at www.cdc.gov/hiv/resources/guidelines/index.htm:

- *A Guide to Primary Care for People With HIV/AIDS*
- *A Guide to the Clinical Care of Women With HIV*
- *Adults and Adolescent Treatment Guidelines*
- *Appendix: Recommendations to Help Patients Avoid Exposure to or Infection From Opportunistic Pathogens*
- *Co-Infection Guidelines*
- *Guidelines for Prevention and Treatment of Opportunistic Infections in HIV-Infected Adults and Adolescents*
- *Interim Guidance—HIV-Infected Adults and Adolescents: Considerations for Clinicians Regarding Swine-Origin Influenza A (H1N1) Virus*

- *MMWR: Guidelines for the Prevention and Treatment of Opportunistic Infections Among HIV-Exposed and HIV-Infected Children*
- *Pediatric Treatment Guidelines*
- *Perinatal Guidelines*
- *Sexually Transmitted Diseases Treatment Guidelines*
- *Tuberculosis Treatment Guidelines*

HIV DISEASE

PATIENT EDUCATION

Related to the Overall Treatment Plan/Disease Process

☐ After diagnosis, patients need to be educated regarding what it means to be HIV positive (they are infected with the HIV virus) versus what AIDS is (their immune system has been affected and they are at risk for life-threatening infections).

☐ Patients need education regarding the chronicity of HIV treatment. The clinician may make an analogy of HIV disease to diabetes; diabetics need insulin for the rest of their life and patients with HIV disease must take their medications daily for the rest of their lives.

☐ HIV-infected patients need to be vaccinated with the recommended adult vaccines, including an annual **influenza vaccine**.

☐ Symptoms of opportunistic infections should be discussed so that patients receive early treatment.

Specific to the Drug Therapy

☐ Highly active antiretroviral therapy (HAART) is a combination of medications and all should be taken together as prescribed to decrease viral load.

☐ Adherence to HAART is critical to prevent the development of drug resistance.

Reasons for Taking the Drug(s)

☐ Prevention of serious complications from AIDS.

☐ Prevention of transmission of infection to the uninfected (public health issue).

Drugs as Part of the Total Treatment Regimen

☐ Importance of seeking treatment when symptoms appear.

☐ Patients need routine preventive care, including lipid monitoring, cardiovascular health screening, cervical cancer screening, STI screening, and immunizations.

Adherence Issues

☐ Importance of following the HAART treatment regimen instructions to prevent resistance and to keep viral loads low.

☐ Importance of contacting the health-care provider if side effects or rash appears.

☐ The potential for drug interactions.

REFERENCES

AmerisouceBergen. (2013). Retrieved January 10, 2013, from http://www

AMFAR (2012). Statistics worldwide. *The Foundation for AIDS Research.* Retrieved January 6, 2013, from http://www.amfar.org/about_hiv_and_aids/facts_and_stats/statistics worldwide/

Ansari, A. F., & Etzel, J. V. (2000). Immune-based therapies for the management of HIV infection: Highly active antiretroviral therapy and beyond. *Journal of Pharmacy Practice, 13,* 515–532.

Barbour, J. D., Wrin, T., Grant, R. M., Martin, J. N., Segal, M. R., Petropoulos, C. J., et al. (2002). Evolution of phenotypic drug susceptibility and viral replication capacity during long-term virologic failure of protease inhibitor therapy in human immunodeficiency virus-infected adults. *Journal of Virology, 76,* 11104–11112.

Bennett, J. A. (2003). Historical overview of the HIV pandemic. In C. Kirton (Ed.), *ANAC's core curriculum for HIV/AIDS nursing* (2nd ed., pp 22–29). Thousand Oaks, CA: Sage.

Bessesen, M., Ives, D., Condreay, L., Lawrence, S., & Sherman, K. E. (1999). Chronic active hepatitis B exacerbations in human immunodeficiency virus-infected patients following development of resistance to or withdrawal of lamivudine. *Clinical Infectious Diseases, 28,* 1032–1035.

Centers for Disease Control and Prevention (CDC). (1992). 1993 revised classification system for HIV infection and expanded surveillance case definition for AIDS among adolescents and adults. *MMWR Recommendations and Reports, 41*(RR-17). Retrieved January 10, 2013, from http://www.cdc.gov/mmwr/preview/mmwrhtml/00018871.htm

Centers for Disease Control and Prevention (CDC). (1998). Report of the NIH Panel to define principles of therapy of HIV infection and guidelines for the use of antiretroviral agents in HIV-infected adults and adolescents. *MMWR, 47*(RR-5), 1–82.

Centers for Disease Control and Prevention (CDC). (2010a). *HIV/AIDS surveillance report: Cases of HIV infection and AIDS in the United States and dependent areas, 2010s.* Retrieved January 6, 0213, from http://www.cdc.gov/hiv/topics/surveillance/basic.htm

Centers for Disease Control and Prevention (CDC). (2010b). Media release at the 17th Conference on Retroviruses and Opportunistic Infections (CROI), San Francisco. Retrieved January 6, 2013, from http://www.cdc.gov/media/pressrel/2010/r100217.htm

Chen, R. Y., Accortt, N. A., Westfall, A. O., Mugavero, M. J., Raper, J. L., Cloud, G. A., et al. (2006). Distribution of health care expenditures in HIV-infected patients. *Clinical Infectious Diseases, 42*(7), 1003–1010.

Chun, T. W., Engel, D., Berrey, M. M., Shea, T., Corey, L., & Fauci, A. S. (1998). Early establishment of a pool of latently infected, resting CD4(+) T cells during primary HIV-1 infection. *Proceedings of the National Academy of Sciences USA, 95,* 8869–8873.

Chun, T. W., Stuyver, L., Mizell, S. B., Ehler, L. A., Mican, J. A., & Baseler, M. (1997). Presence of an inducible HIV-1 latent reservoir during highly active antiretroviral therapy. *Proceedings of the National Academy of Sciences USA, 94,* 13193–13197.

Colagreco, J. P. (2003). Pathophysiology of HIV infection. In C. Kirton (Ed.), *ANAC's core curriculum for HIV/AIDS nursing* (2nd ed., pp 22–29). Thousand Oaks, CA: Sage.

D'Arminio Monforte, A., Lepri, A. C., Rezza, G., Pezzotti, P., Antinori, A., Phillips, A. N., et al. (2000). Insights into the reasons for discontinuation of the first highly active antiretroviral therapy (HAART) regimen in a cohort of antiretroviral naïve patients. I.CO.N.A. Study Group. Italian Cohort of Antiretroviral-Naïve Patients. *AIDS, 14,* 499–507.

Dragsted, U. B., Gerstoft, J., Pedersen, C., Peters, B., Duran, A., Obel, N., et al. (2003). Randomized trial to evaluate indinavir/ritonavir versus saquinavir/ritonavir in human immunodeficiency virus type 1-infected patients: The MaxCmin1 Trial. *Journal of Infectious Disease, 188,* 635–642.

Dragsted, U. B., Gerstoft, J., Youle, M., Fox, Z., Losso, M., Benetucci, J., et al. (2005). A randomized trial to evaluate lopinavir/ritonavir versus saquinavir/ritonavir in HIV-1-infected patients: The MaxCmin2 trial. *Antiviral Therapy, 10,* 735–743.

Finzi, D., Blankson, J., Siciliano, J. D., Margolick, J. B., Chadwick, K., & Pierson, T. (1999). Latent infection of CD4+ T cells provides a mechanism for lifelong persistence of HIV-1, even in patients on effective combination therapy. *Nature Medicine, 5,* 512–517.

Finzi, D., Hermankova, M., Pierson, T., Carruth, L. M., Buck, C., Chaissond R. E., et al. (1997). Identification of a reservoir for HIV-1 in patients on highly active antiretroviral therapy. *Science, 278,* 1295–1300.

Freeman, E., & Winland-Brown, J. E. (2001). Hematologic and immune problems. In L. M. Dunphy & J. E. Winland-Brown (Eds.), *Primary care: The art and science of advanced practice nursing* (pp 959–1024). Philadelphia: F. A. Davis.

Gallant, J. E., Staszewski, S., Pozniak, A. L., DeJesus, E., Suleiman, J. M., Miller, M. D., et al. (2004). Efficacy and safety of tenofovir DF vs. stavudine in combination therapy in antiretroviral-naïve patients: A 3-year randomized trial. *Journal of the American Medical Association, 292,* 191–201.

Garcia, P. M., Kalish, L. A., Pitt, J., Minkoff, H., Quinn, T. C., Burchett, S. K., et al. (1999). Maternal levels of plasma human immunodeficiency virus type 1 RNA and the risk of perinatal transmission. Women and Infants Transmission Study Group. *New England Journal of Medicine, 341,* 394–402.

Grant, P. M., Taylor, J., Nevins, A. B., Calvez, V., Marcelin, A. G., Wirden, M., et al. (2010). International cohort analysis of the antiviral activities of zidovudine and tenofovir in the presence of the K65R mutation in reverse transcriptase. *Antimicrobial Agents and Chemotherapy, 54*(4), 1520–1525.

Greub, G., Cozzi-Lepri, A., Ledergerber, B., Staszewski, S., Perrin, L., Miller, V., et al. (2002). Intermittent and sustained low-level HIV viral rebound in patients receiving potent antiretroviral therapy. *AIDS, 16,* 1967–1069.

Gulick, R. M., Ribaudo, H. J., Shikuma, C. M., Lalama, C., Schackman, B. R., Meyer, W. A., III, et al. (2006). Three- vs. four-drug antiretroviral regimens for the initial treatment of HIV-1 infection: A randomized controlled trial. *Journal of the American Medical Association, 296,* 769–781.

Health Resources and Services Administration. (2006, February). *Tools for grantees: A pocket guide to adult HIV/AIDS treatment.* Retrieved January 6, 2013, from http://hab.hrsa.gov/tools/HIVpocketguide/PktGDrugTables.htm#DrugTable2

Hirsch, M. S., Brun-Vezinet, F., Clotet, B., Conway, B., Kuritzkes, D. R., D'Aquila, R. T., et al. (2003). Antiretroviral drug resistance testing in adults infected with human immunodeficiency virus type 1: 2003 recommendations of an International AIDS Society-USA Panel. *Clinical Infectious Diseases, 37*(1), 113–128.

Johnson, V. A., Calvez, V., Gunthard, H. F., Paredes, R., Pillay, D., Shafer, R. W., et al. (2011). Update of the drug resistance mutations in HIV-1: 2011. Retrieved January 06, 2013, from https://www.iasusa.org/content/2011-update-drug-resistance-mutations-hiv-1.

Kilby, J. M., & Eron, J. J. (2003). Novel therapies based on mechanisms of HIV-1 cell entry. *New England Journal of Medicine, 22,* 2228–2238.

Kirton, C. (Ed.). (2003). *ANAC's core curriculum for HIV/AIDS nursing* (2nd ed.). Thousand Oaks, CA: Sage.

Matassa, M. (2011). Initiation of antiretroviral treatment protects unifected sexual partners from HIV infection (PHTN 052). Retrieved January 06, 2013, from http://www.hptn.org/web%20documents/PressReleases/HPTN052PressReleaseFINAL5_12_118am.pdf

Mellors, J. W., Rinaldo, C. R., Jr., Gupta, P., White, R. M., Todd, J. A., & Kingsley, L. A. (1996). Prognosis in HIV-1 infection predicted by the quantity of virus in plasma. *Science, 272,* 1167–1170.

Mocroft, A., Vella, S., Benfield, T. L., Chiesi, A., Miller, V., & Gargalianos, P. (1998). Changing patterns of mortality across Europe in patients infected with HIV-1. EuroSIDA Study Group. *The Lancet, 352,* 1725–1730.

Mofenson, L. M., Lambert, J. S., Stiehm, E. R., Bethel, J., Meyer, W. A., & Whitehouse, J. (1999). Risk factors for perinatal transmission of human immunodeficiency virus type 1 in women treated with zidovudine. Pediatric AIDS Clinical Trials Group Study 185 Team. *New England Journal of Medicine, 341,* 385–393.

Moore, R. D., Keruly, J. C., Gebo, K. A., & Lucas, G. M. (2005). An improvement in virologic response to highly active antiretroviral therapy in clinical practice from 1996 through 2002. *Journal of Acquired Immune Deficiency Syndrome, 39,* 195–198.

Moyle, G., Gatell, J., Perno, C. F., Ratanasuwan, W., Schechter, M., & Tsoukas, C. (2008). Potential for new antiretrovirals to address unmet needs in the management of HIV-1 infection. *AIDS Patient Care STDS, 22,* 459–471.

Murray, J. S., Elashoff, M. R., Iacono-Connors, L. C., Cvetkovich, T. A., & Struble, K. A. (1999). The use of plasma HIV RNA as a study endpoint in efficacy trials of antiretroviral drugs. *AIDS, 13,* 797–804.

Nettles, R. E., Kieffer, T. L., Kwon, P., Monie, D., Han, Y., Parsons, T., et al. (2005). Intermittent HIV-1 viremia (blips) and drug resistance in patients receiving HAART. *Journal of the American Medical Association, 293,* 817–829.

NIAID. (2013). National Institute of Allergy and Infectious Disease. *HIV replication cycle.* Retrieved January 06, 0213, from http://www.niaid.nih.gov/topics/HIVAIDS/Understanding/Biology/pages/hivreplicationcycle.aspx

Palella, F. J., Delaney, K. M., Moorman, A. C., Loveless, M. O., Fuhrer, J., & Satten, G. A. (1998). Declining morbidity and mortality among patients with advanced human immunodeficiency virus infection. HIV Outpatient Study Investigators. *New England Journal of Medicine, 338,* 853–860.

Panel on Antiretroviral Guidelines for Adults and Adolescents. (2012, March). *Guidelines for the use of antiretroviral agents in HIV-1-infected adults and adolescents.* Department of Health and Human Services. Retrieved January 06, 2013, from http://aidsinfo.nih.gov/contentfiles/lvguidelines/adultandadolescentgl.pdf

Perinatal HIV Guidelines Working Group. (2009, April). *Public Health Service Task Force recommendations for use of antiretroviral drugs in pregnant HIV-infected women for maternal health and interventions to reduce perinatal HIV transmission in the United States.* Retrieved January 1, 2013, from http://aidsinfo.nih.gov/ContentFiles/PerinatalGL.pdf

Riddler, S. A., Haubrich, R., DiRienzo, A. G., Peeples, L., Powderly, W. G., Klingman, K. L., et al. (2006, August). A prospective, randomized, phase III trial of NRTI-, PI-, and NNRTI-sparing regimens for initial treatment of HIV-1 infection—ACTG 5142 [Abstract THLB0204]. XVI International AIDS Conference, Toronto, Canada.

Rodriguez, B., Sethi, A. K., Cheruvu, V. K., Mackay, W., Bosch, R. J., Kitahata, M., et al. (2006). Predictive value of plasma HIV RNA level on rate of CD4 T-cell decline in untreated HIV infection. *Journal of the American Medical Association, 296,* 1498–1506.

Shulman, N., Zolopa, A., Havlir, D., Hsu, A., Renz, C., Boller, S., et al. (2002). Virtual inhibitory quotient predicts response to ritonavir boosting of indinavir-based therapy in human immunodeficiency virus-infected patients with ongoing viremia. *Antimicrobial Agents & Chemotherapy, 46,* 3907–3916.

Squires, K., Lazzarin, A., Gatell, J. M., Powderly, W. G., Pokrovskiy, V., Delfraissy, J. F., et al. (2004). Comparison of once-daily atazanavir with efavirenz, each in combination with fixed-dose zidovudine and lamivudine, as initial therapy for patients infected with HIV. *Journal of Acquired Immune Deficiency Syndrome, 36,* 1011–1019.

Staszewski, S., Morales-Ramirez, J., Tashima, K. T., Rachlis, A., Skiest, D., Stanford, J., et al. (1999). Efavirenz plus zidovudine and lamivudine, efavirenz plus indinavir, and indinavir plus zidovudine and lamivudine in the treatment of HIV-1 infection in adults. *New England Journal of Medicine, 341,* 1865–1873.

Vittinghoff, E., Scheer, S., O'Malley, P., Colfax, G., Holmberg, S. D., & Buchbinder, S. P. (1999). Combination antiretroviral therapy and recent declines in AIDS incidence and mortality. *Journal of Infectious Diseases, 179,* 717–720.

Weverling, G. J., Lange, J. M., Jurriaans, S., Prins, J. M., Lukashov, V. V., Notermans, D. W., et al. (1998). Alternative multidrug regimen provides improved suppression of HIV-1 replication over triple therapy. *AIDS, 12,* F117–122.

Wheeler, W., Mahle, K., & Bodnar, U. (2007, February). *Antiretroviral drug-resistance mutations and subtypes in drug-naive persons newly diagnosed with HIV-1 infection.* Poster session presented at the annual meeting of the Conference on Retroviruses and Opportunistic Infections, Los Angeles, CA.

Wong, J. K., Hezareh, M., Günthard, H. F., Havlir, D. V., Ignacio, C. C., & Spina, C. A. (1997). Recovery of replication-competent HIV despite prolonged suppression of plasma viremia. *Science, 278,* 1291–1295

World Health Organization. (2012). *Global health observatory.* WHO programs and projects. Retrieved January 06, 2013, from http://www.who.int/gho/hiv/en/index.html

CHAPTER 38

HORMONE REPLACEMENT THERAPY AND OSTEOPOROSIS

Marylou V. Robinson

HORMONE REPLACEMENT THERAPY

Hormone replacement therapy (HRT) may be instituted any time there is loss of the body's ability to produce estrogen and progestin. This would include surgical removal of the ovaries as well as menopause. The term ERT is used to differentiate estrogen-only replacement therapy. General recommendations from the American Academy of Obstetricians and Gynecologists (ACOG), the American Society of Reproductive Medicine, the National Association of Nurse Practitioners in Women's Health, the North American Menopause Society, and the U.S. Preventative Services Task Force (USPSTF), along with the U.S. Food and Drug Administration (FDA), support the use of ERT/HRT for the treatment of moderate to severe menopausal symptoms.

The use of ERT/HRT to treat and prevent other chronic illness, with the exception of osteoporosis, is no longer encouraged (USPSTF, 2013). Consideration of alternative osteoporosis treatments for women who are not also experiencing menopausal symptoms must be made. Current use guidelines for ERT/HRT propose utilizing the lowest dose of hormones for the shortest duration possible to help increase the quality of life and decrease the sometimes dramatically disruptive symptoms of menopause. The Woman's Health Initiative (WHI) results and subsequent guidelines indicate that replacement therapy for up to 5 years is reasonably safe (Writing Group for the Women's Health Initiative [WHI] Investigators, 2002).

The WHI, which was started in 1991 and planned a longitudinal study of participants over 15 years, took the broadest look at all the purported health benefits of HRT and ERT. The HRT arm of the study was stopped in 2002 due to a negative risk-to-benefit ratio showing an increased incidence of heart disease, stroke, thromboembolic events, and breast cancer among women taking HRT agents of conjugated estrogen (Premarin) and medroxyprogesterone. The ERT arm was also stopped early in 2004 because of increased risk of stroke in women taking estrogen only. Age-cohort analysis of the WHI data suggests that the timing of initiation of ERT/HRT may play a role in coronary heart disease (CHD) risks. Women who initiate ERT/HRT at the time of menopause appear to be at less risk to develop CHD related to ERT/HRT use. Experts suggest that lower doses of hormones may be adequate to control the symptoms of menopause and not significantly raise the risk of CHD. See Box 38-1.

Pathophysiology

Between the ages of 42 and 56, most women experience a decline in ovarian hormone function, with the resultant natural cessation of menses. At menarche, the ovary starts production of three steroids: estrogen, progestin, and androgen. These three steroids have a dramatic effect on the brain, hypothalamus, pituitary, and the ovary itself. Sex hormones play an important role in the dynamic process of the formation and remodeling of neuronal circuits and neurotransmitters. The target organs of ovarian steroids are the uterine epithelium, the uterine tubes, the breasts, and the vagina. However, these hormones also play other important roles in the body.

In young women, the predominant hormone produced is 17β estradiol, the most biologically active estrogen. After menopause, there is more estrone, a derivative of estradiol. Adipose tissues have a major role in how much estrone is produced; hence the observed difference in menopausal symptoms can vary in thin versus obese women. Estriol is the least active and shortest-acting estrogen.

There are two major estrogen receptors, α and β. The alpha receptors are more plentiful in the breast, endometrium, and ovary. The beta receptors are found in bone, lung, and kidney and in many supporting tissues all around the body. Estrogen is not a reproductive-only active hormone. Its widespread impact creates the multisystem symptoms of menopause when levels naturally drop at the time of the climacteric.

Physiological Effects of Estrogen

Effects of estrogen on the reproductive system include maturation of reproductive organs; development of secondary sexual characteristics; regulation of menstrual cycle; and endometrial regeneration postmenstruation. Estrogen also affects closure of long bones after the pubertal growth spurt; maintains bone density by decreasing rate of bone resorption through antagonizing the effects of parathyroid hormone (PTH); maintains normal structure of skin and blood vessels through its actions on the endothelial cells in the arterial walls, including the induction of nitric oxide to facilitate vasodilation and oxygen uptake by cells; alters plasma lipids (increased high-density lipoprotein [HDL], slight reduction in low-density lipoprotein [LDL], reduced total cholesterol, increased triglycerides) through its action in the liver; reduces motility of the bowel through its modulation of sympathetic nervous system control over smooth muscle; alters production and activity of selected proteins resulting in higher levels of thyroxine-binding globulin, sex-hormone binding globulin, transferrin, and renin substrate; enhances coagulability of blood by increasing the production of fibrinogen; and facilitates loss of intravascular fluid into extracellular space by its action on the renin-angiotensin-aldosterone cycle (retention of sodium and water by the kidney) resulting in edema and decreased extracellular fluid (ECF) volume. In the brain, estrogen maintains stability of the thermoregulatory center. Decline in this function results in acute activation of the sympathetic nervous system and vasomotor instability, causing hot flashes.

Knowledge of the actions of estrogen on areas of the body beyond the reproductive organs combined with the epidemiological evidence of increased incidence of cardiac and related disorders postmenopause leads to the assumption that the lack of endogenous estrogen might be a major contributing factor to this increased incidence. From that conclusion, it was logical to assume that the administration of exogenous estrogen would prevent this problem. Subsequent randomized controlled trials (RCTs) found some flaws in this assumption and even found that use of replacement hormones increased the cardiovascular risk among women. The Heart and Estrogen/Progestin Replacement Study (HERS) studies found that neither ERT nor HRT increased nor decreased the incidence of CHD. The WHI study was halted early due to findings of a statistically significant increased incidence of CHD, stroke, thromboembolic events, and breast cancer in women taking HRT, and an increased incidence of stroke in women taking ERT. These results challenged the traditional use of ERT and HRT and raised significant clinical questions in the pharmacological management of postmenopausal women. As a result, the use of ERT and HRT to prevent cardiovascular disease is no longer recommended (USPSTF, 2013).

The concerns that having a hysterectomy, even without adding ERT/HRT afterward, could increase CHD appear to have been put partially to rest. The surgical menopause of having one or both ovaries removed has been tracked over 11 years in the SWAN study (Mathews, Gibson, El Khoudray, & Thurston, 2013). No additional heart disease risk, after a short rise after surgery, has come to light. Women over the age of 65 were not enrolled in this analysis. With the risk of CHD being highest after 65, transfer of these findings cannot be made to this overall higher-risk group.

From the PEPI (Post-menopausal Estrogen/Progestin Interventions) study through the WHI, studies looking at bone density and estrogen use consistently support the role of estrogen in the prevention of bone loss. Even relatively low doses of estrogen appear to have a beneficial effect on bone. The use of estrogen to prevent osteoporosis is discussed in detail below.

Physiological Effects of Progestin

Effects of progestin on the reproductive organs include thickening of the endometrium and increasing its complexity in preparation for pregnancy; thickening of cervical mucus; thinning the vaginal mucosa; and relaxation of smooth muscles of the uterus and fallopian tubes. During pregnancy, progestin maintains the thickened endometrium, relaxes myometrial muscles, thickens the myometrium for labor, is responsible for placental development, and prevents lactation until the fetus is born. In the absence of pregnancy, the reduced production of estrogen and progestin by the corpus luteum results in the shedding of the endometrium to produce menstruation. Progestin is also responsible for alveolobular development of the secretory apparatus of the breast. It also has actions outside the reproductive system. It stimulates lipoprotein activity and seems to favor fat deposition; increases basal insulin levels and insulin response to glucose; promotes glycogen storage in the liver; promotes ketogenesis; competes with aldosterone in the renal tubule to decrease Na+ resorption; increases body temperature; and increases ventilatory response to CO_2, resulting in a measurable decrease in $PaCO_2$. The latter occurs only during pregnancy.

Thickening of the endometrium related to estrogen stimulation is thought to increase the risk for endometrial cancer, and studies have supported a direct correlation between ERT use and an increased incidence of endometrial cancer (Thorneycroft, 2004). To prevent this occurrence, progestins have been added to HRT as a way to oppose the effects of estrogen on the endometrium and prevent endometrial hyperplasia. Topical progesterone creams and gels, however, do not reach the serum levels required to provide this protection (Pattimakiel &Thacker, 2011). The endometrial estrogen-related cancer risk is also correlated with estrogen dose and length of exposure. Thin women appear to be at greater risk (Brinton & Felix, 2013). These data, combined with the results of the HRT arm of the WHI, have raised concerns about whether the traditional combination estrogen-progestin therapy in a continuous mode is appropriate and are leading factors that contributed to the recommendations to use the lowest dose for the shortest duration possible, and limit treatment to less than 5 years.

Physiological Effects of Androgens

In the female, small amounts of androgens are produced in the ovary and the adrenal gland. Some are precursors to estrogen (androstenedione), serving as an alternate route to estrogen production. At puberty, androgens contribute to the skeletal growth spurt and growth of pubic and axillary hair, activate sebaceous glands (acne), and play a role in libido. Administration of exogenous androgens during menopause is often related to the role they play in skeletal growth and libido.

Menopausal Changes in Hormones

Perimenopause is the transitional period between reproductive and nonreproductive years. During this time approximately 90% of women experience extreme variability in frequency and quality of menstrual flow (McCance & Huether, 2014). Commonly, women experience a short cycle with a shortened follicular phase, ovulation, and insufficient luteal phase; followed by a long cycle with an extended follicular phase, anovulation, and high estradiol levels in the premenstrual phase; followed by a short follicular phase and an anovulation cycle. Perimenopausal cycles are correlated with elevated and irregular follicle-stimulating hormone (FSH), decreased inhibin, normal luteinizing hormone (LH), and slightly elevated estradiol levels. All of these are associated with reduced follicular genesis. The perimenopausal period may last for up to 10 years in some women, during which time hormone levels continue to fluctuate.

Menopause is a period of time in which no menses occur for 12 consecutive months when estrogen and progestin are low, despite FSH and LH levels that are increased due to lost ovary function. If left intact, the postmenopausal ovary continues to produce androgens. These androgens, as well as those from the adrenal gland, are then converted in fatty tissues into less potent estrogens: estrone and estriol. This peripheral conversion of androgens may vary greatly. This variation in peripheral conversion contributes to the spectrum of menopausal symptoms encountered in practice—some women pass through menopause with limited symptoms, whereas others experience severe vasomotor and vaginal symptoms.

These altered levels of hormones result in the symptoms common to the perimenopausal and postmenopausal period. Vasomotor symptoms, which typically begin during the perimenopausal transition, are actually caused by rapid changes in estrogen levels rather than low levels and tend to abate gradually over time for postmenopausal women. ERT/HRT are effective treatments for these symptoms, and data still support the use of both of these replacement therapies for this indication. Breast tissue involutes, yielding a moderate decrease in mammary tissue during perimenopause, and there is significant reduction in glandular breast tissue with an associated increase in fat deposits and connective tissue. Administration of exogenous estrogen (ERT) and HRT is associated with increased risk for breast cancer; however, the data regarding the relative risk of breast cancer among ERT/HRT users have been inconsistent. For women at increased risk of breast cancer, ERT/HRT is contraindicated. The immediate drop in breast cancer incidence following the WHI report has not been sustained, making some experts doubt the true nature of the breast cancer and estrogen risk (Shapiro, Farmer, Stevenson, Burger, & Mueck, 2012).

The urogenital tract also undergoes changes, but this tends to occur later than the vasomotor symptoms. The uterus atrophies and decreases in size. The vagina narrows, shortens, and loses some of its elasticity. Vaginal walls lose their ability to lubricate quickly. Intercourse may become painful. The vaginal pH increases, contributing to a higher incidence of vaginitis. The vaginal epithelium also atrophies, resulting in vaginal irritation, burning, itching, white discharge, and vaginal bleeding. Dyspareunia also results. Urethral tone declines and is associated with an increased risk for urinary frequency, urgency, and incontinence. Topical estrogen has been effective in helping to relieve these symptoms.

Other postmenopausal changes also occur outside the reproductive system. Bone mineral density is reduced, cardiovascular disorders increase, and the risk for various cancers increases. Some of these increased risks can be associated with normal aging, which makes it difficult to directly correlate them with loss of female hormones. In the past, ERT and HRT have been used in an attempt to prevent these disorders. However, large-scale studies have questioned the efficacy and safety of some of these uses.

After the WHI study, the pendulum has swung back and forth on the issue of whether to recommend ERT/HRT. A consensus statement made by the American Society for Reproductive Medicine, the Asia Pacific Menopause Federation, the Endocrine Society, the European Menopause and Andropause Society, the International Menopause Society, the International Osteoporosis Foundation, and the North American Menopause Society (NAMS) all agree that HRT should be used as the best solution for symptomatic menopause. The dose used should be the lowest possible to achieve a reduction of symptoms for individuals. One size does not fit all (NAMS, 2012).

Pharmacodynamics

Estrogens

Estrogen occurs naturally in the body in three forms: estradiol, estrone, and estriol. Estradiol (17β-estradiol) is the most potent and plentiful and is principally produced by the ovaries. The ovaries also produce estrone. Androgens are converted to estrone in ovarian and peripheral adipose tissue. Estriol is the principle metabolite of estrone and estradiol. Most all of the estrogens prescribed for ERT are estradiol, although there are formulations of estrone as well as combinations of estradiol and estrone.

Estradiol formulations are available as conjugated equine estrogen, which is marketed as Premarin, and as esterified estrogen (Menest). Both are taken orally. Premarin 0.625 mg, the most commonly prescribed dose, was the estrogen used in the WHI. Estradiol is also available in oral, injectable/depo, transdermal, and topical formulations (see Chapter 22). Oral drugs are subject to extensive metabolizing through the liver; this may explain some of their effects on lipids and coagulation factors. In contrast, the topical and transdermal formulations are not subject to first-pass metabolism and so have fewer associated changes in coagulation and changes in lipids. Transdermal meds are considered safer.

Estrone formulations include synthetic conjugated estrogen-A (Cenestin) and synthetic conjugated estrogen-B (Enjuvia). Both of these forms derive their estrogen from plant sources but are still manufactured in a laboratory. Plant-derived estrogens have not been shown to have reduced adverse effects over other estrogen sources.

A complexity of hormone therapy is that each of these chemicals has different interactions with the estrogen receptors in the body. Frustratingly, how likely a drug is to bind to a receptor is not correlated with how "potent" it is in creating a therapeutic change. High-affinity drugs with large amounts of 17β-estradiol can have the same impact as a low dose of a medication with low receptor affinity given over a longer time period. This creates many moving parts hard for nonspecialists to grasp, thereby they tend to prescribe a few medications and "hope for the best." Dissatisfied patients have migrated toward having an individualized dosing regimen provided to them using bioidentical and/or compounded substances.

Progestogens

Medroxyprogesterone (MPA) is the primary exogenous progestin prescribed, either alone or in combination with estrogens. It is a synthetic hormone manufactured and branded as Provera. It was the drug used in combination with estrogen (Prempro) in the WHI. Norethindrone (Aygestin) is another frequently used progestin. Their actions are similar to those of the body's own hormone. Two plant-derived "natural" hormones have FDA approval: micronized progesterone (Prometrium), which is taken orally, and Prochieve (also sold under the brand name Crinone), which is a bioadhesive vaginal gel. Use of the latter for hormone replacement is off-label; it has been approved for use in infertility and secondary amenorrhea. Like synthetic progestins, these "bioidentical" hormones are manufactured in the laboratory, so they are synthetic too.

Prescribers are cautioned not to interchange the name progesterone with progestin. MPA was the progesterone used in Prempro, which became the focus of the WHI warning and subsequent aversion to HRT. The other forms of progestogens have less severe chemical and biological impacts on risks such as cancer and inflammatory changes. MPA has a much higher level of bioavailability. Hence, research underway is trying to clarify if the strong warnings about MPA should also extend to the rest of the drug class. This is complex because the various progestogens differ in the way they interact with the receptors. This variance is the basis for the belief that there will be different breast cancer and cardiovascular endpoints; however, that evidence does not yet exist. What is understood, is that progesterone delivered topically does not generate enough antiproliferative impact on an intact uterus to prevent estrogen-induced hyperplasia (Pattimakiel & Thacker, 2011).

It should be noted that the FDA reserves the term *bioidentical* to substances made in compounding pharmacies. Unfortunately, the literature does not adhere to this definition. The more recent issues of quality and lack of standardization of compounding pharmacies makes use of these medication sources something that requires caution. Compounding has a real benefit for creating doses of ERT/HRT for women who are allergic to peanuts and other tree nuts; the micronized FDA forms of progesterone uses a peanut oil base.

All FDA-approved medications require notification to consumers about potential risky side effects. The compounding pharmacies are not required to do so. Because there are no lengthy precautionary handouts, women can get the impression they are somehow safer than the FDA drugs. This is inherently false, because many of the compounding recipes use the exact same ingredients as found in the formulary drugs, including the medications of concern in the WHI. Unlike the WHI medications, the other formulations of estrone, estradiol, and nonconjugated estrogens and other progestins have not been placed under the same level of scrutiny. The lack of longitudinal research cannot be falsely assumed to mean they have less risk (Flies, Ko, & Pruthi, 2011). Determination of less risk cannot be based on shorter-term observational studies. Likewise, there is no reason to believe these drugs offer higher risk. Prescribers are cautioned to counsel patients that we do not know the risk profile.

The American Society of Reproductive Medicine and ACOG have doubts that there are any real benefits from using these products and believe there are some risks associated with quality and purity issues. There are no known head-to-head studies. The major menopause societies do not recommend their use. Off-label use of medications brings inherent legal risk as well. The addition of substances such as DHEA, thyroid hormone, and androgens creates a more complex interaction with a women's physiology that has not been evaluated in controlled studies.

Goals of Treatment

The aim of ERT and HRT is to provide relief from symptoms associated with menopause. Under this general umbrella, the goals are to:

- Prevent or reduce vasomotor symptoms
- Prevent or reduce vaginal atrophy associated with estrogen decline
- Reduce the risk for osteoporosis
- Ensure that the benefits of ERT/HRT outweigh the risk associated with treatment by providing comprehensive pretreatment evaluation of contraindications and risk, and assisting women in making informed decisions about therapy

Treatment of menopausal symptoms and reduction of postmenopausal bone loss with hormone therapy, by prescription medications or herb supplements, have risks that require careful selection and screening of patients. Each woman should be assessed for the presence and severity of vasomotor and vaginal symptoms and screened for contraindications to therapy and predisposing diseases/risks that would increase the likelihood of an adverse event(s). Patient education requires comprehensive discussion of the current risk and benefits of therapy, the current indications for therapy (as these indications are evolving), review of practice recommendations regarding lowest effective dose for the shortest duration of time, and requirements for interval screening and follow-up while on therapy. Clinicians should be prepared to discuss details of the research findings heralded in the media as well as critically appraise an individual's risk for adverse events. A full review of the range of treatment options available, including the option for herbal therapies and the option not to engage in therapy, is critical in the management of women in the perimenopausal to postmenopausal years. The use of ERT/HRT is an intensely personal, emotional decision for many women since the release of the WHI findings. It is no longer acceptable to automatically put all perimenopausal and postmenopausal women on essentially the same drug at essentially the same dose. Individualizing treatment options around patient preference, risk/benefit profiles, and research findings will continue to shape clinical practice.

Clinicians need to assist patients in making rational decisions about the use of medication therapy in menopause. To assist both the prescriber and the patient in making informed choices, the following questions should be considered: What are the personal benefits of using ERT or HRT? How severe are the symptoms—and what are the key symptoms that need to be treated? What are the risks specific to this individual patient's situation? What health history, lifestyle, or family genetic factors could influence the safety of ERT/HRT therapy? Does the patient wish to investigate pharmaceutical options at this time? What alternative options—such as sleep aids, bisphosphonates, antidepressants, herbal preparations, or lifestyle changes—would be appropriate alternatives to ERT/HRT?

For women who elect to use ERT/HRT, annual risks, benefit assessments, and quality-of-life issues need to be considered each year when prescriptions are renewed for perimenopausal and postmenopausal hormonal therapy. In addition, nonpharmacological behaviors such as weight loss, smoking cessation, reduced alcohol intake, regular exercise, and healthy dietary habits need to be encouraged at all office visits.

Rational Drug Selection

General consensus recommendations from the leading national organizations of clinicians who care for women, along with those of the U.S. Preventative Services Task Force and the FDA, were presented earlier in this chapter. The consensus supports the use of ERT/HRT for the treatment of moderate to severe menopausal symptoms using the lowest dose of hormones for the shortest duration possible.

In general, the following recommendations concerning HRT or ERT can be made:

1. Use the lowest dose that relieves the symptoms for the shortest time frame. The optimal time frame appears to be up to 5 years.
2. Individualize the choice of drug and dose based on the woman's risk profile.
3. Monitor women at least annually for changes in risk profile, development of adverse effects, and continued need for therapy.
4. Only start HRT at the time of menopause onset. A disproportionate number of adverse effects in the WHI occurred in women who were postmenopause several years when HRT was initiated and/or restarted.

Historically, ERT/HRT had been used to treat conditions other than symptomatic management of menopausal symptoms. Prescribers should understand that outdated information might still be found in older references and Web sites and be able to counter the requests for supplements other than those currently approved. The nonvasomotor and nonvaginal historical reasons for initiating ERT/HRT are briefly outlined below.

Cardiac Disease Prevention

Because women have traditionally been regarded as "protected" from cholesterol and CV events compared to men, ERT and HRT were promoted to extend this "protection" beyond menopause. Evidence demonstrates the opposite: ERT/HRT should not be used to prevent CHD and care should be used in prescribing it to women who have cardiac risk factors (see below).

Osteoporosis Prevention

HRT and ERT have both consistently demonstrated a decreased risk for osteoporosis and hip fracture. Estrogen-containing therapies continue to be indicated for the prevention and treatment of osteoporosis in postmenopausal women with menopausal symptoms and risk for bone loss. HRT is not used solely for the prevention or treatment of osteoporosis. In women without concurrent vasomotor menopausal symptoms, therapy should be undertaken with other osteoporosis agents because of the risks associated with hormonal treatments and the excellent track record of these agents in sustaining bone density. Osteoporosis and its treatment are discussed later in this chapter. Hormones and osteoporosis agents can be used together for severe cases.

Cognitive Performance, Sleep Disturbance, and Skin Changes

Data on the effects of HRT or ERT on cognitive changes associated with Alzheimer's disease, on insomnia, and on skin changes such as wrinkles are inconsistent. The Women's Health Initiative Memory Study (WHIMS), a substudy of WHI (Chlebowski et al, 2003) reported an increased risk of developing probable dementia in postmenopausal women 65 years of age or older during 5.2 years of treatment with daily conjugated estrogen 0.625 mg alone and during 4 years of treatment with daily conjugated estrogen 0.625 mg combined with MPA 2.5 mg, relative to placebo. It is unknown whether this finding applies to younger postmenopausal women. The "protection" against an aging brain is not supported.

Relief of Perimenopausal and Postmenopausal Symptoms

Relief of menopausal symptoms can be dramatic after the initiation of hormonal therapy. The benefits of short-term hormone use may very well outweigh the small risk over a short time. Women may report feeling more in control of their bodily functions, exhibit improved emotional stability, and reestablish sleep patterns. Dyspareunia and vaginal irritation due to vaginal atrophy improve. Urogenital tissue response to estrogen treatment often relieves urinary urgency. A small percentage of women using ERT/HRT report headaches, fluid retention, breast tenderness, and erratic menses.

The various formulations of estrogen are discussed in Chapter 22. For women who have no objections to estrogens from animal sources, conjugated equine estrogen (Premarin) is available in doses from 0.3 mg to 1.25 mg. Suppression of hot flashes has been shown to be best at 0.625 mg, followed by 0.45 mg and 0.3 mg/d (Liu, 2004). Vasomotor symptoms begin to decrease by week 2 of therapy and reach maximal effect by week 8 of therapy. Dosage increases should not occur, however, until at least a 6 to 8 week interval to give the drug time to reach maximal effect at the dose.

When initiating therapy for any age group, begin with low doses (0.3 mg) every other day for 2 months. Next, increase the estrogens to daily use for another 2 months. Progestin must be included in the treatment regimens above if the patient has a uterus. If symptoms such as bleeding or breast pain do not occur, increase the estrogen to 0.625 mg daily if vasomotor symptoms or vaginal atrophy have not resolved. Some women may need only the lower estrogen dosages as long as they have adequate diets.

Micronized estradiol (Estrace, Gynodiol) is the only bioidentical estrogen-alone product available in pill form. It is available in 0.5 mg to 2 mg. Suppression is found at 1 mg and 2 mg doses. The typical regimen is 1 mg taken daily. The lower dose (0.5 mg) has been used for osteoporosis prevention and is less useful for vasomotor symptom relief. Because of the risks associated with hormone therapy, alternative agents should be considered if osteoporosis is the primary goal of therapy.

For women who prefer estrogens derived from plant sources, estrone-based drugs are available. Conjugated-synthetic estrogen-A (Cenestin) is available in doses from 0.3 mg to 1.25 mg. Patients should be started with Cenestin 0.45 mg daily. Subsequent dosage adjustment may be made based on the individual patient response. This dose should be reassessed periodically by the health-care provider. The lowest effective dose of Cenestin for the treatment of moderate to severe vasomotor symptoms has not been determined. The majority (77%) of women randomized to Cenestin required a total daily dose of 1.25 mg to relieve vasomotor symptoms, whereas the remaining 23% required 0.625 mg or less. By week 8, the vasomotor symptoms were significantly decreased. Conjugated-synthetic estrogen-B (Enjuvia) is available in doses of 0.625 mg to 1.25 mg, with the lower dose producing relief in many women. Estropipate (Ogen, Ortho-EST) is also derived from plant sources and available in 0.75 mg to 6 mg tablets. Following the rule to use the lowest dose to control symptoms, the dosing regimen should start at 0.75 mg.

Several ERT/HRT formulations are available in transdermal delivery systems for the indication of managing vasomotor and urogenital menopausal symptoms. The major advantage of this formulation is its once- or twice-weekly application. A very positive advantage is that topical agents avoid the "first-pass effect," which dramatically decreases the negative effects of generating bad lipid profiles. A potential disadvantage is the incidence of skin irritation (20% to 40%) in users of a patch delivery system. Menostar is a transdermal patch that delivers a very low dose (0.014 mg) of estradiol. It is indicated only for osteoporosis prevention in women without a uterus or in combination with a progestin periodically (every 6 to 12 months) during therapy to prevent endometrial hyperplasia.

Complementary and Alternative Therapies

Phytoestrogens and herbal therapies abound for relief of peri- and postmenopausal symptoms. There is a high level of use of complementary and alternative medicine (CAM) therapies across ethnicities and cultures. The data supporting these treatments for symptom relief are discussed in detail in the chapter on herbals and alternative medicine. Prescribers are directed to the NIH CAM Web site for the most accurate and evidence-based recommendations. Of note, the polyphenols in green tea, already recognized for their antioxidant effects, may be an active ingredient explaining why women who drink green tea appear to have a slower progression of postmenopausal bone loss (Shen, Yeh, Cao, Chyu, & Wang, 2012). This is not certain evidence.

Phytoestrogens

Phytoestrogens are plant compounds that are functionally or structurally related to endogenous estrogens and their active metabolites. They may be agonistic, partially agonistic, or antagonistic with estrogen receptors. Isoflavones are phytoestrogens that are found largely in soy and red clover. Supplemental soy is of no benefit over placebo, especially in the anticipated bone health or suppression of vasoactive effects (Amato et al, 2013). Studies have been inconsistent in demonstrating efficacy of red clover–based products in improving hot flashes and other menopausal symptoms. Black cohosh, gingko biloba, and evening primrose oil have shown no increased efficacy in treating hot flashes in placebo-controlled trials. Most bioidentical estrogens are derived from soy. The FDA warns that these products are not regulated, and cautions that women who are consuming amounts sufficient to achieve effective symptom relief from a phytoestrogen may also experience significant estrogenic stimulation of the endometrium and breast and be at similar risk for adverse events as are those women who use pharmaceutical agents.

Botanicals/Herbals

Plants are used therapeutically in the form of herbs, oils, pills, teas, and tinctures. They may be classified as dietary supplements. The herbal preparations approved for treatment of menopausal symptoms by the German Commission E include black cohosh root and chaste tree fruit. Liu and colleagues (2001) evaluated eight botanicals for estrogenic activity. They found that red clover, hops, and chasteberry had significant binding affinities with estrogen receptors. Dong quai and licorice had weak binding. Asian ginseng, North American ginseng, and black cohosh displayed no binding to estrogen receptors. Langer (2005) reported that black cohosh failed to relieve vasomotor symptoms. This finding was replicated by the National Center for Complementary and Alternative Medicine at the National Institutes of Health; black cohosh failed to show that it reduces the frequency and severity of hot flashes and night sweats in menopausal and perimenopausal participants. Chasteberry contains hormone-like substances with antiandrogenic effects. It also has significant binding affinities for both estrogen-receptor alpha and estrogen-receptor beta. Studies regarding the efficacy of chasteberry have shown symptom reduction; however, questions regarding study design limit the ability to draw clinical conclusions.

For further information on these herbal remedies, the reader is referred to Chapter 10, the German Commission E, and the National Center for Complementary and Alternative Medicine.

Nonhormonal Medications

Several nonhormonal medications have demonstrated benefit in reducing menopausal symptoms. Selective serotonin reuptake inhibitors (SSRIs) (discussed in Chap. 29) and clonidine (Chap. 14) have mixed reported relief of vasomotor symptoms and sleep disturbance. The GLOW study demonstrated the increased fracture risk with SSRI medications after 5 years of use (Aldachi, 2013). The serotonin-norepinephrine reuptake inhibitors (SNRI) have more evidence to support a reduction in the impact on vasomotor symptoms but without a statistically significant actual reduction in intensity. Gabapentin holds promise as a true hot flash reduction medication (Hall, Frey, & Soares, 2011). The North American Menopause Society has published a comprehensive review of alternative treatments for vasomotor symptoms.

Prevention and Management of Vulvovaginal Atrophy and Dryness

In addition to the vasomotor symptoms associated with menopause, the decline in estrogen causes the vaginal mucosa and vulvar skin to become thin and atrophic. The result is discomfort, itching, dyspareunia, and increased cases of vaginitis. Low-dose (0.3 to 0.625 mg) oral ERT with estrogen from both plant and animal sources has been shown to decrease vaginal pH, thus reducing vaginal infections. Estrogen also thickens and revascularizes the vaginal epithelium, increases the number of superficial cells, and reverses vaginal atrophy (Liu, 2004).

Vaginal application of estrogen also produces these positive effects, and improvement in symptoms can be seen in as few as 2 weeks of treatment. Low-dose vaginal estrogens (in ring or cream form) have a less stimulating effect on the endometrial tissue and, therefore, have a reduced risk for endometrial hyperplasia compared to the oral forms. Estrace is a bioidentical vaginal cream approved for the treatment of vaginal and urinary symptoms. The usual doses for all the creams include nightly application at first, followed by a 2 to 3 times a week regimen if symptoms are controlled. Topical application using vaginal rings and vaginal tablets may be preferred to creams in some patients because of the ease of use and a perception that these options are less "messy" than the creams. The Estradiol ring (Femring) is inserted and changed only every 90 days. The total amount of estrogen to which the body is exposed is less with the topical formulations, which may be a consideration for women who have risk factor concerns with ERT.

Studies reported by Thorneycroft (2004) found no evidence of increased risk of CHD, breast cancer, or endometrial cancer with the use of vaginal ERT. There was a slight increase in endometrial hyperplasia with higher doses, so it might be prudent to periodically withdraw patients treated with vaginal ERT, which includes estradiol tablets more than 10 micrograms twice a week, an estradiol ring more than 7.5 micrograms, and estradiol creams more than 0.5 g per week. Any bleeding must be worked up. There are no long-term studies of use without progestin supplementation. An alternative is to use micronized progesterone 200 mg for 12 days a month, which will be followed by a withdrawal bleed. The lower risk of endometrial hyperplasia with vaginal products does not eliminate the need to consult with oncology for women who have had breast cancer or other estrogen-positive cancers.

A new drug, ospemifene (Osphena) has the FDA indication to also assist in vaginal issues, specifically dyspareunia (FDA, 2013). The mechanism of action is as both an estrogen agonist *and* antagonist, dependent on the tissues it is impacting. It is an alternative when estrogen-based medications are not tolerated, patients prefer not to use a "messy" cream, or the medications are considered to be risky in the presence of localized lesions that could be precancerous. Ospemifene has a Black-Box Warning that it might thicken uterine linings, which would predispose the patient to endometrial cancer, a risk not associated with low-dose topical estrogen medications. The drug was not studied in combination with progestins because the original developers considered it more akin to a SERM type of medication. It is also linked to a risk of thromboembolization. Therefore, the FDA has required all estrogen Black-Box Warnings be placed on this drug. Preclinical studies assumed an antagonistic effect on breast tissue and an agonist effect on bone (like a SERM), but there is no clinical trial evidence to support or deny this.

Reduced Risk for Colon Cancer

Colorectal cancer is the third most common cancer in women in the United States and the third most common cause of cancer death in women (Thorneycroft, 2004). Since this cancer is also associated with aging, it clearly is a cancer to be considered with menopause. Reduction in colon and rectal cancers are correlated with both postmenopausal ERT and HRT use and the doses that help with vasomotor symptoms also provide that benefit. The decrease appears to be approximately 40% and the WHI showed a statistically significant reduction. Women with a family/genetic history of colon cancer would benefit from this therapy. These drugs are not indicated for this sole indication.

Increased Risk for Breast Cancer

Data regarding the effects of HRT and ERT on breast cancer are inconsistent and controversial (Shapiro et al, 2012). The WHI evidence suggests that a progestin receptor may be involved in invasive breast cancer; the arm of the study with just estrogen supplements did not have the same breast cancer incidence of the estrogen plus progestin arm of the study (Chlebowski et al, 2003, 2013). No evidence exists that ERT or HRT directly initiates a neoplastic process, but they may be promoters, increasing the rate of division of neoplastic cells. Based on all the available data, it seems prudent to carefully monitor all women on ERT/HRT for breast cancer through annual office evaluation and mammography.

The use of ERT/HRT is contraindicated in women with a history of breast or gynecological cancers and those with first-degree family members with breast cancer. Duration and timing of therapy also seems to be a factor in breast cancer risk. If HRT is started at the very beginning of menopause, breast cancer risk is higher in part due to the continued levels of natural hormone in addition to the drugs (Chlebowski et al, 2013). Women with extended use, especially therapy continued beyond 7 years, are at increased risk.

Advocates of bioidentical hormones have claimed that this cancer risk is not associated with the use of medications other than conjugated estrogens and medroxyprogesterone. The FDA, leading menopause societies, cancer centers, and endocrine specialties do not endorse this claim, stating that it is not backed by evidence (Flies et al, 2011; Stunkel et al, 2012). There have been no head-to-head studies; nor have there been longitudinal studies of women on these selections of medications to lend evidence to the claims. However, the FDA does list bioidentical approved medications that are widely used by many. The different physiological impacts of progestins on the body are cited as creating better quality of life and less cardiovascular risk by proponents of these newer medications that were not included in the WHI research that halted much of the HRT therapies taken by women (Holtorf, 2009).

Increased Risk for Endometrial Cancer

There is a clear and consistent increased risk for endometrial cancer in women with a uterus who are treated with unopposed ERT. To help decrease this risk, progestin has been added to hormone treatment options for women with an intact uterus to help prevent endometrial hyperplasia and cancer. The use of unopposed estrogen in a woman with a uterus is contraindicated. Further discussion occurs in the progestin section below.

Risk for CHD

The first indications that early assumptions about ERT/HRT and improved cardiovascular health might not be true happened years before the WHI. The PEPI study, conducted in 1995 (Writing Group of the PEPI Trial, 1996), started to question this initial hypothesis of a level of "protection" with supplements. Although the drugs tested (estrogen alone, estrogen with MPA, and estrogen with micronized progestin) increased HDL, lowered LDL, and fibrinogen levels and had no adverse effect on blood pressure, these apparently positive CHD risk factors did not translate into decreased CHD events. The ERA (Estrogen Replacement and Atherosclerosis) studies (Herrington et al, 2000; Hodis et al, 2003) contributed to the same conclusion. HERS was the first large randomized trial that looked at reduction in mortality by using menopausal estrogens. Women with CHD had higher adverse events and incidence of death during therapy. Women without cardiovascular disease showed modest benefit but not until the fourth and fifth years of therapy. The definitive study was the WHI, which stopped the HRT arm of its study earlier than planned based on an increased risk for CHD versus possible benefits of HRT. The ERT arm, which included women who did not have a uterus, failed to show statistically significant benefits in prevention of CHD. It is worth noting that the ERT arm of the study was subsequently halted early because of increased incidence of stroke.

The age and years of postmenopause in the WHI study have raised the possibility that the adverse cardiovascular findings may be related to the length of time that the normal hormone balance had been interrupted prior to initiation of hormone therapy and the vascular capacity to respond. Meta-analysis of age-adjusted cohorts and other studies suggest that the risk of CHD might be substantially less in women who initiate ERT/HRT early in perimenopause and menopause (Langer, 2005). Progestin has been shown to block estrogen receptors, which might interfere with nitric oxide production in the endothelial cells and diminish the beneficial effects of estrogen. Questions remain as to the reasons that HRT is associated with increased risk over ERT alone. These questions need to be answered by further research.

It is important to note that oral estrogens are associated with increased levels of C-reactive protein (CRP), a factor associated with increased CHD risk in women (Mosca, Barret-Connor, & Kass Wenger, 2011). Importantly, there is no increased risk of heart attack and stroke with transdermal and intravaginal preparations.

Increased Stroke and Thromboembolic Event Risk

Increased risk for thromboembolic events has been a long-standing concern related to hormone replacement, whether estrogen alone or in combination with progestins. The WHI found significantly increased risk for stroke in post-menopausal women for both ERT and HRT. For HRT the risk was apparent in each decade of age, but for ERT the risk appeared to emerge after age 60 (Langer, 2005). The risk for venous thromboembolic disease, including pulmonary embolism, was doubled in women in the HRT arm, with no difference based on age. There was a nonsignificant increase by about one-third with ERT alone (Anderson et al, 2003, 2004). The risk of a thromboembolic event is greatest in the first year after initiating therapy.

Progestin Therapy

Progestin therapy alone is used for contraception in younger women with menorrhagia. It is also used in the perimenopausal and postmenopausal period in combination with estrogen to prevent endometrial hyperplasia that increases the risk for endometrial cancer. It is not 100% protective. Endometrial biopsy results from the HOPE trial (Liu, 2004) indicate that there was a 3.17% incidence of hyperplasia in the 0.3 mg (Premarin) group versus 27.27% hyperplasia in the 0.625 mg group at 2 years.

Different types of progestogens not only have differing effects on the endometrium, they also have differing effects on estrogen-associated benefits to lipids. Norethindrone acetate has been shown to reverse these benefits on HDL cholesterol while still offering effective endometrial protection. MPA and micronized progestin do not attenuate the effects of estrogen on lipid levels. Norgestimate improves HDL to a level intermediate between MPA and micronized progestin, while also providing good endometrial protection (Langer, 2005).

Combination Therapy with Estrogen and Progestins

Although HRT is as effective as ERT in preventing the uncomfortable symptoms sometimes associated with menopause, reducing the risk of colon cancer, and reducing the risk for osteoporosis and hip fracture, it is not more effective in these areas. The risks associated with HRT are discussed in the ERT section above. Given the studies that indicate a role in increased risk for CHD, it is prudent to avoid HRT, especially in women with CHD risk factors. For this reason, the only specific indication discussed for combination therapy will be the prevention of endometrial hyperplasia and cancer in a menopausal woman with an intact uterus.

Decreased Risk for Endometrial Cancer

Combinations of estrogen and progestin are used when the uterus is intact. Research has consistently demonstrated the risk for endometrial cancer in direct correlation with unopposed ERT in women who have an intact uterus (Brinton & Felix, 2013; Thorneycroft, 2004). The risk also increases substantially the longer the ERT is used and persists for 5 or more years after ERT has been discontinued. Although this effect appears to be dose-related, with higher hyperplasia associated with higher estrogen doses, the risk remains for all dose levels of ERT. To prevent this increased incidence of hyperplasia and cancer, progestin, which reduces the buildup of endometrial tissue, is added to the treatment regimen.

There are several combination therapies for use in menopause. The following regimens have been prescribed and all provide effective prevention of endometrial cancer:

1. Estrogen (0.625 mg) plus medroxyprogesterone acetate (MPA) 2.5 mg daily (Prempro)
2. Estrogen (0.625 mg) plus micronized progesterone 100 mg daily
3. Estrogen (0.625 mg) daily plus MPA 10 mg for 10 to 12 days
4. Estrogen (0.625 mg) daily plus MPA 5 mg for 14 days (Premphase)
5. Estrogen (0.625 mg) daily plus micronized progesterone 200 mg for 12 days (PEPI)
6. Estrogen (0.625 mg) for days 1 to 25 plus MPA days 16 to 25 (the first regimen used, which has the disadvantage of more hot flashes)
7. Estrogen (0.625 mg) plus progestin Monday through Friday (may experience more hot flashes)

Continuous Versus Cyclical (Sequential) Patterns

The most common reason women give for discontinuing HRT is irregular and unpredictable vaginal bleeding. Continuous regimens (1 and 2 above) eliminate monthly withdrawal bleeding, but they are associated with a higher rate of breakthrough bleeding, especially during the first 6 months of therapy. This is most likely to occur in women who have recently become postmenopausal because endogenous production of estrogen is more labile from cycle to cycle in these women. Currently available data suggest that the best profile for a positive risk/benefit ratio for all indications for ERT/HRT accrue when therapy is started near the time of menopause onset. This unwanted side effect may create a problem for many women.

To deal with breakthrough bleeding issues, cyclical or sequential therapy was introduced. These regimens (3 through 7 above) are preferred until endogenous hormone production stabilizes, typically 2 to 3 years after menopause. Differences in potency of various progestins result in differences in rates of bleeding. The PEPI study tested MPA and micronized progestin side by side and found that the micronized progestin was associated with less bleeding during the first 6 months than either the continuous or cyclical MPA (Lindenfeld & Langer, 2002). With any formulation of progestin, breakthrough bleeding decreases substantially after the first 6 months and both drugs produced effective protection from endometrial cancer.

Brinton and Felix (2013) have uncovered a pattern of endometrial cancer risk correlated with how progestins are taken. Continuous-dose patterns appear to confer lesser risk compared to women who did not take any progestin. Interestingly, heavier women had the lowest risk with dosing more than 25 days a month. Women on cyclic dosing for less than 10 days monthly had the highest risk of cancer. There has yet to be a response concerning the safety of intermittent dosing.

Testosterone Therapy

When traditional HRT/ERT is not successful in suppressing hot flashes (only a 28% reduction typically in the WHI) and improving sex drive, estrogen in combination with testosterone has been used empirically. Peripheral conversion of androgens may augment ERT and reduce hot flashes. Masculinizing adverse effects such as lower voice and increased facial and body hair can occur when testosterone is used alone. These adverse effects may not regress after testosterone is withdrawn. Traditionally, testosterone has been used topically (2%) in Aquaphor or petrolatum for vulvar "dystrophies." See the chapters concerning women's health drugs for other treatments for vulvovaginitis.

Available formulations are the following:

1. Esterified estrogen 0.625 mg plus testosterone 1.25 mg
2. Esterified estrogen 1.25 mg plus testosterone 2.5 mg (this higher estrogen is used in post-oophorectomy patients under 49 years of age)
3. Conjugated estrogens 0.625 mg plus testosterone 5 mg
4. Conjugated estrogens 1.25 mg plus testosterone 10 mg

Figure 38-1 presents a treatment algorithm for HRT/ERT.

Monitoring

Women taking hormonal therapy for menopausal symptoms have similar adverse effects and precautions no matter what the estrogen source and the route of administration. Annual complete history, physical examination, and mammogram are needed to evaluate for changes in risk profiles that may indicate a need to alter treatments and screen for early adverse effects of therapy. Liver function tests need to be done at baseline, along with a lipid profile, and repeated annually if abnormal. Authorities agree that all postmenopausal bleeding requires uterine biopsy. Laboratory monitoring of the precise estradiol level (E2) needed to bring vasomotor symptoms under control is not yet available. The available laboratory tests to measure estradiol vary widely and are deemed not reliable to measure the true level of hormone with any replicable accuracy (Rosner, Hankison, Sluss, Vesper, & Wierman, 2013). Importantly, many prescribers of compounded ERT/HRT use a saliva test to monitor how much of each hormone is needed and make dosage changes based on these lab values. The prescriber is directed to the laboratory literature that considers this form of hormone-level testing to be extremely unreliable. Variance in hormone levels in saliva can vary in just a few hours, with diet and even time of day. Collection methods are fraught with unreliable results; replication of values is poor at best (Flies, Ko, & Pruthi, 2011). The FDA does not endorse its use. Symptom endpoints are the things to monitor, not levels of hormones.

Outcome Evaluation

Women may present for treatment complaining of heavy menses. When the bleeding problem is serious enough to cause a drop of 2 g of hemoglobin within one menstrual cycle, management usually requires specialty care. The patient may need a dilation and curettage. It is not uncommon for fibroids and hyperplasia to cause this degree of bleeding. Both conditions will require referral and surgery.

Postmenopausal bleeding—that is, bleeding of any degree after 12 or more months of amenorrhea—needs an evaluation that includes history, physical, pelvic examination, mammogram, pelvic ultrasound, and endometrial biopsy. Laboratory tests are necessary to rule out bleeding disorders and endocrine disease. Biopsy uncovers endometrial cancers.

Frequently, older women present with symptoms of urinary incontinence or chronic bladder infections. If there is blood in the urine (even as few as 8 to 10 RBCs per high-powered field) and the culture is negative, the patient will need a urological evaluation. Because older women who have not been on ERT/HRT have cervical atrophy, performing an endometrial biopsy in the office is too painful. If all of the work-up demonstrates no disease, then local topical therapy is within the primary care scope to support urethral and vaginal tissue health.

Patient Education

Patient education should include a discussion of information related to the overall treatment plan as well as that specific to the drug therapy, reasons for taking the drug, drugs as part of the total treatment regimen, and adherence issues. Media attention to the WHI has led to some misinformation about ERT/HRT. Patients may present to the clinic very fearful about beginning this therapy or wondering if they should stop therapy, even when they have been on such therapy for years without incident. Providers need to inform patients that hormonal therapy has a role postmenopause, but that role is limited and therapy should be undertaken based on symptoms and risk assessment. (See Patient Education box on page 1114.)

OSTEOPOROSIS

Osteoporosis is a worldwide phenomenon. A white woman older than 50 years has more than a 40% chance of having such a fracture during the rest of her life (International Osteoporosis Federation [IOF], 2012). The lifetime risk for men and nonwhite women is less, but it is still substantial and rising in groups such as Hispanic women. Osteoporosis is the most important underlying cause of these fractures, especially in older adults. Using the World Health Organization's definition, there are roughly 10 million Americans older than 50 years with osteoporosis and an additional 34 million with low bone mass (osteopenia) of the hip, which puts them at risk for osteoporosis, fractures, and the complications associated with them. As the life expectancy of women reaches the mid-80s, osteopenia in perimenopausal women does not bode well for bone health of many seniors, especially among white and Asian women in industrial societies (IOF, 2012; National Institute of Arthritis and Musculoskeletal and Skin Diseases [NIAMSD], 2010b). By age 65, at least 6% of men have dual-energy x-ray absorptiometry-determined osteoporosis (Qaseem et al, 2008).

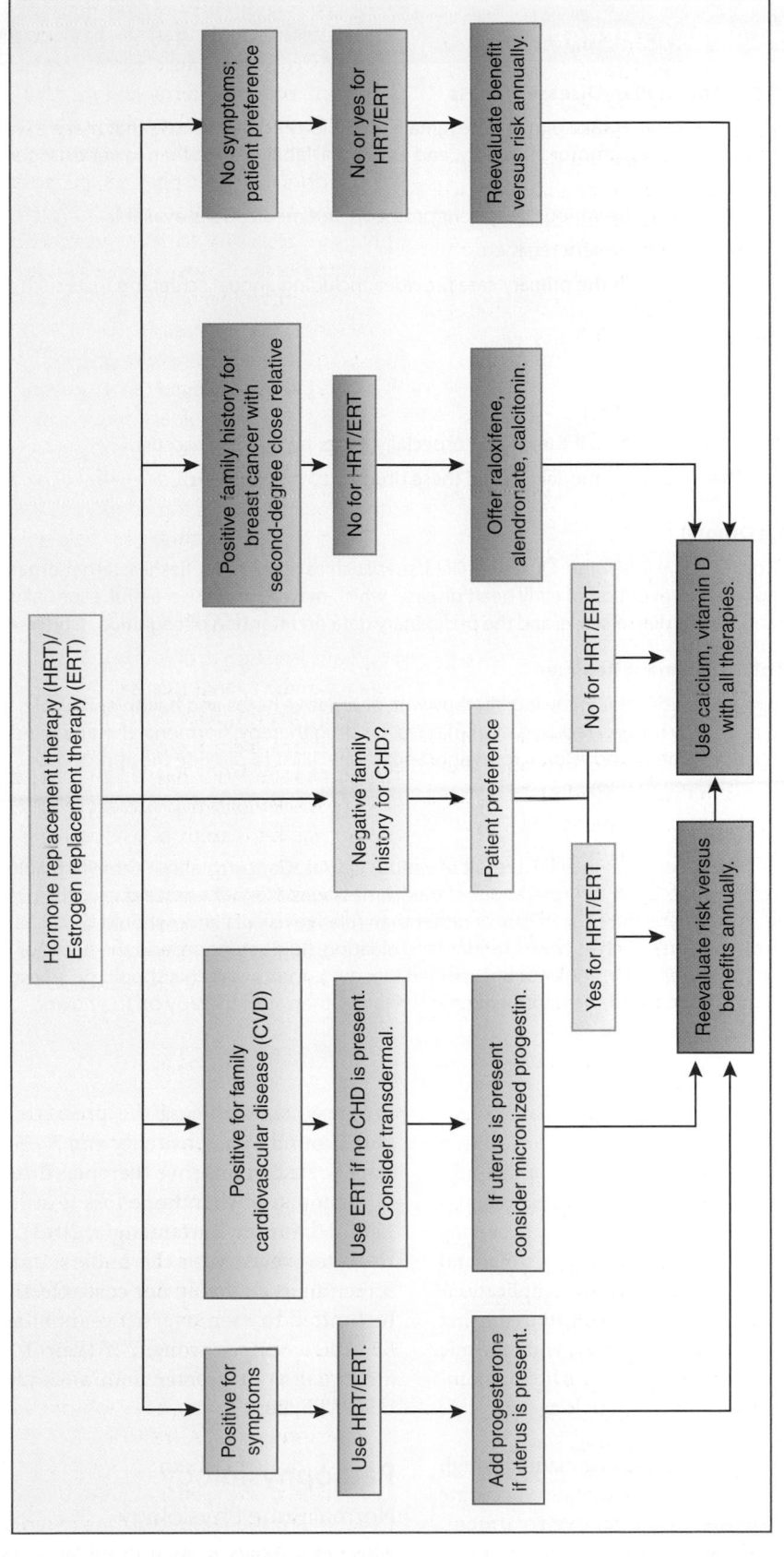

Figure 38–1. Treatment algorithm: Hormone replacement therapy/estrogen replacement therapy.

HORMONE REPLACEMENT THERAPY

Related to the Overall Treatment Plan/Disease Process

☐ Pathophysiology of the changes that take place in the female physiology at menopause that make a woman vulnerable to atrophy of the genital organs, vasomotor instability, and emotional lability, and when lower estrogen levels cause undesirable lipid patterns

☐ Role of lifestyle modifications and the various treatment protocols and medications available

☐ Importance of adherence to the treatment regimen

☐ Need for regular follow-up visits with the primary care provider, including annual screening tests such as mammography

Specific to the Drug Therapy

☐ Reasons for the drug's being given

☐ Doses and schedules for taking the drug

☐ Possible adverse effects and what to do if they occur, especially if uterine bleeding occurs

☐ Interactions between other treatment modalities and these drugs

Reasons for Taking the Drug(s)

Additional information includes the following: Quality-of-life issues such as relief of hot flashes; target organ atrophy prevention; treatment of osteoporosis; prevention of early heart disease, which may be more successful, especially in families who have a hereditary tendency for cardiac disease; and the preliminary data on retention of cognition, which seems promising.

Drugs as Part of the Total Treatment Regimen

The total treatment regimen includes the following: therapy with alternative herbs and healthier lifestyle, which may relieve symptoms but have not proved to bestow reduced morbidity, as has drug therapy; hormonal therapy is indicated for vaginal atrophy and bladder outlet syndrome; and referral to an appropriate specialist to provide the appropriate care when adverse effects occur as a result of estrogen therapy.

Adherence Issues

Nonadherence to the treatment regimen may be a result of various causes. Concerns about the WHI results should be discussed with correction of any inaccurate interpretations of media messages. Nonadherence due to the possible risk of cancer should be discussed, and the absolute risk of cancer rather than relative risk of cancer should be calculated annually. The possibility of minor discomforts, such as breast tenderness, bloating, fluid retention, and the need for follow-up visits, should be discussed prior to therapy. If irregular or unexpected bleeding occurs, patients should be advised to contact their health-care provider for modifications to the treatment regimen rather than stop therapy on their own.

The direct costs of caring for patients who have osteoporotic fractures are estimated to range up to $20 billion each year and that does not take into consideration the indirect costs in lost productivity and wages for the patient and family. With over 75% of fragility fractures actually occurring after age 65 (Bischoff-Ferrari et al, 2012), the personal and medical costs skyrocket. The risk of death from complications associated with a hip fracture approaches 25% within the first year of the incident; this is increased for those with chronic disease. Over 50% of hip fracture patients have lifelong mobility issues, with 25% requiring admission to long-term care (NAMS, 2012).

Real improvements in bone health can be made through assessment of risk factors, preventive strategies, accurate early diagnosis of osteoporosis, and effective treatment. This section will focus on drugs used for prevention and treatment of osteoporosis with special emphasis on their use in women who are postmenopausal. There is no reliable method of determining when menses will stop; however, research is underway: the "SWAN" study that is making progress in narrowing the prediction to around 2 years with around 85% sensitivity and 77 % specificity. Having a target date can improve therapies directed at the first years of menopause when bone loss is at its height (Greendale, Ishii, Huang, & Karlamangia, 2013). Knowing this needs to be tempered with the understanding that widespread screening is probably not cost-effective. Screening should be limited to men over 70 years of age, women over age 65, and younger women if their 10-year fracture risks are equal to or greater than a 65-year-old without risks (USPSTF, 2011).

Pathophysiology

Normal Bone Physiology

The bony skeleton is created by a process that changes throughout a person's lifetime. The underlying process is *remodeling*, which occurs in three phases. Phase 1 (activation) occurs when a stimulus (e.g., hormone, drug, vitamin, or physical stressor) activates the bone cell precursors in a localized area of bone to form osteoclasts. In phase 2 (resorption), the osteoclasts excavate (resorb) bone, leaving behind a cavity that follows the longitudinal axis of the haversian system in compact bone and parallels the trabeculae in spongy bone. Phase 3 (formation) then results in the laying down of new bone by osteoblasts lining the walls of the cavity. Successive layers of bone are laid down until the cavity is filled. The entire process takes about 3 to 4 months.

In order for this process to work, osteoblasts and osteoclasts must communicate with each other. A protein called osteoprotegrin (OPG) may be the key in this conversation. OPG binds to OPG-ligand, preventing the action of osteoclasts and stimulating the action of osteoblasts. The balance between OPG and OPG-ligand appears to control bone resorption and growth. The development of drugs to affect the balance between these two may help in the future to treat disease associated with bone loss.

During childhood and adolescence, the process is one of modeling, which allows for the formation of new bone at one site and the removal of older bone from another site within the same bone. This process allows bones to increase in size and to shift in space. Later in life, the process becomes one of remodeling when existing bone is resorbed and replaced without an increase in the total amount of bone. This process occurs throughout life and becomes dominant by the time the bone reaches peak mass, typically in one's early 20s. Most of the adult skeleton is replaced about every 10 years.

Peak bone mass is determined largely by genetic factors. Other factors that contribute to bone health include diet, endocrine status, and physical activity. A number of diseases and certain drugs and toxic agents can cause or contribute to development of bone loss including chronic use of thyroid supplements, glucocorticoids, proton pump inhibitors and SSRI medications (Table 38-1).

The growth of bone, its response to mechanical stressors, and its role in storage of minerals is dependent on the proper functioning of circulating hormones that respond to changes in serum calcium and phosphorus levels. If calcium or phosphorus levels are low, parathyroid hormone (PTH) stimulates osteoclasts to resorb bone, and calcium and phosphorus are released into the bloodstream. PTH also stimulates the intestines to absorb more calcium and the kidneys to activate more vitamin D to facilitate this absorption. The kidney is also stimulated to reabsorb calcium back into the bloodstream. Disease processes in any of these organ systems can produce osteoporosis. Estrogens also play a role in bone remodeling by reducing the bone-resorbing action of PTH. The reduction in estrogen found with menopause is a significant factor in the increased risk for osteoporosis seen in postmenopausal women.

Table 38–1   Medical Conditions and Drugs That Increase the Risk for Development of Osteoporosis

Medical Conditions		
AIDS/HIV	Hemophilia	Parathyroid tumor
Amyloidosis	Inflammatory bowel disease	Pernicious anemia
Ankylosing spondylitis	Type 1 diabetes mellitus	Rheumatoid arthritis
COPD	Lymphoma and leukemia	Severe liver disease
Congenital porphyria	Malabsorption syndromes	Sprue
Cushing's syndrome	Mastocytosis	Stroke (CVA)
Eating disorders	Multiple myeloma	Thalassemia
Gastrectomy	Multiple sclerosis	Thyrotoxicosis
Hemochromatosis	Hyperparathyroidism	Hypogonadism
Drugs		
Aluminum and *excess use of antacids*	Gonadotropin-release hormones	Progesterone (long acting)
Anticonvulsants (phenobarbital; phenytoin; carbamazepine)	Immunosuppressants like cyclosporine and tracroloimis	*Aggressive treatment of hypothyroidism with thyroxine*
Cytotoxic drugs like chemotherapy and methotrexate	Lithium	Tamoxifen and aromatase inhibitors
Glucocorticosteroids equivalent to 5 mg of prednisone or greater for at least 3 months	Long-term heparin use	Total parenteral nutrition
Warfarin use for >1 year	*Selective serotonin reuptake inhibitors*	*Proton pump inhibitors used >1 year*
ACTH	*Gonadatropin-releasing hormone agonists*	

COPD = chronic obstructive pulmonary disease; CVA = cerebrovascular accident.
   Source: Adapted from *Osteoporosis and Asian American Women, Osteoporosis and African American Women,* and *Osteoporosis and Hispanic Women, Osteoporosis Handout on Health* (all from NIAMSD documents, 2010, 2011); NIH, 2011, Qaseem et al, 2008; and University of Texas, 2008.

Bone Loss (Osteoporosis)

Bone loss occurs when the balance between osteoclastic activity and osteoblastic activity is altered. Figure 38-2 shows the changes within cancellous bone as a consequence of bone loss. Osteoporosis is a generalized metabolic disease characterized by decreased bone mass as a result of this imbalance. The World Health Organization definition of osteoporosis is having a bone density 2.5 standard deviations below the average adult peak bone mass. The bone that remains is histologically and biochemically normal, but there is not enough of it to maintain skeletal integrity and mechanical support. The disease can be generalized, involving major portions of the axial skeleton, or regional, involving one segment of the appendicular skeleton. Both spongy and compact bone are lost, but the spongy bone loss exceeds the compact bone loss (McCance & Huether, 2014). The end result is fractures—vertebral, hip, and wrist fractures are the most common.

There are several well-known risk factors for osteoporosis, such as family history, slight build, fair complexion (Scandinavian), age, diets low in calcium and vitamin D, and minimal sun exposure. Table 38-2 shows these and other risk factors including those for fractures secondary to osteoporosis. There are also a wide variety of diseases and certain drugs and toxic agents that can cause or contribute to development of osteoporosis. Factors associated with increased risk for osteoporosis in men (NIH, 2011) include (but are not limited to) the following:

- Being older than 70 years of age
- Glucocorticoid use of 5 mg or greater for 3 months or longer
- Anticonvulsants including phenobarbital, phenytoin, and carbamazapine
- Long-term proton pump inhibitor use for more than 1 year
- Body weight less than 70 kg or weight loss more than 10% compared with usual young adult or adult weight in recent years
- Heavy tobacco use or consuming more than 14 drinks of alcohol per week
- Sedentary lifestyle
- Deficits in vitamin D or calcium intake

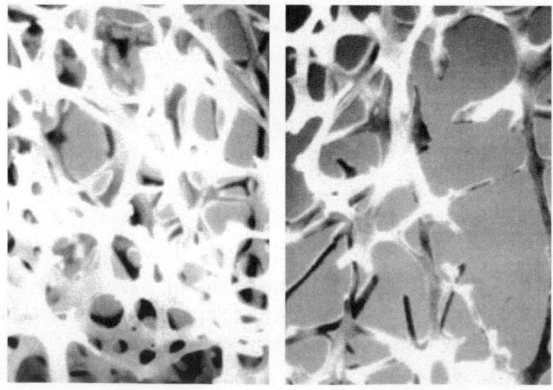

Normal   Osteoporotic

Figure 38-2. Micrographs of normal and osteoporotic bone.

Table 38–2 Risk Factors for Osteoporosis and Resultant Fractures

Risk Factors for Osteoporosis

- Thin, small-boned frame
- Estrogen deficiency <45 yr
- Advanced age (62 in women, >70 in men)
- Diet low in calcium and vitamin D
- White and Asian ancestry (African American and Hispanic women are at lower but significant risk)
- Cigarette smoking
- Alcohol intake >2 drinks per day
- Limited physical activity/sedentary lifestyle

Risk Factors for Fracture Secondary to Osteoporosis

- Personal history of fracture as an adult
- History of fragility fracture in a first-degree relative
- Low body weight (57.7 kg for women, 70 kg for men)
- *Weight loss of >10% in recent years*
- *Height loss of 1.5 in.*
- Use of oral corticosteroid therapy for >3 mo
- Hormone deprivation therapy used for >1 year as treatment for prostate cancer
- Impaired vision
- Dementia
- Recent falls

Source: Adapted from *Osteoporosis and Asian American Women, Osteoporosis and African American Women,* and *Osteoporosis and Hispanic Women* (all from NIAMSD documents, 2010); Qaseem et al, 2008; and University of Texas, 2008.

- Prostate cancer therapy
- Undiagnosed low testosterone

Osteoporosis is typically not diagnosed in men until a fracture occurs because there is no set screening triggers as there are for women (USPSTF, 2011). As in women, small stature and being of the white race are risks. The antihormone therapies for prostate cancer are akin to the increased risk of bone loss with the antihormone therapies used for women with breast, ovarian, and uterine cancers.

For women, the same is true with the following exceptions or additions: the age is greater than 62, the body weight is less than 57.7 kg or body mass index (BMI) less than 21 kg/m2, and there is a history of hip fracture in a parent or a personal history of fracture after menopause (Qaseem et al, 2008). These and other risk factors are shown in Table 38-2.

Ethnic Differences

The bone density of various ethnic groups varies as does their risk for osteoporosis. The National Institute of Arthritis and Musculoskeletal and Skin Diseases (2010a, b, c) published some data about these differences. Tools are available to assess osteopenia and osteoporosis risk at http://www.shef.ac.uk/FRAX.

African American Women

Although African American women tend to have higher bone mineral density than white women throughout life, they are still at significant risk for osteoporosis (NIAMSD, 2010a).

The misperception that it does not occur in this population can delay prevention and treatment. As African American women age, their risk for hip fracture doubles approximately every 7 years and they are more likely to die from the hip fracture than are white women. Diseases prevalent in this population, such as sickle cell disease and lupus, can increase the risk for developing osteoporosis. Most African American women consume 50% less calcium than the Recommended Dietary Allowance (RDA), placing them at risk related to poor calcium intake. This is compounded by the fact that 75% of all African Americans are lactose intolerant, so they avoid milk and other dairy products that are excellent sources of calcium.

Asian Women

Studies show that Asians share many of the risk factors that apply to white women and are at high risk for developing osteoporosis. Compared to white women, Asian women tend to consume less calcium, in part because 90% of Asians are lactose intolerant. Although they generally have lower hip fracture rates than do white women, the prevalence of vertebral fracture is as high (NIAMSD, 2011b).

Hispanic Women

The prevalence of osteoporosis in Hispanic women is similar to that of white women. Ten percent of Hispanic women 50 years and older are estimated to have osteoporosis, and 49% are estimated to have bone mass that is low, but not low enough for a diagnosis of osteoporosis (NIAMSD, 2010c). The incidence of hip fracture in this population is on the rise. In addition, this population also consumes less calcium, probably also related to lactose intolerance. Finally, Hispanic women are twice as likely to develop diabetes as are white women, which may increase their risk for bone loss.

Pharmacodynamics

The results of the Women's Health Initiative called into question the use of estrogen for the sole indication of osteoporosis prevention and treatment due to the risks for cardiovascular adverse responses. Estrogens prevent osteoporosis by reducing the bone-resorbing action of PTH. Estrogen receptors have been found in bone, which validates the hypothesis that estrogen may have direct effects on bone remodeling.

Raloxifene (Evista) is a selective estrogen receptor modulator (SERM) approved for preventing and treating postmenopausal osteoporosis, as a well as prevention of estrogen-receptor-positive (ER positive) breast cancer. Because it selectively activates certain estrogen pathways in bone and has antiestrogen effects on the uterus and breast, raloxifene reduces the resorption of bone with less risk for cardiovascular effects. Most of the effect is on reduction of vertebral fractures by 34%; other site fracture reduction is insignificant.

This drug also has positive effects on lipid metabolism by decreasing total and LDL cholesterol levels. It does not affect other lipid fractions. SERMs are associated with hot flashes because they do not impact natural estrogen-level variations (Zhang, Simondsen, & Kelesar, 2012). Some early menopausal women discontinue therapy because of this adverse effect. There is some risk of postmenopausal uterine cancer development over time. SERMS also contribute to thromboembolic events. The other SERM class medications do not have the same degree of bone density effect as raloxifene.

Bisphosphonates also reduce bone resorption by adhering tightly to bone and inhibiting osteoclastic activity. Although no drug is free of adverse effects, bisphosphonate adverse effects are largely gastrointestinal (GI) in nature and not associated with the same life-threatening consequences seen with estrogen. The exception is the risk atrial fibrillation risk even in those without prior cardiovascular disease. This is more common in the IV formulations (Sharma et al, 2013). Bisphosphonates are listed by all guidelines as first-line therapy. Bisphosphonates are discussed in more detail in Chapter 21. In extreme cases they can be used in combo with SERMs.

Natural calcitonin balances parathyroid hormone by shutting down osteoclastic activity and increasing osteoblastic activity in the presence of hypercalcemia. Low serum calcium levels increase the secretion of endogenous calcitonin, with a resulting small decrease in serum calcium. All previously marketed calcitonin drugs were pulled off the market due to cancer-associated risks.

Teriparatide (Forteo) is a synthetic PTH derived from recombinant DNA technology. Its bone actions are identical to that of human PTH. Unlike other drugs used to treat osteoporosis in which the action is to prevent bone breakdown, this drug acts to stimulate bone formation. In once-daily doses, it does this through preferential stimulation of osteoblastic activity over osteoclastic activity. Most of its anabolic effects occur within the first 6 months of therapy. This drug is only recommended for postmenopausal women who are at high risk for fracture and to increase bone mass in men with primary or hypogonadal osteoporosis who are at high risk for fracture and cannot use other bone medications. It is taken only for 2 years. It can cause orthostatic hypotension within 4 hours of the dose and hypercalcemia. Of note, it has an increased risk for osteosarcoma development that must be closely monitored. It cannot be taken by patients with Paget's disease, those who have had external beam or implanted skeletal radiation or a history of bone metastasis.

Denusomab (Prolia), a human antibody against the tumor necrosis factor RANKL, inhibits osteoclast survival and function. Its use is typically reserved for those who do not respond to bisphosphonate therapy or for cancer patients with bone metastasis. It can be injected twice yearly with a significant (69%) reduction of new vertebral fracture and the very positive reduction (40%) of hip fractures. This newer and very expensive medication is under scrutiny for reports of osteonecrosis of the jaw, increases in sepsis, and unanticipated deaths at levels higher than the bisphosphonates.

Calcium and vitamin D are also critical to bone formation and are generally recommended as complementary agents in the prevention and treatment of osteoporosis. However, the

U.S. Preventive Services Task Force has not found evidence that higher doses of vitamin D over 400 IU and 1 g of calcium lessens fracture risk in patients without a documented vitamin D deficiency (Nestle & Nesheim, 2013). This appears to counter the meta-analysis done by Bischoff-Ferrari and associates (2012), which linked high doses of vitamin D (800 IU) to fracture prevention in older people. The USPSTF states many of the studies were of questionable methodology, leaving the recommendations to be unreliable.

Of the 600 to 1,000 mg of calcium consumed daily, only 100 to 250 mg are absorbed from the gut. In the steady state, renal excretion of calcium and phosphate balances intestinal absorption. The movement of calcium and phosphate across the intestinal lining is closely regulated. Intestinal diseases can disrupt this balance. Hormonal regulation of calcium, mentioned earlier, greatly affects calcium metabolism. Ions such as sodium and fluoride also have an impact on calcium balance. Inadequate vitamin D can produce a decrease in calcium absorption from the intestine and an increase in parathyroid hormone, both of which may lead to bone loss and fractures. Serum levels of vitamin D for optimal bone health are 30 to 100 ng/mL. Deficiency occurs when the amount is less than 20 ng/mL. Drugs taken for other diseases, such as thiazides for hypertension, also affect calcium metabolism. Patients with low levels should be supplemented, but those at normal levels do not have additional benefits with higher doses (Nestle & Nesheim, 2013). Vitamin D supplements come in two active forms: D25-dihydroxy and D1,25-dihydroxy. The latter is the more biologically active. The D3 is formed in the skin or comes in supplements and is converted to D25-dihydoxy in the liver. D2 is a plant-synthesized vitamin that is absorbed from the diet or a supplement and is changed into D1, 25-dihydroxy in the kidney.

It is known that calcium supplementation without vitamin D does not reduce fracture rates (Nestle & Nesheim, 2013). Calcium supplements can also increase the incidence of kidney stones. In addition, there is concern that excess serum calcium deposits into soft, vascular plaque, which makes the plaque less able to regress in the face of statin therapy. These adverse issues should be tempered with the knowledge that taking calcium cuts overall mortality in women compared with women who do not take the supplements (Langsetmo et al, 2013).

Goals of Treatment

The ideal goal of treatment for osteoporosis is that the pharmacological therapy be inexpensive, safe, and effective. Nonpharmacological therapy (and prevention) includes an appropriate exercise program. The best treatment for osteoporosis is prevention. Developing a healthy lifestyle while building bone mass is the most cost-effective strategy. Excessive dieting and exercise or fad diets that are deficient in essential nutrients contribute to reduced bone mass.

Prevention of osteoporosis includes a low-impact aerobic exercise program; however, excessive exercise is not good because stress fractures may result. For treatment of osteoporosis,

weight-bearing activity such as brisk walking (20 min, 3 to 4 times/wk) is ideal. Resistance training (lifting weights or using strength-training machines) is a slow process, so programs should start low and work up over a period of months.

Of new importance is keeping belly fat down to a minimum. Not only is this a cardiac risk factor, but abdominal obesity is now recognized as contributing to less than ideal bone mass (Cohen, 2013). The myth that carrying extra weight strengthens bones has been overturned. The purported mechanical stress for bone growth is probably eliminated by the circulating cytokines and decreased insulin-like growth factors, which results in boss loss. This visceral adiposity is a negative factor for bone health. Additional support for this newly recognized risk factor is a study that measured decreased structural bone health using a new in vivo tool that measures microscopic cracks (Farr et al, 2014). Diabetic women with normal DEXA scans were found to have significant loss of bone strength and quality. This OsteoProbe tool, however, is not in wide use.

Rational Drug Selection

Estrogen Therapy

There is a direct correlation between rate of bone loss in menopausal women and estradiol levels. Bone resorption has also been shown to be highest in the first postmenopausal year. Women in the immediate postmenopausal years are the ones who are most in need of protection from osteoporosis (Greendale et al, 2013).

A head-to-head trial comparing the effects of alendronate alone, conjugated equine estrogen alone, and a combination of the two, found that while both the alendronate and estrogen alone significantly increased bone mineral density (BMD), the combination was better than either alone for bone health (Greenspan et al, 2002); however, the risks of hormone therapy overshadow the added benefit, so it is not used except in extreme cases. This study also looked at stopping therapy after 2 years by switching women who had been on the drugs to placebo. Those on alendronate alone who were switched to placebo had no change in BMD. However, the women initially on estrogen who were switched to placebo had a significant decrease in BMD, almost to baseline levels, within 1 year. The same results are expected in women who react to the WHI study data and stop taking estrogen.

Even though the WHI raised concerns about the risk for coronary events, stroke, pulmonary emboli, and breast cancer in women who took a combination of estrogen and progesterone, it is important to note that the number of hip and vertebral fractures was lower at a statistically significant rate for women taking the combination and for women taking estrogen alone. The addition of progestin to estrogen therapy did not produce a significant difference in BMD. The findings from the WHI have led women's health specialists, the USPSTF, and the FDA to recommend that estrogen products not be considered first-line therapy for the prevention and treatment of osteoporosis unless a woman is also experiencing vasomotor or vaginal atrophy menopausal symptoms. When ERT alone is chosen, low-dose therapy has been shown to produce a positive effect on BMD, even though the dose-related response is less. Lower doses also produce less risk for endometrial hyperplasia in women with an intact uterus; however, unopposed oral estrogen in these women is contraindicated.

Balancing these risks and the availability of other drugs to prevent and treat osteoporosis should be discussed with women, who can then make an informed decision about whether or not to use estrogen. Prescribing information is presented earlier in this chapter. Long-term efficacy of taking estrogen in lower doses for prevention of osteoporosis remains unknown at this time.

Calcium Therapy

A major goal of the use of calcium and vitamin D is increased bone health. Bone buildup is largely complete by the time one is a young adult. To assure a sufficient degree of bone density in adulthood, active promotion of adequate levels of calcium and vitamin D should begin with children and adolescents.

Most guidelines suggest supplementation with calcium and vitamin D both for prevention of osteoporosis and as part of the treatment protocol, especially if screening suggests vitamin D deficiency. Supplementation with vitamin D to an acceptable level of greater than 30 ng/mL before initiating bisphosphonate therapy is recommended.

The wholesale use of calcium and vitamin D supplements for the community-dwelling postmenopausal woman is no longer endorsed by the USPSTF (2013). The evidence only supports use being limited to institutionalized elders over 65 or those who have demonstrated a fragility fracture. The use of vitamin D is still endorsed as a falls risk preventative; hence, those with a prior fracture, high falls risk, and with demonstrated deficiencies are the only patients now being encouraged to take these supplements. The long-term, automatic use of calcium and vitamin D supplementation has not reduced the risk of fractures in those in the community without fracture histories (Nestle & Nesheim, 2013).

When indicated, calcium is the least expensive drug used in osteoporosis therapy. Generic calcium carbonate (Tums) costs pennies a day and contains the most elemental calcium per dose. It should be taken with food to enhance absorption because acid is needed for maximal absorption. Calcium citrate contains less elemental calcium but is better absorbed and may be preferred by patients with reduced gastric acid production (e.g., older adults) or high gastric pH such as those on proton pump inhibitors or histamine2 (H2) blockers because it does not require acid for absorption (NIAMSD, 2011). Calcium formulations should be taken with vitamin D to improve the uptake of the calcium.

For those with osteoporosis risk and osteopenia, dietary sources are encouraged. The typical American diet provides 600 to 1,000 mg calcium daily. The best calcium sources are dairy products and certain vegetables such as broccoli. Whole milk is not recommended for infants after 12 months of age, but yogurt and cheese can be introduced in the infant diet

after 6 months of age (Office of Dietary Supplements, 2013). Yogurt has more than 400 mg per 8-oz serving and broccoli has 150 mg. The average absorption of calcium from dietary sources is only 10% to 12%. Vitamin D is necessary for optimal absorption. Table 38-3 shows the recommended dietary calcium intake in the United States by age. This includes the maximum recommended dosing; overintake is potentially harmful. What remains unclear is the dosing for obese patients. It is understood that Vitamin D absorption is reduced up to 40% (Dihaliwal, Mikhail, Feurerman, & Aloia, 2014), but dosing recommendations specific to the population were not found.

Calcium supplementation is economical. Table 38-4 presents information on available calcium preparations. When increased demand after menopause exceeds the typical dietary intake (1,200 mg), calcium alone as a supplement is not enough to prevent or treat osteoporosis. Patients need

Table 38–3 Recommendations for Adequate Dietary Calcium Intake in the United States

Age	Calcium Intake (mg/d)	Upper Intake Levels (mg)
0–6 months	200	1,000
7–12 months	260	1,500
1–3 years	700	2,500
4–8 years	1000	2,500
9–18 years	1300	3,000
19–50 years	1,000 for men 1200 for women	2,500
50 to >70 years	1,200	2,000

Based on the Office of Dietary Supplements (NIH, 2013). Verified with USPSTF 2013 guidelines.

Table 38–4 Calcium Preparations

Drug	Active Calcium	How Supplied
Calcium acetate	25%	1,000 mg tabs (250 mg calcium)
Calcium carbonate	40%	650 mg tablets (260 mg calcium)
Calcium citrate	21%	950 and 2,376 mg in tablets (200 and 500 mg calcium)
Calcium gluconate	9.3%	500, 650, 975 mg and 1 g tablets (45 mg calcium)
Calcium lactate	13%	325 and 650 mg tablets (42.5 mg and 84.5 mg calcium)
Tricalcium phosphate	39%	1,565.2 mg tablets (600 mg calcium)

Source: Wolters Kluwer Health, 2011, *Drug facts and comparisons*. St. Louis, MO: Wolters Kluwer Health, Inc.

pharmacotherapy, used in conjunction with vitamin D, exercise, and avoidance of certain lifestyle behaviors.

If patients complain of constipation with calcium in combination with carbonate, other formulations need to be substituted. The presence of milk allergy and lactose intolerance can also greatly affect the amount of calcium in the diet and make supplementation mandatory.

Calcium is always ingested in combination with other ions. Depending on which ion, the dose may need to be given away from mealtimes to avoid reduced absorption. Most calcium supplements in combination are only 40% to 50% active, so the practitioner needs to calculate the number of tablets depending on the size of tablet. A 600 mg Tums tablet has 240 mg of active calcium, and five Tums tablets fulfill the requirements for a postmenopausal woman.

Bisphosphonate Therapy

Indications

Primary and Secondary Prevention

NICE (2011a) recommends alendronate (Fosamax) for *primary prevention* in women over 70 years who have an independent risk factor for fracture and for women over 75 years with more than two risk factors. This drug is recommended by NICE (2011b), USPSTF (2011), and the Canadian Consensus Conference for women who are over 65 years and who are confirmed to have osteoporosis (Reid et al, 2009). This drug has also been studied in men, as has risendronate. Ibandronate (Boniva) is recommended as second-line therapy in *primary prevention* for postmenopausal women over 65 years of age with prior vertebral fractures. The American College of Physicians (Qaseem et al, 2008) also recommends that providers consider drug therapy for men and women who are at risk for developing osteoporosis but does not specifically state which drugs to use. The NICE (2011b) guidelines also discuss *secondary prevention*. They recommend the same drugs in the same order for this purpose but limit this recommendation to postmenopausal women who have osteoporosis and have sustained a clinically apparent osteoporotic fragility fracture.

There may be positive outcomes for hip replacement patients who start bisphosphonates after implant surgery. There is a correlation between duration and adherence to bisphosphonate therapy and a 59% reduction in the risk for the need for revision surgery. This positive impact was not found for patients who had already been on bisphosphonates (Prieto-Alhambras et al, 2014).

Patients may present with osteopenia, a precursor to osteoporosis. If the patient has other risk factors for osteoporosis and is found to be osteopenic (bone density of 1 to 2.5 standard deviations below the average adult peak bone mass), treatment with a bisphosphonate may be indicated for prevention of osteoporosis; however, there are doubts whether this is the best choice for those without prior fracture. Osteopenia is not a disease state (Kanis et al, 2013). The debate whether osteopenia should be treated has moved toward an individualized risk-to-benefit ratio discussion that must be undertaken between patient and provider.

Adverse Effects

The adverse effects of bisphosphonate and other bone agent therapies are covered in more detail in Chapter 21. The important risk-to-benefit ratio discussion must include the very, very low rate of osteonecrosis of the jaw and the rare subtrochanteric femoral fractures. Atrial fibrillation development is linked with zoledronic acid use. The media has broadcast these issues with the implication that most patients are at risk. The reality is that the benefit and protection from avoidance of a hip fracture dramatically overshadows the low risks (Black et al, 2010; Rizzoli et al, 2011).

Suggestions are being made that a "drug holiday" should be scheduled after a period of 3 to 5 years of bisphosphonate use (McClung, 2013). The binding of the medication with the bone is long-term; therefore, it is probably still effective over the next 3 to 5 years. Considering the small potential of adverse events, arranging a temporary cessation of drug use over 2 years is being touted as keeping the good qualities of mortality reduction and continuing to support bone health. Those on long-term steroid therapy are probably not good candidates for a drug holiday (McClure et al, 2013).

Treatment of Postmenopausal Women

Among the bisphosphonates, alendronate (Fosamax), risendronate (Actonel), ibandronate (Boniva), and zoledronic acid (Zometa) are all approved for preventing and treating postmenopausal osteoporosis. Studies have been done in large numbers of postmenopausal women with low bone mineral density in varying lengths of time from 2 to 10 years. In each study, the number of symptomatic fractures was reduced. Risendronate was helpful for women who had demonstrated osteoporosis. Ibandronate studied in osteoporotic women or those at high risk showed a reduced rate of vertebral fractures, whereas alendronate, risendronate and zoledronic acid have demonstrated the ability to reduce both hip and vertebral fractures. Zoledronic acid is selected when prior oral bisphosphonate use has not retarded bone loss on scans or when oral agents are not well tolerated.

Dosage schedules vary among guidelines but generally have lower doses for prevention and higher ones for osteoporosis treatment. Patients with a history of GI bleeding, peptic ulcer disease, and gastroesophageal reflux disease (GERD) are not good candidates for bisphosphonates because of the esophageal irritation common with this drug class.

Treatment of Men

Treatment for men who are age 70 or older and who are diagnosed with osteoporosis or have a high risk for hip fracture is similar to that of women. Alendronate is the drug recommended as first-line therapy. In the event of bisphosphonate intolerance, men do not have the option of using estrogen or anti-estrogen therapy.

Treatment of Men and Women Taking Corticosteroid Therapy

Both alendronate and risendronate are approved for use by men and women with glucocorticoid-induced osteoporosis (Watts et al, 2010) as first-line therapy (*Drug Facts and*

Comparisons, 2009; ICSI, 2011). The corticosteroid dose mentioned is equivalent to 5 mg/d of prednisone for a duration of 3 or more months. Chapter 21 provides more information on these drugs, including their dosing.

Cost Versus Dosing Schedule

Because the cost is approximately the same for all oral drugs that have gone generic, the convenience of once-monthly dosing may favor ibandronate. Obviously, the required infusion center costs associated with the zoledronic acid places it in a much higher cost tier. The cost and convenience of bisphosphonates should also be compared with much lower costs for estrogen and estrogen-progestin therapies (as appropriate). ERT/HRT dosing is typically daily.

Adequate supplementation with calcium and vitamin D is necessary before initiating therapy, and some newer formulations have either vitamin D or calcium included. No dosage adjustment is necessary as long as renal function remains between 35 and 60 mL/minute. Creatinine levels must be checked prior to any zoledronic acid infusion.

Reports that generic bisphosphonates, especially alendronate, are causing more GI side effects than the branded version have surfaced (Kanis et al, 2012). If true, that means more patients will be nonadherent to the plan. Substitution with the brand-name drug will increase costs; however, so will the costs of avoidable fractures if the patient refuses therapy.

Selective Estrogen Receptor Modulators

Raloxifene

Raloxifene (Evista) is a selective estrogen receptor modulator (SERM) approved to treat osteoporosis. Postmenopausal women with established osteoporosis had a statistically significant reduction in vertebral fractures when taking 60 mg to 120 mg of raloxifene at the 3-year mark, but at 8 years this difference disappeared. There was, however, a marked reduction in the incidence of invasive breast cancer in women taking this drug for the same period.

Though considered an alternative to tamoxifen as a breast cancer antagonist, raloxifene is not as powerful as the other SERM drugs for that indication. Postmenopausal women taking raloxifene versus placebo had a lower risk for cardiovascular events, most likely secondary to lowered serum LDL. It is indicated for prevention and treatment of osteoporosis in women who do not want to use or are unable to take estrogen therapy. It shares with estrogen the precaution to avoid use in women who have previously had a deep vein thrombus or embolism. SERMs only block estrogen binding, but free serum estrogen remains in the system (Zhang et al, 2012); therefore, they cannot comfortably be taken by pre- or perimenopausal women due to the presence of higher levels of natural estrogen and subsequent intolerable hot flashes.

Guidelines do not recommend raloxifene for *primary prevention* of osteoporotic fragility fracture in postmenopausal women but do list it as a second-line drug for secondary therapy. It is also second-line therapy for women without thrombotic risk who are at increased risk for breast cancer.

Bazedoxifene and others

Bazedoxifene in combination with a conjugated equine estrogen (Duavee) is a SERM plus estrogen combination marketed primarily for dyspareunia treatment. The SERM component of bazedoxifene is protective for the uterus from the estrogen component. It has positive bone health and reduction of menopausal hot flash characteristics as well. Most SERMS have vertebral bone improvement indications; Duavee has shown improvement in hip density. The FDA has indicated it be used for bone health for postmenopausal women with significant risk of bone loss. It carries all the contraindications and risks of any other estrogen-containing medication.

Raloxifene appears to work better in younger patients; bazedoxifene appears to work better as the risk for more fractures increases. These findings are not established until there is longer term use of bazedoxifene.

Adverse Reactions

When compared with estrogen and progesterone, raloxifene's adverse reactions were in the areas of more hot flashes, genital and urinary infection, and chest pain. HRT, by contrast, demonstrated more vaginal bleeding, breast pain, and flatulence. Bazedoxifene plus estrogen carries similar side effects of both of these drug classes.

A previous history of venous thromboembolic events such as deep vein thrombosis, pulmonary embolism, and retinal artery embolism is a contraindication for use of SERMs. Patients with multiple risk factors for osteoporosis should receive BDM assessments to evaluate their need for this drug.

Patients need to be warned that these drugs should be discontinued 72 hours prior to prolonged bedrest and to avoid inactivity while traveling by car or plane. Women need to know that raloxifene medication will not stop hot flashes; in fact, it could trigger hot flashes at the beginning of therapy.

Cost and Dosing Schedule

The dose of raloxifene is 60 mg daily without regard to meals. The cost for a 1-month supply is about the same as for bisphosphonates but over twice the cost of estrogen. It must be taken daily. Bazedoxifen plus estrogen is also a daily medication which comes in 0.45 mg/20 mg and 0.625 mg/20 mg doses. As a brand name drug the cost is higher than most generics. Concurrent supplements of calcium and vitamin D daily are still needed with all SERM medications.

Human Parathyroid Hormone

Teriparatide (Forteo) is the only drug in this class and has limited indications. It is reserved for women at high risk of fracture, including those with very low bone mineral density with a previous vertebral fracture and who are unable to take a bisphosphonate or have had an unsatisfactory response to other therapies. It should be used only after evaluation by a specialist. A prospective, placebo-controlled trial in a large number of women with postmenopausal osteoporosis whose average age was 70 years found a statistically significant decrease in the incidence of vertebral fracture. The doses used in this study were 20 mcg to 40 mcg once daily for 21 months. The safety and efficacy of this injectable drug have not been evaluated beyond 2 years of treatment. It is very costly and has some possible cancer-causing long-term effects. With its very limited indications, it is a third-line drug in treating osteoporosis.

Combination Therapy

Additive effects on bone mineral density tests have been found with alendronate plus raloxifene combinations and in estrogen plus bazedoxifene (Duavee); however, evidence that this will reduce fractures at a higher level is still not established. There is some concern that this combination of two different reabsorptive agents could suppress bone turnover to the point that fracture might actually be increased. This concern is echoed when a bisphosphonate is followed by a PTH medication or denosumab (Kanis et al, 2013). Early studies imply that SERM therapy after PTH analogue may increase the benefit gained from the original analogue impact (Kanis et al, 2013). Teriparatide and bisphosphonates did not have added value. The combination of teriparatide and denosumab after 1 year of therapy had much more positive impact than each used separately (Tsai et al, 2013). This is especially encouraging due to the increase in the femoral neck and hip density. However, the suspicion that bone formation is suppressed as evidenced by newer biomarkers of bone turnover has the experts withholding full endorsement of this therapy (Tsai et al, 2013).

Comparisons

Estrogen is effective in preventing fractures but has cardiovascular and cancer risks. Most SERMs are also effective in preventing fractures, have less cardiovascular risk, and actually reduce the risk for breast cancer, unless mixed with estrogen. They still carry the thromboembolic risks. All require daily dosing. Bisphosphonates are effective in preventing fractures and have once-weekly or once-monthly dosing. They do not have breast cancer reduction characteristics. Bisphosphonates are listed as first-line therapy for osteoporosis in all the guidelines. Estrogen and SERMs are secondary medications for osteoporosis. Synthetic PTH meds have specific indications and carry cost issues and possible cancer risks. Calcium, especially when combined with vitamin D, is central to prevention of osteoporosis and the resultant fractures. They are inexpensive and should be used even if other drugs are chosen. Vitamin D alone is ineffective for osteoporosis treatment or risk reduction (Aloia et al, 2013) Finally, low-impact weight-bearing exercise is critical to prevention of osteoporosis. It should be noted that tamoxifen is a SERM, but contributes to bone loss in premenopausal women. Table 38-5 shows comparison of fracture reduction by class. Figure 38-3 depicts an algorithm for the prevention of osteoporosis in patients without the disease, and Figure 38-4 presents a treatment algorithm for osteoporosis.

Table 38–5 Fracture Risk Reduction Comparisons

	Vertebral Fracture Reduction	Non-Vertebral Reduction
Bisphosphonates		
Alendronate	48%	50% spine and hip
Ibandronate	50%	29.9%
Risendronate	36%	41%–49%
Zoledronic acid	70&	41% hip
Anabolic Hormone		
Teriparatide	65%	53%
Estrogenic Hormone		
Estrogen		34% combined hip and vertebral
Rank Ligand Inhibitors		
Denosumab	68%	
Selective Estrogen Receptor Modulators		
Raloxifen	30%–55%	
Estrogen plus Bazedoxifene	1.5%	1.21%

Based on information from Wright (2011) and manufacturer resources.

Monitoring

Before beginning treatment for osteoporosis, rule out common treatable disorders that can also cause low bone density. These include hyperparathyroidism, vitamin D deficiency, hyperthyroidism, and renal disease. Tests for these disorders are serum calcium and albumin, 25-hydroxy vitamin D, TSH, and serum creatinine levels, respectively. Serum creatinine levels are drawn prior to initiating therapy.

Measurement of bone mineral density is the most accurate predictor of fracture risk and efficacy of these drugs. Each 10% change below peak bone mass is associated with a doubling of the fracture risk for patients with osteoporosis. Dual-energy x-ray absorptiometry (DEXA) is the gold standard by which bone mineral density and therapy are monitored, but a quantitative computed tomography (QCT) can be used. Initial evaluation with these scans can also suggest when a disease process other than aging is the probable cause of the bone loss (Table 38-6).

Once therapy has been established, DEXA is repeated 1 to 2 years later to determine progress. Only the dual-energy DEXA can be used to monitor progression after therapy is initiated. How often to repeat DEXA at later dates is controversial (Rosen & Drezner, 2013). According to the American Association of Clinical Endocrinologists (AACE) (Watts, et al, 2010), DEXA should be used for the following:

1. Women who are estrogen-deficient, to make decisions about therapy

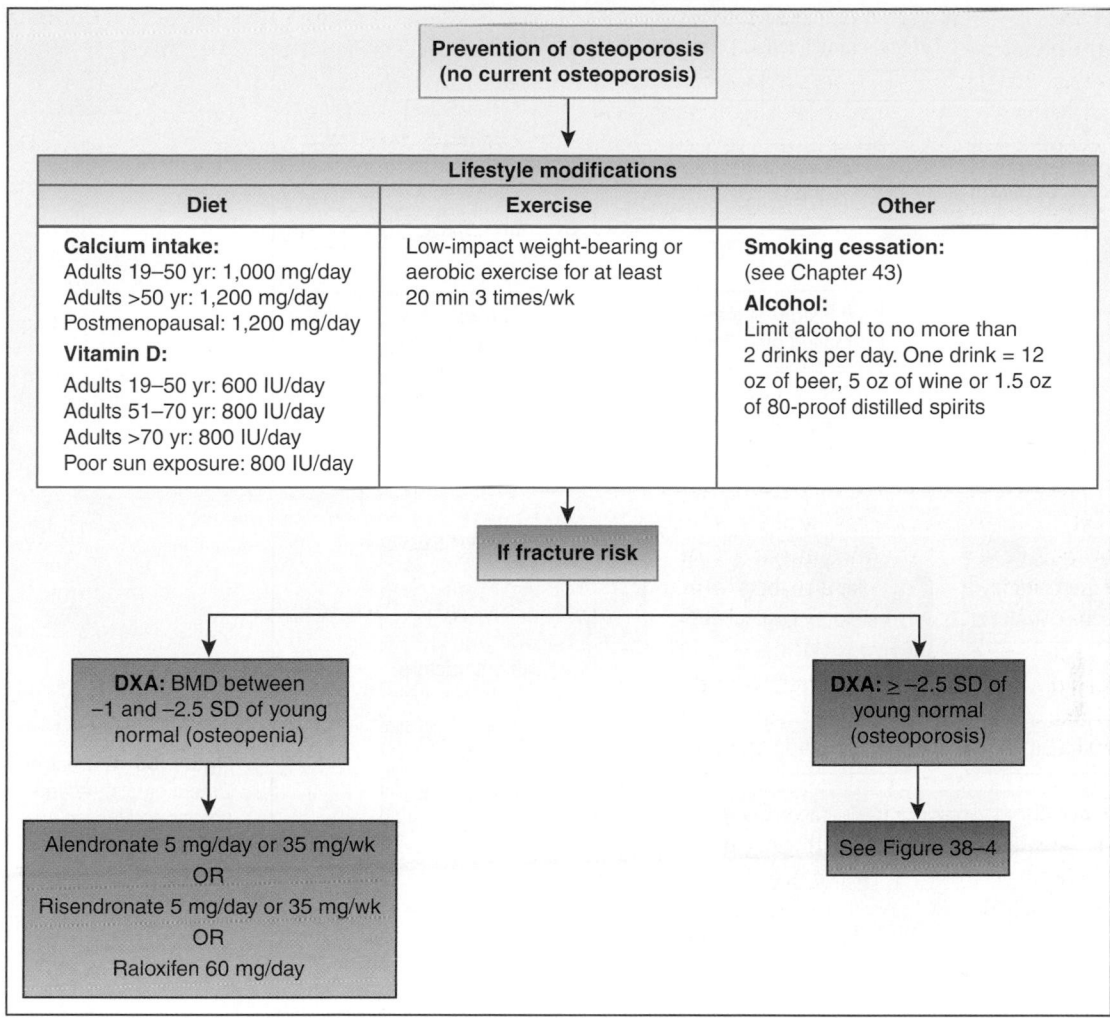

Figure 38–3. Prevention of osteoporosis in patients without the disease.

2. Women who have vertebral abnormalities or osteopenia detected on x-ray, to confirm the diagnosis
3. Patients who are being treated for osteoporosis, to monitor for treatment efficacy
4. Patients receiving long-term glucocorticoid therapy, to guide therapy to preserve bone mass
5. Patients with asymptomatic primary hyperthyroidism or other diseases associated with high risk for osteoporosis, to make therapy decisions.
6. All women 40 years and older who have sustained a fracture
7. All women older than 65 years

ICSI (2011) adds the following risk factors:

1. Body weight less than 127 lb or BMI less than or equal to 20
2. Current smoker
3. Surgical menopause before 40 years
4. On hormone replacement for more than 10 to 15 years
5. Premenopausal women with amenorrhea for more than 1 year
6. Anyone with severe loss of mobility (unable to ambulate outside one's dwelling without a wheelchair) for more than 1 year

Table 38-5 lists methods for bone density measurements. The use of heel scans sometimes found in health fairs and shopping malls can give a false sense of security; the heel is one of the densest bones in the body and requires quite a bit of skeletal bone loss elsewhere before it typically becomes less dense. A "good" heel scan can create an impression of sound bone health, when the opposite is true. Imaging studies of the chest, extremities, and spine can easily uncover occult bone density issues even when obtained for nonbone health reasons.

Estrogen

Estrogen requires the same monitoring when prescribed for osteoporosis as it does when it is used for ERT/HRT. Obtain annual renal function tests on all patients older than 65 years and on those with potentially reduced renal function, such as patients with diabetes.

Calcium

The use of calcium alone for supplementation rarely needs blood test follow-up, but treatment of conditions with vitamin D and high-dose calcium can induce high levels in serum and then in the kidneys.

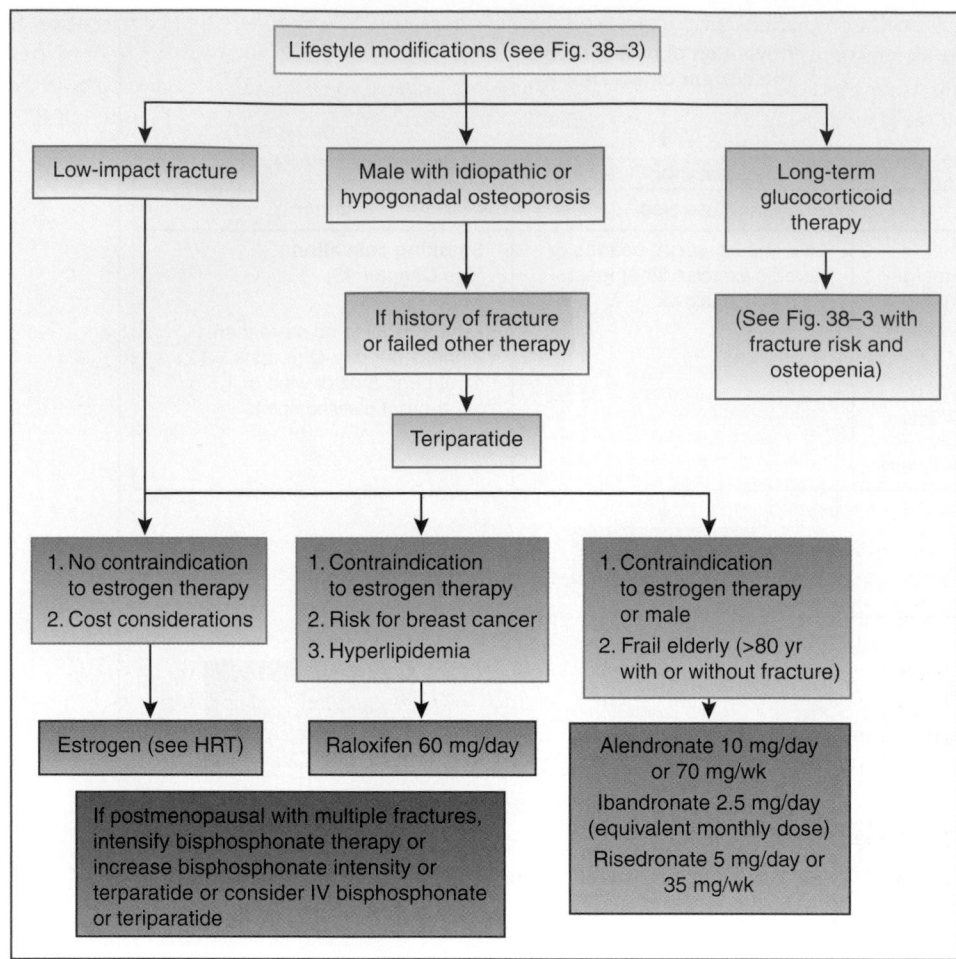

Figure 38–4. Treatment algorithm: Osteoporosis. (Adapted from *Osteoporosis and African American Women; Osteoporosis and Asian American Women; Osteoporosis and Hispanic Women* [all from NIAMS documents, 2005]; and National Osteoporosis Foundation, 2004, *Physician's Guide*.)

Bisphosphonates

Monitoring of bisphosphonates is aimed at electrolyte measurement, renal function, and GI symptoms of patients older than 65 years, and of those with multiple medical conditions.

Dosage alterations or contraindications to using specific bisphosphonates occur with serum creatinine levels above 2.5 mg/dL or creatinine clearance less than 30 mL/min. Because bisphosphonates inhibit intestinal calcium transport, careful monitoring of serum calcium should be done during therapy. Phosphate, magnesium, and potassium should also be monitored because these electrolytes may be altered by bisphosphonate administration.

SERMs

Evaluation of therapy with SERM therapy can be done every 2 years with DEXA, but beneficial effects may be demonstrated as early as 1 year after therapy. Other monitoring is similar to that of estrogen.

Outcome Evaluation

Osteoporosis is expected to begin 2 to 5 years after menopause in women not using ERT/HRT. Assess patients who have had fractures, unusual bone pain, high-risk physical characteristics, or a history of systemic cortisone use. The

Table 38–6 Common Methods for Bone Density Measurements

Test	Sites Measured	Comments
Dual energy x-ray absorptiometry (DEXA)	Spine, hip, total body	Limitations: misdiagnoses low bone mass in patients with arthritis, spinal deformity, or prior spinal surgery
Peripheral dual energy x-ray absorptiometry (P-DEXA)	Wrist, finger, heel	Limitations: older adults who tend to have arthritis in these sites (see above). Omits several areas (vertebra and hip) that are common sites of osteoporosis in this age group. Cannot be used to measure progress of therapy.
Quantitative computed tomography (QCT)	Spine and hip	Good with spinal issues. Limitations: machine must be recalibrated between uses; higher radiation
Ultrasound	Heel, tibia, finger	Limitations: new, younger, no x-ray

advanced practice nurse can begin this evaluation with a history and physical examination, laboratory tests, and imaging studies. If any of these tests or imaging studies indicates acute bone pathology, referral for specialty care is indicated.

Patients who have other medical conditions and multiple medications to manage are candidates for consultation or referral. Consider referral if more than one consultation is made with the specialist over medication choices. After therapy is established and the patient is not having adverse drug effects, most primary care providers handle routine monitoring.

OSTEOPOROSIS

PATIENT EDUCATION

Patient education should include a discussion of information related to the overall treatment plan as well as that specific to the drug therapy, reasons for taking the drug, drugs as part of the total treatment regimen, and adherence issues. Patients who have taken teriparatide should take advantage of the voluntary patient registry to help track the rare occurrence of osteosarcoma.

Related to the Overall Treatment Plan/Disease Process

☐ Pathophysiology of the dynamic relationship between the osteoclasts and osteoblasts in the process of bone metabolism to help the patient understand how the lack of estrogen begins a cascade of events ending with the increased risk of osteoporosis in the early years after cessation of menses. For men, discussion of the role of other factors is important.

☐ The role of excessive intake of alcohol, nicotine, and caffeine and low intake of calcium and vitamin D as modifiable risks for osteoporosis and how nondrug treatments such as diets high in calcium and vitamin D, exercise, and avoidance of the high-risk lifestyles can help to prevent osteoporosis.

☐ An understanding of how knowledge of family history, ethnicity, and genetic characteristics helps to identify patients with nonmodifiable risk factors for osteoporosis.

☐ Importance of adherence to the treatment regimen

☐ Importance of supplementing the diet with additional calcium (up to 1,500 mg) and vitamin D (800 mg) to the osteoporosis therapy

☐ Self-monitoring of symptoms

☐ What to do when symptoms worsen

☐ Need for regular follow-up visits with the primary care provider and for screening tests such as BMDs every 2 years.

Specific to the Drug Therapy

☐ Reason for the drug(s) to be taken and anticipated action in the disease process

☐ Doses and schedules for taking the drug(s)

☐ Possible adverse effects and what to do if they occur

☐ Interactions between other treatment modalities and these drugs

Reasons for Taking the Drug(s)

Patient education specifically for osteoporosis should include the following: that prevention of osteoporosis is more successful than having to treat it later, especially in those who have a hereditary tendency for bone loss disease; treatment of fractures is far more expensive than drug therapy; and postmenopausal fractures are associated with early loss of independent living and reduced life expectancy.

Drugs as Part of the Total Treatment Regimen

The total treatment regimen includes lifestyle modification: healthy diet, dietary supplements, and exercise. However, these lifestyle modifications may not be enough, especially in older patients. Some form of drug therapy is usually necessary. A variety of therapies are available, and selection of estrogen versus nonestrogen therapy is possible with the same results for prevention and treatment of spine, hip, and wrist fractures associated with osteoporosis.

Adherence Issues

Adherence issues include the following:

☐ Media reports about disease and drug therapies have an increasing impact on patients and primary care practices.

☐ Membership in health maintenance organizations may affect the choice of drugs patients will receive.

☐ Patients' fears or issues about drug therapy may not be based on facts.

☐ Drug therapy educational handouts should be available to patients and their families.

☐ Monitoring appointments are problematic if patients are homebound or transportation is difficult.

REFERENCES

Aloia, M., Dihaliwal, R., Shieh, A., Mikhail, M., Islam, S., & Yeh, J. (2013). Calcium and vitamin D supplementation in postmenopausal women. (2013). *Journal of Clinical Endocrinology & Metabolism. 98*(1), E1702–E1709.

Amato, P. Young, R., Steinberg, F., Murray, M., Lewis, R., Cramer, M., et al. (2013). Effect of soy isoflavone supplementation on menopausal quality of life. *Menopause, 20*(4), 443–447. doi: 10.1097/gme.0b013e318275025e

American College of Rheumatology. (2004). Concomitant teriparatide plus raloxifene for the treatment of postmenopausal osteoporosis: Results from a randomized placebo-controlled trial. www.rheumatology.org/press/2004

Anderson, G., Judd, H., Kaunitz, A., Barad, D., Beresford, S., Pettinger, M., et al. (2003). Effects of estrogen plus progestin on gynecologic cancers and associated diagnostic procedures: The Women's Health Initiative Randomized Trial. *Journal of the American Medical Association, 290*(13), 1739–1748.

Anderson, G., Limacher, M., Assaf, A., Bassford, T., Beresford, S., Black, H., et al. (2004). Effects of conjugated equine estrogen in postmenopausal women with hysterectomy: The Women's Health Initiative randomized trial. *Journal of the American Medical Association, 291,* 1701–1712.

Bischoff-Ferrari, H., Willett, W., Orav, E., Lips, P., Meurnier, P., Lyons, R., et al. (2012). A pooled analysis of vitamin D dose requirements for fracture prevention. *New England Journal of Medicine, 367*(1), 40–49. doi: 10.1056/NEJMoa1109617

Black, D., Kelly, M., Genant, M., Palermo, L., Eastell R., Bucci-Rechtweg, C., & HORIZON Pivotal Fracture Trial Steering Communitee (2010). Bisphosphonates and fractures of the subtrochanteric or diphyseal femur. *New England Journal of Medicine, 362*(19), 1761–1771.

Brinton, L., & Felix, A. (2013). Menopausal hormone therapy and risk of endometrial cancer. *Journal of Steroid Biochemistry and Molecular Biology.* doi:10.16/j.sbmb.2013.05.001 epub ahead of print 13 May 2013.

Chlebowski, R., Hendrix, S., Langer, R., Stefanick, M., Gass, M., Lane, D., et al. (2003). Influence of estrogen plus progestin on breast cancer and mammography in healthy postmenopausal women: The Women's Health Initiative Randomized Trial. *Journal of the American Medical Association, 289*(24), 3243–3253.

Chlebowski, R., Manson, J., Anderson, G., Cauley, J., Aragaki, A., Stefanick, M., et al. (2013). Estrogen plus progestin and breast cancer incidence and mortality in the women's health initiative observational study. *Journal of the National Cancer Insitute, 105*(7), e1–e10. doi:10.1093/jnci/dit043

Cohen, A., Dempster, D. Reckers, R., Lappe, J., Zhou, H., Zwaheln, A., et al. (2013). Abdominal fat is associated with lower bone formation and inferior bone quality in healthy premenopausal women: A transiliac bone biopsy study. *Journal of Clinical Endocrinology & Metabolism.* e pub ahead of print 20 Mar 2013. doi:10.1210/jc.2013-1047

Dihaliwal, R., Mikhail, M., Feurerman, M., & Aloia, A, (2014). The vitamin D dose response in obesity. *Endocrine Practice. 20*(12), 1258–1264.

Farr, J., Drake, M., Amin, S., Melton, L., McCready, L., & Khosla, S. (2014). In vio assessment of bone quality in postmenopausal women with type 2 diabetes. *Journal of Bone and Mineral Research. 29*(4), 787–795.

Flies, J., Ko, M., & Pruthi, S. (2011). Bioidentical hormone therapy. *Mayo Clinic Proceedings, 86*(7), 673–680.

Greendale, G., Ishii, S., Huang, M., & Karlamangia, A. (2013) Predicting the timeline to the final menstrual period: The study of women's health across the nation. *Journal of Clinical Endocrinology & Metabolism, 98*(4), 1483–1491. doi:10.1210/jc.2012-3732

Greenspan, S., Emkey, R., Bone, H., Weiss, S., Bell, N., Downs, R., et al. (2002). Significant differential effects of alendronate, estrogen or combination therapy on the rate of bone loss after discontinuation of treatment of postmenopausal osteoporosis: A randomized, double-blind, placebo-controlled trial. *Archives of Internal Medicine, 137*(11), 875–883.

Hall, E., Frey, B., & Soares, C. (2011). Non-hormonal treatment strategies for vasomotor symptoms: A critical review. *Drugs, 71*(3), 287–304.

Herrington, D., Reboussin, D., Brosnihan, K., Sharp, P., Shumaker, S., Snyder, T., et al. (2000). Effects of estrogen replacement on the progression of coronary artery atherosclerosis (ERA). *New England Journal of Medicine, 343*(8), 522–529.

Hodis, H., Mack, W., Azen, S., Lobo, R. A., Shoupe, D., Maher, P. R., et al. (2003). Hormone therapy and the progression of coronary artery atherosclerosis in postmenopausal women. *New England Journal of Medicine, 349*(6), 535–545.

Holtorf, K. (2009). The bioidentical hormone debate: Are bioidentical hormones (estradiol, estriol, and progesterone) safer or more efficacious than commonly used synthetic versions in hormone replacement therapy? *Postgraduate Medicine, 121*(1), 73–85.

Institute for Clinical Systems Improvement (ICSI). (2011). *Diagnosis and treatment of osteoporosis.* Bloomington, MN: www.ICSI.org/osteoporosis

International Osteoporosis Foundation (IOF). (2012). Facts and statistics about osteoporosis and its impact. http://www.iofbonehealth.org

Kanis, J., McClosky, E., Johanssen, H., Cooper, C., Rizzoli, R., & Reginster, J. (2013). European guidance for the diagnosis and management of osteoporosis. *Osteoporosis International, 24*(1), 23–57.

Kanis, J., Reginster, J., Kaufman, J., Ringe, J., Adachi J., Hiligmann, M., et al. (2012). A reappraisal of generic bisphosphates in osteoporosis. *Osteoporosis International, 23,*13–221.

Langer, R. (2005). Postmenopausal hormone therapy. *CME Bulletin of the American Academy of Family Physicians, 4*(1), 1–10.

Langsetmo, L., Berger. C., Kreiger, N., Kovacs, C., Hanly, D., Jamal, S., et al. (2013). Calcium and vitamin D intake and mortality: Results from the Canadian multicenter osteoporosis study (CaMos). *Journal of Clinical Endocrinology & Metabolism.* epub 23 May. doi:10.1210/jc.2013-1516

Lindenfeld, E., & Langer, R. (2002). Bleeding patterns of hormone replacement therapies in the postmenopausal estrogen and progestin interventions trial. *Obstetrics and Gynecology, 100,* 853–863.

Liu, J. (2004). Use of conjugated estrogens after the Women's Health Initiative. *The Female Patient, 29,* 8–13.

Liu, J., Burdette, J., Xu, H., Gu, C., vanBreemen, R., Bhat, K., et al. (2001). Evaluation of estrogenic activity of plant extracts for the potential treatment of menopausal symptoms. *Journal of Agricultural and Food Chemistry, 49,* 2472–2479.

Mathews, K., Gibson, C., El Khoudray, S., & Thurston, R. (2013). Changes in cardiovascular risk factors by hysterectomy status with and without oophorectomy: SWAN Study of Woman's Health Across the Nation. *Journal of the American College of Cardiologists,* 2013 epub ahead of print 22 May. doi:10.1016/jacc2013.04.042

McCance, K. L., & Huether, S. E. (2014). *Pathophysiology: The biologic basis for disease in adults and children* (7th ed.). St Louis, MO: Elsevier.

McClure, M., Harris, S., Miller, P., Bauer, D., Davison, K., Dian, L., et al. (2013). Bisphosponate therapy for osteoporosis: Benefits, risks, and drug holiday. *American Journal of Medicine, 126*(1), 13–20.

Mosca, L., Barret-Connor, E., & Kass Wenger, N. (2011). Sex/gender differences in cardiovascular disease prevention: What a difference a decade makes. *Circulation, 124*(19), 2145–2154.

National Institute for Health and Clinical Excellence (NICE). (2011a). *Alendronate, etidronate, risedronate, raloxifene and strontium ranelate for the primary prevention of osteoporotic fragility fractures in postmenopausal women.* London, England: National Institute for Health and Clinical Excellence (NICE). www.guideline.gov/summary/summary.aspx

National Institute for Health and Clinical Excellence (NICE). (2011b). *Alendronate, etidronate, risedronate, raloxifene, strontium ranelate and teriparatide for the secondary prevention of osteoporotic fragility fractures in postmenopausal women.* London, England: National Institute for Health and Clinical Excellence (NICE). www.guideline.gov/summary/summary.aspx

National Institute of Arthritis and Musculoskeletal and Skin Diseases (NIAMSD). (2010a). *Osteoporosis and African American women.* www.niams.nih.gov/bone/hi/osteoporosis

National Institute of Arthritis and Musculoskeletal and Skin Diseases (NIAMSD). (2010b). *Osteoporosis and Asian American women.* www.niams.nih.gov/bone/hi/osteoporosis

National Institute of Arthritis and Musculoskeletal and Skin Diseases (NIAMSD). (2010c). *Osteoporosis and Hispanic women.* www.niams.nih.gov/bone/hi/osteoporosis

National Institute of Arthritis and Musculoskeletal and Skin Diseases (NIAMSD). (2011). *Osteoporosis handout on health.* www.niams.nih .gov/bone/osteoporosis

National Institute for Health Osteoporosis and Related Bone Diseases (2011). *National Resource Center review.* www.niams.nih.gov/Health-Information/ Bone/Osteoporosis/Conditions-Behaviors /Osteoporosis

Nestle, M., & Nesheim, M. (2013). To supplement or not to supplement: The US Preventive Services Task Force [USPSTF] recommendations on calcium and vitamin D. *Annals of Internal Medicine,158*(9), 701–702.

North American Menopause Society (NAMS). (2012). The 2012 hormone therapy position statement of the North American Menopause Society. *Menopause, 19*(3), 257–271.

Office of Dietary Supplements NIH. (2013). *Dietary supplement fact sheet: Calcium—Health professional fact sheet.* www.ods.od.hih.gov/factssheets/ Calcium-HealthProfessional

Pattimakiel, L., & Thacker, H. (2011). Bioidentical hormone therapy: Clarifying the misconceptions. *Cleveland Clinic Journal of Medicine, 78,*(12), 829–836.

Qaseem, A., Snow, V., Shekelle, P., Hopkins, R., Jr., Forciea, M., Owens, D., the Clinical Efficacy Assessment Subcommittee of the American College of Physicians. (2008). Screening for osteoporosis in men: A clinical practice guideline from the American College of Physicians. *Annals of Internal Medicine, 148*(9), 680–684

Prieto-Alhambra, D., Lalmohamed, A., Abrahamsen, B., Arden, N., de Boer, A., Vestergaard, P., et al. (2014). Oral bisphosphonate use and total knee/hip implant survival: Validation of results in an external population-based cohort. *Arthritis & Rheumatology. 66*(11), 3233–3240.

Reid, R. L., Blake, J., Abramson, B., Khan, A., Senikas, V., & Fortier, M. (2009). SOGC Clinical practice guideline: Menopause and osteoporosis update 2009. *Journal of Obstetrics and Gynecology Canada, 31*(1), S34–S41.

Rizzoli, R., Akesson, K., Boouxsein, M., Kanis, J., Napoli, N., Papapoulos, S., et al. (2011). Subtrochanteric fractures after long-term treatment with bisphosphonates; A European society on clinical and economic aspects of osteoporosis and osteoarthritis, and the International Osteoporosis Foundation Working Group report. *Osteoporosis International, 22*(2), 373–390.

Rosen, H., & Drezner, M. (2012, 10 Oct). Overview of the management of osteoporosis in postmenopausal women. *UpTo Date.* Retrieved November 2012.

Rosner, W., Hankison, S., Sluss, P., Vesper, H., & Wierman, M. (2013). Challenges to the measurement of estradiol: An Endocrine Society position statement. *Journal of Clinical Endocrinolgy & Metabolism, 98*(4), 1376–1387.

Shapiro, S., Farmer, R., Stevenson, J., Burger, H., & Mueck, A. (2012). Does hormone replacement therapy (HRT) cause breast cancer? An application of causal principles to three students, part 5. Trends in breast cancer incidence in relation to the use of HRT. *Journal of Family Planning and Reproductive Health Care, 38*(12), 102–109. doi:10.1136/jfprhc-2012-100508

Sharma, A., Chatterjee, S., Cubab-Zadeh, A., Goyal, S., Lichstein, E., Ghosh, J., et al. (2013). Risk of serious atrial fibrillation and stroke with use of bisphosphonates. Chest 144(4), 1311–1322.

Shen, C., Yeh, J., Cao J., Chyu, M., & Wang, J. (2012). Green tea and bone health. *Pharmacological Research, 64*(2), 155–161.

Stunkel, C., Gass, M., Manson, J., Lobo, R., Pal, L., Rebar, R., et al. (2012). A decade after the women's health initiative—the experts do agree. *Menopause, 19*(8), 846–847. doi:10.1097/gme.0b013e3182622f2

Thorneycroft, I. (2004, February). Unopposed estrogen and cancer. *The Female Patient* (Suppl.), 19–26.

Tsai, J., Uihlein, A., Lee, H., Kumbhani, R., Siwla-Sackman, E., McKay, E., et al. (2013). Teriparatide and denosumab, alone or combined, in women with postmenopausal osteoporosis: The DATA study randomized trial. *The Lancet.* doi:10.1016/S0140-60856(13)60856-9; published online ahead of print 15 May 2013.

University of Texas, School of Nursing, Family Nurse Practitioner Program. (2008). Risk factor assessment for osteoporosis and/or increased fracture risk in men. Austin, TX: University of Texas, School of Nursing. www.guideline.gov/summary/summary.aspx

U.S. Food and Drug Administration[FDA] (2013, 26 Feb). *FDA approves ospemifene for postmenopausal women experiencing pain during sex.* FDA News Release 26 Feb, 2013.

United States Preventative Services Task Force [USPSTF] (2011). Screening for osteoporosis. *Annals of Internal Medicine, 154*(5), 1–40.

United States Preventative Services Task Force [USPSTF]. (2013). Menopausal hormone therapy for the primary prevention of chronic conditions. *Annals of Internal Medicine, 158*(1), 47–54.

Watts, N., Bilezikian, J., Camacho, P., Greenspan, S., Harris, S., Hodgson, S., et al. (2010). American Association of Clinical Endocrinologists medical guidelines for clinical practice for the diagnosis and treatment of postmenopausal osteoporosis: Executive summary. *Endocrinology Practice, 16*(6), 1016–1019.

Wolters Kluwer Health. (2011). *Drug facts and comparisons.* St. Louis, MO: Wolters Kluwer Health.

Wright, W. (2011). Quantifying fracture risk. Advance for NPs & Pas. XX (X) 31-37.

Writing Group for the Women's Health Initiative (WHI) Investigators. (2002). Risks and benefits of estrogen plus progestin in healthy postmenopausal women. *Journal of the American Medical Association, 288*(3), 321–323.

Writing Group of the PEPI Trial. (1996). Effects of hormonal therapy on bone mineral density: Results from the post-menopausal estrogen/ progestin interventions (PEPI). *Journal of the American Medical Association, 276*(17), 1394–1396.

Zhang, Y., Simondsen, K., & Kelesar, J. (2012). Exemestane for primary prevention of breast cancer. *American Journal of Health System Pharmacy, 69*(16), 1384–1388.

HYPERLIPIDEMIA

Marylou V. Robinson

Cardiovascular diseases (CVD) are the major cause of death in the United States. Almost 500,000 people die each year from heart attacks, most commonly related to coronary artery disease (CAD). The care focus is expanding beyond just CAD or coronary heart disease (CHD) to include CVD issues of peripheral vascular disease and strokes as equally important endpoints for evaluating therapeutic effect. One-third of the American population is considered to be at high risk for CVD. The perfect storm of an obesity epidemic, uncontrolled hypertension, metabolic syndromes, and rampant consumption of nutritionally risky diets combined with high stress and lack of regular exercise are all components of the problem. This chapter focuses upon the major contributor of cholesterol to the pathological picture.

Atherosclerosis is characterized by deposits of cholesterol and lipoproteins in artery walls. Three major classes of lipoproteins are found in the serum of fasting individuals: low-density lipoproteins (LDL), high-density lipoproteins (HDL), and very-low-density lipoproteins (VLDL). Guidelines for identifying risk for CAD and CVD have traditionally focused on serum cholesterol levels above 200 mg/dL, fasting triglyceride TG levels above 150 mg/dL, and LDL levels above 100 mg/dL. The newest guidelines place a stronger emphasis upon individual risk factors with lifestyle and pharmacological therapies individualized to reduce that risk. In the classic Framingham studies, a 10% decrease in serum cholesterol level was associated with a 2% decrease in the incidence of CVD morbidity and mortality. Other studies have confirmed, in men and women who were initially free of CHD, a direct relationship between levels of LDL cholesterol and the rate of new-onset CHD. Early trials with HMG-CoA reductase inhibitors (statins) indicated that a 1% decrease in LDL cholesterol reduces the risk of CVD by about 1% (National Cholesterol Education Program [NCEP], 2001). However, these studies and risk tools were not reflective of the true American population because they did not include African Americans and women. Frequently, healthier cohorts of individuals were enrolled in longitudinal studies to monitor the onset of CVD risks in the population. The current guidelines attempt to be more inclusive of the average population.

The management of hyperlipidemia presented is based on the 2013 guidelines of the American College of Cardiology and the American Heart Association but also reflects the anticipated therapeutic shifts that will evolve from developing perspectives over time and the publication of the JNC-8 and Obesity guidelines (JNC-8, 2014; Stone et al, 2013). Chapters 14 and 16 provide specific information on the drugs used.

PATHOPHYSIOLOGY

Serum fat and cholesterol are carried in the circulation in complexes of lipids and proteins called lipoproteins. Fat is transported as TG and phospholipids, and cholesterol is transported in free and esterified forms. Most of the cholesterol in plasma is carried in LDLs. High concentrations of LDLs are associated with an increased risk of CVD. Serum lipoproteins are formed via two pathways: dietary, or exogenous, and liver synthesis, or endogenous.

Exogenous Pathway

After a meal, fat and cholesterol are absorbed by the intestinal cells, esterified into TG and cholesterol, and then packaged into chylomicrons, which are transported via the lymphatic system to the thoracic duct where they enter the venous circulation. Activated endothelial lipoprotein lipase then hydrolyzes the TG into free fatty acids and glycerol, which are removed from the circulation for use by fat and muscle cells. Surface cholesterol is transferred to HDLs. The chylomicrons shrink during this process and become remnants that are removed from the circulation by apolipoprotein (apo) E after it binds to a liver receptor. Antihyperlipidemic pharmacotherapy focuses on the pathway in which fats are absorbed, transported, and metabolized. Medications that affect the absorption of fat and cholesterol in the intestine are classified as bile acid-binding resins, and medications that increase lipolysis of TG are classified as fibric acid derivatives. Lifestyle modifications also affect the absorption, transport, and metabolism of fats through this pathway.

Endogenous Pathway

VLDLs are synthesized and secreted by the liver into the circulation and contain TG and some cholesterol. VLDL is hydrolyzed to free fatty acids and glycerol by lipoprotein lipase in the capillary endothelium. Fat and muscle cells absorb the fatty acid and glycerol. About 50% of the VLDL remnants are taken up by apo B and E receptors in the liver, and the other 50% stays in the circulation and becomes intermediate-density lipoproteins (IDLs). IDLs are then enriched with cholesterol by hepatic triglyceride lipase to become LDLs, which carry about 75% of the circulating cholesterol. LDLs circulate for 2 to 3 days and are removed for use by all types of tissue.

LDL receptors in the liver are downregulated by the presence of LDL; therefore, one mechanism for lowering LDLs is pharmacotherapy that increases the number of LDL receptors in the liver (bile acid-binding resins, statins). Drugs that inhibit VLDL synthesis in the liver (niacin, fibric acid derivatives) also reduce LDLs via the endogenous pathway.

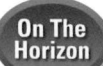 **On The Horizon**

Drugs in the pipeline are seeking to interfere with the synthesis of PCSK9 (proprotein convertase subtilisin/kexin type 9) in the liver. This liver protein is part of the natural synthesis of cholesterol in the body. If blocked with a targeted RNA particle, cholesterol levels drop (Fitzgerald et al, 2013).

Atherogenesis

There are four main types of lipoproteins: VLDLs, IDLs, LDLs, and HDLs. The lipoproteins that contain apo B100 have been identified as the vehicles that facilitate transport of cholesterol into the arterial wall, leading to atherogenesis. LDLs, which make up 60% to 70% of the total serum cholesterol, are the major culprit in this inflammatory-mediated process. LDL levels are increased in individuals who consume large amounts of saturated fats and/or cholesterol, who have defects in the hepatic LDL receptor (familial hypercholesterolemia), or who have a polygenic form of increased LDLs. The relationship of elevated LDL cholesterol to the development of CVD is a multistep process beginning relatively early in life (McCrindle, Kwiterovich, McBride, Daniels, & Kavey, 2012; National Heart, Lung, and Blood Institute [NHLB], 2011).

When serum LDL levels exceed a threshold of 100 mg/dL, they cross the arterial wall and become embedded in the arterial lumen. In the arterial lumen, LDLs undergo oxidation, are taken up by macrophages, and form a plaque known as a fatty streak. The severity is related to the degree of inflammatory changes and metabolites to include Lipoprotein-Associated Phospholipase A2(Lp PLA_2). Atherosclerotic plaques are made up of foam cells, which are transformed macrophages and smooth muscle cells filled with cholesterol. Glycation of lipoproteins in poorly controlled diabetes also contributes to foam cell generation. Arterial hypertension accelerates this process. HDL suppresses the foam cell production, resulting in an anti-inflammatory response. The role of HDL may have less significance than previously believed, with the exception of when it increases after baseline values were very low (Vogel, 2013); but more evidence is needed to move away from all efforts to raise serum HDL levels.

The second step of atherogenesis involves the formation of scar tissue over the fatty plaque in the arterial wall. This formation is called a fibrous plaque. Over time, fibrous plaques become unstable and are prone to rupture, causing potentially life-threatening luminal thromboses. Plaque rupture or erosion is responsible for most acute coronary events (e.g., myocardial infarction, unstable angina, and coronary death). Elevated LDL cholesterol provides fatty substrate for plaque formation, and the larger the plaque, the more unstable it will be.

HDLs, which make up 20% to 30% of total serum cholesterol, function as acceptors of free cholesterol as it passively diffuses from cells. This reverse transport is the mechanism by which cholesterol may be removed from atherosclerotic plaques. Figure 39-1 shows the relationship of lipid metabolism to atherosclerotic plaque formation. Apo A-I and A-II are the major apos in HDL. The level of apos and HDLs are proposed to be inversely related to CVD risk. As serum HDL and apo levels increase, it is believed atherogenesis decreases.

Although LDLs are the lipoprotein toward which therapy has been traditionally directed, some experts believe the ratio of total cholesterol to HDL to be a more powerful predictor of atherosclerotic CVD risk. Strong epidemiological evidence links low levels of HDL cholesterol to increased coronary

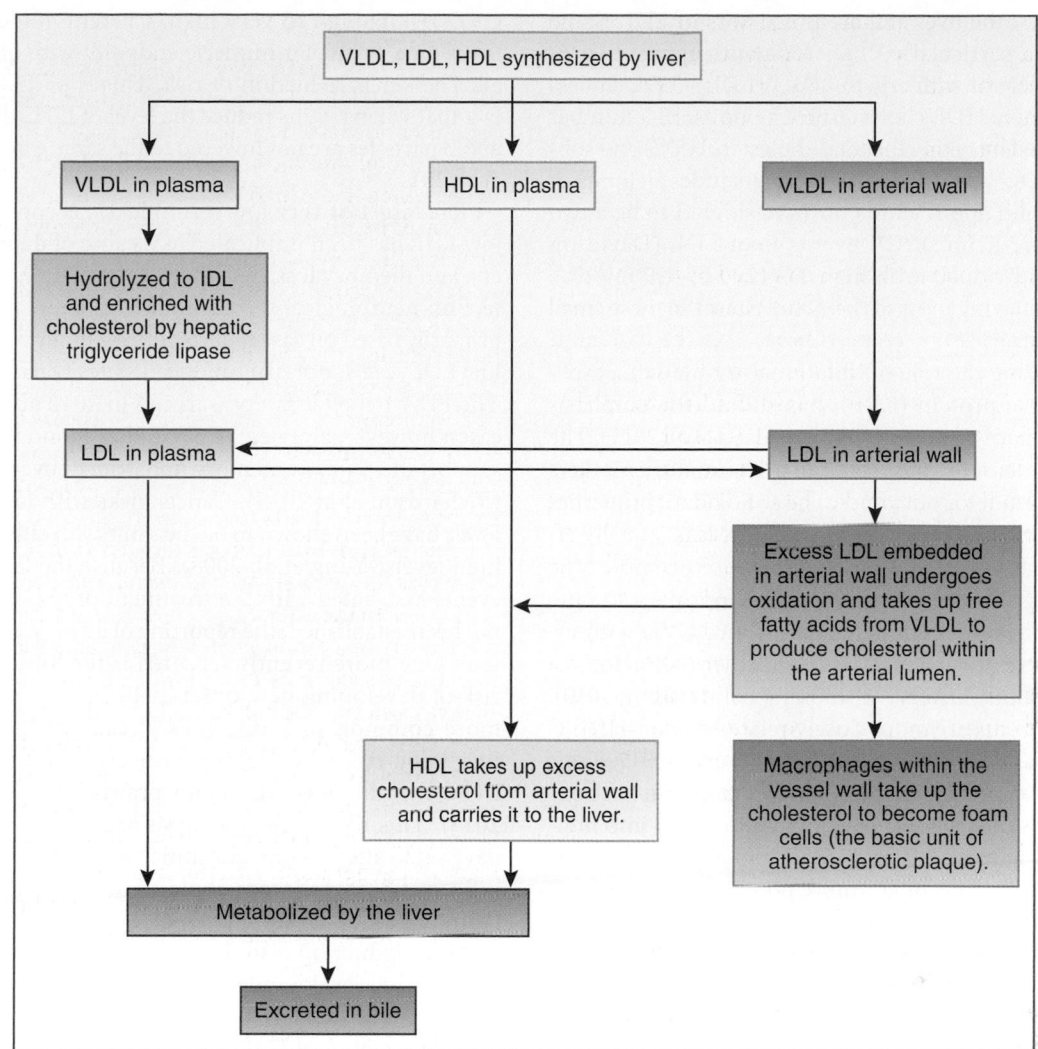

Figure 39–1. Relationship of lipid metabolism to atherosclerotic plaque formation. Excess LDL embedded in the arterial wall undergoes oxidation and takes up free fatty acids from VLDL to produce cholesterol within the arterial lumen. If the excess cholesterol is not taken up by HDL and carried to the liver, macrophages within the vessel wall create atherosclerotic plaque from this excess cholesterol.

morbidity and mortality, and low levels are consistently shown to be an independent risk factor for CVD. However, high values do not confer the reduction in risk once hoped for (Vogel, 2013). Factors that contribute to low HDL are shown in Table 39-1. Each of these factors has been a target of therapy, but results have not been stellar. Drugs that may raise HDL levels include nicotinic acid (niacin), fibrates, and statins. There are drugs in development that specifically target increasing HDL levels, but they have not had major successes yet in preliminary clinical trials.

To make the divisions of "good and bad" more complex, newer research has determined that HDL can "go bad" and become dysfunctional if oxidized by myeloperoxidase. This would reverse the typical "cleansing" function of HDL; it would instead harden and become part of a dangerous arthroma (Huang et al, 2014). Because the HDL testing cannot yet discriminate between "good " versus "bad" forms of the HDL, no therapeutic decisions or options are available at this time.

Table 39–1 Factors That Contribute to Low HDL Cholesterol Levels

Cigarette smoking
Drugs: beta blockers, anabolic steroids, progestational agents
Elevated serum triglycerides
Genetic factors (approximately 50% of cases)
Overweight and obesity (probably most important)
Physical inactivity
Type 2 diabetes mellitus
Very high carbohydrate intake (>60% of total energy intake)

Source: Adapted from the *Third Report of the Expert Panel on Detection, Evaluation and Treatment of High Blood Cholesterol in Adults,* 2001. Rockville, MD: National Institutes of Health, National Heart, Lung, and Blood Institute.

VDDL Levels

VLDLs are triglyceride-rich lipoproteins that contain 10% to 15% of the total serum cholesterol. The major apos of VLDL are apo B100; apo C I, II, and III; and apo E. VLDLs are produced by the liver and are precursors of LDL. Some forms of VLDL, particularly VLDL remnants, appear to promote atherosclerosis similarly to LDL. VLDL + LDL cholesterol is called non-HDL cholesterol. The non-HDL number can be calculated by taking the total cholesterol (TC) and subtracting the HDL. Non-HDL cholesterol includes all lipoproteins that contain apo B and is now considered to be a two times better predictor of CV events than LDL (Davidson et al, 2011). Individuals with high TG (200 to 499 mg/dL), also present as having most of their cholesterol in these small VLDL remnants.

Understanding the role of inflammatory markers, especially C-reactive protein (CRP), has shifted the emphasis away from primarily treating LDL (Davidson et al, 2011). The JUPITER trial demonstrated that the inflammatory markers are more important for outcomes. The antioxidant properties of statin medications may turn out to be at least equally effective as their antilipid effects. This evidence prompted the Food and Drug Administration (FDA) to approve statin use (specifically, Crestor) in individuals without CVD with increased CRP levels over 2 mg/L and one other risk factor like HTN, strong family history, or smoking habits (FDA, 2010). Even cardiac events are more closely related to non-HDL-C than are LDL and apo B levels (Boekholdt et al, 2012). This is especially true in diabetics. This newer emphasis on non-LDL risk prediction is now formally incorporated into individual risk guidelines (Ansell, 2012). Lipid experts claim the non-HDL levels will become a more potent predictor of risk than the LDL (Boekholdt et al, 2012). This would be a shift in who gets treatment. Using 2001 guidelines, someone with a normal LDL but high non-HDL would not be treated; in the 2013 guidelines, they would be treated after consideration of all other cardiovascular risk factors.

Elevated TG is also recognized as an independent risk factor for CVD. TGs are closely linked with metabolic syndrome and diabetes. TG levels greater than 150 mg/dL should be treated once the LDL interventions are undertaken. If the initial medications do not subsequently reduce TG, then pharmacotherapy to directly address TGs must be considered to handle this other non-HDL risk. If TGs are over 150 mg/dL, the measurement of LDL is less accurate, making therapeutic judgments more complex. Isolated TG elevations cannot be treated with statins alone; they should be treated with fibrates, niacin, or omega-3s (Berglund et al, 2012).

GOALS OF TREATMENT

The therapeutic goal for the management of hyperlipidemia is to reduce morbidity and mortality from CVD by reducing atherogenesis. Research suggests that at least a 30% to 40% decrease in LDL levels needs to be achieved to reach this goal (Grundy et al, 2004). Because LDL cholesterol levels below 100 mg/dL throughout life are associated with very low risk for CVD, they were traditionally termed "optimal"; however, several major clinical trials published since the ATP III guidelines have indicated that an LDL goal of lower than 70 mg/dL may be a reasonable therapeutic option for patients when

CVD risk is high to very high. Current guidelines do not focus on a particular numeric endpoint with one size fitting all. The key is reduction of risk. This is partially due to the fact that when statins reduce the level of LDL, the athrogenic apo B particles are not lowered to the same extent (Davidson et al, 2011).

The target of very low serum levels is contentious. Very low LDL has been implicated as a cause of depression, anxiety, and memory loss. Serum levels of LDLs may have an effect on neurological serotonin levels. These concerns were primarily based on case reports with naturally occurring extra-low LDL levels, not drug-induced states (Zhang et al, 2005). The FDA issued a safety warning in 2012 about these rare cases; however, a review of 57 studies found no evidence to support the claim of memory impairment over the long term (Richardson et al 2013). Cancer risks with low serum LDL levels have been shown to be the same with either high or low lipid levels (Yang et al, 2008). Because the level of adverse events associated with the treatment of hyperlipidemia has not been established, the reporting of any CV event is important. One more recently reported is the low, but potential, risk of developing new-onset diabetes with statins. This is more common in individuals already at high borderline metabolic risk when taking rosuvastin and a less obvious trend with the less efficacious pravastatin (Navarese et al, 2013). This recent meta-analysis and a 2012 FDA warning have yet to alter therapeutic initiatives because the risk of significant CV issues from cholesterol is significantly higher than the risk of developing DM.

Lipid reduction also decreases the primary risk of non-hemorrhagic stroke and is also effective in secondary prevention of subsequent ischemic strokes (Elkind, 2013). Each 39 mg reduction of LDL decreases the relative risk of stroke by 21%. This is why strokes have been added as a hard-stop endpoint for calculating cardiovascular risk.

Atherogenesis occurs even when serum LDL cholesterol levels are 100 to 129 mg/dL, especially with higher inflammatory markers (Davidson et al, 2011). Atherogenesis proceeds at a significant rate when LDL levels are 130 to 159 mg/dL; such levels are termed "borderline high." Markedly accelerated atherogenesis occurs at levels of 160 to 189 mg/dL (high) and over 190 mg/dL (very high). Davidson and associates (2011) rank CRP levels of 1.0 to 3.0 mg/L as conferring intermediate risk and high risk at greater than 3.0 mg/L, even without links to high LDL.

Confirmed by log-linear data, a clear increased risk of CVD exists in populations who have higher serum LDL levels (NCEP, 2001). Unfortunately, an independent relationship between LDL reduction and actual percentage of risk reduction is unclear. Data that specify how much a reduction in serum level LDLs decreases how much risk of CVD are not available. The reports of relative risk reduction are extrapolations from the data, not actual endpoints. Early clinical benefits of statin therapy are now recognized to be lipid-independent! This is likely related to the reduction of vessel endothelial inflammation (pleiotrophy) of this drug class.

Atherosclerosis can be identified on gross pathological examination of coronary arteries in adolescence and early adulthood (McCrindle et al, 2012; NHLB, 2011). The cholesterol level in young adulthood predicts the development of CVD later in life. Prospective studies with long-term follow-up have found that elevated serum cholesterol and more rapid changes in BMI in the teenage years (Attard, Herring, Howards, & Gordon-Larsen, 2013) and early adulthood predicted an increased incidence of CVD in middle age. Traditional clinical intervention with LDL-lowering therapy in adult patients with advanced coronary atherosclerosis results in a short-term risk reduction aiming to stabilize plaque and prevent acute coronary syndromes. In contrast, LDL-lowering earlier in life slows atherosclerotic plaque development, the foundation for unstable plaque. This provides a rationale for long-term lowering of serum LDL cholesterol using both public health and clinical approaches (see Children and Adolescents section below).

A 20 year longitudinal study supports a "legacy" effect after just 5 years of statin therapy (Packard, 2014). A cohort of men aged 45 to 64 were given statin therapy and matched with patients who were not started on medications. There was a reduction of 31% in the incidence of non-fatal MI and deaths from CVD in the statin group. Another 10 year study of a subset of the Framingham cohort age 35 to 55 years old without prior CVD demonstrated a 39% of increased CVD even with only slightly elevated cholesterol levels (Navar-Boggan et al, 2015). Their original risk was less than 4.4% and grew to a 16.5% risk in 10 years. Both of these studies underscore early, aggressive therapy has real outcomes.

Though raising HDL levels has been postulated to be a goal, the evidence is not there to make it the primary goal. When LDL levels drop, HDL frequently rises. The positive impact is more likely to be the lowering of LDL, not a direct impact of raising HDL. Even a meta-analysis of genetic studies monitoring cohorts of the population that have higher rates of naturally occurring HDL does not translate into significant MI risk reduction (Voight et al, 2012).

RATIONAL DRUG SELECTION

Hyperlipidemia presents a problem in therapeutic management because patients are usually asymptomatic until damage to the cardiovascular system occurs. Central aspects of treatment are lifestyle modifications, especially dietary, which include the reduction of elements that are often perceived as "making food taste good." Finally, patients often want a prescription for a drug that will "cure" the problem, which currently is not a realistic treatment option. The drugs that are prescribed for hyperlipidemia are added to the therapeutic plan after lifestyle management has failed because the medications available can potentially produce serious adverse events. For effective management of hyperlipidemia, the treatment protocol must be palatable and low cost and have the fewest possible side effects. The factors to consider before developing a treatment plan are the presence or the absence of CVD, any associated risk factors, specific patient variables

and desires, patient interest, plus a realistic consideration of a cost–benefit ratio.

The level of individual risk has become a cornerstone of the new guidelines. The following sections blend the new guidelines with the decades of evidence of all risk factors for the prescriber to consider when selecting medications. The higher the CV risk, the more aggressive the statin treatment recommendations in the new guidelines. Any risk prediction over 7.5% is now earmarked as needing a discussion about whether to start statin therapy (Goff et al, 2013). The guidelines are not intended to be static and absolute, but only to serve as the stepping-stone for individualized decision making.

Risk Stratification

Multiple patient variables based on risk profiles are considered in setting individual goals for lipoprotein levels. The guidelines highlighting a 7.5% risk level are not meant to be absolute standards for starting medications, but only a trigger point for consideration of personal risks. These risks fall into modifiable and nonmodifiable categories. The modifiable risk factors such as diet, smoking behavior, and exercise are targets of therapy through lifestyle modifications. Nonmodifiable risk factors include age, gender, race, and family history. Both categories of risk factors are part of the calculation of overall risk for CVD. Table 39-2 presents the major risk factors for CVD exclusive of the serum LDL.

Five factors are considered contributory to low risk and negative risk for CVD: not smoking, normal BP, normal weight, normal glucose metabolism, and low cholesterol levels. Public education programs of the 1980s and 1990s contributed to measurable decreases in cardiac disease rates in the United States. This progress is waning with the advent of the obesity epidemic; the only positive trend is that a lower percentage of the population smokes than did in the 1970s (Ford, Li, Zhao, Peason, & Capewell, 2009). Currently, only 7.5% of patients are able to achieve the five low-risk factors, a percentage that has dropped from the 10.5% of adults studied in 1994 (Ford et al, 2009). In addition to encouraging patients not to smoke, advanced practice nurses need to place emphasis on helping patients achieve optimal weight, BP, and glucose metabolism and to exercise. The reported positive trend of having lower levels of lipids across the population must be tempered with the understanding that levels have been successfully reduced in higher-risk patients by the wide use of statins (Carroll, Kit, Lacher, Shero, & Mussolino, 2012). Unfortunately, the reported reduction of exercise in youth will skew that trend toward reversal. The good news of pediatric cancer survival rates has also created a new risk group of early onset cardiovascular disease patients. There is a 9% decrease in arterial health in the survivors (Steinberger et al, 2012).

A gradient potential of CVD risk has been delineated in the literature over the past decade. CVD risk equivalents include diabetes, metabolic syndrome, symptomatic carotid artery disease, peripheral arterial disease with an ankle/brachial index less than 0.9, abdominal aortic aneurysm, and

Table 39–2 Major Risk Factors for Coronary Heart Disease (CHD) (Exclusive of LDL Cholesterol)

Risk Factor	Positive Risk	Negative Risk
Age	Male: ≥45	Male: <45
	Female: ≥55	Female: <55
Family history	Premature CHD (MI or sudden death before 55 yr in father or other male first-degree relative or before 65 yr in mother or female first-degree relative)	No family history of CHD
Cigarette smoking	Current smoking (any cigarette smoking in past month)	Nonsmoker
Hypertension	BP ≥140/90 mm Hg or on antihypertensive medication	Normotensive
HDL cholesterol	HDL ≤40 mg/dL	HDL ≥60 mg/dL
Diabetes mellitus	Presence, especially if poorly controlled	Absence

BP = blood pressure; HDL = high-density lipoprotein; MI = myocardial infarction.

Source: Adapted from the *Third Report of the Expert Panel on Detection, Evaluation and Treatment of High Blood Cholesterol in Adults,* 2001. Rockville, MD: National Institutes of Health, National Heart, Lung, and Blood Institute.

a 10-year risk of myocardial infarction/coronary heart disease (MI/CHD) death. The newly developed Pooled Cardiovascular Risk Calculator (http://myamericanheart.org/cvriskcalculator) does not take all of these risks into consideration, which has created rebuttals to its full adoption. Some experts believe that the 2013 guidelines recommend treatment for too many people. Approximately 45 million more Americans are now being considered as at risk for CVD and within the guideline-recommended parameters for use of statins. Some experts say this is without merit (Ridker & Cook, 2013). Others believe there is significant overestimation of risk up to 154% (DeFillippis et al, 2015). The guideline authors counter these arguments with an emphasis upon an individualized personal risk evaluation with discussions of the risks between patient and provider. They insist this goes beyond making provider-centric decisions based on lipid values or only on calculated scores. They also suggest that most of these patients were undertreated by prior guidelines because primary prevention of the first CV is the best goal. The guideline authors have also provided a list of factors that require future consideration for guideline revision that include some of the major objections to the 2013 publication (Table 39-3).

The biggest area of contention is the recommendation for treatment for individuals with mild disease. The newly selected 7.5% risk of CVD over the next 10 years is a major change from the 10% to 20% risk considerations of the Framingham score era. There are experts who are concerned that the risk of statin adverse events may outweigh any future benefit in this group. Abramson, in the *British Medical Journal* (2013), calculates that 140 individuals in this category must take a statin to prevent one heart attack. He goes on to state 1 out of every 5 of those patients might encounter an adverse effect. So the informed discussion must consider that numeric in order that the decision to treat be based on actual statistical evidence. The guidelines provide a list of risk factors that might trigger statin use in this population during those therapy decisions (see Table 39-4).

The REGARDS study (Reasons for Geographic and Racial Differences in Stroke) (Muntner et al, 2014) has provided a positive endorsement of the new risk calculator. This

Table 39–3 Factors to Be Considered in Future Guidelines

1. Specifics on TG therapy
2. The non-HDL impact on decision making
3. LDL particle marker roles in diagnosis and treatment
4. Role of imaging study results in treatment decisions
5. Refining the optimal time frame and age for initiating therapy
6. Determining statin impact of specific subgroups like CKD and HF patients
7. Evaluation of longitudinal adverse effect impacts of medications
8. Inclusion of subgroups of patients typically excluded or underrepresented in RCTs (e.g., HIV, transplant patients, ethnic populations)
9. Impact of genetic testing and pharmacogenetic implications

Source: Adapted from Stone et al. (2013, Nov 12). *2013 ACC/AHA Guideline on the Treatment of Blood Cholesterol.* http://circ.ahajournals

Table 39–4 Individualized Considerations When Risk Assessment Places Patient in Uncertain Category for Pursuing Statin Therapy

Factor	Support Raising Risk Score	No Support for Revising Risk Score
Family Hx early CVD	Male <55 yr or Female < 65yr (1-degree relative)	CV event after age 65 or no history in family of CVD
hs-CRP (C-reactive protein)	>2 mg/L	<2 mg/L
Coronary calcium score	>75th percentile or 300 Angstrom units	<75th percentile or 300 units
Ankle-Brachial Index (ABI)	<0.9	>0.9

Source: Adapted from the ACC/AHA 2013 Guidelines.

prospective population-based study went beyond stroke outcomes to also include CHD and nonfatal MI. The actual occurrence of adverse outcomes in patients in the lowest risk category were "spot on" with the predicted risk calculated from the new guidelines; interestingly, the highest risks appeared to be overestimated. This was attributed to the fact that over 40% of the highest-risk cohort were started on statins and thereby reduced the incidence of bad outcomes (Muntner et al, 2014).

CVD tends to cluster in families. A positive family history of clinical CVD or sudden death in first-degree male relatives before age 55 or first-degree female relatives before age 65 is an important risk factor. The family history should include relatives with the presence or absence of high cholesterol levels, nonlipid risk factors, and the age of onset of each risk factor. This information provides data to assess for inherited lipoprotein disorders.

Ethnicity is also now a recognized risk factor for CHD. For the first time, there are recommended treatment algorithms for lipid management based on race and gender differences in risk factors (Stone et al, 2013). Genetic constitution may result in the need for special attention to certain portions of the treatment algorithm. These features are discussed under specific variables below. Dietary considerations are also of concern (Nettleton, Polak, Tracy, Burke, & Jacobs, 2009).

High Risk: CVD or CV Risk Equivalent

Patients at high risk are those with clinical evidence of CVD or with CV risk equivalents. The literature suggests that having coronary disease substantially increases future risk of another coronary event; this risk increases even more in the presence of elevated cholesterol levels. In women with existing CVD, the rates of new coronary events are similar to those of men. In older adults, new events occur with higher frequency than in younger adults with similar cardiac histories. The authors of the 2013 guidelines consider anyone over the age of 62 as having high risk simply on age alone (Goff et al, 2013). The benefits of lipid lowering in patients with established CVD have been repeatedly demonstrated in clinical studies. Patients without CVD but who have angina, claudication, stroke, TIA, electrocardiogram (ECG) abnormalities, or previous coronary revascularization procedures (Knatterud et al, 2000) have similar risk rates to those of patients who have existing CVD. These softer endpoints, however, are not included in the first edition of the Pooled Cardiovascular Risk tool. Only the endpoint risks for the first "hard" cardiovascular event within the next 10 years are included in the 2013 guidelines. The rationale is that treatment will be targeted toward the individuals most likely to benefit from cholesterol reduction. The hard-stop events include nonfatal myocardial infarction, cardiovascular associated death, or a stroke.

Coronary calcium scores are sometimes considered in various discussions of risk. It has been assumed that the more dense form may be more dangerous. The presence of calcium in the deposits indicates long-term presence, with the higher degree of calcification (the CAC score) being assumed to be hazardous. This has come under scrutiny recently (Criqui et al, 2014). It is becoming understood that the volume of the plaque, not the density, may be more predictive of CV events. Prescribers are referred to the newest evidence published on the CAC scoring systems recommendations.

Of note in the 2013 guidelines is a recommendation *not* to use statins in advanced heart failure patients. It is recognized that this disease state is a frequent comorbidity with lipid disorders; however, there is no evidence that statins impact mortality in this population (Goff et al, 2013; Stone et al, 2013). Any benefit is in early disease when lipid reduction might be helpful; once heart failure is advanced, these drugs have limited to no benefit.

Patients with diabetes are included in this high-risk category, but the presence of diabetes is considered a CV equivalent, not a hard ASCVD event. The absolute risk for first major coronary events for patients with type 2 diabetes approximates that for nondiabetic patients with clinical CVD (Haffner, Lehto, Ronnemaa, Pyorala, & Laasko, 1998; Malmberg et al, 2002). The benefit of lowering LDL cholesterol in patients with type 2 diabetes is well supported. Type 2 diabetics are in this high-risk category because they have an increased MI case fatality rate. In one study, death occurred in 45% of men with diabetes and 35% of women with diabetes, compared to 38% for men and 25% for women without diabetes (Miettinen et al, 1998). In an effort to forestall a high risk of CV events in DM patients over age 40, the newest Canadian guidelines urge use of statins, even if patients have no other risk factors (CDA, 2013). The American Diabetes Association 2015 standards recommend moderate statin doses for patients without overt CVD and high doses for those with established disease (ADA, 2015).

Some authors are concerned that the presence of prediabetes is not directly addressed in the 2013 American guidelines. Others are concerned that specific CRP levels are not strongly emphasized (Ridker & Cook, 2013). The guideline authors counter that any new scoring system will be imperfect, just as the old system was. When considering that the 10-year risk of 7.5% to 10% is still an imperfect process, only a few individuals will actually have a cardiac event and others may have had it prevented, but there is no way to measure that effect.

The cost effectiveness of treating the high-risk groups was established even when drug therapy involved expensive brand names. With the advent of most medications in generic formulations, there is no longer any viable argument against more aggressive therapy based on cost. LDL-lowering drug therapy is also cost-effective for primary prevention in patients with CVD risk equivalents.

Lower Risk: Zero or One Risk Factor

It should be noted that the lower-risk group still has cardiac event risk, although the risk is lower than in groups deemed to have high risk. Data from multiple research trials support that lowering LDL cholesterol is important even for those without CVD. Given that clinical trial participants were likely to be healthier than the general population and that event rates likely will increase as the patient ages, an event rate of 20% per decade presents a minimum estimate of absolute annual risk for those with moderately elevated cholesterol levels.

Patients traditionally considered at low risk for CVD are those with LDL cholesterol levels below 100 mg/dL, HDL cholesterol levels above 60 mg/dL, a total cholesterol-to-HDL ratio below 4.5, VLDL cholesterol levels of 50 to 100 mg/dL, or fasting TG of 150 to 200 mg/dL, no clinical evidence of CVD, and fewer than two risk factors (Brugsts et al, 2009). These optimal numbers reflect zero risk factors but do not provide a true "zero risk" for anyone. It should be remembered that this serum level is only one factor in risk assessment and that a more holistic picture of personal risk needs to be addressed when considering whether pharmacy interventions are indicated. Statin therapy is typically not used in this population.

Asymptomatic patients now have a separate guideline (Brugsts et al, 2009; Greenland et al, 2010) that addresses the cost-effectiveness of using testing to uncover occult disease. History taking, calculating risk scores, and standard lipid testing are approved. CRP testing is not approved for screening women under 60 or men under 50 in this category. Going beyond those basics—including liproprotein measurements, echocardiography, stress testing, and CT angiography for calcium deposit evaluation—is not recommended. If DM is a comorbidity, the recommendations accelerate the screening to include these things on an individual basis.

Treatment Algorithms

Lifestyle Modifications

Lifestyle modifications are the core of treatment for hyperlipidemia. Most cholesterol experts advocate a two-pronged approach for reducing CVD risk: the population approach and the clinical approach. The focus of the population approach includes working with the media so that information from healthcare providers is valued and considered credible. A public health success story of a 58% decrease in trans-fat consumption over the past decade is credited to this effort (Carroll et al, 2012; Doell, Folmer, Lee, Honigfort, & Carberry, 2012). Current legislation to ban all trans-fat in American food products will continue this trend. Further population-based foci includes promoting U.S. Dietary Guidelines using pamphlets/handouts; promoting regular physical activity, up to 30 minutes on most days of the week; ensuring that weight, height, and waist circumference are measured at least annually; providing access to body mass index (BMI) tables in the waiting and exam rooms; ensuring that all adults 20 years and older have their blood cholesterol measured and their results explained; ensuring that all adults have their BP measured and their results explained in keeping with current HTN guidelines; making antismoking literature available; and asking all patients about their smoking habits at every office visit.

Clinical approaches have similar foci as the population-based approach but are directed at specific patients. Clinicians should promote targeted changes in individual lifestyle to produce significant reductions in a patient's risk. These include promoting regular physical activity based on the patient's cardiac status, age, and other factors; teaching about weight management, including 10% weight-loss goals for patients who are overweight (Mente, deKoning, Shannon, & Anand, 2009); following the "treating tobacco use and dependence" guideline (U.S. Department of Health and Human Services, 2000); and promoting the Therapeutic Lifestyle Changes (TLC) during follow-up visits.

The general aim of dietary therapy is to lower cholesterol levels while still maintaining a nutritionally adequate eating pattern. Research has demonstrated that the benefits of eating a heart-healthy and blood-glucose-reducing diet extends across all ethnic groups (Nettleton et al, 2009). It is now understood also be a major factor affecting secondary prevention and is considered a near equivalent to drug therapy (Naci & Ioannidis, 2013). Essential components of the TLC diet are the following:

- Avoidance of heavily saturated fats
- Plant stanols/sterols 2 g/d; plant sterols block cholesterol absorption
- Increased viscous (soluble) fiber to 10 to 25 g/d; viscous fibers increase bile-acid losses
- Total calories adjusted to maintain desirable body weight and prevent weight gain

One group of authors notes that a combination of plant sterols and viscous fiber "is the dietary equivalent of combining a bile acid-binding resin and a statin" (Jenkins, Kendall, & Marchie, 2005).

Patients might elect to follow a high-protein Atkins-style diet to have a greater initial weight loss; however, proteins can be heavy in fats and increase the cortisol hormones that increase CRP, a hallmark of dyslipidemia (Ebbeling et al, 2012). Providers should caution not to exclude only one type of food group; balance is required. There are no "bad foods." For years, eggs were demonized as the major source of dietary cholesterol. Newer research indicates eating eggs might increase CVD risk but primarily in those patients who are already diabetic (Rong et al, 2013). This was a restricted-scope review, but it gives insight into overturning a one-size-fits-all myth about cholesterol sources. Education should show that not all calories are "created equal," in terms of health impacts; however, there is no longer an emphasis on low vs. high glycemic index foods.

Alcohol ingestion is also related to CVD. Observational studies consistently show a J-shaped relationship between alcohol consumption and total mortality. Case-control, cohort, and ecological studies indicate lower risk for CVD at low-to-moderate alcohol intake. A moderate amount of alcohol is no more than 1 ounce of ethanol (e.g., 24 oz beer, 10 oz wine, or 2 oz whiskey) for men. Women and lighter-weight men should consume no more than half this amount. There are purported cardiovascular benefits related to rational alcohol intake in men older than 45 years and women older than 55 years. The beneficial mechanism associated with moderate alcohol use is unknown but may be related to an increase in HDL cholesterol and apo A1 and modest improvement in hemostatic factors (NCEP, 2001).

The dangers of overconsumption of alcohol are well known. Patients with levels of alcohol consumption in excess of a moderate amount present with adverse effects that include HTN, arrhythmia, and myocardial dysfunction. Alcohol excess also promotes pancreatitis and liver dysfunction. Because up to 10% of adults in the United States misuse alcohol, care should be taken about advice given related to alcohol intake, with disadvantages clearly delineated.

Dietary sodium, potassium, and calcium are also not mentioned in the macronutrient recommendations. Recommendations about these minerals are found in Chapter 9. Counter to popular belief, multivitamin intake does not alter CHD risk patterns except in those with nutritional deficits (Fortmann, Burda, Senger, Lin, & Whitlock, 2013).

Lifestyle modifications take time and are part of the treatment regimen whether the patient is being treated with medications or not. Modifications involve active assistance from the health-care team. Figure 39-2 shows the steps in achieving therapeutic lifestyle changes. Even though treating to LDL goal is no longer the standard, if the LDL cholesterol levels have not been lowered after 3 months of TLC, the decision must be revisited as to whether to consider adding drug therapy. Many patients with hyperlipidemia also have HTN. The 2013 lipid guideline supports the new JNC-8 recommendations (2014).

Drug Therapy

The new guidelines identify four groups most recommended to receive statin therapy. These are outlined in Table 39-5.

These are groups deemed most likely to benefit because they typically have higher risk equivalents. Dependent upon degree of risk, a low to high intensity of treatment is recommended (Table 39-6).

CVD and CV Risk Equivalents

For patients with CVD and CV risk equivalents, the type and intensity of LDL-lowering drug therapy is determined by the baseline LDL level plus the entire holistic consideration of personal risks. The 2013 recommendations for high and low statin therapy are based on how much of a lipid-lowering effect is desired and also how fast it should be reduced. Those requiring more than a 50% reduction in lipids are started on a high-dose and high-intensity statin; the moderate level is suggested for those needing a 30% to 50% reduction; and lower doses are expected to gain less than a 30% reduction in LDL (Stone et al, 2013). Figure 39-3 shows the therapeutic approach for this group of patients.

Because novice prescribers desire more specifics in helping them grasp how to evaluate and treat lipid levels, the old ATP III levels are included in Table 39-7 and Table 39-8 as basic reference points and the therapeutic algorithms are referenced in Figures 39-4, 39-5, and 39-6. It is *imperative* that a treatment to a numeric goal orientation *not* be adopted, nor is the inclusion in this text meant to suggest that it be adopted.

Persons with baseline LDL cholesterol at or above 130 mg/dL generally will require LDL-lowering drugs to

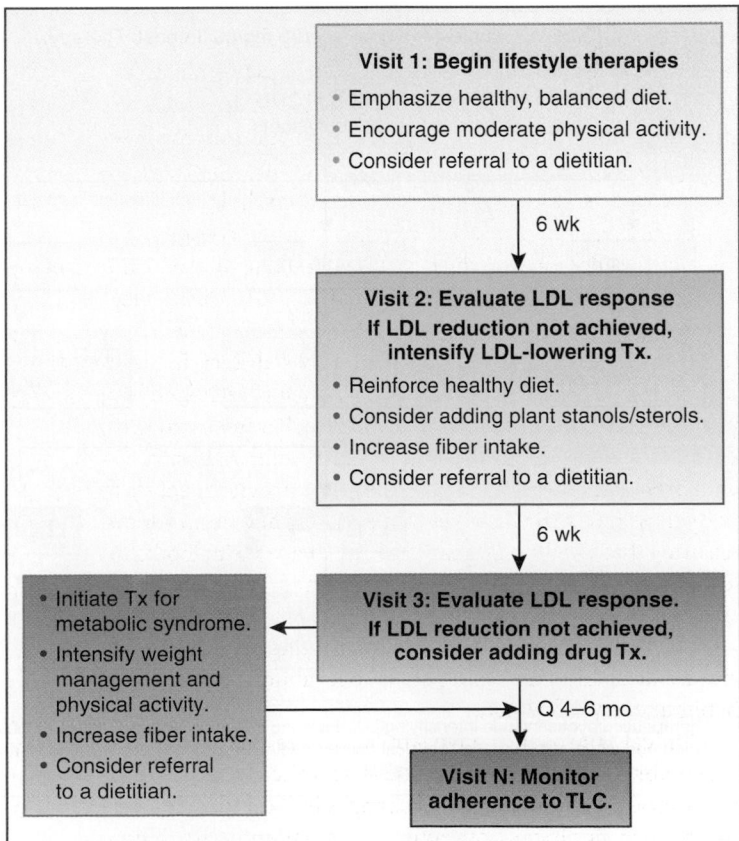

Figure 39-2. Model of steps in Therapeutic Lifestyle Changes (TLC).

Table 39–5   The Four Statin Benefit Groups

Evidence of clinical ASCVD
Primary LDL >190 mg/dL
DM patients with LDL 70–189 mg/dL without clinical ASCVD
    (age 40–75)
Patients age 40–75 without DM or ADCVD with a 10 yr risk of 7.5% or
    higher and LDL of 70–189 mg/dL

Source: Adapted from the ACC/AHA 2013 Guidelines.

Table 39–6   Definitions of High-to Low-Intensity Statin Treatment

High-Intensity Rx Daily	Moderate-Intensity Rx Daily	Low-Intensity Rx Daily
Est. 50% reduction in LDL	Est. 30%–49% reduction LDL	Less than 30% reduction
Atorvastatin (40–80)mg daily	Atorvastatin (10–20) mg	Fluvastatin 20–40 mg
Rosuvastatin (20–40)mg daily	Fluvastatin 40 mg twice	Lovastatin 20 mg
	Fluvastatin XL 80 mg	Pitavastatin 1 mg
	Lovastatin 40 mg	Pravastatin 10–20 mg
	Pitavastain (2–4) mg	Simvastatin 10 mg
	Pravastatin (40–80) mg	
	Rosuvastatin (5–10) mg	
	Simvastatin (20–40) mg	

Presented in alphabetical order, not order deemed best.
    Source: Adapted from 2013 ACC/AHA Guidelines.

achieve LDL cholesterol levels below 100 mg/dL, so drug therapy (usually with a statin) is initiated simultaneously with TLC. Newest guidelines still recommend that the LDL cholesterol for high-risk patients be under 100 mg /dL in the most extreme cases. Though the use of drugs for this population may be central to their therapy, in cases where the patient has metabolic syndrome, dietary therapy is intensified early in the program, with an increased effort to lose excess weight and increase physical activity. If the patient also has elevated TG, a lipid-lowering agent that focuses on that abnormality may be considered. Table 39-9 outlines the classification of TG level, which did not change with the 2013 lipid guidelines.

Zero or One Risk Factor

Individuals in the group with zero or one risk factor usually have a 10 year CV risk of less than 10%. The traditional goal for this patient group is LDL cholesterol levels lower than 160 mg/dL to reduce long-term risk for CVD; the new goal is a progressive reduction toward that level. TLC is initiated and continued for 3 months. After 6 weeks, the LDL panel is redrawn and dietary enhancers of LDL lowering (e.g., plant stanols/sterols and viscous fiber) are increased if needed. After 3 months, another LDL panel is drawn. If LDL cholesterol has lowered, TLC therapy is continued. For LDL cholesterol of 160 to 189 mg/dL, drug therapy is optional. The presence of influential factors such as smoking, poorly controlled HTN, or very low HDL, suggests the risks are not low and drug therapy should be initiated. If the LDL cholesterol remains above 190 mg/dL despite TLC therapy, drug therapy

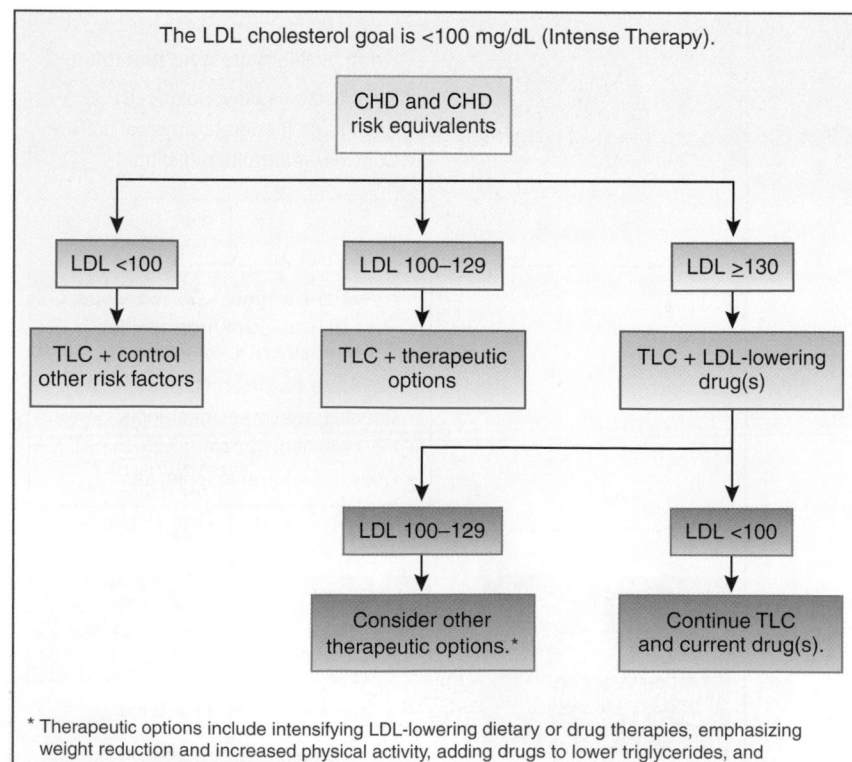

* Therapeutic options include intensifying LDL-lowering dietary or drug therapies, emphasizing weight reduction and increased physical activity, adding drugs to lower triglycerides, and intensifying control of other risk factors (ATP III).

Figure 39–3. Traditional therapeutic approaches for patients with CHD or CHD risk equivalents.

Table 39–7 ATP III Classification of LDL Cholesterol (reference only)

LDL Cholesterol Level (mg/dL)	Category
<100	Optimal
100–129	Near or above optimal
130–159	Borderline to high
160–189	High
>190	Very high

Source: Adapted from the *Third Report of the Expert Panel on Detection, Evaluation and Treatment of High Blood Cholesterol in Adults,* 2001. Rockville, MD: National Institutes of Health, National Heart, Lung, and Blood Institute.

Table 39–8 ATP III Low-Density Lipoprotein Goals (reference only)

LDL Cholesterol Patient Category	Goal (mg/dL)
Coronary heart disease (CHD) or CHD risk equivalent	<100
Multiple (two or more) risk factors	<130
Fewer than two risk factors	<160

LDL cholesterol goal for multiple-risk-factor patients with a 10 year risk higher than 20% is less than 100 mg/dL.

Source: Adapted from the *Third Report of the Expert Panel on Detection, Evaluation and Treatment of High Blood Cholesterol in Adults,* 2001. Rockville, MD: National Institutes of Health, National Heart, Lung, and Blood Institute.

is the more likely treatment option. Some patients may present with very high LDL cholesterol levels (e.g., greater than 220 mg/dL). These individuals usually have a genetic form of hyperlipidemia that cannot be treated adequately with TLC alone.

Drug Therapy

The choice of the pharmacotherapy is heavily weighted toward statins but can also be based on the specific elevated lipoprotein involved. There is a strong trend away from the non-statin lowering medications without specific indications. Detailed discussion of each drug class is provided in Chapter 16.

1. Statins allow most high-risk patients to attain lowered serum LDL levels. Patients treated with a statin may also see a modest decrease in serum TG and an increase in serum HDL. Long-term studies have shown statins to be generally safe and effective. Most compendiums list LDL-lowering agents according to their impact on serum LDL levels. From greatest to lowest impact on serum LDL, the drugs are ranked as follows: rosuvastatin, atorvastatin, simvastatin, lovastatin, pravastin, and fluvastatin. The newest statin, pitivastatin, has an LDL-lowering effect that falls within the list's midrange.

   In many trials, fewer than half of patients with CVD were able to achieve the desired serum LDL cholesterol goal of 100 mg/dL on standard doses of statins (Sacks, et al, 2000). These patients may require relatively high doses of statins (Cannon, 2005; Nissen et al, 2004) if it

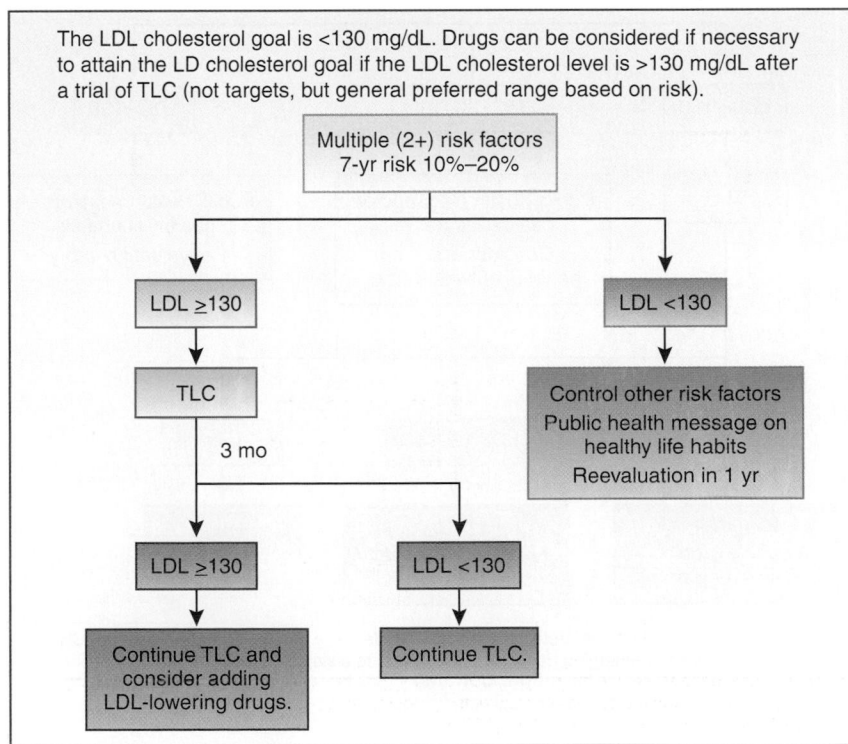

Figure 39–4. Traditional approaches for patients with multiple risk factors and 10 year CHD risk 10% to 20%.

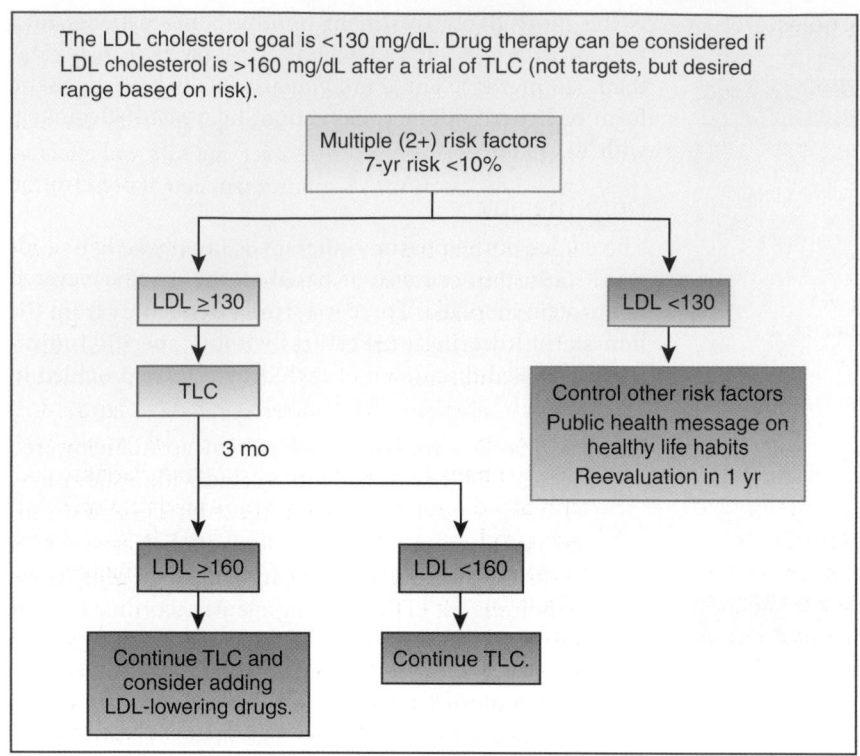

Figure 39–5. Traditional approaches for patients with multiple risk factors and 10 year CHD risk less than 10%.

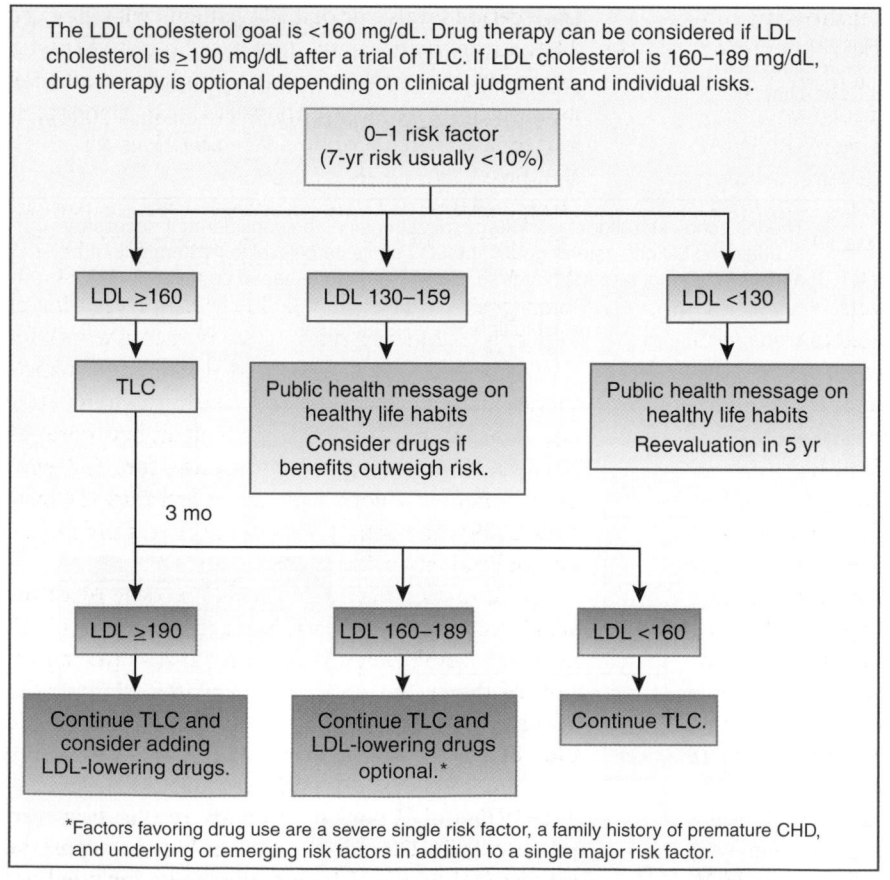

Figure 39–6. Traditional approaches for patients with 0 or 1 risk factor.

Table 39–9   Classification of Triglyceride Levels

Triglyceride Level (mg/dL)	Category
<150	Normal
150–199	Borderline to high
200–499	High
≥500	Very high

Source: Adapted from the *Third Report of the Expert Panel on Detection, Evaluation and Treatment of High Blood Cholesterol in Adults,* 2001. Rockville, MD: National Institutes of Health, National Heart, Lung, and Blood Institute.

is determined that pursuing this goal has an increased personal benefit that outweighs the risk of adverse lipid therapy events.

If patient response to a prescribed agent is not adequate after 3 months, the patient should have the statin dosage increased, be switched to a different agent, or be considered for combination drug therapy. A 2009 systematic review comparing combination therapies to maximum doses of single agents (Sharma et al, 2009) reported very weak evidence that combination therapies offer anything additional regarding mortality and MI and CVA survival. Medications used in combination therapy all have individually established data confirming that they are helpful in cholesterol reduction. The STELLAR trial results on monotherapy tempered the expectation that massive changes in cholesterol levels would result as dosages of drugs were increased. Typically, only a 6% reduction in TC is expected when the dosage of a statin is increased (Jones et al, 2003). Monotherapy does not always address all sources of dyslipidemia. It should be remembered that increasing the dose also increases the risk of adverse events.

2. Nicotinic acid (niacin) was always touted as effective in lowering total cholesterol and triglyceride levels and raising HDL levels. More recent studies that fail to support CV endpoint improvements such as stroke and MI have contributed to a moving away from its use in lipid management (MERCK, 2012; Vogel, 2013). In addition, difficult-to-tolerate side effects such as nausea and flushing have contributed to this trend. However, others believe that with selective low dosing when combining a niacin product with a bile acid-binding resin, patients can lower VLDL and LDL and reduce the side effects of the niacin. Slow-release nicotinic acid (Niaspan) has been studied as another way to reduce the side effects of niacin while still getting therapeutic blood levels of nicotinic acid as well as combining it with premedication of aspirin, but this has not proven to be clinically useful. Nicotinic acid is best for treating patients who have elevated total cholesterol and TG and low HDL levels who cannot tolerate statins. Because nicotinic acid is a vitamin and sold over the counter (OTC), the U.S. Food and Drug Administration (FDA) has issued a statement on using OTC products as a substitute for prescribed cholesterol-lowering drugs, including nicotinic acid. The FDA concluded that the nature of hypercholesterolemia and its potential sequelae are such that OTC use of these drugs is not a safe and effective means for treating this condition in lieu of prescription treatment.

3. Bile acid-binding resins have a strong record of efficacy and safety and are most useful for patients with moderately elevated LDL levels and a low CVD risk profile who are unable to reduce their LDL by TLC alone. Many young adult men and premenopausal women fit the profile appropriate for treatment. Bile acid-binding resins are often used as monotherapy for women who are pregnant or may become pregnant. Patients with combined familial hyperlipidemia who find nicotinic acid products not tolerable may benefit from a combination treatment that includes a bile acid-binding resin plus niacin plus statin.

4. Fibric-acid derivatives are effective triglyceride-lowering drugs that may modestly lower LDL and raise HDL for some patients. Because these drugs usually do not produce substantial reductions in LDL cholesterol, they are not appropriate for effective lowering of LDL levels as a primary LDL-lowering agent. They can be valuable in combination with a statin for patients with very high triglyceride levels, for diabetic patients with elevated TG and good renal function, and for patients with familial dysbetalipoproteinemia. Prudent monitoring and caution is used for increased risk of myopathies and hypoglycemia. Fibric-acid derivatives do have a significant GI side effect profile.

5. Drug combinations are commonly used for patients with more than one lipoprotein abnormality. For patients with elevated LDL and TG below 200 mg/dL, the main goal of treatment is to lower LDL levels first as hypertriglyceridemia does not carry the same risk for CVD as elevated LDL cholesterol levels. Combination therapy can be achieved by ordering two separate agents or by ordering more convenient, but more expensive, single-dosage formulations. Hard CV endpoint benefits are not evident in the literature (Sharma et al, 2009); however, quality of life effects and reduction of lipids are evident.

Combinations of statins with low-dose nicotinic acid have been used for patients at high risk for CVD; however, combining the powerful LDL-lowering action of the statins with the postulated triglyceride-lowering and HDL-raising properties of nicotinic acid did not achieve the major vascular event reduction in the AIM HIGH Study (MERCK, 2012). The HPS2-THRIVE study's poor preliminary results, however, triggered MERCK to pull its niacin-based drug off the market (MERCK). Neither study design included patients with severely low HDL levels, so future analysis may provide insight as to whether niacin has a niche population impact. It should be noted that niacin did increase HDL during these studies but is now considered to have more adverse risk than positive effect except in severe lipid disorders. The niacin in the HPS2-THRIVE study was mixed with an antiflushing agent previously untested in combination with niacin in a major trial, which may have been the issue with achieving endpoints.

The FDA has approved the orphan drugs mipomersen (FDA, 2013) and lomitapide (FDA, 2012b) for treatment of severe forms of familial hyperlipidemia. Mipomersen is a weekly injection associated with a 24% reduction in LDL. Lomitapride is an oral medication in a new class of drugs that inhibits bowel enzymes that help manufacture cholesterol in the liver. It lowered LDL by 47% in a small trial. Both drugs are used as adjuvant therapy with statins plus low-dose niacin as the most efficacious and practical combination for the treatment of combined familial hyperlipidemia.

The combination of statins and fibrates carries an increased risk of myopathy. Treatment with this combination should be undertaken carefully with frequent patient monitoring for symptoms of myopathy. Any reported myopathy symptoms should be followed up with creatinine kinase (CK) testing. The agent should be discontinued if the CK is greater than 10 times the upper limit of normal. The combo does decrease lipid levels; however, the hard endpoints of CV mortality do not improve when compared to just statins alone (ACCORD, 2010).

6. Alternative treatments have a role in managing elevated lipids; however, the Physicians Health Study has shown daily vitamin and supplement therapy does not reduce CV events in "healthy male adults" (Sesso et al., 2012). Omega-3 fatty acids have a place in treating very high triglyceride levels (greater than 500 mg/dL) in adult patients. Omega-3 fatty acid treatment results in HDL levels that are clinically unaffected and LDL levels that may actually rise. Many lipid experts have moved away from recommending their use after a meta-analysis did not find any primary, nor secondary, benefit in CVD (or cancer) prevention (Rizos, Nitzani, Bika, Kostapanos, & Elisaf, 2012). However, they did not find any harm in using them.

Omacor is a prescription formulation that is a more concentrated (840 mg) and quality-controlled source of both the eicosapentanoic acid (EPA) and docosahexaenoic acids (DHA) than those found in OTC supplements (avg 200 to 500 mg). Omacor has the same "fish burp" side effect as its OTC counterparts but may be more tolerable to patients because of its twice-a-day dosing schedule. Concerns about mercury content that surround OTC fish oil products are lessened because Omacor is a regulated drug and not a nutritional product.

There are omega-3 carboxylic acids now approved for cases of high trigylcerides that do not respond to primary interventions. The EVOLVE study (Epanova for Lowering Very High Trigylcerides) gained approval in a subclass of omega-3 medications that have both EPA and DHA components. The full picture of pancreatitis risk and cardiovascular outcomes is still unknown. This medication joins icosapant ethyl (Vascepa), approved in 2012, for the same severe lipid disorder. Due to the complexity of the pathophysiology underlying resistant triglyceride levels, it is recommended to prescribe these medications in consultation with a lipid specialist.

Red yeast rice, an alternative therapy for hyperlipidema, appears to mimic statin medications. The FDA has issued warnings about some formulations of this product that contain the prescription drug lovastatin. Manufacturers claim the yeast growing on their product is the naturally occurring chemical on which lovastatin is based. The unregulated production and packaging of these products makes them unsuitable as a substitute for prescription drug therapy, especially in the era of options that include less expensive generic drug formulations. The omega-3 found in flax and nuts (ALA) does not lower TG, but has other healthy fiber benefits.

Additional Patient Variables

Children and Adolescents

Atherosclerosis can begin in childhood (McCrindle et al, 2012; NHLB, 2011). Up to 25% of children and adolescents have cholesterol levels above 200 mg/dL. Most cases of elevated cholesterol are related to the same environmental factors that result in adult hyperlipidemia. Genetic disorders of lipid metabolism occur in 0.% to 1% of the population. Children with such disorders often have total cholesterol levels 1.5 to 3 times higher than normal. Approximately 80% of these children will experience symptomatic CVD at an age younger than 20 years.

There is controversy about when and whether to screen children for lipid issues (Newman, Pletcher, & Hulley, 2012). The diagnostic rate is thankfully low, but the value to children previously undiagnosed with familial disorders is significant (McCrindle et al, 2012). Limiting screening only to those with known family history does not reflect the reality that many pediatric medical histories do not include an in-depth family medical history or the history is unknown. Testing of children with cutaneous xanthomas is highly suggested. The European Atherosclerosis Society has published newly understood prevalence of familial disorders at levels much greater than previously appreciated (Cuchel et al, 2014). This has increased the testing of more first-degree relatives of known cases.

Optimal cholesterol levels in children are lower than in adults because longer duration of elevated lipid levels theoretically translates into longer-term opportunity for vascular wall changes (NHLB, 2011). Total cholesterol should be below 170 mg/dL (LDL less than 100 mg/dL). Borderline cholesterol levels are 170 to 199 mg/dL, and high cholesterol levels are 200 mg/dL or above. LDL greater than or equal to 130 mg/dL is considered hyperlipidemia in children (NHLB, 2011). Figure 39-7 shows the treatment algorithm for children.

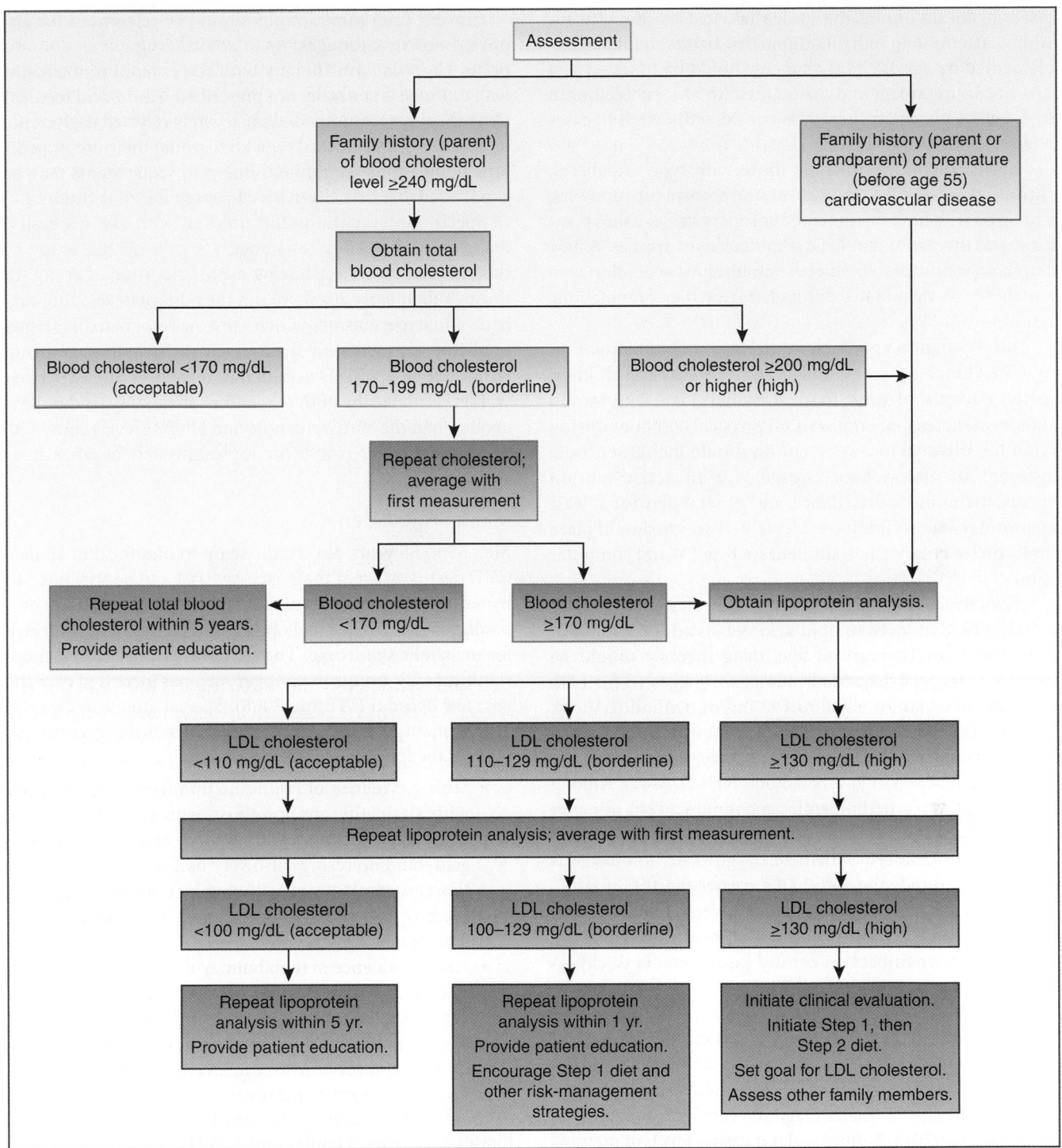

Figure 39–7. Management of blood cholesterol in children.

In children, as with adults, the goal is primary prevention. Lifestyle modifications mirror the TLC for adults. In infants, the diet should include breastfeeding and late introduction of solid foods. The use of whole milk until age 1 to provide required fatty acids for neurological development is still recommended; however, children should be switched to 2% milk and transitioned to skim milk by age 2 (Daniels & Greer, 2008). Framingham or newer pooled risk scores do not exist for children; the scores start at age 20 years. Unlike the adult risk probabilities over the next 10 years as the determinant

for therapy, the pediatric risk includes more of a lifetime risk perspective with the intent to prevent early onset CVD. For children, family histories become key, and children with male parents, grandparents, uncles, or siblings having premature CVD (angina, MI, stroke or sudden cardiac death before age 55) or with female relatives with histories before age 65 are considered to have increased risk.

Reduction in CVD risk factors, such as passive smoking, sedentary lifestyle, and excessive weight, and appropriate management of hypertension, obesity, and diabetes are all essential in childhood dyslipidemias, just as they are for adults. Attention to individual smoking habits should be implemented by age 10. TLC changes should be initiated as a first line of treatment and maintained for at least a 6 month trial, before pharmacotherapy is considered, except in cases of distinct high risk.

High-risk children include those with type 1 diabetes, chronic renal disease, and cancer and transplant survivors, and those who have documented coronary vessel issues post-Kawasaki disease or familial dyslipidemia syndromes. A new emphasis is now placed on obese children who develop type 2 diabetes, as they may exhibit characteristics of metabolic syndrome.

The population approach for therapy includes attention to school lunch programs and alerting parents and children to the dangers of junk food. Providers can take strong stands on increasing emphasis on physical activities during school. Individual focus prevention should include encouragement of after-school engagement in active-motion events, including sports, dance, and general play for at least 60 minutes a day (Gidding et al, 2009). Parents should place limits on sedentary entertainment such as TV and computer games.

When drug therapy is considered, consultation with a pediatrician experienced in lipid disorders is advised; for children less than 10 years of age, drug therapy should be managed by specialists. Medications are suggested for LDL levels greater than or equal to 190 mg/dL without CV risk factors; LDL greater than or equal to 160 with one personal risk or strong family risk; and LDL greater than or equal to 130 mg/dL and two high-risk factors (NHLD, 2011). Among the available antihyperlipidemics, nicotinic acid has a history of established safety in children younger than 18 years. Statins are useful in children with heterozygous or homozygous familial hyperlipidemia with LDLs greater than 500 mg/dL. Long-term use has not revealed any adverse impact on development, but the population taking medications is very limited. Positive impact on carotid intima media thickness mirrors that found in adults.

Very few children should have to take medications after TLC interventions are implemented. Goals for treatment and lipid-lowering impact are similar to those for adults. Monitoring protocols are also the same. Age of initiation of statin pharmacotherapy for males is age 10 years and for females at the onset of menses. Tanner scales measure levels of maturation in children, and the general guide for initiating drug therapy is a Tanner II level of maturation (Daniels & Greer, 2008). Pubescent adolescent females should follow the treatment guidelines for women of childbearing age as discussed later in this chapter. Treatment should consider use of contraception because of the potential teratogenic properties of lipid agents; however, contraceptives also increase lipid levels. Limited studies have not demonstrated alterations in continued maturation, menstrual cycles, or hormone levels in girls who have taken statins for familial dyslipidemias; however, these studies were only 1 to 2 years in duration and did not monitor long-term effects.

Current drug monographs should be referenced for approved pediatric dosages. As in adults, drug interactions do occur. Combination therapy with the exception of a statin with estimibe is generally not prescribed. Fibric-acid medications are only recommended for severely elevated triglyceride levels (>500), but clinical data concerning their use in pediatric populations are limited. Bile-acid sequestrants may be a more suitable first alternative for prepubescent children.

Specific interventions for children with HTN, obesity, diabetes, and insulin resistance are outside the scope of this chapter. However, having a BMI elevation after age 15 through their early 20s increases the odds of developing diabetes and hypertension, which are now recognized as strong predictors for increased cardiovascular risk in this age group (Attard et al, 2013). Dyslipidemic responses are associated with HTN above the 95th percentile for age and gender, BMI greater than the 85th percentile and Hb A1c levels above 7.0. Readers are referred to those topical headers in other areas of the text.

Middle-Aged Men

Men 35 to 65 years old comprise up to one-third of all new CVD deaths. Most of their excessive risk can be attributed to hyperlipidemia, HTN, and cigarette smoking. Men are also predisposed to abdominal obesity, which increases their risk for metabolic syndrome. The frequency of earlier and more significant CV events in younger men has increased over the past few decades (Wilson, 2008). Special attention for cholesterol management in middle-aged men includes consideration of the following:

* Strong evidence of risk reduction from LDL lowering with statin therapy for those with CVD or CV risk equivalents exists. Combination of statin and bile-acid–binding resin is also very useful.
* Fibrates or nicotinic acid may be used as second-line therapy for lipid lowering in men with low HDL and atherogenic dyslipidemia.
* High prevalence of metabolic syndrome requires intensive TLC.
* Factors favoring drug therapy include higher end of age range, obesity, cigarette smoking, positive family history, and very low serum levels of HDL.

Women

Elevated cholesterol levels confer CVD risk in women as well as in men, but the correlation to CVD is lower for women before age 55. Until that age, women are at lower risk for CVD than their male counterparts, in part because of their higher estrogen levels. After age 55, the most common cause of death in both men and women is cardiovascular disease. Cholesterol levels tend to be higher in older women than they are in men. Women younger than 45 years are discussed in the Younger Adults section, and women older than 75 years are discussed in the Older Adults section. This section refers to women in the 45- to 75-year age range.

CVD rates for women approximate those of men only after menopause. The reason for this disparity is not fully understood. The patterns of risk factors often differ between men and women. BP, LDL cholesterol, and TG rise at an earlier age in adult men than they do in women. At puberty, HDL cholesterol levels decrease in males, but not in females. Because a 10 mg/dL difference in HDL cholesterol may account for a 20% to 30% difference in CVD rates, this difference over the adult life span could account for a large portion of the gender disparity.

Although the presence of bioidentical and conjugated equine estrogen is postulated to raise HDL levels, the results of the Women's Health Initiative study raised serious questions about supplemental or replacement estrogen plus medroxyprogesterone acetate (MPA); HRT is no longer recommended for raising HDL as a primary endpoint (Grady et al, 2009; Rossouw et al, 2002).

Women's CV health risks are generally underappreciated by both providers and patients, although a significant public health outreach to educate both populations has shown gains toward clinical treatment parity with men. Parity, however, has not been reached (Mosca, Barrett-Conner, & Kass Wenger, 2011). The validity of Framingham scores are questioned because the population of women included in the analysis was mostly under age 50 and on average fairly healthy. Data were also gathered without much consideration to ethnicity and metabolic syndrome, which has greater and earlier impact on CVD in women (Gleeson & Crabbe, 2009). The risk of a black woman's death being due to CVD is equal to that of a white male. The prevalence of DM in Hispanic women and HTN in blacks makes the risk for women to be much greater than previously considered (Mosca et al, 2011).

The past decade of research has strengthened the addition of novel markers to gain a better appreciation of CVD risk in women. The Reynolds Risk Score (Ridker, Buring, Rifai, & Cook, 2007) is one tool that incorporates novel markers such as CRP, but it has not been validated extensively in diverse populations (Gleeson & Crabbe, 2009). It has been recently suggested that the Reynolds score may underestimate the risk in women by 21% (DeFillippis et al, 2015). Other novel markers such as homocysteine, coronary artery calcification, and functional capacity tests (including cardiac recovery profiles after exercise) are touted as providing a more refined evaluation of actual risk in women. Mosca's team (2011) has identified that a history of pregnancy-induced hypertension, gestational diabetes and/or pre-eclampsia might double the vascular risks of women in later years. Women with strong family histories of early CVD should be more aggressively treated. Those with higher CRP levels and a risk of metabolic syndrome should also be included in the more aggressive treatment plans (Mosca et al, 2011).

Special attention for cholesterol management in women 45 to 75 years includes consideration of the following:

- For women with CVD or CV risk equivalents (including diabetes), statins are as useful in CV risk reduction via LDL lowering as they are for men. All secondary prevention trials with these drugs have included women.

- Control of risk factors by antihypertensive drugs and beta blockers is indicated. Evidence for use of aspirin in women under age 65 has come under scrutiny, but those with high risk are still encouraged to take it if the individualized adverse risk of taking aspirin is lower than the potential benefit (Mosca et al, 2011).

- Clinical trials of LDL lowering demonstrate increased survival in women but may not be as effective in reducing stroke risks (Brugts et al, 2009).

- LDL-lowering drugs are indicated for women with multiple risk factors

- HRT is not recommended for primary LDL lowering or HDL balance.

Older Adults

Most new CVD events and most coronary deaths occur in older adults (men older than 65 years, women older than 75 years) because they have accumulated more coronary atherosclerosis than have younger age groups. Lowering CVD risk by reducing total cholesterol, and specifically LDL levels, is critical in this population. Angiographic studies have shown that even advanced coronary atherosclerosis may respond to reductions in cholesterol; CV events are reduced even after only a few weeks or months of statin therapy (Tsunekawa et al, 2001). Framingham risk scores are less robust for predicting risk in older adults and measurements of atherosclerosis. Considering that CVD is more prevalent in the older population, more individuals will benefit from risk reduction than in other age groups. Other factors such as concomitant chronic diseases (e.g., congestive heart failure, dementia, advanced cerebrovascular disease, or active malignancy), social circumstances, chronological and functional age, and polypharmacy should be taken into account. Financial considerations must be taken into account, but in an era of Medicare drug plans and low-cost generics, these considerations have decreased in importance. Older adults who are otherwise healthy should have therapy if they present with elevated lipid levels.

How aggressive the therapy is depends, as it does in younger adults, on the degree of CVD risk. As with younger people, the CVD risk reduction occurs in 6 to 12 months, even in those with long-standing disease. No statistically significant differences in side-effect profiles have been noted in elders enrolled in studies. Benefits are still evident after age 75 (Savarese et al, 2013).

The same algorithm based on CVD risk is used in elders; however, older adults are less likely to achieve the reduction in cholesterol with diet therapy alone and are more likely to require some drug therapy. Statins are the first-line drug treatment used in this age group because they are well tolerated in this population. Most statins can be taken once daily and do not add much complexity to already existing treatment regimens. Niacin is not recommended because the side effects of orthostasis are not well tolerated, especially in older patients who may also be on other drugs that can produce BP changes. There is evidence niacin may increase stroke risk (MERCK, 2012). Bile-acid–binding resins have risks for impaction and constipation and are not a good choice for older people. Special attention for cholesterol management in older adults includes:

- Prevalence of diabetes, a CV risk equivalent, is markedly increased in the older population.
- Emphasis should be given to TLC, especially dietary changes, but drugs are more likely to be needed. Elders with poor appetites and risk of malnutrition are not candidates for strict dietary enforcement.
- Consideration for drug interactions related to polypharmacy is important. Elders may be at higher risk for muscle toxicity when statins are mixed with macrolides and other antibiotics. Thiazide diuretics are associated with increasing hyperlipidemic patterns and might be substituted for by another class of drugs. Providers should consider statins with less cytochrome P450 competition, such as pitavastatin.
- Patients with very limited life expectancy due to other diseases probably do not benefit from antihyperlipidemic drug therapy. Strict enforcement of TLC is also unnecessary.

Young Adults

CVD is rare in this age group except for patients with severe risk factors such as familial hypercholesterolemia, heavy cigarette smoking, and diabetes. Unfortunately, CVD is becoming more common as the obesity and metabolic syndrome epidemic grows. Long-term predictive studies (NCEP, 2001) have shown that elevated cholesterol found in young adults predicts a higher rate of premature CVD in middle age. For this reason, control of risk factors is important in young adults as primary prevention.

The NCEP (2001) recommends doing lipid profiles beginning at age 20. Such early testing provides an opportunity to begin the public health approach to primary prevention. All young adults must be informed if they are at risk for premature CVD so that they can consider actions to prevent or postpone its occurrence. Finally, patients with cholesterol levels in the upper quartile of the population are clearly at high long-term risk and TLC intervention should begin at the earliest possible age. Most young adults with very high LDL cholesterol (greater than 190 mg/dL) are possible candidates for cholesterol-lowering drugs; however, prudence should be exercised in prescribing cholesterol-lowering drugs to young women.

The following recommendations are made based on the Pregnancy Categories:

- Nicotinic acid and fibric acid derivatives are Pregnancy Category C. Risks and benefits should be carefully weighed before giving these drugs to pregnant women.
- All statins are Pregnancy Category X and should not be given to women who have the potential to become pregnant without strong counseling.
- No pregnancy category has been assigned to the bile-acid–binding resins. Women of childbearing age with elevated cholesterol are best managed with lifestyle modifications. If this is not effective, they should probably be referred to a lipid specialist.

- All antihyperlipidemics should be avoided during breastfeeding.

Special attention for cholesterol management in young adults beyond those listed above for women include consideration of the following:

- Persons with heterozygous familial hypercholesterolemia may develop very premature CVD and require intensive LDL-lowering therapy. To achieve a level of less than 100 mg/dL usually requires both TLC and drug therapy.
- CVD is accelerated in this group for patients with type 1 diabetes or in very heavy cigarette smokers. Clinical judgment is required to determine the LDL goal here.
- Most young adults will not meet the multiple risk factors criteria. Non-LDL risk factors in this age group carry a higher long-term risk and should be the focus of management.

African Americans

HMG-CoA reductase gene variance among ethnic groups shows an interesting, more protective lipid phenotype than in other ethnic groups (Chen et al, 2009); however, African Americans have the highest overall CVD mortality rates and the highest out-of-hospital coronary death rates of any other ethnic group in the United States, particularly at young ages. Although the reasons for this excess CV risk have not been fully elucidated, it can be explained in part by the high prevalence and suboptimal control of coronary risk factors. Hypertension, left ventricular hypertrophy, diabetes, cigarette smoking, obesity, and physical inactivity are all more prevalent in African Americans than in whites. The predictability of standard risk factors for CHD by the Framingham risk assessment tool is somewhat suspect due to the fact that African Americans were not heavily represented in the baseline sample; however, the risk of death and other serious consequences is disproportionately higher in African Americans. This might be caused by higher CRP levels (Cushman et al, 2009). The 2013 guidelines do address the black population. The REGARDS study also has better insights into racial differences (Muntner et al, 2014).

Certain differences between African Americans and whites require special attention:

- African American men often have a high normal baseline level of creatinine kinase. The CK level should be documented before starting a statin.
- Hypertension, a powerful CVD risk factor, is more common in African Americans than whites. If present, left ventricular hypertrophy should be considered in the patient treatment plan because it is a powerful predictor of cardiovascular deaths.
- Obesity, especially abdominal obesity, is twice as common in African American women as compared to white women. Metabolic syndrome is a risk factor for CVD.
- Type 2 diabetes, an independent CV risk factor, is more prevalent in African Americans than whites.

- African Americans with established CVD are at particularly high risk for cardiac death. The new cholesterol guidelines have taken this into consideration and agree there is higher cardiovascular risk in this population. Patients from this ethnic group should be educated about this fact when discussing cardiac risks and the decision to start lipid-lowering therapy.
- African Americans are more likely to have multiple risk factors; therefore, LDL-lowering drugs are warranted when LDL is greater than 130 mg/dL after a TLC trial, especially when individualized family cardiovascular event histories are involved.

Hispanic Americans

Hispanic Americans are a heterogeneous ethnic group with origins in many different countries. The genetic researchers have found two general haplotypes that affect lipid processing; one was associated with higher risk factors of overall higher TC, TG, and LDL levels with low HDL levels, whereas the other type had much lower risks (Chen et al, 2009). CHD and cardiovascular disease are about 20% lower among adult Hispanics than among whites (NCEP, 2001) despite the increased prevalence of diabetes, obesity, lower HDL levels, and higher triglyceride levels. While these concomitant conditions may raise Hispanics' CV risk score, the Framingham tool has not been validated in this group and probably overestimates the risk (D'Agostino, Grundy, Sullivan, Wilson, for the CHD Risk Prediction Group, 2001). There are no special considerations for cholesterol management for Hispanic Americans at this time.

Native Americans (American Indians)

Data from the Indian Health Service indicate that cardiovascular disease rates are increasing in Native Americans. Native Americans were not included in the original studies on the metabolism of statins. CVD incidence rates among Native American men and women were almost twice as high as those in the biracial Atherosclerosis Risk in Communities Study (Howard et al, 1999). In addition to increased rates of CVD, cardiovascular events in Native Americans appeared more often to be fatal.

The significant independent predictors of cardiovascular disease common to both Native American men and women were diabetes, age, LDL levels, albuminuria, and HTN. The increasing incidence of CVD may be related to the increasing prevalence of diabetes in this population. As with the Hispanic population, the Framingham tool appears to overestimate the risk of CVD. Nonetheless, efforts to reduce cholesterol and other CV risk factors are important because there is a higher incidence of CVD and a higher mortality rate in this population. Despite limited data suggesting some differences, there is no separate algorithm for Native American populations.

Asian and Pacific Islanders

There is limited information on the risks and benefits of lipid management for the reduction of CVD and cardiovascular disease in the Asian and Pacific Islander populations. The Honolulu Heart Program is an ongoing prospective study of CHD and stroke in a cohort of Japanese American men living in Hawaii. In this study, CHD and cardiovascular mortality are lower than in the general U.S. population and the Framingham tool appears to overestimate the actual risk. The increased incidence of diabetes in native Hawaiians and Pacific Islanders has not generated a separate algorithm. Some providers question whether alternative BMI charts should be used to determine actual risk levels. It should be noted that familial forms of lipid disorders are more highly prevalent than in many other population groups (Cuchel et al, 2014).

Chinese Americans were included in the recent lipid genetic studies (Chen et al, 2009). Even though this population typically has the lowest BMIs when compared to other racial groups, they have high cardiovascular disease rates. East Asians also have a very high prevalence of coronary disease at younger ages in the absence of standard risk factors. This may be related to the high prevalence of insulin resistance, metabolic syndrome, and diabetes in this population at a lower BMI than in whites. For these reasons, general guidelines recommend that special attention be given to early detection of CV risk factors in Asian populations, with emphasis on metabolic syndrome and diabetes. The treatment plan should place increased emphasis on intensive TLC implementation. Of note, low BMI is also associated with increased risk in the Asian population (Chen et al, 2013).

The peoples of India and Bangladesh, carry more body fat than Europeans and other Asians in the same BMI range, yet unexpectedly have a lower rate of CV events until the BMI range of 35 (Chen et al, 2013). The BMI cut points for risk may not apply to this population and need to be considered during personalized risk discussions concerning statin use.

Concomitant Disease States

Drugs used to treat hyperlipidemia may improve the management of some diseases and worsen others. It is not within the scope of this text to discuss all possible diseases that may coexist with hyperlipidemia, but common diseases that may be impacted as a result of drug selection for the treatment of hyperlipidemia are discussed here.

Diabetes Mellitus

Diabetes mellitus is a CV risk equivalent, so the ideal therapeutic treatment goal for LDL cholesterol levels in diabetic patients, particularly type 2, is less than 100 mg/dL. TLC should be started immediately in all patients presenting with diabetes or prediabetes. Most patients with diabetes will require LDL-lowering drugs to achieve target serum LDL levels below 100 mg/dL. If the patient also has high TG, which is common for type 2 diabetics, non-HDL cholesterol becomes a secondary target for therapy. After serum LDL levels are in a desirable range, the focus of treatment can change to reducing serum TG levels. Nicotinic acid has been shown to have a favorable effect on diabetic dyslipidemia. Unfortunately, nicotinic acid can cause increased insulin resistance. Given in low doses, nicotinic acid produces limited deterioration in glucose control and no changes in glycated hemoglobin levels.

The first line of treatment is intensive TLC plus medications. Maximal control of nonlipid risk factors such as HTN and hyperglycemia are also a focus of management. The drugs of choice for treating HTN in patients with diabetes are angiotensin-converting enzyme (ACE) inhibitors or angiotensin II receptor blockers (ARBs).

Statins are usually the drugs of choice for lowering serum LDLs. Statins are generally well tolerated in this population and have the advantage of lowering VLDL as well. Bile-acid–binding resins can also be used to lower serum LDLs, but they do not reduce serum VLDL, a lipid fraction commonly elevated in diabetics. Diabetic patients taking bile-acid–binding resins should have TG checked regularly because these medications can elevate serum TG levels.

Additional special attention for lipid management in patients with diabetes includes consideration of the following:

- Fibrates are well tolerated and do not worsen hyperglycemia, but they are best used in patients with lowered LDL cholesterol levels.
- If TG are greater than 200 mg/dL, the non-HDL goal is less than 130 mg/dL.
- Control of nonlipid risk factors is central to management in this population. Metformin may help lower hyperglycemia and facilitate weight loss. Insulin, sulfonylureas, metformin, and glitazones all lower TG. Control of hyperglycemia may eliminate the need for a fibrate medication.

Metabolic Syndrome

Patients with metabolic syndrome have an increased risk for coronary disease. There has been a brief surge of interest in what was called "the obesity paradox" whereby CV survival appeared to be paradoxically better in overweight individuals. This "paradox" has been put to rest after a statistical review demonstrated that it did not exist (Tobias et al, 2014). Elevated TG present one factor within a set of risk factors in patients who are obese (especially abdominal obesity), sedentary, have low HDL cholesterol, are hypertensive, and have fasting blood glucose levels at or above 110 to 125 mg/dL. Expert opinion suggests starting metformin even before diabetes is formally diagnosed for the best long-term outcomes. Some patients may be concerned about media reports that statins induce the conversion of metabolic syndrome into full DM. They should be shown that the benefits of CV risk reduction significantly outweigh the low risk of converting to full glucose intolerance (Walters et al, 2013). In studies with Lipitor, development of DM is related to high doses, but this is considered a class effect in patients with two or more risk factors for CVD. It is also considered something that was probably inevitable and not necessarily triggered by the medication and more likely a genetic trait.

The major focus of management for metabolic syndrome is intensive TLC. Restricting alcohol and avoiding a high-carbohydrate diet form the foundation for triglyceride control in this population. Statins are the drugs of choice because they lower both serum LDL and VLDL remnants. In the presence of low serum HDL cholesterol, nicotinic acid

is an alternative therapy used when the serum LDL cholesterol goal has already been achieved. Fibrates can be considered as an alternative option for the treatment of elevated TG.

Hypothyroidism

Untreated hypothyroidism often presents with symptoms that include hypercholesterolemia. Clinically, patients present with elevated cholesterol, high LDL, and mild VLDL elevation. Every patient found to have elevated cholesterol (LDL greater than 160 mg/dL) should be screened for hypothyroidism. Treatment of the primary problem, hypothyroidism, should be initiated and serum lipid levels should be reevaluated after thyroid levels are normal.

Hypertension

HTN and hyperlipidemia commonly occur together. Patients with concomitant HTN and hypercholesterolemia should have both conditions treated aggressively because these two risk factors act synergistically, greatly increasing CVD risk. Management of HTN is discussed in Chapter 40. Lifestyle modifications are the first approach to treatment of both hypertension and hypercholesterolemia. The Dietary Approaches to Stop Hypertension (DASH) diet for HTN also works for hyperlipidemia. Weight control, exercise, lowering sodium consumption, and smoking cessation are lifestyle changes that should be stressed to patients with both disorders.

Diuretics are still considered first-line therapy for HTN with the JNC-8. Thiazide diuretics are the most commonly prescribed agents for HTN. Higher doses of these drugs can cause modest and often transient increases in serum LDL cholesterol and TG, with little or no adverse effects on HDL cholesterol. The effects of loop diuretics are similar to those of thiazides, but serum HDL cholesterol levels are generally lower in patients on furosemide. This may not be a drug effect, but a reflection on the more advanced CV issues of those needing loop diuretics.

Calcium channel blockers, ACE inhibitors, and aldosterone antagonists have little effect on serum lipids. Beta blockers without intrinsic sympathomimetic activity (ISA) tend to reduce HDL cholesterol, increase TG, and have variable effects on total serum cholesterol. These effects are minimal, and should not play a role in the selection of a beta blocker for treating hypertension. ISA beta blockers combined with alpha$_1$ beta blockers (labetalol and carvedilol) have no appreciable effect on lipid levels. Alpha$_1$ blockers and centrally acting agonists provide minimal, beneficial effects on blood lipids by decreasing LDL cholesterol.

Nicotinic acid can cause orthostatic hypotension and should be used with caution in patients who are being treated with antihypertensives that have this same side effect. None of the other classes of drugs used to treat hyperlipidemia have a direct effect on blood pressure. Bile-acid–binding resins may decrease absorption of antihypertensive medications, so their administration should be separated by giving the antihypertensive 1 hour before or 4 hours after the bile-acid–binding resin. Statins have no specific interactions with antihypertensive agents.

Chronic Renal Disease (CKD)

There is an independent relationship between renal disease and CV issues. If CKD patients have eGRF greater than 60 mL/min/1.73m², statins are known to be of benefit. The concerns about individuals with renal function occur as renal function is lost. There are more adverse events as GFR drops; however, statins are not stopped because over a quarter of the deaths in this population are CV related. Use of statins is considered very beneficial. When patients progress to dialysis, however, there is little benefit. Starting individuals on new statin therapy when they are placed on dialysis is not a recommendation (Goff et al, 2013). Fibrates may have a role in mild to moderate disease with a demonstrated risk reduction of 30% and mortality reduction of 40% (Jun et al, 2012).

Cost

In today's health-care environment, the cost-effectiveness of therapy is always an issue. The aggregate cost of CVD in the United States is anticipated to be over $800 billion per year for medication, treatment, and lost wages by the year 2030 according to the authors of the newest cholesterol guidelines. Prevention of CVD could greatly reduce this economic burden, and the management of cholesterol levels is one way to prevent CVD.

Patients in high-risk categories have the greatest likelihood of significant benefit from cholesterol reduction. In men 35 to 64 years and women 35 to 54 years with established CVD, intervention with standard doses of statins has been estimated to save significant amounts of money otherwise spent on CVD events in untreated patients. In older men and women, the cost–benefit ratios are even better. From a public health perspective, the cost of cholesterol treatment is clearly justified for older patients. Patients at lower risk for CVD have a less favorable cost–benefit ratio. For this group, the ratio of cost to savings depends on the drug therapy chosen. When evaluating patients on an individual basis, even low-risk patients may benefit from cholesterol reduction therapy. The more recent links between low to moderate lipid levels in middle-aged adults to higher risk for development of Alzheimer's disease increases the urgency for earlier and more aggressive treatment of hyperlipidemia beyond just CVD issues (Solomon, Kivipelto, Wolozin, Zhou, & Whitner, 2009).

Reduction of major risk factors, like smoking and limited physical activity, have the best cost–benefit ratio for public health and the individual patient. When drug therapy is chosen, the cost includes laboratory assessment and monitoring as well as the price of the medication. Historically, the greatest expense was drug cost. With the marketing of generic drugs, costs associated with the treatment of hyperlipidemia have been reduced significantly. Many major drug companies offer low-cost or free brand-name medications for those with restricted incomes.

MONITORING

The treatment goals must be expanded beyond targeted LDL levels of the ATEP III and become more individualized. The absolute number is not so much the focus as is the percentage of reduction and process toward a better CV risk profile. This trend favors the movement toward changing practice to eliminate the requirement for fasting prior to lipid lab draws (Doran et al, 2014). It appears there may be no clinically significant difference in fasting vs. non-fasting values; however, this recommendation is yet to be substantiated by vigorous research.

Some experts still recommend also including inflammatory marker control, non-HDL targets, HDL-C levels, TG, and peripheral vascular prevention and stroke prevention targets (Ridker & Cook, 2013). For the first time in the 2013 guidelines, a strong emphasis upon patient involvement in therapeutic decision making and lifestyle interventions to include weight control, exercise, smoking cessation, and taking a long-term look at risk rather than just reacting to disease states. Of critical importance to nurse prescribers is that a laboratory value is not the goal; the reduction of risk and the prevention of CV events is the true target.

Monitoring for effectiveness of dietary therapy involves weight loss, BMI reduction, and lipid lowering. Drug therapy is not usually initiated until a 3-month trial of dietary therapy has been completed; the exception is concurrent drug therapy for those patients with DM or metabolic syndrome. Selection of an agent to treat a lipid disorder is based on a minimum of two lipoprotein levels done 1 to 4 weeks apart during maximum dietary therapy and on individualized risk. This provides a baseline for future evaluation of whether a drug needs to be added to improve treatment efficacy. Baseline lab data (liver function, ALT or AST, and CK) should be gathered before drug treatment begins. Serial monitoring of liver labs are no longer indicated for most patients. Specific diagnostic tests for monitoring each drug class are discussed in Chapter 16.

With good medication and adherence to lifestyle changes, patients should show a lowering of cholesterol within 4 to 6 weeks of initiating therapy. Levels of serum LDL cholesterol should be evaluated 6 to 8 weeks after initiating therapy. Nicotinic acid is the exception to this rule, with repeat measurements done when the patient's prescribed dose has been stable for 4 to 6 weeks. For all of these drugs, a second measurement of LDL cholesterol levels is done 6 weeks after the first measurement. A minimum of two measurements is used for establishing the efficacy of the treatment plan. For all treatment regimens, if the dose of a drug is increased, or another drug is added to the treatment regimen, the patient's laboratory data should be evaluated in another 6 to 8 weeks. An aggressive increase in dosing is recommended for those at highest risk for CVD per the new guidelines. After the desired LDL cholesterol range is reached, patients should be followed at 8 to 12 week intervals for 1 year. After 1 year of therapy, during which the patient's response to the treatment regimen has been established and there is no evidence of toxicity, patients should be followed at 4 to 6 month intervals. Myopathies tend not to surface until 9 months into therapy. Evaluation of CK levels after the baseline period is not indicated unless there are symptoms.

Intermittent monitoring of HDL and non-HDL levels is a practice that provides a clearer picture of the actual CVD risk status for the patient but may not be covered by insurance. Apo levels and Lp-PLA$_2$ can be measured, but this is very expensive. These tests are not recommended by experts for anyone other than those with high risk (Davidson et al, 2011). They have not been demonstrated to be reliable for treatment decisions. Simple calculation of the non-HDL levels can give an indication of apo levels. Attention to reductions in the C-reactive protein levels is more critical if measuring treatment effect. There is not great evidence to re-screen nonrisk patients for CRP levels if the baseline was normal and no other situational changes occur that trigger suspicion that levels have gone up.

OUTCOME EVALUATION

Long-term cholesterol control requires lifelong adherence to a treatment regimen. If accompanied by weight loss and other successful TLC achievements, the medications can be considered for reduction. Discontinuation of treatment is quickly followed by a return of the cholesterol to pretreatment levels without other interventions. Achieving long-term clinical control requires the same interest and attention from the patient and the provider as was given to the initial evaluation and treatment plan. Effective use of follow-up visits and skillful employment of adherence-enhancing techniques are required, including nurturing the patient–provider relationship. The primary care provider can manage hyperlipidemia in most patients. Severe forms of hypercholesterolemia that do not respond to general guideline therapies require consultation with a lipid specialist.

Prescribers may need to intervene with administrators and insurance companies, which retain a prescriptive approach to absolute LDL levels to determine "quality" of care. Absolute levels are no longer recommended as performance standards (Stone et al, 2013).

PATIENT EDUCATION

Patient education should include a discussion of the overall treatment plan and the role of medication therapy. Patients who understand the reasons for their drug therapy may show improved adherence to their medication regimens. Careful education helps clarify that risk scores can provide a false sense of health for those with lab levels of "near" risk. The numbers are not absolutes; both provider and patient should err on the side of caution when deciding on therapeutic alternatives when faced with higher risks.

Patients should be made aware that the tendencies for muscle toxicity appear to run in families. Patients should inquire about statin tolerance issues in their older relatives to establish if a potential family risk for myopathies exists. The onset of muscle pain can occur immediately but frequently does not appear for several months. Reinforcement about reporting myalgias should be addressed with patients at every follow-up appointment.

Some patients may question the reports about cognitive impairment or short-term memory issues, which are now recognized to be reversible after statin treatment is discontinued. Issues with memory may be more associated with life stressors and not the drugs (FDA, 2012a). Of greater import is that even mildly elevated lipids in midlife are linked to dementia in older age (Solomon et al, 2009). The reduction of significant CV events increases the probability of a high quality of elder years as well.

HYPERLIPIDEMIA

PATIENT EDUCATION

Related to the Overall Treatment Plan and Disease Process

☐ Pathophysiology of lipid disorders and their long-term effects on cardiovascular morbidity and mortality

☐ Role of lifestyle modification, especially dietary therapy, in improving outcomes and keeping the number and cost of required drugs down

☐ Importance of adherence to the treatment regimen

☐ Need for regular follow-up visits with the primary care provider

Specific to the Drug Therapy

☐ Reason for the drug(s) being given and the anticipated action of the drug(s) on the disease process

☐ Doses and schedules for taking the drug(s)

☐ Possible adverse reactions, how to prevent them, and what to do if they occur

☐ Interaction between lifestyle modifications and the drug(s)

Reasons for Taking the Drug(s)

Patient education about specific drugs is provided in Chapter 16. Specific information related to hyperlipidemia includes the reasons for drug(s) being taken: Antilipidemics are given to reduce morbidity and mortality from the leading cause of death in the United States—cardiovascular disease. Discuss the risk of cardiovascular disease with the patient while maintaining the potential for good quality of life with adequate treatment.

HYPERLIPIDEMIA—cont'd

PATIENT EDUCATION

Drugs as Part of the Total Treatment Regimen

The expectations should be clear about what the drugs can and cannot do. Drugs are supplements to dietary and other lifestyle modifications, not substitutes for them. Lipid disorders are chronic conditions. Lifestyle modifications and drug regimens need to be incorporated into patients' everyday lives. Discontinuation of treatment will result in return of lipids to pretreatment levels.

Adherence Issues

Nonadherence to the treatment regimen may increase patients' risk for cardiovascular morbidity and reduce their life expectancy. Health-care providers should be aware of potential problems with adherence, discuss the importance of adherence at each follow-up visit, and assist patients in removing barriers to adherence, such as lack of social support and fear of side effects. Utilization of other health team members, especially the dietitian, should be maximized. Patient education booklets available from the American Heart Association and the National Cholesterol Education Program may supplement dietary instruction.

REFERENCES

ACCORD Study Group. (2010). Effects of combination lipid therapy in type 2 diabetes mellitus. *New England Journal of Medicine, 362*, 1563–1574.

American Diabetes Association (ADA). (2015). Standards of medical care in diabetes 2015. *Diabetes Care, 38*, (1 Suppl.), S1-S94.

Ansel, B. J. (2012). Managing residual CVD risk: The role of HDL cholesterol. Part 2 of a 3-part newsletter. *HDL and Atherogenesis*. National Lipid Association. www.cme.corner.com

Attard, S., Herring, A., Howards, A., & Gordon-Larsen, P. (2013). Longitudinal trajectories of BMI and cardiovascular disease risk: The national longitudinal study of adolescent health. *Obesity, 21* (11), 2180–2188. doi: 10.1002/oby.20569

Berglund, L., Burnzell, J., Goldberg, A., Golderberg, I., Sacks, F., Murad, M., et al. (2012). Evaluation and treatment of hypertriglyceridemia: An endocrine society clinical practice guideline. *Journal of Clinical Endocrinology and Metabolism, 97*(9), 2969–2989. doi: 10.1210/jc2011-3213

Boekholdt, S., Arsenault, D., Mora, S., Pedersen, T., LaRosa, J., Nestel, P., et al. (2012) Association of LDL cholesterol, non-HDL cholesterol, and apolipoprotein B levels with risk of cardiovascular events among patients treated with statins: A meta-analysis. *Journal of the American Medical Association, 307*(2), 1302–1309.

Brugsts, J., Yetgin, F., Hoeks, S., Gotlo, A., Shepard, J., Westendorp, R., et al. (2009). The benefits of statins in people without established CV disease but with CV risk factors: A meta-analysis of randomized controlled trials. *British Medical Journal, 338*, b2376–b2384.

Canadian Diabetes Association (CDA) Clinical Practice Guidelines Expert Committee. Canadian Diabetes Association. (2013). Clinical practice guidelines for the prevention and management of diabetes in Canada. *Canadian Journal of Diabetes, 37*(1 Suppl), S1–S212.

Cannon, C. P. (2005). The IDEAL cholesterol: Lower is better. *Journal of the American Medical Association, 294*(19), 2492–2494.

Carroll, M., Kit, B., Lacher, D., Shero, S., & Mussolino, M. (2012). Trends in lipids and lipoprotein in US Adults, 1988–2010. *Journal of the American Medical Association, 308*(15), 1545–1554.

Chen, Y. C., Chen, Y. D., Li, X., Post, W., Herrington, D., Polak, J. F., et al. (2009). The HMG-CoA reductase gene and lipid and lipoprotein levels: The multi-ethnic study of atherosclerosis. *Lipids, 44*(8), 733–743.

Chen, Y., Copeland, W., Vedanthan, R., Grant, E., Lee, J., Gu, D., et al. (2013). Association between body mass index and cardiovascular disease mortality in east Asians and south Asians: Pooled analysis of prospective data from the Asia Cohort Consortium. *British Medical Journal, 347*, f1546.

Criqui, M., Denenberg, J., Ix, J., McClelland, R., Wassel, C., Rifkin, D., et al. (2014, 15 Jan). Calcium density of coronary artery plaque and risk of incident cardiovascular events. *Journal of the American Medical Association, 311*(3), 271–278. doi: 10.1001/jama.2013.282535

Cuchel M., Bruckert, E., Ginsberg, H., Raal, F., Santos, R., Hegele, R., et al. (2014). Homozygous familial hypercholesterolaemia: New insights and guidance for clinicians to improve detection and clinical management. A position paper from the Consensus Panel on Familial Hypercholesterolaemia of the European Atherosclerosis Society. *European Heart Journal. 35*(32), 2146–2157.

Cushman, M., McClure, L., Howard, V., Jenny, N., Lakoski, S., & Howard, G. (2009). Implication of increased C-reactive protein for cardiovascular risk stratification in black and white men and women in the U.S. *Clinical Chemistry, 5*(9), 1627–1636.

D'Agostino, R., Grundy, S., Sullivan, L., Wilson, P., for the CHD Risk Prediction Group. (2001). Validation of the Framingham coronary heart disease prediction scores: Results of a multiple ethnic groups investigation. *Journal of the American Medical Association, 286*, 180–187.

Daniels, S., & Greer, F. (2008). Lipid screening and cardiovascular health in childhood. *Pediatrics, 122*, 198–208.

Davidson, M., Ballantyne, C., Jacobson, T., Vittner, V., Braun, L., Brown, A., et al. (2011). Clinical utility of inflammatory markers and advanced lipoprotein testing: Advice from an expert panel of lipid specialists. *Journal of Clinical Lipidology 5*(5), 338–367.

DeFillippis, A., Young, R., Carrubba, C., McEvoy, J., Budoff, M., Blumenthal, R.....Blaha, M. (2015). An analysis of calibration and discrimination among multiple cardiovascular risk scores in a modern multi-ethnic cohort. *Annals of Internal Medicine, 162*(4), 266–275.

Doell, D., Folmer, D., Lee, H., Honigfort, M., & Carberry, S. (2012). Updated estimates of trans fat intake by the US population. *Food Additives & Contaminants: Part A, 29*(6), 861–874.

Doran, B., Guo, Y., Xu, J., Weintraub, H., Mora, S., Maron, D., et al. (2014). Prognostic value of fasting versus nonfasting low-density lipoprotein cholesterol levels on long-term mortality. *Circulation, 130*(7), 546–553.

Ebbeling, C., Swain, J., Feldman, H., Wong, W., Hachey, D., Garcia-Lago, et al. (2012). Effects of dietary composition on energy expenditure during weight loss maintenance. [New Balance Foundation Obesity Prevention center at Boston Children's Hospital]. *Journal of the American Medical Association, 307*(24), 2627–2634.

Elkind, M. (2013, 21 Nov). Cholesterol and primary prevention of stroke. https://secure. quantimed.com

Fitzgerald, K., Frank-Kamenetsky, M., Shulga-Morskaya, S., Liebow, A., Bettencourt, B., Sutherland, J., et al. (2013). Effect of an RNA interference drug on the synthesis of proprotein covertase subtililsin/kexin type 9 (PCK9) and the concentration of serum LDL cholesterol in healthy volunteers: A randomized, single-blind, placebo-controlled phase I trial. *The Lancet*. Published online October 3, 2013, at http://dx.doi.org/10.1016/S0140-6736(13)61914-5 9

Food and Drug Administration (FDA). (2010, 9 Feb). *Questions and answers for healthcare professionals: CRESTOR and the JUPITER trials.*

www.fda.gov/Drugs/DrugSafety/PostmarketDrugSafetyInformation forPatientsandProviders/ucm 199891.htm

Food and Drug Administration (FDA). (2012a, 28 Feb). *FDA Drug Safety Communication: Important safety label changes to cholesterol-lowering statin drugs.* www.fda.gov/Drugs/DrugSafety/ucm293101.htm

Food and Drug Administration (FDA) (2012b, 6 Dec). *FDA approves new orphan drug for rare cholesterol disorder.* www.fda.gov/newsevents/ Newsroom/PressAnnouncements/ucm333285.htm

Food and Drug Administration (FDA) (2013, 29 Jan). *FDA approves new orphan drug Kynamro to treat inherited cholesterol disorder.* www.fda.gov/ newsevents/Newsroom/PressAnnouncements/ucm337195.htm

Ford, E., Li, D., Zhao, G., Peason, W., & Capewell, S. (2009). Trends in the prevalence of low risk factor burden for cardiovascular disease among United States adults. *Circulation, 120,* 1181–1188.

Fortmann, S., Burda, B., Senger, C., Lin, J., & Whitlock, E. (2013). Vitamin and mineral supplements in the primary prevention of cardiovascular disease and cancer: An updated systematic evidence review for the U.S. Preventive Services Task Force. *Annals of Internal Medicine, 159*(12), 824–834.

Gidding, S., Lichtenstein, A., Faith, M., Karpyn, J., Manella, B., Popkin, J., et al. (2009). Implementing American Heart Association pediatric and adult nutrition guidelines: A scientific statement from the American Heart Association Nutrition Committee of the Council on Nutrition, Physical Activity and Metabolism, Council on Cardiovascular Disease in the Young, Council on Arteriosclerosis, Thrombosis and Vascular Biology, Council on Cardiovascular Nursing, Council on Epidemiology and Prevention, and Council for High Blood Pressure Research. *Circulation, 119*(8), 1161–1175.

Gleeson, D., & Crabbe, D. (2009). Emerging concepts in cardiovascular disease risk assessment: Where do women fit in? *Journal of the American Academy of Nurse Practitioners, 21,* 480–487.

Goff, D., Lloyd-Jones, D., Bennett, G., Coady, S., D'Agostino, R., Gibbons, R., et al. (2013, Nov 12). 2013 ACC/AHA guideline on the assessment of cardiovascular risk: A report of the American College of Cardiology/ American Heart Association task force on practice. *Circulation,* http:// circ.ahajournals. org/content/early/2013/11/01.cir.0000437741. 48606.98 .citation

Grady, D., Wenger, N., Herrington, D., Khan, S., Furberg, C., Hunninghake, D., et al, for the Heart and Estrogen/Progestin Replacement Study Research Group. (2000). Postmenopausal hormone therapy increases risk for venous thromboembolic disease: The Heart and Estrogen/ Progestin Replacement Study. *Archives of Internal Medicine, 132,* 689–696.

Greenland, P., Alpert, J., Beller, G., Benjamin, E., Budoff, M., Fayad, Z., et al. (2010). 2010 ACCF/AHA guideline for assessment of cardiovascular risk in asymptomatic adults: Executive summary. *Journal of the American College of Cardiology, 56*(25), 2182–2199.

Grundy, S., Cleeman, J., Merz, C., Brewer, B., Jr., Clark, L., Hinninghake, D., et al, for the Coordinating Committee of the National Cholesterol Education Program. (2004). Implications of recent clinical trials for the National Cholesterol Education Program Adult Treatment Panel III guidelines. *Circulation, 110,* 227–239.

Haffner, S., Lehto, S., Ronnemaa, T., Pyorala, K., & Laasko, M. (1998). Mortality from coronary heart disease in subjects with type 2 diabetes and in nondiabetic subjects with and without prior myocardial infarction. *New England Journal of Medicine, 339,* 229–234.

Howard, B., Lee, E., Cowan, L., Devereaux, R., Galloway, J., Go, O., et al. (1999). Rising tide of cardiovascular disease in American Indians: The Strong Heart Study. *Circulation, 99,* 2389–2395.

Huang, Y., DiDonato, J., Levison, B., Schmidt, D., Li, L., Wu, Y., et al. (2014). An abundant dysfunctional apolipoprotein A1 in human artheroma. *Nature Medicine, 20*(2), 193–203. doi: 10.1038/nm.3459

Jenkins, D., Kendall, C., & Marchie, A. (2005). Diet and cholesterol reduction. *Annals of Internal Medicine, 142,* 793–795.

JNC-8. (2014). Evidence-based guideline for the management of high blood pressure in adults: Report from the panel members appointed to the eight joint national committee. *Journal of the American Medical Association,* published online 18 Dec 2013. doi: 10.1001/jama.2013 .284427

Jones, P., Davidson, M., Stein, E., Bays, H., McKenney, J., Miller, E., et al. (2003). Comparison of the efficacy and safety of rosuvastatin versus atorvastatin, simvastatin, and pravastatin across doses. (STELLAR trial). *American Journal of Cardiology, 92,* 152–160.

Jun, M., Zhu, B., Tonelli, M., Jardine, M. J., Patel, A., Neal, B., et al. (2012). Effects of fibrates in kidney disease: A systematic review and meta-analysis. *Journal of the American College of Cardiology, 60*(20), 2061–2071. doi: 10.1016/j.jacc.2012.07.049

Knatterud, G., Rosenberg, Y., Campeau, L., Geller, N., Hunninghake, D., Forman, S., et al. (2000). Long-term effects on clinical outcomes of aggressive lowering of low-density lipoprotein cholesterol levels and low-dose anticoagulation in the Post Coronary Bypass Graft trial. *Circulation, 102,* 157–165.

Malmberg, K., Yusuf, S., Gerstine, H., Brown, J., Zhao, F., Hunt, D., et al, for the OASIS Registry Investigators. (2002). Impact of diabetes on long-term prognosis in patients with unstable angina and non-Q-wave myocardial infarction: Results of the OASIS (Organization to Assess Strategies for Ischemic Syndromes) Registry. *Circulation, 102,* 1014–1019.

McCrindle, B., Kwiterovich, P., McBride, P., Daniels, S., & Kavey, R. (2012). Guidelines for lipid screening in children and adolescents: Bringing evidence to the debate. *Pediatrics, 130*(2), 353–356.

Mente, A., deKoning, L., Shannon, H., & Anand, S. (2009). A systematic review of the evidence supporting a causal link between dietary factors and coronary heart disease. *Archives of Internal Medicine, 169*(7), 659–669.

MERCK (2012, Dec 20). *Merck announces HPS2-THRIVE study of Predaptive (extended release niacin/laropiprant) did not achieve primary endpoint.* www.thrivestudy.org/press-release

Miettinen, H., Lehto, S., Salomaa, V., Maonen, M., Niemela, M., Haffner, S., et al, for the FINMONICA Myocardial Infarction Register Study Group. (1998). Impact of diabetes on mortality after the first myocardial infarction. *Diabetes Care, 21*(1) 69–75.

Mosca, L., Barrett-Conner, E., & Kass Wenger, N. (2011). Sex/Gender differences in cardiovascular disease prevention: What a difference a decade makes. *Circulation, 124*(19), 2145–2154.

Muntner, P., Colantonio, L., Cushman, M., Goff, D., Howard, G., Howard, V., et al. (2014). Validation of the atherosclerotic cardiovascular disease pooled cohort risk equations. *Journal of the American Medical Association, 311*(14), 1406–1415. doi:10.1001/jama.2014.2630

Naci, H., & Ioannidis, J. (2013). Comparative effectiveness of exercise and drug intervention on mortality outcomes; meta-epidemiological study. *British Medical Journal, 347,* f15577.

National Cholesterol Education Program (NCEP). (2001). *Third report of the expert panel on detection, evaluation, and treatment of high blood cholesterol in adults* (Adult Treatment Panel III). Rockville, MD: National Institutes of Health, National Heart, Lung and Blood Institute.

National Heart, Lung and Blood Institute (NHLB). (2011). Expert panel on integrated guidelines for cardiovascular health and risk reduction in children and adolescents. *Pediatrics, 128*(5 Suppl), 213–256.

Navar-Boggan, A., Peterson, E., D'Agostino, R., Neely, B., Sniderman, A. & Pencina, M. (2015). Hyperlipidemia in early adulthood increases long-term risk of coronary heart disease. *Circulation, 131*(5), 451–458.

Navarese, E., Buffon, A., Andreotti, F., Kozinski, M., Welton, N., Faiszak, T., et al. (2013). Meta-analysis of impact of different types and doses of statins on new-onset diabetes mellitus. *American Journal of Cardiology, 111*(8), 1123–1130.

Nettleton, J. A., Polak, J. F., Tracy, R., Burke, G. L., & Jacobs, D. R., Jr. (2009). Dietary patterns and incident cardiovascular disease in the Multi-Ethnic Study of Atherosclerosis. *American Journal of Clinical Nutrition, 90*(3), 647–654.

Newman, T., Pletcher, M., & Hulley, S. (2012). Overly aggressive new guidelines for lipid and lipoprotein screening in children: Evidence of a broken process. *Pediatrics, 130*(2), 349–352.

Nissen S. E., Tuzcu, E. M., Schoenhagen, P., Brown, B. G., Ganz, P., Vogel, R. A., et al, REVERSAL Investigators. (2004). Effect of intensive compared with moderate lipid-lowering therapy on progression of coronary atherosclerosis: A randomized controlled trial. *Journal of the American Medical Association, 291*(9), 1071–1080.

Richardson, K., Schoen, M., French, B., Umsheid, C., Mitchell, M., Arnold, S., et al. (2013). Statins and cognitive function: A systematic review. *Annals of Internal Medicine, 159*(10), 688–697. doi: 10.7326/0003-4819-159-10-20131190-0007

Ridker, P. M., Buring, J. E., Rifai, N., & Cook, N. R. (2007). Development and validation of improved algorithms for the assessment of global cardiovascular risk in women: The Reynolds Risk Score. *Journal of the American Medical Association, 297*(6), 611–619.

Ridker, P., & Cook, N. (2013). Statins: New American guidelines for prevention of cardiovascular disease. *The Lancet, 382*(9907), 1762–1765.

Rizos, E., Nitzani, E., Bika, E., Kostapanos, M., & Elisaf, M. (2012). Association between omega-3 fatty acid supplementation and risk of major cardiovascular disease events: A systematic review and meta-analysis. *Journal of the American Medical Association, 308*(10), 1024–1033.

Rong, Y., Chen, L., Zhu, T., Song Y., Yu., M., Shan, Z., et al. (2013). Egg consumption and risk of coronary heart disease and stroke: Dose-response meta-analysis of prospective cohort studies. *British Medical Journal, 3460*, e8539–e8552.

Rossouw, J., Anderson, G., Prentice, R., LaCroix, A., Kooperberg, C., Stefanick, M., et al (Writing Group for the Women's Health Initiative). (2002). Risks and benefits of estrogen plus progestin in healthy postmenopausal women: Principle results from the Women's Health Initiative randomized controlled trial. *Journal of the American Medical Association, 288*(3), 321–333.

Sacks, F., Tonkin, A., Shepherd, J., Braunwald, E., Cobbe, S., Hawkins, C., et al, for the Prospective Pravastatin Pooling Project Investigators Group. (2000). Effect of pravastatin on coronary disease events in subgroups defined by coronary risk factors: The Prospective Pravastatin Pooling Project. *Circulation, 102*, 1893–1900.

Savarese, G., Gotto, A., Paolillo, S., D'Amore, C., Losco, T., Musella, F., et al. (2013). Benefits of statins in elderly subjects without established cardiovascular disease: A meta-analysis. *Journal of the American College of Cardiology, 62*(22), 2090–2099.

Sesso, H., Christen, W., Bubes, V., Smith, J. P., MacFadyen, J., ... & Gaziano, J. (2012). A randomized trial of multivitamin in the prevention of cardiovascular disease in men: The Physicians Health Study II. Presentation at American Heart Association Scientific Session 5 Nov 2012, Los Angeles, CA.

Sharma, M., Ansari, M. T., Abou-Setta, A. M., Soares-Weiser, K., Ooi, T. C., Sears, M., et al. (2009). Systematic review: Comparative effectiveness and harms of combinations of lipid-modifying agents and high-dose statin monotherapy. *Annals of Internal Medicine, 151*(9), 622–630.

Solomon, A., Kivipelto, M., Wolozin, B., Zhou, J., & Whitner, R. (2009). Midlife serum cholesterol and increased risk of Alzheimer's and vascular dementia three decades later. *Dementia and Geriatric Cognitive Disorders, 28*(1), 75–80.

Steinberger, J., Sinaiko, A., Kelly, A., Leisenring, W., Steffen, L., Goodman, P., et al. (2012). Cardiovascular risk and insulin resistance in childhood cancer survivors. *Journal of Pediatrics, 160*(3), 494–499.

Stone, N., Robinson, J., Lichtenstein, A., Merz, C., Blum, C., Echel, R., et al. (2013, Nov 12). 2013 ACC/AHA guideline on the treatment of blood cholesterol to reduce atherosclerotic cardiovascular risk in adults: A report of the American College of Cardiology/American Heart Association task force on practice guidelines. *Circulation.* http://circ.ahajournals. org/content/early/2013/11/01.cir.0000437738.63853.7a.citation

Tobias, D. K., Pan, A., Jackson, C. L., O'Reilly, E. J., Ding, E. L., Willett, W. C., et al. (2014, Jan 16). Body-mass index and mortality among adults with incident type 2 diabetes. *New England Journal of Medicine, 370*(3), 233–244. doi: 10.1056/NEJMoa1304501

Tsunekawa, T., Hayashi, T., Kano, H., Sumi, D., Matsui-Hirai., H., Takur, N., et al. (2001). Cervistatin, a hydroxymethylglutaryl coenzyme a reductase inhibitor, improves endothelial function in elderly diabetic patients within 3 days. *Circulation, 104*(4), 376–379.

U.S. Department of Health and Human Services. (2000, June). *Treating tobacco use and dependence: A systems approach. Clinical Practice Guideline.* Washington, DC: Public Health Service, U.S. Department of Health and Human Services.

Vogel, R. A. (2013, Dec 30). HDL raising: A good hypothesis gone bad. *Internal Medicine News.* Report from the Snowmass 2013 Cardiology Conference.

Voight, B. F., Peloso, G. M., Orho-Melander, M., Frikke-Schmidt, R., Barbalic, M., Jensen, M. K., et al. (2012, Aug 11). Plasma HDL cholesterol and risk of myocardial infarction: A Mendelian randomisation study. *The Lancet, 380*(9841), 572–580. doi: 10.1016/S0140-6736(12)60312-2

Walters, D., Ho, J., Boekholdt, M., DeMicco, D., Kastelein. J., Messig, M., et al. (2013). Cardiovascular event reduction versus new-onset diabetes during atorvastatin therapy: Effect of baseline risk factors for diabetes. *Journal of the American College of Cardiology, 61*(2), 148–152. doi: 10:1016/jack 2012: 09 042

Wilson, P. (2008). Progressing from risk factors to omics. *Circulation: Cardiovascular Genetics, 1*(12), 141–146.

Yang, X., So, W., Ko, G. T., Ma, R. C., Kong, A. P., Chow, C. C., et al. (2008). Independent associations between low-density lipoprotein cholesterol and cancer among patients with type 2 diabetes mellitus. *Canadian Medical Association Journal, 179*(5), 427–347.

Zhang, J., McKeown, R. E., Hussey, J. R., Thompson, S. J., Woods, J. R., & Ainsworth, B. E. (2005). Low HDL cholesterol is associated with suicide attempt among young healthy women: The Third National Health and Nutrition Examination Survey. *Journal of Affective Disorders, 89*(1), 25–33.

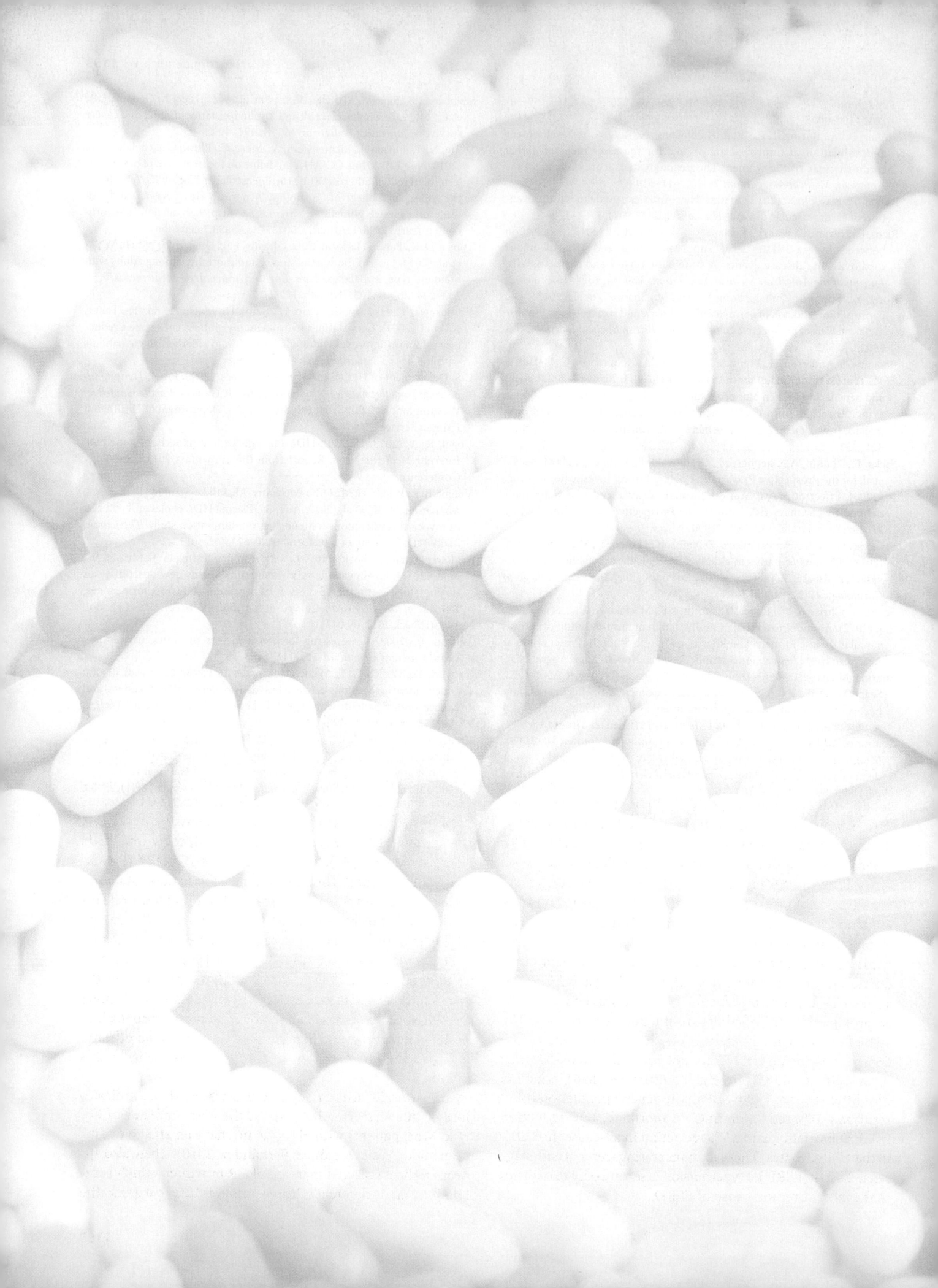

HYPERTENSION

Marylou V. Robinson

Hypertension (HTN) is the most common cardiovascular disease in the United States, and it is also a problem worldwide. The World Health Organization (World Health Report, 2012) reports that 1 out of 3 adults worldwide have suboptimal blood pressure (SBP). Suboptimal blood pressure is thought to be the number-one attributable risk for death throughout the world. According to the 2013 JNC-8 (Eighth Joint National Committee) guideline, blood pressures above 140/90 mm Hg for the general population is considered suboptimal. For nonfrail elders over the age of 60, blood pressure of 150/90 mm Hg is the new cut point (James et al, 2014).

Although the past two decades have seen considerable reduction in deaths from coronary heart disease (CHD) and stroke (CVA), control rates for HTN are still unacceptable. Approximately 30% of adults are still unaware of their HTN, 40% of individuals who have HTN are not in treatment, and 66% of those being treated are not controlled to blood pressures less than 140/90 mm Hg. It is estimated that a reduction of as little as 5 mm Hg of SBP in the general population could result in a 14% reduction in CVA mortality, a 9% reduction in CHD mortality, and a 7% reduction in all-cause mortality in the United States. There is an increasing trend in end-stage renal disease (ESRD). Hypertension is second only to diabetes as the most common cause of ESRD.

PATHOPHYSIOLOGY

Systemic arterial pressure is a function of stroke volume, heart rate, and total peripheral resistance. Alterations in any of these factors result in changes in blood pressure. The major organs involved in regulation of blood pressure are the heart (heart rate [HR] and stroke volume [SV]), the sympathetic nervous system (SNS), total peripheral resistance (TPR), and the kidney (extracellular fluid volume and secretion of renin). Disease processes that affect stroke volume and heart rate include any that increase extracellular fluid volume, the activity of the SNS, or plasma norepinephrine levels and those that produce cardiac rhythm disturbances. Disease processes that affect total peripheral resistance include any that narrow the arteriolar radius or increase blood viscosity. Figure 40-1 shows the relationship of these factors to blood pressure control. In both normotensive and hypertensive patients, blood pressure is maintained by moment-to-moment adjustments in this system.

BP naturally drops at night with sleep. Evidence indicates loss of this nocturnal BP "dip" is the best predictor of CV risk. Most patients with HTN do not have an effective "dip" (Hermida, Ayala, Mojón, & Fernández, 2010). There also appears to be a seasonal increase of BP in winter, which is related to an individual's home temperature patterns: the

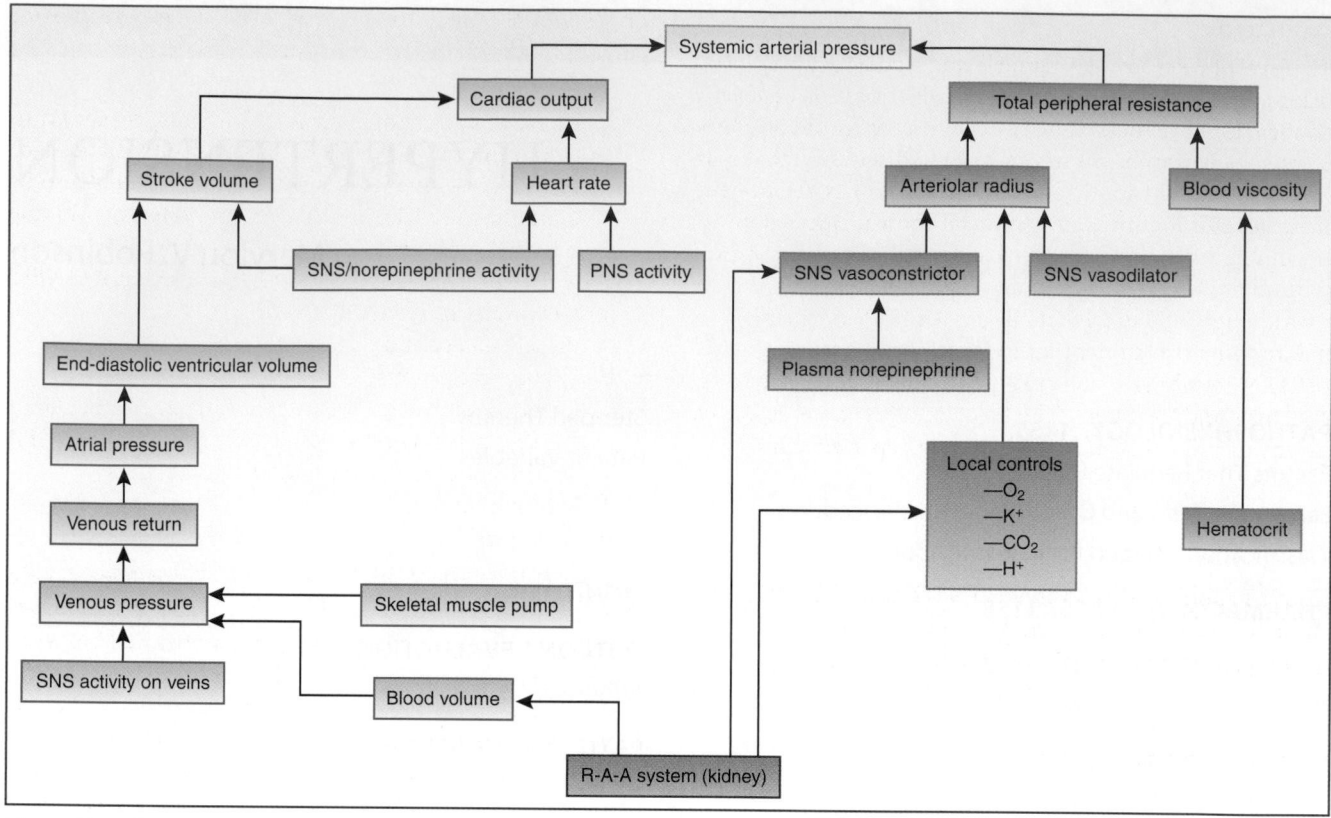

Figure 40–1. Regulation of blood pressure. Systemic arterial pressure is determined by cardiac output and total peripheral resistance. Increases in cardiac output or total peripheral resistance increase systemic arterial pressure, and decreases in these factors decrease systemic arterial pressure. Antihypertensive drugs act at one or more of these anatomical sites of blood pressure control.

warmer the home, the lower the BP. The clinical significance of this is yet to be determined (Modesti et al, 2013).

Factors That Regulate Blood Pressure

Baroreceptors

Change in BP is sensed by baroreceptors located in the carotid arteries and the arch of the aorta. They are sensitive to stretch so that, when stimulated by an increase in BP, they send inhibitory impulses to the sympathetic vasomotor center in the brainstem. Inhibition of efferent nerves in the SNS that innervate cardiac and vascular smooth muscle results in decreased heart rate, decreased force of contraction, and vasodilation of peripheral arterioles. At the same time, increased parasympathetic nervous system (PNS) activity further reduces HR via the vagus nerve. Decreased BP results in a reverse process. This system works well in the maintenance of BP during normal activities; however, in the presence of long-standing HTN, the baroreceptors adapt to the elevated BP levels and "reset" what the body accepts as "normal" BP. Diminished responsiveness to these baroreceptors is one of the most significant cardiovascular effects of aging and a major factor in the lifetime risk of HTN.

Endothelial Factors

In addition to the actions of baroreceptors, vascular endothelium has the ability to produce vasoactive substances and

growth factors. Nitric oxide, an endothelium-derived relaxing factor, helps maintain low arterial tone at rest and inhibits growth of the smooth muscle layer. The vascular endothelium also produces local vasodilators such as prostacyclin and endothelium-derived hyperpolarizing factor. Endothelin, also secreted by the vascular endothelium, is an extremely potent vasoconstrictor and also stimulates vascular smooth muscle growth. Growth of vascular smooth muscle is associated with atherosclerosis and the thickening seen with prolonged exposure to high BP. Endothelial dysfunction may contribute to these changes. Prevention or reversal of endothelial dysfunction may become an important therapeutic area in the future.

Kidneys

The kidneys contribute to BP control by regulation of the renin-angiotensin-aldosterone system. Renin, secreted by the juxtaglomerular apparatus in the kidney, converts angiotensinogen to angiotensin I. Angiotensin I is then converted by angiotensin-converting-enzyme (ACE) in the lungs to angiotensin II, which affects BP in two different ways. Angiotensin II is a potent vasoconstrictor and increases TPR. In addition, it stimulates the adrenal gland to produce aldosterone, which promotes sodium and water retention, thereby increasing extracellular fluid volume. Evidence suggests that angiotensin II also stimulates growth of vascular smooth muscle and may contribute to atherosclerosis and HTN.

Genetic Influences

The level of BP is strongly familial, and studies of rare genetic disorders affecting BP have led to the identification of genetic abnormalities associated with several rare forms of HTN. Genetic polymorphisms have also been discovered that may harbor genes contributing to primary HTN. To date, none of these genetic abnormalities has been shown, either alone or in combination, to be responsible for a clinically significant portion of HTN in the general population.

Although 90% to 95% of all cases of HTN are primary in nature with no identifiable cause, there are identifiable causes of HTN in which a cure may be effected by appropriate diagnosis and treatment. The focus of this chapter is on the diagnosis and management of primary hypertension.

Laboratory Tests and Other Diagnostic Procedures

Confirmation of a diagnosis of HTN is based on BP elevation documented at three different times. Standard measurement techniques, including out-of-office or home blood pressure measurements, can be used when confirming an initially elevated blood pressure and for all subsequent measures during follow-up and treatment (Institute for Clinical Systems Improvement [ICSI], 2012). Children over 3 years of age who are seen in a medical setting should have their BP measured at least once during every health-care visit. The preferred method for children is auscultation; the correct measurement requires using a cuff that is appropriate to the size of the child's upper arm (National Heart, Lung and Blood Institute [NHLBI], 2011).

The "JNC-8" published in late 2013 did not come from the original National Heart, Lung and Blood Institute, which authored the previous JNC recommendations; however, this new document is frequently referenced as the JNC-8 in the literature. The testing recommendations for the initial diagnosis of HTN of the JNC-7, listed below, were not altered and so are included in this chapter as a reliable reference. The recommended tests are used for therapeutic decision making and baseline values for determination of progression or stabilization of the systemic impact of HTN:

1. A 12-lead ECG.
2. Urinalysis, including urinary albumin or albumin/creatinine ratio. For those patients with diabetes or renal disease, the latter test of albumin should also be done annually. The presence of albuminuria, including microalbuminuria, even in the setting of a normal glomerular filtration rate (GFR), is associated with increased cardiovascular risk.
3. Blood glucose and hematocrit.
4. Serum potassium.
5. Creatinine and the corresponding estimated GFR. There is a strong relationship between decreased GFR and increases in CV morbidity and mortality.
6. Serum calcium.
7. Lipid profile.

Elevated levels of high-sensitivity C-reactive protein (HS-CRP), homocysteine, and heart rate may also be considered in patients with cardiovascular disease (CVD) but without other risk factors. Analysis of data from the Framingham Heart Study cohort demonstrated that those with an LDL-C value within the range associated with low CVD risk, but who had an elevated HS-CRP, had a higher risk of CVD compared to those with a low CRP and a high LDL-C. This was especially true in women; however, reduction in CRP has not led to better outcomes (Mosca et al, 2011). Elevations in homocysteine have also been associated with higher CVD risk but not as strongly as the HS-CRP (Ahluwalia et al, 2013). Treating elevated homocysteine has not resulted in decreased CVD risk, however.

Classification of Blood Pressure for Adults

BP readings have been classified according to a progressive risk of end-organ disease and poor outcomes. The higher the classification, the higher the CV risk. Table 40-1 shows the BP readings that fall into each of these categories per the

Table 40–1 Blood Pressure Classifications and Management

Classification	Systolic BP (mm Hg)	Diastolic BP (mm Hg)	Lifestyle Modification	No Compelling Indication (Drug Therapy)	Compelling Indication (Drug Therapy)
Normal	<120	<80	Encourage	No antihypertensive drug	Drug for compelling indication
Prehypertension	120–139	8–89	Yes	No antihypertensive drug	Drug for compelling indication
Hypertension stage 1	140–159	90–99	Yes	Thiazide-type diuretic for most. May consider ACEI, ARB, CCB, or combination.	Drug(s) for compelling indication. Other antihypertensive drugs
Hypertension stage 2	≥160	≥100	Yes	Two-drug combinations for most. Usually thiazide-type diuretic and ACEI or ARB, or BB, or CCB.	Drug(s) for compelling indication. Other antihypertensive drugs.

ACEI = angiotensen-converting enzyme inhibitor; ARB = angiotensin receptor blocker; BB = beta blocker; CCB = calcium channel blocker.
  Source: ACCF/AHA, 2011; James et al, 2014 Arnett et al, 2014).

JNC-7standards, which were not altered by the JNC-8 (James et al, 2014). This classification is based on the average of two or more properly measured seated BP readings on each of two or more office visits.

The JNC-7 first introduced the evidence that there is a degree of lifetime CV risk associated with BP levels previously thought to be normal. The previously termed "normal" BP of 120/80 changed to a BP reading that is now considered "top of normal." Consistent readings over 120/80 are now scrutinized but not treated with medications until over the new cut points. The JNC-7 introduced a new term: *prehypertension.* This level of BP ranges from 120 to 130 SBP and/or 80 to 89 diastolic blood pressure (DBP). The JNC-8 did not change that range, but softens the requirement to bring a person treated with medications down to less than the previously required 120/80 ideal.

Prehypertension is not directly addressed as a factor in the JNC-8, but importantly was not rejected as a consideration of risk. Prehypertensive individuals benefit from early intervention to adopt healthy lifestyles that might reduce BP, decrease the rate of progression to hypertensive levels as the individual ages, or prevent HTN completely. Longitudinal data obtained from the Framingham Heart Study indicate that BP values in the 130 to 139/85 to 89 ranges are associated with a more than 2-fold increase in relative risk for CVD compared to those with BP below 120/80. This is no longer an absolute goal. Consideration is extended to include persons who had adverse effects such as weakness and orthostasis and thus were less likely to adhere to treatment patterns; therefore, a decrease in BP below 140/90 with strict adherence to the 120/80 goals previously touted is no longer recommended.

Long-term studies show that there are noteworthy differences in those treated and not treated for HTN. The more comorbid the risk factors, the worse the outcomes. For patients less than 65 years of age, the SBP has the best predictive value for poor outcomes regardless of the DBP. For elders, increases in SBP also increase mortality, especially when there are large pulse pressures. The larger the CV risk, the more impact therapy can have. This means that treating mild HTN does not improve outcomes as dramatically as lowering higher BP values. However, the Framingham studies have indicated the long-term impact of HTN on all-cause mortality is understood to be very beneficial no matter the baseline value (American College of Cardiology Foundation/American Heart Association [ACCF/AHA], 2011).

PHARMACODYNAMICS

Because primary HTN has no identifiable cause, the treatment necessarily depends on interfering with normal physiological mechanisms that regulate BP by means of six classes of drugs. The new guidelines emphasize the ACE/ARB family of medications plus diuretics before any other drug group in most cases, which is a change from prior practice (James et al, 2014). How the medications work is discussed below.

Diuretics lower BP by depleting the body of sodium and reducing extracellular fluid volume. Agents that act in the renin-angiotensin-aldosterone system (RAAS) reduce pressure by decreasing sodium and water retention (aldosterone action), by decreasing vasoconstriction (angiotensin direct action), and by increasing vasodilation (bradykinin action). Adrenergic blockers and other drugs acting on the SNS lower blood pressure by reducing peripheral vascular resistance, inhibiting cardiac contractility, and increasing venous pooling in capacitance vessels. Calcium channel blockers act as vasodilators to reduce pressure by relaxing vascular smooth muscle, thereby dilating resistance vessels and increasing the area over which blood must flow, and through their negative inotropic activity to reduce cardiac output. Direct vasodilators produce the same effect as the calcium channel blockers on vascular smooth muscle. Centrally acting agents produce vasodilation mainly through reduction in norepinephrine. The latter two classes are used only in specific situations in which other classes are not appropriate or effective. It is unusual that treatment with any one drug class can achieve the blood pressure goal and so combinations of two or more drug classes are common. More detailed discussions of the pharmacokinetics and pharmacodynamics of each of these classes of drugs are in Chapters 14 and 16.

GOALS OF TREATMENT

The first goal of HTN management is reduction in CV risk. The positive relationship between hypertension and CV risk has been long established. The presence of each additional risk factor is assumed to compound the risk from HTN. Figure 40-2 shows the 10 year risk of classic considerations for coronary heart disease (CHD) related to the major risk factors of total serum cholesterol, serum high-density lipid (HDL) level, smoking, diabetes, and left ventricular hypertrophy (LVH).

Easy and rapid calculation of a Framingham or the new pooled CV risk tool may assist in demonstrating the benefits of treatment to patients. Treatment is initiated for individuals with blood pressure greater than 140/90 in the general population and above 150/90 in elders. Management of any other risk factor beyond HTN is essential and should follow the established guidelines. A positive relationship has also been shown between HTN and end-organ damage to the eyes, brain, and kidneys. The second goal is prevention of this end-organ damage. To meet these two goals, the following are needed:

1. Prevent the rise of BP with age. The prevalence of HTN increases with advancing age (see the Pathophysiology section above) to the point at which more than 50% of adults aged 60 to 69 years and 75% of those aged 70 years and older have HTN. The age-related rise in SBP is the primary cause for this increase.
2. Improve control of HTN to below 140/90 mm Hg in adults and below 150/90 in those greater than age 60 are the new targets. Treating HTN to these targets is associated with a decrease in CV disease complications.

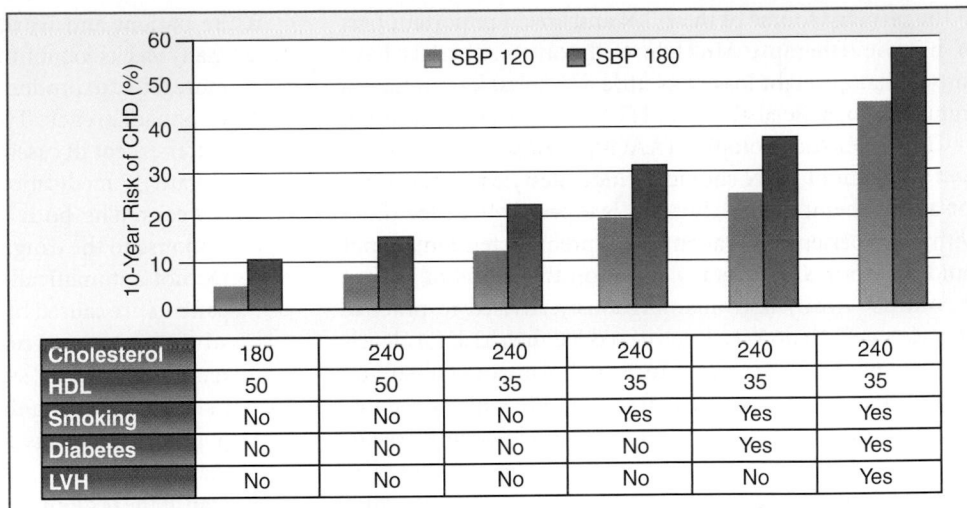

Figure 40–2. Ten-year risk for CHD by SBP and presence of other risk factors. *(Source: Adapted from Anderson, K., Wilson, P., Odell, P., & Kannel, W. [1991]. An updated coronary risk profile: A statement for health professionals.* Circulation, *83, 356–362.)*

Cholesterol	180	240	240	240	240	240
HDL	50	50	35	35	35	35
Smoking	No	No	No	Yes	Yes	Yes
Diabetes	No	No	No	No	Yes	Yes
LVH	No	No	No	No	No	Yes

Under previous American Diabetes Association guidelines for patients with concurrent HTN and diabetes or renal disease, the BP goal was less than 130/80 mm Hg. (The 2015 recommendation is to keep current with the JNC-8 guideline value of 140/90. This decision was made to decrease confusion and to facilitate increased numbers of patients who maintain therapy.) Control should not be relaxed for patients who have been treated to lower target levels based on the JNC-7 if they are not having adverse effects (James et al, 2014).

3. Increase recognition of the importance of controlling isolated systolic hypertension (ISH), as it is the most lethal hypertensive phenotype. Because most persons with HTN, especially those older than 50 years, will achieve control of their DBP once the SBP goal is reached, the primary focus should be on obtaining the SBP goal.

4. Improve recognition of the importance of prehypertension on the development of HTN. Individuals with SBP between 120 and 139 mm Hg and DBP between 80 and 89 mm Hg have a significantly higher risk for developing uncontrolled HTN. Changes in lifestyle are critical.

5. Reduce ethnic, socioeconomic, and regional variations in HTN diagnosis and treatment by improving opportunities for well-tolerated, affordable treatment options, including lifestyle modifications and access to care. The 2013 guidelines specifically address the black population as to the recommended choice of first-line drugs.

6. Recognize that HTN is not only an issue in middle age and older patient groups. It has a real presence in the preadolescent and younger adult population as well. Early intervention can increase long-term outcomes and quality of life in the later years.

Barriers to Goal Achievement

These goals are attainable for a large percentage of patients with HTN with the treatment regimens recommended by the guidelines. Barriers to achievement of these goals include insufficient health education by health-care providers, lack of reimbursement for health education services, and lack of healthy food choices in many schools, worksites, and restaurants. Another factor is nonadherence to the treatment regimen. Chapter 6 focuses on factors that address these and other barriers to health. This chapter discusses treatment regimens that can enable people to control their BP.

RATIONAL DRUG SELECTION

Hypertension presents a unique problem in therapeutic management. It is usually a lifelong disease but is asymptomatic until end-organ damage occurs. For this reason, providers often find themselves prescribing lifestyle modifications or drugs that have disturbing adverse reactions to treat a problem that does not make the patient feel ill. For effective management, the choice of treatment should be low in cost, limited in complexity, and with the fewest possible adverse reactions. Hence the 2013 guidelines allow a more flexible target goal to provide for the maximum number of individuals to achieve at least some hypertension reduction because the lower targets of the JNC-7 may have created a proportion of the population who rejected treatment based on side effects. Management is based on classification of HTN, the presence of comorbid risk factors, and specific patient variables. First, this chapter discusses lifestyle management and stepped therapy, including initial monotherapy, stepping up to multiple drugs, and stepping down when possible. This is followed by specific variations.

Algorithm for Management of Hypertension

Lifestyle Modifications

Of patients with HTN, 30% to 65% are obese, a problem frequently compounded by high sodium intake, sedentary lifestyle, and excessive use of alcohol (American Association of Clinical Endocrinologists [AACE] Hypertension Task Force, 2006). Lifestyle modifications directed at correcting these contributing factors may benefit the patient regardless of the primary course of the HTN and are an important part of first-line therapy. Multiple well-controlled trials have shown that a weight loss of as little as 5 to 10 kg can have a significant beneficial effect on HTN (American Association of Clinical Endocrinologists [AACE], 2006).

Treatment of HTN should include lifestyle modifications for all treatment groups, but this is especially true for those with prehypertension. Patients with prehypertension are not candidates for drug therapy based on their level of BP but should be "firmly and unambiguously advised to practice lifestyle modification in order to reduce their risk for developing hypertension in the future" (Chobanian et al, 2003). Table 40-2 summarizes the lifestyle modifications recommended in several guidelines. Lifestyle modifications are encouraged to reduce BP, prevent or delay the onset of HTN, improve the efficacy of any drug therapy, and decrease cardiovascular risk. Combining two or more lifestyle modifications can achieve better results than one alone. Making "exercise" an additional vital sign is advocated by the Kaiser Medical System (Coleman et al, 2012). Unfortunately, almost 15% of those heart patients who have already sustained an MI or stroke elect not to engage in any lifestyle changes (Teo et al, 2013).

Stepped Therapy

Patients with all stages of HTN who are not able to achieve a BP below 140/90 mm Hg require drug therapy. Once the decision is made to begin drug therapy at the 150/90 cut point, initial drug choices are based on the presence or absence of compelling indications from concurrent disease processes. Figure 40-3 shows the treatment protocol for hypertension management based on JNC-7 and still maintained in the JNC-8. As a general rule, the following suggestions can lead to progress in achieving the BP goal in a primary care population:

1. Set an appropriate therapeutic BP goal based on individual patients and their compelling indications.

2. Be patient and work on attaining the BP goal over many weeks to months. Moving to lower BP quickly is more likely to produce side effects to the drugs that lead to nonadherence. There is no evidence that faster is better except in cases of extreme values.

3. Titrate BP medications no more often than every 4 to 6 weeks. The body needs time to demonstrate full response to the drug.

4. Do not automatically assume symptoms reported by patients are caused by the drug. What may appear to be adverse responses may have other reasons for occurrence. Assigning all symptoms to drug effects may result in changing a drug that is actually working well. Antihypertensive drugs alleviate more adverse responses than they cause.

5. Plan at the beginning of therapy for the use of more than one drug. A single drug is not likely to provide BP control to goal level if the patient is more than 15/10 mm Hg higher than the goal. Explaining to the patient early in treatment the likelihood of more than one drug decreases the risk for nonadherence.

6. Do not ignore ISH in the elderly. Treat to goal SBP in older adults even if DBP is normal, but go more slowly. Titrate to the target of 150/90.

7. Extracellular fluid volume may need to be controlled in order to achieve BP goals. Include a diuretic in any treatment regimen that includes more than one agent.

(Adapted from ADVANSTAR Medical Economics Healthcare Communications [2004], Reducing cardiovascular risk factors. *Patient Care for the Nurse Practitioner: ACE Activity.* Sponsored by Pfizer Inc.)

Initial Drug Therapy

For most patients, the lowest dose of the initial drug should be used to prevent adverse reactions and too much or too abrupt a reduction in blood pressure. The dose is then slowly

---

Table 40–2 Lifestyle Modifications

- Lose weight. Loss of as little as 10 lb may significantly reduce blood pressure.

- Limit alcohol intake to no more than 1 oz (30 mL) ethanol (e.g., 24 oz beer, 10 oz wine, 2 oz 100-proof whiskey) per day or 0.5 oz (15 mL) ethanol per day for women and lighter-weight people.

- Increase aerobic physical activity to 30 to 45 min most days of the week. Obese or low-activity patients may need to start with as little as 3 min of activity per day and increase the activity by 1 min each day until the desired 30 to 45 min is achieved.

- Reduce sodium intake to no more than 100 mmol (2,400 mg of sodium or 6 g of sodium chloride) per day. This can often be achieved by not adding salt during cooking or on the table and by watching hidden sources of salt such as canned foods.

- Maintain adequate intake of dietary potassium (approximately 90 mmol per day).

- Maintain adequate intake of dietary calcium and magnesium for general health.

- Stop smoking. The low doses of nicotine found in nicotine replacement therapy (NRT) do not significantly affect blood pressure, and NRT may be used as needed to aid in smoking cessation.

- Adopt the Dietary Approaches to Stop Hypertension (DASH) diet, which is high in fruits, vegetables, and low-fat dairy products as well as low in dietary cholesterol, saturated fat, and total fat.

Source: Adapted from the National High Blood Pressure Education Program. (2003). *Seventh Report of the Joint National Committee on Prevention, Detection, Evaluation, and Treatment of High Blood Pressure.* Rockville, MD: National Institutes of Health; National Heart, Lung and Blood Institute.

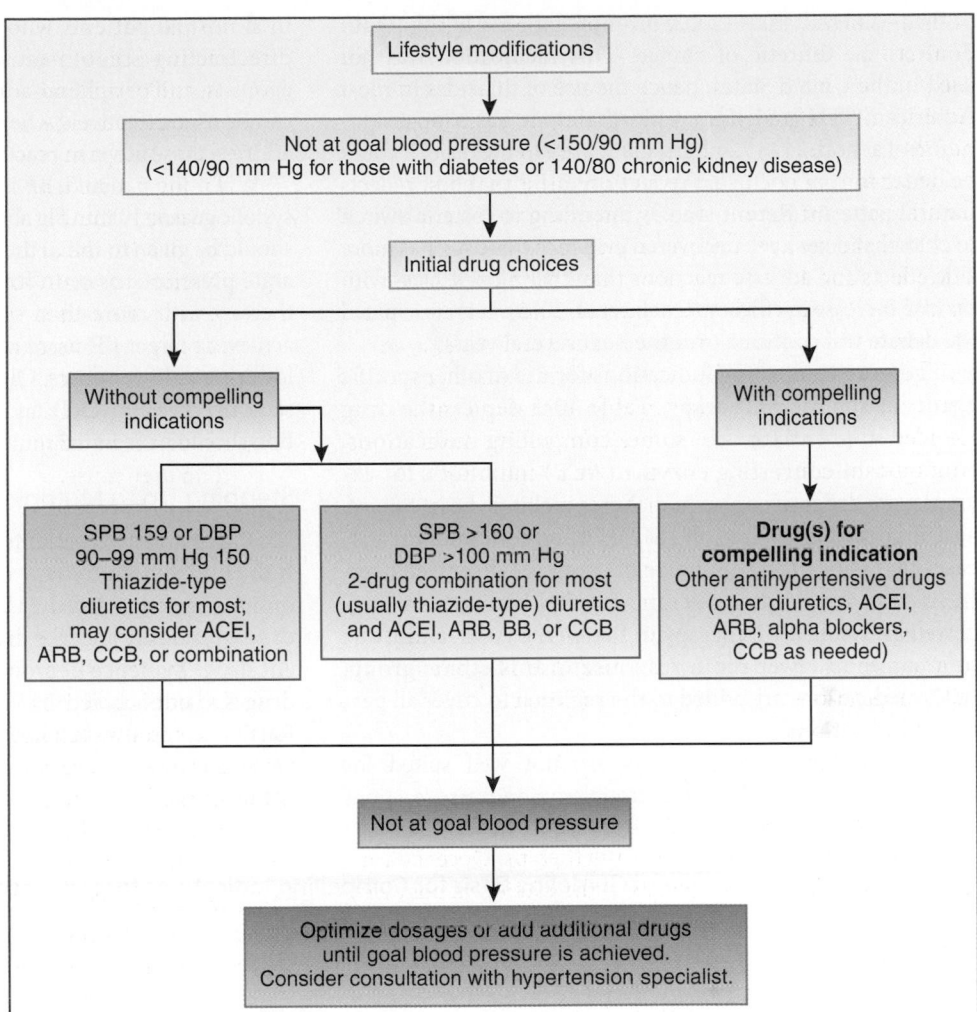

Figure 40–3. James et al. (2014). 2014 evidence-based guideline for the management of high blood pressure in adults: Report from the panel members appointed to the eighth joint national committee (JNC-8). *Journal of the American Medical Association.* 311(5), 507-520. doi: 10.1001/jama. 2013.284427

titrated upward, based on patient response. If BP remains uncontrolled after 1 to 2 months, the next dosage level should be prescribed. The ideal drug should provide 24 hours of efficacy with at least 50% of the peak effect remaining at the end of the 24 hours. Long-acting formulations are preferred over short-acting because (1) adherence is better with once-daily dosing; (2) for many agents, fewer tablets mean lower cost; (3) control of hypertension is smoother; and (4) the risk of sudden death, heart attack, and stroke because of abrupt changes in blood pressure is lessened.

When the decision is made to begin drug therapy and there are no clear indications for another type of drug, a thiazide-type diuretic has been typically chosen because in the landmark ALLHAT study comparing diuretics with other classes of antihypertensive drugs, diuretics were unsurpassed in preventing CV complications of HTN (Wright et al, 2009). Despite this, diuretics are often underused. Of more concern is that use is declining over time, especially in African Americans who show some of the best data for efficacy (Gerber et al, 2013). New evidence suggests closer consideration of BMI and general fluid status when prescribing diuretics. Those who are obese (a significant percentage of HTN patients) have good response to diuretics. Those who are thin or tend to have lower fluid volume conditions

(e.g., dehydration) are now recognized to have potentially worse outcomes on diuretics (Weber et al, 2013). Those patients would be started on an ACE or calcium channel blocker as their initial therapy.

Current practice guidelines do not recommend beta blockers as first-line therapy because they are weaker antihypertensive agents when it comes to stroke prevention. Some negative evidence in 2005 against atenolol as contributing to increased CV event risk has been overturned by a major meta-analysis that demonstrates a similar effect and risk rate for atenolol and metoprolol (Parker et al, 2012). Beta blockers remain best used as a second or add-on drug.

Chapter 16 discusses specific diuretics and their appropriate use and dosing. In general, the lowest dose that achieves the target BP is best because higher doses are more likely to produce more potassium loss without significant improvement in BP control. The choice of diuretic should be based on level of kidney function. For estimated GFRs higher than the mid 40 mL/min range, a thiazide diuretic should be used; loop diuretics are not as effective as thiazides in this setting. For GFRs that are lower than the mid-40 mL/min range, loop diuretics, sometimes in combination with metolazone, are more appropriate and are most effective when dosed twice daily.

The ALLHAT study (2002) promoted the use of chlorthalidone as the diuretic of choice. This medication was not used in the United States; hence the use of thiazides in most American HTN guidelines. Chlorthalidone has a longer duration of action, 24 to 72 hours, giving rise to the belief it could be better for the nocturnal reduction in BP that best reflects natural patterns. Recent studies intending to foster a switch to chlorthalidone have uncovered evidence this drug has more side effects and adverse reactions than the thiazide class with no true increase in efficacy (Dhalla et al, 2013). It is anticipated the debate will continue over the next several years.

There are compelling indications for use of other specific agents as the initial therapy. Table 40-3 depicts the drug choices appropriate for some compelling indications. Angiotensin-converting enzyme (ACE) inhibitors, for example, are drugs of choice in diabetes mellitus, heart failure, and myocardial infarction (MI). Other concomitant diseases that may affect the choice of drugs are discussed later. In African Americans, calcium channel blockers are suggested as first line BP therapy in lieu of the ACE family due to a common lower renin response in this ethnic group. ACE medications are added to the regimen to cover all pertinent indications.

Some antihypertensive drugs are not well suited for monotherapy because they cause troublesome adverse reactions in almost all patients who take them. These drugs include direct-acting smooth-muscle vasodilators, central alpha$_2$ agonists, and peripheral-adrenergic antagonists. These drugs can be used effectively when combined with other drugs that address these adverse reactions.

When the patient's BP is more than 20 mm Hg above the systolic goal or 10 mm Hg above the diastolic goal, consideration should be given to initial therapy with two drugs, either as separate prescriptions or in fixed-dose combinations. Beginning therapy with more than one drug increases the chances of achieving target BP more rapidly and may produce more BP lowering at lower doses. Older adults, those at risk for orthostatic hypotension (OH), and diabetics with autonomic dysfunction should have initial multidrug therapy begun with caution.

Stepping Up to Multiple Drugs

Most hypertensive patients will require two or more drugs. If the initial monotherapy drug choice is inadequate, several options are considered: (1) maxing out the dose of the first drug, (2) adding another drug, or (3) substitution of a different drug. Evidence demonstrates that addition of a second drug is a better choice than raising the dose of the initial drug. Raising doses always increases the risks and impacts of adverse effects. A synergistic effect of using two drugs together is the standard practice, but three or more may be needed.

Table 40–3 Clinical Trial and Guideline Basis for Compelling Indications for Individual Drug Classes

Compelling Indication*	Recommended Drugs						Clinical Trial Basis†
	Diuretic	**BB**	**ACEI**	**ARB**	**CCB**	**Aldo ANT**	
Heart failure	•	•	•	•		•	ACC/AHA Heart Failure Guideline, MERIT-HF, COPERNICUS, CIBIS, SOLVD, AIRE, TRACE, ValHEFT, RALES, CHARM
Postmyocardial infarction		•	•			•	ACC/AHA Post-MI Guideline, BHAT, SAVE, Capricom, EPHESUS
High risk of coronary disease	•	•	•		•		ALLHAT, HOPE, ANBP2, LIFE, CONVINCE, EUROPA, INVEST
Diabetes	•	•	•	•	•		NKF-ADA Guideline, UKPDS, ALLHAT
Chronic kidney disease			•	•			NKF Guideline, Captopril Trial, RENAAL, IDNT, REIN, AASK
Recurrent stroke prevention	•		•				PROGRESS

ACEI = angiotensin-converting enzyme inhibitor; Aldo ANT = aldosterone antagonist; ARB = angiotensin receptor blocker; BB = beta blocker; CCB = calcium channel blocker.

*Compelling indications for antihypertensive drugs are based on benefits from outcome studies or existing clinical guidelines; the compelling indication is managed in parallel with the BP.

†Conditions for which clinical trials demonstrate benefit of specific classes of antihypertensive drugs used as part of an antihypertensive regimen to achieve BP goal to test outcomes.

Source: National High Blood Pressure Education Program. (2003). *The Seventeenth Report of the Joint National Committee on Prevention, Detections, Evaluation, and Treatment of High Blood Pressure*. Rockville, MD: National Institutes of Health; National Heart, Lung and Blood Institute.

Dosing of multiple drugs is implemented on an aggressive schedule when the baseline BP is over 160/90.

The provider must make sure the HTN is actually not controlled on the solo medication. "Pseudo resistance" can trick the provider into upping a dose or adding medications when the actual cause is poor adherence, lifestyle factors, and an irregular/improper dosing schedule (Wright, Rutecki, & Bellone, 2013). OTC meds, NSAID use, an emergency dosing of steroids, or the start of a mental health medication or contraceptives can all appear to be a nonresponse to antihypertensive medication. Taking a rigorous history including very specific questioning as to times and methods of ingestion can reveal nonadherence. Reviewing refill patterns will also provide clues as to adherence. Considering that nearly 40% of patients do not keep to the therapeutic plan within the first year, this potential must be uncovered prior to adding a second medication (Wright et al, 2013).

If the patient is tolerating the first choice well, a second drug is added from another class. The JNC-8 recommends that if an ACE was the first choice, then a diuretic should be added; likewise, if the diuretic was the first choice, an ACE should be added (James et al, 2014). The choice of the second drug may also be influenced by how it might affect the adverse reaction profile of the first drug or by how well these drugs have been shown to work together in clinical studies. An adequate dose of hydralazine results in compensatory tachycardia and salt and water retention. The addition of a beta-adrenergic blocker prevents the tachycardia, and the addition of a diuretic prevents salt and water retention. An ACE inhibitor and a nondihydropyridine calcium channel blocker may reduce proteinuria in a patient with diabetes better than either drug alone. If a diuretic was not chosen as the first drug, it is usually indicated as the second-step drug because its addition will enhance the effects of most other agents.

Drug formulations that include combinations of medication may permit the best of both worlds; the patient takes just one pill or capsule yet receives the benefit of two drugs, and the combination may cost less than the individual components prescribed separately. The downside is that fixed-dose ratios prevent customization of the regimen. Table 40-4 provides information of selected combinations of drugs frequently used in therapy.

If the patient is having significant adverse reactions or no response from the initial drug, an agent from another class is substituted. For example, a persistent cough may be annoying enough that a patient will not continue to take an

Table 40–4 Common Combinations of Antihypertensive Drugs

Combination*	Fixed-Dose Combination (mg)†	Brand Name
ACEIs and CCBs	Amlodipine/benazepril hydrochloride (2.5/10, 5/10, 10/20)	Lotrel
	Enalapril maleate/felodipine (5/5)	Lexxel
	Trandolapril/verapamil (2/180, 1/240, 2/240, 4/240)	Tarka
ACEIs and diuretics	Benazepril/hydrochlorothiazide (5/6.25, 10/12.4, 20/12.5, 20/25)	Lotensin HCT
	Captopril/hydrochlorothiazide (25/15, 25/25, 50/15, 50/25)	Capozide
	Enalapril maleate/hydrochlorothiazide (5/12.5, 10/25)	Vaseretic
	Lisinopril/hydrochlorothiazide (10/12.5, 20/12.5, 20/25)	Prinzide
	Moexipril HCL/hydrochlorothiazide (7.5/12.5, 15/25)	Uniretic
	Quinapril HCL/hydrochlorothiazide (10/12.5, 20/12.5, 20/25)	Accuretic
ARBs and diuretics	Candesartan cilexetil/hydrochlorothiazide (16/12.5, 32/12.5)	Atacand HCT
	Eprosartan mesylate/hydrochlorothiazide (600/12.5, 600/25)	Teveten/HCT
	Irbesartan/hydrochlorothiazide (150/12.5, 300/12.5)	Avalide
	Losartan potassium/hydrochlorothiazide (50/12.5, 100/25)	Hyzaar
	Telmisartan/hydrochlorothiazide (40/12.5, 80/12.5)	Micardis/HCT
	Valsartan/hydrochlorothiazide (80/12.5, 160/12.5)	Diovan/HCT
BBs and diuretics	Atenolol/chlorthalidone (50/25, 100/25)	Tenoretic
	Bisoprolol fumarate/hydrochlorothiazide (2.5/6.25, 5/6.25, 10/6.25)	Ziac
	Propranolol LA/hydrochlorothiazide (40/25, 80/25)	Inderide
	Metoprolol tartrate/hydrochlorothiazide (50/25, 100/25)	Lopressor HCT
	Nadolol/bendrofluthiazide (40/5, 80/5)	Corzide
	Timolol maleate/hydrochlorothiazide (10/25)	Timolide
Centrally acting drug and diuretic	Methyldopa/hydrochlorothiazide (250/15, 250/25, 500/30, 500/50)	Aldoril
	Reserpine/chlorothiazide (0.125/250, 0.25/500)	Diupres
	Reserpine/hydrochlorothiazide (0.125/25, 0.125/50)	Hydropres
Diuretic and diuretic	Amiloride HCl/hydrochlorothiazide (5/50)	Moduretic
	Spironolactone/hydrochlorothiazide (25/25, 50/50)	Aldactone
	Triamterene/hydrochlorothiazide (37.5/25, 50/25, 75/50)	Dyazide, Maxzide

*Drug abbreviations: ACE = angiotensin-converting enzyme inhibitor; ARB = angiotensin receptor blocker; BB = beta blocker; CCB = calcium channel blocker.

†Some drug combinations are available in multiple fixed doses. Each drug dose is reported in milligrams.

ACE inhibitor. Because they do not affect the kallikrein system, angiotensin II receptor blockers (ARBs) do not produce this cough, nor do they commonly have the problem with angioedema that is a contraindication to the use of an ACE inhibitor. Individuals who do have angioedema with an ACE should not be started on an ARB (Van Rinjinsoever, Kwee-Zuiderwijk & Feenstra, 1998). DRIs can still produce the cough and angioedema, so they may not be the best substitute either. Because the hemodynamic effects are similar, an ARB may be substituted for the ACE inhibitor. Documentation of equal long-term cardiac and renal protection for patients with systolic dysfunction and diabetic nephropathy has now been demonstrated for some ARBs, but they are not used in combination for extra effect; this only produces extra adverse effects, especially on the kidney.

Strong consideration should be given to administration of the medication with the longer half-life at night (Hermida et al, 2010; Wright et al, 2013). This circadian congruent approach yields better outcomes and lower adverse events because it helps return the nocturnal "dip" typically lost in HTN.

Stepping Down

Although HTN is generally accepted to be a lifelong disease, after it has been controlled effectively for at least 1 year, a decrease in the dosage and number of antihypertensive drugs may be considered. The reduction should be deliberate, slow, and progressive and accompanied by vigilant BP monitoring. Step-down therapy is often successful for patients who also are making lifestyle modifications. Any patient whose drugs have been discontinued should have regularly scheduled follow-up visits because BP usually rises again to hypertensive levels within months to years after the drugs have been stopped. This return of HTN is especially common in the absence of continued improvements in lifestyle. If adherence to lifestyle modifications is not likely, maintaining a low-dose antihypertensive drug may be preferable to complete discontinuance of all drugs.

Patient Variables

The prevalence of hypertension varies with age, gender, race, education, and many other variables. Some of these variables also affect the clinical use and dosing of specific antihypertensive medications. Some of these variables are covered in Table 40-5.

Children and Adolescents

The U.S. Preventive Services Task Force (USPSTF) (2013) does not recommend for or against routine BP screening for pediatric patients. This runs counter to the suggestions of the American Academy of Pediatrics, National Heart, Lung and Blood Institute, Bright Futures, and the National High Blood

Table 40–5 Drug Choice Based on Concomitant Disease States

Disease State	Drug Choice
Compelling Indications Unless Contraindicated	
Diabetes mellitus (type 1) with proteinuria	ACE inhibitors
Heart failure	ACE inhibitors Diuretics
Isolated systolic hypertension (older adults)	Diuretics (preferred) CCB (long-acting DHP)
Myocardial infarction	Beta blockers (non-ISA) ACE inhibitors (with systolic dysfunction)
May Have Favorable Effects on Comorbid Conditions	
Angina	Beta blockers CCB
Atrial tachycardia and fibrillation CA (non-DHP)	Beta blockers CCB (non-DHP)
Cyclosporine-induced hypertension (caution with the dose of cyclosporine)	CCB
Diabetes mellitus (types 1 and 2) with proteinuria	ACE inhibitors (preferred) CCB
Diabetes mellitus (type 2)	Diuretics (low dose)
Dyslipidemia	Alpha blockers
Essential tremor	Beta blockers (non-CS)
Heart failure	Carvedilol Losartan potassium

Table 40–5   Drug Choice Based on Concomitant Disease States—cont'd

Disease State	Drug Choice
Hyperthyroidism	Beta blockers
Migraine	Beta blockers (non-CS) CCB (non-DHP)
Myocardial infarction	Diltiazem hydrochloride Verapamil hydrochloride
Osteoporosis	Thiazides
Preoperative hypertension	Beta blockers
Prostatism (BPH)	Alpha blockers
Renal insufficiency (caution in renovascular hypertension and creatinine 265.2 mmol/L or higher [3 mg/dL])	ACE inhibitors
May Have Unfavorable Effects on Comorbid Conditions (May Be Used With Special Monitoring Unless Contraindicated)	
Bronchospastic disease	Beta blockers
Depression	Beta blockers Central alpha agonists Reserpine (contraindicated)
Diabetes mellitus (types 1 and 2)	Beta blockers Diuretics (high dose)
Dyslipidemia	Beta blockers (non-ISA) Diuretics (high dose)
Gout	Diuretics
Heart block (second and third degree)	Beta blockers (contraindicated) CCB (non-DHP) (contraindicated)
Heart failure	Beta blockers (except carvedilol) CCB (except amlodipine besylate, felodipine)
Liver disease	Labetalol hydrochloride Methyldopa (contraindicated)
Peripheral vascular disease	Beta blockers
Pregnancy	ACE inhibitors (contraindicated) Angiotensin II receptor blockers (contraindicated)
Renal insufficiency	Potassium-sparing agents
Renovascular disease	ACE inhibitors Angiotensin II receptor blockers

ACE = angiotensin-converting enzyme; CCB = calcium channel blockers; CS = cardiac specific; DHP = dihydropyridine; non-ISA = nonintrinsic sympathomimetic action.

Pressure Education Program. Prescribers dealing with children should consider individual risk factors when determining whether uncovering the current 5% rate of HTN in children is within the beneficial target of the particular child they are caring for.

Definitions of hypertension in children and adolescents (age 1 to 17 years) take into account age and height by sex using a percentile system rating for acceptable levels. Blood pressure in the 90th to less than 95th percentile or blood pressure exceeding 120/90 (even if less than 90th percentile) is considered prehypertension in children. Blood pressure in the 95th to 99th percentile is considered hypertension stage 1, and greater than the 99th percentile plus 5 mm Hg is considered

hypertension stage 2 (NHLBI, 2011). Table 40-6 shows the values consistent with a diagnosis of hypertension for girls and boys based on age and height. Per the 2005–2010 analysis of the National Health and Nutrition Examination Surveys (NHANES), males are less likely to have ideal BP as teens (78% versus 90%) even though females have higher cholesterol levels and lower physical activity scores (Shay et al, 2013).

An identifiable cause for the hypertension is more likely in younger children than it is in adults, and such causes should always be sought. The recreational use of OTC cold medications, illegal purchase of stimulants to help with study sessions, and anabolic steroid abuse must be considered even

Table 40–6 Max Blood Pressure Readings in Children and Adolescents (mm Hg) by Height at 95th Percentile to Diagnose HTN

Age	Girls 50th Percentile for Height	Girls 75th Percentile for Height	Boys 50th Percentile for Height	Boys 75th Percentile for Height
3	107/67	108/68	109/65	110/66
6	111/74	113/74	114/74	115/75
12	123/80	124/81	123/81	125/82
17	129/84	130/85	136/87	138/87

Source: Adapted from Expert Panel on Integrated Guidelines for Cardiovascular Health and Risk Reduction in Children and Adolescents. (2011). Rockville, MD: National Institutes of Health; National Heart, Lung and Blood Institute.

in grade-school children. Comorbid conditions such as DM 1 or 2, chronic kidney disease (CKD), and a history of glomerulonephritis or Kawasaki disease should trigger monitoring prior to age 3 and medication treatment. Children with ambiguous genitalia need closer monitoring for a strong link with adrenal HTN causes. Those who had umbilical vein catheterizations have links to renal causes of HTN. Children born with cardiac defects typically have a cardiac structural cause for the HTN (Mattoo, 2013; Mitchell et al, 2002). Treat all symptomatic children (headache, CV decompensation, intolerance of physical activity) with medications. Children at stage 2 HTN and those with hyperlipidemia, glucose intolerance, and/or CKD should also be started on medications prior to awaiting lifestyle impacts. Referral to a pediatric hypertension specialist is recommended.

Chronic HTN is becoming more common in adolescence and is generally associated with obesity, sedentary lifestyle, sleep apnea, and a positive family history of HTN and other CVDs. Like adults, children with HTN develop end-organ damage, and appropriate assessment for this damage should occur; however, the negative impact may not be overtly evident for decades. Echocardiography is recommended as a primary tool for evaluating these age groups before the overt conditions arise. One study uncovered LVH in 3% to 40% of children without obvious symptoms (Brady, Fivish, Flynn, & Parekh, 2008). Renal ultrasound is recommended to rule out an occult renal source of HTN.

Lifestyle modifications, especially weight management and increased physical activity, are initially used, with drug therapy reserved for higher levels of BP or for inadequate response to lifestyle modifications. Though weight loss is demonstrated to be helpful, the strong association between weight reduction and lowered BP is not as pronounced in children (Mattoo, 2013). Diet modification is in order, especially considering that less than 1% of U.S. teens have an "ideal diet score" (Shay et al, 2013). Adolescents with BP below the 95th percentile should adopt healthy lifestyles similar to those of adults combating prehypertension. Although the choice of drugs is similar to that for adults, dosages in children should be smaller and adjusted very carefully. The U.S. Food and Drug Administration (FDA) has published guidelines for pediatric labeling including dosages; this information is published at the FDA website (http://www.fda.gov). Not all hypertensive medications have pediatric approval. The prescriber must verify the most current dosing schedules. ACE inhibitors and ARBs should not be prescribed for pregnant or sexually active girls because of their teratogenic effects (American College of Obstetricians and Gynecologists [ACOG], 2012).

Uncomplicated HTN alone is not sufficient reason to restrict asymptomatic children from participating in physical activities, because exercise may actually lower blood pressure. Family counseling should include the known link between secondhand smoke and the arteriosclerotic changes in children (Mattoo, 2013).

Older Adults

The number of Americans aged 65 and older is increasing faster than that of any other age group. Hypertension is very common in older adults, occurring in 60% to 71% of the population older than 60 years. Among older adults, SBP increases almost linearly with age and is a better predictor of coronary heart disease (CHD), cardiovascular disease (CVD), heart failure, end-stage renal disease (ESRD), and all-cause mortality than is DBP, which increases until about age 55 and then declines. An even better predictor is pulse pressure (SBP minus DBP), which indicates reduced vascular compliance in large arteries. Evidence of this increased risk has led to recognition of the importance of treating ISH in older adults rather than accepting increased blood pressure as a "normal" part of aging. BP control rates (less than 150/90 mm Hg) are only about 20% in older adults with HTN, largely related to poor control of SBP. Benefits of treatment in this age group have been consistently demonstrated in large randomly controlled trials (RCTs) to include reduction of stroke and heart failure. These benefits do not increase when the BP is held under 140/90; hence, the relaxed number for older adults used in the JNC-8. The choice of initial agent is less important than the degree of BP reduction achieved as long as the risk of falls is also considered. The only exceptions to drug selection are the ACE and ARB groups, which are no longer recommended for those over the age of 75 (James et al, 2014).

This recommendation is based on the risks of hyperkalemia and renal considerations.

As in younger patients, therapy should begin with lifestyle modifications. Older adults respond especially well to salt intake reduction and weight loss because they are prone to sodium retention and volume excess. If lifestyle modifications do not achieve the BP goal, drug therapy should begin. In general, the initial dose should be about half that used in younger patients. Use of specific drugs is similar to that recommended in the general algorithm and for individuals with compelling reasons. Thiazide diuretics are recommended because they have been shown in RCTs to reduce morbidity and mortality and because they are less expensive for patients, who are often on fixed incomes. While considering the comments on orthostatic hypotension below, diuretics are still considered especially as a second add-on choice (ACCF/AHA, 2011). Thiazide diuretics are particularly useful for ISH because of their greater effects on SBP than on DBP. Morbidity and mortality are both improved in older adults when SBP is reduced, if DBP is held stable at between 85 and 90 mm Hg.

It is important to monitor potassium levels with the drugs, especially if the patient is also on digoxin. Even mild hypokalemia may be problematic for older adults with coronary artery disease (CAD). Drug combinations that include both a thiazide diuretic and a potassium-sparing diuretic are useful for patients who have repeated episodes of hypokalemia.

The BP goal for older adults is not the same as it is for younger patients. Any reduction in BP has some benefit; and the closer to the ideal goal, the better for the nonfrail elders with the highest risk. More latitude can be given for those with low risk. Among the most frail, there is no link between mortality risk and BP readings (Odden, Peralta, Haan, & Covinsky, 2012). Special considerations should be given to problems with orthostatic hypotension (OH) and cognitive dysfunction related to older adults.

Orthostatic Hypotension (OH)

Measurement of BP in older adults requires consideration of the possibility of pseudohypertension caused by excessive vascular stiffness. In addition, older adults are more likely to experience orthostatic changes, and their BP should be measured standing as well as in the lying position if symptomatic. OH is associated with an increase in age-adjusted mortality; there is a strong correlation between OH and premature death as well as increased numbers of falls and fractures. Severe volume depletion, baroreflex dysfunction, and autonomic insufficiency are common problems in some older adults. Certain vasodilator antihypertensives (e.g., alpha blockers and alpha beta blockers) as well as diuretics and nitrates may exacerbate this problem. Health-care providers should be alert to potential OH symptoms and adjust drug therapy accordingly.

Cognitive Dysfunction and Dementia

Cognitive impairment and dementia occur more commonly in people with HTN. Progression of cognitive impairment may be reduced with effective treatment of the HTN. Narrowing and sclerosis of small penetrating arteries in the subcortical regions of the brain are often found on autopsy of patients with chronic HTN. These changes may contribute to hypoperfusion, loss of autoregulation, compromise of the blood–brain barrier and white matter demyelination, micro infarction, and cognitive decline. Calcium channel blocker therapy might assist in slowing the decline of cognitive function. It does appear that central alpha$_2$ agonists make cognitive dysfunction worse and so should be avoided or, if there is a compelling reason for their use, used with extreme caution. Visual hallucinations have been cited in rare case reports with ACE inhibitors (Doane & Stults, 2013).

Women

There are no demonstrated clinical differences between men and women related to BP outcomes or responses to therapy; this includes elderly women (ACCF/AHA, 2011). Traditional guidelines most likely underestimate a woman's actual risk (Mosca et al, 2011). Women do have some unique variables related to hypertension: sexual dimorphism of BP and HTN prevalence, menopause, use of oral contraceptives and hormone replacements, and pregnancy. Black women shoulder a higher disease burden than the general population. Wu and associates (2014) have documented an increased risk of psoriasis in women who have used beta blockers for more than 6 years, but not with any other drug group.

Sexual Dimorphism and HTN Prevalence

Women have lower SBP levels than men during early adulthood, but the opposite is true after the sixth decade. The prevalence of HTN in women follows this dimorphism. The highest prevalence of HTN occurs in elderly black women, with the rate being more than 75% in black women older than 75 years (Mosca et al, 2011).

Women may have a higher rate of "white coat" hypertension in which the office value differs from a home BP report. If such patients (male or female) do not demonstrate endorgan symptoms, then a 24-hour BP monitoring test can determine if HTN actually does exist. An alternative is having the BP taken at various times of the day at fire stations, health clubs, pharmacies, or health and wellness kiosks. Some patients who do have HTN use the excuse of "white coat" to avoid taking medications.

Menopause

The effect of menopause on BP is controversial. Longitudinal studies have not shown a rise in BP, whereas cross-sectional studies have found significantly higher SBP and DBP in postmenopausal women versus premenopausal women. When there is a rise, it is often attributed to estrogen withdrawal, overproduction of pituitary hormones, weight gain, or a combination of these or other undefined neurohormonal influences. Studies of hormone replacement therapy (HRT) in postmenopausal women have been inconsistent in findings about changes in BP. Overall, HRT-related change in BP is mainly modest and does not preclude HRT use except in individuals with unusually strong responses to the hormones. It is not wise to treat the BP changes with an antihypertensive because HRT use is not a life-critical medication.

Oral Contraceptives

Women taking oral contraceptives have a small but detectable increase in both SBP and DBP, but these are usually within the normal range. Relative risk for HTN is significantly increased (RR = 1.8) in current users compared to those who have never used oral contraceptives. A strong correlation has also been found in HTN risk for women who smoke and take oral contraceptives. Women older than 35 years who smoke should be discouraged from using oral contraceptives and highly encouraged to stop smoking. If HTN develops in women taking oral contraceptives, then these drugs should be discontinued with counseling to consider a nonmedicated form of birth control (IUD, surgery). Blood pressure can return to normal after an initial rise in the first few months. Oral contraceptives are often prescribed on a yearly basis, but a more prudent approach may be to prescribe them semiannually so that BP can be checked every 6 months in high-risk women.

Pregnancy

Hypertensive disorders in pregnancy are a major cause of maternal, fetal, and neonatal morbidity and mortality. Hypertension during pregnancy is classified into five categories:

1. Chronic hypertension: Hypertension that is present and observable before pregnancy or diagnosed before the 20th week of pregnancy. The goal of management for chronic HTN in pregnant women is to minimize short-term risks while avoiding therapy that compromises the fetus. Women in stage 1 HTN are considered at low risk for cardiovascular complications during pregnancy and are best managed by lifestyle modifications only. A meta-analysis of 45 RCTs of treatment with a variety of antihypertensives in stage 1 and stage 2 HTN in pregnancy showed a direct relationship between treatment-induced drops in mean arterial pressure and the proportion of small-for-gestational-age infants. It appears judicious to carefully consider whether to continue antihypertensive drugs during pregnancy with a specialist. In all cases, treatment should be reinstituted if the BP reaches 150 to 160 systolic or 100 to 110 diastolic (ACOG, 2012). Drug selection is then based on the safety of the fetus. Table 40-7 summarizes some treatment options. Methyldopa has been studied the most and is typically recommended for women whose chronic hypertension is first diagnosed in pregnancy. Beta-adrenergic blockers are equally effective and are safe during the second and third trimesters, but their use in the first trimester has been associated with growth retardation in the fetus. Labetalol is equally effective as methyldopa and has fewer side effects. If the hypertension is diagnosed before the pregnancy, diuretics and some antihypertensives may be continued. Chapters 14 and 16 delineate safety issues in pregnancy for various HTN drugs. ACE inhibitors, ARBs, and DRI should never be used in pregnancy.

2. Preeclampsia: Preeclampsia is a pregnancy-specific condition primarily seen in first-gestation mothers. It involves HTN and proteinuria (greater than 300 mg/24 h) after 20 weeks' gestation. Preeclampsia rarely disappears on its own and usually worsens with time. It may be superimposed on existing chronic hypertension. Because of the risk for development of eclampsia, treatment includes bedrest (although strict bedrest is not recommended) (ACOG, 2012), control of BP, seizure prophylaxis, and timely delivery. Antihypertensive therapy is prescribed only for maternal safety

Table 40–7 Antihypertensives in Pregnancy

The report of the NHBPEP Working Group on High Blood Pressure in Pregnancy permits continuation of drug therapy in women with chronic hypertension (except for angiotensin-converting enzyme [ACE] inhibitors). In addition, angiotensin II receptor blockers should not be used during pregnancy. In women with chronic hypertension with diastolic levels of 100 mm Hg or greater (lower when end-organ damage or underlying renal disease is present) and in women with acute hypertension when levels are 150 mm Hg or greater, the following drugs are recommended:

Acceptable Drug	Comments
Alpha beta blockers	Labetalol (C) is equally effective as methyldopa but has fewer adverse responses.
Beta blockers	Atenolol (C) and metoprolol (C) appear to be safe and effective in late pregnancy; labetalol (C) also appears to be effective.
Calcium antagonists	Potential synergism with magnesium sulfate may lead to precipitous hypotension (C).
Central alpha agonists	Methyldopa (C) is the recommended drug of choice.
Direct vasodilators	Hydralazine (C) is the parenteral drug of choice, based on its long history of safety and efficacy.
Diuretics	Diuretics (C) are recommended for chronic hypertension if prescribed before gestation or if patients appear to be salt-sensitive; they are not recommended in pre-eclampsia.

ACE inhibitors (D) and angiotensin II receptor blockers (D) may result in fetal abnormalities including death; these drugs should not be used in pregnancy.

Pregnancy Category C = adverse effects in animals; no controlled trials in humans; use if risk appears justified. Pregnancy Category D = positive evidence of fetal risk.

Source: From the National High Blood Pressure Education Program. (2003). *Seventh Report of the Joint National Committee on Prevention, Detection, Evaluation, and Treatment of High Blood Pressure.* Rockville, MD: National Institutes of Health; National Heart, Lung and Blood Institute.

because it does not improve perinatal outcomes and may adversely affect utero-placental blood flow. Drug selection depends on time of delivery. If delivery is more than 48 hours away, methyldopa, labetalol, or calcium channel blockers are acceptable. If delivery is imminent, parenteral agents such as hydralazine or labetalol may be used.

3. Chronic HTN with superimposed preeclampsia: This classification is treated like preeclampsia.

4. Gestational HTN: This classification involves HTN without proteinuria occurring after 20 weeks' gestation. It is a temporary diagnosis and requires careful monitoring as it may evolve into preeclampsia. Some bedrest may be useful, but there is insufficient evidence to make a recommendation about the usefulness of salt restriction (ACOG, 2012). HTN that does not resolve in the post-delivery months is treated as new-onset HTN.

5. Transient HTN: This is a retrospective diagnosis and BP is normal by 12 weeks' postpartum. It may be predictive of future primary HTN.

Pregnancy with HTN should generate at least a consultation with a specialist. If the mother returns to the clinic for nonpregnancy-related primary care, attention to BP levels may uncover a need for urgent return to the specialist or for telephonic consultation to coordinate dose adjustments.

Racial and Ethnic Minorities

The prevalence of HTN and the degree of control to target BP among different racial and ethnic groups varies. Native Americans have the same or slightly higher prevalence rates as the white population. Hispanics have the same to slightly lower prevalence rates, despite their increased incidence of obesity and type 2 diabetes mellitus. Asians have the same prevalence and appear to be more responsive to HTN drugs than whites.

The prevalence of hypertension in African Americans is among the highest in the world (Brown, 2006). An estimated 30% of all deaths in this population are attributable to HTN, which develops at younger ages than it does in whites. The average BP is also much higher despite the fact that most black men take multiple medications (Miedema, 2014). The higher rate of severe HTN results in more end-organ damage. The African American stroke rate is 80% higher, the heart disease mortality 50% higher, and the HTN-related ESRD is 320% higher than that of the general population. Many African Americans have the comorbidities of type 2 diabetes or HTN, with up to 14% of adults having both disorders.

In general, this population has lower renin activity, and so the RAAS is thought not to play a major role. Monotherapy with ACE inhibitors is less effective because of this low renin activity; however, in combination with diuretics the therapeutic outcomes are equal (Gerber et al, 2013). In the presence of diabetes mellitus, ACE inhibitors should be used for their renal protective properties. In the presence of MI, ACE continues to be a strong contender to help with HF and left ventricular remodeling protection.

The underlying pathology associated with hypertension in African Americans is thought to be salt sensitivity (Brown, 2006). This increased sensitivity to salt, along with the high prevalence in this population of obesity, cigarette smoking, and type 2 diabetes mellitus, means that lifestyle modifications are especially efficacious. Salt intake should be reduced to less than 6 g per day, and weight should be reduced, if necessary, to approach ideal body weight. If these modifications do not result in achievement of the BP goal, diuretics have been proved in RCTs to reduce morbidity and mortality and are the first agents of choice unless there are compelling reasons to choose another drug class (Gerber et al, 2013).

Calcium channel blockers are recommended as first-line therapy for African Americans (James et al, 2014). The Atherosclerosis Risk in Communities (ARIC) study found, however, that ACE medications are the most commonly prescribed for this group (Miedema, 2014). Monotherapy with most beta-adrenergic blockers is less effective than in whites but should still be used for the post-MI mortality benefit. Despite noted differences in BP response at the population level, race alone is a poor predictor of BP response to any particular class of drugs if they are given in adequate doses and with sufficient time to work. The interracial differences with any drug class are abolished when the drug is combined with a diuretic. Many Americans, both African American and others, have a mixed genetic background, so an assumption of negative response should not preclude the use of any drug class. Individual response monitoring is the key to an optimal therapeutic plan.

The high prevalence of stage 2 hypertension in the African American population means that multidrug therapy is common, which may result in a higher prevalence of adverse responses. For the proportion of African Americans who do not trust the white-dominated medical system, these adverse effects—related to drugs that treat a disease that exists for them only because a medical device (the blood pressure cuff) tells them they have it—increase their distrust, especially when these adverse responses include personal problems such as impotence. All plans should consider racial and ethnic minorities' traditional foods that are high in salt and fat composition.

Racial differences in adverse responses to antihypertensive drugs may occur even in monotherapy. African Americans and Asians, for example, have a 3- to 4-fold higher risk of angioedema (ALLHAT, 2002; Wright et al, 2009), and more cough has been attributed to ACE inhibitors than in whites (Elliot, 1996; Gerber et al, 2013). Unfortunately, insufficient numbers of Mexican Americans and other Hispanic Americans, Native Americans, or Asian/Pacific Islanders have been included in most of the major clinical trials to make strong recommendations about their responses to individual antihypertensives.

Adherence to dietary recommendations also may vary by ethnicity. In a study of nearly 6,000 adults aged 45 to 84 years, there was a significant variation in Dietary Approaches to Stop Hypertension (DASH) goal attainment among ethnic groups (Gao et al, 2009). Chinese Americans were more likely to meet cholesterol goals but less likely to meet magnesium and potassium goals. African Americans and Hispanics had more problems with calcium intake and had less goal attainment related to saturated fat and magnesium.

Concomitant Diseases and Therapies

Antihypertensive drugs may improve the management of some diseases and worsen that of others (Table 40-5). Selection of an antihypertensive that also treats a concomitant disease can simplify the overall therapeutic regimen, reduce cost, and increase the likelihood of adherence. It is not within the scope of this chapter to discuss all possible diseases that may coexist with HTN, but the most common diseases that benefit from appropriate selection of an antihypertensive are discussed below.

Cerebrovascular Disease

The risk of complications of cerebrovascular disease, including CVA and dementia, increases as a function of BP levels. Contrary to popular belief, most ischemic strokes occur in individuals with prehypertension or stage 1 HTN. No specific drug has been proven to be clinically superior to all others for stroke prevention. Management of BP during an acute stroke is not within the scope of this text. Posthospitalization care should be coordinated with specialty services to set new target BP goals, which might be higher than prestroke targets. Treatment is instituted with a goal to reduce BP gradually.

Coronary Artery Disease

Coexisting CAD and hypertension place patients at especially high risk for cardiovascular morbidity and mortality. Antihypertensive therapy is essential and its benefits well established. Blood pressure should be reduced to a goal of 140/90 mm Hg, with lower BP desirable in patients with angina. Excessively rapid lowering of BP, however, may result in reflex tachycardia and sympathetic stimulation so should be avoided. Lowering DBP below 55 to 60 mm Hg has been associated with increased CV events, including MI (Odden et al, 2012). Antihypertensive drugs that have reflex tachycardia and sympathetic stimulation as adverse reactions (alpha-adrenergic blockers, nitrates, and peripheral vasodilators) are generally avoided. Long-acting calcium channel blockers and beta-adrenergic blockers are especially helpful to patients with concomitant angina. Short-acting calcium channel blockers should not be used. After MI, beta-adrenergic blockers with intrinsic sympathomimetic activity are considered the "gold standard" because they reduce the risk of subsequent MI. This is less definitive for those STEMI patients with lower risks (Nakatani et al, 2013). These recommendations are based on older research done in the pre-reperfusion era (Bangalore et al, 2014). There is increased risk of cardiogenic shock and HF with beta blockers; therefore, this currently espoused quality care indictor is being reviewed. Current guides do not differentiate between the two types of beta blockers. ACE inhibitors and ARBs are also useful after MI, especially with concomitant left ventricular (LV) dysfunction, to prevent heart failure and mortality and reduce ventricular remodeling.

Stable Angina and Silent Ischemia

Therapy in these disorders is directed toward preventing MI and death, reducing symptoms of angina, and preventing the occurrence of ischemia. Unless contraindicated, drug therapy should begin with a beta-adrenergic blocker. Beta-adrenergic blockers reduce symptoms, improve mortality, and reduce cardiac output and heart rate, which decreases myocardial oxygen demand. If angina and BP are not controlled by beta-adrenergic blockers alone, or if these drugs are contraindicated, a long-acting calcium channel blocker may be used. These drugs decrease total peripheral resistance, which leads to reduction in BP and wall tension. Non-dihydropyridine calcium channel blockers also decrease heart rate, but when combined with a beta-adrenergic blocker they may produce severe bradycardia or high degrees of heart block. Therefore, dihydropyridine calcium channel blockers are preferred for combination therapy with a beta-adrenergic blocker. If angina is still not controlled, a nitrate or Relenza can be added. Chapter 28 further discusses the management protocol for angina.

Left Ventricular Hypertrophy

Left ventricular hypertrophy (LVH) is a cardiac adaptation to the increased afterload generated by persistent hypertension. LVH is a major independent risk factor for sudden cardiac death, MI, stroke, and other cardiovascular events. In addition to lifestyle modification with salt reduction and weight loss (Coxson et al, 2013), antihypertensive drugs (except direct vasodilators such as hydralazine and minoxidil) are capable of reducing left ventricular mass and wall thickness and reducing cardiovascular risks. ACE inhibitors have been demonstrated to be the most effective in reducing LV mass in patients with LV hypertrophy. Beta-adrenergic blockers had the least reduction in mass, and intermediate effects occurred with diuretics and calcium channel blockers. The ARB class, but not the DRIs (Gheorghiade et al, 2013), has a similar profile to that of ACE inhibitors. Reduction of LV mass is associated with lower overall CVD risk. The combination of an ACE inhibitor and a diuretic has proved to be most effective in regressing LVH and reducing cardiovascular risks.

Heart Failure

Hypertension is the major cause of LV failure in the United States. Control of BP with lifestyle modifications and drug therapy improves myocardial function and reduces the risk for heart failure and cardiovascular mortality. HTN precedes the development of heart failure in approximately 90% of patients; this is most important in African Americans and older adults. CAD is the cause of heart failure in approximately two-thirds of heart failure patients. A variety of neurohormonal systems, especially the RAAS and SNS, are activated by the LV dysfunction seen in heart failure. Such activation may lead to abnormal ventricular remodeling, further LV enlargement, and reduced cardiac contractility. This progression can be significantly reduced by effective therapy.

New York Class I–III heart failure is a compelling indication for the use of ACE inhibitors. In Class IV failure associated with renal disease, the ACE inhibitor might become counterproductive. The alpha- and beta-adrenergic blocker carvedilol (Coreg) has also been shown to be beneficial when used alone or combined with an ACE inhibitor. The dihydropyridines amlodipine (Norvasc) and felodipine (Plendil) have been demonstrated to be safe for treating angina and hypertension in patients with advanced LV dysfunction when they are used in addition to ACE inhibitors, diuretics, or beta-adrenergic blockers, but other calcium channel blockers are not recommended for these patients. Aldosterone antagonists in low doses (12.5 to 25 mg daily) may provide additional benefits for patients with severe LV dysfunction. Chapter 36 discusses the treatment of heart failure in more detail.

Renal Parenchymal Disease

Hypertension may result from any form of renal disease that reduces the number of functioning nephrons, leading to salt and water retention and then to increased extracellular fluid (ECF) volume. Evaluation of renal function in hypertensive patients should include serum creatinine levels (even small elevations reflect large losses in glomerular filtration rate) and urinalysis to detect proteinuria or hematuria. Reversible causes of renal failure should always be sought out and treated. Newest predictions suggest that over half of the population between age 30 to 64 have risks for developing chronic kidney disease (CKD). Currently 13.2% of the population fall into a reduced renal functional pattern. It is anticipated that 14.4% will have documented CKD by 2020 and 16.7% by 2030 (Hoerger et al, 2015).

Blood pressure goals for patients with CKD also reflect the JNC-8 level. The goal is to maintain below 140/90. Injury to renal tissues does occur with BP above 150/90, but values of 140/80 are more tolerated than previously understood (Peralta et al, 2012). One study included within the JNC-8 guidelines did demonstrate improved renal status with a BP under 130/80 (Klahr et al, 1994), but the JNC recommendation is that if side effects of lowered BP interferes with adherence, the risk of CV adverse effects from HTN must be the primary consideration. Sodium restriction is still recommended for these patients, with a dietary restriction of potassium and phosphorus when creatinine clearance is below 30 mL/min. Consultation with renal specialists may determine lower individualized targets. CKD patients without proteinuria can use ACE, ARB, beta blockers or thiazide diuretics. GFR values below 30 require close re-evaluation of medications used. The JNC-8 recommendation for ACE/ARB medications comes without regard to race.

All classes of antihypertensive drugs are effective, and multiple drugs may be needed. ACE inhibitors have been the most effective in patients with diabetic nephropathy, proteinuria of 1 g or more per 24 hours, and renal insufficiency. Interestingly, ACE inhibitors as a drug class may not have a renal protective effect on CKD patients who do not have proteinuria (Mann, 2013). In patients with serum creatinine levels of 3 mg/dL or more, ACE inhibitors should be used with caution. Thiazide diuretics are not effective with renal insufficiency manifested by serum creatinine levels of 2.5 mg/dL or more; the loop diuretics such as furosemide (Lasix) are needed, often at relatively large doses. Potassium-sparing diuretics should be avoided in renal insufficiency.

Renovascular Disease

Clinical clues to renovascular disease include (1) onset of HTN before age 30 or recent onset of severe HTN after age 55; (2) an abdominal bruit, particularly if it continues into diastole and is lateralized; (3) accelerated or resistant HTN; (4) recurrent (flash) pulmonary edema; (5) renal failure of uncertain etiology; (6) coexisting diffuse atherosclerotic vascular disease, especially in heavy smokers; and (7) acute renal failure precipitated by antihypertensive therapy, especially with ACE inhibitors or ARBs. Patients with renovascular disease may require surgical interventions to stabilize their BP. No specific antihypertensive medications are recommended. Sometimes none are needed postsurgery.

Diabetes Mellitus

HTN is disproportionately increased in diabetics. Persons with HTN are 2.5 times more likely to develop diabetes within 5 years (American Diabetes Association [ADA], 2015). Coexistence of HTN and diabetes is especially concerning because both have strong links to CVD, CVA, progression to renal disease, and diabetic retinopathy. A reduction of as little as 10 mm Hg in SBP has been associated with average reductions in diabetes-related mortality by 15%, MI by 11%, and retinopathy and nephropathy by 13%. The rate of decline in diabetic nephropathy is believed to be related to a continuous function of arterial pressure. Antihypertensive drug therapy should be initiated early, along with lifestyle modifications (especially weight loss), to reach a blood pressure goal between 140/90 and 150/90 mm Hg for all patients with diabetes mellitus. The ADA in 2015 elected to use JNC-8 guideline values because the ACCORD trial (Cushman et al, 2010), which originally highlighted the issues of DM and HTN, did not reveal a real difference in outcomes for either the 140 or 150 cut point. Most DM patients need two or more drugs to reach the goal of maintaining below 140/90.

ACE inhibitors, ARBs, beta-adrenergic blockers, calcium channel blockers, and diuretics in low doses are preferred because of their lower effects on glucose metabolism, lipid profiles, and renal function. Of this group, ACE inhibitors are

> **On The Horizon**
>
> Renal GFR values that incorporate cystatin C levels become more reliable and uncover renal impairment earlier than the standard measurements. This can dramatically increase the number of patients requiring renal dosing of medications (Inkler et al, 2012).

considered best because of their demonstrated reduction in risk for diabetic nephropathy (AACE, 2006; ADA, 2015). They work well alone but are more effective when combined with a thiazide diuretic. This fact is confounded by evidence that thiazide diuretics worsen blood glucose control in some patients and can increase the likelihood of developing diabetes in insulin-resistant patients (AACE, 2006).

If ACE inhibitors are not well tolerated, ARBs may be considered, but not in combination. Both drug groups need to be reduced or stopped when renal function (GFR) drops below 30 mL/min. Beta-adrenergic blockers are beneficial as part of multidrug therapy, but their value as monotherapy is less clear. The third-generation beta blockers such as nebivolol or drugs that block both alpha and beta receptors such as carvedilol may prove to be most beneficial. These agents cause vasodilation and may increase insulin sensitivity (AACE, 2006). Other beta-adrenergic blockers have an adverse effect on peripheral blood flow, prolong hypoglycemia, and mask most hypoglycemic symptoms. The diaphoresis of hypoglycemia is not masked. If there is a compelling reason for a patient with diabetes to use beta blockers, they should be combined with a diuretic.

Calcium channel blockers have also been shown to have some degree of renal protection and are most helpful as part of multidrug therapy. The non-dihydropyridine calcium channel blockers (diltiazem and verapamil) may reduce microalbuminuria to an extent comparable with ACE inhibitors, but the dihydropyridine calcium channel blockers may increase it. The DRIs do not have a renal protective effect (Parving et al, 2012).

Metabolic Syndrome

Metabolic syndrome is a constellation of CV risk factors related to HTN, abdominal obesity, dyslipidemia, and insulin resistance. The prevalence of this syndrome is highly age-dependent; only 7% of adults 20 to 29 years demonstrate metabolic syndrome, whereas 40% or more of Americans older than 60 years demonstrate it. The risk for fatal CHD is increased 4-fold and for CVD is increased 2-fold for individuals with this syndrome, even after adjustment for age. Patients with this syndrome also have a 5- to 9-fold increased risk for developing diabetes. The cornerstone of clinical management of metabolic syndrome in adults is lifestyle modification. Most patients with this syndrome fall into the prehypertension or stage 1 hypertension categories. If BP exceeds 150/90 mm Hg, drug therapy is indicated based on the general hypertension treatment algorithm.

Many obese patients also have sleep apnea. Obstructive apnea increases CV risk. Referral to a sleep study center may demonstrate a HTN benefit from CPAP or nocturnal O_2 therapy (Park, Ramar, & Olson, 2011).

Dyslipidemia

Lifestyle modifications are the first approach to treatment of both dyslipidemia and HTN. Emphasis is placed on control of weight; reducing the excess intake of sodium, saturated fat, cholesterol, and alcohol; and increasing physical activity. When drug therapy is chosen, drug effects on lipid metabolism are the primary consideration. Alpha-adrenergic blockers may decrease serum cholesterol to a limited degree and increase HDL. ACE inhibitors, ARBs, calcium channel blockers, and central adrenergic agonists have neutral effects on lipids. Beta-adrenergic blockers increase triglycerides transiently and reduce levels of HDLs. They are chosen mainly for patients with previous MIs who need their protective effects against sudden cardiac death and recurrent MI. In high doses, thiazide and loop diuretics can cause at least short-term increases in levels of cholesterol, triglycerides, and low-density lipids (LDLs); typically, this effect does not persist. Dietary modifications can reduce some of these effects. Low doses of thiazide diuretics do not produce these lipid effects and can be safely used. The risks for cerebrovascular and coronary events are reduced equally in persons with normal lipid levels and those with elevated lipid levels. Lowering lipid levels also reduces CV risks that are shared in common with HTN. Selection of appropriate cholesterol-lowering drugs is discussed in Chapters 16 and 39.

Respiratory Diseases

Hypertension is relatively common in acute asthma and may be related to exuberant treatment with beta agonists or systemic corticosteroids. Bronchial reactivity is unchanged by ACE inhibitors, which are safe for most patients with asthma. If the patient is one of the 10% to 15% who experience the adverse effect of a cough, ARBs are an alternative. Beta-adrenergic blockers and alpha- and beta-adrenergic blockers may exacerbate asthma and should not be used unless there are compelling reasons for doing so.

Many over-the-counter (OTC) drugs used as decongestants and cold and asthma remedies contain a sympathomimetic drug that can raise blood pressure. They are generally safe when taken in limited doses by patients who are controlled on antihypertensive therapy. Cromolyn sodium, ipratropium bromide, or corticosteroids by inhalation can be used safely for nasal congestion by patients with hypertension.

Clarithromycin (Biaxin) is a macrolide antibiotic commonly prescribed for respiratory infections. Several adverse reactions of concern to hypertensive patients have come to light recently. One of these is the increased risk of cardiovascular morbidity and mortality (Schembri et al, 2013), which is compounded by statin toxicity when combined with clarithromycin (Patel et al, 2013). Clarithromycin has also been linked to acute renal failure in patients on calcium channel blockers (Fleet et al, 2013). The other macrolides do not appear to have these same drug interactions.

Surgery Patients

Beta blockers used to carry a warning to hold prior to surgical procedures. This was modified in 2009 by the American College of Cardiology and the American Heart Association to include only severely ill patients and those undergoing cardiac-specific surgery (Fleishmann et al, 2009). Additionally, adding beta blockade to patients undergoing surgery was considered potentially beneficial. This has been a contentious issue, however, because some studies have documented CV problems even during noncardiac surgeries (Patel et al, 2013). Prescribers who have patients requiring surgical care should therefore consult the surgeon or anesthesiologist for their suggestions about use in the days leading up to a planned procedure requiring sedation.

Cost

The cost of antihypertensive drug therapy should be considered in drug selection, especially for patients who require multiple drugs. In most cases, generic formulations are acceptable and cheaper than brand-name counterparts. Nongeneric agents are usually more expensive. If the branded agent is equally effective and there are no compelling reasons for its use, cost might be a major factor in choosing the initial therapy. If the branded agent is more effective or there is a compelling reason for its use, cost should be a secondary consideration. Using combinations can also reduce drug cost. Table 40-4 lists some of the more common drugs found in combination tablets. Shopping at different sources to check prices is often worthwhile. Some higher-dose and lower-dose tablets cost the same, and the tablet can be divided to reduce cost.

Treatment costs include not only the price of the drug but also the price of any routine or special laboratory tests, supplemental therapies, clinic visits, and time lost from work for clinic visits. Maintaining contact with a patient and regularly checking BP are important factors in adherence, but they can also add to cost. Teaching the patient how to do home BP monitoring and using telecommunication or e-mail to maintain contact can reduce unnecessary visits.

In an era of cost-consciousness, the cost of treating HTN is always under scrutiny. Managed-care agencies can be reminded, however, that the cost of HTN management that results in good control is lower than the avoidable cost of hypertension-associated heart disease, stroke, and renal failure, which may result in expensive hospitalizations. RCTs have shown that these reductions occur in a relatively short period of time and are sustained for years (Bitton, Choudry, Matlin, Swanton, & Strank, 2013).

MONITORING

The most important monitoring parameter is BP measurement. Equipment used to monitor BP should be regularly inspected and validated. The operator should be trained and regularly retrained in the appropriate technique and the proper patient positioning. Caffeine, exercise, and smoking should be avoided for at least 30 minutes prior to measurement. The person should be seated in a chair (not on the examination table) for at least 5 minutes with feet on the floor and arm supported at heart level. An appropriately sized cuff (cuff bladder encircling at least 80% of the arm) should be used. At least two measurements are taken and the average recorded. The health-care provider should provide to patients verbally and in writing their specific BP numbers and the BP goal of their treatment.

Home or clinic blood pressure measurement in the early morning before the patient has taken the antihypertensive drug(s) provides data about the adequacy of management related to the increase in blood pressure after arising. Measurement in the late afternoon or evening helps to monitor control across the day. Because the stress of a clinic visit may result in higher blood pressure readings in the clinic, blood pressure goals based on home monitoring are usually lower than those based on clinic monitoring. Less-than-optimal BP readings should not lead to the assumption that medication therapy is ineffective. Some cases can be traced to nonadherence to the plan. Uncovering barriers to treatment is part of monitoring. Telemonitoring has been shown to improve patient outcomes (Kerby et al, 2012).

OUTCOME EVALUATION

Evaluation of hypertensive patients has three objectives: (1) to assess lifestyle and identify other cardiovascular risk factors or concomitant disorders that may affect prognosis and guide treatment, (2) to reveal identifiable causes of HTN, and (3) to assess the presence or absence of target organ damage and CVD. Figure 40-2 shows a treatment protocol for HTN management. Evaluation against a reasonable range of BP values occurs throughout the protocol. The main indications for substitution of a drug from a different class are no response and troublesome adverse reactions to initial drug therapy. Specific drugs to substitute have been previously discussed. When a substitution does not result in achievement of the target BP range, drugs from other classes are continually added until the goal is reached.

Goals in children have not been established by evidence other than expert opinion. Targets below the 95th percentile are typical except for children with major CV risk and DM, which drops the target to below the 90th percentile. Adult treatment recommendations are suggested for those under age 30 with DBP above 90 (James et al, 2014).

When standard therapy is not successful in achieving goal BP (refractory hypertension), when a secondary cause of the hypertension is suspected, when the patient has complex concomitant conditions, or when renal failure worsens even with adequate control, referral to an HTN specialist is appropriate (Stafford, Will & Brooks-Gumbert, 2012). Severe HTN (SBP greater than 180 mm Hg and DBP greater than 120 mm Hg) can exist without major end-organ damage and require consultation for care. Referral for immediate hospitalization is indicated with evidence of a hypertensive urgency (DBP greater than 110 mm Hg) or hypertensive emergency (DBP greater than 120 mm Hg) associated with retinal hemorrhages, bulging optic disks, mental status changes, new-onset heart or renal failure, and unstable angina (Stafford et al, 2012).

Laboratory data and other monitoring parameters related to specific drugs are discussed in Chapters 14 and 16 for each drug class. Annual evaluations for target organ damage should include a 12-lead electrocardiogram (ECG), urinalysis, complete blood count (CBC), blood chemistry (potassium, sodium, creatinine, fasting glucose, total cholesterol), and HDL levels. Optional tests include creatinine clearance, 24-hour urine protein, LDL levels, thyroid-stimulating hormone levels, and limited echocardiography if signs of systemic organ dysfunction are noted on examination. For patients with diabetes, microalbuminuria and glycosylated hemoglobin studies are essential. Physical examination includes fundoscopic examination, neurological examination, and assessment of heart and lung sounds, peripheral pulses, and bruits. It is recommended that HTN patients have a formal ophthalmology exam at baseline and annually.

Adherence Issues

Lack of adherence to a therapeutic regimen to control BP is unfortunately very common. Several factors in HTN management foster this nonadherence. It is hoped that a less stringent acceptable blood pressure range for adults with average risk will improve adherence statistics. Lifestyle modification is a foundation of HTN management, and difficulty in achieving and maintaining lifestyle changes is well documented. Adverse drug reactions and drug costs are also factors in nonadherence. Sexual dysfunction, fatigue, and depression are common adverse reactions to several classes of antihypertensive drugs. A systematic team approach that uses health professionals and community resources can assist in providing the necessary education, support, and follow-up to improve adherence. The ultimate improvement in adherence is related to the patients having a positive experience with, and trust in, their health-care provider. Better communication improves outcomes and empathy builds trust. Table 40-8 details some activities that can improve adherence. Chapter 6 has additional material on improving positive outcomes.

PATIENT EDUCATION

Patient education should include a discussion of information related to the overall treatment plan as well as that specific to the drug therapy, reasons for taking the drug, drugs as part of the total treatment regimen, and adherence issues. Though severe salt reduction is no longer considered necessary for most patients, Americans have an excessive sodium intake in their diet (Bayer, Johns, & Galen, 2012; Coxson et al, 2013). Keeping a diet diary and then identifying specific reductions that can be accomplished more easily can help. Prepared baby and toddler foods are very heavy in sodium content, requiring parents to read the labels very carefully when selecting products.

Population-based predictive models of limiting sodium to only 1,500 mg/d (U.S. Dietary guidelines; 2010), from the usual 3,600 mg/d, would reduce CV deaths by over 20% over a 10 year period (Coxson et al, 2013). The key is to teach patients about hidden sources of sodium in the diet, as well as to have them self-monitor their general response to salt. If a load causes increased edema, then salt reduction becomes a more important part of the therapeutic plan.

Table 40–8 Factors to Improve Adherence to Therapy

- Be aware of signs of patient nonadherence to antihypertensive therapy and monitor for them.
- Establish the goal of therapy jointly with the patient: to reduce blood pressure to nonhypertensive levels with minimal or no adverse effects.
- Educate patients about the disease and involve them and their families in its treatment; have them measure blood pressure at home.
- Maintain regular contact with patients; consider telecommunication.
- Keep treatment regimen as inexpensive and simple as possible.
- Encourage lifestyle modifications and provide support for them.
- Integrate drug regimen into routine activities of daily living.
- Prescribe drugs according to pharmacological principles, favoring long-acting formulations.
- Be willing to stop unsuccessful therapy and try a different approach.
- Anticipate adverse reactions and adjust therapy to prevent, minimize, or ameliorate them.
- Continue to add effective and tolerated drugs, stepwise, in sufficient doses to achieve the goals of therapy while reducing the likelihood of adverse reactions.
- Encourage a positive attitude about achieving therapeutic goals.
- Use nurse case management and a team approach.

Source: Adapted from the National High Blood Pressure Education Program. (2003). *Seventh Report of the Joint National Committee on Prevention, Detection, Evaluation, and Treatment of High Blood Pressure.* Rockville, MD: National Institutes of Health; National Heart, Lung and Blood Institute.

HYPERTENSION

PATIENT
EDUCATION

Related to the Overall Treatment Plan and Disease Process

☐ Pathophysiology of hypertension and its long-term effects on target organs

☐ Role of lifestyle modifications in improving prognosis and keeping the number and cost of required drugs down

☐ Importance of adherence to the treatment regimen

☐ Self-monitoring of blood pressure

☐ Indications of target organ damage

☐ Need for regular follow-up visits with the primary care provider

Specific to the Drug Therapy

☐ Reason for taking the drug(s) and the anticipated action of the drug(s) on the disease process

☐ Doses and schedules for taking the drug(s)

☐ Possible adverse reactions and what to do when they occur

☐ Coping mechanisms for complex and costly drug regimens

☐ Interaction between lifestyle modifications and these drugs

Reasons for Taking the Drug(s)

Patient education about specific drugs is provided in Chapters 14 and 16. Specific information related to hypertension includes the reasons for taking the drugs. Antihypertensive drugs are given to reduce mortality and decrease target organ damage. Some drugs do both; most do one or the other. The expectations should be clear about what the drugs can and cannot do. Hypertension is a chronic condition that rarely develops in a short space of time and is not likely to be corrected in a short space of time, if at all. Patients with hypertension must understand the lifelong nature of the disorder and the need to incorporate the treatment regimen into their everyday lives. The risk of target organ damage must be discussed, but hope must be maintained, and the potential for a good quality of life with adequate treatment must be emphasized.

Drugs as Part of the Total Treatment Regimen

The total treatment regimen includes salt reduction and avoidance of excessive fluid intake. Diuretics reduce fluid volume and may interact with dietary sodium reduction, resulting in orthostatic hypotension (OH). Care should be taken not to reduce salt and fluid too quickly. Patients should be taught to report signs and symptoms of fluid volume deficit. Sodium reduction may lead some patients to seek salt substitutes that have potassium as part of their contents. For patients taking ACE inhibitors or ARBs, this choice can result in excessively high potassium levels. Such salt substitutes should be avoided. Nonsalt herbal seasoning is more appropriate.

Vasodilators can produce OH. Tell patients to rise slowly from a supine position to permit the body to redistribute body fluids.

Regular aerobic exercise such as walking or cycling can improve blood pressure control. Gradually increased, regular exercise may lead to improvement in blood pressure level and reduce the drug(s) needed.

Adherence Issues

Nonadherence with the treatment regimen may reduce life expectancy and affect the functioning of target organs. Health-care providers should be aware of the potential problem of nonadherence, discuss the importance of adherence at each follow-up visit, and assist patients in removing barriers to adherence, such as the complexity and cost of the treatment regimen and the presence of adverse reactions.

REFERENCES

ADVANSTAR Medical Economics Healthcare Communications. (2004). Reducing cardiovascular risk factors, patient care for the nurse practitioner: A ce activity. Sponsored by Pfizer, Inc.

Ahluwalia, N., Blacher, J., Szabo, D. E., Faure, P., Hercberg, S., & Galan, P. (2013, Mar 26). Prognostic value of multiple emerging biomarkers in cardiovascular risk prediction in patients with stable cardiovascular disease. *Atherosclerosis, S0021-9150*(13), 00193-7. Epub ahead of print. doi: 10.1016/j.atherosclerosis.2013.03.017

ALLHAT Officers and Coordinators for the ALLHAT Collaborative Research Group. (2002). Major outcomes in high-risk hypertensive patients randomized to angiotensin-converting enzyme inhibitor or calcium channel blocker vs diuretic: The Antihypertensive and Lipid-Lowering Treatment to Prevent Heart Attack (ALLHAT). *Journal of the American Medical Association, 288,* 2981–2997.

American Association of Clinical Endocrinologists (AACE) Hypertension Task Force. (2006). American Association of Clinical Endocrinologists medical guidelines for clinical practice for the diagnosis and treatment of hypertension. *Endocrine Practice, 12*(2), 193–222.

American College of Cardiology Foundation/American Heart Association (ACCF/AHA). (2011). Expert consensus document on hypertension in the elderly. *Circulation, 123*(21), 2434–2506. doi: 10.1161/CIR.0b013e31821daaf6

American College of Obstetricians and Gynecologists. (2012). ACOG Practice Bulletin No. 125. Chronic hypertension in pregnancy. *Obstetrics and Gynecology, 119*, 396–407.

American Diabetes Association (ADA). (2015). Standards of medical care in diabetes 2015 *Diabetes Care, 38* (1): S1–S94.

Arnett, D., Goodman, R., Halperin, J., Anderson, J., Parekh, A., & Zoghbi, W. (2014). AHA/ACC/HHS strategies to enhance application of clinical practice guidelines in patients with cardiovascular disease and comorbid conditions. *Journal of the American College of Cardiology. 64*(17), 1851–1856.

Bangalore, S., Makani, H., Radford, M., Thakur, K., Toklu, B. Katz, S., et al. (2014). Clinical outcomes with beta blockers for myocardial infarction: A meta-analysis of randomized trials, *American Journal of Medicine, 127*(10),939–953.

Bayer, R., Johns, D., & Galen, S. (2012). Salt and public health contested science and the challenge of evidence-based decision making. *Health Affairs, 31*(12), 2738–2746. doi: 10.1377/hlthaff.2012.0554

Bitton, A., Choudry, N., Matlin, O., Swanton, K., & Strank, W. (2013). The impact of medication adherence on coronary artery disease costs and outcomes: A systematic review. *American Journal of Medicine, 126*(4), 357e&–357e27. doi: 10.1016/j.amjmed.2012.09.004

Brady, T., Fivish, B., Flynn, J., & Parekh, R. (2008). Ability of blood pressure to predict left ventricular hypertrophy in pediatric hypertension. *Journal of Pediatrics, 152*(1), 73–78. doi: 10.1016/j.jpeds.2007.05.053

Brown, M. (2006). Hypertension and ethnic group. *British Medical Journal, 332*(7545), 833–836.

Brown, N., Ray, W., Snowden, M., & Griffin, M. (1996). Black Americans have an increased rate of angiotensin converting enzyme inhibitor-associated angioedema. *Clinical Pharmacology Therapy, 60*, 8–13.

Coleman, K. J., Ngor, E., Reynolds, K., Quinn, V. P., Koebnick, C., Young, D. R., et al. (2012, Nov). Initial validation of an exercise "vital sign" in electronic medical records. *Medicine &Science in Sports & Exercise, 44*(11), 2071–2076. doi: 10.1249/MSS.0b013e3182630ec1

Chobanian, A., Bakris, G., Black, H., Cushman, W., Green, L., Izzo, J., et al, National High Blood Pressure Coordinating Committee. (2003). Seventh Report of the Joint National Committee on Prevention, Detection, Evaluation, and Treatment of High Blood Pressure. *Journal of the American Medical Association, 289*, 2560–2571.

Coxson, P., Cook, N., Joffres, M., Hong, Y., Orenstein, D., Schmidt, S., et al. (2013, Mar). Mortality benefits from US population-wide reduction in sodium consumption: projections from 3 modeling approaches. *Hypertension, 61*(3), 564–570. doi: 10.1161/HYPERTENSIONAHA.111.201293. Epub 2013 Feb 11.

Cushman, W., Evans, G., Byington, R., Goff, D., Grimm, R., Cutler, J., et al, Action to Control Cardiovascular Risk in Diabetes Study Group. (ACCORD) (2010). Effects of intensive glucose lowering in type 2 diabetes. *New England Journal of Medicine, 36*(17):1575–1585.

Dalal, P., Varma, D., & Hegazym, H. (2013, Nov). Do beta-blockers increase perioperative cardiac morbidity? *Chest, 144*(4-meeting abstracts 0:166A). doi:10.1378/chest 1704913

Dhalla, I., Gomes,T., Yao, Z., Nagge, J., Persaud, N., Hellings, C., et al. (2013). Chlorthalidone versus hydrochlorothiazide for the treatment of hypertension in older adults: A population-based cohort study. *Annals of Internal Medicine, 158*(6), 447–455.

Doane, J., & Stults, B. (2013). Visual hallucinations related to angiotensin-converting enzyme inhibitor use: Case reports and review. *Journal of Clinical Hypertension, 15*(4), 230–233. doi: 10.1111/jch.12063

Elliot, W. (1996). Higher incidence of discontinuance of angiotensin converting enzyme inhibitors due to cough in black subjects. *Clinical Pharmacology Therapy, 60*, 582–588.

Flack, J., Sica, D., Bakris, G., Brown, A., Ferdinand, K., Grimm, R., Jr., ... & Jamerson, K. (2010). Management of high blood pressure in blacks: An update of the hypertension in blacks consensus statement. *Hypertension, 56*(5), 780–800. doi: 10.1161/HYPERTENSIONAHA.110.152892

Fleet, J., Shariff, S., Bailey, D., Gandhi, S., Juurlink, D., Nash, D., et al. (2013, Jul 11). Comparing two types of macrolide antibiotics for the purpose of assessing population-based drug interactions. *British Medical Journal* Open, *3*(7), pii: e002857.

Fleischmann, K., Beckman, J., Buller, C., Calkins, H., Fleisher, L., Freeman, W., et al. (2009). 2009 ACCF/AHA focused update on perioperative beta blockade. *Journal of the American College of Cardiology, 54*(22), 2102–2128.

Gao, S., Fitzpatrick, A., Psaty, B., Jiang, R., Post, W., Cutler, J., et al. (2009). Suboptimal nutritional intake for hypertension control in 4 ethnic groups. *Archives of Internal Medicine, 169*(7), 702–707.

Gerber, L. M., Mann, S. J., McDonald, M. V., Chiu, Y. L., Sridharan, S., & Feldman, P. H. (2013, Feb). Diuretic use in black patients with uncontrolled hypertension. *American Journal of Hypertension, 26*(2), 174–179. doi: 10.1093/ajh/hps029. Epub 2012 Dec 28.

Gheorghiade, M., Böhm, M., Greene, S. J., Fonarow, G. C., Lewis, E. F., Zannad, F., et al. (2013). Effect of aliskiren on postdischarge mortality and heart failure readmissions among patients hospitalized for heart failure: The ASTRONAUT randomized trial. *Journal of the American Medical Association, 309*(11), 1125–1135. doi: 10.1001/jama.2013.1954

Hermida, R., Ayala, D., Mojón, A., & Fernández, J. (2010, Sept). Influence of circadian time of hypertension treatment on cardiovascular risk: Results of the MAPEC study. *Chronobiology International, 27*(8), 1629–1651. doi: 10.3109/07420528.2010.510230

Hoerger, T., Simpson, S., Yarnoff, B., Pavkov, M., Burrows, N., Saydah, et al, (2015). The future burden of CKD in the United States: A simulation model for the CDC CKD initiative. *American Journal of Kidney Diseases. 65*(3), 403–411.

Inkler, L., Schmid, C., Tighiouart, H., Heckfeldt, J., Feldman, H., Greene, T., et al, for the CKD-EPI Investigators. (2012, July). Estimating glomerular filtration rate from serum creatinine and cystatin C. *New England Journal of Medicine, 367*, 20–29. doi: 10.1056/NEJMoa1114248

Institute for Clinical Symptoms Improvement (ICSI). (2012, Nov 30). Hypertension diagnosis and treatment.

James, P., Oparil, S., Carter, B., Cushman, W., Dennison-Himmelfarb, C., Handler, J., et al. (2014). 2014 evidence-based guideline for the management of high blood pressure in adults: Report from the panel members appointed to the eighth joint national committee (JNC-8). *Journal of the American Medical Association, 311*(5), 507–520. doi: 10.1001/jama.2013.284427

Kerby, T., Asche, S., Maciosek, M., O'Connor, P., Sperl-Hillen, J., & Margolis, K. (2012, Oct). Adherence to blood pressure telemonitoring in a cluster-randomized clinical trial. *Journal of Clinical Hypertension (Greenwich), 14*(10), 668–674. doi: 10.1111/j.1751-7176.2012.00685.x. Epub 2012 Jul 26.

Klahr, S., Levey, A., Beck, G. , Caggiula, A., Hunsicker, L., Kusek, J., et al. 1994). Modification of diet in renal disease study group. The effects of dietary protein restriction and blood pressure control on the progression of chronic renal disease. *New England Journal of Medicine, 330*(13), 877–884.

Mann, J. (2013). Overview of hypertension in acute and chronic kidney disease. In *UptoDate*. Waltham, MA: UptoDate. Retrieved from http://www.uptodate.com/contents/overview-of-hypertension-in-acute-and-chronic-kidney-disease

Mattoo, T. (2013). Evaluation of hypertension in children and adolescents. In *UpToDate*. Waltham, MA: UptoDate. Retrieved from http://www.uptodate.com/contents/evaluation-of-hypertension-in-children-and-adolescents

Miedema, M. (2014, Nov). Atherosclerosis risk in communities update. Presentation at the American Heart Association Scientific Sessions 7–11 Nov, Chicago Il.

Mitchell, B., Gutin, B., Kapuku, G., et al. (2002). Left ventricular structure and function in obese adolescents: Relations to cardiovascular fitness, percent body fat, and visceral adiposity, and effects of physical training. *Pediatrics, 109*(5), e73–e83.

Modesti, P., Morabito, M., Massetti, L., Rapi, S., Orlandini, S., Mancia, G., et al. (2013). Seasonal blood pressure changes: An independent relationship with temperature and daylight hours. *Hypertension, 61*(4), 908–914. doi 10.161/HYPERTENSIONAHA.111.00315

Mosca, L., Benjamin, E., Berra, K., Beazanson, J., Dolor, R., Lloyd-Jones, D., et al. (2011). Effectivenss-based guildelines for the presention of cardiovascular disease in women—2011 update. *Circulation, 123*(11), 1243–1262. doi 10.1151/CIR.0b013e820faaf8

Nakatani, D., Sakata, Y., Suna, S., Usami, M., Matsumoto, S., Shimizu, M., et al. Osaka Acute Coronary Insufficiency Study (OACIS) Investigators. (2013). Impact of beta blockade therapy on long-term mortality after ST-segment elevation acute myocardial infarction in the percutaneous coronary intervention era. *American Journal of Cardiology, 111*(4), 457–464. doi: 10.1016/j.amjcard.2012.10.026

National Cholesterol Education Program. (2002). Third report of the Expert Panel on Detection, Evaluation, and Treatment of High Blood Cholesterol in Adults (Adult Treatment Panel III): Final report. *Circulation, 106,* 3143–3421. Retrieved March 8, 2011, from http://www .nhlbi.nih.gov/ guidelines/cholesterol

National Heart, Lung and Blood Institute (NHLBI). (2011*). Expert Panel on integrated guidelines for cardiovascular health and risk reduction in children and adolescents summary report.* www. nhlbi.nih.gov/guidelines.current.htm

National High Blood Pressure Education Program (NHBPEP). (2003). *Seventh Report of the Joint National Committee on Prevention, Detection, Evaluation, and Treatment of High Blood Pressure* (JNC-7). Rockville, MD: National Institutes of Health; National Heart, Lung and Blood Institute.

National Kidney Foundation Guideline. (2012). Kidney Disease Outcome Quality Initiative (KDOQI): Clinical practice guidelines for diabetes and chronic kidney disease: *American Journal of Kidney Disease, 60*(5), 850–886.

Odden, M., Peralta, C., Haan, M., & Covinsky, K. (2012). Rethinking the association of high blood pressure with mortality in elderly adults: Impact of frailty. *Archives of Internal Medicine, 172*(15), 1162–1168. doi: 10.1001/ archinternmed.2012.2555

Park, G., Ramar, K., & Olson, E. (2011). Updates on definition, consequences and management of obstructive sleep apnea. *Mayo Clinic Proceedings, 86*(6), 549–555. doi 10.4065.mcp.2010.8010

Parker, E., Margolis, K., Trower, N., Magid, D., Heather, M., Tavel, H., et al. (2012). Comparative effectiveness of two beta-blockers in hypertensive patients. *Archives of Internal Medicine, 172*(18), 1406–1412. doi: 10.101/ archinternmed.2012.4276

Parving, H., Brenner, B., McMurray J., de Zeeuw, D., Haffner, S., Solomeon, S., et al. (2012). Cardiorenal endpoints in a trial of aliskiren for type 2 diabetes ALTITUDE study. *New England Journal of Medicine. 367*(23), 2204–2213. doi: 10.1056/NEJ/Moa1208799

Patel, A., Shariff, S., Bailey, G., Juurlink, D., Gandhi, S., Mamdani., M., et al. (2013, Jun 18). Statin toxicity from macrolide antibiotic coprescription: A population based cohort study. *Annals of Internal Medicine, 158*(12), 869–876.

Schembri, S., Williamson, P., Short, P., Singanayagam, A., Akram, A., Taylor, J., et al. (2013, Mar 20). Cardiovascular events after clarithromycin use in lower respiratory tract infections: Analysis of two prospective cohort studies. *British Medical Journal, 346,* f1235. doi 10.1136/bmj/f1235

Shay, C., Ning, H., Daniels, S., Rooks, C., Gidding, S., & Lloyd-Jones, D. (2013). Status of cardiovascular health in US adolescents: Prevalence estimates from the National Health and Nutrition Examination surveys (NHANES 2005–2010). *Circulation, 127*(13), 1369–1376. doi: 10.1161/ circulationaha.113.0015559

Sowers, J., & Bakris, G. (2000). Antihypertensive therapy and the risk of type 2 diabetes mellitus. *New England Journal of Medicine, 342,* 969–970.

Stafford, E., Will, K., & Brooks-Gumbert, A. (2012) Management of hypertensive urgency and emergency. *Clinician Reviews, 22*(10), 20–26.

Teo, K., Lear, S., Islam, S., Money, P., Dehghan, M., Li, W., et al. (2013). Prevalence of a healthy lifestyle among individuals with cardiovascular disease in high-, middle-, and low-income countries: The Prospective Urban Rural Epidemiology (PURE) study. *Journal of the American Medical Association, 309*(15), 1613–1621. doi: 10.1001/jama2013.3519

U.S. Preventive Services Task Force [USPSTF]. (2013). Screening for primary hypertension in children and adolescents. *Pediatrics, 132*(5), 907–914.

Van Rinjinsoever, E., Kwee-Zuiderwijk, W., & Feenstra, J. (1998). Angioneurotic edema attributed to the use of losartan. *Archives of Internal Medicine, 158,* 2063–2065.

Weber, M., Jamerson, K., Bakris, G., Weir, M., Zappe, D., Zhang,Y., et al. (2013). Effects of body size and hypertension treatments on cardiovascular event rates: Subanalysis of the ACCOMPLISH randomized controlled trial. *The Lancet, 381*(9866), 537–545. doi: org/10.1016/S0140-6736 (12)61343-9

World Health Report. (2012, May). New data highlight increases in hypertension, diabetes incidence. Geneva, Switzerland: World Health Organization.

Wright, B., Rutecki, G., & Bellone, J. (2013). Resistant hypertension: An approach to diagnosis and treatment. *Consultant, 53*(1), 9–18.

Wright, J., Jr., Probstfield, J., Cushman, W., Pressel, S., Cutler, J., Davis, B., et al. for the ALLHAT Collaborative Research Group. (2009). ALLHAT findings revisited in the context of subsequent analyses, other trials, and meta-analyses. *Archives of Internal Medicine, 169*(9), 832–842.

Wu, S., Han, J., Li, W-Q., & Qureshi, A., (2014). Hypertension, antihypertensive medication use and risk of psoriasis. *Journal of the American Medical Association. 154*(9), 957–963.

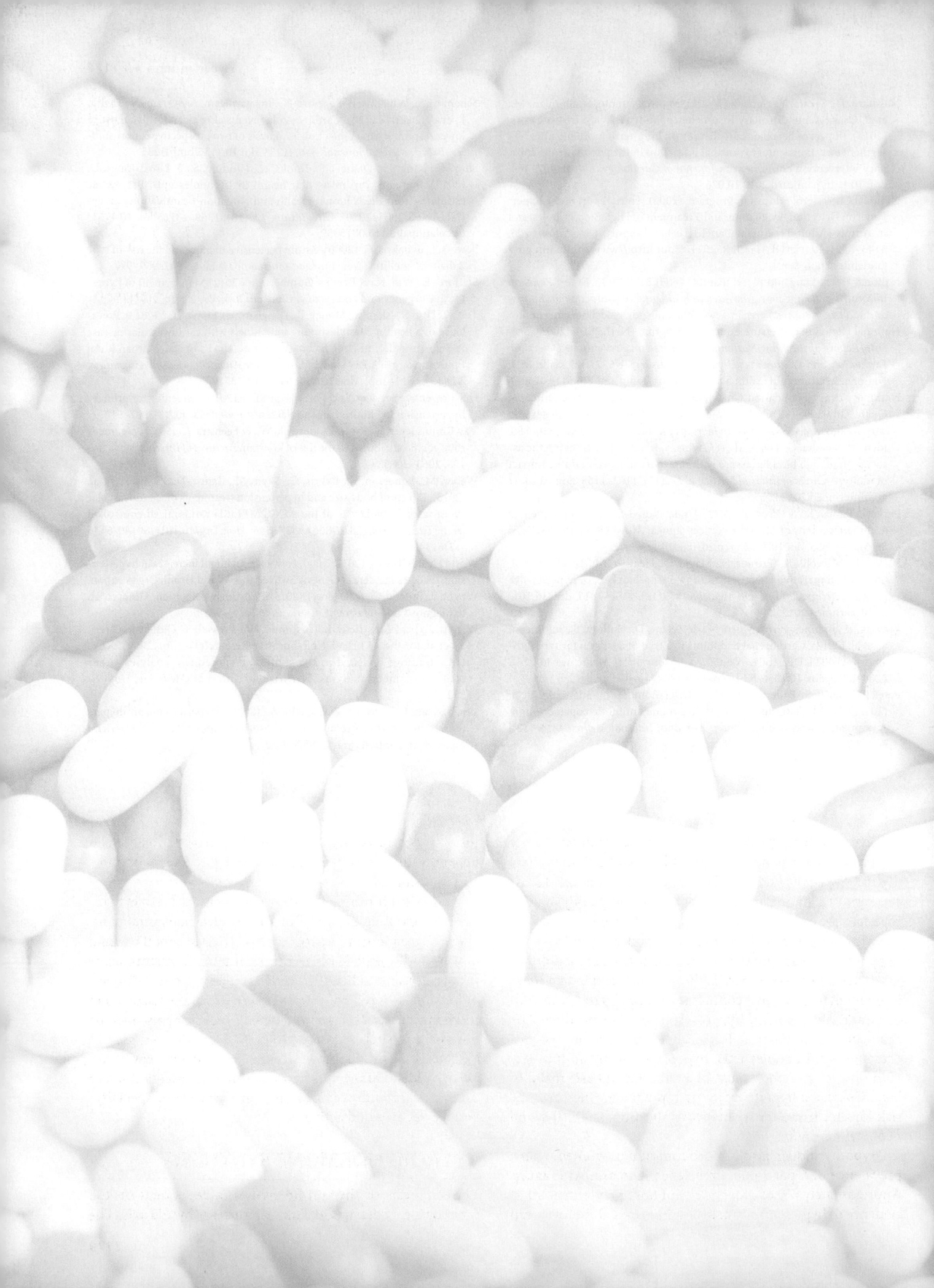

CHAPTER 41

HYPERTHYROIDISM AND HYPOTHYROIDISM

Marylou V. Robinson

Thyroid disorders are among the most common disease processes seen in primary care. About 5% of U.S. adults have thyroid disease or take thyroid drugs. Untreated thyroid disease can result in long-term complications in every body system, especially the cardiovascular system. Most thyroid disorders involve thyroid gland malfunction, but secondary hypothyroid or hyperthyroid issues can stem from pituitary axis interruptions.

Hyperthyroidism is seen in 2% of women and in one-tenth as many men. It is most common from age 20 to 40. In children and older adults, hyperthyroidism can produce cardiomegaly and heart failure. Elders are also at risk for osteoporosis. In adolescents, hyperthyroidism can interfere with normal growth because of alterations in basic metabolism. Untreated hyperthyroidism in pregnancy increases the risk for first-trimester spontaneous abortion, stillbirths, and neonatal mortality.

Hypothyroidism also is more common in women, with a prevalence of 6 per 1,000. Prevalence increases with aging. Approximately 5% of older adults of both genders manifest evidence of hypothyroidism. In children, hypothyroidism can result in decreased mental and physical growth. In adults, it increases the risk for heart disease related to altered lipoprotein metabolism.

Treatment for these two disorders includes lifestyle management and drug therapy. Pharmacological management includes thyroid hormones to treat hypothyroid conditions and antithyroid agents such as propylthiouracil, methimazole (Tapazole), and radioactive iodine (I^{131}) or strong iodine solutions for hyperthyroid states. These drugs are discussed in detail in Chapter 21. Symptom management may also include other drugs, such as beta blockers, which are discussed in Chapter 14. This chapter discusses the management of hyperthyroidism and hypothyroidism that is usually done in primary care and provides only an overview of specialty-based directives and activities.

THYROID HORMONE SYNTHESIS

The synthesis of thyroid hormones is dependent on the functioning of the hypothalamic-pituitary-thyroid axis. The secretion of thyrotropin-releasing hormone (TRH) by the hypothalamus in response to cold, stress, and decreased levels of thyroxine (T4) stimulates the synthesis of thyroid-stimulating hormone (TSH) by the anterior pituitary. TSH, in turn, stimulates the thyroid gland to produce thyroid hormones. Thyroid hormones (T4 and triiodothyronine [T3]) are synthesized from iodine and tyrosine molecules by follicular cells in the thyroid gland.

Dietary iodine of about 100 to 150 mcg/d is required for normal thyroid hormone production. In the United States, adequate iodine is found in foodstuffs and in iodized salt. In the past 20 years, food manufacturers have switched to more noniodized salt in frozen meals and bread products. Per the National Health and Nutrition Examination Survey (NHANES) 2007–2008, U.S. average consumption is still adequate; however, 8.8% of the population has moderate to severe iodine deficiency, including an estimated 14.6% of women of reproductive age, especially non-Hispanic black women (Caldwell, Miller, Wang, Jain, & Jones, 2008).

Dietary iodine absorbed from the gastrointestinal tract is carried in the blood as iodide. When it reaches the thyroid gland, it is actively taken up by the iodide pump, located at the base of the thyroid follicles. The iodide pump is controlled by the serum iodide concentration; low concentration increases pump activity and high concentration inhibits it. The iodide is then oxidized within seconds by the thyroid peroxidase enzyme and binds to tyrosine residues in thyroglobin to form monoiodotyrosine and diiodotyrosine. The coupling of these two iodides forms T4 or T3, which is then stored in the thyroglobin.

The thyroid gland mainly produces T4. About 20% of T3 is synthesized and released from the thyroid gland. The remainder is converted from T4 to T3 peripherally when additional thyroid hormone is needed. Conversion of T4 to T3 is stimulated by cold temperatures and stress. Conversion is inhibited by acute and chronic illness, starvation, and some drugs (Table 41-1). Practitioners must, therefore, consider the role of medications, stress, and other disease states when evaluating patients with newly diagnosed thyroid imbalances. T4 and T3 in plasma are reversibly bound to protein, mainly thyroxine-binding globulin. Only a small portion (0.04% of total T4 and 0.4% of total T3) exists in a free form; however, only this free form is clinically active. The amount of active thyroid hormone in the plasma produces a feedback loop that inhibits or further stimulates TRH and TSH secretion to decrease or increase thyroid hormone production.

THYROID FUNCTION TESTS

Several tests can be used to evaluate thyroid function. These tests and their normal values are listed in Table 41-2. The most commonly used tests in primary care are TSH and free T4 values. Serum TSH measurement is the single most reliable test to diagnose the common forms of hypothyroidism and hyperthyroidism. The sensitive or ultrasensitive forms of the TSH test should be used to avoid missing subclinical conditions. Subclinical conditions exist when TSH is normal but free thyroxine (FT4) and free triiodothyronine (FT3) are abnormal. The growing recognition of circadian changes in TSH release have not yet generated normal values based on the time of day for lab testing purposes (LaFranchi, 2012).

Altered serum TSH confirms the diagnosis in all patients with primary hypo- or hyperthyroidism, but it will not reliably identify all hypothyroid patients with secondary (central)

Table 41–1 Drug Effects on Thyroid Function

Drug	Effect on Thyroid Function
Amiodarone	• Releases iodine as drug is metabolized • Inhibits peripheral conversion of T4 to T3 • Can produce thyrotoxicosis in previously euthyroid patients • Can produce hypothyroidism in auto-immune patients
Carbamazepine	Increases metabolism of T4, resulting in decreased total T4
Estrogen	Increases thyroid-binding globulin levels
Glucocorticoids	Impair basal and TRH-stimulated TSH concentration
Levodopa	Chronic administration displaces thyroid hormone from thyroid-binding globulin, resulting in suppressed TSH response
Lithium	Blocks iodine uptake by thyroid gland, resulting in decreased hormone production
Phenytoin	• Decreases TSH response to TRH by 50% • Enhances cellular uptake and metabolism of T4, resulting in decreased total T4
Propranolol	Inhibits peripheral conversion of T4 to T3
Salicylates (in doses >4 g/d)	Suppress TSH response by inhibiting binding of T4 and T3 to thyroid-binding globulin
Theophylline	Beta-adrenergic stimulation of hypothalamus results in increased TSH response
Tyrosine kinase inhibitors	Suppress thyroid function

TRH = thyroid-releasing hormone; TSH = thyroid-stimulating hormone.

Table 41–2   Adult Thyroid Function Tests

Test	Normal Value	Values in Hyperthyroidism	Values in Hypothyroidism
Free thyroxine index (FT4I)	1.3–4.2	High	Low
Free triiodothyronine index (FT3I)	22–56	High	Normal or low
Free T4 (FT4)	0.7–1.86 ng/dL (9–24 pmol/L)	High	Low
Free T3 (FT3)	0.2–0.52 ng/dL (3–8 pmol/L)	High	Low
Thyrotropin-stimulating hormone (TSH)	0.3–5 microUnits/mL	Low	High
Thyrotropin-releasing hormone (TRH)	>6 microUnits/mL in serum TSH 45 min after injection; blunted TSH response (<2 microUnits/mL) in patients >40 yr	No response	Low exaggerated rise

disturbances wherein TSH values may be atypically low, normal, or elevated. When pituitary or hypothalamic disease is suspected as the cause of hypothyroidism, FT4 concentrations should be measured in addition to TSH. When less-sensitive TSH tests are the only ones available, FT4 and FT3 measurement can give additional information to validate the TSH (Garber et al, 2012).

Adult values should not be used to monitor children. Recommended pediatric target values for TSH range from 0.5 to 2.0 mUL and for T4 they range from 9 to 13 μg/dL (LaFranchi, 2012). Age variances are available from clinical labs; therefore, the practitioner is directed to the local laboratory reference values to evaluate pediatric patients.

Abnormal results from other laboratory tests may also suggest hypo- or hyperthyroidism. Hypercholesterolemia, hyponatremia, anemia, elevated creatinine kinase and lactate dehydrogenase, and hyperprolactinemia all suggest possible hypothyroidism. Elevated calcium, alkaline phosphatase, and/or hepatocellular enzymes suggest hyperthyroidism. These laboratory findings justify thyroid function tests, especially if they are sustained for 2 weeks or more, occur in combination, or occur in patients with increased risk for thyroid disease (Bahn et al, 2011; Garber et al, 2012).

Thyroid abnormalities can present with the development of enlarging thyroid tissues called goiters. This tissue growth may be euthyroid (normal functioning), collections of sub-functioning tissue, or focal cellular growths (nodules) that may produce excess amounts of thyroid hormone. The trigger for excess growth may be autoimmune processes or abnormal cellular disturbances. Goiter size or presence of palpable nodules does not correlate with underlying function. Moreover, abnormalities can exist without goiter presence. Generally, the work-up for a goiter will include serum thyroid antibody screens and a baseline ultrasound. Calling the endocrinology team and requesting which exact tests are required before the initial consultation will preclude unnecessary repetition of blood draws.

Suspicion of cancer or determining whether nodules are "hot" or "cold" in terms of production of excess hormone is confirmed with thyroid scanning. The radioisotope I[123] dose and residual radiation levels used for these tests does not

trigger the same precautions linked with I[131] used to treat hyperthyroidism. In cases that are not urgent, individuals previously on levothyroxine may be switched to liothyronine to deplete the organ of hormone for 2 to 6 weeks prior to the scan. Ideally, the person stops all hormones for the last 2 weeks in order to facilitate the iodine uptake capacity of the thyroid. A synthetic hormone, thyrotropin alpha (Thyrogen), can be given to lessen hypothyroid-like symptoms of hormone withdrawal. Thyrogen does not interfere with iodine uptake but might cause false-negative results in some individuals compared to the earlier standard practice of inducing a short-term hypothyroid state (New York Thyroid Center, 2011). Timing of scans and dosing of medications should be coordinated with the endocrinology team.

SCREENING

The U.S. Preventive Services Task Force (2010–2011) found that the evidence is insufficient to recommend for or against routine screening for thyroid disease in adults. Testing can detect subclinical thyroid disease in people without symptoms of thyroid dysfunction, but the evidence is poor that treating these individuals changes their health status. Screening high-risk groups such as postpartum women, people with Down syndrome, and older adults is more likely to find subclinical disease, but the progression of subclinical thyroid disease to overt disease in patients without a history of prior thyroid issues is not clearly established.

Subclinical hypothyroidism is associated with poor obstetrical outcomes and poor cognitive development in children; nonetheless, the American College of Obstetricians and Gynecologists (ACOG, 2007, reaffirmed 2010), the American Thyroid Association (ATA), and the American Association of Clinical Endocrinologists (Garber et al, 2012) all state that screening tests in asymptomatic pregnant women is not warranted. TSH measurement before pregnancy in women of childbearing age with known thyroid disease is recommended.

No thyroid function tests should be performed unless disease is suspected by the presence of symptoms or suspicion of undiagnosed disease, including in the elderly, those with new cardiovascular or mental health issues, and extreme fatigue. Asymptomatic patients should not be screened unless they fall into specific risk groups. In pediatrics, those with failure to thrive or accelerating behavioral or growth issues should be screened.

TSH is suppressed in the critically ill patient, so values obtained in the hospital are not reliable for screening. Also, values for post-acute care patients can spike for a few months during recovery. Anorexic patients may have thyroid gland involution, so their TSH values are also at risk for unreliable diagnosis (Garber et al, 2012). Previously euthyroid patients started on amiodarone will typically have a fluctuations in thyroid levels for 3 to 6 months without overt symptoms. These alterations usually return to normal except in individuals with prior autoimmune diseases who require closer monitoring for a more sustained hyperthyroid condition. These fluctuations should not be considered for treatment unless symptomatic just like other causes of subclinical changes. Do not stop the amiodarone.

HYPERTHYROIDISM

Pathophysiology

Thyrotoxicosis, or hyperthyroidism, occurs when the feedback loop fails and excessive levels of thyroid hormone are circulating. Extreme thyrotoxicosis is called thyroid storm, a life-threatening condition beyond the scope of this text. The cause of excessive secretion may be a hyperfunctioning thyroid nodule, toxic diffuse goiter (Graves' disease), anterior pituitary disorders, toxic multinodular goiter, excess thyroid supplementation, or iodine-induced disease, including amiodarone therapy (Bahn et al, 2011). Identifiable risk factors for hyperthyroid dysfunction include diabetes mellitus, pernicious anemia, primary adrenal insufficiency, vitiligo, leukotrichia (prematurely gray hair), and drugs or compounds that contain iodine or affect iodine metabolism. Viruses and pregnancy are two of many conditions that can trigger thyroiditis.

By far, the most common hyperthyroid etiology (60% to 90% of all cases) is Graves' disease. Graves' disease is an autoimmune disorder characterized by generation of abnormal immunoglobulin G (IgG) autoantibodies to thyroid peroxidase and thyroglobulin. The antibodies bind to the TSH receptors, activating excessive glandular growth and hormone production. Normally, any hyperfunction of the thyroid gland would lead to suppression of TSH and TRH; however, in autoimmune conditions, the feedback system is altered.

The hyperfunction of the thyroid gland with Graves' disease results in a dramatic increase in iodine uptake and subsequent systemic metabolism. The thyroid gland becomes more vascular and enlarges, forming a goiter. A disproportionate increase in T3 production is a hallmark of longer-term overstimulation of the gland. The overproduction leads to a decreased concentration of thyroid-binding globulin and increased circulating levels of free hormone. These hormone levels are responsible for the many thyrotoxic symptoms.

The clinical features of hyperthyroidism are attributable to metabolic effects of increased circulating hormone. Typical effects include heat intolerance and heightened sensitivity to sympathetic nervous system stimulation. Table 41-3 shows the most common systemic effects of hyperthyroidism. Treatment goals are to diminish negative cardiovascular effects while returning the patient to a euthyroid state.

Ophthalmopathy

Many patients with Graves' disease experience ocular symptoms. These symptoms include functional abnormalities

Table 41–3 Systemic Effects of Hyperthyroidism

Body System	Clinical Manifestation	Underlying Mechanism
Cardiovascular	Increased cardiac output, decreased peripheral vascular resistance, tachycardia at rest, arrhythmias	Increased metabolism and need to dissipate heat
Respiratory	Dyspnea and reduced vital capacity	Weakness of respiratory muscles
Gastrointestinal	• Increased appetite with concurrent weight loss	Increased utilization of carbohydrates, proteins, and fats to support rapid metabolism
	• Diarrhea, nausea, vomiting, abdominal pain	Increased peristalsis and cholesterol conversion salts
	• Decreased serum lipid levels	Malabsorption of fat, fat stores depleted for energy, increased excretion of cholesterol in feces
	• Decreased tissue stores of glucose, protein, and vitamins	Increased glucose utilization, use of protein as energy source, and impaired conversion of B vitamins to their coenzymes, causing an increased need for water- and fat-soluble vitamins
Integumentary	• Excessive sweating, flushing, warm skin	Need to dissipate heat
	• Temporary hair loss; hair fine, soft, and straight; nails grow away from nail beds	Hyperdynamic circulatory state
Reproductive	Oligomenorrhea or amenorrhea in women; impotence or decreased libido in men	Hypothalamic or pituitary disturbances; increased production of sex hormone–binding globulin

Table 41–3   Systemic Effects of Hyperthyroidism—cont'd

Body System	Clinical Manifestation	Underlying Mechanism
Neurological	• Restlessness, short attention span, fatigue, insomnia, emotional lability	Alteration in cerebral metabolism
	• Ocular manifestations, including decreased blinking and fine tremor of the lid	Hyperactivity of sympathetic nervous system
Musculoskeletal	• Hypercalcemia	Excessive bone resorption
	• Loss of muscle mass	Excessive protein catabolism
Endocrine	• Enlarged gland; systolic or continuous bruit of thyroid gland	Hyperactivity of the gland and increased circulation to support that hyperactivity
	• Diminished sensitivity to exogenous insulin	Increased insulin degradation

(e.g., lid lag with upward or downward gaze) related to hyperactivity of the sympathetic nervous system (McCance & Huether, 2014). Other changes involve orbital and periorbital edema and altered fat deposition. More than half of adult Graves' disease patients develop the characteristic wide-eyed stare with protrusion of the globe (exophthalmus). These ocular concerns can exist in tandem. The provider must recognize that the absence of classic exophthalmus does not negate the need for ophthalmological consultation. Ocular changes can result in damage to the cornea, the retina, and optic nerve, any of which may lead to blindness (McCance & Huether, 2015).

Thyroid-related eye issues are caused by a mechanism different from the one that causes hyperthyroidism. Twenty percent of patients with eye involvement that predates the treatment of their hyperthyroidism experience an exacerbation after treatment is initiated. Successful treatment of hyperthyroidism does not necessarily improve eye conditions, but treatment-induced hypothyroidism increases the risk for worsening the eye disorders. Radioactive iodine has the highest risk for post-treatment hypothyroidism, with up to 50% of patients becoming hypothyroid. Antithyroid drugs are much less likely to result in post-treatment hypothyroidism and are often chosen in preference to radiation for patients with ophthalmopathy (Ross, 2012). Patients are also advised to wear sunglasses, use artificial tears, elevate the head of their bed, and use corneal protectors for severe exophthalmos when sleeping. Bedtime diuretics may also be prescribed (Bahn et al, 2011). Consultation with an ophthalmologist experienced in the treatment of orbital disease is required in the management of these cases, because extensive testing, including orbital ultrasonography, CT scanning, or MRI imaging may be necessary. Treatment may include corticosteroids, retro-orbital irradiation, or surgical intervention.

Myxedema

A small number of patients with Graves' disease experience pretibial myxedema (Graves' dermopathy), characterized by subcutaneous swelling of the anterior portions of the leg and in the hands, with bumpy, erythematous skin. This puts skin integrity at risk. This form of myxedema is not synonymous with myxedema coma from profound hypothyroidism.

Pharmacodynamics

Antithyroid drugs reduce the production of thyroid hormones. Propylthiouracil and methimazole inhibit the synthesis of new thyroid hormone by the thyroid gland but do not inactivate existing or stored hormone. Propylthiouracil also inhibits the peripheral conversion of T4 to T3. Neither of these drugs treats the underlying pathophysiology of hyperthyroidism. Resumption of hormone synthesis occurs quickly after these drugs are withdrawn, because iodine is no longer blocked from use.

A treatment typically requires 6 to 12 months for total reversal of hyperthyroid symptoms. Some authorities advocate high-dose therapy; others favor low doses. Relapse rates are higher in those taking lower doses. Higher doses increase the probabilities for development of post-treatment hypothyroidism. This sequela may not surface for several years. Dosing is covered in Chapter 21.

Trials have shown no clinical outcome differences when methimazole is compared with propylthiouracil; however, the concerns of hepatic toxicity with propylthiouracil have resulted in a withdrawal of the indication for use in children and for those with hepatic issues (U.S. Food and Drug Administration [FDA], 2009, 2010). Methimazole should be preferentially used in almost all cases. Adherence is significantly better for patients on methimazole owing to its once-daily dosing schedule.

Beta blockers address the symptoms of hyperthyroidism by decreasing the response to sympathetic stimulation and are used as adjunct therapy to control uncomfortable or unhealthy tachycardia. Low doses are all that are typically needed, with early-onset symptom management evident. The most commonly prescribed drugs in this class are propranolol, because of its short half-life, and atenolol, because of its once-daily dosing. Patients with unstable hypoglycemia and severe reactive airways dependent on rescue inhalers may do better on the cardio-selective beta blockers such as atenolol. These drugs are gradually withdrawn as the patient becomes euthyroid.

Iodides block peripheral conversion of T4 to T3 and inhibit hormone release. Potassium iodine is mainly used for preoperative preparation before thyroid surgery. Not only are the levels of circulating hormone reduced but the vascularity of the tissue is also lessened. Dilution in fruit juices can make iodides more palatable and protect the teeth from discoloration. Administration with meals minimizes GI irritation.

Goals of Treatment

The goal of therapy for adult patients with hyperthyroidism is correction of the hypermetabolic state, with a minimum of adverse reactions and with the smallest incidence of resultant hypothyroidism. This means symptom relief and normalization of TSH and FT4 levels. Beta blockers can reduce symptomatic effects in the short term, but definitive therapy usually requires at least the addition of an antithyroid agent or surgery.

Rational Drug Selection

Three main avenues of treatment are used for patients with hyperthyroidism: (1) antithyroid drugs, (2) radioactive iodine, and (3) surgery. Radioactive iodine and the antithyroid drugs are also discussed in Chapter 21. Iodides are sometimes useful as supplemental suppressive drugs or for individuals who refuse I[131] or cannot tolerate surgery. Presurgical use of iodides is indicated for those with cardiovascular compromise or for the elderly. Such use also decreases the immediate post-operative spike in hyperthyroid symptomatology experienced by many.

Lifestyle Management

Lifestyle management is primarily related to diet. The thyroid gland requires adequate amounts of iodine to produce thyroid hormones. Patients should be taught how to recognize iodine sources in their diets. These include iodized salt; seafood products, especially shellfish; and seaweed or kelp. The labels of vitamin supplements that have minerals and many over-the-counter (OTC) cold medications, especially cough syrups, should be screened for iodine.

The potential for nutritional deficits is the major concern, related to the hypermetabolic state. A high-calorie (4,000 to 5,000 kcal/d) diet may be necessary to satisfy hunger and prevent tissue breakdown. To provide this number of calories, six meals a day may be required, as well as snacks that are high in protein; carbohydrates; minerals; and vitamins, particularly vitamins A and B$_6$ and ascorbic acid. Caffeinated fluids and highly seasoned food should be avoided because they augment the tachycardia and hot flushing symptoms of hyperthyroidism. Because hyperthyroid states deplete bone calcium, supplementation is advised to reduce the risk of osteopenia. Children will require caloric-dense foods to maintain weight.

Other lifestyle concerns include providing adequate rest and avoiding external sources of stress, including work, domestic issues, and undue worry. Circulating catecholamines have more intensive cardiovascular effects in the presence of excessive thyroid hormone. Risks for triggering angina and dysrhythmias are heightened. Insomnia is made worse by any heat intolerance or sweating. Relaxation therapy and yoga are potentially helpful interventions. Climate control, especially during hot weather, can reduce the burden of feeling hot.

Drug Therapy

Choices in drug therapy are based on patient variables (severity of the disease, duration of the disease, age of the patient, pregnancy, and the likelihood of patient adherence to the treatment regimen) and on drug-related variables. Figure 41-1 depicts some drug choices based on these variables.

The Institute for Safe Medication Practices (2008) has issued an alert not to use the abbreviation PTU for propylthiouracil on prescription forms. The abbreviation has led to fatal confusion with the brand-name drug Purinethol (mercaptopurine), which is used for oncology patients.

Preoperative Preparation

Primary care providers should coordinate dosing and tapering schedules of any thyroid drugs with the endocrine and surgical teams. Preoperative administration of antithyroid drugs is common to avoid precipitating post-operative thyroid storm. The addition of potassium iodide to beta blocker therapy produces more rapid and greater pre-operative control. This combination is especially useful for patients who must undergo surgery fairly quickly and for those who fail to achieve control (resting pulse less than 90 beats/min) on beta blockers alone. The iodide dose is mixed in a full glass of fruit juice, water, broth, or milk 3 times a day for 10 days pre-op.

Patient Variables

Severity of Disease

Antithyroid drugs are prescribed with the intent of achieving spontaneous remission of the disease. Patients most likely to achieve remission are those with mild disease and small goiters (Bahn et al, 2011). Methimazole is the initial drug of choice because of the hepatic risks of propylthiouracil (FDA, 2010), its faster action, and reduced interference with I[131] therapy (Bahn et al, 2011). Because these drugs do not inhibit the action of existing or stored thyroid hormone, full clinical response typically takes 4 to 8 weeks with either drug.

Adult patients with severe disease may require 400 mg daily of propylthiouracil (maintenance doses are typically 100 to 150 mg daily). Methimazole is similarly initiated at the higher doses as well. One advantage to methimazole is that doses may be divided and given every 8 hours if not well tolerated or once-daily dosing may be tried. Pediatric patients receive 0.25 to 1 mg/kg/day of methimazole. If methimazole cannot be taken or is ineffective, then propylthiouracil is dosed at 0.25mg/kg/day.

Once control of symptoms and appropriate levels of thyroid hormone production are achieved, the doses of both drugs can be tapered to the lowest amount needed to maintain a euthyroid state. Treatment is continued for 12 to 24 months and then stopped to see if a relapse occurs. Relapse is more common for patients treated less than 12 months. Patients who fail to achieve control of symptoms with antithyroid drugs,

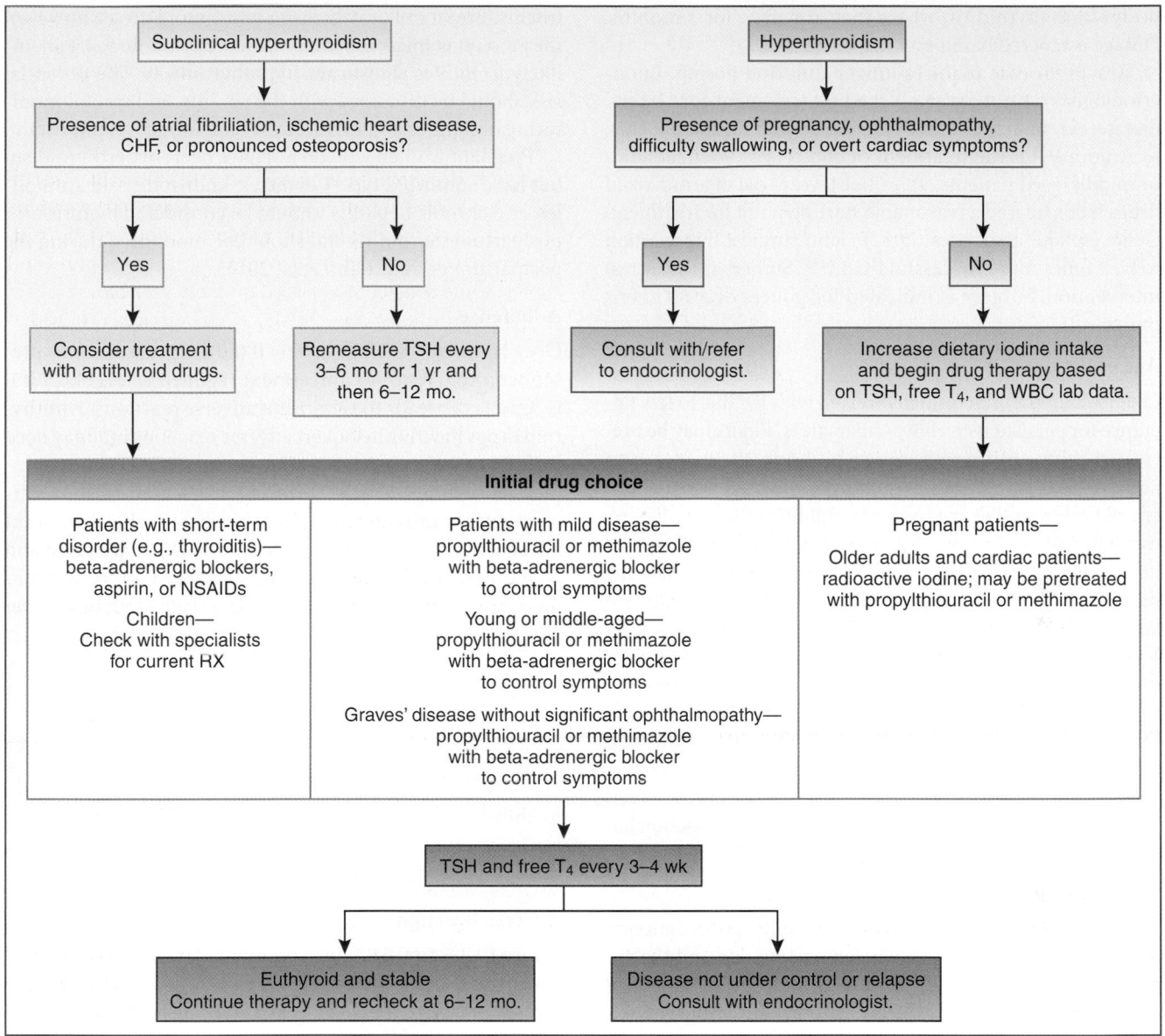

Figure 41–1. Drug therapy algorithm: Hyperthyroidism.

who are unable to tolerate the therapy, or who experience a relapse after completion of therapy are candidates for radioactive iodine or surgery.

In severe thyrotoxic states, adjuvant treatment with iodides may be needed. Excess iodine limits the activity of thyroid peroxidase, thus decreasing iodide oxidation and rapidly blocking the release of T3 and T4 from the thyroid. Patients with Graves' disease are more sensitive to the inhibitory effects of iodine than are healthy individuals. The inhibitory effects of iodides, however, are short-term in some individuals. Potassium iodide is given orally as Lugol's solution (8 mg/drop) or as saturated solution of potassium iodide (SSKI; 35 to 50 mg/drop). The dose of Lugol's solution is 3 to 5 drops, and for SSKI it is 1 drop, both given 3 times a day.

Duration of Disease

Beta blockers without concurrent thioamides provide excellent symptomatic relief for transient disorders (e.g., thyroiditis)

because spontaneous remission is the rule. Atenolol offers the advantages of fewer adverse reactions, based on its beta₁ selectivity and once-daily dosing for patients who are less adherent if the regimen is too complex. Propranolol offers the advantage of peripheral blockage of T4 conversion to T3.

Some patients with long-standing hyperthyroidism may be relatively resistant to the effects of beta blockers, so larger and more frequent doses may be necessary. Propranolol is the drug most widely used, with the usual starting dose at 80 to 160 mg/d. Larger doses (360 to 480 mg/d) are sometimes necessary. Adequate doses of these drugs are determined by measuring resting and exercising heart rates and degree of symptom relief. These drugs can be tapered and discontinued once the patient is no longer symptomatic.

Aspirin, NSAIDs, and corticosteroids are also used in subacute thyroiditis to control inflammatory symptoms. Steroids inhibit conversion of T4 to T3, but consistent evidence of any therapeutic help is lacking. These drugs are equally useful for postpartum thyroiditis, where they are given for 3 months. Dosage is tapered based on symptom relief.

Graves' disease requires longer-duration dosing. Endocrinologists do not agree on the best treatment for Graves' disease, except in the case of older adults and cardiac patients, for whom I^{131} is the treatment of choice. For younger adult or middle-aged patients, an initial 1-year trial of antithyroid drugs is considered a reasonable starting point for treatment. Genovese and associates (2012) claim surgical intervention to be 3 times more successful than I^{131}. Surgery is the fastest intervention. Surgery is indicated for goiters over 80 grams in size.

Age of Patient

Older adults are preferentially treated with I^{131} due to less tolerance for persistent cardiovascular stress. Elders may be pretreated with antithyroid drugs to bring them closer to euthyroid status before I^{131} therapy is initiated. Most endocrinologists prefer drug therapy in childhood Graves' disease, waiting until age 10 for I^{131} therapy. Propylthiouracil-related hepatic toxicity has triggered the recommendation that only methimazole be used in pediatrics (FDA, 2009). Treatment lasts 6 to 18 months; most patients are treated for at least 1 year. As with adults, relapse is less likely with the longer duration of therapy. A major difference is that pediatric specialists prefer treating to a full hypothyroid state to avoid the potential toxicity of needing an additional antithyroid course of medication in the future and a potential for a lower risk for subsequent thyroid tumors (Rivkees & Dinauer, 2007). This desire for full suppression of thyroid function has driven the increased use of I^{131} therapy in children.

Pregnancy

Hyperthyroidism during pregnancy presents special concerns best managed collaboratively by an obstetrician and the endocrinology team. Antithyroid drugs are the treatment of choice but are Pregnancy Category D. Methimazole is lipid-soluble and not protein bound, so it freely crosses the placenta and breast epithelium and is associated with birth defects when used in the first trimester (FDA, 2010). Propylthiouracil, conversely, is 80% to 90% protein bound and ionized at physiological pH. Although it can cause fetal harm, it is preferred in pregnant women because its pharmacokinetics make it less likely to cross the placenta. The lowest possible dose is used to keep the mother's thyroid function at the upper limit of normal. Pregnancy itself has an ameliorating effect on Graves' disease, so the dose of the drug required usually decreases as the pregnancy progresses. In some cases, the drug can be withdrawn 2 to 3 weeks before delivery if laboratory values indicate improved functioning.

Pregnant women with Graves' disease may transfer large amounts of thyroid-stimulating antibody to the fetus and induce fetal thyrotoxicosis. The infant's pediatric provider should be informed of the mother's hyperthyroidism and treatment of this disorder during pregnancy. The infant's thyroid function should be tested at birth.

Postpartum patients who are receiving thioamides should consult their child's provider before choosing to nurse their infants. Breast milk can transfer antithyroid drugs; however, the amount is small, especially with propylthiouracil, and unlikely to induce significant hypothyroidism. The potential risk should be discussed with the parents, and careful monitoring of mother and infant for several months is important.

Pregnant women who do not have overt hyperthyroidism but have comorbid type 1 diabetes, known thyroid antibodies, and chronic hepatitis, should be considered high risk for postpartum thyroiditis and should be monitored during the postpartum period (Bahn et al, 2011).

Adherence

Drug treatment is effective only if the drugs are taken as prescribed. Adherence to a treatment regimen is less likely if it is complex or leads to significant adverse reactions. Antithyroid drugs have limited overt adverse reactions but may need to be taken 3 times daily, making the treatment regimen complex. This complexity is especially problematic if the treatment regimen also involves a beta blocker that has significant adverse reactions and must also be taken 3 times daily, but on a different schedule. To facilitate adherence, both methimazole and atenolol can be given once daily. Both have fewer adverse reactions than other drugs in their classes.

Drug-Related Variables

Cost

The actual retail price of the thioamides can vary significantly. Propylthiouracil prices are typically affordable, but methimazole is one-third lower in price. Therapy extends for weeks or months. I^{131} therapy is more expensive than drug therapy but lower in cost than surgery.

Adverse Reactions

A rare (0.3% to 0.6%) but potentially fatal complication of antithyroid drug therapy is agranulocytosis. The risk increases with age, beginning at about age 40, and is dose-independent for propylthiouracil and dose-dependent for methimazole. Patients taking less than 30 mg/d of methimazole typically do not experience this adverse reaction, making it the safer of the two drugs. The propylthiouracil hepatic concerns also make methimazole a safer alternative for all age groups, especially those with polypharmacy.

Monitoring

Monitoring therapy includes attention to clinical status and thyroid function test results. Clinical status is assessed by watching weight, degree of heat tolerance, appetite, anxiety level, energy level, resting heart rate, and skin texture and temperature. For patients with ophthalmopathy, assessment also includes changes in visual acuity, increasing corneal dryness, and adherence to suggestions such as use of sunglasses. Ophthalmic appointments should be scheduled frequently to monitor for complications that can include cataract development, corneal scarring, and retinal detachments.

The same tests that are used to diagnose hyperthyroidism are used to monitor the effectiveness of treatment. The amount of circulating thyroid hormone is monitored by changes in TSH and free T4. Initially, patients are seen every 3 to 4 weeks, with levels drawn until the patients are euthyroid. TSH may remain low for several weeks after actual euthyroid status is achieved. Once normal, the frequency of visits decreases, with testing of TSH only, and clinical evaluation is done at 3 and 6 months and then annually, based on symptom relief (Bahn et al, 2011). TSH provides the earliest evidence of overtreatment or development of hypothyroidism.

Pregnant patients are usually monitored at each visit because the progression of pregnancy is associated with altered thyroid hormone production. Dosage adjustments are commonly required. Pregnant patients with Graves' disease may have thyroid-stimulating antibodies in their circulation that can cross the placenta and affect the fetus. Measurement of maternal thyroid-stimulating antibody may be useful to assess potential fetal risk.

Though routine monitoring of white blood cell (WBC) counts is not necessary, it is important during the first 4 months of thioamide therapy, especially in those over age 40 with any febrile illness (Bahn et al, 2011). Mild leukopenia is common but does not require discontinuance of the drug. Leukocyte counts below 1,500 mm³ are indications for stopping therapy. Agranulocytosis usually occurs within 2 months and rarely beyond 4 months after initiation of therapy. Onset is rapid, so it is prudent to obtain a baseline WBC count before initiating therapy.

Special monitoring for I¹³¹ patients is not indicated. Half of the dose is gone in a week. After 2 months only 1% remains in the body. Long-term effects do not appear to include localized, or distant, cancers related to the radiation exposure (Sisson, et al, 2011), even in children (Rivkees & Dinaur, 2007).

Outcome Evaluation

Figure 41-1 shows the drug treatment protocol for hyperthyroidism. Evaluation is based on reduction of clinical symptoms and normalization of TSH and free T4 levels. The main indications for substituting surgery or I¹³¹ are a patient's failure to achieve control of symptoms with antithyroid drugs, an inability to tolerate the therapy, and relapse after completion of therapy. Having persistently high antibody titers after discontinuation of an antithyroid drug is predictive of relapse. Postmenopausal women should be screened for any associated bone loss.

Consultation with or referral is appropriate when:

1. Patients require surgery or I¹³¹
2. Hyperthyroidism occurs during pregnancy and lactation or when those on antithyroid drugs become pregnant
3. Patients develop ophthalmopathy or visual impairment
4. Patients have an obstruction to swallowing or desire post-treatment cosmetic improvement
5. Patients with heart failure, rapid atrial fibrillation, or angina need a cardiology consultation

Patient Education

Patient education should include discussion of information related to the overall treatment plan, as well as that specific to the drug therapy. Understanding the reasons for taking the drug, the expected duration of therapy, and anticipated side effects can help with adherence issues. Patients need to anticipate weight gain if they do not adjust diets to a normal metabolic rate. They should have lifelong monitoring of thyroid function.

Patients receiving I¹³¹ should be instructed on dietary and OTC sources of iodine, such as multivitamins with minerals and cough syrups. They require education that reduced levels of iodine before scans and treatments facilitate better I¹³¹ uptake. Patients should delay return to work and limit use of public transportation for a day to limit radiation exposure of others. In the home and at work, individuals are instructed to keep others at arm's length—a distance of about 3 feet—for the next 2 to 3 days. Forcing fluids to help excrete the ions and flushing toilets twice to reduce residual elements in the reservoir also is suggested for 2 to 3 days. Eating utensils should not be shared. Disposable plates and utensils are recommended, which will preclude the need to wash dishes separately. Sleeping alone and avoiding close personal contact, especially with infants and pregnant women, should be practiced for 5 to 11 days. Saliva, vaginal secretions, tears, and sweat are possible sources of contamination during that period. Those patients receiving very high doses for cancer treatment are given a wallet card to carry in the highly unlikely chance of setting off radiation detection alarms at some worksites and federal buildings (Sisson et al, 2011).

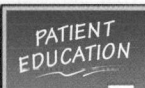

HYPERTHYROIDISM

Related to the Overall Treatment Plan and Disease Process

> Understanding the pathophysiology of hyperthyroidism and its prognosis
> Role of iodine intake in thyroid hormone production
> Importance of adherence to the treatment regimen
> Need to take the drug for at least 1 year
> Indications of relapse or complications that need to be reported
> Importance of discussing pregnancy or the potential for pregnancy with the primary care provider
> Need for regular follow-up visits with the primary care provider

Specific to the Drug Therapy

> Discussion of the reasons for taking the drug(s) and the anticipated action of the drug(s) on the disease process. It is especially important to inform the patient that antithyroid drugs take 4 to 8 weeks to have a noticeable effect.
> Doses and schedules for taking the drug(s)
> Possible adverse reactions and what to do when they occur
> Patient education specific to antithyroid drugs is provided in Chapter 21.
> Patient education specific to beta-adrenergic blockers is provided in Chapter 14.

SUBCLINICAL HYPERTHYROIDISM

Subclinical hyperthyroidism is characterized by a serum TSH level less than 0.5 microUnits/mL and normal FT4 and FT3. Exogenous TSH suppression or endogenous production of thyroid hormones appears to be sufficient in this disorder to keep FT4 and FT3 levels normal but to suppress pituitary TSH production and secretion. It can be the result of high-dose glucocorticoids or iodine deficiency. It is estimated that up to 25% of concurrent estrogen replacement patients might fall into this category, with smokers at even greater risk. Self-medication with "natural thyroid health supplements" can be the cause. The clinical significance is the potential for progression to overt hyperthyroidism, exacerbation of any concurrent cardiac problems, and a decrease in bone mineral density if it is more than a transient situation. It is more commonly found in regions with iodine deficiency.

Professionals differ on their views as to whether to screen for and/or treat this disorder. Patients with subclinical hyperthyroidism attributable to nodular thyroid disease warrant treatment. Postmenopausal women, who are already at risk for osteoporosis, are also treated. In older adults, the relative risk for atrial fibrillation increases 3-fold for those with subclinical hyperthyroidism, so treatment is prudent. In most patients, no treatment is necessary unless the source of the disorder is exuberant exogenous hormone replacement. In that case, dosage adjustment is indicated (Bahn et al, 2011).

Patients with subclinical hyperthyroidism should have periodic clinical and laboratory assessments. Persistent rather than transient hormonal abnormalities are more often associated with clinical problems. Data are unreliable about an association with dementia risk. Suppressed TSH is also linked with sleep disturbances; however, many patients report enhanced well-being at these levels. If sustained TSH suppression (less than 0.1 microUnits/mL) is established for those on replacement therapy, then dosage reduction is appropriate to avoid long-term consequences.

HYPOTHYROIDISM

Pathophysiology

The underlying mechanisms that cause hypothyroidism can be primary or secondary. Primary disorders include the following:

- Defective hormone synthesis resulting from autoimmune thyroiditis, endemic iodine deficiency, or antithyroid drugs that were used to treat hyperthyroidism
- Congenital defects or loss of tissue after treatment for hyperthyroidism

Secondary causes of hypothyroidism, which are less common, include conditions that cause either pituitary or hypothalamic failure. In secondary disorders, the TSH response is inadequate so that the gland is normal or reduced in size, with both T3 and T4 synthesis equally reduced.

Primary hypothyroidism is based on the hypothalamic-pituitary-thyroid gland feedback system and occurs when the hypothalamus responds to a decreased thyroid hormone level with an increase in TRH, resulting in increased TSH secretion, which in turn stimulates thyroid gland enlargement, goiter formation, and preferential synthesis of T3 over T4. Of all patients with hypothyroidism, 95% have primary thyroid disease.

Primary Disease

Hashimoto's thyroiditis is an immune-mediated disorder in which all components of the thyroid gland are injured, but especially the TSH receptors. Antibodies generated to attack glandular antigens impair TSH response, hormone synthesis, and hormone release. Some patients have mild disease and may remain euthyroid; approximately 70% go on to develop permanent hypothyroidism.

Postpartum thyroiditis with hypothyroid characteristics affects up to 7% of postpartum women. Antibody production in this disorder peaks 3 to 4 months after delivery and then declines. Symptoms resolve spontaneously in 95% of patients, and most return to euthyroid states without therapy.

Subacute thyroiditis is an inflammation of the thyroid often preceded by a viral infection. It is accompanied by fever, tenderness, and enlargement of the gland. Elevated levels of thyroid hormone are due to the release of stored thyroglobin related to the inflammatory process. Symptoms last 2 to 4 months. Anti-inflammatory agents such as NSAIDs may be used to address the inflammation. Beta blockers are used to reduce tachycardia. There is usually spontaneous remission of the disorder, but it can become chronic.

Congenital hypothyroidism occurs in infants as a result of absent thyroid tissue (thyroid dysgenesis in 90% of cases) and hereditary defects in thyroid hormone synthesis. It is more common in females. Because thyroid hormone is essential for embryonic growth, especially of brain tissue, an infant with no T4 during fetal life will be mentally impaired. This condition can be modulated with administration of T4 immediately after birth. Capillary blood screening of all infants in the United States and Canada before discharge from the hospital or birthing center tests for this disorder. Infants suspected of the disorder are referred immediately to a pediatric endocrinologist. Infants may be initially asymptomatic due to maternal T4 levels.

Endemic iodine deficiency has not been a problem in the United States since the early 1900s. Iodized table salt largely eliminated this form of hypothyroidism. The recent return to home gardens and preferential shopping for local produce might create subsets of patients in the traditional goiter regions of the Great Lakes and across the northern tier of states.

Secondary Disease

Secondary hypothyroidism most commonly is a result of a pituitary disorder. The net result is inadequate TSH production, resulting in poor production of both T3 And T4. Commonly associated pituitary disorders linked with secondary hypothyroidism include Cushing's syndrome, acromegaly, and pituitary adenomas. Other secondary causes include the administration of drugs that reduce thyroid hormone production (see Table 41-1) and the treatment of hyperthyroidism.

Regardless of the etiology, the clinical features of hypothyroidism are attributable to the metabolic effects of decreased circulating levels of thyroid hormone. The patient develops a low basal metabolic rate, cold intolerance, lethargy, and a slightly lowered body temperature. Table 41-4 shows the most common systemic effects of hypothyroidism.

Long-standing undertreated hypothyroidism often results in myxedema, a condition similar to the pretibial myxedema seen in Graves' disease. It is a result of connective tissues being separated by an increased amount of protein and mucopolysaccharides. These protein complexes bind water, producing pitting, boggy edema, especially around the eyes, hands, and shins and in the supraclavicular fossae. They also produce thickening of the tongue and the laryngeal-pharyngeal membranes, resulting in thick, slurred speech and hoarseness. The medical emergency of myxedema coma can occur, signaling severe hypothyroidism. Signs and symptoms include hypoventilation, hypotension, hypoglycemia, and lactic acidosis. Older adults with vascular disease and untreated hypothyroidism are especially at risk. This critical care state is beyond the scope of this text.

Pharmacodynamics

For patients who are clinically hypothyroid, replacement therapy with thyroid hormones is indicated. Administration of synthetic thyroid hormones (levothyroxine [T4], liothyronine [T3], and liotrix [a 4:1 or 3:1 mixture of T4 and T3]) produces the same effects on body tissues as the body's own thyroid hormones, including the negative feedback required to reduce further secretion of TSH. Dosing schedules for these drugs are provided in Chapter 21. These drugs are inexpensive and relatively free of adverse reactions, but there are conditions in which they are contraindicated or to be used with caution.

Goals of Treatment

The therapeutic goal for patients with hypothyroidism is correction of the hypometabolic state and normalization of

Table 41–4 Systemic Effects of Hypothyroidism

Body System	Clinical Manifestation	Underlying Mechanism
Cardiovascular	Reduced stroke volume and heart rate (reduced cardiac output); increased peripheral vascular resistance to maintain blood pressure; decreased blood flow to tissue; sinus bradycardia; ECG changes	Decreased metabolic demands and loss of regulatory and rate-setting effects of thyroid hormone
Hematologic	Decreased red blood cell mass (normocytic/normochromic anemia); macrocytic anemia associated with B_{12} deficiency and inadequate folate or iron absorption	Decreased basal metabolic rate and oxygen requirements, decreased production of erythropoietin. Possible association between thyroid hormone and hematologic response to B_{12}
Respiratory	Dyspnea, hypoventilation, CO_2 retention	Myxedematous changes in respiratory muscles
Gastrointestinal	Decreased appetite, constipation, weight gain, fluid retention; decreased protein metabolism (lightly positive nitrogen balance); decreased glucose absorption; elevated serum lipid levels	Decreased metabolic demand; reduced peristaltic activity; increased capillary permeability to proteins; depressed insulin degradation; depressed lipid synthesis and degradation
Renal	Increased total body water; reduced erythropoietin production; dilutional hyponatremia	Reduced blood flow and glomerular filtration rate, leading to decreased excretion of water
Integumentary	Dry, flaky skin; dry, brittle hair; reduced growth of nails and hair; slow wound healing; myxedema; cool skin	Reduced sweat and sebaceous gland secretion; increased hyaluronic acid binds water and causes a puffy appearance; decreased circulation to skin; reduced tissue regeneration
Reproductive	Anovulation, decreased libido, high incidence of spontaneous abortion in women; decreased libido and oligospermia in men	Increased estriol formation in women, decreased androgen secretion in men, decreased levels of sex hormone–binding globulin in both genders
Neurologic	Confusion, slow speech and thinking; memory loss; hearing loss; night blindness; slow; clumsy movements; cerebellar ataxia	Decreased cerebral blood flow, resulting in cerebral hypoxia
Musculoskeletal	Muscle and joint aching and stiffness; reduced deep tendon reflexes; increased bone density	Decreased innervation of muscles; decreased bone formation and resorption
Endocrine	Increased TSH production; decreased cortisol turnover rate but normal serum cortisol levels	Impaired thyroid hormone synthesis; decreased deactivation of cortisol

ECG = electrocardiogram; TSH = thyroid-stimulating hormone.

TSH and T4 levels with a minimum of adverse reactions. Adequate hormone replacement should improve fatigue, facilitate weight loss, and reduce cardiovascular and neurological complications.

Rational Drug Selection

Thyroid hormones were originally ground-up thyroid glands of animals. Such preparations are still available today. Because the pharmacokinetics and concentration of hormones in these drugs are highly variable, they have been replaced in practice with synthetic formulations. Patients may prefer the "natural" forms like Armour. There are also OTC "natural" supplements that sometimes contain actual thyroid hormones. The focus of this chapter is the synthetic thyroid hormones.

Drug Therapy

Patients develop the symptoms of hypothyroidism slowly and are often quite low in thyroid hormone before they are diagnosed. These patients have adapted to a low level of hormone and become very sensitive to the effects of synthetic thyroid hormone replacement. Treatment, therefore, should be gradual. The first signs of clinical response to therapy are a modest weight loss, an increase in pulse rate, and resolution of constipation. Other symptoms, such as myxedema, cardiovascular problems, and elevated creatinine kinase levels, take more time to improve. Most patients feel better in about 2 weeks, with clinical resolution occurring in about 3 months.

All of the synthetic forms of thyroid hormone have been successfully used to treat hypothyroidism. Drug choice is based on patient and drug variables. Figure 41-2 depicts the treatment algorithm based on these variables. All patients with TSH greater than 10 microUnits/mL should be treated (Garber et al, 2012).

Patient Variables

Age and Gender

Women older than 50 with markedly elevated TSH levels (greater than or equal to 10 microUnits/mL) have the highest risk for complications from hypothyroidism, such as cardiac conditions associated with altered lipid metabolism. Research evidence is not sufficient to recommend or discourage treatment for patients with lower TSH levels, but the best option is to treat patients with symptoms and previously recognized lipid or CV disorders.

Men, younger women, and patients with a mildly elevated TSH level (6 to 9 micro Units/mL) have a lower risk for complications. At a minimum, these patients should have TSH levels drawn every 2 to 5 years to see if the disease progresses to the point at which treatment is appropriate. Symptomatic patients should be treated.

The most common presentation in pediatrics is a goiter. The disease should be considered when slowing growth patterns, decreasing school performance, and delayed puberty are evident. Children with genetic disorders like Down, Turner, or Klinefelter syndromes need closer screening. One-third of childhood head and neck cancer survivors develop thyroid disorders (LaFranchi, 2012). Because children clear T4 faster than adults, dosages are typically higher.

Pregnancy

Untreated overt hypothyroidism during pregnancy may increase the incidence of maternal hypertension, pre-eclampsia, anemia, postpartum hemorrhage, cardiac ventricular dysfunction, spontaneous abortion, fetal death or stillbirth, low birth weight, and possibly abnormal fetal brain development (Garber et al, 2012). Evidence from a population-based study suggests that even mild, asymptomatic, untreated maternal hypothyroidism during pregnancy may have an adverse effect on cognitive function in the offspring. These outcomes can be avoided by thyroid hormone replacement. Because thyroid hormones are Pregnancy Category A, replacement is advised for all pregnant women even with mild disease. Therapy begun before pregnancy should not be stopped. The increased metabolic rate common to pregnancy often requires higher doses. Increasing a patient's maintenance dose by 25% usually provides adequate coverage. TSH levels should then be checked in 4 weeks to determine the need for any further dosage adjustment. ATA, AACE, and ACOG all recommend levothyroxine, because the combination T4 and T3 medications lower maternal TSH levels, potentially resulting in fetal neurological suppression.

Concomitant Diseases

Concomitant disease state patients should be comanaged with the endocrine team. Thyroid hormone replacement is generally contraindicated after recent *myocardial infarction*. If hypothyroidism is a complicating or causative factor of the cardiac problem, judicious use of small doses may be indicated in consultation with cardiology. *Coronary artery disease* may worsen when thyroid hormones are given because the increased heart rate increases oxygen demand by the heart muscle and decreases the oxygen supply by decreasing the diastolic filling time. The lowest possible dose is used, with careful monitoring for indications of worsening cardiovascular disease. Although both levothyroxine and liothyronine have content stability, liothyronine is 3 to 4 times more active than levothyroxine, making it more likely to produce cardiotoxicity. In patients with *angina*, the initiation of thyroid hormone replacement may precipitate unstable angina. Beta-adrenergic blockers may be concurrently administered to decrease this risk.

Long-term use of levothyroxine therapy in women has been associated with decreased bone density in the hip and spine. Postmenopausal women with *osteoporosis* and not on estrogen replacement require the lowest effective doses and scheduled DEXA screens (see Chaps. 21 and 38).

Approximately 10% of patients with *type 1 diabetes mellitus* develop chronic thyroiditis, with an insidious onset of subclinical hypothyroidism (Garber et al, 2012). Up to 25% of women with this disorder will develop postpartum thyroiditis. Patients with diabetes should be routinely examined for the development of goiter and altered TSH levels. Levothyroxine is the drug of choice.

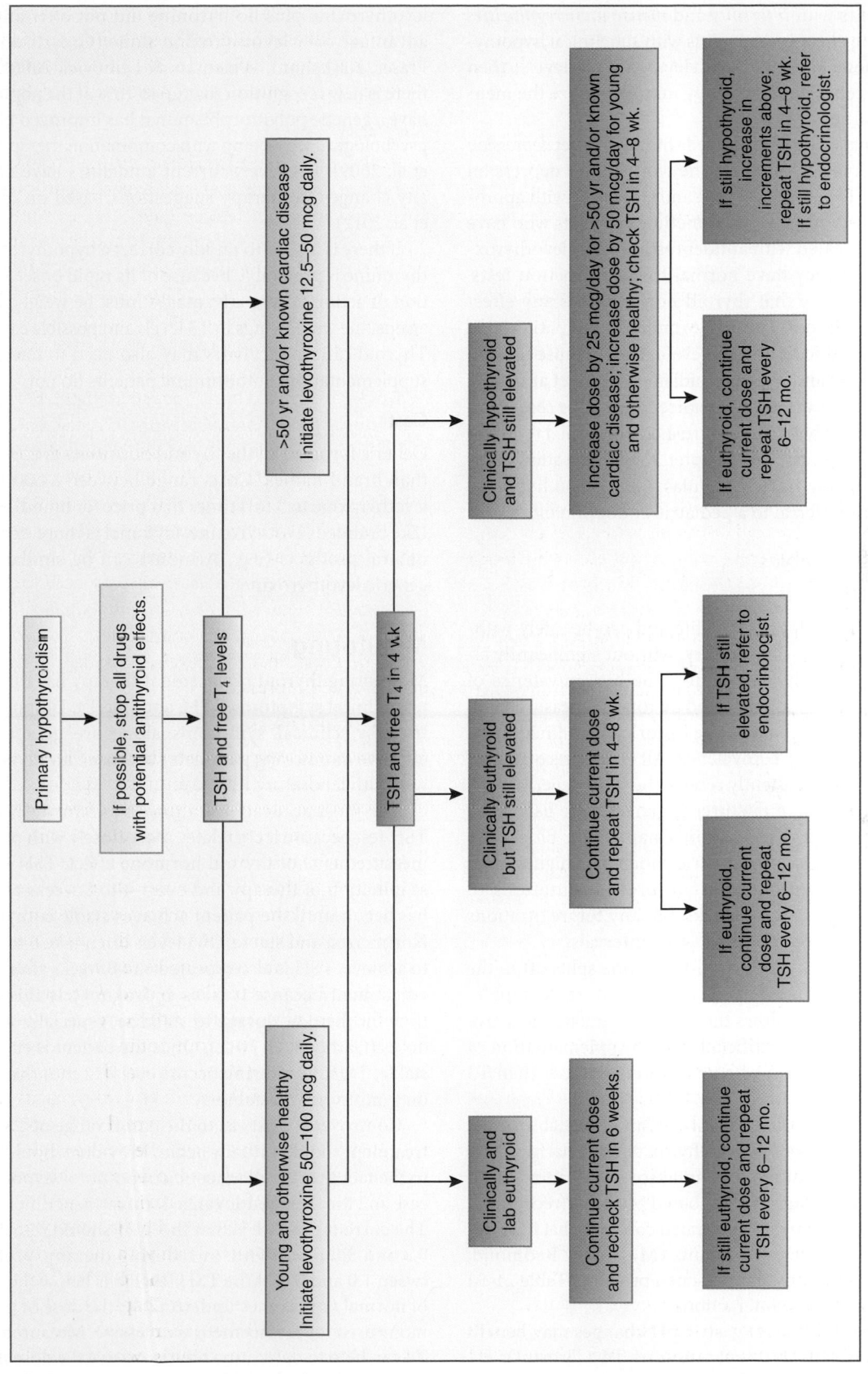

Figure 41–2. Drug therapy algorithm: Hypothyroidism.

Some patients with *infertility* and *menstrual irregularities* have underlying chronic thyroiditis with subclinical hypothyroidism. If these patients have elevated TSH levels, then levothyroxine replacement therapy may normalize the menstrual cycle and restore fertility.

A few patients who are diagnosed with new-onset *depression* have primary hypothyroidism. The work-up for depression should include TSH measurement and treatment with appropriate doses of levothyroxine. Sometimes patients who have depression are treated with antidepressants plus levothyroxine even though they have normal thyroid function tests. There is no evidence that thyroid hormone has any effect on depression without TSH abnormalities. All patients on lithium require periodic thyroid evaluation because lithium may induce goiter and hypothyroidism (Garber et al, 2012).

Levothyroxine is the drug of choice for treating *congenital hypothyroidism*. Tablets may be crushed and added to infant formula. This is discussed in Chapter 21 with the added caution concerning soy-based formulas. Congenital hypothyroidism requires referral to a pediatric endocrinologist.

Drug-Related Variables

Pharmacokinetics

Levothyroxine has a longer half-life and can be safely withheld for up to 2 weeks, if necessary, without significantly altering the patient's thyroid status. The bioequivalence of levothyroxine preparations is based on total T_4 measurement, which some specialty groups have historically claimed is not the same as therapeutic equivalence. All groups recommend the patient should consistently receive the same generic product from the same manufacturer if generics are used. The dosing variables are discussed in Chapter 21. Elders are started on lower doses and pediatric patients on higher ones. Due to metabolic and steady-state profiles, titrations in dosage initially occur after 4 weeks, but any future titrations should occur at no sooner than 6 week intervals.

T4 is not clinically active until the iodine splits off in the peripheral tissues to form T3. It is more natural to supplement T4, because this allows the body to regulate the active hormone level without artificially high supplementation of T3. When T4 absorption or conversion is suspect, then T3 becomes a rational choice.

Malabsorptive states and patient age can change absorption of thyroid hormone. Because levothyroxine has a narrow therapeutic range, small differences in absorption can result in clinical changes. The surge in soy-based products (recognized for potential thyroid impact) generated concerns that have not come to fruition, except for infants (Messina & Redmond, 2006). Drug interactions also present a problem. Table 21-34 in Chapter 21 lists these interactions.

Those with known large gastric pH changes may benefit from the liquid capsule preparation of T4 (Tirosint). H2 blockers and PPI drug use have not been demonstrated to alter absorption (Garber et al, 2012).

There has been a resurgence of interest in the use of combination thyroid hormones to treat hypothyroidism. A 2006 meta-analysis concluded that physiological combinations of levothyroxine plus liothyronine did not offer any objective advantage over levothyroxine alone (Groszinski-Glasberg, Fraser, Nashshoni, Weizman, & Leibovici, 2006). However, there is new recognition that up to 16% of the population may have a genetic polymorphism that has improved physical and psychological well-being with combination therapy (Panicker, et al, 2009). However, current guidelines have not adopted any changes to therapy suggestions based on this (Garber et al, 2012).

If there is a need to rapidly correct a hypothyroid state, liothyronine is preferable because of its rapid onset and dissipation of action. These advantages must be weighed, however, against the wide swings in T3 levels and possible cardiotoxicity. Thyroid cancer survivors may also need to have higher T3 supplementation; autoimmune patients do not.

Cost

Generic forms of all the thyroid hormones are less expensive than brand names. Costs range between $4.00 for generic levothyroxine to 3 to 4 times that price for brand-name drugs. Like branded levothyroxine, Cytomel is more expensive, but natural products (e.g., Armour) can be similar in cost to generic levothyroxine.

Monitoring

Monitoring thyroid replacement therapy has three parameters: clinical symptoms, TSH, and free T4. Despite some controversy, clinical symptoms alone are generally not an effective monitoring parameter because they do not correlate well with laboratory findings.

The most accurate monitoring parameter is a sensitive TSH test because it correlates most closely with physiological measurements of thyroid hormone effect. TSH is evaluated at initiation of therapy and every 4 to 8 weeks after therapy has begun until the patient achieves stable euthyroid status. Normalized and stable TSH levels often take 6 to 12 months to achieve. TSH is also repeated 6 to 8 weeks after any dosage adjustment because it takes approximately this amount of time for the new dosage to stabilize, especially with smaller doses (Garber et al, 2012). Once the patient is euthyroid and stable, TSH monitoring occurs every 12 months, depending on symptoms and stability.

Controversy exists as to the cutoff range of TSH at which treatment should initially begin. Providers should be attuned to the fact that the diagnostic cut point for hypothyroid disease and the therapeutic range for treatment differ in practice. The current practice is that the TSH should remain between 0.3 and 3.0 microUnits/mL during therapy, preferably between 1.0 and 2.0. If the TSH level falls below the lower limit of normal or becomes undetectable, the dose of thyroid hormone used for replacement is excessive. Measurement of free T4 can help to determine how excessive the dose is. FT4 may correlate poorly with physiological status during the initial therapy period. It is more reliable once the patient is stable (e.g., after 12 months).

Levothyroxine is the easiest to monitor with standard TSH and free T4 laboratory measurements of thyroid function.

Monitoring liothyronine therapy is more difficult; it is best monitored as a TSH suppressor. Liotrix offers no clear monitoring benefit over either of these other drugs on any of these parameters. During pregnancy, elevated estrogen increases thyroid-binding globulin levels, which alters total T4 values but not FT4. During pregnancy, both TSH and FT4 levels are evaluated to determine appropriate replacement dosage. Tests are done at 8 weeks and 6 months of gestation. The goal is to normalize TSH and maintain FT4 at the upper limits of normal. Women with hypothyroidism who become pregnant may have their thyroid function change. In general, the dosage of thyroid hormone may need to be increased, and these patients should have their serum TSH level evaluated every 6 weeks during pregnancy and in the postpartum period to ensure that the dose of levothyroxine is appropriate.

Anemia is a frequent concomitant disease with hypothyroidism. A complete blood count (CBC) should be drawn at initiation of therapy. After a thorough work-up of any anemia to assess for other possible causes (e.g., iron deficiency, blood loss, vitamin B_{12} or folic acid deficiency), hypothyroidism should be treated with standard thyroid hormone replacement. Management of anemia, including monitoring parameters, is discussed in Chapter 27.

Other common concomitant disorders that require monitoring include hypercholesterolemia and hypertension. T4 supplementation modulates the lipid disturbances triggered by low thyroid levels. Management of these disorders, including monitoring parameters, is discussed in Chapters 39 and 40. Planned weight loss to control lipids and blood pressure may trigger less need for thyroid supplementation.

Outcome Evaluation

Figure 41-2 shows the drug treatment protocol for hypothyroidism. Evaluation is based on reduction of clinical symptoms such as goiter size and normalization of TSH and FT4 levels. Although most health-care providers can diagnose and treat hypothyroidism, certain situations suggest referral to a clinical endocrinologist experienced in the spectrum of thyroid disease:

- Patients age 18 years or under
- Patients unresponsive to therapy
- Pregnant and lactating patients
- Cardiac patients
- Presence of goiter, nodule, or other structural changes in the thyroid gland
- Presence of autoimmune or other endocrine diseases
- Failure to achieve control of symptoms or normalized TSH within 12 months by standard doses despite patient adherence to the treatment regimen
- Relapse after a period of stability on a standard dose
- Pending surgery; careful anesthesia planning is required because clearance of anesthetics is reduced

Patient Education

Patient education should discuss the overall treatment plan, reasons for taking the drug, dietary considerations, and the negative aspects of keeping TSH levels too low. Patients need to be aware of the typical permanence of drug therapy. Thyroid products are best taken 1 hour before breakfast or at least 2 hours after an evening meal. Coffee can decrease absorption of T4 by 27% to 30%. Some individuals are sensitive to a large intake of cabbage and other goiterogenic products.

SUBCLINICAL HYPOTHYROIDISM

Subclinical hypothyroidism refers to mildly increased serum TSH levels in the setting of normal FT4 and FT3. It is a common disorder, ranging from 4% to 10% of the adult population, with increased frequency in women, older adults, and those

---

HYPOTHYROIDISM

PATIENT EDUCATION

Related to the Overall Treatment Plan and Disease Process

Understanding the pathophysiology of hypothyroidism and its prognosis.

Role of iodine intake in thyroid hormone production.

Importance of adherence to the treatment regimen.

Length of time the drug will need to be taken. For those with thyroiditis, this may be less than 12 months. For many with primary hypothyroidism, the treatment will be lifelong. The patient should be informed not to stop taking the drug without first consulting the health-care provider.

Indications of relapse or complications that need to be reported.

Importance of discussing pregnancy or the potential for pregnancy with the primary care provider.

Need to wear a medical identification bracelet stating that patient is taking thyroid hormone replacement and to inform any provider who sees him or her that this is the case. This is especially important if this provider prescribes any new drugs for the patient.

Need for regular follow-up visits with the primary care provider, which will include laboratory monitoring of thyroid function to determine the status of the hypothyroidism and any needed dosage adjustments of the drug therapy.

Specific to the Drug Therapy

Discussion of the reasons for taking the drug(s) and the anticipated action of the drug(s) on the disease process. It is especially important to inform the patient that thyroid hormone replacement may take 4 to 8 weeks to have a noticeable effect.

Doses and schedules for taking the drug(s).

Possible adverse reactions (e.g., rapid heart rate, cardiac arrhythmias, chest pain, insomnia, diarrhea, or heat intolerance) and what to do when they occur.

Additional patient education specific to thyroid hormones is provided in Chapter 21.

with higher dietary iodine intake (NHANNES III). Subclinical hypothyroidism is usually asymptomatic and discovered on routine thyroid screening. The most common cause is Hashimoto's disease. Progression to overt hypothyroidism is reported to vary from 3% to 20%.

Potential risks for this condition, besides progression to hypothyroidism, include cardiovascular disease, hyperlipidemia, and neuropsychiatric effects. The ATA and ACCE (Garber et al, 2012) recommend treatment for patients with TSH levels of 5 to 10 microUnits/mL who also have goiter or positive thyroid peroxidase antibodies. These patients have the highest rate of conversion to overt hypothyroidism. Lower than full replacement doses are needed. As with overt hypothyroidism, the target TSH level should be between 0.3 and 3.0 microUnits/mL. Once this level is achieved, an annual evaluation is sufficient.

REFERENCES

American College of Obstetricians and Gynecologists (ACOG). (2007, Oct 1; reaffirmed 2010). *Routine thyroid screening not recommended for pregnant women* [Press Release]. http://www.acog.org

Bahn, R., Burch, H., Cooper, D., Garber, J., Greenlee, M. C., Klein, I., et al. (2011). Hyperthyroidism and other causes of thyrotoxicosis: Management guidelines of the American Thyroid Association and American Association of Clinical Endocrinologists. *Endocrinology Practice, 17*(3). Epub ahead of print, e1–e65.

Caldwell, K., Miller, G., Wang, R., Jain, R., & Jones, R. (2008). Iodine status of the U.S. population. National Health and Nutrition Examination Survey 2003–2004. *Thyroid, 18*(11), 1207–1214.

Garber, J., Cobin, R., Gharib, H., Hennesey, J., Klein, I., Mechanick, J., et al. (2012). Clinical practice guideline for hypothyroidism in adults: Cosponsored by the American Association of Clinical Endocrinologists and the American Thyroid Association. *Thyroid, 22*(12), 1200–1235.

Genovese, B., Noureldine, S., Gleeson, E., Tufano, R., & Dandil, E. (2012, Sep 7). What is the best definitive treatment for Grave's disease? A systematic review of the existing literature. *Annals of Surgical Oncology*, published online, e1–e8.

Grozinski-Glasberg, S., Fraser, A., Nashshoni, E., Weizman, A., & Leibovici, L. (2006).Thyroxine-triiodothyronine combination therapy versus thyroxine monotherapy for clinical hypothyroidism: Meta-analysis of randomized controlled trials. *Journal of Clinical Endocrinology & Metabolism, 91*(7), 2592–2599.

Institute for Safe Medication Practices (ISMP). (2008, May 22). Mix-ups with propylthiouracil and purinethol. *ISMPNewletter.*

LaFranchi, S. (2012). Acquired hypothyroidism in childhood and adolescence. In D. Ross & M. Mitchell (Eds.), *UpToDate*. Waltham, MA: *UpToDate*. Retrieved from http://www.uptodate.com/contents/acquired-hypothyroidism-in-childhood-and-adolescence

McCance, K., & Huether, S. (2014). *Pathophysiology: The biological basis for disease in adults and children* (7th ed.). St. Louis, MO: Mosby.

Messina, M., & Redmond, G. (2006). Effects of soy protein and soybean isoflavones on thyroid function in healthy adults and thyroid patients: A review of the relevant literature. *Thyroid, 16*(3), 249–258.

New York Thyroid Center. (2011). Radioactive iodine. http://www. Columbiathyroidcenter.org

Panicker, V., Saravanan, P., Vaidya, B., Evans, J., Hattersley, A., Frayling, T., et al. (2009). Common variation in the DIO2 gene predicts baseline psychological well-being and response to combination thyroxine plus triiodothyronine combination therapy versus thyroxine monotherapy in hypothyroid patients. *Journal of Clinical Endocrinology and Metabolism, 94*(5), 1623–1629.

Rivkees, S. & Dinaur, C. (2007). An optimal treatment for pediatric Graves's disease is radioiodine. *Journal of Clinical Endocrinology and Metabolism. 92*(3) 797–800.

Ross, D. (2012). Treatment of hypothyroidism. In D. Cooper (Ed.), *UpToDate*. Waltham, MA: *UpToDate*. Retrieved from http://www.uptodate.com/contents/treatment-of-hypothyroidism

Sisson, J., Freitas, J., McDougall, I., Dauer, L., Hurley, J., Brierley, J., et al. (2011, Apr 4). Radiation safety in the treatment of patients with thyroid diseases by radioiodine 131I: Practice recommendations of the American Thyroid Association. *Thyroid*, (4), 335–346. Erratum, June 21 (6), 689.

U.S. Food and Drug Administration (FDA). (2009). *Propylthiouracil-induced liver failure*. Retrieved June 5, 2009, from http://www.fda.gov/Drugs/DrugSafety/PostmarketDrugSafetyInformationfor PatientsandProviders/ucm162701

U.S. Food and Drug Administration (FDA). (2010). *FDA Drug Safety Communication: New boxed warning on severe liver injury with propylthiouracil*. Retrieved April 21, 2010, from http://www.fda.gov/Drugs/DrugSafety/PostmarketDrugSafetyInformationfor PatientsandProviders/ucm209023.htm

U.S. Preventive Services Task Force. (2010, July). *Screening for thyroid disease: Recommendation statement*. www.uspreventiveservicestaskforce.ogr/recommendations.htm.

PNEUMONIA

Anne Hedger

Pneumonia affects more than 5 million people a year in the United States, making it one of the more commonly seen medical problems and the eighth leading cause of death in the United States; yet there has been a significant decrease in death rates relative to previous years (National Center for Health Statistics, 2011). As in most bacterial illnesses, those patients at the extremes of age are most severely affected, with infants and older adults often requiring hospitalization and IV antibiotics. Pertinent issues in managing health-care–associated pneumonia (HCAP) include the increased risk of infection from drug-resistant isolates of the usual community-acquired pathogens and an increased risk of infection with less common, usually hospital-associated pathogens (Mandell et al, 2007).

ADULT PATIENTS WITH PNEUMONIA

Pathophysiology

Pneumonia develops when an organism invades the lung parenchyma and the host defenses are depressed. Bacterial pneumonia results when the lung's primary defense mechanisms are altered, either by a viral infection or by immunological problems. Chronically ill patients of all ages are more prone to pneumonia, usually because of their underlying medical problem. There may be other origins of pneumonia besides bacterial organisms, such as viral, fungal, rickettsial, and parasitic organisms; inflammatory processes; and inhalation of toxic substances.

Pneumonia should be considered in any patient who presents with respiratory symptoms such as cough, dyspnea, or sputum production. Fever or abnormal breath sounds, such as crackles, would strengthen the suspicion of pneumonia. Chest radiographs assist in confirming the diagnosis of pneumonia versus other respiratory disorders such as lung abscess or tuberculosis (Mandell et al, 2007). However, given the limitations of diagnostic testing, most community-acquired pneumonia (CAP) is still treated empirically (Mandell et al, 2007).

The predominant organism found in pneumonia depends on the age and health status of the patient. For all ages (except neonates), *Streptococcus pneumoniae* is the organism most commonly found in pneumonia (Mandell et al, 2007). *S. pneumoniae* is identified as the causative organism in 60% to 75% of adults with bacterial pneumonia, based on sputum culture. Nontypeable *Haemophilus influenzae* and *Moraxella catarrhalis* are common pathogens in patients with underlying lung disease. *Staphylococcus aureus* has become a common co-pathogen in influenza-associated pneumonia. *Mycoplasma pneumoniae,* a pathogen difficult to detect on Gram's stain or culture, is another common cause of pneumonia. In many patients viruses are the cause of pneumonia; viruses are identified in 18% to 36% of pneumonia cases (Mandell et al, 2007). It must be noted that the responsible organism is not identified in up to 50% of patients with CAP (American Thoracic Society [ATS], 2001). Table 42-1 lists the common pathological agents for CAP at different ages.

In the past, practitioners attempted to determine the most likely pathogen by the clinical presentation of the patient, using terms like *typical* and *atypical*. Typical infections were those caused by *S. pneumoniae, H. influenzae, S. aureus,* or gram-negative bacteria. The presentation of typical pneumonia included fever, chills, yellow or green sputum, pleuritic chest pain, and lobar consolidation on chest x-rays; the presentation of atypical pneumonia included a gradual onset of cough, no or scant sputum, low-grade fever, myalgias, arthralgias, and lack of consolidation on x-rays. It was thought that patients with atypical pneumonia most likely had *M. pneumoniae, Legionella pneumophila,* or a viral infection. In clinical practice, these classifications have little usefulness, as numerous studies have shown that few reliable clinical features distinguish between the different bacterial pathogens (ATS, 2001).

Goals of Treatment

The ultimate goal of treatment for all patients is the return to the respiratory status they had before the illness. Initially, patients who are responding to empirical antibiotic therapy should show improved clinical condition in 48 to 72 hours. Fever should resolve in 2 to 4 days, and leukocytosis usually resolves by day 4 of treatment (ATS, 2001; Mandell et al, 2007). The patient's chest x-ray may actually deteriorate, however, and not return to baseline for weeks or months. In previously healthy adults younger than age 50 years, 66% of patients with pneumonia return to baseline chest x-rays within 4 weeks. In older patients or those who have previously had respiratory or other chronic illness, only 26% of patients have normal chest x-rays by the fourth week of treatment (ATS, 2001). Children may require 6 to 8 weeks for the chest x-ray to return to normal (Bradley et al, 2011). Therefore, a clear chest x-ray may not be the best indicator of successful treatment initially. The best indicator of improvement in clinical status is that the overall clinical manifestations of pneumonia (e.g., fever and increased white blood cell [WBC] count) should improve. Older patients, those with multiple coexisting illnesses, and those with increased severity of disease will have delayed resolution of clinical signs and symptoms (level II evidence) (ATS, 2001).

Rational Drug Selection

Clinical Guidelines

In 1993, the American Thoracic Society (ATS) issued guidelines for the initial management of adults with CAP that discuss the diagnosis, assessment of severity, and initial antimicrobial therapy; these guidelines were revised and updated in 2001. In 2007, the Infectious Diseases Society of America and the American Thoracic Society published a consensus document on the management of community-acquired pneumonia (Mandell et al, 2007). The original ATS guidelines published in 2001 are similar to those used in Europe and Canada and break down the treatment into severely ill and not severely ill patients, patients who require hospitalization, and those who require intensive care unit (ICU) hospitalization (ATS, 2001; Mandell et al, 2007; Riley, Aronsky, & Dean, 2004). These categories include the following:

1. Previously healthy outpatients with no history of cardiopulmonary disease and no modifying factors such as risk for drug-resistant streptococcal pneumonia (DSRP) (excludes those with HIV).
2. Outpatients with cardiopulmonary disease (congestive heart failure or chronic obstructive pulmonary disease [COPD]), diabetes, liver or renal disease, alcoholism, malignancies, asplenia, immunosuppression, use of antimicrobials in the past 3 months, and/or modifying factors (risk factors for DSRP [age greater than 65] or gram-negative bacteria).

Table 42–1   Community-Acquired Pneumonia: Common Pathogens by Age

Age	Common Pathogens
Neonates	Coliform bacteria, cytomegalovirus, enterovirus, group B streptococci, herpes virus, *Mycoplasma hominis, Ureaplasma urealyticum*
Infants 4–16 weeks	Cytomegalovirus, influenza virus, parainfluenza virus, respiratory syncytial virus (RSV), *Chlamydia trachomatis, Haemophilus influenzae, Staphylococcus aureus, Streptococcus pneumoniae, U. urealyticum*
Children up to 5 years	Adenovirus, group A streptococci, influenza virus, RSV, *H. influenzae, S. aureus, S. pneumoniae*
Children over 5 years through adolescence	Influenza virus, varicella, *Chlamydia pneumoniae, H. influenzae, Legionella pneumophila, Mycoplasma pneumoniae, S. pneumoniae*
Adults group I: no cardiopulmonary disease and no modifying factors	Respiratory viruses, *C. pneumoniae, H. influenzae, M. pneumoniae, S. pneumoniae;* other (1%): endemic fungi, *Legionella* spp., *Mycobacterium tuberculosis, S. aureus*
Adults group II: with cardiopulmonary disease and/or modifying factors	Aerobic gram-negative bacilli, respiratory viruses, *H. influenzae, S. aureus, S. pneumoniae* (including DSRP); other (1%): endemic fungi, *Legionella Moraxella catarrhalis, M. tuberculosis, Mycoplasma pneumoniae,* mixed infection

DSRP = drug-resistant streptococcal pneumonia; RSV = respiratory syncytial virus.

3. Inpatients not admitted to the ICU who have the following:
   a. Cardiopulmonary disease and/or other modifying factors, such as having recently stayed at a nursing home.
   b. No cardiopulmonary disease and no other modifying factors.
4. ICU-admitted patients who have the following:
   a. No risks for *Pseudomonas aeruginosa*
   b. Risks for *P. aeruginosa*

Basically, the practitioner needs to take into consideration the comorbidities of the patient (cardiopulmonary disease), the severity of the illness at initial presentation, and the treatment setting (outpatient or hospital). In the 1993 ATS guidelines, age was a factor in decision making, but studies have found that age alone has little impact on the bacterial etiology of pneumonia (ATS, 2001). The only exception is that patients over age 65 are at risk for DSRP, which automatically places them in group 2, but age does not affect susceptibility to other organisms. Because most primary care practitioners are in the ambulatory setting, the first two categories, which cover the treatment of the outpatient, are discussed here.

In selecting treatment, the practitioner must also decide whether to treat the patient on an outpatient basis or in a hospital. The presence of any one of the following warrants admission to a hospital: respiratory rate greater than 30, temperature above 101°F, a PaO_2 less than 60 mm Hg, or a $PaCO_2$ greater than 50 mm Hg on room air. Age over 65 years, presence of coexisting illnesses such as COPD, diabetes mellitus, and chronic renal failure, congestive heart failure, chronic liver disease, alcohol abuse, and malnutrition all increase mortality of pneumonia and should warrant consideration for initial treatment as an inpatient (ATS, 2001). A severity-of-illness scale such as CURB-65 may be used to guide hospital admission decision making. The CURB-65 criteria evaluate confusion, uremia, respiratory rate, low blood pressure, and age 65 years or greater; patients with a score of 2 or above require either hospitalization or intensive home health services (Mandell et al, 2007). Even in the absence of any of these complicating factors or findings, the severity of the overall clinical picture may warrant hospitalization.

If the patient can be treated on an outpatient basis, the practitioner, using the ATS guidelines, determines the appropriate treatment based on the modifying factors that increase the risk of infection with specific pathogens. The treatment decision is based on the slightly different organisms found in each group. Figure 42-1 is an outpatient treatment algorithm for adults with CAP.

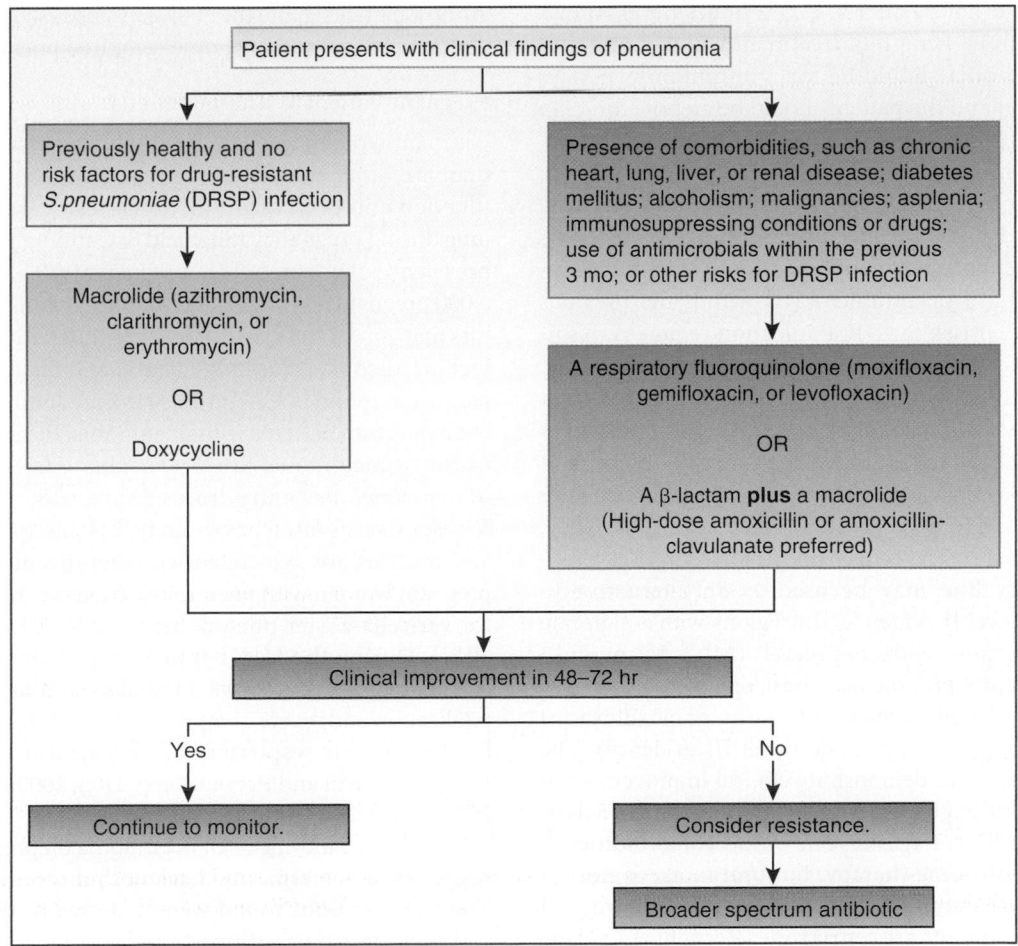

Figure 42–1. Treatment algorithm: Outpatient treatment of adults with community-acquired pneumonia.

Dosing Regimen

Initial empirical therapy for the previously healthy outpatient with no cardiopulmonary disease, no antibiotics in the past 3 months (no risk for DRSP), and no modifying factors (group 1) is to treat with an advanced-generation macrolide (level I evidence), such as azithromycin or clarithromycin, with doxycycline (level III evidence) a second choice if the patient is allergic or intolerant to macrolides. Erythromycin is the least expensive macrolide, whereas the ATS guidelines note that the newer macrolides have a lower incidence of gastrointestinal (GI) side effects and require fewer doses, improving the likelihood of patient compliance with therapy (Mandell et al, 2007). Azithromycin 500 mg on day 1, followed by 250 mg/d for days 2 to 5 is one choice (about $25 per course of treatment with generic medication), with clarithromycin 250 to 500 mg twice a day for 7 to 10 days (about $73 for 10 days of treatment, either strength) also an appropriate choice. Erythromycin 500 mg given PO qid for 7 to 10 days is the least expensive (about $17 for 7 days of treatment). Patients may also be prescribed erythromycin 333 mg tid (about $16 for 10 days) or 500 mg bid ($15 for 10 days). If patients have GI upset from the erythromycin at a dose of 500 mg qid, they may respond to 250 mg of erythromycin given qid.

The patient should begin to exhibit clinical response in 48 to 72 hours; therefore, unless the patient is deteriorating, treatment should not be altered for 72 hours (level III evidence) (ATS, 2001). Length of treatment with community-acquired pneumonia should be for a minimum of 5 days (level I evidence) and the patient should be afebrile for 48 to 72 hours with vitals signs, including oxygen saturation, within normal limits (Mandell et al, 2007).

Presence of comorbidities, such as chronic heart, lung, liver, or renal disease; diabetes mellitus; alcoholism; malignancies; asplenia; immunosuppressant conditions or use of immunosuppressant drugs; use of antimicrobials within the previous 3 months; or other risk for DRSP infection requires a respiratory fluoroquinolone such as moxifloxacin, gemifloxacin, or levofloxacin (Mandell et al, 2007). An alternative treatment in patients with comorbidities is a beta lactam *plus* a macrolide (level I evidence). High-dose amoxicillin (1 gm tid) or amoxicillin/clavulanate (Augmentin) is the preferred choice (Mandell et al, 2007). Alternatives include cefpodoxime, cefuroxime, or parenteral ceftriaxone followed by oral cefpodoxime. Doxycycline may be used as an alternative to the macrolide (level II evidence). In regions with a high rate (125%) of infection with high-level (MIC 16 mg/mL) macrolide-resistant *S. pneumoniae,* consider use of a respiratory fluoroquinolone (levofloxacin, gemifloxacin, or moxifloxacin) or a beta lactam plus a macrolide (level III evidence). The patient should begin to demonstrate clinical improvement in 48 to 72 hours and length of treatment is a minimum of 5 days.

If the patient is over age 60 years or has comorbidities, is stable enough for home therapy, but oral intake is not assured, home parenteral therapy is an option. The drugs of choice for these patients are ceftriaxone (Rocephin) 1 g daily via IV or IM or levofloxacin 500 mg IV daily. Consider adding a macrolide to ceftriaxone for coverage against atypical pathogens if indicated. Once clinical response is observed, the patient is switched to oral therapy, as described previously. Although parenteral therapy is expensive, it is still much more cost-effective than a hospital stay.

Patient Variables

Patient With Nursing Home–Acquired Pneumonia

Pneumonia is a common illness among patients residing in nursing homes, with a significant 30-day morbidity rate of 10% to 30% (Mills, Nelson, Winslow, & Springer, 2009). Patients with nursing home–acquired pneumonias are classified by the ATS guidelines as group 2 patients, with nursing home residence considered a modifying factor. *S. pneumoniae* is the most common pathogen in nursing home–acquired pneumonia (up to 48%), but patients may also have *S. aureus* (up to 33%), *H. influenzae* (up to 22%), aerobic gram-negative pathogens, Enterobacteriaceae, *Mycobacterium tuberculosis,* and certain viral agents (adenovirus, respiratory syncytial virus [RSV], and influenza) (Mills et al., 2009). Anaerobes should be considered if the patient has poor dentition or a swallowing disorder (ATS, 2001; Muder, Agahbabian, Loeb, Solot, & Higbee, 2004). These pathogens should be part of the differential for treating a patient who resides in a long-term care facility, yet the ATS recommends that nursing home patients should be initially treated in the same fashion as other group 2 patients. Note the 2007 consensus statement does not directly address nursing home–acquired pneumonia.

Pregnant Patient With Pneumonia

Pregnant women are at a slightly higher risk for infections than are other women because of diminished lymphocyte function and decreased functional residual capacity of the lung during pregnancy (Sheffield & Cunningham, 2009). The prevalence of pneumonia in pregnancy is 0.5 to 1.5 cases per 1,000 pregnancies (Sheffield & Cunningham, 2009). Risk factors that appear to be associated with antepartum pneumonia include anemia, prior lung disease, and illicit drug use. The pathogens found in CAP are also the predominant pathogens in antepartum patients with pneumonia; the main pathogens causing pneumonia are *S. pneumoniae, H. influenzae, M. pneumoniae,* and viruses (Larson & Powrie, 2014). Viruses such as influenza (both type A and type B), varicella, and measles are associated with significant morbidity for pregnant women with pneumonia. Maternal mortality is high for varicella-zoster pneumonia, at 40% (Larson & Powrie, 2014). During the H1N1 influenza pandemic of 2009, infected pregnant women were found to be at high risk for hospitalization and severe complications, specifically pneumonia leading to acute respiratory distress syndrome (Centers for Disease Control and Prevention [CDC], 2009; Jamieson et al, 2009; Sheffield & Cunningham, 2009).

A review of the effects of pneumonia on pregnant patients suggests that maternal and fetal morbidity remain a concern. The complications found were maternal death, fetal death, and preterm labor, with preterm labor rates as high as 44% in some studies (Sheffield & Cunningham, 2009). Pregnant women with pneumonia may require hospitalization, treatment with the appropriate antimicrobial/antiviral, and consultation with a perinatologist as occult onset of preterm labor may occur (Larson & Powrie, 2014). Antibiotic therapy for the pregnant patient is similar to treatment of other adults with CAP: the macrolides erythromycin, azithromycin, and clarithromycin are safe during pregnancy, although erythromycin or azithromycin is the first choice, as each is Pregnancy Category B, whereas clarithromycin is Pregnancy Category C. Sheffield and Cunningham (2009) report a 99% treatment success rate among previously healthy pregnant women treated with macrolides. Doxycycline, a tetracycline, is not used during pregnancy because it may cause discoloration of deciduous teeth in neonates. Fluoroquinolones are avoided during pregnancy due to concerns for fetal malformations, based on animal studies. Women with comorbid conditions or recent antibiotics should be treated with a beta lactam plus a macrolide (Larson & Powrie, 2014; Mandell et al, 2007).

Prevention of viral causes of pneumonia is key to the health of the pregnant patient. The patient who has not previously had varicella should receive the varicella vaccine prior to planning a pregnancy (measles/mumps/rubella [MMR] cannot be given during pregnancy). The pregnant or postpartum patient should receive an influenza vaccine in the fall of the year, and any patient with a chronic medical condition should receive a pneumococcal vaccine.

Lifestyle Modifications

Although the mainstay of treatment is antibiotic therapy, other measures improve outcome. Adequate hydration enables the patient to liquefy any secretions present. Also, patients who are ill with pneumonia often are anorectic and have decreased fluid intake, so education regarding "pushing" fluids is helpful. Rest is one aspect of therapy that younger, working patients may have a hard time accepting. Encouraging patients to not work for a few days will speed the healing process. Tobacco smoke irritates the lungs and increases the coughing associated with the pneumonia. The patient and other household members should refrain from smoking.

Monitoring

The practitioner needs to monitor the patient's clinical status closely. Early identification of the need for hospitalization will enhance the outcome of the illness. The patient's fever, respiratory status, hydration, and activity tolerance all need to be monitored for early signs of either improvement or deterioration.

Outcome Evaluation

As previously mentioned, the patient needs to be monitored for response to empirical antibiotic therapy. The patient should become afebrile in 2 to 4 days. Leukocytosis most often resolves by the fourth day of treatment. Radiographic improvement usually requires more time and is not an indicator of improvement. If the chest x-ray worsens yet the patient

shows clinical improvement, that is the natural progression of the disease. Up to 15% of patients do not respond to appropriate initial empiric antibiotic therapy (Mandell et al, 2007). In severe CAP, if the radiographic findings worsen *and* the clinical picture worsens, then that is a predictor of increased morbidity and mortality (ATS, 2001; Mandell et al, 2007).

If no improvement in clinical status occurs within 72 hours, the practitioner needs to consider that the pathogen is not being treated appropriately. Two possibilities exist. One is that the antibiotic chosen is not treating the pathogen. Another consideration is that the pathogen is resistant to the antibiotic chosen. In an era of increasing antibiotic resistance, the practitioner is always choosing between the narrowest treatment spectrum and the shotgun approach to treatment. There are more powerful oral antibiotics available than those the ATS recommends for empirical therapy, but if all practitioners routinely overprescribe them, then resistance will soon develop. Therefore, the prudent practice is to start with the recommendation and save the broader-spectrum antibiotics for true cases of resistance.

Patient Education

Patient education related to pneumonia should focus on the following:

1. The patient should understand that pneumonia might be bacterial, viral, or mycoplasmal and the expected course of improvement for each. The patient should know that the initial clinical picture might not clearly indicate what type of pathogen is causing the pneumonia. The response to treatment will help to clarify the pathogen.
2. The patient should understand the antibiotic that is prescribed, including expected adverse reactions, drug interactions, and length of treatment.
3. Lifestyle modifications, such as increased hydration, smoking cessation, and rest, should all be discussed.
4. Symptoms of worsening status should be described and the patient told to notify the practitioner or seek urgent care if symptoms worsen rather than improve. Patients should be told to expect clinical improvement in 48 to 72 hours.

Patient education should also focus on prevention.

PEDIATRIC PATIENTS WITH PNEUMONIA

Pneumonia in the pediatric patient can cause the infant or child to become quite ill very rapidly. In the postneonatal period (28 days through 11 months after birth), pneumonia is the seventh highest cause of death in the United States (National Center for Health Statistics, 2011). Specific pathogens are more likely at certain ages (Bradley et al, 2011). In children, treatment is determined by the organism most likely to be causing the pneumonia or by positive cultures for a specific organism. Children may be treated on an outpatient basis if their clinical condition is stable. Indications for hospitalization in children beyond early infancy include moderate to severe respiratory distress, failure to respond to oral antibiotics, lobar consolidation in more than one lobe, immunosuppression, empyema, abscess or pneumatocele, or underlying cardiopulmonary disease. Pneumonia is the second highest reason for admission through the emergency department in children and adolescents, following just behind asthma in a 2004 Healthcare Cost and Utilization Project (Merrill & Owens, 2007). This section focuses on the outpatient treatment of pneumonia in children. Neonates (children less than 30 days old) with pneumonia require hospitalization, with few exceptions; therefore, this group is not discussed in this chapter.

Pathophysiology

S. pneumoniae is the most common cause of bacterial pneumonia in children of all ages (Bradley et al, 2011). The pneumococcal vaccine has demonstrated a decreased overall incidence and prevalence of invasive pneumococcal disease and pneumococcal pneumonia (CDC, 2012b). Following the introduction of PCV7 in 2000, the rates of invasive pneumococcal disease in children less than 5 years of age decreased from 80 cases per 100,000 to less than 1 case per 100,000 by 2007. Subsequently, the replacement of PCV7 with PCV13 in 2010 was approved by the Food and Drug Administration (FDA) on the basis of studies that demonstrated safety and ability comparable to that of PCV7 to elicit antibodies (CDC, 2012b) and remains recommended for all children younger than 59 months old. In children, the most common organisms after *S. pneumoniae* vary according to age (see Table 42-1).

S. pneumoniae is rarely found in neonates, whereas perinatal infection from group B streptococci is often the leading pathogen in this age group. *C. trachomatis,* another perinatal infection, can occur in 5% to 20% of 3 to 16 week-old infants whose mother has untreated disease at the time of birth. Viral infections should also be considered, with mixed viral-bacterial pneumonia identified in up to 30% of children hospitalized with pneumonia (Bradley et al., 2011; Michelow et al, 2004). In a study of children less than age 5 years with radiologically confirmed community-acquired pneumonia diagnosed in the emergency department, the viral pathogens identified were the following: respiratory syncytial virus (RSV) accounted for 23.1%; human metapneumovirus, 8.3%; adenovirus, 3.4%; influenza A, 2.9%; and parainfluenza, 2.9% (Wolf et al, 2010). The clinical findings or age can often differentiate among the pathogens that cause pneumonia in children.

Goals of Treatment

The goals of treatment for pediatric patients with pneumonia are the same as the goals for adults with pneumonia.

Rational Drug Selection

Patient Variables

Infants With Chlamydial Pneumonia

Infants who are 2 to 19 weeks old and who present as afebrile, with a repetitive staccato cough and tachypnea, cervical adenopathy, and rales, are likely to have chlamydial pneumonia (American Academy of Pediatrics [AAP], 2012a). Wheezing is rare. Chest x-ray will show hyperinflation and bilateral diffuse infiltrates. The patient may also have nasal stuffiness and otitis media. Diagnosis is confirmed by detecting chlamydia-specific immunoglobulin M (IgM) in serum (1:32 or greater is diagnostic) (AAP, 2012a).

Drug Therapy

The standard treatment for infants with confirmed chlamydial pneumonia is erythromycin (EryPed) 50 mg/kg daily for 14 days or oral azithromycin (Zithromax) 20 mg/kg/d for 3 days (AAP, 2012a; Bradley et al, 2011). These infants can usually be treated as outpatients if they are able to eat and maintain hydration. An association between the use of erythromycin and hypertropic pyloric stenosis in infants less than 6 weeks of age has been reported. The AAP *Redbook* notes there is limited data on the use of azithromycin to treat chlamydial infections in infants (AAP, 2012a). The AAP continues to advise use of erythromycin for treatment of diseases caused by *C. trachomatis*, and recommends any cases of pyloric stenosis associated with the use of erythromycin or azithromycin be reported to Medwatch (AAP, 2012a). A diagnosis of *C. trachomatis* infection in an infant should prompt treatment of the mother and her sexual partner(s). See Table 42-2 for drugs commonly used with patients with CAP.

Children With Bacterial Pneumonia

Bacterial pneumonia in children usually occurs as a secondary infection following a viral infection. Primary bacterial

Table 42–2 ❋ Drugs Commonly Used: Community-Acquired Pneumonia

Drug	Dose	Length of Treatment	Strengths Available	Comments
Amoxicillin (Amoxil, Trimox)	*Adults and children ≥16 yr:* 875 mg q12h or 500 mg q8h *Children:* 80–100 mg/kg/d divided bid or tid	*Adults:* 7–14 days *Children:* 7–14 days	Tablets: 500, 875 mg Capsules: 250, 500 mg Chewable tablets: 125, 200, 250, 400 mg Powder for suspension: 50, 125, 200, 250, 400 mg/5 mL	
Amoxicillin/clavulanate (Augmentin)	*Adults:* 875 mg q12h *Children <3 mo:* 30 mg/kg/d of amoxicillin divided q12h *Children >3 mo:* 80–90 mg/kg/d of amoxicillin divided q12h Use Augmentin ES-600 formula or combine Augmentin and amoxicillin to equal amoxicillin 80–90 mg/kg/d	10–14 days for all patients	Tablets: 250 mg amoxicillin with 125 mg clavulanate, 500 mg amoxicillin with 125 mg clavulanate, 875 mg amoxicillin with 125 mg clavulanate Chewable tablets: 125 mg amoxicillin with 31.25 mg clavulanate, 200 mg amoxicillin with 28.5 mg clavulanate, 250 mg amoxicillin with 62.5 mg clavulanate, 400 mg amoxicillin with 57 mg clavulanate Suspension: 125 mg amoxicillin with 31.25 mg clavulanate/5 mL, 200 mg amoxicillin with 28.5 mg clavulanate/5 mL, 250 mg amoxicillin with 62.5 mg clavulanate/5 mL, 400 mg amoxicillin with 57 mg clavulanate/5 mL, 400 mg amoxicillin with 57 mg clavulanate Augmentin ES-600 600 mg amoxicillin with 42.9 mg clavulanate per 5 mL	Children's dose is based on amoxicillin content. Because of the clavulanate content, two 250 mg tablets are not the same as one 500 mg tablet. Because of the different clavulanate levels in the suspensions, it is not appropriate to dose the 125 or the 250 mg/5-mL suspensions twice a day. Children should not be given the 250 mg tablet until they are >40 kg. In children, if combining Augmentin and amoxicillin, do not exceed 6.4 mg/kg/d of clavulanate.
Azithromycin (Zithromax)	*Adults:* 500 mg on day 1, then 250 mg daily for days 2–5 *Children:* day 1, 10 mg/kg, followed by 5 mg/kg on days 2–5	5 days	Capsules: 250 mg, Z-pak: six 250 mg tablets with instructions for daily dosing Suspension: 100, 200 mg/5 mL	
Ceftriaxone (Rocephin)	*Adults:* 1–2 g every 12–24 h *Children:* 50–100 mg/kg/d up to 2 g/d	Based on clinical response, switch to oral therapy when able	Powder for Injection: 250 mg, 500 mg 1 g	Broad spectrum Expensive but less expensive than hospitalization
Erythromycin base (E-Mycin, Ery-Tab)	*Adults:* 250–500 mg q6h or 333 mg q8h or 500 mg q12h *Children:* 30–50 mg/kg/d divided into tid dosing	*Adults:* 7–14 days *Children:* 10–14 days	Tablets: 250, 333, 500 mg	Should be taken with food to decrease GI upset
Erythromycin estolate (Ilosone)	*Adults:* 250–500 mg q6h or 333 mg q8h or 500 mg q12h *Children:* 30–50 mg/kg/d divided into tid dosing	*Adults:* 7–14 days *Children:* 10–14 days	Tablets: 500 mg Capsules: 250 mg Suspension: 125, 250 mg/5 mL	Should be taken with food to decrease GI upset

Continued

Table 42–2 ❀ **Drugs Commonly Used: Community-Acquired Pneumonia—cont'd**

Drug	Dose	Length of Treatment	Strengths Available	Comments
Erythromycin ethylsuccinate (E.E.S., EryPed)	*Adults:* 400–800 mg q6h–12h *Children:* 30–50 mg/kg/d divided in q6h *or* q12h dosing	*Adults:* 7–14 days *Children:* 10–14 days	Tablets: 400 mg Chewable tablets: 200 mg Drops: 100 mg/2.5 mL Suspension: 200, 400 mg/ 5 mL	Should be taken with food to decrease GI upset
Gatifloxacin (Tequin)	*Adults ≥18 yr:* 400 mg daily	7–14 days	Tablets: 400 mg	Expensive
Levofloxacin (Levaquin)	*Adults:* 500 mg once a day	7–14 days	Tablets: 250, 500 mg Injection: 500 mg	Expensive
Moxifloxacin (Avelox)	*Adults ≥18 yr:* 400 mg once a day	7–14 days	Tablets: 400 mg	Expensive
Ofloxacin (Floxin)	*Adults ≥18 yr:* 400 mg q12h	10 days	Tablets: 400 mg	Expensive
Sparfloxacin (Zagam)	*Adults ≥18 yr:* 400 mg PO day 1 then 200 mg PO daily for 10 days	10 days	200 mg tablets	Expensive

pneumonia is less common. The viral infection affects the lung defenses, setting the stage for secondary bacterial infection. Prior to universal PCV7 vaccination, the pathogen was identified as *S. pneumoniae* in 73% of bacterial pneumonia cases and in 24% to 33% of all cases of childhood pneumonia (Michelow et al, 2004).

The prevalence of *S. pneumoniae* is decreasing, but it remains the leading cause of bacterial pneumonia in children, especially in those under age 5 (Su-Ting & Tancredi, 2010). The emergence of drug-resistant *S. pneumonia* is increasingly prevalent (CDC, 2012b). The clinical findings may include the following: fever (usually high), cough, shaking and chills, tachypnea, tachycardia, cyanosis, fine crackles (rales), decreased breath sounds, abdominal pain, and vomiting. Oxygen saturation less than 94% may be present. Symptoms can worsen suddenly, and children can become quite ill. Definitive diagnosis of a bacterial infection is difficult to obtain without positive culture on sputum aspirate, although a chest x-ray demonstrates lobar consolidation (Bradley et al, 2011). Blood cultures are not routinely necessary in nontoxic, fully immunized children managed in the outpatient setting but are recommended if these children fail to demonstrate clinical improvement or if there is clinical deterioration after initiation of antibiotic therapy (Bradley et al, 2011). A complete blood count is no longer recommended for routine outpatient management of pneumonia but may be warranted if the pneumonia presentation is severe (Bradley et al, 2011). If pneumatoceles are seen on chest x-ray, suspect staphylococcal pneumonia.

Drug Therapy

If *S. pneumoniae* is the suspected organism based on the clinical picture in previously healthy, appropriately immunized infants, preschool, school-aged, and adolescent children, high-dose amoxicillin (90 mg/kg daily, divided in two doses) is the drug of choice for 7 to 10 days of outpatient treatment

(Bradley et al, 2011)). If highly resistant pneumococci are in the community, the practitioner may choose between IV or IM ceftriaxone (50 mg/kg in one daily dose) or cefotaxime (150 mg/kg/d every 8 hours) followed by appropriate oral therapy after 1 or 2 doses (Bradley et al, 2011). Vancomycin has not been shown to be more effective than a third-generation cephalosporin with DRSP, yet is recommended if clinical, laboratory, or imaging characteristics are consistent with an infection caused by *S. aureus* (Bradley et al, 2011). Patients who are treated early in the course of the illness usually respond to high-dose amoxicillin. *S. pneumonia* may be resistant to macrolides (AAP, 2009c) but are recommended for CAP caused by atypical pathogens (Bradley et al, 2011). Macrolides are not considered first-line therapy for children under age 5 due to the most common pathogen being either *pneumococcus* or a virus (Bradley et al, 2011).

If *S. aureus* is the confirmed or highly suspected organism, the preferred oral regimen for methicillin-susceptible cases is cephalexin (75 to 100 mg/kg/d in 3 to 4 doses) or an alternative of clindamycin (30 to 40 mg/kg/d in 3 to 4 doses), with cefazolin, oxacillin, clindamycin, or vancomycin in hospitalized cases (Bradley et al, 2011). Vancomycin would be added to the regimen if methicillin-resistant *S. aureus* (MRSA) is suspected. Patients with *S. aureus* pneumonia are usually quite ill and require hospitalization for at least a few days. They may require a chest tube if there is significant empyema.

Children and Adolescents With Mycoplasma Pneumonia

Mycoplasma pneumonia is the most common type in children over age 5 years, with approximately 10% of school-age children presenting with symptoms consistent with atypical or mycoplasma infection (AAP, 2012b). The disease is usually mild. The typical history includes upper respiratory symptoms, fever, dry cough, malaise, sore throat, headache, and possibly chills. Symptoms often last for 3 to 4 weeks (AAP, 2012b). A maculopapular rash may develop in up to 10% of children with mycoplasma pneumonia (AAP, 2012b). *M. pneumoniae* may be associated with asthma exacerbation. The patient may have been treated with amoxicillin for "bronchitis" without improvement. Chest x-ray reveals bronchovascular markings with areas of atelectasis. A polymerase chain reaction (PCR) test for *M. pneumoniae* is the standard, with 80% to 100% sensitivity and specificity, as a culture may take up to 21 days (AAP, 2012b). Serum cold hemagglutinin titers are nonspecific and only positive in 50% of children with mycoplasma pneumonia (AAP, 2012b).

Drug Therapy

Mycoplasma pneumonia is usually mild and will resolve without treatment, although observation data indicate children will have a shorter duration of symptoms and fewer relapses if treated with an antimicrobial (AAP, 2009b). The treatment of choice for mycoplasma pneumonia is a macrolide. The preferred oral treatment is azithromycin (10 mg/kg on day 1 and 5 mg/kg on days 2 through 5), though as an alternative clarithromycin (15mg/kg/day in 2 doses) or erythromycin (40 to 50 mg/kg daily is given qid or tid or, for larger children, 333 mg PO tid for 10 days) is an option (AAP, 2012b; Bradley et al, 2011). Erythromycin is inexpensive and provides good coverage for other atypical organisms. Azithromycin (Zithromax) is also packaged in a "Z-pak," a 5-day dose pack for older children or children over 50 kg; printed on the package are instructions to take two 250 mg capsules on day 1 and one capsule daily thereafter. Because mycoplasmas lack a cell wall, they are inherently resistant to beta lactam agents.

Monitoring

Patients with bacterial pneumonia need to be monitored closely for clinical improvement or deterioration. If children are being treated with the appropriate antibiotic, they often show rapid improvement, much faster than adults. Children can also deteriorate rapidly, and any infant or young child who is not hospitalized needs to be seen in the clinic the following day for reassessment. Recommendations are that families receive clear instructions regarding the symptoms of deterioration in respiratory status.

If cultures are drawn, results are usually available in 24 hours, and the practitioner needs to determine (1) if the appropriate antibiotic has been chosen and (2) the level of resistance the organism has to the chosen antibiotic. If the patient is improving clinically, there is no need for repeat blood counts or cultures. If the patient is not improving or the clinical condition worsens, a chest x-ray can determine if effusions or empyema are developing. Routine chest radiographs are not recommended for the confirmation of suspected CAP in pediatric patients well enough to be treated in the outpatient setting but should be obtained in those with suspected or documented hypoxemia, significant respiratory distress, those who have failed initial antibiotic therapy, and those who are being admitted (Bradley et al, 2011).

Patients with mycoplasma pneumonia should be monitored for clinical improvement. The cough may last for weeks after the infection is treated. *M. pneumoniae* can spread to the blood, central nervous system, heart, skin, and joints, so monitoring for these complications is prudent. A child with sickle cell disease who contracts mycoplasma pneumonia develops a more severe pulmonary disease than the average child.

All children with pneumonia need monitoring of their hydration status. Nutritional intake should also be assessed in infants who may be ill for a few days. The parents' ability to successfully administer medication and their ability to monitor their child's status are essential to the successful outpatient treatment of children with pneumonia.

Outcome Evaluation

Like the adult patient, the child with pneumonia must be monitored for response to the antibiotic therapy. The child should become afebrile in 24 to 48 hours. There may be a residual cough for weeks, which should lessen with time. If the child's clinical status fails to improve in 48 to 72 hours, then the treatment plan must be reconsidered. There may be bacterial resistance to the antibiotic, or the patient might have mycoplasma pneumonia, which requires a macrolide antibiotic.

Patient Education

Patient education when a child has bacterial pneumonia focuses on the following:

1. How to assess the child's respiratory status and signs of respiratory deterioration. Clear instructions, such as "If breathing over __ breaths per minute, call the practitioner," help parents monitor their child at home.
2. A clear plan of where the parents should take a child whose status worsens during the evening or night. Given the variable insurance rules regarding after-hours care, the practitioner needs to explain to parents how to access high-quality pediatric after-hours care in the event of deterioration in the child's status. Not all urgent-care clinics are equipped to handle a child in respiratory distress, and an emergency room is probably the best place for the child to be assessed. Use of the emergency 911 system for respiratory distress should be discussed with families, with clear guidelines given as to what constitutes respiratory distress.
3. How to administer medication appropriately. Make sure the parents have a medicine syringe to accurately administer the oral medications. Some medications must be taken on an empty stomach and others must be taken with food, and the parents need to be reminded about any special instructions regarding the administration of the antibiotic.
4. The parents need to know how to assess hydration and what parameters are expected for urine output. Instructions that clearly define minimum output are the easiest to understand; for example, "Your infant should have a wet diaper every 6 to 8 hours at a minimum."

REFERENCES

ACIP Adult Immunization Work Group. (2013). *Advisory Committee on Immunization Practices (ACIP): Recommended immunization schedule for adults aged 19 Years and older—United States, 2013. Morbidity and Mortality Weekly Report (MMWR), 62*(01), 9–17. Retrieved from http://www.cdc.gov/mmwr/pdf/wk/mm62e0128.pdf

ACIP Childhood/Adolescent Immunization Work Group. (2013). *Advisory Committee on Immunization Practices (ACIP): Recommended immunization schedule for persons aged 0 through 18 Years—United States, 2013. Morbidity and Mortality Weekly Report (MMWR), 62*(01), 2–8. Retrieved from http://www.cdc.gov/mmwr/preview/mmwrhtml/su6201a2.htm

American Academy of Pediatrics (AAP). (2012a). *Chlamydia trachomatis.* In L. K. Pickering (Ed.), *Red book: 2012 Report of the Committee on Infectious Diseases* (29th ed., pp 276–281). Elk Grove Village, IL: American Academy of Pediatrics. Retrieved from http://aapredbook.aappublications.org/content/1/SEC131/SEC158/SEC161.body

American Academy of Pediatrics (AAP). (2012b). *Mycoplasma pneumoniae* and other *Mycoplasma* species infections. In L. K. Pickering (Ed.), *Red book: 2012 Report of the Committee on Infectious Diseases* (29th ed., pp 518–521). Elk Grove Village, IL: American Academy of Pediatrics. Retrieved from http://aapredbook.aappublications.org/content/1/SEC131/SEC223.body?sid=726d791b-d269-4fdb-9a88-a8e6552f9b37

American Academy of Pediatrics (AAP). (2012c). Pneumococcal infections. In L. K. Pickering (Ed.), *Red book: 2012 Report of the Committee on Infectious Diseases* (29th ed., pp 571–582). Elk Grove Village, IL: American Academy of Pediatrics. Retrieved from http://aapredbook.aappublications.org/content/1/SEC131/SEC241.body?sid=cfa4eb5f-a037-4392-b582-1eea63cb8765

American Academy of Pediatrics (AAP). (2012d). Staphylococcal infections. In L. K. Pickering (Ed.), *Red book: 2012 Report of the Committee on Infectious Diseases* (29th ed., pp 653–658). Elk Grove Village, IL: American Academy of Pediatrics. Retrieved from http://aapredbook.aappublications.org/content/1/SEC131/SEC263.body?sid=6aa390d0-0d24-4ee3-b166-3613961e8ce1

American Thoracic Society (ATS). (2001). Guidelines for the management of adults with community-acquired pneumonia: Diagnosis, assessment of severity, antimicrobial therapy and prevention. *American Journal of Respiratory and Critical Care Medicine, 163*, 1730–1754.

Bradley, J. S., Byington, C. L., Shah, S. S., Alverson, B., Carver, E. R., Harrison, C., et al. (2011). The management of community-acquired pneumonia in infants and children older than 3 months of age: Clinical Practice Guidelines by the Pediatric Infectious Diseases Society and the Infectious Diseases Society of America. *Clinical Infectious Diseases, 53* (7), e25–e76. Retrieved from http://cid.oxfordjournals.org/content/53/7/e25

Centers for Disease Control and Prevention (CDC). (2009). Interim guidance: Considerations regarding 2009 H1N1 influenza in intrapartum and postpartum hospital settings. Retrieved from http://www.cdc.gov/h1n1flu/guidance/obstetric.htm

Centers for Disease Control and Prevention (CDC). (2012a). *Use of 13-valent pneumococcal conjugate vaccine and 23-valent pneumococcal polysaccharide vaccine for adults with immunocompromising conditions: Recommendations of the Advisory Committee on Immunization Practices (ACIP). Morbidity and Mortality Weekly Report (MMWR), 61*(40), 816–819. Retrieved from http://www.cdc.gov/mmwr/preview/mmwrhtml/mm6140a4.htm

Centers for Disease Control and Prevention (CDC). (2012b). Chapter 11: Pneumococcal manual for the surveillance of vaccine-preventable diseases. Retrieved from http://www.cdc.gov/vaccines/pubs/surv-manual/chpt11-pneumo.html

Centers for Disease Control and Prevention (CDC). (2013). *Use of 13-valent pneumococcal conjugate vaccine and 23-valent pneumococcal polysaccharide vaccine among children aged 6–18 years with immunocompromising conditions: Recommendations of the Advisory Committee on Immunization Practices (ACIP). Morbidity and Mortality Weekly Report (MMWR), 62*(25), 521–524. Retrieved from http://www.cdc.gov/mmwr/preview/mmwrhtml/mm6225a3.htm

Jamieson, D. J., Honein, M. A., Rasmussen, S. A., Williams, J. L., Swerdlow, D. L., Biggerstaff, M. S., & Novel Influenza A H1N1 Pregnancy Working Group (2009). H1N1 2009 influenza virus infection during pregnancy in the USA. *The Lancet, 374*, 451–458.

Larson, L., & Powrie, R. (2014). Treatment of respiratory infections in pregnant women. *UpToDate.* Waltham, MA: Wolters Kluwer. Retrieved from http://www.uptodate.com/contents/treatment-of-respiratory-infections-in-pregnant-women

Mandell, L. A, Wunderink, R. G., Anzueto, A., Bartlett, J. G., Campbell, G. D., Dowell, S. F., et al. (2007). Infectious Diseases Society of America/American Thoracic Society consensus guidelines on the management of community-acquired pneumonia in adults. *Clinical Infectious Disease, 44* (2 Supp.), S27–S72.

Merrill, C. T., & Owens, P. L. (2007). *Reasons for being admitted to the hospital through the emergency department for children and adolescents, 2004.* HCUP Statistical Brief #33. Agency for Healthcare Research and Quality, Rockville, MD. Retrieved from http://www.hcup-us.ahrq.gov/reports/statbriefs/sb33.pdf

Michelow, I. C., Olsen, K., Lozano, J., Rollins, N. K., Duffy, L. B., Zeiger, T., et al. (2004). Epidemiology and clinical characteristics of community-acquired pneumonia in hospitalized children. *Pediatrics, 113*, 701–707.

Mills, K., Nelson, A. C., Winslow, B. T., & Springer, K. L. (2009). Treatment of nursing home-acquired pneumonia. *American Family Physician, 79*(11), 976–982.

Muder, R. R., Agahbabian, R. V., Loeb, M. B., Solot, J. A., & Higbee, M. (2004). Nursing home-acquired pneumonia: An emergency department treatment algorithm. *Current Medical Research and Opinion, 20*(8), 1309–1320.

National Center for Health Statistics. (2011). National vital statistics report. *Deaths: Final data for 2009, 60*(3). Retrieved from http://www.cdc.gov/nchs/data/nvsr/nvsr60/nvsr60_03.pdf

Ramsey, P. S., & Ramin, K. D. (2001). Pneumonia in pregnancy. *Obstetrics and Gynecology Clinics of North America, 28*(3), 553–569.

Riley, P. D., Aronsky, D., & Dean, N. C. (2004). Validation of the 2001 American Thoracic Society criteria for severe community acquired pneumonia. *Critical Care Medicine, 32*(12), 2398–2402.

Sheffield, J. S., & Cunningham, F. G. (2009). Community-acquired pneumonia in pregnancy. *Obstetrics & Gynecology, 114*(4), 915–922.

Su-Ting, T. L., & Tancredi, D. J. (2010). Empyema hospitalizations increase in U.S. children despite pneumococcal conjugate vaccine. *Pediatrics, 125*(1), 26–33.

Wolf, D. G., Greenberg, D., Shemer-Avni, Y., Govon-Lavi, N., Bar-Jiv, J., & Dagan, R. (2010). Association of human metapneumovirus with radiologically diagnosed community-acquired alveolar pneumonia in young children. *Journal of Pediatrics, 156*(1), 115–120.

SMOKING CESSATION

Benjamin J. Miller

The current rate of adults over age 18 years who smoke cigarettes in the United States is 18%, representing a steady decline in smoking rates from a high of 41.9% in 1965 (National Center for Health Statistics, 2013). Tobacco is the leading cause of preventable illness and death in the United States, contributing to more than 443,000 deaths annually, including an estimated 49,000 deaths from secondhand exposure (National Cancer Institute, National Institute of Health, 2012). Tobacco use contributes to the development of cancers, cerebrovascular disease, cardiovascular disease, dental disease, gastrointestinal (GI) disorders, and respiratory disease, making it the most preventable health problem in developed countries. Smokers who do not quit by age 35 have a 50% chance of dying from a tobacco-related disease.

Patients' tobacco use needs to be addressed by all primary care providers, especially those who care for children; the 2006 National Survey on Drug Use & Health indicated that 7.1% of middle school students and 23.2% of high school students use tobacco in some form (Centers for Disease Control [CDC], 2012). Secondhand or environmental exposure to tobacco smoke also poses a health hazard to nonsmokers, and the health-care provider plays an important role in educating parents of young children about the effects of secondhand smoke. Education about secondhand smoke should be used as an opportunity to offer tobacco cessation to the smoking family member, thereby decreasing the health risks for the whole family.

A review of the physiological and psychological process of addiction will assist the health-care provider in understanding the rationale for pharmacological intervention. Tobacco smoke contains many different chemicals, many of them known health hazards (ammonia, formaldehyde, carbon monoxide, benzene, arsenic, and lead). The addictive component in tobacco is nicotine. Nicotine has all the components of an addictive substance, similar to those of heroin, in which "addiction is characterized by compulsive drug seeking and use, even in the face of negative health consequences" (National Institute on Drug Abuse, 2006).

The many forms of tobacco include cigarettes, pipes, cigars, smokeless tobacco, electronic cigarettes, and snuff, and patients can be addicted to any of them (see Box 43-1). The health-care provider needs to assess if the patient is using any form of tobacco and address cessation in the patient's plan of care. Although behavioral modification also plays an essential role in quitting, it is discussed only briefly as a component of the treatment plan because this chapter focuses on pharmacological management. According to a recent meta-analysis of 38 studies with more than 15,000 participants, the success rate of smoking cessation will increase by 16% with combined behavioral therapy/pharmacological management versus pharmacological management alone (Stead & Lancaster, 2012).

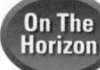

TOBACCO-CESSATION THERAPIES

The future looks promising for tobacco-cessation therapies. Currently, a sublingual form of nicotine replacement, in a 2 mg or 4 mg dose, is available in Europe and Canada. Scientists are also investigating the potential of a vaccine that stimulates antibodies that block nicotine receptors in the brain and will be used to prevent relapse in smokers who quit. A recent study examining nicotine vaccinations found the vaccines were safe and well tolerated; however, insufficient antibodies developed that would lead to a significant long-term effect on relapse prevention (Tonstad et al, 2013).

PATHOPHYSIOLOGY

Nicotine is a naturally occurring substance that is soluble in water and lipids. It is readily absorbed from many sites, including the lungs, mucosa, skin, and GI tract.

Nicotine Delivery

Nicotine is absorbed rapidly from tobacco smoke into the pulmonary circulation. It is then transported via the bloodstream to the brain, where it reaches the nicotine cholinergic receptors in 10 to 15 seconds after a puff. The mean time to peak concentration in the bloodstream is 7 to 8 minutes. Each puff contributes to maintaining the nicotine concentration. With each cigarette averaging 10 puffs, the pack-a-day smoker reinforces the blood nicotine level 200 times per day, with each puff providing distinct reinforcement of the habit. Smokeless tobacco is absorbed more slowly from the oral or nasal cavity.

BOX 43–1 **ELECTRONIC CIGARETTES**

Electronic cigarettes or e-cigarettes are growing in popularity as an alternative to traditional tobacco use, with U.S. sales expected to exceed $1 billion in 2013. E-cigarettes are battery-operated devices that deliver nicotine via inhaled vapor, eliminating the harmful tars and carbon monoxide. At present, there is considerable controversy over the health implications of e-cigarettes, which has attracted the attention of the FDA and the CDC (Sutfin, McCoy, Morrell, Hoeppner, & Wolfson, 2013).

Because of the ability to regulate the nicotine content, there may be a role for e-cigarettes in nicotine replacement therapy and tobacco cessation. In a small study of 86 tobacco users, the use of 18 mg of nicotine resulted in a significant decrease in withdrawal symptoms compared to a control group (Dawkins, Turner, Hasna, & Soar, 2012). These data suggest there may be a future role for e-cigarettes; however, no evidence-based recommendations can be made at this time. Further study of the potential toxic effects of e-cigarette chemicals is warranted before large scale studies occur.

Nicotinic Receptors

The neuronal nicotinic receptors appear to be complex, with the complexity contributing to the different responses to nicotine agonists. Chronic use of nicotine results in an increased number of brain nicotinic receptors, which appears to be an important factor in the development of tolerance of and dependence on nicotine.

Nicotine has both stimulant and depressant effects in the central nervous system (CNS). The stimulant effect is exerted mainly at the cortex, producing increased alertness and cognitive performance. Nicotine activates the nucleus accumbens "reward" system in the limbic system, causing increased extracellular fluid dopamine levels in the region. This increases the "reinforcing" quality of nicotine. IV administration of nicotine activates neurohormonal pathways, releasing acetylcholine, norepinephrine, dopamine, serotonin, vasopressin, beta endorphins, growth hormone, and adrenocorticotropic hormone (ACTH).

Nicotine Withdrawal Syndrome

Nicotine withdrawal syndrome is characterized by craving, nervousness, irritability, impatience, hostility, labile mood, difficulty in concentrating, restlessness, and anxiety. Physical symptoms include decreased heart rate, increased appetite, and weight gain averaging 8 to 11 pounds (Aubin, Farley, Lycett, Lahmek, & Aveyard, 2012). Somatic complaints such as myalgia, headache, constipation, and fatigue are common. The urge to smoke is closely related to low blood nicotine levels, which bring on early morning withdrawal symptoms. The smoker may not be smoking to achieve the effects of nicotine but rather to avoid withdrawal symptoms.

GOALS OF TREATMENT

A critical step in treatment of tobacco use is identifying patients who are ready to quit. Every health-care encounter should encompass screening for tobacco use and assessment for the readiness to quit. The initial intervention for treatment of tobacco use includes the Advise, Assess, and Refer (AAR) approach, which involves a conversation with the patient, assessing readiness to quit, and then giving the patient a referral to a tobacco treatment specialist or local tobacco quit line. In a recent study by Vidrene and colleagues (2013), a novel approach to smoking treatment focuses on making a referral to a tobacco quit line that contacts the patient, which resulted in a 13-fold increase in treatment compared to those who were given information and asked to make a call.

The goal of tobacco cessation treatment is the complete discontinuation of tobacco. It can be achieved either "cold turkey" without pharmacological intervention or by using nicotine replacement therapy, which is then gradually reduced over time to zero. If bupropion (Zyban) is used, the goal is for the patient to be tobacco-free at the end of the 7 to 12 weeks of therapy. Twelve weeks is the recommended treatment length if varenicline (Chantix) is prescribed.

RATIONAL DRUG SELECTION

The pharmacological management of tobacco cessation involves three different treatment modalities: nicotine replacement therapy, the antidepressant bupropion, and the nicotine receptor partial agonist varenicline. The combination of bupropion and nicotine replacement via a nicotine patch or lozenge may provide higher long-term rates of smoking cessation (Jorenby et al, 1999; Piper et al, 2009; Steinberg et al, 2009); however, one recent study suggests there is no superiority of combined therapy when controlling for behavioral modification (Stapleton et al, 2013). All of the nicotine replacement therapy products deliver nicotine to the CNS at a lower dose and slower rate than do tobacco cigarettes, and all the products can double quit rates (Abramowicz, 2003). Varenicline (Chantix) has a reported a continuous abstinence rate of 43.9% after 9 to 12 weeks of therapy (Garrison & Dugan, 2009).

Nicotine Replacement Therapy

Nicotine replacement therapy comes in five different forms: gum, lozenge, transdermal patch, inhaler, and nasal spray. The gum and transdermal patch Nicotrol, the transdermal patch Habitrol, and the lozenge Commit are available over-the-counter (OTC); the inhaler (Nicotrol Inhaler) and the spray (Nicotrol NS) are by prescription. Although the patient can self-treat with the OTC products, the health-care provider should educate the patient regarding their proper use to ensure successful treatment. Nicotine replacement does not achieve the same peak levels of nicotine as does smoking, but it does achieve a level high enough to suppress nicotine withdrawal symptoms. Nicotine replacement therapy is recommended for patients who smoke more than 20 cigarettes per day (one pack), patients who smoke within 30 minutes of awakening in the morning, and patients who have tried to quit previously and have failed because of strong withdrawal symptoms and craving within the first week of quitting. Cooper and colleagues (2004) found that patients treated with nicotine replacement therapy combined with nonpharmacological interventions (behavioral counseling or telephone intervention contact) reported greatest adherence to treatment.

Nicotine polacrilex gum is Pregnancy Category C, and transdermal nicotine is Pregnancy Category D, as nicotine is associated with decreased fetal breathing movements, probably caused by decreased placental perfusion. Nicotine replacement therapy is contraindicated for people with a hypersensitivity to nicotine and should be used with caution in persons immediately after myocardial infarction (MI) and in patients with life-threatening arrhythmias and severe or worsening angina pectoris because of increases in heart rate.

Nicotine Gum

Nicotine gum improves smoking cessation rates by 40% to 60% compared with controls through 12 months of follow-up. The active ingredient in nicotine gum (Nicorette) is nicotine polacrilex, a nicotine resin complex. The nicotine is bound to an ion-exchange resin that is released only during chewing. The medication is administered when the patient places a piece of gum in his or her mouth and chews slowly five to eight times, until a peppery taste appears. The patient then "parks" the gum in the buccal space. Intermittent chewing and parking the gum over a period of 30 minutes promotes slow buccal absorption. Chewing too quickly causes an excess amount of nicotine to be released into the bloodstream, producing nausea, throat irritation, and hiccoughs. The patient should avoid smoking while chewing nicotine gum because toxicity symptoms may occur (nausea, vomiting, and headache). Nicotine gum should not be the first-line choice for patients with temporomandibular joint (TMJ) disease or peptic ulcer disease on account of adverse effects.

Nicotine polacrilex gum takes 30 minutes to reach its peak serum concentration. The patient who is just beginning a tobacco-cessation program should chew one piece of 2 or 4 mg gum per hour. Abstinence rates appear to be higher when the patient chews the gum on a fixed schedule of every hour or every 2 hours. The patient who smokes more than 25 cigarettes per day should be started on the 4 mg dose initially and not exceed the maximum number of pieces per day of gum (30/d of 2 mg, 20/d of 4 mg). Acidic foods (coffee, soft drinks, juice) interfere with the buccal absorption of nicotine from nicotine polacrilex and should be avoided for 15 minutes before, during, and after chewing the gum.

After the patient has successfully quit smoking for 6 weeks, a gradual weaning of the gum dosage should begin. Suggestions for a gradual withdrawal of treatment are as follows:

1. Weeks 7 to 9, chew one piece of gum every 2 to 4 hours.
2. Weeks 10 to 12, chew one piece of gum every 4 to 8 hours.
3. After 12 weeks, discontinue nicotine gum and suggest substituting sugarless gum if needed.

Online support for quitting smoking is available from the brand-name drug manufacturer at www.nicorette.com; the program includes tools for dealing with cravings and lapses.

Nicotine Lozenge

Nicotine polacrilex lozenge (Nicorette Lozenge) is indicated as an adjunct in smoking-cessation therapy. The usual dose is either a 2 mg or 4 mg lozenge, based on how early in the day the smoker smoked the first cigarette. If a smoker has the first cigarette of the day 30 minutes or more after awakening, then the 2 mg lozenge is indicated. The 4 mg lozenge is used if the smoker has the first cigarette within 30 minutes of arising. The lozenge dissolves over 20 to 30 minutes with peak serum levels of nicotine reached in 20 to 30 minutes after the lozenge dissolves in the mouth. The patient should not chew or swallow the lozenge because there is a significant first-pass metabolism that will decrease bioavailability (Abramowicz, 2003). The patient should use 1 lozenge every 1 to 2 hours for the first 6 weeks, at least 9 lozenges per day with a maximum of 20 lozenges per day. Dosing should taper based on a set schedule similar to that for nicotine polacrilex gum:

1. Weeks 1 to 6, one lozenge every 1 to 2 hours.
2. Weeks 7 to 9, one lozenge every 2 to 4 hours.
3. Weeks 10 to 12, one lozenge every 4 to 8 hours.

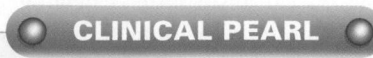

CLINICAL PEARL

Nicotine Gum
Patients complain about the taste of the nicotine gum. Suggest that the patient try the flavored variety, which patients seem to tolerate better.

The patient should not eat or drink for 15 minutes before or while the lozenge is dissolving in the mouth. There may be a tingling sensation in the mouth as the lozenge dissolves. Online quitting support is available at http://www.nicorette.com/.

Nicotine Transdermal System

The transdermal nicotine system, or "patch," provides a slow, cutaneous absorption of nicotine over many hours. The patch is applied to clean, nonhairy skin on the upper body or upper arm when the patient wakes up. Peak nicotine levels occur in 2 to 6 hours (brand-dependent) and then gradually decrease. Once the patch is removed, nicotine levels in the blood reach a nondetectable level in 10 to 12 hours in nonsmokers. There are different strengths of patches available and patches that are for 16-hour and for 24-hour use, allowing for dose regulation (Table 43-1). The 16-hour patch works well for the light to average smoker but is not effective for early morning withdrawal symptoms. The 24-hour patch provides a steady-state blood level of nicotine, with minimum peaks and troughs, and avoids morning withdrawal symptoms. The disadvantage of the 24-hour patch is that there are more adverse effects, including sleep disruption. Evaluating the patient's smoking habit and determining if early morning withdrawal is an issue will enable the provider to recommend the best transdermal system for the patient. Transdermal nicotine approximately doubles 6- to 12-month abstinence rates over those produced by placebo interventions.

The transdermal nicotine system has the advantage of delivering a steady-state level of nicotine that prevents nicotine withdrawal symptoms while allowing the smoker to work on the behavioral aspects of quitting. Unlike nicotine gum, the patch has the advantage of not reinforcing the oral aspects of smoking. Patients appreciate the ease of administration and once-daily dosing. Weaning off the transdermal nicotine system is accomplished by decreasing the dose of the patch on a scheduled basis. Longer duration of use and weaning, rather than abrupt withdrawal of the nicotine patch, had the greatest effectiveness in a review of nicotine replacement for smoking cessation (Silagy, Lancaster, Stead, Mant, & Fowler, 2004).

One disadvantage of the nicotine patch is that patients report they are unable to self-regulate the dose if they are exhibiting withdrawal symptoms. This makes the patch less effective for highly dependent smokers, and a highly dependent smoker who is started on a transdermal nicotine system should be started on a high-dose, 24-hour system to decrease withdrawal symptoms. The patient *must* refrain from smoking while using the nicotine patch because life-threatening dysrhythmias or acute myocardial infarction may occur.

The most common adverse effect of the nicotine patch is skin irritation, with 35% to 47% of patients reporting some skin irritation during clinical trials. Advising the patient to change the site every day and not to reuse the site within a week can minimize this problem. The amount of skin irritation differs with the brand and dose used, so a change may alleviate the problem. If the patient exhibits symptoms of sleep disturbance or insomnia while using the transdermal nicotine system, first determine whether the patient has signs of too high a dose or early morning withdrawal. Delayed onset of sleep is usually associated with too high a dose and early awakening is associated with withdrawal symptoms. The provider can either switch the patient from the 24-hour to the 16-hour patch to decrease the dose or, if the patient is already using the 16-hour patch, decrease the dose. If withdrawal is the problem, then increase the patch from a 16-hour to a 24-hour or increase the dose of the patch. The patient needs to be aware that some adjustment of the dose may be necessary to provide effective relief of symptoms with minimum adverse effects. Advise the patient to report any adverse effects so that adjustments can be made.

Other adverse effects observed include symptoms of nicotine toxicity (headache, nausea, and vomiting) with higher-dose patches and with smoking while using a patch. If symptoms of toxicity occur, remove the patch and flush the skin area with water. *Do not use soap,* which increases nicotine absorption from the site. Nicotine will continue to be delivered into the bloodstream for a number of hours because there is a deposit of nicotine under the skin. Patients should report any symptoms of toxicity immediately to their healthcare provider. Generic transdermal nicotine is available at substantial savings to the patient.

Nicotine Nasal Spray

Nicotine nasal spray (Nicotrol NS) is an inhaled form of nicotine replacement therapy. The usual dose is 1 to 2 sprays in each nostril per hour, not to exceed 5 doses (10 sprays) per

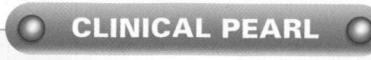

CLINICAL PEARL

Nicotine Patch
Advise patients to dispose of used nicotine patches out of the reach of children or animals. Enough nicotine is left in a *used* patch to lead to toxic levels in a child or small animal.

Table 43–1 🔗 Drugs Commonly Used: Smoking Cessation

Drug	Strength Available	Dosage	Comments
Nicotine Gum			
Nicotine polacrilex (Nicorette)	2, 4 mg	If smoking <20–25 cigarettes/d: chew one 2 mg piece every 1–2 h (at least 9/d), max of 30/d If smoking >20–25 cigarettes/d: chew one 4 mg piece every 1–2 h (at least 9/d), max of 20/d After 6 wk decrease dose to 1 every 2–4 h for 3 wk, then 1 piece every 4–8 h for 3 wk, and then discontinue Alternative: After 6 wk, gradually wean the dose by decreasing one piece of gum/d every 4–7 days	Abstinence rates are higher if gum is chewed on a scheduled basis, rather than prn. Acidic foods and drinks interfere with absorption, so they should be avoided during and for 15 min before and after chewing nicotine gum. The use of nicotine gum for longer than 6 mo is not recommended.
Nicotine Transdermal Patch			
Habitrol (OTC)	21 mg/d 14 mg/d 7 mg/d	If >10 cigarettes/d: 21 mg/d for first 6 wk, 14 mg/d for next 2 wk, and 7 mg/d for final 2 If ≤10 cigarettes/d: 14 mg/d for 6 wk, then 7 mg/d for final 2–4 wk *Length of treatment:* 8–12 wk	24-h patch Apply to clean, nonhairy area on upper body or upper arm upon waking. Rotate application site.
Nicoderm CQ (OTC)	21 mg/d 14 mg/d 7 mg d	21 mg/d for first 6 wk, 14 mg/d for next 2 wk, and 7 mg/d for final 2 wk *Low-dose regimen:** 14 mg/d for 6 wk, then 7 mg/d for final 2–4 wk *Length of treatment:* 8–12 wk	24-h patch Apply to clean, nonhairy area on upper body or upper arm upon waking. May remove after 16–24 h.
Nicotrol Step-Down Patch (OTC)	15 mg/6 h 10 mg/16 h 5 mg/16 h	15 mg/16 h for first 6 wk, 10 mg/16 h for 2 wk, then 5 mg/16 h for final 2 wk *Alternative:* Use 15 mg/16 h patch daily for 6 wk, then discontinue *Length of treatment:* 10 wk	16-h patch Apply to clean, nonhairy area on upper body or upper arm upon waking. Remove after 16 h (before bed).
Prostep (OTC)	22 mg/d 11 mg/d	22 mg/d for 4–8 wk, then 11 mg/d for 2–4 wk *Low-dose regimen**: 11 mg/d for 4–8 wk *Length of treatment:* 6–12 wk	24-h patch Apply to clean, nonhairy area on upper body or upper arm upon waking.
Nicotine Nasal Spray			
Nicotrol NS (Rx)	0.5 mg/spray 1 dose = 1 mg, or 1 spray in each nostril	Start with 1–2 doses (2–4 sprays)/h, max of 5 sprays/h, 40 sprays/d *Length of treatment:* max 3 mo	Can be used ad lib. Advise patient not to sniff, inhale, or swallow the spray.
Nicotine Inhaler			
Nicotrol inhaler (Rx)	10 mg/cartridge (4 mg nicotine delivered)	Patient puffs on mouthpiece frequently and continuously for 20 min. Initially, begins with at least 6 cartridges/d (max 16 cartridges/d) for the first 3–6 wk. Gradually decrease over 12 wk *Length of treatment:* max 6 mo	Provides oral stimulation similar to smoking.
Nicotinic Receptor Partial Agonists			
Varenicline (Chantix)	Strength: 0.5, 1.0 mg	*Patients ≥18 yr:* 0.5 mg PO daily for the first 3 d, then 0.5 mg bid days 4–7. On day 8 increase to 1.0 mg bid. *Length of treatment:* 12 wk; may continue for another 12 wk	Start 1 wk before quit date. Take on full stomach with a glass of water. Reduce dose if intolerable nausea or other side effects occur. Monitor closely for signs of mood change or suicide ideation.
Antidepressant			
Bupropion (Zyban) (Rx)	150 mg tablet	*Patients ≥ 18 yr:* Begin 150 mg/d 1–2 wk prior to quit date. Increase dose to 150 mg bid (at least 8 h apart) after 3 d. *Length of treatment:* 7–12 wk	May be combined with nicotine replacement. Avoid bedtime dosing, which may cause insomnia. Do not use with other forms of bupropion. Monitor closely for signs of mood change or suicide ideation.

*Low-dose therapy is used for patients weighing less than 100 lb, patients with cardiovascular disease, and patients who smoke one-half pack per day or less.

    OTC = over the counter.

hour and not to exceed 40 doses (80 sprays) per day. The advantage to nicotine nasal spray is rapid achievement of peak blood levels, with peak levels reached in 4 to 15 minutes after a single 1 mg (2 spray) dose. This speed is advantageous for patients who report severe withdrawal symptoms because the rate of absorption into the bloodstream is similar to that of smoking cigarettes, providing immediate relief of withdrawal symptoms through self-administration. Patients can have a sense of control over their nicotine cravings.

Patients need to be instructed *not to inhale, swallow, or sniff* the spray, unlike many other inhaled medications. The most common adverse effect is nasopharyngeal and ocular mucosa irritation. The use of nicotine nasal spray can cause serious arrhythmias and elevated blood pressure and should be avoided immediately after MI because it may cause angina. If the patient is experiencing any cardiac symptoms, then nicotine nasal spray (Nicotrol NS) can be abruptly discontinued, an advantage of this delivery system over the longer-acting nicotine products.

With nicotine nasal spray, there is potential for abuse, as patients report a "head rush" and the sensation of feeling good, similar to that of cigarette smoking. Careful monitoring of the use of nicotine spray and advising patients of the potential for replacing their cigarette addiction with an addiction to the nicotine spray can help to avoid this problem. Three months is the recommended maximum length of treatment with nicotine nasal spray.

Nicotine Inhaler

The nicotine (Nicotrol) inhaler is a unique delivery method of nicotine replacement therapy in that the medication stimulates the act of smoking a cigarette. The inhaler consists of two parts, a cartridge containing 10 mg of nicotine (4 mg of delivered drug) and a mouthpiece. The patient puffs continuously on the inhaler for 20 minutes, providing the nicotine equivalent of two cigarettes. The patient should use at least 6 cartridges per day for 3 to 6 weeks. A maximum of 16 cartridges is used for the first 12 weeks. After 12 weeks the dose is reduced gradually, with a maximum of 6 months of treatment. Adverse effects include coughing, mouth and throat irritation, and dyspepsia.

Antidepressants

Antidepressants are thought to be helpful in smoking cessation because of the relationship between depressed mood and smoking behavior. During tobacco withdrawal, patients often exhibit depressed and anxious moods. Several antidepressants, including bupropion, doxepin, and nortriptyline, have been shown to be effective in smoking cessation. This chapter discusses bupropion (Zyban), currently the only antidepressant approved by the U.S. Food and Drug Administration (FDA) for smoking cessation.

Bupropion

Bupropion is chemically unrelated to other antidepressants, and the mechanism by which it enhances the ability to abstain

from smoking is unknown. It is presumed that bupropion's action as a weak inhibitor of neuronal uptake of dopamine and norepinephrine accounts for its ability to assist in smoking cessation. Bupropion is started 1 to 2 weeks before the quit-smoking date. The patient begins taking 150 mg daily for 3 days and then increases the dose to 150 mg twice a day at least 8 hours apart, avoiding bedtime dosing. On the quit day, the patient can quit cold turkey or use a nicotine replacement therapy along with the bupropion. Bupropion and the nicotine patch are a successful combination, more successful than the nicotine patch alone. Therapy continues for 7 to 12 weeks, although treatment may be extended an additional 12 weeks up to 6 months if smoking cessation is successful. If the patient has not made significant progress toward quitting by week 7 of treatment, it is unlikely he or she will successfully quit during the attempt and bupropion (Zyban) should be discontinued.

Bupropion is contraindicated in patients with seizure disorders, bulimia, and anorexia nervosa and within 14 days of the use of monoamine oxidase inhibitors (MAOIs). Bupropion should not be used in patients with a history of stroke, brain tumor, brain surgery, or history of closed head injury (Abramowicz, 2003). Frequency of dosing is reduced in patients with renal failure, as the drug and drug metabolites may accumulate. Bupropion should be used with caution in patients with hepatic cirrhosis, with the dose decreased to 150 mg every other day. Although it is Pregnancy Category B, it is not recommended during pregnancy or for use in children under age 18. Nondrug treatments should be tried first in pregnant patients. If used with nicotine replacement therapy, the patient should be monitored for hypertension. Bupropion is the active ingredient in Wellbutrin, used to treat depression. The concurrent use of bupropion (Zyban) and Wellbutrin is contraindicated. The most frequent adverse effects of bupropion are insomnia (40%), dizziness (10%), and dry mouth (10%). Constipation is also a reported adverse effect, and the patient should be advised to increase fiber and fluid intake during treatment.

Bupropion is the active ingredient in the antidepressant Wellbutrin and as such has received a Black-Box Warning regarding increased risk of suicide ideation and suicidality in children, adolescents, and young adults. Zyban is not approved for smoking cessation in children under 18 years of age. Patients prescribed Zyban should be monitored closely for signs of suicide ideation when treatment is started.

Nicotinic Receptor Partial Agonists

Varenicline (Chantix) was approved by the FDA in 2006 as a pharmacological aid to quit smoking. Varenicline is a partial agonist/antagonist with affinity and selectivity for alpha(4) beta(2) (α4β2) nicotinic acetylcholine receptors. Its mechanism of action appears to be its action as an agonist on the α4β2 receptors, as well as an antagonist preventing nicotine from binding to the receptors. Varenicline is highly selective to the α4β2 and is moderately selective to the 5-HT3 receptor.

By preventing binding of nicotine to the nicotinic receptors, there is less dopaminergic reinforcement and reward for smoking, as well as decreased withdrawal symptoms with smoking cessation. The patient experiences reduced cravings and decreased satisfaction with smoking.

To begin smoking cessation therapy with varenicline (Chantix), the patient chooses a quit date and varenicline is started 1 week before the scheduled quit date. Varenicline reaches steady state in 4 days from the onset of therapy. A titration of varenicline up to 1 mg twice a day is required, with the manufacturer suggesting a schedule of 0.5 mg once a day for the first 3 days, then 0.5 mg twice a day on days 4 to 7. The dose may be increased to 1 mg twice a day on day 8 and continue throughout treatment. Varenicline is administered with a full glass of water after eating. Treatment should continue for 12 weeks. If the patient has successfully quit smoking, treatment with an additional 12 weeks of therapy is thought to increase the long-term likelihood of abstinence.

Nausea is the most common adverse effect reported when taking varenicline, with 16% to 41% of patients reporting nausea compared to placebo in double-blind trials (Garrison & Dugan, 2009). Patients also report insomnia and headache at higher rates than placebo when taking varenicline. The most concerning adverse effect of varenicline has been found in post-marketing surveillance related to changes in behavior, agitation, depressed mood, suicidal ideation, and actual suicidal behavior (FDA, 2008). These concerns prompted a modification of the label highlighting a warning regarding neuropsychiatric symptoms and noting that Chantix was not studied in patients with preexisting serious psychiatric illness such as schizophrenia, bipolar disorder, and major depressive disorder, therefore safety in these patients had not been established.

Varenicline (Chantix) is Pregnancy Category C and is not recommended for pregnant or nursing women. Varenicline should not be prescribed for children under 18 years of age. Pharmacokinetic properties of varenicline in a small study ($N = 16$) of the elderly appears to be similar to those in younger adults, although as a renally eliminated drug, dosing may need to be adjusted in older patients with decreased renal function.

Alpha$_2$ Adrenergic Agonists

Clonidine has been used as a second-line treatment for smoking cessation, although this is not an approved indication by the FDA. Clonidine is available in tablets and patch and may be used in patients who refuse or cannot tolerate nicotine replacement, varenicline, or bupropion. The starting dose is 0.1 mg/d, increasing slowly to a maximum of 0.3 mg/d. Side effects are the same as if using clonidine for hypertension: dry mouth, sedation, dizziness, and hypotension (Abramowicz, 2003).

Combination Therapy

The Agency for Health Care Policy and Research (AHCPR) has published *Smoking Cessation: Clinical Practice Guidelines* (Fiore et al, 2008), which recommends that the provider consider combining multiple first-line medications (level A evidence) for smoking cessation:

- Long-term (more than 14 weeks) nicotine patch plus other nicotine replacement therapy (NRT) (gum and spray)
- The nicotine patch plus the nicotine inhaler
- The nicotine patch plus bupropion SR (sustained release)

Steinberg and colleagues (2009) evaluated the use of triple-medication therapy (nicotine patch at 21 mg/d, nicotine oral inhaler to be used as needed, and bupropion 150 mg/d) in medically ill smokers, including those with cardiovascular disease, chronic pulmonary disease, cancer, hypertension, diabetes, and current pulmonary infection. The study found that patients who used a combination of nicotine patch, nicotine inhaler, and bupropion had a 16% higher abstinence rate at 6 months than did those who used nicotine patch alone (35% versus 19% [CI 1% to 31%]), with no higher incidence of adverse effects (Steinberg et al, 2009). This study is significant because it addresses the concerns of providers about prescribing smoking-cessation medications to patients with chronic illness, as well as validating the use of combination therapies.

Nonpharmacological Treatment of Nicotine Addiction

The AHCPR *Smoking Cessation: Clinical Practice Guidelines* recommends a number of nonpharmacological interventions (Fiore et al, 2008):

1. Smoking-cessation interventions should include either individual or group counseling. There is strong evidence (level A) that a combination of medication and counseling is more effective than is either method alone.
2. Smokers should be offered access to support through a telephone hot line, help line, or online support group, when feasible, as a self-help intervention.
3. Smoking-cessation interventions should include problem solving, skills training, relapse prevention, and stress management to increase cessation success rates.

The provider needs to consider quit rates and cost-effectiveness when determining what nonpharmacological smoking cessation therapy to recommend. Higher quit rates are found with more intensive therapies and use of multiple therapies, for example, combining behavioral counseling and individualized computer reports (Lerman, Patterson, & Berrettini, 2005; Ramon & Bruguera, 2009), a combination of counseling and pharmacological therapies, or a combination of pharmacological therapies (Fiore et al, 2008).

Other nonpharmacological therapies include hypnosis, acupuncture, and massage. Self-massage of the ear or hand with circular or stroking motions decreases feelings of anxiety, depressed mood, withdrawal cravings, and craving intensity in smoking patients attempting to quit (Hernandez-Reif, Field, & Hare, 1999). Relaxation and exercise are also central to smoking-cessation therapy to counter the anxiety that is associated with nicotine withdrawal and to decrease the amount of weight gained during cessation. The successful treatment of the smoker who desires to quit will include a variety of treatment modalities, both pharmacological and nonpharmacological.

Patient Variables

Pregnant Women

A pregnant woman who smokes places herself and her fetus in danger. Smoking is associated with low birth weight and prematurity, as well as increased perinatal mortality. Smoking cessation during pregnancy is ideal for the developing fetus. Pregnant smokers are advised to quit smoking without the use of nicotine replacement therapy. The benefits and risks of nicotine replacement therapy have not been studied on pregnant patients, but the risk of smoking is thought to outweigh the short-term risk of low-dose nicotine replacement. Therefore, the FDA has classified nicotine gum as a Pregnancy Category C medication; the transdermal patch and inhaled forms continue to be classified as Pregnancy Category D. The manufacturer of Nicorette gum continues to recommend that nonpharmacological measures be used first. Bupropion (Zyban) and varenicline (Chantix) are not recommended during pregnancy.

Children

Children should never receive nicotine replacement products, bupropion, or varenicline for tobacco cessation. Their use is usually experimental, and children are rarely addicted to nicotine. Primary education about tobacco use is the appropriate method to be used with children who may be tempted to smoke. Toxic levels of nicotine are reached quickly in children, and all nicotine products should remain out of their reach. Adults should be advised to dispose of used nicotine patches in a safe manner so that children cannot touch or play with the used patch.

Adolescents

Adolescent patients pose a challenge because most adult smokers began as teenage smokers. The American Academy of Pediatrics, in *Guidelines for Adolescent Preventive Services* and *Bright Futures: Guidelines for Health Supervision of Infants, Children, and Adolescents,* recommends screening for tobacco use beginning at the 11- to 14-year-old well-child care visit (Hagan, Shaw, & Duncan, 2008). Physically and psychologically, adolescents can be addicted to tobacco (Prokhorov, Pallonen, Fava, Ding, & Niaura, 1996). The peer group norm can lead teens to use tobacco, even when they know it is illegal and a poor choice for them to make. Tobacco-cessation programs in this age group need to be geared

toward identifying the teen smoker early and providing support for quitting.

The provider who identifies a teen smoker who is ready to quit can choose a variety of options. It is essential for the teen to have a peer support group of other teen nonsmokers. Many schools have drug and alcohol counselors who organize support groups in the school. There has been minimal research in adolescents regarding nicotine replacement therapy. Because adolescent smokers report the same nicotine withdrawal and cravings as do adults, a teenager who smokes 20 or more cigarettes per day warrants the trial use of nicotine replacement. Transdermal nicotine replacement has been studied in adolescent patients and may be the best choice for treatment.

● CLINICAL PEARL ●

Constipation and Tobacco Cessation
Many patients experience constipation during tobacco cessation as the stimulating effects of nicotine on the GI system are decreased. Increased dietary fiber, increased fluids, and use of a bulk-producing laxative (Metamucil or Citrucel) or osmotic laxative (Miralax) will help with this problem.

Buying tobacco products is illegal for adolescents under age 18, although a study of 4,078 adolescents found that 50% of respondents stated they could easily access nicotine replacement products (Klesges, Johnson, Somes, Zbikowski, & Robinson, 2003). Writing a prescription for the product and having the parent purchase the product will allow the patient access to nicotine replacement therapy legally. The adolescent needs to have clear directions regarding not smoking while using nicotine replacement and the symptoms of nicotine toxicity. Careful education and monitoring of the patient throughout therapy will decrease adverse outcomes.

MONITORING

The patient needs to be monitored closely during all phases of tobacco cessation. As patients begin therapy, they need to be monitored for signs of nicotine withdrawal or, in the case of nicotine replacement, nicotine toxicity (see Box 43-2). The dose of nicotine replacement can be adjusted up or down, based on a patient's clinical symptoms. As patients are weaned down on the dose of nicotine replacement (every 2 to 3 weeks), they need to be monitored for increasing withdrawal symptoms. After patients are weaned off nicotine replacement, they need to be continually assessed as to their abstinence from tobacco. It is not unusual for patients to

---

BOX 43–2 NICOTINE POISONING

Nicotine poisoning is a concern if children or pets ingest nicotine replacement products. There has been a rise in nicotine poisonings since e-cigarettes have appeared on the market (Chatham-Stephens et al, 2014). Ingesting even a small amount of nicotine may be toxic to young children. Symptoms of nicotine poisoning include nausea, vomiting, increased salivation, headache, and sweating. Seizures and respiratory failure may occur (Toxnet, 2014). Treatment for nicotine poisoning for mild toxicity is supportive (IV fluids, observation). Treatment for severe toxicity includes IV fluids, airway support, and mechanical ventilation, with atropine given for bradycardia or muscarinic signs (Toxnet, 2014).

---

relapse, and the health-care provider needs to provide support for their repeated attempts to quit.

Patients who are using varenicline for tobacco cessation need to be monitored for neuropsychiatric symptoms such as changes in behavior, agitation, depressed mood, suicidal ideation, and suicidal behavior. Patients and family members need to be informed to stop taking varenicline and report symptoms to their health-care provider immediately.

Smoking alters the metabolism of several medications, and patients taking them need to be monitored closely and the dosage of their medications adjusted accordingly as they successfully quit. Both smoking and nicotine can increase circulating cortisol and catecholamines. Patients taking adrenergic agonists (isoproterenol, phenylephrine) or adrenergic blockers (beta blockers) must be monitored closely as they decrease their nicotine dependence. Smoking may reduce the diuretic effects of furosemide and reduce cardiac output, and smoking cessation may reverse these actions. Glutethimide (Doriden) absorption may be decreased with smoking cessation. First-pass metabolism of propoxyphene (Darvocet) may be decreased with smoking cessation. Smoking cessation potentiates theophylline, insulin, pentazocine, oxazepam, tricyclic antidepressants (e.g., imipramine), caffeine, and acetaminophen. Careful assessment of medications that the patient is taking prior to beginning a tobacco-cessation program will decrease the adverse effects during cessation.

OUTCOME EVALUATION

The goal of tobacco cessation is for the patient to be nicotine free at the end of treatment. Understanding that nicotine is highly addictive and that there are behavioral patterns ingrained in a smoker's habit can help define successful treatment. The patient who quits smoking cold turkey and is successful over the long term clearly has a positive outcome. The patient who uses nicotine replacement, bupropion, or varenicline for a number of weeks and then is tobacco-free for a long period of time (more than 12 months) also has a positive outcome.

The reality of tobacco-cessation treatment is that many patients relapse. Recognizing that many smokers quit for a while 2 or 3 times before successfully achieving long-term cessation will enable the patient and the provider to view any period of abstinence as one step closer to long-term success. By supporting patients during this process and assuring them that they are not failures if they begin smoking again, the health-care provider preserves an environment in which patients can again attempt quitting when they are ready.

PATIENT EDUCATION

Patient education should include a discussion of information related to the overall treatment plan as well as that specific to the drug therapy, reasons for taking the drug, drugs as part of the total treatment regimen, and adherence issues.

Patients should be taught that there is a relationship between smoking cessation and development of mouth ulcers, not related to the smoking-cessation medications. Forty percent of quitters develop mouth ulcers in the first 2 weeks after quitting, with most ulcers (60%) resolving by 4 weeks. The more dependent quitters are more likely to report ulcers (McRobbie, Hajek, & Gillison, 2004).

Educational Resources

Many resources pertaining to tobacco cessation are available for providers and patients. The American Lung Association (ALA) has local chapters that can provide posters; written educational materials to promote tobacco cessation; and materials for the Great American Smokeout, an annual anti-smoking event. Both the American Cancer Society (ACS) and the American Heart Association (AHA) have local chapters that can also provide educational materials to health-care providers. There are Web sites devoted to tobacco cessation that health-care providers can access. The key AHCPR *Clinical Guidelines* are available at http://www.ahrq.gov/clinic/tobacco. Smoking support information with links to multiple resources is available at the ALA Web site, http://www.lungusa.org. At the RxList Web site, http://www.rxlist.com, the provider can type in a medication and print or e-mail the patient information about the medication. With the abundance of resources available to the health-care provider, patient education should be easily incorporated into the care of the patient.

SMOKING CESSATION

PATIENT
EDUCATION

Related to the Overall Treatment Plan/Disease Process

☐ Education regarding the physical and psychological aspects of tobacco addiction

☐ Role of lifestyle modifications

☐ Importance of adherence to the treatment regimen

☐ Need for regular follow-up visits with the primary care provider

Specific to the Drug Therapy

☐ Doses and schedules for taking the drug

☐ Possible adverse effects and what to do if they occur

☐ Interactions between other treatment modalities and these drugs

Reasons for Taking the Drug(s)

These drugs are given to help a person stop smoking. The medications that are used for smoking cessation need to be used as prescribed; overuse or underuse will increase treatment failure or lead to adverse effects. The patient needs to understand the danger of nicotine toxicity, know the symptoms, and have clear instructions to cease the medication and notify the health-care provider. The patient must not smoke while using a nicotine replacement. Nicotine replacement products, even after they are used, can be toxic to children and to pets; therefore, all of the products need to be handled carefully and disposed of properly after use.

Drugs as Part of the Total Treatment Regimen

The total treatment regimen includes nonpharmacological strategies. Nonpharmacological strategies such as relaxation, acupuncture, massage, exercise, and group therapy should be discussed and patients encouraged to incorporate multiple strategies to help them be successful.

A weight gain of 5 to 8 lb is common during tobacco cessation. Patients need to avoid strict diets during tobacco cessation and increase exercise during cessation treatment. After they have been tobacco-free for a few months, they can then work on weight reduction. Encouraging exercise during treatment will decrease the amount of weight gained.

Adherence Issues

Patients should know that having quit before and resumed their habit does not predict that they cannot be successful and that patients often quit for a while and then lapse 2 or 3 times before they succeed.

Many patients need external motivation to be successful at tobacco cessation. Identifying each patient's motivation and reminding her or him of it at each visit will assist patients in refocusing their goals when they feel like giving up. Common motivators include the health of their children or spouse and their own health. Pointing out the cost savings of quitting smoking, which can add up to over $250 a month for a pack-a-day smoker in New York City, where cigarettes are $9.00 a pack, can also help patients focus on their goal. Have them place a photo of what they will buy with their savings in a prominent place (the refrigerator or bathroom mirror) as a reminder.

REFERENCES

Abramowicz, M. (Ed.). (2003). Drugs for tobacco dependence. *Treatment Guidelines from the Medical Letter, 1*(10), 65–68.

Aubin, H.-J., Farley, A., Lycett, D., Lahmek, P., & Aveyard, P. (2012). Weight gain in smokers after quitting cigarettes: Meta-analysis. *British Medical Journal, 345.* doi: 10.1136/bmj.e4439

Centers for Disease Control (CDC). (2012). Current tobacco use among middle and high school students—United States 2011. *Morbidity and Mortality Weekly Report (MMWR), 61*(31), 581–585.

Chatham-Stephens, K., Taylor, E., Melstrom, P., Bunnell, R., Wang, B., & Apelchier, J. G. (2014). Notes from the field: Calls to poison centers for exposures to electronic cigarettes—United States, September 2010–February 2014. *Morbidity and Mortality Weekly Report (MMWR), 63*(13), 292–293. http://www.cdc.gov/mmwr/preview/mmwrhtml/mm6313a4.htm

Cooper, T. V., DeBon, M. W., Stockton, M., Klesges, R. C., Steenbergh, T. A., Sherrill-Mittleman, M., et al. (2004). Correlates of adherence with transdermal nicotine. *Addictive Behaviors, 29,* 1565–1578.

Cromwell, J., Bartosch, W. J., Fiore, M. C., Hasselblad, V., & Baker, T. (1997). Cost effectiveness of the clinical practice recommendation in the AHCPR guidelines for smoking cessation. *Journal of the American Medical Association, 278,* 1759–1766.

Dawkins, L., Turner, J., Hasna, S., & Soar, K. (2012). The electronic-cigarette: Effects on desire to smoke, withdrawal symptoms and cognition. *Addictive Behaviors, 37*(8), 970–973. doi: http://dx.doi.org/10.1016/j.addbeh.2012.03.004

Fiore, M. C., Jaén, C. R., Baker, T. B., Bailey, W. C., Benowitz, N. L., Curry, S. J., et al. (2008). Treating tobacco use and dependence: 2008 update. *Clinical practice guideline.* Rockville, MD: U.S. Department of Health and Human Services, Public Health Service.

Garrison, G. D., & Dugan, S. E. (2009). Varenicline: A first-line treatment option for smoking cessation. *Clinical Therapeutics, 31*(3), 463–491.

Hagan, J. F., Shaw, J. S., & Duncan, P. M. (Eds.). (2008). *Bright futures: Guidelines for health supervision of infants, children, and adolescents* (3rd ed.). Elk Grove Village, IL: American Academy of Pediatrics.

Heishman, S. J., Balfour, D. J. K., Benowitz, N. L., Hatsukami, D. K., Lindstrom, J. M., & Ockene, J. K. (1997). Society for Research on Nicotine and Tobacco: Conference summary. *Addiction, 92*(5), 615–633.

Hernandez-Reif, M., Field, T., & Hare, S. (1999). Smoking cravings are reduced by self-massage. *Preventive Medicine, 28*(1), 28–32.

Hjalmarson, A., Nilsson, F., Sjöström, L., & Wiklund, O. (1997). The nicotine inhaler in smoking cessation. *Archives of Internal Medicine, 157,* 1721–1728.

Hurt, R. D., Offord, K. P., Croghan, I. T., Croghan, G. A., Gomez-Dahl, L. C., Wolter, T. D., et al. (1998). Temporal effects of nicotine nasal spray and gum on nicotine withdrawal symptoms. *Psychopharmacology, 140,* 98–104.

Jimenez-Ruiz, C., Kunze, M., & Fagerstrom, K. O. (1998). Nicotine replacement: A new approach to reducing tobacco-related harm. *European Respiratory Journal, 11,* 473–479.

Jorenby, D. E., Leischow, S. J., Nides, M. A., Rennard, S. I., Johnston, J. A., Hughes, A. R., et al. (1999). A controlled trial of sustained-release bupropion, a nicotine patch, or both for smoking cessation. *New England Journal of Medicine, 340*(9), 685–691.

Klesges, L. M., Johnson, K. C., Somes, G., Zbikoswki, S., & Robinson, L. (2003). Use of nicotine replacement therapy in adolescent smokers and nonsmokers. *Archives of Pediatric and Adolescent Medicine, 157*(6), 517–522.

Krawiec, J. V., & Pohl, J. M. (1998). Smoking cessation and nicotine replacement therapy: A guide for primary care providers. *American Journal for Nurse Practitioners, 2*(1), 15–33.

Lerman, C., Patterson, F., & Berrettini, W. (2005). Treating tobacco dependence: State of the science and new directions. *Journal of Clinical Oncology, 23*(2), 311–323.

McRobbie, H., Hajek, P., & Gillison, F. (2004), The relationship between smoking cessation and mouth ulcers. *Nicotine & Tobacco Research, 6*(4), 655–659.

National Cancer Institute, National Institute of Health. (2012). Tobacco facts. *Tobacco statistics snapshot.* Bethesda, MD: National Institute of Health. Retrieved November 27, 2013, from http://www.cancer.gov/cancertopics/tobacco/statisticssnapshot

National Center for Health Statistics. (2013). *Health, United States, 2008. With Chartbook on trends in the health of Americans.* Hyattsville, MD: U.S. Department of Health and Human Services. Retrieved November 27, 2013, from http://www.cdc.gov/nchs/data/hus/hus08.pdf#063

National Institute on Drug Abuse. (2006). Tobacco addiction. *National Institute on Drug Abuse: Research report series* (NIH Publication No. 06-4342). Retrieved March 8, 2011, from http://www.nida.nih.gov/ResearchReports/Nicotine/Nicotine.html

Piper, M. E., Smith, S. S., Schlam, T. R., Fiore, M. C., Jorenby, D. E., Fraser, D., et al. (2009). A randomized placebo-controlled clinical trial of 5 smoking cessation pharmacotherapeutics. *Archives of General Psychiatry, 66*(11), 1253–1262.

Prochazka, A. V., Weaver, M. J., Keller, R. T., Fryer, G. E., Licari, P. A., & Lofaso, D. (1998). A randomized trial of nortriptyline for smoking cessation. *Archives of Internal Medicine, 158,* 2035–2039.

Prokhorov, A. V., Pallonen, U. E., Fava, J. L., Ding, L., & Niaura, R. (1996). Measuring nicotine dependence among high-risk adolescent smokers. *Addictive Behaviors, 21*(1), 117–127.

Ramon, J. M., & Bruguera, E. (2009). Real world study to evaluate the effectiveness of varenicline and cognitive-behavioural interventions for smoking cessation. *International Journal of Environmental Research and Public Health, 6,* 1530–1538. doi: 10.3390/ijerph6041530

Schneider, N. G., Lunell, E., Olmstead, R. E., & Fagerström, K. (1996). Clinical pharmacokinetics of nasal nicotine delivery: A review and comparison to other nicotine systems. *Clinical Pharmacokinetics, 31*(1), 65–80.

Silagy, C., Lancaster, T., Stead, L., Mant, D., & Fowler, G. (2004). Nicotine replacement therapy for smoking cessation. *Cochrane Database of Systematic Reviews,* 3. Art. No.: CD000146. doi:10.1002/14651858. CD000146.pub2

Stapleton, J., West, R., Hajek, P., Wheeler, J., Vangeli, E., Abdi, Z., et al. (2013). Randomized trial of nicotine replacement therapy (NRT), bupropion and NRT plus bupropion for smoking cessation: Effectiveness in clinical practice. *Addiction, 108*(12), 2193–2201. doi: 10.1111/add.12304

Stead, L. F., & Lancaster, T. (2012) Behavioral interventions as adjuncts to pharmacotherapy for smoking cessation. *Cochrane Database of Systematic Reviews* Dec 12;12:CD009670. doi: 10.1002/14651858.CD009670.pub2.

Steinberg, M. B., Greenhaus, S., Schmelzer, A. C., Bover, M. T., Foulds, J., Hoover, D. R., et al. (2009). Triple-combination pharmacotherapy for medically ill smokers: A randomized trial. *Annals of Internal Medicine, 150*(7), 447–454.

Sutfin, E. L., McCoy, T. P., Morrell, H. E. R., Hoeppner, B. B., & Wolfson, M. (2013). Electronic cigarette use by college students. *Drug and Alcohol Dependence, 131*(3), 214–221. doi: http://dx.doi.org/10.1016/j.drugalcdep.2013.05.001

Tonstad, S., Heggen, E., Giljam, H. Lagerback, P. A., Tonnesen, P., Wikingsson, L. D. et al. (2013). Niccine®, a nicotine vaccine, for relapse prevention: A phase II, randomized, placebo-controlled, multicenter clinical trial. *Nicotine and Tobacco Research, 15*(9), 1492–1501.

ToxNet. (2014). *Nicotine.* http://toxnet.nlm.nih.gov/

U.S. Food and Drug Administration (FDA). (2008). *FDA issues public health advisory on Chantix: Agency requests that manufacturer add new safety warnings for smoking cessation drug.* Bethesda, MD: U.S. Food and Drug Administration. Retrieved March 8, 2011, from http://www.fda.gov/NewsEvents/Newsroom/PressAnnouncements/2008/ucm116849.htm

Vidrine, J., Shete, S., Cao, Y., Greisinger, A., Harmonson, P., Sharp, B., et al. (2013). Ask-advise-connect: A new approach to smoking treatment delivery in health care settings. *Journal of the American Medical Association Internal Medicine, 173*(6), 458–464. doi: 10.1001/jamainternmed.2013.3751

Ward, B. W., Schiller, J. S., & Freeman, G. (2013, Sept). *Early release of selected estimates based on data from the January–March 2013 National Health Interview Survey.* National Center for Health Statistics. Retrieved November 27, 2013, from www.cdc.gov/nchs/nhis.htm

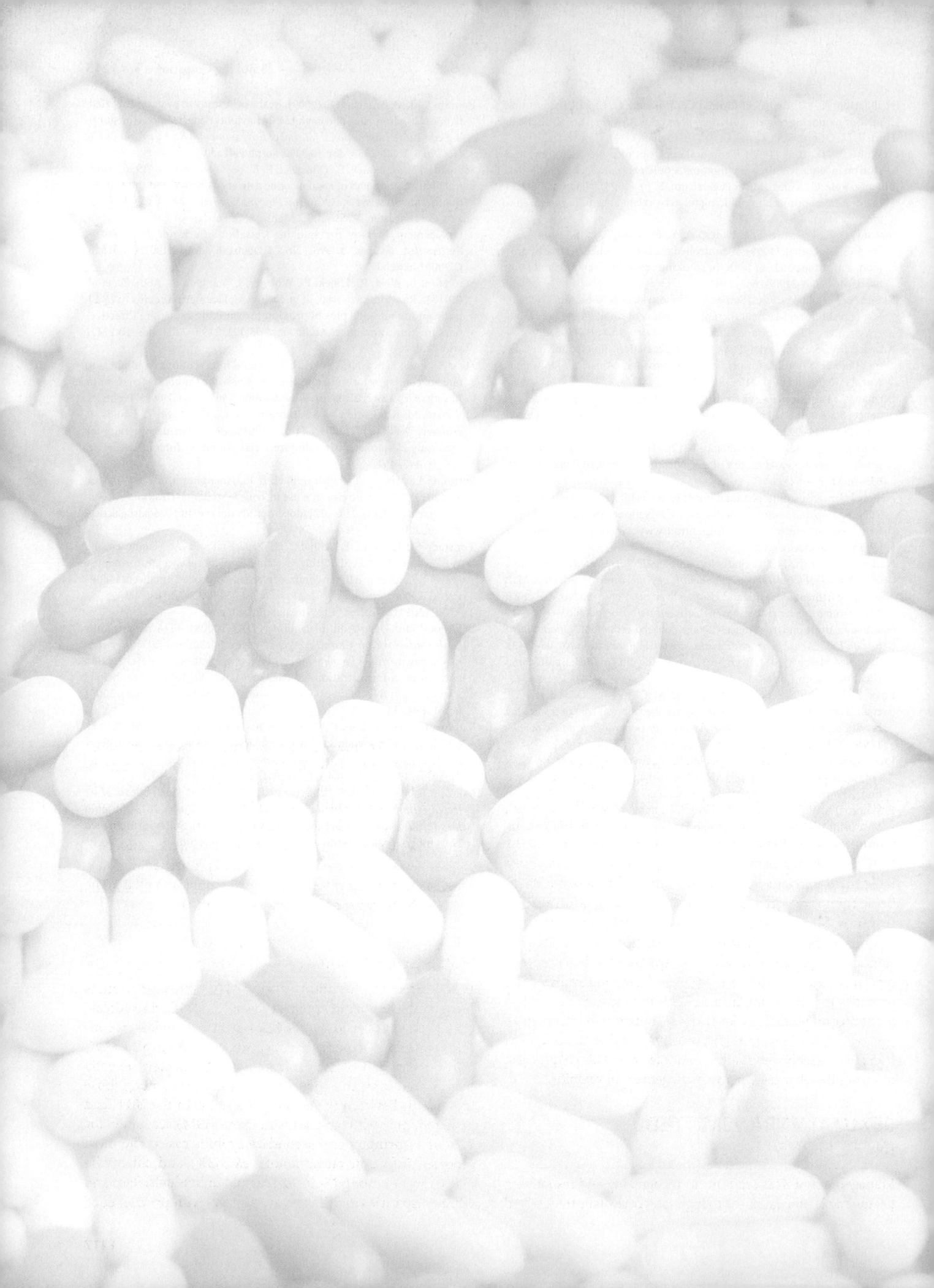

CHAPTER 44

SEXUALLY TRANSMITTED INFECTIONS AND VAGINITIS

Theresa Granger

Two common conditions seen by nurse practitioner providers are sexually transmitted infections (STIs) and vaginitis. The Centers for Disease Control and Prevention (CDC) has surveillance teams across the United States (West, Midwest, Northeast, and Southern regions) monitoring sexually transmitted infection rates. From this surveillance, the CDC collects demographic, regional, and infection rate data and provides treatment recommendations for those infections being monitored. In addition, due to the nationwide mandatory provider reporting of many of the sexually transmitted infections to the CDC, their recommendations remain the gold standard for patient and partner treatment of STIs. This chapter synthesizes the most recent CDC information available and provides the nurse practitioner with the most current treatment recommendations for sexually transmitted infections.

Vaginitis is an inflammation of the vagina that may be caused by STIs or may be the result of other factors. This chapter also discusses the pharmacological management of vaginitis.

SEXUALLY TRANSMITTED INFECTIONS

Management of STIs requires (a) recognizing and responding to vulnerable populations with high rates of sexually transmitted infections, (b) an understanding of drug resistance, and (c) an awareness of the escalating costs of treatment to the patient and to the health-care system. The estimated cost to our health-care system to monitor and treat infected individuals is approximately $17 billion dollars annually (CDC, 2011). In 2012, there were 1,422,976 cases of *Chlamydia trachomatis* infection, 334,826 cases of gonorrhea, 15,667 cases of primary and secondary syphilis, and 322 cases of congenital syphilis reported to the CDC (CDC Division of STD Prevention, 2014).

Populations at Risk

When screening for and treating STIs, nurse practitioners must be able to identify populations most at risk. The adolescent, young adult, and gay and bisexual male populations continue to be among those highest at risk. According to the CDC (2011), over half of the estimated 19 million new sexually transmitted infections occurring annually are among those individuals between the ages of 15 and 24. In the 2011 data gathered, men who have sex with men (MSM) accounted for 72% of all primary and secondary syphilis cases. The most reported infection rates, gonorrhea (62%) and chlamydia (71%), occur among 15- to 24-year-old individuals. Race and ethnic disparities in STI rates are present, with prevalence of chlamydia, gonorrhea, and syphilis all higher in the black population (CDC Division of STD Prevention, 2014).

The number of patients requiring services for STIs has increased in proportion to those who are sexually active. Not every infected individual chooses to seek treatment. The reasons why those infected with STIs do not seek treatment vary and can be complicated. For example, homophobia and social stigma may be some reasons why certain high-risk groups (MSM) fail to seek appropriate care and treatment (CDC, 2011). Thus, it is important for the nurse practitioner to remain as empathetic and nonjudgmental as possible when treating vulnerable individuals.

Viral STIs such as the human papilloma and herpes simplex viruses are incurable and tend to produce lifelong periods of exacerbations and remissions. Women are at high risk for infertility if certain sexually transmitted infections remain untreated. This can pose a treatment challenge for the nurse practitioner because many of these infections can be "silent" and do not produce many symptoms until complications have occurred. Thus, it is important for nurse practitioners to screen early and often in susceptible, high-risk individuals.

Sexual health history is critical in order to determine the risk of STI. It has been suggested that many providers do not routinely obtain a sexual history (Swygard & Cohen, 2012). When conducting a health history, questioning the patient using the 5 P approach can be helpful in identifying patients at risk: (1) Partners, (2) Prevention of pregnancy, (3) Protection from STDs, (4) Practices, and (5) Past history of STDs (CDC, 2010, p 3).

STI as Precursor to Cancer

Scientific identification of the viral genotype of human papilloma virus (HPV) has enabled primary care providers to view cancer of the cervix in women and anus in men and women as an STI. Although more than 30 types of HPV can infect the genital tract, genotypes 16, 18, 31, 33, and 35 have been strongly associated with cervical neoplasia, with 16 and 18 being the most prevalent (CDC, 2010). Within the past decade, cervical cancer screening rates have increased and mortality rates have decreased (CDC, 2012b). This has been attributed to women receiving cervical cancer screening via Pap tests at regular intervals. According to the data analyzed by race and ethnicity, cervical screening rates are highest among the black (80%), white (75%), and Hispanic (75%) groups. Blacks have the highest cervical cancer death rates. Because most HPV infections are asymptomatic, early diagnosis and treatment of suspicious lesions are essential to prevent the spread of potentially cancerous lesions.

In 2009, the American College of Obstetricians and Gynecologists (ACOG) revised its cancer screening guidelines to recommend that the first cervical screening be performed at 21 years of age. Rescreening can be less frequent than previously recommended (ACOG, 2009; Wright et al, 2007). However, nurse practitioners should be aware of the fact that these guidelines are for women considered to be average risk (CDC, 2012c). Risk factors that may indicate the need for more frequent screening include HIV infection; immunosuppression; history of diethylstilbestrol (DES) exposure in utero; and abnormal Pap test results such as cervical intraepithelial neoplasia (CIN) 2, CIN 3, or history of cervical cancer.

HIV is another form of cancer that can be transmitted sexually. The mechanism of action behind the interrelated nature of sexually transmitted infections can be complex. Gonorrhea, chlamydia, and syphilis are thought to facilitate the transmission of HIV infection (CDC, 2010) in susceptible individuals. The incidence of syphilis is highest in those infected with HIV. Genital ulcerations can also increase HIV risk (Swygard & Cohen, 2012).

Hepatitis C is an example of another virus that can be transmitted sexually that has the potential to cause liver cancer and other complications. At-risk individuals should be routinely tested and receive counseling on how to prevent contracting the virus and how to prevent spreading the virus to others (CDC, 2012a).

Pathophysiology

The pathogenic potential of the viruses and bacteria capable of causing STIs and overall general discomfort depends on several factors. Age of host, sex of patient, number of sexual partners, pregnancy, immune system status, and coexisting infections are examples of the numerous factors to be considered when managing STIs. Age of the host is, perhaps, one of the most important factors for the nurse practitioner to consider.

Prepubertal, lactating, and postmenopausal women lack the vaginal effects of estrogen (Markusen & Barclay, 2003). This estrogen deficit results in a thin vaginal mucosa and vaginal epithelium. As a result, the vaginal area becomes more susceptible to infection and trauma. In addition to lacking the effects of estrogen, the pH of the vagina can be abnormally high (5.0 to 7.0) for some women and the normally acidogenic flora of the vagina may be replaced by mixed flora, which predisposes to infection. The normally acidic environment of the vagina (pH 3.5 to 4.1) promotes growth of the normal flora and helps prevents growth of infectious or irritative organisms. Although most women grow between three and eight types of bacteria, which are considered part of the "normal flora," lactobacilli and corynebacteria are the most common organisms (Markusen & Barclay, 2003). Treatments such as antibiotic therapy or behaviors such as having multiple sex partners triggers a nonphysiological response, and the "normal flora" of the vagina becomes disturbed enough to produce pathological symptoms. Postmenopausal women may experience vulvovaginal pain as a direct result of decreased estrogen production, which results in a thin, superficial epithelium. Some of the irritative symptoms may also be caused by infection. This reduced layer of epithelial cells can make the woman more vulnerable to infection and trauma (atrophic vaginitis). Infection can be from a woman's own perineal bacterial flora, and trauma can be a result of normal sexual relations. Other common irritants to the vaginal ecosystem are "forgotten" tampons, douches, contraceptive preparations, diabetes mellitus, and even stress.

In women, STIs are a common cause of vaginitis. Presenting symptoms often include discharge and vaginal irritation. However, it is important to note that not all vaginitis is infectious and that those infected with an STI are often asymptomatic. The differential diagnosis of vaginal discharge is presented in Table 44-1. Treatments for infectious vaginitis that may be acquired without sexual contact as well as for noninfectious vaginitis are discussed later in this chapter.

Genital contact between people is required for transmission of most STIs, although fomite transmission (such as through vibrators, toilet seats, and bath towels) can occur with hardier organisms. Women tend to experience more morbidity than men because of the secretions deposited into the vaginal vault during intercourse. This does not mean that men are not without risk. Transmission from one partner to the other can be facilitated or impeded by alterations in vaginal pH, the presence of inflammation caused by spermicides, and the mucosal integrity of either partner. Bacteria and viruses can invade the mucosal lining of the oral, genital, or anal tract. All bodily secretions, especially blood, have the potential to transmit infection from human to human.

Goals of Treatment

There are four main goals of STI treatment. There is ample literature to validate that STIs are preventable through safe sexual behavior. Therefore, the first goal of therapy is to educate patients about high-risk behaviors and screen those at risk. As a form of primary prevention, vaccinations should also be offered to eligible individuals. Currently, only two vaccines providing protection against viral STIs are available (hepatitis B and HPV vaccines). Prevention of long-term sequelae due to unsafe sex practices and, where possible, eradicating the responsible organism(s) are the second goals of therapy. Potential complications of STIs are tubal occlusion leading to infertility and ectopic pregnancy, neonatal morbidity and mortality caused by transmission during pregnancy and parturition, genital cancers, and possible exposure to HIV because of its association with other STIs. The third goal of therapy is to choose the most specific, cost-effective drug that has the best regimen for adherence, after verifying pregnancy status in all women of childbearing age. The fourth goal of therapy is to reduce morbidity and provide comfort for those chronic conditions that are not curable.

Rational Drug Selection

Guidelines

Treatment for STIs is based on national guidelines recommended by the CDC (2010). Nurse practitioners and other health-care providers play a crucial role in the diagnosis, treatment, and counseling of STIs. The treatment information presented in this chapter is consistent with the CDC's *Sexually Transmitted Diseases Treatment Guidelines.* Specific treatments for STIs mentioned in this chapter are outlined in Table 44-2. The CDC guidelines in their entirety can be accessed from the following Web site: http://www.cdc.gov/STD/treatment/. There are new CDC guidelines being published in 2015.

Syphilis

Syphilis is a systemic disease caused by *Treponema pallidum* that has been present in society for centuries. Syphilis is spread by direct contact of the mucosal tissue with infected lesions. Diagnostic symptoms may present as early as 5 days and as late as 90 days after exposure to the organism. Primary syphilis infection presents with ulcer or chancre at the site of infection. Secondary infection manifestations include rash, mucocutaneous lesions, adenopathy, and neurologic complications. Not all vaginal "warts" are attributed to HPV disease; anogenital condylomata lata are a common symptom of secondary syphilis as well as a generalized papulosquamous eruption.

Table 44–1 Differential Diagnosis of Vaginal Discharge

Discharge Appearance	Symptoms	pH	Diagnostic Tests	Microscope Findings	Disease/ Syndrome
White, curdy	+ Burn, itch	<4.5	Culture/KOH	Budding yeast hyphae	Moniliasis Candidiasis
Mucopurulent, thick	+ Irritating	Normal	DNA/culture	WBCs >10/hpf	GC/Chlamydiasis
Thin, white, odor	+ Itch, odor a big issue	>4.5	+Amine/culture-change in vaginal flora	"Clue cells" (coccoid bacteria that obscure epithelial cell borders)	Bacterial vaginosis (BV)
Blood-tinged, purulent	+ Itch, dysuria, foul odor	<4.5	Wet mount = + Trichomonads	Trichomonads >10 WBCs/hpf	Trichomoniasis
Nonspecific, white	+ Pruritus, burn	3.5–4.5	Culture reports change in normal flora	4 + *Lactobacillus*	Cytological
Scanty, may be white or yellow	+ Burn, sore, cracks	>5–7	Culture is negative	Several epithelial cells	Atrophic
White	None	3.8–4.2	Not necessary	1–2 + *Lactobacillus*	Normal

Table 44–2 ✹ Drugs Commonly Used: Sexually Transmitted Infections

Pathogen	First Choice	Alternative Choice
Bacterial Pathogens Syphilis, primary, secondary, and early latent (tertiary)	Benzathine penicillin G *Adults including pregnant women:* 2.4 million units (IM) in a single dose *Children:* 50,000 units/kg in one dose up to the adult dose of 2.4 million units	Pregnant patients allergic to penicillin should be desensitized. Nonpregnant: use doxycycline 100 mg bid for 14 days *or* tetracycline 500 mg qid for 14 days.
Syphilis, late latent or unknown	3 weekly doses of benzathine penicillin G 2.4 million units (total 7.2 million units) *Children:* 50,000 units/kg IM weekly for 3 weeks (total 150,000 units/kg up to adult dose of 7.2 million units)	Pregnant patients: 2.4 million units of benzathine penicillin weekly × 3 weeks
Gonococcal infections (uncomplicated infections of cervix, urethra, and rectum)	Ceftriaxone 250 mg intramuscular single-dose injection *plus* azithromycin 1 g orally in a single dose *or* doxycycline 100 mg orally twice daily × 7 days (azithromycin is recommended over doxycycline)	Cefixime 400 mg orally in a single dose *plus* azithromycin 1 g orally in a single dose *or* doxycycline 100 mg orally twice daily × 7 days (test-of-cure in 1 week). If patient has severe cephalosporin allergy: increase azithromycin to 2 g orally in a single dose (monitor for nausea and vomiting).
Gonococcal infections (pharynx)	Ceftriaxone 250 mg intramuscular single dose injection *plus* azithromycin 1 g orally in a single dose or doxycycline 100 mg orally twice daily for 7 days	Note: Do not use oral cefixime
Chlamydia (adults and adolescents)	Azithromycin 1 g orally in a single dose *or* doxycycline 100 mg twice daily for 7 days	Erythromycin base 500 mg orally 4× daily for 7 days *or* erythromycin ethylsuccinate 800 mg orally 4× a day for 7 days *or* ofloxacin 300 mg orally twice daily for 7 days *or* levofloxacin 500 mg orally once daily for 7 days
Chlamydia (pregnancy)	Azithromycin 1 g orally in a single dose *or* amoxicillin 500 mg orally 3× daily for 7 days	Erythromycin base 500 mg orally 4× a day for 7days *or* erythromycin ethylsuccinate 800 mg orally 4× a day for 7 days *or* erythromycin ethylsuccinate 400 mg orally 4× a day for 7 days *or* erythromycin base 250 mg orally 4× a day for 14 days
Chancroid	Azithromycin 1 g orally in a single dose *or* ceftriaxone 250 mg single-dose intramuscular injection *or* ciprofloxacin 500 mg orally twice daily for 3 days *or* erythromycin base 500 mg PO 3× daily for 7 days	Ciprofloxacin is not for patients under 18 years of age or for those who are pregnant *or* lactating
Granuloma inguinale (donovanosis)	Doxycycline 100 mg orally twice daily for at least 3 weeks or until ulcers have completely healed	Ciprofloxacin 750 orally twice daily for 3 weeks *or* erythromycin base 500 mg orally 4× a day for 3 weeks *or* azithromycin 1 g orally weekly for 3 weeks *or* trimethoprim-sulfamethoxazole one double-strength (160 mg/800 mg) tablet orally twice daily for 3 weeks. Note: Treat for a minimum of 3 weeks. Continue treatment until all lesions have healed.
Lymphogranuloma venereum	Doxycycline 100 mg orally twice daily for 21 days Do not use doxycycline in pregnant *or* lactating women	Erythromycin base 500 mg orally 4× daily for 21 days
Bacterial vaginosis	Metronidazole 500 mg orally twice daily for 7 days *or* clindamycin cream 2% 5 g intravaginally (one applicator) at bedtime for 7 days *or* metronidazole gel 0.75% 5 g (one applicator) intravaginally at bedtime for 5 days *Pregnant women:* metronidazole 500 mg bid for 7 days *or* metronidazole 250 mg tid for 7 days *or* clindamycin 300 mg bid for 7 days	Tinidazole 2 g orally once daily for 2 days *or* tinidazole 1 g orally once daily for 5 days *or* clindamycin 300 mg orally twice daily for 7 days *or* clindamycin ovules 100 mg intravaginally at bedtime for 3 days
Viral Pathogens Herpes Simplex types 1 and 2	**First Episode** Acyclovir 400 mg orally 3× daily for 7–10 days *or* acyclovir 200 mg orally 5× daily for 7–10 days *or* famciclovir 250 mg orally 3× daily for	**Recurring Episodes** Treatment for recurrent genital herpes can be administered either episodically to ameliorate or shorten duration of lesions or continuously as

Table 44–2 ❁ **Drugs Commonly Used: Sexually Transmitted Infections—cont'd**

Pathogen	First Choice	Alternative Choice
	7–10 days *or* valacyclovir 1 g twice a day for 7–10 days Note: Treatment can be extended if complete healing does not occur after 10 days of therapy.	suppressive therapy to reduce frequency of recurrences. Episodic therapy: Acyclovir 400 mg orally 3× times daily for 5 days *or* acyclovir 800 mg orally twice daily for 5 days *or* acyclovir 800 mg orally 3× times daily for 2 days *or* famciclovir 125 mg orally twice daily for 5 days *or* famciclovir 1 g orally twice daily for 1 day *or* valacyclovir 500 mg orally twice daily for 3 days *or* valacyclovir 1 g orally once a day for 5 days. Suppression is same dosage but given: acyclovir 400 mg orally twice daily; famciclovir 250 mg orally twice daily; valacyclovir 500 mg once daily; valacyclovir 1 g once daily.
Human Papillomavirus		
Human papillomavirus (HPV) (vaginal)	Due to the risk of vaginal perforation and fistula formation, cryotherapy is not recommended in the vaginal area. TCA or BCA 80%–90% in small amounts should be applied directly to wart area. Use talc, sodium bicarbonate, or liquid soap to remove unreacted acid. Repeat weekly if needed.	Cervical lesions: Biopsy lesions and refer for treatment.
Human papillomavirus (HPV) (external genital)	Patient-applied treatments (can be expensive for the patient): 1. Podofilox 0.5% solution or gel. Apply with cotton swab to visible warts twice a day for 3 days followed by 4 days of no treatment. Repeat for up to four cycles. 2. Imiquimod 5% cream. Apply once daily at bedtime three times a week for up to 16 weeks. Wash treatment area with soap/water 6 to 10 hours after application. 3. Sinecatechin 15% ointment. Apply 0.5 cm strand of ointment to each wart three times daily. Do not use for more than 16 weeks. Provider-applied treatments 1. Cryotherapy (only for the nurse practitioner who has been specially trained) 2. Pedophyllin resin 10%–25% applied to each wart. Wash preparation off 1–4 hours after application. Can repeat weekly if needed (do not use if patient is pregnant). 3. Trichloroacetic acid (TCA) or bichloroacetic acid (BCA) 80%–90% (widely used, but have not been widely studied; use with caution). Apply weekly if needed. Neutralize acid with soap or sodium bicarbonate. 4. Surgical removal.	Urethreal meatus warts 1. Cryotherapy with liquid nitrogen 2. Podophyllin 10%–25% in compound tincture of benzoin. Repeat weekly if needed. (Do not use during pregnancy.) Anal warts 1. Cryotherapy with liquid nitrogen
Fungal Pathogen	**Intravaginal**	**Oral**
Candidia albicans	Over-the counter agents: Butoconazole 2% cream 5 g for 3 days Clotrimazole 1% cream 5 g for 7–14 days Clotrimazole 2% cream 5 g for 3 days Miconazole 2% cream 5 g for 7 days Miconazole 4% cream 5 gfor 3 days Miconazole 100 mg vaginal suppository for 7 days Miconazole 200 mg vaginal suppository for 3 days Miconazole 1,200 mg vaginal suppository for 1 day Tioconazole 6.5% ointment 5 grams as a single dose Prescription Agents: Butoconazole 2% cream (single dose) 5 g intravaginally for 1 day	Fluconazole 150 mg orally as a single-dose tablet. Note: Cream and ointments may weaken condoms and diaphragms.

Continued

Table 44–2 ❈ **Drugs Commonly Used: Sexually Transmitted Infections—cont'd**

Pathogen	First Choice	Alternative Choice
	Nystatin 100,000 unit vaginal tablet for 14 days Terconazole 0.4% cream 5 g for 7 days Terconazole 0.8% cream 5 g for 3 days Terconazole 80 mg suppository for 3 days	

Pathogen	First Choice	Alternative Choice
PROTOZOAN PATHOGEN		
Trichomoniasis	Metronidazole 2 g orally as a single dose or tinidazole 2 g orally as a single dose	Metronidazole 500 mg orally twice a day for 7 days
ECTOPARASITIC PATHOGENS		
Pubic lice	Permethrin 1% cream rinse applied to affected areas, wash off in 10 minutes *or* pyrethrins with piperonyl butoxide applied to affected areas and washed off in 10 minutes	Alternative regimens: Malathion 0.5% lotion applied for 8–12 hours, then washed off *or* ivermectin 250 mcg/kg orally repeated in 2 wk The use of ivermectin is contraindicated in pregnancy, lactation, and children.
Scabies	Permethrin cream 5% applied to all areas of body from neck down and washed off 8–14 hours after application *or* ivermectin 200 mcg/kg orally, repeated in 2 weeks Permethrin is the preferred agent.	Lindane 1% 1 oz of lotion or 30 g of cream applied in a thin layer to affected areas. Wash off after 8 hours. Note: Lindane is not recommended as first-line therapy because of toxicity and risk of seizures. Only use if pt. cannot tolerate other therapies. Lindane should *not* be used immediately after a bath or shower, or in persons with dermatitis, women who are pregnant/lactating, and children <2 yr.

BCA = bichloroacetic acid; TCA = trichloroacetic acid.

Source: Adapted from *Sexually transmitted diseases treatment guidelines* (2010). Atlanta, GA: Centers for Disease Control and Prevention.

Tertiary infections with syphilis present with cardiac, neurological, ophthalmic, auditory, or gummatous lesions. Neurosyphilis may occur at any stage but most commonly presents in the latent stage.

Treatment of latent syphilis is intended to prevent occurrence or progression of late complications. Latent infections lack clinical symptoms and are detected by serological testing. Misdiagnosis or delayed diagnosis is possible because of the low level of suspicion in many family practice settings. All patients with syphilis should be tested for HIV (CDC, 2010).

All women should be screened for syphilis early in pregnancy, with many states mandating screening with the first prenatal visit (CDC, 2010). Untreated syphilis infections can lead to infection of the fetus or perinatal death. In communities and populations with a high prevalence of syphilis, patients are screened at 28 to 32 weeks' gestation and at delivery to avoid possible neonatal transmission (CDC, 2010). The high-risk category for repeated screening is described as a person who has a history of multiple sex partners, a history of current or recent STIs, a user of street drugs (Hatcher, Trussell, & Kowal, 2008), or men who have sex with men (MSM) (CDC, 2010).

Parenteral penicillin G (rather than oral penicillin) has been used effectively for more than 50 years and is the preferred drug for the treatment of all stages of syphilis. Dosing information can be found in Table 44-2. Patients who are allergic to penicillin may be treated with 14 days of doxycycline or tetracycline. Doxycycline causes less gastrointestinal upset

and for this reason may have better compliance rates than tetracycline (CDC, 2010).

Parenteral penicillin G is the only therapy with documented efficacy for syphilis during pregnancy, with dosing being the same as for nonpregnant patients (CDC, 2010). Pregnant women with syphilis in any stage who report penicillin allergy should be desensitized and treated with penicillin.

Gonorrhea

First isolated in 1879, the gram-negative intracellular diplococcus *Neisseria gonorrhoeae* can be transmitted through the urethra, rectum, pharynx, vagina, or eye. In the United States, an estimated 700,000 new *N. gonorrhoeae* infections occur each year (CDC, 2010) with the highest reported cases being in the southern region of the United States. Men tend to be symptomatic when infected (Swygard & Cohen, 2012). Many infected women have no symptoms until complications, such as pelvic inflammatory disease (PID), have occurred (CDC, 2010). The incubation period can be 2 days to 2 weeks. Patients infected with gonorrhea are often co-infected with chlamydia. This finding led to the recommendation that patients being treated for gonorrhea also need treatment for chlamydia (CDC, 2010). The reverse statement is also true, that patients being treated for chlamydia should receive treatment for gonorrhea. Table 44-2 outlines the specific treatment regimen recommended for the treatment of gonorrhea.

Complications of gonococcal infection include PID, tubal scarring, infertility, ectopic pregnancy, salpingitis, or disseminated gonococcal (GC) infection. Disseminated GC infection is characterized by pustular dermatitis, asymmetrical arthralgia, tenosynovitis, or septic arthritis. An infected pregnant woman is at risk for endometritis after procedures such as therapeutic abortions, chorionic villus sampling, or dilation and curettage. Between 30% and 50% of newborns of women with GC cervicitis develop GC conjunctivitis. In addition, gonococcal infections may facilitate the transmission of HIV infection (CDC, 2010).

Due to the increased resistance to fluoroquinolones across the United States, the drug class is no longer recommended for the treatment of gonorrhea (CDC, 2012). In addition, it is important for nurse practitioners to remember that co-infection with chlamydia and syphilis often occurs. For these reasons, the CDC recommends combination treatment with ceftriaxone IM or oral cefixime, plus either oral azithromycin or doxycycline. Combination treatment should eradicate co-existing organisms. Azithromycin is the preferred agent over doxycycline. Persons with severe cephalosporin allergies should be treated only after consultation with an infectious disease specialist (CDC, 2010).

Pregnant patients are treated with ceftriaxone 250 mg IM or cefixime 400 mg orally. Pregnant patients may also be treated with high-dose azithromycin (2 g) if they cannot tolerate cephalosporins (CDC, 2010). However, azithromycin in high doses can cause nausea and vomiting in all individuals.

Sexual partners require treatment, including those without symptoms, if they had sexual contact with the patient during the 60 days preceding the onset of symptoms or diagnosis of the infection (Swygard & Cohen, 2012). To prevent reinfection, patients and their partners should abstain from intercourse until therapy is completed. Women have a high rate of reinfection in the 6 months after treatment. Recommendations include retesting men and women 3 months after treatment regardless of whether the sex partner has been treated (CDC, 2010; Swygard & Cohen, 2012). Rescreening in 12 months after the initial diagnosis has been made is also recommended. A test-of-cure in 1 week is recommended if oral cefixime is used to treat infections of the cervix, urethra, and rectum (CDC, 2012d).

Chlamydia

The most commonly reported sexually transmitted infection in the United States is *Chlamydia trachomatis* (often termed *chlamydia*) with approximately 1.8 million infections annually (Torrone, Papp, & Weinstock, 2014). *C. trachomatis* is an often asymptomatic disease that causes serious sequelae, such as PID, ectopic pregnancy, and infertility. In susceptible individuals, chlamydia infections can facilitate the transmission of HIV infection (CDC, 2010). Some women who have uncomplicated cervical infections already have subclinical upper reproductive tract infections. Asymptomatic infection is common among both men and women. However, the rate of infection in women is over twice that of reported cases in men (CDC, 2010). Currently, economically disadvantaged women ages 16 to 24 years of age are at the highest risk, with one in seven sexually active non-Hispanic black women ages

14 to 24 years infected with chlamydia in 2012 (Torrone et al, 2014).

As explained previously, co-infection with gonorrhea often occurs. Therefore, dual therapy for gonorrhea and chlamydial infections is the treatment standard for both men and women. This chapter outlines the treatment recommendations for adolescents and adults. Treatment of the infection in infants is not discussed.

The CDC recommended treatment for chlamydia infection is outlined in Table 44-2. Azithromycin as a single dose or doxycycline for 7 days are the recommended regimens (CDC, 2010). Either treatment is efficacious, although the single-dose azithromycin may have a higher compliance rate (CDC, 2010), but it carries a higher risk of nausea and vomiting.

Pregnant women are treated with either azithromycin or amoxicillin (see Table 44-2). Doxycycline is contraindicated in pregnancy. Alternative therapy with erythromycin is recommended for pregnant women, but adverse reactions and gastrointestinal side effects make it a less desirable option.

Except in pregnant women or in those who have been noncompliant, a test-of-cure (repeat testing 3 weeks after completing therapy) is not recommended for persons treated with the recommended or alternative regimens (CDC, 2010). High-risk, pregnant individuals should be retested during the third trimester to decrease the possibility of the infection being passed during delivery. Pregnant women should have follow-up testing after treatment and should be retested 3 months after treatment (CDC, 2010). The majority of post-treatment infections result from reinfection. To minimize transmission, persons being treated for chlamydia should be instructed to abstain from sexual intercourse for 7 days after single-dose therapy or until completion of a 7-day regimen. Treatment of sex partners will also help to minimize the risk of reinfection.

All sexual partners in the past 60 days should be tested and treated. The most recent partner, even if more than 60 days has elapsed, should be evaluated. Expedited partner therapy is recommended to decrease reinfection (CDC, 2010).

Chancroid

Chancroid, caused by *Haemophilus ducreyi,* is endemic in some areas of the United States and is common in many of the world's poorest regions, such as areas of Africa, Asia, and the Caribbean (WHO, 2010). Co-infection with HIV, syphilis, and herpes simplex virus (HSV) can occur. Diagnosis is difficult because of the lack of available and sensitive testing media. As a result, treatment is initiated when the following criteria are satisfied: (1) one or more painful ulcers, (2) negative tests for syphilis and HSV, and (3) the appearance of ulcers with suppurative inguinal adenopathy.

Chancroid usually starts as a small papule that rapidly becomes pustular and then eventually ulcerates. The ulcer enlarges and begins to develop ragged and uneven borders and is surrounded by an erythematous rim. Unlike syphilis, chancroid lesions are tender. Treatment recommendations include oral azithromycin or ceftriaxone (IM) or oral ciprofloxacin or erythromycin (CDC, 2010). Pregnant women are treated with azithromycin, ceftriaxone, or erythromycin. Ciprofloxacin is contraindicated in pregnancy. Patients should be re-examined 3 to 7 days after therapy is started (CDC, 2010). Ulcers usually improve symptomatically after 3 days but may take up to 2 weeks to heal. Although treatment is successful, there still may be significant scarring. Poor response to treatment may indicate the patient is co-infected with another STI, has HIV, or the pathogen is resistant. Healing may be slower for uncircumcised men with ulcers under their foreskin.

In those men who are uncircumcised or who have HIV, response to treatment may be suboptimal. Therefore, patients should have HIV testing at the time of chancroid diagnosis (CDC, 2010). Follow-up is recommended because lack of response may indicate presence of HIV disease due to the fact that chancroid is considered a cofactor for HIV transmission. Patients should be retested for syphilis and HIV at 3-month intervals after the diagnosis of chancroid if the initial test results were negative (CDC, 2010). If the lymphadenopathy is fluctuant, incision and drainage may be necessary to enhance healing.

Sexual partners should be examined and treated if they have had sexual contact with the patient in the 10 days preceding diagnosis.

Granuloma Inguinale (Donovanosis)

Granuloma inguinale is a rare, genital ulcerative disease caused by the intracellular gram-negative bacterium *Klebsiella granulomatis* (formerly known as *Calymmatobacterium granulomatis*). This infection results in painless, slow-progressing ulcers without lymphadenopathy that bleed easily on contact. Granuloma inguinale usually affects the skin and mucous membranes in the genital region and results in nodular lesions that progress to large, beefy lesions that are difficult to heal. The ulcers progressively expand and are locally destructive. The mode of transmission of granuloma inguinale primarily occurs through sexual contact; however, it may have low infectious capabilities because repeated exposure is necessary for clinical infection to occur. Additionally, granuloma inguinale may also be obtained through the fecal route or by passage through an infected birth canal (CDC, 2006). Most infections are endemic in tropical and developing areas of India, Papua New Guinea, central Australia, and southern Africa.

The treatment for granuloma inguinale is outlined in Table 44-2. The current recommended antibiotic treatment is doxycycline (CDC, 2010). Alternatives include ciprofloxacin, erythromycin, azithromycin, or trimethoprim/sulfmethoxazole. Treatment is a minimum of 3 weeks or until all lesions have completely healed (CDC, 2010). Relapse is common within 6 to 18 months despite the best therapy. Although treatment stops the progression of lesions, prolonged therapy may be required to permit granulation and re-epithelialization of the ulcers. Sex partners should have clinical signs and symptoms prior to initiation of therapy.

Lymphogranuloma Venereum

Lymphogranuloma venereum (LGV) is caused by *C. trachomatis* serovars L1, L2, or L3. LGV infection manifestations share characteristics with chancroid, such as unilateral tender lymphadenopathy and self-limited genital ulcers. Homosexual men may present with proctocolitis and women with perianal inflammation, with the complication being strictures or fistulas. LGV can become an invasive systemic infection, and if it is not treated early, LGV proctocolitis may lead to chronic, colorectal fistulas and strictures.

The treatment for lymphogranuloma vereneum is outlined in Table 44-2. The diagnosis is made serologically and the recommended treatment is doxycycline. An alternative treatment is erythromycin base (CDC, 2010). Pregnant women are treated with erythromycin. Local lesions (buboes) may require incision and drainage. Patients may need further testing to rule out the high rate of coexisting STIs. Sexual partners who had contact with the patient in the past 60 days should be examined and treated (CDC, 2010).

Bacterial Vaginosis

Accounting for approximately 50% of all vaginitis cases in women, bacterial vaginosis (BV) is the most prevalent of vaginal infections (Sobel, 2012a). BV is caused by a replacement of the normal hydrogen-peroxide-producing lactobacilli present in the vaginal flora by an overgrowth of organisms such as *Prevotella* spp., *Mobiluncus* spp., *Gardnerella vaginalis,* or *Mycoplasma hominis.* The normally acidic vaginal environment is important in preventing the overgrowth of other organisms, which tends to occur when the pH is raised. Relapses and recurrences of the infection are common.

Although BV is not considered an STI, the majority of women infected are sexually active. Women with BV are also at risk for other sexually transmitted illnesses. BV is associated with having multiple sex partners, douching, and lack of vaginal lactobacilli. BV has caused endometritis and PID after invasive procedures such as endometrial biopsy, intrauterine device insertion, cesarean delivery, hysterectomy, and therapeutic abortion. Bacterial vaginosis is also a risk factor for contracting HIV, HSV-2, gonorrhea, and chlamydia (Sobel, 2012a).

BV can be diagnosed by the use of clinical criteria or Gram's stain criteria and must include three of the four following signs and symptoms (CDC, 2010): (1) a homogeneous, white, noninflammatory discharge that smoothly coats the vaginal walls; (2) a vaginal pH greater than 4.5; (3) a positive whiff test (fishy odor) with 10% potassium hydroxide (KOH); or (4) the presence of "clue cells" (vaginal epithelial cell peppered with coccoid bacteria) under high-power microscopy. The Pap smear is not reliable for the diagnosis of BV (Sobel, 2012a). In addition, obtaining cultures is also not reliable because there is no bacteria diagnostic of BV.

Due to the fact that asymptomatic women tend to spontaneously improve, treatment should be reserved for symptomatic women (Sobel, 2012a). However, nurse practitioner providers should use clinical judgment and individualize treatment to each patient and patient situation. Treatment of asymptomatic, pregnant women preparing to undergo termination of pregnancy is recommended.

The recommended metronidazole regimens are outlined in Table 44-2. Metronidazole orally, metronidazole gel, or clindamycin cream are the current CDC (2010) recommendations. Topical vaginal metronidazole is thought to be as effective as oral metronidazole (Sobel, 2012a). Vaginal clindamycin cream may be less effective than the metronidazole regimen. However, the drug provides an option for women unable to have metronidazole. It is important to note that clindamycin cream can weaken condoms, especially those made with latex. The use of probiotics to treat BV is controversial, and there is no current evidence to support this as a treatment option (Sobel, 2012a).

When mixed with alcohol, metronidazole has the potential to cause disulfiram-like reactions. Alcohol should not be consumed during or for at least 1 day following completion of metronidazole therapy (American Society of Health-System Pharmacists, 2010; CDC, 2010). Clindamycin cream is oil-based and may weaken latex condoms and diaphragms. Due to the fact that treatment of the sex partner has not been shown to be effective in preventing recurring infections, routine treatment of sexual contacts is not recommended. BV during pregnancy is associated with premature rupture of membranes, preterm labor, preterm birth, and postpartum endometriosis. For this reason, pregnant women should be screened for BV once the diagnosis of pregnancy is made. Current data do not support the use of topical agents to treat BV during pregnancy. There has been evidence to show adverse events after the use of clindamycin cream. For this reason, treatment of BV in the pregnant woman should be oral, rather than topical, with a medication that is safe during pregnancy. Oral metronidazole can be safely prescribed for pregnant women with bacterial vaginosis (CDC, 2010).

Due to the frequent relapses and reinfection that can occur, it is important for the nurse practitioner to have a treatment regimen available, as many women will need suppressive therapy (Sobel, 2012a). Current experts feel that three documented episodes of BV in the past 12 months make a woman a candidate for long-term treatment with metronidazole gel: 0.75% twice weekly for 4 to 6 months. Vaginal boric acid (not oral) 600 mg for 21 days, along with oral metronidazole for 7 days, is another treatment option.

Vulvovaginal Candidiasis

Vulvovaginal candidiasis (VVC) may be caused by several yeast species, although *Candida albicans* is the most common. It is estimated that 75% of women will have at least one episode of VVC, and 40% to 45% will have two or more episodes (CDC, 2010). For many women, a recent history of antibiotic use is most often the cause. The patient with chronic recurrent infections should be screened for diabetes (Sobel, 2012b). Candida vaginitis is not considered a sexually transmitted infection. However, sexually active women can be at risk for contracting the infection. Table 44-2 outlines the treatment for candida vaginitis.

Vulvar itching with a history of "cottage cheese-like" discharge are the primary complaints seen in those having the infection. The diagnosis for VVC in a woman can be made by wet preparation (saline, 10% KOH), Gram's stain, or culture. In addition, a low vaginal pH (4 to 4.5) can help to distinguish candida from other vaginal infections (bacterial vaginosis or trichomonas, for example) (Sobel, 2012b).

The azoles as a drug class are among the most effective treatments, with oral and topical treatments being equally effective (Sobel, 2012b). However, many women prefer oral treatment over topical. Oral fluconazole is available as a generic medication and may be cheaper than topical treatments. Oral azole agents stimulate the cytochrome P450 (CYP450) enzyme system in the liver and have potential drug interactions with calcium channel antagonists, cisapride, warfarin, oral hypoglycemic agents, phenytoin, protease inhibitors, theophylline, and rifampin.

The recommended creams and suppositories for the treatment of VVC are oil-based and may weaken latex condoms and diaphragms. Self-medication with over-the-counter (OTC) preparations is advised only for women who have been previously diagnosed with VVC and who have a recurrence of the same symptoms. Those patients experiencing severe pruritus may benefit from the temporary use (48 hours) of a low-potency topical steroid (Sobel, 2012b).

VVC often occurs during pregnancy. Only topical azole therapies, applied for 7 days, are recommended for use by pregnant, symptomatic women. Oral azoles are contraindicated in pregnancy.

Severe vulvovaginitis, characterized by extensive vulvar erythema, edema, excoriation, and fissure formation, may not clear with standard short therapy. Thus, longer doses may be needed. In severe cases, 7 to 14 days of topical therapy, or fluconazole 100 mg, 150 mg, or 200 mg orally every third day for a total of 3 doses, can be used (CDC, 2010). Oral fluconazole (100 mg, 150 mg, or 200 mg) weekly for 6 months can also be used for suppression of the infection (CDC, 2010; Sobel, 2012b). Due to the lack of data demonstrating effectiveness, the use of probiotics is not recommended (Sobel, 2012b).

Herpes Simplex Virus Type 1 and Herpes Simplex Virus Type 2

Genital herpes is incurable and tends to be recurrent although the periods of exacerbation and remission are highly variable. Two serotypes of HSV have been identified: HSV-1 and HSV-2. Most recurrences are a result of HSV-2. At present, approximately 50 million people have genital HSV infection. Most persons infected with HSV-2 have not been diagnosed and shed the virus in the genital tract without obvious symptoms (CDC, 2010). HSV-2 infections can also cause recurrent BV (Swygard & Cohen, 2012). Table 44-2 outlines the treatment of genital herpes.

Due the recurring nature of extremely painful vesicles during outbreaks, restoring and preserving quality of life is important in the patient with genital herpes. Suppressive therapy is recommended for patients experiencing six or more outbreaks each year. Most patients experience fewer episodes after 1 year of suppressive therapy. However, suppressive treatment can be effective in patients with less frequent attacks. Suppressive antiviral therapy reduces, but does not eliminate, subclinical viral shedding. Systemic treatment with oral acyclovir, famciclovir, and valacyclovir are the mainstays of treatment for genital herpes. Antiviral therapy for recurrent genital herpes can be administered episodically or continuously as suppressive therapy. Episodic therapy is effective in shortening the duration of outbreaks if started within the first 24 hours of lesion outbreaks or during the prodromal phase (burning, itching, and tingling) that often precedes outbreaks. In order for the antiviral treatment to be effective, the nurse practitioner provider should supply the patient receiving episodic treatment for HSV with a prescription to self-medicate immediately when symptoms begin. Consider reassessing the need for suppressive therapy annually by temporarily discontinuing the drug to see if outbreaks occur.

Patients with HIV infection or those who are immuno-compromised due to other causes may have prolonged or severe, painful episodes of genital, perianal, or oral herpes. Drug choices and dosing for HSV in the HIV patient are the same as for those with a first episode (or initial outbreak). Episodic or suppressive therapy with oral antiviral agents is beneficial.

Perinatal transmission of HSV is low (less than 1%) in women who have a history of genital HSV, but because recurrent herpes is common in pregnant women there is concern for transmission to the neonate at birth (CDC, 2010). The safety of acyclovir, valacyclovir, and famciclovir in pregnant women has not been well established. However, acyclovir can be administered orally to pregnant women with first-episode genital herpes or severe recurrent herpes (CDC, 2010). Perinatal transmission of HSV is 30% to 50% if women are infected near delivery and can be life-threatening; therefore protected sex is necessary if sex partners are infected (CDC, 2010). Cesarean delivery does not ensure protection from HSV-2 infection. Pregnant women with HSV require careful management by an obstetrical specialist during pregnancy and delivery.

Human Papillomavirus

According to the CDC, by the age of 50 more than 80% of American women will have contracted at least one strain of genital HPV. Both men and women can be carriers of HPV (CDC, 2010). Most HPV infections are asymptomatic or not visible but can lead to the development of anogenital cancers. For this reason, aggressive screening and treatment is often warranted, particularly in high-risk individuals. Reports indicate that more than 40 viral types can infect the genital area in men and women. HPV types 6 and 11 are considered low risk and cause 90% of all genital warts. Patients with visible warts may be infected with several types simultaneously.

HPV types (16, 18, 31, 33, and 35) are associated with cervical neoplasia and detected through the Pap smear process in women (CDC, 2010). HPV types 16 and 18 cause approximately 70% of cervical cancers. Lesions may be penile, scrotal, cervical, vaginal, urethral, oral, or perianal. Table 44-2 outlines the treatment for HPV.

Genital warts are usually flat, papular, or pedunculated growths on the genital mucosa. Diagnosis of genital warts is made by visual inspection and may be confirmed by biopsy. Biopsy is recommended in certain circumstances (for example, if the diagnosis is uncertain; the lesions do not respond to standard therapy; the disease worsens during therapy; the patient is immunocompromised; or warts are pigmented, indurated, fixed, bleeding, or ulcerated).

The application of 3% to 5% acetic acid usually turns HPV-infected genital mucosal tissue to a whitish color. However, acetic acid application is not a specific test for HPV infection, and the specificity and sensitivity of this procedure for screening have not been defined. Therefore, the routine use of this procedure for screening to detect HPV infection is not recommended (CDC, 2006). However, those clinicians who are experienced in the management of genital warts have determined that this test is useful for identifying flat genital warts.

In addition to the external genitalia (that is, penis, vulva, scrotum, perineum, and perianal skin), genital warts can occur on the uterine cervix and in the vagina, urethra, anus, and mouth. Intra-anal warts are observed predominantly in patients who have had receptive anal intercourse. These warts are distinct from perianal warts, which can occur in men and women who do not have a history of anal sex. Genital warts are usually asymptomatic, but depending on the size and anatomical location, lesions can be painful, friable, or pruritic.

HPV types 16, 18, 31, 33, and 35 are found occasionally in visible genital warts and have been associated with external genital squamous intra-epithelial neoplasia. These HPV types also have been associated with vaginal, anal, and cervical intra-epithelial neoplasia (CIN). They have also been associated with anogenital and some head and neck squamous cell carcinomas. Patients who have visible genital warts are frequently infected simultaneously with multiple HPV types (CDC, 2006). Management of HPV involves removing warts if the patient is symptomatic due to location, size, and number of warts and monitoring for the development of cancer cells especially in patients with abnormal Pap test results.

The primary goal of treating visible genital warts is the removal of the warts. In the majority of patients, treatment can induce wart-free periods. If left untreated, visible genital warts might resolve spontaneously, remain unchanged, or increase in size or number. Treatment possibly reduces, but does not eliminate, HPV infection. So far, existing data indicate that currently available therapies for genital warts might reduce, but probably do not eradicate, HPV infections.

The patient's symptoms, number of warts, where the warts are on the body, and size of warts are some of the factors that need to be considered in selecting a treatment modality. Other factors include cost of treatment, patient preference, the experience of the provider, and access to wart morphology. In general, warts located on moist surfaces or areas such as the armpits, underneath pendulous breasts, groin, creases of the neck, or skinfolds respond better to topical treatment than do warts on skin surfaces that are drier. The majority of patients will need more than one treatment and most respond within 3 months of therapy. Treatment regimens are classified as either patient-applied or provider-applied.

For external genital warts, the CDC (2010) recommends patient-applied therapy with podofilox 0.5% solution or gel or imiquimod 5% cream. These therapies need to be applied several times a week and can be costly. Provider-applied management includes cryotherapy with liquid nitrogen or cryoprobe or podophyllin resin 10% to 25% in a compound tincture of benzoin or trichloroacetic acid (TCA) or bichloroacetic acid

(BCA) 80% to 90%. An alternative provider-applied management includes the use of intralesional interferon or laser surgery. Surgical referral should be considered by the nurse practitioner when the size, number of warts, ineffective response to topical treatments, and location of warts make it difficult to treat effectively. Imiquimod, podophyllin, and podofilox should not be used during pregnancy. Because genital warts can proliferate and become friable during pregnancy, many specialist recommend their removal during pregnancy.

There is no evidence to suggest that one treatment is superior to another. Only trained nurse practitioners should administer cryotherapy. Treatment regimens should be changed if warts do not resolve in three to six treatments. Treatment of these lesions may result in chronic pain syndromes of the vulva, but these are extremely rare. In the absence of genital warts or cervical squamous intra-epithelial lesion (SIL), the CDC does not recommend treatment for subclinical genital HPV infection.

Currently in the United States, two vaccines to prevent HPV infection are currently on the market: Gardasil and Cervarix (CDC, 2010). Cervarix (a bivalent vaccine) provides protection against HPV types 16 and 18 and is licensed for use in females 11 to 25 years of age. Gardasil (a quadrivalent vaccine) provides protection from HPV types 6, 11, 16, and 18 and is licensed for both males and females ages 9 to 26 years. These vaccines can be costly, but children and adolescents less than 19 years of age can receive assistance through the Vaccines for Children (VFC) program (http://www.cdc.gov/vaccines/programs/vfc/index.html). A nine-valent HPV vaccine (HPV9) is currently undergoing FDA review for approval and protects against HPV strains 6, 11, 16, 18, 31, 33, 45, 52, and 58.

Trichomoniasis

Trichomonas spp. are protozoa, and protozoan infections require a different therapeutic approach. Men are rarely symptomatic but may harbor *Trichomonas* in the prostate gland for years if left untreated. Many women have a malodorous, yellow-green vaginal discharge with vulvar irritation. However, some women have minimal discharge and may be asymptomatic. An increase in vaginal pH in women may increase the risk of *Trichomonas* infection in men (Swygard & Cohen, 2012).

The availability of rapid testing has increased the sensitivity and specificity significantly compared to the use of microscopy, which requires provider experience and immediate evaluation of wet prepared slides to capture the classic *Trichomonas* movement. The diagnosis is therefore often missed because wet mounts must be viewed quickly. The wet-prep method is not a sensitive test in men (CDC, 2010; Swygard & Cohen, 2012). Urine sediment microscopy may frequently demonstrate this organism fortuitously. Table 44-2 outlines the treatments for trichomoniasis.

The treatment regimen for trichomoniasis includes oral metronidazole or tinidazole (CDC, 2010). Patients need to be advised to avoid consuming alcohol during treatment with metronidazole. In doing so, a disulfiram reaction may occur. Rescreening for *T. vaginalis* 3 months after treatment may be

considered in sexually active women, due to a high (17%) reinfection rate (CDC, 2010).

Pregnant women who are infected with vaginal trichomoniasis are at risk of preterm labor, premature rupture of membranes, and low birth weight (CDC, 2010). Treatment for symptomatic women or asymptomatic women in any stage of pregnancy is oral metronidazole (CDC, 2010). The safety of tinidazole in pregnancy has not been well evaluated. Pregnant women should be followed up in 1 month.

Sexual partners should be treated for trichomoniasis and patients should be instructed to abstain from intercourse until both partners are treated and asymptomatic (CDC, 2010).

Pediculosis Pubis (Genital Lice)

Pediculosis pubis (i.e., genital lice), commonly called crabs, is an ectoparasitic infection that is treated differently based on where the lice are found (e.g., scalp, body, or the pubic area). Pubic lice are generally sexually transmitted, with teenagers and young adults being those most commonly affected (Goldstein & Goldstein, 2011).

The organism is genetically programmed to attach to hair of different diameters. Considerable resistance to medication for treatment of head lice has been seen, but pediculosis can be eradicated by the methods listed in Table 44-2. Pubic itching is the primary complaint and the organism can be resistant to treatment (Goldstein & Goldstein, 2011). Retreatment in one week of symptomatic individuals is recommended.

Pubic lice may be treated with pyrethrins: permethrin 1%, pyrethrin lotion, or shampoo. Advise the patient to thoroughly saturate hair with the medication. Leave medication on for 10 minutes, then thoroughly rinse off with water. Dry off with a clean towel (CDC, Division of Parasitic Diseases, 2008a; Goldstein & Goldstein, 2011). Reapply in 7 days if needed.

Resistance to pediculicides is becoming more frequent and widespread. Malathion 0.5% lotion or oral ivermectin are reasonable options and may be used when treatment failure is believed to have occurred or if resistance is suspected (CDC, 2006; Goldstein & Goldstein, 2011). Further discussion of the treatment of body lice is included in Chapter 32.

According to Goldstein & Goldstein (2011), sexual partners should be treated at the same time to avoid reinfection. Treatment of nonsexual contacts is not needed.

Decontamination of household and personal items with hot washing or dry-cleaning is usually adequate. Pubic lice cannot live away from the body for more than 72 hours, and fumigating the home is not necessary if the above-mentioned methods are observed.

Scabies

Sarcoptes scabiei is the parasite involved in scabies. The most common predominant symptom is severe, nocturnal pruritus. After a person is infested with scabies for the first time, sensitization can take up to several weeks to develop. Pruritus can then occur within 24 hours following a subsequent infestation. Direct contact from person to person is needed to contract the parasite (Goldstein & Goldstein, 2012). Scabies can be passed sexually in adults, but adults and particularly children may become infected by sleeping on infected sheets in motels and hotels. If scabies has been contracted via sexual contact, the skin adjacent to the nipples, periumbilical area, waist, genitalia, buttocks, and thighs is commonly affected. Although it is possible to obtain skin scrapings from patients, the diagnosis can be made through history and physical examination alone. Table 44-2 outlines the treatments for scabies.

Permethrin 5% cream (Elimite, Acticin) is the drug of choice for the treatment of scabies, especially in pregnant women or young children. The cream is massaged into the skin from the neck to the soles of the feet. It should be left on for 8 to 14 hours and then washed off in the shower. A repeat application in 1 to 2 weeks is recommended (Goldstein & Goldstein, 2012).

Oral ivermectin is another alternative. The use of ivermectin is not recommended in pregnant or lactating women, and children (Goldstein & Goldstein, 2012). However, ivermectin is considered the drug of choice for nursing home outbreaks or when topical treatment is not practical. Ivermectin may need to be repeated in 2 weeks. Ivermectin is not active against nits. Topical ivermectin (Sklice) is not currently approved for scabies treatment.

Although treatment with lindane is an option, the routine use of this treatment is discouraged due to the adverse-effect profile. Lindane can cause seizures and is contraindicated in pregnant women and children.

The itching experienced due to a scabies infection can be quite severe. Therefore, in addition to eradicating the mite, treatment with antihistamines and topical low- or medium-dose corticosteroids to control the itching can be helpful (Goldstein & Goldstein, 2012). Nonsedating antihistamines can be used during the day. Sedating antihistamines can be used at night, which will also aid in sleep.

Bedding and clothing should be decontaminated or removed from body contact for at least 72 hours. Patient education is important when treating ectoparasitic infections. The rash and pruritus of scabies can persist for up to 2 weeks after treatment. Sexual contacts and family members may be in the incubation period (4 weeks). For this reason, all family members and close contacts need simultaneous treatment to prevent recurrence. Reinfection from family members or fomites might occur in the absence of appropriate contact treatment and decontamination of bedding and clothing. The treatment of scabies is discussed in depth in Chapter 32.

Special Treatment Situations

The following sections describe certain treatment situations that warrant special consideration: pregnant women and adolescents, those with pelvic inflammatory disease (PID), sexual assault victims, men who have sex with men, and women who have sex with women. Delay in treatment of PID or treatment with the wrong antibiotic can result in continued spread of the organism. A woman who presents for care with signs of PID needs treatment as though she has all types of infection, including gonorrhea, chlamydia, and BV. The sexual assault victim needs urgent evaluation, with testing, prophylactic antibiotics, and emergency contraception offered.

Pregnancy

All pregnant women and their sexual partners should be asked routinely about STIs, counseled about the possibility of perinatal infection, and ensured prompt access to treatment. At the first prenatal visit, women should be screened for syphilis, HBsAg, chlamydia, gonorrhea, and hepatitis C and should receive a Pap test (CDC, 2010; Swygard & Cohen, 2012). Pregnant women should be screened for HIV in the first and third trimesters (CDC, 2010).

A pregnant woman with an STI requiring treatment may present as a treatment challenge for the nurse practitioner. Consultation with an expert or referral for treatment is recommended. All women of childbearing age should have a documented pregnancy test before beginning any treatment. Ciprofloxacin, ofloxacin, and doxycycline are all contraindicated in pregnancy.

Children

STIs in children, if acquired after the neonatal period, should raise the index of suspicion about the possibility of child abuse. Sexual abuse is the most frequent cause of gonococcal infection in preadolescent children (CDC, 2010). Specially trained nurse practitioners or other health providers must perform extensive evaluation and referral to a child abuse specialist in order to effectively evaluate and treat this population.

The use of fluoroquinolones in children younger than 18 years is generally not recommended. Therapy with this particular class of drugs has caused articular cartilage damage in some studies utilizing young animals.

Adolescents

Adolescents have the highest risk for acquiring HPV, chlamydia, and gonorrhea. Reasons cited for these risks include (1) engaging in frequent unprotected intercourse, (2) being biologically more susceptible to infection, (3) having partnerships of limited duration, and (4) difficulty gaining access to care.

Adolescents in most states can consent to the confidential diagnosis and treatment of STIs. In these states, nurse practitioners need to be aware that screening, treatment, and counseling for STIs can be provided to adolescents without parental consent or knowledge. Nurse practitioners should check the appropriate state laws. The CDC resources for this can be found online: http://wwwn.cdc.gov/nndss/script/downloads.aspx.

Pelvic Inflammatory Disease

Delay in treatment of STIs and other diseases (bacterial vaginosis) can result in pelvic inflammatory disease (PID) and infertility. Pelvic inflammatory disease, by definition, is an acute infection of the upper genital tract (Wiesenfeld, 2012). Organisms that cause PID can be sexually transmitted (*N. gonorrhoeae*, chlamydia, and bacterial vaginosos), part of the normal flora (*G. vaginalis* and *Haemophilus influenzae*), or can be atypical agents (cytomegalovirus and *Mycoplasma hominis*) not generally associated with sexual activity.

PID is difficult to diagnose due to (1) the wide variation in signs and symptoms and (2) the fact that more than one organism may be involved. Empirical treatment of PID should be initiated if the following minimum criteria are met and no other cause for the symptoms (e.g., appendicitis) can be found: (1) uterine/adnexal tenderness or (2) cervical motion tenderness. Additional criteria that support the diagnosis of PID include (1) oral temperature higher than 38.3°C, (2) abnormal cervical or vaginal mucopurulent discharge, (3) presence of white blood cells upon saline microscopy examination, (4) elevated erythrocyte sedimentation rate, (5) elevated C-reactive protein, and (6) laboratory-documented cervical infection with gonorrhea or chlamydia.

Treatment for PID is a multidrug regimen that provides empiric, broad-spectrum coverage of the most likely pathogens. The nurse practitioner who suspects PID must begin treatment immediately to avoid the life-altering complications that can occur. Prevention of long-term complications has been linked directly with immediate administration of appropriate antibiotics. A woman who presents for care with signs and symptoms suggestive of PID needs to be treated as if she has all types of infection. A pregnancy test should be obtained and the results known before beginning treatment. All pregnant women with PID should be hospitalized and treated with intravenous antibiotics. In addition, a woman may need intravenous antibiotics and/or hospitalization if her temperature is high or if she cannot tolerate oral drugs (due to nausea and vomiting).

The outpatient treatment for mild to moderate PID includes a single intramuscular dose of cefoxitin 2 g plus a single dose of oral probenecid 1 g plus oral doxycycline 100 mg twice daily for 14 days. Metronidazole orally 500 mg twice a day for 14 days should also be added. An expert should be consulted when treating the penicillin-allergic patient with PID (Wiesenfeld, 2012). The primary care nurse practitioner should hospitalize and refer all patients with severe pelvic inflammatory disease as well as all pregnant women with PID regardless of the severity of infection.

The transition from IV therapy to oral therapy can usually be initiated within 24 hours of clinical improvement. Consider changing patients who fail to respond to oral therapy within 72 hours to parenteral therapy. The PID patient should show substantial clinical improvement within 3 days after initiation of therapy. Patients who do not improve within this time period usually require hospitalization, additional diagnostic testing, and surgical intervention.

Sexual Assault

Trichomoniasis, bacterial vaginosis, gonorrhea, and chlamydial infection are the most frequently diagnosed infections among women who have been sexually assaulted. Screening and treating sexual assault victims requires specialized training. Except in rare cases, evaluation and treatment of sexual assault victims should not be attempted by untrained providers (Bates, 2012). The information presented in this section is directed toward adults and does not include the treatment of sexual assault/abuse in children. In addition, the information is not meant to replace the specialized training needed to treat these patients.

Testing for chlamydia and gonorrhea via nucleic acid amplification testing and wet mount for bacterial vaginosis, trichomoniasis, and candida is recommended (Bates, 2012). Testing for HIV, hepatitis, and syphilis should also be considered. A pregnancy test should be done in all women of childbearing age and emergency contraception should be offered. Empiric treatment for gonorrhea, chlamydia, and trichomoniasis is recommended. Prophylactic treatment for HIV is controversial but should also be considered.

Sexual assault victims should be evaluated for ingestion of date rape and other drugs via blood and urine samples. In certain cases, hair samples can also be used. Alcohol and benzodiazepines are drugs commonly used (Bates, 2012).

The date rape drug Rohypnol (flunitrazepam) is available illegally in the United States. This drug has been associated with an increased incidence of adolescent date rape (American Academy of Pediatrics [AAP], 2009). Flunitrazepam, a very rapid onset benzodiazepine with amnesic properties, is a tasteless drug that can go undetected if added to any drink (Kosten, 2009). The tasteless properties of these drugs make the victim incapable of protecting him- or herself. Due to the amnesic properties of the drug, the sexual assault victim is unable to remember the events of the incident after the drug effects have worn off. These drugs, in the amounts most commonly used, produce intoxication and can produce fatalities if used with other respiratory depressants (such as large amounts of alcohol or opioids).

Men Who Have Sex With Men

The CDC (2010) recommendations include at least annual STI screening (or 3- to 6-month intervals for those at high risk) for HIV, syphilis, urethral/rectal/pharyngeal gonorrhea, chlamydia, and HBsAg in men who have sex with men (MSM).

Vaccinations against hepatitis A and B are recommended for all MSM in whom previous infection or immunization cannot be documented. Men should be offered the HPV quadrivalent vaccine, regardless of their sexual orientation.

The same STI treatment principles applied to heterosexuals are relevant to men having sex with men. If the nurse practitioner treats for gonorrhea, then treatment for possible co-infection with chlamydia should be prescribed. The reverse statement is also true.

Women Who Have Sex With Women

CDC (2010) data on women who have sex with women is limited. However, it is important to consider this population when screening for and treating sexually transmitted infections. A great majority of women have also had sex with men (Carroll, 2013). Screening for STIs should be performed in symptomatic women (Swygard & Cohen, 2012). The rates of screening for cervical cancer among these women are lower than that of heterosexual women.

Bacterial vaginosis is more common among women with female partners. For this reason, treatment of female partners is recommended. Sexual acts using shared penetrative devices (including hands and fingers) present a possible means for the transmission of infected cervico-vaginal secretions. Transmission of HPV (including the types attributed to cancer) can occur through skin-to-skin or skin-to-mucosa contact (Carroll, 2013).

Hepatitis

Serological testing is necessary for all suspected cases of hepatitis. In the United States almost half of all reported hepatitis A cases have no specific risk factors identified. However, among adults with identified risk factors, the majority of cases are among MSM, persons who use illegal drugs, and international travelers (CDC, 2006). Only about 1.8% of patients die from liver disease as a result of hepatitis A, but there is considerable morbidity, well worth the cost and inconvenience of two vaccine injections. Currently two products are available for the prevention of hepatitis A (HAV) infection: hepatitis A vaccine and immune globulin (Ig) for IM administration. No specific treatment therapy is available for persons with acute hepatitis A or B; treatment is supportive.

Chronic infections of hepatitis B occur in 1% to 6% of infected adults; however, they occur in 90% of infected newborns. The risk for premature death from either cirrhosis or hepatocellular carcinoma among persons infected with hepatitis B is between 15% and 25% (CDC, 2006). Hepatitis B virus (HBV) is passed through vertical transmission. Sexual transmission among adults accounts for most HBV infections in the United States. Prevention aimed at several groups is necessary. Prevention strategies include screening all pregnant women, vaccinating all newborns, vaccinating older children at high risk (e.g., Alaskan Natives, Pacific Islanders) and residents in households with first-generation immigrants from countries that have high levels of endemic disease, vaccinating children aged 11 and 12 who do not fit into the preceding categories, and vaccinating teens and adults at high risk (sexual behaviors confer increased risk). Hepatitis A and B are the only vaccines available for preventable hepatitis diseases. There is no vaccine for hepatitis C.

Two products have been approved for hepatitis B prevention: hepatitis B immune globulin (HBIG) and hepatitis B vaccine. HBIG provides 3 to 6 months of temporary protection from hepatitis B infection. There are two monovalent hepatitis B vaccines for use in adolescents and adults: Recombivax HB and Engerix-B. There is also a combination vaccine of hepatitis A and B for use in adults, Twinrix. See Chapter 19 or www.cdc.gov/vaccines for more information.

Hepatitis C virus (HCV) is the most common chronic blood-borne infection in the United States. HCV transmission occurs by direct percutaneous exposure to infected blood, as well as by occupational, perinatal, and sexual exposure. Sexual transmission of HCV accounts for up to 15% to 20% of HCV infections (CDC, 2007a). Furthermore, co-infection with HIV increases the risk for sexual transmission of HCV. Newly infected persons with HCV commonly are either asymptomatic or have a mild clinical illness and may not seek medical care. HCV RNA can be detected within 1 to 3 weeks of exposure. Chronic HCV infections develop in 60% to 85% of HCV-infected persons. Of these, 60% to 70% have evidence of active liver disease. No vaccine is available for

HCV, and prophylaxis with immune globulin is not effective in preventing HCV infection after exposure (CDC, 2006).

HIV

The immunosuppressive pathology of HIV predisposes some infected individuals to STIs. HIV affects the immune system, which in turn has an impact on diagnostic testing and evaluation of some of these infections. In addition, those infected with HIV often have a suboptimal response to treatment or present as treatment failures when infected with an STI. As a result, HIV-infected patients who have concurrent STI infections may require longer, more aggressive courses of therapy. When included as part of the treatment recommendations, nurse practitioners should consider prescribing suppressive therapy (HSV vaccine) sooner rather than later. Treatment of HIV infection is covered in Chapter 37.

Penicillin Allergy

Individuals infected with an STI but who have an allergy to penicillin also present as a treatment challenge. There are no CDC recommendations or proven alternatives to penicillin for the treatment of neurosyphilis, congenital syphilis, or syphilis in pregnant women. Penicillin is also the treatment of choice in HIV-infected patients. However, the administration of penicillin to those allergic to the drug can cause severe, immediate anaphylaxis, which can be fatal. As a general rule, penicillin should never be used in penicillin-allergic patients. Those patients needing penicillin should be referred to allergy specialists who can safely perform allergy skin testing and acute desensitization to eliminate anaphylactic sensitivity.

Monitoring

Drug sensitivity, patient intolerance, and noncompliance with drugs requiring multiple daily doses frequently necessitate use of alternate drugs. Although treatments for most STIs are quite effective, follow-up is necessary, particularly in high-risk or noncompliant individuals. Each nurse practitioner should use clinical judgment when deciding who and when to screen and rescreen. Generally speaking, experts recommend rescreening in women and men at 3-month intervals because recurrence is common with many of these infections (Swygard & Cohen, 2012).

Viral STIs present a challenge for most health-care providers. Patient education, appropriate viral testing, and evaluation of possible concurrent infections are necessary components of any management. It is important to be sure that all sexual partners have been treated and that the organism in question has either been eradicated or brought under control. Asymptomatic partners may be resistant to treatment and may require education and assistance from the local health department.

Laboratories are required by law to report most STIs to the state, so patients need to know that they will be contacted for verification of treatment. In addition, nurse practitioner providers should educate themselves about which sexually transmitted infections they are legally required to report. This information can be found on the CDC's National Notifiable Diseases Surveillance System Web site: wwwn.cdc.gov/nndss/default.aspx.

Although it may improve treatment and recurrence rates, partner-delivery of patient medications is not recommended and is not legal in many states (Swygard & Cohen, 2012). Partners of those infected patients should be evaluated and promptly treated.

Outcome Evaluation

Infection in the genital tract with chlamydia or gonorrhea, if not treated in a timely manner, may ascend and invade the fallopian tubes, thus causing life-threatening PID and sepsis. Patients and their sexual partners should abstain from intercourse until 7 days after a single-dose treatment or upon successful completion of treatment (Swygard & Cohen, 2012).

A pregnant patient with an untreated STI may spontaneously abort and hemorrhage. Sepsis and bleeding require hospitalization and parenteral therapy. Consultation and referral to a gynecologist must be completed swiftly to prevent further complications. The specialist, in turn, will need information that only the nurse practitioner may possess: the patient's full past medical history, laboratory findings, previous treatments, and drug allergies.

Patient Education

Patient education should include a discussion of information related to the overall treatment plan as well as that specific to the drug therapy, reasons for taking the drug, drugs as part of the total treatment regimen, and potential compliance issues (Box 44-1). Partner education is also important to consider. Assessment of the barriers to drug adherence need to be explored and discussed with the patient.

VAGINITIS

Vagnitis symptoms among women are extremely common which often results in self-diagnosis and treatment with

---

BOX 44–1 VACCINE-PREVENTABLE SEXUALLY TRANSMITTED INFECTIONS

Many of the sexually transmitted infections are vaccine preventable (HAV, HBV, and HPV). Due to growing public health concerns, escalating costs of treatment, and lack of insurance, preventing infections is, in most cases, easier and less expensive than treatment. Whenever possible, patients should be educated early and often regarding the type of vaccines that they would be successful candidates to receive. Currently, there is no approved vaccine available for hepatitis C virus (HCV). Prophylaxis treatment after exposure to the virus has not been shown to be effective (CDC, 2010).

---

over-the-counter agents (Sobel, 2012c). The three diseases most frequently associated with vaginal discharge are trichomoniasis, bacterial vaginosis, and candidiasis (CDC, 2010; Sobel, 2012c). *C. trachomatis* and *N. gonorrhoeae* are less frequent causative organisms. Other, less common causes are cervicitis, atrophic vaginitis, foreign body resulting in secondary infection, irritants, and allergies (Sobel, 2012c). Treatment without an appropriate history and examination is not recommended as self-diagnosis can be inaccurate.

Diagnosing vaginal discharge and vulvar conditions requires a thorough history and examination of the area affected. Not all practitioners are adept at microscopy; however, microscopy skills are essential for a proper diagnosis of the patient with vaginitis. The diagnosis may be elusive without prompt examination of vaginal discharge.

This chapter earlier discussed the most common STIs and their treatment. Vaginal infections can be sexually transmitted, but some may also be acquired without sexual contact: VVC, some types of bacterial vaginosis, cytolytic vaginosis, atrophic vaginitis with secondary bacterial infection, and some types of streptococcal infections. *Staphylococcus aureus,* found in toxic shock syndrome, is associated with foreign bodies (tampons) inadvertently left during menses. Treatment of vulvovaginal infections is discussed separately from those vulvovaginal conditions that present with vaginal burning, pruritus, and dyspareunia, yet are not infectious.

Pathophysiology

Normal vaginal discharge contains desquamated vaginal epithelial cells, cervical secretions, lactic acid, and bacteria that are both anaerobic and aerobic. Vaginal microflora, predominantly *Lactobacillus,* appear under the microscope as unclumped, rod-like organisms. Estrogen fluctuations, age influence, and infections may alter the delicate balance. The most common infections are due to bacteria, yeast, and parasites. Conditions not covered earlier in the chapter are discussed here.

Cytolytic Vaginosis

In cytolytic vaginosis, an overgrowth of *Lactobacillus* occurs late in the menstrual cycle. It is frequently treated as a chronic yeast infection. Diagnosis is made by absence of *Trichomonas,* hyphae, clue cells, and white blood cells under microscopy. The pH may be as low as 3.5, and treatment is aimed at raising the pH rather than eradicating all bacteria. Treatments that involve douching of medications are discouraged. Instead, patients are encouraged to make vaginal suppositories from clear gelatin capsules (size 0) filled with sodium bicarbonate (baking soda) and dose twice weekly in the last week of the menstrual cycle.

Atrophic Vaginitis

Atrophic vaginitis with secondary infection occurs due to estrogen deficiencies. As a result, the thinned vaginal epithelium

SEXUALLY TRANSMITTED INFECTIONS

PATIENT EDUCATION

Related to the Overall Treatment Plan/Disease Process

☐ Importance of routine Pap smears in women and testicular self-examinations (TSE) in men

☐ Prevention of high-risk sexual behaviors

☐ Avoidance of sexual intercourse until the organism is either eradicated (bacterial) or under control (viral)

☐ Include immunization against selected STDs as part of treatment regimen

Specific to the Drug Therapy

☐ Many OTC products are available to treat symptoms.

☐ Douching is no longer recommended because of the potential for pelvic infection and destroying the normal flora of *Lactobacillus*.

☐ BV must be diagnosed and treated on the same day in patients suspected of being pregnant (BV may cause preterm labor).

☐ Importance of assessment of pregnancy status in all women of childbearing years *before* prescribing

☐ Choosing a generic agent that has daily or twice-daily dosing increases patient compliance with treatment.

Reasons for Taking the Drug(s)

☐ Prevention of serious complications such as PID and infertility

☐ Prevention of transmission of infection to the uninfected (public health issue)

☐ Prevention of dyspareunia, which affects normal sexual relations

Drugs as Part of the Total Treatment Regimen

☐ Importance of seeking treatment when symptoms appear

☐ Importance of culturing asymptomatic young persons (aged 15 to 24) every 6 months

Adherence Issues

☐ Importance of following the labeled instructions to totally eradicate the infection

☐ Importance of finishing the full course of antibiotics

☐ Importance of contacting the health-care provider if side effects or rash appears

☐ The potential for drug interactions (the macrolides with antifungal, systemic antifungals, and birth control pills)

---

has reduced defenses against common perineal bacteria. Culturing is necessary, as well as microscopy. See Table 44-2 for treatment once the infecting organism is diagnosed and Table 44-3 for treatment of the underlying atrophic conditions.

Toxic Shock Syndrome

S. aureus associated with toxic shock syndrome (TSS) can be life-threatening. A patient with TSS requires immediate referral for hospitalization. *S. aureus* commonly colonizes skin and mucous membranes in humans. TSS has been associated with use of tampons and intravaginal contraceptive devices in women and occurs as a complication of skin abscesses or surgery. Risk groups include menstruating women, women using barrier contraceptive devices, persons who have undergone nasal surgery, and persons with postoperative staphylococcal wound infections (CDC, 2007). Some women harbor *S. aureus* in their normal vaginal secretions but experience no symptoms until using tampons sets up an anaerobic climate. Criteria for making this diagnosis and

treatment are based on CDC guidelines and include four of the following five diagnostic criteria: fever of 38.9°C (102°F) or higher, presence of a diffuse macular erythroderma, desquamation 1 to 2 weeks after onset of illness (palms and soles), hypotension (orthostatic changes of 15 mm Hg diastolic pressure or syncope), and involvement of three or more organ systems (GI, muscular, mucous membrane, renal, hepatic, hematological, and central nervous system [CNS]) (CDC, 2007).

Noninfectious Vaginal Conditions

Noninfectious vaginal conditions may result from the following:

1. Normal cyclical hormonal changes, which occur at midcycle under high estrogen levels, and premenses, which is under progestin dominance. The changes in amount of vaginal secretions may concern some women, and microscopy may be necessary to reassure the patient and to rule out pathological organisms.

Table 44–3   Treatment for Noninfectious Vulvovaginal Conditions

Condition	Drug Used	Nondrug Treatment
Chemical or other irritants, spermicidals, douching solutions	Systemic steroid burst Medrol Dosepak	Avoid products with color and fragrance. Always use sanitary pads. Treat urinary incontinence with hygiene and disposable pads. Referral to urology for surgical correction.
Allergic, hypersensitivity, contact dermatitis, lichen simplex, foreign body	Steroid burst if severe reaction occurs Topical preferred over systemic	Avoidance and education about use of excessive hygiene measures. Use of Crisco (vegetable shortening) and avoidance of detergents in older women.
Desquamative inflammatory vaginitis (steroid responsive)	If short course is helpful, consult about length of therapy; need tissue diagnosis	Avoid harsh scrubbing, soaps, and other over-the-counter vaginal products.
Erosive lichen planus	Steroids are usually necessary; need tissue diagnosis and consult or refer	Avoid excessive hygiene measures; there are "vulvar" specialists in gynecology.
Collagen vascular disease, Behçet's and pemphigus syndromes	Refer aggressive and painful lesions for diagnosis and treatment May use low-dose (25–50 mg) tricyclic antidepressants for pain control	Support groups may be helpful for some patients.
Hormonal Changes (normal responses)		
1. Midcycle	None	If culture and microscopy clear, then educate and reassure patient.
2. After intercourse	None	If culture and microscopy are clear, then educate and reassure.
3. Atrophic	Vaginal lubricants and moisturizers are first-line treatments. In women without a history of breast cancer, low-dose vaginal estrogen therapy is preferred over systemic estrogen therapy: ≤50 mcg estradiol or <0.3 mg conjugated estrogens/ ≤0.5 g cream.	May require 3–6 mo of therapy for full therapeutic benefit. Can use topical treatments indefinitely. All postmenopausal women experiencing vaginal bleeding should be evaluated for cancer.
Epithelial disorders (previously called dystrophies), lichen sclerosus (white lesions)	Clobetasol 0.05% ointment daily at night for 6–12 weeks and then 1–3 times per week for maintenance.	Biopsy is required for diagnosis. Support group may be helpful for some patients. Women are at high risk for developing squamous cell cancer of the vulva. Steroid creams should be avoided because they can contain irritants not found in ointments.

Sources: Bachmann, G., & Santen, R. J. (2012). *Treatment of vaginal atrophy*. Retrieved from www.uptodate.com. Doseck, J., & Stern, L. (2009). Treatment options for bacterial vaginosis. *Clinical Advisor for Nurse Practitioners, 12*(11); Stewart, E. G. (2011). *Vulvar lichen sclerosus*. Retrieved from www.uptodate.com. Thompson, I. M., Teichman, J. M., Elston, D. M., & Sea, J. (2010). Noninfectious penile lesions. *Journal of the American Academy of Family Physicians, 81*(2).

2. Irritant or allergic products, such as those found in hygiene and contraceptive products (e.g., spermicides and latex).
3. Atrophic conditions, such as those associated with the postpartum period and breastfeeding and those associated with postmenopausal vaginal atrophy.

Other Conditions

Less common and more worrisome are inflammatory, collagen, and epidermal sclerosing conditions, which are commonly diagnosed in older women: inflammatory conditions related to trauma from excessive washing, wiping, and scratching; inflammatory conditions reflecting collagen-vascular disease; and inflammatory conditions associated with white or pigmented lesions that may be dysplastic or cancers.

Goals of Treatment

The goals of treatment are to treat the infection or inflammation, prevent reinfection, and prevent complications of the infection or inflammation. The infection cannot be treated without an accurate diagnosis. Patients often call the office numerous times for prescriptions for yeast infections, yet frequently they do not have monilial vaginitis. Telephone diagnoses run the risk of being incorrect. As a result, patients often spend money on ineffective medications. In addition, prescribing an ineffective antibiotic exposes the patient to potential side effects, adverse effects, and drug-drug interactions.

For patients aged 15 to 24, there is a probability the complaint is related to a sexually transmitted infection. For patients age 50 to 70, vaginal symptoms are more often related to atrophy of the genital tissues, vulvar presentation of collagen-vascular disease, or cancer. However, sexually transmitted infections can still occur in the geriatric population. The prudent nurse practitioner should include these infections as part of the differential diagnosis of the geriatric women with vaginal complaints, particularly those women with new sexual partners.

Reinfection occurs when the etiology of the vaginal irritation is not known. If lack of estrogen is making the vaginal tissues thin and vulnerable to bleeding, then treatment with an antibiotic alone allows the infection to recur. Treatment with vaginal estrogen or the vaginal ring thickens the vaginal epithelium and permits natural defenses (intact mucous membranes) to prevail.

Complications of the infection can occur when symptoms of itching and irritation go untreated and the affected tissues thicken and lose elasticity (lichenification). When vulvar tissues become inflamed and heal, they often shrink in size so that the vagina will not allow sexual penetration. Early and aggressive treatment of conditions such as lichen sclerosus delays permanent hardening of the epidermis and dermal layers of the vulva.

Rational Drug Selection

Guidelines

Treatment of STI infections is guided by the CDC but should not replace nurse practitioner clinical judgment. Treatment for nuisance infections may vary according to severity of patient symptoms or health-care provider preference.

All recommended treatments have the potential to be costly for the patient and for the health-care system and are not without side effects, adverse effects, and drug-drug interactions (Lexicomp, 2013). For example, the concurrent use of penicillin G with tetracycline, erythromycin, and doxycycline is not recommended. In addition, penicillin and doxycycline both have the potential to interfere with estrogen-containing oral contraceptives. For this reason, a backup method of contraception is recommended. The use of erythromycin with oral azoles is not recommended due to the cardiac adverse effects that can occur. Metronidazole in both oral and gel preparations has the potential to cause seizures. Finally, ciprofloxacin has been known to cause tendonitis and tendon rupture in all age groups. Photosensitivity reactions can also occur and patients should be educated to take precautions when in the sun.

Cost

Many fungal infections are easily eradicated with topical antifungals such as miconazole, which is available OTC. Maximizing the use of OTC agents is a more cost-effective approach for the patient, especially for those without insurance, to cover the cost of a written prescription.

Patient Variables

There are many variables to consider when preparing a patient treatment plan. Generic drugs are more cost-effective for the patient. Prescribing the shortest possible course of treatment

with an agent that has the potential to cause the least amount of side effects and drug-drug interactions will also improve compliance rates. Oral medications are often preferred over vaginal creams and suppositories, which can be messy and uncomfortable for the patient.

Drug Variables

Many vulvovaginal conditions can successfully be treated topically, thus avoiding the potential side effects and adverse effects of oral medications. Use of intravaginal antibiotics and antifungals generally does not affect the absorption of oral contraceptives or other medications that patients may be taking. Low-dose topical steroids can be used for longer periods without suppressing the adrenal gland and reducing total body immunity. When used around vaginal tissues, low-dose topical steroids are preferred over higher, more potent doses due to the potential adverse effects that can occur.

Monitoring

There are many factors to consider when screening, rescreening, and performing test-of-cures. When in doubt, the nurse practitioner should rescreen. Nurse practitioners should use clinical judgment and individualize the approach used while being mindful of the recommended guidelines and available resources. Over-the-phone treatment is not recommended. Experts do not advise treating the patient and his/her partner without conducting an appropriate history and physical examination.

Outcome Evaluation

When a patient has a dermal condition that the practitioner has not seen before, a consultation or referral is strongly recommended. Consultation is also necessary when pigmented or white lesions are seen during examination. If patients remember that they were born with pigmented lesions (birthmarks), then biopsy is generally not necessary.

When patients do not respond to initial or follow-up treatments, consider referral. If the provider is not adept or comfortable with vulvar biopsies, then referral for specialty care is necessary. When conditions of the vulva appear in the very young (patients aged 1 to 12), in the older adult (patients age 60 or older), or in the pregnant patient, referral is recommended.

Patient Education

When treating the patient with an STI, extensive education is often needed and should be thoroughly documented in the patient's medical record. Patient education should include a discussion of information related to the overall treatment plan as well as that specific to the drug therapy, reasons for taking the drug, drugs as part of the total treatment regimen, and adherence issues.

VAGINITIS

PATIENT EDUCATION

Related to the Overall Treatment Plan/Disease Process

☐ Knowledge of many causes of vaginal irritation, ranging from allergy to inflammatory conditions associated with local and systemic disease

☐ Knowledge of the physiological changes in vaginal epithelium from age 12 to 50

☐ Hygiene issues such as types of clothing for underwear, wiping correctly, and emptying bladder before and after intercourse

Specific to the Drug Therapy

☐ Many OTC products that were previously under prescriptive authority are available to treat symptoms and are still efficacious.

☐ Douching is no longer recommended because of the potential for pelvic infection and its destruction of the normal flora of *Lactobacillus*.

Reasons for Taking the Drug(s)

☐ Prevention of dyspareunia, which affects normal sexual relations

☐ Control of miserable chronic conditions like lichen sclerosus

Drugs as Part of the Total Treatment Regimen

☐ Importance of seeking treatment when symptoms first appear to obtain the correct diagnosis

☐ Drug treatment early may prevent long-term morbidity (atrophy, sclerosis, and cancers).

Adherence Issues

☐ Importance of following the labeled instructions to totally eradicate the infection

☐ Importance of contacting the health-care provider if side effects or rash appears

☐ Potential for drug interactions (the macrolides with antifungal, systemic antifungals, and birth control pills)

REFERENCES

American College of Obstetricians and Gynecologists (ACOG). (2009). New ACOG cervical cancer screening recommendations. Retrieved from http://www.acog.org/departments/dept_notice.cfm?recno=20&bulletin=5021

American Society of Health-System Pharmacists. (2010). *AHFS drug information*. Bethesda, MD: Author.

Bates, C. K. (2012). Evaluation and management of adult sexual assault victims. Retrieved from www.uptodate.com

Carroll, N. M. (2013). Medical care of women who have sex with women. Retrieved from www.uptodate.com

Centers for Disease Control and Prevention (CDC). (2007). Toxic-shock syndrome: 1997 case definition. (Updated July 26, 2007.) Retrieved from http://www.cdc.gov/ncphi/od/ai/casedef/toxicsscurrent.htm

Centers for Disease Control and Prevention, Division of Parasitic Diseases. (2008a). Pubic lice infestation. Retrieved from http://www.cdc.gov/lice/pubic/index.html

Centers for Disease Control and Prevention, Division of Parasitic Diseases (CDC). (2008b). Scabies. Retrieved from http://www.cdc.gov/scabies/treatment.html

Centers for Disease Control and Prevention (CDC). (2009). *Trends in reportable sexually transmitted diseases in the United States, 2008: National surveillance data for chlamydia, gonorrhea, and syphilis*. Atlanta, GA: Centers for Disease Control and Prevention. Retrieved from http://www.cdc.gov/STD/stats08/trends.htm

Centers for Disease Control and Prevention (CDC). (2010). Sexually transmitted treatment guidelines, 2010. *Morbidity and Mortality Weekly Report, 59*(RR-12), 1–116.

Centers for Disease Control and Prevention (CDC). (2011). *CDC fact sheet: STD trends in the United States*. Retrieved from http://www.cdc.gov/std/stats11/trends-2011.pdf

Centers for Disease Control and Prevention (CDC). (2012a). *Hepatitis C information for health professionals*. Retrieved from http://www.cdc.gov/hepatitis/HCV/index.htm

Centers for Disease Control and Prevention (CDC). (2012b). *Cervical cancer*. Retrieved from http://www.cdc.gov/cancer/cervical/index.htm

Centers for Disease Control and Prevention (CDC). (2012c). *Cervical cancer screening guidelines for average risk women*. Retrieved from http://www.cdc.gov/cancer/cervical/pdf/guidelines.pdf

Centers for Disease Control and Prevention (CDC). (2012d). *Update to CDC's sexually transmitted diseases treatment guidelines, 2010: Oral cephalosporins no longer a recommended treatment for gonococcal infections. Morbidity and Mortality Weekly Report, 61*(31), 590–594.

Centers for Disease Control and Prevention Division of STD Prevention (2014). *Sexually transmitted disease surveillance 2012*. Atlanta, GA: US Department of Health and Human Services, CDC, National Center for HIV/AIDs, Viral Hepatitis, STD and TB Prevention. Retrieved from http://www.cdc.gov/std/stats12/surv2012.pdf

Goldstein, A. O., & Goldstein, B. G. (2011). *Pediculosis pubis and pediculosis ciliaris*. Retrieved from www.uptodate.com

Goldstein, B. G., & Goldstein, A. O. (2012). *Scabies*. Retrieved from www.uptodate.com

Goroll, A., May, L., & Mulley, A. (2010). *Primary care medicine* (6th ed.). Philadelphia: Lippincott.

Harper, D. (2009). Clinical diagnosis of vaginitis was moderately accurate in symptomatic women. *Evidence-Based Medicine, 14*(3), 88.

Hatcher, R., Trussell, J., & Kowal, D. (2008). *Contraceptive technology* (19th ed.). New York: Ardent Media.

Judlin, P. (2010). Current concepts in managing pelvic inflammatory disease. *Current Infectious Diseases, 23*(1), 83–87.

Katzung, B. (2009). *Basic and clinical pharmacology* (11th ed.). Norwalk, CT: Appleton & Lange.

Kisa, S., & Taskin, L. (2009). Validity of the symptomatic approach used by nurses in diagnosing vaginal infections. *Journal of Clinical Nursing, 18*(7), 1059–1068.

Kosten, T. R. (2009). Drugs of abuse. In B. G. Katzung (Ed.), *Basic & clinical pharmacology* (11th ed.). San Francisco: McGraw-Hill.

Lexi-Comp Online, AHFS Essentials Online; (2013, Feb 5). Hudson, OH.

Markusen, T. E., & Barclay, D. L. (2003). Benign disorders of the vulva and vagina. In A. H. DeCherney & L. Nathan (Eds.), *Current obstetric & gynecologic diagnosis & treatment.* San Francisco: McGraw-Hill.

Montgomery, K., & Bloch, J. (2010). The human papillomavirus in women over 40: Implications for practice and recommendations for screening. *Journal of the American Academy of Nurse Practitioners, 22*(2), 92–100.

Paavonen, J. (2006). Update vulvodynia: A therapeutic challenge. *Women's Health, 2*(2), 289–296.

Partnership for Prevention. (2007). *Preventive care: A national profile on use, disparities and health benefits.* Washington, DC: Partnership for Prevention.

Secor, R. (1997). Vaginal microscopy: Refining the nurse practitioner's technique. *Clinical Excellence for Nurse Practitioners, 1*(1), 29–34.

Setterfield, J. F., Neill, S., Shirlaw, P. J., Theron, J., Vaughan, R., Escudier, M., et al. (2006). The vulvovaginal gingival syndrome: A severe subgroup of lichen planus with characteristic clinical features and a novel association with the class II HLA DQB1*0201 allele. *Journal of American Academy of Dermatology, 55*(1), 98–113.

Sobel, J.D. (2012a). *Bacterial vaginosis.* Retrieved from www.uptodate.com/contents/bacterial-vaginosis

Sobel, J.D. (2012b). *Candida vulvovaginitis.* Retrieved from http://www.uptodate.com/contents/candida-vulvovaginitis

Sobel, J. D. (2012c). *Evaluation of women with symptoms of vaginitis.* Retrieved from http://www.uptodate.com/contents/approach-to-women-with-symptoms-of-vaginitis

Swygard, H., & Cohen, M. S. (2012). *Screening for sexually transmitted infections.* Retrieved from www.uptodate.com

Torrone, E., Papp, J., & Weinstock, H. (2014). Prevalence of *Chlamydia trachomatis* genital infection among persons aged 14–39 years—United States, 2007–2012. *Morbidity and Mortality Weekly Report, 63*(38), 834–838.

U.S. Preventive Services Task Force. (2002). *Guide to clinical preventive services* (3rd ed.). Baltimore: Williams & Wilkins.

Wallace, L., Scoular, A., Hart, A. G., Reid, M., Wilson, P., & Goldberg, P. D. (2008). What is the excess risk of infertility in women after genital chlamydia infection? A systematic review of the evidence. *Sexually Transmitted Infections, 84,* 171–175.

Wiesenfeld, H.C. (2012). *Treatment of pelvic inflammatory disease.* Retrieved from www.uptodate.com

World Health Organization (WHO). (2006). *Viral cancers: Human papillomavirus. Initiative for Vaccine Research (IVR).* Retrieved from http://www.who.int/vaccine_research/diseases/viral_cancers/en/

Wright, T. C., Massad, L. S., Dunton, C. J., Spitzer, M., Wilkinson, E. J., & Solomon, D. (2007). 2006 consensus guidelines for the management of women with abnormal cancer screening tests. *American Journal of Obstetrics & Gynecology, 197*(4), 346–355.

Zhao, C., Florea, A., & Austin, R. (2010). Clinical utility of adjunctive high-risk human papillomavirus DNA testing in women with Papanicolaou test findings of atypical glandular cells. *Archives of Pathology & Laboratory Medicine, 134*(1), 103–108.

TUBERCULOSIS

Teri Moser Woo

Tuberculosis (TB) presents a serious threat to global health, with 8.6 million people developing TB and 1.3 million deaths in 2012 (World Health Organization [WHO], 2013). Nearly one-third of the world population is infected with Mycobacterium tuberculosis. In 1993, the World Health Organization (WHO) declared a global emergency concerning TB, the number-one infectious disease killer worldwide. WHO has a goal to reduce prevalence of and deaths from TB by 50% by 2015 compared to a 1990 baseline, and eliminate TB as a public health problem by 2050 (WHO, 2013). By 2012, the TB mortality rate had decreased by 45%, but the prevalence rate has only dropped by 37% worldwide (WHO, 2013).

In the past 20 years, TB incidence in the United States decreased significantly from 10.4 cases per 100,000 in 1992 to 3.2 cases per 100,000 in 2012 (Centers for Disease Control and Prevention [CDC], 2013a). Yet TB continues to present a significant health problem; in 2012 there were 9,945 TB cases reported to the Centers for Disease Control and Prevention (CDC) from all 50 states, the District of Columbia (DC), and the U.S.-affiliated Pacific Islands (CDC, 2013b).

TB infection rates vary among racial and ethnic populations in the United States, with Asians having the highest rate of 18.9 cases per 100,000 in 2012 compared to 0.8 cases per 100,000 persons identifying themselves as white (CDC, 2013a). The majority of cases of TB in the United States in 2012 were in foreign-born persons (CDC, 2013b).

Canada reported 1,686 cases of new active or recurrent TB in 2012 (Public Health Agency of Canada, 2014). The majority of cases (64%) of TB in Canada are among foreign-born people. Canadian-born aboriginal people have a higher incidence (21.2% of cases) of TB than Canadian-born non-aboriginal peoples (11.8% of cases) (Public Health Agency of Canada, 2014).

In the United States, federal funding for TB programs decreased in the 1970s, with states and the federal government spending less money on TB prevention. Because of decreased funding and the growing worldwide HIV epidemic, the emergence of drug-resistant TB was inevitable. In the 1990s, the U.S. Congress increased funding for TB, and the CDC established three National Model TB Centers (in San Francisco, Newark, and New York City) and a National Tuberculosis

Surveillance Network. The CDC Division of Tuberculosis Elimination has developed and funded from 2013 through 2017 five Regional TB Training and Medical Consultation Centers to provide education and consultation to TB programs and providers in all 50 states and U.S. territories.

Acquired resistance to TB medications stems from inadequate or inappropriate prescribed treatment regimens or from patient noncompliance. Surveillance indicates cases of multidrug-resistant (resistance to at least isoniazid and rifampin) TB decreased from 2.5% of TB cases in 1993 to 1.1% in 2012. Cases of extensively drug-resistant (XDR) TB (resistance to isoniazid and rifampin plus resistance to any fluoroquinolone and at least one of three injectable second-line anti-TB drugs [i.e., amikacin, kanamycin, or capreomycin]) decreased from ten cases in 1993 to two cases in 2012 (CDC, 2013b). In Canada, 9.5% of TB isolates were resistant to at least one first-line antituberculosis drug in 2009, predominately (85%) isoniazid (INH), and 1.4% of isolates were resistant to multiple drugs (Public Health Agency of Canada, 2010).

Global data indicate 3.6% of newly diagnosed TB cases and 20% of cases in those who were previously treated for TB had multiple-drug-resistant (MDR) TB (WHO, 2013). The problem of MDR TB is worldwide, with the highest rates of MDR TB in eastern Europe and central Asia; MDR TB accounts for up to 20% of new cases and 50% of those previously treated (WHO, 2013). WHO is concerned with MDR TB and has partnered with the International Union Against Tuberculosis and Lung Disease (IUATLD), and the Bill and Melinda Gates Foundation to develop a Call to Action, including a goal of universal access to MDR/XDR-TB diagnosis and treatment by 2015.

Both the diagnosis and treatment of TB have become complex. Diagnostic criteria depend not only on the results of testing but also on the patient's immigration and immune status. Multidrug regimens that vary according to the patient's risk factors require the practitioner to be familiar with a wide variety of treatment regimens. Compliance with long treatment courses is an issue in the treatment of TB. Noncompliance leads to the emergence of drug-resistant TB. This chapter addresses the treatment of TB and strategies to increase compliance with the treatment regimen, as well as the drug regimen used for TB prevention.

PATHOPHYSIOLOGY

TB is an infectious disease caused by *M. tuberculosis,* an organism that is inhaled into the alveolus, where it is ingested by the pulmonary macrophage. The bacilli multiply and spread to local pulmonary areas and to extrathoracic organs via the lymphatic system. The infected macrophage releases a substance that attracts T lymphocytes. The infected macrophage presents antigens from the phagocytosed bacilli to the lymphocytes, producing a series of committed immune effector cells. This causes a delayed hypersensitivity and, combined with the newly activated macrophages, leads to intracellular killing of the bacilli and granuloma formation.

M. tuberculosis and most of the other mycobacteria grow quite slowly, with a doubling time of 18 hours. Thus, skin test reactivity does not occur until 4 to 6 weeks after infection,

with longer intervals noted. Colonies on culture media do not appear for 3 to 5 weeks, creating delays in culture confirmation and testing for drug susceptibility.

Infection is spread almost exclusively by aerosolization of contaminated lung secretions. This organism primarily affects the pulmonary tissue, although extrapulmonary TB is not uncommon, especially in immunocompromised patients. Patients with cavitary lung disease cough frequently and, therefore, are particularly infectious. The aerosolized droplets can remain suspended in room air for many hours. The skin and respiratory mucous membranes of a healthy, normally exposed person are resistant to invasion. The problem occurs with heavy or prolonged exposure to an infected or immunocompromised person. The very young and the very old or debilitated are also more susceptible because of decreased host defenses.

Pulmonary TB presents with the classic symptoms of TB: cough with productive, purulent secretions, often with blood streaks. Other symptoms include wide temperature variations, malaise, fatigue, wasting, chest pain, and dyspnea. Sweating, including night sweats, is common.

Extrapulmonary TB presents with a more problematic set of symptoms, often mimicking other diseases. Lymphatic TB may present initially as unilateral, painless, cervical lymphadenopathy. TB bacilli can also settle in the genitourinary tract, bones or joints, meninges, gastrointestinal (GI) tract, and pericardium. When these extrapulmonary sites are infected, the symptoms are often vague and difficult to define. The suspicion of TB and intradermal testing as part of a work-up for other diseases may lead to a quicker diagnosis. Also of concern is that the tuberculin skin test can be negative 20% to 25% of the time. Appropriate biopsy and culture of affected tissues or cerebrospinal fluid—which usually require consultation with a specialist in infectious diseases—increase the likelihood of an accurate diagnosis.

GOALS OF TREATMENT

The initial goal of treatment in TB is an accurate diagnosis. This requires a practitioner who understands the current guidelines for screening and puts TB high on the differential list for any pulmonary or other illness with vague presenting symptoms. A second goal is the patient's completion of the recommended therapy, because failure to complete therapy can lead to drug-resistant TB. Finally, the effectiveness of treatment must be evaluated. Effective treatment of TB is not only intended to treat the sick patient but also to prevent the transmission of *M. tuberculosis* to the public.

Patients who have positive sputum cultures at the beginning of treatment should have monthly cultures, and the culture should convert to negative. A final chest x-ray is needed for documentation of baseline for future films, but the x-ray is not as important as the sputum examination (American Thoracic Society [ATS], 2003).

In patients with radiographic abnormalities consistent with TB, an effort should be made to establish a diagnosis via sputum culture. The CDC and the Canadian guidelines recommend that three sputum specimens should be obtained if pulmonary involvement is suspected (CDC, 2003a; Canadian Thoracic Society and The Public Health Agency of Canada, 2013). Nucleic acid amplification tests for the diagnosis of TB and to determine drug resistance is sensitive and provides a more rapid result than traditional culture. Bronchoscopy may be necessary to obtain an accurate diagnosis. If presumptive treatment is the only option, the key indicators for response to therapy are the chest x-ray findings. Improvement should be noted within the first 3 months of therapy. If there is no improvement, then either resistance or inaccurate diagnosis must be considered. The CDC recommends that all patients with TB have testing for HIV infection at the time treatment is initiated, if not earlier (CDC, 2003a).

RATIONAL DRUG SELECTION

Risk Stratification

Although anyone may become infected with TB, some populations are identified as being at greater risk: children up to age 4 years, the infirm elderly, and immunocompromised patients, including those with HIV infection or AIDS and organ transplant recipients. Foreign-born people are also at higher risk, accounting for 63% of U.S. TB cases in 2011 (CDC, 2013b) and 64% percent of Canadian cases (Public Health Agency of Canada, 2014). The top five countries of origin for foreign-born TB cases from 2000 to 2012 were Mexico, the Philippines, India, Vietnam, and China (CDC, 2013c). Canadian statistics reflect the immigration patterns of the country, with the world regions of the Western Pacific, Southeast Asia, and Africa accounting for the highest prevalence of foreign-born TB cases (Canadian Thoracic Society and The Public Health Agency of Canada, 2013). In the United States and Canada, certain populations are identified as being at higher risk, specifically medically underserved, low-income populations, including high-risk racial or ethnic minority populations; people who are homeless; blacks; Hispanics; and Native Americans/Canadian aboriginal peoples. Nonwhite patients have a peak incidence of TB between ages 25 and 44, significantly younger than that of whites, which is over age 70. Residents of long-term-care facilities (nursing homes, prisons, and mental institutions) are also at higher risk.

Screening

Targeted screening for TB is usually based on the patient's presenting with an identified risk factor. In some areas of the country, routine TB testing is part of all health maintenance visits because of an increased incidence of TB in the area. Patients identified as being at risk are those with compromised immune systems (e.g., HIV-positive or undergoing immunosuppressive therapy or prolonged adrenocorticosteroid therapy), close contacts of patients with newly diagnosed infectious TB, injection drug users known to be HIV seronegative, foreign-born persons from high-prevalence countries, medically underserved low-income populations, and residents and staff of long-term-care facilities or prisons. All health-care providers should be screened routinely.

Two screening methods for TB may be used, the tuberculin skin test (TST) or interferon-gamma release assays (QuantiFERON-TB Gold test and T-SPOT.TB test). The most commonly used screening test is an intradermal injection of TB protein antigens (such as purified protein derivative [PPD]). In 48 to 72 hours, an induration response is considered positive, based on the population being tested. The CDC in the United States and Public Health Agency of Canada have slightly different criteria for positive tuberculin skin test results. The CDC (2012) states that for adults and children with HIV infection, close contacts of people with infectious TB and patients with fibrotic lesions on chest x-ray (especially in upper lung regions), an induration of 5 mm or more is considered positive. A reaction of 10 mm or more is considered positive for other high-risk adults and children, including infants and children under age 4. For people not considered at risk for TB infection, a reaction of 15 mm or more is considered positive.

The Canadian criteria for a positive skin test are the following: an induration of 5 to 9 mm is considered positive in patients with HIV infection, close contacts of contagious cases within the past 2 years, children suspected of having TB, patients with abnormal chest x-ray with fibronodular disease or immune suppression, and patients with end-stage renal disease; a greater than 10 mm induration is positive in all other cases (Canadian Thoracic Society and The Public Health Agency of Canada, 2013).

In 2005, the U.S. Food and Drug Administration (FDA) approved QuantiFERON-TB Gold as an aid in diagnosing *M. tuberculosis* infection, both latent and active (Mazurek et al, 2005). Health Canada approved QuantiFERON-TB in 2006. The QuantiFERON-TB Gold (QFT-G) is an enzyme-linked immunoassay (ELISA) test that tests for the proteins present in *M. tuberculosis* that are absent from bacille Calmette-Guérin (BCG) vaccines (Mazurek et al, 2005). The T-SPOT. TB test is an in vitro immunoassay test that measures T cells primed to *M. tuberculosis* antigens; it was FDA-approved in 2008 (Oxford Immunotec, 2014). A positive QFT-G or T-SPOT test should be treated in the same manner as a positive TST: the patient needs a medical evaluation, including a chest x-ray, to rule out latent versus active TB infection.

A new, fully automated test, Xpert MTB/RIF, has been developed and is being recommended by WHO for initial screening in patients with suspected MDR-TB or HIV/TB (WHO, 2013b). Xpert MTB/RIF can detect TB and rifampin-resistant TB, with results available within 24 hours. The test is expected to triple the number of drug-resistant cases of TB identified and double the number of TB cases diagnosed in HIV patients. Development and rollout of the testing worldwide is being partially funded by the Bill and Melinda Gates Foundation to keep the costs within the ability of resource-poor countries to use the technology (WHO, 2013b).

Drug Therapy for Infectious Tuberculosis

Treatment of infectious TB requires the practitioner to apply three basic principles, as recommended by the ATS,

CDC, and the Infectious Diseases Society of America (CDC, 2003b):

1. Treatment regimens must contain multiple drugs to which the organisms are susceptible.
2. The drugs must be taken regularly.
3. Drug therapy must continue for a sufficient period of time.

Another fundamental principle of managing TB patients is never to add a single drug to a failing treatment regimen (ATS, 2003).

Many combinations of drugs and frequencies of administration are possible, but the initial phase of treatment is critical to prevent drug resistance and improve outcomes. Treatment for TB has two phases: the first phase or initiation phase (bactericidal or intensive phase), which lasts for 2 months, and the continuation phase (sterilizing phase), which lasts for 4 to 7 months (Blumberg, Leonard, & Jasmer, 2005). This chapter discusses the treatment regimens that may be used. As newer medications are approved, these regimens may change, but the basic principles remain (Table 45-1).

Table 45–1 Drug Regimens for Culture-Positive Pulmonary Tuberculosis Caused by Drug-Susceptible Organisms

Initial Phase			Continuation Phase			Rating (Evidence)		
Regimen	Drugs	Interval and Doses‡ (Minimal Duration)	Regimen	Drugs	Interval and Doses‡ (Minimal Duration)	Range of Total Doses (Minimal Duration)	HIV–	HIV+
1	INH RIF PZA EMB	7 d/wk for 56 doses (8 wk) or 5 d/wk for 40 doses (8 wk)⁵	1a	INF/RIF	7 d/wk for 126 doses (18 wk) or 5 d/wk for 90 doses (18 wk)⁵	182–130 (26 wk)	A (I)	A (II)
			1b	INH/RIF	Twice weekly for 36 doses (18 wk)	92–76 (26 wk)	A (I)	A (II)*
			1c**	INH/RPT	Once weekly for 18 doses (18 wk)	74–58 (26 wk)	B (I)	E (I)
2	INH	7 d/wk for 14 doses (2 wk). Then twice weekly for 12 doses (6 wk) or 5 d/wk for 10 doses (2 wk).⁵ Then twice weekly for 12 doses (6 wk)	2a	INH/RIF	Twice weekly for 36 doses (18 wk)	62–58 (26 wk)	A (II)	B (II)*
	RIF PZA EMB		2b**	INH/RPT	Once weekly for 18 doses (18 wk)	44–408 (26 wk)	B (I)	E (I)
3	INH RIF PZA EMB	Three times weekly for 24 doses (8 wk)	3a	INH/RIF	Three times weekly for 54 doses (18 wk)	78 (26 wk)	B (I)	B (II)
4	INH RIF	7 d/wk for 56 doses (8 wk) or 5 days/wk for 40 doses (8 wk)⁵	4a	INH/RIF	7 d/wk for 217 doses (31 wk) or 5 d/wk for 155 doses (31 wk)⁵	273–195 (39 wk)	C (I)	C (II)
	EMB		4b	INH/RIF	Twice weekly for 62 doses (31 wk)	118–102 (39 wk)	C (I)	C (II)

EMB = ethambutol; INH = isoniazid; PZA = pyrazinamide; RIF = rifampin; RPT = rifapentine.

*Definitions of evidence ratings: A = preferred; B = acceptable alternative; C = offer when A and B cannot be given; E = should never be given.

†Definition of evidence ratings: I = randomized clinical trial; II = data from clinical trials that were not randomized or were conducted in other populations; III = expert opinion.

‡When DOT is used, drugs may be given 5 d/wk and the necessary number of doses adjusted accordingly. Although no studies compare five with seven doses, extensive experience indicates this would be an effective practice.

§Patients with cavitation on initial chest radiograph and positive cultures at completion of 2 months of therapy should receive a 7 months' continuation phase (31 weeks either 217 doses [daily] or 62 doses [twice weekly]).

⁵Five-day-a-week administration is always given by DOT. Rating for 5 d/wk regimens is A III.

#Not recommended for HIV-infected patients with CD4+ cell counts <100 cells/mcL.

**Options 1c and 2b should be used only in HIV-negative patients who have negative sputum smears at the time of completion of 2 months of therapy and who do not have cavitation on initial chest radiograph (see text). For patients started on this regimen and found to have a positive culture from the 2-month specimen, treatment should be extended an extra 3 months.

Source: Centers for Disease Control and Prevention. (2003). Treatment of tuberculosis, American Thoracic Society, CDC, and Infectious Diseases Society of America. *Morbidity and Mortality Weekly Report, 52*(RR-11).

There are several combination drugs available to treat TB. Combination tablets offer ease of dosing with one tablet, but may be more expensive than single-ingredient tablets. Rifater tablets contain 120 mg rifampin, 50 mg isoniazid, and 300 mg pyrazinamide and cost $259 for 60 tablets. Rifamate or IsonaRif capsules contain 300 mg rifampin and 150 mg isoniazid and the generic form costs $60 for 60 capsules, which is a 30-day supply for adults. In comparison, rifampin 300 mg capsules cost $47 for 60 capsules, and isoniazid 300 mg tablets are $8 for 60 tablets, for a total of $55 for a 30-day supply. The $200 difference in cost is significant for clients who must pay all or a large part of their drug costs. The ATS (2003) guidelines note that no evidence supports combination medications over single-ingredient drugs, although the combination drugs may be preferable if directly observed therapy (DOT) is not used.

Six-Month Regimen

A 6-month regimen is recommended for patients who adhere to treatment and have fully susceptible organisms. This regimen consists of 2 months of four-drug therapy administered daily: isoniazid (INH), rifampin (RIF), pyrazinamide (PZA), and ethambutol (EMB), followed by 4 months of INH and RIF. Alternative regimens for the first 2 months of therapy include the same four drugs (INH, RIF, PZA, and EMB) given (regimen 2) daily for 2 weeks followed by twice weekly for 6 weeks; or (regimen 3) three times a week for 8 weeks (CDC, 2003a). This four-drug therapy is effective even when the infecting organism is resistant to INH. Dosing for the continuation phase (after the initial 2 mo) should consist of INH and RIF (regimen 1) daily, (regimen 2) twice weekly, and (regimen 3) three times weekly for 4 months (CDC, 2003a). Streptomycin is substituted for EMB in children too young to be monitored for visual acuity.

This 6-month treatment can be used in patients who have HIV infection and patients who are not infected with HIV. Patients who have HIV infection should be monitored for treatment response, and their therapy should be prolonged if the response is suboptimal. The continuation phase of treatment should be followed for an additional 3 months for patients who have cavitation on the initial or follow-up chest radiograph and are still culture-positive after the initial 2 months of treatment (CDC, 2003a).

Nine-Month Regimen

A 9-month regimen of INH and RIF may be used for patients who cannot take PZA or who have isolates resistant to PZA. EMB (streptomycin in young children) should also be included in the treatment protocol for the first 2 months, followed by INH and RIF given either daily or twice weekly for 7 months (CDC, 2003a). Dosages for the drugs commonly used for treatment and prevention are shown in Table 45-2.

Table 45–2 ❈ Drugs Commonly Used: Tuberculosis

			Doses*			
Drug	**Preparation**	**Adults/ Children†**	**Daily**	**1 ×/wk**	**2 ×/wk**	**3 ×/wk**
First-Line Drugs						
Isoniazid (INH)	Tablets (50, 100, 300 mg); elixir (50 mg/5 mL); aqueous solution (100 mg/mL) for IV or IM injection	*Adults* (max)	5 mg/kg (300 mg)	15 mg/kg (900 mg)	15 mg/kg (900 mg)	15 mg/kg (900 mg)
		Children (max)	10–15 mg/kg (300 mg)	—	20–30 mg/kg (900 mg)	—
Rifampin (RIF)	Capsule (150, 300 mg); powder may be suspended for oral administration; aqueous solution for IV injection	*Adults‡* (max)	10 mg/kg (600 mg)	—	10 mg/kg (600 mg)	10 mg/kg (600 mg)
		Children (max)	10–20 mg/kg (600 mg)	—	10–20 mg/kg (600 mg)	—
Rifabutin	Capsule (150 mg)	*Adults‡* (max)	5 mg/kg (300 mg)	—	5 mg/kg (300 mg)	5 mg/kg (300 mg)
		Children	Appropriate dosing for children is unknown	Appropriate dosing for children is unknown	Appropriate dosing for children is unknown	Appropriate dosing for children is unknown

Continued

Table 45–2 ✿ Drugs Commonly Used: Tuberculosis—cont'd

Drug	Preparation	Adults/ Children[†]	Daily	1 ×/wk	2 ×/wk	3 ×/wk
			Doses*			
Rifapentine	Tablet (150 mg, film coated)	*Adults*	—	10 mg/kg (continuation phase) (600 mg)	—	—
		Children	Not approved for use in children	Not approved for use in children	Not approved for use in children	Not approved for use in children
Pyrazinamide (PZA)	Tablet (500 mg, scored)	*Adults* :	1,000 mg	—	2,000 mg	1,500 mg
		Wt: 40–55 kg	1,500 mg	—	3,000 mg	2,500 mg
		Wt: 56–75 kg	2,000 mg	—	4,000 mg	3,000 mg
		Wt: 76–90 kg	15–30 mg/kg	—	50 mg/kg (2.5 g)	—
		Children (max)	(2.0 g)			
Ethambutol (EMB)	Tablet (100, 400 mg)	*Adults*	800 mg	—	1,600 mg	1,200 mg
		Wt: 40–55 kg	1,200 mg	—	2,800 mg	2,000 mg
		Wt: 56–75 kg	1,600 mg	—	4,000 mg	2,400 mg
		Wt: 76–90 kg	15–20 mg/kg	—	50 mg/kg (2.5 g)	—
		Children[§] (max)	daily (1.0 g)			
Second-Line Drugs						
Cycloserine	Capsule (250 mg)	*Adults* (max)	10–15 mg/kg/d (1.0 g in 2 doses), usually 500–750 mg/d in 2 doses[¶]	No data to support intermittent administration	No data to support intermittent administration	No data to support intermittent administration
		Children (max)	10–15 mg/kg/d (1.0 g/d)	—	—	—
Ethionamide	Tablet (250 mg)	*Adults** (max)	15–20 mg/kg/d (1.0 g/day), usually 500–750 mg/d in a single daily dose or 2 divided doses*	No data to support intermittent administration	No data to support intermittent administration	No data to support intermittent administration
		Children (max)	15–20 mg/kg/d (1.0 g/d)	No data to support intermittent administration	No data to support intermittent administration	No data to support intermittent administration
Moxifloxacin	Tablets (400 mg): aqueous solution (400 mg/250 mL) for IV injection	*Adults*	400 mg daily	No data to support intermittent administration	No data to support intermittent administration	No data to support intermittent administration
		Children	‡‡	‡‡	‡‡	‡‡
Gatifloxacin	Tablets (400 mg); aqueous solution (200 mg/20 mL; 400 mg/40 mL) for IV injection	*Adults*	400 mg daily	No data to support intermittent administration	No data to support intermittent administration	No data to support intermittent administration
		Children	§§	‡‡	‡‡	‡‡

Table 45–2 ✿ **Drugs Commonly Used: Tuberculosis—cont'd**

		Doses*				
Drug	Preparation	Adults/ Children†	Daily	1 ×/wk	2 ×/wk	3 ×/wk
Bedaquiline	Tablets (100 mg)	Adults	400 mg qd for 2 weeks followed by 200 mg 3 times a week for 22 weeks			400 mg qd for 2 weeks followed by 200 mg 3 times a week for 22 weeks

*Dose per weight is based on ideal body weight. Children weighing more than 40 kg should be dosed as adults.

†For purposes of this document, adult dosing begins at age 15 years.

‡Dose may need to be adjusted when there is concomitant use of protease inhibitors or nonnucleoside reverse transcriptase inhibitors.

§The drug can likely be used safely in older children but should be used with caution in children less than 5 years of age in whom visual acuity cannot be monitored. In younger children, EMB at the dose of 15 mg/kg/d can be used if there is suspected or proven resistance to INH of RIF.

¶*Note:* Although this is the dose recommended generally, most clinicians with experience using cycloserine indicate that few patients can tolerate this amount. Serum concentration measurements are often useful in determining the optimal dose for a given patient.

#The single daily dose can be given at bedtime or with the main meal.

**Dose: 15 mg/kg/d (1 g) and 10 mg/kg in persons more than 59 years of age (750 mg). Usual dose: 750–1,000 mg administered IM or IV, given as a single dose 5–7 d/wk and reduced to two or three times per week after the first 2–4 months or after culture conversion, depending on the efficacy of the other drugs in the regimen.

††The long-term (more than several weeks) use of levofloxacin in children and adolescents has not been approved because of concerns about effects on bone and cartilage growth. However, most experts agree that the drug should be considered for children with tuberculosis caused by organisms resistant to both INH and RIF. The optimal dose is not known.

‡‡The long-term (more than several weeks) use of moxifloxacin in children and adolescents has not been approved because of concerns about effects on bone and cartilage growth. The optimal dose is not known.

§§The long-term (more than several weeks) use of gatifloxacin in children and adolescents has not been approved because of concerns about effects on bone and cartilage growth. The optimal dose is not known.

Source: Centers for Disease Control and Prevention. (2003). Treatment of tuberculosis, American Thoracic Society, CDC, and Infectious Diseases Society of America. *Morbidity and Mortality Weekly Report, 52*(RR-11).

Drug Therapy for Drug-Resistant Tuberculosis

Drug-resistant TB has been increasing worldwide for the past 20 years. Microbial resistance to anti-TB drugs may be either primary or acquired. Primary resistance occurs in the patient who has never been treated for TB. Risk factors for primary resistance include exposure to a patient who has drug-resistant TB, immigration from a country with a high prevalence of drug-resistant TB, and a greater than 4% incidence of resistant TB in the community.

Acquired or secondary resistance occurs in a patient who has been previously treated for TB. Poorly or inadequately treated TB is the leading cause of secondary resistance, with prevalence of MDR TB greater than 20% of new diagnosed cases and 50% of those previously treated for TB (WHO, 2013). Extensively resistant TB (resistant to multiple second-line drugs) is found in 9.6% of MDR TB globally and in 1.1% of cases in the United States (CDC, 2013b; WHO, 2013). Extensively resistant TB is resistant both to isoniazid and rifampin and to any fluoroquinolone drug and at least one of three second-line injectable drugs (amikacin, kanamycin, or capreomycin). Drug resistance can be proved only by susceptibility testing.

For treatment of drug- or multidrug-resistant TB, the administration of at least two drugs to which susceptibility has been demonstrated is recommended. For isolated INH

resistance, the 6-month, four-drug (INH, RIF, EMB, PZA) protocol is recommended (ATS, 2003).

If INH resistance is documented in a patient on a 9 month regimen (without PZA), then INH should be discontinued. If EMB was included in the initial regimen, then treatment with RIF and EMB should continue for a minimum of 12 months. If the initial treatment did not include EMB, then testing for drug susceptibility should be repeated, and INH needs to be discontinued and two new drugs should be added. The regimen may need to be adjusted when drug susceptibility test results are available.

If a patient is resistant to multiple first-line drugs (INH, RIF, EMB, PZA), then at least three new drugs that the organism is susceptible to should be administered. These second-line drugs include capreomycin (Capastat), cycloserine (Seromycin), EMBionamide (Trecator), kanamycin (Kantrex), para-aminosalicylic acid (Sodium P.A.S.), levofloxacin (Levaquin), and moxifloxacin (Avelox) (see Table 45-2). This regimen should be followed until sputum cultures are clear; then the patient should have 12 months of two-drug therapy. Often, 24 months of therapy are given to patients who have TB that is resistant to multiple first-line drugs. Patients with resistant TB should have their medications administered via DOT (Box 45 1).

Bedaquiline fumarate (Sirturo) has received a provisional approval from the U.S. Food and Drug Administration for use as part of a four-drug regimen for laboratory-confirmed

---

BOX 45–1 DIRECTLY OBSERVED THERAPY

Directly observed therapy (DOT) reduces the risk of developing drug resistance. In DOT, the patient is required to take all of the medication in front of a health-care or other service provider. The Centers for Disease Control and Prevention (CDC), the American Thoracic Society (ATS), and the World Health Organization (WHO) recommend the widespread or universal use of DOT in the treatment of TB. DOT has been demonstrated to ensure the highest degree of compliance with the medication regimen. Compliance with DOT can be increased in many ways, including convenient clinic times and locations and incentives such as food, clothing, bus or carfare money, and gifts.

---

pulmonary MDR TB in adults (Mase, Chorba, Loube, & Castro, 2013). Bedaquiline (400 mg) is given once a day for 2 weeks, followed by 200 mg three times a week for 22 weeks (Mase et al, 2013). The effectiveness and safety of treatment beyond 24 weeks have not been studied.

Second-line treatment usually requires injectable medications, which complicates the treatment regimen. Fluoroquinolones such as levofloxacin, moxifloxacin, and gatifloxacin are all active against *M. tuberculosis*. Based on the evidence so far, levofloxacin is the preferred oral fluoroquinolone for treating drug-resistant TB or when first-line agents cannot be used because of intolerance (CDC, 2003b). Patients with extensively resistant TB require broader coverage including parenteral cycloserine (Seromycin) and a fluoroquinolone. In a recent study of 48 patients with extensively resistant disease, patients were prescribed an average of 5.3±1.3 antimycobacterial agents for which either susceptibility had been documented or the duration of prior exposure had not exceeded 1 month and susceptibility had not been tested, leading to a 60% cure rate (Mitnick et al, 2008). Any patient whose TB demonstrates resistance must be seen by an infectious disease specialist who treats patients with TB. Inadequate treatment is one of the leading causes of secondary resistant TB.

Algorithm

Treatment of TB begins with an accurate diagnosis. Once a screening test for TB is considered positive, treatment begins, even if a definitive diagnosis of TB has not been made. Therapy may be altered, based on the patient's risk factors or on the sensitivity of the organisms to the medications being used. DOT should be considered at any point of therapy based on patient history and local drug-resistance pattern. A treatment algorithm is presented in Figure 45-1.

Extrapulmonary Tuberculosis

Extrapulmonary TB is often difficult to diagnose. Once a bacteriological examination has determined a diagnosis of TB, the treatment is basically the same as for pulmonary TB. Although little research has been done regarding the effectiveness of shortened treatment for extrapulmonary TB, the ATS guidelines (2003) recommend 6 to 9 months of therapy as probably effective. Infants and children with miliary TB, bone or joint TB, and TB meningitis should receive 12 months of therapy.

Response to treatment is more difficult to monitor in patients with extrapulmonary TB than in those with pulmonary TB and must often be determined based on clinical and radiographic improvement. Bacteriological evaluation of extrapulmonary sites often requires invasive procedures to evaluate treatment. Referral to an infectious disease specialist is usually necessary to ensure optimal treatment.

Patient Variables

Pregnancy and Lactation

TB infection during pregnancy presents in the same manner as does TB in nonpregnant patients. The clinical symptoms include cough, weight loss, fever, malaise and fatigue, and hemoptysis. Eighty-five percent of patients have upper lobe disease; extrapulmonary TB is rare in pregnant patients. TB screening during pregnancy is recommended for all patients. Positive results are the same as for nonpregnant patients. Patients who have active untreated TB at the time of delivery need to be placed in respiratory isolation and separated from their infants. Therefore, it is best to treat TB prior to delivery.

The initial treatment regimen for pregnant women is INH and RIF. EMB should be included unless INH resistance is unlikely. The length of therapy is 6 months. Pyridoxine (vitamin B_6) 25 mg/d should be added to the regimen in pregnant or lactating patients to decrease the incidence of peripheral neuropathy associated with INH (ATS, 2003).

Pregnant patients have a 2.5-fold higher risk of INH-induced hepatitis than other patients (Riley, 1997). RIF may also be associated with maternal hepatitis. Monthly monitoring of liver function tests will detect any change in liver function indicating hepatitis.

INH, RIF, and EMB all cross the placenta, but these drugs have not been demonstrated to have teratogenic effects (ATS, 2003). Streptomycin and other aminoglycosides are contraindicated because of harmful effects on the fetus, including congenital deafness and altered ear development. Streptomycin is Pregnancy Category D.

PZA is recommended for routine use in pregnant women by WHO, but the drug has not been used routinely in the United States due to a lack of safety studies. Some U.S. public health officials are using PZA in pregnant women without reported adverse effects (CDC, 2003a). If PZA is not included in the initial treatment regimen, then 9 months of therapy needs to be considered.

Breastfeeding is not contraindicated during treatment. Small amounts of INH and RIF are excreted into breast milk, but these amounts are well below the therapeutic dose. EMB and PZA are both excreted in very small amounts as well. The risk of toxic reactions in the infant may be further minimized

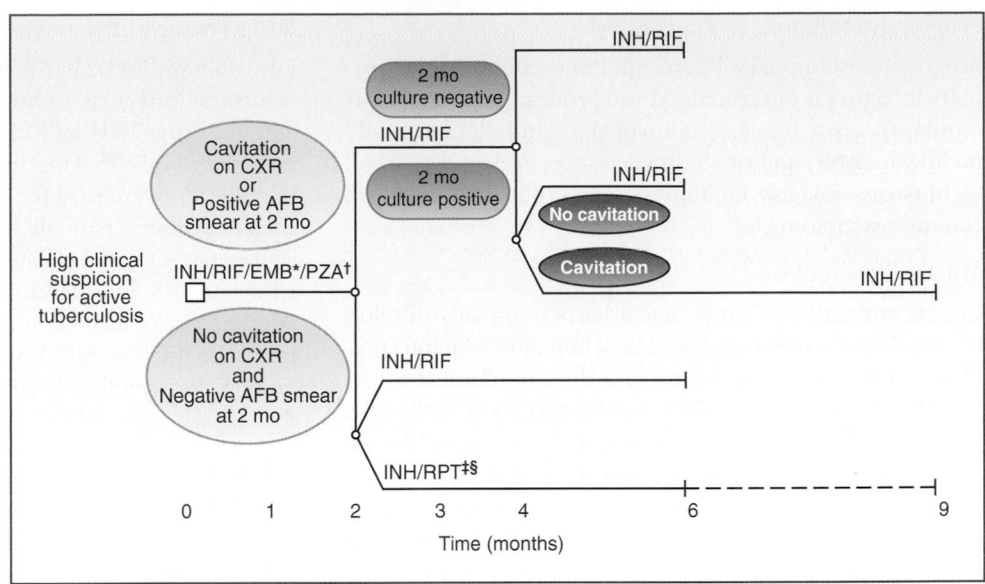

Figure 45–1. Treatment algorithm for TB.

Patients in whom tuberculosis is proved or strongly suspected should have treatment initiated with isoniazid, rifampin, pyrazinamide, and ethambutol for the initial 2 months. A repeat smear and culture should be performed when 2 months of treatment have been completed. If cavities were seen on the initial chest radiograph or the acid-fast smear is positive at completion of 2 months of treatment, the continuation phase of treatment should consist of isoniazid and rifampin daily or twice weekly for 4 months to complete a total of 6 months of treatment. If cavitation was present on the initial chest radiograph and the culture at the time of completion of 2 months of therapy is positive, the continuation phase should be lengthened to 7 months (total of 9 months of treatment). If the patient has HIV infection and the CD4+ cell count is <100/μL, the continuation phase should consist of daily or 3 times weekly isoniazid and rifampin. In HIV-uninfected patients having no cavitation on chest radiograph and negative acid-fast smears at completion of 2 months of treatment, the continuation phase may consist of either once weekly isoniazid and rifapentine, or daily or twice weekly isoniazid and rifampin, to complete a total of 6 months (bottom). Patients receiving isoniazid and rifapentine, and whose 2-month cultures are positive, should have treatment extended by an additional 3 months (total of 9 months).

*EMB may be discontinued when results of drug susceptibility testing indicate no drug resistance.

†PZA may be discontinued after it has been taken for 2 months (56 doses).

‡RPT should not be used in HIV-infected patients with tuberculosis or in patients with extrapulmonary tuberculosis.
§Therapy should be extended to 9 months if 2-month culture is positive.

CXR = chest radiograph; EMB = ethambutol; INH = isoniazid; PZA = pyrazinamide; RIF = rifampin; RPT = rifapentine.

Source: American Thoracic Society, CDC, and Infectious Diseases Society of America (2003). Treatment of Tuberculosis. MMWR, 52 (RR11), 1–77.

if the mother breastfeeds just prior to taking a dose of TB medication. Breastfeeding does not provide effective treatment for active or latent TB infection in a nursing infant; therefore, newborns should be evaluated for congenital TB (ATS, 2003; Public Health Agency of Canada, 2013). Pyridoxine (vitamin B₆) 25 mg/d is recommended in lactating women taking INH (ATS, 2003).

Pediatric Patients

Primary Pulmonary Tuberculosis

Children pose challenges in the treatment of TB because older infants and children may present with a positive screening test and are asymptomatic yet may have primary pulmonary TB. A chest x-ray may be normal or demonstrate minimum abnormalities (infiltrates with hilar adenopathy). WHO published guidelines for diagnosis of TB in children, which include the following: (1) careful history, including TB contacts; (2) clinical examination, including growth assessment; (2) TB skin test; (3) bacteriological confirmation whenever possible; (4) chest x-ray for pulmonary TB or evaluation for extrapulmonary TB (lymph node biopsy, lumbar puncture if meningitis is suspected, etc.); and (5) HIV testing in high-prevalence areas (WHO, 2006).

Obtaining sputum cultures for confirmatory diagnosis is difficult in young children; use of drug susceptibility testing from the presumed source case can guide the choice of drugs in children (CDC, 2003a). If drug resistance is suspected or if no source case is available, attempts to isolate organisms via three morning gastric lavages, bronchoalveolar lavage, or tissue biopsy should be considered. In infants and children under age 3 years with primary pulmonary infection, the disease may be progressive and merge with miliary TB or progressive central nervous system (CNS) disease to produce TB meningitis. Children under age 13 years usually have paucibacillary pulmonary disease (low organism numbers), and cavitating disease is rare (less than 6% of cases) (WHO, 2006). Primary infection in older children and adolescents presents with an upper lobe infiltrate and cavitation without calcification. Progressive disease does occur in immunocompromised children of all ages.

Progressive Pulmonary Tuberculosis

Progressive pulmonary TB in children occurs when the primary infection is not contained and produces bronchopneumonia or when the lesions involve a whole lobe (usually middle or lower) and cavitation develops. Weight loss, fever, night sweats, malaise, hemoptysis, and productive cough are common symptoms.

Miliary Tuberculosis

Infants and children under age 3 years frequently develop miliary TB, which is widespread dissemination with infection of multiple organs. The lesions are the size of millet seeds, thus the name *miliary* TB. The infant or child is quite ill, often with a sudden onset, and may have a high fever, weakness, malaise, anorexia, hepatosplenomegaly, and night sweats. A chest x-ray reveals diffuse miliary infiltrates. A tuberculin skin test (PPD) may be nonreactive as a result of anergy. The child may need a liver or bone marrow biopsy to determine an accurate diagnosis.

Tuberculosis Meningitis

TB meningitis is the most serious complication of TB. It usually occurs in young children (younger than 5 years) and within 6 months of primary infection. The disease has three stages: prodromal (lasts 1 wk), neurological involvement, and then increasing neurological involvement resulting from increasing intracranial pressure. The skin test (PPD) is positive in two-thirds of cases, but anergy may be present in very ill patients.

Drug Therapy

Drug therapy for pediatric patients depends on the infection or disease category, as noted in Table 45-3. The standard anti-TB drugs INH and RIF are used for asymptomatic infection and for 6 to 9 months. Multidrug regimens, as noted in Table 45-3, are used for progressive disease. EMB may be used in pediatric patients if risk of drug-resistant organisms is present (ATS, 2003). DOT should be used for all children with TB (ATS, 2003). If children are not able to swallow pills, administrating medications requires crushing the pills, and tolerance must be monitored. Parents should not be relied on to correctly administer TB treatment.

Adverse Reactions

RIF and INH can be administered to children safely, with minimal adverse reactions. Patients should be monitored for liver function alterations, especially if the patient presents with a flu-like illness. Pyridoxine deficiency associated with INH can be prevented in infants, children, and adolescents with 25 mg/d of vitamin B_6 supplementation (ATS, 2003; Public Health Authority of Canada, 2009). EMB is an effective drug, but its main limitation is ocular toxicity, which causes optic neuritis, leading to blurred vision, color blindness, and visual field constriction. Although the visual changes associated with EMB are reversible, it should not be prescribed to children under age 6 years whose visual changes cannot be accurately monitored. Streptomycin can be used in children in place of EMB, but it is used for only a short time (12 weeks or less), and patients should be monitored for

Table 45–3 Treatment of Tuberculosis in Infants, Children, and Adolescents

Disease Category	Drug Therapy	Comments
Asymptomatic infection (positive skin test only)	*9-mo regimen:* INH-susceptible: INH daily	Twice-weekly therapy may be used if daily therapy is not feasible.
	INH-resistant: RIF daily	Children with INH-resistant TB should be treated for 12 mo.
Pulmonary disease	*6 mo regimen:* INH, RIF, and PZA daily for first 2 mo, followed by 4 mo of INH and RIF daily *or* INH, RIF, and PZA daily for 2 mo, followed by 4 mo of INH and RIF twice weekly *9 mo regimen:* 9 mo of INH and RIF daily *or* 1 mo of INH and RIF daily, followed by 8 mo of INH and RIF twice weekly	If drug resistance is a concern, then a 4-drug regimen is used (INH, RIF, PZA, and ETH or streptomycin) for the first 2 mo.
Extrapulmonary TB (meningitis, miliary, bone, and joint)	*12-mo regimen:* INH, RIF, PZA, and streptomycin daily for 2 mo, followed by 10 mo of INH and RIF daily or INH, RIF, PYZ, and streptomycin daily, followed by INH and RIF twice weekly	4-drug therapy is used for the first 2 mo of treatment, until drug susceptibility is known.
Extrapulmonary TB (other than meningitis, miliary, bone, or joint)	Same as for pulmonary disease	

ETH = ethionamide; INH = isoniazid; PZA = pyrazinamide; RIF = rifabutin.

DOT (directly observed therapy) should be used for all children with tuberculosis. Parents should not be relied on to administer medications (CDC, 2003a).

ototoxicity and nephrotoxicity. PZA is used in multidrug therapy in children and has few adverse reactions.

Newborn Infants

Management of the newborn infant whose mother (or other household contact) has TB is based on individual considerations. Infants born to mothers with active disease are at high risk for TB in the first year of life (CDC, 2003a). Unfortunately, in infants, the skin test may not be positive until age 6 months.

If the mother has a positive PPD but no evidence of active disease, then the family and household contacts must be investigated. If no evidence of active disease is found in the mother or extended family, the infant needs to have a Mantoux (5 TU PPD) skin test at 4 to 6 weeks of age and at 3 to 4 months of age. If the TB status of household contacts cannot be evaluated, the infant may be started on INH (10 mg/kg/d).

If the mother has newly diagnosed TB but is not contagious at delivery, the newborn infant requires a chest x-ray and Mantoux test at age 4 to 6 weeks. If these are negative, then the child is monitored at age 3 to 4 months and again at 6 months with repeat Mantoux skin tests. INH is started at birth and discontinued at 3 to 4 months (some sources say 6 months) if the PPD is negative and the family has no active disease. The infant should receive INH even if the initial chest x-ray and PPD are negative because cell-mediated immunity of a degree sufficient to mount a significant reaction to skin testing can develop as late as age 6 months in an infant infected at birth. The mother may breastfeed. The infant should be examined carefully at monthly intervals. In cases of poor compliance, maternal positive sputum, or uncertain supervision, the infant may be given bacille Calmette-Guérin (BCG) vaccine. BCG does not prevent TB but may decrease the severity of the disease.

If the mother has active disease and is contagious at the time of delivery, the infant and mother should be separated until the mother is no longer contagious. The infant is managed the same as if the maternal disease were not contagious at the time of delivery.

If the mother has hematogenous spread of TB (bone, meningitis, or miliary TB), congenital TB is possible. If the infant is suspected of having congenital TB, INH is given for 6 months. If the PPD is positive at 6 months, then the INH is continued until age 9 months. As for any mother with active disease at delivery, a chest x-ray and Mantoux skin test should be done shortly after birth, and the infant should be monitored closely, with monthly assessments.

The HIV-Positive Patient

In 2012, 1.1 million (13%) of the 8.6 million patients worldwide who were HIV-positive developed TB (2013a). There were 320,000 deaths from TB among HIV-infected persons worldwide in 2012 (WHO, 2013a). In the early stages of HIV infection, the clinical manifestations of TB are similar to those of a normal host. As the T-lymphocyte count decreases, changes occur:

1. A steady reduction in the percentage of patients will have a positive TB skin test, decreasing to 10% to 20% in patients with advanced AIDS.

2. Extrapulmonary TB increases, with 60% to 80% of patients with CD4 counts below 50 demonstrating extrapulmonary infection.

3. Changing patterns of disease are noted on chest x-ray, although 56% of HIV/AIDS patients with TB still present with upper lobe disease (Refaie, Chaudry, Alfakir, & Khan, 2010).

The treatment regimen for patients with HIV infection or AIDS as well as TB is the same as it is for uninfected adults (6 mo regimen, with initial 2 mo, four-drug [INH, RIF, PZA, and EMB] phase followed by 2 mo of INH and RIF). Two exceptions to this recommendation for the patient who is HIV-positive are that (1) once-weekly RIF should not be used in any HIV-infected patient, and (2) twice-weekly INH-RIF or rifabutin should not be used for patients with CD4 counts lower than 100/mcL.

Patients who are HIV-positive with TB have lower mortality if they are on antiretroviral therapy during treatment for TB (CDC, 2013d). It is recommended that antiretroviral therapy be started within 2 weeks of starting TB treatment in patients with CD4 counts less than 50 cells/mm^3. Therefore, patients with HIV infection or AIDS are usually on multiple drugs besides the anti-TB medication, requiring dosage adjustment and monitoring for interactions between the medications. RIF is known to alter the liver's metabolism of many drugs, leading to treatment failure or suboptimal response in the patient on multiple antiretroviral medications. A complex drug interaction also takes place between RIF and protease inhibitors that can create a therapeutic challenge, possibly leading to changes in the antiretroviral regimen. All HIV-infected patients who are undergoing treatment with isoniazid should be on pyridoxine (vitamin B$_6$) 25 to 50 mg daily or 50 to 100 mg twice weekly to reduce the occurrence of isoniazid-induced side effects in the central and peripheral nervous system.

Providing an optimal outcome to a patient with HIV infection or AIDS with TB will require referral to an infectious disease specialist. Recommendations regarding treating HIV-infected patients with TB change frequently as new antiretroviral agents are introduced; providers can find up-to-date information at the CDC's Division of Tuberculosis Elimination site (http://www.cdc.gov/tb/).

MONITORING

Patients with positive pretreatment sputum for *M. tuberculosis* are best monitored by repeat sputum cultures monthly until sputum cultures are negative. After 2 months of treatment with INH and RIF, more than 80% of patients who had positive sputum cultures at the beginning of treatment should have converted to negative. Patients should be monitored monthly and should have a sputum smear and culture at the end of the course of treatment. DOT should be considered for all cases of TB.

Radiographic monitoring is not as important as sputum examination during the course of treatment (ATS, 2003). At the completion of treatment, a chest x-ray should be done to provide a baseline for comparison with any future films.

In patients with negative pretreatment sputum yet having radiographic findings consistent with TB, an extensive effort to make a microbiological diagnosis is necessary. These patients most likely need medical evaluation by a pulmonologist. Bronchoscopy to perform biopsies and bronchoalveolar lavage should be considered to confirm the diagnosis of TB. If presumptive treatment is started without sputum cultures, then the chest x-rays should be repeated. Failure to show improvement of the lesions on the chest film after 3 months of therapy strongly suggests a misdiagnosis or a lesion that is an old TB lesion (not currently active).

Adverse Reactions to the Medications

Patients should also be monitored for adverse reactions to the medications used to treat TB by means of a baseline measurement of hepatic enzymes, bilirubin, serum creatinine, a complete blood count (CBC), and platelet count. Patients who are taking PZA require a baseline serum uric acid. A baseline ophthalmology examination for visual acuity and a red-green color examination are required for patients on EMB. These baseline tests are used to determine any underlying abnormality that would affect the treatment regimen. Children generally do not require baseline laboratory tests, except visual acuity, unless they have some underlying medical condition that may complicate the treatment regimen.

INH has a Black-Box Warning regarding the development of severe and sometimes fatal hepatitis, even after many months of treatment. The risk is age-related, with the highest incidence in persons aged 50 to 64 years (23 cases per 1,000). Increased risk for hepatitis is associated with daily alcohol use, chronic liver disease, and IV drug use. Black and Hispanic women, as well as any woman during the postpartum period who takes INH, may have increased risk of developing fatal hepatitis. All patients taking INH should have monthly symptom reviews to screen for hepatitis. Symptoms to screen for include unexplained anorexia, nausea, vomiting, dark urine, icterus, rash, persistent paresthesias of hands or feet, fatigue, weakness, fever longer than 3 days, or abdominal tenderness especially in the right upper quadrant. Liver enzymes should be measured in patients over age 35 years prior to starting INH and then periodically throughout treatment.

Once treatment is begun, patients are monitored clinically for adverse reactions. They usually do not need routine laboratory tests unless laboratory abnormalities are present prior to beginning therapy. Patients should be told of the symptoms associated with the most common adverse reactions to the medications. They should report all flu-like illness immediately and see their health-care provider at least monthly during treatment. At the monthly visit, the provider should ask specific questions regarding adverse reactions to the medication and follow any positive answer with confirming laboratory tests.

Adult patients treated for TB are at risk for peripheral neuropathy associated with INH therapy; therefore, they also need 25 to 50 mg per day of pyridoxine (vitamin B_6) to decrease the likelihood of developing this serious but avoidable adverse reaction.

OUTCOME EVALUATION

Because of the lengthy treatment time for TB and the increased incidence of resistant organisms found with inadequate treatment, health-care providers should include both the actual sputum culture evaluation and the patient's compliance with the medication regimen in judging the success of the treatment. Ideally, the patient will have TB-free sputum within the first 2 months of treatment and a clear sputum culture throughout the rest of the treatment. After treatment, no standard follow-up is required. If a patient is immunosuppressed, reevaluation is suggested 6 months after treatment has been completed. Any relapse is most likely to occur within the first 2 years after treatment.

PATIENT EDUCATION

Extensive patient education is essential to successful TB treatment. Administration should be explained, including the instructions to take isoniazid on an empty stomach because food reduces bioavailability. The patient must also understand the purpose for the long, multidrug treatment regimen and be a partner in the process. Compliance is a major issue in TB treatment; therefore, all teaching should have the underlying theme of taking all medication as scheduled. The lengthy treatment requires that education be repeated and reviewed at the monthly visits. Because patients may be illiterate or understand little English, education should be presented in a variety of media, such as videotapes in a patient's primary language. Peer health counselors may also be helpful in educating patients with TB.

PREVENTION OF TUBERCULOSIS

Most patients infected with the tubercle bacillus never develop active TB. Approximately 90% to 95% of those infected are able to mount an immune response that prevents active TB infection (CDC, 2005). The goal of preventive therapy is early identification of patients at risk of developing active TB so that they can be treated with drugs to prevent their conversion to active disease. Patients at risk for developing active TB include those who have been newly exposed to persons with active TB, those who convert from negative to positive on indirect testing, and those who have dormant infections that are at risk for reactivation (Jereb et al, 2011).

Skin testing with PPD or Mantoux is a necessary screening test to determine if the patient has been infected. Evaluation of the results of the skin test is based on the likelihood of infection and the risk of active TB if infection has occurred. If the patient is HIV-positive or has fibrotic lesions on chest x-ray, a reaction of 5 mm or more is considered positive. A reaction of 10 mm or more is considered positive in other at-risk patients, including infants and children. In patients who are not in any high-risk category or high-risk environment, a result of 15 mm or more is considered positive. The interferon-gamma release assays (QuantiFERON-TB Gold test and T-SPOT.TB test) may also be used to detect TB and results are available within 24 hours. A positive result indicates a patient has been infected; additional evaluation is necessary to determine if the disease is latent or active. Further evaluation would include chest x-ray, HIV testing, and other testing determined by patient risk status.

Patients are considered high risk if they have the following medical conditions: diabetes mellitus, prolonged therapy with adrenocorticosteroids, immunosuppressive therapy, hematological or reticuloendothelial diseases such as leukemia or Hodgkin's disease, injection drug use by a patient known to be HIV-seronegative, end-stage renal disease, and any clinical presentation that consists of substantial rapid weight loss or chronic malnutrition. A person who is in a high-incidence group with a skin test reaction of 10 mm or more is a candidate for preventive therapy, even without any of these risk factors. High-incidence groups include foreign-born people from high-prevalence countries; medically underserved, low-income populations; and residents of long-term-care facilities.

Pathophysiology

Most cases of TB in the United States and Canada occur from reactivation of latent infection acquired at an earlier time, months or years before, when the patient's immune system was able to mount a sufficient defense. The patient has no outward sign of ever having been infected by TB. All that remains to identify that the patient was exposed to TB is a positive tuberculin skin test or interferon-gamma release assays (QuantiFERON-TBGold test and T-SPOT.TB test). Reactivation, leading to active infection, occurs in patients who, for whatever reason, cannot muster a sufficient immune response.

Drug Therapy

The preferred drug therapy for TB prevention consists of a combination of INH and rifapentine (CDC, 2013e). The treatment, referred to as the "12 Dose Regimen," consists of INH 15 mg/kg (maximum 900 mg) and rifapentine (RPT) 900 mg (for adults more than or equal to 50 kg) administered once weekly utilizing DOT (CDC, 2011). INH may also be used as self-administered monotherapy to treat latent TB. INH is given in a single daily dose of 300 mg for adults and 10 to 15 mg/kg for children, not to exceed 300 mg. Or INH may be given as a twice-weekly dose of 10 to 15 mg/kg (maximum 900 mg/dose) in adults and 20 to 30 mg/kg (maximum 900 mg/dose) for children (CDC, 2013e). DOT is recommended for twice-weekly INH dosing.

The standard length of treatment for monotherapy with INH is 9 months (CDC, 2013e; Jereb et al, 2011). Patients who are HIV positive should receive 12 months of therapy. The preferred therapy in children age 2 years to 11 years is 9 months of INH (CDC, 2011). Shortened 2 month therapy that combines RIF and PZB is no longer recommended because of high rates of hospitalization and death from liver injury associated with the treatment (CDC, 2003b). Treatment regimens for latent TB are found in Table 45-4.

The INH should be dispensed in monthly allotments, with the patient's compliance monitored at least monthly. For patients who may have questionable adherence, DOT is recommended. If resources prohibit daily DOT, then INH may be given twice a week at the dose of 15 mg/kg, utilizing DOT to monitor adherence.

Prior to beginning drug therapy with INH or RIF/RPT, evaluate the patient as follows:

1. Exclude active TB by both radiographic and bacteriological tests. All patients with a positive skin test require a chest x-ray to rule out pulmonary TB. If the chest x-ray is consistent with pulmonary TB, then an extensive evaluation to rule out active disease is necessary. Bacteriologic studies of the sputum and comparisons with old x-rays are helpful in gaining a clear clinical picture of when the patient has active disease. Because of the risk of developing INH resistance when only INH is used for active disease, patients with any suspicion of active disease should be started on multidrug therapy until the final diagnosis is clarified.
2. Determine if the patient has a history of adequate TB preventive therapy.
3. Determine if the patient has had prior INH therapy to decide if the patient has had adequate drug therapy.
4. Look for any contraindications to the administration of INH therapy: previous INH-induced hepatitis, history of severe INH reactions, or liver disease of any etiology.

Table 45–4   Latent TB Treatment Regimens

Drug	Duration	Dosing Schedule	Total Number of Doses
Isoniazid (INH) and rifapentine	3 months	Once weekly*	12
INH	9 months	Daily	270
		Twice weekly*	76
INH	6 months	Daily	180
		Twice weekly*	52
Rifampin	4 months	Daily	120

Derived from Centers for Disease Control and Prevention (CDC). (2013e). Latent TB infection. Retrieved from http://www.cdc.gov/tb/topic/treatment/ltbi.htm

*Directly Observed Therapy recommended.

5. Identify patients who require special cautions. They include patients over age 35 years as well as patients with daily alcohol use, previous problems with INH therapy, current chronic liver disease, and injection drug use. Other patients requiring cautions include pregnant women and patients at higher risk for developing fatal hepatitis (women, particularly black and Hispanic women). Hepatitis risk is also increased in the postpartum period.

Monitoring

Patients receiving preventive TB therapy with INH or via DOT with weekly INH/RPT should be monitored at least monthly. At monthly visits, the health-care provider should carefully assess the patient's compliance and ask the patient about symptoms of adverse effects of INH, specifically liver damage. A standardized form should be used to evaluate the patient for symptoms of liver damage, including unexplained anorexia; nausea; vomiting; dark urine; icterus; rash; persistent paresthesias of the hands and feet; persistent fatigue, weakness, or fever for more than 3 days' duration; and abdominal tenderness. If these or other signs or symptoms occur during preventive therapy, patients should contact their health-care provider immediately.

Of those receiving INH therapy, 10% to 20% will have mildly abnormal liver enzymes, which usually resolve even if the INH is continued. Patients over age 35 years have the highest frequency of hepatitis; therefore, a baseline transaminase should be obtained before therapy is begun for such patients, and the study should be repeated monthly during therapy. If values are greater than 3 to 5 times normal, then INH should be discontinued. Other patients at risk for developing hepatitis are those who have chronic liver disease, those who inject drugs, and those who use alcohol daily. Monthly liver function tests are not a substitute for monthly clinical evaluations of the patient on preventive therapy.

Outcome Evaluation

The success of preventive TB therapy is determined by the absence of active disease and by whether the patient has been compliant with the prescribed drug treatment. Because patients who are receiving preventive therapy often do not feel ill or have any overt symptoms, compliance with the long treatment regimen is even more difficult than it is for patients with active TB.

Patient Education

Education for patients receiving preventive TB therapy is similar to education for those receiving treatment for active TB. The key difference is stressing the need for months of treatment to a patient who often has no symptoms and feels well. Education should occur in the patient's primary language and at an appropriate literacy level. Patients must understand that adherence to the treatment regimen is essential, and the health-care team cannot emphasize it enough.

On The Horizon | **DRUGS IN THE PIPELINE**

Significant TB drug research has been spawned by the Global Alliance for TB Drug Development, which was established in 2000 to address the need for new and better TB drug treatment (www.tballiance.org). Child-appropriate formulations of the standard four-drug therapy (isoniazid + rifampin + pyrazinamide + ethambutol) are currently in development and undergoing phase I clinical trials, as current formulations require either crushing of tablets or cannot easily be measured in the mg/kg dose required for infants less than 5 kg. The following are currently in early phase II trials:

- A combination of bedaquiline, clofazamine, and PA-824 in a less than 4-month, all-oral regimen for MDR TB. PA-824 is a nitroimidazole, a novel antibacterial class.
- A combination of bedaquiline, pyrazinamide, and PA-824 in a less than 4-month, all-oral regimen for MDR TB.
- A combination of bedaquiline, clofazimine, pyrazinamide, and PA-824 in a less than 4-month, all-oral regimen for MDR TB.
- A combination of bedaquiline, clofazimine, and pyrazinamide in a less than 4-month, all-oral regimen for MDR TB.

Late phase II trials include a combination of PA-824, moxifloxacin, and pyrazinamide that is showing promise for curing TB and some forms of MDR TB in 4 months using an oral regimen that can be administered in a fixed dose. Phase III trials include investigation of a combination of isoniazid, rifampin, pyrazinamide, and moxifloxacin that is demonstrating promise in shortening the length of TB treatment from 6 months to 4 months. Another phase III trial is investigating a combination of ethambutol, rifampin, pyrazinamide, and moxifloxacin in a 4-month regimen to treat TB.

The Global Alliance continues to focus funds and scientific energy toward developing drugs that simplify and shorten treatment regimens, are effective against MDR TB, are compatible with antiretroviral therapies for HIV, and expand the pediatric formulations available.

TUBERCULOSIS

Related to the Overall Treatment Plan and Disease Process

☐ A clear description of the pathophysiology and mode of transmission of TB: patients need to understand that they can be infectious to their close contacts if they do not receive adequate treatment.

☐ A thorough outline of the complete treatment regimen, including an estimated length of time for treatment: patients need to know up front that they will be receiving months and possibly more than a year of treatment.

☐ Importance of adherence to the treatment regimen.

☐ Importance of regularly scheduled follow-up appointments.

Specific to the Drug Therapy

☐ A written plan of the medication schedule is essential, especially with multidrug regimens.

☐ Possible adverse effects of the medications and the importance of reporting immediately to the health-care provider any vague, flu-like symptoms.

Reasons for Taking the Drug(s)

☐ The drugs are given to prevent or eliminate infection by *M. tuberculosis*.

Drugs as Part of the Total Treatment Regimen

Tuberculosis medications are a part of the total treatment regimen, which also includes strict pulmonary care.

Adherence Issues

Extensive patient education is essential to successful treatment. The patient must understand the purpose for the long, multidrug treatment regimen and be a partner in the treatment. Adherence is a major issue; therefore, all teaching should have the underlying theme of taking all medication as scheduled. The long period of treatment requires education that is repeated and reviewed at the monthly visits. To teach patients who may be illiterate or who understand English only minimally, education should be conducted in a variety of media, such as videos in the patient's primary language. Peer health counselors may also help to educate patients with TB. DOT may enhance compliance with and adherence to therapy.

REFERENCES

American Thoracic Society (ATS). (2003). American Thoracic Society/Centers for Disease Control and Prevention/Infectious Diseases Society of America: Treatment of tuberculosis. *American Journal of Respiratory and Critical Care Medicine, 167,* 603–662.

Blumberg, H. M., Leonard, M. K., & Jasmer, R. M. (2005). Update on the treatment of tuberculosis and latent tuberculosis infection. *Journal of the American Medical Association, 293*(22), 2776–2784.

Cain, K. P., Haley, C. A., Armstrong, L. R., Garman, K. N., Wells, C. D., Iademarch, M. F., et al. (2007). Tuberculosis among foreign-born persons in the United States: Achieving tuberculosis elimination. *American Journal of Respiratory and Critical Care Medicine, 175,* 75–79.

Canadian Thoracic Society and The Public Health Agency of Canada (2013). *Canadian tuberculosis standards, 7th edition.* Ottawa, ON: Public Health Agency of Canada. Retrieved from http://www.respiratoryguidelines.ca/tb-standards-2013

Centers for Disease Control and Prevention (CDC). (2003a). Treatment of tuberculosis, American Thoracic Society, CDC, and Infectious Diseases Society of America. *Morbidity and Mortality Weekly Report, 52*(RR-11), 1–77.

Centers for Disease Control and Prevention (CDC). (2003b). Update: Adverse event data and revised American Thoracic Society/CDC recommendations against the use of rifampin and pyrazinamide for treatment of latent tuberculosis infection—United States, 2003. *Morbidity and Mortality Weekly Report, 52*(31), 735–739.

Centers for Disease Control and Prevention (CDC) (2011). Recommendations for use of isoniazid-rifapentine regimen with direct observation to treat latent *Mycobacterium tuberculosis* infection. *Morbidity and Mortality Weekly Report, 60*(48), 1650–1653.

Centers for Disease Control and Prevention (CDC) (2012). *Tuberculin skin testing.* Retrieved from http://www.cdc.gov/tb/publications/factsheets/testing/skintesting.htm

Centers for Disease Control and Prevention (CDC). (2013a). *TB incidence in the United States, 1953–2012.* Retrieved from http://www.cdc.gov/tb/statistics/tbcases.htm

Centers for Disease Control and Prevention (CDC). (2013b). *Tuberculosis in the United States: National Tuberculosis Surveillance System Highlights from 2012.* Retrieved from http://www.cdc.gov/tb/statistics/surv/surv2012/default.htm

Centers for Disease Control and Prevention (CDC). (2013c). *Reported tuberculosis in the United States, 2012.* Retrieved from http://www.cdc.gov/tb/statistics/reports/2012/default.htm

Centers for Disease Control and Prevention (CDC). (2013d). *Managing drug interactions in the treatment of HIV-related tuberculosis.* Retrieved from http://www.cdc.gov/tb/publications/guidelines/TB_HIV_Drugs/default.htm

Centers for Disease Control and Prevention (CDC). (2013e). *Latent TB infection.* Retrieved from http://www.cdc.gov/tb/topic/treatment/ltbi.htm

Dasgupta, K., & Menzies, D. (2005). Cost-effectiveness of tuberculosis control strategies among immigrants and refugees. *European Respiratory Journal, 25,* 1107–1116.

Global Alliance for TB Drug Development. (2013). *TB drug portfolio.* Retrieved from http://www.tballiance.org

Haddad, M. B., Wilson, T. W., Ijaz, K., Marks, S. M., & Moore, M. (2005). Tuberculosis and homelessness in the United States, 1994–2003. *Journal of the American Medical Association, 293*(22), 2762–2766.

Jereb, J. A., Goldberg, S. V., Powell, K., Villarino, M. E., LoBue, P., & Division of Tuberculosis Elimination, National Center for HIV, Viral Hepatitis, STD and TB Prevention. (2011). Recommendations for use of an isoniazid-rifapentine regimen with Direct Observation to treat latent

Mycobacterium tuberculosis infection. *Morbidity and Mortality Weekly Report, 60*(48), 1650–1653.

LoBue, P., Sizemore, C., & Castro, K. G. (2009). Plan to combat extensively drug-resistant tuberculosis recommendations of the federal Tuberculosis Task Force. *Morbidity and Mortality Weekly Report, 58*(RR03), 1–43.

Manangan, L., Elmore, K., Lewis, B., Pratt, R., Armstrong, L., Davison, J., et al. (2009). Disparities in tuberculosis between Asian/Pacific Islanders and non-Hispanic Whites, United States, 1993–2006. *International Journal of Tuberculosis and Lung Disease, 13*(9), 1077–1085.

Mase, S., Chorba, T., Loube, P. & Castro, K. (2013). Provisional CDC guidelines for the use and safety monitoring of bedaquiline fumarate (Sirturo) for the treatment of multidrug-resistant tuberculosis. *Morbidity and Mortality Weekly Report (MMWR), 62*(RR09), 1–12.

Mazurek, G. H., Jereb, J., LoBue, P., Iademarco, M. F., Merchock, B., & Vernon, A. (2005). Guidelines for using QuantiFERON-TB Gold test for detecting *Mycobacterium tuberculosis* infection, United States. *Morbidity and Mortality Weekly Report, 54*(RR-15), 49–55.

Mitnick, C. D., Shin, S. S., Seung, K. J., Rich, M. L., Atwood, S. S., Furin, J. J., et al. (2008). Comprehensive treatment of extensively drug-resistant tuberculosis. *New England Journal of Medicine, 359*(6), 563–574.

Oxford Immunotec (2014). *The T-SPOT.TB test.* Retrieved from http://oxfordimmunotec.com/international/products-solutions/t-spot-tb/t-spot-tb-test/

Public Health Agency of Canada (2009). *Tuberculosis: Information for health care providers. 4th edition.* Ottawa, ON: Public Health Agency of Canada.

Public Health Agency of Canada. (2014). *Tuberculosis in Canada 2012.* Ottawa, ON: Public Health Agency of Canada. Retrieved from http://www.phac-aspc.gc.ca/tbpc-latb/pubs/tbcan12pre/index-eng.php

Rafaie, T., Chaudry, F. A., Aflakir, M., & Khan, M. A. (2010). Chest x-ray presentation of pulmonary tuberculosis in patients with HIV/AIDS. *American Journal of Respiratory and Critical Care Medicine, 181,* A1787.

Riley, L. (1997). Pneumonia and tuberculosis in pregnancy. *Infectious Disease Clinics of North America, 11*(1), 119–133.

World Health Organization (2013a). *Global tuberculosis report.* Geneva, Switzerland: World Health Organization. Retrieved from http://www.who.int/tb/publications/global_report/en/

World Health Organization (2013b). *Tuberculosis Diagnostics Xpert MTB/RIF Test.* Retrieved from http://who.int/tb/features_archive/factsheet_xpert.pdf

CHAPTER 46

UPPER RESPIRATORY INFECTIONS, OTITIS MEDIA, AND OTITIS EXTERNA

Teri Moser Woo

Upper respiratory infections (URIs) are the most common minor acute illnesses seen in primary care. The most common secondary infections seen with viral URIs are sinusitis and, in children, otitis media (OM). Practitioners encounter these illnesses countless times among their patients and should be aware of the pathogens commonly found and the pharmacological and nonpharmacological management of these illnesses. This chapter discusses the pharmacological management of these acute illnesses, as well as the management of otitis externa (OE).

VIRAL UPPER RESPIRATORY INFECTION

Viral URIs, also known as common colds, are the most frequent disease seen in a primary care practice and also the number-one cause of absenteeism from work and school. The frequency of viral URIs varies with age, with adults averaging 2 to 3 colds a year (Chow et al, 2012) and children aged 1 to 5 averaging 7 or 8 (Friedman & Sexton, 2009). Infants have an average of 6 or 7 colds per year, but being in day care increases their incidence of colds to 9 to 11 in the first year of life. Overall, the common cold accounts for 22 million missed school days and 20 million missed workdays in the United States due to caring for an ill child. (Bramley, Lerner, & Sames, 2002). The total economic cost of the common cold is estimated to be more than $40 billion, when costs of medical care, medications (including OTC medications), and loss of productive work time are factored in (Fendrick, Monto, Nightengale, & Sarnes, 2003).

A viral URI usually starts with the symptoms of nasal congestion, rhinorrhea, malaise, and scratchy throat. The nasal discharge typically starts out thin and clear and then thickens and progresses to a green or yellow color. Respiratory symptoms generally peak in severity on days 3 to 6 and then improve but may persist for 10 to 12 days (Wald et al, 2013). Generalized muscle aches may be present, but fever is usually absent in adults. Young children may have a low-grade fever for 24 to 48 hours (Wald et al, 2013). Fever in adults or a high fever (greater than or equal to 39°F) in children suggests influenza or a secondary infection, such as sinusitis or OM. URI symptoms are irritating but not severe. More severe symptoms should be investigated for secondary infection or other bacterial infection. Most patients are symptom-free in 7 to 10 days from the beginning of the illness.

Pathophysiology

The rhinovirus is the most common cause of the common cold (American Academy of Pediatrics [AAP], 2012a). There are more than 100 serotypes of rhinovirus (AAP, 2012a); therefore, even though immunity is produced by rhinoviral infections, the patient can quickly become infected with another strain of rhinovirus. The common story heard in the clinic is that the patient has just gotten over a cold and now it has come back. Other viruses causing the common cold include, but are not limited to, adenovirus, respiratory syncytial virus, parainfluenza virus, influenza viral strains and human metapneumovirus (Pappas & Hendley, 2009). These viruses are transmitted between people by airborne droplets or by direct transmission of the virus in secretions via hand contact.

Goals of Treatment

Viral URIs are self-limiting and require no treatment other than symptomatic relief; therefore, the major goal in treating a patient with a viral URI is relieving irritating symptoms, specifically nasal congestion.

Rational Drug Selection

Drug Therapy

Although viral URI (the common cold) is a self-limited disease that requires no treatment, a huge industry touts nonprescription medications for treatment of colds. First, note that antibiotics have no place in the treatment of the common cold. Using antibiotics for a viral infection increases the likelihood of antimicrobial resistance to secondary bacterial infections that may occur in the upper respiratory tract. Antihistamines have not been shown to alter the course of a common cold, yet many over-the-counter (OTC) cold preparations contain some form of antihistamine, probably for their "drying" effect.

The mainstay of pharmacological management for a cold is the decongestant, either systemic or topical. Decongestants cause vasoconstriction of the capillaries in the nasal mucous membranes. This results in shrinkage of the mucous membrane, which promotes drainage and decreases the nasal stuffiness that accompanies a URI. Dosing of common decongestants can be found in Table 46-1. Topical decongestants

Table 46–1 ❁ Drugs Commonly Used: Viral Upper Respiratory Infections

Drug	Adult Dose	Pediatric Dose	Strengths Available	Comments
Oral Decongestants				
Pseudoephedrine HCl (Sudafed, Genafed, Pseudo Tabs, Pediacare)	60 mg q4–6h Extended release: 120 mg q12h	*Children 6–12 yr*: 30 mg q4–6h	Tablets: 30, 60 mg	Adults: do not exceed 120 mg in 24 h
		Children 2–5 yr: 15 mg q4–6h *Infants–2 yr*: 1 mg/kg or 0.1 mL/kg of 7.5 mg/ 0.8 mL drops	Extended release: 120 mg Liquid: 15 mg/5 mL, 30 mg/5mL Drops: 7.5 mg/0.8 mL Capsules: 60 mg	Children: do not exceed 4 doses/d *Not recommended in children under age 4 yr
Pseudoephedrine sulfate (Afrin, Drixoral Non-Drowsy)	120 mg q12h	Not for use in children <12 yr	Extended release: 120 mg	Do not crush or chew
Phenylephrine (Sudafed PE)	*Adults*: 10 mg q4h Maximum of 60 mg/24 h	*Children 2–6 yr*: 2.5–5 mg every 12 h *Children >6 yr*: 5–10 mg q12h	Tablet: 10 mg Chewable tablet: 10 mg Dissolving tablet: 10 mg	*Decongestants are not recommended in children <age 4 yr
Topical Decongestants				
Phenylephrine HCl (Neo-Synephrine, Nostril, Sinex, Alconefrin, Rhinall)	2–3 sprays each nostril; repeat q3–4h	*Children 6–12 yr*: 2 sprays each nostril q4h *Children >6 mo*: 1 to 2 drops each nostril q3h	Spray: 0.125%, 0.16%, 0.25%, 0.5%, 1% Drops: 0.25%, 0.5%, 1%	Do not use for longer than 3 d because of rebound congestion; rarely used in young children.
Oxymetazoline HCl (Afrin, 12 Hour Nasal, Dristan Long Lasting, Allerest 12 Hour, Afrin Children's Nose Drops)	2 or 3 sprays or drops of 0.05% solution in each nostril bid or q10–12h	*Children ≥6 yr*: 2 or 3 drops of 0.025% solution in each nostril bid, morning and evening	Solution: 0.05%, 0.025%	Do not use for longer than 3 d because of rebound congestion. Do not use in children <6 yr.

(Afrin, Neo-Synephrine) may be helpful for temporary relief of congestion without causing systemic side effects. Topical decongestants may be used safely for up to 3 consecutive days. Prolonged use of topical decongestants will lead to rebound congestion. Analgesics such as acetaminophen (Tylenol), aspirin, and ibuprofen (Motrin) can be given for malaise.

Due to concerns about the use of pseudoephedrine to manufacture methamphetamine, a number of states have decreased access to OTC pseudoephedrine. Some states have declared pseudoephedrine a prescription medication; Oregon made it a Schedule III drug. In 2006, the Combat Methamphetamine Epidemic Act was incorporated into the USA Patriot Act, requiring special handling of pseudoephedrine, ephedrine, and phenylpropanolamine, all precursors to methamphetamine. The law requires precursors to methamphetamine to be placed behind the pharmacy counter nationwide to restrict access. Retailers must ask for purchaser identification and limit the amount of drug purchased to a 30-day supply. Providers need to be aware of the changing laws in their state or province of practice and provide a prescription for pseudoephedrine as needed. Many manufacturers have begun to create new products that replace the pseudoephedrine with phenylephrine (Sudafed PE), a decongestant that cannot be used to manufacture methamphetamine (see Table 46-1).

The use of cough and cold medications in young children, specifically children under age 5 years, has become an area of significant debate. The safety of cough and cold medications, specifically those containing decongestants, has been questioned after reports of deaths in infants taking cold medications (Taverner & Latte, 2007). Decongestants also have questionable efficacy in children. A *Cochrane Review* of the use of decongestants to treat nasal congestion associated with the common cold found a small (6%) but statistically significant improvement in congestion in adults but insufficient evidence regarding effectiveness in children (Taverner & Latte, 2007). A second *Cochrane Review* found no evidence supporting the efficacy of systemic decongestants or antihistamine-decongestant combinations in the treatment of URI in children younger than age 5 years (DeSutter, van Driel, Kumar, Lesslar, & Skrt, 2012).

In October 2007, a U.S. Food and Drug Administration (FDA) panel recommended that all pediatric cough and cold medications be relabeled as not indicated for use in children under age 4 years. This led to a voluntary withdrawal of infant drop formulations of cough and cold medications from the market in October 2007. This withdrawal of infant formulations of OTC cough and cold medications has resulted in a reduction (1,248 visits versus 2,790 visits) in emergency department visits related to adverse events in children younger than age 2 years (Shehab, Schaefer, Kegler, & Budnitz, 2010).

Nonpharmacological Therapy

Nonpharmacological therapy or lifestyle management includes increasing fluid intake, using nonmedicated cough drops, using nasal saline spray or drops to decrease the viscosity of nasal secretions, and rest. Patients and parents or other family members need to be reminded that anorexia is often associated with the common cold and that fluids often need to be forced on the ill person to maintain adequate hydration. Infants who are congested often cannot breathe and drink liquids from the bottle or breast at the same time; therefore, their fluid intake may be inadequate. Parents need to be encouraged to suction the infant's nose with a nasal bulb syringe to clear secretions before the infant eats or drinks. Nasal saline spray is also beneficial in thinning secretions at all ages to make blowing or bulbing secretions more effective. Patients can make their own saline solution by adding a quarter tsp salt to 8 oz warm water. If a dropper is not available, patients can use a cotton ball saturated with saline solution to squeeze three or four drops into each nasal passage. Many patients are overcommitted and overworked and must be reminded of the restorative powers of rest. Encouraging patients to take a day or two off from work is much more effective than prescribing an unnecessary antibiotic.

Monitoring

The patient with a viral URI should be monitored for signs of secondary bacterial infection. Monitor decongestant use in cardiac patients, who may have increased hypertension from the added vasoconstriction caused by oral decongestants. Older adults are more likely to have adverse reactions from decongestants.

Outcome Evaluation

Secondary bacterial infections may complicate the common cold. The most common complication in adults is sinusitis, which occurs in approximately 0.5% to 2.5% of colds (Friedman & Sexton, 2009). In children, sinusitis is a common secondary infection in 6% to 7% of colds (Wald et al, 2013), as is OM, which occurs in about 10% to 50% of children with colds (Pelton & Leibovitz, 2009). Some children appear more apt to get OM as a secondary infection, possibly because differences in middle ear and eustachian tube anatomy predispose them to ear infections or because of the number of bacterial otopathogens present in the nasopharynx. Children in day care tend to have more otopathogens present in the nasopharynx and therefore may be more likely to develop otitis media when they have a URI (Pelton & Leibovitz, 2009). Adults may not get acute otitis media as often as do children, but 50% to 80% of adults will develop eustachian tube dysfunction after a rhinovirus or influenza infection (Friedman & Sexton, 2009).

This chapter discusses sinusitis and otitis media, common complications of URI. Another complication of viral URIs is exacerbation of asthma symptoms, occurring in 30% to 50% of the colds acquired by people with asthma. See Chapter 30 for asthma management.

Patient Education

Patient education for a viral URI is centered on symptomatic treatment and proper dosing of decongestants. Parents should be educated about avoiding the use of cough and cold medications in children, especially those age 4 years and younger. Patients need to be assured that most URIs resolve in 7 to 10 days and that very little can be done to shorten the course of the disease. Antibiotics are not necessary for viral infections, and education regarding the signs and symptoms of a secondary bacterial infection needs to be provided.

SINUSITIS

Diagnosis of sinusitis is based on clinical symptoms and the course of the illness. Any persistent URI lasting longer than 10 days without any clinical improvement is likely to be bacterial sinusitis (Chow et al, 2012). Severe symptoms such as high fever (greater than or equal to 39°F), facial pain, or purulent nasal discharge that last 3 to 4 consecutive days may be bacterial sinusitis (Chow et al, 2012; Wald et al, 2013). Likewise, patients may experience "double-sickening," that is, a worsening of symptoms such as new onset of fever, headache, or an increase in purulent nasal discharge that was previously improving (Chow et al, 2012; Wald et al, 2013).

In adults, three symptoms have high specificity and sensitivity for diagnosing acute sinusitis: purulent rhinorrhea, facial pain or pressure, and nasal obstruction (Chan & Kuhn, 2009). Patients may have a headache that worsens when they bend over, and they may have a cough that is worse at night. A sudden worsening of symptoms after improvement is also suggestive of sinusitis (Chan & Kuhn).

Children have subtler symptoms. Because their frontal sinuses are not completely developed until they are 10 years old, children often do not have the classic frontal headache of sinusitis. Children may vomit due to gagging on mucus. Children have colds more frequently than do adults. Therefore, a careful history of whether the symptoms have actually been prolonged or whether the patient has a new viral URI is essential.

Children and adults alike may have puffy eyes and a cough that worsens when they lie down. Radiological studies are of questionable validity because sinus images look the same for a viral URI as for a sinus infection (Wald et al, 2013). A contrast-enhanced CT should be obtained if orbital or intracranial extension of sinusitis is suspected (Chow et al, 2012). In children, a contrast-enhanced MRI or CT is ordered to rule out orbital or intracranial extension (Wald et al, 2013).

Sinus infections can be either acute or chronic. Chronic sinusitis is defined as signs and symptoms consistent with sinusitis that last 8 to 12 weeks and is confirmed via endoscopy or CT imaging (Chan & Kuhn, 2009; Desrosiers et al, 2011). Multiple (3 or 4) episodes of acute bacterial sinusitis per year suggest chronic sinusitis and require referral to a specialist for confirmation (Chow et al, 2012).

Pathophysiology

The most common bacterial organisms found in acute sinusitis are *Streptococcus pneumoniae, Haemophilus influenzae, Moraxella catarrhalis,* and, more rarely, *Staphylococcus. Staphylococcus,* gram-negative enteric organisms

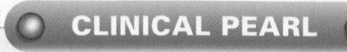

CLINICAL PEARL

Nutritional or herbal therapy

Nutritional or herbal therapy is often thought to decrease symptoms of the common cold. In the 1970s, Linus Pauling first brought forward the idea that vitamin C prevents and alleviates episodes of the common cold. Although this has still not been scientifically proven, many patients continue to take vitamin C at the first sign of a cold.

Zinc lozenges have also been proposed as a treatment for the common cold. It is thought that zinc ions inhibit rhinovirus replication in vitro. In a systematic review of seven randomized controlled trials (RCTs) (754 patients total), two of the studies suggested reduced duration and severity of upper respiratory infection (URI) symptoms (Marshall, 2000). Another review of 14 placebo-controlled trials published from 1966 to 2000 found that one well-designed study showed improvement with the use of zinc nasal gel (Caruso, Prober, & Gwaltney, 2007). In a more recent RCT, a group of patients took a 13.3 mg zinc lozenge every 2 to 3 hours while awake and had a significantly shorter duration of cold symptoms (4.0 days versus 7.1 days; *P* less than 0.0001), shorter duration of cough (2.1 days versus 5.0 days), and nasal discharge (3.0 versus 4.5 days) than did the placebo control group (Prasad, Beck, Bao, Snell, & Fitzgerald, 2008). In light of these studies, zinc lozenges may decrease URI symptoms in some patients. Zinc nasal gels (Zicam) should be avoided after reports of permanent anosmia and an FDA warning to avoid their use.

Another common herbal therapy that patients may be using for their cold symptoms is echinacea. Echinacea is widely used in Europe for the prevention and treatment of colds and flu. Its use is increasing in the United States. A number of European studies have demonstrated the immune-enhancing properties of echinacea, specifically increasing T-cell activity and interferon. Among European providers, echinacea is the leading herbal recommendation for the prevention of colds and flu. It is available in tablet, liquid, and tea bag form. The correct dosage is 900 mg daily divided into two or three doses, or 40 drops of the juice 3 times a day. Length of therapy should not exceed 8 weeks. There are no reported side effects at the recommended dosages. It appears to be safe during pregnancy and lactation. The only true contraindication is having a progressive systemic disease such as tuberculosis or multiple sclerosis or an autoimmune illness. Echinacea is a relative of the daisy; therefore, patients who are allergic to daisies should also avoid any form of echinacea.

and anaerobic bacteria, are more common in chronic sinusitis. Rarely, the causative organism in chronic sinusitis is fungal, with *Aspergillus* the most common fungus found. Patients who are immunocompromised develop severe infection, even invasive infections with eye, mouth, and brain extensions. Culture of the nasal mucosa is not helpful in determining the causative agent in sinusitis. If the patient is not responding to therapy, sinus aspiration or endoscopic aspiration is the only accurate way to determine the organism involved; both procedures require referral to an otolaryngologist.

Goals of Treatment

The overall goal for the treatment of sinusitis is absence of infection, demonstrated by the patient's freedom from all symptoms of a sinus infection.

Rational Drug Selection

Given the most likely organisms to be found in both children and adults, the first choice for antibiotic therapy in acute sinusitis is amoxicillin with or without clavulanate (Chow et al,

2012; Wald et al, 2013). The Infectious Disease Society of America recommends prescribing standard-dose amoxicillin-clavulanate for bacterial sinusitis and high-dose amoxicillin-clavulanate (2 g orally twice daily or 90 mg/kg/d orally twice daily) in patient at risk for resistance (age younger than 2 years or older than 65 years, recent hospitalization or antimicrobial use, day care attendance) (Chow et al, 2012). The AAP guidelines recommend standard-dose amoxicillin (45 mg/kg/d) as first-line therapy unless the local resistance pattern for *S. pneumonia* is greater than 10%; then high-dose amoxicillin is prescribed (Wald et al, 2013). Amoxicillin is inexpensive and well tolerated (Table 46-2). For adults, the dose is 500 mg given 3 times a day, and in children, the daily dose is 45 mg/kg/d for standard dose and 80 to 90 mg/kg/d for high dose, divided in two to three doses. The usual length of treatment is 5 to 7 days in adults and 10 to 14 days in children (Chow et al, 2012).

Table 46–2 ❖ Drugs Commonly Used: Sinusitis and Otitis Media

Drug	Dose	Length of Treatment	Strengths Available	Comments
Amoxicillin (Amoxil, Trimox)	*Adults and children >20 kg:* 500 mg q8h *Children:* 80–90 mg/kg/d divided in 3 doses	Sinusitis: 10–14 days or until 7 d after symptom-free (may need 21 d of treatment) Otitis media: 7–10 d; children <2 yr: 10 d	Capsules: 250, 500 mg Chewable tablets: 125, 200, 250, 400 mg Powder for suspension: 50, 125, 200, 250, 400 mg/5 mL	First choice for non–penicillin allergic patients. Higher doses may be used for children who have recently been on antibiotics or in day care, up to 90 mg/kg/d.
Amoxicillin and clavulanate (Augmentin)	*Adults:* 500 mg q12h or 250 mg q8h *Children <3 mo:* 30 mg/kg/d of amoxicillin divided q12h *Children >3 mo, <40 kg:* 25–45 mg/kg/d of amoxicillin divided q12h (use 200 mg/5 mL or 400 mg/5 mL suspension) *or* 20–45 mg/kg/d of amoxicillin if using 125 mg/5 mL or 250/5 mL suspension dosed every 8 h. Drug-resistance dosing: 80–90 mg/kg/d divided every 12 h. Use Augmentin ES or a 7:1 bid formulation.	5–14 d for all patients	Tablets: 250 mg amoxicillin & 125 mg clavulanate; 500 mg amoxicillin & 125 mg clavulanate; 875 mg amoxicillin & 125 mg clavulanate Chewable tablets: 125 mg amoxicillin & 31.25 mg clavulanate; 200 mg amoxicillin & 28.5 mg clavulanate; 250 mg amoxicillin & 62.5 mg clavulanate; 400 mg amoxicillin & 57 mg clavulanate Suspension: 125 mg amoxicillin & 31.25 mg clavulanate/5 mL; 200 mg amoxicillin & 28.5 mg clavulanate/5 mL; 250 mg amoxicillin & 62.5 mg clavulanate/5 mL; 400 mg amoxicillin & 57 mg clavulanate/5 mL; 400 mg amoxicillin & 57 mg clavulanate (Augmentin ES = 600) amoxicillin 600 mg/5 mL and 42.9 mg clavulanate/5 mL (Augmentin ES = 600) amoxicillin 600 mg/5 mL & 42.9 mg clavulanate/5 mL	Children's dose is based on amoxicillin content. Because of the clavulanate content, two 250 mg tablets are *not* the same as one 500 mg tablet. Because of the different clavulanate levels in the suspensions, it is not appropriate to dose the 125 mg/5 mL or the 250 mg/5 mL suspensions bid. Children should not be given the 250 mg tablet until they are >40 kg. High-dose amoxicillin/ clavulanate requires use of a formula of 600 mg amoxicillin/ 42.9 mg clavulanate per 5 mL.
Cefdinir (Omnicef)	*Adults ≥13 yr:* 300 mg q12h or 600 mg q24h *Children:* 14 mg/kg/d in 1 or 2 doses	AOM: 5–10 d Sinusitis: 10 d	Capsules: 300 mg Suspension: 125 mg/5 mL 250 mg/5 mL	Do not use for type 1 Penicillin = allergic patients (urticaria of anaphylaxis). Adjust dosing for renal insufficiency.
Cefpodoxime (Vantin)	*Adults:* 200 mg q12h *Children:* 10 mg/kg/d divided q12h (max dose 400 mg)	5–14 d	Tablets: 100 mg, 200 mg Suspension: 50 mg/5 mL, 100 mg/5 mL	Broad spectrum

Continued

Table 46–2 ❀ Drugs Commonly Used: Sinusitis and Otitis Media—cont'd

Drug	Dose	Length of Treatment	Strengths Available	Comments
Cefprozil (Cefzil)	*Adults and children >12 yr:* 500 mg q12h *Children:* 30 mg/kg/d divided into 2 doses 12 h apart	10–14 d	Tablets: 250 mg, 500 mg Suspension: 125 mg/5 mL, 250 mg/5 mL	Broad-spectrum coverage
Ceftibuten (Cedax)	*Adults:* 400 mg once daily *Children:* 9 mg/kg/d in 1 daily dose	10 d	Tablets: 400 mg Suspension: 90 mg/5 mL, 180 mg/5 mL	Must be given on an empty stomach.
Ceftriaxone (Rocephin)	*Children:* 50 mg/kg given as 1 IM dose (maximum of 1 g/dose)	One dose only	Powder for injection: 250 mg, 500 mg, 1 g	May be used as 1-time dose for otitis media in children. Very expensive compared with amoxicillin. Broad spectrum
Cefuroxime (Ceftin)	*Adults and children >12 yr:* 250 mg or 500 mg q12h *Children:* 30 mg/kg/d given q12h up to 1,000 mg/d	10 d	Tablets: 125, 250, 500 mg Suspension: 125 mg/5 mL Note: Tablets and suspension are *not* bio-equivalent and are *not* substitutable on a mg-for-mg basis	Prolonged half-life in patients with renal failure. Suspension must be given with food. Broad spectrum Expensive

The AAP guidelines include the option of observing the patient for 3 days before starting antibiotics (Wald et al, 2013). Antibiotics are started if there is no improvement in symptoms or if the patient worsens during the observation period.

If the adult patient is allergic to penicillin, doxycycline (100 mg PO bid or 200 mg daily) or a respiratory fluoroquinolone, such as levofloxacin (500 mg daily) or moxifloxacin (400 mg daily) may be prescribed. Children with penicillin allergy may be treated with a third-generation cephalosporin, including cefdinir (14 mg/kg/d), cefuroxime (30 mg/kg/d), or cefpodoxime (10 mg/kg/d).

If the patient is worsening or not improving after 72 hours, bacterial resistance needs to be considered. For sinusitis that fails to improve after a week of first-line therapy, the drugs of choice are high-dose amoxicillin-clavulanate (Augmentin) or in adults a respiratory fluoroquinolone (levofloxacin, moxifloxacin) (Chow et al, 2012; Wald et al, 2013). Fluoroquinolones should not be prescribed for children or adolescents because of the potential for adverse reactions, which is discussed further in Chapter 24. Children treated with amoxicillin who fail to improve are treated with high-dose amoxicillin-clavulanate (80 to 90 mg/kg/d of amoxicillin component), cefdinir (14 mg/kg/d), cefuroxime (30 mg/kg/d), or cefpodoxime (10 mg/kg/d) (Wald et al, 2013). Failure to respond indicates either misdiagnosis of sinusitis or resistance. Although radiological evaluation is not indicated in patients initially diagnosed with sinusitis, failure to improve warrants either computed tomography (CT) or MRI to confirm diagnosis. Consultation with an otolaryngologist may also be warranted to determine the need for sinus aspiration to guide antimicrobial choice (Chow et al, 2012; Wald et al, 2013).

Chronic sinusitis is defined by 8 to 12 weeks of symptoms and the documentation of inflammation either by examination or radiographic findings (Desrosiers et al, 2011; Rosenfeld et al, 2014). Amoxicillin-clavulanate is the drug of choice in chronic sinusitis; adults may also be treated with a respiratory fluoroquinolone. Patients with chronic sinusitis may also need a short course of inhaled or oral corticosteroids, both of which have no proven efficacy in acute sinusitis (Chan & Kuhn, 2009; Desrosiers et al, 2011). Hypertonic or isotonic saline washes are a critical part of chronic sinusitis treatment. Patients who fail to respond to antibiotics may need referral to an otolaryngologist. Other causes for chronic sinusitis need to be considered, including allergies and immunodeficiency (Rosenfeld et al, 2014). Figure 46-1 provides an algorithm for the treatment of sinusitis.

Monitoring

Patients who are being treated with antibiotics for sinusitis need to be monitored for adverse reactions to the antibiotics and for their response to treatment. They should begin to respond in 3 to 4 days. If there is no improvement in clinical symptoms, then bacterial resistance must be considered.

Outcome Evaluation

Sinusitis symptoms should resolve after 7 days of treatment. Chronic or recurrent sinusitis requires a referral to an otolaryngologist. Often, surgical intervention is needed to provide adequate drainage from the sinuses. Untreated sinusitis can lead to invasive disease such as orbital cellulitis or brain involvement. These are both medical emergencies and fortunately rare, usually seen only in immunocompromised patients. As with viral URIs, acute or chronic sinusitis may exacerbate asthma.

Patient Education

Nonprescription management includes decongestants, either topical or systemic, to improve nasal obstruction. Patients

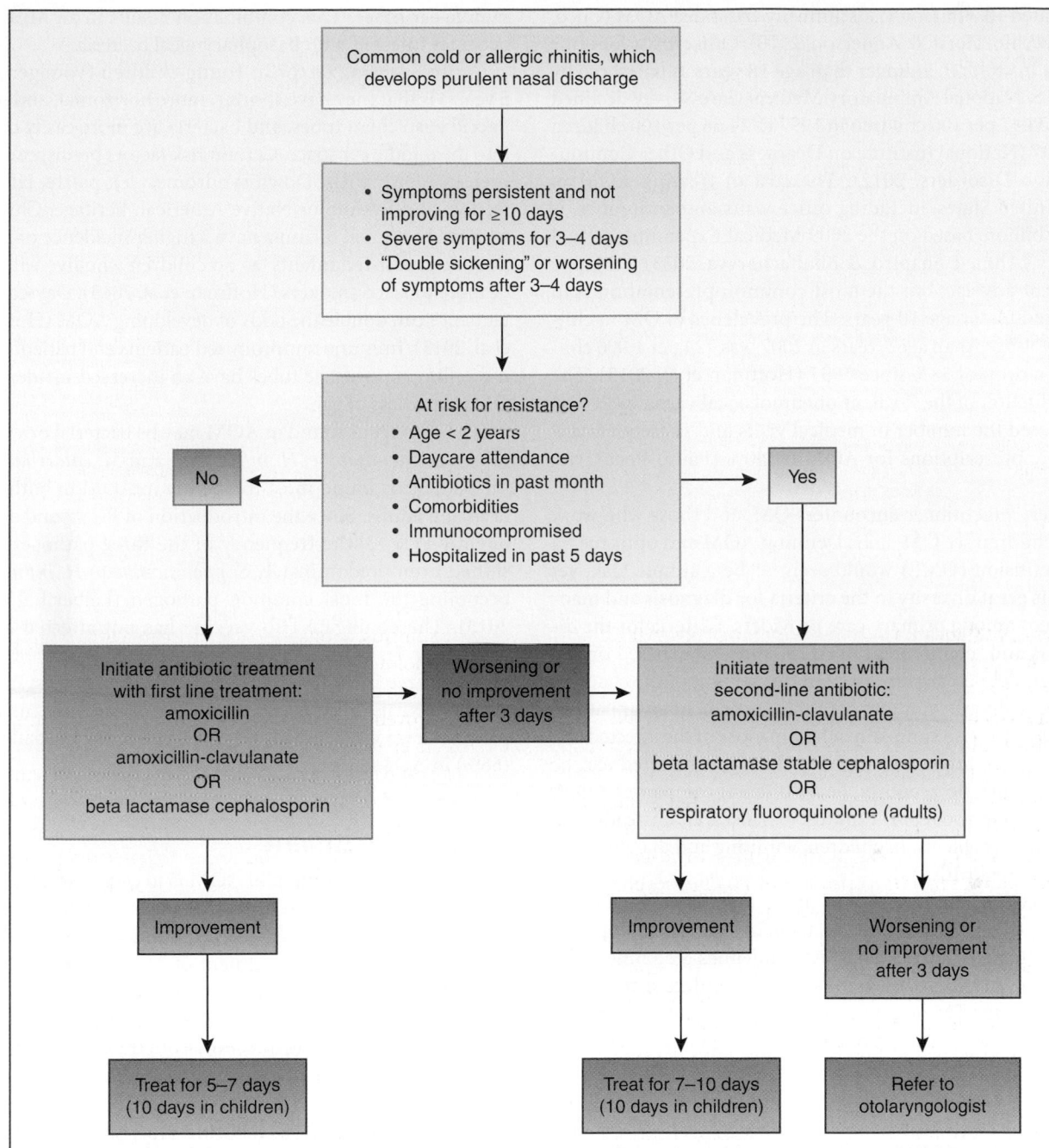

Figure 46–1. Algorithm for treatment of sinusitis.

should be warned against long-term use of topical decongestants, but they can be very helpful in providing symptomatic relief during the few days it takes to respond to antibiotics. Saline nasal spray or wash prevents crusting of secretions in the nasal cavity, facilitating removal of secretions. Adequate hydration is essential in liquefying secretions. The facial pain and headache associated with sinusitis can be severe, and the patient should be encouraged to take acetaminophen or ibuprofen for pain. A warm pack to the frontal and maxillary sinuses often provides pain relief. Running a humidifier at night can alleviate the dry mouth caused by mouth breathing during sleep. Breathing in hot steam often helps clear nasal passages, but caution patients about burns.

Sinusitis causes the air passages in the sinuses to become swollen and blocked and to trap air. Therefore, sinusitis poses a hazard to patients who dive because of the changing air pressures in the sinuses, and diving is contraindicated. Patients who are planning to fly or to drive over mountain ranges can use topical decongestants prior to the trip to prevent the pain associated with the changing air pressures in the air trapped in the sinuses.

OTITIS MEDIA

The most common reason for which children in the United States receive antibiotics is acute otitis media (AOM); an estimated 10.3 million visits annually are coded AOM (Coco, Vernacchio, Horst, & Anderson, 2010). Office visits for otitis media in children younger than age 18 years as measured by the U.S. National Ambulatory Medical Care Survey declined from 34.47 per 100 children in 1997 to 24.66 per 100 children in 2007 (National Institute on Deafness and Other Communication Disorders, 2012). The cost of treating AOM in the United States, including office visits and antibiotics, is $2.88 billion, based on the 2009 Medical Expenditure Panel Survey (Ahmed, Shapiro, & Bhattacharyya, 2013). OM may occur at any age, but the most common presentation is in children under age 10 years. The prevalence of OM in children younger than age 3 years in 2007 was 724 per 1,000 children, a drop of 38% since 1997 (Hoffman et al, 2013). The introduction of the 7-valent pneumococcal vaccine (PCV7) decreased the number of medical visits and subsequent antibiotic prescriptions for AOM by 40% (Falup-Pecurariu, 2012).

Every practitioner encounters OM, and those who work with children see OM daily. Defining AOM and otitis media with effusion (OME) would seem to be a simple task, yet there is great diversity in the criteria for diagnosis and management among primary care providers. Criteria for the diagnosis and management of AOM and OME, based on the AAP guidelines, are discussed in this section of the chapter.

The hallmark symptom of OM is ear pain, often unilateral. Patients may also complain of hearing loss in the affected ear. Preverbal children may tug or poke at the affected ear, be irritable, and sleep poorly. Fever often accompanies AOM. Patients may also report tinnitus, dizziness, an unsteady gait, or balance problems. In children, vomiting and diarrhea may be associated with OM.

According to the AAP guidelines, the diagnosis of AOM is a clinical one based on a spectrum of signs and symptoms (Lieberthal et al, 2013). The AAP guidelines recommend diagnosing AOM in children with (1) moderate to severe bulging of the TM or new onset of otorrhea not due to acute otitis externa or (2) mild bulging of the TM and recent (less than 48 hours) onset of ear pain or intense erythema of the TM; and (3) no diagnosis of AOM in children who do not have middle ear effusion (MEE) (Lieberthal et al, 2013). OME is fluid in the middle ear without any signs or symptoms of acute illness. Erythema is nonspecific, and AOM should never be diagnosed on the basis of tympanic membrane (TM) color alone, as the TM can redden from crying or a fever. Fluid in the middle ear (MEE) is assessed by observing white or yellow fluid, observing the air/fluid level, observing air bubbles, or noting decreased TM movement via pneumatic otoscopy. A thin-walled bulla is seen with bullous myringitis, a very painful form of AOM.

Pathophysiology

AOM occurs when there is a combination of eustachian tube dysfunction, which blocks the flow of secretions from the middle ear to the pharynx, and negative pressure developing in the middle ear, which causes reflux of bacteria into the middle ear space. This combination results in an MEE that becomes infected with nasopharyngeal bacteria.

A predisposing factor in young children (younger than 5 years) is that they have shorter, more horizontal, and more flaccid eustachian tubes, and bacteria are more easily drawn into the middle ear space. Certain risk factors predispose children to AOM: URIs, Down syndrome, cleft palate, HIV infection, and Eskimo or Native American heritage. Children who are bottle-fed formula have a higher incidence of AOM than do breast-fed infants, as do children who live with one or more tobacco smokers (Hoffman et al, 2013). Day-care attendance can double the odds of developing AOM (Hoffman et al, 2013). Immunocompromised patients and patients with indwelling nasogastric tubes have an increased incidence of OM, regardless of age.

The pathogens found in AOM may be bacterial or viral in origin. *S. pneumoniae, H. influenzae,* and *M. catarrhalis* are the pathogens found most frequently in AOM in both children and adults. Since the introduction of PCV7 and subsequently PCV13, the frequency of the three pathogens has shifted from predominately *S. pneumoniae* to *H. influenzae* becoming the most common pathogen (Leiberthal et al, 2013). The conjugate Hib vaccine has not affected AOM caused by *H. influenzae* because approximately 90% of *H. influenzae* in AOM is nontypeable. Viruses (respiratory syncytial virus, rhinovirus, coronavirus, adenovirus, and parainfluenza virus) are found alone (4%) or as a copathogen (66%) in AOM cases (Lieberthal et al, 2013).

Goals of Treatment

The goal for the treatment of AOM is to clear infection from the middle ear fluid with the use of antibiotics. If the antibiotic chosen is effective against the pathogen, then the infection clears. Because the treatment of AOM is empiric based on the most commonly found pathogens, a change of antibiotic is necessary at times to treat the infection. The goal remains the same: clearing infection from the middle ear fluid.

Rational Drug Selection

Guidelines

There is much controversy regarding the treatment of OM. In 2004, the AAP and the AAFP issued a joint clinical practice guideline for the diagnosis and treatment of AOM, which provides an evidence-based approach to caring for the child aged 2 months to 12 years with uncomplicated AOM. The guideline was updated by the AAP in 2013 (Leiberthal et al, 2013).

The AAP recommendations are the following:

1. Diagnosis of AOM includes the following criteria: spectrum of symptoms: (1) moderate to severe bulging of the TM or new onset of otorrhea not due to acute otitis externa; (2) mild bulging of the TM and recent (less than 48 hours) onset of ear pain or intense erythema of the TM; and (3) no diagnosis of AOM in children who do not have middle ear effusion (MEE).

2. Pain must be assessed and adequate pain management provided.

3a. Antibiotic therapy should be prescribed for severe AOM in children aged 6 months or older. Symptoms of severe AOM include: moderate or severe otalgia, otalgia for at least 48 hours, or temperature great than 39°C (102.2°F).

3b. Antibiotics should be prescribed for nonsevere bilateral AOM in young children (6 months to 23 months).

3c. For nonsevere unilateral AOM in children 6 to 23 months of age, an antibiotic or initial observation may be prescribed with close follow-up within 48 to 72 hours, based on a joint decision with the parent(s) or caregiver. Antibiotic therapy is started if the child worsens or fails to improve in 48 to 72 hours.

3d. An antibiotic or observation should be offered for nonsevere AOM (unilateral or bilateral) in children age 24 months or older based on joint decision making with the parent(s) or caregiver. Antibiotic therapy is started if the child worsens or fails to improve in 48 to 72 hours.

4a. If treating with an antibiotic, amoxicillin is the first choice for most children if they have not received amoxicillin in the last 30 days. Amoxicillin should be dosed at 80 to 90 mg/kg/d. Patients with penicillin allergy may be treated with cefdinir (14 mg/kg/d), cefuroxime (30 mg/kg/d divided bid), cefpodoxime (10 mg/kg/d divided bid), or ceftriaxone (50 mg/d IM or IV for 1 to 3 days).

4b. Patients who have had amoxicillin in the past 30 days, those with concurrent conjunctivitis, or those who warrant coverage for beta lactamase–positive *H. influenzae* and *M. catarrhalis*, should be prescribed amoxicillin-clavulanate (90 mg/kg/d of amoxicillin and 6.4 mg/kg/d of clavulanate in two divided doses) as the drug of choice.

4c. If the patient fails to respond to an initial management option (3a, 3b, or 3c) within 48 to 72 hours, the clinician must reassess the patient to confirm AOM and exclude other causes of illness. If initially managed with observation, then antibiotics should be started. If an antibiotic was initially prescribed, then the antibiotic should be changed.

5. Clinicians should encourage prevention of AOM according to the Advisory Committee on Immunization Practices (ACIP) through the reduction of risk factors such as recommending pneumococcal conjugate vaccine and annual influenza vaccine to all children, breastfeeding for the first 6 months of life, and reducing exposure to tobacco smoke.

Figure 46-2 provides an algorithm for treating OM.

Antimicrobial Resistance

The emergence of antimicrobial resistance among respiratory pathogens has caused primary care providers to reevaluate their routine use of antibiotics for all illnesses, especially OM.

Almost 100% of *M. catarrhalis* produces beta lactamase, which can be resistant to amoxicillin and other penicillins (AAP, 2012b). *H. influenzae,* another beta lactamase producer, is 30% to 40% resistant to amoxicillin (AAP, 2012c). At one point in the early 2000s, up to 20% of *S. pneumoniae* was resistant and 20% was intermediately resistant to penicillin, but more recent studies indicate 92% of pneumococci is susceptible to penicillin (Centers for Disease Control and Prevention, 2008). The decrease in resistance is the reason amoxicillin remains the first-line treatment for acute otitis media.

S. pneumoniae is also resistant to the common macrolides erythromycin (35.3% resistance), azithromycin (35.3% resistance), and clarithromycin (35.2% resistance) (Jenkins & Ferrell, 2009). Resistant *S. pneumoniae* is more common among children who are in day care, have recurrent AOM, are younger than 2 years, or have been recently treated with beta lactamase antibiotics (Leiberthal et al, 2013). In light of this increasing resistance among common OM pathogens, the provider needs to decide carefully whether an antibiotic is necessary and, in the case of treatment failure, consider the possibility of resistant bacterial strains. The common antibiotics and their dosages used for OM are listed in Table 46-2.

Dosing Regimen

Amoxicillin remains the first-line drug of choice for AOM in spite of resistance per the AAP guidelines for the management of AOM (Lieberthal, et al, 2013). Amoxicillin is dosed at 80 to 90 mg/kg/d, which raises the concentration in the middle ear fluid to be effective against intermediate and resistant strains of *S. pneumoniae.* Conversely, patients who have had repeated episodes of AOM or have been on antibiotics in the past 30 days should be treated with beta lactamase–stable amoxicillin/clavulanate or beta lactamase–stable cephalosporin if allergic to penicillin. Table 46-3 discusses antibiotic treatment options for AOM in patients who have been on antibiotics recently.

Length of Treatment

Length of treatment has also been investigated in recent years. In the United States, AOM has traditionally been treated for 10 days with antibiotics. There are few controlled studies to support the practice. Compliance and completion of the 10-day regimen have also been an issue. A number of studies have compared outcomes after 5 or 7 days of antibiotics versus 10 days. For patients over age 5 years, a shortened 5-day course of treatment is probably adequate (Lieberthal et al, 2013). Children age 2 to 5 years may be treated for 7 days, and children under age 2 years or with severe symptoms are treated for 10 days (Leiberthal et al, 2013).

Watchful Waiting (No Antibiotics)

With the guidelines recommending a period of "watchful waiting" for 48 to 72 hours in low-risk patients, providers must have confidence in their decision to not treat with antibiotics. Providers are concerned not only about the prudence

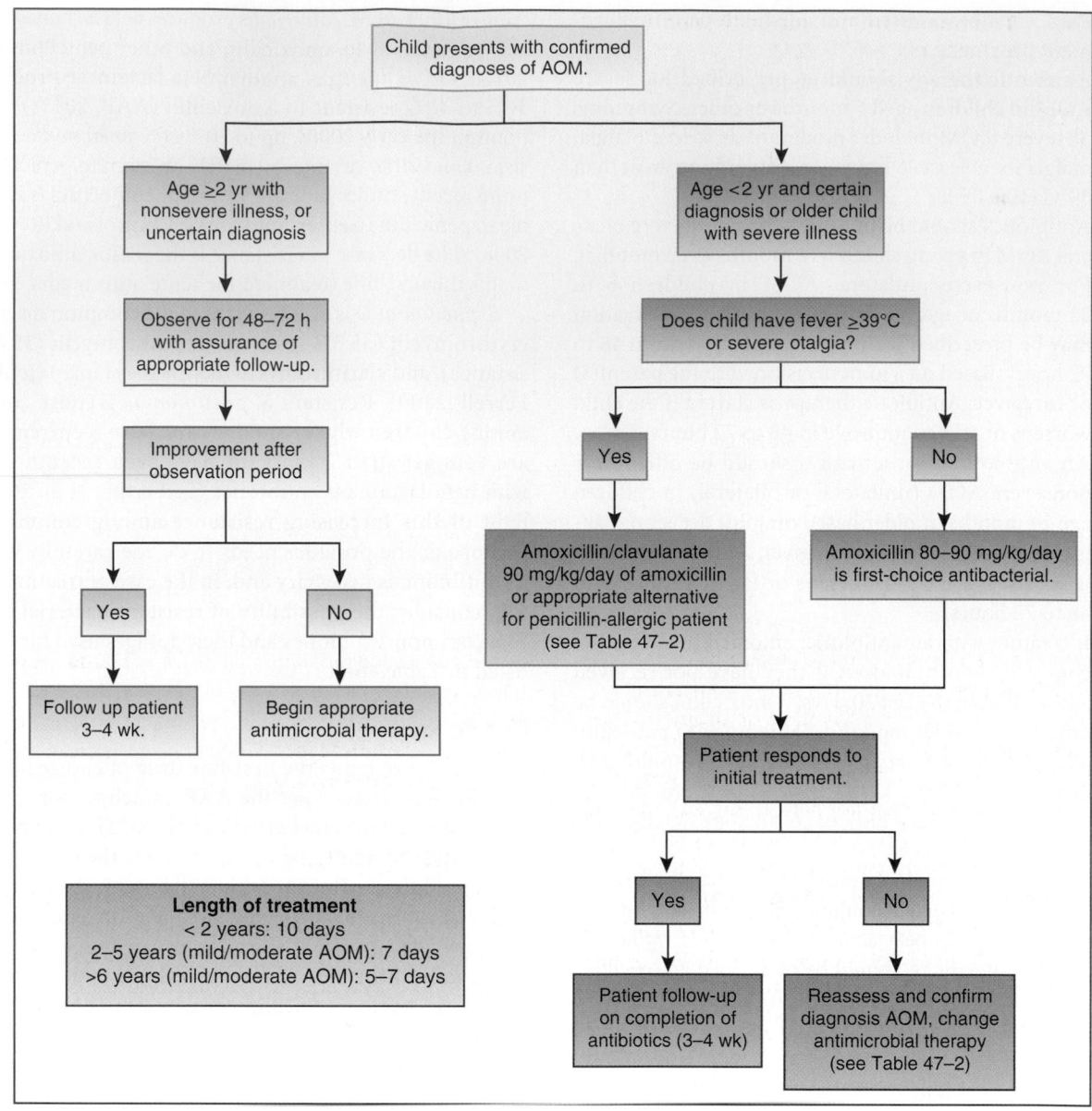

Figure 46–2. Algorithm for treatment of AOM.

of the treatment but also about the acceptance of watchful waiting by parents of children with OM.

Acceptance of watchful waiting among parents of children with AOM has been evaluated. A *Cochrane Review* of 10 studies examining delayed antibiotics for respiratory infections including AOM indicates delayed antibiotic prescription slightly reduces parent satisfaction compared to immediate antibiotics (87% versus 92%) (Spurling, Del Mar, Dooley, & Foxlee, 2007). A study examining the AAP recommendation of watchful waiting indicates that although antibiotic prescribing in children under age 2 years decreased 21% to 26%, parental sick days increased 13% to 14% (Meropol, Glick, & Asch, 2008). The increase in parental sick days may be a reason for decreased parental satisfaction with watchful waiting.

Providing a "safety-net" prescription for parents to fill after an initial period of observation or watchful waiting is an option for the treatment of AOM. Initial observation of

AOM for 48 to 72 hours has been a recommendation of the Dutch College of General Practitioners for almost 30 years (Culpepper & Froom, 1997). Using these guidelines, Dutch children have outcomes at 2 months similar to those of children from other countries treated with antibiotics. Meropol and colleagues (2008) found that using the watchful waiting approach reduced antibiotic use 67% in children aged 2 to 12 years. The pediatric provider needs to educate parents about the rationale for initial observation of AOM and provide adequate pain relief during the observation period to ensure success with this approach.

Pain Relief

Regardless of whether the patient receives antibiotics, all children require pain relief for the first 24 to 72 hours of treatment. Adequate dosing of acetaminophen (15 mg/kg per dose) or ibuprofen (5 to 10 mg/kg per dose) is necessary.

Table 46–3 Treatment Options for Otitis Media

Temperature >39°C (102.2°F) and Severe Otalgia; or <age 2 years	Initial Treatment	Alternative Treatment (if Penicillin Allergy)	Antibiotic Treatment After 48–72 h of Failure of Initial Antibiotic Treatment
No	High-dose amoxicillin (80–90 mg/kg/d in 2 divided doses)		Amoxicillin-clavulanatea (90 mg/kg/d of amoxicillin, with 6.4 mg/kg/dof clavulanate [amoxicillin to clavulanate ratio, 14:1] in 2 divided doses)
		Cefuroxime, Cefdinir	
		Cefpodoxime	
		Cefriaxone (IM)	
		Cefixime	
Yes	High-dose amoxicillin/ clavulanate (80–90 mg/kg/d)	IM ceftriaxone OR Clindamycin (30–40 mg/kg per day in 3 divided doses) plus third-generation cephalosporin	IM ceftriaxone × 3 d or tympanocentesis

Source: From Lieberthal et al, 2013.

It is the provider's responsibility to determine the dose of analgesic that ensures adequate pain relief. Topical analgesia (Auralgan otic solution, a combination of antipyrine, benzocaine, and u-polycosanol 410 otic solution) can be applied. In a study of children aged 5 years or older who were being adequately dosed with acetaminophen (15 mg/kg), the study patients who received Auralgan reported lower ear pain scores than did the control group who received the placebo (olive oil). A number of the study patients reported dramatic and immediate reductions in pain (Hoberman, Paradise, Reynolds, & Urkin, 1997). Some providers stock Auralgan in the clinic to provide immediate pain relief for their OM patients. Auralgan should never be used before the provider observes an intact TM.

Monitoring

Monitoring the effectiveness of the treatment chosen, either to prescribe antibiotics or to provide symptomatic care for the first 2 to 3 days, is essential to the optimal outcome for the patient. Patients may still experience pain with OME, even if the appearance of the TM improves. Patients with persistent symptoms or failure to improve in 48 to 72 hours should be reexamined to determine whether the initial plan (whether antibiotics were prescribed or not) needs to be reevaluated (Leiberthal et al, 2013).

If symptoms resolve, patients younger than 2 years of age should be reexamined in 8 to 12 weeks after beginning antibiotics, with the understanding that, at 4 weeks, there is a 40% chance that fluid is still present in the middle ear and that effusions can last up to 3 months (Leiberthal et al, 2013). Older children (older than 2 years) without language or learning problems can be followed at their next scheduled well-child exam, or sooner if there are concerns (Klein & Pelton, 2009). Older children with known language or learning problems should be examined 8 to 12 weeks after the AOM.

Antibiotics are not appropriate for the initial treatment of OME, and there is controversy regarding their use at all for this indication, even after 3 months of persistent effusion. Persistent effusion beyond 3 months is an indication for a referral to an otolaryngologist.

Outcome Evaluation

The patient should be evaluated 8 to 12 weeks from the beginning of treatment to determine if the infection is completely resolved. The provider may choose to evaluate the patient sooner, with the understanding that some MEE may remain.

Patient Education

Two areas have to be covered in educating patients and families about the use of antibiotics for AOM: the proper use of the prescribed antibiotic and the predicted course of the infection once antibiotics are started. The instructions regarding the antibiotic dosage and timing of doses must be clear, and any questions regarding the medication answered. Expected adverse reactions, such as the mild diarrhea that may accompany many of the antibiotics, must be discussed. Patients and family members should be aware that the expected course of the ear infection, once antibiotics are started, is some symptomatic relief in 24 to 48 hours. Use of acetaminophen or ibuprofen for pain relief is necessary during this initial period to provide comfort. Parents should be encouraged to give their children a dose of ibuprofen or acetaminophen just before bedtime because children seem to complain of greater ear pain at night during the healing stages. Patients who are still having significant pain after 48 hours should be reexamined for the possibility of a resistant organism. Bacterial resistance ought to be mentioned, and the patient should be encouraged to complete the course of medication to prevent the development of antibacterial resistance to a partially treated organism.

OTITIS EXTERNA

OE (external OM) is an acute infection that causes an inflammatory reaction in the external auditory canal. It is also known as swimmer's ear.

The patient generally presents with severe ear pain, which may have begun as itching and irritation. The pain is generally unilateral and localized to the ear. Manipulation of the pinna or tragus causes moderate to severe pain, a finding that is usually absent in OM. The TM is normal in OE, but the external auditory canal may be swollen such that the TM is difficult to visualize. Malignant OE is found in patients with diabetes and presents as severe cellulitis due to *Pseudomonas aeruginosa.*

Pathophysiology

Trauma or prolonged exposure to moisture predisposes to infection. The chlorine in swimming pools kills the normal flora in the external ear canal, which allows growth of pathogens. The most common organism found is *P. aeruginosa,* followed by *Staphylococcus aureus.*

Goals of Treatment

The goal of treatment of OE is resolution of the infection, pain control, and prevention of recurrence.

Rational Drug Selection

Topical therapy delivers a high concentration of the antimicrobial to the infected tissue, significantly more than can be delivered via systemic antimicrobial treatment (Rosenfeld et al, 2014). The medications used in the treatment of OE include combination products (Cortisporin, Cipro HC) that contain a corticosteroid (hydrocortisone) and antibiotic(s) (neomycin, polymyxin B, ciprofloxacin), antibiotic alone (gentamicin, ofloxacin), and acetic acid or alcohol drops (Otic Domeboro, Burow's Otic, Vosol, Vosol HC).

The medication of choice is antibiotic/steroid eardrops, which combine an antibiotic(s) and an anti-inflammatory such as neomycin sulfate, polymyxin B, and hydrocortisone (Cortisporin Otic); ciprofloxacin and hydrocortisone (Cipro HC Otic); or ciprofloxacin and dexamethasone (Ciprodex). Eyedrops can be used for external otitis, including tobramycin and dexamethasone (Tobradex eyedrops), gentamicin and prednisolone (Pred-G), and sulfacetamide and prednisolone (Vasocidin solution).

Acid and alcohol solutions may also be used. Common products are Otic Domeboro and Burow's Otic, which contain 2% acetic acid in aluminum acetate solution. Another acid solution, Vosol Otic, contains 2% acetic acid solution and 3% propylene glycol. These solutions reduce inflammation and are antibacterial and antifungal.

Treatment consists of irrigation and antibiotic eardrops. The medication of choice is antibiotic/steroid eardrops, with cost and convenient dosing factored into decision making because all are equally effective (Rosenfeld et al, 2014). The routine dosing is three to four drops administered 4 times a day. Suspension formulations are less ototoxic than solution preparations of eardrops. A cotton wick may be necessary if the ear canal is extremely swollen. For severe cellulitis, parenteral antistaphylococcal and antipseudomonal antibiotics are necessary. Pain can be severe but patients should have relief with topical therapy and should only need NSAIDs for pain. Some patients with severe pain may need a combination product that contains an opioid (oxycodone or hydrocodone) in the short term to provide relief of pain while undergoing treatment (Rosenfeld et al, 2014).

Monitoring

The patient should begin to experience relief from pain in 3 or 4 days. Reevaluation in 1 week determines if the patient is clinically improving. Referral to a dermatologist or otolaryngologist may be necessary if there is no improvement or if symptoms worsen in spite of treatment.

Outcome Evaluation

To evaluate the effectiveness of OE treatment, the provider determines if the infection is resolved after treatment with antibiotic/steroid eardrops.

Patient Education

Educate the patient to prevent OE by avoiding pooling of water in the ears and by using a mildly acidic solution after swimming. Patients can instill three to four drops of a 1:1 solution of water and white vinegar or 70% ethyl alcohol. Commercially available products (EarSol, Swim-Ear) can also be used. Earplugs may be helpful for avoiding developing external otitis.

Explain proper irrigation of debris prior to instillation of eardrops to ensure that the medication contacts the affected area. Swimming should be avoided until external otitis has cleared, ideally for 7 to 10 days (Rosenfeld et al, 2014). Monitoring for increasing severity is essential to detect cellulitis early in the diabetic patient. The patient may take ibuprofen or another analgesic for the first 24 to 48 hours of treatment to provide pain relief.

REFERENCES

Ahmed, S., Shapiro, N. L., & Bhattacharyya, N. (2013). Incremental health care utilization and costs for acute otitis media in children. *The Laryngoscope, 124*(1), 301–305.

American Academy of Pediatrics (AAP). (2012a). Rhinovirus infections. In L. K. Pickering (Ed.), *Red book: 2012 Report of the Committee on Infectious Diseases* (29th ed., pp 619–620). Elk Grove Village, IL: American Academy of Pediatrics. Retrieved from http://aapredbook.aappublications.org/content/1/SEC131/SEC250.body

American Academy of Pediatrics (AAP). (2012b). *Moraxella cararrhalis* infections. In L. K. Pickering (Ed.), *Red book: 2012 Report of the Committee on Infectious Diseases* (29th ed., p 513). Elk Grove Village, IL: American Academy of Pediatrics. Retrieved from http://aapredbook.aappublications.org/content/1/SEC131/SEC221.body

American Academy of Pediatrics (AAP). (2012c). *Haemophilus influenzae* infections. In L. K. Pickering (Ed.), *Red book: 2012 Report of the Committee on Infectious Diseases* (29th ed., pp 345–352). Elk Grove Village, IL: American Academy of Pediatrics. Retrieved from http://aapredbook .aappublications.org/content/1/SEC131/SEC186.body

Caruso, T. J., Prober, C. G., & Gwaltney, J. M. (2007). Treatment of naturally acquired common colds with zinc: A structured review. *Clinical Infectious Disease, 45*(5), 569–574.

Centers for Disease Control and Prevention (CDC). (2008). Effects of new penicillin susceptibility breakpoints for Streptococci pneumonia—United States, 2006–2007. *Morbidity and Mortality Weekly Report, 57*(50), 1353–1355.

Chow, A. W., Benninger, M. S., Brook, I., Brozek, J. L., Goldstein, E. J. C., Hicks, L. A., et al. (2012). ISDA clinical practice guideline for acute bacterial rhinosinusitis in children and adults. *Clinical Infectious Disease, 54*(8):e72–e112. doi: 10.1093/cid/cir1043.

Coco, A., Vernacchio, L., Horst, M., & Anderson, A. (2010). Management of acute otitis media after publication of the 2004 AAP and AAFP clinical practice guideline. *Pediatrics, 125*(2), 214–220.

Desrosiers, M., Evans, G. A., Keith, P. K., Wright, E. D., Kaplan, A., Bouchard, J., et al. (2011). Canadian clinical practice guidelines for acute and chronic rhinosinusitis. *Allergy, Asthma & Clinical Immunology,* 7(2), 1-38 doi:10.1186/1710-1492-7-2

DeSutter, A., van Driel, M., Kumar, A., Lesslar, O., & Skrt, A. (2012). Oral antihistamine-decongestant-analgesic combinations for the common cold. *Cochrane Database of Systematic Reviews (Online), 2*CD004976.

Falup-Pecurariu, O. (2012). Lessons learned after the introduction of the seven valent-pneumococcal conjugate vaccine toward broader spectrum conjugate vaccines. *Biomedical Journal, 35*(6), 450–456.

Fendrick, A. M., Monto, A. S., Nightengale, B., & Sarnes, M. (2003). The economic burden of non-influenza-related viral respiratory tract infection in the United States. *Archives of Internal Medicine, 163*(4), 487–494.

Hoffman, H. J., Daly, K. A., Bainbridge, K. E., Casselbrant, M. L. O., Homoe, P., Kvestad, E., et al. (2013). Panel 1: Epidemiology, natural history and risk factors. *Otolaryngology—Head and Neck Surgery, 148*(4S), E1–E25. doi: 10.1177/0194599812460984

Jenkins, S. G., & Farrell, D. J. (2009). Increase in pneumococcus macrolide resistance, United States. *Emerging Infectious Diseases, 15*(8), 1260–1264. Retrieved from http://www.cdc.gov/EID/content/15/8/1260.htm

Lieberthal, A. S., Carroll, A. E., Chonmaitree, T., Ganiats, T. G., Hoberman, A., Jackson, M. A., et al. (2013). Diagnosis and management of acute otitis media, *Pediatrics, 131,* e964–e999.

Marshall I. (2000). Zinc for the common cold. *Cochrane Database Systematic Reviews,* (2):CD001364.

National Institute on Deafness and Other Communication Disorders. (2012). *Ambulatory care visits with a diagnosis of otitis media.* Retrieved from http://www.nidcd.nih.gov/health/statistics/Pages/officevisits.aspx

Pelton, S., & Leibovitz, E. (2009). Recent advances in otitis media. *Pediatric Infectious Disease Journal, 28*(10), S135–S137.

Rosenfeld, R. M., Schwartz, S. R., Cannon, C. R., Roland, P. S., Simon, G. R., Kumar, K. A., et al. (2014). Clinical practice guideline: Acute otitis externa. *Otolaryngology—Head and Neck Surgery, 150*(1S), A1–S24.

Shehab, N., Schaefer, M., Kegler, S., & Budnitz, D. (2010). Adverse events from cough and cold medications after a market withdrawal of products labeled for infants. *Pediatrics, 126*(6), 1100–1107.

Siegel, R. M., Kiely, M., Bien, J. P., Joseph, E. C., Davis, J. B., Mendel, S. G., et al. (2003). Treatment of otitis media with observation and a safety-net antibiotic prescription. *Pediatrics, 112*(3), 527–531.

Taverner, D., & Latte, J. (2007). Nasal decongestants for the common cold. *Cochrane Database of Systematic Reviews (Online),* 1, Art. No.: CD001953.

Wald et al. (2013). Clinical Practice Guideline for the Diagnosis and Management of Acute Bacterial Sinusitis in Children Aged 1 to 18 Years. *Pediatrics,* 132; e262–e280.

URINARY TRACT INFECTIONS

Erin Anderson

U rinary tract infections (UTIs) are responsible for 8.27 million office visits per year (1.41 million men; 6.86 million women) (Litwin & Saigal, 2007). UTIs are more common in women because the short female urethra provides easy access to the bladder for bacteria (Griebling, 2007a). The lifetime risk of a woman developing a UTI is 60.4%, with one-third of women diagnosed with a UTI by age 18 years (Griebling, 2007a). UTIs also occur in men, who have a 13.6% lifetime risk, with most UTIs related to urinary tract obstructions, such as benign prostatic hypertrophy, which is reflected in the increased incidence of UTI as men age (Griebling, 2007b). UTIs affect 2.6% to 3.4% of children annually, with a childhood risk of developing a UTI 2% for boys and 8% for girls (Freedman, 2007). In infant males, circumcision decreases the risk of developing a UTI, with the rate in the first 6 months of life in uncircumcised boys 12 times higher than in circumcised boys (Freedman, 2007). Vesicoureteral reflux, constipation, and dysfunctional voiding all increase the risk for UTI in children (Freedman, 2007).

Most patients with UTIs do not experience long-term complications from these disorders. Those who do usually have a comorbid condition such as vesicoureteral reflux, renal stones, neurogenic bladder, diabetes, or obstruction. This chapter discusses the management of uncomplicated UTIs in otherwise healthy patients who do not have these comorbid conditions and who do not have retention catheters inserted.

PATHOPHYSIOLOGY

A complex interaction between host and microbial factors leads to UTIs. The anatomy and physiology of the genitourinary tract offer protective defenses against UTIs, although certain factors may increase risk for developing a UTI in certain populations. Likewise, behavioral factors may contribute to developing UTIs.

Host Factors

Anatomy and Physiology of the Genitourinary Tract

The bladder has unique intrinsic defenses against infection. Periodic washout, by voiding, of the bacteria that perpetually colonize the urethra is one of the main defense mechanisms. The bladder also deters microbial adherence to the mucosa through the antibacterial properties of the urinary bladder epithelium. Patients who have repeated UTIs appear to have altered bladder epithelial cells that facilitate adherence of bacteria to the mucosa rather than deter it. The low pH and high osmolality of urea and secretions from the uroepithelium and a competent urethral valve that prevents backflow also decrease UTIs. The longer urethra and prostatic secretions decrease the risk of infection in men.

These defense mechanisms are severely limited if residual urine is regularly present after voiding. Pregnancy increases the risk for UTIs because of pressure on the bladder from the enlarging fetus, increased incidence of residual urine, and changes in estrogen levels. Genetic factors, including expression of HLA-A3 and Lewis blood group Le(a–b–) or Le(a+b–), may put women at higher risk for developing UTIs (Griebling, 2007a). Estrogen deficiency and concomitant decreased acidification of the vagina, with increased vaginal colonization by *Enterobacteriaceae*, also contribute to increased risk in postmenopausal women. Men who develop benign prostatic hypertrophy (BPH) are at increased risk of developing a UTI due to bladder outlet obstruction (Griebling, 2007b). Fecal and urinary incontinence, lack of estrogen, immunocompromised states—including diabetes mellitus and taking antibiotics for other infections—have been associated with increased risk in the older adult. Any instrumentation of the urinary tract—including catheter placement or cystoscopy—places patients at risk of developing a UTI (Griebling, 2007b).

Behavioral Factors

Sexually active women are at higher risk than sexually inactive women for developing UTIs. Frequency of sexual intercourse, diaphragm or spermicide use, and failure to void within 10 to 15 minutes of coitus have all been associated with a risk for UTIs in women (Griebling, 2007a). Reasons for the increased risk may be urethral trauma, decreased urge to void, and residual urine. Diaphragm or spermicide use also appears to compromise host defense mechanisms to the extent necessary for virulent strains of bacteria to become capable of causing an infection.

Other behavioral factors have been inconsistently associated with UTI and are subject to some controversy. Purposely resisting the urge to void has been associated with UTIs in some studies and not in others. Increased fluid intake has also had an inconsistent association, although it is difficult to find a reason not to suggest adequate fluid intake for a variety of reasons, including increasing bacterial washout through more frequent voiding. Cranberry juice has an "on-again, off-again" history of association with prevention of UTI (Berger, 2005). A recent *Cochrane Review* states new studies show cranberry products are less effective than previously thought (Jepson, Williams, & Craig, 2012). Little evidence indicates that the direction of wiping after bowel movements, the use of oral contraceptives or tampons, or the habit of taking bubble baths or douching contributes to UTIs.

Microbial Factors

Ability of the Bacteria to Adhere to Epithelial Cells

Escherichia coli is responsible for 85% of community-acquired UTIs and 50% of hospital-acquired UTIs. This organism is successful in part because it contains fimbriae that allow attachment to host cell receptor sites on the bladder mucosa. Some women are thought to be genetically susceptible to certain strains of *E. coli* attachment. Other organisms that commonly infect the urinary tract include *Klebsiella, Proteus* (more common in men), *Pseudomonas,* Enterobacter, and *Staphylococcus saprophyticus.*

Virulence of the Organism

Coliforms cultured from women with recurrent UTIs were more virulent than those cultured from patients with first-time infections or from the fecal flora of patients who had no history of UTIs.

Ability of the Organism to Survive the Urinary Tract Environment

Some bacteria are more tolerant of the low pH of urine. Table 47-1 lists the factors shown by research to be associated with the occurrence of UTIs. It also lists those factors that have been inconsistently related to UTIs or not demonstrated by research to be associated with UTIs.

Inflammatory Reaction to Bacteria

Infection with any organism initiates an inflammatory response and the symptoms of cystitis. The inflammatory edema in the bladder wall stimulates stretch receptors, which discharge with even small volumes of urine, producing the urgency and frequency or urination association with UTIs. Prostaglandins released from the mast cell as part of the inflammatory response produce pain. They also increase vascular permeability, which may be exhibited as hematuria.

Diagnosis of UTI is based on symptoms and laboratory data. Presenting symptoms of UTI vary with age, as shown in Table 47-2. Symptom presentation is similar for both men and women. All ages often exhibit dark, cloudy, and malodorous urine. Urethral discharge in men is more commonly associated with sexually transmitted infections (STIs) than with UTIs. STIs are discussed in Chapter 44.

Laboratory data for diagnosis include urinalysis (UA) and urine culture and sensitivity. The most common findings from a clean-catch urine specimen are (1) a positive leukocyte esterase or pyuria (usually greater than five white blood cells [WBCs] per high-power field), which has a sensitivity range of 90% to 100% and a specificity range of 58% to 91%; (2) the presence of bacteria, which has a sensitivity of approximately 81% and a specificity of approximately 83%; (3) and/or a positive dipstick for nitrates. When all are positive, the sensitivity is 99% to 100% and the specificity is up to 92%. The presence of casts or hematuria suggests an upper UTI.

Quantitative urine cultures are the most reliable method for diagnosing UTIs; however, they require trained personnel, are more expensive, and take time to complete, which might lead to postponing treatment of symptomatic patients. Cultures are usually reserved for children and men and for recurrent UTIs in women. Pregnant women should be screened for bacteriuria by urine culture at least once in early pregnancy because this population is at risk for asymptomatic UTI (Institute for Clinical Systems Improvement [ICSI], 2004; Nicolle et al, 2005). Nicolle and

Table 47–1   Factors Associated With Urinary Tract Infections

Host Factors	Microbial Factors	Inconsistent or Not Associated Factors
Anatomical and Physiological		
• Periodic washout with voiding* • Bladder epithelial cells that prevent adherence of bacteria*	• Ability of the organism to adhere to epithelial cells	• Ingestion of cranberry juice* • Purposely resisting the urge to void • Increased fluid intake* • Wiping from front to back after defecation* • Oral contraceptive use • Tampon use • Bubble baths • Douching
• Acid pH of urine* • Osmolality of urine*	• Virulence of the organism	
• Competent urethral valves to prevent backflow of urine* • Pregnancy • Estrogen deficiency • Residual urine • Lack of circumcision in males • Benign prostate hyperplasia	• Ability of the organism to survive the urinary tract environment	
Behavioral		
• Frequent sexual intercourse • Diaphragm use • Spermicide use • Failure to void 10–15 min after coitus • Multiple sexual partners • Anal intercourse • Fecal and urinary incontinence		

*These factors are negatively associated with UTIs and may prevent them.

Table 47–2   Urinary Tract Infection Symptoms by Age

Neonate	Failure to thrive, irritability, fever, hypothermia, sepsis, jaundice, vomiting, acidosis
Infant	Failure to thrive, irritability, fever, hypothermia, sepsis, jaundice, vomiting, acidosis, hematuria, urinary frequency, dysuria
Preschool- or school-age child	Abdominal or suprapubic pain, dysuria, frequency, urgency, enuresis, urinary incontinence
Adult	• Dysuria, frequency, urgency, burning on urination, incontinence, urethral pain, suprapubic pain, low back pain, hematuria • Significant fever is unusual in bladder infections but may occur, along with severe flank pain and costovertebral tenderness, in upper UTIs • Patients with upper UTIs may also demonstrate headache, malaise, nausea, and vomiting • Symptoms are similar for women and men
Older adult	• Same symptoms as adult, but also mental status changes from patient's norm • Urinary incontinence

colleagues (2005) do not recommend screening for or treatment of asymptomatic bacteriuria for premenopausal, nonpregnant women; diabetic women; older persons living in the community; older adults who are institutionalized; or catheterized patients while the catheter is still in place. Older institutionalized adults who exhibit altered mental status from their norm should be screened for UTI, because this symptom may indicate UTI in the absence of other reported symptoms.

PHARMACODYNAMICS

There is a wide range of antimicrobial agents available for treatment of UTIs. They include trimethoprim/sulfamethoxazole

(Bactrim, Septra), nitrofurantoin (Furadantin, Macrodantin), fluoroquinolones (cipro-floxacin [Cipro], gatifloxacin [Tequin], levofloxacin [Lavaquin], ofloxacin [Floxin]), cephalosporins (cephalexin [Keflex], cefixime [Suprax]), and penicillins (amoxicillin [Amoxil], amoxicillin/clavulanate [Augmentin]). The spectrum of antimicrobial activity varies among these agents. Recent studies have shown a slight but generalized decrease in bacterial susceptibility to some of these agents. Each of these is discussed in Chapter 24.

A *Cochrane Review* of the use of cranberries in the treatment of UTIs concluded that cranberry juice is less effective in decreasing the incidence of symptomatic UTIs than previously thought and cannot be recommended at this time to help decrease UTIs over a 12 month period (Jepson et al, 2012). Although there is some evidence that cranberry juice can decrease UTIs, it was not statistically significant and many people quit drinking it (Jepson et al, 2012). These new recommendations were specifically for cranberry juice. Cranberry products (powder, tablets, capsules) have differing amounts of the "active" ingredient and further testing is needed (Jepson et al, 2012). Studies indicate that a substrate in cranberries may exert a bacteriostatic effect by inhibiting the adherence of organisms to the mucosal surface of the bladder. Cranberries also change the surface properties of *E. coli,* preventing it from adhering to the bladder wall (Jepson & Craig, 2008). Symptomatic relief is often provided by urinary analgesics. The primary ingredient in these products is phenazopyridine, an azo dye taken orally that exerts a topical analgesic effect on the urinary tract mucosa when it is excreted into the urine. This dye is available under several different brand names. Azo-Standard, Prodium, Pyridium, Uricalm, and Urogesic all contain phenazopyridine 95 mg.

GOALS OF TREATMENT

Eradication of the causative organism is the primary goal of therapy. Relief of symptoms and prevention of recurrent infections are also therapeutic goals.

RATIONAL DRUG SELECTION

The main focus of this section is appropriate selection and use of drugs to treat both upper and lower UTIs.

Algorithm

This chapter does not discuss the testing involved in the diagnosis of UTIs beyond that needed for treatment decisions. The treatment protocol here assumes accurate diagnosis of the UTI by means of the appropriate diagnostic tools, including laboratory data. Once the diagnosis has been made, treatment regimens are determined.

Treatment of UTIs is directed at the three goals of eradication of organisms, relief of symptoms, and prevention of recurrence. The infecting organism is eradicated with antimicrobial therapy. Treatment for symptom relief often includes urinary

analgesics. Prevention of recurrence may involve prophylactic drug therapy but involves lifestyle management as well.

Drug Therapy

Drug therapy is aimed at eradicating the infecting organism. Appropriate antimicrobial selection is based on drug variables—spectrum of activity of the drug, potential adverse drug reactions, patterns of resistance to the antimicrobial, and cost—and patient variables—age, gender, pregnancy, and the underlying cause of the UTI.

Drug Variables
Spectrum of Activity

Lower-tract UTIs are most commonly caused by gram-negative bacteria (95% of UTIs), with *E. coli* the most prevalent organism (80% of all lower UTIs are caused by *E. coli*) (Wagenlehner, Weidner, & Naber, 2005). Among community-acquired infections, *S. saprophyticus, Klebsiella,* and gram-negative enteric bacilli cause almost all the UTIs not caused by *E. coli.* In children, additional organisms include *Klebsiella* in neonates and *Proteus* in boys. All of the antimicrobial agents mentioned have a spectrum of activity that covers these organisms.

Empirical treatment with trimethoprim/sulfamethoxazole (TMP/SMX, Septra, Bactrim) is the first-line treatment choice when no complicating factors are present and the rate of local resistance rates is less than 20% (Gupta et al, 2011). TMP/SMX has fallen out of favor in spite of its being the recommended first-line drug per guidelines, inexpensive, and effective (Griebling, 2007a; Grover et al, 2007). A 3-day treatment is cost-effective, increases compliance, and reduces risk of developing *Candida* vaginitis (Thomas & Porter, 2007). The recommended dose for treating uncomplicated UTIs in adults is one double-strength tablet bid for 3 days (Hooton & Gupta, 2014a). The dose of TMP/SMZ to treat UTIs in children older than 2 months of age is 6 to 12 mg trimethoprim and 30 to 60 mg sulfamethoxazole/kg/day (Septra or Bactrim) in two divided doses (1 mL suspension per kg/d). Children should be treated with a 10 day regimen. Resistance to TMP/SMZ is seen in patients who have had antibiotic therapy for any reason in the past 3 months or if they have been hospitalized recently.

Nitrofurantoin is an effective treatment for lower UTIs, with a low *E. coli* resistance rate of 2.1% compared to TMP/SMZ, ciprofloxacin, and levofloxacin (Kashanian et al, 2008). It is now being recommended as a first-line therapy for uncomplicated lower UTIs in adult women (Gupta et al, 2011). The Infectious Disease Society guidelines recommend 100 mg bid for 5 days (Gupta et al, 2011); however, ACOG (2008) recommends a 7-day course. The pediatric dose is 5 to 7 mg/kg/d divided every 6 hours for 7 to 10 days. Shortened therapy should not be used in children. Nitrofurantion can be used prophylactically in adults and children who have recurrent UTIs defined as more often than 3 times per year.

Nitrofurantoin is Pregnancy Category B but should be avoided in pregnancy near term, in labor, and during lactation when the infant is less than 1 month of age because of a risk for the infant to develop hemolytic anemia.

Fluoroquinolones, including ciprofloxacin, are highly effective in treating UTIs; however, resistance and overuse are hindering its effectiveness to treat other infections (Gupta, et al, 2011). The American College of Obstetricians and Gynecologists (ACOG) recommends against using fluoroquinolones if the local resistance pattern is sensitive to TMP/SMX (ACOG, 2008). From 2000 to 2010, ciprofloxacin resistance increased from 3% to 17.1% (Sanchez, Master, Karlowsky, & Bordon, 2012). The dose is 250 mg bid for 3 days or ciprofloxacin extended release (Cipro XR) 500 mg daily for 3 days. Note that generic ciprofloxacin is similar in cost to TMP/SMZ, but Cipro XR is significantly more expensive ($4 versus $28 for a 3-day supply). Other fluoroquinolones that may be used as second-line therapy include Gatifloxacin 200 to 400 mg daily and levofloxacin 250 mg daily. Moxifloxacin and gemifloxacin are not approved for use with UTIs because they have poor concentration in the urine. Fluoroquinolone resistance has been steadily increasing, with 24.2% of *E. coli* resistant to ciprofloxacin and 24% resistant to levofloxacin (Kashanian et al, 2008). Cross-resistance occurs with the fluoroquinolones. Fluoroquinolones are not prescribed to children or pregnant women because of concern for adverse effects on joints and cartilage in animal studies. The exception is ciprofloxacin, which has U.S. Food and Drug Administration (FDA) approval as second-line therapy in complicated UTI or pyelonephritis in children.

Beta-lactam antibiotics such as amoxicillin or the cephalosporins (cephalexin, cefpodoxime, cefixime) can be prescribed as second-line therapy to patients who are allergic to sulfa drugs or the fluoroquinolones or as first-line treatment for women who are pregnant. Because 25% to 70% of *E. coli* is resistant to amoxicillin, it should not be used as first-line therapy unless patient factors warrant its use.

Any of these treatments generally sterilizes the urine and produces symptom relief in 24 or fewer hours. Patients who are very symptomatic or have severe burning on urination can have phenazopyridine 200 mg 3 times a day added to their treatment regimen for 2 to 3 days as a urinary analgesic.

Complicating factors in which short-course (3-day) therapy is not appropriate (ICSI, 2002) include the following:

- Symptoms longer than 7 days' duration
- Shaking chills (rigors)
- Flank pain: midback, severe, new-occurring with onset of UTI symptoms
- History of diabetes, pregnancy, immunosuppressed status, renal calculi, renal insufficiency, discharge from hospital or nursing home within the past 2 weeks, four or more UTIs in past year, failure of this drug to treat UTI within the past 4 months, or resident of extended-care facility

For patients with complicating factors, longer treatment protocols are needed or referral may be appropriate. Urine culture should be used to guide therapy.

All of the drugs discussed so far may also be used for prophylaxis. The drug of choice for adults for prophylaxis or for recurrent infections (more than three infections in 1 year) is one single-strength tablet of trimethoprim/sulfamethoxazole daily at bedtime for a minimum of 6 months or a self-administered single dose of two double-strength tablets at symptom onset. For children, the recommended dose of trimethoprim/sulfamethoxazole is 2 mg trimethoprim/10 mg sulfamethoxazole per kg as a single bedtime dose (Craig, et al, 2009). The nitrofurantoin adult dose is 50 to 100 mg at bedtime and for children it is 1 to 2 mg/kg/d in a single dose (Gaylord & Starr, 2009).

Patients with risk factors for STIs, a positive dipstick for leukocyte esterase or hemoglobin, and a negative Gram's stain are likely to have a UTI complicated by *Chlamydia trachomatis*. The recommended drug for these patients is doxycycline (Doxy-Caps, Vibramycin) 100 mg bid for 7 days. The alternative drug is azithromycin (Zithromax) 1 g in a single dose. Azithromycin is the preferred drug if the patient's adherence to the 7-day regimen is questionable.

Upper UTIs (e.g., pyelonephritis) involve the same likely organisms because the infections are most often ascended from a bladder infection; *E. coli* is the identified organism in more than 80% of pyelonephritis cases. Failure of a 3-day course of antimicrobials generally indicates an upper UTI.

Uncomplicated pyelonephritis in adults can usually be treated with an oral antibiotic with a 90% success rate (Ramakrishnan & Scheid, 2005). A pyelonephritis is uncomplicated if it is caused by a typical pathogen in an immunocompetent person with a normal urinary tract (Ramakrishnan & Scheid, 2005). The ICSI recommends ciprofloxacin 500 mg twice a day for 7 to 14 days as the first-line drug for nonpregnant adults (2004). Other fluoroquinolones (gatifloxacin 400 mg daily, levofloxacin 250 mg daily, or ofloxacin 400 mg bid) may also be used. The alternative drugs recommended are amoxicillin/clavulanate or an oral cephalosporin with the treatment extending for 14 days. Pregnant patients should be treated with amoxicillin or amoxicillin/clavulanate and followed closely. Patients with acute pyelonephritis who are not acutely ill or in whom oral therapy can be assured (i.e., not vomiting) may benefit from 1 to 2 g ceftriaxone IM at the time of diagnosis and switched to oral therapy on day 2 of treatment. Acutely ill patients require initiating parenteral therapy in an inpatient observation unit or hospital admission for IV fluids and parenteral antibiotics.

Potential Adverse Drug Reactions

A significant number of patients have allergies to sulfonamides and penicillins. Approximately 15% of patients allergic to penicillin are also allergic to the other class of beta-lactam drugs, cephalosporins. Note: Patients with allergies to other substances such as pet dander and pollens are at high risk for drug allergies. Patients allergic to sulfonamides and penicillins can be treated with nitrofurantoin 50 to 100 mg bid.

Amoxicillin and cephalosporins have a negative effect on bowel flora and often result in diarrhea. This adverse reaction is much less common with trimethoprim, and nitrofurantoin does not affect bowel flora. Patients with bowel disease should be given either of the latter two drugs.

The fluoroquinolones—including ciprofloxacin—that are usually well tolerated have a Black-Box Warning regarding the development of tendonitis and tendon rupture, even after therapy has been completed. The risk is greatest in patients over age 60 years, those on corticosteroid therapy, and patients with previous tendon disorders or who exercise strenuously. Fluoroquinolones may have central nervous system effects, including increased intracranial pressure, dizziness, confusion, tremors, hallucinations, depression, and rarely, suicidal thoughts (Bayer Healthcare Pharmaceuticals, 2009). Patients with a known seizure disorder or a disorder that may predispose them to seizures should not be prescribed fluoroquinolones, because the drugs may lower the seizure threshold. Fluoroquinolones should not be prescribed for pregnant women because of the risk of joint disorders in the fetus and green discoloration of primary teeth developing in newborns. Fluoroquinolones are not the drug of first choice in pediatric patients because of concerns for joint disorders. The only exception is ciprofloxacin, which can be prescribed as second-line therapy in complicated UTIs and pyelonephritis in children ages 1 year to 17 years.

Long-term therapy with nitrofurantoin has been associated with pulmonary fibrosis and peripheral neuropathy. Short-term therapy has not been associated with this problem. If this drug is chosen for prophylaxis, it should be used for no more than 3 months. Nitrofurantoin should not be prescribed to pregnant women at term or during labor because of the risk of hemolytic anemia in the newborn. The drug should also be avoided in lactating women whose infants are less than one month old for the same reason.

Resistance Patterns

Drug resistance to antimicrobial therapy is a major factor in drug selection. In the United States, the resistance of *E. coli* to trimethoprim/sulfamethoxazole is approximately 24% and ciprofloxacin has resistance of 17% (Sanchez et al, 2012). The resistance pattern for nitrofurantoin has remained steady at 1.6% (Sanchez et al, 2012). Resistance to fluoroquinolones among *E. coli* isolates has been increasing; and they should be thoughtfully prescribed.

Resistance patterns vary in other countries. Prais and colleagues (2003) report research data from Israel, the United Kingdom, the Netherlands, and South Africa that show a clear difference in resistance patterns. In all of these countries, however, resistance to trimethoprim/sulfamethoxazole is lower than it is to any other drugs. Nitrofurantoin resistance was less than 10% in all countries studied and only 2% in the United States. Prais and colleagues also found that cephalexin was inadequate to resolve UTI in approximately one-third of cases, but 95% of the organisms were susceptible to cefuroxime axetil and amoxicillin/clavulanate.

Amoxicillin is no longer recommended for empirical therapy in the United States because up to one-third of the UTI organisms are resistant. Providers should be aware of local resistance patterns in their community. Providers can consult with their reference laboratory regarding the antibiogram pattern of resistance. The resistance patterns seen in inpatients may be different from community patterns of resistance.

Cost

Trimethoprim/sulfamethoxazole is the least expensive of the antimicrobials, especially when it can be given for 1 to 3 days. Generic ciprofloxacin is comparable in cost with TMP/SMZ for a 3-day supply, but be aware that brand-name Cipro XR is significantly more expensive than generic ciprofloxacin. Nitrofurantoin is also relatively inexpensive, although the brand-name Macrodantin that has bid dosing is more expensive.

Table 47-3 summarizes antimicrobial recommendations for upper and lower UTIs. Recommendations are included for adults and children. Figure 47-1 depicts the treatment protocol for management of UTIs in adult women.

Table 47–3 ❖ Drugs Commonly Used: Upper and Lower Urinary Tract Infections

Indication	Primary Choices	Alternative Choices
Upper UTIs (Adults)		
Simple, uncomplicated upper UTI Mild to moderately ill	• Ciprofloxacin 500 mg bid for 14 d • Trimethoprim-sulfamethoxazole double-strength 1 tablet bid for 14 d *or* • Ofloxacin 400 mg bid for 14 d • If client status warrants: give 1 to 2 g ceftriaxone IV on day 1, switching to one of the oral medications above on day 2	• Amoxicillin-clavulanate 500 mg bid for 14 d • Cefixime 200 mg bid for 14 d
Lower UTIs		
Simple, uncomplicated lower UTI in adults Symptomatic or asymptomatic and reinfection (single event)	• Trimethoprim-sulfamethoxazole double-strength 1 tablet bid for 3 d *or* • Nitrofurantoin 100 mg bid for 5–7 d • Ciprofloxacin 250 mg bid for 3 d • Ciprofloxacin Extended Release 500 mg daily for 3 d	• Gatifloxacin 200–400 mg daily for 3 d • Levofloxacin 250 mg daily for 3 d

Table 47–3 ❀ Drugs Commonly Used: Upper and Lower Urinary Tract Infections—cont'd

Indication	Primary Choices	Alternative Choices
Simple, uncomplicated lower UTI Serial reinfections (more than 3/yr)	• Trimethoprim-sulfamethoxazole double-strength 1 tablet bid for 3 d with onset of symptoms	• Ciprofloxacin 250 mg bid for 3 d with onset of symptoms
Simple, uncomplicated lower UTI associated with intercourse prophylaxis	• Trimethoprim-sulfamethoxazole double-strength 1 tablet single dose after intercourse	• Ciprofloxacin 250 mg single dose after intercourse
Simple, uncomplicated lower UTI recurrence prophylaxis	• Trimethoprim-sulfamethoxazole double-strength 1 tablet daily at bedtime for at least 6 mo	• Nitrofurantoin 50 mg daily at bedtime for no more than 3 mo
Complicated lower UTI or symptomatic after 3 d of therapy	• Trimethoprim-sulfamethoxazole double-strength 1 tablet bid for 7–14 d • Ciprofloxacin 250 mg bid for 7–14 d	• Nitrofurantoin 100 mg bid for 7–14 d • Ofloxacin 200 mg bid for 7–14 d
Special Considerations		
Risk factors for STD	• Doxycycline 100 mg bid for 7 d	• Azithromycin 1 g single dose
Pregnancy	• Nitrofurantoin 100 mg bid for 7 d	• Amoxicillin 500 mg tid for 7 d • Cefixime 200 mg bid for 7 d
Afebrile children: >1 month	• Trimethoprim-sulfamethoxazole 6 to 12 mg/kg/d trimethoprim plus 30 to 60 mg/kg/d sulfamethoxazole given in 2 divided doses for 10 d in infants > 2 months of age	• Nitrofurantoin 5 to 7 mg/kg/d in 3 or 4 divided doses × 10 d • Amoxicillin 40 mg/kg/d in 2 or 3 divided doses × 10 d if no resistance in the community • Augmentin 40 mg/kg/d of amoxicillin component divided TID × 10 d • Cefixime 8 mg/kg/d • Cephalexin 25 to 50 mg/kg/d in 3 or 4 doses • Cefpodoxime 10 mg/kg/d in 2 divided doses

Febrile UTI in children >1 month of age	• Parenteral antibiotics for first 24 h or until afebrile
	  • Ceftriaxone 50 to 75 mg/kg every 12 to 24 h
	  • Cefotaxime 150 mg/kg/d divided every 6 to 8 h
	  • Ceftazidime 150 mg/kg/d divided every 6–8 h
	• Oral antibiotics are started once the child is afebrile and continued for 10 to 14 d, followed by prophylaxis until radiological workup is complete
	• Oral antibiotic choices are the same as for afebrile UTI	

Estrogen deficiency/postmenopausal female	• Vaginal estrogen cream 0.5–2 g intravaginally daily	
Advanced age	• No treatment if asymptomatic	

Patient Variables

Age

Infants and Children

Signs and symptoms of UTI in infants and very young children are different from those in adults. The likelihood of UTI, especially with fever, increases in these circumstances: a history of crying on urination, foul-smelling urine, altered urination pattern, irritability, vomiting, diarrhea, and failure to

thrive. All infants with fever of unknown origin should have a catheterized urine specimen obtained to rule out a UTI. The most accurate diagnosis of a UTI in a non–toilet-trained child is made with a catheterized urine sample. Bagged urine samples should not be used to diagnose a UTI (American Academy of Pediatrics [AAP], 2011). The common UTI symptoms of dysuria, urgency, frequency, and hesitancy may be present in preschool-age children, but are difficult to discern in this age group. The older the child is, the more likely

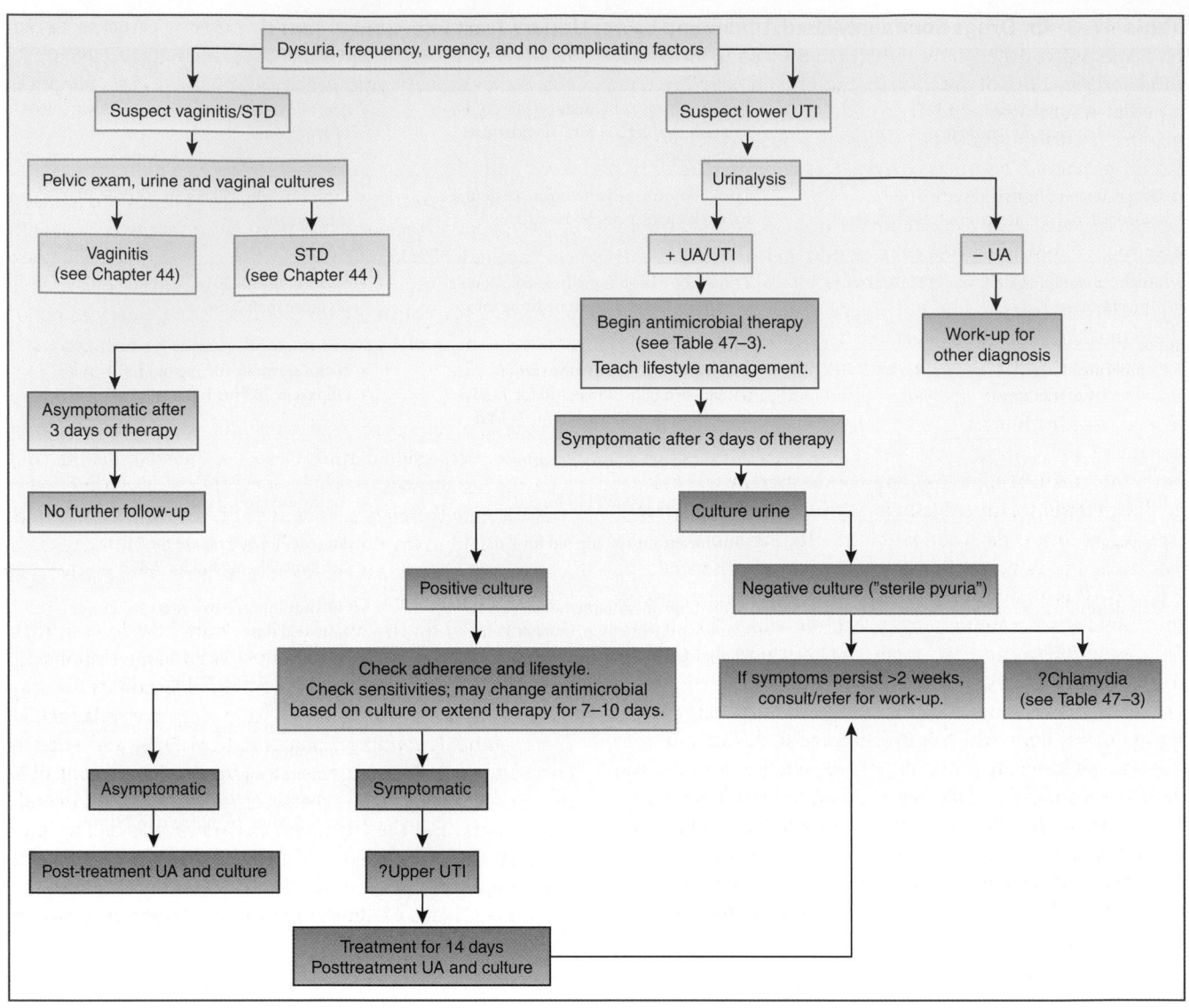

Figure 47–1. Treatment protocol: Urinary tract infections in women.

he or she is to have the "classic" UTI symptoms of dysuria and frequency.

Febrile UTI is treated aggressively in infants and children because fever is often an indication of pyelonephritis (Gaylord & Starr, 2009). Infants and children with febrile UTI should receive parenteral antibiotics for the first 24 hours or until afebrile. Ceftriaxone 50 to 75 mg/kg divided every 12 to 24 hours IV/IM is often used in children older than 3 months because of the convenience of 24-hour dosing. Other appropriate parenteral antibiotic choices are cefotaxime, ceftazidime, ampicillin, or gentamicin (see Table 47-3 for dosing).

All infants and children with febrile UTI are evaluated daily until afebrile. Complicated febrile UTI in children warrants inpatient treatment with IV antibiotics. Symptoms warranting inpatient treatment include high fever, toxic appearance, persistent vomiting, moderate to severe dehydration, and poor compliance (Gaylord & Starr, 2009). In addition, any patient younger than age 6 months who appears toxic should receive initial inpatient treatment for febrile UTI.

The goals for treatment of UTI in infants and children are the same as those for adults, with the exception that a search should be made for anatomical abnormalities of the bladder and kidneys. The AAP (2011) recently changed its guidelines for initial febrile UTI in children aged 2 to 24 months and now recommends a renal ultrasound (RUS) for the first infection and voiding cystourethrography (VCUG) after the *second* febrile UTI, provided the RUS is normal. The AAP recommends a RUS within the first two days of treatment. The rationale is that risk of renal scarring is low after one febrile UTI and the recommendation is meant to prevent unnecessary testing (AAP, 2011).

The new recommendation prompted a response from the section on Urology (Wan et al, 2012) expressing concerns about waiting until the second febrile UTI before obtaining VCUG. It remains to be seen if the AAP guidelines will be revised; however, the guidelines are only for children ages 2 to 24 months and are never a substitute for clinical judgment. In addition, the risk of renal damage increases as the number of recurrences of UTI increases. Children with documented or suspected vesicoureteral reflux, renal scarring, or structural abnormalities of the urinary tract should be referred to a pediatric urologist. Children with an identified renal or bladder stone should also be referred to a pediatric urologist. Children should be on prophylactic antibiotics until the urological evaluation is complete.

Adolescents with pyelonephritis or a second UTI with documented positive urine cultures and no history of recent sexual activity require at least consultation (Gaylord & Starr, 2009). Older children (older than age 5) can be treated with the same drugs as adults, whether they are asymptomatic or symptomatic, but the extent of treatment may need to be 7 to 14 days. In a meta-analysis of published randomized controlled trials in children 0 to 18 years of age comparing long-course (7 to 14 days) with short-course (3 days or less) antibiotic treatment of UTI, long-course therapy was associated with fewer treatment failures with concomitant increase in reinfections, even when studies including subjects with evidence of pyelonephritis were excluded from the analysis. Based on this analysis, Keren and Chan (2002) recommend that clinicians continue to treat children with UTI for 7 to 14 days until more accurate methods of distinguishing upper from lower UTIs in children are available.

Consideration should be given to the effect of the agent chosen on bowel flora, which is highly correlated with diarrhea. Younger children are more likely to experience fluid volume deficits secondary to diarrhea. Among the available drugs, nitrofurantoin has the least effect on bowel flora and amoxicillin has the most effect. The effect of trimethoprim/sulfamethoxazole is only slightly more than that of nitrofurantoin. Figure 47-2 shows the treatment protocol for management of UTIs in children.

Older Adults

Elderly patients are at increased risk for UTIs and asymptomatic bacteriuria. In 1999, UTI was reported as the admitting or current diagnosis in 7.1% of female and 5.6% of male nursing home residents (Griebling, 2007b). Asymptomatic bacteriuria may be present in more than 20% of women over age 80 years and 6% to 15% of men over age 75 years living independently in the community (Fekete & Hooton, 2014). Asymptomatic bacteriuria is defined by the Infectious Diseases Society of America (IDSA) guidelines as two consecutive clean-catch voided urine specimens in women and one clean catch in men with isolation of a single organism in quantitative counts of greater than 10^5 cfu/mL (Fekete & Hooton, 2014).

Asymptomatic bacteriuria is commonly associated with urinary incontinence, multiple medical illnesses, and impairment of mental status. Treatment with antimicrobial therapy is frequently unsuccessful in eradicating the infection and may be associated with the development of more resistant bacteria. Choice of antimicrobial should be based on culture and sensitivity tests rather than done empirically. No treatment is indicated in asymptomatic adults of advanced age unless in conjunction with surgery to correct obstructive uropathy or after removal of an indwelling catheter (Fekete & Hooton, 2014; Nicolle et al, 2005). Changes in mental status, however, may indicate a symptomatic UTI that requires treatment.

Male Gender

Signs and symptoms of UTI are similar in males and females. Urethral discharge in men is more commonly associated with STDs than with a UTI. In children and young men, UTIs are more commonly associated with congenital obstructive disorders. The risk of infection with *E. coli* is increased in homosexual men and heterosexual men with a colonized partner. The rate of UTIs increases in men aged 50 to 65 and parallels the increase in hyperplasia of the prostate gland. Glandular enlargement leads to bladder outflow obstruction and increased residual urine. Older adult men (older than 65) have further prostate enlargement and increased urine residuals. Despite the high prevalence of UTIs in this age group, most remain asymptomatic and seem to be at low risk for serious complications. However, gram-negative sepsis from a UTI can occur and can be life-threatening.

Culture and sensitivity studies should be done in men with a history of UTI. In men, the organisms responsible for infection are slightly different. *E. coli* accounts for only about 25% of their infections. Gram-negative rods such as *Proteus* and *Pseudomonas* account for 50%, and enterococci and coagulase-negative staphylococci are responsible for the remaining 25%. Treatment should be based on culture results, and the treatment period should be for 10 to 14 days, with a follow-up culture drawn. Treatment for men of advanced age is similar to that for women of the same age. Figure 47-3 presents the treatment protocol for males with UTIs.

Pregnancy

Asymptomatic bacteriuria is relatively common, affecting 2% to 7% of pregnancies (Hooton & Gupta, 2014b). It should be treated because eradication of bacteriuria reduces the high incidence of symptomatic UTI that commonly occurs later; treatment may reduce the risk for preterm birth. All pregnant women should be screened for bacteriuria by urine culture at least once early in pregnancy, and they should be treated if the results are positive (Hooton & Gupta, 2014b; Nicolle, et al, 2005). Periodic screening for recurrent bacteriuria should be done following completion of therapy to ensure clearance of the infection and to monitor for any recurrence. Women who are culture negative at early screening do not require additional screening later in pregnancy. Symptoms of UTI should always result in urine testing and treatment if needed throughout pregnancy.

Nitrofurantoin 100 mg bid for 5 to 7 days, amoxicillin/clavulanate 500 mg bid for 3 to 5 days, and cephalosporins (cephalexin 500 mg every 12 hours for 3 to 7 days) are all acceptable during pregnancy (Hooton & Gupta, 2014b). Patients should have a repeat urine culture 1 week after completion of therapy to test for cure and then monthly until delivery.

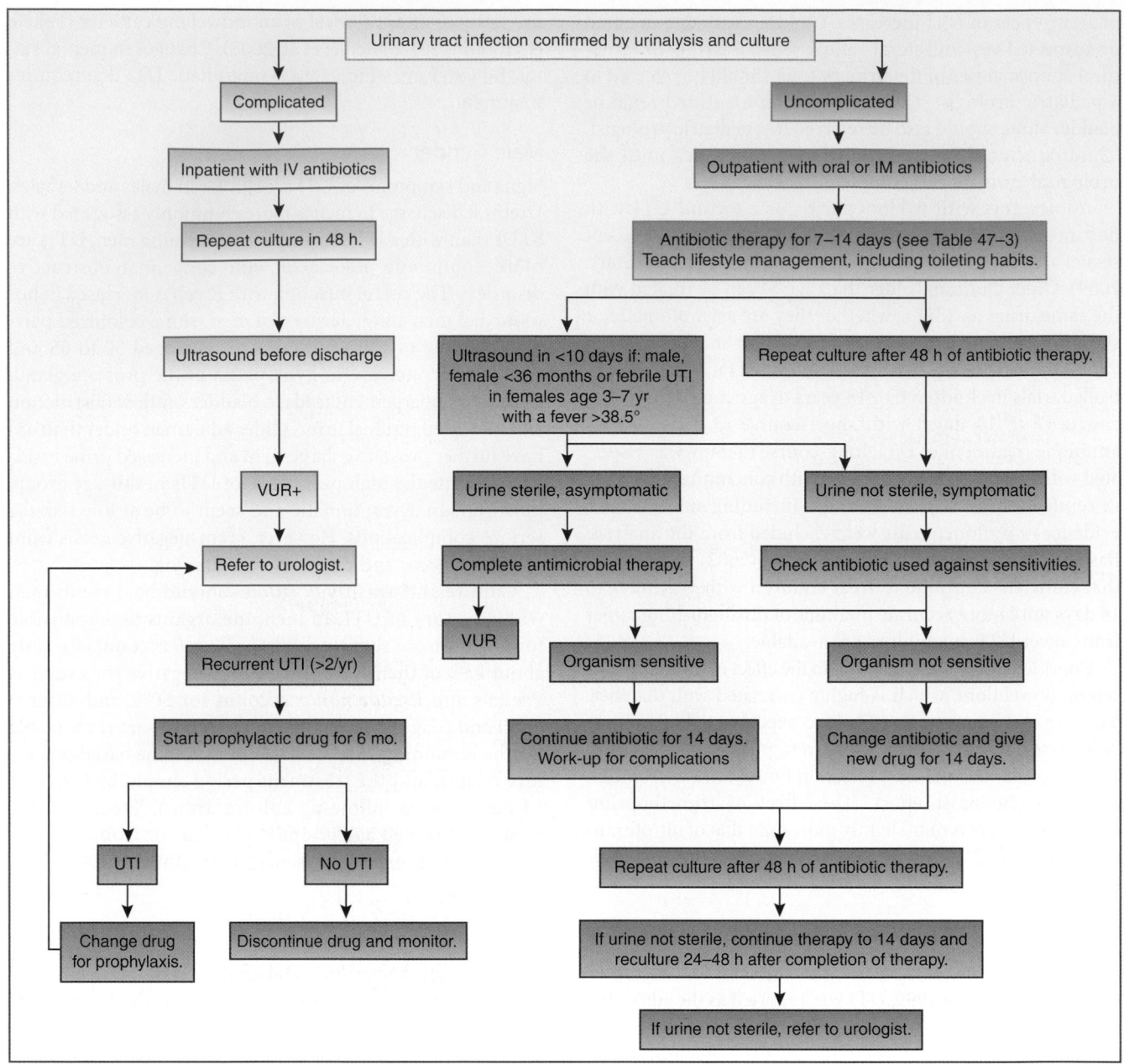

Figure 47–2. Treatment protocol: Urinary tract infections in children.

Underlying Cause

If the UTI should develop in relation to intercourse, trimethoprim/sulfamethoxazole (double-strength, one tablet after coitus) may prevent the UTI. It is effective and inexpensive. A single dose of a fluoroquinolone (see earlier comments) is a second-line choice. It is also effective but more expensive. Patients should also void within 10 minutes after intercourse.

In postmenopausal women, UTIs associated with estrogen deficiency can be reduced by daily application of vaginal estrogen cream 0.5 to 2 g intravaginally.

MONITORING

For lower UTIs in women, a standard UA is cost-effective in diagnosing the disorder. Symptom resolution within 48 hours is considered sufficient monitoring of outcome. If symptoms persist, a urine culture is obtained and any necessary changes in antimicrobial therapy are instituted. For these patients, a follow-up office visit in 10 to 14 days should be scheduled.

For patients with recurrent infections, obtaining and documenting one urine culture is worthwhile, although it is generally unnecessary for women with acute UTI. If the culture is negative despite a positive UA, investigation is needed for organisms that do not grow on standard laboratory media, such as those that cause gonorrhea, chlamydia, and renal tuberculosis. One post-treatment UA is useful to rule out persistent infection or hematuria. Routine UA to test for a cure is generally unnecessary in healthy adult women because all the main antimicrobials used to treat UTIs have 91% and

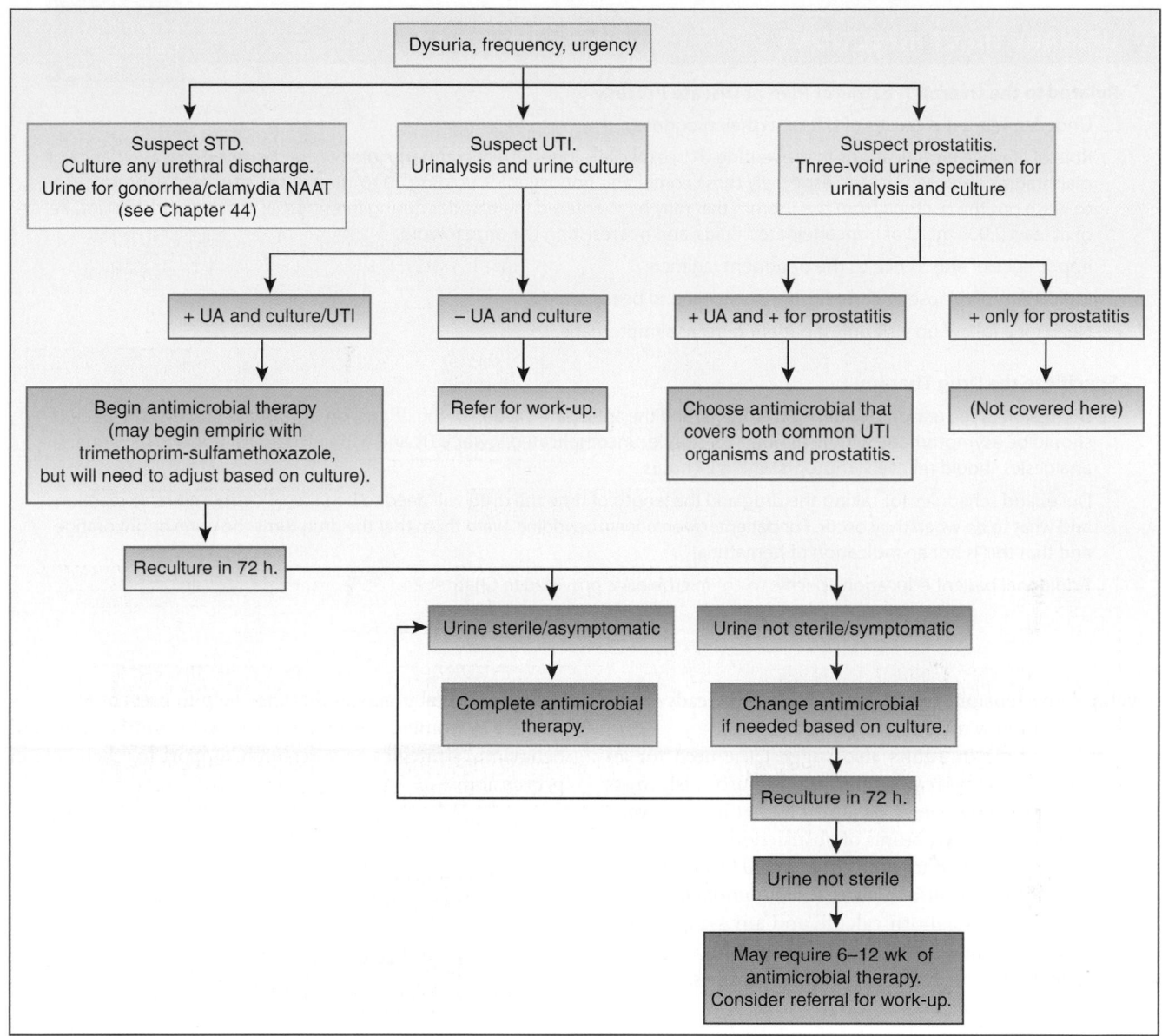

Figure 47–3. Treatment protocol: Urinary tract infections in men.

higher cure rates. Follow-up cultures are appropriate in children, pregnant, and elderly patients. If persistent as opposed to recurrent UTI is suspected, a follow-up UA may be helpful in making this diagnosis.

All children age 5 years and younger need radiological evaluation and appropriate referral to a pediatric urologist. Older children with a simple, uncomplicated UTI require urine culture for diagnosis of the offending organism and a culture after completion of therapy. Failure to produce sterile urine after 14 days of therapy suggests referral.

Pregnant patients with a positive urine culture should have a follow-up urine culture every 2 weeks until delivery and at their postpartum evaluation to validate sterile urine. Reinfections require prophylactic antimicrobial therapy. For upper UTIs, an initial telephone assessment of the patient's symptoms and response to therapy is important within 24 hours. A second assessment with an office visit should occur in 2 to 3 days. If symptoms do not resolve or if they worsen, hospitalization may be required. A urine culture should be done 1 to 2 weeks after therapy in pregnant patients, children, patients who remain symptomatic, and those for whom suppression therapy is being considered. Follow-up cultures are optional for all other patients.

OUTCOME EVALUATION

Neonates, infants, and children under age 5 years who present with clinical and laboratory evidence of UTIs should be referred to a pediatric urologist. The cause is likely to be an anatomical obstructive problem, especially in boys. Although adults do not often have long-term complications from UTIs, 10% of children with reflux nephropathy go on to develop hypertension with bilateral scarring of the kidney within 10 years. Risk for development of end-stage renal disease after UTI is rare in adults but is 1:500 for children who later

URINARY TRACT INFECTIONS

PATIENT EDUCATION

Related to the Overall Treatment Plan or Disease Process

☐ Understanding the causes of UTIs and their prognoses.

☐ Role of lifestyle modifications in preventing UTIs, especially ingestion of cranberry juice or cranberry extract; avoidance of diaphragms and spermicides, especially those containing nonoxynol-9; voiding 10 to 15 minutes after sexual intercourse to wash out the bacteria from the urethra that may have entered the bladder during intercourse; maintaining fluid intake of at least 2,000 mL/d of noncaffeinated fluids; and not resisting the urge to void.

☐ Importance of adherence to the treatment regimen.

☐ Indications of relapse or complications that need to be reported.

☐ Need for a follow-up visit only if patient remains symptomatic.

Specific to the Drug Therapy

☐ Discussion of the reasons for taking the drug(s) and the anticipated action of the drug(s) on the disease process. The patient should be asymptomatic within 48 hours for simple, uncomplicated lower UTIs and within 7 days for upper UTIs. Urinary analgesics should relieve symptoms within 24 hours.

☐ Doses and schedules for taking the drug and the length of time the drug will need to be taken. Possible adverse reactions and what to do when they occur. For patients given phenazopyridine, warn them that the drug turns the urine bright orange and that this is not an indication of hematuria.

☐ Additional patient education specific to antimicrobials is provided in Chapter 24.

develop hypertension. Recurrent UTI in girls leads to increased risk for new infection in pregnancy.

Certain criteria in adults also suggest the need for an aggressive workup that requires referral to a urologist. Gross hematuria; persistent microscopic hematuria between episodes of infection; symptoms of obstruction; a clinical impression of persistent rather than recurrent UTI, or infection with urea-splitting bacteria, such as *Proteus mirabilis,* which are associated with staghorn calculi; and any symptomatic pregnant patients and patients who have a high fever or appear dehydrated or septic suggest referral. These patients may require hospitalization for IV therapy.

If patients remain symptomatic after 3 days of therapy for a simple, uncomplicated lower UTI or after completion of 10 to 14 days of therapy for an upper UTI, a culture should be done to determine the causative organism and a different antimicrobial may be needed.

PATIENT EDUCATION

Patient education should include a discussion of information related to the overall treatment plan as well as that specific to the drug therapy, reasons for taking the drug, drugs as part of the total treatment regimen, and adherence issues. Lifestyle changes to prevent UTIs should be addressed, especially with patients who have recurrent UTIs.

Lifestyle Management

Prevention is the key to management of UTIs. Although lifestyle management may not always prevent UTIs, studies confirm several practices that may help to prevent UTIs, especially in women. The following lifestyle modifications and behavioral strategies have research support for their role in prevention:

1. Avoiding spermicide and diaphragms. Use of these products may cause a change in vaginal pH and flora that increases the potential for vaginal colonization with organisms likely to produce UTIs. Nonoxynol-9 spermicides are especially associated with increased incidence of bacteriuria. The essential first step to UTIs in women is frequently thought to be the colonization of the vaginal introitus.

2. Voiding 10 to 15 minutes after sexual intercourse. Urination washes out the bacteria from the urethra that may have entered the bladder during intercourse.

Additional measures that have inconsistent support but would not be harmful and are likely to be helpful include the following:

1. Ingesting cranberry juice or cranberry extract. Cranberry substrates exert a bacteriostatic effect. Most studies have been done in elderly women, but the same mechanism may prove effective in younger women and in men. There is no evidence for the effectiveness of cranberry in preventing UTIs in children.

2. Maintaining fluid intake of at least 2,000 mL/d of noncaffeinated fluids. Sufficient fluid is necessary to ensure regular voiding throughout the day. Caffeinated fluids have a mild diuretic effect but are less likely to maintain fluid volume balance.

3. Not resisting the urge to void. "Holding" urine may stretch the bladder and cause small breaks in the bladder

mucosal layer that provide entrance for bacteria. Holding also increases the risk for growth of bacteria in residual urine.

4. Avoiding douche products that change the vaginal pH and flora. This practice may decrease the likelihood of vaginal canal colonization.

REFERENCES

American Academy of Pediatrics (AAP). (2011). Urinary tract infection: Clinical practice guideline for the diagnosis and management of the initial UTI in febrile infants and children 2 to 24 months Committee on Quality Improvement: Subcommittee on Urinary Tract Infections. *Pediatrics, 128*(3), 595–610.

Bayer Healthcare Pharmaceuticals. (2009). Cipro [Manufacturer's label]. Retrieved from http://www.univgraph.com/bayer/inserts/ciprotab.pdf

Berger, R. (2005). Cranberries for preventing urinary tract infections. *Journal of Urology, 173*(6), 1988.

Craig, J. C., Ch, B., Simpson, J. M., Williams, G. J., Lowe, A., Reynolds, G. J., McTaggart, S. J., et al. (2009). Antibiotic prophylaxis in recurrent urinary tract infection in children. *New England Journal of Medicine, 361*(18), 1748–1759.

Fekete, T., & Hooton, T. M. (2014). Approach to the adult with asymptomatic bacteriuria. *UpToDate.* Wolters Kluwer. Retrieved from http://www.uptodate.com/contents/approach-to-the-adult-with-asymptomatic-bacteriuria

Freedman, A. L. (2007). Urinary tract infection in children. In M. S. Litwin & C. S. Saigal (Eds.), *Urologic diseases in America* (NIH Publication No. 07–5512, pp 439–457). U.S. Department of Health and Human Services, Public Health Service, National Institutes of Health, National Institute of Diabetes and Digestive and Kidney Diseases. Washington, DC: U.S. Government Printing Office.

Gaylord, N. M., & Starr, N. B. (2009). Genitourinary disorders. In C. E. Burns, A. M. Dunn, M. A. Brady, N. B. Starr, & C. G. Blosser (Eds.), *Pediatric primary care* (pp 866–905). St. Louis, MO: Saunders.

Griebling, T. L. (2007a). Urinary tract infection in women. In M. S. Litwin & C. S. Saigal (Eds.), *Urologic diseases in America* (NIH Publication No. 07–5512, pp 588–617). U.S. Department of Health and Human Services, Public Health Service, National Institutes of Health, National Institute of Diabetes and Digestive and Kidney Diseases. Washington, DC: U.S. Government Printing Office.

Griebling, T. L. (2007b). Urinary tract infection in men. In M. S. Litwin & C. S. Saigal (Eds.), *Urologic diseases in America* (NIH Publication No. 07–5512, pp 621–645). U.S. Department of Health and Human Services, Public Health Service, National Institutes of Health, National Institute of Diabetes and Digestive and Kidney Diseases. Washington, DC: U.S. Government Printing Office.

Grover, M. L., Bracamonte, J. D., Kanodia, A. K., Bryan, M. J., Donahue, S. P., Warner, A., et al. (2007). Assessing adherence to evidence-base guidelines for the diagnosis and management of uncomplicated urinary tract infection. *Mayo Clinic Proceedings, 82*(2), 181–185.

Gupta, K., et al. (2011). International Clinical Practice Guidelines for the treatment of acute uncomplicated cystitis and pyelonephritis in women: A 2010 update by the Infectious Diseases Society of America and the European Society for Microbiology and Infectious Diseases. *Clinic Infectious Diseases 52*(5), e103–e120.

Hooton, T. M., & Gupta, K. (2014a). Acute cystitis in women. *UpToDate Online.* Retrieved from http://www.uptodate.com/contents/acute-uncomplicated-cystitis-and-pyelonephritis-in-women

Hooton, T. M., & Gupta, K. (2014b). Urinary tract infections and asymptomatic bacteriuria in pregnancy. *UpToDate.* Wolters Kluwer. Retrieved from http://www.uptodate.com/contents/urinary-tract-infections-and-asymptomatic-bacteriuria-in-pregnancy

Institute for Clinical Systems Improvement (ICSI). (2004). *Uncomplicated urinary tract infection in women.* Bloomington, MN: ICSI.

Jepson, R. G., & Craig, J. C. (2008). Cranberries for preventing urinary tract infections. *Cochrane Database of Systematic Reviews* (1):CD001321.

Jepson, R. G., Williams, G., & Craig, J. C. (2012). Cranberries for preventing urinary tract infections. *Cochrane Database of Systematic Reviews, CD001321*

Kashanian, J., Hakimian, P., Blute, M., Wong, J., Khanna, H., Wise, G., et al. (2008). Nitrofurantoin: The return of an old friend in the wake of growing resistance. *British Journal of Urology International, 102,* 1634–1637.

Keren, R., & Chan, E. (2002). A meta-analysis of randomized, controlled trials comparing short- and long-course antibiotic therapy for urinary tract infections in children. *Pediatrics, 109*(5), e70.

Litwin, M. S., & Saigal, C. S. (2007). Introduction. In M. S. Litwin & C. S. Saigal (Eds.), *Urologic diseases in America* (NIH Publication No. 07–5512, pp 588–617). U.S. Department of Health and Human Services, Public Health Service, National Institutes of Health, National Institute of Diabetes and Digestive and Kidney Diseases. Washington, DC: U.S. Government Printing Office.

Nicolle, L., Bradley, S., Colgan, R., Rice, J., Schaeffer, A., & Hooton, T. (2005). Infectious Diseases Society of America guideline for the diagnosis and treatment of asymptomatic bacteriuria in adults. *Clinical Infectious Diseases, 40*(5), 643–654.

Prais, D., Straussberg, R., Avitzur, Y., Nussinovitch, M., Harel, L., & Amir, J. (2003). Bacterial susceptibility to oral antibiotics in community acquired urinary tract infection. *Archives of Disease in Childhood, 88,* 215–218.

Ramakrishnan, K., & Scheid, D. C. (2005). Diagnosis and management of acute pyelonephritis in adults. *American Family Physician, 71,* 933–942.

Sanchez, G. V., Master, R. N., Karlowsky, J. A., & Bordon, J. M. (2012). In vitro antimicrobial resistance of urinary *excherichia coli* isolates among U.S. outpatients from 2000–2010. *Antimicrobial Agents and Chemotherapy, 56*(4), 2181–2183.

Wagenlehner, F., Weidner, W., & Naber, K. (2005). Emerging drugs for bacterial urinary tract infections. *Expert Opinion on Emerging Drugs, 10*(2), 275–298.

Wan, J., et al. (2012). Section on Urology response to new guidelines for the diagnosis and management of UTI. *Pediatrics, 129*(4), e1051–1053.

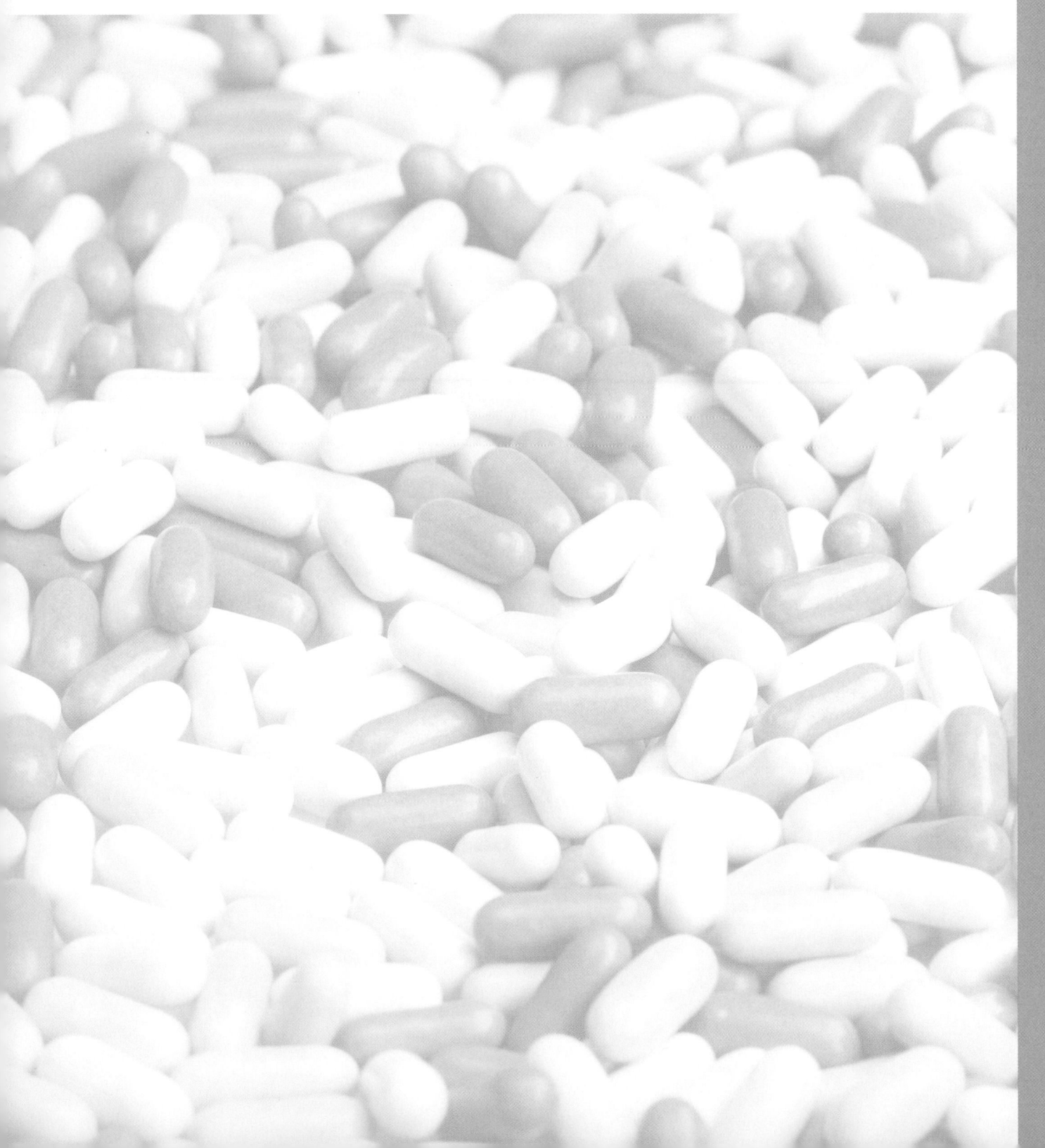

SPECIAL DRUG TREATMENT CONSIDERATIONS

WOMEN AS PATIENTS

Priscilla M. Nodine

Differences in patterns of health and illness between females and males have been well documented. Women tend to pay more attention to changes in health patterns, seeking health care earlier and more often than men. Even when diagnosed with similar medical conditions (such as cardiac disease or Alzheimer's disease), adult women have very different needs for care than do their male counterparts. Adherence to a prescribed medication regimen may be affected by gender, especially if the adverse effects have a particular impact on females (e.g., hirsutism or risk of thromboembolic disorders). This chapter will discuss treatment of common conditions experienced by women as a special population.

To review growth and development briefly, both sexes progress similarly until puberty, when increases in estrogen and progesterone prepare women for fertility and reproduction. Menopause signals the cessation of reproductive capability for females. During puberty, males respond to the influence of increased androgens, triggering a cascade of changes such as increased height, weight, and muscle mass and the genital changes that accompany the ability to reproduce. Whereas females are born with all of their gamete cells already present, sperm production in males begins at puberty and continues throughout their adult lives until levels of testosterone start to wane, usually in their sixth or seventh decade.

Prescribing for women in their childbearing years requires constant awareness of the possibility of pregnancy in order to avoid exposing the developing fetus to potential teratogens. Sexually active women who use birth control also become pregnant. In the United States, 48% of pregnancies are unintended (Finer & Zolna, 2011). Sexual activity (especially if begun early) can lead to lifelong viral infections or silent bacterial infections that scar delicate fallopian tubes and change cervical tissues, contributing to infertility. Early sexual activity in adolescents exposes them to risks of both infection and pregnancy, at a time when their bodies are still growing and their personalities are not yet mature.

Teenage pregnancy is associated with inconsistent prenatal care, smaller infants, and preterm labor. These infants are at high risk for developmental disorders and other medical conditions associated with low birth weight. Neglect and abuse account for 2 deaths per 1,000 healthy infants born to adolescents 15 years or younger, and the risk from sudden infant death syndrome (SIDS) increases (Moos, 2005).

Breastfeeding is another time when prescribing for women requires special care and knowledge. For information on pharmacokinetics about breastfeeding to assist the practitioner in making safe decisions about prescribing, see Chapter 50.

Cultural attitudes, behaviors, and beliefs related to health can affect how a woman responds to and complies with health advice. Caring for women from different cultures requires knowledge of the treatments they will accept, of their personal values and beliefs, and of the customs of their identified cultural group. With the assistance of an interpreter, health-care providers should provide written and verbal instruction to women with language barriers (Davidson, London, Ladewig, & Davidson, 2011). Translation alone may not be an issue. The patients may not understand explanations if they lack basic education in their own country. Cultural influences are discussed in detail in Chapter 7.

During the 1980s, abuse of children and women was recognized as a significant public health problem. Although boys have also been abused, most abuse has been against girls and women. "Domestic violence against women is a major public health concern. Abuse often increases in frequency and severity over time and leads to significant social, psychological, and medical consequences" (Bohn, Tebben, & Campbell, 2004). Intimate partner violence (IPV), which can vary in frequency and severity, is a type of violence that occurs among heterosexual and same-sex couples. IPV is also a serious public health problem (Centers for Disease Control and Prevention, 2013b). Statistics about IPV vary because of differences in the way different data sources define IPV and collect data. In addition, most IPV incidents are not reported to the police; thus, available data underestimate the true extent of the problem (Centers for Disease Control and Prevention, 2013b).

Women are at high risk for violence during pregnancy, a complication that can lead to many other problems: miscarriage, placental abruption, low-birth-weight infants, premature labor or birth, substance abuse, late entry to prenatal care, intrauterine fetal death, and sexually transmitted and urinary tract infections (Bohn et al, 2004; Schoening, Greenwood, McNichols, Heermann, & Agrawal, 2004).

The American Nurses Association (ANA), the Association of Women's Health, Obstetrics and Neonatal Nurses (AWHONN), the American College of Obstetricians and Gynecologists (ACOG), and the American Medical Association (AMA) recommend that practitioners screen all patients for IPV at every encounter with the health-care system, regardless of the reason for which health care is being sought. Routinely asking all women about physical and emotional abuse increases a practitioner's opportunity to uncover the underlying causes of women's physical symptoms or depression, conditions that may be related to some form of abuse

(Schoening et al, 2004). Women are 4 times more likely to report abuse if they are simply asked.

In most of the world, the majority of the older population is comprised of women. This demographic phenomenon has been called the feminization of later life (Ginn, Street, & Arber, 2001). Women's life expectancy in developed countries is an average of 7 years longer than that of men, with the gender gap narrowing to 3 years in developing countries (mostly due to high maternal mortality rates) (United Nations, 2012). The feminization of later life carries consequences that include a high incidence of widowhood, living alone, disability, and poverty. Women are more likely to live alone than are their male counterparts, who frequently marry again. In addition, an increase in chronic illness also accompanies women's longer life spans, including cardiovascular disorders, strokes, diabetes, arthritis, and Alzheimer's disease. Management of chronic illnesses in the face of economic concerns in this vulnerable population presents significant challenge for health-care providers.

In the United States, women are the most impoverished subgroup of society. At both ends of the demographic spectrum, single mothers with children and elderly women are the poorest of the poor (U.S. Department of Health and Human Services, 2005). Lack of health insurance coverage leads many women not to fill prescriptions or to take medications on an altered schedule. Prescribers must adequately assess a patient's financial status and be aware of the possibility that a woman's noncompliance may be primarily economically driven.

Practitioners often neglect the complex needs of older women, maintaining a symptom-specific focus. By age 65, half of all women have two or more chronic conditions (Agency of Healthcare Research and Quality, 2002). The need for polypharmacy that often results from multiple comorbidities necessitates a more holistic approach to these patients' care.

Although defining disability can be a daunting task because of a multitude of components, practitioners need to be aware that about 27 million women in the United States have disabilities, about 1 in 5. Rates are higher in older women, with 50% of women older than 65 living with a disability, most commonly caused by arthritis or rheumatism (National Institute of Health, 2009). Because of their longer life expectancy, women are more likely than men to be disabled, with the most prevalence among women over age 85.

Disability refers to a chronic physical or mental health problem or an impairment that restricts an individual's ability to perform one or more activities (Davidson et al, 2011). Various categories of disabilities include developmental (present before the age of 22), neurological, psychiatric, and sensory. Autoimmune diseases are categorized as neurological disabilities, as is Alzheimer's disease (AD). Psychiatric disabilities include depression, anxiety, panic disorders, and phobias. Women have 50% higher rates than do men of all of these disabling conditions.

As women age, changes in cognitive functioning—learning, memory, concentration, and planning ability—often occur. Clinically apparent cognitive decline is called dementia (Davidson et al, 2011). In the United States, Alzheimer's disease (AD) is the most commonly occurring form of dementia (Plassman et al, 2011). About twice as many women suffer from Alzheimer's disease as men. This sex difference is due in large part to the fact that life expectancy is longer for women, but also women may survive longer than men after initial diagnosis (Plassman et al, 2011).

Acetylcholinesterase inhibitors are the only medications approved by the U.S. Food and Drug Administration (FDA) to treat cognitive dysfunction. Evidence has been conflicting about the effect of estrogen or hormone replacement therapy (HRT) in either prevention or the delay of AD onset in women. Studies have found impaired cognition in older women taking both estrogen and progesterone (Shumaker et al, 2003).

In 2010, the National Institutes of Health (NIH) published a six-goal agenda on women's health that included Goal 2: "Incorporate findings of sex/gender differences in the design and applications of new technologies, medical devices, and therapeutic drugs" (Wood, Blehar, & Mauery, 2011). Research continues to include more women as subjects, but work needs to persist in this area.

In this chapter, the biological and molecular basis for sex-related differences in pharmacokinetics, pharmacodynamics, drug effects, and safety will be discussed based on the current science.

PHARMACOKINETICS AND PHARMACODYNAMICS IN WOMEN

Pharmacokinetics

Gender differences occur in all phases of pharmacokinetics between men and women. Table 48-1 presents some gender differences in pharmacokinetic properties. Women have longer gastric emptying times, which influence the absorption and bioavailability of some drugs. The volume of distribution (Vd) of drugs is dramatically altered by body composition. The higher percentage of body fat means a larger Vd for lipophilic agents (Gandhi, Aweeka, Greenblatt, & Blaschke, 2004; *Women and trials*, 2005). The fat-soluble drug diazepam (Valium) has been observed to have a significantly larger Vd in women, and the water-soluble drug metronidazole (Flagyl) demonstrates a lower Vd, although increased clearance in women accounts for a lower area under the curve (AUC) for this drug in females. Water-soluble fluoroquinolones also have a smaller Vd in women. Both the oral clearance and Vd of prednisolone are significantly lower in women (Gandhi et al, 2004). Tricyclic antidepressants take longer to reach a steady state in women because of the drugs' lipophilic distribution. As a result, women experience more adverse reactions after the drug saturates all the sites in adipose tissues and more active drug remains in the bloodstream.

Gastric levels of alcohol dehydrogenase are lower in women, so a greater fraction of ingested alcohol would be oxidized

Table 48–1   Gender Differences in Pharmacokinetic Parameters

Pharmacokinetic Parameter	Sex-Based Difference
Absorption and bioavailability	• Gastric emptying time is slower in females, mainly related to the effects of estrogen. Drugs absorbed in the stomach will have longer exposure to absorption sites. • Gastric levels of alcohol dehydrogenase are lower in females. Plasma concentrations are greater in females than males after ingestion of similar amounts of alcohol. • Gastric acid secretion, pH, osmolality, electrolyte concentrations, and levels of bile acids and proteins do not vary significantly between sexes.
Distribution	• Females have lower body weights and BMI than males. • Females have a higher proportion of body fat. Lipophilic drugs are more readily absorbed and have relatively greater volumes of distribution than hydrophilic drugs. • Plasma volume is lower in females. Drugs with high volumes of distribution will be more concentrated in the plasma of females. • Organ blood flow is lower in females. • Estrogen is distributed attached to a serum-binding globulin. Exogenous estrogens increase levels of many serum-binding globulins such as corticosteroid-binding globulin and thyroxine-binding globulin resulting in less free drug.
Metabolism	• Studies have been inconsistent in showing differences in CYP450 substrates; the general trend is toward high rates of metabolism for CYP450 3A4 substrates and lower rates for 1A2 and 2D6 substrates. • Females have lower levels of p-glycoprotein and higher rates of drug clearance for drugs that are substrates of p-glycoprotein.
Excretion	• Gender differences in rates of renal excretion of most drugs are probably more related to simple weight differences. • Drugs that are actively secreted by the kidney may show gender differences, but further study is required to demonstrate this difference.

BMI = body mass index.

in men prior to absorption than in women. This is a significant factor behind why blood alcohol levels are disproportionately higher in women after ingestion of similar amounts of alcohol.

Gender-based differences in drug metabolism play a larger role in inter-gender pharmacokinetic differences than any of the other parameters. While hepatic blood flow is lower in women, differences in hepatic enzymes seem to be the major factor in variability. The frequency of variant alleles for the CYP450 system (a major group of enzymes involved in drug metabolism and bioactivation) has been shown to exist both between races and sexes. Studies have shown that CYP 3A4 activity is 24% higher in women (Gandhi et al, 2004) and CYP 1A2 is lower (Davis, 1998). It is acknowledged that some studies demonstrated that the mean amounts of these isoenzymes did not differ (Gandhi et al, 2004), but specific drugs have shown differences. For example, erythromycin is more rapidly cleared in women than it is in men, which is thought to be related to its CYP450 3A4–mediated effect. Orally administered verapamil (Isoptin, Calan) clears more quickly in men than it does in women based in part on its CYP 3A4 metabolism. Higher absolute bioavailability of this drug in women may explain the greater pharmacodynamic effects on blood pressure and heart rate in women. The CYP 2D6 isoenzyme is important in the metabolism of many psychotropic drugs. One study showed that tardive dyskinesia develops more frequently in female Chinese schizophrenics secondary to increased frequency of a defective CYP 2D6 allele in Chinese women (Gandhi et al, 2004).

Propranolol (Inderal) was one of the earliest drugs to show a clear gender difference in metabolic clearance of a drug. Oral doses of this drug had a significantly higher (63%) rate of clearance in men than it did in women (*Women and trials*, 2005). IV doses demonstrated no differences, indicating that this was a hepatic first-pass metabolism issue. Women might be expected, therefore, to show a significantly greater clinical response to oral doses of this drug than men.

The difference in clearance rates among the benzodiazepines can be explained in part by CP450 (oxidative) versus conjugative activity for drug metabolism. Those that undergo oxidative metabolism (alprazolam, diazepam, and midazolam), which is higher in women, are more rapidly metabolized than those that undergo conjugation (chlordiazepoxide, temazepam, and oxazepam), which is lower in women. The gender-related difference in CYP 2D6 activity and p-glycoprotein expression may be an important reason for different responses to antidepressants such as serotonin reuptake inhibitors (*Women and trials*, 2005). Finally, oral contraceptives have been demonstrated to significantly inhibit CYP 2C19 activity, which accounts for many drug interactions with other drugs using this substrate.

Studies aimed at showing differences in drug metabolism based on menopausal status have been inconsistent. Conflicting data exist on whether menopausal status or estrogen and progesterone level in HRT significantly affects drug metabolism and, therefore, no recommendations can be made at this time.

Kleist (2005) reminds us that many of these effects have been subtle and their overall clinical relevance remains to be demonstrated. With the exception of propranolol and verapamil, in which differences in outcome have been clearly significant, and erythromycin, which appears to be more effective in women, the provider should use these data to alter individual drug regimens cautiously.

Excretion of drugs by the kidney depends on weight, body surface area, age, and gender. Renal clearance of drugs that are not actively secreted or reabsorbed is dependent on the glomerular filtration rate, which is directly proportional to weight and consequently higher (on average) in men. Gender differences in excretion, therefore, are thought to be largely related to weight differences. Drugs that are actively secreted by the kidney may show gender-based differences, but further study in humans is necessary to clearly demonstrate this difference (Gandhi et al, 2004).

Pharmacodynamics

Pharmacodynamic differences in drug response based on gender have not been studied to the same extent as pharmacokinetic differences. Pharmacodynamic differences are demonstrated only when the same plasma concentration of a drug in both males and females yields a different pharmacological outcome. The clinical relevance of gender-related differences in pharmacodynamics appears with greater risk for adverse drug responses (1.5% to 1.7% higher) in women (Rademaker, 2001). However, not all drugs that have pharmacokinetic differences have pharmacodynamic differences.

The pharmacokinetic differences seen in prednisolone correlate with increased cortisol and T-helper lymphocyte suppression in women. This difference may be mediated by endogenous estrogen, because increased sensitivity has been found at higher estradiol concentrations, which may translate into clinical differences in postmenopausal women. The pharmacokinetic differences seen in verapamil lead to pharmacological effects of greater reductions in blood pressure and heart rate in women.

Gender differences in response to various analgesics have been well studied. Opiates seem to have a greater analgesic effect in women (Gandhi et al, 2004; *Women and trials*, 2005), but this difference is accompanied by an increase in adverse effects, especially nausea and vomiting. These differences in pharmacological response appear to be due to pharmacodynamic differences, including gender differences in drug-receptor affinity, receptor density, or signal transduction pathways (Gandhi et al, 2004). The effects of several cardiovascular drugs on women are different from their effects on men. Women aged 15 to 50 years have longer QT intervals, making them more vulnerable to cardiac arrhythmias. Macrolide antibiotics cause a woman's heart to repolarize more slowly. Pharmacokinetic differences in females may explain the increased incidence of life-threatening ventricular arrhythmias, which are twice as common in women who are taking erythromycin (*Women and trials,* 2005). Women taking oral anticoagulants (warfarin) or thrombolytic agents (e.g., after myocardial infarction [MI]) have less benefit with respect to mortality but more bleeding episodes (Gandhi et al, 2004; *Women and trials*, 2005). Aspirin is often prescribed for MI and stroke prevention. Randomized trials have shown that although aspirin lowers the risk for ischemic stroke in women, it has little effect on their risk for MI; the opposite is true in men (*Women and trials,* 2005). The exact mechanism for this gender-related difference in outcome has yet to be elucidated.

Many psychotropic drugs appear to exhibit gender-mediated differences in pharmacodynamics. In general, women show both greater improvement in symptoms and more severe adverse reactions with antipsychotics (Gandhi et al, 2004). These effects appear to be related to the anti-dopaminergic actions of estrogens, duplicating the major mechanism of action of typical antipsychotics. These findings have resulted in a trend toward prescribing lower doses for women. Tricyclic antidepressants exhibit both pharmacokinetic and pharmacodynamic differences between genders. Studies have shown that premenopausal women respond better to selective serotonin reuptake inhibitors (SSRIs), and men respond better to tricyclic antidepressants (Anderson, 2005; Davis, 1998). Another example is lithium and its increased bioavailability because of renal excretion. This pharmacokinetic difference can result in levels of this drug that are higher in women. The narrow therapeutic range for this drug means the risk for toxicity is increased in women, though no studies have confirmed this (Grandjean & Aubry, 2009). Drug levels drawn early in therapy may prevent toxicity in drugs, such as lithium, digoxin, and theophylline, which have narrow margins of safety.

Infection with HIV and the development of AIDS are increasing in females, as is the use of antiretroviral drugs. Multiple studies have shown differences in treatment efficacy, toxicity profile, and drug pharmacokinetics between women and men (Gandhi et al, 2004). Women experience more frequent and severe adverse effects with various protease inhibitors, including higher rates of gastrointestinal and neurological adverse effects, with ritonavir secondary to higher plasma concentrations of this drug. They also demonstrate higher rates of allergic reactions and nephrolithiasis with protease inhibitors. Related problems (neuropathy, pancreatitis, and toxicity-driven regimen changes) also occur more often in women (Gandhi et al, 2004). A few studies have shown increased efficacy of antiretrovirals in women compared to men, including slower rates of disease progression and hospital admissions related to HIV disease in women on highly active antiretroviral therapy (HAART) (Hermes et al, 2012; Moore, Sabin, Johnson, & Phillips, 2002). Further discussion of HIV infection and AIDS is found in Chapter 37.

In summary, an increasing number of gender-related differences in pharmacokinetics and pharmacodynamics are emerging. Kleist (*Women and trials,* 2005) warns, however, that these differences generally have not had an impact on drug dosing and most drugs on the market have a wide enough therapeutic index that minor differences usually do not reach clinical significance. Clinical significance can be seen in drugs that have marked gender-specific pharmacokinetic differences and those with narrow therapeutic indices, a steep dose-concentration curve, or both. As more clinical trials include both women and men, more pharmacodynamic and pharmacotherapeutic differences may appear.

FACTORS THAT INFLUENCE MEDICATION ADMINISTRATION

Puberty

Adolescent female athletes may display a combination of symptoms, including amenorrhea, disordered eating, and osteoporosis, called the "female athlete triad" (Gibbs, Williams, & De Souza, 2012). This syndrome is a disruption in normal growth and development caused by inadequate nutrition (caloric intake lower than expenditure) and over exercising (strenuous athletic training). These two behaviors lead to suppression of the hypothalamic-pituitary-ovarian axis, which in turn leads to reduced estrogen levels, amenorrhea, and decreased bone mineralization. Incidence of secondary amenorrhea (defined as absence of menses for 6 months in a girl who has had at least one menstrual period) runs between 10% and 50% in highly trained female athletes. Many young athletes present with primary amenorrhea (absence of menses by age 13 with secondary sex characteristics or absence of menses by age 15 with secondary sex characteristics). Hormonal therapy is not successful with this type of hypogonadism; however, other strategies that decrease the risk for osteoporosis should be incorporated into the routine health care of adolescent females in order to promote positive lifetime habits. Strategies include increasing daily calcium intake and assessing the amount of vitamin D exposure, which can help decrease the risk of osteoporosis. Decreasing the level of physical activity, increasing dietary intake, and increased body mass index (BMI) have been associated with the return of normal menstruation (Arends, Cheung, Barrack, & Nattiv, 2012).

Persistent low levels of estrogen in adolescent women are of concern regarding bone mineralization. Forty percent of bone accrual occurs during adolescence with bone formation continuing up to age 30 years, after which a gradual bone loss begins (Moos, 2005), so building bone during this developmental stage is crucial. Because adolescents have not yet reached peak bone mass, interpreting adolescent bone density measurements should be done appropriately with pediatric/adolescent-specific software that calculates Z scores, rather than T scores. Without appropriate intervention, girls with low bone density may never achieve adequate bone mass and run the risk of fractures and osteoporosis. Bisphosphonates (used to treat osteoporosis in postmenopausal women) are not FDA-approved for use in the teen population and do not appear effective in treating osteoporosis in teens (Dominguez-Bartmess, Tandberg, Cheema, & Szalay, 2012). Adequate calcium intake along with vitamin D can help build bone mass. Successful management of the female athlete triad must be multidisciplinary, requiring the support of coaches, family, trainers, nutritionists, physicians, and counselors (Arends et al, 2012).

Because adolescent diets are often not healthy, strategies that decrease the risk for osteoporosis should be incorporated into the routine health care of adolescent females in order to promote lifetime wellness habits. A daily intake of 1,300 mg of calcium daily is recommended for females aged 9 through 18 years, an amount that can be obtained by drinking three cups of low-fat or skim milk and consuming 8 ounces of low-fat yogurt. If a young woman consistently is unable to meet the recommended daily amount of calcium through diet alone, calcium carbonate (Tums, Caltrate, or Viactiv) should be consumed with food to maximize absorption. Because vitamin D is required for optimal calcium absorption, a daily multivitamin that includes at least 400 IU vitamin D should also be taken (Moos, 2005). Adolescents should also be discouraged from smoking, because smoking has been associated with poor uptake of the nutrients needed to build healthy bone.

Another concern related to bone mineral density (BMD) is long-term use of medroxyprogesterone acetate (Depo-Provera), an injectable form of birth control used by approximately 10% of adolescents. In 2004, the FDA announced a Black-Box Warning for this drug when studies demonstrated an association between long-term Depo-Provera use and significant BMD loss. Because adolescent females have not yet reached their peak BMD, prolonged use of Depo-Provera may put these girls at increased risk for osteoporosis. Mounting evidence suggests bone mass recovery occurs when the drug is discontinued; however, the long-term impact of this drug on BMD throughout a woman's life remains unknown (Harel et al, 2010). The FDA warning indicates that Depo-Provera should not be used as a birth control method for longer than 2 years (Isley & Kaunitz, 2011). Treatment of osteoporosis, including nutrition, is discussed in Chapter 38.

Another concern common in adolescent girls and young women is iron-deficiency anemia (IDA), a condition often related to heavy menstruation. Oral iron supplementation is recommended to replenish iron loss during menstruation. Girls going through puberty may also be avoiding red meat, a good source of iron, in favor of lower-calorie salads and vegetables. Although green, leafy vegetables contain iron, plant sources are not as fully absorbed as the iron found in meats. IDA is discussed in more detail in Chapter 27.

Pregnancy

Extraordinary anatomical and physiological changes occur in a woman's body during pregnancy. Her body changes shape and size, and every organ system modifies its function to create a protective and nurturing environment for the developing fetus (Cunningham & Williams, 2010). Drug absorption through the lungs, skin, and mucous membranes is increased because of increased cardiac output, which peaks at 20 to 24 weeks' gestation. Increases in cardiac output may be 30% to 50% above prepregnancy levels. Plasma volume is 50% higher by the third trimester; most of the volume is in the products of conception.

Clearance of some drugs is altered by these changes. Phenytoin clearance, for example, is increased during the second and third trimesters. The risks/benefits of continuation of anticonvulsants during pregnancy need to be weighed against the real potential risk of seizure activity during pregnancy on the mother and the fetus. Valproate is not recommended in pregnancy because its teratogenicity is higher than other anticonvulsants, in part due to higher levels found in fetal cord blood. Another example of changed metabolism is theophylline, which has increased half-life and volume distribution in the third trimester because of decreased renal clearance (Isoherranen & Thummel, 2013). Other drugs with effects similar to theophylline for asthma are preferred during pregnancy. In general, serum levels of phenytoin, theophylline, and other medications with altered metabolism, if used in pregnancy, need to be monitored.

Iron deficiency anemia (IDA) is one of the most common complications of pregnancy and is primarily due to expansion of plasma volume without equivalent expansion of maternal hemoglobin mass. This condition is called physiologic anemia (Friedman et al, 2012). IDA puts a pregnant woman at risk for susceptibility to infections, fatigue, and an increased chance of pre-eclampsia and postpartum hemorrhage. In addition, a pregnant woman with IDA tolerates even minimal blood loss during birth poorly and may experience delayed healing of an episiotomy, laceration, or cesarean birth incision (Cunningham & Williams, 2010).

Dietary iron is necessary for hemoglobin production, and during pregnancy hemoglobin is vital for transport of oxygen to the growing fetus. Daily iron intake of 30 mg is necessary during pregnancy, with the greatest need for iron intake in the last 20 weeks (Friedman et al, 2012). Stinging nettle (*Urtica dioica*) and chlorophyll are good sources of iron for pregnant women who find it difficult to consume adequate amounts of iron-containing foods. Stinging nettle can be consumed as a cooked green leafy vegetable, added to soups, or drunk as a tea. The tea is prepared by adding boiling water to two teaspoons of the dried or fresh herb and then steeping for several minutes. A woman should drink two cups of tea per day with cinnamon and honey added to improve the taste (Davidson et al, 2011). Table 48-2 lists herbs to avoid in pregnancy.

> ● **CLINICAL PEARL** ●
>
> **Prescribing for adolescents**
> State laws vary regarding consent for treatment of sexually transmitted infections, contraception, and medical record confidentiality in minor patients. Nurse practitioners should become familiar with what health-care services can be provided to minors without parental consent.

The physiologic anemia of pregnancy is commonly treated with ferrous sulfate. This oral preparation should be taken with vitamin C for increased absorption and should be taken after meals to reduce gastrointestinal irritation. Because

Table 48–2 Use of Selected Herbs During Pregnancy

Common Name	Comments
Selected Herbs to Avoid in Pregnancy	
Alder buckthorn	Very potent stimulators of bowel peristalsis known to irritate the uterus in sensitive women that may cause premature labor.
Almond oil	External application to abdomen has been associated with preterm birth.*
Angelica, dong quai	Uterine stimulant or may induce abortion/preterm labor. Dong quai is also an anticoagulant.
Arbor vitae and aloe	Oil-containing plants and essential oils that should not be taken internally during pregnancy.
Autumn crocus	Alkaloid-containing herbs that can be very potent and are best avoided in pregnancy.
Barberry	Uterine stimulant.
Black cohosh	Uterine stimulant.
Blessed thistle	Powerful laxative; may overstimulate digestion and metabolism, causing fluid and electrolyte imbalances.
Blue cohosh	Uterine stimulant.
Cascara sagrada	Powerful laxative; may overstimulate digestion and metabolism, causing fluid and electrolyte imbalance.
Ephedra	Cardiovascular stimulant.
Feverfew	Uterine stimulant.
Ginseng	Thought to affect the hormonal system.
Goldenseal	Uterine stimulant.
Gotu kola	Potential teratogen.
Juniper	Potential teratogen.
Licorice root	Powerful laxative; may overstimulate digestion and metabolism, causing fluid and electrolyte imbalances.
Mugwort	Uterine stimulant.
Pennyroyal	Uterine stimulant.
Senna	Powerful laxative; may overstimulate digestion and metabolism, causing fluid and electrolyte imbalances.
Yarrow root	Uterine stimulant.
Selected Herbs That Appear to Be Safe in Pregnancy†	
Chamomile flowers	May be taken in capsule form or used as a tea or infusion for nausea.
Black haw/cramp bark	Uterine relaxant; used for cramping.
Dandelion greens and root	For anemia.
False unicorn root	Uterine tonic; used with black haw/cramp bark to prevent miscarriage.
Ginger root	For nausea.
Jasmine	Essential oils that can be safely used in aromatherapy during pregnancy. Do not ingest or use internally.
Nettle leaf	Allergy prevention.
Peppermint leaf	For nausea.
Red raspberry leaf	Uterine toner.
Slippery elm bark	Uterine relaxant; used for cramping.

*Facchinetti, F., Pedrielli, G., Benoni, G., Joppi, M., Verlato, G., Dante, G., et al. (2012). Herbal supplements in pregnancy: Unexpected results from a multicentre study. *Human Reproduction, 27*(11), 3161–3167.

†Effectiveness for most of these herbs has not been proven.

women with IDA may be asymptomatic, and because not all pregnant women need large quantities of supplemental iron, monitoring hemoglobin and hematocrit is necessary. To prevent IDA, a prenatal vitamin with an iron supplement of 30 mg/d should be initiated at the first prenatal visit, and pregnant women should be advised to eat an iron-rich diet (Friedman et al, 2012).

Pregnancy may present an opportune time for women to modify unhealthy or high-risk lifestyle behaviors. For example, illicit drug use may be corrected or reduced when patients are motivated by the birth of a child. Although legal, nicotine and alcohol are harmful to the developing fetus.

The use of caffeine during pregnancy remains controversial. At this time, no conclusive evidence links caffeine consumption to birth defects, spontaneous abortion (Davidson et al, 2011), pregnancy duration, condition of newborn (Jarosz, Wierzejska, & Siuba, 2012), or offspring behavior problems at age 5 to 6 (Loomans et al, 2012). Caffeine is found in beverages such as coffee, teas, colas, and some other sodas, in foods such as chocolate, and some over-the-counter (OTC) pain relievers. Caffeine, a central nervous system stimulant, causes mood swings and diuresis and readily crosses the placenta to the fetus, who is unable to metabolize it effectively. Caffeine may cause fetal or newborn cardiac arrhythmias. Some women may choose to avoid caffeine intake during pregnancy altogether. Until more information is available, pregnant women should be counseled about sources of caffeine and advised to limit their consumption to 150 to 300 mg a day or less (ACOG, 2010; Davidson et al, 2011).

Smoking has been linked to higher infertility rates in both men and women. Women who smoke have a higher risk for spontaneous abortion, preterm birth, placenta previa, abruptio placentae, and premature rupture of membranes. The risk is directly related to the number of cigarettes smoked, so any decrease in smoking will improve fetal outcomes. Two main ingredients in cigarette smoke affect the fetus: carbon monoxide and nicotine. Carbon monoxide competes for oxygen binding sites on fetal hemoglobin and nicotine causes vasoconstriction in both the mother and the fetus. The compound effect of these two ingredients is decreased availability and delivery of oxygen to maternal and fetal tissues, including the uterus and placenta (Cunningham & Williams, 2010).

Alcohol causes decreased folic acid and thiamine absorption. Mothers who drink alcohol while pregnant frequently deliver low-birth-weight infants, and they risk their infants' having problems of growth and development associated with fetal alcohol syndrome. To date, no safe level of alcohol consumption during pregnancy has been identified; therefore, women should be counseled to abstain from alcohol during pregnancy (Cunningham & Williams, 2010).

Complementary and alternative therapies, such as the use of medicinal herbs, are currently being evaluated with randomized methodologies to evaluate their efficacy. Many herbs can be useful for treating pregnancy-associated discomforts. Examples include ginger for nausea and vomiting, horse chestnut for varicose veins, and meadowsweet for heartburn (Blumenthal, Goldberg, & Brinckman, 2000; Gottlieb, 2008; Hardy, 2000). Women interested in taking herbs during pregnancy should be advised: (1) to avoid most herbs during the first trimester (except up to 1 g of ginger per day), (2) to avoid standardized or highly concentrated extracts, and (3) not to ingest essential oils (Davidson et al, 2011; Hardy, 2000). Table 48-2 presents selected herbs that are contraindicated during pregnancy and some that may be beneficial.

Menopause

Menopause, a natural passage in a woman's life, is a time of transition that marks the end of a woman's reproductive abilities. Women experience changes in their reproductive, musculoskeletal, and cardiovascular systems as well as vasomotor and cognitive function changes. Despite the significance of these changes, few women going through menopause have engaged in discussion with their health-care provider about menopausal symptoms, risk for chronic disease, or hormone use (Davidson et al, 2011; Smith, 2005).

Many options for managing menopausal symptoms are available, such as the use of exercise, relaxation techniques, massage therapy, acupuncture, herbs, or pharmaceuticals such as HRT (Roush, 2012). Some women are unable or choose not to take HRT and have turned to phytoestrogens, substances with estrogen-like properties found in certain herbs—such as ginseng, black cohosh, dong quai, fenugreek, and licorice—and certain foods—especially carrots, yams, and soy products—with varying efficacy (Roush, 2012). Another menopause treatment option the practitioner should consider is nutritional supplements for a diet rich in calcium and vitamins E, D, and B complex. In addition, menopausal women should avoid foods such as caffeine, alcohol, and spicy foods that can trigger vasomotor symptoms (Davidson et al, 2011). Alternative therapies for symptoms of menopause are presented in Table 48-3; herbal therapies are discussed in Chapter 10, and HRT is discussed in detail in Chapter 38.

Although managing menopausal symptoms is important, it is also vital at this time of life for a woman to achieve and/or maintain good health. Emphasis in the care of women in their 50s should be on health promotion and prevention of the diseases of older age. Classically, after menopause the lipid profile of women changes. The decline in endogenous estrogen removes a protective physiological mechanism that supports higher levels of high-density lipoprotein (HDL) and lowers low-density lipoproteins (LDL). Loss of estrogen places a woman at increased risk for coronary artery disease, hypertension, and stroke (Davidson et al, 2011). In fact, menopausal women "catch up" to men in relation to risks for these diseases and may experience "silent" coronary artery disease, which can become their greatest risk factor for death. Studies show that fewer women than men survive their first heart attack (Davidson et al, 2011). Providers need to educate themselves and their female patients about the signs and symptoms of cardiac disease in women and how the symptoms differ from

Table 48–3   Alternative Therapies for Menopause Symptoms

Symptom	Alternative Therapy and Its Effects
Hot flashes	• **Suggest taking vitamin E 400 bid:** affects blood vessel walls; some women have blood pressure changes; monitor patients with hypertension. • **Suggest taking soy 2 oz:** contains 45 mg phytoestrogens (genistein); may protect from cancer. • **Suggest taking evening primrose 3 oz:** eliminate breast tenderness: stabilizes hormone fluctuations. • **Suggest taking remifemin (black cohosh) 1 tablet bid:** suppresses LH but not FSH; progesterone precursor; reduces hot flashes; used in Germany. • **Suggest taking dong quai:** estrogen precursor. • **Suggest taking bioidentical hormones:** contain equivalent hormones but from plant sources.
Reduced libido (or lack of sex drive)	• **Talk with the patient, sexual counseling/therapy:** ensure that spousal issues are not a hidden factor; if the intimate relationship is not good, menopause may not be the primary problem. • **Investigate sleep issues:** sleep disturbances can cause depression. • **Screen for depression:** depression often associated with altered libido. • **Suggest using alternative therapies listed for weight fluctuation:** improves self-image, which weight gain may hinder; increases energy after minimal weight loss (5 to 10 lb). • **Suggest using alternative therapies for vaginal dryness or soreness:** reduces vaginal dryness and pain; allows for anticipation of positive sensations.
Mood changes (irritability, depression)	• **Take vitamin B₆ (pyridoxine) 1.3 mg daily:** turns amino acids into serotonin, which affects mood. • **Practice meditation, yoga, or prayer:** calms nervous system; stimulates immunity; enhances personal control. • **Obtain adequate sleep:** aids relaxation. • **Improvise stress management techniques:** improves relaxation.
Sleep disturbances	• **Suggest taking valerian root, chamomile, melatonin:** aids relaxation. • **Exercise:** stimulates serotonin production after 40 min; affects mood. • **Decrease intake of or avoid stimulants (caffeine, nicotine, large protein-rich meals):** allows relaxation of nervous system. • **Avoid alcohol:** negatively affects all stages of sleep. • **Meditate, pray:** calms nervous system; stimulates immunity; enhances personal control.
Stress incontinence (urinary)	• **Decrease intake of caffeine beverages and diuretics:** reduces irritated detrusor muscle; results in less urgency. • **Perform Kegel exercises:** strengthens pelvic floor muscles. • **Treat/reduce constipation:** relieves pressure on urethra and bladder. • **Participate in bladder training programs:** reduces incidence of incontinence.
Vaginal dryness or soreness	• **Reduce or avoid use of medications such as antihistamines, decongestants, anticholinergics, and diuretics:** improves tissue moisture. • **Suggest using alternative therapies listed for hot flashes:** increases epithelial lining of vaginal tissues. • **Use water-soluble lubricants daily (e.g., Replens, Astroglide, Lubrin):** facilitates penetration; enhances foreplay (ensure that the patient knows areas to apply for maximum stimulation).
Weight fluctuations	• **Exercise 30 to 60 min daily:** reduces weight gain; stabilizes mood; strengthens muscles; improves balance; stimulates good bone metabolism.

LH = luteinizing hormone; FSH = follicle-stimulating hormone.

those in men, with particular emphasis on the need to seek early treatment. Angina and ischemic heart disease are discussed in Chapter 28. Hypertension is discussed in Chapter 40, and hyperlipidemia in Chapter 39.

Genetics play a role in the diseases that afflict women at midlife, including heart disease, but preventive measures can be taught as well as prescribed. Primary prevention studies demonstrate that diets high in complex carbohydrates, fiber, and protein and low in animal fat are best. Balanced diets such as those recommended in *My Pyramid* (Guenther, Reedy, & Krebs-Smith, 2008) can lead to a lower body mass index (BMI). Normal BMI is considered between 18.5 and 24.9; 25 to 29.9 is considered overweight, and 30 or more is

obese. Persons with a BMI greater than 30 are associated with morbidity and shortened life expectancy.

Exercise is a nonpharmacological health promotion strategy. The exercise does not have to be strenuous, just consistent. Walking, yard work, bicycling, and swimming are all good forms of exercise. Thirty minutes of moderate physical activity for at least 6 days per week is recommended for best health (Leitzmann et al, 2007). Other alternative therapies for menopausal symptoms are listed in Table 48-3.

Other postmenopausal physical changes seen in women are the results of normal human aging and are shared by both sexes. These changes include thinning and graying of the hair, weight gain, drying skin, vision changes associated with presbyopia, and increased healing time for musculoskeletal injuries. Female genitourinary tract changes, affecting the vagina and urinary system, are the result of the cessation of ovarian function and decreased estrogen levels. Loss of the ureterovesicular angle and detrusor muscle instability result in urinary frequency and leakage, with increased residual bladder volume. Breast composition changes from dense glandular tissue to fatty replacement.

Older Age

In this millennium, many women are living as long after menopause as they did before it. Women in every culture live longer than men (Austad, 2006). Race is a major determinant of women's life spans. In the United States, white women have a life expectancy of 80.5 years, in contrast to African Americans, whose life expectancy is 76.1 years (Hoyert, Mathews, Menacker, Strobino, & Guyer, 2006). Cardiovascular disease causes the greatest morbidity and mortality for the aging woman, followed by cancer and cerebrovascular disease (Bertoia, et al, 2012).

Aging women experience more frequent autoimmune disease, which manifests itself in joint and soft tissue pain and deformity. Although the risks for cancer increase with age and an estimated 250,000 new cases of breast cancer are diagnosed in the United States every year, many women never have mammograms because of lack of information, poor access to health care, or insufficient insurance coverage (Peipins et al, 2012). Smoking by women increased during the post–World War II years until the 1970s, which is hypothesized as the reason for increased lung cancer rates for older women. More recently, smoking rates have declined such that 17.9% of U.S. women smoke (Moolgavkar et al, 2012).

FACTORS THAT INFLUENCE POSITIVE OUTCOMES

Factors that produce positive outcomes are discussed in detail in Chapter 6. This section will discuss only those specific to women.

Number of Drugs Taken

Adult women receive more prescription drugs than men of the same age. Women are more apt to take medications for their skin, muscles, urinary tract, ophthalmological and otological problems, fatigue, extremity pain, weight, hypertension, and emotional complaints. Depression and connective tissue diseases are much more common in women. The risk for adverse reactions and drug interactions increases proportionately with the number of drugs being taken concurrently. The overall treatment regimen of each female patient should be regularly reviewed to eliminate any drugs that have "outlived" their usefulness or are duplicates.

Duration of Medication Therapy

Most patients can remember to take medications for a few days, especially if they are feeling ill, but drugs that must be taken daily and for many years are subject to poor adherence rates. Women may find themselves responsible for taking oral contraceptive pills (OCPs) for 10 to 40 years, with other drugs added in from time to time. Adherence with OCP use varies over time, but generally averages between 47% to 74% (Zapata, Steenland, Brahmi, Marchbanks, & Curtis, 2012). Providers who care for women of childbearing age need to be ever cognizant of the risk of pregnancy, even in women who are using contraception.

Strategies to improve compliance, such as taking medications along with other routine activities of daily living, have been shown to work well. Women are frequently the primary caregivers of children and may also care for other family members (spouses, elderly parents, and relatives). The busyness of women's lives can complicate medication administration and decrease adherence.

Fear That Medications Cause Disease

Social networking is frequently the way that women access health information. Through social media they hear about drugs (such as hormones) causing cancer or other disease from the media (e.g., television, newspapers) and from friends and relatives. This information is often sensational and can be inflammatory while being nonspecific. Concerns about exogenous hormones being carcinogenic can drive patient behavior, and it behooves providers to take time to explore them with patients. Education is needed to help women understand the results of studies done when much higher levels of potent estrogen were used in OCP and HRT formulations. Recent studies on the risk of gynecological cancers have shown a large hereditary component in breast cancer, especially when it occurs in women who are premenopausal. Genetic testing is now available for breast and ovarian cancers. Women may have a hard time deciding if they should use hormonal therapies because it is difficult to calculate their own absolute risk. What they hear in the media are relative risks, which refer to populations of women in certain age brackets. The results of the Women's Health Initiative (WHI) continue to be evaluated and clarified. Providers need to read current research and be accurate in their knowledge in this area and share updated data with patients (Nelson, Walker, Zakher, & Mitchell, 2012).

Nutritional Status

Appropriate diet and good nutritional status are necessary for facilitating optimal growth in adolescents and for promoting health and wellness in women of all ages.

Obesity is a growing problem in all segments of the U.S. population. Women are at higher risk than men for eating disorders, which can lead to both overweight and underweight conditions. Many women have weight retention after pregnancy and then start their next pregnancy overweight. Obesity carries with it increased risks of pregnancy complications, infertility, cardiovascular and organ disease, hypertension, and diabetes. Anorexia nervosa and bulimia are complicated disorders with mental, emotional, and physical components that can lead to underweight as well as dental problems, infertility, osteopenia/osteoporosis, organ failure, and death. Of note, depression—more women than men suffer from this chronic mental illness—is the most common comorbidity with both obesity and anorexia (Ward & Hisley, 2009). Treatment for both overweight and underweight women can be challenging, with the best results involving an interdisciplinary team of providers. Polypharmacy can be a hazard in these patients, and prescriber vigilance in monitoring both drugs and changing doses, as weight and other body parameters change, is needed.

Safety of Medications While Breastfeeding

The benefits conferred to infants by breastfeeding, especially in the first year of life, are well described in the literature. Points to be considered in prescribing to lactating mothers are the acidity of breast milk in relation to the pH of plasma, the protein-binding effects of the drug prescribed, the liposolubility of the drug prescribed, and the molecular weight of the drug prescribed. All prescribed medications in the United States have labeling delineating breastfeeding risks. The National Library of Medicine maintains an evidence-based database of the effects of drugs and other chemicals to which breastfeeding mothers might be exposed Called LactMed (http://toxnet.nlm.nih.gov/). The LactMed database provides information on the level of substances in breast milk, effects on the breastfeeding infant, as well as suggested therapeutic alternatives.

Ethnic, Cultural, and Religious Differences

Although women from diverse cultures commonly seek health care more often than do men (this is true in most cultures), many cultures are patriarchies. In patriarchal societies, men make the decisions about birth control, whether women work outside the home, and how much money women receive to run the household. Women may not have the choice to refuse sexual relations. The lack of power and control over their own bodies can generate many somatic complaints. These women patients often present on multiple occasions with what may appear to be nonspecific and unrelated symptoms (Crissman, Adanu, & Harlow, 2012). Pelvic pain and genital pain are frequent complaints, and unplanned pregnancies are not unusual. Adherence to prescribed contraceptive regimens is difficult, if not impossible, for women in many of these situations.

Religion can also raise issues related to the prescribing of medications. If a patient's belief system does not support a treatment that the provider is prescribing, adherence may become a problem. Cultural issues are discussed in detail in Chapter 7.

COMMON PROBLEMS THAT REQUIRE MEDICATIONS

In addition to the array of medical problems shared by both genders—hypertension, cardiovascular disease, diabetes,

---

CLINICAL PEARL

Prescribing in pregnancy and lactation

The pregnancy risk categories (A, B, C, D, X) should be used as a guide only. Category X (known teratogenic effects on the fetus) must be avoided in pregnancy. Category D drugs should be used only in a life-threatening situation (i.e., chemotherapy drugs), as known fetal risks exist. Categories A, B, and C may have some risks. Every prescription drug now provides "Pregnancy Implications" and "Lactation" labeling and these should be read and understood before prescribing.

In 2014 the Food and Drug Administration passed The Pregnancy and Lactation Labeling Rule that will affect all prescription drugs and biological products. The pregnancy risk categories (A, B, C, D, X) will be eliminated and replaced with a summary of risks of using the drug during pregnancy and while breastfeeding. There will be a new section on drug labels titled "Female and Male of Reproductive Potential" that will include information about the need for pregnancy testing, contraceptive recommendations, and drug effects on fertility. All new drugs approved after June 30, 2015, will have the new labeling format (with no A, B, C, D, or X). The new format will be phased in gradually for previously approved drugs.

---

cancer, glaucoma, organ disease, arthritis, mental illnesses, autoimmune disorders, and pain management—specific problems in women that require medications include urinary tract infection and urinary incontinence, sexually transmitted infections and vaginitis, premenstrual disorders, endometriosis, polycystic ovarian syndrome (PCOS), contraception, infertility, menopause, gynecological cancers, osteoporosis, depression, and hypothyroidism. Many of these problems are discussed in the appropriate chapters in Unit III. Problems not discussed in Unit III chapters are included here: menopause, premenstrual syndrome and premenstrual dysphoric disorder, endometriosis, PCOS, HIV/AIDS in pregnancy, and infertility.

CLINICAL PEARL

Prescribing in a diverse culture

Be aware of the common ethnic groups in your patient population. Get to know the cultures. Frequently, community programs that teach cultural awareness and some simple ethnic phrases are available for health-care personnel. Bookstores carry pocket-sized books to facilitate a simple medical interview in different languages.

Menopause

Menopause is a normal physiological process in women, with the mean age of menopause in the United States at 51.3 years (Davidson et al, 2011; Smith, 2005). Several years of gradual decline or erratic levels of endogenous estrogen precede cessation of ovarian function. All women experience changes in their secondary sexual characteristics. Some women barely notice vasomotor instability, whereas hot flashes and insomnia incapacitate others. Estrogen and progesterone may interact at more than 200 receptor sites in a woman's body, so exogenous treatment may affect women in many different ways. Alternative therapies for symptoms of menopause are presented in Table 48-3. When women are postmenopausal and choose to use drug therapy (HRT), absolute risks versus benefits for the individual should be assessed and discussed. Present recommendations are for the lowest amount of drug to be used for the shortest period of time to alleviate problematic symptoms (The North American Menopause Society, 2012). It is recommended that treatment with estrogen and progesterone, for women with a uterus, be for no more than 3 to 5 years due to earlier increased risk of breast cancer, but that estrogen therapy alone, for those without a uterus, can safely be continued longer when the balance of potential benefits and risks is favorable for the individual woman (North American Menopause Society, 2012).

Dysmenorrhea, Premenstrual Syndrome, and Premenstrual Dysphoric Disorder

Women typically have menstrual cycles for about 40 years. Cyclic perimenstrual pain and discomfort (CPPD) is the name of a concept developed by a team of American Women's Health, Obstetric and Neonatal Nurses (AWHONN) nurse-researchers (Collins Sharp, Taylor, Thomas, Killeen, & Dawood, 2002). This concept includes dysmenorrhea, premenstrual syndrome (PMS), and premenstrual dysphoric disorder (PMDD). CPPD can have a significant impact on a woman's quality of life. Nurse practitioners play a vital role in identifying and diagnosing dysmenorrhea, PMS, and the more disabling PMDD and in managing the symptoms of these disorders. Bhati and Bhati (2002) report that as many as 20% to 40% of menstruating women experience one of the disorders.

Dysmenorrhea

Dysmenorrhea, pain shortly before or during menstruation, is one of the most common gynecological complaints. Young adult women (under 20 years old) present most frequently with this complaint, but the condition affects women of all ages. Between 41% to 93% of adolescents experience symptoms; this incidence decreases with age (Zahradnik, Hanjalic-Beck, & Groth, 2010). Primary dysmenorrhea is due to increased myometrial activity, with contractions induced by prostaglandins in the second half of the menstrual cycle. NSAIDS are the first line of drug treatment for women not desiring contraception (Zahradnik et al, 2010) and are particularly effective if begun 2 to 3 days before menses or at the first sign of bleeding. OTC NSAIDs have the same active ingredients (e.g., ibuprofen, naproxen sodium) as prescription drugs; however, the labeled recommended dose for general discomfort may be subtherapeutic for dysmenorrhea. Preparations containing acetaminophen, which is not an NSAID, are ineffective because of the absence of antiprostaglandin

properties. For women who want contraception, oral contraceptive pills (OCPs) are a good therapeutic choice. Decreased prostaglandin synthesis results from an atrophic endometrium (Zahradnik et al, 2010). No single brand of OCP has been shown to be superior for this indication.

> ### CLINICAL PEARL
>
> **Progesterone-only therapies**
> Women who have contraindications to estrogen use need to be counseled that there are several easy-to-use progesterone methods, without estrogen, that offer effective contraception and treatment for dysmenorrhea.

Many nonpharmacological measures can be used to relieve primary dysmenorrhea, and often the best treatment strategies involve using medications and comfort measures along with lifestyle modifications. Complementary and alternative medicines (CAMs) shown to improve symptoms of dysmenorrhea include thiamine (vitamin B_1), magnesium, vitamin E, and omega-3 fatty acids (Zahradnik et al, 2010). Comfort measures, including heat (poultices or heating pads), massage/effleurage, guided imagery, progressive relaxation, yoga, exercise, and meditation, have been successful in managing menstrual discomfort. Decreasing dietary intake of salt, sugar, and red meat in the luteal phase and increasing water intake may reduce edema (Lowdermilk & Perry, 2007).

If dysmenorrheal discomfort is not relieved by one of the NSAIDS, further investigation into the cause of symptoms is required. Secondary dysmenorrhea usually develops later in a woman's life (after age 25) with a prevalence of about 5% (Zahradnik et al, 2010). Pelvic pathology—such as adenomyosis, endometriosis, pelvic inflammatory disease (PID), endometrial polyps, and myomas (fibroids)—is associated with secondary dysmenorrhea (Lowdermilk & Perry, 2007). Many of the relief measures for primary dysmenorrhea are also helpful for women with secondary dysmenorrhea, but treatment is aimed at removal of the underlying pathology.

Premenstrual Syndrome (PMS)

The diagnostic criteria for PMS were written by the ACOG (Davis & Johnson, 2000). Symptoms include irritability, depression, angry outbursts, anxiety, confusion, social withdrawal, and mood swings. Somatic symptoms include fatigue, insomnia, dizziness, headaches, breast tenderness, weight gain, abdominal bloating, edema secondary to water retention, and muscle and joint pain (*Premenstrual syndrome*, 2003). Women often respond to exercising aerobically, decreasing caffeine, reducing salt intake, and taking ibuprofen 500 to 1,000 mg/d during the luteal phase: days 17 to 28 of the menstrual cycle (Frackiewicz & Shiovitz, 2001). Pritham (2002) recommends eating smaller, more frequent meals that are high in complex carbohydrates and fiber; reducing intake of salty foods, sugar, caffeine, chocolate, red meat, dairy products, and alcohol; and increasing the dose of calcium supplementation. She also recommends relaxation techniques, yoga, stress management, and good sleep hygiene. CAM that has been shown to be helpful include calcium, magnesium, vitamin B_6, evening primrose, and chasteberry (Zahradnik et al, 2010).

Premenstrual Dysphoric Disorder

A small subgroup of CPPD patients (2% to 10%) has a more severe form of the disorder: premenstrual dysphoric disorder (PMDD) (Epperson et al, 2012; Qiao et al, 2012). Diagnosis of PMDD is based on criteria established by the American Psychiatric Association (APA, 2013). To meet diagnostic criteria, patients must exhibit five or more symptoms, including at least one "core" symptom. Severely affected women typically have symptoms for 6 to 7 days each cycle. Symptoms of PMDD include the core symptoms of markedly depressed moods, heightened anxiety/tension/edginess/nervousness, affective lability, persistent and marked anger and irritability; plus other symptoms, such as decreased interest in usual activities, marked lack of energy (fatigue, lethargy), hypersomnia or insomnia, difficulty concentrating, appetite changes or cravings, and a subjective sense of being overwhelmed or "out of control," *plus* any of the physical symptoms already described in the PMS section of this chapter (Halbreich, et al, 2012). Symptoms are cyclical, occurring during the luteal phase of the menstrual cycle and are significantly reduced or disappear completely during menstruation. The morbidity of this condition is staggering when one considers that an average woman might have more than 400 cycles between the ages of 14 and 51, depending on the number of pregnancies and how long she breastfeeds. Some women can experience approximately *8 cumulative years* of severe PMDD during their reproductive years!

Pathophysiology

The exact cause of PMS and PMDD is unknown, but clearly multifaceted interactions among the central nervous system, hormones, and other chemical modulators occur. Genetic influences mediated phenotypically through neurotransmitters and neuroreceptors seem to play a large role. Seventy percent of women whose mothers have PMS will have PMS themselves, and a 93% concordance rate occurs in monozygotic twins compared to 44% in dizygotic twins (*Diagnosis and treatment of premenstrual dysphoric disorder,* 2002).

Theories about the pathophysiological cause that are supported in research suggest that PMDD may be caused by altered sensitivity in the serotonergic system to phasic fluctuation in female gonadal hormones. Some of the nutritional interventions are based in studies of the effectiveness of L-tryptophan, a precursor of serotonin, and of pyridoxine, a cofactor in the conversion of tryptophan into serotonin, in relieving PMDD symptoms. The success of SSRIs, which are considered first-line therapy in this disorder (*Diagnosis and treatment of premenstrual dysphoric disorder,* 2002; Frackiewicz & Shiovitz, 2001; Kaur, Gonsalves, & Thacker, 2004), also supports this hypothesis. Prostaglandins appear to play a role in some of the symptoms, and NSAIDs seem to be effective through their action on prostaglandins. Continuous combined oral contraceptive pills with 20 mcg estrogen and 90 mcg of levonorgestrel have been successful at treating symptoms of PMDD (Halbreich et al, 2012).

Treatments

The same lifestyle modifications used with PMS are also useful with PMDD. The outcome most suited to pharmacological therapy in PMDD is symptom reduction. Nutritional, herbal, and drug therapies play a role in this complex disorder. The dosing of selected nutritional, herbal, and drug therapies is presented in Table 48-4.

Nutritional Supplements

Randomized, placebo-controlled trials have shown vitamin B_6 in dosages up to 100 mg per day to benefit patients with premenstrual symptoms and premenstrual depression. Calcium

Table 48–4 Treatment Options for PMDD

Therapy	Dosing	Symptom Improvement
Nutritional Supplements		
Calcium carbonate	1,200–1,600 mg/d	Core symptoms
Magnesium	Up to 500 mg/d	Bloating
Tryptophan	Up to 6 g/d	Insomnia; affective symptoms
Vitamin B_6	Up to 100 mg/d	Core symptoms; depression
Vitamin E	200–400 mg/d	Stabilizes hormonal fluctuations
Herbals		
Evening primrose oil	500 mg daily to 1,000 mg tid	Anti-inflammatory; breast tenderness
Chaste tree berry	30–40 mg/d	Breast engorgement
Drugs (SSRIs)		
Citalopram (off-label)*	10–30 mg/d	All symptoms; fewer side effects than other SRIs

Continued

Table 48–4 Treatment Options for PMDD—cont'd

Therapy	Dosing	Symptom Improvement
Fluoxetine (indication)	20 mg/d	All symptoms; sexual side effects
Paroxetine (indication)	10–30 mg/d	All symptoms; GI and sexual side effects
Sertraline (indication)	50–150 mg/d	All symptoms; GI and sexual side effects
Drugs (Other)		
Alprazolam	0.375–1.5 mg/d	Anxiety and other affective symptoms
Bromocriptine	Up to 2.5 mg tid	Breast engorgement
Clomipramine	25–75 mg/d	All symptoms; anticholinergic effects
Ibuprofen	500–1,000 mg/d	Pain; breast engorgement
Spironolactone	100 mg/d	Water retention

PMDD = premenstrual dysphoric disorder.

carbonate in dosages of 1,200 to 1,600 mg per day reduced core premenstrual symptoms by 48% for 466 patients in one study (*Diagnosis and treatment of premenstrual dysphoric disorder,* 2002). Vitamin E, an antioxidant, reduces affective and physical symptoms in some patients. Finally, magnesium and tryptophan may also benefit PMS/PMDD patients. Nutritional supplements are generally considered second-line therapies, though they may be tried initially by women who are reluctant to take pharmaceuticals.

Herbals

Data on the efficacy and safety of herbal supplements marketed for women with PMS/PMDD have been inconsistent for many products. In addition, manufacturing standards for herbal products are not uniform. Given these caveats, two products based on research are recommended by Bhati and Bhati (*Diagnosis and treatment of premenstrual dysphoric disorder,* 2002). The most studied is evening primrose oil, which may be a precursor for prostaglandin synthesis and so may benefit symptoms associated with prostaglandins. Doses are 500 mg daily to 1,000 mg tid. Chaste tree berry has also been studied, although less so. Doses of 30 to 40 mg per day may benefit breast symptoms because it inhibits prolactin production (Pearlstein, 2012). Studies of vitamin A do not support its use. Other studies do not support the use of other herbals, such as black cohosh.

Drug Therapies

First-line therapy for PMDD is SSRIs. Three of them have been FDA-approved for PMDD: fluoxetine, paroxetine, and sertraline (*Diagnosis and treatment of premenstrual dysphoric disorder,* 2002). Both luteal phase and continuous use are beneficial, but continuous use may be better when cycles are not predictable, such as during peri-menopause (Pearlstein, 2012). Steiner and colleagues (Steiner et al, 2003) looked at fluoxetine efficacy related to affective and occupational functioning rather than physical symptoms. They found it reduced these symptoms relatively quickly at a low dose of 20 mg per day. Although they have been used for PMDD, the

anxiolytics, citalopram and alprazolam, are off-labeled for this indication.

Second-line drug therapy includes tricyclic clomipramine and benzodiazepine. Although they are often helpful, tricyclic clomipramine has anticholinergic side effects and benzodiazepine is associated with tolerance if used long term.

Ibuprofen, spironolactone, and bromocriptine are focused on specific PMS/PMDD symptoms and are useful for patients with those symptoms. Table 48-4 gives doses for these drugs and the types of symptoms they are most effective in relieving.

Gonadotropin-releasing hormone (GnRH) agonists, and danazol, a weak androgen, have been used to treat PMDD (Epperson et al, 2012). GnRH agonists inhibit follicle-stimulating hormone (FSH) and luteinizing hormone (LH), suppressing ovarian steroid hormone production and preventing ovulation. As the effect is equivalent to a medically induced oophorectomy and often requires add-back estrogen and/or progesterone (Epperson et al, 2012), these drugs are best prescribed by a specialist.

Psychotherapeutics

A comprehensive treatment meta-analysis of 22 studies (6 psychotherapeutic; 16 SSRI) found that psychotherapeutics, such as cognitive-behavioral therapy, are as effective as SSRIs and yet both had a small to moderate effect. The authors suggest that a combination of psychotropic and psychotherapeutic treatments may offer improved outcomes, but this has not been studied (Kleinstauber, Witthoft, & Hiller, 2012).

Endometriosis

Endometriosis is primarily a disorder of young women. The incidence is hard to determine in asymptomatic adolescents and fertile women, but it has been estimated that 10% to 15% of reproductive-age women and 2% to 4% of menopausal women have endometriosis. As many as 50% of women evaluated for pelvic pain, infertility, or a pelvic mass are diagnosed with this disorder (McCance & Huether, 2014). The frequency and severity of symptoms do not correlate with the extent or site of the lesions, and as many as 31% of asymptomatic fertile women are found to have endometriosis when undergoing laparoscopy.

Pathophysiology

Endometriosis is the presence of functioning endometrial tissue (called implants) outside the uterus. The cause is unknown, but theories include retrograde menstruation, depressed cytotoxic T-cell response to endometrial cells in ectopic locations, and a genetic hypothesis that proposes abnormal development of epithelial cells of the reproductive organs (McCance & Huether, 2014). Endometriosis appears to have a genetic predisposition; the condition is 6 to 7 times more prevalent in women who have a first-degree relative with endometriosis as compared to the general population (Layman, 2013). Women with early menarche, late menopause, low body mass index, nulliparity, mullerian anomalies, and shorter menstrual cycles are also at higher risk for endometriosis (Schrager, Falleroni, & Edgoose, 2013).

Endometrial implants can occur throughout the body but are most often found on the ovaries, uterine ligaments, rectovaginal septum, and pelvic peritoneum. Other common sites include the surface of the intestines, bladder, vulva and vagina, and the pleural cavity and lungs (McCance & Huether, 2014). Cyclical changes in gonadal hormones result in proliferation of the ectopic endometrium with the subsequent breakdown and bleeding that is part of the normal menstrual cycle. The bleeding produces inflammation with the usual release of inflammatory mediators and macrophage involvement (Capobianco & Rovere-Querini, 2013). Pain occurs in the surrounding tissues and the inflammatory process can lead to fibrosis, scarring, and adhesions, which are the lesions often held responsible for infertility in these women. Symptoms relate to the inflammatory process caused by the bleeding and include pelvic pain, dysmenorrhea, dyspareunia, and, less commonly, constipation and abnormal vaginal bleeding (*Endometriosis—Start with a natural approach*, 2011; McCance & Huether, 2014).

Drug Therapies

The ACOG (1999) issued the following recommendations based on reliable scientific evidence:

- For pain relief, GnRH agonists for at least 3 months or danazol for at least 6 months. Treatment with danazol is about one-third less costly than GnRH agonist treatment.
- When GnRH agonist treatment must continue for some time, "add-back" regimens with progestin, bisphosphonates, or pulsatile parathyroid hormone should be considered to reduce GnRH-induced bone mineral loss.

Pick and Holmes (*Endometriosis—Start with a natural approach*, 2011) recommend less dramatic treatments first. They report a high rate of success with a combination of dietary changes, nutrient support, emotional healing, and alternative therapies such as acupuncture. Their dietary recommendations remove xenoestrogen exposure by eliminating nonorganic dairy products, beef, and chicken; increase nutrient-rich food such as cruciferous vegetables, soy, cold water fish, and fiber; and suggest a lower carbohydrate diet to support healthy insulin metabolism. Supplementation with calcium and magnesium (see PMDD) and omega-3, an essential fatty acid, reduces inflammation. Resveratrol (found in the skin of grapes and other fruit) and epigallocatechin gallate (an antioxidant) have had success in rodent studies (Ricci et al, 2013).

When drugs are chosen, ibuprofen, naprosyn, and other NSAIDs are used to decrease pain and inflammation. Ovulation suppression therapies, such as oral contraceptives, are effective in treating endometriosis pain but do not improve pregnancy rates. To improve pregnancy rates, surgical treatment is recommended (Schrager et al, 2013).

HIV/AIDS in Pregnancy

Women are now the fastest-growing population with HIV infection and AIDS; an estimated 20% of new infections occur in women, and young women aged 25 to 44 accounted for the majority of new HIV infections among women in 2010 (CDC, 2013a). Pregnant women who are HIV-positive face many challenges, such as unpredictable symptoms and prognosis, the potential for maternal to infant transmission, and problematic life circumstances that have the potential to compromise parenting, such as poverty, substance abuse, and the stigma associated with this disease. Despite these challenges, HIV-infected women are no less likely to become pregnant, nor are they more likely to terminate a pregnancy (Kirshenbaum et al, 2004).

Other viral infections, such as herpes and cytomegalovirus, seem to be more prevalent in women infected with HIV than in men (Cunningham & Williams, 2010). HIV-positive women also may have more severe pelvic inflammatory disease than other women, and rates of cervical dysplasia and human papillomavirus (HPV) may be higher in HIV-positive women, with the clinical course accelerated and more frequent recurrence (Lowdermilk & Perry, 2007).

An infected woman can pass the HIV virus to her baby during pregnancy, delivery, or breastfeeding. Triple combined antiretroviral (ARV) therapy during pregnancy greatly reduces the risk of passing the HIV virus to the fetus. Reported rates of mother-to-child transmission are 2% when women begin ARV medication treatment early in pregnancy (Stephenson, 2005). This rate increases to 12% to 13% if treatment is not initiated until labor, delivery, or after birth and shoots up to 25% should women receive no preventive treatment (National Institute of Health, 2013).

Effective counseling, screening, and the use of zidovudine or another highly active antiretroviral therapy (HAART) for infected pregnant women has contributed to the decline in the number of new pediatric AIDS cases. Therefore, the Centers for Disease Control (CDC) recommends universal prenatal counseling and testing for pregnant women (National Institute of Health, 2014). Breastfeeding is not recommended in countries where other good alternatives exist (National Institute of Health). Further discussion of the management of HIV/AIDS is found in Chapter 37.

Infertility

Infertility, defined as the absence of conception despite unprotected sexual intercourse for at least 1 year, has a profound emotional, psychological, and economic impact on the affected couple and society. Women with infertility experience greater psychological symptoms, including depression, anxiety, and poor self-esteem (El Kissi et al, 2013). A serious medical concern, the condition affects the quality of life for about 6% to 10% of reproductive-age couples (CDC, 2012). About 35% of infertility problems are due to a male factor, 45% to a female factor, and the remaining 20% are due to problems with both partners or are unexplained. Incidence of infertility increases with a woman's age, particularly in women older than age 40 (Lobo, Lentz, Gershenson, & Katz, 2012).

Determination of hormone levels, such as prolactin, FSH, LH, estradiol (E2), progesterone, and thyroid, may be necessary to diagnose the cause of absent or irregular menstrual cycles. The clomiphene citrate challenge test (CCCT) can be given to assess ovarian reserves. Couples should undergo an infertility evaluation by a specialist if after 1 year of trying they have been unable to conceive. A woman older than 35 years may be referred earlier, for example, after only 6 to 9 months of unprotected intercourse without achieving conception (Davidson et al, 2011).

Polycystic Ovarian Syndrome

An endocrine imbalance that results in high levels of estrogen, testosterone, and LH with decreased levels of FSH, polycystic ovarian syndrome (PCOS) is associated with a number of problems in the hypothalamic-pituitary-ovarian axis. The ovaries can double in size with multiple follicular cysts, producing excess estrogen. Impaired glucose occurs in about 45% of women with PCOS (Huang & Coviello, 2012), and affected women are at high risk of developing type 2 diabetes and cardiovascular diseases (Huang & Coviello, 2012).

Analgesics may be prescribed for pain management, and regular examination is needed to monitor the symptoms. OCPs may be indicated to suppress functional cysts, if pregnancy is not desired. GnRH analogues may be used to treat hirsutism if OCPs do not improve this distressing symptom. If pregnancy is desired, medications for ovulation induction are usually given (Misso et al, 2013). Insulin and metformin are prescribed to manage the type 2 diabetes, lowering blood glucose and testosterone, which, in turn, can reduce acne, hirsutism, abdominal obesity, and amenorrhea in some women with PCOS (ACOG, 2003; Lord & Wilkin, 2004).

HEALTH PROMOTION, DISEASE PREVENTION, AND SCREENING

Preventive screening and testing save lives by identifying previously undiagnosed conditions and by allowing for early intervention and treatments so that health outcomes are improved. Many simple, preventive measures can be taken by women to reduce morbidity and mortality. These measures include immunizations for pneumonia and influenza and screening for high blood pressure, cholesterol, and blood sugar. Screening tests to identify heart disease, cancers, and diabetes are recommended by the American Cancer Society, the American Diabetes Association, the American Heart Association, the American Academy of Family Physicians, and the U.S. Preventive Services Task Force.

Some preventive health-care screening recommendations for adult women without symptoms of disease should begin at age 18 years and include an eye examination, blood pressure check, and gynecology visits as indicated. PAP testing is recommended at age 21 (National Institute of Health, 2013). Studies on self-breast exams failed to show a benefit and have reported a higher rate of breast biopsies for benign disease (Baxter, 2001; Hackshaw & Paul, 2003), although self-breast exams may prevent mortality from breast cancer (Harvey, Miller, Baines, & Corey, 1997).

Tetanus with pertussis (Tdap) immunizations should be updated, with a pregnant women needing a Tdap with every pregnancy. Anyone in a risk category should complete immunization series for hepatitis A and B. In 2006, the CDC recommended routine vaccination of girls aged 12 to 24 years against HPV (CDC, 2012). Other screening tests should be implemented beginning at age 40 years, such as a breast examination performed by a health-care provider and mammograms (American Cancer Society, 2006). There is no consensus on the frequency of mammograms for women between 40 and 49 years of age; recommendations vary from annually over age 40 (American Cancer Society) to annually over age 50 (Squiers et al, 2011). Providers are urged to individualize recommendations for their patients. Since lung and colon cancers have increased in the past century, patients need to begin screening procedures, such as colonoscopy at age 50 years. Skin examination for cancer should be done every 3 years between ages 20 and 40 and at least annually afterward. Bone mineral density (BMD) testing is recommended for all women aged 65 and older and younger women at risk for osteoporosis. A complete list of preventive health-care screening tests can be found at http://www.womenshealth.gov/.

GAY AND LESBIAN HEALTH

Membership in a sexual minority group is not in and of itself hazardous; however, risk factors may be conferred through the social stress of being different. Homophobia is the socialization of heterosexuals against members of the lesbian, gay, bisexual, and transgendered (LGBT) community. The strain of societal homophobia has been linked to increased rates in smoking, alcohol use, depression, HIV/AIDS, physical violence, and attempted suicide rates among LGBT individuals and occurs at a great cost to society (Goldberg, 2005).

Heterosexist attitudes permeate health-care environments and are manifested through avoidance, inappropriateness, and distance, which create an atmosphere of nondisclosure of important health-related information to health-care providers. The assumption by health-care providers that heterosexuality is the relationship norm and any other variation is deviant makes it difficult and embarrassing for individuals to open up about their sexuality (Schuklenk & Smalling, 2013). Ignorance resulting from heterosexist assumptions has resulted in practitioners erroneously advising lesbians they cannot contract a sexually transmitted infection (STI) from a female partner or that screening for cervical cancer is not required. Evidence has demonstrated that lesbians who have had no history of sexual intercourse with males can have abnormal Pap smears (Goldberg, 2005).

Lesbian health is not completely the same as women's health because their lived experiences in the world are different (Goldberg, 2005). As a group, lesbian and bisexual women are less likely to have health-care insurance or access to health-care services. Those with access to care are less likely than heterosexual women to adequately use preventive health-care services because of fear of discrimination.

Providers have a professional and moral responsibility to treat all people with respect and dignity, regardless of their sexual orientation or preference. Providers working with the gay and lesbian community can use several helpful strategies to promote a positive environment. First and foremost, the provider must be aware of his or her own biases and be open, knowledgeable, and comfortable with sexual differences. This "gay positive" posture creates a safe atmosphere for disclosure of information so that appropriate diagnosis, treatment, and information can be provided to the patient. The provider should also reconsider how health histories are obtained. For example, consider creating a space for the client to document nonheterosexual relationships on written documents and modifying questions used to obtain information regarding sexuality. One method for acknowledging a current relationship status is to ask questions such as, "Are you at present in a relationship?" or "Who is your partner in your relationship?" In addition, an accepting physical environment can be achieved by having pamphlets about lesbian and bisexual health readily available. Finally, providers and others should avoid using euphemisms such as "special friend" when asking about the patient's partner (Goldberg, 2005).

Providers can obtain additional facts and information about gay and lesbian health-care issues from the Lesbian Health and Research Center at http://www.lesbianhealthinfo.org/ or the Gay and Lesbian Medical Association at http://www.glma.org.

REFERENCES

Agency of Healthcare Research and Quality. (2002). *AHTQ focus on research: Healthcare for women*. Washington, DC: Author.

American Cancer Society. (2006). *Cancer facts and figures, 2006*. New York: Author.

American College of Obstetrics and Gynecology (ACOG). (1999, Dec). *ACOG practice bulletin. Medical management of endometriosis. Number 11* (replaces Technical Bulletin Number 184, September 1993).

American College of Obstetrics and Gynecology (ACOG). (2000). Clinical management guidelines for obstetrician-gynecologists. *International Journal of Gynaecology and Obstetrics, 71*(2), 183–196.

American College of Obstetricians and Gynecologists (ACOG). (2003). ACOG practice bulletin. Polycycstic ovary syndrome, Number 41, December 2002. *International Journal of Gynaecology and Obstetrics, 80*(3), 335–348.

American College of Obstetrics and Gynecology (ACOG). (2010). ACOG Committee Opinion No. 462: Moderate caffeine consumption during pregnancy. *Obstetrics and Gynecology, 116*(2, Pt 1), 467–468.

American Psychiatric Association (APA). (2013). *Diagnostic and statistical manual of mental disorders 5th ed.* Association AP, editor. Washington, DC: Author.

Anderson, G. D. (2005). Sex and racial differences in pharmacological response: Where is the evidence? Pharmacogenetics, pharmacokinetics, and pharmacodynamics. *Journal of Women's Health (Larchmt), 14*(1), 19–29.

Arends, J. C., Cheung, M. Y., Barrack, M. T., & Nattiv, A. (2012). Restoration of menses with nonpharmacologic therapy in college athletes with menstrual disturbances: A 5-year retrospective study. *International Journal of Sports Nutrition and Exercise Metabolism, 22*(2), 98–108.

Austad, S. N. (2006). Why women live longer than men: Sex differences in longevity. *Gender Medicine, 3*(2), 79–92.

Baxter, N. (2001). Preventive health care, 2001 update: Should women be routinely taught breast self-examination to screen for breast cancer? *Canadian Medical Association Journal, 164*(13), 1837–1846.

Bertoia, M. L., Allison, M. A., Manson, J. E., Freiberg, M. S., Kuller, L. H., Solomon, A. J., et al. (2012). Risk factors for sudden cardiac death in postmenopausal women. *Journal of the American College of Cardiology, 60*(25), 2674–2682.

Blumenthal, M., Goldberg, A., & Brinckman, J. (Eds.). (2000). *Herbal medicine: Expanded Comission E monographs*. Newton, MA: Integrated Medicine Communications.

Bohn, D. K., Tebben, J. G., & Campbell, J. C. (2004). Influences of income, education, age, and ethnicity on physical abuse before and during pregnancy. *Journal of Obstetrical, Gynecologic, and Neonatal Nursing, 33*(5), 561–571.

Capobianco, A., & Rovere-Querini, P. (2013). Endometriosis, a disease of the macrophage. *Frontiers in Immunology, 4*, 9.

Centers for Disease Control (CDC). (2012). Integrated prevention services for HIV infection, viral hepatitis, sexually transmitted diseases, and tuberculosis for persons who use drugs illicitly: Summary guidance from CDC and the U.S. Department of Health and Human Services. *Morbidity and Mortality Weekly Report, 61*(RR-5), 1–40.

Centers for Disease Control and Prevention (CDC). (2012, updated 7/30/2013). *FastStats: Infertility*. Atlanta, GA: National Center for Health Statistics. Available from: http://www.cdc.gov/nchs/fastats/fertile.htm

Centers for Disease Control and Prevention (CDC). (2013a, accessed 18 Mar 2013). *HIV among women*. Atlanta, GA: CDC. Available from: http://www.cdc.gov/hiv/topics/women/index.htm

Centers for Disease Control and Prevention (CDC). (2013b, 18 Mar). *Intimate partner violence*. Atlanta, GA. Available from: http://www.cdc.gov/violenceprevention/intimatepartnerviolence/index.html

Collins Sharp, B. A., Taylor, D. L., Thomas, K. K., Killeen, M. B., & Dawood, M. Y. (2002). Cyclic perimenstrual pain and discomfort: The scientific basis for practice. *Journal of Obstetrics, Gynecologic and Neonatal Nursing, 31*(6), 637–649.

Crissman, H. P., Adanu, R. M., & Harlow, S. D. (2012). Women's sexual empowerment and contraceptive use in Ghana. *Studies in Family Planning, 43*(3), 201–212.

Cunningham, F. G., & Williams, J. W. (2010). *Williams obstetrics* (23rd ed.). New York: McGraw-Hill Medical.

Davidson, M., London, M., Ladewig, P., Davidson, M. (Eds.). (2011). *Old's maternal-newborn nursing and women's health care across the lifespan* (9th ed.). Upper Saddle River, NJ: Prentice Hall.

Davis, A. J., & Johnson, S. R. (2000; reaffirmed 2008). *Premenstrual syndrome: ACOG Practice Bulletin No.15* (pp 1–9). Washington, DC: American College of Obstetrics and Gynecology.

Diagnosis and treatment of premenstrual dysphoric disorder [database on the Internet]. (2002; cited 14 Mar 2013). Available from: http://www.aafp.org/afp/2002/1001/p1239.html

Davis, W. (1998). Impact of gender on drug response. *Drug Topics*, 91–98.

Dominguez-Bartmess, S. N., Tandberg, D., Cheema, A. M., & Szalay, E. A. (2012). Efficacy of alendronate in the treatment of low bone density in the pediatric and young adult population. *Journal of Bone and Joint Surgery Am, 94*(10), 00751.

El Kissi, Y., Romdhane, A. B., Hidar, S., Bannour, S., Ayoubi Idrissi, K., Khairi, H., et al. (2013). General psychopathology, anxiety, depression and self-esteem in couples undergoing infertility treatment: A comparative study between men and women. *European Journal of Obstetrics, Gynecology, and Reproductive Biology, 167*(2013), 185–189.

Endometriosis—Start with a natural approach [database on the Internet]. (2011, cited 12 Mar 13]. Available from: http://www.womentowomen.com/sexualityandfertility/endometriosis.aspx

Epperson, C. N., Steiner, M., Hartlage, S. A., Eriksson, E., Schmidt, P. J., Jones, I., et al. (2012). Premenstrual dysphoric disorder: Evidence for a new category for DSM-5. *American Journal of Psychiatry, 169*(5), 465–175.

Finer, L. B., & Zolna, M. R. (2011). Unintended pregnancy in the United States: Incidence and disparities, 2006. *Contraception, 84*(5), 478–485.

Frackiewicz, E. J., & Shiovitz, T. M. (2001). Evaluation and management of premenstrual syndrome and premenstrual dysphoric disorder. *Journal of the American Pharmaceutical Association (Wash), 41*(3), 437–447.

Friedman, A. J., Chen, Z., Ford. P., Johnson, C. A., Lopez, A. M., Shander, A., et al. (2012). Iron deficiency anemia in women across the life span. *Journal of Women's Health, 21*(12), 1282–1289.

Gandhi, M., Aweeka, F., Greenblatt, R. M., & Blaschke, T. F. (2004). Sex differences in pharmacokinetics and pharmacodynamics. *Annual Review of Pharmacology and Toxicology, 44*, 499–523.

Gibbs, J. C., Williams, N. I., & De Souza, M. J. (2013). Prevalence of individual and combined components of the female athlete triad. *Medicine & Science in Sports & Exercise 45*(5), 985–996.

Ginn, E., Street, D., & Arber, S. (2001). *Women, work and pensions.* Buckingham, England: Open University Press.

Goldberg, L. (2005). Understanding lesbian experience. *AWHONN Lifelines, 9*(6), 463–467.

Gottlieb, B. (2008). *Alternative cures.* New York: Random House.

Grandjean, E. M., & Aubry, J. M. (2009). Lithium: Updated human knowledge using an evidence-based approach. Part II: Clinical pharmacology and therapeutic monitoring. *CNS Drugs, 23*(4), 331–349.

Guenther, P. M., Reedy, J., & Krebs-Smith, S. M. (2008). Development of the Healthy Eating Index—2005. *Journal of the American Dietetic Association, 108*(11), 1896–1901.

Hackshaw, A. K., & Paul, E. A. (2003). Breast self-examination and death from breast cancer: A meta-analysis. *British Journal of Cancer, 88*(7), 1047–1053.

Halbreich, U., Freeman, E. W., Rapkin, A. J., Cohen, L. S., Grubb, G. S., Bergeron, R., et al. (2012). Continuous oral levonorgestrel/ethinyl estradiol for treating premenstrual dysphoric disorder. *Contraception, 85*(1), 19–27.

Hardy, M. L. (2000). Herbs of special interest to women. *Journal of the American Pharmaceutical Association* (Wash), *40*(2), 234–242; quiz, 327–329.

Harel, Z., Johnson, C. C., Gold, M. A., Cromer, B., Peterson, E., Burkman, R., et al. (2010). Recovery of bone mineral density in adolescents following the use of depot medroxyprogesterone acetate contraceptive injections. *Contraception, 81*(4), 281–291.

Harvey, B. J., Miller, A. B., Baines, C. J., & Corey, P. N. (1997). Effect of breast self-examination techniques on the risk of death from breast cancer. *Canadian Medical Association Journal, 157*(9), 1205–1212.

Hermes, A., Squires, K., Fredrick, L., Martinez, M., Pasley, M., Trinh, R., et al. (2012). Meta-analysis of the safety, tolerability, and efficacy of lopinavir/ritonavir-containing antiretroviral therapy in HIV-1-infected women. *HIV Clinical Trials,13*(6), 308–323.

Hoyert, D. L., Mathews, T. J., Menacker, F., Strobino, D. M., & Guyer, B. (2006). Annual summary of vital statistics: 2004. *Pediatrics, 117*(1), 168–183.

Huang, G., & Coviello, A. (2012). Clinical update on screening, diagnosis and management of metabolic disorders and cardiovascular risk factors associated with polycystic ovary syndrome. *Current Opinion in Endocrinology, Diabetes and Obesity, 19*(6), 512–519.

Isley, M. M., & Kaunitz, A. M. (2011). Update on hormonal contraception and bone density. *Reviews in Endocrine and Metabolic Disorders, 12*(2), 93–106.

Isoherranen, N., & Thummel, K. E. (2013). Drug metabolism and transport during pregnancy: How does drug disposition change during pregnancy and what are the mechanisms that cause such changes? *Drug Metabolism and Disposition, 41*(2), 256–262.

Jarosz, M., Wierzejska, R., & Siuba, M. (2012). Maternal caffeine intake and its effect on pregnancy outcomes. *European Journal of Obstetrics, Gynecology, and Reproductive Biology, 160*(2), 156–160.

Kaur, G., Gonsalves, L., & Thacker, H. L. (2004). Premenstrual dysphoric disorder: A review for the treating practitioner. *Cleveland Clinic Journal of Medicine, 71*(4), 303–321.

Kirshenbaum, S. B., Hirky, A. E., Correale, J., Goldstein, R. B., Johnson, M. O., Rotheram-Borus, M. J., et al. (2004). "Throwing the dice": Pregnancy decision-making among HIV-positive women in four U.S. cities. *Perspectives on Sexual and Reproductive Health, 36*(3), 106–113.

Kleinstauber, M., Witthoft, M., & Hiller, W. (2012). Cognitive-behavioral and pharmacological interventions for premenstrual syndrome or premenstrual dysphoric disorder: A meta-analysis. *Journal of Clinical in Psychology Medical Settings, 19*(3), 308–319.

Layman, L. C. (2013). The genetic basis of female reproductive disorders: Etiology and clinical relevance. *Molecular & Cellular Endocrinology, 370*(1–2) 138–148.

Leitzmann, M. F., Park, Y., Blair, A., Ballard-Barbash, R., Mouw, T., Hollenbeck, A. R., et al. (2007). Physical activity recommendations and decreased risk of mortality. *Archives of Internal Medicine, 167*(22), 2453–2460.

Lloyd, K. B., & Hornsby L. B. (2009). Complementary and alternative medications for women's health issues. *Nutrition in Clinical Practice, 24*(5), 589–608.

Lobo, R. A., Lentz, G. M., Gershenson, D. M., & Katz, V. L. (Eds.). (2012). *Comprehensive gynecology* (6th ed.). Philadelphia, PA: Elsevier Mosby.

Loomans, E. M., Hofland, L., van der Stelt, O., van der Wal, M. F., Koot, H. M., Van den Bergh, B. R., et al. (2012). Caffeine intake during pregnancy and risk of problem behavior in 5- to 6-year-old children. *Pediatrics, 130*(2), 2011–3361.

Lord, J., & Wilkin, T. (2004). Metformin in polycystic ovary syndrome. *Current Opinions in Obstetrics and Gynecology, 16*(6), 481–486.

Lowdermilk, D., & Perry, S. (Eds.). (2007). *Maternity and women's health care.* St. Louis, MO: Mosby/Elsevier.

McCance, K., & Huether, S. (Eds). (2014). *Pathophysiology: The biological basis for disease in adults and children* (7th ed.). St. Louis, MO: Elsevier Mosby.

Misso, M. L., Costello, M. F., Garrubba, M., Wong, J., Hart, R., Rombauts, L., et al. (2013). Metformin versus clomiphene citrate for infertility in non-obese women with polycystic ovary syndrome: A systematic review and meta-analysis. *Human Reproduction Update, 19*(1), 2–11.

Moolgavkar, S. H., Holford, T. R., Levy, D. T., Kong, C. Y., Foy, M., Clarke, L., et al. (2012). Impact of reduced tobacco smoking on lung cancer mortality in the United States during 1975–2000. *Journal of the National Cancer Institute, 104*(7), 541–548.

Moore, A. L., Sabin, C. A., Johnson, M. A., & Phillips, A. N. (2002). Gender and clinical outcomes after starting highly active antiretroviral treatment: A cohort study. *Journal of Acquired Immune Deficiency Syndrome, 29*(2), 197–202.

Moos, M. K. (2005). Have your teenagers had their calcium today? *AWHONN Lifelines, 9*(4), 324–326.

National Institute of Health. (2009). Prevalence and most common causes of disability among adults—United States, 2005. *Morbidity and Mortality Weekly Report, 58*(16), 421–426.

National Institute of Health. (2013). Cervical cancer screening among women aged 18–30 years—United States, 2000–2010. *Morbidity and Mortality Weekly Report, 61*(51–52), 1038–1042.

National Institute of Health, Panel on Treatment of HIV-Infected Pregnant Women and Prevention of Perinatal Transmission. (2014, updated 3/28/14). *Recommendations for use of antiretroviral drugs in pregnant HIV-1-infected women for maternal health and interventions to reduce perinatal HIV transmission in the United States.* Rockville, MD: National Institute of Health. Available from: http://aidsinfo.nih.gov/guidelines

Nelson, H. D., Walker, M., Zakher, B., & Mitchell, J. (2012). Menopausal hormone therapy for the primary prevention of chronic conditions: A systematic review to update the U.S. Preventive Services Task Force recommendations. *Annals of Internal Medicine, 157*(2), 104–113.

The North American Menopause Society (NAMS). (2012). The 2012 hormone therapy position statement of The North American Menopause Society. *Menopause, 19*(3), 257–271.

Pearlstein, T. (2012). Psychotropic medications and other non-hormonal treatments for premenstrual disorders. *Menopause International, 18*(2), 60–64.

Peipins, L. A., Miller, J., Richards, T. B., Bobo, J. K., Liu,. T, White, M. C., et al. (2012). Characteristics of US counties with no mammography capacity. *Journal of Community Health, 37*(6), 1239–1248.

Plassman, B. L., Langa, K. M., McCammon, R. J., Fisher, G. G., Potter, G. G., Burke, J. R., et al. (2011). Incidence of dementia and cognitive impairment, not dementia in the United States. *Annals of Neurology 70*(3), 418–426.

Premenstrual syndrome [database on the Internet]. (2003, cited 12 Mar 2013). Available from: http://www.aafp.org/afp/2003/0415/p1743.html

Pritham, U. A. (2002). Managing PMS & PMDD. Exploring new treatment options. *AWHONN Lifelines, 6*(5), 430–437.

Qiao, M., Zhang, H., Liu, H., Luo, S., Wang, T., Zhang, J., et al. (2012). Prevalence of premenstrual syndrome and premenstrual dysphoric disorder in a population-based sample in China. *European Journal of Obstetrics, Gynecology, and Reproductive Biology, 162*(1), 83–86.

Rademaker, M. (2001). Do women have more adverse drug reactions? *American Journal of Clinical Dermatology, 2*(6), 349–351.

Ricci, A. G., Olivares, C. N, Bilotas, M. A., Baston, J. I., Singla, J. J., Meresman, G. F., et al. (2013). Natural therapies assessment for the treatment of endometriosis. *Human Reproduction, 28*(1), 178–188.

Roush, K. (2012). Managing menopausal symptoms. *American Journal of Nursing, 112*(6), 28–35.

Schoening, A. M., Greenwood, J. L., McNichols, J. A., Heermann, J. A., & Agrawal, S. (2004). Effect of an intimate partner violence educational program on the attitudes of nurses. *Journal of Obstetrical, Gynecological, and Neonatal Nursing, 33*(5), 572–579.

Schrager, S., Falleroni, J., & Edgoose, J. (2013). Evaluation and treatment of endometriosis. *American Family Physician, 87*(2), 107–113.

Schuklenk, U., & Smalling, R. (2013). Queer patients and the health care professional—Regulatory arrangements matter. *Journal of Medical Humanities, 34*(2), 93-99.

Shumaker, S. A., Legault, C., Rapp, S. R., Thal, L., Wallace, R. B., Ockene, J. K., et al. (2003). Estrogen plus progestin and the incidence of dementia and mild cognitive impairment in postmenopausal women: The Women's Health Initiative Memory Study: A randomized controlled trial. *Journal of the American Medical Association, 289*(20), 2651–2662.

Smith, P. E. (2005). Menopause: Assessment, treatment, and patient education. *Nurse Practitioner, 30*(2), 33–38.

Squiers, L. B., Holden, D. J., Dolina, S. E., Kim, A. E., Bann, C. M., & Renaud, J. M. (2011). The public's response to the U.S. Preventive Services Task Force's 2009 recommendations on mammography screening. *American Journal of Preventive Medicine, 40*(5), 497–504.

Steiner, M., Brown, E., Trzepacz, P., Dillon, J., Berger, C., Carter. D., et al. (2003). Fluoxetine improves functional work capacity in women with premenstrual dysphoric disorder. *Archives of Women's Mental Health, 6*(1), 71–77.

Stephenson, J. (2005). Reducing HIV vertical transmission scrutinized. *Journal of the American Medical Association, 293*(17), 2079–2081.

United Nations. (2012). *State of world population 2012*. New York: UNFPA.

U.S. Department of Health and Human Services. (2005). Overview of the uninsured in the United States: An analysis of the 2005 current population survey. In ASPE Issue Brief Sep 22, 2005. Rockville, MD: U.S. Department of Health and Human Services.

Ward, S., & Hisley, S. (Eds.). (2009). *Maternal-child nursing care*. Philadelphia: F.A. Davis.

Women and trials: When is gender a consideration? [database on the Internet]. (2005). Available from: http://www.appliedclinicaltrialsonline.com/appliedclinicaltrials/article/articleDetail.jsp?id=165483&sk=&date=&pageID=5

Wood, S. F., Blehar, M. C., & Maucry, D. R. (2011). Policy implications of a new National Institutes of Health Agenda for Women's Health Research, 2010–2020. *Women's Health Issues, 21*(2), 99–103.

Zahradnik, H. P., Hanjalic-Beck, A., & Groth, K. (2010). Nonsteroidal anti-inflammatory drugs and hormonal contraceptives for pain relief from dysmenorrhea: A review. *Contraception, 81*(3), 185–196.

Zapata, L. B., Steenland, M. W., Brahmi, D., Marchbanks, P. A., & Curtis, K. M. (2012). Patient understanding of oral contraceptive pill instructions related to missed pills: A systematic review. *Contraception. 87*(5), 674-684.

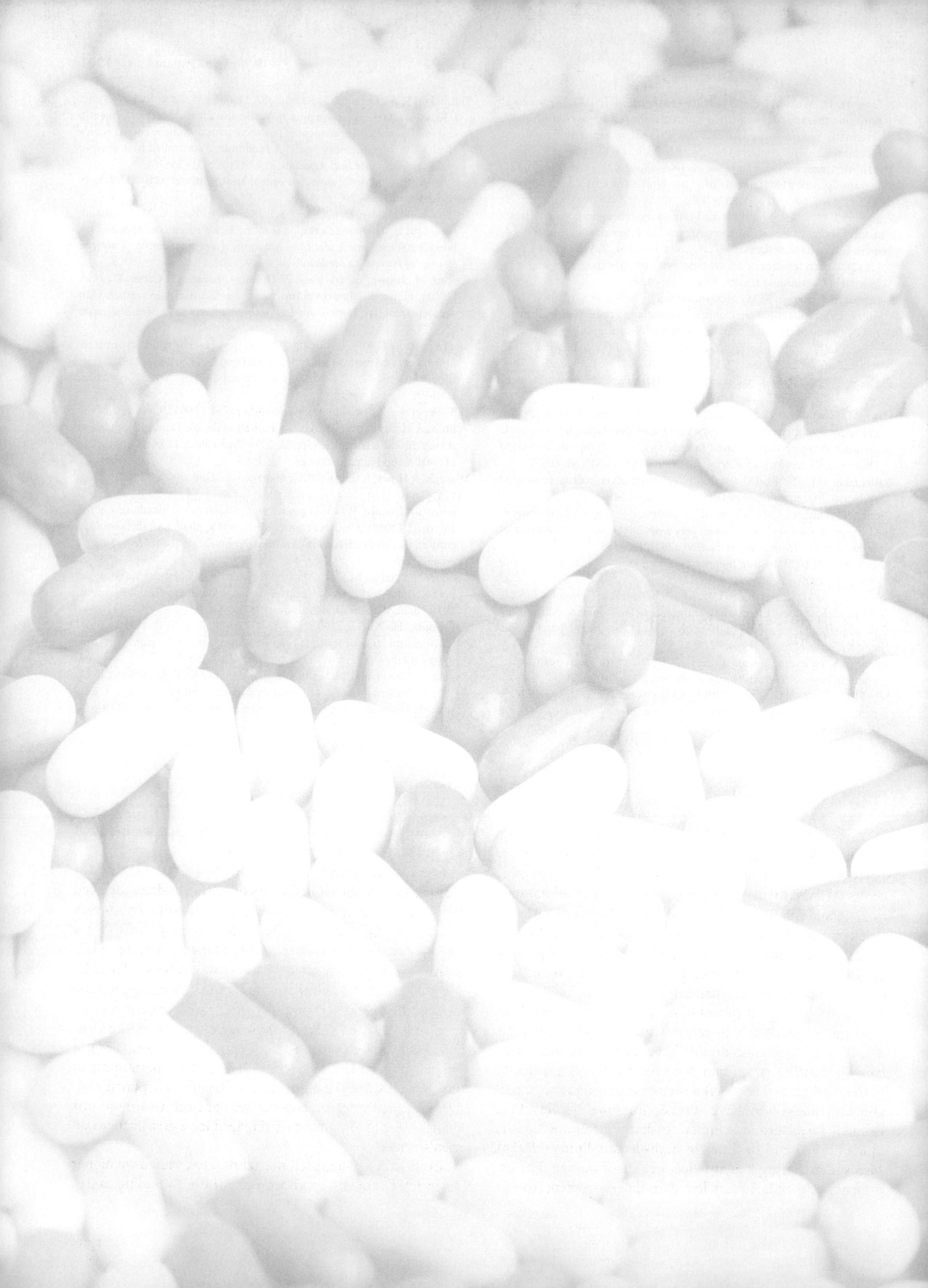

MEN AS PATIENTS

James Raper

Gender-related health disparity across the life span is significant for men. The Men's Health Network (2008) reports a number of disparities between males and females across their life spans. The male fetus is at greater risk for miscarriage and stillbirth, and male newborns have a 25% greater risk of mortality than do female newborns. Three-fifths of sudden infant death syndrome (SIDS) victims are boys. Men are 100% less likely to receive annual examinations and disease prevention services than are women. Men die at higher rates from the top 10 causes of death than do women. Men are 4 times more likely to commit suicide than women are. A total of 33% of men do not have health-care insurance, compared to 28% of women. Men account for 92% of deaths in the workplace. Men have fewer infection-fighting T cells and are thought to have weaker immune systems than women. Testosterone is linked to elevations of low-density lipids (LDLs) and declines in high-density lipids (HDLs). Men suffer hearing loss at twice the rate of women. Life expectancy of men is 5 years less than that of women; women outnumber men 8 to 1 by age 100 years. Clearly, there is a need to address health specific to men.

Some government agencies, such as the Agency for Healthcare Research and Quality (AHRQ), address the need for greater dissemination of information about men's health issues. AHRQ's campaign Real Men Wear Gowns (www.ahrq.gov/realmen/) is an example of how to increase public awareness of the importance of men's health issues. These issues do not fare as well when compared to efforts to promote awareness of disease conditions affecting women. It is common to see diseases affecting women grouped under the identifier of women's health (www.qualityforum.org/Topics/Disparities.aspx). The paucity of literature pertaining to men's health, the glaring absence of health-care policies addressing men's health, and the lack of health-care options available for men underscore the need for a greater focus on men's health.

Even with age-adjusted mortality rates, men have higher death rates compared with women for the 15 leading causes of death in the United States, except for Alzheimer's disease (Williams, 2003). The leading causes of death in men are heart disease, cancer, and unintentional accidents, whereas the leading causes of death in women are heart disease, breast cancer, and stroke (Centers for Disease Control and Prevention [CDC], 2007). According to the U.S. Department of Health and Human Services (2007), men are 2 1/2 times less likely to have seen a doctor than are women. The determinants of men's poorer health status arise from cultural and social beliefs about men, manhood, and masculinity. Although socioeconomic status (SES) is considered the strongest determinant of men's health (Williams, 2003), men from all SES groups are considered disadvantaged as compared with women. Other determinants of men's health are absence of work, marginality, poor emotional processing ability, cumulative adversity over a life span, and access to and use of health services. Little is known about men's perception of health and the influences of masculinity on health-care–seeking behaviors by men (Liburd, Namageyo-Funa, & Jack, 2007).

The cultural concept of masculinity begins with socialization at a young age. Edley and Wetherell (1996) define masculinity as a "shared understanding of what it means to be a man: what one looks like, how one should behave and so forth" (p 185). Masculinity directly affects health care and health-care choices. The socialization of men helps determine to what degree men respond to pain (Braithwaite, 2001), make health-care selections, engage in risk-taking behaviors, achieve effective self-care in the management of type 2 diabetes (Liburd et al, 2007), and adhere to medical plans of care (Brooks, 2001).

Although culture plays a significant role in masculinity, steroid hormones known as androgens affect the development of male-specific phenotype during embryogenesis; in the establishment of sexual maturation at puberty; and in the maintenance of the male reproductive function, spermatogenesis, and sexual behavior during adult life. These steroid hormones also affect a wide variety of functions in nonreproductive tissues, such as bone and skeletal muscle (Matsumoto, Shiina, Kawano, Sato, & Kato, 2008). Testosterone and its active metabolite dihydrotestosterone (DHT) exert most of their effects by binding to the androgen receptor (AR), a ligand-activated transcription factor that results in the control of gene transcription by the interaction of AR with coregulators and specific DNA sequences of androgen-responsive genes of the target cells. Because of the involvement of androgens in a large number of pathological processes, several synthetic steroidal and nonsteroidal AR ligands have been developed and are widely used in clinical applications, including the treatment of male hypogonadism (AR agonists), prostate diseases (AR antagonists), and others.

In this chapter, the basic effects of androgen deficiency on various organ systems; reported improvement of features of metabolic syndrome, bone mineral density, mood and sexual function; and the potential complications of testosterone treatment are presented. Symptoms related to androgen deficiency are presented as psychosomatic complaints, metabolic disorders, and sexual health problems. Patients suffering from one of these three constellations of symptoms may exhibit distinct features in terms of androgen levels, age, and body mass index. In addition to discussing testosterone-related health conditions of men as patients, the chapter discusses other common conditions requiring medication along with racial and cultural differences affecting men's health.

A number of health issues in men respond to pharmacological treatment. The natural decline in testosterone levels as men age or in adolescents with hypogonadism may respond to testosterone therapy. Erectile dysfunction may respond to phosphodiesterase type 5 (PDE-5) inhibitors. Benign prostatic hypertrophy, prostatitis, and male pattern hair loss may also respond to pharmacological intervention.

HYPOGONADISM

Hypogonadism, thought to be one of the main causes of male fertility problems, occurs in an estimated 13 million men in the United States. The exact prevalence is uncertain, because less than 10% of those affected by hypogonadism seek treatment. Hypogonadism refers to the failure of the testes to produce androgen, sperm, or both. Hypogonadism affects a man's fertility because the lack of testosterone makes it difficult for men to properly produce sperm. Furthermore, a low testosterone level can contribute to a low sex drive as well as erectile dysfunction.

Pathophysiology

Circulating testosterone is largely protein bound. The major protein is sex hormone–binding globulin (SHBG) with only 2% present as the biologically active or free fraction. The bioavailable fraction, representing testosterone loosely bound predominantly to serum albumin, is probably more meaningful. Hepatic SHBG production rises with aging and thyroid hormone excess and declines in hyperinsulinemic states (obesity and type 2 diabetes) so that free values may not always be concordant with total testosterone values. The biological effects of testosterone may be mediated directly by testosterone or by its metabolites, 5a-dihydrotestosterone or estradiol (Fig. 49-1).

Classifications

Men with classical hypogonadism are routinely classified into two categories: (1) those with primary hypogonadism (testicular failure) characterized by low testosterone and elevated gonadotropins and (2) those with secondary hypogonadism (hypothalamic-pituitary failure) with low testosterone and low or normal gonadotropins. Interestingly, a third category represents a significant proportion of older men who do not fit into either of the classical categories. These men are typically older and have high gonadotropins and testosterone within the normal range (Harkonen et al, 2003; van den Beld et al, 1999; Wu et al, 2008). This may represent a state of

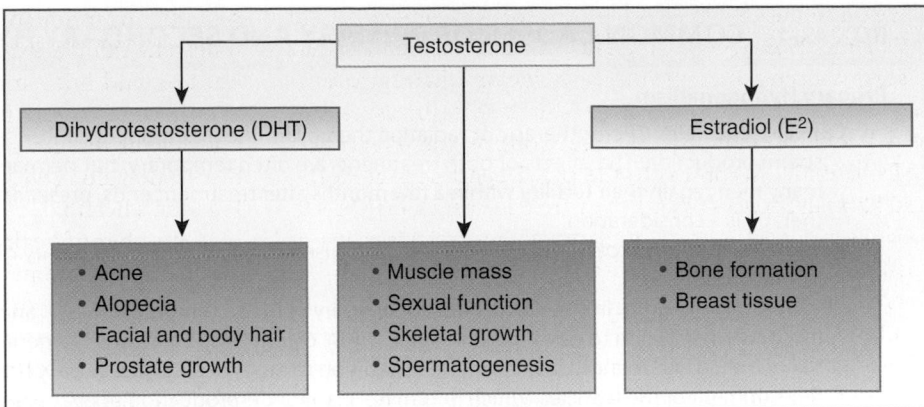

Figure 49–1. Effects of testosterone and its metabolites in men.

compensated, or subclinical, hypogonadism that could eventually develop into overt primary hypogonadism. A similar, well-recognized situation occurs in the pituitary-thyroid axis when high TSH is observed in the face of normal thyroid hormone levels, a hallmark of subclinical hypothyroidism.

Deficient testosterone production can happen at any point during a man's life. Common causes of hypogonadism are displayed in Box 49-1. In some men, hypogonadism is a congenital abnormality, as the deficiency has been present from birth. For other men, the deficiency does not present itself until the onset of puberty. In some cases, a man may not develop the testosterone disorder until well into adulthood.

Testosterone production declines with advancing age; 20% of men older than 60 years and 30% to 40% of men older than 80 years have serum testosterone levels that would be subnormal in their younger adult male counterparts. This physiological decline in circulating testosterone levels is compounded in frequency by permanent disorders of the hypothalamic-pituitary-gonadal axis, including transient deficiency states associated with acute stressful illnesses, such as surgery and myocardial infarction, and the more chronic deficiency states associated with wasting illnesses, such as cancer and AIDS.

The underlying etiologies and clinical management of secondary and primary hypogonadism are different. It may be informative to differentiate older men who are candidates for the diagnosis of late-onset hypogonadism (LOH) into different categories of hypogonadism by coupling testosterone with luteinizing hormone (LH) levels. Specific risk factors or clinical features can differentiate between secondary, primary, and the new subclinical form of compensated hypogonadism (Lee et al, 2009). Age-related symptoms of LOH, such as decreased bone density, energy, muscle mass and strength, erectile function, mood, and libido, are reminiscent of typical androgen deficiency in symptomatic hypogonadism due to pituitary or testicular disease in young men (Snyder, 2004). Other common terms used to describe LOH are andropause, male menopause, and androgen deficiency syndrome of the aging male (ADAM).

Perhaps the minor contribution of adrenal androgens (or androgenic precursors) may substitute for testicular deficiency once the target tissues have been fully developed. Moreover, ingrained behavior patterns may be resistant to androgenic hormone deficiency. Certainly, prolactin excess, testosterone deficiency, or both in men may result in decreased libido and erectile dysfunction. The yield of finding hyperprolactinemia or testosterone deficiency, or both, in patients presenting with these symptoms is generally less than 5%. However, a large survey of patients with erectile dysfunction presenting to a Veterans Affairs center suggested that the prevalence of these abnormalities is substantial, with 18.7% of patients having low testosterone levels and 4.6% with elevated prolactin levels (Bodie, Lewis, Schow, & Monga, 2003).

Signs and Symptoms of Hypogonadism Across the Life Span

In instances of congenital hypogonadism, insufficient amounts of testosterone are produced by the gonads. This causes the developing fetus to have improperly formed external genitals and internal reproductive organs, resulting in the birth of a child whose sex is not entirely clear. Beginning at birth and through infancy, the persistent failure of the testes to descend may be an early manifestation of testicular dysfunction. In addition, a normally formed but hypotrophic penis may provide a clue to an abnormality of the hypothalamic-pituitary-gonadal axis. Later, during puberty, delayed, arrested, or absent testicular growth and secondary sexual characteristic development are hallmarks of pubertal disorders. Males starting puberty with a testosterone deficiency suffer from a variety of symptoms affecting almost every part of their normal growth and development. Because the body does not produce enough testosterone, the voice does not deepen and little muscle mass increase occurs, although there may be some development of the breasts. The penis and testicles also do not develop and mature, the growth of facial hair is inhibited, and arms and legs grow out of proportion to the trunk of the body. Skeletal proportions may be abnormal (eunuchoid) with more than a 5 cm difference between span and height and between pubis-floor and pubis-vertex dimensions. During adulthood, manifestations are generally more subtle.

When hypogonadism presents itself in adulthood, the physical appearance of the man can be significantly altered.

BOX 49–1   COMMON CAUSES OF PRIMARY AND SECONDARY HYPOGONADISM

Primary Hypogonadism

Cancer treatment. Chemotherapy or radiation therapy for the treatment of cancer can interfere with testosterone and sperm production. The effects of both treatments are often temporary, but permanent infertility may occur. Although many men regain their fertility within a few months after treatment ends, preserving sperm before starting cancer therapy is a consideration.

Hemochromatosis. Excess iron in the blood can cause testicular failure or pituitary gland dysfunction, affecting testosterone production.

Klinefelter syndrome. In this congenital abnormality of the sex chromosomes, X and Y, a male has two or more X chromosomes in addition to one Y chromosome. The Y chromosome contains the genetic material that determines the sex of a child and related development. In addition to other defects, the extra X chromosome causes abnormal development of the testicles, which in turn results in underproduction of testosterone.

Mumps orchitis. If a mumps infection involving the testicles (mumps orchitis) occurs during adolescence or adulthood, long-term testicular damage may occur. This may affect normal testicular function and testosterone production.

Normal aging. As men age, testosterone production slowly and continuously decreases. The rate of decline varies greatly among men. As many as 30% of men older than 75 years have a low testosterone level, according to the American Association of Clinical Endocrinologists. The value of treatment is controversial.

Trauma to the testicles. The testicles are prone to injury. Damage to normally developed testicles can cause hypogonadism. Damage to one testicle may not impair testosterone production.

Undescended testicles. Before birth, the testicles develop inside the abdomen and normally move down into their permanent place in the scrotum. Sometimes, one or both of the testicles do not descend at birth. This condition often corrects itself within the first few years of life without treatment. If not corrected in early childhood, it may lead to malfunction of the testicles and reduced production of testosterone.

Secondary Hypogonadism

HIV/AIDS. This virus can cause low levels of testosterone by affecting the hypothalamus, the pituitary, and the testes.

Inflammatory disease. Certain inflammatory diseases, such as sarcoidosis, histiocytosis, and tuberculosis, involve the hypothalamus and pituitary gland and can decrease testosterone production.

Kallmann syndrome. Abnormal development of the hypothalamus can cause hypogonadism. This abnormality is also associated with impaired development of the ability to smell (anosmia).

Medications. Certain drugs and some hormones can affect testosterone production.

Obesity. Being significantly overweight at any age may be linked to hypogonadism.

Opioid users. Commonly prescribed opioids in sustained-action dosage forms usually produce subnormal sex hormone levels, which may contribute to a diminished quality of life for many patients with painful chronic illness.

Pituitary disorders. An abnormality in the pituitary gland can impair the release of hormones from the pituitary gland to the testicles, affecting normal testosterone production. A pituitary tumor or other type of brain tumor located near the pituitary gland may cause testosterone or other hormone deficiencies. Surgery or radiation therapy for the treatment of brain tumor may impair pituitary function and cause hypogonadism.

Normal reproductive functioning may cease, while emotionally a man can exhibit changes similar to those of menopausal women. Symptoms of this type of hypogonadism may include depression, development of male breasts, erectile dysfunction, failure of facial and body hair to grow, increase in body fat, loss of energy, inhibited sexual desire, loss of muscle mass; menopausal emotions including hot flashes, irritability and mood swings; onset of osteoporosis; and shrinking and softening of the testicles.

Hypogonadism affects a man's fertility because the lack of testosterone makes it difficult for men to properly produce sperm. Male factor infertility is likely to be responsible for one-third of the 10% to 15% of couples who are unable to conceive within 1 year of unprotected intercourse. Most of these male-associated cases result from diminished, absent, or faulty spermatogenesis. In addition to abnormal sperm production, other associated conditions causing infertility include obstructive ductal disease, epididymal hostility, immunological disorders, and erectile or ejaculatory dysfunction. Furthermore, a low testosterone level can contribute to a low sex drive as well as erectile dysfunctions.

Older Men

The aging man represents a special case. There is a well-known decline in testosterone production with age in otherwise healthy men. This decline in mean testosterone values can be seen in free testosterone levels, beginning in the mid-40s (some clinicians suggest even earlier), as a consequence of increasing sex hormone–binding globulin levels. The physiological mechanism for this is unknown. Total testosterone levels decline on average beyond 70 years. The diurnal rhythm is lost beyond 60 years. Although testicular size also declines in this age group, spermatogenesis may be well maintained into the 80s or even beyond. Gonadotropin levels tend to rise after 70 years, indicating that the testosterone deficiency is usually primary. Using the criterion of a low testosterone value, and remembering that commercially available tests have considerable variability regarding normal young-adult ranges, an estimated 7% of 40- to 60-year-olds, 22% of 60- to 80-year-olds, and 36% of 80- to 100-year-olds are hypogonadal (Vermeulen & Kaufman, 1995).

Increased longevity and population aging will increase the number of older men with LOH. The condition is common but often underdiagnosed and undertreated. Although controversy remains regarding indications for testosterone supplementation in aging men because of lack of large-scale, long-term studies assessing the benefits and risks of testosterone replacement therapy (TRT), reports indicate that TRT may produce a wide range of benefits for men with hypogonadism that include improvement in body composition, bone density, cardiovascular (CV) disease, cognition, erythropoiesis, libido and sexual function, mood, muscle mass, and quality of life. The ultimate issue as to whether these changes are normal and physiological or should be considered pathological, thus demanding therapy, remains unresolved. Indeed, it is a situation analogous to the ongoing dilemma of hormone replacement therapy for postmenopausal women, although in women the hormonal deficiency state is usually more abrupt and symptomatic.

In the largest double-blind, placebo-controlled interventional study of testosterone replacement in elderly men to date, Srinivas-Shankar and colleagues (2010) report that for intermediate-frail and frail elderly community-dwelling hypogonadal men at least 65 years of age, TRT prevents deterioration in muscle strength and improves body composition and symptom-related quality of life. Furthermore, TRT was associated with improved physical function in older and frailer men, highlighting possible functional consequences of small changes in physical performance.

Diagnosis

A biochemical diagnosis of low testosterone is dependent on accurate measurement. Serum testosterone has a well-known diurnal rhythm that appears to be lost when a man reaches age 60 years. Because testosterone values are 30% or so higher near 8 a.m. versus the later day trough, a testosterone value should be determined first thing in the morning. Although normal testosterone ranges vary among reference laboratories, the usually quoted range for young men is 300 to 1,000 ng/dL. In general, values below 220 to 250 ng/dL are clearly low in most laboratories; values between 250 and 350 ng/dL should be considered borderline low. Because the acute effect of stressful illness may result in a transient lowering of testosterone levels, a

confirmatory early morning specimen should be obtained. Measurement of free testosterone levels or bioavailable testosterone levels, determined adequately in some reference laboratories, may provide additional information. Free testosterone levels may be lower than expected from the total testosterone level as a result of aging and higher than expected in insulin-resistant individuals, such as in the case of obesity. In addition, serum follicle-stimulating hormone (FSH), luteinizing hormone (LH), and prolactin levels should be used to help determine the cause of hypogonadism.

If gonadotropin levels are not elevated, despite clearly subnormal testosterone values, anterior pituitary (thyroid-adrenal) function should be determined by measuring free thyroxine and thyroid-stimulating hormone levels, as well as an early morning cortisol level. A magnetic resonance imaging (MRI) scan of the brain and sella should be considered. An exception to this recommendation is the condition of morbid obesity, in which both total and free testosterone levels are typically low and gonadotropin values not elevated. Hyperprolactinemia, even of a small degree, may also warrant ordering an MRI, because interference of hypothalamic-pituitary vascular flow by space-occupying, stalk-compressing lesions will lead to disruption of the tonic inhibitory influence of hypothalamic dopamine and result in modest hyperprolactinemia (20 to 50 ng/mL range). Semen analysis should be performed when fertility is in question.

TESTOSTERONE REPLACEMENT THERAPY

Pharmacodynamics

Restoring testosterone levels to within the normal range by using testosterone replacement therapy (TRT) can improve many of the effects of hypogonadism (Table 49-1). Gooren (2010) presents a review of clinically based evidence from the past decade that denotes the benefits of TRT on multiple target organs of hypogonadal men. The review provides a comprehensive appraisal of the well-substantiated benefits of clinically indicated TRT and areas that need additional investigation.

Anemia

Endogenous androgens are known to stimulate erythropoiesis; increase reticulocyte count, blood hemoglobin levels, and bone marrow erythropoietic activity in mammals, whereas castration has opposite effects. Hypogonadism results in a 10% to 20% decrease in the blood hemoglobin (Hgb) concentration that can result in anemia. Young hypogonadal men usually have fewer red blood cells and lower Hgb levels than do age-matched controls.

Bone Mineral Density

Osteopenia, osteoporosis, and fracture prevalence rates are higher in hypogonadal men because testosterone plays a major role in bone density (BMD). The prevalence of osteoporosis in hypogonadal males is twice that of those of eugonadal men.

Table 49–1 Postpubertal Hypogonadal-Related Problems and Effectiveness of Testosterone Replacement

Postpubertal Problems Associated With Hypogonadism	Evidence of Improvement With Administration of Testosterone
Decreased bone mineral density	Increased bone mineral density
Decreased cognitive function	Increased cognitive function
Decreased energy, mood, and quality of life	Increased energy, mood, and quality of life
Erectile dysfunction	Increased sexual function
Decreased hematocrit and hemoglobin concentrations	Increased hematocrit and hemoglobin concentrations
Decreased muscle mass	Increased muscle mass
Decreased prostate glands	Increased prostate gland size—prostate symptom score, urine flow rate, and postvoiding residual urine in the bladder after voiding did not change significantly*
Decreased sexual desire	Increased libido

*Snyder et al, 2000.

Bone density in hypogonadal men of all ages increases under appropriately dosed TRT, although normal adult bone mass is not achieved. Testosterone produces this effect by increasing osteoblastic activity and through aromatization to estrogen-reducing osteoclastic activity. Part of testosterone's effect on bone is at least partially indirect, mediated via its aromatization product estradiol. Patients with prostate cancer treated with androgen deprivation therapy have an increased risk of osteoporotic fracture. The role of LOH in bone fracture rate in aging males is not known.

The long-term benefit of TRT requires further investigation. Trials of the effects of TRT on BMD yield mixed results. The pooled results of a meta-analysis suggest a beneficial effect on lumbar spine bone density and equivocal findings on femoral neck BMD. Trials of intramuscular testosterone reported significantly larger effects on lumbar bone density than trials of transdermal testosterone, particularly among patients receiving chronic glucocorticoids. No studies have been powerful enough to show a reduction in fracture risk with TRT.

Cognitive Function

Age-related decreases in testosterone predict an age-related decline in visual and verbal memory. Evidence exists for a correlation between testosterone levels and cognitive performance, such as spatial abilities or mathematical reasoning. Higher free testosterone concentrations are associated with better performance in specific aspects of memory and cognitive function, optimally in men ranging from 35 to 90 years of age, even after adjustment for age, educational attainment, and CV morbidity. Total testosterone does not consistently have the same associations. Suppression of endogenous testosterone synthesis and blockade of the androgen receptor in men undergoing hormonal therapy for prostate cancer result in a beneficial effect on verbal memory but an adverse effect on spatial ability and slowed reaction time. There is no definitive proof of the beneficial effects of restoring testosterone levels to normal in elderly men.

Trials of TRT in men to evaluate its effects on measures of cognitive function and memory are relatively small, are of a short duration, and show mixed results (Beauchet, 2006; Hogervorst, Bandelow, Combrinck, & Smith, 2004). Testosterone treatment in men aged 34 to 70 years improved verbal memory, spatial memory, and constructional abilities in nonhypogonadal men with mild cognitive impairment and Alzheimer's disease (Cherrier, Craft, & Mastsumoto, 2003; Cherrier et al, 2005). In one study of healthy men aged 50 to 90 years, testosterone alone or in combination with the aromatase inhibitor anastrozole improved spatial memory, but verbal memory only improved in testosterone-treated men in the absence of anastrozole (Cherrier et al, 2005). This raises the possibility that part of the effect of exogenous testosterone is mediated by its aromatization to estradiol. Whereas the results from these observational studies are not uniform, it appears that lower free testosterone is associated with poorer outcomes on measures of cognitive function, particularly in older men, and that testosterone therapy in hypogonadal men may have some benefit in cognitive performance.

Lower Urinary Tract Symptoms

In addition to improvement in sexual function, TRT may also improve lower urinary tract symptomatology and bladder functions by increasing bladder capacity and compliance and decreasing detrusor pressure at maximal flow in men with LOH.

Metabolic Syndrome and Type 2 Diabetes

Dyslipidemia-impaired glucose regulation, hypertension, insulin resistance, and obesity (all components of the metabolic syndrome) are also present in hypogonadal men. Lower testosterone levels are associated with surrogate markers for CV disease, including less favorable carotid intimal medial thickness, ankle/brachial index as a measure of peripheral arterial disease, and calcific aortic atheroma. There is a positive correlation between serum testosterone levels and insulin sensitivity in men across the full spectrum of glucose tolerance.

Improvement of insulin sensitivity is noted after TRT. The effects of TRT, diet, and exercise on glycemic control of men with diabetes mellitus indicate a favorable effect. By increasing lean body mass and reducing fat mass, testosterone therapy modulates insulin resistance and risk of metabolic syndrome. The mechanism of the fall in lipids may be related to the decrease in the visceral abdominal fat mass under the influence of testosterone, which inhibit lipoprotein lipase activity and increase lipolysis, with improvement of insulin sensitivity and mobilization of triglycerides from abdominal fat tissue. Hypogonadism is associated with an increased risk of CV disease in men (Muller et al, 2004). However, data are lacking as to whether higher testosterone levels predict reduced incidence of combined nonfatal and fatal major CV events. The inverse correlation between testosterone levels and the severity of coronary artery disease may be related to the fact that low testosterone levels are accompanied by an accumulation of abdominal visceral fat associated with increased CV risk factors, impaired glucose tolerance, and non-insulin-dependent diabetes mellitus (Caminiti et al, 2009).

Cardiovascular Disease

TRT does not increase the incidence of CV disease, myocardial infarction, stroke, or angina. The evidence supports no association between TRT and cardiac events. However, trials of TRT generally have not been designed or adequately powered to detect effects on clinically significant CV events. The outcome of most studies in men report either a favorable or neutral effect of normal testosterone levels on CV disease in men (Caminiti et al, 2009). TRT at physiological concentration increases coronary blood flow in patients with coronary heart disease. Beneficial effects on endothelial function and myocardial ischemia have been demonstrated, but not on CV mortality. Thus, although lower testosterone levels are associated with higher CV risk and mortality in aging men, adequately powered, randomized controlled clinical trials are needed to determine whether TRT will reduce morbidity and mortality from CV disease in hypogonadal or eugonadal men.

Mood and Energy and Quality of Life

Hypogonadal men older than 50 years report decreased quality of life, including common complaints of dysphoria, fatigue, loss of libido, and irritability (Wang et al, 2004; Wang et al, 2000). These symptoms coincide with signs and symptoms of major depression. There is significant inverse correlation between free testosterone levels (but not with total testosterone) and a depression score in elderly men, regardless of age and weight. There are reduced libido and reduced feelings of well-being with hypogonadism; the depressive symptoms during the hypogonadal state are reversed by TRT. Men who received TRT report variable effects on mood, energy, and sense of well-being.

TRT at physiological doses to nondepressed eugonadal men does not result in significant effects on mood (Haren, Wittert, Chapman, Coates, & Morley, 2005; Tricker et al, 1996). In hypogonadal men, testosterone replacement was associated with improved mood and well-being and reduced fatigue and irritability. Randomized controlled trials of TRT in men without or with underlying chronic illness report equivocal improvements in quality-of-life measures, including fatigue and general well-being (Gruenewald & Matsumoto, 2003; Livermann & Blazer, 2004).

For patients with major depression and/or dysthymia, improvement was equal to that achieved with standard antidepressants with significant improvement in the depression inventory score. This effect may be a direct effect of testosterone or related to positive effects of testosterone on weight and/or other anthropometric measures. Additional research is needed to assess the effects of TRT on clinical depression in patients with human immunodeficiency virus. No relationship between testosterone level and depressive symptoms was found in the Massachusetts Male Aging Study (Harkonen et al, 2003; Seidman, Araujo, Roose, & McKinlay, 2001). Gooren (2010) postulates that the discrepancy in the results of the effects of TRT on mood is the result of a genetic polymorphism in the androgen receptor that defines a vulnerable group in whom depression is expressed when testosterone levels fall below a particular threshold.

Muscle Mass and Strength

Aging is accompanied by significant changes in body composition as evidenced by decreased fat-free mass and increased and redistributed fat mass. These changes may impose functional limitations and increase morbidity. Maximal muscle strength correlates with muscle mass independently of age. In men, declining testosterone levels that occur with aging can contribute to these changes by direct effect on muscle cells or by stimulating IGF-1 expression directly and indirectly, leading to increased muscle protein synthesis and growth. There is a correlation between free testosterone concentrations and fat-free mass; however, the correlation with grip strength is not clear.

TRT may reverse age-dependent body composition changes and associated morbidity. TRT improves body composition: a decrease of fat mass and an increase of lean body mass. In many studies, body weight change did not differ significantly (Morley et al, 1993; Page et al, 2005; Sih et al, 1997). TRT was associated with a greater improvement in grip strength than a placebo. Research supports the benefits of TRT on skeletal muscle performance in elderly men with chronic heart failure and its positive effects on the prevention of loss of muscle strength of the lower limbs (Caminiti et al, 2009; Srinivas-Shankar et al, 2010). Although TRT is promising for improving muscle mass in some patients, changes in lower-extremity muscle strength and measures of physical function are inconsistent.

In aging men, positive correlations between testosterone and muscle strength parameters of upper and lower extremities also exist, as measured by leg extensor strength and isometric hand-grip strength (Srinivas-Shankar et al, 2010). Testosterone replacement is positively associated with functional parameters, including the doors test as well as the "get up and go" test and the 5-chair sit/stand test. Although increase in lean body mass has been observed, there is no proof of increase in physical function or in strength of knee extension or flexion. Although a potential role for TRT in the management of frailty exists, whether testosterone replacement improves physical function and other health-related outcomes or reduces the risk of disability, falls, or fractures in older men with low testosterone levels is unknown.

Sexual Desire, Function, and Performance

The prevalence of erectile dysfunction (ED) increases with age. Free testosterone is correlated with erectile and orgasmic function. Compared with younger men, elderly men require higher levels of circulating testosterone for libido and erectile function. Decreased libido, with or without hypogonadism, might be related to other comorbidities or medications.

Men with ED or decreased libido and documented hypogonadism may benefit from TRT. Adequate TRT can restore venous leakage in the corpus cavernosum, a condition that is a frequent factor in ED in elderly men. Research indicates some benefit of TRT on sexual health-related outcomes (Krause, Mueller, & Mazur, 2005). Long-term follow-up of TRT in hypogonadal males indicates that self-assessment of libido is higher with TRT (Bhasin et al, 2010). TRT also enhances libido and the frequency of sexual acts and sleep-related erections (Bhasin et al, 2010). Transdermal TRT is linked to positive effects on fatigue, mood, sexual function, and increases in sexual activity. In the presence of a clinical picture of hypogonadism and borderline testosterone levels, a short therapeutic trial may be reasonable. Evidence indicates that the combined use of testosterone and PDE-5 inhibitors in hypogonadal or borderline eugonadal men have a synergetic effect (Shabsigh, Kaufman, Steidle, & Padma-Nathan, 2004). The combination treatment should be considered in hypogonadal patients with ED failing to respond to either single treatment. Testosterone produces this effect by enhancing the production of nitric oxide synthase.

Testosterone Clinical Use and Dosing

Testosterone replacement therapy is relatively straightforward. See Table 49-2 for testosterone preparations available in the United States. Typically, the depot esters are administered parenterally by an intramuscular (IM) or subcutaneous (SQ) route. Testosterone cipionate (Depo-Testosterone) is the only IM form available in the United States. It is administered once every 2 weeks at a dose of 200 mg in adult men. An SQ slow-release pellet (Testopel) is the other parenteral option. The pellets have 75 mg of testosterone. Usually 8 to 14 pellets are inserted SQ in the buttock area, which then provides coverage for 3 to 6 months (Cavender & Fairall, 2009). A usual dosage for the transdermal or the buccal preparations results in the systemic absorption of 2.5 to 10 mg daily.

If the parenteral IM route is chosen, patients should and can be taught to self-inject. The major disadvantage with the IM parenteral route is that testosterone levels exhibit a sawtoothed pattern, with high-normal or supranormal levels on days 2 to 4 and low-normal or borderline-low trough values before the next injection. Mood, sense of well-being, and libido may vary accordingly in some individuals. Dosages may be adjusted by aiming for midnormal (400 to 600 ng/dL) testosterone levels after 1 week or at the low end (250 to 350 ng/dL) just before the next injection is due at 2 weeks. The insertion procedure for the testosterone pellets is simple with a short learning curve. Limited compliance issues and the elimination of risk of transdermal transmission of drug to others are distinct benefits for the use of pellets. However, disadvantages include wound infection and pellet extrusion, seen in 0.3% to 12% of patients in various studies (Cavender & Fairall, 2009).

Patches are applied daily and are rotated to different sites with minimal risk for skin transmission to others, although use may be limited by site dermatitis. Three hydro-alcoholic gel formulations are currently available in the United States: Androgel (1% or 1.62%), which is applied to the chest or the shoulders; Fortesta (2%), which is applied to the thighs; and

Table 49–2 ❈ Testosterone Preparations Available in the United States for Replacement in the Hypogonadal Male

Drug	Dose
Buccal (Striant)	30 mg to the gum region twice daily (q12h)
Intramuscular Depot esters—testosterone cypionate (Depo-Testosterone), enanthate (Delatestryl), propionate, phenylpropionate, isocaproate, decanoate, acetate	50–400 mg administered every 2–4 weeks
Subcutaneous pellets (Testopel)	10–15 pellets every 3–6 months
Topical gel (AndroGel 1% or 1.62% , Testim)	5–10 mg (1–2 packets/tubes or 1–8 pumps depending on concentration) once a day to clean, dry, intact skin of shoulders and/or upper arms or abdomen
Topical gel (Fortesta 2%)	40 mg (4 pump actuations) applied once daily to the inner and anterior thighs
Topical genital skin patch (Testoderm)	6 mg/d applied to scrotal area and worn for 22–24 h
Topical liquid (Axiron)	30–90 mg (2–4 pumps) once daily to axillae
Topical nongenital skin patch (Androderm)	5 mg/d applied once daily to clean, dry, intact skin of the shoulders, upper arm, or abdomen

Testim 1%, which is applied to the shoulders. A new liquid preparation, Axiron, is applied to the axillae. Because secondary transfer to women and children is possible, it is important to thoroughly wash hands after application and to cover the treated skin with clothing. In 3 to 4 hours, all the medication is absorbed, and the area should then be washed before direct skin contact with others.

Testosterone values become stable within a few days or weeks after initiation of the buccal, liquid, gel, or patch preparation. It should be ascertained whether the preparation was actually used on the day that the sample was drawn. A testosterone value in the midnormal range (400 to 600 ng/dL) is the goal. Although comparable testosterone levels are reached via the patch and the gels, skin reactions at the application site are much more common with patch use. Because of the very high cost associated with transdermal preparations, many insurance plans do not include them on their formularies or require prior authorization. The buccal preparation is difficult for some patients to use because of gum irritation, pain, tenderness, and/or swelling. Alkylated oral androgens should be viewed as potentially hepatotoxic and should not be used. Criteria for the selection of testosterone preparations are summarized in Table 49-3.

Risks and Contraindications

The most controversial issue related to TRT is associated risk (Bassil, Alkaade, & Morley, 2009; Bhasin et al, 2010). Erythrocytosis is a recognized risk of TRT; therefore, hemoglobin (Hgb) and hematocrit (Hct) levels should be checked periodically. Incremental increases are to be expected in the first 6 months of treatment, but an Hgb level higher than 17.5 g/dL, Hct higher than 54%, or both suggests overtreatment or occasionally abuse. Greater increments tend to occur more frequently with the IM preparations than with the transdermal. If the Hct is greater than 54%, therapy is stopped until the Hct decreases to a safe level. The patient should also be evaluated for hypoxia and sleep apnea (Bhasin et al, 2010). Restarting therapy at a reduced dose usually solves problems.

There is a risk of prostate cancer with the use of testosterone replacement. The Endocrine Society lists detection of subclinical prostate cancer and growth of metastatic prostate cancer as known risks of TRT (Bhasin et al, 2010). The Endocrine Society advises avoiding TRT in patients with metastatic prostate cancer or breast cancer (Bhasin et al, 2010). A digital rectal examination and PSA should be monitored throughout therapy. A urological consultation should be obtained if indicated by prostate symptom score, decreased urine flow rate, or postvoiding residual urine.

Additional risks of TRT have been identified. There is evidence of decreased sperm production and infertility reported by the Endocrine Society among men receiving TRT (Bhasin et al, 2010). Boys receiving TRT may experience acne and gynecomastia. The most serious risks of TRT in adolescents are aggressive behavior and premature closure of the epiphyses, leading to permanent short stature (Snyder, 2010).

Consideration of a number of clinical situations makes the risk of TRT an absolute or relative contraindication. Potential risks and contraindications are presented in Table 49-4. Clinical studies in large numbers of patients (either young or old) are limited, so potential risks and benefits should be individualized. Pierorazio and colleagues (2009) report that higher levels of serum-free testosterone are associated with an increased risk of aggressive prostate cancer among older men. Their data highlight the importance of prospective trials to ensure the safety of TRT in men older than age 65.

Drug-Drug Interactions

A total of 111 drugs (467 brand names and generics) are known to interact with testosterone (Drug Information Online, 2012). Of these, five medications have major interactions. The five high-risk medications are anisindione, dicumarol, leflunomide, teriflunomide, and warfarin. Using testosterone with any of these medicines is usually not recommended but may be required in some cases. Dose adjustment may be required for one or both of the interacting medicines. See Chapter 22 for further discussion of drug interactions with reproductive drugs, including testosterone.

Monitoring

The Endocrine Society recommends monitoring the following in men receiving testosterone replacement therapy (Bhasin, et al, 2010):

1. Evaluate the patient 3 to 6 months after treatment is started to determine efficacy in treating symptoms and if there are any adverse effects.

Table 49–3   Comparison of Testosterone Replacement Therapies

	Buccal	Intramuscular	Subcutaneous	Topical Gels & Liquids	Topical Patch
Convenience	Yes	No	Yes, but requires surgical intervention	Yes	Yes
Cost	High	Low	High	Very high	High
Physiological	Yes	No (sawtooth)	Yes	Yes	Yes
Side effects	Local, moderate	Systemic and local	Local, risk of pellet migration or extrusion	Local, minimal	Local, moderate
Stigma	No	No	No	No	Yes

Alkylated oral androgens should be viewed as potentially hepatotoxic and should not be used.

Table 49–4 Contraindications and Associated Potential Risk for Testosterone Replacement Therapy

Parameter	Contraindication vs. Potential Risk
Abnormal digital rectal examination	Contraindication
Breast carcinoma (history or presence)	Contraindication
Elevated levels of prostate-specific antigen	Contraindication
Erythrocytosis	Risk
Exacerbation of sleep apnea	Risk
Gynecomastia	Risk
Hypercoagulable states	Contraindication
Liver toxicity and liver tumor	Risk
Polycythemia (hematocrit >51%)	Contraindication
Prostate carcinoma (history or presence)	Contraindication
Psychopathology	Contraindication
Severe benign prostatic hyperplasia	Contraindication
Severe coronary heart failure (class III or IV)	Contraindication
Skin diseases	Risk
Stimulate growth of prostate cancer and breast cancer	Risk
Testicular atrophy and infertility	Risk
Untreated sleep apnea	Contraindication
Worsen symptoms of benign prostatic hypertrophy	Risk

2. Evaluate the patient's testosterone level 3 to 6 months after starting therapy. The goal is the midnormal range.
   a. Injectable testosterone: measure levels midway between injections.
   b. Transdermal patches: measure levels 3 to 12 hours after applying patch.
   c. Buccal testosterone: measure immediately after applying a new dose.
   d. Testosterone pellets: measure at the end of therapy.
   e. Oral testosterone: measure 3 to 5 hours after ingestion.
3. Evaluate hematocrit at baseline, at 3 and 6 months, then annually.
4. Evaluate bone mineral density after 1 to 2 years of therapy.
5. Evaluate PSA levels and perform a digital rectal exam prior to beginning therapy, at 3 and 6 months, then per age-related guidelines for prostate cancer screening.

Obtain a urological consultation if there are concerns about response to therapy, an increase in PSA levels of greater than 1.4 ng/mL in a 12 month period, or if any prostatic abnormality is palpated on rectal exam (Bhasin et al, 2010).

Patient Education

TRT should not replace healthy lifestyle changes. There has been a significant increase in the initiation of TRT for nonspecific symptoms of LOH in aging, androgen-deficient men. With this increase in TRT, there is a risk of overtreating. While there are many encouraging associations between treatment of androgen deficiency and improvement in rates of morbidity and mortality, much remains unknown about the overall long-term risks and benefits of TRT. It is important to remember that TRT should not replace healthy lifestyle changes, including smoking cessation, regular exercise, weight loss, and diet modifications that may provide the patient symptom resolution. It is important to have a thoughtful dialogue with the patient before the initiation of TRT. This conversation should include thorough disclosure of the risks and benefits of treatment and the limitations of the data as it evolves.

COMMON PROBLEMS THAT REQUIRE MEDICATIONS

Erectile Dysfunction

Erectile dysfunction (ED) is a common sexual problem in men. The incidence increases with age and affects up to one-third of men at some time during their lives. ED causes a substantial negative impact on intimate relationships, quality of life, and self-esteem. Treatment includes phosphodiesterase type 5 (PDE-5) inhibitors or TRT, if appropriate. Penile self-injection and vacuum-assisted erection devices are not discussed in this chapter, as these are usually prescribed by urological specialists. Cognitive behavior therapy and therapy aimed at improving relationships may also help to improve ED (Heidelbaugh, 2010).

Pathophysiology

Normal erections require a complex interaction between hormonal, vascular, neurological, and psychological systems (Spark, 2011). Any disruption in any of these systems may cause ED. Risk factors for ED include chronic illnesses such as diabetes mellitus, hypertension, obesity, dyslipidemia, and cardiovascular disease (Spark, 2011). Smoking and medication use may also contribute to development of ED. Because there is no preferred first-line diagnostic test, in most cases history and physical examination are sufficient to make a diagnosis. Initial diagnostics are usually limited to a fasting serum glucose level and lipid panel, morning total testosterone level, and thyroid-stimulating hormone test. Screening for CV risk factors should be considered in men with ED because symptoms of ED present on average 3 years earlier than symptoms of coronary artery disease (Heidelbaugh, 2010).

Phosphodiesterase Type 5 (PDE-5) Inhibitors

Pharmacodynamics

First-line therapy for ED consists of lifestyle changes, modifying drug therapy that may cause ED, and pharmacotherapy with PDE-5 inhibitors. PDE-5 inhibitors are the most effective oral drugs for treatment of ED, including ED associated with antidepressants, diabetes mellitus, and spinal cord injury. There are three PDE-5 inhibitors available: sildenafil (Viagra), vardenafil (Levitra), and tadalafil (Cialis). One aspect of a normal erection is the release of nitric oxide in the corpus cavernosum during sexual stimulation. Catabolism of cyclic GMP (guanosine monophosphate) is responsible for detumescence. The PDE-5 inhibitors work by blocking the catabolism of cyclic GMP. Blocking cyclic GMP results in an increased number and duration of erections in men with ED.

PDE-5 inhibitors are indicated for the treatment of ED. They vary in onset and duration of action (see Table 49-5 for dosing). Sildenafil and vardenafil have a 4-hour duration of effectiveness. Tadalafil may assist men with ED to have an erection in response to sexual stimulation for up to 36 hours after a single dose. Sildenafil and vardenafil should be taken on an empty stomach, as high-fat meals or alcohol will delay absorption. Tadalafil absorption is not affected by food or alcohol. Sildenafil has the longest safety record of the three (Spark, 2010).

Risks and Contraindications

PDE-5 inhibitors are contraindicated in patients sensitive to any component of the medication.

There is a potential for fatal hypotension if PDE-5 inhibitors are taken concurrently with nitrates (nitroglycerine).

Patients with cardiovascular disease, including acute myocardial infarction, stroke, or life-threatening arrhythmia within the past 6 months should not be prescribed PDE-5 inhibitors. Unstable angina, severe heart failure or prolonged QT, hypotension (systolic blood pressure less than 90 mg Hg), or hypertension (blood pressure greater than 170/110) requires caution in prescribing PDE-5 inhibitors.

Priapism is a rare occurrence. If the patient has an erection lasting longer than 4 hours, he should seek medical care.

Although PDE-5 inhibitors are specific for PDE-5, there have been reports of visual disturbances in some users of PDE-5 inhibitors most likely related to type 6 phosphodiesterase, which is required for the transformation of light into electrical signals.

PDE-5 inhibitors have been associated with rare reports of sudden hearing loss of unknown etiology. The hearing loss is temporary in one-third of patients and ongoing for the remaining patients (Spark, 2010). The U.S. Food and Drug Administration (FDA) is monitoring reports of hearing problems and any new hearing loss in patients who experience hearing problems while taking PDE-5 inhibitors; these cases should be reported to MedWatch (www.fda.gov/safety/medwatch).

Drug-Drug Interactions

The most concerning drug interactions with the PDE-5 inhibitors are the vasodilators, specifically the nitrates or nitroprusside.

Coadministration with alpha blockers may lead to additive hypotension. If coadministration is being considered, the patient should be stable on his dose of alpha blocker before considering PDE-5 inhibitors. The lowest dose of a PDE-5 inhibitor should be used and the patient monitored closely for hypotension.

PDE-5 inhibitors may interact with any of the antihypertensives and cause additive hypotension.

PDE-5 inhibitors should not be given concurrently with class 1A or III antiarrhythmics or drugs that cause prolonged QT interval.

Plasma levels of PDE-5 inhibitors may be increased by CYP3A4 inhibitors.

Monitoring

There is no specific laboratory monitoring for PDE-5 inhibitors. Patients should report symptoms of hypotension and any changes in self-monitored blood pressure readings.

Patient Education

Patients should be educated regarding the proper use of PDE-5 inhibitors. Drug interactions, specifically nitrates and other antihypertensives, should be discussed. Adverse drug reactions including priapism and visual and hearing disturbances should be explained and the patient advised to seek care if these occur.

Table 49–5 ⚇ Dosing Schedule of PDE-5 Inhibitors

Drug Name	How Supplied	Dose
Sildenafil (Viagra)	25, 50, 100 mg tablets	Initial dose 50 mg Take 1 dose as needed 1–4 hours before sexual activity, up to once daily. Decrease dose to 25 mg in patients with hepatic or renal impairment, or coadministration with CYP3A4 inhibitors.
Tadalafil (Cialis)	2.5, 5, 10, 20 mg tablets	As needed dosing: Initial dose 10 mg Take 1 dose as needed before sexual activity. May increase dose to 20 mg. May last up to 36 hours. Higher dose should not be used daily. Daily dosing: 2.5 mg taken at the same time each day. May increase dose to 5 mg daily.
Vardenafil (Levitra)	2.5, 5, 10, 20 mg tablets	Initial dose 10 mg Take 1 dose as needed 1–4 hours before sexual activity, up to once daily. Decrease dose to 5 mg in patients with hepatic or renal impairment, or coadministration with CYP3A4 inhibitors.

Benign Prostatic Hyperplasia

Benign prostatic hyperplasia affects the prostate, a male sex gland beneath the urinary bladder. A donut-shaped gland, the prostate encircles the urinary outlet, or urethra. Contraction of the muscles in the prostate squeezes fluids into the urethral tract during ejaculation. An enlarged prostate is not cancerous but can cause disability and even serious illness if left untreated. When the prostate becomes too large, it presses against the urethral canal and interferes with normal urination. As a result, urine may back up in the kidneys, subsequently damaging them by excessive pressure and contaminated urine. Bladder infections such as cystitis commonly occur as well.

These lower urinary tract symptoms (LUTS) are a common complaint among aging men: 8% of men aged 31 to 40 years, 50% in those aged 51 to 60 years, 70% in those aged 61 to 70 years, and 90% in those aged 81 to 90 years (Laborde & McVary, 2009). The symptoms are often caused by benign prostatic hyperplasia (BPH) and include nocturia, burning, decreased urine flow rates, difficulty in starting and stopping urination, hesitancy, incomplete bladder emptying, pain, progressive urinary frequency, urgency, and urinary frequency. A number of medical treatments for LUTS/BPH exist, such as alpha blockers (discussed in Chapter 14), 5-alpha-reductase inhibitors (discussed in Chapter 22), anticholinergics (discussed in Chapter 14), PDE-5 inhibitors, and combination therapies.

The science of how tadalafil treats ED may explain how it also treats the symptoms of BPH. Whereas tadalafil belongs to a group of medicines called PDE-5 inhibitors, phosphodiesterase type 5 is an enzyme found in many tissues in the body; it helps prevent blood vessels from relaxing and filling up with blood. Blood flow to the penis is necessary to get and keep an erection. Tadalafil blocks PDE-5 and causes smooth muscle and blood vessels in the penis to relax. This relaxation leads to the increased blood flow that is necessary for getting and maintaining an erection. PDE-5 enzymes are also found in the prostate and bladder. Tadalafil inhibits PDE-5 in these tissues as well, but the mechanism of how tadalafil reduces BPH symptoms is not completely understood.

Prostatitis and Male Pelvic Pain Syndrome

Prostatitis and male pelvic pain syndrome combine to form a multifactorial syndrome of largely unknown etiology. Prostatitis can partially or totally block the flow of urine from the bladder, resulting in urine retention. This causes the bladder to become distended, weak, tender, and susceptible to infection due to the increased amount of bacteria in the retained urine.

Prostatitis is classified into a number of subtypes: acute bacterial prostatitis, chronic bacterial prostatitis, inflammatory and noninflammatory chronic pelvic pain syndrome, and asymptomatic prostatitis. Some symptoms of acute prostatitis include fever, chills, frequent urination accompanied by a burning sensation, pain between the scrotum and rectum, fatigue, blood or pus in the urine, lower back pain, and ED. It usually results from a bacterial infection and is common among males between the ages of 20 and 50. Pathogenic organisms can be cultured only in acute and chronic bacterial prostatitis. It is important for men who suffer from any of the symptoms associated with prostatitis to see a health-care provider because the condition may progress to more severe complications, including kidney infection, orchitis (painful swelling of the testicles), and epididymitis (inflammation of the epididymis, a tube along the backside of the testicles). Acute prostatitis is treated with antibiotics, usually fluoroquinolones, for an adequate period of time. Treatment of prostatitis is covered in Chapter 44.

Premature ejaculation (PE) is a common sexual problem, and chronic prostatitis is an important cause of PE. Antimicrobial therapy is useful in the treatment of PE associated with inflammatory prostatitis (Zohdy, 2009).

Ninety percent of patients with prostatitis syndrome, however, suffer not from bacterial prostatitis but from chronic (abacterial) prostatitis/chronic pelvic pain syndrome (CP/CPPS). It remains unclear whether CP/CPPS is of infectious origin, and therefore the utility of a trial of antimicrobial treatment is debatable (Wagenlehner, Naber, Schleipfer, Brähler, & Weidner, 2009). Noninfective forms of prostatitis may be associated with autoimmune disorders. Bladder outlet obstruction and prostate stones may also occur if chronic prostatitis remains untreated.

Hair Loss

Rogers and Avram (2008) provide a comprehensive review discussing the current medications available to treat hair loss and medications currently under investigation. There has been extensive use of minoxidil (2% and 5%) topical solutions. Minoxidil maintains and thickens existing hair and, in some patients, it regrows hair follicles. Minoxidil is also available in a foam preparation. Finasteride is a type II 5-alpha-reductase inhibitor that is used to treat BPH and androgenetic alopecia. Finasteride is an effective inhibitor of type II 5-alpha-reductase, the enzyme responsible for the reduction of testosterone to dihydrotestosterone (see Fig. 49-1). Its effects include increasing the hair growth rate, thickness, and hair count. Clinical use and dosing of minoxidil and finasteride are discussed in depth in Chapter 32.

Medications currently under investigation but not approved for the treatment of hair loss include dutasteride, ketoconazole, and latanoprost. Dutasteride is a potent type I and type II 5-alpha-reductase inhibitor that has shown superior hair count number and growth rate. Ketoconazole is an antifungal medication that has also been shown to promote hair growth. Its exact mechanism in hair loss treatment is poorly understood. In a clinical trial, Inui and Itami (2007) found that ketoconazole topical cream (2%) showed increased vertex hair growth in two of the five patients. Latanoprost is a prostaglandin analogue used for glaucoma and ocular hypertension that was found to encourage eyebrow and eyelash hair regrowth. Although no formal clinical studies exist using latanoprost, it appears to be a promising agent for further investigations.

In addition to the current medications and those under investigation, the field of hair transplantation has evolved considerably. The cosmetic results of contemporary hair transplantation are virtually undetectable. Large, pluggy "punch grafts" have been replaced with natural-appearing follicular unit grafts, which maintain their existing anatomy and with proper technique can match the orientation of surrounding hair follicles. Some of the important factors to consider include age of the patient, pattern of hair loss, and expected future hair loss (Lee & Minton, 2009).

HEALTH PROMOTION, DISEASE PREVENTION, AND SCREENING IN MEN

The top 10 threats to the health of men in the United States include heart disease, cancer, injuries, stroke, chronic obstructive pulmonary disease (COPD), type 2 diabetes, influenza, suicide, kidney disease, and Alzheimer's disease (Mayo Clinic, 2010). Health promotion through preventive screening and testing is very important to preventing mortality and morbidity associated with these threats. Health promotion is about keeping healthy, living a healthy lifestyle, preventing illness, and preventing any existing illness from becoming worse. Immunizations also play an important role in health promotion. A schedule of recommended screening tests and guidelines for men by age is presented in Table 49-6. Immunizations recommended for men of all ages are found in Chapter 19.

ETHNIC AND RACIAL ISSUES

Compared with African American women and white men in the United States, African American men have more health risks and a shorter life span. The U.S. Department of Health and Human Services (2000) reported that African American men live an average 6 years less than African American women and 7 years less than white men. Reducing

Table 49–6   Screening Tests and Immunization Guidelines for Men by Age

Screening Tests	Ages 18–39	Ages 40–49	Ages 50–64	Ages 65 and Older
Blood pressure test	At least every 2 years	At least every 2 years	At least every 2 years	At least every 2 years
Cholesterol test	Start at age 20	Health-care provider to discuss with patient	Health-care provider to discuss with patient	Health-care provider to discuss with patient
Colorectal health (use 1 of these 3 methods): 1. Fecal occult blood test 2. Flexible sigmoidoscopy (with fecal occult blood test) 3. Colonoscopy			Yearly Every 5 years Every 10 years	Yearly; older than age 75, discuss with patients Every 5 years. Older than age 75, discuss with patient Every 10 years. Older than age 75, discuss with patients
Diabetes: blood sugar test	Health-care provider to discuss with patient	Start at age 45, then every 3 years	Every 3 years	Every 3 years
Eye and ear health: complete eye exam	At least once between the ages 20–29 and at least twice between the ages 30–39, or any time there is an eye problem	Get an exam at age 40, then every 2–4 years or as health-care provider advises	Every 2–4 years or as health-care provider advises	Every 1–2 years
Hearing test	Starting at age 18, then every 10 years	Every 10 years	Every 3 years	Every 3 years
General health: full checkup, including weight and height	Patient specific	Patient specific	Patient specific	Patient specific
HIV test	Test once for basic screening and then risk-based screening thereafter	Test once for basic screening and then risk-based screening thereafter	Test once for basic screening and then risk-based screening thereafter	Discuss with patient
Mental health screening	Patient specific	Patient specific	Patient specific	Patient specific
Oral health: dental exam	One or two times every year	One or two times every year	One or two times every year	One or two times every year
Prostate health: digital rectal exam (DRE)		Discuss with patient	Discuss with patient	Discuss with patient
Prostate-specific antigen (PSA) test		Discuss with patient	Discuss with patient	Discuss with patient

Continued

Table 49–6 Screening Tests and Immunization Guidelines for Men by Age—cont'd

Screening Tests	Ages 18–39	Ages 40–49	Ages 50–64	Ages 65 and Older
Reproductive health: testicular exam	Discuss with patient	Discuss with patient	Discuss with patient	Discuss with patient
Sexually transmitted infection (STI) tests	Both partners should be tested for STIs, including HIV, before initiating sexual intercourse	Both partners should be tested for STIs, including HIV, before initiating sexual intercourse	Both partners should be tested for STIs, including HIV, before initiating sexual intercourse	Both partners should be tested for STIs, including HIV, before initiating sexual intercourse
Skin health: mole exam	Monthly mole self-exam; by a health-care provider as part of a routine full checkup starting at age 20	Monthly mole self-exam; by a health-care provider as part of routine full checkup	Monthly mole self-exam; by a health-care provider as part of routine full checkup	Monthly mole self-exam; by a health-care provider as part of routine full checkup
Immunizations				
HPV vaccine	All males 13 through 21 years of age, up to 26 years of age for men who have sex with men.			
Influenza vaccine	Yearly	Yearly	Yearly	Yearly
Meningococcal vaccine	One dose between age 16 years and 21 years.			
Pneumococcal vaccine	High risk patients	High risk patients	High risk patients	One time only
Tetanus-diphtheria booster vaccine	Every 10 years	Every 10 years	Every 10 years	Every 10 years
Zoster (Shingles)			Discuss with patient	Discuss with patient

Source: Adapted from http://www.everydayhealth.com/family-health/mens-health/screening-tests-and-immunizations-guidelines-for-men.aspx.

the life expectancy disparity between African American men and other ethnic groups requires efforts to improve the overall health of these men with an emphasis on factors that influence their health-related behaviors, the role of their health perceptions in perpetuating their behaviors, and strategies to overcome the disadvantages.

Factors such as socialization, structural barriers, and practitioner bias can adversely affect health behaviors and health outcomes in African American men. Young African American males are socialized to accept masculine behavior through strength, dominance, autonomy, and physical aggression into adulthood. Difficulty expressing feelings leads to inner stress and adverse health consequences such as high rates of anxiety disorders and depression. Structural barriers such as poverty and lack of health insurance impede the delivery of health care to African American men. These men hold a disproportional share of part-time, contract, or temporary jobs. Many of these jobs have no associated health-care benefits. Practitioner bias and patronizing attitudes, especially by those who are non-African American, can have a negative impact on African American men's health and heighten perceptions of mistrust. Some providers may inadvertently engage in negative racial stereotyping when caring for African American men and thereby contribute to their patients' negative health perceptions and underuse or delayed use of health-care services.

HEALTH ISSUES FOR MEN WHO HAVE SEX WITH MEN

Health care for gay men and other men who have sex with men (MSM) is a complicated mix of physical, psychosocial, and cultural phenomena that requires provider awareness of the issues. Gay men's health issues are unique and need to be incorporated into clinical practice to provide comprehensive and culturally appropriate care.

HIV Infection and Sexually Transmitted Infections

Although HIV infection and sexually transmitted infections (STIs) are potential major health issues for all people, those issues remain of significant importance to gay men. The continued high rate of newly diagnosed HIV and STI cases signals that many gay men and other MSM are not taking the threat to their health seriously. Additionally, MSM are much more likely to become infected with HIV than their heterosexual counterparts. African American and Latino American MSM have twice the risk for acquiring HIV infection when compared to whites (CDC, 2006b).

Rates of three sexually transmitted infections (STIs)—chlamydia, gonorrhea, and syphilis—remain high in the United States (CDC, 2009). These infections can be cured but can cause serious complications if untreated and can increase the risk of HIV acquisition and transmission. High STI rates among African Americans and teens are particularly alarming, and MSM account for the greatest prevalence of syphilis (CDC, 2009).

Additionally, recreational drug use with substances such as cocaine, ecstasy, inhalants, and methamphetamines influence unsafe sexual behavior in gay men and MSM (CDC, 2009). Many of these recreational drugs are used during "white" or "circuit" party activities in which gay men from various geographical locales gather in one large metropolitan gay community over an extended 2 or 3 day period for the purpose of intense recreation and sexual activity.

Anal Cancer

Anal cancer is increasing in MSM and particularly in HIV-infected MSM. From 1973 to 2000, the incidence of anal cancer (2.1 per 100,000) in the United States increased in the general population for both men (160%) and women (78%). The incidence is substantially higher in MSM, HIV-infected men and women, transplant recipients, and women with cervical squamous intraepithelial lesions. Data collected before the height of the HIV epidemic revealed the incidence of anal cancer in U.S. MSMs to be 35 per 100,000 (Daling, Weiss, & Hislop, 1987; Daling, Weiss, & Klopfenstein, 1982). Estimates now put the incidence among HIV-infected MSM at least twice as high; 70 to 100 per 100,000. The incidence of anal cancer is 17 times higher in gay and bisexual men than it is in heterosexual men (CDC, 2008b).

In view of this increased incidence, there has been considerable discussion about whether regular anal screening using an anal PAP test should be implemented in the MSM population and specifically in the HIV-infected MSM population (CDC, 2008b). In 2011, the Advisory Committee on Immunization Practices (ACIP) recommended routine use of quadrivalent human papillomavirus (HPV) vaccine (HPV4; Gardasil, Merck & Co. Inc.) in boys aged 11 or 12 years. ACIP also recommended vaccination with HPV4 for young men aged 13 through 21 years who have not been vaccinated previously or who have not completed the three-dose series; males aged 22 through 26 years may be vaccinated. These recommendations replaced the 2009 ACIP guidance that HPV4 may be given to males aged 9 through 26 years. For these recommendations, ACIP considered information on vaccine efficacy (including data available since October 2009, on prevention of grade 2 or 3 anal intraepithelial neoplasia [AIN2/3], a precursor of anal cancer), vaccine safety, estimates of disease and cancer resulting from HPV, cost-effectiveness, and programmatic considerations.

Tobacco Abuse

Tobacco abuse continues to plague the gay community. Smoking among gay men occurs in nearly 33% of the population, whereas it remains at around 24% for the general public (CDC, 2006a). There is a paucity of interventions designed to target gay men with tobacco-abuse problems. Because HIV-infected individuals develop significant CV disease, a concerted effort must be taken to curtail smoking in this population. In addition, smokers who survive into later life may be at risk for significant cognitive decline. People who smoked 20 or more cigarettes daily have demonstrated faster declines in their verbal memory and slower visual search skills (Richards, Jarvis, Thompson, & Wadsworth, 2003). Smoking cessation programs designed to target gay men are being implemented slowly, but the need remains great. Smoking cessation is discussed in Chapter 43.

CONCLUSION

Most of the published studies addressing gender influence on health care focus on women's health or low-income and minority groups (Galdas, Cheater, & Marshall, 2005). There is a gap in research pertaining to men's health and an absence of health-care policies addressing men's health. Although men are usually research subjects, they are rarely the subjects of research.

Limited health-care resources; inequitable options available to men in seeking health care; and the absence of policies addressing gender-specific issues such as learning styles, masculinity, influences of testosterone on health, and stereotypical male traits—such as risk-taking behaviors—underscore the need for further studies and better understanding of men's health (Perls, Salzman, & Schaefer, 2006).

REFERENCES

Bassil, N., Alkaade, S., & Morley, J. E. (2009). The benefits and risks of testosterone replacement therapy: A review. *Therapeutics and Clinical Risk Management, 5,* 427–448.

Beauchet, O. (2006). Testosterone and cognitive function: Current clinical evidence of a relationship. *European Journal of Endocrinology, 155,* 773–781.

Bhasin, S., Cunningham, G. R., Hayes, F. J., Matsumoto, A. M., Snyder, P. J., Swerdloff, R. S., et al. (2010). Testosterone therapy in adult men with androgen deficiency syndromes: An Endocrine Society clinical practice guideline. *Journal of Clinical Endocrinology & Metabolism, 95*(6), 2536–2559.

Bodie, J., Lewis, J., Schow, D., & Monga, M. (2003). Laboratory evaluations of erectile dysfunction: An evidence-based approach. *Journal of Urology, 169,* 2262–2264.

Braithwaite, R. (2001). The health status of black men. In R. Braithwaite & S. Taylor (Eds.), *Health issues in the black community* (pp 62–80). San Francisco, CA: Jossey-Bass.

Brooks, G. (2001). Masculinity and men's mental health. *Journal of American College of Health, 49*(6), 285–297.

Caminiti, G., Volterrani, M., Iellamo, F., Marazzi, G., Massaro, R., Miceli, M., et al. (2009). Effect of long-acting testosterone treatment on functional exercise capacity, skeletal muscle performance, insulin resistance, and baroreflex sensitivity in elderly patients with chronic heart failure: A double-blind, placebo-controlled, randomized study. *Journal of the American College of Cardiology, 54,* 919–927.

Cavender, R. K., & Fairall, M. (2009). Subcutaneous testosterone pellet implant (Testopel) therapy for men with testosterone deficiency syndrome: A single-site retrospective safety analysis. *Journal of Sexual Medicine, 6,* 3177–3192.

Centers for Disease Control and Prevention (CDC). (2006a). Cigarette smoking among adults—United States. *Mortality and Morbidity Weekly Report, 56,* 1157–1161.

Centers for Disease Control and Prevention (CDC). (2006b). *HIV and AIDS among gay and bisexual men.* Retrieved November 12, 2012, from http://www.cdc.gov/nchhstp/Newsroom/docs/FastFacts-MSM-FINAL 508COMP.pdf

Centers for Disease Control and Prevention (CDC). (2007). *Top 20.* Retrieved November 12, 2012, from http://cdc.gov

Centers for Disease Control and Prevention (CDC). (2008a). *Sexually transmitted diseases surveillance.* Retrieved November 12, 2012, from http://www.cdc.gov/std/stats08/msm.htm

Centers for Disease Control and Prevention (CDC). (2008b). HPV and men—CDC fact sheet. Retrieved November 12, 2012, from http://www.cdc.gov/std/hpv/stdfact-hpv-and-men.htm

Centers for Disease Control and Prevention (CDC). (2009). NHBS: HIV risk taking and testing behaviors among young MSM. Retrieved November 12, 2012, from http://www.cdc.gov/hiv/topics/msm/ymsm.htm

Centers for Disease Control and Prevention (CDC). (2010). *Screening tests and immunizations guidelines for men.* Retrieved November 12, 2012, from http://www.womenshealth.gov/prevention/men/men.pdf

Centers for Disease Control and Prevention (CDC). (2011). Recommendations on the use of quadrivalent human papillomavirus vaccine in males— Advisory Committee on Immunization Practices (ACIP), 2011. *Morbidity and Mortality Weekly Report, 60,* 1705–1708.

Cherrier, M. M., Craft, S., & Matsumoto, A. H. (2003). Cognitive changes associated with supplementation of testosterone or dihydrotestosterone in mildly hypogonadal men: A preliminary report. *Journal of Andrology, 24,* 568–576.

Cherrier, M. M., Matsumoto, A. M., Amory, J. K., Asthana, S., Bremner, W., Peskind, E. R., et al. (2005). Testosterone improves spatial memory in men with Alzheimer disease and mild cognitive impairment. *Neurology, 64,* 2063–2068.

Chin-Hong, P., & Palefsk, J. (2002). Natural history and clinical management of anal human papillomavirus disease in men and women infected with human immunodeficiency virus. *Clinical Infectious Diseases, 35,* 1127–1134.

Daling, J., Weiss, N., & Hislop, T. (1987). Sexual practices, sexually transmitted diseases, and the incidence of anal cancer. *New England Journal of Medicine, 317,* 973–977.

Daling, J., Weiss, N., & Klopfenstein, L. (1982). Correlates of homosexual behavior and the incidence of anal cancer. *Journal of the American Medical Association, 247,* 1988–1990.

Drug Information Online. (2012). *Testosterone drug interactions.* Retrieved December 4, 2012, from http://www.drugs.com/drug-interactions/testosterone.html

Edley, N., & Wetherell, M. (1996). Masculinity, power and identity. In M. Mac an Ghaill (Ed.), *Understanding masculinities* (pp 185–201). Buckingham, England: Open University Press.

Everyday Health. (2012). *Screening tests and immunization guidelines of men,* Retrieved December 7, 2012, from http://www.everydayhealth.com/family-health/mens-health/screening-tests-and-immunizations-guidelines-for-men.aspx

Galdas, P., Cheater, F., & Marshall, P. (2005). Men and health help-seeking behavior: Literature review. *Journal of Advanced Nursing, 49*(6), 616–623.

Goedert, J., Cote, T., & Virgo, P. (1998). Spectrum of AIDS-associated malignant disorders. *The Lancet, 351,* 1833–1839.

Gooren, L. J. (2010). Androgens and male aging: Current evidence of safety and efficacy. *Asian Journal of Andrology, 12,* 136–151.

Gruenewald, D. A., & Matsumoto, A. M. (2003). Testosterone supplementation therapy for older men: Potential benefits and risks. *Journal of the American Geriatric Society, 51,* 101–115.

Haren, M. T., Wittert, G. A., Chapman, I. M., Coates, P., & Morley, J. E. (2005). Effect of oral testosterone undecanoate on visuospatial cognition, mood and quality of life in elderly men with low normal gonadal status. *Maturitas, 50,* 124–133.

Harkonen, K., Huhtaniemi, I., Makinen, J., Hubler, D., Irjala, K., Koskenvuo, M., et al. (2003). The polymorphic androgen receptor gene CAG repeat, pituitary-testicular function and andropausal symptoms in ageing men. *International Journal of Andrology, 26,* 187–194.

Heidelbaugh, J. J. (2010). Management of erectile dysfunction. *American Family Physician, 81,* 305–312.

Hogervorst, E., Bandelow, S., Combrinck, M., & Smith, A. D. (2004). Low free testosterone is an independent risk factor for Alzheimer's disease. *Experimental Gerontology, 39,* 1633–1639.

Inui, S., & Itami, S. (2007). Reversal of androgenetic alopecia by topical ketoconazole: Relevance of antiandrogenic activity. *Journal of Dermatological Science, 45,* 66–68.

Krause, W., Mueller, U., & Mazur, A. (2005). Testosterone supplementation in the aging male: Which questions have been answered? *Aging Male, 8,* 31–38.

Laborde, E. E., & McVary, K. T. (2009). Medical management of lower urinary tract symptoms. *Reviews in Urology, 11,* S19–S25.

Lee, D. M., O'Neill, T. W., Pye, S. R., Silman, A. J., Finn, J. D., Pendleton, N., et al. (2009). The European Male Ageing Study (EMAS): Design, methods and recruitment. *International Journal of Andrology, 32,* 11–24.

Lee, T. S., & Minton, T. J. (2009). An update on hair restoration therapy. *Current Opinion in Otolaryngology & Head and Neck Surgery, 17,* 287–294.

Liburd, L., Namageyo-Funa, A., & Jack, L. (2007). Understanding "masculinity" and the challenges of managing type-2 diabetes among African-American men. *Journal of the American Medical Association, 99*(5), 550–558.

Liverman, C. T., & Blazer, D. G. (Eds.). (2004). *Testosterone and aging: Clinical research directions.* Washington, DC: National Academies Press.

Matsumoto, T., Shiina, H., Kawano, H., Sato, T., & Kato, S. (2008). Androgen receptor functions in male and female physiology. *Journal of Steroid Biochemistry and Molecular Biology, 109*(3–5), 236–241.

Mayo Clinic. (2010). *Men's health: Preventing your top 10 threats.* Retrieved November 12, 2012, from http://www.mayoclinic.com/print/mens-health/MC00013

Men's Health Network. (2008). *Reports.* Retrieved November 12, 2012, from http://www.menshealthnetwork.org

Morley, J. E., Perry, H. M., III, Kaiser, F. E., Kraenzle, D., Jensen, J., Houston, K., et al. (1993). Effects of testosterone replacement therapy in old hypogonadal males: A preliminary study. *Journal of the American Geriatrics Society, 41,* 149–152.

Muller, M., van den Beld, A. W., Bots, M. L., Grobbee, D. E., Lamberts, S. W., & van der Schouw, Y. T. (2004). Endogenous sex hormones and progression of carotid atherosclerosis in elderly men. *Circulation, 109,* 2074–2079.

Page, S. T., Amory, J. K., Bowman, F. D., Anawalt, B. D., Matsumoto, A. M., Bremner, W. J., et al. (2005). Exogenous testosterone (T) alone or with finasteride increases physical performance, grip strength, and lean body mass in older men with low serum T. *Journal of Clinical Endocrinology and Metabolism, 90,* 1502–1510.

Perls, T., Salzman, B., & Schaefer, S. (2006, June). Why do men die at a younger age than women, and what can be done about it? *Patient Care,* 20–28.

Pierorazio, P. M., Ferrucci, L., Kettermann, A., Longo, D. L., Metter, E. J., & Carter, H. B. (2009). Serum testosterone is associated with aggressive prostate cancer in older men: Results from the Baltimore Longitudinal Study of Aging. *BJU International, 105*(6), 824–829.

Rhoden, E. L., & Morgentaler, A. (2004). Risk of testosterone-replacement therapy and recommendations for monitoring. *New England Journal of Medicine, 350*(5), 482–492.

Richards, M., Jarvis, M. J., Thompson, N., & Wadsworth, M. E. (2003). Cigarette smoking and cognitive decline in midlife: Evidence from a prospective birth cohort study. *American Journal of Public Health, 93,* 994–998.

Rogers, N., & Avram, M. (2008). Medical treatments for male and female pattern hair loss. *Journal of the American Academy of Dermatology, 59,* 547–566.

Seidman, S. N., Araujo, A. B., Roose, S. P., & McKinlay, J. B. (2001). Testosterone level, androgen receptor polymorphism, and depressive symptoms in middle-aged men. *Biological Psychiatry, 50,* 371–376.

Shabsigh R., Kaufman, J. M., Steidle, C., & Padma-Nathan, H. (2004). Randomized study of testosterone gel as adjunctive therapy to sildenafil in hypogonadal men with erectile dysfunction who do not respond to sildenafil alone. *Journal of Urology, 172,* 658–663.

Sih, R., Morley, J. E., Kaiser, F. E., Perry, H. M., III, Patrick, P., & Ross, C. (1997). Testosterone replacement in older hypogonadal men: A 12-month randomized controlled trial. *Journal of Clinical Endocrinology and Metabolism, 82,* 1661–1667.

Snyder, P. J. (2004). Hypogonadism in elderly men: What to do until the evidence comes. *New England Journal of Medicine, 350,* 440–442.

Snyder, P. J. (2010). Testosterone treatment in male hypogonadism. *UpToDate Online.* Retrieved November 12, 2012, from http://www.uptodate.com

Snyder, P. J., Peachey, H., Berlin, J. A., Hannoush, P., Haddad, G., Dlewati, A., et al. (2000). Effects of testosterone replacement in hypogonadal men. *Journal of Clinical Endocrinology and Metabolism, 85,* 2670–2677.

Spark, R. F. (2011). Overview of male sexual dysfunction. *UpToDate Online.* Retrieved November 12, 2012, from http://www.uptodate.com/contents/overview-of-male-sexual-dysfunction

Srinivas-Shankar, U., Roberts, S. A., Connolly, M. J., Adams, J. E., Oldham, J. A., & Wu, F. C. (2010). Effects of testosterone on muscle strength, physical function, body composition, and quality of life in intermediate-frail and frail elderly men: A randomized, double-blind, placebo-controlled study. *Journal of Clinical Endocrinology and Metabolism, 95*(2), 639–650.

Tricker, R., Casaburi, R., Storer, T. W., Clevenger, B., Berman, N., Shirazi, A., et al. (1996). The effects of supraphysiological doses of testosterone on angry behavior in healthy eugonadal men—a clinical research center study. *Journal of Clinical Endocrinology and Metabolism, 81*(10), 3754–3758.

U.S. Department of Health and Human Services. (2000). *National statistics reports.* Retrieved November 12, 2012, from http://www.hhs.gov

van den Beld, A., Huhtaniemi, I. T., Pettersson, K. S., Pols, H. A., Grobbee, D. E., de Jong, F. H., et al. (1999). Luteinizing hormone and different genetic variants, as indicators of frailty in healthy elderly men. *Journal of Clinical Endocrinology and Metabolism, 84,* 1334–1339.

Vermeulen, A., & Kaufman, J. M. (1995). Aging of the hypothalamic-pituitary-testicular axis in men. *Hormone Research, 43,* 25–28.

Wagenlehner, F. M. E., Naber, K. G., Schleipfer, T., Brähler, E., & Weidner, W. (2009). Prostatitis and male pelvic pain syndrome: Diagnosis and treatment. *Deutsches Ärzteblatt International, 106,* 175–183.

Wang, C., Cunningham, G., Dobs, A., Iranmanesh, A., Matsumoto, A. M., Snyder, P. J., et al. (2004). Long-term testosterone gel (AndroGel) treatment maintains beneficial effects on sexual function and mood, lean and fat mass, and bone mineral density in hypogonadal men. *Journal of Clinical Endocrinology and Metabolism, 89,* 2085–2098.

Wang, C., Swerdloff, R. S., Iranmanesh, A., Dobs, A., Snyder, P. J., Cunningham, G., et al. (2000). Transdermal testosterone gel improves sexual function, mood, muscle strength, and body composition parameters in hypogonadal men. *Journal of Clinical Endocrinology and Metabolism, 85,* 2839–2853.

Williams, D. (2003). The health of men: Structured inequalities and opportunities. *American Journal of Public Health, 93*(5), 724–731.

Wu, F. C., Tajar, A., Pye, S. R., Silman, A. J., Finn, J. D., O'Neill, T. W., et al. (2008). Hypothalamic-pituitary-testicular axis disruptions in older men are differentially linked to age and modifiable risk factors: The European Male Aging Study. *Journal of Clinical Endocrinology and Metabolism, 93,* 2737–2745.

Zohdy, W. (2009). Clinical parameters that predict successful outcome in men with premature ejaculation and inflammatory prostatitis. *Journal of Sexual Medicine, 6,* 3139–3146.

PEDIATRIC PATIENTS

Teri Moser Woo

Pediatric patients present a special challenge to the primary care practitioner; they are constantly changing, both physiologically and developmentally. The practitioner who is making a treatment decision must consider the parent and the family situation, as well as the patient, in determining if the treatment will be appropriate. In addition, information on use of medications in children is evolving as new studies regarding efficacy and safety of medications in children are published. This chapter presents the factors that the prescriber will need to consider to safely prescribe to children.

HISTORICAL PERSPECTIVE ON PEDIATRIC PRESCRIBING

Federal Drug Regulation

Drug regulation in the United States has often been moved forward after tragedies have occurred that directly involved children. Regulation began with the passage of the Federal Food and Drug Act of 1906, which was enacted because children had died from ingesting tainted food products and soldiers had died from ingesting adulterated quinine. This law, known as the Wiley Act, prohibited the manufacture and interstate shipment of adulterated and misbranded foods and drugs. In 1938, the next major legislation, the federal Food, Drug, and Cosmetic Act, was enacted. It was passed as the result of continued adulteration of products, including sulfanilamide, which had caused more than 100 deaths in children because of the diethylene glycol used in the elixir. For the first time, documentation of drug safety was mandated. This act also mandated truthful labeling and established the new drug application process that required toxicology testing prior to drugs being promoted and distributed. In 1962, the Harris-Kefauver Amendment was passed, prompted by the births of thousands of deformed infants whose mothers had taken the sedative thalidomide. This amendment mandated preclinical animal trials before testing drugs in humans. It also established three phases of clinical testing: phase I establishes safety and pharmacokinetics; phase II establishes initial effectiveness and dose range; phase III conducts comparative clinical trials.

Although the Harris-Kefauver Amendment increased the safety of new drugs coming onto the market, it also slowed new drug development, increasing the time from investigational new drug to new drug approval to 8 or 9 years. In 1972, an over-the-counter (OTC) drug review process was begun to enhance the safety and labeling of nonprescription medications. In 1986, the Child Vaccine Act was passed requiring patients/parents be informed regarding the vaccines they are being given. In spite of all of these laws, as late as the 1990s the percentage of approved drugs that contained no labeling information for children was approximately 70%.

The next major legislation that affected children was the U.S. Food and Drug Administration (FDA) Modernization Act of 1997. The act had two main components pertaining to pediatrics. First, the FDA could require in writing that the manufacturer submit data on pediatric patients for drugs that appeared to have a pediatric use. Previously, drugs were approved for use in adults and the pediatric prescribing information happened later. This law mandated that the FDA require the pediatric data up front. Second, pharmaceutical companies were rewarded by a 6-month extension on any patent if they voluntarily tested the medications for safety in children. The FDA Modernization Act was challenged by the drug companies and overturned in 2002, a setback for pediatric drug safety.

Best Pharmaceuticals for Children Act

Fortunately, the American Academy of Pediatrics and other groups concerned with pediatric drug safety went before Congress and the result was the passage in 2003 of the Best Pharmaceuticals for Children Act (BPCA). This reinstated the pediatric exclusivity rule, giving a 6-month extension on patents if a manufacturer studies a given drug in children. It also established a mandate for an annual list of drugs requested to be studied. Experts in pediatrics are consulted and a list is developed for priority testing. In addition, the Pediatric Research Equity Act (PREA) was signed into law in December 2003. It requires that all applications for new active ingredients, new indications, new dosage forms, new dosing regimens, and new routes of administration must contain a pediatric assessment unless the sponsor has obtained a waiver or deferral of pediatric studies. The BPCA was renewed in 2007 and became permanent in 2012 under the Food and Drug Administration Safety and Innovation Act. The outcome so far of these major moves toward pediatric drug safety has been 469 studies completed between September 2007 and November 2013.

As of June 2014, 512 drugs have been relabeled or newly labeled for pediatric use (FDA, 2014). As more studies are completed, we will have a clearer picture of the safety and efficacy of the drug prescribed, and pediatric providers will have to do less off-label prescribing of medications. When a relabeled drug contains the statement "Safety and effectiveness have not been established," it really means that the drug is either not safe or not effective in children as determined by pediatric studies. Providers can find current information regarding drug label changes at the FDA Web site: http://www.fda.gov in the Pediatric Product Development section.

Pediatric exclusivity, which grants a 6-month extension on the patent if drugs are studied in children, has been successful in ensuring most new drugs are at least evaluated for use in children. Wharton and colleagues (2014) examined 401 pediatric exclusivity requests and found that from 1998 to 2012 there were 189 studies completed and 173 drugs received new pediatric labeling. Of note is that Wharton and colleagues found efficacy was not established for 78 of the drugs studied. The economic benefit of the 6-month market exclusivity is weighed not only in additional profits for the manufacturer of the drug but in improved outcomes for pediatric patients (Vernon, Shortenhaus, Mayer, Allen, & Golec, 2012). Another exciting development in pediatrics is an international movement toward improving pediatric drug safety. The World Health Organization (WHO) launched the "make medicines child size" campaign in December 2007 to raise awareness and encourage medication development for children younger than age 12 years (WHO, 2010). A global alliance in pediatric pharmacology has been formed and pediatric pharmacologists from more than 30 countries have met to share information from pharmacokinetic and pharmacodynamic studies and avoid unnecessary duplication of studies (Koren, Reider, & MacLeod, 2009). The WHO publishes a *Model List of Essential Medicines for Children* with over 200 medicines to be used as a reference for countries to develop their own national pediatric essential medications lists (WHO, 2013).

> The Pediatric Trials Network is funded by the Best Pharmaceuticals for Children Act via the Eunice Shriver National Institute of Child Health and Human Development (NICHD). The purpose of the Pediatric Trials Network (PTN) is to create an infrastructure to study critical drugs and diagnostic devices in children to improve labeling for pediatric use. The PTN will conduct 16 trials over the next 5 years, adding to critical information on pediatric drug safety and efficacy. For more information see PTN's website, www.pediatrictrials.org.

PHARMACOKINETIC AND PHARMACODYNAMIC DIFFERENCES IN CHILDREN

Pharmacokinetics

Drug absorption, metabolism, and excretion can vary throughout infancy and early childhood. Even at puberty, there are differences in drug clearance between girls and boys as drug clearance rates reach adult levels. As more is learned about the metabolic pathways in the adult liver, more knowledge is gained about how to study the differences in children. Past disasters caused by lack of understanding about the physiology of newborn metabolism have led to caution regarding the use of medications in infants. Gray baby syndrome caused by inadequate glucuronidation of chloramphenicol, which led to dangerous drug accumulation, and sulfonamide-induced kernicterus (caused by displacement of bilirubin from plasma proteins by sulfonamides) are two such disasters that have been hard lessons in the use of medication in newborns. Well-designed pharmacokinetics studies in the newborn and careful therapeutic drug monitoring have improved our knowledge of neonatal pharmacology, yet care is essential when any new therapy is tried.

Drug Absorption

Drug absorption can be affected in children more than it is in adults by three factors: (1) the blood flow at the site of administration (intramuscular [IM] or subcutaneous [SC] administration), (2) gastrointestinal (GI) function, and (3) thin stratum corneum.

Neonates have more variability in the blood flow to the muscles, especially ill newborns, and poor blood flow can lead to delayed or variable absorption of medications. If perfusion suddenly improves, there can be a rapid absorption of the medication from the muscle, leading to possible toxic levels. Care should be taken when administering potentially toxic drugs such as cardiac glycosides, aminoglycoside antibiotics, and anticonvulsants IM to ill infants.

GI function is variable in neonates and young infants. Gastric acid function begins soon after birth and gradually increases over several hours. In premature infants, gastric acid secretion occurs more slowly and takes up to 4 days to reach normal levels. Gastric pH does not reach adult values until 20 to 30 months. Gastric emptying time is prolonged, reaching adult values by 6 to 8 months, meaning medications absorbed from the stomach may therefore have increased absorption. The neonate also has slow and irregular peristalsis, and medications absorbed primarily from the small intestine should be monitored for potentially toxic levels. It is known that the neonate has decreased oral absorption of acetaminophen, phenobarbital, and phenytoin, whereas ampicillin and penicillin G have increased bioavailability when taken orally. Diarrhea, a common ailment in young children, lessens the extent of absorption from the intestine, causing decreased drug levels.

The developmental changes in gastric function alter drug absorption in a fairly predictable manner. The oral bioavailability of acid labile compounds (beta-lactams) is increased and the oral bioavailability of weak organic acids (phenobarbital and phenytoin) is decreased. Basic drugs, such as diazepam and theophylline, have increased absorption. Gastric motility greatly alters the absorption of drugs with limited water solubility (phenytoin and carbamazepine) (Kearns, 2000; Kearns et al, 2003; Rakhmanina & van den Anker, 2006).

It is well known that infants and young children have a thin stratum and larger body surface area in relation to size and this affects topical absorption of medication. Children absorb topical medications more readily than do adults, leading to the systemic toxicity seen with topical medication use, for example, lidocaine or diphenhydramine. Most providers are familiar with the concern for systemic absorption of topical corticosteroids in children, with systemic Cushingoid symptoms or HPA (hypothalamic-pituitary-adrenal-axis) suppression developing with topical use.

Due to BPCA and pharmacokinetic studies that indicated HPA-axis suppression or adrenal suppression in children, a number of topical corticosteroids have been relabeled. Diprolene (diprosone) cream, ointment, and lotion are not recommended for use in children younger than 12 years due to HPA-axis suppression. In addition, Diprolene AF and Elocon (mometasone) lotion are not recommended, although Elocon cream and ointment may be used in children as young as 2 years. In an open-label study of Lotrisone (clotrimazole and betamethasone dipropionate) cream for the treatment of tinea pedis, 17 of 43 (39.5%) patients (12 to 16 years) demonstrated adrenal suppression as determined by cosyntropin testing. In an open-label study of Lotrisone cream for the treatment of tinea cruris, 8 of 17 (47.1%) patients (12 to 16 years) demonstrated adrenal suppression by cosyntropin testing. Lotrisone has been relabeled and is not recommended for children younger than 17 years and not recommended for diaper dermatitis; previously it was not recommended for children younger than 12 years. Cutivate (fluticasone) ointment has been similarly relabeled to be used only in adults (U.S. Food and Drug Administration, 2010).

Distribution

There are clear changes in body composition in neonates, infants, children, and adolescents. Newborns have total body water (TBW) of 80%, which drops over the first few months to TBW of 60% at 6 months; therefore, infants require higher doses of hydrophilic drugs. Infants also have a decreased volume of distribution for lipid-soluble drugs. Infants younger than 6 months have decreased plasma proteins available for drug binding, which will cause elevated levels of unbound medication. Providers need to monitor for drug toxicity even if there is normal or low plasma concentration of total drug. Phenytoin is one example of this, as it is only 80% to 85% bound in infants and 94% to 98% bound in adults (Kearns, 2000; Kearns et al, 2003).

The ratio of fat to lean muscle also shifts throughout childhood with a shift toward decreased total body fat in adolescence, a shift of approximately 50% in males between ages 10 and 20 years. Consequently, lean body mass increases more in males. The shift in females is less dramatic, shifting from 28% to 25% from ages 10 to 20 years (Kearns, 2000; Rakhmanina & van den Anker, 2006). Due to these changes, it may be difficult to predict pharmacokinetics of some drugs during pubertal growth. Medications that the patient takes chronically, such as seizure medications, need to be monitored closely during pubertal growth.

Metabolism

Phase I Enzymes

The pathways of drug metabolism develop variably over the first year of life and may be influenced by medications that induce drug-metabolizing enzymes (e.g., phenobarbital). In adults, much has been learned about the cytochrome P450 (CYP450) enzymes, and much is still unknown. The exact developmental pattern is not known for all of the CYP450 isoenzymes although our knowledge is increasing rapidly. It is known that CYP 3A7 is active during gestation and is the most active isoenzyme at birth. CYP 3A7 disappears at a few weeks of life but may remain active in 5% of people (Kearns, 2000; van den Anker, 2010).

Studies of CYP450 1A2 using caffeine as the test substrate demonstrate limited metabolic clearance in the newborn. CYP 1A2 reaches adult levels at 4 months and then exceeds adult levels at 1 to 2 years throughout childhood. At puberty (Tanner stage II), clearance begins to decline to adult levels, in girls sooner than in boys. Diseases such as cystic fibrosis (CF) can affect CYP1A2 activity and CF patients may need higher doses of medications metabolized via the CYP1A2 pathway. There are many medications that are metabolized via the CYP1A2 enzymes, including theophylline, erythromycin, cimetadine, phenobarbitol, phenytoin, carbamazepine, clarithromycin, and others. Foods that are affected by the CYP1A2 pathway are grapefruit juice, cruciferous vegetables, and charbroiled foods—foods not commonly eaten by children, but the provider should be aware of these food interactions. Cigarette smoking also affects CYP1A2 enzymes and providers should inquire if patients taking medications are smoking because it may affect therapeutic levels of medication, including a number of seizure medications. In practice, this implies that drug dosages need to be adjusted as a child goes through phases of CYP1A2 maturation; higher dosages may be needed from 1 year until puberty and therapeutic drug levels will need to be monitored as a child goes through puberty.

CYP 2D6 is absent in the fetal liver and 0% to 5% active at birth. At 1 month of age CYP 2D6 has 20% adult activity and reaches adult activity at age 3 to 5 years of age (Kearns, 2000; van den Anker, 2010). There is significant genetic variability in CYP 2D6 activity. Up to 20% of Africans of Ethiopian descent are 2D6 ultrametabolizers, whereas 3.4% to 6.5% of African Americans are ultrametabolizers (FDA, 2012). Among Caucasians 3.6% to 6.5% are ultrametabolizers. CYP 2D6 ultrametabolizers may be at risk for respiratory depression after taking codeine because they metabolize codeine to morphine at a greater than predicted rate, leading to elevated morphine levels. In 2012, the FDA issued an advisory regarding prescribing codeine to children.

Additionally, 5% to 10% of Caucasians and 1% to 2% of Asians are poor CYP 2D6 metabolizers. Many psychotropics, including SSRIs, are inhibitors of CYP 2D6, leading to prolonged half-life, and even small doses may not be tolerated by poor metabolizers. Antiseizure medications such as carbamazepine, topiramate, and lamotrigine will require careful monitoring in poor metabolizers.

The isoenzyme CYP3A4 is the most abundant CYP isoform and undergoes a maturational process similar to CYP1A2. CYP3A4 has low activity at birth and reaches 30% to 40% of adult levels by 1 month. By 6 months, it is at full adult levels and exceeds adult levels at 1 to 4 years. At puberty it decreases to adult levels. The CYP3A4 enzymes are used to metabolize more than 20 commonly used pediatric medications, including carbamazepine, prednisone, oral contraceptives, macrolides, NSAIDS, antihistamines, and others. The implications for pediatric practice include monitoring when prescribing more than one drug metabolized by CYP3A4 enzyme and monitoring during developmental changes.

Recent studies recognize that the small intestine is a major site of drug metabolism because it contains enterocytes in the bowel mucosa, which have CYP450 drug metabolism enzymes. This information enhances our knowledge of drug metabolism, but there may be large interindividual variation in the capacity of the small bowel to metabolize drugs.

Phase II Enzymes

Phase II enzymes are responsible for synthesis of water-soluble compounds. There is less information available on phase II activity in children. UDP glucuronosyltransferase (UGT) is responsible for the glucuronidation of hundreds of hydrophobic compounds. It is known that morphine is metabolized by UGT 2B7. It is known from morphine studies in neonates that premature infants (gestational age 24 to 37 weeks) have a much lower plasma clearance of morphine than children 1 to 16 years. It is thought that morphine clearance reaches adult levels at 2 to 6 months, although some children do not reach adult levels until 3 years (Blake, Castro, Leeder, & Kearns, 2005; Kearns, 2000; Rakhmanina & van den Anker, 2006). There appear to be ethnic variations in thiopurine methyltransferase (TPMT) activity; Koreans, for example, do not reach adult activity levels until 7 to 9 years. Little is known about the phase II enzymes in children, but the knowledge base is growing. Commonly used medications such as acetaminophen, morphine, propofol, and caffeine are metabolized via the phase II enzymes, and providers need to be aware of developmental as well as possible ethnic variations.

One essential consideration from our knowledge thus far is that, during times of great physiological change (the premature, the neonate, puberty), there are likely to be major changes in pharmacokinetics. More variability among individuals and within the individual is likely during these periods. Careful monitoring of therapeutic drug levels is critical to safe outcomes. In the neonatal period, frequent adjustments may be necessary because of the rapid changes the neonate is undergoing. A drug dosage that is at a therapeutic level in a 9-year-old girl has to be carefully monitored as she proceeds through puberty to ensure that she will not develop toxic levels as her drug clearance reaches adult levels.

Drug metabolism is an area in which the BPCA and Pediatric Research Equity Act (PREA) studies have expanded our knowledge. For example, females aged 8 to 11 years have higher therapeutic levels of fluvoxamine (Luvox) compared to boys the same age. The studies indicate that girls need lower doses of fluvoxamine (FDA, 2014). Likewise, pharmacokinetic studies of oxcarbazepine (Trileptal) in children have determined clearance decreases with age, to the point that children aged 2 to younger than 4 years may require up to twice the dose per body weight compared to adults, and children aged 4 to 12 years may require a dose 50% higher per weight than adults (FDA, 2014). Pharmacokinetic studies of levetriacetam (Keppra) found clearance increased with increased body weight; adults have a 40% higher clearance than do children. Hence, prescribers need to be aware of nonlinear pharmacokinetics seen with some pediatric medications and prescribe and monitor accordingly.

Excretion

Drug excretion rates are affected by the lower glomerular filtration rate in newborns, which is only 30% to 40% of adult values. By age 6 to 12 months, the glomerular filtration rate reaches adult values (per unit surface area). Drugs that depend on renal excretion are cleared more slowly in neonates. Drug dosages and dosing intervals in newborns are adjusted accordingly for medications such as ampicillin, aminoglycoside antibiotics, and digoxin. Renal blood flow is also reduced in neonates and reaches adult levels at approximately 9 months.

Pharmacodynamics

There are pharmacodynamic differences between children and adults that need to be taken into consideration in prescribing for children. Like much medical knowledge, information on the differences between children and adults has been gained from an unexpected outcome in children in response to a medication that is safe for adults. The classic examples are antihistamines and barbiturates, which may cause hyperactivity rather than sedation when given to children. Another classic example is tetracycline, which deposits in developing teeth and causes permanent stains. Systemic corticosteroids stunt linear growth if taken for long periods, as well as producing all of the same adverse reactions found in adults. Some medications, such as isoniazid, are less toxic in children than they are in adults.

Another concern in children is the vehicle in which the medication is administered or the formulation of the vehicle. Children have sometimes had toxic or unexpected results not from the medication, but from the additives or preservatives used. As recently as the 1980s, benzyl alcohol, a preservative used in drugs, was discovered to cause "gasping syndrome" when medications containing it were administered to newborns.

Topical ointments and creams are routinely prescribed to adults and children, yet there is a major difference between adults and children in the absorption rates from the skin. Infants and children have a thinner stratum corneum that allows medications to be more readily absorbed. Compared with older children and adults, infants have a larger skin surface area that is capable of greater weight-adjusted absorption of hydrophilic drugs. Occlusive dressings can increase the absorption of medications, which is of particular concern regarding corticosteroids in the diaper area. The plastic coating on the diaper can cause occlusion, thereby increasing absorption and producing systemic steroid effects.

DEVELOPMENTAL ASPECTS OF PEDIATRIC MEDICATION ADMINISTRATION

With adults, the provider can assume that, if reasonably clear instructions are given, the patient will take the medication as prescribed. With children, many added variables affect administration of the medication and compliance with the medication regimen. The first consideration is the developmental level of the child and the amount of parental control at each developmental level. This section addresses these differences and suggests strategies for improving compliance at each age level.

Breastfed Infants

Breastfeeding an infant the first year of life is beneficial both physically and emotionally to the infant. Therefore, when prescribing medications to a lactating woman, the practitioner needs to be aware of which medications can be used safely and which are contraindicated (Box 50-1). The most up-to-date, peer-reviewed, and easily accessible resource is the LactMed database at the National Library of Medicine TOXNET Web site (http://toxnet.nlm.nih .gov/index.html). LactMed is searchable by drug name and gives recommendations for prescribers with updated safety information.

BOX 50–1   PRESCRIBING TO LACTATING WOMEN

Prescribing medications for lactating women should be undertaken with the same caution as prescribing for pregnant women. Assume that any drug prescribed will, in some amount, be found in the breast milk. Therefore, knowledge regarding safety of medications for lactating women is essential for all primary care practitioners. When prescribing, take the following steps:

1. Review the safety of the drug during lactation.
2. If the drug is relatively safe, discuss the risks with the mother and explain the symptoms of drug toxicity.
3. Explain that the drug should be taken just after nursing or before infant's sleep.
4. Measure drug concentrations in milk or infant's serum when toxicity is likely.
5. Monitor the infant for signs of pharmacological action or drug toxicity.
6. Report any symptoms or signs of drug toxicity to the American Academy of Pediatrics, Committee on Drugs.

A few medications are absolutely contraindicated in lactating women (see Table 50-1). Contraindications include antineoplastic drugs because of immediate or delayed toxicity in the infant. Weekly use of methotrexate for rheumatic disease is acceptable during lactation, but the infant needs to be monitored closely, with routine laboratory analysis of complete blood count with differential, liver enzymes, and renal function essential to infant safety. Another contraindication to breastfeeding

Continued

BOX 50–1 PRESCRIBING TO LACTATING WOMEN—cont'd

is iodine-containing radioactive medications used in nuclear medicine studies. In this case, temporary cessation of breast-feeding ("pump and dump") is indicated. The length of time before resumption of breastfeeding is determined by the half-life of the radiopharmaceutical agent.

Drugs that should be avoided include lithium and oral contraceptives, yet both have been used in lactating women. Lithium is excreted in breast milk at about 40% of the concentration of maternal serum, and milk and infant serum levels are approximately equal. If, for maternal health reasons, lithium needs to be prescribed, the infant's serum lithium level needs to be monitored closely. The main contraindication to oral contraceptives containing estrogen is that they may decrease milk supply. An oral contraceptive with low estrogen levels can be prescribed once the milk supply is well established (more than 6 weeks' postpartum), but the first choice should be a progestin-only oral contraceptive. Decreased milk supply should be discussed with the mother as an adverse effect of estrogen-containing oral contraceptives prior to prescribing.

All illicit drugs are contraindicated in lactating women, specifically cocaine, heroin, and methamphetamine. Infants exposed to cocaine via breast milk may show signs of toxicity (irritability, tremors, increased startle response). Cocaine metabolites can be found in breast milk for up to 36 hours after the mother's last dose. Heroin enters breast milk and can cause neonatal depression. Amphetamines are excreted in breast milk and cause excitation in the infant. Methamphetamine poses an additional concern because some of the chemicals used to manufacture the illicit drug are toxic to both mother and infant, specifically lead, which is quite harmful to the infant. Any drug use during lactation should be explored and the mother encouraged to discontinue breastfeeding if illicit drug use is a concern.

Alcohol and **tobacco** are two commonly used legal drugs that can affect the breastfed infant. Alcohol passes freely into breast milk and reaches levels close to maternal serum levels. High levels of alcohol in the breast milk put the infant at risk for sedation and cause a reduction in the maternal milk-ejecting response. There is controversy regarding maternal alcohol use during lactation. It is probably safe for the mother to ingest small amounts of alcohol timed just after a feeding, when levels in the milk are the lowest possible. Tobacco is a concern because of both secondhand smoke exposure and the nicotine that passes into breast milk. Nicotine passes freely into breast milk, and therefore the breastfed infant is exposed to this toxin. If a nicotine replacement patch is used for maternal smoking cessation, then the nicotine blood levels and therefore breast milk levels are lower than with smoked tobacco.

Because drugs are almost never tested for use in lactating women prior to their release onto the market, questions regarding their safety during breastfeeding always exist. Understanding some basic principles regarding the transfer of drugs into breast milk and their pharmacokinetic actions helps the practitioner make decisions about safe prescribing. The practitioner should have ready reference to the most current information available about drugs during lactation, including *Drug Facts and Comparisons; Drugs in Pregnancy and Lactation* by Biggs, Freeman, and Yaffe; and *Teratogen Information Services,* available from your local Poison Control Center.

The National Library of Medicine TOXNET (Toxicology Data Network) maintains a peer-reviewed, searchable online database of drugs in lactation: LactMed (http://toxnet.nlm.nih.gov/index.html).

Drug Excretion in Breast Milk

The mammary gland can be viewed as an elimination organ in relation to maternal medication ingestion. Like other elimination organs, the properties of the medication determine how much of the medication will be in the breast milk. Because breast milk is more acidic than plasma, basic compounds (beta blockers) may be slightly more concentrated in the milk, and the concentration of acidic compounds (penicillins and NSAIDs) in the milk will be lower than plasma levels (Berlin & Briggs, 2005). Protein binding also affects the transfer of medications into breast milk. Highly plasma protein–bound drugs have a lower amount of drug available to transfer into milk because only the free drug is available for transfer. Liposolubility also affects the ability of drugs to cross the alveolar cells by diffusion and enter the milk. Another factor is the molecular weight of the drug: drugs with high molecular weight are transferred less easily into milk than drugs with lower molecular weight.

Factors Influencing an Infant's Exposure to Drugs in Breast Milk

A number of factors must be accounted for in determining the infant's exposure to a drug (Table 50-1). The following variables

encompass physiological processes in both the infant and the mother that influence the effects of a drug on the infant:

1. Maternal pharmacokinetics has a great impact on the level of drug found in breast milk; the higher the drug concentration in the maternal plasma, the higher the concentration of that drug in the milk. Pregnant women have altered pharmacokinetics in the last trimester of gestation. Failure to monitor doses and decrease medication dosages appropriately after delivery may lead to toxic effects in both the mother and the breastfed infant. A higher maternal drug dose or decreased clearance leads to increased amounts of a drug in breast milk.

2. The infant suckling pattern can determine the level of drug found in breast milk. The time of the feeding in relation to the maternal dosing determines how much of the drug is in the breast milk. A drug with a short half-life, given to the mother right after feeding, decreases the amount of drug the infant is exposed to. Likewise, drugs with a long half-life increase the infant's exposure to the drug. Infant suckling time and the number of feedings also have an impact on drug exposure. Some infants nurse for long periods or very

Table 50–1   Effects of Commonly Prescribed Medications on Infants During Lactation

Drug	Effect on Infant	Comments
Acetaminophen	Minimal	Found in breast milk. No adverse reactions reported. Safer than aspirin when lactating.
Amoxicillin (all penicillins)	Minimal	Excreted in breast milk in low concentrations. May cause mild diarrhea in infant.
Amoxicillin-clavulanate (Augmentin)	Minimal	Excreted in breast milk. Infant may have diarrhea.
Amphetamine	Unknown	It is not known if levels prescribed for medical indications affect the neurological development of the infant.
Aripiprazole	Unknown	Maternal doses up to 15 mg daily produce low levels in milk. Avoid in nursing women until more information is available.
Asenapine	Unknown	Avoid until more information is available.
Aspirin	Minimal, rare complication of bleeding or metabolic acidosis	Excreted in breast milk. Low dose (75–162 mg daily) may be considered as antiplatelet therapy for breastfeeding women. Avoid breastfeeding for 1–2 h after a dose to minimize effects on the infant.
Atenolol	Moderate to significant	Excreted in breast milk in a milk to plasma (M:P) ratio of 1.5:6.8 (one patient had an estimated dose of 0.13 mg atenolol per feeding with a maternal dose of 100 mg/d). Cyanosis and bradycardia have been reported in breastfed infants with maternal intake of 100 mg/d. **Use with caution. Avoid in infants younger than 3 months of age.**
Caffeine	Minimal	Excreted in breast milk. If mother has one cup of coffee, the infant probably ingests 1.5–3.1 mg of caffeine. Caffeine has a long half-life in young infants (82 h in term newborn, 14.4 h in 3–4.5/2-mo-old infants, and 2.6 h in 6-mo-old infants). Probably safe in small amounts, with variable reaction based on individual infant.
Bromocriptine	Minimal	Used to suppress lactation.
Carbamazepine	Moderate	Infants have measurable carbamazepine levels. Monitor the infant for jaundice, drowsiness, adequate weight gain, and developmental milestones, especially in younger, exclusively breastfed infants (LactMed).
Chloramphenicol	Significant	**Avoid while lactating.** Possible bone marrow suppression.
Cascara	Moderate	Excreted in breast milk. Causes colic and diarrhea in the infant. **Avoid.**
Cephalosporin antibiotics	Minimal	Excreted in small amounts in milk. Probably safe.
Chlorpromazine	Probably minimal	Excreted in breast milk. Monitor infant for drowsiness and developmental milestones.
Citalopram	Minimal	Excreted in breast milk. Monitor infant for sedation or fussiness. OK if required by mother. Consider a trial of escitalopram, which appears safer.
Codeine	Minimal; infant may experience lethargy	Excreted in breast milk. Limit use to 4 d and keep dose low. Newborns particularly sensitive to effects of maternal codeine use (LactMed).
Diazepam (all benzodiazepines)	Significant; infant may experience lethargy; apnea reported	Infants metabolize benzodiazepines more slowly than adults; accumulation of toxic levels of drug is possible. **Avoid in nursing mothers** other than a single dose for procedures (LactMed).
Dicumarol	Minimal	Excreted in breast milk in **inactive** form. May want to monitor infant's prothrombin time.
Digoxin	Minimal	Small amounts excreted in breast milk. Probably safe.
Duloxetine	Minimal, not well studied	Dose in milk is low. Monitor infant for drowsiness, weight gain, and developmental milestones.

Continued

Table 50–1 Effects of Commonly Prescribed Medications on Infants During Lactation—cont'd

Drug	Effect on Infant	Comments
Ergot	Significant; infant may experience vomiting, diarrhea, peripheral vasoconstriction	**Contraindicated** in lactation. May suppress lactation.
Escitalopram	Minimal	Maternal doses up to 20 mg/d produce low levels in breast milk. Safer than citalopram.
Fluoroquinolones	Unknown	Small amounts in breast milk. Little information available. Use an alternate drug for which safety information is available (LactMed).
Fluoxetine	Moderate	Colic, irritability, feeding and sleep disorders, slow weight gain. If mother requires fluoxetine, lactation is not a reason to stop. Monitor the infant.
Fluconazole	Minimal	Fluconazole is excreted in breast milk at concentrations similar to plasma. Safe.
Fluvoxamine	Minimal	Maternal doses up to 300 mg/d produce low levels in milk.
Furosemide	Minimal or unknown	Excreted in breast milk. Use with close monitoring of the infant.
Gold salts	Significant hepatonephrotoxicity	**Contraindicated** in lactation. May be excreted in milk after therapy is discontinued.
Heparin, LMW heparin	Minimal	Not excreted in breast milk in significant amounts.
Iodine (radioactive)	Significant; may cause thyroid suppression in the infant	**Contraindicated.** Maternal testing requiring radioactive iodine requires breast milk to be discarded according to the half-life of the drug.
Isoniazid (INH)	Minimal; possibility of pyridoxine deficiency developing in the infant	Milk levels same as maternal plasma levels. Observe infant for adverse effects. Probably safe. Nursing mothers who are taking isoniazid should take 25 mg of oral pyridoxine daily.
Lithium	Moderate	Lithium may be used in full-term infants if monitored closely. Consider monitoring infant serum lithium levels, serum creatinine, BUN, and TSH every 4–12 wk during breastfeeding. Lithium toxicity may occur if elimination is impaired, as in infant dehydration, prematurity, or the immediate newborn period (LactMed).
Macrolide antibiotics	Minimal	All macrolides are minimally excreted in breast milk. Monitor infant for diarrhea and *Candida* infection.
Methadone	Significant	May be used under close medical supervision at doses of less than 100 mg/d. Infants receive 1%–3% of maternal dose. Infant may exhibit signs of withdrawal if methadone is discontinued abruptly or if breastfeeding is discontinued abruptly.
Metoprolol	Minimal	Excreted in very small amounts in breast milk. Infant consuming 1 L breast milk will get <1 mg metoprolol.
Metronidazole	Unknown	Milk levels similar to maternal plasma levels. Half-life in breast milk 8–10 h. Long-term systemic therapy produces measurable amounts of metronidazole in infant's serum and the effects are unknown. Nursing mothers should express and discard milk during and for 24–48 h after single-dose treatment. Topical and vaginal application is probably safe.
Olanzapine	Minimal	Doses up to 20 mg/d not detected in infant serum. Limited information available. Monitor the infant for drowsiness and developmental milestones, especially if other antipsychotics are used concurrently (LactMed).
Oral contraceptives	Minimal to moderate	Hormones are released into breast milk. May cause jaundice and breast enlargement in the infant. Estrogen compounds suppress lactation, decreasing the quantity and quality of breast milk. Use progestin-only preparations ("minipill") or wait until milk supply is well established (>6 wk postpartum) to use combined forms.
Paroxetine	Minimal	Minimal levels in breast milk. Preferred drug in lactating women (LactMed).

Table 50–1   Effects of Commonly Prescribed Medications on Infants During Lactation—cont'd

Drug	Effect on Infant	Comments
Phenobarbital	Moderate; lethargy in the infant	Excreted in breast milk. Monitor infant for lethargy and feeding problems.
Phenytoin	Minimal	Low levels in breast milk. Probably safe.
Prednisone	Moderate	Excreted in breast milk and may suppress growth and interfere with exogenous steroid production in the infant. Low maternal doses (<20 mg/d) probably safe. Larger doses for a short time may not harm the infant. It is best to time the medication dose just after a feeding and wait 3–4 h for next feeding.
Propranolol	Minimal	Excreted in breast milk in amounts too small to have any effect.
Propoxyphene (removed from U.S. market)	Minimal; possible lethargy	Excreted in small amounts in breast milk.
Propylthiouracil	Minimal	Little PTU passes into breast milk. Doses up to 450 mg/d may be safe. Take dose of PTU just after nursing and wait 3–4 h to minimize infant dose. Monitor CBC, T4, and TSH if any suspicion of adverse effects.
Risperidone	Unknown	Maternal doses up to 6 mg/d produce low levels in milk. Little information available. Other agents may be preferred especially in the newborn or preterm infant.
Radioactive material	Significant; carcinogenic	**Contraindicated**
Sertraline	Minimal	Low levels of sertraline in breast milk, so amounts ingested by infant are small. One of the preferred antidepressants during lactation.
Spironolactone	Minimal	Very small amounts (0.2%) of metabolite of mother's daily dose are excreted in breast milk. Safe for use with breastfeeding.
Tetracycline	Moderate; discolored teeth	Excreted in breast milk, M:P ratio of 0.6–0.8. **Avoid when lactating.** Use safer antibiotics.
Warfarin	Minimal	Excreted in breast milk in inactive form. Safe during breastfeeding.
Ziprasidone	Unknown	Avoid while breastfeeding until more information available.
Zolpidem	Minimal	Low levels excreted in breast milk. Short-acting.

frequently, which will increase the amount of drug that the infant ingests.

3. Infant pharmacokinetics also plays an important role in how maternal medication use affects the breastfed infant. As mentioned at the beginning of this chapter, gastric acid production and gastric emptying time are decreased and variable in neonates. The volume of distribution in infants is greater because of their greater total body water and their lower body fat. Infants also have significant differences in drug metabolism by the liver, as previously mentioned. Renal excretion, too, is altered in younger infants, which can affect their overall clearance rate of drugs. All of these factors need to be considered in prescribing to a lactating woman, especially if the breastfed infant is very young (less than 1 month old).

4. Susceptibility to a drug's effects can vary among infants. There is some dose-related predictability to a drug's effects that are related to the pharmacological properties of the drug. In some infants, however, there are unique effects that are not dose-related and instead are idiosyncratic and therefore unpredictable. This reaction is fortunately uncommon but must be considered if an infant is demonstrating some effects of maternal drug use.

5. The milk to plasma (M:P) drug ratio affects the infant's exposure to a medication because the infant's clearance of the drug affects the overall exposure. Even drugs with a low M:P ratio may produce a toxic level if the infant is unable to effectively excrete the drug.

Infants

Infants are totally dependent on their parents to administer their medication. Although the infant may balk at the taste of a medication, the parent is still in control of administering it. Intervention at this age is aimed at teaching parents or caregivers how to properly administer the medication. Parents need to be edified and encouraged as they take on the role of administering and monitoring a child's medication. Many parents are nervous the first time they give their child medication. Thorough education ensures better medication compliance.

Medication dosing errors by parents are common; 39.4% of parents made a measurement error in a study of 287 parents enrolled in the emergency department after their child was prescribed liquid medication (Yin et al, 2014). Discussing the reason for the medication, the dose, how to draw up the medication in milliliters, the length of treatment, medication administration tips, and expected and unexpected adverse effects (e.g., the mild diarrhea that is expected with some antibiotics) should increase a parent's comfort with administering medications. Written instructions are essential at all ages but especially for the infant, because the parent is more likely to be fatigued and less likely to retain instructions given orally. Dosing medications for parental convenience increases compliance. Ask parents if they are working outside their home and who else may be administering the medication. A medication with fewer daily doses may be indicated if the child is in a day-care setting or has multiple caregivers.

○ CLINICAL PEARL ○

Infants

- Parents are often unsure how to administer medication to an infant. While the parents are in the clinic with the child, the practitioner should address this issue and demonstrate how to do it. For ease of administration, use a medication syringe and insert the syringe into the mouth along the inner cheek. To decrease choking, advise parents to squirt small amounts (1 mL) of medication at a time into the inner buccal space. Wait until the infant swallows, and then administer another small amount until all the medication is administered. Direct parents not to administer the medication directly over the tongue, which increases choking and allows the infant more easily to spit out the medication.
- Advise parents to check with the pharmacist before mixing any medication with formula or breast milk; some medications are bound with the calcium or other ingredients in the formula, causing them to be less effective.
- Breastfed infants often choke and sputter when medications are first administered because these infants are used to only the feel of the breast in their mouths. Warning parents of this response and teaching them proper technique will help them gain confidence in medication administration.
- Giving acetaminophen in suppository form is an option if administering oral medications to the infant is difficult. The practitioner can demonstrate this procedure, which works well in breastfed infants especially.

Toddlers and Preschoolers

Toddlers and preschoolers are beginning to exert their independence, and administering medications to this age group can be a challenge, even a battlefield. Even the most experienced parent can have difficulty administering oral medications to a toddler. The key to success with this age group is to discuss medication administration with the parent prior to prescribing and, if possible, choose a medication that poses the fewest problems with administration. Doses per day, palatability, and dosage forms should be taken into consideration. If the toddler is resistant to taking medication, prescribe a once- or twice-daily medication if possible. Using chewable formulations, if the child has molars, can increase compliance because the child can self-administer the medication. Using higher concentrations of medication, if possible, to decrease the volume administered can be helpful. By 2 or 3 years, children can often begin to self-administer oral medication by using a vertical medication spoon or medicine cup. Parents can help a child practice this skill with juice or another liquid before taking the medication. Discussing administration of the prescribed medication while the family is still in the clinic is essential. Ask the parent what has worked in the past to ease medication administration and what has not worked. Listen to parents; they know their child and can anticipate what will ease the medication administration.

School-Age Children

Giving medication to school-age children is often easier than it is in other age groups. Developmentally, they are industrious and eager to learn. It is essential to include the child in the decision-making process, if possible. Let the child choose the formulation. Does he or she want liquid, chewable tablets, or pills to swallow? Some liquid medication doses become large in volume as the child gets to school age (e.g., trimethoprim-sulfamethoxazole and prednisone), so advise parents and the child who chooses a liquid formulation of this fact. Be sure the child can swallow pills before prescribing them. Some medications can be crushed and mixed with highly viscous fluid (e.g., chocolate syrup). Check with the pharmacist prior to suggesting this if you are not familiar with a medication. Teaching with this age group should be aimed at both the parent and the child. Children need to know the rationale for prescribing a particular medication. They are being taught in school to avoid "drugs," and they need clarification about helpful medication and illicit drugs. Schools have varying regulations regarding administration of medication at school. If possible, avoid school-hour dosing to simplify the medication regimen.

Adolescents

Adolescent patients often administer their own medications. The compliance rates vary with this age group. Some teenagers are excellent at medication self-administration, and others are poorly compliant. The adolescent is developmentally entering the period of formal operational thinking, characterized by propositional thinking and abstract reasoning. Younger adolescents may still be in the concrete-thinking stage, and their interactions with the health-care provider may reflect this stage rather than the abstract thought process of older teenagers.

Although adolescents may be able to self-administer medication and appear to be capable of the task, they may vary in their sophistication regarding medication use. The practitioner needs to form an alliance with teenagers and ask their perspective regarding their medications. Do they have an opinion regarding the medication? What schedule will work best with their lifestyle? Teenagers appreciate having their opinions taken into consideration as treatment is planned. When a medication history is taken with the parent present, the teenager may not be completely truthful. Practitioners need to be aware of the laws of the state in which they practice and, when treating teenagers, maintain confidentiality if necessary. Teenagers, too, must understand the confidentiality laws of their state and at what age they are able to receive confidential treatment. Parents often struggle with letting teenagers self-administer medications. The practitioner needs to be skilled at assisting family members as they move from parent-controlled to child- or teen-controlled medication administration. This transition varies by family.

FACTORS THAT INFLUENCE POSITIVE OUTCOMES

Compliance or adherence with the medication regimen is an issue for all patients. Pediatric patients pose a unique dilemma because the practitioner has to address both the child's compliance and the parent's, plus possibly that of other caregivers. The many factors that influence adherence include length of medication regimen; number of medications prescribed; the medication interval, palatability, cost, and family issues. The practitioner needs to consider all of these issues when prescribing to ensure successful treatment.

There is little agreement over the definitions of *compliance* and *noncompliance*. Is anything less than full compliance considered noncompliance? If the therapeutic outcome is adequate, is less than full compliance with the treatment regimen acceptable? Dose omission and delay are the most common dosing errors, yet other forms of noncompliance may occur, including failure to fill the prescription, incorrect dosing or dosing intervals, and discontinuation of the medication prior to the recommended time.

A systematic review and meta-analysis of 46 studies of antibiotic misuse found a mean compliance rate of 62.2% (95% confidence level, 56.4% to 68.0%), although this study was not specific to pediatric patients (Kardas, Devine, Golembesky, & Roberts, 2005). In a review of the literature related to pediatric medication compliance, Winnock, Lucas, Hartman, and Toll (2005) found compliance ranged from 11% to 93% in the more than 250 articles they reviewed. Adherence to prescribed treatment regimen was measured in a retrospective cohort study of 24,438 Medicaid patients (89.39% under age 18 years) that found the overall adherence rate to be 11.74% (Tan et al, 2013). A study of adolescent females (aged 14 to 17 years) taking oral contraceptives pills (OCPs) found 45% of coital events were protected by OCPs (Woods et al, 2006). Clearly, medication adherence is less than ideal in children and adolescents.

Specific Factors That Influence Compliance

Long-Term Medication Regimens

Chronic illness, often including a daily medication regimen, presents a number of problems for the family. Adherence to daily preventive therapy for asthma is generally poor, with one large cohort study of 18,456 children enrolled in Medicaid reporting average adherence of 20% for inhaled corticosteroids and 28% for leukotriene inhibitors (Herndon, Mattke, Evans Cuellar, Hong, & Shenkman, 2012). Adherence to ADHD medication based on Medicaid prescription claims in Texas ($n = 62,789$) ranged from 9.8% (short-acting stimulants) to 25.8% (nonstimulants) (Barner, Khoza, & Oladapo, 2011). Even patients for whom noncompliance can be life-threatening are not taking their medications as prescribed. Children with sickle cell disease were found to have a refill rate for their daily medications of 58.4% (Patel, Lindsey, Strunk, & DeBaun, 2010). Of 104 adolescents prescribed antiretroviral treatment for HIV, 65.4% reported full adherence, with nonadherance associated with higher viral load (Chandwani et al, 2012). Risk factors for medication nonadherence after pediatric heart transplantation (median age 6 years) includes adolescent age at transplant, black race, Medicaid insurance, and ventilator or ventricular assist device support at transplant (Oliva et al, 2013).

Number of Medications Prescribed

The number of medications prescribed can have an impact on compliance with the regimen. The more medications that are prescribed, the lower the compliance rate is. Keeping medication schedules simple increases the likelihood of success for the treatment.

Medication Interval

Medication interval has a significant impact on the success of the treatment, especially given the number of families with both parents working and more children in day care. Children who are in school or have parents who are both working may not receive their medications as often as recommended if they are taking any medication that needs to be administered more than twice a day.

◉ CLINICAL PEARL ◉

Electrolyte solutions

- Pediatric electrolyte solutions are often not well accepted by children. One trick is to use electrolyte popsicles (Pedialyte) or freeze the bottled solution into homemade popsicles. The cold taste seems to be better accepted.

- Sugar-free Kool-Aid or another drink mix sweetened with Nutrasweet can be added to unflavored electrolyte solutions to make the taste of the electrolyte solution more acceptable to children.

Palatability

Palatability is often overlooked as a reason for noncompliance, yet in children it is a critical factor in medication compliance. Studies comparing the taste of a variety of antibiotics (Holas, Chiu, Notario, & Kapral, 2005; Powers, Gooch, & Oddo, 2000) determined that some antibiotics were ranked better tasting than others, with the cephalosporins (cefindir, cefixime, cephalexin, and cefaclor) ranked as the best tasting overall. Dicloxacillin ranked the worst for taste. Although no published reports studied taste differences between brand-name and generic preparations, anecdotal reports from parents and patients suggest that brand-name preparations taste better. Of medications with the same efficacy profile, the best tasting is the easiest to administer to young children.

Cost

The cost of the medication needs to be addressed for patients who are not adequately insured for prescriptions. The cost of common antibiotics prescribed for otitis media range from $4 to more than $100 to treat a 15-kg child for 10 days. Prescribing an expensive antibiotic for a family who cannot afford to fill the prescription places the family in an uncomfortable position. Simply asking the family if they have insurance to cover the medication and then problem solving with them if they do not will increase the likelihood that the family will fill the prescription. For example, if an antibiotic is indicated, check the retail $4 list first to determine if the medication is available. If possible, give the family a few days of medication samples to defray the cost of the treatment if a less expensive medication is not available. Knowing which pharmacies in the local area are the least expensive or calling ahead for a price check before sending the family to the pharmacy is helpful. A family who knows the approximate amount that the medication will cost will not be surprised when the prescription is filled.

Family Issues

Family issues affect the family's ability to comply with the prescribed treatment regimen. Families in which both parents are working and therefore have limited time with their children have more problems with complex treatment regimens. Lack of social support can leave a parent isolated and make parenting more stressful. Parental fatigue is often overlooked as a factor in treatment outcomes. Parents who are fatigued can easily miss medication doses; even those who are usually well organized can miss medication doses when they are tired. Disruptive and dysfunctional families may have difficulty in following the plan of treatment because of the chaos present in the home. Another family situation that needs to be addressed when clinical improvement is less than satisfactory is parental use of the child's medications. For example, a child may be prescribed stimulants for attention deficit-hyperactivity disorder, and a parent or other family member may be abusing the child's medication. This is a situation no practitioner wants to encounter, yet there should always be some index of suspicion when the family history is not clear. All of these issues need to be accounted for when the practitioner is prescribing a medication and during follow-up on the patient's progress. They often present in an unclear fashion, and ferreting out the reason for noncompliance with the treatment regimen may take some time.

Improving Compliance in the Pediatric Patient

When poor compliance is identified, it is essential to address this issue and determine strategies with the patient and parent to improve the success of the treatment regimen. There are a variety of methods to improve the success of the treatment regimen, but first it is necessary to make sure that the diagnosis is accurate and that the drug therapy is beneficial.

Medication Concentration

Medication concentration can be adjusted in some of the liquid preparations. The practitioner can choose to prescribe a more concentrated form when a parent has difficulty administering medications to a patient. Many of the antibiotics come in different strengths, and giving one-half teaspoon is easier than administering a full teaspoon. Prednisone comes in two different strengths, as well as in tablets that can be crushed. By involving the parents in the decision to use a more concentrated form of a medication, you are allowing them some control over the treatment regimen, and they may therefore be more likely to administer the medication that is prescribed.

Written Versus Oral Instructions

Most practitioners should address the issue of written versus oral instructions in their own practice. Giving written instructions along with the oral directions will improve compliance. This is especially important for over-the-counter medications such as acetaminophen and ibuprofen. Parents need to understand the different formulations and dosing by weight, and every parent should have a weight-based dosing chart (Box 50-2).

Self-Monitoring Calendars

Self-monitoring calendars should be a standard in the treatment of preschool and school-age children. Children can apply a sticker or color in a box as each dose is taken. Parents should be involved in the process and set a reward for completion of the medication regimen. In acute illness such as otitis media, in which the patient will be returning to the clinic, the practitioner may offer a reward for a full calendar. Children with chronic illness, who are often on long-term medication, need to have a set reward for a certain number of days of successfully taking their medication. Parents need to take an active role in medication calendar usage, and they, too, should be praised for their participation in the medication regimen.

BOX 50–2 PRESCRIBING OVER-THE-COUNTER PAIN MEDICATIONS FOR PEDIATRIC PATIENTS

Pain in children can range from teething pain to pain associated with otitis media. Parents often ask the practitioner about using acetaminophen or ibuprofen for the treatment of pain in children. For the safety of their children and the efficacy of the medication, parents should be taught how to administer over-the-counter (OTC) pain medications properly.

The two most commonly used analgesics in pediatric patients are acetaminophen and ibuprofen. Aspirin should never be given to children for acute pain management due to the risk of Reye syndrome, and the practitioner should teach parents this rule.

Acetaminophen can be administered orally or rectally (suppository), and it peaks in 30–60 minutes. Dosage for children is 10–15 mg/kg/dose q4–6h.

Ibuprofen is effective for pain control and has an additive anti-inflammatory effect, which appears to provide better pain control in acute otitis media than acetaminophen. The correct dosage is 5–10 mg/kg/dose q6–8h. Ibuprofen should not be administered by parents to children under age 6 months because immature kidneys are unable to excrete it, leading to increased risk of toxicity and renal damage. All children receiving ibuprofen should be well hydrated to prevent renal damage. Avoid ibuprofen if fluid intake is decreased.

Although acetaminophen and ibuprofen provide good pain relief for mild to moderate pain and both have antipyretic effects, ibuprofen may be the drug of choice for night pain associated with otitis media because of its longer duration. Both drugs are equally easy to administer, although ibuprofen is not available in suppository form. Combining acetaminophen and ibuprofen in an alternating schedule for fever or pain is not recommended in the outpatient setting. One or the other, properly dosed, should be used. The goal of antipyretic therapy is not to reduce temperature to normal, but to decrease discomfort associated with fever.

Give parents a dosing chart with their child's dose based on weight. The different strengths of acetaminophen must be dosed correctly.

Telephone/E-mail Reminders

Telephone or e-mail reminders are helpful in increasing compliance, especially if the parent is leaving the clinic with multiple prescriptions. A quick telephone call or e-mail allows the parent to clarify the treatment regimen and reinforces teaching that took place in the clinic.

Mobile Phone Medication Adherence Apps

There are a number of mobile phone apps available for reminding patients to take medications. In a review of 160 unique medication reminder apps, Dayer, Heldenbrand, Anderson, Gubbins, and Martin (2013) identified attributes to compare apps, including online data entry, cloud data storage, complex medication instructions (taper schedules, etc.), ability to export data, tracking missed doses, and the ability for the provider or pharmacist to input data. A medication regimen does not have to be complex in order to use a reminder app. For example, an app can be used to help remind adolescent females to take their daily oral contraceptive pill.

Contracts and Reinforcement Programs

Contracts or reinforcement programs may be necessary if compliance continues to be a problem. The practitioner, the patient, and the family need to be in agreement about the goals of the treatment contract and the consequences of noncompliance. A case conference may be necessary to involve other disciplines in the treatment. A home visit may provide information that leads to an altered treatment program that will be better tolerated by the family. The role of the practitioner is to attempt to simplify the medication treatment and

CLINICAL PEARL

Improving compliance with ophthalmic preparations

- Administration of ophthalmic preparations to toddlers and preschoolers is often difficult, and the incidence of noncompliance increases with each dose that is a battle to administer. Parents can safely restrain the child to administer eye medications as follows:

  1. Sit on the floor with the child sitting on the floor between the parent's legs.
  2. Place the child's feet near the parent's feet and the child's head between the parent's thighs.
  3. Slip the child's arms under the parent's thighs and, with the legs, hold the child's head and arms still.

  The parent then has both hands free to administer the eye medication. Although this procedure may sound drastic, it is a quick way for a parent to administer the medication when no other adult is around to assist with a squirming, resistant child.

- Older preschoolers and school-age children often cooperate with administration of eyedrops if they are told to lie back and close their eyes. Eyedrops can then be applied to the inner corner of the eyes (while the eyes are closed). Next, children are told to open their eyes, without any head movement. The medication rolls into the eye when the eye is opened. This is much easier than the bull's-eye approach of trying to get children to keep their eyes open for squeezing in drops.

still have an adequate therapeutic outcome. This goal should be shared with the patient and family.

Childhood Obesity Influences Outcomes

Over the past 30 years pediatric overweight and obesity have steadily increased. Approximately 17% of children and adolescents age 2 years to 19 years are obese (Centers for Disease Control and Prevention, 2013). Little is known about pharmacokinetic differences in obese children. Small studies on pediatric oncology patients indicate doxorubicinol, but not doxorubicin, clearance is decreased in patients with body fat greater than 30% (Thompson et al, 2009). Volume of distribution may be altered, particularly for lipid-soluble drugs. Obese children with nonalcoholic fatty liver disease may have altered metabolism of drugs, but large studies have not been conducted.

For the obese patient, the prescriber needs to decide whether to calculate the dose based on actual body weight or ideal body weight. When young children weigh as much as an adult, dosing quickly becomes a challenge. Although body weight may be consistent in an adult, liver and kidney functions are still at the chronological age of the child. Currently, no guidelines are available for dosing obese children, other than not to exceed adult doses of most medications. Studies are in progress and until guidelines are published, the nurse practitioner prescriber will need to use clinical judgment and monitor the patient closely for adverse effects if dosed by weight and efficacy if dosed by age.

REFERENCES

Barner, J. C., Khoza, S., & Oladapo, A. (2011). ADHD medication use, adherence, persistence and cost among Texas Medicaid children. *Current Medical Research and Opinion, 27*(2 Suppl), 13–22.

Berlin, C. M., & Briggs, G. G. (2005). Drugs and chemicals in human milk. *Seminars in Fetal & Neonatal Medicine, 10,* 149–159.

Blake, M. J., Castro, L., Leeder, J. S., & Kearns, G. L. (2005). Ontogeny of drug metabolizing enzymes in the neonate. *Seminars in Fetal and Neonatal Medicine, 10,* 123–138.

Centers for Disease Control and Prevention. (2013). Childhood overweight and obesity. Retrieved from http://www.cdc.gov/obesity/childhood/index.html

Chandwani, S., Koenig, L. J., Sill, A. M., Abramowitz, S., Conner, L. C., & D'Angelo, L. (2012). Predictors of antiretroviral medication adherence among a diverse cohort of adolescents with HIV. *The Journal of Adolescent Health: Official Publication of the Society for Adolescent Medicine, 51*(3), 242–251.

Conroy, S., & McIntyre, J. (2005). The use of unlicensed and off-label medicines in the neonate. *Seminars in Fetal & Neonatal Medicine, 10,* 115–122.

Dayer, L., Heldenbrand, S., Anderson, P., Gubbins, P. O., & Martin, B. C. (2013). Smartphone medication adherence apps. *Journal of the American Pharmacy Association, 53*(2), 172–181.

Giacoia, G. P., & Mattison, D. R. (2005). Newborns and drug studies: The NICHD/FDA drug development initiative. *Clinical Therapeutics, 27*(6), 796–813.

Hanley, M. J., Abernathy, D. R., & Greenblatt, D. J. (2010). Effect of obesity on the pharmacokinetics of drugs in humans. *Clinical Pharmacokinetics, 49*(2), 71–87.

Herndon, J. B., Mattke, S., Evans Cuellar, A., Hong, S. Y., & Shenkman, E. A. (2012). Anti-inflammatory medication adherence, healthcare utilization and expenditures among Medicaid and children's health insurance program enrollees with asthma. *Pharmacoeconomics, 30*(5), 397–412.

Holas, C., Chiu, Y. L., Notario, G., & Kapral, D. (2005). A pooled analysis of seven randomized crossover studies of the palatability of cefdinir oral suspension versus amoxicillin/clavulanate potassium, cefprozil, azithromycin, and amoxicillin in children aged 4 to 8 years. *Clinical Therapeutics, 27*(12), 1950–1960.

Kardas, P., Devine, S., Golembesky, A., & Roberts, C. (2005). A systematic review of misuse of antibiotic therapies in the community. *Journal of Antimicrobial Agents, 26*(2), 106–113.

Kearns, G. L. (2000). Impact of developmental pharmacology on pediatric study design: Overcoming the challenges. *Journal of Allergy and Clinical Immunology, 106,* S128–S138.

Kearns, G. L., Abdel-Rahman, S. M., Alander, S. W., Blowey, D. L., Leeder, S. L., & Kauffman, R. E. (2003). Developmental pharmacology—drug disposition, action, and therapy in infants and children. *New England Journal of Medicine, 349*(12), 1157–1167.

Koren, G., Reider, M., & MacLeod, S. M. (2009). The global alliance for pediatric pharmacology: The future is here and now. *Paediatric Drugs, 11*(1), 4–5.

National Library of Medicine. (2014). Drugs and lactation data base (LactMed). Retrieved from http://toxnet.nlm.nih.gov/cgi-bin/sis/htmlgen?LACT

Oliva, M., Singh, T. P., Gauvreau, K, Vanderpluym, C. J., Bastardi, H. J., & Almond, C. S. (2013). *Impact of medication non-adherence on survival after pediatric heart transplantation in the U.S.A. 32*(9), 881–888.

Patel, N. G., Lindsey, T., Strunk, R. C., & DeBaun, M. R. (2010). Prevalence of daily medication adherence among children with sickle cell disease: A 1-year retrospective cohort analysis. *Pediatric Blood & Cancer, 55*(3), 554–556.

Powers, J. L., Gooch, W. M., III, & Oddo, L. P. (2000). Comparison of the palatability of the oral suspension of cefdinir vs. amoxicillin/clavulanate potassium, cefprozil and azithromycin in pediatric patients. *Pediatric Infectious Disease Journal, 19*(12 Suppl), S174–S180.

Rakhmanina, N. Y., & van den Anker, J. N. (2006). Pharmacological research in pediatrics: From neonates to adolescents. *Advanced Drug Delivery Reviews, 58,* 4–14.

Stephenson, T. (2005). How children's responses to drugs differ from adults'. *British Journal of Clinical Pharmacology, 59*(6), 670–673.

Tan, X., Al-Dabagh, A., Davis, S. A., Lin, H. C., Balkrishman, R., Chang, J., et al. (2013). Medication adherence, healthcare costs and utilization associated with acne drugs in Medicaid enrollees with acne vulgaris. *American Journal of Clinical Dermatology, 14*(3), 243–251.

Thompson, P. A., Rosner, G. L., Matthay, K. K., Moore, T. B., Bomgaars, L. R., Ellis, K. J., et al. (2009). Impact of body composition of pharmacokinetics of doxorubicin in children: A Glaser Pediatric Research Network study. *Cancer Chemotherapy Pharmacology, 64,* 243–251.

U.S. Food and Drug Administration (FDA). (2009a). The story of the laws behind the labels: Part 1: 1906 Food and Drugs Act. Retrieved from http://www.fda.gov/AboutFDA/WhatWeDo/History/Overviews/ucm056044.htm

U.S. Food and Drug Administration (FDA). (2009b). The story of the laws behind the labels: Part 2: 1938 Federal Food, Drug and Cosmetic Act. Retrieved from http://www.fda.gov/AboutFDA/WhatWeDo/History/Overviews/ucm056044.htm

U.S. Food and Drug Administration (FDA). (2009c). The story of the laws behind the labels: Part 3: 1962 Drug Amendments. Retrieved from http://www.fda.gov/AboutFDA/WhatWeDo/History/Overviews/ucm056044.htm

U.S. Food and Drug Administration (FDA). (2010). Milestones in food and drug law history. Retrieved from http://www.fda.gov/AboutFDA/WhatWeDo/History/Milestones/

U.S. Food and Drug Administration (FDA). (2014). Pediatric labeling changes through June 12, 2014. Retrieved from http://www.fda.gov/downloads/ScienceResearch/SpecialTopics/PediatricTherapeuticsResearch/UCM163159.pdf van den Anker, J. N. (2010). Developmental pharmacology. *Developmental Disabilities Research Reviews, 16,* 233–238.

Vernon, J. A., Shortenhaus, S. H., Mayer, M. H., Allen, A. J., & Golec, J. H. (2012). Measuring the patient health, societal and economic benefits of US pediatric therapeutics legislation. *Pediatric Drugs, 14*(5), 283–294.

Wharton, G. T., Murphy, M. D., Avant, D., Goldsmith, J. V., Chal, G., Rodriguez, W. J., et al. (2014). Impact on Pediatric Exclusivity on drug labeling and demonstration of efficacy. *Pediatrics.* Published online July 14, 2014.

Winnock, S., Lucas, D. O., Hartman, A. L., & Toll, D. (2005). How do you improve compliance? *Pediatrics, 115,* e718–e724.

Woods, J. L., Shew, M. L., Tu, W., Ofner, S., Ott, M. A., & Fortenberry, J. D. (2006). Patterns of oral contraceptive pill-taking and condom use among adolescent contraceptive pill takers. *Journal of Adolescent Health, 39*(3), 381–387.

World Health Organization (WHO). (2010). Make medicines child size. Retrieved from http://www.who.int/childmedicines/en/

World Health Organization (WHO). (2013). *WHO Model List of Essential Medicines for Children,* 4th list. Retrieved from http://www.who.int/medicines/publications/essentialmedicines/4th_EMLc_FINAL_web_8Jul13.pdf

Yin, H. S., Dreyer, B. P., Ugboaja, D. C., Sanchez, D. C., Paul, I. M., Moreira, H. A., et al. (2014). Unit of measurement used and parent medication dosing errors. *Pediatrics, 07.* Published online July 14, 2014.

GERIATRIC PATIENTS

Joan M. Nelson

Prescribing medications and predicting responses to these medications by older adults can be difficult because clinical drug trials often limit enrollment by age. Age-related changes in pharmacokinetics and pharmacodynamics can cause different responses to medications than those seen in the younger adult population. Older adults are at increased risk of adverse drug reactions as a result of the fact that they take more medications and due to the biological effects of aging and chronic diseases. Medication under- and overutilization by this population has been shown to increase the number of hospitalizations and emergency room visits, to worsen cognitive functioning, and to contribute to falls. Several large national initiatives geared toward reducing these catastrophic effects have been launched and will be discussed in this chapter.

DEMOGRAPHICS

The United States is rapidly aging. In 1900, only 2% of the U.S. population were age 65 and older, but by the year 2008 over 13% were older than 65. The U.S. Census Bureau anticipates that by the year 2030, older adults will comprise one-fifth of the U.S. population (The Federal Interagency Forum on Aging-Related Statistics, 2010). The rate of growth in the "old old" population of adults over the age of 85 is rising even faster. In the decade from 1990 to 2000, this population rose by over a million people, an increase of 25% of all people over 85 years of age in the United States (CensusScope, 2000). The dramatic rise in the older population results from both the increased birthrate during the time the baby boomers, who are now entering old age, were born and because of increased life expectancy. In 1960, people who survived to age 65 could expect to live another 14.5 years, whereas currently, at age 65, the life expectancy is an additional 18.5 years. At age 85, a woman can expect an additional 6.8 years of life and a man is likely to survive another 5.7 years (Federal Interagency Forum on Aging-Related Statistics, 2010).

In adults over the age of 85, females outnumber males by a ratio of 3:1 and are, therefore, more likely to live alone than older males. Although only 10% of U.S. older adults live below the poverty level, members of ethnic minority populations are far more likely to live in poverty than Caucasians. Twenty-seven percent of older African American women and 20% of older Hispanic women live below the poverty level. Average prescription drug costs for older Americans were $2,107 in 2004, making it difficult for many older adults to purchase required medications (The Federal Interagency Forum on Aging-Related Statistics, 2010). Increased chronic illness, commonly seen with aging, is associated with higher prescription drug costs.

Diseases Associated With Aging

The most common chronic conditions among older adults are hypertension, arthritis, heart disease, cancer, and diabetes. Sixty percent of people over 85 have deficits in hearing and 28% have visual loss. These conditions cause functional losses; a staggering 47% of women over the age of 65 report some deficits in functional status (The Federal Interagency Forum on Aging-Related Statistics, 2010). These functional losses can make it difficult for older adults to manage their own medication administration due to an inability to read drug labels, see pill colors, and remember to take and order the medications in a timely manner.

Pharmacological Issues in Aging

Older adults comprise 13% of the population and use about one-third of all prescription and over-the-counter (OTC) drugs sold in the United States. One-third of older adults use three or more prescription drugs in conjunction with three or more dietary supplements (Nahin et al, 2009). This number is markedly higher for hospitalized patients or those living in nursing homes or assisted living facilities. Polypharmacy is not always inappropriate in this population of clients who have multiple chronic illnesses, but increased numbers of medications carry increasing risks. Budnitz, Lovegrove, Shehab, and Richards (2011) examined a large national database to discover that almost 100,000 Americans over the age of 65 were admitted to the emergency department (ED) annually, between 2007 and 2009 due to adverse drug events. Over half of these admissions were for patients over the age of 80 and four specific classes of medications accounted for over two-thirds of these ED visits: warfarin, insulin, oral hypoglycemic medications and oral antiplatelet medications.

PHYSICAL CHANGES ASSOCIATED WITH AGING

The physical changes associated with aging are responsible for some of the unique prescribing rules and drug effects seen with older adults. In this chapter, some of these physiological changes and their impact on pharmacokinetics and pharmacodynamics will be reviewed.

Mental Changes

Mental changes in the healthy older adult are minimal. Although white brain matter does begin to deteriorate at about 60 years, an inability of the older adult to function independently is not a normal part of the aging process. Disease processes are the culprits that rob older adults of the ability to think clearly and maintain independence. Both acute (hypoglycemia, infection, electrolyte imbalances, and many others) and chronic diseases, such as Alzheimer's disease and cerebrovascular accidents, may impair a person's mental status.

Cerebral blood flow, brain mass, and neurotransmitter concentrations are reduced as we age (Esiri, 2007), causing older adults to be more susceptible to the neurological side effects of drugs than younger people. These pharmacological effects can cause delirium, a reversible cognitive impairment. Younger people will likely respond to an infective process with fever, whereas older adults, who have reduced immunologic function and reduced ability to generate a fever, will often present with confusion.

Sensory Changes

Sight

Almost one-third of adults over the age of 65 have some impairment in their ability to see (Hartford Institute for Geriatric Nursing, 2005). Presbyopia results from a loss of elasticity in and thickening of the lens, which impairs near vision. Conditions that become increasingly prevalent with age, such as cataracts, glaucoma, and macular degeneration, can create difficulties for the patient in self-management of medications and can restrict the pharmacological choices available to treat the patient's medical condition in order to prevent worsening of the eye disease. Visual loss also makes it difficult for patients to manage their own medication or provide their own transportation and causes them to be increasingly dependent upon others.

Hearing

About one-third of adults over the age of 65 have some level of hearing loss, especially in the high-frequency range, and the incidence of hearing impairment increases with each decade (McCance & Huether, 2014). Cerumen impaction, seen in over one-third of older adults, further impairs hearing. Older adults have drier cerumen and are more likely to use hearing aids, which contribute to impaction (Roland et al, 2008).

Older adults may have lost their hearing gradually and be unaware that they are not fully hearing what is spoken. Missing one or two words in the instructions for a prescribed drug could have devastating consequences.

Smell and Taste

The senses of smell and taste decline with aging and are further impaired with the use of medications (Hartford Institute for Geriatric Nursing, 2005). These sensory losses may impair appetite and nutritional status. Lack of dietary iron or the B vitamins can lead to atrophic changes of the oral mucosa, resulting in dry mouth and a change in taste.

Some older adults may complain of a burning mouth and tongue. Local trauma, poor nutrition, diabetes, or anemia can cause these symptoms. Chapter 50 discusses the role of taste and texture in the willingness of children to take certain drugs. Older adults also respond to taste and texture in taking oral suspensions.

Peripheral Sensation

Peripheral neuropathy, which can significantly increase fall risk, occurs in 28% of adults aged 70 to 79 and 35% of adults aged 80 and older (Vinik, Strotmeyer, Nakave, & Patel, 2008). Problems with circulation, vitamin deficiencies, and diabetes can aggravate an age-related loss of peripheral nerve function. Many classes of medications further contribute to fall risk, especially in the frail older adult. Prescribing requires a careful assessment of risk versus benefit of these agents.

Musculoskeletal Changes

Musculoskeletal changes associated with aging range from impaired manual dexterity, which can prevent older adults from opening medication containers, to mobility problems, which can keep them from getting to the pharmacy. These musculoskeletal changes can cause older adults to experience difficulty with drug administration and adherence. Mobility problems, including disorders affecting gait, limb function, manual dexterity, and driving, can threaten the independence and functioning of older adults, specifically their adherence to drug therapy.

Neurological diseases, such as cerebrovascular disease, Parkinson's disease, and motor neuron disease, can lead to increased difficulties in the practical application of drug treatments. Such problems may range from the inability to visit the health-care provider's office to the inability to open the childproof containers.

Immobility from joint deformity, pain, and impaired manual dexterity may make activating inhalers or nebulizers or applying eye drops difficult to perform. Some medications may dramatically improve patients' mobility (e.g., medications to treat Parkinson's disease), but others may dramatically exacerbate mobility problems (e.g., antihypertensives, tricyclic antidepressants).

PHARMACOKINETIC CHANGES

Absorption and Distribution

Older adults undergo normal age-related changes in the body that affect the action of bioactive substances. General absorption of drugs is not dramatically different in the older adult compared to the younger population for the vast majority of prescribed and OTC medications. Oral drugs are absorbed by the gastrointestinal (GI) tract. With aging, the GI tract produces less acid as fewer parietal cells are generated, but the change is too small to be clinically relevant. However, this small change does become clinically significant in the presence of drugs that compound this problem, such as proton pump inhibitors (Blume, Donath, Warnke, & Schug, 2006). There is decreased active transport of some drugs, causing decreased bioavailability.

Total body fat increases with age, whereas subcutaneous fat decreases (Hughes et al, 2004). Frail, older adults can have very little subcutaneous fat, which can reduce the absorption of transdermal drugs. This can be clinically important when managing pain with transdermal systems.

Distribution of drugs can be dramatically changed with age. Aging results in a reduction of lean muscle mass by about 20% and total body water by 10% to 15%, causing changes in the distribution of many drugs (Paddon-Jones, Short, Campbell, Volpi, & Wolfe, 2008). Pharmaceutical agents primarily distributed in lean body mass or body water may reach higher serum concentrations in older adults, resulting in magnified effects compared to similar doses in younger adults. Water-soluble drugs, such as lithium and digoxin, can have a smaller volume of distribution, resulting in a higher peak plasma concentration at normal dosages due to the lower ratio of water to fat in the body of the older adult. (Zagaria, 2005). This is especially important for drugs with narrow therapeutic ranges. Increased bioavailability is also apparent with drugs administered IM, which are often highly water soluble.

Lipid-soluble drugs, such as benzodiazepines, have a higher tendency to accumulate in adipose tissue, resulting in lowered serum concentrations. This accumulation in the adipose tissue can result in a prolonged duration of action due to an increased half-life. The result is a less intense immediate medication effect as well as a prolonged or unpredictable effect in the older adult.

Normal aging also results in a decrease, by as much as 20%, in serum albumin levels. Albumin is the primary drug-binding protein in the plasma. The consequence of these lowered serum albumin levels is fewer protein molecules available for binding to the drug and higher levels of free, unbound drug. It is free drug that exerts the physiological effect, so the result of decreased albumin is an increased potential for drug toxicity. This problem can be aggravated by poor nutrition, age-related liver changes, or the competition of multiple medications for protein-binding sites. With decreased binding ability, drug doses need to be reduced in order to prevent deleterious effects.

Metabolism and Excretion

Aging results in a decrease in both liver size and blood flow (Woodhouse & Wynne, 1988). Drug clearance by the liver depends on hepatic blood flow and enzyme activity. Acetylation and conjugation do not change appreciably with age. Oxidative metabolism through the cytochrome P450 (CYP450) system does decrease with aging, resulting in a decreased clearance of some drugs.

The oxidative reactions of phase I metabolism decline secondary to these changes in the liver, resulting in decreased drug clearance and an increase in half-life for agents such as amitriptyline, morphine, and propranolol that rely on high rates of blood flow through the liver for extraction (Zagaria, 2005). In contrast, phase II metabolism is relatively unaffected by age, so that benzodiazepines such as temazepam and oxazepam, which are metabolized through phase II conjugation reactions, are better tolerated than diazepam, metabolized through phase I reactions. Reduction in metabolism is more pronounced in malnourished or frail elders.

First-pass metabolism is also decreased so that drugs like propranolol and verapamil, which undergo first-pass metabolism, have increased bioavailability in older adults. On the other hand, pro-drugs which rely on first-pass metabolism for activation, will act more slowly in older adults (Wilkinson, 1997).

Most drugs are eliminated through the kidney. The human kidney loses about 1% of its function every year, beginning at age 30, so that by age 80 there is generally a 50% decline in renal function. Dosing guidelines are available to help providers make appropriate adjustments for renal impairment. Examples of drug classes for which there is evidence of age-related reduction in clearance include antihypertensives, fibrates, sedative/hypnotic, and anxiolytic medications (Aronoff et al, 2007). Disease processes may be more of a factor in the reduction of renal function than normal aging. Diabetes and hypertension, for example, have been found to be powerful determinants of renal dysfunction in the very old (Wasen et al, 2004).

Determination of normal renal function is not easily established in the older adult. Although serum creatinine is the most reliable and easiest test to determine renal function in younger persons, it is an unreliable marker in older adults. Renal function tests are affected by poor nutrition and reduced lean muscle mass. Adequate protein ingestion is a requirement for evaluating accurate blood urea nitrogen levels, and adequate muscle mass is a requirement for determining accurate serum creatinine levels. Creatinine clearance evaluated with the Cockcroft-Gault equation (discussed in Chapter 2) is the best method for this evaluation (Zagaria, 2005). Although it is the most accurate method of evaluation, this equation still has limitations, especially in frail elders for whom it may overestimate creatinine clearance.

Table 51-1 presents common pharmacokinetic and pharmacodynamic age-related changes and the drug implications.

Table 51–1   Common Pharmacokinetic and Pharmacodynamic Changes in Older Adults

Pharmacokinetic Process	Changes in Older Adults	Implications
Absorption	Change not clinically significant	
	Oral drugs: Decreased acid production by parietal cells; delayed gastric emptying; reduced blood flow to GI tract. IM drugs: Decreased lean muscle mass.	Use of drugs that have same action as aging change may increase problem to level of clinical significance.
Distribution	Increased fat stores	Lipid-soluble drugs have greater Vd and longer half-lives.
	Decreased body water	Water-soluble drugs have smaller Vd and higher peak plasma levels.
	Decreased serum albumin levels	Decreased drug-protein binding; increased levels of free drug. Especially a problem for drugs with high protein-binding percentages. Changes onset and duration of action of highly tissue-bound drugs as well.
Metabolism	Decreased hepatic blood flow	Less first-pass effect so increased amount of drugs that have high first-pass breakdown and decreased amount of pro-drugs that require first-pass activation.
	Decreased CYP450 system function	Decreased metabolic clearance of drugs. Decreased metabolism of some drugs. Altered drug-drug interactions.
Excretion	Decreased renal mass and GFR Decreased tubular secretion	Decreased renal clearance of drugs. May require dosage adjustments. Treat older adults as if they had renal impairment.
Pharmacodynamic changes	Reduced thermoregulatory ability	Increased hypothermia risk. Direct effect on phenothiazines, BDZs, TCAs, and narcotics.
	Impaired baroreceptor function and altered fluid status	Postural hypotension with antihypertensives, TCAs, MAOIs, antihistamines.

BDZs = benzodiazepines; GI = gastrointestinal; MAOIs = monoamine oxidase inhibitors; TCAs = tricyclic antidepressants; Vd = volume of distribution.

PHARMACODYNAMIC CHANGES

Aside from the pharmacokinetic changes, one of the characteristics of old age is a progressive decline in counterregulatory (homeostatic) mechanisms and altered receptor sensitivity. Pharmacodynamic changes of aging involve increased sensitivity to drugs such as anticoagulants, and cardiovascular and psychotropic drugs due to common physiological changes in the cardiac and neurological systems. Decreased elasticity in the blood vessels and reduced heart rate responsiveness to the demands of exercise increase the risk for orthostatic hypotension in older adults. Reductions in cerebral blood flow and neurotransmitter concentrations enhance the neurological effects of pharmacological agents (Mangoni & Jackson, 2004). The results of this decline include less mitigation of drug effects, more intense drug reactions than those experienced by younger patients, and a higher rate and intensity of adverse effects (Zagaria, 2005).

Reflex tachycardia, commonly seen with vasodilator therapy, is often blunted, possibly due to dampened baroreceptor response. Caution must be exercised with the use of anticholinergic medications because older adults are very sensitive to adverse drug effects related to this class of medications. These adverse effects include cognitive impairment, hallucinations, dry mouth, blurred vision, glaucoma, constipation, nausea, urinary retention, and tachycardia.

Narcotic and psychoactive drugs can cause oversedation, confusion, and respiratory depression and distort the patient's sense of balance. Drugs that lower blood pressure may cause orthostatic hypotension. Some drugs used to treat diabetes are more likely to produce hypoglycemia. Diuretics carry an increased risk for fluid and electrolyte imbalances. Nonsteroidal anti-inflammatory drugs (NSAIDs) are more likely to produce GI bleeding, cognitive impairment, fluid overload, and hypertension. Coumarin anticoagulants have a greater effect on clotting factor synthesis such that required warfarin doses are generally lower in older adults compared to younger adults. Some over-the-counter (OTC) cold remedies with anticholinergic side effects may cause the patient with glaucoma to experience vision loss secondary to the increase of intraoptic pressure and commonly cause urinary retention and constipation.

Paradoxically, some older adults are less sensitive to certain drugs (Masoodi, 2008). For example, when compared to younger patients' reactions, older adults may have a decreased response to a beta blocker (propranolol), resulting in smaller reduction in heart rate or only a mild increase in heart rate in response to a beta agonist (epinephrine).

PHARMACOTHERAPEUTICS

The advanced practice nurse needs to consider the possibility of drug-disease interactions, drug-drug interactions, and drug-metabolism interactions when planning and monitoring drug therapy in the older adult. The onset of any new symptom in an older person should raise suspicion of an adverse drug reaction (ADR).

Older adults are at higher risk for drug interactions, not only because of physiological changes but also because of the medication practices of both health-care providers and patients. Nonadherence with drug therapy, either intentional or unintentional, is reported in up to 50% of older adults (Hughes et al, 2004). Health-care providers must be aware of the many compounding factors that create complexity in prescribing for the older adult population.

Polypharmacy

Polypharmacy is the concurrent use of several different drugs; the number of drugs constituting "polypharmacy" varies throughout the literature but is generally considered to be 5 to 10 medications, including OTC and herbal products. Polypharmacy alone does not necessarily create a problem. The problem begins when more drugs are prescribed than are clinically indicated or warranted. Polypharmacy becomes an issue for older adults when a medication regimen includes overlapping drugs for the same therapeutic effect. Another serious concern is the prescription of optional drugs for an effect that could be managed by nonpharmacological approaches. Other situations contributing to polypharmacy include the use of drugs prescribed to treat the adverse effects of other drugs rather than to treat the underlying problem, and drugs whose benefit is marginal at best. Failure to consider the patient's goals of care can also lead to overzealous use of medications in cases where limited life expectancy may make many medications inappropriate (Mitchell et al, 2009).

Polypharmacy contributes to ADRs, drug-drug interactions, decreased adherence to drug regimens, unnecessary drug expenses, and poor quality of life for the patient (Barat, Andreasen, & Damsgaard, 2001; Gray, Mahoney, & Blough, 2001; Gurwitz et al, 2003; Masoodi, 2008; Patel, 2003).

Multiple factors contribute to polypharmacy in the older adult. Older adults are more likely than younger patients to have multiple comorbidities managed by multiple providers. Disease-specific clinical practice guidelines often suggest multiple medications, which may interact with medications recommended by the guidelines for patients' other conditions.

Several steps can be taken to reduce polypharmacy (Bergman-Evans, 2004):

- Obtain a complete drug history and review current drugs (prescription and others) every 6 months. Look for drugs without indications and discontinue. (Many drugs must be tapered rather than abruptly discontinued to avoid serious withdrawal symptoms).

 CLINICAL PEARL

Start low, go slow
The Golden Rule of geriatrics: Start low, go slow, but go! Treat the problem, starting at lower dosages, and titrate up slowly over a longer period of time than for a younger person. Evaluate for ADRs before they become serious and costly.

- Avoid prescribing when the benefit is questionable. Consider the age of the patient and the stage of the disease when evaluating the benefit of prescription drug use.
- Evaluate for duplications in drug therapy. Simplify the regimen by using drug combinations or by prescribing single drugs that will provide multiple therapeutic effects whenever possible. The use of combination drugs improves adherence when compared to dual therapy.
- Review the medication list for drugs prescribed for an ADR. If these exist, explore whether the original drug can be withdrawn or changed to avoid this reaction. Avoid treating adverse reactions/side effects with more drugs. Treat the underlying condition, rather than the symptoms, if possible.
- Prescribe lifestyle changes and other nondrug therapies whenever possible. These may require support from family and other health-care providers.
- Clearly understand the difference between manifestations of the aging process and the disease state that must be treated.

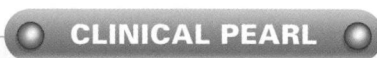

CLINICAL PEARL

Avoiding ADRs

The first step in avoiding ADRs is to establish risk predictions. Polypharmacy is only part of the picture. Take into account age, gender, multiple comorbidities, body weight, renal and hepatic failure, and previous drug reactions. Avoid medications that create unnecessary risk for patients who are determined to be at high risk for ADR.

Adverse Drug Reactions

Because the prevalence of prescription medication use among older adults increases with advanced age, older adults are 2 to 3 times more at risk for ADRs. Older adults account for about one-quarter of emergency room visits and half of all hospitalizations due to ADRs (Budnitz et al, 2006). Risk of ADRs can be predicted based on the number of medications a patient takes and whether he or she has suffered a previous ADR (Onder et al, 2010).

Poor medication practices of older adults can also contribute to ADRs. Examples of poor practices include using another's medications, changing the medication regimen without notifying the provider, and neglecting to inform the provider about all therapies being utilized. Preventable ADRs are most commonly associated with the use of anticoagulants, atypical antipsychotics, loop diuretics, opioids, ACE inhibitors, antiplatelet agents, antidepressants, benzodiazepines, insulin, and laxatives (Gurwitz et al, 2005).

Providers can help to reduce ADRs with appropriate drug prescribing, monitoring, and dosing. Consistent use of the "start low, go slow" axiom will help reduce potential problems. Start with the lowest dose that will provide a therapeutic effect and titrate upward at a slower rate than is used with younger adults. Monitoring older adult patients closely for deterioration in function (including physiological) and cognition is also necessary. Computerized order entry and electronic decision support tools with computer alerts may help to reduce ADRs.

Medications should be reconciled with the patient's pill bottles and drug list at each visit. Medication lists should be reviewed to see if there is an indication for each drug and if any can be discontinued. The advanced practice nurse should check to see if any medications can be substituted with nonpharmacological therapy or a safer drug. The dosing schedule should be made as simple as possible. Providers, on the other hand, need to ensure that all health conditions are being optimally treated and should not avoid the use of drugs with known benefit (Scott, Gray, Martin, & Mitchell, 2012).

Involving the patient in his or her care can also help to reduce ADRs. Some ways that patients who are competent to manage their own medications can play a role in reducing ADRs include:

- Maintaining a current and accurate drug record, including allergies and previous ADRs. This list should include generic and brand names of medications to avoid duplication.
- Bring a "brown bag" including all herbal and dietary supplements, OTC, and prescription medications to each clinic visit.
- Ask for a patient information sheet for each medication and review drug-drug interactions and contraindications.
- Use a medication organizer or "pill box."
- Make an appointment with the primary care provider as soon as possible after transitioning care from a hospital or rehabilitation center so that medications can be reconciled.

The Centers for Disease Control and Prevention (CDC) has developed a medication safety program with information for patients about high-risk medications and medication safety strategies that is available at www.cdc.gov/medicationsafety/. The Food and Drug Administration (2012) is spearheading a multiagency effort called the "Safe Use Initiative" that aims to coordinate efforts in order to improve the safe use of medications and to prevent harm caused from medication errors, abuse, and misuse. The American Pharmacists Association and the National Association of Chain Drugstores Foundation (2008) have created a service model to help with medication management.

Drug-Drug and Drug-Food Interactions

Empirical data about drug-drug interactions in community-living older adults are very likely underestimated. Pharmacological interventions contribute significantly to the treatment of diseases; however, ADRs also occur more frequently with the increased use of pharmacological treatments. Drug-drug interactions are a significant contributor to hospital and emergency room visits for ADRs (Juurlink, Mamdani, Kopp, Laupacis, & Redelmeier, 2003).

Interactions can also occur between prescription drugs and OTC medications and herbal remedies. These nonprescription remedies should also be included on the comprehensive medication list maintained by the older adult.

Drug-food interactions are also important, so a dietary assessment should be done. The patient is the best source of information about any ADRs he or she might have experienced. Ask about allergies and adverse reactions to both medications and foods. Drug-drug and drug-food interactions are presented throughout this book in each drug class.

During the drug history assessment, providers need to inquire directly regarding the use of OTC drugs, herbs, and vitamins. Specific questions should be asked in the review of systems that relate to the common ADRs that older adults experience (e.g., constipation). Providers should also instruct older adults to maintain a current medication list. This list should be kept accessible for use by emergency care providers.

Drug-disease interactions may also occur. Patients with Parkinson's disease have increased risk for drug-induced confusion. NSAIDs can exacerbate heart failure and reduce the effect of other drugs used to treat hypertension. Urinary retention may occur in older adults with benign prostatic hyperplasia if they take decongestants or anticholinergic drugs. Table 51-2 highlights some frequently occurring drug-drug interactions that can lead to adverse drug reactions.

Alternative Medicines

Utilization of alternative medicines is worth investigating, and knowledge about this area is valuable. Several reputable drug information sources now provide data about these drugs and these are discussed in Chapter 10. Diverse cultures, fads, and advertising have combined to make alternative medicines more prevalent now in the American culture. Use of complementary therapies is very common in older adults. Some common herbs and alternative therapies include the following:

- "Anti-aging" DHEA (dehydroepiandrosterone) and growth hormone
- Ginkgo biloba to prevent or treat dementia
- Saw palmetto to relieve the symptoms of benign prostatic hyperplasia
- Chondroitin sulfate and glucosamine sulfate for osteoarthritis
- St. John's wort and SAMe (S-Adenosyl-L-Methionine) to treat depression

Many practitioners utilize herbal medications, but the practice is very diverse and complicated. If the practitioner has only a limited knowledge of herbal medications or cultural practices, opening the dialogue with the older adult to understand the patient's practices will help in avoiding the adverse reactions of polypharmacy. Contact with a local person who is knowledgeable concerning these topics will help the practitioner prescribe and recommend appropriate treatment. Chapter 7 deals with cultural influences on pharmacotherapeutics.

Assessment

Assessing functional ability may be one of the most important steps in evaluating appropriate pharmaceutical interventions.

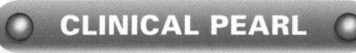

CLINICAL PEARL

Medication review

Have the older adult bring all the drugs he or she is taking, including herbs, vitamins, and OTC drugs, in a brown bag to the annual visit. This will enable you to see all the drugs and to determine if there are overlapping drugs that could be eliminated, combinations that could reduce the total number of drugs, or drugs prescribed by other providers that the patient failed to mention. It also helps to evaluate the patient's knowledge of the drugs, including why the drug is being taken and if he or she understands the ADRs.

Using a thorough and quick checklist at each clinic visit with older adult patients provides an accurate evaluation of their understanding of the drugs and their ability to manage the regimen. Box 51-1 is a questionnaire that may be used for this assessment.

Table 51–2 Selected Common Drug-Drug Interactions in Older Adults

Drug	Drug	Interaction
Warfarin	Macrolides, trimethoprim-sulfamethoxazole, fluoroquinolones, metronidazole, acetaminophen	Changes in INR
Warfarin	NSAIDS, fish oil, garlic, ginseng, gingko, ginger, vitamin E	Increased bleeding risk
Potassium-sparing diuretics	ACE inhibitors	Hyperkalemia
Cholinesterase inhibitors	Anticholinergic medications	Antagonistic effects
Sinemet	Antipsychotic agent	Antagonistic effects
Clonidine	Beta-blockers	Bradycardia and heart block and antagonistic effects
Glyburide	Trimethoprim-sulfamethoxazole	Hypoglycemia
Digoxin	Clarithromycin	Digitalis toxicity

| BOX 51–1 | QUESTIONNAIRE FOR ASSESSING MEDICATION MANAGEMENT |

- Did you bring all of your medications with you?
- List your medications, and tell me how you take them.
- Do you have any new eye drops, either over the counter or from your eye doctor?
- What over-the-counter medications are you taking, such as food supplements, vitamins, laxatives, pain relievers, and herbal or natural products?
- What medicine or herbs do you use for headaches, muscle aches or pains, nausea, or constipation?
- Do you have any problems opening the bottles?
- Do you sometimes skip some of the medicine? Why?
- What do you do when you run out of your pills?
- At what time of the day do you take your pills, and do you do this the same every day?
- How do you remember to take your pills? Do you use a pill box?
- How do you tell the difference between your medications (size, color)?
- What questions do you have about your medications?
- Do you have any difficulty paying for your medications?
- Who sets up and orders your medications?

Older adults' abilities to manage activities of daily living and their cognitive status and social systems are strong indicators of their ability to manage pharmaceutical interventions. Several assessment tools developed specifically for use with older adults include the Katz Index of Independence in Activities of Daily Living (ADLs), the Lawton Instrumental Activities of Daily Living (IADLs), the Folstein Mini Mental Status Exam (MMSE), and the Geriatric Depression Scale (GDS). These tools are short, quick, and provide evidence-based assessment data for the evaluation of an older adult's overall functional ability (see Clinical Pearl, "Resources").

In addition, assessing older adults' sensory functions (sight, hearing, taste, touch) is important because of the possible impairments that occur with aging that may affect the patient's ability to manage a medication regimen. An accurate functional assessment helps assess risk behaviors, prevent catastrophic events triggered by ADRs or inadvertent misuse of medications, and improve a patient's quality of life.

Cognitive function must also be assessed. The MMSE or Mini-Cog (see "Try This" resource listing below) can be used to evaluate cognitive function. Several tools have been developed and tested in order to help assess a patient's ability to manage medications, but there is currently insufficient evidence to support the use of any one specific tool (Elliott & Marriott, 2009). The Medication Management Ability Assessment (MMAA) (Patterson et al, 2005) is a 1-hour assessment and the Medication Assessment Instrument (MAT)

(Schmidt & Lieto, 2005) takes about 15 minutes to administer. Both assessments require the patient to set up a day's supply of a simulated medication regimen. The Drug Regimen Unassisted Grading Scale (DRUGS) (Edelberg, Shallenberger, & Wei, 1999) and Medication Management Instrument for Deficiencies in the Elderly (MedMaIDE) (Orwig, Brandt, & Gruber-Baldini, 2006) assess the patient's ability to set up his or her own medications and take 15 and 30 minutes, respectively, to administer. These assessments can help to highlight barriers to optimal medication management and help to identify resources to combat these barriers.

CLINICAL PEARL

Resources

- A helpful resource to evaluate the quality and content of herbs and supplements: National Center for Complementary and Integrative Health https://nccih.nih.gov/
- Helpful assessment tools: Try This and How to Try This Series—Resources for the care of older adults, including assessment tools and instructions for the proper use of those tools: http://consultgerirn.org/

Adherence

Adherence problems fall into two categories: intentional and unintentional. Intentional lack of adherence can occur because of doubt about the drug or its validity to treat the problem, lack of motivation, poor acceptability of the drug or the provider, poor tolerability of the drug and its effects, advice from others, dislike of the formulation, or financial concerns. Many older adults live on fixed incomes and have limited drug coverage in their health insurance plan. The Medicare Prescription Benefit (Medicare Part D) is a good first step, but it does not cover all drugs or the full cost of a drug. Some generic and OTC drugs are available on the $4.00 list, offered at many pharmacies, but this list is limited. Some older adults engage in "intelligent nonadherence" (Hindi-Alexander & Throm, 1987). They believe they are making an informed or valid decision to stop the drug or change the dose, but they fail to discuss it with their provider.

Unintentional nonadherence can occur because instruction about the drug and its use was poor or lacking altogether; the drug dosing regimen is complex and the older adult has some degree of cognitive, visual, or auditory impairment or dysphagia; the drug container is difficult to use; or the older adult has decreased mobility and may not be able to get to a pharmacy to fill the prescription. All of these are compounded if the person lives alone and has no family support.

Older adults often require small doses, but the dexterity needed to halve tablets may be a problem. Providers can help by prescribing the lower dose or by having the pharmacy halve the tablets for the patient and put them in blister packs. Pharmacies may change the company that supplies their generic drugs. The new generic may be a different color or shape. Whereas ordering generics can save the older adult money—sometimes a great deal of money—older adults often use color and shape to keep track of their medications. If a change is required, special attention needs to be taken to assure that they know about the new drug and that it is the same medication as they were previously taking. Taping one old tablet and one new tablet on a paper together with the instructions may be helpful.

A variety of other methods can be used to improve adherence. Calendars, charts, medication boxes, measured-dose systems, and other memory aids are helpful. Planning drug administration around daily activities or at the beginning of the day can serve as a memory aid and increase adherence. Home delivery of drugs can be arranged. Regimens can be simplified. Caregivers and home-health visits can be supplied if needed. Chapter 6, "Factors That Foster Positive Outcomes," has other suggestions as well.

Exciting innovations to improve monitoring of adherence are on the horizon. The Food and Drug Administration has just approved a tiny ingestible sensor, made of silicon, which can be incorporated into the drug tablet or capsule and is able to relay information to a disposable patch that is applied to the patient's skin. Information about time of ingestion as well as physiological data such as temperature, heart rate, and respiratory rate are relayed to the patch, which communicates with a handheld mobile device for information display (Pullen, 2012).

Advice to Prescribers

Some practical guidelines that can be applied in most settings to facilitate drug therapy include the following:

1. While writing a prescription, assess potential problems that may create unintentional medication nonadherence. Can the patient open and remove the tablets from the childproof bottle or the prepackaged blister packs? Can the patient being asked to take half a tablet see the tablet well enough and have the manual dexterity to break or cut the tablet in half?

2. If an inhaler has been prescribed, does the older adult have the manual dexterity, cognitive function, and inhalation volume to activate the inhaler? Older adults require the use of a spacer (Aerochamber) in order to receive the fully inhaled dose from an MDI. Breath-activated inhalers (BAIs), which deliver the drug upon inhale without requiring the patient to push on the canister, have been developed to assist the patient with manual dexterity problems.

3. Home medication assessments of frail older adults may reveal drug administration problems, including incorrect dosages, incorrect frequency, use of expired drugs, and drug omission. Home visits could lead to improved pharmaceutical interventions and adherence. With the recent changes in Medicare reimbursement, the nurse practitioner can be reimbursed for such a home visit.

4. Utilize a pharmacist who has educational information and the ability to check for potential drug-drug interactions or duplications that can arise with medications from multiple prescribers.

Self-Medication Practices

The majority of minor, acute illnesses are treated independently, by patients, without consulting a primary care provider (World Health Organization [WHO], 2007). The current cohort of older adults grew up in a time when they went to the local druggist with their health/illness problems and together they decided on a drug/potion solution. They often also asked family members who were considered to be knowledgeable in the area of the problem or who had had similar symptoms. Health-care providers were considered "consultants" not "controllers" of their health/illness and its management.

In addition to use of prescribed drugs, older adults commonly use other products such as OTC drugs, herbal remedies, and dietary supplements. About half of community-dwelling, older American women use at least one dietary supplement (Qato, Alexander, Conti, Johnson, Schumm, & Lindau, 2008). There is a widespread misperception among the general public that OTC drugs and dietary supplements are generally safe.

Self-prescribing of potentially dangerous OTC medications, use of someone else's prescribed medication, over- or underuse of prescribed medications, and underreporting of drug side effects are common problems among older adults that contribute to adverse drug reactions (Neafsey et al, 2011). Box 51-2 presents poor medication practices commonly seen in older adults.

Inappropriate Prescribing: Drugs to Be Avoided in Older Adults

Medication toxic effects and drug-related problems can have profound medical and safety consequences for older adults and economically affect the health-care system. Beers, Ouslander, Rollingher, Reuben, and Beck (1991) first produced a list of explicit criteria for determining inappropriate medication use in the elderly. The list was updated in 1997 and again in 2003 and 2012 (American Geriatric Society [AGS], 2012; Beers, 1997; Fick et al, 2003).

Commonly referred to as the Beers Criteria, the authors have determined that medications found to be in conflict with these criteria should be discontinued, unless compelling evidence exists for their use in the older adult (AGS, 2012; Bergman-Evans, 2004; Fick et al, 2003). The decision to list

---

BOX 51–2 POOR DRUG PRACTICES COMMONLY SEEN IN OLDER ADULTS

- Using another's medications or remedies.
- Changing the prescribed medication regimen without informing the provider.
- Utilizing self-care practices based on no or poor information.
- Neglecting to inform the health-care provider about all therapies being utilized.
- Hoarding medications.

drugs and to rate them as "high concern" or "low concern" was made by a group of experts using the Delphi method. Drugs rated "high concern" included those that should be generally avoided in persons 65 years or older because they are ineffective or they pose unnecessarily high risk for older persons and a safer alternative is available. Drugs rated "low concern" included those that should not be used in older persons known to have specific medical conditions. These medications include long-acting benzodiazepines, sedatives, long-acting oral hypoglycemics, analgesics, antiemetics, and gastrointestinal antispasmodics. The comprehensive list of medication potentially inappropriate for use in older adults may be accessed at www.americangeriatrics.org/files/documents/beers/2012BeersCriteria_JAGS.pdf (AGS, 2012). It is imperative to seek out safer alternatives for those medications with a narrow therapeutic range, very slow elimination rates, or for which elimination is dependent on kidney function.

The Beers Criteria have been criticized over lack of evidence to support their effectiveness at reducing adverse drug events and reducing costs of care and because drugs known to cause adverse drug events are omitted from the list (O'Mahoney, et al, 2010). The Screening Tool of Older Persons' Prescriptions (STOPP) and the Screening Tool to Alert to Right Treatment (START) are new, validated tools for identification of inappropriate prescribing in the older adult that are suggested for use in conjunction with the Beer's Criteria (O'Mahoney et al, 2010). These criteria were developed by a consensus panel in the United Kingdom and Ireland, using the Delphi process, and have been shown to have good interrater reliability. Drugs to be avoided using the STOPP criteria and started using the START criteria are listed by body system.

About half of hospitalized older adults and one-fourth of community-dwelling older adults (Gallagher, Ryan, Byrne, Kennedy, & O'Mahoney, 2008) were found to lack one or more medicines that were known to be potentially beneficial, such as aspirin in patients with known coronary artery disease. The START criteria list these types of medications that should be used in older adults with specific conditions. In a study comparing hospital admissions of older adults in Europe due to the use of potentially inappropriate medications, violations of STOPP criteria were found to lead to these hospitalizations more often than violations of the Beers Criteria (Gallagher & O'Mahoney, 2008; Hamilton, Gallagher, Ryan, Byrne, & O'Mahoney, 2011). These results may differ geographically since medications on the Beers list include those more frequently used in the United States, whereas those on the STOPP list are biased toward those generally used in Europe. The American Geriatrics Society therefore recommends the use of both sets of criteria (AGS, 2012).

TRANSITIONS OF CARE AND CARE SETTINGS

According to the Institute of Medicine report (IOM), medication errors due to poor communication results in approximately 98,000 patient deaths per year (IOM, 2000). Of the 4,000 sentinel events from the last decade, the Joint Commission concluded that 60% were the direct result of ineffective communication, and of these, 70% resulted in patient death (Leonard, Graham, & Bonacum, 2004). Good communication is especially critical in the care of the older adult, who often has multiple specialists and frequently transitions from care setting to care setting. Frail older adults often live in independent living or assisted living facilities but may transition to emergency departments, hospitals, and skilled nursing facilities during periods of illness. Transitions between care settings represent periods of patient vulnerability, especially for older adults for whom comorbid illness, functional impairment, and multiple caregivers can compound complexity and compromise safety.

Each setting has its own unique challenges for the medical prescriber. A description of several of the living environments available for older adults and the personnel involved in each is critical to understanding these challenges.

- Private homes: Many older adults remain independent in their own homes and may require informal assistance from family, friends, and neighbors in order to pick up medications from the pharmacy, order medications, set up pill boxes, etc. After seeking the patient's permission, it may be as important to communicate the plan of care and information about medications ordered to the informal caregiver as it is to the patient. Investigation of limitations related to availability of care is important; for example, an adult child may only be available to help the patient acquire medications on his or her day off from work, so alternative plans may need to be made for medications needed more urgently.

- Home care is sometimes available as adjuvant care for the homebound older adult and can be provided as skilled or unskilled care. Skilled care, provided by a nurse or licensed physical or speech therapist, is reimbursed by Medicare for a limited period of time following a hospitalization, with the goal of restoring baseline functioning. Occasionally, the patient will be able to receive skilled services for a longer period of time as long as the "skilled need" continues to exist. Examples of skilled needs include wound care, IM injections, and catheter changes (Centers for Medicare and Medicaid Services [CMS], 2012).

- Many frail older adults have no "skilled needs" but do need help with instrumental activities of daily living. If the older person has no available family or friends to provide these services, they often utilize home caregivers and pay out of pocket for this care. These caregivers may change over time and have no nursing or medical training. The prescriber may need to communicate with these caregivers, who are charged with administering and organizing the patient's medications. It is important to remember that information should be provided in a manner appropriate for a lay audience. When soliciting information about the patient's health status from these caregivers, it is important to remember that they are not trained health-care providers.

- Patients who live independently and self-manage their medications will benefit from a simplified medication regimen, including the substitution of long-acting medication for drugs requiring multiple daily doses and combination pills, when available. Medications that interfere with cognitive functioning should be avoided. Patients should be encouraged and taught to use pill boxes that are divided by days of the week and times of day. Coordinating medication administration with key daily activities like mealtimes, grooming routines, etc. can help patients remember to take medications appropriately.

- Independent living facilities provide individual apartments for seniors with no nursing or medical assistance. These facilities usually include an option for dining within the facility and provide transportation services to shopping and entertainment. The health-care provider will encounter the same limitations when providing care in these facilities as with patients who live in private homes. These apartments are, essentially, private homes with a few additional, nonmedical services.

- Assisted living facilities (ALF) exist as small group homes with 4 to 8 residents or as large facilities with over 100 residents that provide assistance with activities of daily living and 24-hour supervision. They generally share a philosophy toward providing a home-like, rather than a medical, environment and are not licensed as health-care facilities. ALFs are regulated by states, resulting in variable standards and admission criteria across the nation. Availability of nursing support in assisted living varies widely; some of the larger facilities have 24-hour nursing care, whereas most have a licensed practical nurse available for part of the day on weekdays only. Smaller facilities rarely have a nurse on staff.

- Residents of ALFs take an average of 9 to 10 medications (Young et al, 2008). Some patients self-administer medications, in which case provider concerns are similar to those associated with private homes or independent living facilities. Most patients living in ALFs require some help with medication management, however. Requirements for training of personnel who may administer medications in ALFs vary by state, but the majority of states allow nonlicensed personnel to administer some medications. Colorado, for example, allows medications to be administered by an unlicensed Qualified Medical Administration Person (QMAP), who records the administration on a medication administration record (MAR). QMAPs are not permitted to make any assessments or evaluations or exercise judgment related to these medications and may not administer injectable medications, including insulin. Written prescriptions for all medications, including OTC medications, dietary supplements, and herbal supplements must be provided in order for the QMAP to legally administer the drug or product. QMAPs receive one day of instruction related to medication administration and then take an exam that includes a practicum and a written portion (Department of Regulatory Agencies [DORA], 2008).

- Ninety percent of ALF residents have some level of cognitive impairment (Zimmerman et al, 2007), which is often the reason for moving into the ALF. In these cases, the prescriber is dependent upon the ALF staff to recognize and report symptoms that may signal disease. Since older adults often present with atypical signs and symptoms of disease, the untrained caregiver may miss and fail to report significant changes in health status. These caregivers may also call to insist upon treatment for a symptom expressed by a frail older adult when, at times, the risk of treatment for this vulnerable patient outweighs the benefit. Providers may have unrealistic expectations related to the caregivers' knowledge and ability to monitor for potential drug side effects. Specific orders for monitoring of vital signs related to drug effects will need to be provided to ALF staff. Careful communication and mutual understanding between prescribers and ALF staff is crucial to optimal care provision.

- Prescribers must remember to write prescriptions for all medications, including supplements and OTC medications, and to fax these prescriptions to the assisted living facility in order to ensure that patients living in this environment will actually be able to receive the drugs that are ordered. Any dose change or order for a new medication as substitute for another must be accompanied with an order to discontinue the initial dose or medication in order to avoid duplicative therapy. Prescribers must recognize the limited knowledge and experience of QMAPs and provide adequate additional instruction related to medications ordered. The provider must be knowledgeable about limits in the QMAPs' ability to administer injectable medications and monitor side effects of the drug.

- It is not uncommon to see patients leave their primary care provider's office with a prescription in hand for a given medication. The patient may pick up the medication from the pharmacy and return to the assisted living facility only to learn that the drug may not be administered, since there is no order for the ALF staff to administer it. Messages communicated to the patient related to dose or drug changes are insufficient to create this change if the medication is managed by the facility.

- Skilled nursing facilities (SNFs) are sometimes called "rehabilitation" because they provide short-term care after hospitalization in order to help the patient return to baseline functioning or learn to function with newly acquired deficits. They also provide professional staff for monitoring, treating, and evaluating a health condition. SNF care is not available when care needs are strictly custodial (ADL and IADL support) (CMS, 2012). SNF stays are reimbursable by Medicare with escalating co-pays for longer stays. SNFs are highly regulated by the Centers for Medicare and Medicaid Services as health-care facilities. CMS requires oversight of medication use by a licensed pharmacist and administration of medications only by nursing staff, who are also charged with monitoring for ADRs. CMS requires pharmacists and providers to collaborate to ensure that each medication is associated with a diagnosis, dosages and duration of use of medications are consistent with manufacturer guidelines, nonpharmacological interventions are used as substitutions or adjuvants to pharmacological therapy, medication side effects are considered as potential causative agents for newly emerging symptoms, and that appropriate drug monitoring is performed (Long Term Care Professional Leadership Council, 2009).

- Prescribers working with patients in SNFs should be prepared to collaborate with pharmacists and to participate in quality improvement activities related to improving medication administration practices and patient safety. Queries by pharmacists related to drug substitutions, discontinuations, and monitoring are commonplace in this setting. As with ALFs, prescribers need to be sure to write discontinuation orders when substituting one drug for another or when changing medication dosages.

- Long-term care (LTC), or "nursing home" care, is utilized by people whose care needs exceed those that can be provided in the home or in assisted living facilities. Twenty-four-hour nursing care is provided and regulated by CMS in the same way that SNF care is regulated, but LTC costs are not covered by Medicare. Issues with prescribing are similar for LTCs and SNFs.

GENERAL PRINCIPLES FOR PRESCRIBING FOR OLDER ADULTS

Chapters 1 and 3 provide information about rational drug selection for the general population. All of these recommendations are valid for older adults but some are especially important for this population:

- Before prescribing, collect a complete drug history— including herbs, vitamins, and nonprescription drugs that the patient is taking. Ask specifically about the latter categories, because older adults may not consider these to be drugs.

- Evaluate if drug therapy is required. Determine if the problem can be treated with nonpharmacological interventions or if it can be resolved by removing unnecessary drugs from the patient's medication regimen. Discontinue drugs when possible if the benefit is unclear or the adverse effects of the drug result in nonadherence.

- Avoid a drug if the benefit is marginal or if a nonpharmacological alternative exists. This is especially true of high-cost newer drugs. Determine if the newer drug provides some unique benefit and if the benefit of adding an additional drug to the medication regimen is sufficient to justify the cost, the increased complexity of the regimen, and the risk of adverse reactions.

- When therapy is deemed appropriate, start low and go slow. However, do not fail to prescribe appropriate therapy in doses that are sufficient to resolve or treat the problem.

- Evaluate if the drug and its formulation are appropriate for older adults based on the normal physiological changes associated with aging. Check the Beers and the STOPP criteria to ensure the drug is appropriate to use in this population.

- Use single daily-dose regimens or the simplest effective regimen. Avoid polypharmacy wherever possible.

- Limit the use of prn drugs.

- Consider all new drugs as a therapeutic trial; stop the drug if it is ineffective.

- Attempt to prescribe a drug that will treat more than one existing problem (e.g., an ACE-inhibitor to treat hypertension, heart failure, and/or as renal protection in diabetes).

- Provide legible written instructions and follow up on adherence to the treatment regimen.

- Consider the unique nature of individuals in terms of their diseases, comorbid conditions, and experiences with medications when prescribing.

REFERENCES

American Geriatrics Society (AGS). (2012). American Geriatrics Society updated Beers criteria for potentially inappropriate medication use in older adults. *Journal of the American Geriatrics Society,* doi: 10.1111/j.1532-5415.2012.03923.x.

Aronoff, G. R., Berns, J. S., Brier, M. E., et al. (2007). *Drug prescribing in renal failure: Dosing guidelines for adults* (5th ed.). Philadelphia: American College of Clinicians.

Barat, I., Andreasen, F., & Damsgaard, E. M. (2001). Drug therapy in the elderly: What doctors believe and patients actually do. *British Journal of Clinical Pharmacology, 51,* 615–622.

Beers, M. H. (1997). Explicit criteria for determining potentially inappropriate medication use by the elderly. *Archives of Internal Medicine, 157,* 1531–1536.

Beers, M. H., Ouslander, J. G., Rollingher, J., Reuben, D. B., & Beck, J. C. (1991). Explicit criteria for determining inappropriate medication use in nursing home residents. *Archives of Internal Medicine, 151,* 1825–1832.

Bergman-Evans, B. (2004). *Improving medication management for older adult clients.* Gerontological Nursing Interventions Research Center, Research Dissemination Care. Iowa City, IA: University of Iowa.

Blume, H., Donath, F., Warnke, A., & Schug, B. S. (2006). Pharmacokinetic drug interaction profiles of proton pump inhibitors. *Drug Safety, 29*(9), 769–784.

Budnitz, D. S., Lovegrove, M. C., Shehab, N., Richards, C. L. (2011). Emergency hospitalizations for adverse drug events in older Americans. *New England Journal of Medicine, 365,* 2002–2012.

Budnitz, D. S., Pollock, D. A., Weidenbach, K. N., et al. (2006). National surveillance of emergency department visits for outpatient adverse drug events. *Journal of the American Medical Association, 296,* 1858–1866.

CensusScope. (2000). *Age distribution, 2000.* Retrieved August 2, 2012, from http://www.CensusScope.org

Centers for Medicare and Medicaid Services (CMS). (2012). *Medicare and home health care.* Accessed August 8, 2012, from http://www.medicare.gov/publications/pubs/pdf/10969.pdf

Centers for Medicare and Medicaid Services (CMS). (2012). *Medicare coverage of skilled nursing facility care.* Accessed August 8, 2012, from http://www.medicare.gov/publications/pubs/pdf/10153.pdf

Department of Regulatory Agencies (DORA). 2008. *2008 Sunset review: Administration of medications by unlicensed persons.* Accessed August 8, 2012, from http://www.dora.state.co.us/opr/archive/2008Medication Administration.pdf

Edelberg, H. K., Shallenberger, E., & Wei, J. Y. (1999). Medication management capacity in highly functioning community-living older adults: Detection of early deficits. *Journal of the American Geriatrics Society, 47*(5), 592–596.

Esiri, M. M. (2007). Ageing and the brain. *The Journal of Pathology, 211*(2), 181–187. doi: 10.1002/path.2089

Federal Interagency Forum on Aging-Related Statistics. (2010). *Older Americans 2010: Key indicators of well-being.* Washington, DC: U.S. Government Printing Office. Retrieved August 2, 2012, from http://www.agingstats.gov/agingstatsdotnet/Main_Site/Data/2010_Documents/Docs/OA_2010.pdf

Fick, D., Cooper, J., Wade, W., Waller, J., McClean, J., & Beers, M. (2003). Updating the Beers Criteria for potentially inappropriate medication use in older adults. *Archives of Internal Medicine, 163,* 2716–2724.

Food and Drug Administration. (2012). *Safe Use Initiative: Collaborating to reduce preventable harm from medications.* Accessed August 9, 2012, from http://www.fda.gov/Drugs/DrugSafety/SafeUseInitiative/default.htm

Gallagher, P., & O'Mahoney, D. (2008). STOPP (Screening Tool of Older Persons' potentially inappropriate Prescriptions): Application to acutely ill elderly patients and comparison with Beers' criteria. *Age and Ageing, 37,*673–679, doi: 10.1093/ageing/afn197

Gallagher, P., Ryan, C., Byrne, S., Kennedy, J., & O'Mahoney, D. (2008). Screening Tool of Older Persons' potentially inappropriate Prescriptions (STOPP) and Screening Tool to Alert doctors to Right Treatment (START): Validation and application to hospitalised elderly patients. *Age and Ageing, 37,* 56.

Gray, S. L., Mahoney, F. E., & Blough, D. K. (2001). Medication adherence in the elderly patients receiving home health services following hospital discharge. *Annals of Pharmacotherapy, 35,* 539–545.

Gurwitz, J. H., Field, T. S., Harrold, L. R., Rothschild, J., Debellis, K., Seger, A. C., Cadoret, C., Fish, L. S., Garber, L., Kelleher, M., & Bates, D. W. (2003). Incidence and preventability of adverse drug events among older persons in the ambulatory setting. *Journal of the American Medical Association, 289,* 1107–1116.

Gurwitz, M. D., Field, T., Judge, J., Rochon, P., et al. (2005). The incidence of adverse drug events in two large academic long-term care facilities. *American Journal of Medicine, 118,* 251.

Hamilton, H., Gallagher, P., Ryan, C., Byrne, S., & O'Mahoney, D. (2011). Potentially inappropriate medications defined by STOPP criteria and the risk of adverse drug events in older hospitalized patients. *Archives of Internal Medicine, 171*(11), 1013–1019. doi:10.1001/archinternmed.2011.215

Hartford Institute for Geriatric Nursing. (2005).*Want to know more: Sensory changes.* Accessed August 4, 2012, at http://consultgerirn.org/topics/sensory_changes/want_to_know_more/

Hindi-Alexander, M. C., & Throm, J. (1987) Compliance or noncompliance: That is the question! *American Journal of Health Promotion, 1*(4), 5–11.

Hughes, V. A., Roubenoff, R., Wood, M., Frontera, W. R., Evans, W. J., & Fiatarone Singh, M. A. (2004). Anthropometric assessment of 10-y changes in body composition in the elderly. *The American Journal of Clinical Nutrition, 80,* 475–482.

Institute of Medicine (IOM). (2000). *To err is human: Building a safer health system.* Washington, DC: The National Academy Press.

Juurlink, D. N., Mamdani, M., Kopp, A., Laupacis, A., & Redelmeier, D. A. (2003). Drug-drug interactions among elderly patients hospitalized for drug toxicity. *Journal of the American Medical Association, 289*(13), 1652.

Leonard, M., Graham, S., & Bonacum, D. (2004). The human factor: The critical importance of effective teamwork and communication in providing safe care. *Quality Safe Health Care, 13*(Suppl), i85–i90.

Long Term Care Professional Leadership Council. (2009). *The medication use process.* Retrieved August 8, 2012, from http://www.achca.org/content/pdf/LTCPLC_Stmt3_MedUseProcess_081031.pdf

Masoodi, N. A. (2008). Polypharmacy: To err is human, to correct divine. *British Journal of Medical Practitioners, 1*(1), 6–9.

McCance, K. L., & Huether, S. E. (2014). Pathophysiology. *The biologic basis for disease in adults and children* (7th ed.). Maryland Heights, Missouri: Mosby Elsevier.

Mitchell, S. L., Teno, J. M., Kiely, D. K., Shaffer, M. L., Jones, R. N., Prigerson, H. G., et al. (2009). The clinical course of advanced dementia. *New England Journal of Medicine, 361*(16), 1529.

Nahin, R. L., Pecha, M., Welmerink, D. B., Sink, K., DeKosky, S. T., & Fitzpatrick, A. L. (2009). Concomitant use of prescription drugs and dietary supplements in ambulatory elderly people. *Journal of the American Geriatrics Society, 57*(7), 1197–1205.

National Center for Health Statistics. (2009). *Health, United States, 2009: With special feature on medical technology.* Hyattsville, MD: U.S. Government Printing Office.

Neafsey, P. J., M'lan, C. E., Ge, M., Walsh, S. J., Lin, C. A., & Anderson, E. (2011). Reducing adverse self-medication behaviors in older adults with hypertension: Results of an e-health clinical efficacy trial. *Ageing International, 36*(2), 159–191.

O'Mahoney, D., Gallagher, P., Ryan, C., Byrne, S., Hamilton, H., Barry, P., et al. (2010). STOPP and START criteria: A new approach to detecting potentially inappropriate prescribing in old age. *European Geriatric Medicine, 1*(1), 45–51.

Onder, G., Petrovic, M., Tangiisuran, B., Meinardi, M. C., Markito-Notenboom, W. P., Somers, A., et al. (2010). Development and validation of a score to assess risk of adverse drug reactions among in-hospital patients 65 years or older: The GerontoNet ADR risk score. *Archives of Internal Medicine, 170*(13), 1142.

Orwig, D., Brandt, N., & Gruber-Baldini, A. L. (2006). Medication management assessment for older adults in the community. *Gerontologist, 46*(5), 661–668.

Paddon-Jones, D., Short, K. R., Campbell, W. W., Volpi, E., & Wolfe, R. R. (2008). Role of dietary protein in the sarcopenia of aging. *The American Journal of Clinical Nutrition, 87*(5), 1562S–1566S.

Patel, R. (2003). Polypharmacy and the elderly. *Journal of Infusion Nursing, 26*(3), 166–169.

Patterson, T. L., Lacro, J., McKibbin, C. L., Moscona, S., Hughs, T., & Jeste, D. V. (2005). Medication management ability assessment: Results from a performance-based measure in older outpatients with schizophrenia. *Journal of Clinical Psychopharmacology, 22*(1), 11–19.

Pullen, L. C. (2012 Aug 3). FDA approves digestible microchips to be placed in pills. *Medscape Diabetes and Endocrinology News.* Accessed August 8, 2012, from http://www.medscape.com/viewarticle/768665?src=nldne

Roland, P. S., Smith, T. L., Schwartz, S. R., Rosenfeld, R. M., Ballachanda, B., Earll, J. M., et al. (2008). Clinical practice guideline: Cerumen impaction. *Otolaryngology–Head and Neck Surgery, 139,* S1–S21.

Schmidt, K. S., & Lieto, J. M. (2005). Validity of the Medication Administration Test among older adults with and without dementia. *American Journal of Geriatric Pharmacotherapeutics, 3*(4), 255–261.

Scott, I. A., Gray, L. C., Martin, J. H., & Mitchell, C. A. (2012). Minimizing inappropriate medications in older populations: A 10-step conceptual framework. *American Journal of Medicine, 125*(6), 529–537.

Vinik, A. I., Strotmeyer, E. S., Nakave, A. A., & Patel, C. V. (2008). Diabetic neuropathy in older adults. *Clinical Geriatric Medicine, 24*(3), 407–435. doi: 10.1016/j.cger.2008.03.011

Wasen, E., Isoaho, R., Mattila, K., Vahlberg, T., Kivela, S., & Irjala, K. (2004). Renal impairment associated with diabetes in the elderly. *Diabetes Care, 27*(11), 2648–2653.

Wilkinson, G. R. (1997). The effects of diet, aging and disease-states on presystemic elimination and oral drug bioavailability in humans. *Advanced Drug Delivery Reviews, 15*(27), 129–159.

Woodhouse, K. W., & Wynne, H. A. (1988) Age-related changes in liver size and hepatic blood flow. The influence on drug metabolism in the elderly. *Clinical Pharmacokinetics, 15,* 287–294.

World Health Organization (WHO). (2007). *Responsible self-care and self-medication: A worldwide review of consumer surveys.* Accessed August 4, 2012, at http://www.wsmi.org/pdf/wsmibro3.pdf

Young, H. M., Gray, S. L., McCormick, W. C., et al. (2008). Types, prevalence, and potential clinical significance of medication administration errors in assisted living. *Journal of the American Geriatrics Society, 56,* 1199–1205.

Zagaria, M. (2005). The effects of aging on drug efficacy: Drug pharmacodynamics and pharmacokinetics. *U.S. Pharmacist, 30*(5), 54–57.

Zimmerman, S., Sloane, P. D., Williams, C. S., et al. (2007). Residential care/assisted living staff may detect undiagnosed dementia using the Minimum Data Set Cognition Scale (MDS-COGS). *Journal of the American Geriatrics Society, 55,* 1349–1355.

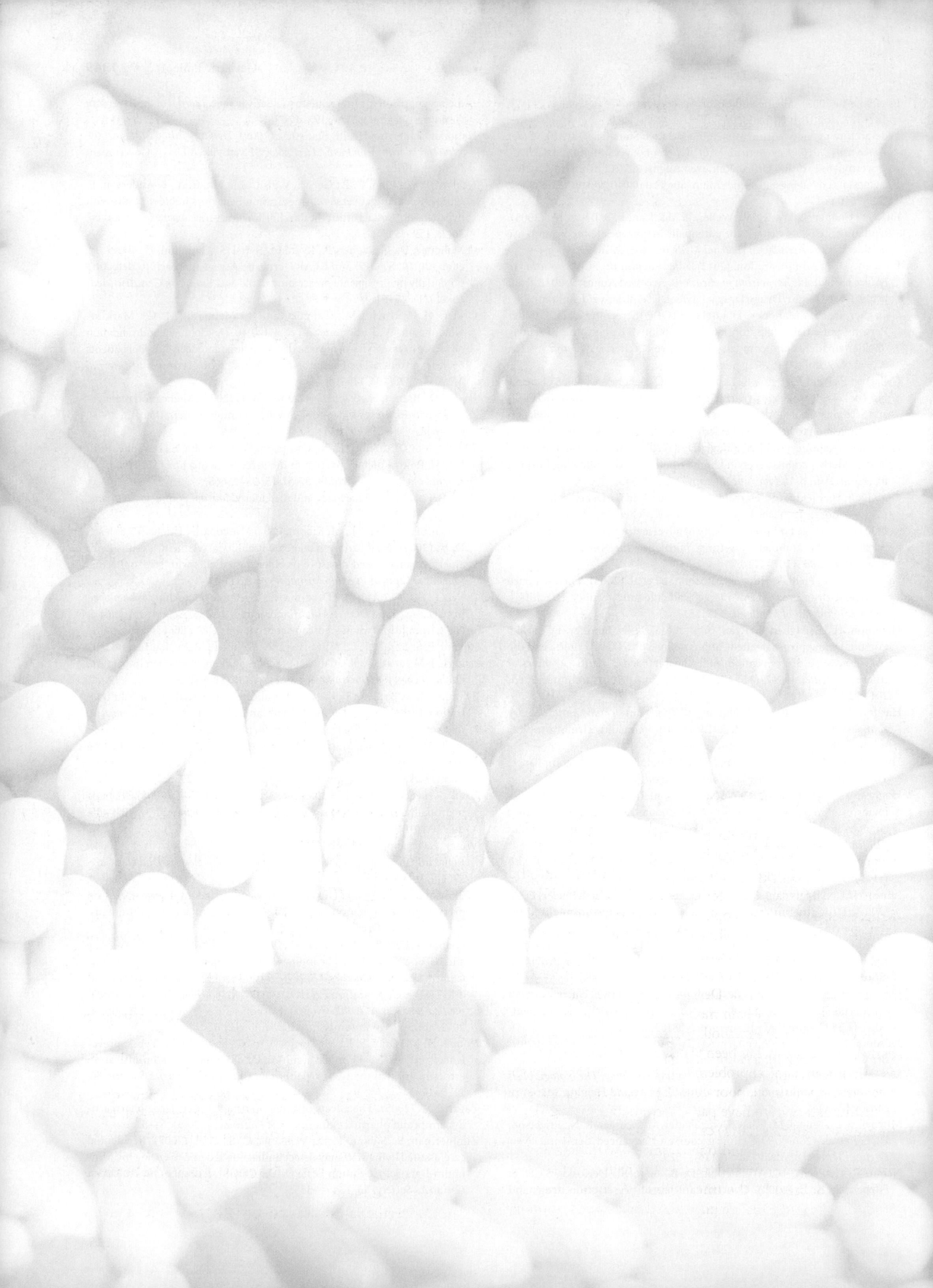

CHAPTER 52

PAIN MANAGEMENT: ACUTE AND CHRONIC PAIN

Ruth L. Schaffler

OVERVIEW OF PAIN CONCEPTS

Pain is the most common reason people seek health care (Centers for Disease Control [CDC], 2013; National Institutes of Health [NIH], 2013) not only in the United States but worldwide (Brennan, Carr, & Cousins, 2007; Scholten, Nygren-Krug, & Zucker, 2007); people expect pain relief when seeking treatment. Brennan and colleagues (2007) and Fishman (2007) declared pain management as a human right but also stated that a standard of care for pain management is neither an absolute science nor is it free of risk. Despite research that has increased the understanding of pain management and has broadened knowledge of effective methods to assess and manage pain, undertreatment of pain has been widely reported in the literature as a significant clinical problem (Wu & Raja, 2011). Failure to treat pain is unethical, poor clinical practice, and a violation of the human right to have pain appropriately managed. The Institute of Medicine (2011) called for examining pain as a national health problem and transforming the understanding, prevention, assessment, and treatment of pain.

Pain is defined by the International Association for the Study of Pain (IASP) as "an unpleasant sensory and emotional experience associated with actual or potential tissue damage, or described in terms of such damage, or both"; however, pain is a subjective complaint. IASP (2012) updated a taxonomy of pain terms that have specific application to the perception of pain:

- Allodynia—pain from a stimulus that does not normally produce pain
- Analgesia—absence of pain in response to stimulation that would normally be painful
- Causalgia—a syndrome of sustained burning pain after a traumatic nerve lesion
- Dysesthesia—an unpleasant abnormal sensation, whether spontaneous or evoked
- Hyperalgesia—increased pain from a stimulus that normally provokes pain
- Hyperesthesia—increased sensitivity to stimulation
- Hyperpathia—a painful syndrome characterized by an abnormally painful reaction to a stimulus, especially a repetitive stimulus, as well as an increased threshold
- Hypoalgesia—diminished pain response to a normally painful stimulus
- Hypoesthesia—decreased sensitivity to stimulation

- Neuralgia—pain in the distribution of a nerve or nerves
- Neuritis—inflammation of a nerve or nerves
- Neuropathic pain—pain caused by a lesion or disease of the somatosensory nervous system
- Neuropathy—a disturbance of function or pathological change in a nerve: in one nerve, mononeuropathy; in several nerves, mononeuropathy multiplex; if diffuse and bilateral, polyneuropathy
- Nociception—the neural process of encoding noxious stimuli
- Nociceptive pain—pain that arises from actual or threatened damage to nonneural tissue and is due to the activation of nociceptors
- Nociceptor—a high-threshold sensory receptor of the peripheral somatosensory nervous systems that is capable of transducing and encoding noxious stimuli
- Paresthesia—an abnormal sensation, whether spontaneous or evoked
- Sensitization—increased responsiveness of nociceptive neurons to their normal input and/or recruitment of a response to normally subthreshold inputs

Suffering is an emotional reaction to pain and can be manifested by feelings of helplessness or hopelessness (Schaffler, 2007). Understanding of these terms can help the practitioner assess the pain symptoms, consider causality, and develop the best pain management plan for patients with specific presentations.

Pain can be either acute or chronic and is generally classified according to duration of symptoms and the presence or absence of sympathetic nervous system activity. Acute pain is associated with tissue injury and resolves when healing occurs and is subcategorized as physiological. Chronic pain lasts more than 6 months, well beyond the expected time of injury healing, and is subcategorized as pathological. Table 52-1 identifies the differences between the two pain categories. Each will be discussed in depth.

The Experience of Pain

Pain is a subjective experience with both sensory and emotional components, a uniquely personal experience that virtually all people encounter at some point during their lifetime. The IASP definition of pain recognizes that pain is a perception and, as such, may or may not correlate to a source of injury that can be identified. Stimulation in the nociceptive system, the physiological mechanisms of pain, can occur with a disease process without a specific injury being present. In other cases, pain may not be related to a physical process, which indicates the influence of emotional and psychological factors that produce subjective reports of pain.

McCaffery (1972) defined pain as "Whatever the experiencing patient says it is and exists whenever he says it does" (p 8). It is important that the patient's statements about pain are believed by the practitioner as an initial step in pain management. A comprehensive assessment is imperative but the practitioner should also understand the nature of the patient's pain in terms of etiology, pathophysiology, relevant comorbid conditions, and the impact of the pain on activity and quality of life when making treatment decisions. Melzack and Casey (1968) developed a model for pain levels in terms of a hierarchy with three components:

- Sensory-Discriminative—the location, intensity, and quality of pain
- Motivation-Affective—depression or anxiety associated with the pain
- Cognitive-Evaluation—the patient's thoughts about the significance of the pain

These components influence the descriptions and importance of the pain experience that need to be acknowledged and explored.

Pain Threshold and Pain Tolerance

Pain threshold is the lowest point at which a nociceptive stimulus is perceived as pain. The perception of pain varies widely among patients and even within the individual at times. Perceptual dominance, the experience of intense pain in one location, is likely to increase the threshold in other areas. An example might be a trauma patient with multiple injuries who perceives only one injury as painful. The significance of pain as a threat to well-being may also influence the pain

Table 52–1 Comparisons of Acute and Chronic Pain

	Acute	Chronic
Etiology	Physiological	Pathological
Onset	Sudden	Gradual development
Localization	Generally well identified	Less easy to differentiate
Duration	Generally self-limiting with healing	Lasts beyond 6 months
Character	Varies, more overt signs	Varies, fewer overt signs
Temporal pattern	Varies, symptoms correctable	Varies, symptoms persistent
Associated symptoms	Physical and psychological (anxiety or irritability)	Physical and psychological (depression, insomnia, lethargy)
Prognosis	Complete relief in most cases	Complete relief generally not achieved

threshold. A patient experiencing chest pain may perceive pain as significant if the patient believes he or she is having a heart attack and is threatened with disability or death.

Pain tolerance is the amount of intensity or time a patient will endure before taking steps to relieve the pain. Past experience with pain is a factor in the patient's evaluation of the current pain experience. Tolerance to painful stimuli may decrease over time and can be influenced by anger, fear, lack of sleep, or other cognitive factors. Tolerance may increase with the use of medications, recreational drugs or alcohol, distraction, applications of heat and/or ice, herbs or alternative therapies such as acupuncture or hypnosis, cultural beliefs or expectations, or religious activities.

Neurological Basis of Pain

Anatomy and Physiology

The information in this section comes from Nelson-Marsh and Banasik (2010) and the American Medical Association's (2013a) online CME course entitled Pain Management.

The portions of the nervous system involved in the sensation and perception of pain can be divided into three areas:

- *Afferent pathways* are composed of nociceptors (pain receptors) in the peripheral tissues that respond to injury or inflammation. When cells are damaged, phospholipids in the cell membrane are broken down by the phospholipase A enzyme and converted to arachidonic acid. Further breakdown of arachidonic acid by another enzyme, cyclooxygenase (COX), forms prostaglandins. Nociceptors are sensitized by prostaglandins and lower the pain threshold. Other chemical mediators alter the membranes of the pain receptors—among them are bradykinins, histamine, cannabinoids, neurotensin, lactate, K^+, H^+ and others—to affect depolarization and transmission of the pain impulse. When depolarization of the nociceptors occurs, the impulse is sent along afferent neurons, A-delta fibers and C-fibers, to the spinal cord. A-delta fibers are myelinated, respond to mechanical and mechanico-thermal stimuli, have a fast conduction velocity, and have small reception fields, which allow for precise pain location. C-fibers represent approximately 70% of the fibers carrying thermal and chemical pain impulses, are unmyelinated, have a much slower conduction velocity, and less location-specific pain perception. The afferent pathway terminates in the dorsal horn of the spinal cord. Nociceptors that are stimulated transmit impulses through collateral branches to the central nervous system.
- *The central nervous system* is involved in interpretation of pain signals. Pain fibers bifurcate when they enter the spinal cord through the posterior nerve roots and ascend as well as descend several segments to form the tract of Lissauer, where interneurons carry the impulse across the cord to the contralateral ascending anterolateral tract to the brain. The substantia gelatinosa is a key anatomical region within the cord and has multiple synapses. Within this region pain impulses can be

intensified or blocked. Neurotransmitters such as Substance P, GABA, cholecystokinin, somatostatin, calcitonin-gene-related peptide, and excitatory amino acids (glutamate) bind to the neurons in the pathway in the spinal cord to transmit the impulses to the brain. Glutamate binding to *N*-methyl-D-aspartate (NMDA) receptors is thought to produce a kind of pain memory so that if repeated mild stimulation of C-fiber occurs, the stimulus can be perceived as painful and may be a mechanism that contributes to chronic pain syndromes. The synapses in the cord can become points of pain modulation through endogenous or exogenous means.

The anterolateral tract has two divisions, the neospinothalamic tract and the paleospinothalamic tract. The neospinothalamic tract transmits A-delta fibers quickly to the thalamus. Despite fewer synapses, the pain signal is received without the emotional component. C-fibers travel mainly through the paleospinothalamic tract, which has more synapses but the pain signal travels more slowly. The tract projects into the medulla and reticular activating systems, which alert, arouse, and elicit pain recognition and pain-related behaviors (Fig. 52-1).

Discrimination and localization of pain occur in a portion of the thalamus. Use of a dermatomal map may be helpful for isolating sources of neurological pain. The medulla and hypothalamus activate coping responses such as the release of catecholamines and corticosteroids and physical responses such as increased heart rate and blood pressure. Complex modulations of pain transmission occur in other regions of the brain as well. Because the pain impulses arrive in the brain at two different speeds several seconds apart, the phenomenon of "double pain" sensation occurs.

- *Efferent pathways* are responsible for modulating the pain sensation. The pathway is composed of fibers that connect the reticular formation, midbrain, and substantia gelatinosa in the dorsal horn of the spinal cord. Neurons in these regions converge and interact to inhibit the transmission of pain signals through chemical mediation.

Within the brainstem nucleus is an area known as the raphe magnus that receives input from two other areas, the periaqueductal gray (PAG) area in the midbrain, which is rich in endogenous opioids (endorphins and enkephalins) considered the body's pain killers, and the rostral pons in the brainstem. Endorphins are neuropeptides that inhibit transmission of pain impulses within the spinal cord and brain. Enkephalins are found in the brain neurons; they are weaker than endorphins but more potent than morphine and last longer. Dynorphins found in the hypothalamus, PAG, and dorsal horn of the spinal cord are potent endorphins that impede pain signals but can also incite pain. Endomorphins are peptides formed in the brain that have high affinity for morphine receptors and cause vasodilation due to release of nitric acid from endothelial cells. When the PAG is stimulated, these opioids are released; concurrent serotonin release

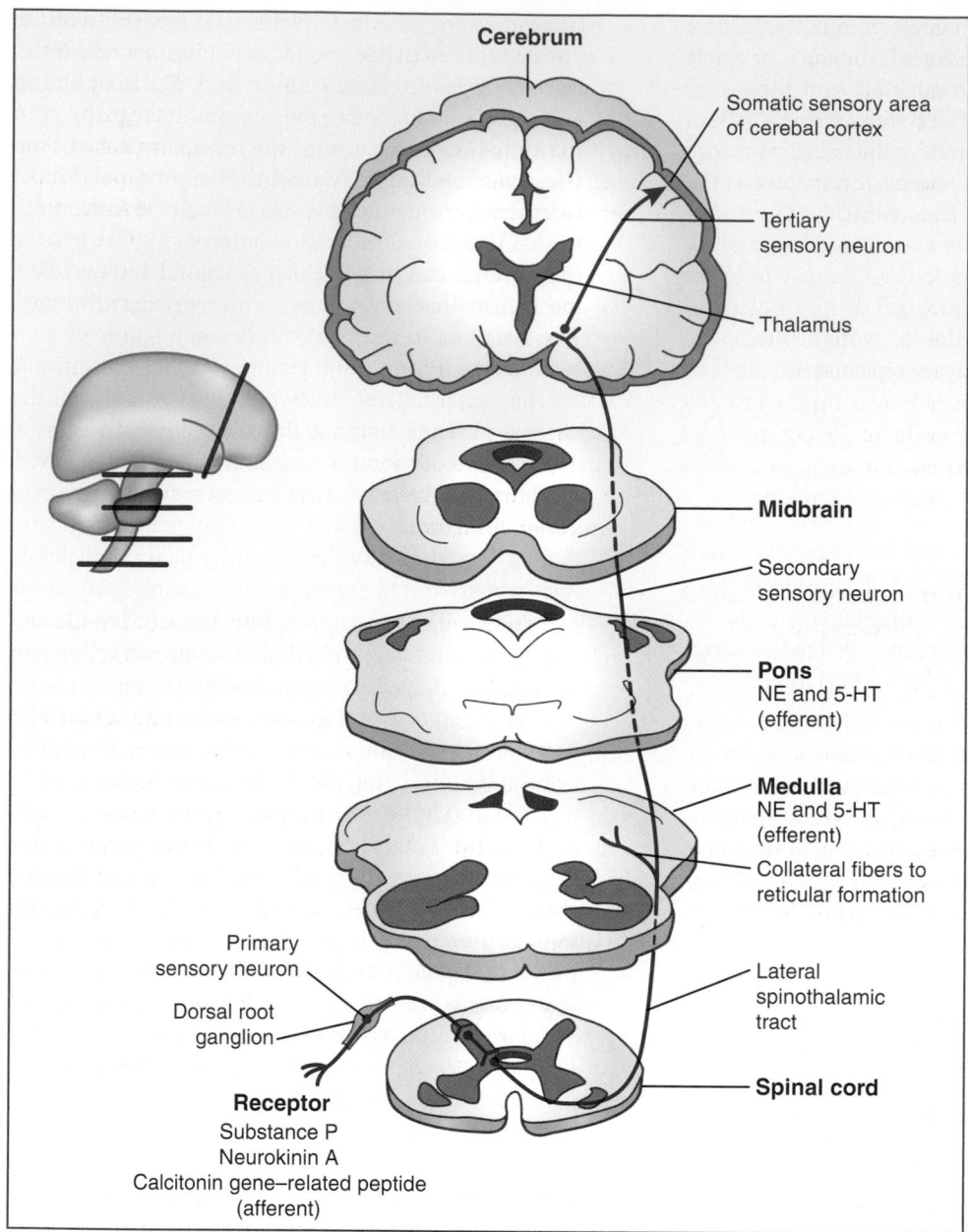

Figure 52–1. Anatomy of pain transmission.

Labels in figure:

Cerebrum

Somatic sensory area of cerebal cortex

Tertiary sensory neuron

Thalamus

Midbrain

Secondary sensory neuron

Pons
NE and 5-HT (efferent)

Medulla
NE and 5-HT (efferent)

Collateral fibers to reticular formation

Primary sensory neuron

Dorsal root ganglion

Lateral spinothalamic tract

Spinal cord

Receptor
Substance P
Neurokinin A
Calcitonin gene–related peptide
(afferent)

sends analgesic signals to the raphe magnus. Neurons projecting from the rostral pons to the raphe magnus secrete norepinephrine, which also has an analgesic effect.

Pain Modulation

The brain, spinal cord, and peripheral tissues contain opioid receptors— mu (μ), kappa (κ), and delta (δ)—to modulate pain perceptions. The μ and κ receptors have primary analgesic activity; other functions of the μ receptors are euphoria and respiratory depression, and the κ receptors produce sedative effects. The δ receptors have less analgesic activity but do have antidepressant effects. The μ and δ receptors are also responsible for physical dependence. Sigma (σ) receptors are no longer considered opioid receptors because they produce stress-related depression and dysphoria as well as other psychomimetic effects rather than analgesia; they are targets for drugs like phencyclidine (PCP) (Trescot, Datta, Lee, & Hansen, 2008).

In addition to CNS activity, the pituitary gland contains high levels of β-endorphins, which are believed to be released in times of pain or stress. The adrenal glands also release endogenous opioids as a stress response but these endorphins, which are released into the bloodstream, cannot effectively cross the blood–brain barrier, so the effects occur in the periphery. Endorphins are found in nerve endings, immune-related cells, and the CNS. Endorphins are released in times of stress, extreme physical exertion, acupuncture, or intercourse to raise the amount of endorphins circulating in the bloodstream. All endorphins attach to opiate receptors, so increased amounts raise the pain threshold.

Special Populations

The pain assessment should include a detailed history of the pain characteristics; symptom treatment prior to the visit; the impact on function and well-being, sleep, medical and/or psychiatric conditions; and current medications. A complete physical examination should be conducted with a focus on the neurological and musculoskeletal systems to identify sensory and functional deficits. A review of the medical record will ascertain previous conditions and diagnostic test results that may contribute to the current pain complaint. Thorough data collection will help formulate a working diagnosis for the etiology of the pain and a plan for best treatment of the underlying cause and related symptoms.

The undertreatment of pain in the very young, the elderly, and in minority populations has been reported for decades. An inability to adequately report pain may contribute to lack of attention by the practitioner to evaluate the potential for pain. Understanding the multifactorial sources of pain is necessary to provide best practices in pain management.

Pediatric Patients

Neuroscientists have concluded that the nervous system is sufficiently developed before birth, which dispels the myth that infants are incapable of sensing pain. The inflammatory response is quite robust in infants and young children and can produce a greater neural response following noxious stimuli, yet enzyme systems that metabolize drugs are immature in preterm infants and neonates. Pain-producing events can have a significant impact on a young nervous system that can have lasting effects and produce a lower pain threshold for months (American Medical Association [AMA], 2013c). Older children tend to have higher pain thresholds, but responses are highly individualized.

Older Adults

Adults over age 65 can have multiple causes of pain that may not be adequately identified, which increases the risk for inadequate pain management. With aging come physiological changes in anatomy and the underlying neurophysiological mechanisms of pain along with comorbid conditions (Gibson & Helme, 2001), which can increase the pain threshold. Pain, particularly persistent pain, can be common in older adults, especially in those over age 85, most commonly due to arthritis. Older people are often reluctant to report pain for multiple reasons, and assessment can be a challenge especially in the presence of cognitive decline. The practitioner may need to clarify the words used by older adults to describe their discomfort as they are more apt to dismiss pain as part of the aging process or disease progression and may fear additional tests as well as costs.

Cognitive Impairment

Dementia and other cognitive impairments are more common in the elderly but can occur at any age. Mental capacity that is reduced does not mean physiological responses to pain are also reduced. Pain assessment becomes a challenge when patients are unable to clearly communicate their symptoms and needs. Pain that is poorly managed can result in behaviors that mimic psychological disorders, and misdiagnoses may lead to inappropriate treatment decisions.

Agitation, mood changes, withdrawal from activity, or other behavioral disturbances can be indicators of pain or distress but may not be recognized as such. The Mini Mental Status Examination (Folstein, Folstein, & McHugh, 1975) is an effective tool to screen for cognitive impairment and has been used extensively. Access to pain assessment tools for patients with dementia can be obtained through the Alzheimer's Disease Association at http://www.alz.org. The Checklist of Nonverbal Pain Indications (Feldt, 2000) is a more recent tool that specifically measures pain behaviors in cognitively impaired adults. Another useful tool, the Pain Assessment in Advanced Dementia (PAINAD) Scale, measures breathing, vocalization, facial expression, body language, and consolability in noncommunicative patients (Warden, Hurley, & Volicer, 2003). Additional pictorial pain scales used with young children can also be used to assess patients with communication limitations.

Comorbid Chronic Illnesses

Older adults are more prone to having comorbid conditions such as arthritis, cardiovascular disease, or diabetes requiring pharmacological therapy. NSAIDs used for the mild to moderate pain of arthritis have the potential for interaction with commonly prescribed drugs such as antihypertensive and antidiabetic medications. The risk of serious gastrointestinal (GI) side effects and renal toxicity are also contributors to complications. In addition, the aging process alters organ function important for the absorption, distribution, metabolism, and elimination of drugs. Patients should be carefully screened for GI disorders, hepatic and renal function, hypothyroidism, and adrenal function. NSAIDs are contraindicated in those with a history of GI bleeding. Patients with endocrine deficiencies are at risk for prolonged and exaggerated responses to opiates. Kidney dysfunction alters drug elimination, so dosing of analgesics is critical to avoid toxicity.

Pregnancy

In general, pregnant women should avoid the use of medications. The safe use of analgesics during pregnancy has not been well established and most are in Pregnancy Category C or D, indicating the practitioner should carefully weigh the benefits of therapy against the risk of fetal harm. Because research has demonstrated no fetal risk, acetaminophen, naproxen, oxycodone, and topical anesthetics are in Category B. If a pregnant woman is addicted to opiates, the newborn is subject to respiratory depression or excessive sedation in addition to drug withdrawal symptoms. The Food and Drug Administration (FDA) relabeled all extended-release and long-acting opioid analgesics in 2013 to add a boxed warning cautioning that maternal use may cause neonatal opioid withdrawal syndrome (FDA, 2013).

Substance Abuse

The overuse of alcohol or prescription or recreational drugs is a prevalent societal issue. Any practitioner who treats acute or chronic pain is likely to face the dilemma of selecting appropriate treatment for a known or suspected substance abuser who presents with a complaint of pain. Chronic over-use of addictive substances alters the brain's neurochemistry, neurotransmission, and interactions within the reward structures in the frontal cortex that control motivation, memory, impulse, and craving. Problems in the frontal cortex lead to altered judgment, impulsivity, and a dysfunctional need for gratification. Development of these brain structures are still in process into adolescence and young adulthood, an important factor to consider when assessing the history and possible early exposure to addictive substances. Genetics also plays a significant role in the likelihood of addiction. Cultural factors can influence how a patient develops behaviors in a desire to be socially accepted within a group.

Addictive behaviors can be characterized as the inability to abstain from the drug of choice, impaired behavioral control, craving for drugs, inability to recognize significant problems with behaviors or relationships, or dysfunctional emotional responses (American Society of Addiction Medicine [ASAM], 2011). Pseudoaddiction is described as addiction-like behaviors such as "clock-watching" that occur when pain is undertreated. A distinction can be made between addiction and pseudoaddiction when eliciting history and pain assessment data because patients with pseudoaddiction no longer exhibit these drug-related behaviors when pain is effectively treated (AMA, 2013c, 2013d).

When considering prescribing potentially abusable drugs, the American Academy of Pain Medicine and the American Society of Addiction Medicine (2001) recommend using the following definitions to determine the degree of substance abuse disorder:

- *Addiction* is a primary, chronic, neurobiological disease, with genetic, psychosocial, and environmental factors influencing its development and manifestations. It is characterized by behaviors that include one or more of the following: impaired control over drug use, compulsive use, continued use despite harm, and craving.
- *Physical dependence* is a state of adaptation that is manifested by a drug class-specific withdrawal syndrome that can be produced by abrupt cessation, rapid dose reduction, decreasing blood level of the drug, and/or administration of an antagonist.
- *Tolerance* is a state of adaptation in which exposure to a drug induces changes that result in a diminution of one or more of the drug's effects over time.

Patients with addiction are often extremely anxious about insufficient receipt of pain medications in association with trauma, disease, or surgery, which may influence how they express their pain. Practitioners should assure these patients that acute pain will be adequately treated despite the addiction (AMA, 2013d). Those who are opioid-dependent may require higher doses to reduce acute pain due to higher tolerance. Decision making about choice of drug, dosing, and scheduling should be shared to provide the patient with a sense of control and satisfaction that pain relief will be achieved.

ACUTE PAIN

Acute pain can be due to mechanical or thermal stimulation of nociceptive receptors in somatic or visceral tissues. Symptoms are of sudden onset and generally disappear when healing occurs.

Pathophysiology

Acute pain may be somatic, visceral, referred, neuropathic, or psychogenic in origin. A patient may experience single or multiple types of pain. Afferent neurons, A-delta fibers and C-fibers, are found in the skin, muscle, connective tissues, joints, and in some visceral tissues. A-delta fibers are myelinated and respond to thermal and mechanical sources; stimuli are fast-traveling and highly localized. C-fibers are unmyelinated and are activated by multiple sources; stimuli are poorly localized and impulses travel more slowly than through A-delta fibers.

Somatic pain involves skin, joints, bone, muscle, or connective tissue and is generally localized and described as aching, throbbing, stabbing, squeezing, stinging, pinching, or sharp. Examples might be burns, arthritis, or metastatic bone pain. Somatic pain responds well to NSAIDs, acetaminophen, corticosteroids, opiates, and topical applications of anesthetics, cold, or heat. *Visceral* pain arises from hollow organs and is often described as dull, aching, and burning, gnawing, or cramping sensations. Tissue damage to organs such as the heart produces complaints of sharp, stabbing, or throbbing pain and other descriptors similar to somatic pain. The use of opiates, NSAIDs, and corticosteroids are useful for this type of pain.

Referred pain can be perceived at a more distant site; some patterns are clinically relevant. Examples might be pain referred to the right shoulder from inflammation of the gallbladder or pain in the groin due to ureteral colic (Fig. 52-2).

Neuropathic pain is felt along dermatomes and can originate in central or peripheral nerves (Fig. 52-3). It is described as tingling, prickling, burning, or shock-like. Examples of this type of pain might be neuropathy due to herpes zoster or trigeminal neuralgia, or radiculopathy in an extremity from compression on a spinal nerve root.

More problematic is a report of pain that has no identifiable physiological etiology. The phenomenon of *psychogenic* pain is often seen in patients with psychiatric conditions or psychosocial disorders. Psychogenic pain can be a component of acute pain or caused by an array of reactive psychosocial disturbances. Assessment is complex and the practitioner should evaluate both the pain component and the psychiatric problem. The neurotransmitters norepinephrine and serotonin play a role in depression but also modulate sensitivity to pain in the efferent pathways. For psychologically based pain, traditional analgesics are not indicated (Agency for Healthcare Research and Quality [AHRQ], 2011).

Signs and Symptoms

Acute pain is typically associated with stimulation of the nociceptors arising from tissue injury. Signs and symptoms

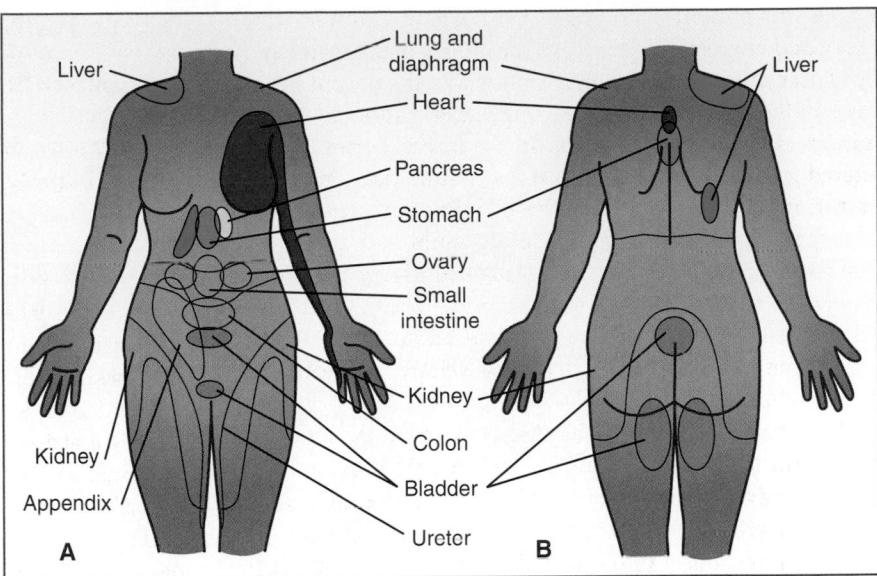

Figure 52–2. Referred pain sites.

include both physiological responses in the sympathetic nervous system and behaviors used to express pain. The practitioner should be alert to physiological responses, which include increased heart rate and blood pressure, increased respiratory rate, dilated pupils, diaphoresis, and pallor as blood flow to the skin decreases. Elevation of blood sugar can occur. Gastric motility and blood flow to the viscera decrease and can produce nausea and vomiting. Behavioral signs can range from stoicism and stillness to demonstrative expressions such as grimacing, moaning, crying, guarding, rocking, or pacing (Table 52-2).

Pain management is dependent on a detailed pain history and appropriate physical examination. Information about the onset, location, duration, characteristics, aggravating or relieving factors, and self-treatment is essential. Information regarding characteristics and intensity can be obtained through the use of pain scales. The numeric pain scale measures pain intensity on a 0 to 10 scale with 0 being no pain straight line with dichotomous endpoints. The patient marks a point on the line that correlates to the pain intensity and then the length of the line to the mark is measured in millimeters. The Brief Pain Inventory (BPI) is multidimensional and includes four pain intensity scales and seven scales that measure the pain impact on activity, mood, relationships, sleep, and quality of life (Daut, Cleeland, & Flanery, 1983). The McGill Pain Questionnaire (MPQ) is a tool that assesses three pain dimensions—sensory, affective, and evaluative—in sets of words the patient chooses that describe the pain, which, in turn, may suggest to the practitioner the underlying etiology (Melzack, 1975).

A review of past medical records and diagnostic studies should be included in the pain assessment. It is also important to obtain a history of potential substance abuse, which typically begins by asking about past or current smoking and use of alcohol and progresses to specific questions about recreational and prescription drug use. Other data may

include the patient's mood, coping strategies, and pain interference with activities of daily living. The practitioner should develop a working diagnosis for the pain etiology and a plan of care that may include additional diagnostic studies and treatments.

Pain assessment in infants and children younger than 18 months can be a challenge due to their inability to verbally express their discomfort. Validated pain scales for preterm and term infants can be used to monitor behaviors. The Premature Infant Pain Profile (Stevens, Johnston, Petryshen, & Taddio, 1996) and the CRIES Postoperative Pain Scale (Grunau, Johnston, & Craig, 1990) combine physiological measurements along with facial expressions to determine the degree of pain. The FLACC (Face, Legs, Activity, Cry and Consolability) Scale (Merkle, Shayvitz, Voelpel-Lewis, & Malviya, 1997) is a behavioral scale that can be used in children 2 months to 7 years in age. A pain score is calculated after observing the child for 5 minutes. Children as young as 18 months may be able to indicate their discomfort; children ages 3 to 4 years and older have acquired words they can use to report the pain location and describe its characteristics. They can generally use self-report pain scales such as the Wong-Baker Faces Scale (Hockenberry & Wilson, 2012), the Oucher Scale (Beyer, Denyes, & Villaruel, 1992), or the Poker Chip Scale (Hester, Foster, & Kristensen, 1990). School-age children may be able to use adult scales such as the Numeric Rating Scale or the Visual Analog Scale. Questionnaires have also been developed for children with chronic pain and include the Children's Comprehensive Pain Questionnaire (Ross & Ross, 1990) and the Varni-Thompson Pediatric Pain Questionnaire (Varni, Thompson, & Hanson, 1987).

Practitioners should take a thorough pain history and assess for pain as a routine part of the elderly patient's visit. The physical exam should focus on the musculoskeletal and neurological systems. Functional and range of motion testing

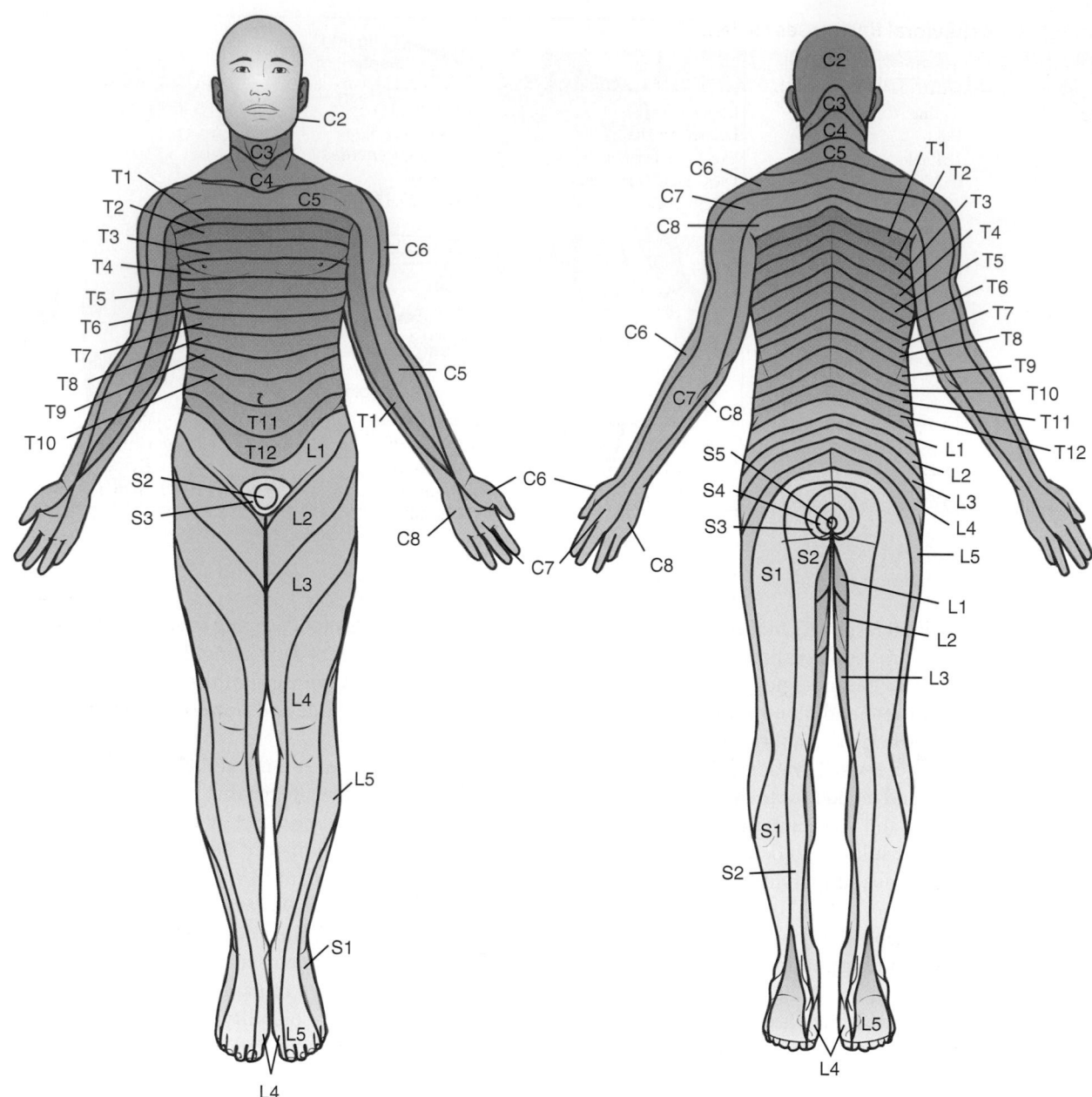

Levels of principal dermatomes

C5	Clavicles	**T10**	Level of umbilicus
C5, 6, 7	Lateral parts of upper limbs	**T12**	Inguinal or groin regions
C8, T1	Medial sides of upper limbs	**L1, 2, 3, 4**	Anterior and inner surfaces of lower limbs
C6	Thumb	**L4, 5, S1**	Foot
C6, 7, 8	Hand	**L4**	Medial side of great toe
C8	Ring and little fingers	**S1, S2, L5**	Posterior and outer surfaces of lower limbs
T4	Level of nipples	**S1**	Lateral margin of foot and little toe
		S2, 3, 4	Perineum

Figure 52–3. Spinal dermatomes.

should be included in the pain assessment. Cognitive ability is also an important part of the assessment process; look for new or worsening symptoms along with evaluation for depression or anxiety, which can accompany persistent pain. Using common visual analog or numeric rating scales are useful but geriatric pain assessment tools may better assist in the overall assessment of pain in the elderly. Patients with cognitive deficits may do better with the Faces Scale or other pictures. Pain has a significant impact on quality of life in the older adult and should not be overlooked.

Table 52–2 Behavioral Responses to Pain

Age Group	Vocalizations	Facial Expressions	Body Movements	Coping Strategies
Infants	Crying Fussy Irritable	Lowered brows Drawn together Eyes closed (young infant) Eyes open (older infant) Mouth open	Generalized body responses; rigid or thrashing (young infant) Localized body response; withdraws stimulated area (older infant)	Oral stimulation (sucking) Crying Fetal position
Toddlers/ Preschoolers	Crying Screaming Asks to stop painful stimulus Points to area of pain	Eyes closed or open Furrowed brow	Physical resistance Uncooperative Restless Clinging	Oral stimulation Crying while sleeping (toddlers) Rocking Lying still or being active (preschoolers)
School age	Crying Verbalizing pain Quality, location, duration	Withdrawn facial expression Furrowed brow	Muscle rigidity Gritted teeth Clenched fists Splinting/guarding Lying still	Verbal stalling Being active or lying still Talking about the pain Using distraction techniques Sleeping Playing or watching television
Adolescents	Verbalizing pain Crying	Withdrawn Eyes closed Furrowed brow	Muscle tension and body control Splinting/guarding Lying still	Verbalizing pain Taking medication or initiating actions to relieve pain Sleeping Lying still
Adults	Groaning Moaning Sobbing Grunting Shouting Praying Crying out for help	Frowning Staring Furrowed brow Teeth clenching	Thrashing Tossing Rocking Muscle rigidity	Protective behaviors Posturing Massaging
Elderly	Sighing Moaning Grunting Chanting Praying Crying for help	Eyes squeezed closed Withdrawn look Furrowed brow Staring	Rocking Clutching side rails Muscle rigidity	Wandering Rubbing Guarding

Source: Schaffler, R. (2007). Pain management. In K. Hoyt & J. Selfridge-Thomas (Eds.), *Emergency nursing core curriculum* (6th ed., p 148). St. Louis, MO: Saunders. Reprinted with permission.

Pharmacodynamics

The use of nonopioid and opioid analgesics is the primary intervention to reduce or alleviate pain. Anti-inflammatory drugs and opiates are the two primary classes used to treat acute pain (Table 52-3). Corticosteroids also have value in reducing inflammation. In addition to analgesics, nonpharmacological strategies may also be used such as physical therapy, massage therapy, complementary and alternative medicine (CAM), and biofeedback or other behavioral or psychological interventions.

Anti-Inflammatory Drugs

Pain is commonly caused by inflammation at the cellular level. Anti-inflammatories are often the first-line drugs to manage acute pain symptoms and are generally administered orally. This class of drugs interrupts the chemical mediators released from destruction of cell membranes at the site of injury. The COX enzyme discussed earlier is the target of these drugs, which include salicylates, acetaminophen, and nonsteroidal anti-inflammatory (NSAID) agents. Although the exact mechanism of NSAIDs is not known, it is believed they inhibit the action of the COX enzyme and the production and synthesis of prostaglandins, thus reducing inflammation and pain.

The COX enzyme consists of three currently identified isoenzymes. COX-1 is continuously present (constitutive) in all body cells and tissues with concentration in the endothelium; in platelets to cause aggregation; in the stomach to regulate acid and mucous production; and in the microvasculature, glomerulus, and collecting ducts in the kidney to regulate water excretion. COX-2 is not normally present in tissues but rapidly increases in concentration when inflammation is present

Table 52–3 Common Analgesics Used for Pain Relief

Classification	Drug	Indication	Contraindications	Side Effects	Route
Nonopioids	Acetaminophen (Tylenol, APAP and others)	Mild to moderate pain	Hypersensitivity; active liver disease or severe dysfunction; alcoholism	Generally safe and well tolerated; unsafe with hepatic dysfunction or acute toxicity, gastric upset, bleeding, prolonged prothrombin time; CNS and metabolic toxicity at high dosages or with prolonged use	Oral, rectal
	Salicylates (aspirin products)	Mild to moderate pain	Hypersensitivity; bleeding disorders; vitamin K deficiency; peptic ulcer disease; do not administer to children with flu-like symptoms because of its risk of Reye's syndrome		Oral, rectal
	NSAIDs (ibuprofen, indomethacin, ketorolac, naproxyn, diclofenac, celecoxib)	Mild to moderate pain	Hypersensitivity to NSAIDs or aspirin; active GI bleeding or ulcer disease; severe hepatic or renal disease; not recommended during pregnancy	GI symptoms, bleeding; hepatitis; rash; headache	Oral, IM, IV
Selected Analgesic Adjuncts	Gabapentin (Neurontin)	Neuropathic pain and fibromyalgia	Hypersensitivity; lactation	Confusion, depression, drowsiness; vertigo, ataxia; dry mouth	Oral
	Pregabalin (Lyrica)				Oral
	Tramadol (Ultram)	Moderate to moderately severe pain	Hypersensitivity; alcohol intoxication, CNS depression; opioid dependency; pregnancy, lactation	Seizures, dizziness, somnolence, GI symptoms, serotonin syndrome	Oral
Opioids	Codeine	Mild to moderate pain	Hypersensitivity; severe respiratory depression; severe renal, hepatic, or pulmonary disease; pregnancy; alcoholism; MAO inhibitor therapy within past 2–4 weeks; lactation; use cautiously in head trauma	Sedation, confusion; Respiratory depression, apnea; hypotension; nausea/vomiting; constipation; urinary retention; seizures	Oral, rectal
	Fentanyl (Sublimaze)	Moderate to severe pain; procedural sedation			IV, IM, transdermal, transmucosal
	Hydromophone (Dilaudid)	Moderate to severe pain			Oral, IM, IV, subcutaneous
	Morphine sulfate	Moderate to severe pain			Oral, rectal, IM, IV, subcutaneous, transdermal patch
	Oxycodone (Oxycontin, Percocet, Percodan, Tylox)	Moderate to severe pain			Oral, rectal
	Hydrocodone (Lortab, Vicodin, Ibudone)	Moderate to severe pain			Oral
	Oxymorphone (Opana)	Moderate to severe pain			Oral, IM, IV, subcutaneous
	Meperidine (Demerol)	Moderate to severe pain			Oral, IM, IV, SC
	Tapentadol (Nucynta)	Moderate to severe pain			Oral
	Methadone (Dolophine)	Severe pain; suppress withdrawal symptoms in opioid detoxification			Oral, IM, subcutaneous

Table 52–3   Common Analgesics Used for Pain Relief—cont'd

Classification	Drug	Indication	Contraindications	Side Effects	Route
Local Anesthetics/ Analgesics	Lidocaine (Xylocaine, Mepivacaine, Carbocaine) Procaine (Novocaine) Tetracaine (Pontocaine)	Infiltration, nerve blocks, topical, relief of pain of procedures or dermatological conditions	Hypersensitivity; use cautiously in severe hepatic disease, heart failure, respiratory depression, shock, or heart block; pregancy or lactation; geriatric or patients weighing less than 50 kg (110 lb)	Seizures, cardiovascular collapse; anaphylaxis; CNS toxicity, confusion, drowsiness Readily absorbed through mucous membranes Safety of patch not established in children	Topical, patch, infiltrate, mucosal
	LET (Lidocaine, epinephrine, tetracaine) EMLA cream (2.5 % lidocaine + 2.5% prilocaine)	Safer than TAC because it does not containe cocaine)			
	Capsaicin (Capzasin. Zostrix, Icy Hot, Salonpas)	Minor pain from arthritis sprains, herpes zoster, or diabetic neuropathy	Hypersensitivity to hot peppers Not for use near open skin or in eyes	BP increase, cough, transient burning sensation	Topical, transdermal patch

Adapted from Schaffler, R. (2007). Pain management. In K. Hoyt & J. Selfridge-Thomas (Eds.), *Emergency nursing core curriculum* (6th ed., pp 153–155). St. Louis, MO: Saunders.

(inducible). COX-3 has been more recently identified and is located only in the CNS within the blood–brain barrier. The properties of COX-3, also inducible, are to mediate central analgesia and to provide antipyretic activity.

Nonselective NSAIDs inhibit both COX-1 and COX-2 isoenzymes; the ratio varies by drug. COX-1 inhibition decreases the availability of gastroprotective prostaglandins, which is a primary factor in the development of adverse GI effects, particularly erosion and bleeding. Specific COX-2 inhibition is increased with celecoxib (Celebrex), currently the only drug on the market in this class, but which carries a Black-Box Warning of increased risk for cardiovascular events.

NSAIDS, as a class, bind to plasma proteins tightly, and interactions with other drugs commonly occur when they compete for binding sites. For example, platelet action is blocked by aspirin and other NSAIDs, which may have an effect on low-dose aspirin use associated with cardiovascular disease. The decision to initiate NSAID therapy must include consideration of the risk:benefit ratio.

Opioids

Opioids act on both central and peripheral pain receptors, most notably the μ and κ receptors, to inhibit the transmission and perception of pain impulses. Opioids are further classified according to their binding action at opioid receptor sites. Full agonists are the most widely prescribed and include morphine, codeine, hydrocodone, oxycodone, fentanyl, hydromorphone, methadone, and meperidine. Partial agonists (e.g., buprenorphine) have decreased activity at the μ sites, and mixed agonist-antagonists (e.g., butorphanol, nalbuphine) have action that can either bind or block opiates at receptor sites. Most have an analgesic ceiling that relates to

opioid-related side effects. Opioids have a high abuse potential and can cause withdrawal symptoms, especially in patients who are physically dependent on agonist opioids.

Agonist drugs can be further classified into categories based on duration of action. Short-acting opioids (4 to 6 hours), like morphine, require more frequent dosing to maintain a therapeutic effect. Long-acting opioids (8 hours or more) have long half-lives and release the drug more slowly. Examples include extended-release preparations of oxycodone, oxymorphone, morphine, and fentanyl and long-acting agents like methadone; these drugs may be preferred when managing chronic pain.

Adverse effects at the μ sites include euphoria, which is an incentive for abuse and contributes to dependence, as well as undesired effects of respiratory depression, constipation, and urinary retention. Tramadol is non-narcotic but acts on μ receptors to produce centrally acting analgesia. This drug also inhibits the reuptake of serotonin and norepinephrine, which provides dual-action pain relief. Sedation is produced at the κ sites without the other side effects. Naloxone is an antagonist for both μ and κ receptors and is the agent of choice for reversing the effects of opioids.

Goals of Treatment

The goal of treatment for acute pain is complete relief. In some cases, this may not be possible, so reduction may be a more realistic outcome. In either case, pain management with the least amount of adverse effects is desirable.

Addiction and Dependency

Opiates carry a high risk for tolerance, dependence, and abuse but are still appropriate to use for pain management with monitoring. Practitioners should be aware of the red flags for addiction or dependency, which include the following:

- Concurrent use of alcohol or illicit drugs used for recreation
- Frequent need for dose escalations
- Multiple episodes of prescription loss
- Seeking prescriptions from multiple providers
- Prescription forgery
- Selling prescription drugs or buying from unauthorized sources
- Resisting change in therapy from pills to other modalities

Screening for substance abuse risk can be done with the use of questionnaires. Two popular tools are the CAGE-AID and the Drug Abuse Screening Test (DAST).

- CAGE-AID (Brown & Rounds, 1995) asks if the patient has ever
  - Felt you ought to cut down on your drinking or drug use?
  - Had people annoy you by criticizing your drinking or drug use?
  - Felt bad or guilty about the consequences of your drinking or drug use?
  - Had a drink or used drugs first thing in the morning to steady your nerves or to get rid of a hangover (eye-opener)?

Scoring for item responses are "0" for no and 1 for "yes." While the normal cutoff for this tool is two positive answers, it is recommended that primary care practitioners lower the threshold to one positive answer to identify more patients who may have a substance abuse disorder.

The DAST questionnaire (Gavin, Ross, & Skinner, 1989) has been found useful in screening for drugs of abuse other than alcohol. The tool consists of 28 questions:

- Have you used drugs other than those required for medical reasons?
- Have you abused prescription drugs?
- Do you abuse more than one drug at a time?
- Can you get through the week without using drugs?
- Are you always able to stop using drugs when you want to?
- Do you abuse drugs on a continuous basis?
- Do you try to limit your drug use to certain situations?
- Have you had "blackouts" or "flashbacks" as a result of drug use?
- Do you ever feel bad about your drug abuse?
- Does your spouse (or parents) ever complain about your involvement with drugs?
- Do your friends or relatives know or suspect you abuse drugs?
- Has drug abuse ever created problems between you and your spouse?
- Has any family member ever sought help for problems related to your drug use?
- Have you ever lost friends because of your use of drugs?
- Have you ever neglected your family or missed work because of your use of drugs?

- Have you ever been in trouble at work because of drug abuse?
- Have you ever lost a job because of drug abuse?
- Have you gotten into fights when under the influence of drugs?
- Have you ever been arrested because of unusual behavior while under the influence of drugs?
- Have you ever been arrested for driving while under the influence of drugs?
- Have you engaged in illegal activities in order to obtain drugs?
- Have you ever been arrested for possession of illegal drugs?
- Have you ever experienced withdrawal symptoms as a result of heavy drug intake?
- Have you had medical problems as a result of your drug use (e.g., memory loss, hepatitis, convulsions, bleeding, etc.)?
- Have you ever gone to anyone for help for a drug problem?
- Have you ever been in a hospital for medical problems related to your drug use?
- Have you ever been involved in a treatment program specifically related to drug use?
- Have you been treated as an outpatient for problems related to drug abuse?

A score of 1 is recorded for each "yes" answer except for items 4, 5, and 7, for which a score of 1 is given for a "no" answer. A total score of 12 or more is considered to be indicative of a substance abuse problem.

When substance abuse is suspected or detected, a pain contract may be appropriate. Opioids have been implicated in accidental death or even suicide due to overdose, particularly in combination with alcohol or other drugs. Setting clear expectations and responsibilities is critical to achieve mutually set treatment goals.

Rational Drug Selection

An algorithm for the management of acute pain is seen in Figure 52-4. Drug selection should be made based on the overall severity of the pain, side-effect profile, and the suspected source of pain. Nonopioids can provide effective relief for many types of acute pain and inflammation. Salicylates, acetaminophen, and NSAIDs are useful for somatic, dental, arthritic, traumatic, and post-operative pain of mild to moderate intensity. They differ from opioids in that they inhibit prostaglandin formation, have antipyretic properties, and are not associated with dependence or addiction. Regular use of nonopioids carries risks for bleeding and has potential for interaction with other drugs that may be taken on a regular basis (see Chapter 25).

Researchers (Coxib and Traditional NSAID Trialists' Collaboration, 2013) recently conducted a meta-analysis of more than 600 studies showing the effects of long-term (1-year) use of NSAIDs. Findings included a significant increase in major vascular and coronary events, including death, occurring with long-term use of high-dose coxibs and

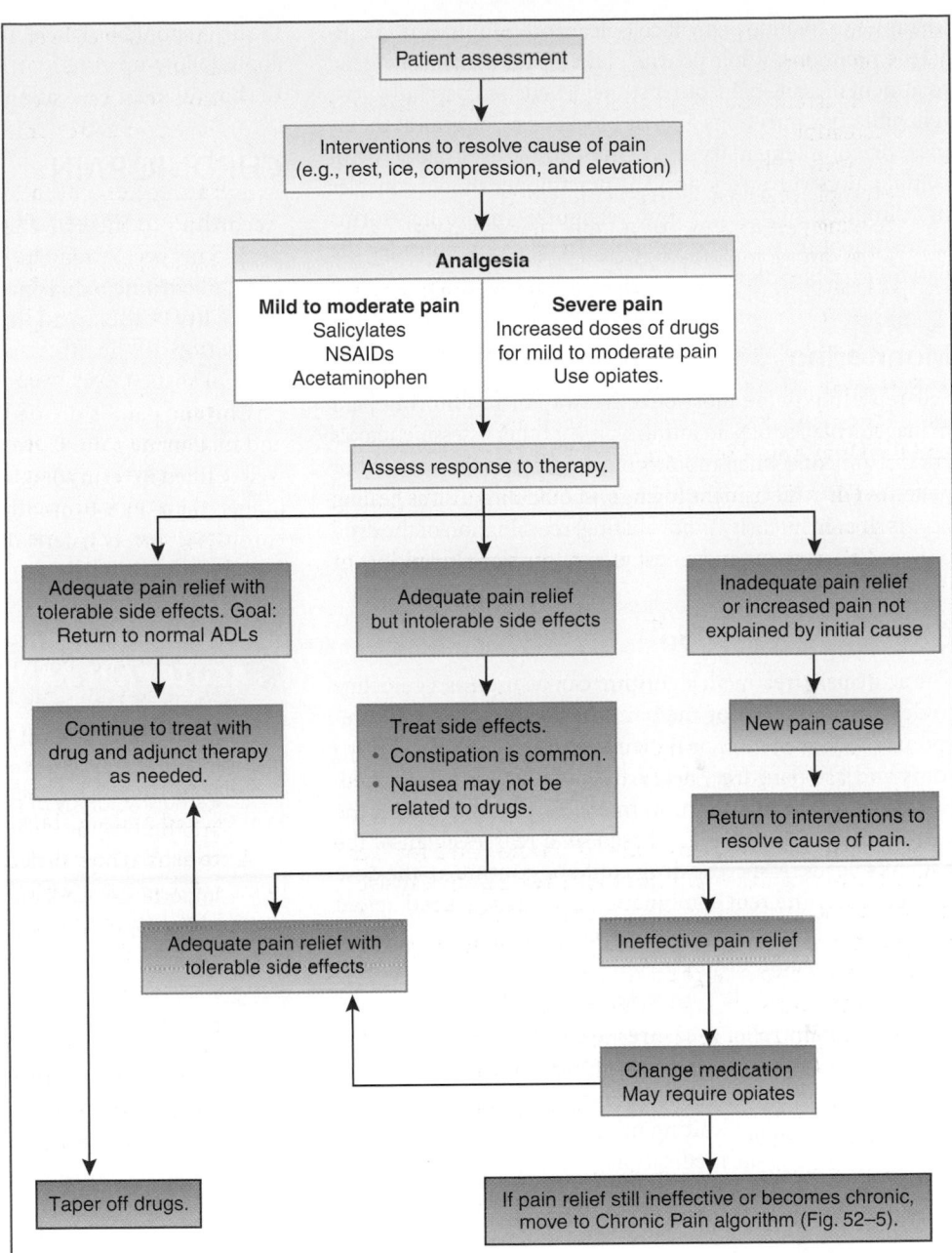

Figure 52–4. Acute pain management algorithm.

diclofenac; ibuprofen significantly increased coronary events but not vascular; and naproxen showed no increased risk for vascular or coronary events. The risk of heart failure was nearly doubled with all NSAIDs, and all NSAIDs increased GI complications. The practitioner should keep this information in mind when choosing to prescribe NSAIDs. Coxibs and diclofenac should be avoided in patients with known heart disease and cautiously in patients with high risk for coronary or vascular events.

Opioids are meant for short-term use and should be reserved for moderate to severe acute pain that is not well controlled with nonopioid analgesics. This therapeutic class of drugs carries risk for potential tolerance or abuse, and pain management should be monitored as to drug effect and pain reduction. The best choices for moderate pain are codeine,

oxycodone, and hydrocodone, usually in combination with acetaminophen or aspirin. Morphine, oxycodone, hydromorphone, oxymorphone, or fentanyl are better choices for severe pain. Hydromorphone in high doses is more potent than morphine and could be considered in special cases. Meperidine is no longer a favorable drug to use for pain management due to its degradation to neurotoxic metabolites and association with tremors, delirium, and seizures. Neuropathic pain can be effectively treated with anticonvulsants such as gabapentin and pregabalin, which are analgesic adjuncts that bind to calcium channels in CNS tissue and stabilize neuronal membranes, thus interfering with the transmission of pain impulses rather than binding to opioid receptors.

There is no single approach for the use of drugs to manage pain. Treatment requires skillful application of multimodal therapies to include pharmacological and nonpharmacological interventions. While pharmacotherapy is a mainstay in the treatment of acute pain, other strategies such as psychological, rehabilitative, injections and/or blockades, behavioral therapies, or complementary medicine can be used alone or in combination with analgesics. The practitioner should consider the simplest approaches but recognize that other forms of treatment may also be valuable. In all cases, consider the patient variables discussed earlier.

Monitoring

Self-reporting is the most effective way of monitoring pain management. Use of pain rating scales or other assessment tools are instrumental when monitoring trends in pain intensity or patterns. For acute pain the intensity should diminish as healing occurs. If pain intensity is not abating, reevaluation of the drug or dose should occur and a new plan of care developed.

Outcome Evaluation

The acute pain treatment algorithm can be used as a guideline to develop and monitor the pain management plan and responses to treatment. For patients who have relief of symptoms and are pain free, no further treatment is indicated. For those who remain symptomatic, further changes in the treatment plan can be made based on a reassessment of the patient's needs. A specific drug could be continued, the dose changed, or a different combination of nonopioid and opioid drugs could be used. Nonpharmacological therapies could also be tried. Questions to consider at this phase of treatment could be:

- What pain relief measures are currently being used? Should additional or different measures be tried?
- When is the pain medication being used? Is it timely? Is the individual waiting until the pain becomes severe before taking the medication? Fixed intervals have been shown to be more effective in controlling pain than "as-needed" dosing.
- Does the individual believe the treatment plan is effective? There tends to be a placebo effect for pain treatment and if a patient believes a drug will be effective, it likely will be; and if he or she believes a drug will not be effective, the expected outcome will likely not occur.

If the response to initial or readjusted therapy is not successful, or if complications related to the pain source arise, the individual may need consultation with a specialist. If the complications are related to the pain medication, referral to a pain specialist may be prudent, especially in the case of dependency or addiction, even if pain relief is accomplished.

Patient Education

The practitioner should provide education about the drug, its side effects, dosing regimen, and the expected length of time the drug should be taken. The patient should also be informed about follow-up visits, particularly if complications occur. See the box "Patient Education: Acute Pain Management."

CHRONIC PAIN

According to the IOM (2011) report, nearly 120 million people in the United States suffer from chronic pain. The effect of chronic pain is profound on ability to function and on quality of life. In addition, chronic pain leads to higher utilization of health care, lost productivity, and other societal costs.

Chronic pain is divided into categories of nonmalignant and malignant pain. Chronic pain, unlike acute pain, is less well defined in terms of its onset and duration. It usually lasts longer than 3 to 6 months. Pain can also be classified as chronic if it meets criteria of lasting a month beyond the usual

---

ACUTE PAIN MANAGEMENT — PATIENT EDUCATION

Related to the Overall Treatment Plan and Disease Process

☐ Pathophysiology of pain and its cause (where appropriate), at a level the patient can understand, to explain how the drugs work.

☐ Importance of adherence to the treatment regimen.

☐ Indications for contacting the health-care provider when pain relief is ineffective.

☐ Need for follow-up visit(s) with the primary care provider.

Specific to the Drug Therapy

☐ Reasons for taking the drug(s) and the anticipated action of these drug(s) in pain relief.

☐ Doses and schedules for taking the drug(s), including early round-the-clock dosing of drugs.

☐ Possible adverse reactions and what to do if they occur.

Reasons for Taking the Drug(s)

☐ Patient education about specific drugs is provided in Chapters 15 and 25. The explanations should be clear about what pain drugs can and cannot do.

Drugs as Part of the Total Treatment Regimen

☐ Role of both pharmacological and nonpharmacological treatments for pain and their interconnection.

Adherence Issues

☐ The fact that most acute pain can be resolved should be stressed. The importance of that resolution to avoid the development of chronic pain should be addressed.

☐ Adherence to the drug regimen is important to resolving acute pain.

course of an illness or injury, is associated with chronic pathological conditions, or if it is recurrent over weeks or months (AMA, 2013b). Recurrent pain can be a hallmark of certain disorders, such as headaches, inflammatory arthritis, dysmenorrhea, inflammatory bowel disease, musculoskeletal disorders, or sickle cell disease. Recurrent acute pain can also occur in patients with cancer or AIDS related to the disease processes, treatments, or both. When acute episodes occur in the presence of otherwise controlled underlying pain, it is known as breakthrough pain. The focus in this section will be on nonmalignant pain.

Pathophysiology

Pain experts have endorsed a key concept that when pain is persistent, it should be conceptualized as its own illness (AMA, 2013g). Pain that is present most of the time can be due to a variety of pain syndromes. The underlying cause is not always identifiable. Chronic pain is not generally associated with sympathetic activity seen in the presence of acute pain. The body has become accustomed to the pain and the nervous system has been desensitized to noxious stimuli. Changes occur over time in nerve terminals, dorsal root ganglion, afferent fibers, and the CNS, thus increasing stimulation of C-fibers and decreasing the production of endorphins. Persistent pain causes physiological adaptation over time so that blood pressure along with heart and respiratory rates remain normal. Responses to chronic pain vary and have fewer overt signs but tend to be more psychological than physical.

The origins of persistent, nonmalignant pain are often multifactorial. The etiology of chronic pain is described as nociceptive, neurogenic, or psychogenic. Chronic pain is difficult to assess in that there are often no overt signs of tissue injury, nerve damage, or inflammation.

Nociceptive Pain

Nociceptive pain infers some sort of tissue damage or inflammation to somatic or visceral tissues. In the case of chronic pain, the damage may be ongoing and insidious. Ongoing tissue injury or inflammation leads to neurochemical and neurophysiological changes that affect the nervous system, leading to persistent input along afferent neurons from a specific source as discussed earlier.

Neurogenic Pain

The underlying cause of neurogenic pain is damage to neural tissues in the central nervous system, the peripheral nervous system, or both. Characteristics of neurogenic pain are varied but are usually expressed as burning, tingling, or electric shock sensations. Neuropathic pain syndromes can also be accompanied by allodynia, hyperalgesia, hyperpathia, or referred pain. Neuralgia occurs as a result of injury to a peripheral nerve from infection or disease. Classic examples are post-herpetic neuralgia and diabetic neuropathy.

The origins of neurogenic pain are not as clear as somatic pain. Injury to a peripheral axon can result in altered nerve morphology where multiple nerve sprouts generate increased activity within weeks after the injury. These nerve sprouts can form neuromas. The areas of increased sensitivity also have changes in sodium receptor concentrations, which make them more sensitive to stimuli. Tinel's sign, a pain or tingling response to tapping over a nerve, is often positive. Over time, atypical cross-connections are developed between somatic and efferent nerves and nociceptors, which alter transmission of pain impulses. Nerve sprouts may also occur in the dorsal horn of the spinal cord following a peripheral injury. These changes also occur at sites of demyelinzation. Reports of pain may or may not be out of proportion to overt signs of injury. If peripheral injury is most likely, interventions such as release of entrapped nerves, anesthetic injection, or resection of a neuroma should be considered. In the case of a CNS injury, as seen with spinal cord trauma, there is little information about the processes that cause central pain syndromes.

Psychogenic Pain

The term *psychogenic pain* is generally used when there seems to be no physiological evidence of the source of pain, and the pain becomes predominantly unremitting due to psychological factors. There is a complex relationship between pain perception and psychological factors. Persistent pain can induce changes in mood, coping abilities, or behavior changes. Some patients develop these in the presence of chronic pain while others have underlying comorbid psychiatric disturbances that become exaggerated when pain is unrelieved. All patients who present with suspected psychogenic pain may be inappropriately labeled and stigmatized, so it is imperative to conduct both physical and psychological assessments before making a judgment.

Pharmacodynamics

NSAIDs and opioids are commonly prescribed for patients with chronic pain. Due to an added psychological factor associated with chronic pain, patients who exhibit signs of depression or anxiety may require medications such as SNRIs or TCAs to manage those symptoms. Patients with neurogenic pain may benefit from the use of anticonvulsants.

The transmission of pain impulses is inhibited by the presence of norepinephrine in the rostral pons and serotonin in the PAG. These neurotransmitters also play a role in mood stabilization. Decreased levels of norepinephrine and serotonin are common in depression. SNRIs inhibit the reuptake of serotonin and norepinephrine into nerve terminals thus making more of the transmitter available at the synapses.

Originally developed to treat depression, TCAs are now more commonly used to treat neuropathic pain syndromes and insomnia, which can accompany chronic pain. Full analgesic effect may take several weeks or months. TCAs also block the reuptake of norepinephrine and serotonin but have a more significant side-effect profile due to their additional blockage of histaminergic, dopaminergic, adrenergic, and muscarinic receptors. Of particular note is the risk for dysrhythmias and suicidal thoughts.

Goals of Treatment

The goal of treatment for all pain is elimination. In cases of chronic pain this is less likely to occur and a more realistic goal might be to reduce the pain to a tolerable level to maximize function and quality of life. As with acute pain management, it is desirable to meet treatment goals with minimum side effects. A comprehensive approach is needed and multimodal forms of pain relief should be incorporated into the plan of care. Mutual decision making between the patient and practitioner should be employed when choosing the drug, dosing, pain relief goals, and follow-up. Spiritual and cultural factors should be incorporated into the plan to make pain management patient-centered.

Pawar and Garten (2010) concluded that children should have chronic pain managed in the same manner as adults. Treatment is aimed at the underlying cause and associated symptoms. Oral medication is preferred and on a scheduled rather than a prn basis. It is important to consider the neurodevelopmental age of the child as well as to know how to assess pain in different age groups so that the most effective treatment plan can be implemented. A young infant may have a central respiratory problem, so opioid use should be minimized. A toddler or older child may require less medication and use play or other distraction methods to cope with pain. No analgesia should be withheld from a child due to practitioner bias or insufficient assessment.

Rational Drug Selection

An algorithm for the management of chronic pain is depicted in Figure 52-5. Treatment is not solely based on the use of drugs. Multimodal interventions are available to attain the treatment goal of reducing chronic pain while maintaining maximum function.

Lifestyle Modifications

Chronic pain frequently requires lifestyle modifications. Weight loss can be helpful in those who are overweight. Achievement of ideal body weight may not be possible but even small, incremental weight losses can be of benefit to reduce stress on muscles and joints. An increase in physical activity can help with weight loss as well as maintenance of mobility. Exercise has also been shown to have a positive effect on mood and sleep. A progressive plan of exercise should be developed to improve flexibility, strength, balance, and endurance. Walking and resistance training are low-impact exercises that are suitable for patients with chronic pain; activity can be increased based on the patient's tolerance and allows the patient to have an active role in the treatment plan.

Rehabilitative methods can improve physical functioning. Physical therapy, occupational therapy, ice, heat, massage, and aquatic therapy are useful for many types of pain but particularly for fibromyalgia.

Cognitive-Behavioral Interventions

The Institute for Clinical Systems Improvement (2011) recommended several strategies for managing chronic pain. There are a number of independent activities that do not require a specialist, such as relaxation techniques, meditation, imagery, diaphragmatic breathing, and muscle relaxation exercises. Interventions that would likely require a therapist include biofeedback, hypnosis, guided imagery, and counseling. The patient's family members as well as the practitioner can be powerful reinforcers of wellness behaviors that are beneficial to overall well-being. The patient should be encouraged to make progress visits with the practitioner on a regularly scheduled basis rather than only when the pain is out of control.

Drug Therapy

In 1986, the World Health Organization (WHO) developed a conceptual analgesic ladder to help guide the management of pain. Initially developed for cancer pain, it has since been more broadly used in the treatment of all types of pain. The ladder consists of three steps: (1) nonopioids + adjuvants such as antidepressants or antiepileptics that do not have primary indications for pain management, (2) adding an opioid for mild to moderate pain, and (3) adding a stronger opioid for moderate to severe pain. Use of these principles can help the practitioner and patient select the best treatment plan based on the overall severity of the pain and the desired outcomes.

Anti-Inflammatories

As discussed in the acute pain section, anti-inflammatory drugs can be quite useful to reduce mild to moderate pain and inflammation. NSAIDs are often the first-line drugs of choice in Step 1 of the analgesic ladder, but all carry risk of serious adverse effects, especially in the elderly who are more likely to have comorbid conditions. The patient's risk for cardiovascular disease, GI bleeding, and renal dysfunction should be assessed before recommending this class of drugs. The risk for renal insufficiency increases with chronic NSAID use, especially in diabetics. Piroxicam and indomethacin are of high risk in older adults due to CNS side effects, GI bleeding, and drug-induced hepatitis. Naproxen may be safer than diclofenac and ibuprofen when the risk of cardiovascular disease is high. Celecoxib also carries a Black-Box Warning about cardiovascular disease and should be used with caution. One specific drug should *not* be considered for chronic pain—ketorolac (Toradol)—which is meant only for short-term use that should not exceed 5 days. Acetaminophen may be a good choice for older adults but liver function should be monitored with long-term use. All patients should be cautioned to read labels for common OTC remedies also containing acetaminophen to avoid accidental overdosing.

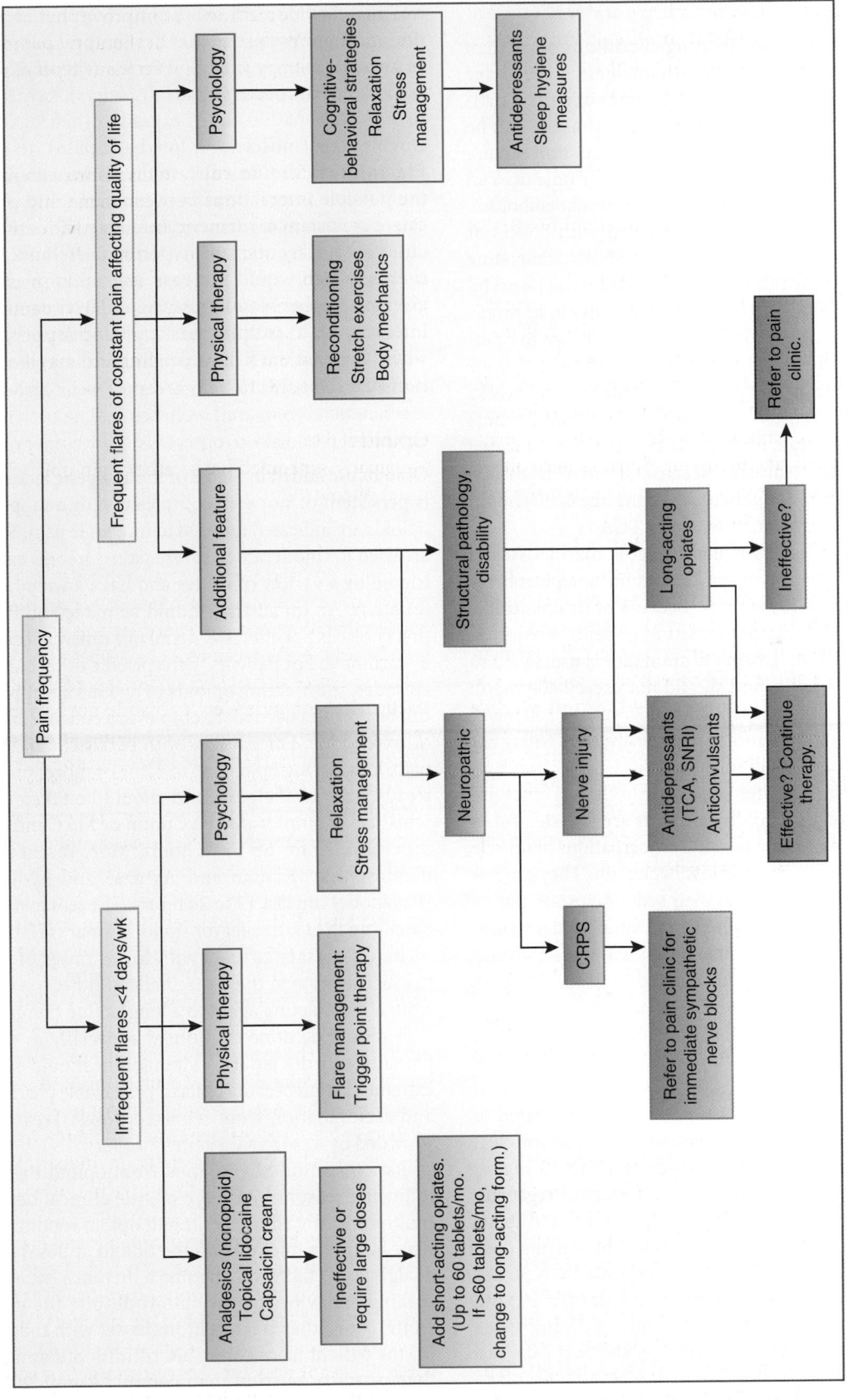

Figure 52-5. Chronic pain management algorithm.

Adjuvant Analgesics

Adjuvant drugs are used for treating conditions other than pain. However, in combination with analgesics, they have a synergistic effect to reduce multiple types of pain. Corticosteroids such as prednisone and dexamethasone can be helpful in relieving the discomfort of inflammation but are generally used short-term for this purpose. Chronic use can cause adrenal suppression, GI bleeding, or thromboembolism.

Depression or anxiety can be managed with SNRIs or TCAs along with pain modulation. Of the SNRIs, duloxetine (Cymbalta) 30 mg daily (titrated to 60 mg daily) can be useful for diabetic peripheral neuropathy with results in approximately 1 week; venlafaxine (Effexor) has also shown to be effective at doses of 150 to 225 mg daily. TCAs are effective for several types of neuropathic pain but can take up to 6 weeks for full analgesic effect. Avoid amitriptyline in older adults due to its anticholinergic effects. TCAs are contraindicated in patients with heart disease because sudden death can occur. A baseline ECG for patients over the age of 40 should be obtained prior to treatment with any TCA.

Tramadol (Ultram) is a nonopioid analgesic that binds to the μ receptor and has weak opioid and serotonin-norepinephrine reuptake inhibitor (SNRI) activity. Because of its opioid-like activity, tramadol should not be used in patients recovering from narcotic addiction. Dosing of tramadol is usually 50 to 100 mg every 4 to 6 hours and should not exceed 400 mg/d; the maximum dose in patients older than 75 years is 300 mg/d. Seizures and serotonin syndrome are adverse effects. Safety has not been established in children.

Cyclobenzaprine or other skeletal muscle relaxants are useful for fibromyalgia. Muscle relaxants are also helpful in the short-term management of acute exacerbations of muscle spasms associated with chronic low back pain. They are not helpful for long-term use due to their sedating properties.

Topical applications of anesthetics or capsaicin can be useful for neuropathic pain at peripheral sites without significant systemic effects. Other drug classes for neuropathic pain include anticonvulsants; gabapentin (Neurontin) and pregabalin (Lyrica) are recommended for diabetic neuropathy, post-herpetic neuralgia, and fibromyalgia. Gabapentin is more efficacious than TCAs in treating post-herpetic neuralgia. It is initially dosed at 300 mg 3 times a day and titrated to 900 to 1,800 mg 3 times a day; it is a suitable drug for children over the age of 3 at initial doses of 10 to 15 mg/kg 3 times a day and titrated based on age and weight. Pregabalin also has anxiolytic effects, which are helpful for mood stabilization in patients with neuropathic pain. The starting dose of pregabalin for the pain of diabetic neuropathy is 50 mg 3 times a day, then titrated over the next 7 days to 100 mg 3 times a day. The dose for fibromyalgia is 75 mg twice a day initially, then may be increased over the next 7 days to 150 mg twice a day.

Patients may also wish to use complementary or alternative therapies for chronic pain relief. Herbal preparations are not regulated nor do they undergo the rigorous testing done on pharmaceuticals; however, they may play a role in treating chronic pain conditions. Internet consumers can find multiple Web sites that list "natural pain killers" such as turmeric (fibromyalgia), feverfew (rheumatoid arthritis), eucommia (connective tissue disorders), kava kava (arthritis and neuropathic pain), capsaicin (neurogenic pain), or Devil's claw (muscle and low back pain), to name a few. Practitioners should educate themselves about herbs and the possible interactions between herbs and pharmaceuticals. For instance, turmeric interacts with anticoagulants, antidiabetic agents, antihypertensives, and hepatotoxic agents, which would increase the risk of bleeding, hypoglycemia, higher blood pressure, and liver damage; feverfew interacts with antiplatelets and antidepressants, which would increase the risk of bleeding and may worsen depression (Ulbricht, 2011).

Opioids

Opioids are added in Step 2 of the analgesic ladder when pain is persistent or not well controlled with nonopioids. Step 2 opioids are indicated for mild to moderate pain; Step 3 opioids are used for moderate to severe pain. Opioids can be administered by a variety of routes and have a wide range of drug duration. An initial trial should be made and if the drug of first choice is not effective, a trial of a different opioid or route is warranted. For patients with episodic or breakthrough pain episodes, short-acting opioids (4 to 6 hr) are appropriate and can be taken as needed. Examples are codeine, hydrocodone, or oxycodone. For patients with persistent and unrelenting pain, long-acting opioids (8 to 12 hr or more) provide a more steady state of analgesia and should be taken on a regular schedule. Examples are OxyContin or MS Contin, which can provide relief for up to 12 hours. More recent preparations of morphine (Kadian and Avinza) and hydromorphone (Palladone) can last 12 to 24 hours. The fentanyl transdermal patch can provide relief for up to 72 hours (Hattori, n.d.).

It is necessary to start with lower doses of opioids and gradually titrate to the desired effect. If necessary to convert from a short-acting agent to a long-acting opioid, the transition should be done cautiously, especially in opioid-naïve patients and the elderly. Methadone should be used with extreme caution because of its unpredictable pharmacokinetics and accumulation from repeated doses. Treatment is best provided by a pain management expert.

Patients should be weaned from opioid therapy for the following reasons: (1) there is little clinical benefit despite multiple dosing adjustments and opioid rotation, (2) the patient has poor tolerance to the opioid at doses required for analgesia, (3) there are ongoing adherence issues (e.g., drug-seeking behaviors or diversion) despite the use of a pain contract or other treatment limits set with the patient, and (4) the patient has a comorbid condition that makes opioid therapy more harmful than helpful (Argoff, 2011). Downward tapering of drug doses should be done over time by decreasing the opioid dose by 10% of the original dose each week over several weeks. Abrupt cessation or rapid tapering can precipitate seizures or withdrawal symptoms. Switching from a long-acting opioid to a short-acting one may also be helpful because some patients may do better with lower potency drugs.

To decrease the possibility of nonadherence to the treatment plan, limit the opioid supply to 7 days at the new dose during tapering. Monitor the patient during the withdrawal period for signs of abstinence syndrome, such as nausea, diarrhea, muscle pain, and myoclonus. These symptoms can be managed with clonidine (Catapres) 0.1 to 0.2 mg every 6 hours or a clonidine patch 0.1 mg over 24 hours weekly during the transition period (Washington State Agency Medical Directors' Group, 2007). Mild withdrawal symptoms may last up to 6 months after opioids have been discontinued; although the symptoms may be unpleasant, they are not serious. The patient should be monitored for behavioral changes during the tapering process and appropriate management strategies utilized.

In general, Schedule II controlled substance prescriptions are written for a 30-day supply (subject to state laws and insurance carriers) without refills, which would ordinarily require an office visit for renewal. The Drug Enforcement Administration (2006) revised its regulations to allow multiple prescriptions for Schedule II drugs in some cases, authorizing a total of a 90-day supply under the following conditions: the practice of writing multiple prescriptions is permissible under applicable state laws, the practitioner indicates on each prescription the earliest date the prescription can be filled, and the practitioner concludes there is no risk of aberrant behavior or drug abuse. Schedule III and IV controlled substances may be refilled if authorized on the prescription. These prescriptions may only be refilled up to 5 times within 6 months of the original issue date; after that time a new prescription is required.

RECLASSIFICATION OF HYDROCODONE AS SCHEDULE II

In 2013 the U.S. Food and Drug Administration (FDA) recommended that the U.S. Drug Enforcement Administration (DEA) reclassify hydrocodone from a Schedule III to a Schedule II drug due to the misuse and abuse of the drug. In October 2014 the DEA reclassified hydrocodone, the most prescribed opioid in the United States, as a Schedule II drug.

Monitoring

Periodic assessment should be made of patients treated for chronic pain. Assessment of progress toward goal attainment should include documentation of pain intensity, functional ability, and quality of life. The practitioner should observe mood, affect, and coping abilities along with a physical examination. If the patient's status is stable, these assessments can be brief; if worsening conditions or complications are encountered, a more in-depth assessment is necessary.

The practitioner should always assess for changing conditions and the risk of aberrant behaviors. For patients with a high risk of aberrant drug use, such as patients who are only interested in obtaining oral pills or who "run out" of medication before the 30-day period, other strategies should be utilized. For instance, urine drug screens or frequent follow-up visits with pill counts could be initiated. A pain contract that clearly identifies goals, expectations, and responsibilities of both patient and practitioner may be useful for patients who have a history of substance abuse or fall in the high-risk category. Comanagement with or referral to an addiction specialist could also be arranged.

Outcome Evaluation

Goals of treatment should be negotiated when therapy begins and a baseline of acceptable pain level should be established. The outcome may not be total pain relief but should aim to restore as much function as possible. Quality of life is also a mainstay of therapy. Since psychological effects of chronic pain are prevalent, assessing mood and coping skills is also important. It is difficult to use physiological measures but other indicators such as sleep, appetite, amount of physical activity, participation in work or hobbies, and social relationships can give insight into the success or failure of the treatment plan.

Patient Education

As with treatment of acute pain, the individual should be educated about the specific choice of drug or combination drug therapy to address chronic pain, dosing regimens, and realistic goals about pain management. Complete relief may be an unrealistic expectation, yet there are not only drugs but also adjunct and alternative therapies that can be helpful in reducing the pain to an acceptable level. Common side effects with long-term use of an opioid should be explained along with adverse effects. Differences between drug dependence, tolerance, and addiction should be reviewed because many patients are fearful that addiction will occur. The practitioner should assure the individual's report of pain is believed and that there are multiple modalities that can address the pain as well as the accompanying symptoms. Establishing a therapeutic partnership for the control of chronic persistent and recurrent pain is key. See "Patient Education, Chronic Pain Management."

CHRONIC PAIN MANAGEMENT

PATIENT EDUCATION

Related to the Overall Treatment Plan and Disease Process

☐ Pathophysiology of pain and its cause (where appropriate), at a level the patient can understand, to explain how the drugs work.

☐ Role of lifestyle modification in improving prognosis and keeping the number and cost of required drugs and other treatments down.

☐ Indications for contacting the health-care provider when pain relief is ineffective.

☐ Need for follow-up visit(s) with the primary care provider.

Specific to the Drug Therapy

☐ Reasons for taking the drug(s) and the anticipated action of these drug(s) in pain relief.

☐ Doses and schedules for taking the drug(s), including round-the-clock dosing of drugs.

☐ Possible adverse reactions and what to do if they occur.

☐ Coping mechanisms to deal with the complex and costly treatment regimens.

Reasons for Taking the Drug(s)

☐ Patient education about specific drugs is provided in Chapters 15 and 25. The explanations should be clear about what pain drugs can and cannot do.

☐ Patient should be made aware that the drug(s) may need to be taken over a long period of time, so interventions to reduce adverse reactions and reporting them when they occur are important.

Drugs as Part of the Total Treatment Regimen

☐ Role of both pharmacological and nonpharmacological treatments for pain and their interconnection.

Adherence Issues

☐ The fact that most chronic pain cannot be resolved should be addressed.

☐ Adherence to the drug regimen is important to improving chronic pain.

☐ Adherence to lifestyle issues is equally important.

☐ Discussion of ways to remove barriers to adherence should occur.

REFERENCES

Agency for Healthcare Research and Quality. (2011). Pain management guideline. Retrieved from http://www.guideline.gov/content.aspx?id=9744

American Academy of Pain Medicine, American Pain Society, and the American Society of Addiction Medicine. (2001). Definitions related to the use of opioids for the treatment of pain: Consensus statement. Retrieved from http://www.asam.org/advocacy/find-a-policy-statement/view-policy-statement/public-policy-statements/2011/12/15/definitions-related-to-the-use-of-opioids-for-the-treatment-of-pain-consensus-statement

American Medical Association (AMA). (2013a). Pain management Module 1: Pathophysiology of pain and pain assessment. Retrieved from http://ama-cmeonline.com/pain_mgmt/printversion/ama_painmgmt_m1.pdf

American Medical Association (AMA). (2013b). Pain management Module 2: Overview of management options. Retrieved from http://ama-cmeonline.com/pain_mgmt/printversion/ama_painmgmt_m2.pdf

American Medical Association (AMA). (2013c). Pain management Module 3: Barriers to pain management and pain in special populations. Retrieved from http://ama-cmeonline.com/pain_mgmt/printversion/ama_painmgmt_m3.pdf

American Medical Association (AMA). (2013d). Pain management Module 4: Assessing and treating pain in patients with substance abuse concerns. Retrieved from http://ama-cmeonline.com/pain_mgmt/printversion/ama_painmgmt_m4.pdf

American Medical Association (AMA). (2013e). Pain management Module 5: Assessing and treating pain in older adults. Retrieved from http://ama-cmeonline.com/pain_mgmt/printversion/ama_painmgmt_m5.pdf

American Medical Association (AMA). (2013f). Pain management Module 6: Pediatric pain management. Retrieved from http://ama-cmeonline.com/pain_mgmt/printversion/ama_painmgmt_m6.pdf

American Medical Association (AMA). (2013g). Pain management Module 7: Assessing and treating nonmalignant pain: An overview. Retrieved from http://ama-cmeonline.com/pain_mgmt/printversion/ama_painmgmt_m7.pdf

American Society of Addiction Medicine. (2011). Definition of addiction. Retrieved from http://www.asam.org/for-the-public/definition-of-addiction

Argoff, C. (2011). Discontinuing opioid therapy: Developing and implementing an "exit strategy." *Pain Management Today eNewsletter, 1*(10). Retrieved from http://newsletter.qhc.com/JFP/JFP_pain041411.htm

Beyer, J., Denyes, M., & Villaruel, A. (1992). The creation, validation, and continuing development of the Oucher: A measure of pain intensity in children. *Journal of Pediatrics, 7,* 335–346.

Brennan, F., Carr, D., & Cousins, M. (2007). Pain management: A fundamental human right. *Anesthesia and Analgesia, 105*(1), 205–221.

Brown, R., & Rounds, L. (1995). Conjoint screening questionnaire for alcohol and other drug abuse: Criterion validity in a primary care practice. *Wisconsin Medical Journal, 94*(3), 135–140.

CAGE-AID.(n.d.). Retrieved from http://www.hopkinsmedicine.org/johns_hopkins_healthcare/downloads/CAGE%20Substance%20Screening%20Tool.pdf

Centers for Disease Control (CDC). (2013). *Health, United States, 2012: With special feature on emergency care.* National Center for Health Statistics: Hyattsville, MD. Library of Congress Catalog Number 76–641496.

Coxib and Traditional NSAID Trialists' Collaboration. (30 May 2013). Vascular and upper gastrointestinal effects of non-steroidal anti-inflammatory drugs: Meta-analyses of the individual participant data from randomized trials. *The Lancet.* doi: 10.1016/S0140-6736(13)60900-9

Daut, R., Cleeland, C., & Flanery, R. (1983). Development of the Wisconsin Brief Pain Questionnaire to assess pain in cancer and other diseases. *Pain, 17,* 197–210.

Drug Enforcement Administration. (2006). *Practitioner's manual: An informational outline of the Controlled Substances Act.* U.S. Department of Justice: Drug Enforcement Administration.

Feldt, K. (2000). The Checklist of Nonverbal Pain Indicators (CNPI). *Pain Management Nursing, 1*(1) 13–21.

Fishman, S. M. (2007). Recognizing pain management as a human right: A first step. *Anesthesia and Analgesia, 105*(1), 8–9.

Folstein, M., Folstein. S., & McHugh, P. (1975). "Mini-mental state." A practical method for grading the cognitive state of patients for the clinician. *Journal of Psychiatric Research, 12*(3), 189–198. doi:10.1016/0022-3956(75)90026-6 .PMID 1202204

Gavin, D., Ross, H., & Skinner, H. (1989). Diagnostic validity of the Drug Abuse Screening Test in the assessment of DSM-III drug disorders. *British Journal of Addiction, 84*(3), 301–307.

Gibson, S., & Helme, R. (2001). Age-related differences in pain perception and report. *Clinical Geriatric Medicine, 17,* 433–456.

Grunau, R., Johnston, C., & Craig, K. (1990). Neonatal facial and cry responses to invasive and non-invasive procedures. *Pain, 42,* 295–305.

Hattori, M. (n.d,) Short-acting vs. long-acting opioids for chronic persistent pain. Retrieved from http://www.saintfrancismemorial.org/Medical_Services/198690

Hester, N., Foster, R., & Kristensen, K. (1990). Measurement of pain in children: Generalizability and validity of the Pain Ladder and the Poker Chip Tool. In D. Tyler & E. Krane (Eds.), *Pediatric pain, Vol. 15* (pp 70–84). New York: Raven Press.

Hockenberry, M., & Wilson, D. (2012). *Wong's essentials of pediatric nursing* (9th ed.). St. Louis, MO: Elsevier.

Institute of Medicine (2011). Relieving pain in America: A blueprint for transforming prevention, care, education, and research. Retrieved from http://www.iom.edu/Reports/2011/Relieving-Pain-in-America-A-Blueprint-for-transforming-Prevention-Care-Education-Research.aspx

International Association for the Study of Pain. (2012). IASP taxonomy. Retrieved from http://www.iasp-pain.org/AM/Te mplate.cfm?Section=Pain_Definitions

Institute for Clinical Systems Improvement. (2011). Assessment and management of chronic pain. Bloomington, MN: Author. Retrieved from https://www.icsi.org/_asset/bw798b/ChronicPain.pdf

Melzack, R. (1975). The McGill Pain Questionnaire: Major properties and scoring methods. *Pain, 1,* 277–299.

Melzack, R., & Casey, K. (1968). Sensory, motivational, and central control determinants of pain: A new conceptual model. In D. Kensahalo (Ed.), *The skin senses* (pp 423–429). Springfield, IL: C. Thomas.

Merkle, S., Shayvitz, J., Voelpel-Lewis, T., & Malviya, S. (1997). The FLACC: A behavioral scale for scoring postoperative pain in young children. *Pediatric Nursing, 23,* 293–297.

McCaffery, M. (1972). *Nursing management of the patient with pain.* Philadelphia: Lippincott.

National Institutes of Health. (2013). NIH fact sheets: Pain management. Retrieved from http://report.nih.gov/NIHfactsheets/ViewFactSheet.aspx?csid=57

Nelson-Marsh, J., & Banasik, J. (2010). Pain. In L. Copstead & J. Banasik (Eds.), *Pathophysiology* (4th ed., pp 1105–1121). St. Louis, MO: Saunders.

Pawar, D., & Garten, L. (2010). Pain management in children. In IASP's *Guide to pain management in low resource settings* (pp 255–268). Seattle, WA: International Association for the Study of Pain. Retrieved from http://www.iasp-pain.org/AM/Template.cfm?Section=Home&Template=/CM/ContentDisplay.cfm&ContentID=12197

Ross, D., & Ross, S. (1990). Children's comprehensive pain questionnaire. In P. McGrath (Ed.), *Pain in children: Nature, assessment, and treatment* (pp 68–70). New York: Guilford Press.

Schaffler, R. (2007). Pain management. In K. Hoyt & J. Selfridge (Eds.), *Emergency Nursing Core Curriculum,* (6th ed., pp 142–157). St. Louis, MO: Saunders.

Scholten, W., Nygren-Krug, H., & Zucker, H. (2007). The World Health Organization paves the way for action to free people from the shackles of pain. *Anesthesia and Analgesia, 105*(1), 1–4.

Stevens, B., Johnston, C., Petryshen, P., & Taddio, A. (1996). A Premature Infant Pain Profile: Development and initial validation. *Clinical Journal of Pain, 12,* 13–22.

Trescot, A., Datta, S., Lee, M., & Hansen, H. (2008). Opioid pharmacology. *Pain Physician, Special Issue 11,* S133–S153. Retrieved from http://www.painphysicianjournal.com/2008/march/2008;11;S133-S153.pdf

Ulbricht, C. (2011). *Davis's pocket guide to herbs and supplements.* Philadelphia: F.A. Davis.

Varni, J., Thompson, K., & Hanson, V. (1987). The Varni-Thompson pediatric pain questionnaire: Chronic musculoskeletal pain in juvenile rheumatoid arthritis. *Pain, 28,* 29–38.

Warden, V., Hurley, A., & Volicer, L. (2003). Development and psychometric evaluation of the pain assessment in advanced dementia (PAINAD) Scale. *Journal of the American Medical Directors Association, 4*(1), 9–15.

Washington State Medical Directors' Group. (2010). Interagency guideline on opioid dosing for chronic non-cancer pain. Retrieved from http://www.agencymeddirectors.wa.gov/Files/OpioidGdline.pdf

World Health Organization (WHO. (1986). *Cancer pain relief. With a guide to opioid availability* (2nd ed.). Geneva: World Health Organization.

World Health Organization (WHO). (2012). Persisting pain in children. Retrieved from http://whqlibdoc.who.int/publications/2012/9789241548120_Physicians&Nurses.pdf

Wu, C. L., & Raja, S. N. (2011). Treatment of acute postoperative pain. *The Lancet, 377,* 2215–2225.

Index

Page numbers followed by *b* indicate boxes or boxed material; *f,* figures; *t,* tables.